C000230548

THE PHARMACEUTICAL CODEX

ELEVENTH EDITION

Amendments and Corrigenda

Page xx
(Amendments to the British Pharmaceutical Codex 1973): *after* the entry relating to amendments to items on page 738 of the B.P.C. 1973 *insert*
"Page 742
Ferrous Sulphate Mixture and **Ferrous Sulphate Mixture, Paediatric**—formulae: *amend* the amount of Ascorbic Acid in both preparations *to* 2 g"

Page 28
Amiloride Hydrochloride—Identification, ULTRAVIOLET ABSORPTION: *amend to* "In 0.1N hydrochloric acid, maxima at 284 nm (E1%, 1 cm = 550), and 362 nm (E1%, 1 cm = 610)."

Page 38
(Amoxycillin Trihydrate)—AMOXYCILLIN MIXTURE, description: *amend to* "a suspension of amoxycillin trihydrate in a suitable flavoured vehicle which may be coloured."

OTHER PREPARATIONS—INJECTION: *amend* "amoxycillin trihydrate" *to* "amoxycillin sodium"

Page 111
Brilliant Green—Identification. TESTS. 2: *delete* "1 ml of hydrochloric acid and"

TESTS. 3, line 1: *amend to* "To 10 ml of a 0.05% solution add 1 ml of hydrochloric acid and 200 mg of zinc . . ."

Page 182
(Chlorpheniramine Maleate)—Metabolism, EXCRETION, line 4: *amend to* "increase in urinary flow and by decreased urinary pH . . ."

Page 193
Cimetidine—Determination in body fluids, HIGH PRESSURE LIQUID CHROMATOGRAPHY—line 3: *delete* "148" and *insert* "1148"

Metabolism, FURTHER INFORMATION—line 4: *delete* "1149" and *insert* "1148"

Actions and uses—paragraph 1: *add* "It is important to exclude malignancy before commencing treatment with cimetidine."

Paragraph 2, line 4: *after* "4 weeks" *insert* "(6 weeks in gastric ulceration)"

Precautions: *delete* the second sentence of paragraph 2 and the whole of paragraph 3 and *insert* "Cimetidine may potentiate the action of anticoagulants administered orally."

Page 198
Citronella Oil—Refractive index, Ceylon oil: *for* "1.408" *read* "1.480"

Page 396
(Glycine)—Actions and uses, line 4: *for* "15%" *read* "1.5%"

Page 584
Nandrolone Phenylpropionate—Identification, INFRA-RED ABSORPTION: *amend to* "Major peaks at 703, 1173, 1241, 1259, 1675, and 1728 cm^{-1} (see Appendix 2a: Infra-red Spectra)."

Page 603
Norethynodrel—Identification, ULTRAVIOLET ABSORPTION: *delete* entry

Page 607
Nutmeg—Actions and uses: *amend to* "Nutmeg is a carminative and a flavouring agent."

Page 675
(Pharmacy Practice)—Hospital Pharmacies: *add* the following "In the United Kingdom, pharmaceutical operations (other than dispensing) in National Health Service Hospitals are subject to the provisions of Health Services Circular HSC (IS) 128, 1975."

Page 855
(Stilboestrol)—Actions and uses, last paragraph: *delete* "carcinoma of the prostrate and". At the end *add* "In the treatment of prostatic carcinoma it is customary to start with a dose of 1–3 mg daily and increase the dose, usually to 10–20 mg daily, according to the patient's response."

Page 893
(Fabric Absorbents)—OTHER FABRIC ABSORBENTS, lines 4 and 5: *delete* "They are occasionally used in error as a simple wound dressing"

Page 894
Fabric and Fibrous Compound Absorbents—NON-WOVEN FILMATED SWABS—lines 4–7: *amend* sentence commencing in line 4 *to* "They can be used for general swabbing and cleansing and as a protection on dry clean wounds."

Page 900
Medicated Bandages—ZINC PASTE BANDAGE, line 4: *amend* "Viscopaste BP7®" *to* "Viscopaste PB7®"

Page 914
Tar, Coal, Preparations—COAL TAR PAINT, formula and directions for preparation: *amend to*

"Coal tar .. .. 100 g
Acetone .. .. to 1000 ml
Disperse the coal tar in 700 ml of the acetone, allow to stand for one hour, filter if necessary, and add sufficient acetone to produce 1000 ml."

Page 1025
(Infra-red Spectra)—Spectrum for NANDROLONE PHENYLPROPIONATE, *substitute the following diagram:*

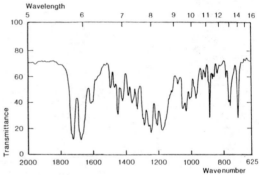

NANDROLONE PHENYLPROPIONATE - KBr disk
703,1173,1241,1259,1675,1728

THE
PHARMACEUTICAL
CODEX

Incorporating the British Pharmaceutical Codex

ELEVENTH EDITION

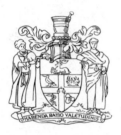

Prepared in the Department of Pharmaceutical
Sciences of The Pharmaceutical Society of Great Britain
and published by direction of the Society's Council

LONDON
THE PHARMACEUTICAL PRESS
1979

Copyright © 1979
The Pharmaceutical Society of Great Britain

No part of this book may be reproduced or utilised in
any form or by any means, including photocopying,
without written permission from the publisher

First published 1979
Reprinted 1983

ISBN 0 85369 129 0

THE PHARMACEUTICAL PRESS
1 Lambeth High Street, London SE1 7JN
Reprinted in the USA

Contents

THE COUNCIL OF THE
PHARMACEUTICAL SOCIETY OF GREAT BRITAIN
1978–9

President: J. E. Balmford, F.P.S.

Vice-President: D. N. Sharpe, F.P.S.

Treasurer: J. C. Bloomfield, O.B.E., F.P.S., F.B.O.A., J.P.

L. Adamson, B.Sc., M.B., Ch.B., M.R.C.S., L.R.C.P., M.R.C.P., M.R.C.Psych.
J. P. Bannerman, M.P.S.
Professor A. H. Beckett, D.Sc., Ph.D., F.P.S., F.R.I.C.
T. G. Booth, B.Pharm., Ph.D., F.P.S.
D. J. Dalglish, B.Sc., M.P.S.
W. M. Darling, O.B.E., F.P.S.
Jill Gilbert, M.P.S.
Joyce M. Gilbert, B.Pharm., F.P.S.
C. R. Hitchings, B.Pharm., M.Sc., M.P.S.
W. H. Howarth, M.P.S., J.P.
J. P Kerr, F.P.S.

Estelle J. M. Leigh, F.P.S.
A. G. M. Madge, F.P.S.
J. A. Myers, B.Pharm., F.P.S., LL.B., D.P.A., A.C.I.S.
R. W. Odd, M.P.S.
T. E. Owen, M.P.S.
Christine M. Puxon, M.B., Ch.B., M.R.C.S., L.R.C.P., M.D.(Obst.), F.R.C.O.G., Barrister-at-Law
J. M. T. Ross, F.P.S.
S. E. Smith, M.A., D.M., B.Ch., Ph.D., D.A.
C. C. B. Stevens, O.B.E., LL.B., F.P.S.
G. Walker, B.Pharm., M.P.S.

Secretary and Registrar: D. F. Lewis, O.B.E, F.P.S., Barrister-at-Law

CODEX REVISION COMMITTEE

Chairman: Professor P. Turner, M.D., B.Sc., F.R.C.P.

J. E. Balmford, F.P.S.
Professor A. H. Beckett, D.Sc., Ph.D., F.P.S., F.R.I.C.
Professor J. W. Fairbairn, D.Sc., Ph.D., B.Sc., F.P.S., F.L.S.

Professor R. J. Fitzpatrick, Ph.D., B.Sc., M.R.C.V.S.
J. W. Hadgraft, F.P.S., F.R.I.C.
D. C. Garratt, D.Sc., Ph.D., F.R.I.C., M.Chem.A.

K. W. Youings, F.P.S.

Secretary to the Committee: G. R. Brown, B.Pharm., B.Sc., F.P.S.
Director of Revision: S. C. Jolly, B.Pharm., B.Sc., M.P.S., C. Chem., F.R.I.C.
General Editors: R. G. Todd, F.P.S.; A. Wade, B.Pharm., M.Phil., F.P.S.

Actions and Uses Subcommittee

Chairman: Professor P. Turner, M.D., B.Sc., F.R.C.P.

G. Bryan, F.P.S.
E. C. Huskisson, B.Sc., M.B., B.S., M.R.C.P., M.R.C.S.
E. S. Johnson, B.Sc., Ph.D., M.B., B.S., M.R.C.S., L.R.C.P.
M. H. Lader, Ph.D., M.D., M.R.C.S., L.R.C.P.
J. G. Lewis, D.Sc., M.D., F.R.C.P.
F. Prescott, Ph.D., M.Sc., M.R.C.P., F.R.I.C.
L. Priest, M.Sc., B.Pharm., F.P.S.
I. D. Ramsay, M.D., M.R.C.P.
Professor J. D. Williams, M.D., M.R.C.Path.

Secretaries to the Committee: G. R. Brown; Jasmine Miller

Analytical Chemistry Subcommittee

Chairman: D. C. Garratt, D.Sc., Ph.D., F.R.I.C., M.Chem.A.

B. Baker, B.Pharm., M.Phil., M.P.S.
*C. G. Butler, B.Pharm., Ph.D., M.P.S., F.R.I.C.
C. Daglish, Ph.D., B.Pharm., F.P.S., F.R.I.C.
T. Duffy, B.Sc., Ph.D., M.P.S.
J. Edmond, B.Pharm., M.P.S.
A. G. Hill, F.R.I.C.
J. V. Jackson
N. Nix, B.Sc., F.R.I.C.
G. F. Phillips, M.Sc., F.R.I.C.
I. Senior, B.Sc., A.R.I.C.

Secretary to the Committee: E. S. Greenfield

Pharmaceutical Chemistry Subcommittee

Chairman: Professor A. H. Beckett, D.Sc., Ph.D., F.P.S., F.R.I.C.

J. W. Bridges, B.Sc., Ph.D.
L. F. Chasseaud, B.A., Ph.D.
R. F. Long, B.Sc., Ph.D., A.R.I.C.
G. F. Phillips, M.Sc., F.R.I.C.
Professor T. F. Slater, Ph.D., D.Sc., F.R.I.C., F.I.Biol.
Professor R. L. Smith, D.Sc., Ph.D., B.Pharm.

Secretary to the Committee: E. S. Greenfield

Pharmacognosy Subcommittee

Chairman: Professor J. W. Fairbairn, D.Sc., Ph.D., F.P.S., F.L.S.

W. E. Court, M.Pharm., Ph.D., F.P.S., F.L.S.
D. F. Cutler, Ph.D., B.Sc., F.L.S., D.I.C.
A. M. Humphrey, B.Sc., A.R.C.S.
J. D. Phillipson, M.Sc., Ph.D., M.P.S., F.L.S.
Professor E. J. Shellard, B.Pharm., Ph.D., F.P.S., F.R.I.C., F.L.S.
A. A. Williams

Secretary to the Committee: K. B. K. Davis

Pharmacy Subcommittee

Chairman: J. W. Hadgraft, F.P.S., F.R.I.C.

J. E. Balmford, F.P.S.
C. W. Barrett, M.Pharm., M.P.S.
D. Ganderton, Ph.D., B.Pharm., M.P.S.
A. W. Newberry, F.P.S.
Professor D. A. Norton, B.Sc., F.P.S., F.I.Biol., D.B.A., A.C.T.(Birm.)
J. R. Phillips, F.P.S.
G. Smith, Ph.D., B.Sc., F.P.S.
Margaret A. Steane, B.Sc., M.Pharm., M.P.S.

Secretary to the Committee: K. B. K. Davis

Formulation Panel: G. Smith, Ph.D., B.Sc., F.P.S. (*Chairman*), T. M. Jones, B.Pharm., Ph.D., M.P.S., A.R.I.C., A. W. Newberry, F.P.S., and S. A. Wood.

Secretary: W. Lund

*Deceased, September, 1976

Preface

In 1903 the Council of the Pharmaceutical Society decided to produce a book of reference supplying authoritative guidance to those engaged in the prescribing and dispensing of medicines throughout the British Empire. The first edition of this book was published in 1907 under the title The British Pharmaceutical Codex, and it has since been revised and extended in scope in 1911, 1923, 1934, 1949, 1954, 1959, 1963, 1968, 1973, and 1979. Monographs on surgical dressings were first introduced in a Supplement published in 1922. Analytical standards were added to certain monographs in 1934 and greatly extended in 1949. Subsequently, as a result of investigations in the Laboratories of the Pharmaceutical Society and in collaboration with members of the subcommittees of the Codex Revision Committee, many preparations were reformulated in metric units and rational standards were introduced for preparations that could be made extemporaneously in the pharmacy.

The Codex and its companion volume the British Veterinary Codex played a leading part in introducing modern analytical methods into published standards, notably polarography (1959), complexometry for the analysis of compound preparations of calcium, magnesium, etc. (1963), column chromatography (1965), and gas–liquid chromatography (1965). Reference standards (authentic materials used to control analytical procedures) were introduced in 1963.

The British Pharmaceutical Codex was designed to supplement the information in the British Pharmacopoeia by providing information on actions, uses, undesirable effects, etc. of pharmacopoeial substances and preparations and by providing in addition formulae and standards for a range of materials that were not included in the pharmacopoeia. For the convenience of users, new editions of the B.P. and B.P.C. were published simultaneously from 1963 onwards. The standards in both publications were accepted for the purposes of the U.K. Food and Drugs Act and were recognised under the Medicines Act 1968. Nevertheless, the Medicines Commission subsequently recommended (in its Annual Report for 1972) that there should be only one compendium of standards for all medicines in the United Kingdom, and that this should be the British Pharmacopoeia; as a consequence, the provision of Codex standards has been discontinued. A major reconstruction of the Codex has therefore been undertaken by the Codex Revision Committee with a view to maintaining and increasing its value to users. The resulting publication differs very strikingly from its predecessors and it has been decided that there should be some appropriate change in the title of the book.

This eleventh Codex, now known as The Pharmaceutical Codex, has been prepared by the Codex Revision Committee by direction of the Council of the Pharmaceutical Society, which acknowledges its great indebtedness to all members of the Committee and its subcommittees for the expert knowledge they have contributed and the valuable time they have so freely given. The membership of the Codex Revision Committee and of its subcommittees is given on pages vi and vii.

K. B. K. Davis, M.P.S., and E. S. Greenfield, members of the editorial staff of the Department of Pharmaceutical Sciences, have acted as secretaries to the committees and assisted with editorial work throughout the revision and reconstruction process. Analytical work, including the preparation of some 240 infra-red spectra, was carried out in the Laboratories of the Pharmaceutical Society. Problems relating to pharmaceutical technology and formulation have been investigated in the laboratory by W. Lund, F.P.S., assisted by Marjorie Lynch, B.Sc., M.P.S., and Carol A. Farley, B.Sc., M.P.S. Assistance in the preparation of the text and in editorial work was given by P. Forbes, B.Sc., K. G. Marriott, M.Sc., C.Chem., M.R.I.C., M.I.Inf.Sc., and Jasmine Miller, B.Sc., M.P.S., and J. R. Greenfield, B.Sc., M.B., B.S., M.R.C.S., L.R.C.P., helped to prepare the entries describing diseases and related topics. Elizabeth J. Hunter typed most of the manuscript, and Jennifer M. Hallson, B.Pharm., M.P.S., Linda Hanrahan, W. Harman, B.Sc., Susan A. Jones, B.Pharm., M.P.S., and Pamela Morley, B.Pharm., M.P.S., also helped in preparing the text and in reading the proofs. Thanks are also due to the publications manager B. J. M. O'Malley, F.P.S., for guidance in relation to printing and many other aspects of publication.

The British Pharmacopoeia Commission has given advice on those analytical standards of the British Pharmaceutical Codex 1973 that were considered to require amendment. The Commission has continued its valued cooperation in respect of other matters, and thanks are due to members of the Secretariat of the Commission for advice on various points arising during the preparation of this edition. The Codex Revision Committee gratefully acknowledges the cooperation and advice it has received from other sections of the Department of Health and Social Security, the Ministry of Agriculture, Fisheries and Food, various overseas health authorities, the Tropical Products Institute, the Faculty of Ophthalmologists, the Association of the British Pharmaceutical Industry, numerous pharmaceutical manufacturers, and pharmacists in hospital and general practice. Thanks are due to the Home Office Central Research Establishment, Aldermaston, for permission to reproduce the infra-red spectra in Appendixes 2b and 2c, and to Dr A. C. Moffat for his cooperation in this matter.

A number of experts provided help in drafting some of the major new entries, notably F. Alexander, A. J. M. Bailey, Barbara J. Boucher, R. F. Branch, G. C. Brander, A. W. Brown, T. Chard, G. B. Cox, S. F. M. Davies, P. M. Dean, the late Katherine Dormandy, A. Goldberg, T. W. Groves, P. J. Houghton, E. C. Hulse, G. I. C. Ingram, A. F. Lant, D. E. Lovett, J. S. Malpas, Sir William Maycock, J. W. Paterson, P. M. F. Sambrook, J. Sanford, Alison Smithies, J. E. Stark, D. C. Taylor, T. D. Turner, G. N. Volans, J. B. Walsby, J. A. Walker-Smith, and R. Watkins.

Introduction

The Pharmaceutical Codex is intended to be an encyclopaedia of drug information for pharmacists and others who are engaged in work involving the preparation and use of medicines and medicinal preparations. The information given in the entries on drugs, other pharmaceutical substances, and formulated products has been considerably expanded compared with previous editions of the British Pharmaceutical Codex, as also have a number of the sections dealing with types of pharmaceutical preparations. In addition, a large number of new entries giving information on diverse subjects of pharmaceutical, clinical, chemical, and analytical interest have been added.

For ease of reference, the entries are presented in an alphabetical arrangement and preparations of drugs, previously described in a separate formulary section, are now appended to the appropriate drug monographs.

The preparations that are included are those that have official standards, including those described in the B.P. or B.P.C. 1973. The British Pharmacopoeia Commission has agreed (in its Annual Report for 1973) to provide standards to support formulae appearing in the British National Formulary, and therefore preparations of the B.N.F. 1976–78 have also been included. Information about other (non-official) preparations containing not more than two ingredients is briefly given. A few official preparations have been omitted, generally because they are no longer available or are going out of use.

The following are some of the principal new features of this edition.

Diseases and conditions. The causes, signs, symptoms, and treatment, including drug treatment, are given for many common diseases. Entries are also included for conditions such as pregnancy and subjects such as contraception in which drug treatment may be involved.

Expanded entries on medicinal substances. The monographs on drug substances included in the previous edition have been expanded and reorganised so as to cater for the increasing interest of pharmacists in clinical matters, and to give more detailed information on stability and other pharmaceutical and analytical aspects.

A new feature is the inclusion of references to published literature which may be helpful to the reader who wishes to follow up particular topics of interest. Many monographs now include information on metabolism and bioavailability. Where appropriate, information on paediatric dosage is included. Most drug entries have a section headed "Identification" which includes chemical tests and spectrophotometric and chromatographic data, and many cite useful references to the literature under the heading "Determination in body fluids".

Pharmaceutics. There are entries on pharmaceutical topics such as pharmacy practice, diluents, incompatibility, intravenous additives, radiopharmaceuticals, packaging, stability, storage, and sterilisation.

Clinical pharmacy. New entries have been included on advice to patients, paediatric dosage, and dosage in renal failure. There is a major entry on metabolism which covers the absorption, distribution, and elimination of drugs and thereby provides background information for the new matter added under the heading "metabolism" in the entries for many drugs. The current interest in bioavailability is reflected in an entry that reviews the development of bioavailability studies.

Analysis. General information is included in entries which describe chromatographic and spectrophotometric techniques, and some 320 infra-red spectra have been included in reduced facsimile as an aid to identification. Entries which define dissociation constants, partition coefficients, and solubility, also include information on how these parameters are determined.

Surgical dressings. The information on uses of surgical dressings has been greatly enlarged. Dressings are usually classified according to their construction, but in this edition a new system of classification has been introduced. It is based on the features that are of greatest importance to the user, mainly performance of particular functions. The text is arranged with materials used for a particular purpose grouped together so as to assist in the logical selection of dressing types according to the user's requirements.

Pesticides. As in previous editions a number of insecticides and similar products used in human medicine are the subject of entries in this Pharmaceutical Codex; products used for sheep and cattle in the form of washes and dips, some of which were included in the British Veterinary Codex, are likewise included. In this edition a general entry on pesticides has been added giving information mainly from the point of view of their use in crop protection. Although these substances cannot be considered as medicines since they are not applied directly to persons or animals, pharmacists are frequently asked for information on the properties and uses of agricultural and horticultural pesticides, and the Codex Revision Committee therefore decided that general information on these products should be included. The entry also includes brief statements on the properties of more than a hundred substances used as insecticides, fungicides, herbicides, rodenticides, nematocides, and molluscicides.

Veterinary information. A short description is given of the veterinary uses, doses, and official preparations of the substances described in the British Pharmacopoeia (Veterinary) 1977.

General Notices

Legal Aspects

Substances and their preparations described in The Pharmaceutical Codex may be subject to legal control in the United Kingdom or in other parts of the world in which The Pharmaceutical Codex is used. This control may be concerned with preparation, labelling, and standards.

In the United Kingdom, regulations under the Medicines Act 1968 require the licensing of the manufacture of medicinal products and the examination of new products by the Committee on Safety of Medicines before they are marketed. It should not be assumed that medicinal products prepared in accordance with the recommendations of The Pharmaceutical Codex will necessarily have been approved by the Committee on Safety of Medicines.

Licence to manufacture substances or products protected by Letters Patent is neither conveyed nor implied by the inclusion of information on such substances in The Pharmaceutical Codex.

Trade Marks

Names printed in italic type followed by the symbol® are or have been used as proprietary names in the United Kingdom. These names may in general be applied only to products supplied by the owners of the trade marks.

Standards for Articles and Preparations of The Pharmaceutical Codex

The standards in certain publications including the British Pharmaceutical Codex are recognised in the U.K. Medicines Act 1968.[1] However, the Medicines Commission, an advisory body appointed under the Act, has recommended that in the United Kingdom there should be only one compendium of standards, namely the British Pharmacopoeia.[2] The Council of the Pharmaceutical Society has reluctantly accepted that recommendation and agreed that analytical standards would no longer be included in any future publication issued by the Society. It has received an assurance that all British Pharmaceutical Codex standards of continuing value will in due course be incorporated in the British Pharmacopoeia. There will therefore be an interim period during which certain standards of the British Pharmaceutical Codex 1973 will continue to be official pending their incorporation in the Pharmacopoeia. This Pharmaceutical Codex is intended to update the British Pharmaceutical Codex 1973 as a formulary and general reference book but does not supersede that volume in respect of any standards not taken into the British Pharmacopoeia.

[1] In the United Kingdom a medicinal product ordered under a name that is at the head of a monograph in one of the recognised publications, or an approved synonym, must comply with the appropriate standard given in a recognised publication. When the publication to be used is not specified in the prescription or order it must comply with the standard in the "appropriate current monograph". The sequence in which publications are searched to find the appropriate current monograph is essentially the European Pharmacopoeia, British Pharmacopoeia, British Pharmaceutical Codex, in that order of precedence. For full details see Medicines Act 1968, section 65, or J. R. Dale and G. E. Appelbe, *Pharmacy Law and Ethics*, 2nd edition, London, Pharmaceutical Press, 1979, p. 136.

[2] Nevertheless, the standards of the European Pharmacopoeia will continue to be the official standards applicable within the United Kingdom, as required under Article 1 of the Convention on the Elaboration of a European Pharmacopoeia (1964).

In the view of the Department of Health and Social Security this Pharmaceutical Codex does not constitute a British Pharmaceutical Codex for the purpose of sections 65 and 103 of the Medicines Act. The expression "British Pharmaceutical Codex" or the abbreviation "B.P.C." without qualification, when used to indicate the composition and quality of a medicinal product, therefore refers to the 1973 edition. If articles or preparations are ordered under the names used as titles in this volume, either without qualification or with the qualification "Pharmaceutical Codex" or "P.Cx." they must comply with any relevant standards in the "appropriate current monograph" as defined in section 65 of the Medicines Act. The volume that should be consulted is indicated in the text, and is correct at the time of going to press, but it should be realised that the "appropriate current monograph" may change with the subsequent publication of volumes of the European Pharmacopoeia and the British Pharmacopoeia.

Health and Safety

This book is intended to be used by trained persons, and care must be exercised in the interpretation of statements concerning the actions, uses, and other clinical effects of medicinal substances, so that due consideration is given to the implications and limitations of any particular statement or description. Processes and tests described should be performed in suitable premises by personnel with adequate training and equipment. Care should be taken to ensure the safe handling of all chemical or biological materials, and particular attention should be given to the possibility of allergy, fire, explosion, or poisoning (including inhalation of toxic vapours) occurring. Particular hazards exist in the preparation of radioactive materials, vaccines, and certain other products. Cautionary notes have been included in a number of entries, but the possibility of danger should always be kept in mind when handling medicinal substances.

Manufacture

When making products in accordance with recipes given in the text, the ingredients must comply with the official standard or, where there is no official standard, must be of good commercial quality suitable for medicinal and pharmaceutical use.

The instructions given for compounding medicinal products are suitable when relatively small quantities, such as those specified in the recipe, are made by a pharmacist in general practice. Deviations from these instructions are permitted, provided that the products do not differ significantly from those produced when the methods of The Pharmaceutical Codex are applied to the quantities in the recipe. When so indicated, colouring and flavouring agents may be added, provided that the materials used are permitted for colouring or flavouring food in the country in which the product is intended to be used.

Temperatures

Unless otherwise indicated, temperatures are expressed in degrees Celsius (centigrade).

Measures

Unless otherwise indicated, measurements are intended to be made at 20°. Measures are to be graduated at 20°.

Percentage Strengths

Percentage strengths are expressed as w/w, w/v, v/v, or v/w, and represent the number of grams or millilitres of substance in 100 g or 100 ml of the product. Unless otherwise stated, solutions of solids in liquids are expressed as percentage w/v, of liquids in liquids as percentage v/v, of liquids in solids as percentage v/w, and of gases in liquids as percentage w/w.

Crude Drugs

VARIETIES. The description of a crude drug is designed to include those commercial varieties considered suitable for medicinal use. Frequently these commodities have distinctive names related to their country of origin or to some individual peculiarity. In order to provide useful information about commodities that are acceptable for medicinal use, they are named and briefly described in the paragraph headed "Varieties". In this context the term "variety" is not necessarily equivalent to the botanical "varietas".

SUBSTITUTES AND ADULTERANTS. Substances referred to under this heading have occurred in admixture with the genuine drug or as a complete counterfeit. They may contain active principles related to those in the genuine drug, but more frequently they are useless or dangerous materials.

POWDERING. When a batch of a crude drug is ground and sifted no portion of the drug shall be rejected. However, the final tailings may be withheld if an approximately equal weight of tailings from a previous batch has been added before grinding.

Essential Oils

Certain essential oils are liable to deteriorate on keeping. This deterioration is accompanied by increase in viscosity, and by changes in the quality of the odour and in other properties. Oils that have deteriorated are not suitable for pharmaceutical or medicinal use.

Syrup

When syrup is used for the dilution of elixirs, linctuses, and mixtures, as described in the relevant entries, there is the possibility of incompatibility between these preparations and any preservatives used in the syrup. Investigations in the Laboratories of the Pharmaceutical Society have provided indications of incompatibility between the following preparations and syrup preserved with hydroxybenzoate esters: methadone linctus, noscapine linctus, paediatric opiate squill linctus, paediatric belladonna and ephedrine mixture, ferrous sulphate mixture, paediatric ferrous sulphate mixture, potassium citrate mixture, paediatric sodium bicarbonate mixture, and sodium citrate mixture.

Labelling

Recommendations for labelling are included in some entries, but it is recognised that these recommendations may need to be modified according to circumstances. All medicinal substances and preparations should be labelled in accordance with legal requirements, which usually require, among other things, batch markings of manufactured items. Warning statements required by law should take precedence over corresponding Pharmaceutical Codex recommendations. For example in some countries certain articles are required to be labelled "not to be taken" where the Pharmaceutical Codex recommends the expression "for external use only", and in some countries the term "flammable" is used in place of "inflammable".

Explanation of Terms Used

WATER-BATH. This term means a bath of boiling water, unless water at some other temperature is indicated by the context.

APPROPRIATE PHARMACEUTICAL ADJUVANTS. This term means additives such as antoxidants, and buffering, dispersing, suspending, wetting, and preserving agents, but it does not include flavouring and colouring agents.

Atomic and Molecular Weights

Molecular weights are based on the Table of Relative Atomic Weights 1975, published by the International Union of Pure and Applied Chemistry and based on the ^{12}C scale. Values for selected elements are given in the entry on Weights and Measures.

Solutions

When preparing solutions for the purpose of tests, water should be used as the solvent unless otherwise stated.

Reagents

Reagents for use in tests should be of normal quality for laboratory use. Titles of reagent solutions are printed in *italic* type and the solutions are described in Appendix 1.

Physical Characteristics of Chemical Substances

When a range is quoted for the value of a physical characteristic such as weight per millilitre, refractive index, moisture content, etc., the figures are not to be interpreted as standards, although they are generally in agreement with current standards at the time of going to press.

Determination in Body Fluids

The methods referred to in the references quoted under the heading "Determination in body fluids" in the monographs on medicinal substances are not intended to be recommended methods. These references are intended to be used as a guide to the literature on the particular subject.

Analytical Data

Information about the interpretation of data given under the headings "Dissociation constant", "Ultraviolet absorption", "Infra-red absorption", and "Thin-layer chromatography" in the monographs on medicinal substances, is given in the main entries which describe these topics.

Chloroform

The restrictions on the use of chloroform in the United Kingdom, mentioned briefly on page 175, are given in the Medicines (Chloroform Prohibition) Order 1979, Statutory Instrument 1979 No. 382.

Amendments to the British Pharmaceutical Codex 1973

A number of amendments to the monographs of the British Pharmaceutical Codex 1973 have been published from time to time, either in the British Pharmaceutical Codex Supplement 1976, in amendment leaflets, or in *The Pharmaceutical Journal*. For the convenience of analysts and others who may continue to use the British Pharmaceutical Codex 1973 for information on standards the following pages contain details of all the amendments which apply to standards and formulations of the British Pharmaceutical Codex 1973. They are intended to be read in conjunction with the British Pharmaceutical Codex 1973 and the Supplement 1976.

The standards for some substances of the British Pharmaceutical Codex 1973 have been replaced by standards published subsequent to 1973 by the British Pharmacopoeia Commission and by the European Pharmacopoeia Commission, and these are noted below. The amendments to standards issued since 1973 have been adopted on the advice of the British Pharmacopoeia Commission. No further amendments to the B.P.C. 1973 will be issued by the Council of the Pharmaceutical Society after the publication of this Pharmaceutical Codex.

1. Changes in standards

In the United Kingdom, the following substances, standards for which were included in the British Pharmaceutical Codex 1973, Part 1, must now comply with the requirements of the European Pharmacopoeia:

Cellacephate	Heavy Kaolin
Charcoal	Phenazone
Chloramine	Piperazine Hydrate
Ephedrine	Polysorbates 20, 60, 80
Ethylmorphine Hydrochloride	Sodium Thiosulphate

The following substances, which were described in the British Pharmaceutical Codex 1973, Part 1, must now comply with the requirements of the British Pharmacopoeia:

Bephenium Hydroxynaphthoate	Isoprenaline Hydrochloride
Caraway Oil	Physostigmine Sulphate
Cardamom Oil	Pilocarpine Hydrochloride
Calcium Sodium Lactate	Terpineol
Catechu	Thiabendazole
Chloramphenicol Sodium Succinate	Titanium Dioxide
Chloroxylenol	Trimeprazine Tartrate
Cinnamon Oil	

The following substance which was described in the British Pharmaceutical Codex 1973, Part 2, must now comply with the requirements of the British Pharmacopoeia:

Scorpion Venom Antiserum

The following preparations, which were described in the British Pharmaceutical Codex 1973, Part 6, must now comply with the requirements of the British Pharmacopoeia:

Atropine Sulphate Eye-drops	Methyl Salicylate Liniment
Cetrimide Cream	Methyl Salicylate Ointment
Chloramphenicol Sodium Succinate Injection	Noradrenaline Injection
Chlorhexidine Cream	Noradrenaline Solution, Strong, Sterile
Chloroform and Morphine Tincture	Phenytoin Capsules
Chloroxylenol Solution	Physostigmine Eye-drops
Co-trimoxazole Tablets, Paediatric	Pilocarpine Eye-drops
Homatropine Eye-drops	Thiabendazole Tablets
	Trimeprazine Tablets

2. Amendments to British Pharmaceutical Codex 1973

Page xxxv
Authentic Specimens—3rd paragraph: *amend to* "Where Authentic Specimens (*A.S.*) or British Chemical Reference Substances (*B.C.R.S.*) are referred to in the assays and tests of the British Pharmaceutical Codex, the British Pharmacopoeia Chemical Reference Substance (*B.P.C.R.S.*) should be used. British Pharmacopoeia Chemical Reference Substances are available from the British Pharmacopoeia Commission Laboratory, Government Buildings (Block 2), Honeypot Lane, Stanmore HA7 1AY, England.
European Pharmacopoeia Chemical Reference Substances (*E.P.C.R.S.*) are available from the European Pharmacopoeia Commission, Annexe Jacoutot, 1, Rue Boecklin, 67000 Strasbourg, France."

Page 23
Ammonium Bicarbonate—CHLORIDE: *amend* "10 parts per million" *to* "70 parts per million"

Page 45
(Benethamine Penicillin)—CONTENT OF TOTAL PENICIL-LINS: *amend* "*benzylpenicillin sodium B.C.R.S.*" *to* "*benzylpenicillin sodium E.P.C.R.S.*"

Page 71
(Dried Calcium Sulphate)—ACIDITY OR ALKALINITY: *amend* "6.5" *to* "6.0"

Page 86
Cephaloridine—Solubility: *amend* "in 12 parts of water" *to* "in 5 parts of water"

Page 262
Lavender Oil—Solubility: *amend* "English oil, in 3 parts of alcohol (30 per cent)" *to* "English oil, in 3 parts of alcohol (80 per cent)"

Page 376
Phenylmercuric acetate—POLYMERCURATED BENZENE COMPOUNDS, line 3: *amend* "2 g" *to* "about 0.8 g"

Page 438
Senna Leaf—CONTENT OF TOTAL ANTHRAQUINONE GLY-COSIDES, lines 14–15: *amend* "0.05 ml of *hydrochloric acid*" *to* "0.1 ml of 2N hydrochloric acid"
Lines 15–16: *amend* "two successive 15-ml portions" *to* "three successive 15-ml portions"
Line 22: *amend* "on a water-bath" *to* "in a water-bath"
Line 32: *amend* "10.0 ml" *to* "20.0 ml"
Line 38: *amend* "210" *to* "200"

Page 468
Below the monograph on "Squill" *insert* the monograph on "Squill, Indian" of the British Pharmaceutical Codex Supplement 1976, page xix

Page 471
Prepared Storax—ACID VALUE: *amend to* "52 to 76"
SAPONIFICATION VALUE: *amend to* "160 to 190"
LOSS ON DRYING: *delete* the test

Page 472
(Prepared Storax)—CONTENT OF TOTAL BALSAMIC ACIDS: *amend to* "Not less than 28.5 per cent determined by the method for Benzoin (page 49)"

Page 566
Rubella Vaccine (Live Attenuated)—introductory paragraph, line 3: *amend* "Water for Injections" *to* "a suitable sterile liquid"

Page 600
Diameter and tensile strength of stainless steel sutures—heading of third and fourth columns: *amend to* "Average breaking force on a straight pull (kgf)"

Page 613
Domette Bandage—introductory paragraph, line 3: *after* "cotton" *insert* "or rayon or of combined cotton and rayon yarn"

Page 614
(Domette Bandage)—FABRIC: *delete* this paragraph

Open-wove Bandage—introductory paragraph: *amend to* "Open-wove Bandage consists of cloth of plain weave, in which the warp threads are of cotton and the weft threads are of cotton or rayon or of combined cotton and rayon yarn."
DESCRIPTION: *amend* "Cotton cloth" *to* "Cloth"

Page 621
Paraffin Gauze Dressing—introductory paragraph, line 3:

amend "with yellow soft paraffin" *to* "with yellow or white soft paraffin"
Line 7: *amend* "yellow" *to* "the"
Line 9: *delete* "yellow"
Line 11: *delete* "yellow"
DESCRIPTION, line 4: *amend* "Yellow Soft Paraffin" *to* "Yellow Soft Paraffin or White Soft Paraffin"
ETHER-SOLUBLE EXTRACTIVE, line 1: *amend* "Not less than 200 g per m²" *to* "Not less than 100 g per m²"

Page 624
Standard Dressing No. 10, No. 11 and No. 12—DESCRIPTION: *add* the following:
"The Euflavine Lint may be replaced by Absorbent Lint impregnated with about 0.1 per cent of aminacrine hydrochloride or chlorhexidine hydrochloride (or the equivalent amount of the gluconate), or about 0.15 per cent of domiphen bromide. The medicated lint complies with the appropriate standard for content of antiseptic given in Appendix 27 (pages 916–17)."

Labelling – *add*: "In addition, the name and proportion of antiseptic (other than euflavine) in the lint is stated on the label."

Page 625
Standard Dressing No. 13, No. 14 and No. 15—DESCRIPTION, line 12: *after* "page 626," *insert* "or for Cotton and Rayon Gauze,"

Page 627
Absorbent Gauze, X-ray-detectable—introductory paragraph, line 2: *delete* "absorbent"
DESCRIPTION, line 1: *amend* "Absorbent gauze" *to* "Gauze"
Line 5: *delete* "absorbent"
Line 6: *after* "(13 Light)," *insert* "or for Cotton and Rayon Gauze"

Page 628
Above the heading "GAUZE PADS" *insert* the monograph on "Cotton and Rayon Gauze" of the British Pharmaceutical Codex Supplement 1976, page xvii
Gauze Pad—introductory paragraph, line 1: *delete* "absorbent"
DESCRIPTION, line 1: *delete* "absorbent"
Line 3: *after* "page 626," *insert* "or for Cotton and Rayon Gauze,"

Page 629
Gauze and Capsicum Cotton Tissue—Standard for the gauze, DESCRIPTION: *after* "page 626," *insert* "or for Cotton and Rayon Gauze"
YARN; etc: *after* "page 626" *add* ", or under Cotton and Rayon Gauze"
Gauze and Cellulose Wadding Tissue—Standard for the gauze, DESCRIPTION; etc: *after* "page 626" *add* ", or under Cotton and Rayon Gauze"

Gauze and Cotton Tissue—Standard for the gauze, DESCRIPTION; etc: *after* "page 626" *insert* ", or under Cotton and Rayon Gauze"

Page 630
Absorbent Lint—SYNONYMS: *delete* "Absorbent Cotton Lint; Cotton Lint; Lint"
Introductory paragraph, line 1: *delete* "cotton"
Line 2: *after* "plain weave," *insert* "in which the warp threads are of cotton and the weft threads are of cotton or rayon or of combined cotton and rayon yarn,"
DESCRIPTION: *amend* "Cotton cloth" *to* "Cloth"

Page 635
Calico, Unbleached—introductory paragraph: *amend to* "Unbleached Calico consists of unbleached cloth of plain weave, in which the warp threads are of cotton and the weft threads are of cotton or rayon or of combined cotton and rayon yarn."
DESCRIPTION, line 1: *delete* "cotton"

Page 653
Vitamins A and D Capsules—formula: *amend* the quantity of vitamin D *to* 400 Units and the quantity of vitamin-A activity *to* 4000 Units

Page 654
(Vitamins A and D Capsules)—method of preparation: *add* "The capsule shells may be coloured."
CONTENT OF VITAMIN-A ACTIVITY: *amend* "3750 to 5250 Units" *to* "3500 to 4700 Units"
CONTENT OF VITAMIN D: *amend* "375 to 525 Units" *to* "350 to 470 Units"

Vitamins Capsules—method for preparation: *add* "The capsule shells may be coloured."

Page 656
Betamethasone Valerate Cream—Note, second paragraph, line 4: *delete* "or with Buffered Cream"

Buffered Cream—formula: *amend* "Citric Acid" to "Citric Acid Monohydrate"

Page 657
Cetomacrogol Cream—*Formula B*: *amend* "Thiomersal...0.02 g" *to* "Benzyl Alcohol...15.0 g" and *amend* the quantity of Purified Water, freshly boiled and cooled, *to* 682.7 g.

Page 658
Fluocinolone Cream—introductory paragraph: *amend to* "Fluocinolone Cream is a dispersion of Fluocinolone Acetonide in a suitable water-miscible basis containing a mixture of benzyl alcohol, methyl hydroxybenzoate, and propyl hydroxybenzoate as the preservative system."

Page 665
Hydrocortisone and Neomycin Ear-drops—CONTENT OF HYDROCORTISONE ACETATE: *amend* "hydrocortisone acetate B.C.R.S." to "hydrocortisone acetate E.P.C.R.S."

Page 671
Ephedrine Elixir—CONTENT OF EPHEDRINE HYDROCHLORIDE, line 11: *amend*: "0.1N hydrochloric acid" *to* "1N hydrochloric acid"

Page 672
Isoniazid Elixir—formula: *amend* "Citric Acid" *to* "Citric Acid Monohydrate"

Page 677
Streptomycin Elixir, Paediatric—formula: *amend* "Citric Acid" *to* "Citric Acid Monohydrate"

Page 679
Liquid Paraffin and Magnesium Hydroxide Emulsion—formula: *amend* the quantity of Magnesium Hydroxide Mixture *to* 735 ml and the quantity of Chloroform Spirit *to* 15 ml.
CONTENT OF MAGNESIUM HYDROXIDE: *amend* the limits *to* 5.1 to 7.0 per cent w/w.

Page 680
Peppermint Emulsion, Concentrated—in the formula and

in the first and second lines of the method of preparation: *amend* "Quillaia Liquid Extract" *to* "Polysorbate 20"

Page 685
Squill Liquid Extract—formula: *after* "Squill" *insert* "or Indian Squill"
WEIGHT PER ML: *delete* this requirement
TOTAL SOLIDS: *delete* this requirement

Page 688
Adrenaline Eye-drops, Neutral—fourth and fifth lines: *amend* "and other adjuvants" *to* "or other suitable stabilising agents"

Page 692
Hypromellose Eye-drops—formula: *after* "Hypromellose 4500" *insert* ", or 4000, or 5000"

Page 695
Sulphacetamide Eye-drops—formula and method of preparation: *amend* as described in the British Pharmaceutical Codex Supplement 1976, page 38–39.

Page 709
(Injections)—first line: *amend* "500 ml" *to* "50 ml"

Page 710
(Benethamine Penicillin Injection, Fortified)—CONTENT OF BENZYLPENICILLIN SODIUM: *amend* "benzylpenicillin sodium B.C.R.S." *to* "benzylpenicillin sodium E.P.C.R.S."
CONTENT OF TOTAL PENICILLINS: *amend* "benzylpenicillin sodium B.C.R.S." *to* "benzylpenicillin sodium E.P.C.R.S."

Page 711
(Benzathine Penicillin Injection, Fortified)—CONTENT OF BENZYLPENICILLIN POTASSIUM: *amend* "benzylpenicillin sodium B.C.R.S." *to* "benzylpenicillin sodium E.P.C.R.S."
CONTENT OF BENZATHINE PENICILLIN, lines 9 and 10: *amend* "wash the combined ethereal extracts with three successive 5-ml portions of water" *to* "wash the combined ethereal extracts with successive 5-ml portions of water until the washings are neutral to *litmus paper*,"
Line 14: *amend* "glacial acetic acid" *to* "anhydride-free glacial acetic acid"
CONTENT OF TOTAL PENICILLINS: *amend* "benzylpenicillin sodium B.C.R.S." *to* "benzylpenicillin sodium E.P.C.R.S."

Page 713
Dextrose Injection, Strong—first paragraph: *delete* the words "or by filtration"
ACIDITY: *amend* "6.5" *to* "5.5"
Standard: *add* the following test: "5-HYDROXYMETHYLFURFURAL AND RELATED SUBSTANCES. Dilute 2.0 ml to 250 ml with water and measure the extinction of a 1-cm layer of the solution at the maximum at about 284 nm; the extinction is not more than 0.25."

Page 716
Phenol Injection, Oily—CONTENT OF PHENOL, line 4: *amend*: "10 g" *to* "8 g"

Pages 716–717
Phenytoin Injection: *replace* the monograph by the new monograph of the British Pharmaceutical Codex Supplement 1976, pages 39–40.

Page 722
Codeine Linctus, Diabetic—formula: *amend* "Citric Acid" *to* "Citric Acid Monohydrate"

Page 723
Ipecacuanha and Squill Linctus, Paediatric—WEIGHT PER ML: *delete* this requirement.

Noscapine Linctus—formula: *amend* "Citric Acid" *to* "Citric Acid Monohydrate"

Page 724
Pholcodine Linctus, Strong—formula: *amend* "Citric Acid" *to* "Citric Acid Monohydrate"

Simple Linctus—formula: *amend* "Citric Acid" *to* "Citric Acid Monohydrate"

Page 725
Squill Linctus, Opiate—method of preparation: *amend* "disperse 0.5 g of Powdered Tragacanth" *to* "disperse 0.1 g of xanthan gum or 0.5 g of Powdered Tragacanth" *Add* "If xanthan gum is used, a high-speed stirrer is required in order to disperse the material." WEIGHT PER ML: *delete* this requirement.

Tolu Linctus, Compound, Paediatric—formula: *amend* "Citric Acid" *to* "Citric Acid Monohydrate"

Page 733
(Formaldehyde Lozenges)—formula: *amend* "Citric Acid" *to* "Citric Acid Monohydrate"

Hydrocortisone Lozenges—DISINTEGRATION TIME: *amend to* "Carry out the method of the British Pharmacopoeia for the Disintegration Test for Tablets, using 5 lozenges and water at 25°. None of the 5 lozenges disintegrates in less than 10 minutes." CONTENT OF HYDROCORTISONE: line 5, *amend* "0.02 mg" *to* "0.02 g"

Page 734
(Penicillin Lozenges)—CONTENT OF BENZYLPENI-CILLIN: *amend* "*benzylpenicillin sodium B.C.R.S.*" *to* "*benzylpenicillin sodium E.P.C.R.S.*" and *amend* "benzylpenicillin sodium B.C.R.S." *to* "benzylpenicillin sodium E.P.C.R.S."

Page 735
(Mixtures)—above "**Labelling**" *add*: **Manufacture of mixtures.** A number of monographs provide a complete formula and directions for preparing a mixture that is directed to be recently prepared. Manufacturers may add suitable preservatives and stabilising agents to these mixtures to extend the shelf life, but the preparations should not otherwise differ significantly in appearance and composition from mixtures prepared as directed in the monographs. The requirements under "Standard" must be complied with and the added substances must not interfere with the analytical methods given in the monographs.
Labelling—under section "A" *add*: The label on the container of a mixture directed to be recently prepared, but to which suitable preservatives and stabilising agents have been added states:
(1) the name and concentration of the added adjuvants; and
(2) the date after which the preparation is not intended to be used.

Aluminium Hydroxide and Belladonna Mixture—*amend* "It should be recently prepared" *to* "It must be freshly prepared"
Standard: *delete* the requirements

Page 738
Belladonna and Ipecacuanha Mixture, Paediatric: *amend*

"It should be recently prepared" *to* "It must be freshly prepared"
Standard: *delete* the requirements

Cascara and Belladonna Mixture: *amend* "It should be recently prepared" *to* 'It must be freshly prepared".
Standard: *delete* the requirements

Page 743
Fusidic Acid Mixture—second footnote: *amend to* "This mixture should not be diluted. The general direction given under Mixtures that the preparation should be diluted so that the dose is contained in 5 ml does not apply to this mixture; it may be necessary for a dose of 2.5 ml to be measured by the patient in a 5 ml spoon; if a dose smaller than 2.5 ml is required, the dose should be measured by means of a graduated pipette."

Page 745
Kaolin Mixture, Paediatric—RESIDUE ON IGNITION: *amend* "14.3 to 19.1" *to* "13.4 *to* 18.0"

Page 747
Magnesium Trisilicate and Belladonna Mixture—*replace* the monograph by the following:
Belladonna Tincture .. .. 50 ml
Magnesium Trisilicate Mixture.. .. to 1000 ml
It must be freshly prepared.
Labelling. A direction to shake the bottle should be given on the label.
Dose. 10 to 20 millilitres.

Page 750
Potassium Citrate Mixture—formula: *amend* "Citric Acid" *to* "Citric Acid Monohydrate"

Page 751
Potassium Citrate and Hyoscyamus Mixture—formula: *amend* "Citric Acid" *to* "Citric Acid Monohydrate", and *amend* "It should be recently prepared" *to* "It must be freshly prepared"
Standard: *delete* the requirements

Page 753
Sodium Citrate Mixture—formula: *amend* "Citric Acid" *to* "Citric Acid Monohydrate"

Page 754
Succinylsulphathiazole Mixture, Paediatric: *add* the following formula and method, which is suitable for the extemporaneous preparation of the mixture:
Succinylsulphathiazole, in fine
  powder .. .. 100 g
Light Kaolin, or Light Kaolin
  (Natural) .. .. 60 g
Sodium Carboxymethylcellulose 50 .. .. 10 g
Maize Starch .. .. 20 g
Amaranth Solution .. .. 10 ml
Benzoic Acid Solution .. .. 20 ml
Chloroform Spirit .. .. 50 ml
Raspberry Syrup .. .. 200 ml
Water (see B.P.C. 1973, page 642) to 1000 ml
Stir a suspension of the starch in 125 ml of Water into about 350 ml of boiling Water. Maintain the temperature until the mixture becomes translucent, and cool rapidly. Triturate the sodium carboxymethylcellulose 50, the succinylsulphathiazole, and the light kaolin with the raspberry syrup to form a smooth paste; add gradually, with constant stirring, the starch mucilage, the benzoic acid solution, the amaranth solution, the chloroform spirit, and sufficient Water to produce the required volume.
It should be recently prepared.

Sulphadimidine Mixture, Paediatric: *add* the following formula and method, which is suitable for the extemporaneous preparation of the mixture:

Sulphadimidine, in fine powder	100 g
Sodium Carboxymethylcellulose 50	10 g
Maize Starch	20 g
Amaranth Solution	10 ml
Benzoic Acid Solution	20 ml
Chloroform Spirit	50 ml
Raspberry Syrup	200 ml
Water (see B.P.C. 1973, page 642) to	1000 ml

Stir a suspension of the starch in 125 ml of Water into about 350 ml of boiling Water. Maintain the temperature until the mixture becomes translucent, and cool rapidly. Triturate the sodium carboxymethylcellulose 50 and the sulphadimidine with the raspberry syrup to form a smooth paste; add gradually, with constant stirring, the starch mucilage, the benzoic acid solution, the amaranth solution, the chloroform spirit, and sufficient Water to produce the required volume.

It should be recently prepared.

Page 765

Squill Oxymel—formula: *after* "Squill" *insert* "or Indian Squill"

Coal Tar Paint—formula: *amend* "Benzene, nitration grade of commerce" *to* "Industrial Methylated Spirit"

Standard: *delete* the requirement

Page 766

Mastic Paint, Compound—formula: *amend to*

Mastic	400 g
Castor Oil	12.5 ml
Acetone	} of each
Industrial Methylated	equal
Spirit	volumes to 1000 ml

Page 769

Pastilles—formula: *amend* "Citric Acid" *to* "Citric Acid Monohydrate"

Page 780

Amaranth Solution—*replace* the monograph by the following:

A solution containing 1 per cent w/v of amaranth, food grade of commerce, with 20 per cent v/v of chloroform spirit, and 25 per cent v/v of glycerol, in purified water.

Page 781

Benzoic Acid Solution—in the formula: *insert* "to" *before* "1000 ml"

Page 788

(Intraperitoneal Dialysis Solutions)—footnote on Intraperitoneal Dialysis Solution (Acetate), last line: *amend* "lactate" *to* "acetate"

Page 791

Tartrazine Solution, Compound: *replace* the monograph by the following:

SYNONYM: Liquor Flavus

A solution containing 0.75 per cent w/v of tartrazine, food grade of commerce, and 0.1 per cent w/v of sunset yellow FCF, food grade of commerce, with 20 per cent v/v of chloroform spirit and 25 per cent v/v of glycerol, in purified water.

Pages 794–5

Adrenaline and Atropine Spray, Compound—Standard, CONTENT OF ADRENALINE ACID TARTRATE: *amend* the method of determination *to* "Dilute 5 ml to 250 ml with water; to 25 ml of this solution add 10 ml of *solution of standard pH 4.0* and dilute to 50 ml with water.

To 10 ml of this solution add 8 ml of 0.02N iodine, allow to stand for 10 minutes, add 2 ml of 0.1N sodium thiosulphate, mix well, and measure the extinction of a 1-cm layer at the maximum at about 492 nm. Repeat the procedure using 25 ml of a 0.016 per cent w/v solution of *adrenaline acid tartrate B.P.C.R.S.* in place of the 25 ml of sample solution. From the two extinctions calculate the amount of adrenaline acid tartrate in the sample."

CONTENT OF PAPAVERINE HYDROCHLORIDE: *amend* the method of determination *to* "To 20 ml add 1 ml of *dilute sulphuric acid* and extract with six successive 20-ml portions of *chloroform*, washing each extract with the same mixture of 10 ml of water and 0.05 ml of *dilute sulphuric acid* and reserving the acid solution and washings. Filter the chloroform extracts through cotton wool covered with a layer of *anhydrous sodium sulphate*, wash the residue with *chloroform*, and evaporate the combined filtrate and washings just to dryness on a water-bath.

Dissolve the residue in 40 ml of *glacial acetic acid*, with the aid of gentle heat, add 10 ml of *mercuric acetate solution* and titrate with 0.1N perchloric acid using *crystal violet solution* as indicator. Each ml of 0.1N perchloric acid is equivalent to 0.03759 g of $C_{20}H_{22}ClNO_4$."

Page 800

Lemon Syrup—formula: *amend* "Citric Acid" *to* "Citric Acid Monohydrate"

Page 801

Squill Syrup—WEIGHT PER ML: *delete* this requirement

Page 807

Belladonna and Phenobarbitone Tablets—CONTENT OF PHENOBARBITONE, line 5: *amend* "half a tablet" *to* "5 tablets"

Page 809

Calcium with Vitamin D Tablets—method of preparation: *add* "In making this preparation, the calcium sodium lactate may be replaced by calcium lactate, using 300 milligrams of calcium lactate for each 450 milligrams of calcium sodium lactate. Alternatively, a suitable quantity of a mixture of calcium sodium lactate with calcium lactate may be used."

Page 821

(Benzoin Tincture, Compound)—line 7: *amend* "0.890 g" *to* "0.880 g"

Page 823

Squill Tincture—formula: *after* "Squill" *insert* "or Indian Squill"

WEIGHT PER ML: *delete* this requirement

TOTAL SOLIDS: *delete* this requirement

Squill Vinegar—formula: *after* "Squill" *insert* "or Indian Squill"

WEIGHT PER ML: *delete* this requirement

TOTAL SOLIDS: *delete* this requirement

Page 829

Reagents and Solutions—*after* Acetic Acid, Glacial, *insert* the following:

Acetic Acid, Glacial, Anhydride-free: *glacial acetic acid* which complies with the following additional requirement:

ACETIC ANHYDRIDE. To 1 ml in a small porcelain dish add 0.1 ml of a reagent prepared by acidifying a 0.5 per cent w/v solution of *ferric chloride* in *alcohol (95 per cent)* with 0.05 ml of *hydrochloric acid* and saturating the solution with *hydroxylammonium chloride*. Evaporate the mixture to dryness; no violet colour is produced.

Anhydride-free glacial acetic acid may be prepared by fractionally distilling 1000 ml of *glacial acetic acid* to which has been added 3 g of *benzylamine*.

Page 833

Celite 545: amend the statement *to* "a flux-calcined diatomaceous earth obtainable from Johns-Manville Company Ltd, Hull, North Humberside."

Page 834

Chloride Solution, Standard—line 4: *amend* "0.5μg" *to* "5 μg"

Page 836

Digoxin Solution, Standard: *amend* "digoxin B.C.R.S." *to* "digoxin E.P.C.R.S."

Page 838

Fluorine Solution, Standard—line 4: *amend* "0.5 μg" *to* "5 μg"

Page 843

Phosphate Buffer pH 7.0, Glycerinated: *amend* "0.02M" *to* "0.2M", and *amend* "0.02N" *to* "0.2N"

Phosphoric Acid Solution, Standard: *amend* "2.777 g" *to* "0.2777 g"

Page 846

Sodium Chloride 0.0004M—line 3: *before* "dilute 20 ml" *insert* "dilute 1 ml of the solution to 100 ml and then"

Page 848

(Reagents and Solutions)—*above* the heading "Standard pH, Solution of" *insert* the following:

Sodium Zincate Solution: dissolve a quantity of *sodium hydroxide*, equivalent to 180 g of NaOH, in about 200 ml of water, heat the solution gently and, whilst stirring continuously, slowly add 80 g of *zinc oxide*. When all the zinc oxide has been added, boil until the solution becomes clear or only slightly turbid; cool, add 200 ml of water, stir well, cool to room temperature and dilute to 500 ml with water. Filter the solution through a sintered-glass filter (British Standard Grade No. 2) before use.

Sodium Zincate Solution, Dilute: to 1 volume of *sodium zincate solution* add, with stirring, 2 volumes of water and mix well. This solution should be used within 24 hours of preparation.

Page 849

Thioacetamide Reagent: *amend* "0.4 per cent" *to* "4 per cent"

Page 851

Dioctyl Sodium Sulphosuccinate, 0.005M—line 3: *amend* "1000 ml" *to* "100 ml"

Pages 852–853

C. AUTHENTIC SPECIMENS AND BRITISH CHEMICAL REFERENCE SUBSTANCES: *Delete* this section

Page 856

(Appendix 3, Ultraviolet Absorption for Identification)—Potassium Sorbate, under Extinction: *amend* "0.72" *to* "0.89"

Page 858

Aminobenzoic Acid—MOBILE PHASE: *add* "Shake together, allow to separate, and use the lower layer."

Page 859

(Aminobenzoic Acid Lotion)—MOBILE PHASE: *add* "Shake together, allow to separate, and use the lower layer."

Page 862

(Deoxycortone Pivalate)—*Limit Test for Related Foreign Steroids,* SOLUTION (2): *amend* "cortisone acetate B.C.R.S." *to* "cortisone acetate E.P.C.R.S." and *amend* "deoxycortone acetate B.C.R.S." *to* "deoxycortone acetate E.P.C.R.S."

Page 874

Reference Solutions: *amend* "Hydrocortisone acetate B.C.R.S." *to* "Hydrocortisone acetate E.P.C.R.S."

Page 877

Aluminium Magnesium Silicate: *amend* "1.25 g" *to* "3.3 g"

Page 886

Lead Solution (A), Standard: *after* "1000 ml" *insert* "and dilute 10 ml of this solution to 1000 ml with water."

Page 887

(Lead in Bismuth Carbonate)—left-hand column, line 26: *before* "standard lead" *insert* "dilute"

Page 912

Uniformity of Diameter of Tablets and Lozenges—Co-trimoxazole Paediatric Tablets: *amend* "8.0 to 8.5" *to* "7.5 to 8.0"

Page 917

(Appendix 27, Examination of Surgical Dressings)—CONTENT OF DOMIPHEN BROMIDE, lines 1 and 2: *after* "0.08 to 0.20 per cent," *insert* "calculated with reference to the air-dry material and" *Method 1*, second paragraph, *amend to*: "Add 40 ml of water and 0.2 ml of *bromophenol blue solution*, titrate with 2N sodium hydroxide until a blue or green colour is produced and then add 5 ml in excess; add 3.0 g of *anhydrous sodium acetate* and 10 ml of *chloroform*, shake the mixture and titrate with a 0.014 per cent w/v solution of *purified sodium lauryl sulphate* in water until the chloroform layer changes to colourless or yellow."

Method II, penultimate line: *amend* "35 ml" *to* "40 ml"

CONTENT OF EUFLAVINE, line 2: *after* "$C_{14}H_{14}ClN_3$" *insert* "and with reference to the air-dry material"

Page 919

Culture Media, lines 15–16: *amend* "Transfer 50-ml, 100-ml, or 150-ml portions, as appropriate," *to* "Transfer appropriate volumes (*see* below under QUANTITIES TO BE USED IN THE TEST)"

Test Procedure for Dressings other than Paraffin Gauze Dressing: *amend* the statement under "QUANTITIES TO BE USED IN THE TEST. 1. *Culture medium:*" *to*: "Use a volume just sufficient to ensure that the test portion becomes saturated and remains completely below the surface of the medium during the test; generally, this volume will be between 20 and 150 ml depending upon the absorbency and volume of the test portion."

Page 920

In the table at the top of the right-hand column, in the entry for more than 500 packages, *amend* the number to be taken *to* "2 per cent or 20 packages whichever is the less"

3. Amendments to British Pharmaceutical Codex Supplement 1976

Page 42
(Sodium Chloride and Dextrose Powder, Compound)—
above **Labelling**, *insert* the following:
Standard
PRESENCE OF DEXTROSE. 1. Heat; it melts, swells up, and burns, evolving the odour of burnt sugar.
2. Heat with *potassium cupri-tartrate solution*; a copious precipitate of cuprous oxide is produced.
PRESENCE OF POTASSIUM. 0.5 g complies with reaction D characteristic of potassium, given in the British Pharmacopoeia, Appendix V.
PRESENCE OF SODIUM. 0.2 g complies with reaction B and 0.7 g complies with reaction C characteristic of sodium, given in the British Pharmacopoeia, Appendix V.
CONTENT OF POTASSIUM. 1.70 to 1.88 per cent w/w, calculated as K, determined by method I of the British Pharmacopoeia, Appendix XIA, for flame photometry, an accurately weighed quantity, dissolved in a suitable volume of water, being used; use *potassium solution FP*, diluted if necessary with water, for the standard solutions.
CONTENT OF SODIUM. 1.74 to 1.92 per cent w/w, calculated as Na, determined by method I of the British Pharmacopoeia, Appendix XIA, for flame photometry, an accurately weighed quantity, dissolved in a suitable

volume of water, being used; use *sodium solution FP*, diluted if necessary with water, for the standard solutions.
CONTENT OF SODIUM BICARBONATE. 3.24 to 3.58 per cent w/w, calculated as $NaHCO_3$, determined by the following method: Dissolve an accurately weighed quantity of the powder, equivalent to about 0.07 g of sodium bicarbonate, in water, and titrate with 0.1N hydrochloric acid using *methyl orange solution* as indicator; each ml of 0.1N hydrochloric acid is equivalent to 0.00840 g of $NaHCO_3$.
CONTENT OF TOTAL CHLORIDE. 2.85 to 3.15 per cent w/w, calculated as Cl, determined by the following method:
Dissolve about 2 g, accurately weighed, in water, and titrate with 0.1N silver nitrate using *potassium chromate solution* as indicator; each ml of 0.1N silver nitrate is equivalent to 0.003545 g of Cl.
At the end of the monograph, *add* the following: When Sodium Chloride and Dextrose Powder, Compound, Small Size, is ordered, a powder of identical composition containing 8.8 grams in each single-unit container is supplied. The powder is dissolved, as described under "Uses", in sufficient water, recently boiled and cooled, to make 200 millilitres (7 fluid ounces) of solution. Sodium Chloride and Dextrose Powder, Compound and Sodium Chloride and Dextrose Powder, Compound, Small Size may be flavoured.

The Pharmaceutical Codex

Abbreviations

see under WEIGHTS AND MEASURES

Abnormalities of Metabolism, Inborn

see under FRUCTOSAEMIA, GALACTOSAEMIA, PHENYL-KETONURIA, and PORPHYRIA

Abortion

Abortion is the termination of pregnancy before the foetus is viable.

Spontaneous abortion is abortion which occurs without external stimuli. In the early weeks of pregnancy, spontaneous abortion is usually due to ovofoetal factors, such as foetal abnormalities, but in later weeks it is usually due to maternal factors, such as abnormalities of the genital tract.

Threatened abortion is uterine bleeding in the presence of an apparently intact pregnancy. The usual treatment is rest in bed for a few days or until the bleeding stops.

Inevitable abortion occurs when in addition to vaginal bleeding in early pregnancy there are uterine contractions accompanied by pain, and passage of foetal or placental tissue. Soon after the onset of symptoms abortion occurs. If abortion is incomplete (products of conception remain in the uterus) it may be completed by curettage.

Missed abortion is the retention of products of conception within the uterus for a prolonged period after the death of the foetus. There is cessation of growth or diminution in the size of the uterus. The pregnancy test becomes negative but there is no expulsion of uterine contents. Complete abortion is achieved by stimulation of the uterus with oxytocin or prostaglandins or by curettage.

Habitual abortion is repeated spontaneous abortion. The usual criterion is the occurrence of three consecutive, spontaneous, unexplained abortions, usually in a subject who has never had a successful pregnancy. Causes of habitual abortion include endocrine and metabolic disease, anatomical uterine abnormalities, and incompetence of the internal cervical os. Defective function of the corpus luteum is a common cause and progestogens have been used to maintain the uterine endometrium. Suturing of the internal os may prevent abortion in cases of incompetent os.

Therapeutic abortion is the elective termination of pregnancy. Its legality varies in different countries. In the United Kingdom under the Abortion Act 1967 abortion may only be legally induced if two registered medical practitioners form in good faith an opinion (i) that the continuance of the pregnancy would involve risk to the life of the pregnant woman greater than if the pregnancy were terminated, or (ii) that it would involve risk of injury to the physical or mental health of the pregnant woman greater than if the pregnancy were terminated, or (iii) that it would involve risk of injury to the physical or mental health of any existing children of the pregnant woman's family greater than if the pregnancy were terminated, or (iv) that there is a substantial risk that if the child were born it would suffer from such physical or mental abnormalities as to be seriously handicapped.

In early pregnancy, that is, before 12 weeks' gestation, complete abortion is usually achieved by dilatation of the cervix followed by manual or suction curettage. Later in pregnancy, abortion is achieved by intra-amniotic infusion of hypertonic sodium chloride or dextrose injection, or by stimulation of the uterus with oxytocin or prostaglandins. Pregnancy may also be terminated by hysterotomy.

Acacia

The air-dried gummy exudation flowing naturally from and obtained by incision of the stem and branches of *Acacia senegal* (L.) Willd. (Fam. Leguminosae), a small tree widely distributed in north, east, and west Africa. It may also be derived from certain other species of *Acacia* of African origin growing in Africa or elsewhere.

OTHER NAMES: Acac.; Acaciae Gummi; Gum Acacia; Gum Arabic

A standard is given in the European Pharmacopoeia Vol. I

Varieties. Many varieties occur in commerce, but the most esteemed is that collected in Kordofan, the best varieties of which are sun-bleached and yellowish-white in colour.

It may occur as "bleached druggists' acacia". This is produced by exposing tears to the hot sun for several weeks while workers remove pieces of bark and yellow tears. The resulting gum consists of almost white friable tears covered with numerous small fissures. However, this quality is now seldom available and for pharmaceutical purposes the use of unbleached gum of good quality is permitted.

The best qualities of Nigerian and Senegal gum are also suitable for pharmaceutical use. They are more transparent than the bleached Kordofan gum and contain occasional pieces of vermiform shape.

Constituents. Acacia is composed chiefly of the calcium, potassium, and magnesium salts of arabic acid which is a highly branched polysaccharide with uronic groups. It has an approximate molecular weight of 250 000. Acid hydrolysis with 2% v/v sulphuric acid yields mainly D-galactopyranose, L-arabofuranose, L-rhamnopyranose, and D-glucuronic acid, in the approximate molar ratio of 3:3:1:1. The basic structure consists of a main chain of $(1 \rightarrow 3)$-linked β-D-galactopyranose units, each of which bears a side chain at the C-6 position consisting predominantly of two $(1 \rightarrow 6)$-linked β-D-galactopyranose units terminated by a $(1 \rightarrow 6)$-linked β-D-glucuronic acid unit.

It also contains small amounts of 4-O-methyl-D-glucuronic acid, diastase, and a peroxidase system. Peroxidase is sensitive to heat, and, although present in unground acacia, may be destroyed when grinding the material to powder.

It yields about 2.7 to 4% of ash, which consists chiefly of the carbonates of calcium, potassium, and magnesium.

Description. UNGROUND DRUG. Rounded or ovoid tears, about 5 to 40 mm in diameter; tears yellowish-white to pale amber, sometimes with a pinkish tint; either brittle and opaque from the presence of numerous minute fissures, often broken into angular fragments with glistening surfaces, or transparent, breaking with difficulty, and exhibiting a conchoidal fracture.

It is almost odourless with a bland and mucilaginous taste.

POWDERED DRUG: Powdered Acacia. A white or yellowish-white powder possessing the odour, taste, and characteristic reactions of the unground drug.

Solubility. Almost entirely soluble in 2 parts of water, forming a slightly acid solution or mucilage which is not glairy; practically insoluble in alcohol.

Adulterants and substitutes. Many dark-coloured kinds of gum arabic occur in commerce and are used for various industrial purposes.

Gum acacia of Indian origin is obtained from numerous species of *Acacia* and from plants of other families unrelated to Leguminosae; the commercial article collected locally is therefore of a very mixed character and consists of tears of different sizes and colours, the majority being dark brown.

Other possible adulterants are agar, dextrin, starch, sterculia, and tragacanth.

When in powder and treated with *ruthenium red solution*, staining of the powder indicates the presence of agar or sterculia.

On dissolving in water and adding *lead acetate solution* the development of a cloudiness indicates the presence of agar or tragacanth as does the production of a crimson or olive-green colour when 0.02N iodine is added to a sample in powder. When a solution in water, previously boiled and cooled, is treated with 0.1N iodine, the production of a blue or reddish-brown colour indicates the presence of starch or dextrin.

Hygroscopicity. At relative humidities between 25 and 65%, the equilibrium moisture content of powdered acacia at 25° is between about 8 and 13%, but at relative humidities above about 70%, it absorbs substantial amounts of moisture.

Storage. It should be stored in a cool dry place. Powdered acacia should be stored in airtight containers.

Identification. 1. A solution in water is laevorotatory. 2. Shake a 5% solution in water with 0.5 ml of *dilute hydrogen peroxide solution* and 0.5 ml of *guaiacum tincture* and allow to stand for a few minutes; a deep blue or bluish-green colour develops.

Uses. Acacia in solution in water is used as a suspending agent, usually with tragacanth, in mixtures containing resinous tinctures or powders which do not readily disperse. A mucilage may be prepared by dissolving 40 g of acacia tears, previously rinsed, in 60 ml of chloroform water. The mucilage deteriorates rapidly on storage. Solutions of acacia have a remarkably low viscosity, a 30% w/v aqueous solution having a typical viscosity of only 200 centipoises (0.2 Pa.s), but they have a marked activity as a protective colloid, hence their use to stabilise particulate dispersions. Viscosity may be increased by incorporation of tragacanth as indicated above.

Acacia is an effective oil-in-water emulsifying agent, forming a rigid interfacial film which is stable in the presence of electrolytes and high hydrogen ion concentration. The gum, in powder, is used for emulsifying fixed and volatile oils and liquid paraffin. One part of gum will emulsify 4 parts of fixed oil or liquid paraffin, 2 parts of water being used to produce the primary emulsion; volatile oils require twice the proportion of gum and water. The primary emulsion may be prepared by dispersing the gum in the oil in a mortar, adding the water in one quantity and triturating thoroughly until the white viscous primary emulsion is formed; the emulsion may then be diluted with more of the aqueous phase, any electrolytes being added, in solution, just before making up to volume. Alternatively, a mucilage is prepared by rapidly triturating the acacia with the specified quantity of water and the oil is added in small portions; after each addition the mixture is triturated thoroughly to produce the primary emulsion; the procedure for completing the preparation is then the same as for the first method. The two methods are known respectively as the dry- and wet-gum methods. If mechanical aids are used to produce an emulsion, the amount of gum may need to be appreciably reduced to produce an emulsion of the required viscosity.

Acacia is used in lozenge manufacture as a firm binder that imparts a mucilaginous texture and slow dissolution characteristics which are necessary for preparations to be dissolved slowly in the mouth.

For tablet manufacture, it has been largely superseded because of cost, the possibility of contamination, and a tendency to prolong the disintegration time of the product. On the other hand granulation problems may be resolved in some cases by the sticky nature of acacia solutions. When used in tabletting, visual examination of the powder should be made and samples showing dark particles should be rejected as these will show on the tablet surface after compression. It is now possible to obtain commercially acacia powder prepared by spray-drying, which eliminates "bitterness".

Acacia is used in combination with gelatin to form complex coacervates. By control of the dispersed state, temperature, and pH, and addition of desolvating agents, these colloidal mixtures can be used to micro-encapsulate drugs to ease handling or to control dissolution rate.

Acacia contains peroxidase enzymes which cause incompatibility with some drugs. These enzymes may be destroyed by heating to 100°.

Because acacia is a natural product, the gum is frequently contaminated with micro-organisms. *Escherichia coli* and salmonellae may be present. Any process for reducing microbial contamination should be such that the emulsifying and suspending properties of the gum are not impaired.

Preparation

Acacia is an ingredient of compound tragacanth powder.

Acepromazine Maleate

2-Acetyl-10-(3-dimethylaminopropyl)phenothiazine hydrogen maleate

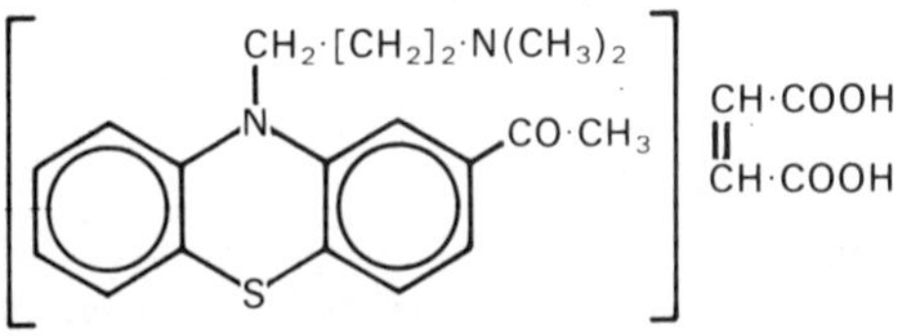

$C_{23}H_{26}N_2O_5S = 442.5$

OTHER NAMES: Acetylpromazine Maleate

Large Animal Immobilon® (with etorphine hydrochloride)

A standard is given in the British Pharmacopoeia (Veterinary)

Description. A yellow crystalline odourless powder with a bitter taste.

Solubility. Soluble, at 20°, in 27 parts of water, in 13 parts of alcohol, and in 3 parts of chloroform; very slightly soluble in ether.

Acidity. A 1% solution has a pH of 4 to 4.5.

Moisture content. Not more than 1%, determined by drying at 105°.

Sterilisation. Solutions for injection are sterilised by heating in an autoclave or by filtration.

Storage. It should be protected from light.

Identification. TESTS. 1. Dissolve about 5 mg in 2 ml of sulphuric acid; a yellow colour is produced. Warm for 2 minutes; the colour changes to deep orange.
2. Dissolve about 200 mg in a mixture of 3 ml of water and 2 ml of *sodium hydroxide solution*, and extract with three successive 3-ml portions of ether; to the aqueous solution add 2 ml of *bromine solution AsT*, warm in a water-bath for 10 minutes, heat to boiling, cool, add 5 drops of the solution to a solution of 10 mg of resorcinol in 3 ml of sulphuric acid, and heat in a water-bath for 15 minutes; a bluish-black colour develops.

MELTING-POINT. About 137°.

ULTRAVIOLET ABSORPTION. In 0.1N hydrochloric acid, maxima at 244 nm (E1%, 1cm = 550) and 280 nm (E1%, 1cm = 410).

Veterinary uses. Acepromazine is used in animals as a tranquilliser and motion-sickness remedy. It is also used in premedication for anaesthesia. The usual dose by intramuscular or slow intravenous injection for horses, cattle, sheep, and pigs is the equivalent of 50 to 100 micrograms of acepromazine per kilogram body-weight and for dogs and cats the equivalent of 125 to 250 micrograms per kilogram body-weight. The dose by mouth for dogs and cats is the equivalent of 1 to 3 milligrams of acepromazine per kilogram body-weight as a tranquilliser and the equivalent of 1 milligram per kilogram body-weight for motion sickness.

Preparations

ACEPROMAZINE INJECTION (*Syn.* Acepromazine Maleate Injection): a sterile solution of acepromazine maleate in water for injections. The acidity of the solution is adjusted to pH 5 by the addition of sodium hydroxide. The solution is sterilised by heating in an autoclave or by filtration.

Available in 10-ml units containing acepromazine maleate equivalent to 2 mg of acepromazine per ml and in 20-ml units containing acepromazine maleate equivalent to 10 mg of acepromazine per ml.

A standard for this injection is given in the British Pharmacopoeia (Veterinary)
Containers: see the entry on Injections for general information on containers.
Labelling: see the entry on Injections for general information on labelling. In addition, the label on the container should state the amount of the medicament as the equivalent amount of acepromazine in 1 ml.
Storage: it should be protected from light.

ACEPROMAZINE TABLETS (*Syn.* Acepromazine Maleate Tablets): available as tablets containing acepromazine maleate equivalent to 10 and 25 mg of acepromazine; they may be coated with sugar or other suitable material.

A standard for these tablets is given in the British Pharmacopoeia (Veterinary)
Containers, Labelling, and *Storage:* see the entry on Tablets for general information on containers, labelling, and storage. Containers should be airtight and light resistant.

ETORPHINE AND ACEPROMAZINE INJECTION: a sterile solution of etorphine hydrochloride and acepromazine maleate, with sodium chloride and a suitable preservative, in water for injections. The acidity of the solution is adjusted to pH 4. It is sterilised by heating in an autoclave or by filtration. Available in 10-ml vials containing 2.45 mg of etorphine hydrochloride and 10 mg of acepromazine maleate per ml.

A standard for this injection is given in the British Pharmacopoeia (Veterinary)
Containers and *Labelling:* see the entry on Injections for general information on containers and labelling.
Storage: it should be protected from light.

Acetaminophen

see PARACETAMOL

Acetarsol

3-Acetamido-4-hydroxyphenylarsonic acid

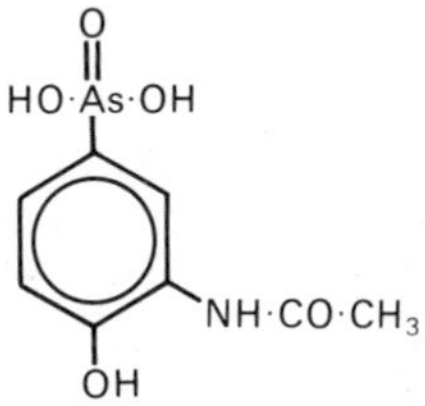

$C_8H_{10}AsNO_5 = 275.1$

OTHER NAMES: Acetarsone; *Stovarsol*®; *SVC*®

A standard is given in the British Pharmacopoeia 1973

Description. A white crystalline odourless powder with a faintly acid taste.

Solubility. Very slightly soluble in water; practically insoluble in alcohol and in dilute acids; soluble in dilute alkalis.

Dissociation constants. pK$_a$ 3.73, 7.9, 9.3.

Identification. TESTS. 1. Dissolve 200 mg in 2 ml of 1N sodium hydroxide, add 2 ml of sulphuric acid and 2 ml of alcohol (95%), and heat; the odour of ethyl acetate is produced.
2. To a solution of 1 g in 10 ml of *sodium hydroxide solution* add 10 ml of water and 2 g of sodium dithionite and heat in a water-bath for 20 minutes; a yellow precipitate is produced. Decant; the precipitate is soluble in excess *sodium hydroxide solution.*

MELTING-POINT. About 240°, with decomposition.

INFRA-RED ABSORPTION. Major peaks at 784, 823, 887, 1400, 1419, and 1538 cm^{-1} (see Appendix 2a: Infra-red Spectra).

Metabolism. ABSORPTION. Readily absorbed after oral administration.

DISTRIBUTION. Small amounts are stored in the liver and other tissues and it also enters the cerebrospinal fluid.

EXCRETION. Rapidly excreted in the urine.

Actions and uses. Acetarsol is used in the treatment of intestinal amoebiasis, but it has been largely replaced by less toxic drugs. The dose for the treatment of intestinal amoebiasis is 250 milligrams twice daily for 10 days, usually in conjunction with emetine or another amoebicide. The oral dose for children under one year is 5 to 10 milligrams per kilogram body-weight, 1 to 5 years 60 to 100 milligrams, and 6 to 12 years 120 milligrams.
Acetarsol has been used locally in the treatment of vaginal trichomoniasis but toxic amounts may be absorbed and safer drugs are available.

Undesirable effects. Gastro-intestinal disturbances, urticaria, and erythema may occur. Excessive use of vaginal preparations may cause arsenical poisoning; this rarely happens after oral administration.

Contra-indications. It is contra-indicated in liver disease and kidney disease.

Poisoning. For the treatment of anaphylactoid reactions, subcutaneous injections of adrenaline should be given. The toxic effects of arsenic, such as exfoliative dermatitis and arsenical encephalopathy, may be treated by intramuscular injections of dimercaprol.

Preparations

ACETARSOL PESSARIES (*Syn.* Acetarsol Vaginal Tablets): for each pessary take:

Acetarsol	..	..	..	..	..	250 mg
Anhydrous dextrose	..	..	..	..	320 mg
Starch	..	..	..	..	..	350 mg

Mix, and prepare by moist granulation and compression as described in the entry on Tablets. Acetarsol pessaries may be prepared with any other suitable basis, including an effervescent basis.
A standard for these pessaries is given in the British Pharmaceutical Codex 1973
Containers and *Storage:* see the entry on Tablets for general information on containers and storage.
Advice for patients: the pessaries should be inserted high into the vagina without previously moistening them with water, preferably at night. The prescribed course should be completed.

OTHER PREPARATIONS available include TABLETS containing acetarsol 30 and 250 mg.

Acetazolamide

N-(5-Sulphamoyl-1,3,4-thiadiazol-2-yl)acetamide

$$CH_3 \cdot CO \cdot NH \underset{N \underline{\quad\quad} N}{\overset{S}{\diagup\diagdown}} SO_2 \cdot NH_2$$

C$_4$H$_6$N$_4$O$_3$S$_2$ = 222.2

OTHER NAME: *Diamox* ®

A standard is given in the British Pharmacopoeia 1973

Description. A fine, white or yellowish-white, crystalline, odourless, tasteless powder.

Solubility. Very slightly soluble in water; soluble, at 20°, in 400 parts of alcohol and in 100 parts of acetone; practically insoluble in ether, in chloroform, and in carbon tetrachloride.

Dissociation constants. pK$_a$ 7.2, 9.0 (25°).

Identification. TESTS. 1. Triturate 500 mg with 5 ml of water and 1 ml of 1N sodium hydroxide, and add 200 mg of zinc powder and 10 drops of hydrochloric acid; hydrogen sulphide is evolved.
2. To a small quantity add 5 ml of water, 3 drops of 1N sodium hydroxide, and 2 drops of *copper sulphate solution*; a bluish-green colour or precipitate is produced.
3. Dissolve 100 mg in 5 ml of *sodium hydroxide solution*, add 5 ml of a solution containing 1% of hydroxyl-ammonium chloride and 0.8% of copper sulphate, mix and heat the pale yellow solution in a water-bath for 5 minutes; a clear bright yellow solution is produced with no heavy precipitate or dark brown colour.

MELTING-POINT. About 258°.

ULTRAVIOLET ABSORPTION. In 0.1N hydrochloric acid, maximum at 265 nm (E1%, 1cm = 475).

INFRA-RED ABSORPTION. Major peaks at 671, 704, 1176, 1316, 1538, and 1667 cm^{-1} (see Appendix 2b: Infra-red Spectra).

Determination in body fluids. GAS CHROMATOGRAPHY. In blood, plasma, or saliva—S. M. Wallace *et al.*, *J. pharm. Sci.*, 1977, **66**, 527.

HIGH PRESSURE LIQUID CHROMATOGRAPHY. In plasma: a short review of other methods is also included— W. F. Bayne *et al.*, *J. pharm. Sci.*, 1975, **64**, 402.

ENZYME INHIBITION. In plasma—G. J. Yakatan *et al.*, *Analytica chim. Acta*, 1976, **84**, 173.

Metabolism. ABSORPTION. Readily absorbed after oral administration.

BLOOD CONCENTRATION. After an intravenous dose of 1.4 mg/kg, plasma concentrations of free drug of 0.5 to 13 μg/ml are obtained; effective plasma concentrations are in the range 10 to 15 μg/ml; after an oral dose of 500 mg, peak plasma concentrations of about 25 μg/ml are attained within 2 to 3 hours.

HALF-LIFE. Plasma half-life, about 2 to 6 hours.

DISTRIBUTION. Acetazolamide binds tightly to carbonic anhydrase and will accumulate in tissues in which this enzyme is present, particularly in red blood cells and the renal cortex; it enters the cerebrospinal fluid, crosses the placenta, and is secreted in milk; *protein binding*, 90 to 95% bound to plasma proteins.

METABOLIC REACTIONS. Acetazolamide does not appear to be metabolised in the body.

EXCRETION. 70 to 90% of a dose is excreted in the urine as unchanged drug in 24 hours; the drug is excreted by active transport processes and its renal clearance is increased if the urine is alkaline; small amounts of the drug are excreted in the bile.

FURTHER INFORMATION. Concentrations in plasma— W. F. Bayne et al., J. pharm. Sci., 1975, **64**, 402; absorption in rats—R. D. Schoenwald and R. L. Ward, J. pharm. Sci., 1976, **65**, 677; see also T. H. Maren, Physiol. Rev., 1967, **47**, 595.

Actions and uses. Acetazolamide produces diuresis by specifically inhibiting carbonic anhydrase. It was formerly used as a diuretic but is now used to reduce intra-ocular pressure in the treatment of glaucoma. It acts on the renal tubules, and when the rate at which carbonic acid is formed is reduced by the inhibition of carbonic anhydrase, hydrogen- and sodium-ion exchange is greatly reduced. As a result, bicarbonate resorption is incomplete and there is an increased volume of alkaline urine.

Acetazolamide is of limited value as a diuretic because, if it is given continuously, the decrease of bicarbonate ion in the extracellular fluid and the increase in hydrogen ion gradually overcomes the effect of carbonic anhydrase inhibition, and produces a metabolic acidosis. Renal compensation thus occurs, most of the filtered bicarbonate is resorbed, and diuresis ceases, but a mild degree of metabolic acidosis may persist. Therefore, the effect of subsequent doses on consecutive days diminishes and diuresis ceases by the sixth day. Carbonic anhydrase is inhibited for 6 hours by a single dose of 250 milligrams of acetazolamide.

In glaucoma, the initial dose is 500 milligrams, followed by 250 milligrams every 6 hours; when the intra-ocular tension is normal, the maintenance dosage is 250 milligrams 2 or 3 times daily.

As a diuretic, 250 to 500 milligrams of acetazolamide has been given by mouth once daily or every other day.

Undesirable effects. Large doses of acetazolamide may cause drowsiness and numbness and tingling of the face and extremities. If potassium bicarbonate is given with acetazolamide, renal stone formation may occur.

Preparations

ACETAZOLAMIDE TABLETS: available as tablets containing 250 mg of acetazolamide.

A standard for these tablets is given in the British Pharmacopoeia 1973

Containers and Storage: see the entry on Tablets for general information on containers and storage. Containers should be airtight.

Advice for patients: daily doses should preferably be taken in the morning. When used in glaucoma, treatment should not be discontinued without the advice of the prescriber. The tablets may cause drowsiness; persons affected should not drive or operate machinery. Alcohol should be avoided.

OTHER PREPARATIONS available include CAPSULES containing acetazolamide 500 mg in a slow-release formulation; and an INJECTION reconstituted from vials of powder containing acetazolamide sodium equivalent to acetazolamide 500 mg.

Acetic Acid, Glacial

$CH_3 . CO_2H = 60.05$

OTHER NAME: Glac. Acet. Acid

A standard is given in the British Pharmaceutical Codex 1973

Description. A translucent crystalline mass, or, at temperatures above its crystallising-point, a clear colourless liquid; odour pungent. It crystallises at about 15°.

Solubility. Miscible with water, with alcohol, with chloroform, and with most fixed and volatile oils.

Weight per ml. At 20°, 1.048 to 1.051 g.

Boiling-point. About 117°.

Dissociation constant. pK_a 4.8 (25°).

Storage. It should be stored in airtight containers.

Uses. Glacial acetic acid is used to prepare dilute acetic acids and strong ammonium acetate solution. It has been used for the destruction of warts.

Poisoning. A stomach tube or emetics should not be used. The acid must be neutralised as quickly as possible and large quantities of water or milk should be given if there is a delay in obtaining a suitable alkali. Calcium hydroxide in water and magnesium hydroxide mixture are good antidotes; carbonates should be avoided if possible, as they lead to the liberation of carbon dioxide and the consequent risk of perforation. If perforation is suspected nothing should be given by mouth.

After neutralisation of the acid, demulcents such as milk, raw eggs, or a vegetable oil, such as olive oil, should be given, and shock should be treated by warmth and an intravenous infusion if required. Morphine should be given for the relief of pain and prednisolone may be given in a dosage of 60 milligrams daily to reduce oesophageal stricture.

Glacial acetic acid burns should be treated immediately by flooding with water, followed by the application of sodium bicarbonate or chalk in powder, or by sodium bicarbonate or saline packs.

Preparations

ACETIC ACID: may be prepared by diluting 1 part by weight of glacial acetic acid with 2 parts by weight of purified water or by suitably diluting a pure commercial acetic acid, usually one containing 80% of $C_2H_4O_2$. It contains 33% w/w of $C_2H_4O_2$.

A standard for acetic acid is given in the British Pharmacopoeia 1973

Uses: it has a mild expectorant action. It is administered by mouth, usually in linctuses as oxymel or squill oxymel. Applied externally, it has an irritant action and has been used in liniments.

DILUTE ACETIC ACID:

Acetic acid	182 g
Purified water, freshly boiled and cooled	818 g

Mix. Dilute acetic acid contains 6% w/w of $C_2H_4O_2$.

A standard for dilute acetic acid is given in the British Pharmacopoeia 1973

OXYMEL:

Acetic acid	150 ml
Purified water, freshly boiled and cooled	150 ml
Purified honey	to 1000 ml

Mix thoroughly.

A standard for oxymel is given in the British Pharmaceutical Codex 1973

Dose: 2.5 to 10 millilitres.

OTHER PREPARATION: acetic acid is an ingredient of squill oxymel.

Acetomenaphthone

2-Methylnaphthalene-1,4-diyl diacetate

$C_{15}H_{14}O_4 = 258.3$

OTHER NAMES: *Amisyn*® (with nicotinamide); *Chilblain Treatment Dellipsoids D27*® (with nicotinic acid); *Pernivit*® (with nicotinic acid)

A standard is given in the British Pharmacopoeia 1973

Description. A white crystalline powder which is odourless or has a slight odour of acetic acid and has a bitter taste.

Solubility. Very slightly soluble in water and in cold alcohol; soluble in 3.3 parts of boiling alcohol; soluble in acetic acid.

Identification. TEST. To about 50 mg add 5 ml of 0.1N sodium hydroxide, warm for a few minutes, cool, add a few drops of *hydrogen peroxide solution* and then sufficient *dilute hydrochloric acid* to neutralise the solution, filter, and wash the filter with water; dissolve 0.5 mg of the residue in 5 ml of alcohol (95%) and add 2 ml of *strong ammonia solution* followed by a few drops of ethyl cyanoacetate; a violet colour is produced. Add 5 ml of *sodium hydroxide solution*; a brownish-yellow colour is produced. The violet colour is destroyed on the addition of acid or on exposure to sunlight.

MELTING-POINT. About 113°.

ULTRAVIOLET ABSORPTION. In dehydrated alcohol, maxima at 285 nm (E1%, 1cm = 250) and 322 nm (E1%, 1cm = 37).

Actions and uses. Acetomenaphthone has actions, uses, and undesirable effects similar to those described under Phytomenadione, but it acts more slowly.

As a prophylactic against haemorrhagic disease of the newborn 5 to 10 milligrams may be given daily for one week before delivery. For the treatment of haemorrhagic disease of the newborn phytomenadione is preferred.

For the pre-operative treatment of obstructive jaundice doses of 10 to 20 milligrams are given daily for one week.

Preparations

ACETOMENAPHTHONE TABLETS: available as tablets containing 5 and 10 mg of acetomenaphthone. They may be sugar-coated.

A standard for these tablets is given in the British Pharmacopoeia 1973

Containers and *Storage:* see the entry on Tablets for general information on containers and storage. Containers should be airtight.

OTHER PREPARATIONS available include TABLETS containing acetomenaphthone 10 mg with nicotinamide 50 mg and tablets containing acetomenaphthone 7 mg with nicotinic acid 25 mg.

Acetone

Propan-2-one *or* dimethyl ketone

$$CH_3 \cdot CO \cdot CH_3$$

$C_3H_6O = 58.08$

A standard is given in the British Pharmaceutical Codex 1973

Description. A clear, colourless, inflammable, mobile, volatile liquid with a characteristic odour.

Solubility. Miscible with water, with alcohol, with methyl alcohol, with ether, and with chloroform.

Weight per ml. At 20°, 0.789 to 0.791 g.

Refractive index. About 1.359.

Storage. It should be stored in airtight containers in a cool place.

Identification. TESTS. 1. To 1 ml of a 0.5% v/v solution in water add 1 ml of *sodium nitroprusside solution*, 2 ml of 1N sodium hydroxide, and a slight excess of acetic acid; a deep red colour is produced which changes to violet on dilution with water.

2. To 10 ml of a 0.1% v/v solution in alcohol (50%) add 1 ml of *2-nitrobenzaldehyde solution*, followed by 1 ml of *sodium hydroxide solution*, allow to stand for about 2 minutes, and acidify with acetic acid; a bluish-green colour is produced.

3. To 1 ml add 1 ml of a 4% solution of sodium hydroxide, warm, and add 3 ml of 0.1N iodine; a yellow precipitate of iodoform is produced.

BOILING-POINT. About 56°.

Determination in body fluids. ULTRAVIOLET ABSORPTION. In blood or urine—V. C. Klendshoj and M. Feldstein, *Can. J. med. Technol.*, 1955, **17**, 74.

INFRA-RED ABSORPTION. In blood—R. D. Stewart *et al.*, *Nature Lond.*, 1961, **191**, 1008.

GAS CHROMATOGRAPHY. In breath—M. D. Trotter *et al.*, *Clinica chim. Acta*, 1971, **35**, 137.

Metabolism. ABSORPTION. Absorbed through the lungs and skin.

METABOLIC REACTIONS. Oxidation, or utilised in the body as acetate or formate.

EXCRETION. Excreted in the urine and through the lungs; large doses are mainly excreted unchanged but small doses are excreted mainly as carbon dioxide; about 7% of doses of up to 2 mg/ml in rats is exhaled unchanged.

Uses. Acetone is used as a solvent for organic substances, including resins, fats, and pyroxylin, and in some solutions used for film-coating tablets. It should not be used as a solvent for iodine, with which it forms a volatile compound which is extremely irritating to the eyes. On account of its low boiling-point it is a suitable menstruum for extracting thermolabile substances from crude drugs. It is an ingredient of some preparations for cleansing the skin before operations.

Acne

Acne (Acne vulgaris) is a papular affection of the skin characterised by the presence of comedones (blackheads) resulting from an excessive secretion from the sebaceous glands and blockage and infection of the pilosebaceous ducts due to hyperkeratosis. The subsequent retention of sebum results in the formation of the characteristic pustule. Acne occurs most commonly in adolescence and is found mainly on the face, neck, shoulders, chest, and ears. It is brought about either by an androgen–oestrogen imbalance or by excessive reactivity of the pilosebaceous glands to circulating androgens.

Treatment usually consists in cleansing the skin with detergent solutions having antiseptic properties and the application of antiseptic creams or lotions, including sulphur, neomycin, and peroxides. Antibacterial agents may also be given by mouth, especially tetracycline, clindamycin, and occasionally co-trimoxazole and erythromycin. It may be a month or more before real improvement occurs and in some instances antibiotic therapy may be necessary for periods as long as two or more years.

Local applications of sulphur ointments and creams may cause peeling and occasionally aggravate the condition. The use of abrasive creams has been recommended but their efficacy has not been proved.

Since the excretion of sebum is regulated in response to circulating androgens, treatment with oestrogens may be used in refractory cases but large doses are required and their other effects may be troublesome.

Diet is not considered to be a causative factor.

Acrocyanosis

Acrocyanosis is characterised by a persistent symmetrical cyanosis of the hands and less commonly the feet caused by spasm of the small arterioles of the skin. The skin sweats profusely and has an uneven blue and red discoloration which is more persistent than in Raynaud's disease.

Treatment may be unnecessary, but vasodilator drugs such as nicotinic acid may be used for cosmetic reasons.

Addison's Disease

Addison's disease is due to chronic hypofunction of the adrenal cortex. It is characterised by progressive lassitude, weight loss, hypotension, dusky pigmentation of the skin, and gastro-intestinal disturbances including anorexia, nausea, diarrhoea, and rarely steatorrhoea.

The adrenal insufficiency may be due to adrenal atrophy often attributable to autoimmune processes or to destruction of the adrenals, for example, by tuberculosis or secondary deposits of neoplastic tissue particularly of the bronchus. Total adrenalectomy for the treatment of Cushing's syndrome may also result in Addison's disease.

Adrenal failure secondary to panhypopituitarism results in a deficiency of glucocorticoid and androgenic secretions but not of aldosterone; the symptoms are similar to though milder than those of Addison's disease and pigmentation of the skin does not occur.

Addison's disease is treated by replacement therapy with corticosteroids chosen to provide a suitable balance of glucocorticoid and mineralocorticoid activity, as described under Cortisone Acetate.

Adrenal Insufficiency, Acute

Acute adrenal insufficiency is an acute deficiency of corticosteroid hormones due either to adrenal haemorrhagic necrosis caused by an overwhelming infection or to an exacerbation of Addison's disease by stress, infections, or withdrawal of maintenance therapy. It may also be precipitated by too rapid withdrawal of steroids used in the treatment of other conditions and therefore withdrawal of steroids should always be gradual.

Acute adrenal insufficiency is rapid in onset and characterised by weakness, apathy, nausea, vomiting, diarrhoea, and peripheral vascular collapse followed by oliguria and, in the absence of treatment, death.

Intravenous administration of corticosteroids such as hydrocortisone (cortisol) and fluid replacement therapy are required to overcome the acute adrenal crisis. Replacement treatment with corticosteroids as for Addison's disease may be required subsequently, and dosage should be adjusted as necessary. During surgery or infection and in times of stress the requirements for corticosteroids by the body are increased, and dosage should therefore be increased accordingly.

Adrenaline

(R)-1-(3,4-Dihydroxyphenyl)-2-methylaminoethanol or (R)-3,4-dihydroxy-α-methylaminomethylbenzyl alcohol

$C_9H_{13}NO_3 = 183.2$

OTHER NAMES: Adren.; Epinephrine; Epirenamine; Eppy®; Levorenin; Simplene®

A standard is given in the British Pharmacopoeia 1973

Adrenaline is an active principle of the suprarenal gland.

Description. A white or creamy-white, sphaerocrystalline, odourless powder.

Solubility. Very slightly soluble in water; practically insoluble in alcohol, in ether, in chloroform, in liquid paraffin, and in many other organic solvents; readily soluble in solutions of mineral acids and of alkali hydroxides, but not in solutions of ammonia or of alkali carbonates.

Dissociation constants. pK_a 8.7, 10.2, 12 (20°).

Stability. Adrenaline and adrenaline acid tartrate darken slowly on exposure to air and light. Adrenaline is degraded in aqueous solution by racemisation to biologically inactive substances; a red discoloration is produced by adrenochrome and other coloured products. The reactions are catalysed by hydrogen ions and by hydroxyl ions. Solutions are most stable at pH 3.2 to 3.6. Adrenaline reacts with salts of sulphurous acid to form a derivative of sulphonic acid which is biologically inactive. This interaction may be important in those pharmaceutical preparations in which the oxygen content is low and the molar ratio of sodium metabisulphite to adrenaline approaches unity; in medicines in which an excess of adrenaline is present, interaction with sodium metabisulphite reduces the biological activity only very slightly. Solutions containing adrenaline and sodium metabisulphite can be stabilised by the addition of boric acid provided that the oxygen content is low; stabilisation is due to chelation of adrenaline by the boric acid and the degree of chelation is enhanced by an increase in pH.

FURTHER INFORMATION. Stability in aqueous solution—G. B. West, *J. Pharm. Pharmac.*, 1950, **2**, 864. Stability of adrenaline injection—K. Backe-Mansen *et al.*, *Acta pharm. suec.*, 1966, **3**, 269; P. Lundgren and S. Strom, *Acta pharm. suec.*, 1966, **3**, 273. Interactions between adrenaline and sulphites—L. C. Schroeter, *Sulfur Dioxide, Applications in Food, Beverages, and Pharmaceuticals*, London, Pergamon Press, 1966; B. R. Hajratwala, *J. pharm. Sci.*, 1975, **64**, 45. Stabilisation of solutions of adrenaline and sodium metabisulphite and boric acid—S. Riegelman and E. Z. Fischer, *J. pharm. Sci.*, 1962, **51**, 206 and 210.

Incompatibility. Adrenaline and adrenaline acid tartrate are incompatible with oxidising agents, alkalis, copper, iron, silver, zinc, and other metals, gum, and tannin. Interaction with sulphites is discussed under Stability above.

Storage. It should be stored in airtight containers, preferably in an atmosphere of nitrogen, protected from light.

Identification. TESTS. 1. To a neutral or faintly acid solution add a few drops of a 0.25% solution of ferric chloride; an emerald-green colour develops. Add *sodium bicarbonate solution* gradually; the colour changes first to blue and then to red.
2. To one drop of a 1% solution in acetic acid (1%) add 1 drop of *copper sulphate solution* followed by 1 drop of 2N sodium hydroxide; a green colour changing to greenish-brown is produced.
3. Dissolve a few mg in 5 ml of *solution of standard pH 4.0*, add 1 ml of 0.1N iodine, mix, allow to stand for 5 minutes, and then add 2 ml of 0.1N sodium thiosulphate; a deep red colour is produced.

MELTING-POINT. About 212°, with decomposition.

ULTRAVIOLET ABSORPTION. In 0.1N hydrochloric acid, maxima at 221 nm (E1%, 1cm = 305) and 281 nm (E1%, 1cm = 159).

INFRA-RED ABSORPTION. Major peaks at 945, 1224, 1258, 1279, 1420, and 1496 cm⁻¹ (see Appendix 2a: Infra-red Spectra).

Determination in body fluids. GAS CHROMATOGRAPHY. In plasma, serum, or urine: adrenaline and noradrenaline —H. G. Lovelady and L. L. Foster, *J. Chromat.*, 1975, **108**, 43.

SPECTROFLUORIMETRY. In plasma: adrenaline and noradrenaline—J. F. O'Hanlon jun. *et al.*, *Analyt. Biochem.*, 1970, **34**, 568. In urine: adrenaline and noradrenaline—A. Pekkarinen and M.-E. Pitkanen, *Scand. J. clin. Lab. Invest.*, 1955, **7**, 1.

Metabolism. ABSORPTION. Rapidly destroyed in the gastro-intestinal tract after oral administration, and any unchanged drug which is absorbed is rapidly metabolised by the liver; the effects of adrenaline after subcutaneous administration are produced within 5 minutes and appear more slowly than those achieved by intramuscular administration.

BLOOD CONCENTRATION. Endogenous plasma concentrations in normal subjects are in the range 30 to 160 pg/ml.

DISTRIBUTION. Rapidly taken up by the heart, spleen, several glandular tissues, and adrenergic nerves; only metabolites are detectable in the cerebrospinal fluid; adrenaline readily crosses the placenta; *protein binding,* about 50% bound to plasma proteins.

METABOLIC REACTIONS. Rapidly metabolised by oxidative deamination and *O*-methylation followed by reduction or glucuronic acid or sulphate conjugation.

EXCRETION. 73 to 95% of an intravenous dose is excreted in the urine; of the excreted material about 80% is excreted as *O*-methyl metabolites and 2% as catechol metabolites and only 1% is excreted as unchanged drug; the major urinary metabolite is 4-hydroxy-3-methoxymandelic acid (HMMA); other metabolites include 4-hydroxy-3-methoxyphenylacetic acid (HVA), conjugated metadrenaline, and 4-hydroxy-3-methoxyphenylglycol along with minor amounts of dihydroxymandelic acid in free or conjugated form and N-methyladrenaline.

FURTHER INFORMATION. See J. Axelrod, The formation, metabolism, uptake, and release of noradrenaline and adrenaline, *The Clinical Chemistry of Monoamines*, H. Varley and A. H. Gowenlock (Eds), London, Elsevier Publishing Company, 1963, p. 5; A. Danon and J. D. Sapira, The binding of noradrenaline and adrenaline to human serum albumin, *J. Pharmac. exp. Ther.*, 1972, **182**, 295.

Actions and uses. Adrenaline acts on the effector cells of the sympathetic system. Some effector cells that respond to sympathetic-nerve stimulation are stimulated by adrenaline; others are inhibited. At these sites two kinds of receptor are assumed and called, for convenience, alpha and beta as described under Adrenergic Receptors. Adrenaline and ephedrine show both alpha- and beta-receptor effects, noradrenaline primarily alpha-receptor effects, and isoprenaline, orciprenaline, salbutamol, and terbutaline mostly beta-receptor effects. Salbutamol acts mainly on the beta-receptors in the bronchi and the respiratory tract and the cardiac beta-receptors are relatively little affected.

Adrenaline is particularly effective in the treatment of bronchial asthma and may be life-saving in status asthmaticus. It relaxes the constricted bronchial musculature and also reduces bronchial oedema by inducing local vasoconstriction. It is of value in allergic states such as angioneurotic oedema and urticaria, in anaphylactic shock of any origin, and often in serum sickness. When extrasystoles are present, adrenaline should not be used because of the risk of inducing ventricular fibrillation.

The vasoconstrictor action of adrenaline is used to diminish the absorption and localise the effects of local anaesthetics and to reduce local haemorrhage. For these purposes a concentration of 1 in 200000 of adrenaline should not be exceeded if more than 50 millilitres is to be injected; higher concentrations such as 1 in 100000 to 1 in 50000 are used in dentistry, but the total quantity of adrenaline injected should not exceed 500 micrograms. Solutions of local anaesthetics containing adrenaline should not be used for producing anaesthesia in digits, because the profound ischaemia produced may lead to gangrene. Adrenaline need not be used with cocaine. For the control of capillary bleeding the local application of a 1 in 5000 solution is usually effective.

Applied to mucous membranes, adrenaline produces ischaemia by constricting the peripheral vessels; it therefore relieves turgescence and is of value in hay fever and laryngeal, nasal, and ophthalmic inflammation; for these purposes, however, phenylephrine is usually preferred.

Noradrenaline or metaraminol is to be preferred to adrenaline as a vasoconstrictor for restoring peripheral vascular collapse.

Adrenaline is usually administered as a single dose of 200 to 500 micrograms by subcutaneous or intramuscular injection, or by inhalation of a fine mist through the mouth; it is almost ineffective when swallowed. In extreme emergency it may be given intravenously in dilute solution and in reduced dosage. It is usually administered as the acid tartrate.

Undesirable effects. In therapeutic doses adrenaline may cause toxic effects such as anxiety, fear, tremor, headache, and palpitations.

Precautions and contra-indications. Adrenaline should not be used in hyperthyroidism or coronary insufficiency, or in the presence of ventricular hyper-excitability produced by chloroform, halothane, cyclo-propane, digitalis, mercurial diuretics, or quinidine.

Drug interactions. The pressor actions of adrenaline are enhanced by drugs which block its neuronal uptake, for example, tricyclic antidepressants such as amitriptyline and adrenergic blocking drugs such as bethanidine, debrisoquine, and guanethidine.

Preparations

NEUTRAL ADRENALINE EYE-DROPS: a sterile solution containing 1% of adrenaline, with sodium metabisul-phite, 8-hydroxyquinoline sulphate, or other suitable stabilising agents, in a borate buffer solution. The pH of the solution is adjusted to 7.4 by the addition of sodium hydroxide. The air in the container is replaced by nitrogen or other inert gas after filling.
A standard for these eye-drops is given in the British Pharmaceutical Codex 1973
Containers and *Labelling:* see the entry on Eye-drops for general information on containers and labelling.
Storage: it should be stored in a cool place, protected from light.
Advice for patients: see the entry on Eye-drops for general information on the use of eye-drops. When used in conjunction with pilocarpine or another miotic, the miotic should be instilled first and neutral adrenaline eye-drops used 5 to 10 minutes later. Treatment should not be discontinued without the advice of the prescriber. With prolonged usage, staining of the sclera may occur. The eye-drops should not be used if the solution is discoloured.

NEUTRAL VISCOUS ADRENALINE EYE-DROPS: a sterile solution containing 1% w/v of adrenaline with *N*-acetylcysteine, ammonium lactate, hydroxyethylcellu-lose, and benzalkonium chloride, or with other suitable stabilising, buffering, and preservative agents, in purified water. The pH of the solution is adjusted to 6.5 by the addition of strong ammonia solution. The air in the containers is replaced by nitrogen or other inert gas after filling.
Containers and *Labelling:* see the entry on Eye-drops for general information on containers and labelling.
Storage: it should be stored in a cool place, protected from light.
Advice for patients: see above under Neutral Adrenaline Eye-drops.

OTHER PREPARATIONS of adrenaline and its salts available include various compound antirheumatic creams, and inhalations for the relief of bronchospasm.

Adrenaline Acid Tartrate

(*R*) - *N* - Methyl - β,3,4 - trihydroxyphenethylammonium hydrogen tartrate

$C_9H_{13}NO_3,C_4H_6O_6 = 333.3$

OTHER NAMES: Adren. Tart.; Adrenaline Tartrate;

Adrenalinii Tartras; Epinephrine Bitartrate; *Medihaler-Epi*®
A standard is given in the European Pharmacopoeia Vol. I

Description. A white to greyish-white, crystalline, odourless powder.

Solubility. Soluble, at 20°, in 3 parts of water and in 520 parts of alcohol; very slightly soluble in ether and in chloroform.

Dissociation constant. See under Adrenaline.

Acidity. A 5% solution has a pH of 3 to 4.

Stability; Incompatibility; Storage. See under Adrenaline.

Sterilisation. Solutions are sterilised by heating in an autoclave or by filtration.

Identification. TEST. Dissolve 300 mg in 10 ml of water containing 100 mg of sodium metabisulphite, make al-kaline with *dilute ammonia solution*, and allow to stand for 1 hour at 4°; filter, wash the filter with three 2-ml portions of water, then with 5 ml of alcohol followed by 5 ml of ether, and dry *in vacuo* for 3 hours. The residue complies with the tests for Adrenaline.

MELTING-POINT. About 150°, with decomposition.

ULTRAVIOLET ABSORPTION. In 0.1N hydrochloric acid, maxima at 220 nm (E1%, 1cm = 165) and 281 nm (E1%, 1cm = 88).

Determination in body fluids; Metabolism. See under Adrenaline.

Actions and uses. Adrenaline acid tartrate has the actions, uses, and undesirable effects described under Adrenaline; 1.8 milligrams of adrenaline acid tartrate is approximately equivalent to 1 milligram of adrenaline. The usual dose is 0.4 to 1 milligram by subcutaneous injection as a single dose.

Precautions and contra-indications; Drug inter-actions. As for Adrenaline.

Veterinary uses. Adrenaline acid tartrate is a sympa-thomimetic. It is used as a vasoconstrictor to control limited bleeding from mucous membranes and has been given by injection to control haemorrhage or cardiac collapse. However, intravenous injection may give rise to cardiac arrhythmias especially when used in conjunc-tion with certain anaesthetics. The usual dose for horses and cattle is 8 to 16 micrograms per kilogram body-weight by subcutaneous or intramuscular injection and 4 to 8 micrograms per kilogram body-weight by slow intra-venous injection. The usual dose for dogs is 10 to 30 micrograms per kilogram body-weight by subcu-taneous, intramuscular, or slow intravenous injection.

Preparations

ADRENALINE INJECTION (*Syn.* Adrenaline Tartrate Injection):

Adrenaline acid tartrate ..	..	..	..	180 mg
Sodium metabisulphite ..	..	..	..	100 mg
Sodium chloride ..	..	..	..	800 mg
Water for injections	..	..	..	to 100 ml

Dissolve the sodium metabisulphite in 10 ml of the water and add the adrenaline acid tartrate. Dissolve the sodium chloride in 75 ml of the water. Mix the two solutions and add sufficient of the water to produce the required volume. Sterilise by heating in an autoclave or by filtration. Adrenaline injection contains the equivalent of adrenaline, 1 in 1000 (1 mg per ml).

A standard for this injection is given in the British Pharmacopoeia 1973

Containers: see the entry on Injections for general information on containers.

Labelling: see the entry on Injections for general information on labelling. In addition, the label on the container should state the amount of the medicament as "Adrenaline 1 in 1000".

Storage: it should be protected from light.

ADRENALINE SOLUTION (*Syn.* Adrenaline Tartrate Solution):

Adrenaline acid tartrate	1.8 g
Chlorocresol	1.0 g
Sodium metabisulphite	1.0 g
Chlorbutol	4.0 g
Sodium chloride	8.0 g
Purified water, freshly boiled and cooled	to 1000.0 ml

Dissolve the sodium metabisulphite in 100 ml of the water and add the adrenaline acid tartrate. Dissolve the chlorbutol and the chlorocresol in 750 ml of the water with the aid of gentle heat, cool, and dissolve the sodium chloride in the solution. Mix the two solutions and add sufficient of the water to produce the required volume. Adrenaline solution contains the equivalent of 1 in 1000 (1 mg per ml) of adrenaline.

When Liquor Adrenalinae Hydrochloridi or Solution of Adrenaline Hydrochloride is prescribed or demanded, Adrenaline Solution may be dispensed or supplied.

A standard for this solution is given in the British Pharmacopoeia 1973

Containers: see the entry on Injections for general information on containers with special reference to glass containers.

Storage: it should be stored in well-filled airtight containers, protected from light.

COMPOUND ADRENALINE AND ATROPINE SPRAY:

Adrenaline acid tartrate	8 g
Atropine methonitrate	1 g
Papaverine hydrochloride	8 g
Sodium metabisulphite	1 g
Chlorbutol	5 g
Propylene glycol	50 ml
Purified water, freshly boiled and cooled	to 1000 ml

Adrenaline and atropine compound spray contains the equivalent of about 1 in 225 (4.5 mg per ml) of adrenaline.

A standard for this spray is given in the British Pharmaceutical Codex 1973

Containers: see the entry on Sprays for general information on containers.

Storage: it should be stored in well-filled airtight containers, protected from light.

Advice for patients: the spray solution should be used with an atomiser and inhaled through the mouth. Excessive use of the spray should be avoided.

OTHER PREPARATIONS available include an AEROSOL INHALATION containing adrenaline acid tartrate 15 mg per ml providing 280 micrograms of adrenaline acid tartrate per metered dose.

Adrenaline acid tartrate is an ingredient of lignocaine and adrenaline injection; procaine and adrenaline injection; and zinc sulphate and adrenaline eye-drops.

Adrenergic Receptors

Adrenergic receptors (Adrenoceptors) may be divided into two main groups, alpha and beta.

Effects mediated by alpha-receptors include vasoconstriction of peripheral and splanchnic arterioles, dilatation of the pupils, inhibition of the movements of the stomach, intestine, and bladder, and liberation of glucose from the liver. These effects are usually blocked by alpha-adrenergic-blocking agents such as phenoxybenzamine, phentolamine, thymoxamine, and tolazoline; this group also includes indoramin.

Effects mediated by beta-receptors are generally concerned with inhibitory effects, an important exception being the stimulatory effect on the heart; effects include vasodilatation of the blood vessels supplying skeletal muscle, and of coronary vessels, acceleration of the heart rate, increase in the force of cardiac contractions, and relaxation of uterine and bronchial muscles.

The beta-receptors may be subdivided into beta-1-receptors mediating the rate and force of cardiac contraction, and beta-2-receptors mediating bronchial relaxation and vasodilatation of coronary and skeletal muscle arterioles. The beta-receptors can be blocked by propranolol and similar drugs.

Substances with generalised adrenergic-receptor-stimulating effects include adrenaline, amphetamine, dexamphetamine, ephedrine, mephentermine, phenylpropanolamine, and pseudoephedrine.

Substances with predominantly alpha-receptor-stimulating effects include metaraminol, methoxamine, noradrenaline, and phenylephrine.

Substances with predominantly generalised beta-receptor-stimulating effects include isoprenaline, orciprenaline, and terbutaline.

Substances with predominantly beta-2-receptor-stimulating effects include salbutamol.

Advice for Patients

It is desirable that patients should be given adequate advice to enable them to use their medicines safely and effectively, and pharmacists may therefore need to amplify or clarify any advice that has been given by the prescriber or manufacturer of a dispensed medicine or by the manufacturer of a medicine sold in the pharmacy so as to ensure that the patient is aware of a suitable dosage schedule and knows the correct way of using the medicine. Patients may be reminded that they should seek advice if they have reason to believe that the medicine is causing undesirable reactions or if it is not having the intended effect.

Patients should be encouraged to keep medicines out of the reach of children, to destroy any medicines that are left over and no longer needed, and not to share prescribed medicines or pass them to other persons for whom they may not be appropriate.

The general advice given above may need to be supplemented by information relating to the particular medicine being supplied. Warnings may be given with medicines that stain clothing, urine or faeces, cause drowsiness, or interact with foods or with household medicines. The more important of these matters are summarised in the paragraphs headed "advice for patients" appearing in the entries for medicinal preparations. Relevant information given under Storage and Labelling should also be given to the patient. The advice given is not necessarily applicable in all circumstances and will need to be modified if it appears to conflict with the intentions of the prescriber.

Information useful for answering enquiries from patients may also be found in the paragraphs headed Actions and uses, Precautions, Undesirable effects, and Drug interactions.

Since requirements for patient advice vary considerably according to the circumstances of the case and the custom of the country concerned the pharmacist should use the information with discretion. In particular, any special directions given by the prescriber should be respected.

Pharmacists dispensing medicines should ensure that the patient has noted and fully understood the prescriber's instructions, and may give such additional advice as may be considered necessary to ensure that the maximum benefit is obtained from the medicine and that hazards are reduced to a minimum. When supplying non-prescription medicines pharmacists may provide general advice on the lines indicated above, related to the needs of the individual patient and give advice on problems that may arise when other medicines are also being taken. The statements in the entries on medicinal preparations have been framed to give limited information for the preparations generally prescribed since the patient will be receiving some advice from the physician. For those preparations that are usually obtained without prescription, advice is given in rather more detail; for analgesics, cough mixtures etc. it is suggested that medical advice should be sought after a period since if the treatment has not been successful the underlying condition may need medical attention.

Advice for patients may be given verbally or on labels or leaflets as considered appropriate. In the United Kingdom, warning cards are issued by pharmacists with monoamine-oxidase inhibitors and certain medicines that interact with aspirin, namely, coumarin anticoagulants, phenindione, and methotrexate. Identification cards are sometimes issued to diabetics and haemophiliacs and to patients being treated with corticosteroids in high dosage or over a long period.

Aerosol Inhalations

An aerosol inhalation consists of a solution or suspension of a medicament in a mixture of inert propellants which is held under pressure in an aerosol dispenser, which consists of a suitable container fitted with a special metering valve. In the case of a solution, the medicament is dissolved in a solvent (co-solvent) which is miscible with the propellants. The particle size of the medicament in a suspension and the droplet size of a solution must be controlled so that, when the aerosol is inhaled, the medicament reaches the region of the respiratory tract where it is intended to be deposited. Substances of low boiling-point suitable for use as propellants are described in the entry on Propellants. The preparation may also contain surface-active agents, stabilising agents, and other adjuvants.

Use. The aerosol dispenser is fitted with an adapter in order to facilitate the transfer of the preparation into the body through the mouth (an oral adapter being used) or through the nose (a nasal adapter being used). One form of oral adapter consists of a plastic tube, open at both ends, containing an integral spray nozzle into which fits the valve stem; the nozzle is designed so that when the valve is actuated, the dose is delivered from the open end of the plastic tube which forms the mouthpiece; the nozzle end of the plastic tube may be shaped so that it supports the aerosol dispenser in the correct position in the adapter, the tube usually being angled in the centre so that when the mouthpiece is correctly placed in the mouth, the aerosol dispenser is held vertically, either in an inverted position, which is the more usual, or in an upright position, in accordance with the manufacturer's instructions. The metering valve is actuated by finger pressure on the base of the container forcing the top of the valve stem against an inner wall of the adapter. Another form of oral adapter incorporates a mechanism which automatically applies pressure to the valve stem when actuated by the reduced pressure created when the patient inhales through the mouthpiece.

In use, actuation of the metering valve releases an appropriate quantity of the preparation in the form of an aerosol of appropriate droplet size, a portion of which becomes deposited on the inner surface of the adapter and the remainder issues from the open end of the adapter. The quantity of medicament available to the patient with each spray is therefore less than the quantity released by the valve.

To use the assembled unit, the patient exhales as fully as possible, inserts the open end of the adapter into his mouth or nostril as appropriate, and inhales, at the same time actuating the valve. The orally inhaled medicament is usually intended to be deposited in the bronchial or upper pulmonary regions.

Aerosol inhalations are potent preparations and care should be taken to ensure that the patient is fully aware of this. Any leaflet or card which is enclosed in the package and gives all the necessary instructions for using the unit should be issued with the appliance and the patient should be advised verbally to read all the directions before use.

Containers. They should be supplied in containers of metal or of glass protected with a plastic coating; this coating also serves to protect the user if the glass fractures. Aerosol dispensers should comply with the relevant part of British Standard 3914.

Labelling

A. The label on the pressurised container should indicate:

(1) the name of the preparation and, where applicable, the strength of the preparation expressed as the weight of active ingredient(s) per millilitre,

(2) the amount(s) of active ingredient(s) available to the patient each time the valve is actuated, and

(3) a warning indicating that the container is pressurised and must be kept away from heat, including the sun, and must not be punctured, broken, or incinerated even when apparently empty.

In addition, the label or marking on the container or the label or marking on the adapter gives, in a position such that the directions are visible when the unit is assembled for use,

(4) a direction to shake the container before use, if applicable,

(5) a warning that the patient should adhere strictly to and not exceed the prescribed dosage,

(6) a direction to read the instructions on the enclosed card or leaflet before use, and

(7) an indication of the correct aspect of the container in use.

B. A leaflet or card should be included in the package giving:

(1) the directions for the correct use of the preparation,

(2) the recommended dosage schedule,

(3) the maximum number of doses that may be taken in 24 hours,

(4) the directions for keeping the unit clean, and

(5) the directions for the disposal of the used or partly used container.

C. The label or wording on the carton should give:

(1) the name of the preparation,

(2) the amount(s) of active ingredient(s) available to the patient each time the valve is actuated,

(3) the expected number of times the valve can be actuated before the container becomes empty,

(4) the date after which the preparation is not intended to be used, if applicable,

(5) a direction to read the instructions enclosed before use, and

(6) sufficient space for the pharmacist to add any additional label without obscuring any directions that the patient needs to read.

Storage. Aerosol inhalations should be stored in a cool place but protected from frost. Aerosol dispensers must be protected from heat, including the sun, because they may explode, even when apparently empty.

African Horsesickness Vaccine, Living

A freeze-dried preparation containing a mixture of several antigenically distinct modified strains of horsesickness virus. It is reconstituted immediately before use with an appropriate volume of a suitable sterile liquid.

A standard is given in the British Pharmacopoeia (Veterinary)

Storage. The dried vaccine should be protected from light and stored at 2° to 8° when it may be expected to retain its potency for at least 12 months. It should be used immediately after reconstitution.

Veterinary uses. It is administered to horses, mules, and donkeys, by subcutaneous injection, for prophylaxis of African horsesickness.

Albumin Fraction (Saline), Human

A solution of the proteins of liquid human plasma containing albumin and some globulins that retain their solubility on heating. It exerts a colloidal osmotic pressure equivalent to that of pooled liquid human plasma containing 5.2% w/v of protein. It contains no fibrinogen and only traces of gamma globulin.

OTHER NAME: Human Plasma Protein Fraction

A standard is given in the British Pharmacopoeia 1973

Human albumin fraction (saline) is obtained from pooled liquid human plasma and may be prepared by precipitation with organic solvents such as alcohol under controlled conditions of pH, ionic strength, and temperature.

No bactericide or antibiotic is added at any stage during preparation. Freeze-drying or other suitable treatment is used to remove residual solvent. The resultant protein is dissolved in water, and sodium caprylate or other suitable substances are added to stabilise it to heat and sodium chloride to adjust the concentration of sodium ions to about 150 millimoles per litre at pH 7.0.

The solution is sterilised by filtration and distributed aseptically into containers which are then sealed to exclude micro-organisms and heated to and maintained at 59.5° to 60.5° for 10 hours to prevent the transmission of hepatitis B.

Finally, the containers are incubated for not less than 14 days at 30° to 32° and examined visually for signs of microbial contamination.

Human albumin fraction (saline) is a clear amber-coloured liquid and contains not less than 4.3% w/v of protein, 130 to 160 millimoles of sodium ions, not more than 15 millimoles of citrate ions, and not more than 2 millimoles of potassium ions per litre. It has a pH of 6.7 to 7.3.

Storage. It should be protected from light and stored at a temperature between 2° and 25°. It should not be used if it has become turbid or contains a deposit.

Actions and uses. Human albumin fraction (saline) is used in the same way as reconstituted plasma for the purposes described under Plasma, Human, Dried.

Albumin Fraction (Saline), Human, Dried

Freeze-dried human albumin fraction (saline). Before drying, the solution in the final containers is heated to and maintained at 59.5° to 60.5° for 10 hours to prevent the transmission of hepatitis B.

A standard is given in the British Pharmacopoeia 1973

Dried human albumin fraction (saline) is a cream-coloured powder which, when dissolved in a volume of water equal to the volume of water for injections stated on the label, yields a solution that contains not less than 4.3% w/v of protein, 130 to 160 millimoles of sodium ions, not more than 15 millimoles of citrate ions, and not more than 2 millimoles of potassium ions per litre.

Storage. It should be stored in an atmosphere of nitrogen, in sterile containers sealed to exclude micro-organisms and moisture, at a temperature below 25°, and protected from light. It should not be used if after adding water a gel forms or solution is incomplete. The solution should be used immediately after reconstitution and should be discarded if not used within 3 hours.

Actions and uses. Dried human albumin fraction (saline) is used for the purposes described under Plasma, Human, Dried.

Albumin, Human

A solution in water of human albumin containing a low proportion of salt.

A standard is given in the British Pharmacopoeia 1973

Human albumin is obtained from pooled human plasma and may be prepared by precipitation with organic solvents such as alcohol, under controlled conditions of pH, ionic strength, and temperature. No bactericide or antibiotic is added at any stage during preparation. Freeze-drying or other suitable treatment is used to remove residual solvent.

The resultant protein is dissolved in water, and sodium caprylate or other suitable substances are added to stabilise it to heat at pH 7.0.

The solution is sterilised by filtration and distributed aseptically into containers which are then sealed to exclude micro-organisms. The solution is then heated to and maintained at 59.5° to 60.5° for 10 hours to prevent the transmission of hepatitis B.

Finally, the containers are incubated for not less than

14 days at 30° to 32° and examined visually for signs of microbial contamination.

Human albumin is a clear amber to deep orange-brown liquid and contains 15 to 25% w/v of protein and not more than 0.65 millimole of sodium ions, not more than 0.05 millimole of potassium ions, and not more than 0.1 millimole of citrate ions per g of protein. It has a pH of 6.7 to 7.3.

Storage. It should be protected from light and stored at 2° to 25°. It should not be used if it has become turbid or contains a deposit.

Actions and uses. Human albumin is used when it is desired to administer relatively large amounts of protein in a small volume and with minimal amounts of sodium and potassium.

It has been used in the treatment of certain liver disorders such as cirrhosis in which hypoalbuminaemia occurs; its value for this purpose is uncertain, but benefit to patients with predominantly peripheral oedema has been reported. It has also been used in nephrotic nephritis with the object of inducing diuresis, but its value has not been established.

Human albumin is also used to restore a depleted blood volume. Additional fluid should be given by mouth if the patient is dehydrated. The amount of human albumin transfused and the rate at which it is given depend on the patient's age and general condition, the state of his circulatory system, and the indication for its use.

Albumin, Human, Dried

Freeze-dried human albumin prepared from human albumin with a protein concentration not exceeding 10% w/v. Before drying, the solution in the final containers is heated to and maintained at 59.5° to 60.5° for 10 hours to prevent the transmission of hepatitis B.

A standard is given in the British Pharmacopoeia 1973

Dried human albumin is a cream-coloured powder. When dissolved in a volume of water equal to the volume of water for injections stated on the label the solution contains 24.0 to 26.0% w/v of protein and not more than 0.65 millimole of sodium ions, not more than 0.05 millimole of potassium ions, and not more than 0.1 millimole of citrate ions per g of protein.

Storage. It should be stored in an atmosphere of nitrogen, in sterile containers sealed to exclude micro-organisms and moisture, at 2° to 25°, protected from light. It should not be used if after adding water a gel forms or solution is incomplete. The solution should be used immediately after reconstitution and should be discarded if not used within 3 hours.

Actions and uses. Dried human albumin is used for the purposes described under Albumin, Human.

Alclofenac

4-Allyloxy-3-chlorophenylacetic acid

$C_{11}H_{11}ClO_3 = 226.7$

OTHER NAME: *Prinalgin* ®

A standard is given in the British Pharmacopoeia Addendum 1978

Description. A white or slightly yellowish-white odourless powder.

Solubility. Very slightly soluble in water; soluble, at 20°, in 3 parts of alcohol, in 4 parts of chloroform, and in 6 parts of ether.

Identification. MELTING-POINT. About 91°.

ULTRAVIOLET ABSORPTION. In 0.1N hydrochloric acid, maximum at 281 nm (E1%, 1cm = 78); in alcohol (95%), maxima at 228 nm (E1%, 1cm = 344), 282 nm (E1%, 1cm = 82), and 290 nm (E1%, 1cm = 75).

INFRA-RED ABSORPTION. Major peaks at 933, 1238, 1260, 1410, 1428, and 1691 cm⁻¹ (see Appendix 2a: Infra-red Spectra).

THIN-LAYER CHROMATOGRAPHY. See under Thin-layer Chromatography, System 3.

Metabolism. ABSORPTION. Readily absorbed after oral administration.

BLOOD CONCENTRATION. After oral doses of 5.3 mg/kg and 1 g, peak plasma concentrations of 13 μg/ml and 136 μg/ml respectively, are attained in 1 to 4 hours; peak concentrations in synovial fluid are attained in 2 hours after an oral dose of 1 g and reach 32 μg/ml.

HALF-LIFE. Plasma half-life, measured during the first 6 hours after an oral dose, about 75 minutes.

DISTRIBUTION. Readily enters the synovial fluid; *protein binding,* about 99% bound to plasma proteins.

METABOLIC REACTIONS. Mainly glucuronic acid conjugation along with some conjugation with glycine, de-allylation to form 3-chloro-4-hydroxyphenylacetic acid and hydroxylation at the aliphatic double bond to form 3-chloro-4-(2,3-dihydroxypropyloxy)phenylacetic acid which may be methylated.

EXCRETION. 85 to 90% of an oral dose is excreted in the urine in 24 to 48 hours, 18% as the glucuronic acid conjugate.

FURTHER INFORMATION. Simultaneous pharmacokinetics of alclofenac in plasma and synovial fluid in patients with rheumatoid arthritis—G. M. Thomas *et al., Curr. med. Res. Opinion,* 1975, **3**, 264; chemical and biological background to alclofenac—L. F. Wiggins, *Curr. med. Res. Opinion,* 1975, **3**, 241.

Actions and uses. Alclofenac is an analgesic with minor anti-inflammatory properties and has the actions and uses described under Ibuprofen. The usual dosage is 1 gram 3 times a day, which may be reduced according to the response of the patient to 500 milligrams 3 times a day.

Undesirable effects. Alclofenac may give rise to allergic reactions and gastro-intestinal upsets. Rashes, which may occasionally be severe, may occur and vasculitis has been reported.

Precautions. As for Ibuprofen. Alclofenac should be withdrawn immediately if a rash develops, which is usually within the first week of treatment.

Preparation

ALCLOFENAC CAPSULES: consisting of alclofenac, in powder, which may be mixed with a suitable inert diluent, enclosed in a hard capsule. Available as capsules containing 500 mg of alclofenac.

A standard for these capsules is given in the British Pharmacopoeia Addendum 1978
Containers and *Storage*: see the entry on Capsules for general information on containers and storage.
Advice for patients: the capsules should preferably be taken after meals.

Alcohol (95 per cent)

A mixture of ethyl alcohol (ethanol), $CH_3.CH_2OH$, and water.

A standard is given in the British Pharmacopoeia 1973

Description. A clear, colourless, mobile, volatile liquid with a characteristic spirituous odour and a burning taste. It is readily inflammable, burning with a blue smokeless flame.

Solubility. Miscible with water, with ether, and with chloroform; when mixed with water, contraction of volume and rise of temperature occur.

Specific gravity. 0.8119 to 0.8139 (20°/20°).

Boiling-point. About 78°.

Dilute alcohols. Dilute alcohols of various strengths may be prepared by diluting the appropriate volume of alcohol (95 per cent) to 1000 ml with purified water as specified in the following table. Before the final adjustment of volume is made, the mixture is cooled to the same temperature, about 20°, as that at which the alcohol (95 per cent) was measured.

Strength of dilute alcohol required (% v/v)	Volume of alcohol (95%) to be diluted to 1000 ml (ml)	Specific gravity (20°/20°)
90*	947	0.8289 to 0.8319
80	842	0.8599 to 0.8621
70	737	0.8860 to 0.8883
60	632	0.9103 to 0.9114
50	526	0.9314 to 0.9326
45	474	0.9407 to 0.9417
25	263	0.9694 to 0.9703
20	210	0.9748 to 0.9759

* Rectified Spirit

Proof spirit. Proof spirit (Spiritus Tenuior) is defined legally as "that which at the temperature of 51° by Fahrenheit's thermometer weighs exactly twelve–thirteenth parts of an equal measure of distilled water". It has a specific gravity (60°/60° F) of 0.9198 and contains about 57.1 per cent v/v or 49.2 per cent w/w of C_2H_6O. Spirits are described in terms of so many degrees over or under proof (O.P. or U.P.), according to the quantity of distilled water which must be added to, or deducted from, 100 volumes of the sample in order to produce spirit of proof strength. The "Proof Gallon" is the unit of alcohol for revenue purposes. Bulk gallons of "over proof" alcohol may be converted into "proof gallons" by multiplying by the factor

$$\frac{100 + \text{the number of degrees over proof}}{100},$$

and "under proof" alcohol by the factor

$$\frac{100 - \text{the number of degrees under proof}}{100}.$$

An alternative method of indicating spirit strength is sometimes used on the labels of alcoholic beverages. The strength is given as a number of degrees, proof spirit being taken as 100°; for example, a spirit stated to be "70°" would be 30° under proof and would contain 70 per cent of proof spirit. Alcohol (95 per cent) corresponds to about 66° over proof, and 100 volumes thus contain about as much C_2H_6O as 166 volumes of proof spirit. If 100 volumes of alcohol (95 per cent) are diluted to 166 volumes with water, the resulting spirit is of approximately proof strength.

Sterilisation. Alcohol is sterilised by heating in sealed ampoules in an autoclave or by filtration.

Storage. It should be stored in airtight containers, in a cool place.

Identification. TESTS. 1. Place 5 drops in a small beaker, add 1 ml of *potassium permanganate solution* and 5 drops of *dilute sulphuric acid*, and cover the beaker immediately with a filter paper moistened with a recently prepared solution of 100 mg of sodium nitroprusside and 500 mg of piperazine hydrate in 5 ml of water; an intense blue colour is produced on the filter paper, the colour becoming paler after a few minutes.
2. To 5 ml of a 0.5% solution add 1 ml of 0.1N sodium hydroxide, and then slowly add 2 ml of *iodine solution*; the odour of iodoform develops and a yellow precipitate is produced.

Determination in body fluids. COLORIMETRY. In blood or urine—K. J. Roos, *Clinica chim. Acta*, 1971, **31**, 285.

GAS CHROMATOGRAPHY. In blood—P. Blume *et al.*, *Analyt. Biochem.*, 1973, **54**, 429.

REVIEW. Determination in breath—M. F. Mason and K. M. Dubowski, *J. forens. Sci.*, 1976, **21**, 9.

Metabolism. ABSORPTION. Readily absorbed after oral administration but absorption may be delayed by the presence of food; alcohol vapour is rapidly absorbed in the lungs.

BLOOD CONCENTRATION. After an oral dose of about 800 mg/kg administered in water over a 5-minute period, a blood concentration of about 1 mg/ml is attained within 30 minutes, which declines at the rate of about 0.1 mg/ml per hour; fructose, galactose, and sorbitol, administered before the intake of alcohol, appear to reduce the blood alcohol concentration; following an intravenous infusion of 720 ml of an 8% v/v solution of alcohol for 2 hours, peak capillary blood concentrations of 0.6 to 0.8 mg/ml are attained at the time the infusion is stopped; chronic consumption of alcohol or the administration of chlorpromazine or haloperidol appear to stimulate an increase in the rate of disappearance of alcohol from blood.

HALF-LIFE. Dose dependent.

DISTRIBUTION. Rapidly distributed throughout the total body water, crosses the placenta, and is secreted in milk in small amounts.

METABOLIC REACTIONS. Metabolised in the liver by oxidation; it is converted to acetaldehyde and further metabolised; some of the unchanged alcohol may be conjugated with sulphate or glucuronic acid; the rate of oxidative metabolism appears to be increased by fructose; there may be a racial variation in the ability to metabolise alcohol; Eskimos and North American Indians, for example, may metabolise alcohol much more slowly than other races.

EXCRETION. Excreted through the lungs as unchanged alcohol, acetaldehyde, and carbon dioxide; unchanged alcohol and its sulphate and glucuronide conjugates are excreted in the urine and after an oral dose of 800 mg/kg, about 750 mg is excreted unchanged in the urine in 2 hours as unchanged alcohol.

FURTHER INFORMATION. Metabolism of alcohol in various racial groups—L. J. Bennion and Ting-Kai Li, *New Engl. J. Med.*, 1976, **294**, 9 and D. Fenna *et al.*, *Can. med. Ass. J.*, 1971, **105**, 472; influence of psychotic drugs on concentration of alcohol in blood—H. Casier *et al.*, *Arzneimittel-Forsch.*, 1966, **16**, 1505; effect of oral administration of various sugars on concentration of alcohol in blood—E. R. Clark *et al.*, *J. Pharm. Pharmac.*, 1973, **25**, 319; metabolism of alcohol and its metabolic effects—R. D. Hawkins and H. Kalant, *Pharmac. Rev.*, 1972, **24**, 67; effect of alcohol on drug metabolism —M. H. Kater *et al.*, *J. Am. med. Ass.*, 1969, **207**, 363; metabolism in the liver—H. I. D. Thieden, *Acta pharmac. tox.*, 1975, **36**, Suppl. 1; concentration in the blood during constant-rate intravenous infusion—P. K. Wilkinson *et al.*, *Clin. Pharmac. Ther.*, 1976, **19**, 213; concentrations in blood of fasting and non-fasting adults —P. K. Wilkinson *et al.*, *J. Pharmacokinet. Biopharm.*, 1977, **5**, 41.

Actions and uses. The action of alcohol on the central nervous system is depressant and is most marked on the cerebral cortex and on its inhibitory functions. By masking hesitancy, circumspection, and self-criticism, alcohol in small doses may appear initially to stimulate, especially in surroundings which are conducive to excitement; without such an environment its action is usually hypnotic. The effect of small amounts may be to postpone the onset of fatigue and to increase the work done, as long as the task involved is simple.

Alcohol is rapidly absorbed when taken by mouth, but only 10 to 15 millilitres is metabolised per hour; this and the action of alcohol on the central nervous system limit its food value, but it is useful in illness and convalescence when appetite is deficient and the assimilation of ordinary food is impaired. It also produces peripheral vasodilatation which increases heat loss.

Preparations containing high concentrations of alcohol irritate the stomach and produce gastritis if taken habitually, but small amounts adequately diluted help digestion by inhibiting emotions such as anxiety and anger.

Concentrations of 80% or more are sometimes injected into ganglia or around nerve trunks to destroy them and to relieve severe and chronic pain.

Solutions containing from 2.5 to 10% of alcohol, with about 5% of dextrose, in water for injections are used by intravenous infusion as a source of calories in malnutrition and post-operatively. The rate of administration should not exceed the equivalent of 15 millilitres of alcohol per hour.

Alcohol is a valuable solvent and preservative. In appropriate strengths it is used in the manufacture of tinctures, spirits, and many other galenical preparations. For external use, industrial methylated spirit and surgical spirit may be used.

It has a bactericidal action against most vegetative organisms at concentrations between 60 and 95% v/v but it is not effective against bacterial spores. A concentration of 70% v/v is considered to be the optimum for bactericidal action. Dilutions of alcohol in concentrations above 20% v/v are also used as preservative solvents in galenical manufacture.

Scalp lotions or shampoos containing 50% or more of alcohol should be labelled to indicate that they are inflammable and should not be used, nor the hair dried, near a fire or naked flame.

Undesirable effects. The consumption of small amounts of alcohol impairs the ability of an individual to carry out tasks involving discrimination or selection; accuracy is diminished and the amount of work done may be reduced, even though the subject feels particularly efficient. Such loss of efficiency is important when the control of mechanically propelled vehicles is concerned and in some countries the concentration of alcohol in the blood of drivers may be subject to legal limits.

A limited tolerance to the action of alcohol on the brain may develop and addiction to alcohol usually involves tolerance to other aliphatic narcotics and anaesthetics. Alcohol increases, sometimes dangerously, the intensity and duration of action of barbiturates and increases the sedative action of antihistamine drugs.

Alcohol crosses the placenta and, while moderate intake does not affect the foetus, large amounts taken immediately before parturition may cause neonatal respiratory depression. Alcohol is secreted in the milk and the consumption of large amounts should be avoided when breast feeding.

Alcohol must be avoided by patients taking disulfiram.

Dependence. Dependence of the barbiturate-alcohol type is described under Drug Dependence.

Poisoning. In acute alcoholic poisoning, the stomach should be washed out and respiration sustained, if depressed, by artificial respiration.

Fructose may be given by the intravenous infusion of 500 millilitres of a 40% solution over a period of 30 minutes to accelerate the elimination of alcohol from the blood. This treatment may cause retrosternal pain, epigastric discomfort, and acidaemia requiring correction by the intravenous administration of an appropriate quantity of sodium bicarbonate injection.

Preparation

SPIRIT EAR-DROPS:

Alcohol (95%)	50 ml
Water for preparations .. .. to	100 ml

In making this preparation the alcohol (95%) may be replaced by industrial methylated spirit, provided that the law and the statutory regulations governing the use of industrial methylated spirit are observed.

A standard for these ear-drops is given in the British Pharmaceutical Codex 1973

Containers and *Labelling:* see the entry on Ear-drops for general information on containers and labelling.

Alcohol, Dehydrated

$CH_3 . CH_2OH = 46.07$

OTHER NAMES: Absolute Alcohol; Ethanol

A standard is given in the British Pharmacopoeia 1973

Description. A clear, colourless, mobile, volatile, very hygroscopic liquid with a characteristic spirituous odour and a burning taste; it burns readily with a blue smokeless flame.

Solubility. Miscible with water, with ether, and with chloroform; when mixed with water, contraction and a rise of temperature occur.

Specific gravity. 0.7904 to 0.7935 (20°/20°).

Storage. It should be stored in airtight containers, in a cool place.

Identification. See under Alcohol (95 per cent).

Determination in body fluids. See under Alcohol (95 per cent).

Metabolism. See Alcohol (95 per cent).

Uses. Dehydrated alcohol is used as a solvent and dehydrating agent and for the destruction of nerve tissue.

Alginic Acid

A polyuronic acid composed of residues of D-mannuronic and L-guluronic acids in linear or very slightly branched chains which have $\beta 1 \rightarrow 4$ linked units in long sequences of each unit. It has an equivalent weight of about 200.

A standard is given in the British Pharmaceutical Codex 1973

Alginic acid is obtained chiefly from algae belonging to the Phaeophyceae, mainly species of *Laminaria*.
The algae from which alginic acid is obtained grow in large quantities off the west coasts of Scotland and Ireland. A small proportion of the acid groups of alginic acid may be neutralised with sodium carbonate in order to produce a more granular and less bulky material.

Description. A white to pale yellowish-brown, odourless, tasteless powder.

Solubility. Practically insoluble in water and in organic solvents; soluble in solutions of alkali hydroxides.

Acidity. A 3% dispersion in water has a pH of 1.5 to 3.5.

Moisture content. Not more than 18%, determined by drying at 105°.

Sterilisation. It is sterilised by heating in an autoclave. Solutions of soluble alginates may be similarly sterilised. Some loss of viscosity usually occurs in solutions prepared from sterilised alginic acid and in sterilised alginate solutions to an extent which varies according to the nature of the other substances present.

Identification. TESTS. 1. To about 5 mg add 5 ml of water, 1 ml of a freshly prepared 1% solution of naphthoresorcinol in alcohol (95%), and 5 ml of hydrochloric acid; boil for 3 minutes, cool, add 5 ml of water, and extract with 15 ml of ether. Repeat the test without the sample; the ether extract from the sample exhibits a deeper purple colour than that from the blank.
2. To 5 ml of a 0.5% solution in 0.1N sodium hydroxide add 1 ml of *calcium chloride solution*; a voluminous gelatinous precipitate is formed.

Uses. Alginic acid is used as a tablet disintegrant and binder; it is preferably incorporated by a dry-mixing process.

Allergic Rhinitis and Hay Fever

Allergic rhinitis is characterised by nasal congestion, nasal discharge, watering of the eyes, and sneezing. It is caused by an allergic reaction in the nasal mucosa which provokes oedema and excessive secretion. Hay fever is a seasonal form of allergic rhinitis due to sensitivity to various pollens, but perennial forms also occur due to sensitivity to allergens from house-dust mites, fungal spores, animal hair, etc.
Desensitisation or local treatment with sodium cromoglycate are possible forms of prophylaxis. Symptomatic treatment may involve oral administration of antihistamines, local use of a nasal decongestant such as ephedrine hydrochloride, and eye-drops to relieve conjunctival irritation. Corticosteroids may also be used topically and, in severe cases, by injection.
Substances used in the treatment of allergic rhinitis and hay fever include antihistamines, corticosteroids, ephedrine, phenylephrine, pseudoephedrine, and sodium cromoglycate.

Allopurinol

1*H*-Pyrazolo[3,4-*d*]pyrimidin-4-ol

$C_5H_4N_4O = 136.1$

OTHER NAME: *Zyloric*®

A standard is given in the British Pharmacopoeia 1973

Description. A white, microcrystalline, odourless, tasteless powder.

Solubility. Very slightly soluble in water and in alcohol; practically insoluble in ether and in chloroform; soluble in solutions of alkali hydroxides.

Identification. TESTS. 1. Dissolve 50 mg in 5 ml of *dilute sodium hydroxide solution*, add 1 ml of *alkaline potassium mercuri-iodide solution*, boil, and allow to stand; a yellow flocculent precipitate is produced.
2. Dissolve a few mg in 5 ml of 0.1N sodium hydroxide and add 3 ml of *lithium and sodium molybdophosphotungstate solution* and 5 ml of a 20% solution of sodium carbonate; a grey-blue colour is produced.

MELTING-POINT. It has no definite melting-point; above 300° it darkens and, at an indefinite high temperature, it chars and decomposes.

ULTRAVIOLET ABSORPTION. In 0.1N hydrochloric acid, maximum at 250 nm (E1%, 1cm = 550).

INFRA-RED ABSORPTION. Major peaks at 917, 1219, 1235, 1351, 1587, and 1695 cm⁻¹ (see Appendix 2b: Infra-red Spectra).

Determination in body fluids. HIGH PRESSURE LIQUID CHROMATOGRAPHY. In serum—R. Endele and G. Lettenbauer, *J. Chromat.*, 1975, **115**, 228. In plasma or urine—M. Brown and A. Bye, *J. Chromat.*, 1977, **143**, 195.

Metabolism. ABSORPTION. Absorbed after oral administration.

BLOOD CONCENTRATION. During therapy with 300 mg administered once daily or in divided doses of 100 mg thrice daily, plasma concentrations of alloxanthine, the major metabolite, of 3 to 19 µg/ml and 5 to 15 µg/ml, respectively, are attained after 1 week.

HALF-LIFE. Plasma half-life, about 2 hours for allopurinol and 20 to 30 hours for alloxanthine.

DISTRIBUTION. Alloxanthine may accumulate in renal function impairment; *protein binding*, does not appear to be bound to plasma proteins.

METABOLIC REACTIONS. Rapidly oxidised to alloxanthine which is an active metabolite.

EXCRETION. Less than 10% of a dose is excreted unchanged in the urine whilst 45 to 65% is excreted as alloxanthine.

ENZYME INHIBITION. Allopurinol inhibits the metabolism of mercaptopurine to 6-thiouric acid and therefore potentiates the activity of mercaptopurine.

FURTHER INFORMATION. Renal clearance of alloxanthine, the chief metabolite of allopurinol—G. B. Elion *et al.*, *Am. J. Med.*, 1968, **45**, 69; allopurinol and gouty hyperuricaemia; efficacy of a single daily dose—G. P. Rodnan *et al.*, *J. Am. med. Ass.*, 1975, **231**, 1143.

Actions and uses. Allopurinol, by inhibiting xanthine oxidase, reduces the formation of uric acid from mono- and di-substituted purines. Serum levels of hypoxanthine and xanthine, however, remain low because of their high renal clearance rates and because of their re-entry into purine metabolic processes. Serum and urine levels of uric acid therefore fall and are maintained at normal levels so long as therapy is continued regularly.

Acute attacks of gout may be precipitated in the early stages of therapy, particularly if the drug is started in full dosage, but after some weeks or months attacks become infrequent and finally stop altogether; tophi also gradually diminish in size and may finally disappear.

Allopurinol is useful, not only in reducing the incidence of attacks of gout, lessening tophi, and rendering plasma uric acid levels normal, but also in reducing the incidence of urinary calculi and possibly in preventing damage to the kidneys. Impaired renal function is therefore not a contra-indication, but rather an added indication in suitable cases, whereas uricosuric agents may become ineffective in advanced renal failure. The kidneys of patients about to undergo treatment for conditions likely to release large amounts of uric acid into the circulation, such as deep X-ray or cytotoxic therapy for lymphosarcoma, polycythaemia, or leukaemia, are best protected by allopurinol started before such therapy commences and continued throughout it.

Allopurinol should not be used in the treatment of acute gout.

It prevents elevation of plasma uric acid levels in thiazide-treated patients and allows such treatment to be given to patients with gout and congestive heart failure when diuresis is an essential part of treatment. If allopurinol alone is not enough to restore normal levels of plasma uric acid, a uricosuric agent, such as probenecid or sulphinpyrazone, may be given in addition, but this should only occasionally be necessary.

Treatment is continuous and it is best to start with small doses such as 50 milligrams 2 or 3 times a day to prevent precipitation of acute attacks of gout and to increase the dose by 50 milligrams daily every week until the serum uric acid level is in the normal range. An effective final dosage is usually between 300 and 600 milligrams daily in divided doses. To prevent acute attacks of gout in the early stages of treatment 500 micrograms of colchicine may be given 2 or 3 times a day.

Allopurinol may be used for the prevention of uric acid nephropathy due to excessive nucleoprotein catabolism in neoplastic disease, especially during treatment with X-rays or cytotoxic drugs. The usual dosage is 600 milligrams daily in divided doses for adults or 10 to 20 milligrams per kilogram body-weight for children, beginning 2 or 3 days before the X-irradiation or cytotoxic treatment and reducing to about half these doses if prolonged treatment is necessary to control the serum uric acid level.

Undesirable effects. Toxic effects are uncommon and are rarely severe. They include maculopapular rashes, pruritus, nausea, and, very rarely, vomiting, diarrhoea, abdominal pain, malaise, fever, and headaches.

Drug interactions. It enhances the action of azathioprine and mercaptopurine.

Preparation

ALLOPURINOL TABLETS: available as tablets containing 100 and 300 mg of allopurinol.

A standard for these tablets is given in the British Pharmacopoeia 1973

Containers and *Storage:* see the entry on Tablets for general information on containers and storage. Containers should be airtight.

Advice for patients: the tablets should preferably be taken after meals. Adequate fluid intake should be maintained.

Almond Oil

The fixed oil obtained by cold expression from the seeds of *Prunus amygdalus* Batsch. var. *dulcis* (DC.) Koehne (sweet almond) or of *P. amygdalus* Batsch. var. *amara* Focke (bitter almond) (Fam. Rosaceae). Both varieties are cultivated in countries bordering on the Mediterranean Sea and in the U.S.A.; supplies are derived mainly from bitter almond.

OTHER NAME: Oleum Amygdalae

A standard is given in the British Pharmacopoeia 1973

Constituents. Almond oil consists of glycerides, the fatty acid constituents of which are chiefly oleic acid and smaller amounts of linoleic, palmitic, and myristic acids.

Description. A pale yellow oil with a slight characteristic odour. Almond oil remains clear after exposure to a temperature of $-10°$ for 3 hours and does not congeal until the temperature has been reduced to about $-18°$.

Solubility. Very slightly soluble in alcohol; miscible with ether, with chloroform, and with light petroleum.

Weight per ml. At 20°, 0.910 to 0.915 g.

Refractive index. 1.470 to 1.473.

Adulterants and substitutes. Apricot-kernel oil, peach-kernel oil, cottonseed oil, sesame oil, and arachis oil may be present.

Shake vigorously 5 ml for 1 minute with 1 ml of a freshly prepared mixture of equal parts by weight of sulphuric acid, fuming nitric acid, and water, kept cool while cautiously mixed; a whitish mixture is produced; the development of a pink colour after 15 minutes indicates the presence of apricot-kernel oil or peach-kernel oil.

Mix 2.5 ml with 2.5 ml each of amyl alcohol and a 1% solution of precipitated sulphur in carbon disulphide and heat in a closed tube by immersing in boiling water; the development of a pink or red colour within 30 minutes indicates the presence of cottonseed oil.

Shake 2 ml with 1 ml of a 1% solution of sucrose in hydrochloric acid; the development of a pink colour in the acid layer on standing indicates the presence of sesame oil if the colour is more intense than that produced by repeating the test without the sucrose.

Reflux 1 ml with 5 ml of 1.5N alcoholic potassium hydroxide for 10 minutes and mix with 50 ml of alcohol (70%) and 0.8 ml of hydrochloric acid; if a turbidity appears above 4° when cooled slowly, arachis oil may be present. This is confirmed as follows: reflux 5 g of the oil in a 250-ml conical flask with 25 ml of 1.5N alcoholic potassium hydroxide for 10 minutes, add to the hot solution 7.5 ml of acetic acid and 100 ml of alcohol (70%) containing 1 ml of hydrochloric acid, and maintain the temperature of the mixture at 12° to 14° for one hour; filter, and wash with the same mixture of alcohol (70%)

and hydrochloric acid at 17° to 19°, until the washings give no turbidity with water; dissolve the precipitate in the smallest possible quantity (25 to 70 ml) of hot alcohol (90%), cool, and allow to stand for 3 hours at 15°; if any crystals appear, filter, and wash at 15° with about half the volume of alcohol (90%) used for crystallisation, and finally with 50 ml of alcohol (70%); dissolve the crystals in warm solvent ether, evaporate off the solvent, and dry the residue at 105°; a melting-point higher than 71° with respect to the residue or the product after recrystallisation of the residue from alcohol (90%) indicates the presence of arachis oil.

Sterilisation. It is sterilised by dry heat.

Storage. It should be stored in well-filled airtight containers.

Actions and uses. Almond oil has properties similar to those of olive oil. It is used in emollient preparations for the skin, as a vehicle for oily injections, and to soften wax in the ear. The usual dose by mouth is 15 to 30 millilitres.

Preparation

Almond oil is an ingredient of oily phenol injection.

Aloes

The solid residue obtained by evaporating the liquid which drains from the leaves cut from various species of *Aloë* (Fam. Liliaceae). It is known either as Barbados aloes or as Cape aloes, according to origin. The juice is concentrated by spontaneous evaporation, or more generally by boiling, and poured into boxes or other suitable receptacles; on cooling, it solidifies. Slow cooling produces the hepatic (crystalline) variety and rapid cooling the vitreous (amorphous) variety.

OTHER NAMES: Aloe; Aloe Barbadensis; Aloe Capensis

A standard is given in the European Pharmacopoeia Vol. III

Varieties. Cape aloes is prepared in Cape Province from various species, mainly *A. ferox* Mill. and its hybrids. Barbados aloes (more correctly referred to as Curaçao aloes) is obtained from *A. barbadensis* Mill. on the islands of Curaçao, Aruba, and Bonaire; it was formerly produced on the island of Barbados.

Constituents. Aloes contains the pale yellow crystalline substance barbaloin, a 10-glucopyranosyl derivative of aloe-emodin anthrone (10-deoxyglucosyl-9,10-dihydro-1,8-dihydroxy-3-hydroxymethyl-9-oxoanthracene).   In Barbados aloes this is accompanied by isobarbaloin, little of which is found in Cape aloes; there is also present in Cape aloes an amorphous β-barbaloin and aloinosides A and B. Aloinoside B is an 11-mono-α-L-rhamnoside of barbaloin.

Other constituents of aloes are resin and aloe-emodin (9,10-dihydro-1,8-dihydroxy-3-hydroxymethyl-9,10-dioxoanthracene). The resin of Cape aloes may partly consist of capaloresinotannol combined with *p*-coumaric acid; the resin of Curaçao aloes contains also barbaloresinotannol combined with cinnamic acid; these resins may be associated with condensation products of anthraquinones and anthranols.

Good Barbados aloes may yield up to 30% of crystallisable aloins and Cape aloes about 20%.

Description. UNGROUND DRUG. *Macroscopical characters:* Cape aloes: dark brown or greenish-brown glassy masses; thin fragments transparent, exhibiting a yellowish or reddish-brown tinge; fracture clean and glassy. It has a distinctive, somewhat acid, odour.

Barbados aloes: dark chocolate-brown, usually in opaque masses; fracture dull, waxy, uniform, and frequently conchoidal; occasional specimens vitreous. It has a penetrating characteristic odour reminiscent of iodoform and a nauseous and bitter taste.

Microscopical characters: mounted in *lactophenol*: Cape aloes composed of fragments, usually amorphous but sometimes having embedded crystals; Barbados aloes appearing as fragments containing numerous acicular crystals.

POWDERED DRUG: Powdered Aloes. A yellowish-brown to dark reddish-brown powder, possessing the diagnostic microscopical characters, odour, and taste of the unground drug.

Adulterants and substitutes. Socotrine aloes occurs in hard dark-brown or nearly black opaque masses, with an uneven porous fracture and an unpleasant cheesy odour. It is prepared to a certain extent on the island of Socotra, but probably more largely on the African and possibly on the Arabian mainland, from the leaves of *A. perryi* Baker; it is imported usually in a pasty condition in kegs, and subsequent drying is necessary. The nitric acid test, described under Identification (test 2), produces a pale brownish-yellow colour; the copper sulphate test is negative, indicating absence of isobarbaloin. Zanzibar aloes is livery-brown and has a nearly smooth, slightly porous fracture; its odour is slight and not disagreeable. It is usually imported in masses partly covered with leaves, or in skins. The nitric acid test gives a yellowish-brown colour; the copper sulphate test for isobarbaloin, as for Socotrine aloes, is negative. Natal aloes, believed to be derived from *A. spectabilis* Reynolds, has been imported; it resembles Cape aloes in odour, but is opaque; when the powder is mixed with sulphuric acid and the vapour of nitric acid blown over it, a deep blue coloration is produced.

Solubility. Almost entirely soluble in alcohol (60%).

Identification. 1. Shake 100 mg, in powder or small pieces, with 10 ml of *ferric chloride solution* mixed with 5 ml of hydrochloric acid and immerse in a water-bath for about 10 minutes; filter immediately, cool the filtrate, and extract with 10 ml of carbon tetrachloride; separate the carbon tetrachloride layer, wash with 5 ml of water, and shake with 5 ml of *dilute ammonia solution*; a rose-pink to cherry-red colour is produced in the ammoniacal layer (presence of anthraquinone derivatives).

2. Prepare a 1% solution by boiling aloes with water until almost completely dissolved, adding kieselguhr, and filtering until clear. Add 0.2 g of borax to 5 ml of the filtrate and dissolve by boiling; a few drops of the resulting solution gives a green fluorescence when added to water (presence of anthranols). Another portion of the filtrate gives a copious pale yellow precipitate when mixed with an equal volume of freshly prepared *bromine solution* (presence of aloin). Mix 5 ml of the filtrate with 2 ml of nitric acid; that prepared from Cape aloes gives a yellowish-brown colour passing rapidly to a vivid green; with Barbados aloes, the colour is a deep brownish-red. Dilute 1 ml of the filtrate to 10 ml with water, add 1 drop of *copper sulphate solution*, 0.5 ml of *brine*, and 1 ml of alcohol (95%), and warm gently; Barbados aloes gives a reddish-violet colour and Cape aloes a faint evanescent violet tint (presence of isobarbaloin).

Actions and uses. Aloes is a purgative. It is administered by mouth and after absorption is excreted partly into the colon and partly in the urine. The usual dose is 100 to 200 milligrams and takes from 8 to 12 hours to produce an effect, but doses up to 300 milligrams are sometimes given. Antispasmodics may be given to prevent griping. Aloes colours urine red. It has been largely replaced by safer purgatives.

Undesirable effects. Aloes causes some pelvic congestion.

Precautions and contra-indications. Aloes should not be given when there is intestinal irritation, or to pregnant women. In nursing mothers it may be excreted in the milk.

Preparation

Aloes is an ingredient of compound benzoin tincture.

Aloxiprin

A polymeric condensation product of aluminium oxide and aspirin.

OTHER NAME: *Palaprin Forte®*

Description. A white tasteless powder.

Solubility. Practically insoluble in water; it hydrolyses rapidly in alkaline media but much less rapidly in acid media.

Actions and uses. Aloxiprin is an analgesic, antipyretic, and anti-inflammatory substance. After administration by mouth it is hydrolysed in the alkaline conditions of the small intestine, releasing aspirin which is responsible for the activity of the compound.
It is used for the relief of pain and inflammation in rheumatic disease. As it is slowly absorbed it is suitable for regular long-term use rather than for the occasional relief of pain. The usual dose is 100 milligrams per kilogram body-weight daily in divided doses. 600 milligrams of aloxiprin is approximately equivalent to 500 milligrams of aspirin.

Undesirable effects. As for Aspirin but it causes less tendency to gastric disturbance and it does not give rise to occult bleeding.

Precautions and contra-indications. The use of aloxiprin in conjunction with anticoagulant drugs should be avoided as it may increase the risk of haemorrhage. It is contra-indicated in patients who are hypersensitive to aspirin.

Poisoning. As for Aspirin.

Preparations

Preparations available include TABLETS containing aloxiprin 600 mg.

Alpha Tocopheryl Acetate

α-Tocopheryl acetate

$C_{31}H_{52}O_3 = 472.8$

OTHER NAMES: *Ephynal®* (*dl*-α-tocopheryl acetate); α-Tocopherol Acetate; α-Tocopheroli Acetas; *Vita-E®* (*d*-α-tocopheryl acetate)
Dystosel® (with potassium selenate)

A standard is given in the European Pharmacopoeia Vol. III Supplement

There are a number of isomeric forms of α-tocopheryl acetate. The natural form is *RRR*-α-tocopheryl acetate or *d*-α-tocopheryl acetate which has a potency of approximately 1.36 units of vitamin-E activity per milligram. Synthetic *all-rac*-α-tocopheryl acetate or *dl*-α-tocopheryl acetate is also available commercially; it has a potency of approximately 1 unit per milligram. In the paragraphs on actions and uses and veterinary uses the doses are expressed in milligrams of *dl*-α-tocopheryl acetate.

Description. A clear, slightly greenish-yellow, viscous, oily, odourless liquid.

Solubility. Practically insoluble in water; soluble in alcohol, in chloroform, in solvent ether, and in fixed oils.

Weight per ml. 0.949 to 0.963 g.

Refractive index. 1.494 to 1.498.

Storage. It should be stored in airtight containers, protected from light.

Identification. TEST. Dissolve about 200 mg in 2 ml of alcohol (95%), add 4 drops of nitric acid, and heat on a water-bath for 5 minutes; the colour changes from yellow to brick-red.

ULTRAVIOLET ABSORPTION. In alcohol (95%), maximum at 284 nm (E1%, 1cm = 43).

Actions and uses. Alpha tocopheryl acetate has vitamin-E activity and is more active than other tocopherols. It has been used in a number of conditions stated to be due to vitamin-E deficiency but its value in these conditions has not been established. The usual dose in the treatment of vitamin-E deficiency is 3 to 15 milligrams. Infants, in whom vitamin-E deficiency may possibly cause haemolytic anaemia, may be given up to 10 milligrams per kilogram body-weight daily. Supplements of alpha tocopheryl acetate are of value in the rare syndrome of abetalipoproteinaemia.
Alpha tocopheryl acetate has also been used in other conditions such as intermittent claudication in doses up to 600 milligrams daily.
It is used as an antioxidant in oils and fats. It is usually effective in a concentration of 0.001 to 0.05%. Its effectiveness can be enhanced by the addition of an oil-soluble antioxidant synergist such as lecithin.

Veterinary uses. Alpha tocopheryl acetate is used in conjunction with potassium selenate in the prevention and treatment of vitamin-E deficiencies, particularly nutritional myopathies of young cattle and sheep. The usual dose is up to 5 milligrams per kilogram body-weight by mouth or by injection daily. Doses of 100 to 500 micrograms per kilogram body-weight daily are used for the prevention of deficiency.

Preparations

Preparations available include CAPSULES containing alpha tocopheryl acetate 75, 200, and 400 units (approximately 55, 147, and 294 mg of *d*-α-tocopheryl acetate respectively), a veterinary INJECTION containing potassium selenate equivalent to selenium 1.5 mg and α-tocopherol acetate 68 units per ml in 50-ml vials, an OINTMENT containing alpha tocopheryl acetate 30 units (approximately 22 mg of *d*-α-tocopheryl acetate) per g, and TABLETS containing alpha tocopheryl acetate 75 units (approximately 55 mg of *d*-α-tocopheryl acetate), and 3 mg, 10 mg, 50 mg, and 200 mg of *dl*-α-tocopheryl acetate.

Alphadolone Acetate

3α,21-Dihydroxy-5α-pregnane-11,20-dione 21-acetate

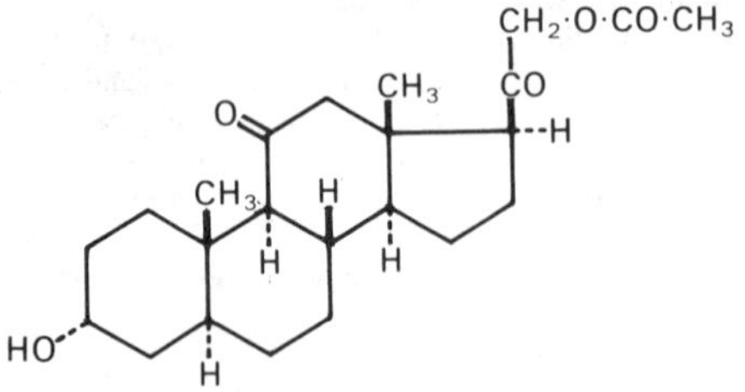

$C_{23}H_{34}O_5 = 390.5$

OTHER NAMES: *Althesin*®; *Saffan*® (both with alphaxalone)

Description. A white crystalline odourless powder.

Solubility. Practically insoluble in water; soluble in alcohol, in acetone, and in chloroform.

Incompatibility. For administration by intravenous infusion, solutions for injection may be mixed with dextrose injection (5%) or with sodium chloride injection.

Storage. It should be protected from light.

Identification. MELTING-POINT. About 178°.

ULTRAVIOLET ABSORPTION. In alcohol (95%), maximum at 289 nm (E1%, 1cm = about 2).

INFRA-RED ABSORPTION. Major peaks at 1010, 1228, 1278, 1375, 1710, and 1758 cm^{-1} (see Appendix 2a: Infrared Spectra).

THIN-LAYER CHROMATOGRAPHY. See under Thin-layer Chromatography, System 10.

Metabolism. *Protein binding*, 20 to 40% bound to plasma proteins in man.

EXCRETION. After an intravenous dose to rats, 60 to 70% is excreted in the faeces and 20 to 30% in the urine in 5 days; 60% of a dose is excreted in the bile in 3 hours; alphadolone appears to be rapidly excreted in man.

FURTHER INFORMATION. Clinical, pharmacological, and pharmacokinetic studies—R. N. Brogden *et al.*, *Drugs*, 1974, **8**, 87; metabolism and excretion—K. J. Child *et al.*, *Postgrad. med. J.*, 1972, **48**, *Suppl.* 2, 37.

Actions and uses. Alphadolone acetate is a steroid anaesthetic having about one-half the anaesthetic activity of alphaxalone. It is included in intravenous preparations of alphaxalone to improve the solubility of the latter.

Undesirable effects; Precautions; Contra-indications. As for Alphaxalone.

Preparations

Preparations available include an INJECTION and a veterinary injection containing alphadolone acetate 3 mg with alphaxalone 9 mg per ml in 5- and 10-ml ampoules.

Alphaxalone

3α-Hydroxy-5α-pregnane-11,20-dione

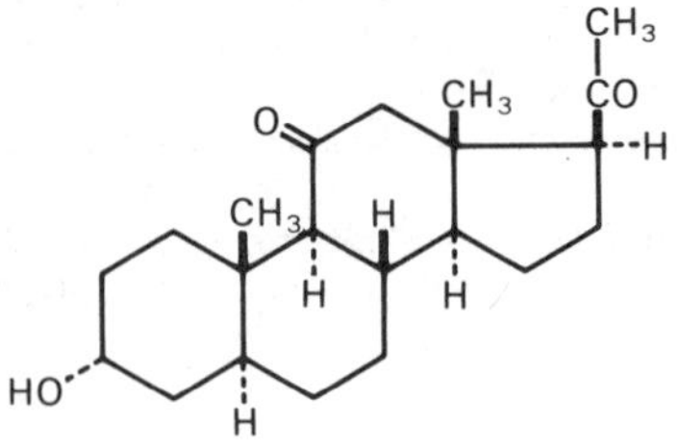

$C_{21}H_{32}O_3 = 332.5$

OTHER NAMES: *Althesin*®; *Saffan*® (both with alphadolone acetate)

Description. A white crystalline odourless powder.

Solubility. Practically insoluble in water; soluble in alcohol, in acetone, and in chloroform.

Stability. It may be precipitated from solution at low temperatures. Once formed such precipitates may be difficult to re-dissolve.

Incompatibility. For administration by intravenous infusion, solutions for injection may be mixed with dextrose injection (5%) or with sodium chloride injection.

Identification. MELTING-POINT. About 168°.

ULTRAVIOLET ABSORPTION. In alcohol (95%), maximum at 293 nm (E1%, 1cm = about 2).

INFRA-RED ABSORPTION. Major peaks at 1149, 1219, 1266, 1354, 1389, and 1695 cm^{-1} (see Appendix 2b: Infrared Spectra).

THIN-LAYER CHROMATOGRAPHY. See under Thin-layer Chromatography, System 10.

Determination in body fluids. GAS CHROMATOGRAPHY. In plasma—M. Dubois *et al.*, *Br. J. Anaesth.*, 1975, **47**, 902.

Metabolism. BLOOD CONCENTRATION. After an intravenous dose of 0.7 mg/kg of alphaxalone, a plasma concentration of about 1 μg/ml is obtained by 2 minutes falling to 70 ng/ml by 1 hour.

HALF-LIFE. In the rat, the plasma half-life is 7 minutes after an intravenous dose.

DISTRIBUTION. In the rat, alphaxalone is widely distributed throughout the tissues and is found in the central nervous system within 1 minute; highest concentrations appear in the liver; alphaxalone crosses the placenta; *protein binding*, 20 to 40% bound to plasma protein in man.

METABOLIC REACTIONS. In the rat, hydroxylation and glucuronic acid conjugation.

EXCRETION. After an intravenous dose to rats, 60 to 70% is excreted in the faeces and 20 to 30% in the urine in 5 days; 75% of the dose is excreted in the bile in 3 hours; the major metabolite in the bile appears to be the glucuronide of 2α-hydroxyalphaxalone; in man, alphaxalone appears rapidly in the urine, about 80% of a dose being excreted by this route in 5 days.

FURTHER INFORMATION. Clinical, pharmacological, and pharmacokinetic studies—R. N. Brogden *et al.*, *Drugs*, 1974, **8**, 87; metabolism and excretion—K. J. Child *et al.*, *Postgrad. med. J.*, 1972, **48**, *Suppl.* 2, 37; metabolism in man—L. Strunin *et al.*, *Br. J. Anaesth.*, 1974, **46**, 319.

Actions and uses. Alphaxalone is a steroid possessing anaesthetic properties and is used for the induction and maintenance of general anaesthesia. It is administered by the intravenous injection of a solution containing in addition alphadolone acetate which has a small anaesthetic effect but which is included to increase the solubility of the alphaxalone in the solvent.

The usual dose of a solution containing 9 milligrams of alphaxalone and 3 milligrams of alphadolone acetate per millilitre is 0.05 to 0.07 millilitre per kilogram body-weight by slow intravenous injection; this dose is usually adequate for the induction of anaesthesia in adults and children, but young children usually require the upper dose. A single dose rapidly induces anaesthesia with a normal duration of about 5 to 15 minutes. For the maintenance of anaesthesia for short operations, incremental doses of the intravenous injection are given. For longer operations, 25 millilitres of the intravenous solution is diluted in 250 millilitres of sodium chloride injection or dextrose injection (5%) and infused at the rate of 10 to 20 millilitres per hour.

Premedication with intravenous analgesics should be used when painful operations are to be carried out as alphaxalone and alphadolone acetate possess little analgesic activity. Recovery from maintenance anaesthesia may be prolonged, particularly when several doses of analgesics have been given.

Undesirable effects. Coughing, hiccoughing, salivation, transient flushing, muscle twitching, laryngospasm, shivering, and clonic contractions may occur. Euphoria, depression, nausea, and vomiting may occur during recovery from anaesthesia. Severe undesirable effects such as deep red or purple flushing, low blood pressure, pallor, sweating, and respiratory difficulty may occasionally occur.

Precautions. The jaw should be supported to prevent obstruction of the airway, as relaxation of the jaw occurs during anaesthesia.

Contra-indications. Alphaxalone should not be administered to patients who have experienced severe reactions to it or to patients with hepatic insufficiency.

Preparations

See above under Alphadolone Acetate.

Alprenolol Hydrochloride

N-[3-(2-Allylphenoxy)-2-hydroxypropyl]isopropylammonium chloride

$C_{15}H_{24}ClNO_2 = 285.8$

A standard is given in the British Pharmacopoeia 1973

Description. Odourless colourless crystals or white crystalline powder, with a bitter taste followed by a sensation of numbness.

Solubility. Soluble, at 20°, in less than 1 part of water, in 2 parts of alcohol, and in 3 parts of chloroform; practically insoluble in ether.

Acidity. A 5% solution in water has a pH of 5.5 to 6.5.

Incompatibility. It is incompatible with alkalis.

Sterilisation. Solutions are sterilised by heating in an autoclave or by filtration.

Storage. It should be stored in airtight containers, protected from light.

Identification. TEST. Dissolve about 300 mg in 10 ml of water, make alkaline with *dilute sodium hydroxide solution*, and extract with two 5-ml portions of solvent ether, wash the mixed extracts with water until they are free from alkali, dry the solution over anhydrous sodium sulphate, filter, and evaporate to dryness; the residue melts at about 58°.

MELTING-POINT. About 109°.

ULTRAVIOLET ABSORPTION. In alcohol (95%), maxima at 271 nm (E1%, 1cm = 65), and at 277 nm (E1%, 1cm = 60).

Determination in body fluids. GAS CHROMATOGRAPHY. In plasma—T. Walle, *J. pharm. Sci.*, 1974, **63**, 1885.

Metabolism. ABSORPTION. Readily absorbed after oral administration.

BLOOD CONCENTRATION. After a single oral dose of 200 mg, peak plasma concentrations of 80 to 150 ng/ml are attained in 1 to 2 hours; during therapy with daily doses of 600 mg, steady-state plasma concentrations of 11 to 150 ng/ml are attained; up to a tenfold variation in peak concentration may occur as a result of individual variations; therapeutically effective concentrations are in the range 50 to 100 ng/ml.

HALF-LIFE. After oral or intravenous doses, about 2 hours.

DISTRIBUTION. Apparent volume of distribution, about 200 litres; in rats, concentrations of 50 to 100 times that in the blood are found in the heart, lungs, liver, and skeletal muscles; *protein binding*, about 85% bound to plasma proteins.

METABOLIC REACTIONS. Extensive first pass metabolism; almost completely metabolised to 4-hydroxyalprenolol, which is active, and to desisopropylalprenolol.

EXCRETION. Most of a dose is excreted in the urine with less than 2% excreted as unchanged drug and 90% as metabolites in 72 hours.

FURTHER INFORMATION. Pharmacological effects and serum levels of orally administered alprenolol—B. Åblad *et al.*, *Eur. J. clin. Pharmac.*, 1972, **5**, 44; absorption, distribution, and excretion of alprenolol—N.-O. Bodin *et al.*, *Acta pharmac. tox.*, 1974, **35**, 261; pharmacokinetics and pharmacodynamics of alprenolol—P. Collste *et al.*, *Eur. J. clin. Pharmac.*, 1976, **10**, 85 and 89; pharmacokinetics and biopharmaceutics of alprenolol—C. Regardh, *Acta pharmac. tox.*, 1975, **37**, Suppl. 1.

Actions and uses. Alprenolol hydrochloride is a beta-adrenoceptor blocking agent with actions and uses similar to those described under Propranolol Hydrochloride. It has also a slight sympathomimetic action.

For the treatment of cardiac arrhythmias it is given by mouth in doses of 100 to 200 milligrams daily in divided doses but larger amounts up to 400 milligrams daily in divided doses may be given if necessary; the usual dose by slow intravenous injection is 2 to 5 milligrams.

In the treatment of angina pectoris and arterial hypertension 200 milligrams gradually increased if necessary to 800 milligrams may be given daily in divided doses.

Undesirable effects. As for Propranolol Hydrochloride.

Precautions. It should be administered with caution to patients with a history of bronchial asthma or heart failure.

Preparations

ALPRENOLOL INJECTION: a sterile solution of alprenolol hydrochloride in water for injections. It is sterilised by heating in an autoclave or by filtration.
A standard for this injection is given in the British Pharmacopoeia 1973
Containers and *Labelling:* see the entry on Injections for general information on containers and labelling.
Storage: it should be protected from light.

ALPRENOLOL TABLETS: containing alprenolol hydrochloride.
A standard for these tablets is given in the British Pharmacopoeia 1973
Containers and *Storage:* see the entry on Tablets for general information on containers and storage. Containers should be airtight and light resistant.
Advice for patients: the tablets should preferably be taken before meals. Treatment should not be discontinued without the advice of the prescriber.

Alum

$AlK(SO_4)_2, 12H_2O = 474.4$

OTHER NAMES: Alumen; Potash Alum; Potassium Aluminium Sulphate

A standard is given in the European Pharmacopoeia Vol. I

Description. Odourless, colourless, transparent, crystalline masses or a granular powder, with a sweetish, astringent taste. When heated, it melts and, at about 200°, loses its water of crystallisation with the formation of the anhydrous salt.

Solubility. Soluble in water and in glycerol; practically insoluble in alcohol.

Acidity. A 10% solution has a pH of 3 to 3.5.

Incompatibility. It is incompatible with borax, alkali hydroxides and carbonates, phosphates, salts of calcium, lead, and mercury, and tannin.

Storage. It should be stored in airtight containers.

Actions and uses. Alum precipitates proteins and is a powerful astringent. It is now seldom given by mouth. Dilute solutions (1 to 4%) have been used as astringent mouth-washes and gargles but they have a destructive action on the teeth; a 2% solution has been used for application to the skin to reduce excessive perspiration. Stronger solutions (5 to 10%) are used to harden the skin, especially of the feet. Alum, either powdered or as a strong solution, is used as a styptic for minor cuts and abrasions.
Alum, diluted with 6 parts of purified talc, has been used as a foot powder.

Aluminium Glycinate

A partly hydrated, basic aluminium glycinate.

$C_2H_6AlNO_4 = 135.1$

OTHER NAMES: Dihydroxyaluminium Aminoacetate; Dihydroxyaluminium Glycinate; *Robalate®*

Prodexin® (with magnesium carbonate); *Glycinal®* (with magnesium trisilicate)

A standard is given in the British Pharmacopoeia Addendum 1975

Description. A white or almost white odourless powder.

Solubility. Practically insoluble in water and in organic solvents; soluble in dilute mineral acids and in solutions of alkali hydroxides.

Acidity or alkalinity. A 4% suspension has a pH of 6.5 to 7.5.

Moisture content. Not more than 12%, determined by drying at 130°.

Storage. It should be stored in airtight containers.

Identification. TESTS. 1. Mix 1 g with 25 ml of 0.5N hydrochloric acid and heat gently until a clear solution is formed; reserve half of the solution. The solution gives the reactions of aluminium.
2. To 2 ml of the solution reserved in Test 1 add 3 drops of liquefied phenol, shake, and then add without shaking 5 ml of *dilute sodium hypochlorite solution*; a blue colour is produced.
3. Dissolve 840 mg of citric acid in 8 ml of 1N sodium hydroxide and dilute to 20 ml with water. To 10 ml of this solution add about 100 mg of the sample followed by 0.5 ml of a 0.1% solution of ninhydrin in methanol and warm; a purple colour is produced.

Actions and uses. Aluminium glycinate is a slow-acting antacid with actions and uses similar to those described under Aluminium Hydroxide Gel.
The usual dose is 1 to 2 grams, repeated in accordance with the needs of the patient, and it is administered as a suspension or by allowing the tablets to dissolve slowly in the mouth. As it may cause constipation it is frequently given in conjunction with a mildly laxative antacid such as magnesium carbonate.

Undesirable effects. As for Aluminium Hydroxide Gel.

Preparations

Preparations available include a MIXTURE containing aluminium glycinate 500 mg in 5 ml, TABLETS containing aluminium glycinate 900 mg with magnesium carbonate 100 mg and peppermint flavouring, and tablets containing aluminium glycinate 750 mg with magnesium trisilicate 250 mg and peppermint flavouring.

Aluminium Hydroxide Gel

An aqueous suspension of hydrated aluminium oxide containing varying quantities of basic aluminium carbonate. It contains about 4% of Al_2O_3.

OTHER NAMES: *Aludrox®*; Alum. Hydrox. Gel; Alum. Hydrox. Mixt.; Aluminium Hydroxide Mixture

A standard is given in the British Pharmacopoeia 1973

Aluminium hydroxide gel may be prepared by the interaction in aqueous solution of an aluminium salt and a suitable alkali such as ammonium carbonate or sodium carbonate and washing the precipitate. A suitable preservative, such as 0.5% w/w of sodium benzoate, and, as a flavouring agent, 0.015% v/v of peppermint oil are added; saccharin sodium may be added as a sweetening agent.

Description. A white viscous suspension from which small amounts of clear liquid may separate on standing; it may exhibit thixotropic properties.

Alkalinity. A 50% dilution in water has a pH of not more than 7.5.

Storage. It should be stored at a temperature not exceeding 25°; it should not be allowed to freeze.

Actions and uses. Aluminium hydroxide gel is a useful slow-acting antacid; it is mildly astringent and may therefore cause constipation. It adsorbs small quantities of phosphate and vitamins from the gastro-intestinal tract, but this is probably of little significance unless the diet is low in these substances.

Aluminium hydroxide gel is used in the treatment of peptic ulcer and hyperchlorhydria; it may be administered diluted with water or milk. In peptic ulcer it is given every 2 to 4 hours just after food; during convalescence it is given every 4 hours.

Aluminium hydroxide gel, diluted with 2 to 3 parts of water, may also be given by intragastric drip, the rate of flow being from 15 to 20 drops a minute throughout the day.

The usual dose for an adult is 7.5 to 15 millilitres, repeated in accordance with the needs of the patient. Aluminium hydroxide gel is used in large doses, up to 100 millilitres daily, to reduce the absorption of phosphate in hypoparathyroidism and renal osteodystrophy. Its constipating action may be counteracted by giving magnesium hydroxide or magnesium trisilicate with it.

Undesirable effects. Aluminium hydroxide gel diminishes the absorption of the tetracyclines from the gut and is therefore pharmacologically incompatible with them.

Preparations

ALUMINIUM HYDROXIDE AND BELLADONNA MIXTURE:

Belladonna tincture	100 ml
Chloroform spirit ..	50 ml
Aluminium hydroxide gel	to 1000 ml

It must be freshly prepared.

Containers: see the entry on Mixtures for general information on containers. It should be supplied in wide-mouthed bottles.

Labelling: a direction to shake the bottle should be given on the label.

Advice for patients: the mixture may be taken alone, or with water or other fluid, between meals. It should not be used for longer than a few days without medical advice.

Dose: 5 millilitres suitably diluted.

OTHER PREPARATIONS available include numerous compound preparations in which aluminium hydroxide gel is an ingredient.

Aluminium Hydroxide Gel, Dried

It consists mainly of hydrated aluminium oxide, together with varying quantities of basic aluminium carbonate.

OTHER NAMES: *Aludrox®*; Aluminium Hydroxide Powder; Dried Alum. Hydrox. Gel

A standard is given in the British Pharmacopoeia 1973

Dried aluminium hydroxide gel may be prepared by drying under suitable conditions the precipitate formed by the interaction in aqueous solution of an aluminium salt with ammonium carbonate or sodium carbonate.

Description. A fine white odourless powder containing some aggregates.

Solubility. Practically insoluble in water and in alcohol; soluble in dilute mineral acids and in excess of caustic alkalis.

Alkalinity. A 4% suspension has a pH of not more than 10.

Stability. Heating to temperatures much in excess of 30° results in gradual dehydration and loss of therapeutic value; partial loss of neutralising activity may occur during tabletting.

Hygroscopicity. At relative humidities between about 15 and 70%, the equilibrium moisture content at 25° is between about 17 and 20%, but at relative humidities above 75%, the powder absorbs substantial amounts of moisture.

Storage. It should be stored in airtight containers at a temperature not exceeding 25°.

Actions and uses. Dried aluminium hydroxide gel has the actions, uses, and undesirable effects described under Aluminium Hydroxide Gel.

The usual dose for an adult is 0.5 to 1 gram, repeated in accordance with the needs of the patient.

Preparations

ALUMINIUM HYDROXIDE TABLETS: for each tablet take:

Dried aluminium hydroxide gel	500.0 mg
Lactose	150.0 mg
Sucrose	150.0 mg
Starch	200.0 mg
Peppermint oil	0.004 ml

Mix the solid ingredients and granulate by moist granulation as described in the entry on Tablets; dry the granules at a suitable temperature, which should not exceed 30° if a drying oven is used, mix with the peppermint oil previously dissolved in a small quantity of alcohol (95%), and prepare by compression.

A standard for these tablets is given in the British Pharmacopoeia 1973

Containers and *Storage:* see the entry on Tablets for general information on containers and storage. Containers should be airtight. The tablets should be stored at a temperature not exceeding 25°.

Labelling: a direction to chew the tablets before they are swallowed should be given on the label.

Dose: 1 to 2 tablets.

Advice for patients: the tablets may be chewed half an hour after meals. They should not be used for longer than a few days without medical advice.

OTHER PREPARATIONS available include numerous compound preparations in which dried aluminium hydroxide gel is an ingredient. Dried aluminium hydroxide gel is an ingredient of magnesium trisilicate compound tablets.

Aluminium Magnesium Silicate

A native colloidal hydrated aluminium magnesium silicate (saponite) freed from gritty particles.

OTHER NAME: *Veegum®*

A standard is given in the British Pharmaceutical Codex 1973

A number of different grades are available which are distinguished by the degree of alkalinity and the viscosity of an aqueous dispersion. With an average pharmaceutical grade, the pH of a 4% dispersion in water is about 9 and the viscosity of a 5% dispersion is about 250 centipoises (0.25 Pa.s).

Description. *Macroscopical characters:* odourless, tasteless, small, creamy-white flakes or a creamy-white powder.

Microscopical characters: a powder or flakes varying in shape and in size from about 0.3 to 0.4 mm to 1.0 by 2.0 mm and about 25 to 240 μm thick; many of the flakes are perforated by scattered circular holes about 20 to 50 to 120 μm in diameter. Between crossed polars on a dark field innumerable bright specks are seen scattered over the flakes.

Solubility. Practically insoluble in water, but swells to form a colloidal thixotropic dispersion; practically insoluble in organic solvents.

Moisture content. Not more than 10%, determined by drying at 105°.

Uses. Aluminium magnesium silicate is used, usually at a concentration of between 0.5 and 2.5%, as a suspending, thickening, and emulsion-stabilising agent. Dispersions in water are thixotropic and at a concentration of 10% a firm gel is formed. The viscosity of dispersions is increased by heating, by the addition of electrolytes, and, at higher concentrations, by ageing.

When used in conjunction with other suspending agents such as methylcellulose and sodium carboxymethylcellulose the dispersions produced have an enhanced viscosity; it can also be used in conjunction with natural gums such as acacia.

Aluminium magnesium silicate is also used as a binder and disintegrant in tablets.

Aluminium Phosphate Gel

An aqueous suspension of aluminium orthophosphate. It contains about 7.5% of AlPO$_4$.

OTHER NAMES: *Aluphos*®; Alum. Phos. Gel

A standard is given in the British Pharmacopoeia 1973

Aluminium phosphate gel may be prepared by precipitation from a solution of an aluminium salt by the addition of a suitable alkali phosphate. A suitable preservative is added and peppermint oil, 0.01% v/v, is added as a flavouring agent; saccharin sodium may be added as a sweetening agent.

Description. A white viscous suspension, from which small amounts of clear liquid may separate on standing.

Acidity. A 50% dilution in water has a pH of 5 to 6.

Storage. It should be stored at a temperature not exceeding 30°; it should not be allowed to freeze.

Actions and uses. Aluminium phosphate gel has the actions, uses, and undesirable effects described under Aluminium Hydroxide Gel to which it is a useful alternative for patients on restricted diets low in phosphates because, unlike the hydroxide gel, it does not interfere with the absorption of phosphates.

The usual dose for an adult is 5 to 15 millilitres, repeated in accordance with the needs of the patient.

Aluminium Phosphate Gel, Dried

It consists largely of hydrated aluminium orthophosphate.

OTHER NAMES: *Aluphos*®; Dried Alum. Phos. Gel

A standard is given in the British Pharmacopoeia 1973

Dried aluminium phosphate gel may be prepared by drying under suitable conditions the product of interaction in aqueous solution of an aluminium salt with an alkali phosphate such as sodium phosphate.

Description. A white odourless powder containing some friable aggregates.

Solubility. Practically insoluble in water and in alcohol; soluble in dilute mineral acids; practically insoluble in solutions of alkali hydroxides.

Acidity. A 4% suspension has a pH of 5.5 to 6.5.

Storage. It should be stored at a temperature not exceeding 30°.

Actions and uses. Dried aluminium phosphate gel has the actions, uses, and undesirable effects of Aluminium Phosphate Gel.

The usual dose for an adult is 400 to 800 milligrams, repeated in accordance with the needs of the patient.

Preparation

ALUMINIUM PHOSPHATE TABLETS: containing dried aluminium phosphate gel with peppermint oil as flavouring agent. They contain the equivalent of 400 mg of aluminium phosphate (AlPO$_4$).

A standard for these tablets is given in the British Pharmacopoeia 1973

Containers and *Storage:* see the entry on Tablets for general information on containers and storage. Containers should be airtight. The tablets should be stored at a temperature not exceeding 30°.

Labelling: a direction to chew the tablets before they are swallowed should be given on the label.

Advice for patients: the tablets may be chewed half an hour after meals. They should not be used for longer than a few days without medical advice.

Dose: 1 or 2 tablets.

Aluminium Powder

Al = 26.98154

It consists principally of metallic aluminium in the form of very small flakes, and may be prepared by hammering aluminium in a suitable mill.

A standard is given in the British Pharmaceutical Codex 1973

In addition to metallic aluminium, the powder usually contains an appreciable proportion of aluminium oxide. Aluminium powder is lubricated with stearic acid during manufacture and this lubricant serves to protect the material from oxidation during storage.

Description. A silvery-grey, odourless powder.

Storage. It should be stored in airtight containers.

Actions and uses. Aluminium powder has been used for dusting on the skin around an ileostomy, caecostomy, or colostomy as a protection against proteolytic or irritant discharges. Compound aluminium paste is used similarly by applying it thickly round a fistula or sinus.

Preparation

COMPOUND ALUMINIUM PASTE (*Syn.* Baltimore Paste):

Aluminium powder	..	..	..	..	200 g
Zinc oxide ..	..	..	..	..	..	400 g
Liquid paraffin	..	..	..	..	..	400 g

Mix thoroughly the zinc oxide and the aluminium powder with the liquid paraffin until smooth.

A standard for this paste is given in the British Pharmaceutical Codex 1973

Containers and *Storage:* see the entry on Pastes for general information on containers and storage.

Aluminium Sulphate

A hydrated mixture of the normal salt, $Al_2(SO_4)_3$, with a small proportion of basic aluminium sulphate. It contains a variable quantity of water of crystallisation.

OTHER NAME: Aluminii Sulfas

A standard is given in the European Pharmacopoeia Vol. II

Description. Odourless colourless lustrous crystals or crystalline masses.

Solubility. Soluble, at 20°, in 1 part of water, giving a solution which may be slightly turbid; practically insoluble in alcohol.

Acidity. A 2% solution has a pH of 3 to 4.

Storage. It should be stored in airtight containers.

Actions and uses. Aluminium sulphate has actions similar to those described under Alum but is more astringent than alum. A saturated solution is employed as a mild caustic. Solutions (5 to 10%) have been used as local applications to ulcers and to arrest foul discharges from mucous surfaces.
Aluminium sulphate is also employed in the preparation of aluminium acetate solution, which is used as astringent ear-drops. A 1 in 20 dilution of this solution may be used as an astringent lotion for wet dressing in dermatitis and suppurating wounds.

Preparations

ALUMINIUM ACETATE EAR-DROPS: consisting of aluminium acetate solution (see below).
Containers: see the entry on Ear-drops for general information on containers.

ALUMINIUM ACETATE LOTION:

Aluminium acetate solution .. .. .. 50 ml
Purified water, freshly boiled
  and cooled .. .. to 1000 ml

It must be freshly prepared.
Containers and *Labelling:* see the entry on Lotions for general information on containers and labelling.
Advice for patients: the undiluted lotion should be applied to the skin. The lotion should not be used if a precipitate is present.

ALUMINIUM ACETATE SOLUTION (*Syn.* Burow's Solution; Aluminium Acetate Ear-drops):

Aluminium sulphate .. .. 225 g
Acetic acid .. .. 250 ml
Tartaric acid .. .. 45 g
Calcium carbonate .. .. 100 g
Water for preparations .. .. 750 ml

Dissolve the aluminium sulphate in 600 ml of the water, add the acetic acid and then the calcium carbonate mixed with the remainder of the water, and allow to stand for not less than 24 hours in a cool place, stirring occasionally; filter, add the tartaric acid to the filtered solution, and mix. It contains about 13% of aluminium acetate.
A standard for this solution is given in the British Pharmaceutical Codex 1973
Storage: it should be stored in well-filled containers, in a cool place.

Amantadine Hydrochloride

Tricyclo[3,3,1,1^{3,7}]dec-1-ylammonium chloride

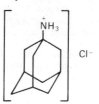

$C_{10}H_{18}ClN = 187.7$

OTHER NAME: *Symmetrel*®

Description. An odourless white crystalline powder with a bitter taste.

Solubility. Soluble in 2.5 parts of water, in 5 parts of alcohol, and in 18 parts of chloroform; practically insoluble in ether.

Acidity. A 20% solution has a pH of 3 to 5.5.

Identification. TEST. Mix 100 mg with 1 ml of pyridine and 100 μl of acetic anhydride, heat to boiling for 10 seconds, pour the hot solution into 10 ml of *dilute hydrochloric acid*, and cool to 5°; a precipitate is produced which, after washing with water and drying at 60° for 1 hour, melts at about 148°.

MELTING-POINT. About 360°, with decomposition.

ULTRAVIOLET ABSORPTION. In 0.1N hydrochloric acid there is no significant absorption in the range 230 nm to 360 nm.

INFRA-RED ABSORPTION. Major peaks at 1089, 1317, 1370, 1458, 1497, and 1503 cm^{-1} (see Appendix 2a: Infra-red Spectra).

Determination in body fluids. GAS CHROMATOGRAPHY. In plasma—P. Biandrate *et al.*, *J. Chromat.*, 1972, **74**, 31.

Metabolism. ABSORPTION. Almost completely absorbed after oral administration.

BLOOD CONCENTRATION. After an oral dose of 4 to 5 mg/kg body-weight, peak plasma concentrations of 0.5 to 0.6 μg/ml are attained within 1 to 4 hours.

HALF-LIFE. Plasma half-life, about 9 to 20 hours.

DISTRIBUTION. Accumulates in renal function impairment; secreted in the milk.

METABOLIC REACTIONS. *N*-methylation in dogs.

EXCRETION. About 85% of an oral dose is excreted unchanged in the urine in 4 days.

FURTHER INFORMATION. Absorption, distribution, and excretion of amantadine hydrochloride—W. E. Bleidner *et al.*, *J. Pharmac. exp. Ther.*, 1965, **150**, 484; accumulation of amantadine hydrochloride in renal insufficiency—T. S. Ing *et al.*, *New Engl. J. Med.*, 1974, **291**, 1257; urinary excretion of amantadine by the elderly—C. Montanari *et al.*, *Eur. J. clin. Pharmac.*, 1975, **8**, 349.

Actions and uses. Amantadine hydrochloride has antiviral activity and is used in the prophylaxis and treatment of infection with influenza type A viruses. It is also used in the treatment of parkinsonism, usually in conjunction with other therapy, and to alleviate pain associated with herpes zoster infection in elderly or debilitated patients.
In the prophylaxis and treatment of influenza caused by type A viruses, the adult dose is 100 milligrams twice daily; the dose for children aged 10 to 15 years is 100

milligrams daily. Treatment of influenza is continued for 5 to 7 days and prophylaxis for as long as protection from influenza is required, usually 7 to 10 days.

In the treatment of parkinsonism 100 milligrams is given daily in conjunction with other therapy increasing after 1 week to 100 milligrams twice daily depending on the patient's condition.

For the alleviation of pain associated with herpes zoster, 100 milligrams is given twice daily, as soon as the condition is diagnosed, for 14 days and continued for a further 14 days if the pain persists.

Undesirable effects. Nervousness, insomnia, dizziness, hallucinations, light headedness, and convulsions may occur.

Precautions. Amantadine should be administered cautiously to patients being treated with central nervous stimulants. Amantadine is secreted in the milk and may cause vomiting, urinary retention, and skin rashes in the infant. Its use in nursing mothers should preferably be avoided.

Contra-indications. Amantadine should not be administered to children under 10 years or to patients with a history of epilepsy or gastro-intestinal disturbances.

Preparations

AMANTADINE CAPSULES: consisting of amantadine hydrochloride, in powder, which may be mixed with a suitable inert diluent, enclosed in a soft capsule. The capsule shells may be coloured. Available as capsules containing 100 mg of amantadine hydrochloride.

Containers and *Storage:* see the entry on Capsules for general information on containers and storage.

Advice for patients: when used as an antiviral agent the prescribed course should be completed. When used in parkinsonism treatment should not be discontinued without the advice of the prescriber. The capsules may affect mental concentration; persons affected should not drive or operate machinery. To avoid insomnia doses should not be taken for several hours before bed time.

OTHER PREPARATIONS available include an ELIXIR containing amantadine hydrochloride 50 mg in 5 ml, diluent syrup, shelf-life of diluted elixir 4 weeks.

Amaranth Solution

A solution containing 1% of amaranth, food grade of commerce, with 20% of chloroform spirit, and 25% of glycerol, in purified water.

Uses. Amaranth is a red dye used in colouring medicines. For dispensing purposes it is generally used in the form of amaranth solution.

Amenorrhoea

see under UTERINE BLEEDING, ABNORMAL

Amethocaine Hydrochloride

2-Dimethylaminoethyl 4-butylaminobenzoate hydrochloride

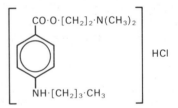

$C_{15}H_{25}ClN_2O_2 = 300.8$

OTHER NAMES: *Anethaine*®; Tetracaine Hydrochloride; Tetracainii Chloridum
Optocol® (with chloramphenicol)

A standard is given in the European Pharmacopoeia Vol. I

Description. A white crystalline odourless powder with a slightly bitter taste followed by local numbness.

Solubility. Soluble, at 20°, in 7.5 parts of water, in 40 parts of alcohol, and in 30 parts of chloroform; practically insoluble in ether.

Acidity. A 1% solution has a pH of 4.5 to 6.5.

Dissociation constant. pK_a 8.5.

Stability. In aqueous solution, amethocaine hydrochloride degrades by hydrolysis to n-butylaminobenzoic acid and 2-dimethylaminoethanol; decarboxylation of n-butylaminobenzoic acid to butylaniline then occurs and the butylaniline oxidises to form various purple-coloured products. The hydrolysis of amethocaine is catalysed by hydrogen ions and hydroxyl ions. At 25°, solutions are most stable at about pH 3.5.

FURTHER INFORMATION. Stability in aqueous solution —H. W. Schmid, *Pharm. Acta Helv.*, 1961, **36**, 423; R. E. Thomas and M. Woodward, *Australas. J. Pharm.*, 1963, **44**, 590.

Sterilisation. Solutions are sterilised by heating in an autoclave, by heating with a bactericide, or by filtration.

Storage. It should be stored in airtight containers, protected from light.

Identification. TESTS. 1. To about 200 mg in 10 ml of water add 1 ml of *ammonium thiocyanate solution*; a white crystalline precipitate is produced which, after recrystallisation from water and drying at 80° for 2 hours, melts at about 131°.
2. Dissolve a small portion in fuming nitric acid, evaporate to dryness, dissolve the residue in acetone, and add *alcoholic potassium hydroxide solution*; a crimson colour is produced (distinction from lignocaine and most other similar anaesthetics).

MELTING-POINT. About 148°, or it may occur in either of two other polymorphic forms, melting at about 134° or at about 139°; mixtures of the forms may melt in the range 134° to 147°.

ULTRAVIOLET ABSORPTION. In 0.1N sulphuric acid, maxima at 229 nm (E1%, 1cm = 509), 281 nm (E1%, 1cm = 55), and 312 nm (E1%, 1cm = 76).

INFRA-RED ABSORPTION. Major peaks at 1126, 1174, 1286, 1345, 1600, and 1688 cm⁻¹ (see Appendix 2a: Infra-red Spectra).

THIN-LAYER CHROMATOGRAPHY. See under Thin-layer Chromatography, System 2.

Determination in body fluids. ULTRAVIOLET SPECTROPHOTOMETRY. In blood—I. Porush et al., J. pharm. Sci., 1965, **54**, 1809.

Metabolism. METABOLIC REACTIONS. Hydrolysed in the body to 4-aminobenzoic acid, and is completely metabolised within 1 hour of injection.

Actions and uses. Amethocaine is a local anaesthetic which is suitable for infiltration, surface, or spinal anaesthesia. Although it is several times more toxic than either procaine by injection or cocaine by application, it is relatively safer because its local anaesthetic action is greater and it can therefore be used in lower concentrations than are normally employed with procaine or cocaine; in addition, it does not produce the idiosyncratic reactions that may arise after the administration of cocaine.

The risk of toxic effects may be reduced by the addition of adrenaline, which delays absorption; solutions containing adrenaline should not, however, be used for inducing anaesthesia in digits, because the profound ischaemia produced may lead to gangrene.

In infiltration and spinal anaesthesia, the action of amethocaine is slower in onset than that of procaine, but is of longer duration.

In ophthalmology, amethocaine hydrochloride is usually employed as a 0.25% solution; the use of solutions stronger than 1% should be avoided as they may result in damage to the cornea. As an analgesic in otorhinolaryngology, a 0.5 to 2% solution is employed; stronger solutions are sometimes used, but it is doubtful whether they are necessary. A 0.5% solution may be used as a throat spray before the introduction of a gastroscope, and a 0.1% solution may be injected into the urethra before the introduction of a catheter or cystoscope. A 1 to 3% ointment is useful in painful conditions of the anus and rectum.

For spinal anaesthesia, 5 to 20 milligrams may be administered as a 0.1 to 0.5% solution. Solutions having a higher density than that of cerebrospinal fluid may be prepared by dissolving the dose in a 6% dextrose injection. Solutions having a density approximately equal to that of cerebrospinal fluid are also used; these are prepared by dissolving 1% of amethocaine hydrochloride in sodium chloride injection or occasionally by dissolving the dose in cerebrospinal fluid. For techniques in which a solution of relatively low density is required, a suitable preparation is a 0.066% solution of amethocaine hydrochloride in water for injections containing 0.5% of sodium chloride.

For infiltration anaesthesia, up to 4 milligrams per kilogram body-weight, with a maximum of 250 milligrams, administered as a 0.03 to 0.1% solution in sodium chloride injection, may be used.

Poisoning. The procedure described under Cocaine should be adopted.

Preparations

AMETHOCAINE EYE-DROPS: a sterile solution containing up to 1% of amethocaine hydrochloride, with 0.1% of sodium metabisulphite and 0.002% w/v of phenylmercuric acetate or nitrate, in purified water. It is prepared by Method A, B, or C described in the entry on Eye-drops.
A standard for these eye-drops is given in the British Pharmaceutical Codex 1973
Containers: see the entry on Eye-drops for general information on containers. This solution is adversely affected by alkali. The eye-drops should preferably be supplied in single-dose containers.

Labelling: see the entry on Eye-drops for general information on labelling.

OTHER PREPARATIONS available include a CREAM containing amethocaine hydrochloride 1%; and a veterinary POWDER containing amethocaine hydrochloride 0.1% with chloramphenicol 0.5%.

Amicarbalide Isethionate

1,3-Bis(3-amidinophenyl)urea di(2-hydroxyethanesulphonate)

$$\left[\begin{array}{c} NH_2C-\phenyl-NH\cdot CO\cdot NH-\phenyl-C{=}NH,\ NH_2 \end{array} \right] \quad 2\ \begin{array}{l} CH_2OH \\ | \\ CH_2\cdot SO_3H \end{array}$$

$C_{19}H_{28}N_6O_9S_2 = 548.6$

OTHER NAME: *Diampron*®

A standard is given in the British Pharmacopoeia (Veterinary)

Description. A white or slightly cream, almost odourless powder with a sweet taste.

Solubility. Soluble, at 20°, in less than 1 part of water and in 250 parts of alcohol; practically insoluble in ether and in chloroform.

Acidity. A 50% solution has a pH of 5 to 7.

Moisture content. Not more than 1%, determined by drying at 105°.

Sterilisation. Solutions for injection are sterilised by filtration.

Identification. TESTS. 1. Dissolve about 100 mg in 10 ml of water and add 1 ml of *dilute sulphuric acid*; a white precipitate is produced.
2. Dissolve about 5 mg in 10 ml of water, add 1 ml of *borate buffer solution* and 1 ml of *glyoxal solution*, and heat on a water-bath for 10 minutes; a magenta colour is produced.

MELTING-POINT. About 202°.

ULTRAVIOLET ABSORPTION. In 0.01N hydrochloric acid, maximum at 232 nm (E1%, 1cm = 650), and an inflection at 257 nm (E1%, 1cm = 500).

Veterinary uses. Amicarbalide isethionate is used in the treatment of cattle redwater due to *Babesia* infection. The usual dosage is 5 to 10 milligrams per kilogram body-weight by subcutaneous or intramuscular injection, repeated if haematuria persists after 24 hours.

Preparation

AMICARBALIDE INJECTION: a sterile solution of amicarbalide isethionate in water for injections. It is sterilised by filtration. Available in 50-ml units containing 500 mg of amicarbalide isethionate per ml.
A standard for this injection is given in the British Pharmacopoeia (Veterinary)
Containers and Labelling: see the entry on Injections for general information on containers and labelling.

Amiloride Hydrochloride

N- Amidino - 3,5 - diamino - 6 - chloropyrazine - 2 - carboxamide hydrochloride dihydrate

$C_6H_9Cl_2N_7O, 2H_2O = 302.1$

OTHER NAMES: *Midamor®*
Moduretic® (with hydrochlorothiazide)

Description. An odourless yellow to greenish-yellow
powder.

Solubility. Soluble in water.

Storage. It should be stored in airtight containers, in a
cool place, protected from light.

Identification. MELTING-POINT. About 286°, with
decomposition.

ULTRAVIOLET ABSORPTION. In 0.1N hydrochloric acid,
maxima at 284 nm (E1%, 1cm = 639), and 362 nm (E1%,
1cm = 699).

INFRA-RED ABSORPTION. Major peaks at 1235, 1515,
1538, 1587, 1639, and 1695 cm^{-1} (see Appendix 2b: Infra-
red Spectra).

Determination in body fluids. SPECTROFLUORIMETRY.
In plasma, serum, or urine—J. E. Baer *et al.*, *J. Pharmac. exp. Ther.*, 1967, **157**, 472; in urine: separation by
thin-layer chromatography—E.Schmid and G. Fricke,
Pharmacol. Clin., 1969, **1**, 110.

Metabolism. ABSORPTION. Incompletely absorbed after
oral administration but the extent of absorption is increased after fasting.

BLOOD CONCENTRATION. After an oral dose of 20 mg,
peak serum concentrations of about 50 ng/ml are attained
by about 3 hours.

HALF-LIFE. Serum half-life, about 6 hours which may be
increased in renal function impairment.

DISTRIBUTION. Volume of distribution, 350 to 480 litres
(determined for ^{14}C-amiloride).

METABOLIC REACTIONS. It does not appear to be metabolised in man.

EXCRETION. 20 to 50% of an oral dose is excreted
unchanged in the urine and about 40% in the faeces in
72 hours.

FURTHER INFORMATION. Kinetics and bioavailability in
man—A. J. Smith and R. N. Smith, *Br. J. Pharmac.*,
1973, **48**, 646; metabolism in man—P. Weiss *et al.*, *Clin.
Pharmac. Ther.*, 1969, **10**, 401.

Actions and uses. Amiloride is a mild diuretic that acts
mainly on the distal part of the distal tubule. It increases
the excretion of sodium and chloride and reduces the
excretion of potassium, whether aldosterone is present
or not. It does not affect the glomerular filtration rate or
inhibit carbonic anhydrase. It begins to act about 2 hours
after administration by mouth and its diuretic action may
last for up to 24 hours.
Amiloride is used in conjunction with thiazide or other
potent diuretics to conserve potassium during diuretic
therapy. In the treatment of congestive heart failure,
hypertension, and hepatic cirrhosis with ascites, the
daily adult dosage is 5 to 10 milligrams by mouth which
may be increased if necessary to 20 milligrams daily.

Undesirable effects. Anorexia, nausea, vomiting,
abdominal distension, constipation, diarrhoea, dryness
of the mouth and thirst, paraesthesia, dizziness, weakness, muscle cramps, orthostatic hypotension, rashes,
pruritus, confusion, and visual disturbances may occur.

Precautions. Patients should be observed for symptoms
of hyperkalaemia, metabolic or respiratory acidosis, electrolyte imbalance, and raised blood urea concentrations,
especially in diabetic, cirrhotic, and elderly patients.

Contra-indications. Amiloride should not be given in
conjunction with potassium supplements or other
potassium conserving drugs, or to patients with hyperkalaemia, anuria, acute renal failure, severe renal
disease, or diabetic nephropathy. It should not be given
to patients with blood urea concentrations over 60 milligrams per 100 millilitres (equivalent to 10 millimoles per
litre) or serum creatinine concentrations over 1.5 milligrams per 100 millilitres (equivalent to 0.13 millimoles
per litre), unless the concentrations of electrolytes and
urea in the blood can be monitored. Amiloride should
not be given during pregnancy or to children.

Preparations

AMILORIDE TABLETS: available as tablets containing 5 mg
of amiloride hydrochloride.
Containers and *Storage:* see the entry on Tablets for
general information on containers and storage. Containers should be airtight and light resistant. The tablets
should be stored in a cool place.
Advice for patients: daily doses should preferably be
taken in the morning. Treatment should not be discontinued without the advice of the prescriber.

OTHER PREPARATIONS available include TABLETS containing amiloride hydrochloride 5 mg with hydrochlorothiazide 50 mg.

Aminoacetic Acid

see GLYCINE

Aminobenzoic Acid

4-Aminobenzoic acid

$C_7H_7NO_2 = 137.1$

OTHER NAMES: *p*-Aminobenzoic Acid; Para-aminoben-
zoic Acid

*A standard is given in the British Pharmaceutical
Codex 1973*

Description. Odourless, white or slightly yellow crystals
or crystalline powder, gradually darkening on exposure
to air and light.

Solubility. Soluble, at 20°, in 200 parts of water and
in 8 parts of alcohol; soluble in solutions of alkali
hydroxides and carbonates.

Dissociation constants. pK_a 2.4, 4.9 (25°).

Incompatibility. It is incompatible with ferric salts and oxidising agents.

Storage. It should be stored in airtight containers, protected from light.

Identification. TESTS. 1. Dissolve 100 mg in 2 ml of *dilute hydrochloric acid* with the aid of heat if necessary, cool in ice, add 4 ml of a 1% solution of sodium nitrite in water and pour the mixture into 2 ml of *2-naphthol solution* containing 1 g of sodium acetate; a bright red precipitate is produced.
2. Dissolve about 50 mg in a mixture of 1 ml of *dilute sodium hydroxide solution* and 1 ml of water and add in the order named, 0.5 ml of *potassium iodide solution*, 0.5 ml of *dilute hydrochloric acid* and 0.5 ml of *sodium hypochlorite solution*; a brown precipitate is produced.

MELTING-POINT. About 187°.

ULTRAVIOLET ABSORPTION. In 0.1N sodium hydroxide, maximum at 265 nm (E1%, 1cm = 1060); in alcohol (95%), maximum at 280 nm (E1%, 1cm = 960).

Actions and uses. Aminobenzoic acid has sunscreening properties and is used as an ingredient in topical preparations for the prevention of sunburn.

Preparation

AMINOBENZOIC ACID LOTION:

Aminobenzoic acid	..	..	..	..		50 g
Glycerol	..	..	..	..	..	200 ml
Alcohol (95%)	..	..	..	..	..	600 ml
Purified water, freshly boiled and cooled	..	..	..	..		to 1000 ml

In making this preparation, the alcohol (95%) may be replaced by industrial methylated spirit, provided that the law and the statutory regulations governing the use of industrial spirit are observed.
A standard for this lotion is given in the British Pharmaceutical Codex 1973
Containers: see the entry on Lotions for general information on containers.
Labelling: see the entry on Lotions for general information on labelling. A caution should be given on the label that the lotion is inflammable and may stain clothing. In addition, the label should state that the preparation discolours slightly on storage.
Storage: it should be protected from light.
Advice for patients: the undiluted lotion should be applied to the skin without friction and allowed to dry every 2 hours and immediately after bathing. See also under Labelling.

Aminocaproic Acid

6-Aminohexanoic acid

$$NH_2 \cdot [CH_2]_5 \cdot COOH$$

$C_6H_{13}NO_2 = 131.2$

OTHER NAMES: EACA; *Epsikapron®*; Epsilon Aminocaproic Acid

A standard is given in the British Pharmacopoeia 1973

Description. Odourless colourless crystals or white crystalline powder, with a bitter taste.

Solubility. Soluble, at 20°, in 1.5 parts of water.

Alkalinity. A 20% solution has a pH of 7.5 to 8.

Dissociation constants. pK_a 4.4, 10.8 (25°).

Incompatibility. Aminocaproic acid solutions may be mixed with sodium chloride injection, dextrose injection (5%), and Ringer's solution. They should not be mixed with solutions containing fructose (laevulose) or with blood preparations.

Sterilisation. Solutions for injection are sterilised by filtration.

Storage. It should be stored in airtight containers.

Identification. MELTING-POINT. About 204°, with decomposition.

INFRA-RED ABSORPTION. Major peaks at 1099, 1316, 1370, 1449, 1538, and 1613 cm^{-1} (see Appendix 2b: Infrared Spectra).

Determination in body fluids. GAS CHROMATOGRAPHY. In serum—T. R. Keucher *et al.*, *Clin. Chem.*, 1976, **22**, 806.

Metabolism. ABSORPTION. Readily absorbed after oral administration.

BLOOD CONCENTRATION. Peak plasma concentrations are attained within 2 hours following oral administration.

HALF-LIFE. Plasma half-life, about 2 hours.

DISTRIBUTION. Widely distributed throughout body fluids.

EXCRETION. About 80% of a dose is excreted in the urine in 12 hours.

Actions and uses. Aminocaproic acid inhibits plasminogen activation in blood and urine and so reduces fibrinolysis and increases the stability of clots when they have been formed. As there are potent plasminogen activators in urine, saliva, and endometrial secretions, aminocaproic acid may be expected to reduce haemorrhage after dental extraction and urinary surgery and in menorrhagia; it may also stabilise internal thrombi once they have been formed.
Aminocaproic acid should only be used where there is free haemorrhage on a mucous surface or as an antagonist to streptokinase. It may be used in haemophilia to reduce bleeding after tooth extraction by preventing lysis of the first formed clot, so avoiding exhaustion of depleted coagulation factors. For this purpose the sockets are rinsed with a sterile 10% solution and plugs moistened with the solution are inserted in the sockets.
Aminocaproic acid may also be useful in limiting the action of streptokinase. It has not been found of established benefit in menorrhagia and most other conditions in which it might be expected to be of value; spontaneous bleeding in haemophilia is not significantly reduced and organising clots may persist in joints and serous cavities. It apparently increases clot colic and retention when the bleeding is in the urinary tract.
Aminocaproic acid is administered by mouth; it may also be administered by slow intravenous injection or by intravenous infusion of a solution diluted with sodium chloride injection or with dextrose injection (5%).
Aminocaproic acid may be given by mouth or by slow intravenous injection in a dose of 100 milligrams per kilogram body-weight 5 times a day. In menorrhagia, 3 grams is given by mouth 4 to 6 times daily for 3 to 6 days. A 0.5% solution is used as a bladder irrigation.

Undesirable effects. Nausea, diarrhoea, and dizziness may occur, but these disappear when the dose is reduced.

Contra-indications. Aminocaproic acid should not be given when there is renal impairment, which increases the risk of overdosage, or to patients taking contraceptive steroids, as this may increase the risk of blood-clot formation.

Preparations

AMINOCAPROIC ACID EFFERVESCENT POWDER: consists of aminocaproic acid in a suitable effervescent basis. Available as sachets containing 3 g of aminocaproic acid with 3 g of basis.
Containers and *Storage:* see the entry on Powders for general information on containers and storage. Containers should be airtight.
Labelling: the label on the container should give the directions for taking the powder.
Advice for patients: the powder should be taken dissolved in water.

AMINOCAPROIC ACID ELIXIR (*Syn.* Aminocaproic Acid Mixture): a solution of aminocaproic acid in a suitable flavoured vehicle. Available as a solution containing 300 mg per ml.
Containers and *Labelling:* see the entry on Elixirs for general information on containers and labelling.

AMINOCAPROIC ACID INJECTION: a sterile solution of aminocaproic acid in water for injections. The acidity of the solution is adjusted to pH 6.5 to 7.5 by the addition of dilute hydrochloric acid. It is sterilised by filtration.
A standard for this injection is given in the British Pharmacopoeia 1973
Containers and *Labelling:* see the entry on Injections for general information on containers and labelling.

Aminophylline

It consists of 78 to 84% of theophylline, about 13% of ethylenediamine, and a variable amount of water. Its composition is approximately represented by the formula $(C_7H_8N_4O_2)_2, C_2H_4(NH_2)_2, 2H_2O$.

OTHER NAMES: *Cardophylin®*; *Phyldrox®*; *Phyllocontin®*; Theophylline and Ethylenediamine; Theophyllinum et Ethylenediaminum
Theodrox® (with dried aluminium hydroxide gel)

A standard is given in the European Pharmacopoeia Vol. II

Description. A white or slightly yellowish powder or granules with a slightly ammoniacal odour and a bitter taste.

Solubility. Soluble, at 25°, in 5 parts of water, the solution usually becoming turbid on standing; practically insoluble in dehydrated alcohol and in ether.
In order to effect complete solution in water, the addition of ethylenediamine or ammonia solution may be necessary.

Stability. It absorbs carbon dioxide from the air with liberation of theophylline. Aqueous solutions absorb carbon dioxide from the air with precipitation of theophylline.

Incompatibility. It is incompatible with acids; with lactose and other sugars, a yellow or brown colour develops on standing; in the presence of copper, solutions develop a blue colour.

Sterilisation. Solutions for injection are sterilised by heating in an autoclave or by filtration, exposure to carbon dioxide and contact with metals being avoided throughout.

Storage. It should be stored in small, well-filled, airtight containers, protected from light.

Identification. TESTS. 1. General test for xanthines: mix a few mg with 5 drops of *strong hydrogen peroxide solution* and 5 drops of *dilute hydrochloric acid* and heat to dryness; a yellow-red residue is obtained. Add 1 drop of *dilute ammonia solution;* the colour changes to red-violet.
2. Dissolve about 1 g in 10 ml of water, add 2 ml of *dilute hydrochloric acid* dropwise and with shaking, filter, and reserve the filtrate; the residue, after washing with water and drying at 105° melts at about 272°.
To the reserved filtrate add 0.2 ml of benzoyl chloride, make alkaline with *dilute sodium hydroxide solution,* shake vigorously, filter, wash the filter with 10 ml of water, and dissolve the residue in 5 ml of hot alcohol, add 5 ml of water and filter; the residue, after washing with water and drying at 105°, melts at about 249°.

ULTRAVIOLET ABSORPTION. In 0.1N hydrochloric acid, maximum at 272 nm (E1%, 1cm = 454).

INFRA-RED ABSORPTION. Major peaks at 741, 1525, 1566, 1625, 1640, and 1667 cm^{-1} (see Appendix 2a: Infra-red Spectra).

THIN-LAYER CHROMATOGRAPHY. See under Thin-layer Chromatography, System 12.

Metabolism (see also the entry on Theophylline). ABSORPTION. More rapidly absorbed than theophylline but its absorption may be delayed by food after oral administration; aminophylline is converted by the gastric juice to theophylline and ethylenediamine; after rectal administration it is erratically absorbed, the absorption being influenced by the type of suppository basis used in the formulation.

BLOOD CONCENTRATION. After an oral dose of 300 mg every 6 hours, serum concentrations of theophylline of 6 to 23 μg/ml are obtained after 1½ to 2 days; after a single oral dose of 450 mg, peak plasma concentrations of about 7 μg/ml are obtained within 1 to 2 hours; after a single rectal dose of 300 mg of aminophylline in solution, serum concentrations of about 5 μg/ml are obtained during the period 1 to 4 hours following administration.

HALF-LIFE. After an intravenous dose of aminophylline, the serum half-life of theophylline is 3 to 9 hours.

DISTRIBUTION. Crosses the placenta.

METABOLIC REACTIONS. Aminophylline is rapidly converted to theophylline which is further metabolised by demethylation and oxidation.

FURTHER INFORMATION. Importance of individual aminophylline elimination rates in the maintenance of therapeutic levels—J. W. Jenne *et al., J. Lab. clin. Med.,* 1970, **76,** 1027; transplacental aminophylline toxicity—T. F.Yeh and R. S. Pilder, *Lancet,* i/1977, 910.

Actions and uses. Aminophylline has actions and uses similar to those described under Theophylline but it is more soluble. It is used in the treatment of bronchial asthma. Its therapeutic action is related to relaxation of bronchial smooth muscle, but it has also been shown to inhibit the release of histamine from mast cells. It may also be used in cases of bronchitis where bronchospasm is present and in the emergency treatment of left heart failure. It dilates the venous circulation and has diuretic and inotropic effects.
Aminophylline is effective when given in doses of 250 to 500 milligrams by slow intravenous injection or in doses of 360 milligrams once or twice daily by rectum

in suppositories. Children up to 1 year may be given 12.5 to 25 milligrams, 1 to 5 years 50 to 100 milligrams, and 6 to 12 years 100 to 200 milligrams once or twice daily by rectum in suppositories.

Intravenous injections should be given over a period of at least 10 to 15 minutes as aminophylline has dangerous central nervous and cardiovascular side-effects which include agitation, convulsions, arrhythmias, and hypotension.

Aminophylline may be given by mouth in doses of 100 to 300 milligrams but it is a gastric irritant and causes nausea and vomiting; choline theophyllinate is therefore preferred.

Aminophylline suppositories are often used at bedtime to abort nocturnal attacks of asthma or left ventricular failure.

Preparations

AMINOPHYLLINE INJECTION (*Syn.* Theophylline and Ethylenediamine Injection): a sterile solution of aminophylline in water for injections free from carbon dioxide. It may be prepared by dissolving theophylline in a solution of ethylenediamine hydrate in water for injections free from carbon dioxide, 870 mg of theophylline being used for each g of aminophylline required. Ethylenediamine hydrate additional to that necessary for the formation of aminophylline may be added but the total amount of ethylenediamine, $C_2H_4(NH_2)_2$, should not exceed 251 mg for each g of anhydrous theophylline, $C_7H_8N_4O_2$, present.

It is sterilised by heating in an autoclave or by filtration. Exposure to carbon dioxide and contact with metals must be avoided throughout.

Available in 10-ml ampoules containing 25 mg of aminophylline per ml and in 2-ml ampoules containing 250 mg per ml.

A standard for this injection is given in the British Pharmacopoeia 1973

Containers and *Labelling:* see the entry on Injections for general information on containers and labelling.

Storage: it should be protected from light.

AMINOPHYLLINE SUPPOSITORIES (*Syn.* Theophylline and Ethylenediamine Suppositories): prepared as described in the entry on Suppositories by incorporating aminophylline in theobroma oil or other suitable basis. Available as suppositories containing 50, 100, 150, and 360 mg of aminophylline.

A standard for these suppositories is given in the British Pharmacopoeia 1973

Containers and *Storage:* see the entry on Suppositories for general information on containers and storage. Containers should be light resistant.

Labelling: the label on the container should state the date after which the suppositories are not intended to be used and the conditions under which they should be stored.

Advice for patients: see the entry on Suppositories for general information on the use of suppositories.

AMINOPHYLLINE TABLETS (*Syn.* Theophylline and Ethylenediamine Tablets): available as tablets containing 100 mg of aminophylline.

A standard for these tablets is given in the British Pharmacopoeia 1973

Containers and *Storage:* see the entry on Tablets for general information on containers and storage. Containers should be airtight and light resistant.

Advice for patients: the tablets should preferably be taken after meals.

OTHER PREPARATIONS available include TABLETS containing aminophylline 100 and 225 mg in a slow-release formulation and tablets containing aminophylline 195 mg with dried aluminium hydroxide gel 260 mg.

Amitriptyline Embonate

3-(10,11-Dihydro-5*H*-dibenzo[*a,d*]cyclohepten-5-ylidene)propyl-*NN*-dimethylammonium 4,4'-methylenebis(3-hydroxynaphthalene-2-carboxylate)

$C_{63}H_{62}N_2O_6 = 943.2$

OTHER NAME: *Tryptizol*®

A standard is given in the British Pharmaceutical Codex 1973

Description. A pale yellow to brownish-yellow odourless powder.

Solubility. Practically insoluble in water; soluble, at 20°, in 8 parts of chloroform and in 6 parts of acetone; very slightly soluble in alcohol.

Moisture content. Not more than 5%, determined by Fischer titration.

Storage. It should be protected from light.

Identification. ULTRAVIOLET ABSORPTION. In a solution prepared by dissolving 20 mg in 20 ml of dichloromethane, adding 20 ml of 0.5N sodium hydroxide, shaking for 2 minutes, centrifuging for 2 minutes, and then diluting 5 ml of the upper aqueous layer to 100 ml with 0.1N sodium hydroxide, maxima at 236 nm (E1%, 1cm = 1940), 277 nm (E1%, 1cm = 180), 288 nm (E1%, 1cm = 200), and 363 nm (E1%, 1cm = 134).

Determination in body fluids; Metabolism. See under Amitriptyline Hydrochloride.

Actions and uses. Amitriptyline embonate has the actions of amitriptyline, as described under Amitriptyline Hydrochloride. Because it is insoluble in water it is almost tasteless and is therefore preferred to the hydrochloride for preparing liquid medicines for oral administration; 1.5 grams of amitriptyline embonate is approximately equivalent to 1 gram of amitriptyline hydrochloride.

Undesirable effects; Precautions and contra-indications; Drug interactions. As for Amitriptyline Hydrochloride.

Preparation

AMITRIPTYLINE MIXTURE (*Syn.* Amitriptyline Embonate Mixture; Amitriptyline Syrup): a suspension of amitriptyline embonate in a suitable coloured flavoured vehicle. When a dose less than or not a multiple of 5 ml is prescribed, the mixture may be diluted, as described in the entry on Mixtures, with syrup. The diluted mixture must be freshly prepared. Available as a suspension containing amitriptyline embonate equivalent to 10 mg of amitriptyline in 5 ml.

A standard for this mixture is given in the British Pharmaceutical Codex 1973

Containers and *Labelling:* see the entry on Mixtures for general information on containers and labelling.

Advice for patients: daily doses should preferably be taken at bedtime. When initiating treatment there may be a time lag of up to 2 weeks before a full therapeutic response is obtained. The mixture may cause drowsiness; persons affected should not drive or operate machinery. Alcohol should be avoided. The mixture may colour the urine blue-green.

Amitriptyline Hydrochloride

3-(10,11-Dihydro-5*H*-dibenzo[*a,d*]cyclohepten-5-yl-idene)propyl-*NN*-dimethylammonium chloride

$C_{20}H_{24}ClN = 313.9$

OTHER NAMES: *Amizol®*; *Domical®*; *Lentizol®*; *Saroten®*; *Tryptizol®*
Limbitrol® (with chlordiazepoxide); *Triptafen®* (with perphenazine)

A standard is given in the British Pharmacopoeia 1973

Description. Odourless colourless crystals or white powder, with a bitter and burning taste followed by a sensation of numbness.

Solubility. Soluble, at 20°, in 1 part of water, in 1.5 parts of alcohol, in 1.2 parts of chloroform, and in 1 part of methyl alcohol; practically insoluble in ether.

Dissociation constant. pK_a 9.4.

Acidity. A 1% solution has a pH of 4.5 to 6.0.

Stability. Oxidation of amitriptyline hydrochloride in aqueous solutions is catalysed by metal-ion contaminants. Disodium edetate is a suitable stabiliser.

FURTHER INFORMATION. Stabilisation of aqueous solutions—R. P. Enever *et al., J. pharm. Sci.*, 1977, **66**, 1087.

Sterilisation. Solutions for injection are sterilised by filtration.

Storage. It should be stored in airtight containers, protected from light.

Identification. TEST. Dissolve about 50 mg in 3 ml of water and add 1 drop of a 2.5% solution of quinhydrone in methyl alcohol; no red colour is produced within 15 minutes (distinction from nortriptyline).

MELTING-POINT. About 197°.

ULTRAVIOLET ABSORPTION. In 0.1N hydrochloric acid, maximum at 241 nm (E1%, 1cm = 453); in alcohol (95%), maximum at 240 nm (E1%, 1cm = 474).

INFRA-RED ABSORPTION. Major peaks at 746, 756, 770, 969, 1441, and 1487 cm⁻¹ (see Appendix 2a: Infra-red Spectra).

Determination in body fluids. ULTRAVIOLET SPECTROPHOTOMETRY. In blood or urine: amitriptyline and nortriptyline—H. E. Hamilton *et al., Analyt. Chem.*, 1975, **47**, 1139. In urine: *N*-oxide metabolite, thin-layer chromatographic separation—G. Santagostino *et al., J. pharm. Sci.*, 1974, **63**, 1690.

GAS CHROMATOGRAPHY. In plasma: amitriptyline and nortriptyline: the 10-hydroxy- and 10,11-dihydroxy-metabolites are stated not to interfere—H. B. Hucker, *J. pharm. Sci.*, 1974, **63**, 296. In serum—amitriptyline and nortriptyline—A. Jørgensen, *Acta pharmac. toxic.*, 1975, **36**, 79; J. E. Wallace *et al., Analyt. Chem.*, 1975, **47**, 1516.

HIGH PRESSURE LIQUID CHROMATOGRAPHY. In plasma—R. R. Brodie *et al., J. Chromat.*, 1977, **143**, 535.

THIN-LAYER CHROMATOGRAPHY. In plasma: amitriptyline and nortriptyline—D. B. Faber, *et al., J. Chromat.*, 1974, **100**, 55.

Metabolism. ABSORPTION. Readily absorbed after oral administration.

BLOOD CONCENTRATION. After an oral dose of 75 mg daily for 6 days, blood concentrations of 40 to 90 ng/ml and about 40 ng/ml for amitriptyline and nortriptyline respectively are attained 12 hours after the last dose; after an oral dose of 100 mg of a sustained release preparation daily, concentrations of 25 to 70 ng/ml are attained for amitriptyline and 60 to 80 ng/ml for nortriptyline; after an oral dose of 75 mg in pelletised form, peak concentrations of 93 ng/ml and 53 ng/ml are attained for amitriptyline and nortriptyline respectively in 6 hours; after an intravenous dose of 25 mg, blood concentrations of about 30 ng/ml are obtained for total amitriptyline and metabolites.

HALF-LIFE. The serum half-life is in the range 9 to 76 hours.

DISTRIBUTION. Rapidly taken up by the tissues; may be secreted in milk; volume of distribution, 450 to 850 litres; *protein binding*, 97% bound to plasma proteins but phenytoin may reduce the extent of binding by displacement.

METABOLIC REACTIONS. Demethylation, hydroxylation, and conjugation with glucuronic acid together with some *N*-oxide formation; the metabolites formed include nortriptyline, didesmethylamitriptyline, their conjugates and their 10-hydroxy derivatives, and amitriptyline *N*-oxide; the formation of hydroxylamines has been shown *in vitro*.

EXCRETION. About 90% of an intravenous dose is excreted in the urine in 1 week, 30 to 40% being excreted in the first 24 hours; of the dose, 1 to 5% is excreted unchanged, 1% is excreted as the *N*-oxide, 27% is excreted as 10-hydroxyamitriptyline mainly as the glucuronide, 41% is excreted as 10-hydroxynortriptyline either free or as the glucuronide, and 6% is excreted as either nortriptyline or desmethylnortriptyline; about 8% of a dose is excreted in the faeces unchanged; no metabolites are detectable in the faeces.

FURTHER INFORMATION. Metabolic fate of amitriptyline in the rat and in man—E. von Eschenhof and J. Rieder, *Arzneimittel-Forsch.*, 1969, **19**, 957; metabolism of amitriptyline—A. H. Beckett and S. Al-Sarraj, *J. Pharm. Pharmac.*, 1973, **25**, 335; urinary excretion of amitriptyline *N*-oxide—G. Santagostino *et al., J. pharm. Sci.*, 1974, **63**, 1690; urinary metabolites of amitriptyline in the dog—H. B. Hucker *et al., Drug Met. Disp.*, 1977, **5**, 132; pharmacokinetics of amitriptyline in man—A. Jørgensen and V. Hansen, *Eur. J. clin. Pharmac.*, 1976, **10**, 337; the biological half-life of amitriptyline—A. Jørgensen and P. Staehr, *J. Pharm. Pharmac.*, 1976, **28**, 62; plasma levels for a pelletised form of amitriptyline—H. B. Hucker *et al., J. clin. Pharmac.*, 1975, **15**, 168.

Actions and uses. Amitriptyline is a tricyclic antidepressant which does not inhibit monoamine oxidase. Its action is believed to be related to its ability to block the re-uptake of released monoamines into pre-synaptic nerve endings. It has anticholinergic actions and sedative properties. It is used to treat patients with depressive illnesses of all but the most severe intensity. It is also effective in reducing the incidence of bed-wetting in some children.

The initial oral daily dosage in adults is usually 75 milligrams either in divided doses or as one dose at night. Depending on the response of the patient, the dosage can be raised to a total of 150 milligrams daily and in some apparently unresponsive cases to 225 milligrams daily or more. A satisfactory response should be evident within 7 to 14 days of attaining the required dose level. When the depressive mood has lifted, dosage can be reduced to 50 to 100 milligrams daily as maintenance therapy and then carefully withdrawn over the next few months. Dosage should be assessed with caution in the elderly. Amitriptyline may be used to control nocturnal enuresis in children but the bed-wetting usually returns when the drug is discontinued. The oral dose for children 6 to 10 years of age is 10 to 20 milligrams daily and for children over 10 years 25 to 50 milligrams daily.

Amitriptyline hydrochloride may also be administered by intramuscular or intravenous injection but oral therapy should be substituted as soon as possible. The usual adult dose is 20 to 30 milligrams 4 times a day by intramuscular or intravenous injection.

Undesirable effects. The most frequently occurring undesirable effects are dryness of the mouth, constipation, tachycardia, and a tendency to perspire. Moderate hypotensive effects and occasional blurring of vision may occur. In addition gastro-intestinal disturbances may occur and a fine tremor is often apparent.

Precautions and contra-indications. Amitriptyline may impair alertness and activities such as driving a car or operating dangerous machinery should then be avoided. Amitriptyline increases sensitivity to alcohol and patients should be warned of this danger. Amitriptyline should be used with caution in patients with cardiac failure, especially when there is evidence of rhythm disturbance, recent myocardial infarction, or epilepsy, and in the presence of liver disease. Because of its anticholinergic activity amitriptyline should be avoided in patients with glaucoma or in those who might develop urinary retention.

Drug interactions. Extreme caution should be exercised when giving amitriptyline hydrochloride to patients who are being treated with a monoamine-oxidase inhibitor, such as isocarboxazid, nialamide, phenelzine, or tranylcypromine, or who have been so treated within the previous 2 weeks.

Like other tricyclic antidepressants it may cause the effects of bethanidine, debrisoquine, guanethidine, and possibly other antihypertensive agents to be attenuated and may give rise to hypertension in patients given local anaesthetics containing adrenaline or noradrenaline.

Preparations

AMITRIPTYLINE INJECTION: a sterile solution of amitriptyline hydrochloride in water for injections. It may contain anhydrous dextrose and a suitable buffering agent. It is sterilised by filtration. Available in 10-ml vials containing 10 mg of amitriptyline hydrochloride per ml. *A standard for this injection is given in the British Pharmacopoeia 1973*

Containers and *Labelling:* see the entry on Injections for general information on containers and labelling.

AMITRIPTYLINE TABLETS: available as tablets containing 10, 25, and 50 mg of amitriptyline hydrochloride; they may be film coated or sugar coated; the coat may be coloured.

A standard for these tablets is given in the British Pharmacopoeia 1973

Containers and *Storage:* see the entry on Tablets for general information on containers and storage. Containers should be airtight.

Advice for patients: daily doses should preferably be taken at bedtime. When initiating treatment there may be a time-lag of up to 2 weeks before a full therapeutic response is obtained. The tablets may cause drowsiness; persons affected should not drive or operate machinery. Alcohol should be avoided. The tablets may colour the urine blue-green.

OTHER PREPARATIONS available include CAPSULES containing amitriptyline hydrochloride 25, 50, and 75 mg in a slow-release formulation, capsules containing amitriptyline hydrochloride equivalent to 12.5 mg of amitriptyline with chlordiazepoxide 5 mg, capsules containing amitriptyline hydrochloride equivalent to 25 mg of amitriptyline (base) with chlordiazepoxide 10 mg; TABLETS containing amitriptyline hydrochloride 10 mg with perphenazine 2 mg, tablets containing amitriptyline hydrochloride 25 mg with perphenazine 2 mg, and tablets containing amitriptyline hydrochloride 25 mg with perphenazine 4 mg.

Ammonia Solution, Strong

An aqueous solution of ammonia, NH_3, which is usually prepared by synthesis from atmospheric nitrogen or may be obtained from the ammoniacal liquors from gas works by distillation with slaked lime. It contains 27 to 30% w/w of NH_3.

OTHER NAME: Liquor Ammoniae Fortis

A standard is given in the British Pharmaceutical Codex 1973

Description. A clear colourless liquid with a strongly pungent and characteristic odour.

Solubility. Miscible with water.

Weight per ml. At 20°, 0.892 to 0.901 g.

Stability. It may be less stable at tropical temperatures (about 30°) and potentially dangerous to handle. A solution containing 27.5% w/w of NH_3 is stated to be safe, but should preferably be diluted to 10% before storage and use at tropical temperatures.

FURTHER INFORMATION. Data concerning the storage and use of ammonia solution at tropical temperatures —A. B. Elliott and P. L. K. Siong, *Malay. pharm. J.*, 1955, **4**, 269.

Incompatibility. It is incompatible with iodine, hypochlorites, salts of heavy metals, notably mercuric chloride and silver salts, alkaloidal salts, and tannins.

Storage. It should be stored in airtight containers, in a cool place.

Actions and uses. Ammonia, when inhaled, irritates the mucosa of the upper respiratory tract and reflexly, through the medulla, causes stimulation of respiration, acceleration of the heart, and rise of blood-pressure; the rationale of the use of smelling-salts depends upon these effects. As a restorative in cases of fainting and collapse it is usually administered as aromatic ammonia spirit.

Applied externally, solutions of ammonia have rubefacient and counter-irritant actions and have been used as ingredients of liniments. Strong ammonia solution is used in the preparation of strong ammonium acetate solution, which is used as a mild expectorant and diuretic.

Precautions. Great care should be taken in handling strong solutions of ammonia, as the vapour may inflame the respiratory tract and cause tracheitis, bronchitis, and pneumonia. Spasm of the glottis with resulting asphyxia may occur. Ammonia burns of the eye should be treated by irrigation with water, followed by drops of liquid paraffin.

Ammonia burns have resulted from treating insect bites and stings with the strong solution and even with the dilute solution, especially if a dressing is subsequently applied.

Poisoning. Vinegar, or any suitable mineral acid well diluted, should be given, followed by demulcent drinks of olive oil. If there is any delay in obtaining a suitable acid large quantities of water or milk should be given. A stomach tube or emetics should not be used. Morphine may be necessary for the relief of pain and the patient should be treated for shock with infusions of plasma or suitable electrolytes if necessary. Tracheotomy may be needed for oedema of the larynx.

Preparations

AROMATIC AMMONIA SOLUTION (*Syn.* Sal Volatile Solution):

Ammonium bicarbonate	25.0 g
Strong ammonia solution	67.5 ml
Nutmeg oil	0.3 ml
Lemon oil	0.5 ml
Alcohol (90%)	37.5 ml
Purified water, freshly boiled and cooled	to 1000.0 ml

Dissolve the ammonium bicarbonate in 800 ml of the water and add the lemon oil and the nutmeg oil previously dissolved in the alcohol, add the strong ammonia solution, and sufficient water to produce the required volume. Add 25 g of sterilised purified talc, shake, allow to stand for a few hours, shaking occasionally, and filter.

A standard for this solution is given in the British Pharmaceutical Codex 1973

Storage: it should be stored in airtight containers, in a cool place.

Dose: 1 to 5 millilitres, diluted with water.

AROMATIC AMMONIA SPIRIT (*Syn.* Spirit of Sal Volatile):

Ammonium bicarbonate	25.0 g
Strong ammonia solution	67.5 ml
Nutmeg oil	3.0 ml
Lemon oil	5.0 ml
Alcohol (90%)	750.0 ml
Purified water, freshly boiled and cooled	to 1000.0 ml

Distil the lemon oil, the nutmeg oil, the alcohol, and 375 ml of the water, reserving the first 875 ml. Distil a further 55 ml, add the ammonium bicarbonate and the strong ammonia solution, and heat on a water-bath to 60° in a sealed bottle of appropriate capacity, shaking occasionally, until solution is complete; cool; filter through cotton wool, mix the filtrate with the reserved portion of the distillate, add sufficient of the water to produce the required volume, and mix.

A standard for this spirit is given in the British Pharmaceutical Codex 1973

Storage: it should be stored in well-filled airtight containers, in a cool place.

Dose: 1 to 5 millilitres, diluted with water.

DILUTE AMMONIA SOLUTION:

Strong ammonia solution	375 ml
Purified water, freshly boiled and cooled	to 1000 ml

When Ammonia Solution or Liquor Ammoniae is prescribed or demanded, Dilute Ammonia Solution is dispensed or supplied.

A standard for this solution is given in the British Pharmaceutical Codex 1973

Storage: it should be stored in airtight containers, in a cool place.

STRONG AMMONIUM ACETATE SOLUTION: may be prepared as follows:

Ammonium bicarbonate	470 g
Glacial acetic acid	453 g
Strong ammonia solution .. a sufficient quantity
Purified water, freshly boiled and cooled	to 1000 ml

Dissolve the ammonium bicarbonate by adding gradually to the glacial acetic acid diluted with 350 ml of the water and add the strong ammonia solution in a quantity such that 1 drop of the resulting solution diluted with 10 drops of purified water gives a full blue colour with 1 drop of *bromothymol blue solution* and a full yellow colour with 1 drop of *thymol blue solution*; about 100 ml of the strong ammonia solution is required. Add sufficient of the water to produce the required volume.

When Ammonium Acetate Solution, Liquor Ammonii Acetatis, Dilute Ammonium Acetate Solution, or Liquor Ammonii Acetatis Dilutus is prescribed or demanded, Strong Ammonium Acetate Solution diluted to 8 times its volume with freshly boiled and cooled purified water is supplied.

A standard for this solution is given in the British Pharmaceutical Codex 1973

Storage: It should be stored in lead-free glass bottles.

Dose: 1 to 5 millilitres.

Ammonium Bicarbonate

$NH_4HCO_3 = 79.06$

OTHER NAME: Ammon. Bicarb.

When Ammonium Carbonate or Ammonii Carbonas is prescribed or demanded, Ammonium Bicarbonate is dispensed or supplied.

A standard is given in the British Pharmaceutical Codex 1973

Description. Slightly hygroscopic white crystals, white fine crystalline powder, or colourless glassy solid with a slightly ammoniacal odour.

Solubility. Soluble, at 20°, in 5 parts of water; practically insoluble in alcohol.

Stability. It volatilises rapidly at 60°, with dissociation into ammonia, carbon dioxide, and water; volatilisation takes place slowly at ordinary temperatures if the substance is slightly moist.

Incompatibility. It is incompatible with acids, iron salts, and salts of alkaline earths.

Storage. It should be stored in airtight containers, in a cool place.

Actions and uses. Ammonium bicarbonate is irritant to mucous membranes and is used in doses of 300 to 600 milligrams as a reflex expectorant. Larger doses cause nausea and vomiting.

Preparations

AMMONIA AND IPECACUANHA MIXTURE (*Syn.* Mistura Expectorans):

Ammonium bicarbonate ..	..	..	..	20 g
Ipecacuanha tincture	..	..	..	30 ml
Concentrated anise water	..	..	..	5 ml
Concentrated camphor water	..	..	..	10 ml
Liquorice liquid extract ..	..	..	..	50 ml
Chloroform water, double-strength	..	..	500 ml
Water for preparations ..	..	..	to 1000 ml

It should be recently prepared.
A standard for this mixture is given in the British Pharmaceutical Codex 1973
Containers and *Labelling:* see the entry on Mixtures for general information on containers and labelling.
Advice for patients: the mixture should not be used for longer than a few days without medical advice.
Dose: 10 to 20 millilitres.

OTHER PREPARATIONS. Ammonium bicarbonate is an ingredient of aromatic ammonia solution, aromatic ammonia spirit, strong ammonium acetate solution, ammonium chloride and morphine mixture, paediatric ipecacuanha and ammonia mixture, and ammoniated rhubarb and soda mixture.

Ammonium Chloride

$NH_4Cl = 53.49$

OTHER NAMES: Ammon. Chlor.; Ammonii Chloridum

A standard is given in the European Pharmacopoeia Vol. I

Description. Odourless colourless crystals or white crystalline powder; taste saline and cooling. On heating it sublimes without melting.

Solubility. Soluble, at 20°, in 2.7 parts of water and in 100 parts of alcohol.

Moisture content. Not more than 1%, determined by drying at 105°.

Incompatibility. It is incompatible with alkalis, carbonates of alkaline earths, and lead and silver salts.

Sterilisation. Solutions are sterilised by heating in an autoclave or by filtration.

Storage. It should be stored in airtight containers.

Actions and uses. Ammonium chloride is rapidly absorbed from the gastro-intestinal tract. The ammonium ion is converted into urea in the liver; the anion thus liberated into the blood stream and extracellular fluids causes a metabolic acidosis and decreases the pH of the urine; this is followed by transient diuresis.
A mild acidosis is produced by the administration of ammonium chloride by mouth in a single dose of 2 grams. This is used to increase the diuretic effect of mercurial diuretics in dosage of up to 6 grams daily in divided doses.
Ammonium chloride is an ingredient of expectorant cough mixtures although it is doubtful whether its irritant

action on the gastric mucous membrane contributes to any expectorant action. The usual expectorant dose for an adult is 0.3 to 1 gram and the dose for children is one quarter to three quarters of the adult dose.
Ammonium chloride is used in the treatment of urinary infections when a low pH is required and to aid the excretion of basic drugs such as amphetamine, in cases of overdosage. It also aids the elimination of lead in lead poisoning. It is occasionally used by intravenous infusion as a one-sixth molar solution (approximately 0.89%) in the treatment of alkalosis.
Large doses should be given in tablets, coated to prevent disintegration in the stomach. Liquorice liquid extract may be used to disguise its taste in liquid medicines.

Undesirable effects. Large doses of ammonium chloride may cause nausea, vomiting, thirst, headache, hyperventilation, progressive drowsiness, mental confusion, and hyperchloraemic acidosis. It is contraindicated in the presence of renal or hepatic disease.

Poisoning. Acidosis and electrolyte loss should be corrected by sodium bicarbonate or sodium lactate given intravenously, and hypokalaemia prevented with potassium salts given by mouth.

Preparations

AMMONIUM CHLORIDE AND MORPHINE MIXTURE (*Syn.* Mistura Tussi Sedativa):

Ammonium chloride	..	..	..	30 g
Chloroform and morphine tincture	..	..	30 ml
Ammonium bicarbonate ..	..	..	..	20 g
Liquorice liquid extract ..	..	..	..	50 ml
Water for preparations ..	..	..	to 1000 ml

It should be recently prepared.
A standard for this mixture is given in the British Pharmaceutical Codex 1973
Containers and *Labelling:* see the entry on Mixtures for general information on containers and labelling.
Advice for patients: the mixture should not be used for longer than a few days without medical advice.
Dose: 10 to 20 millilitres.

AMMONIUM CHLORIDE MIXTURE:

Ammonium chloride	..	..	..	100 g
Aromatic ammonia solution	..	..	..	50 ml
Liquorice liquid extract ..	..	..	..	100 ml
Water for preparations ..	..	..	to 1000 ml

It should be recently prepared.
A standard for this mixture is given in the British Pharmaceutical Codex 1973
Containers and *Labelling:* see the entry on Mixtures for general information on containers and labelling.
Advice for patients: the mixture should not be used for longer than a few days without medical advice.
Dose: 10 to 20 millilitres.

AMMONIUM CHLORIDE TABLETS: may be prepared by moist granulation and compression as described in the entry on Tablets. Available as tablets containing 450 and 500 mg of ammonium chloride; they may be enteric coated and the coat may be coloured.
A standard for these tablets is given in the British Pharmaceutical Codex 1973
Containers and *Storage:* see the entry on Tablets for general information on containers and storage.
Advice for patients: enteric-coated tablets should be swallowed whole; milk and antacids should not be taken within one hour.

Amodiaquine Hydrochloride

4-(7-Chloroquinol-4-ylamino)-2-(diethylaminomethyl)-phenol dihydrochloride dihydrate

2HCl, 2H$_2$O

$C_{20}H_{24}Cl_3N_3O, 2H_2O = 464.8$

OTHER NAME: *Camoquin*® (available in certain overseas countries only)

A standard is given in the British Pharmacopoeia 1973

Description. A yellow odourless crystalline powder with a bitter taste.

Solubility. Soluble, at 20°, in 22 parts of water and in 70 parts of alcohol; very slightly soluble in ether and in chloroform.

Acidity. A 2% solution has a pH of 4.0 to 4.6.

Moisture content. 6 to 10%, determined by drying over phosphorus pentoxide *in vacuo*.

Storage. It should be stored in airtight containers.

Identification. TEST. To 1 ml of a 2% solution add 0.5 ml of *cobalt thiocyanate solution*; a green precipitate is produced.

MELTING-POINT. About 158°.

ULTRAVIOLET ABSORPTION. In 0.1N hydrochloric acid, maxima at 223 nm, 237 nm, and 343 nm (E1%, 1cm = 366).

Determination in body fluids. SPECTROFLUORIMETRY. In plasma or serum—G. M. Trenholme *et al.*, *Bull. Wld Hlth Org.*, 1974, **51**, 431.

Metabolism. ABSORPTION. Readily absorbed after oral administration.

BLOOD CONCENTRATION. After an oral dose of 10 mg/kg, plasma concentrations of 300 to 560 ng/ml are attained in 4 hours; therapeutic concentrations are attained 1 to 2 hours after dosing.

DISTRIBUTION. Widely distributed throughout the tissues; high concentrations are found in the liver, spleen, kidneys, and lungs with smaller amounts in the brain and cerebrospinal fluid; in the blood, higher concentrations are found in red cells than in the plasma.

EXCRETION. Slowly excreted in the urine but the rate may be increased if the urinary pH is decreased.

Actions and uses. Amodiaquine hydrochloride is an antimalarial drug which has actions and uses similar to those described under Chloroquine Phosphate.

A dose equivalent to 200 to 400 milligrams of the base given by mouth once a week is usually adequate for the suppression or so-called prophylaxis of malaria in an adult; 130 milligrams of the hydrochloride is equivalent to 100 milligrams of the base.

A single dose equivalent to 600 milligrams of the base is often sufficient to control a malarial attack, although the equivalent of 400 to 600 milligrams of the base daily for 3 days may be necessary.

The dose in terms of the base for a child corresponding to 600 milligrams of the base for an adult is: up to one year 75 to 150 milligrams; 1 to 5 years, 125 to 250 milligrams; 6 to 12 years, 270 to 450 milligrams.

Amodiaquine has been used for the treatment of chronic discoid lupus erythematosus; a single dose equivalent to 200 milligrams of the base is given daily until the condition is controlled, and thereafter 200 milligrams is given 3 or 4 times a week for maintenance.

Undesirable effects. Undesirable effects are rare with antimalarial doses but it may cause nausea, vomiting, and diarrhoea. Long continued use of the drug may result in blue-grey deposits in the cornea, fingernails, and hard palate. The corneal deposits slowly resolve after stopping treatment.

Preparation

AMODIAQUINE TABLETS: available as tablets containing amodiaquine hydrochloride equivalent to 200 mg of amodiaquine base.

A standard for these tablets is given in the British Pharmacopoeia 1973

Containers and *Storage:* see the entry on Tablets for general information on containers and storage. Containers should be airtight.

Labelling: the label on the container should state the amount of the medicament as the equivalent amount of amodiaquine base.

Advice for patients: the tablets should be taken at regular intervals, preferably after meals. For prophylaxis, doses should be taken during the period at risk and for 4 weeks thereafter. For therapy the prescribed course should be completed.

Amoebiasis

Amoebiasis is caused by infection with *Entamoeba histolytica*. Infection is transmitted by the faecal-oral route. Amoebae present in the lumen or wall of the gut may give rise to dysentery (intestinal amoebiasis) while those present in the liver give rise to liver abscesses (hepatic amoebiasis).

Intestinal amoebiasis is insidious in onset and is characterised by a bloody diarrhoea flecked with mucus. Infection is chronic and diarrhoea may be intermittent and interspersed with periods of constipation. In a few patients there may be an acute watery blood-stained diarrhoea with fever, anorexia, and severe illness due to fulminating necrotising colitis. In this case there is danger of perforation of the bowel leading to peritonitis.

Amoebic liver abscess is caused by death and liquefaction of liver cells surrounding amoebae which have been taken via the hepatic portal system from the gut to the liver.

A wide range of substances is available for the treatment of amoebiasis, and most of them are suitable for use in both intestinal and hepatic forms. They include acetarsol, chloroquine, clioquinol, di-iodohydroxyquinoline, diloxanide furoate, emetine, halquinol, metronidazole, and tetracyclines.

Amoxycillin Trihydrate

(6R)-6-(α-D-4-Hydroxyphenylglycylamino)penicillanic acid trihydrate

$C_{16}H_{19}N_3O_5S$, $3H_2O = 419.5$

OTHER NAMES: *Amoxil®*; *Clamoxyl®*

A standard is given in the British Pharmacopoeia Addendum 1975

Description. A white microcrystalline odourless powder.

Solubility. Soluble, at 20°, in 400 parts of water, in 1000 parts of alcohol, and in 200 parts of methyl alcohol; very slightly soluble in ether, in chloroform, and in fixed oils.

Acidity. A 0.2% solution has a pH of 3.5 to 5.5.

Moisture content. 11.5 to 14%, determined by Fischer titration.

Stability. Unbuffered solutions of the sodium salt are most stable at pH 5.8 and solutions in citrate buffer solution are most stable at pH 6.5.

FURTHER INFORMATION. Kinetic studies on the degradation of amoxycillin solutions—H. Zia *et al.*, *Canad. J. pharm. Sci.*, 1977, **12**, 80.

Storage. It should be stored in airtight containers at a temperature not exceeding 25°.

Identification. TESTS. 1. Mix 2 mg with 2 mg of chromotropic acid sodium salt and 2 ml of sulphuric acid, and immerse in a suitable liquid at 150° for 4 minutes; the solution remains colourless at first, then changes through yellow to violet and finally chars (distinction from certain other penicillins).
2. Mix about 10 mg with 1 ml of water and add 2 ml of a mixture containing 2 ml of *potassium cupri-tartrate solution* and 6 ml of water; a magenta colour is produced immediately.
3. Dissolve 2 drops of aniline in a mixture of 1 ml of hydrochloric acid and 3 ml of water, cool in ice, and add 200 mg of sodium nitrite dissolved in 1 ml of water. Add this mixture, dropwise, to a cold solution containing 100 mg of the sample in 2 ml of *sodium hydroxide solution*; the solution becomes deep cherry red and a copious dark brown precipitate is produced.

ULTRAVIOLET ABSORPTION. In 0.1N hydrochloric acid, maximum at 274 nm (E1%, 1cm = 26); in 0.1N sodium hydroxide, maximum at 292 nm (E1%, 1cm = 59); in alcohol (95%), maximum at 275 nm (E1%, 1cm = 30).

INFRA-RED ABSORPTION. Major peaks at 1248, 1396, 1484, 1583, 1684, and 1775 cm⁻¹ (see Appendix 2a: Infra-red Spectra).

Determination in body fluids. SPECTROFLUORIMETRY. In blood or urine: amoxycillin and its penicilloic acid metabolite—K. Miyazaki *et al.*, *Chem. pharm. Bull.*, *Tokyo*, 1977, **25**, 253.

Metabolism. ABSORPTION. Amoxycillin is stable to gastric acid and 50 to 90% of a dose is absorbed after oral administration; absorption is more complete than that of ampicillin and it is not greatly influenced by the presence of food.

BLOOD CONCENTRATION. After an oral dose of 500 mg, peak serum concentrations of 3 to 20 µg/ml are attained in 1 to 2 hours; detectable concentrations are present after 8 hours; peak concentrations occur earlier in children and infants but later in neonates.

HALF-LIFE. Serum half-life, 1 hour which may be increased to 15 hours in renal failure.

DISTRIBUTION. Enters most tissues and fluids but is not detectable in the cerebrospinal fluid even when the meninges are inflamed; crosses the placenta and small amounts are secreted in the milk; volume of distribution at steady-state serum concentrations, about 0.3 litres/kilogram body-weight; *protein binding*, 15 to 25% bound to plasma proteins.

METABOLIC REACTIONS. Metabolised to inactive metabolites and 10 to 25% appears to be converted to penicilloic acid.

EXCRETION. 35 to 45% is excreted in the urine after an oral dose and about 75% after intramuscular or intravenous doses; urinary excretion is delayed by probenecid and it also occurs more slowly in the newborn; small amounts are excreted in the bile.

FURTHER INFORMATION. Antibacterial and pharmacokinetic properties and therapeutic use of amoxycillin: a review—R. N. Brogden *et al.*, *Drugs*, 1975, **9**, 88; pharmacokinetics of amoxycillin—D. Zarowny *et al.*, *Clin. Pharmac. Ther.*, 1974, **16**, 1045 and B. M. Leng *et al.*, *J. int. med. Res.*, 1976, **4**, 449.

Actions and uses. Amoxycillin is a semisynthetic penicillin which is acid resistant and has a similar antibacterial spectrum to ampicillin. It is, however, better absorbed after oral administration, yielding blood levels approximately twice as high as those obtained with similar doses of ampicillin. More than half the dose is excreted in the urine within 6 hours of administration. Amoxycillin is used for the same purposes as ampicillin and is especially suitable for the treatment of infections of the urinary and respiratory tracts by ampicillin-sensitive organisms. The usual dose is the equivalent of 250 milligrams of amoxycillin for adults, 62.5 milligrams for children up to 1 year, or 125 milligrams from 1 to 10 years, 3 times a day. The dose may be doubled in severe infections. 1.2 grams of amoxycillin trihydrate is approximately equivalent to 1 gram of amoxycillin.

Undesirable effects. Gastro-intestinal disturbances and rashes may occur. Small amounts of amoxycillin excreted in the milk may provoke allergic reactions in breast-fed infants.

Precautions. The precautions against allergy described under Benzylpenicillin should be observed. Patients allergic to other penicillins must be assumed to be allergic to amoxycillin.

Preparations

AMOXYCILLIN CAPSULES: consisting of amoxycillin trihydrate, in powder, which may be mixed with an inert diluent, enclosed in a hard capsule. The capsule shells may be coloured. Available as capsules containing amoxycillin trihydrate equivalent to 250 and 500 mg of amoxycillin.
A standard for these capsules is given in the British Pharmacopoeia Addendum 1975
Containers and *Storage:* see the entry on Capsules for general information on containers and storage. The capsules should be stored at a temperature not exceeding 25°.
Labelling: the label on the container should state the

amount of the medicament as the equivalent amount of amoxycillin. The label should also state the date after which the capsules are not intended to be used and the conditions under which they should be stored.

Advice for patients: the capsules should be taken at regular intervals. The prescribed course should be completed.

AMOXYCILLIN MIXTURE: a suspension of amoxycillin trihydrate in a suitable coloured flavoured vehicle. It is prepared freshly by suspending a powder consisting of the mixed dry ingredients in the specified volume of water for preparations.

When a dose less than or not /a multiple of 5 ml is prescribed, the mixture may be diluted, as described in the entry on Mixtures, with syrup.

Available as a suspension containing amoxycillin trihydrate equivalent to 125 and 250 mg of amoxycillin in 5 ml when reconstituted.

Containers and *Labelling:* see the entry on Mixtures for general information on containers and labelling. The name on the label of the container of the dry powder is "Powder for Amoxycillin Mixture".

Storage: the dry powder should be stored at a temperature not exceeding 25°. The mixture and the diluted mixture should be used within one week of preparation.

Advice for patients: the mixture should be taken at regular intervals. The prescribed course should be completed.

OTHER PREPARATIONS available include an INJECTION reconstituted from vials of powder containing amoxycillin trihydrate equivalent to 0.25, 0.5, and 1 g of amoxycillin, and a MIXTURE containing amoxycillin trihydrate equivalent to 125 mg of amoxycillin in 1.25 ml when reconstituted (paediatric preparation).

Amphetamine Sulphate

($\pm$)-α-Methylphenethylammonium sulphate

$$\left[\begin{array}{c} \overset{+}{N}H_3 \\ | \\ C_6H_5 \cdot CH_2 \cdot CH \cdot CH_3 \end{array} \right]_2 \quad SO_4^{2-}$$

$C_{18}H_{28}N_2O_4S = 368.5$

OTHER NAMES: Amphetamini Sulfas; Amphet. Sulph.

A standard is given in the European Pharmacopoeia Vol. III

Description. A white odourless powder with a slightly bitter taste followed by a sensation of numbness.

Solubility. Soluble, at 20°, in 9 parts of water and in 515 parts of alcohol; practically insoluble in ether and in chloroform.

Dissociation constant. pK_a 9.9 (20°).

Moisture content. Not more than 1%, determined by drying at 105°.

Incompatibility. It is incompatible with alkalis and with calcium salts.

Hygroscopicity. It absorbs insignificant amounts of moisture at 25° at relative humidities up to about 90%.

Sterilisation. Solutions for injection are sterilised by heating in an autoclave or by filtration.

Identification. TESTS. 1. Dissolve 1 g in 50 ml of water, add 10 ml of *sodium hydroxide solution* and 0.5 ml of benzoyl chloride, and shake; add further benzoyl chloride in portions of 0.5 ml until no further precipitate is

produced; the precipitate, after recrystallising twice from alcohol, melts at about 135°.

2. Dissolve a few mg in about 4 ml of water, add 1 ml of 1N hydrochloric acid, 2 ml of *diazotised nitroaniline solution*, 4 ml of 1N sodium hydroxide, and 2 ml of n-butyl alcohol, shake, and allow to separate; a red colour develops in the butyl alcohol layer (distinction from methylamphetamine).

MELTING-POINT. About 300° with decomposition.

ULTRAVIOLET ABSORPTION. In 0.1N sulphuric acid, weak maxima at 251, 257, and 263 nm.

INFRA-RED ABSORPTION. Major peaks at 699, 741, 1111, 1389, 1493, and 1562 cm^{-1} (see Appendix 2b: Infra-red Spectra).

Determination in body fluids. COLORIMETRY. In urine: C. S. Frings *et al.*, *Clin. Chem.*, 1971, **17**, 1016.

ULTRAVIOLET SPECTROPHOTOMETRY. In whole blood, serum, or urine: method will also determine other drugs with a phenethylamino group—J. E. Wallace *et al.*, *Analyt. Chem.*, 1968, **40**, 2207.

THIN-LAYER CHROMATOGRAPHY. In urine: method of differentiation from other primary amino drugs: stated to be no interference from barbiturates, morphine, codeine, quinine, methadone, cocaine, propoxyphene, caffeine, or phenothiazines—R. J. Bussey, and R. C. Backer, *Clin. Chem.*, 1974, **20**, 302.

GAS CHROMATOGRAPHY. In urine—K. Kamei *et al.*, *Chem. pharm. Bull.*, Tokyo, 1973, **21**, 1996.

Metabolism. ABSORPTION. Readily absorbed after oral or rectal administration; amphetamine delays gastric emptying and decreases gastro-intestinal motility and may therefore delay the absorption of other drugs.

BLOOD CONCENTRATION. After an oral dose of 10 to 15 mg of the sulphate peak plasma concentrations of 40 to 50 ng/ml are attained in 1 to 2 hours falling to about 2 ng/ml after 8 to 10 hours; after an intravenous dose of 13 mg of the sulphate, plasma concentrations of 120 to 170 ng/ml are attained in 0.5 to 3.5 minutes.

HALF-LIFE. Influenced by urinary pH values; the plasma half-life is 4 to 6 hours when the urine is acid and much longer when the urine is alkaline. At a urinary pH of 6.7, the plasma half-life may be up to about 34 hours and in subjects whose urinary pH values are uncontrolled the plasma half-life is about 12 hours.

DISTRIBUTION. Rapidly distributed extravascularly and taken up, to some extent, by red blood cells; volume of distribution, 200 to 300 litres; *protein binding*, 20 to 40% bound to plasma proteins.

METABOLIC REACTIONS. Mainly oxidative deamination to form benzyl methyl ketone which is then oxidised to benzoic acid and conjugated with glycine to form hippuric acid; minor reactions include aromatic hydroxylation to form 4-hydroxyamphetamine, an active metabolite; β-hydroxylation, which is stereoselective for the (d)-isomer of amphetamine, to form norephedrine; N-oxidation to form a hydroxylamine derivative; the products of aromatic hydroxylation and N-oxidation may be conjugated with sulphate or glucuronic acid.

EXCRETION. The excretion of amphetamine is pH-dependent; in acid urine, 55 to 85% of a dose is excreted in the urine unchanged and in alkaline urine, 1 to 4% is excreted unchanged and about 50% is excreted as hippuric acid; under uncontrolled urinary pH conditions 15 to 50% of an oral dose is excreted unchanged in the urine; in rats desipramine reduces the amount of

4-hydroxyamphetamine excreted and increases the amount of unchanged drug in the urine; amphetamine is excreted in the saliva in concentrations paralleling those in the blood.

FURTHER INFORMATION. *International Symposium on Amphetamines and Related Compounds*, E. Costa and S. Garratini (Eds), New York, Raven Press and Amsterdam, North Holland Publishing Company, 1970; *Pharmacokinetics and Metabolism of Amphetamines*, T. B. Vree, Nijmegen, Drukkerij Brakkensteine te Nijmegen, 1973; metabolism of amphetamines—A. H. Beckett *et al.*, *J. Pharm. Pharmac.*, 1973, **25**, 708; metabolic fate of amphetamine in man and other species—L. G. Dring *et al.*, *Biochem. J.*, 1970, **116**, 425; blood and urine levels in man—M. Rowland, *J. pharm. Sci.*, 1969, **58**, 508.

Actions and uses. Amphetamine is a sympathomimetic drug with marked central stimulant effects. Like ephedrine, it produces vasoconstriction, inhibition of the motility of the gastro-intestinal tract and of the bladder, and dilatation of the pupil. It is less effective than ephedrine in relaxing bronchial muscle and less liable to increase the heart rate.

Its principle actions are stimulation of the cerebral cortex and the respiratory and vasomotor centres. These actions produce increased motor activity and mental alertness, euphoria, diminished sense of fatigue, and increased wakefulness. In some patients the drug produces insomnia, headache, hyperexcitability, and cardiac and gastro-intestinal disturbances. Large doses are followed by fatigue and mental depression; a rise in blood pressure may also occur.

Amphetamine sulphate is administered by mouth. It is used, usually in conjunction with tricyclic antidepressants, in the treatment of narcolepsy. It was formerly used in depressive states but has now been replaced by other drugs. It has also been used in doses of 5 to 10 milligrams 2 or 3 times daily as an adjunct to the treatment of obesity but it is of doubtful value and should not be used for this purpose because of the danger of creating a state of dependence.

Precautions and contra-indications. Amphetamine sulphate should not be given to patients who are being treated with a monoamine-oxidase inhibitor, such as isocarboxazid, nialamide, phenelzine, or tranylcypromine, or within about 2 weeks of the discontinuation of such treatment.

The indiscriminate use of amphetamine in attempts to increase capacity for work or to overcome fatigue is undesirable, as it may lead to dependence.

Amphetamine is contra-indicated in patients with cardiovascular disease and thyrotoxicosis and in those showing anxiety, hyperexcitability, and restlessness. It may cause a reversal of the effect of antihypertensive drugs.

Dependence. It may give rise to dependence of the amphetamine type as described under Drug Dependence.

Poisoning. A suitable tranquilliser such as chlorpromazine should be administered.

A suitable substance which will render the urine acid, such as ammonium chloride, may be administered during forced diuresis in a sufficient quantity to increase the rate of excretion of amphetamine.

Preparation

AMPHETAMINE SULPHATE TABLETS: available as tablets containing 5 mg of amphetamine sulphate.

A standard for these tablets is given in the British Pharmacopoeia 1973

Containers and *Storage:* see the entry on Tablets for general information on containers and storage. Containers should be airtight.

Advice for patients: they may affect mental concentration; persons affected should not drive or operate machinery. To avoid insomnia, doses should not be taken for several hours before bedtime.

Amphotericin

A mixture of antifungal substances produced by the growth of certain strains of *Streptomyces nodosus*. The crude product of fermentation can be separated into two chemically related active substances which are polyenes. These have been designated amphotericin A, which has the properties of a conjugated tetraene, and amphotericin B, which has the properties of a conjugated heptaene. Amphotericin B is less soluble in water and less stable than amphotericin A, but it is significantly more active *in vivo*. In the United Kingdom the title "Amphotericin" is applied to a substance which contains not less than 85% of amphotericin B. Amphotericin B is a large molecule with a molecular weight of about 920, and it is optically active.

OTHER NAMES: *Fungilin®*; *Fungizone® Mysteclin®* (with tetracycline)

A standard is given in the British Pharmacopoeia 1973

Description. A yellow to orange, odourless, almost tasteless powder.

Solubility. Practically insoluble in water, in alcohol, and in ether; soluble, at 20°, in 625 parts of dehydrated methyl alcohol, in 20 parts of dimethyl sulphoxide, and in 200 parts of dimethylformamide; soluble in propylene glycol.

Acidity or alkalinity. A 3% suspension in water has a pH of 6 to 8.

Moisture content. Not more than 5%, determined by drying at 60° *in vacuo*.

Stability. It is inactivated at low pH values and dilute solutions are light-sensitive. A solution containing 100 micrograms per ml of amphotericin in dextrose injection, stored in darkness, has been shown to be stable for 6 weeks at 5°, but potency is reduced by 2 to 3% in 3 days at 25° and reduced by 10 to 15% on exposure to light.

FURTHER INFORMATION. Stability studies in intravenous solutions—J. F. Gallelli, *Am. J. Hosp. Pharm.*, 1967, **24**, 425.

Incompatibility. It is compatible with dextrose injection. It is precipitated from solution by sodium chloride. Suspensions are sensitive to dissolved ions. It is incompatible with heparin.

Storage. It should be stored in airtight containers at a temperature of 2° to 10°, protected from light. Under these conditions it may be expected to retain its potency without significant deterioration for at least one year.

Identification. TEST. To a small amount of the powder add 1 ml of an 85% w/v solution of phosphoric acid; a deep blue colour is produced.

MELTING-POINT. It gradually decomposes above 170°.

ULTRAVIOLET ABSORPTION. In a solution prepared by dissolving 50 mg in 5 ml of dimethyl sulphoxide, diluting to 50 ml with dehydrated methyl alcohol, and then diluting 2 ml of the solution to 200 ml with the same solvent, maxima at 362 nm, 381 nm, and 405 nm.

Metabolism. ABSORPTION. Amphotericin is poorly absorbed after oral, intramuscular, or subcutaneous administration and is therefore usually administered intravenously; absorption is improved if the drug is administered in colloidal form with sodium deoxycholate.

BLOOD CONCENTRATION. After an oral dose of 3 to 7 g, blood concentrations of 0.1 to 5 μg/ml are obtained; after intravenous injection of about 1 mg/kg body-weight, mean serum concentrations of about 1 μg/ml are obtained within 1 hour.

HALF-LIFE. Plasma half-life, about 24 hours.

DISTRIBUTION. Small amounts of amphotericin enter the cerebrospinal fluid.

EXCRETION. Amphotericin is slowly excreted; only 5% is excreted in the urine in 24 hours; after 7 days up to 40% may be excreted; traces are detectable in the urine after 2 months.

FURTHER INFORMATION. Factors governing serum concentrations—C. M. Kunin, *Ann. intern. Med.*, 1967, **67**, 151; serum concentrations during therapy—B. T. Fields *et al.*, *Appl. Microbiol.*, 1970, **19**, 955.

Actions and uses. Amphotericin is a polyene antibiotic related to nystatin. It has an antifungal action against a wide range of yeasts and fungi. It is used in the treatment of infections by yeast-like organisms, such as cryptococcosis, candidiasis, blastomycosis, and histoplasmosis.

For the treatment of local infections it is used in the form of a mixture containing 100 milligrams per millilitre, tablets containing 100 milligrams, cream, lotion, and ointment containing 3%, lozenges containing 10 milligrams, and pessaries containing 50 milligrams. For the treatment of systemic infections a special grade of amphotericin is usually administered by slow intravenous infusion of a solution containing amphotericin in the form of a water-soluble complex with sodium deoxycholate dissolved in dextrose injection (5%) of pH not less than 4.2. In meningeal infections an aqueous solution containing the equivalent of 250 micrograms per millilitre may be mixed with cerebrospinal fluid in the syringe and given intrathecally if intravenous infusion is not effective. Solutions should be protected from light before and during administration.

For systemic therapy, most treatment regimens of amphotericin aim to achieve a total dose of 3 grams for an adult. Because severe systemic reactions may occur the daily dose should be built up gradually. The total dose given may be limited because of nephrotoxicity and treatment is usually terminated if the blood urea rises over 150 milligrams per 100 ml (25 mmol/litre). Two treatment regimens are used and in each the dose is dissolved in 500 millilitres of dextrose injection (5%) and given intravenously over 3 to 4 hours. The dose is given on alternate days because the compound is excreted slowly. A dose of 1 milligram is given on the first day and the dose built up by 3-milligram amounts until 60 milligrams is given on alternate days. Alternatively, a shorter regimen may be used in which the dose is increased by 20-milligram amounts to a level of 100 milligrams on alternate days. With smaller doses treatment may need to be continued for some months. In view of its toxicity amphotericin should be given by injection only in susceptible types of infection.

Undesirable effects. Unpleasant and potentially dangerous side-effects of systemic treatment are common because dosage must be as high as possible. Headache, anorexia, and fever occur frequently at the beginning of treatment but usually pass off in a few days. The main toxic effect is disturbance of renal function, which should be tested at intervals, and administration of amphotericin should be stopped if progressive deterioration occurs.

Precautions. The injection is irritant to the endothelium of the vein and may be painful. The risk of thrombophlebitis is reduced by frequently changing the site of the injection and reducing the rate of administration. Corticosteroids should not be administered concurrently unless they are necessary to control drug reactions and no corticosteroid should be added to the infusion solution.

Preparations

AMPHOTERICIN CREAM: a dispersion of amphotericin in a suitable water-miscible basis. Available as a cream containing 2.5 and 3% w/w of amphotericin. This cream should not be diluted.

Containers and *Labelling:* see the entry on Creams for general information on containers and labelling.

Storage: see the entry on Creams for general information on storage. It should be stored at room temperature. It should not be allowed to freeze.

Advice for patients: the cream should be applied sparingly to the affected area.

AMPHOTERICIN INJECTION: a sterile solution of amphotericin B–sodium deoxycholate complex, with sodium phosphate and sodium acid phosphate, in water for injections. No bactericide is present, nor should one be added. It is prepared by dissolving the contents of a sealed container which contains the sodium deoxycholate and the buffering agents, in water for injections shortly before use.

For intravenous infusion, the initial solution is diluted with dextrose injection (5%), immediately before use, to produce a solution containing the equivalent of 100 micrograms of amphotericin per ml. The dextrose injection used should have a pH not lower than 4.2. If necessary the pH of the dextrose injection is adjusted, by the addition of 1 to 2 ml of sterile buffer solution containing 4.01% of sodium phosphate and 1.25% of sodium acid phosphate in water for injections, before mixing with the initial amphotericin solution. The buffer solution is sterilised by heating in an autoclave or by filtration.

Available as a powder in vials containing 50 mg (50 000 units) of amphotericin with sodium phosphate, sodium acid phosphate, and approximately 41 mg of sodium deoxycholate.

For intrathecal injection, the contents of the vial are dissolved in sufficient water for injections to provide a solution containing 250 micrograms of amphotericin per ml before admixture with the cerebrospinal fluid.

Containers and *Labelling:* see the entry on Injections for general information on containers and labelling.

Storage: the sealed container should be stored at a temperature between 2° and 10°, protected from light. Protection from light should, if possible, be maintained for all procedures following preparation of the injection, including administration. The injection contains no bactericide and should be used as soon as possible after preparation, but the concentrated solution can be stored for up to 1 week after preparation without appreciable loss of potency provided that it is stored at 2° to 10°.

AMPHOTERICIN LOZENGES: available as lozenges containing 10 mg of amphotericin; they may contain suitable flavouring. Each lozenge weighs about 1 g.

A standard for these lozenges is given in the British Pharmaceutical Codex 1973

Containers: see the entry on Lozenges for general information on containers. Containers should be airtight.

Labelling: the label on the container should state the date after which the lozenges are not intended to be used.

Storage: they should be stored at room temperature, protected from light.

Advice for patients: the lozenges should be allowed to dissolve slowly in the mouth. The prescribed course should be completed.

AMPHOTERICIN MIXTURE: a suspension of amphotericin in a suitable coloured flavoured vehicle. Available as a suspension containing 100 mg of amphotericin per ml. This mixture should not be diluted. The general direction given in the entry on Mixtures that the preparation should be diluted so that the dose is contained in 5 ml does not apply to this mixture; the dose prescribed should be measured by means of a graduated pipette.

Containers and *Labelling:* see the entry on Mixtures for general information on containers and labelling.

Storage: it should be stored in a cool place, protected from light.

Advice for patients: the dose should be retained in the mouth for as long as possible before swallowing. The prescribed course should be completed.

AMPHOTERICIN OINTMENT: a dispersion of amphotericin in a polyethylene and liquid paraffin gel or other suitable anhydrous basis. Available as an ointment containing 3% of amphotericin. This ointment should not be diluted.

Containers and *Labelling:* see the entry on Ointments for general information on containers and labelling.

Storage: it should be stored at room temperature.

Advice for patients: the ointment should be applied sparingly to the affected area.

OTHER PREPARATIONS available include a lotion containing amphotericin 3%, a dental PASTE containing amphotericin 20 mg per gram, PESSARIES containing amphotericin 50 mg, a MIXTURE containing amphotericin 25 mg and tetracycline equivalent to tetracycline hydrochloride 125 mg in 5 ml, and TABLETS, for oral administration, containing amphotericin 100 mg.

Ampicillin

(6R)-6-(α-D-Phenylglycylamino)penicillanic acid

$C_{16}H_{19}N_3O_4S = 349.4$

OTHER NAMES: *Amfipen®*; Anhydrous Ampicillin

A standard is given in the British Pharmacopoeia Addendum 1978

Description. A white microcrystalline odourless powder with a bitter taste.

Solubility. Soluble, at 20°, in 170 parts of water; very slightly soluble in alcohol, in ether, in chloroform, in acetone, and in fixed oils.

Acidity. A 0.25% solution has a pH of 3.5 to 5.5.

Moisture content. Not more than 2%, determined by Fischer titration.

Specific rotation. +280° to +305°, determined on a 0.25% solution.

Dissociation constants. pK_a 2.6, 7.3 (25°).

Hygroscopicity. Absorbs insignificant amounts of moisture at 25° at relative humidities up to about 80%, but under damper conditions it absorbs significant amounts.

Storage. It should be stored in airtight containers at a temperature not exceeding 25°.

Identification. TESTS. 1. Mix 2 mg with 2 mg of chromotropic acid sodium salt and 2 ml of sulphuric acid and immerse in a suitable liquid at 150° for 4 minutes; the solution remains colourless at first, then changes to violet and finally chars (distinction from certain other penicillins).

2. Place 2 drops of a 0.1% solution of ninhydrin on a filter paper and dry at 105°; add 2 drops of a 0.1% solution of the sample and heat for 5 minutes at 105°; a mauve colour is produced.

3. Mix a few mg with 1 ml of water and add 2 ml of a mixture of *potassium cupri-tartrate solution* and 6 ml of water; a magenta-violet colour is produced.

MELTING-POINT. About 200°.

ULTRAVIOLET ABSORPTION. In neutral or acid (pH 5) aqueous solutions and also in methyl alcohol solution, ampicillin exhibits weak maxima at 257, 262, and 268 nm with E1%, 1cm values in the range of 5 to 8. In alkaline aqueous solution (pH 9) the absorption is similar except that the peak at 268 nm disappears.

INFRA-RED ABSORPTION. Major peaks at 1308, 1382, 1497, 1526, 1693, and 1775 cm^{-1} (see Appendix 2a: Infrared Spectra).

Determination in body fluids. ULTRAVIOLET SPECTROPHOTOMETRY. In plasma—L. Angelucci and M. Baldieri, *J. Pharm. Pharmacol.*, 1971, **23**, 471.

SPECTROFLUORIMETRY. In serum or urine—W. J. Jusko, *J. pharm. Sci.*, 1971, **60**, 728; in serum—A. Duerr and H. J. Schatzmann, *Experientia*, 1975, **31**, 503.

Metabolism. ABSORPTION. Ampicillin is acid stable and 30 to 60% of an oral dose is absorbed.

BLOOD CONCENTRATIONS. Peak serum concentrations of 0.8 to 4.0 μg/ml are attained 1 to 2 hours after oral doses of 250 to 500 mg of anhydrate or trihydrate; after an intramuscular injection of 250 to 1000 mg of the trihydrate, serum concentrations of 2 to 5 μg/ml are attained in about 2 hours; after an intramuscular dose of 500 mg of the sodium salt, peak serum concentrations of about 7 μg/ml are attained in 1 hour.

HALF-LIFE. Serum half-life, 1 to 2 hours which is increased in subjects with renal function impairment.

DISTRIBUTION. Ampicillin enters most body cavities, tissues, and fluids except the cerebrospinal fluid unless the meninges are inflamed, in which case large amounts may be detectable in this fluid; ampicillin crosses the placenta and is secreted in the milk; volume of distribution about 20 litres which in subjects with cirrhosis may reach about 60 litres; *protein binding,* about 20% bound to plasma proteins.

EXCRETION. 30 to 50% of an oral or intramuscular dose is excreted in the urine in 6 to 8 hours and up to 70% is excreted in 24 hours; urinary excretion is decreased after the administration of probenecid; ampicillin is excreted in the bile in concentrations up to 4 μg/ml after an oral dose of 250 mg; biliary excretion is increased in subjects with cirrhosis.

FURTHER INFORMATION. Pharmacokinetics of ampicillin —J. T. Doluisio *et al.*, *J. pharm. Sci.*, 1971, **60**, 715 and J. C. K. Loo *et al.*, *Clin. Pharmac. Ther.*, 1974, **16**, 35; comparison of bioavailability and pharmacokinetics after oral and intravenous administration of 3 brands of ampicillin—P. Bolme *et al.*, *Eur. J. clin. Pharmac.*, 1976, **10**, 237; pharmacokinetics of ampicillin in cirrhosis— G. P. Lewis and W. J. Jusko, *Clin. Pharmac. Ther.*, 1975, **18**, 475; ampicillin concentration in joint fluid— E. A. Baciocco and R. L. Iles, *Clin. Pharmac. Ther.*, 1971, **12**, 858; plasma, urine, and bile levels of ampicillin in the dog and in man—F. Bertè *et al.*, *Farmaco, Edn prat.*, 1972, **27**, 205; placental transfer of ampicillin— L.-O. Boréus, *Acta pharmac. tox.*, 1971, **29**, *Suppl.* 3, 250; blood-level studies—P. G. Gooding *et al.*, *Curr. ther. Res.*, 1972, **14**, 43.

Actions and uses. Ampicillin is a semisynthetic penicillin which is acid resistant and can therefore be given orally, while the sodium salt may be given parenterally. It is destroyed by most bacterial penicillinases but it is more effective against non-penicillinase-producing Gram-negative organisms than benzylpenicillin. It is particularly useful against *Haemophilus influenzae* infections but its effectiveness against *Proteus* species and coliform organisms may be slowly diminishing because of replacement of sensitive strains by resistant ones.

Ampicillin is inappropriate for the treatment of staphylococcal infections because it is destroyed by staphylococcal penicillinase and because the minimum inhibitory concentration is higher than that of benzylpenicillin.

The usual oral dose is 1 to 6 grams daily in divided doses every 6 hours. The dose for children under 1 year is one-quarter of the adult dose and for children from 1 to 10 years half the adult dose.

For doses by injection see under Ampillicin Sodium.

Undesirable effects. Ampicillin may give rise to a rash which, unlike that caused by benzylpenicillin, may be of toxic rather than allergic origin and not necessarily a contra-indication to future treatment with ampicillin or another penicillin. Rashes almost invariably result when ampicillin is given to patients with glandular fever. Small amounts of ampicillin excreted in the milk may provoke allergic reactions in breast-fed infants.

Precautions. The precautions against allergy described under Benzylpenicillin should be observed. Patients allergic to other penicillins must be assumed to be allergic to ampicillin.

Veterinary uses. Ampicillin is used in animals in the treatment of infections of the gastro-intestinal, respiratory, and urogenital systems. The usual dosage by mouth for all species is 4 to 12 milligrams per kilogram body-weight twice daily but ampicillin should not be administered by mouth to adult ruminants. The usual dose by intra-uterine administration for the treatment of metritis in cows, ewes, and sows is up to 400 milligrams, repeated if necessary after 2 days.

Preparations

AMPICILLIN CAPSULES: consisting of ampicillin or ampicillin trihydrate in powder, which may be mixed with an inert diluent, enclosed in a hard capsule. The capsule shells may be coloured. Available as capsules containing 50, 250, and 500 mg of ampicillin, or the equivalent amount of ampicillin trihydrate.

A standard for these capsules is given in the British Pharmacopoeia Addendum 1978

Containers and *Storage:* see the entry on Capsules for general information on containers and storage. The capsules should be stored at a temperature not exceeding 25°.

Labelling: when the active ingredient is ampicillin trihydrate, the label on the container should state the amount of the medicament as the equivalent amount of ampicillin. The label should also state the date after which the capsules are not intended to be used and the conditions under which they are to be stored.

Advice for patients: the capsules should be taken at regular intervals, preferably half to 1 hour before meals. The prescribed course should be completed.

AMPICILLIN MIXTURE (*Syn.* Ampicillin Syrup): a suspension of ampicillin or ampicillin trihydrate in a suitable flavoured vehicle. It is prepared freshly by dispersing a powder consisting of the mixed dry ingredients in the specified volume of water for preparations.

When a dose less than or not a multiple of 5 ml is prescribed, the mixture may be diluted, as described in the entry on Mixtures, with syrup; an exception is *Vidopen®* syrup for which the diluent recommended by the manufacturer is freshly boiled and cooled purified water.

Available as a mixture containing 125 and 250 mg of ampicillin, or the equivalent amount of ampicillin trihydrate, in 5 ml when reconstituted.

When strong ampicillin mixture or strong ampicillin syrup is ordered or prescribed, the preparation containing 250 mg of ampicillin, or the equivalent amount of ampicillin trihydrate, in 5 ml when reconstituted is supplied.

A standard for this mixture is given in the British Pharmaceutical Codex 1973

Containers and *Labelling:* see the entry on Mixtures for general information on containers and labelling. The name on the label of the container of the dry powder should be "Powder for Ampicillin Mixture".

Storage: the dry powder should be stored at a temperature not exceeding 25°, protected from light.

The mixture and the diluted mixture should be stored in a cool place and used within one week of preparation.

Advice for patients: the mixture should be taken at regular intervals, preferably half to 1 hour before meals. The prescribed course should be completed.

PAEDIATRIC AMPICILLIN TABLETS: available as tablets containing ampicillin trihydrate equivalent to 125 mg of ampicillin. These tablets may also be prepared from ampicillin.

A standard for these tablets is given in the British Pharmaceutical Codex 1973

Containers and *Storage:* see the entry on Tablets for general information on containers and storage. Containers should be airtight.

Labelling: the label on the container should state the amount of the medicament as the equivalent amount of ampicillin. The label also states the date after which the tablets are not intended to be used and the conditions under which they should be stored.

Advice for patients: the tablets should be taken at regular intervals, preferably half to 1 hour before meals. The prescribed course should be completed.

Ampicillin Sodium

Sodium (6*R*)-6-(α-D-phenylglycylamino)penicillanate $C_{16}H_{18}N_3NaO_4S = 371.4$

OTHER NAMES: *Amfipen®*; *Penbritin®* *Ampiclox®* (with cloxacillin sodium); *Magnapen®* (with flucloxacillin sodium)

A standard is given in the British Pharmacopoeia Addendum 1978

Description. An odourless, hygroscopic, white, crystalline or amorphous powder with a bitter taste.

Solubility. Soluble, at 20°, in 2 parts of water and in 50 parts of acetone; very slightly soluble in chloroform; practically insoluble in ether, in liquid paraffin, and in fixed oils.

Alkalinity. A 10% solution has a pH of 8 to 10.

Moisture content. Not more than 2%, determined by Fischer titration.

Specific rotation. $+258°$ to $+287°$, determined on a 0.25% solution in a 0.02 M solution of potassium hydrogen phthalate.

Stability. In aqueous solution, ampicillin sodium degrades by hydrolysis. Degradation is catalysed by hydrogen ions and by hydroxyl ions. At 35°, the stability in unbuffered solutions is at a maximum at about pH 5.9. Degradation is also catalysed by citrate ions and phosphate ions; in solutions of ampicillin sodium buffered with citric acid and disodium hydrogen phosphate, the pH of maximum stability at 35° is 4.9. When stored at 5°, 90% of the potency may be expected to be retained for 7 days for 1% aqueous solutions of ampicillin sodium and for 24 hours for 5% solutions; solutions containing 10 and 25% of the drug may be expected to retain 80% of their original potency for 24 hours and 6 hours respectively.

A 1% solution of ampicillin sodium, with 0.002% of phenylmercuric nitrate, in water for injections, sterilised by filtration, may be expected to lose approximately 8% of its potency in 7 days at 2° to 10°. Such a solution would be suitable for use as eye- or ear-drops. A 2% preparation of ampicillin or ampicillin sodium, with 25% of liquid paraffin, in white soft paraffin, shows little loss of potency in 1 year's storage at room temperature in a moisture-proof container.

FURTHER INFORMATION. Ear- and eye-drops and eye ointment—B. Lynn, *Chemist Drugg.*, 1967, **187**, 157. Stability in aqueous solution—J. P. Hou and J. W. Poole, *J. pharm. Sci.*, 1969, **58**, 447; C. Larsen and H. Bundgaard, *Arch. Pharm. Chemi. scient. Edn*, 1977, **5**, 201; B. Lynn, *J. Hosp. Pharm.*, 1970, **28**, 71. Stability in intravenous infusions —D. R. Savello *et al.*, *Am. J. hosp. Pharm.*, 1972, **29**, 321; J. Jacobs *et al.*, *J. clin. Path.*, 1973, **26**, 742; J. Ashwin and B. Lynn, *Pharm. J.*, 1975, **214**, 487; G. Stjemström *et al.*, *Acta pharm. suec.*, 1978, **15**, 33.

For further information on the stability and other properties of ampicillin see *Analytical Profiles of Drug Substances*, K. Florey (Ed.), London, Academic Press, 1973, Vol. 2, pp. 1–61.

Incompatibility. In aqueous solution, ampicillin sodium is compatible with streptomycin sulphate but not with a stabilised injection of streptomycin sulphate. Ampicillin sodium equivalent to 500 mg of ampicillin dissolved in 1.5 ml of water is compatible with a solution of 250 000 units of polymyxin B sulphate in 1.5 ml of water, but more dilute solutions are incompatible.

Ampicillin is incompatible with adrenaline, *Aminosol*®, atropine sulphate, calcium chloride, calcium gluconate, chloramphenicol sodium succinate, chlorpromazine hydrochloride, chlortetracycline, erythromycin ethyl succinate, gentamicin sulphate, heparin, hydrallazine hydrochloride, kanamycin sulphate, lincomycin hydrochloride, metaraminol tartrate, noradrenaline, novobiocin, oxytetracycline hydrochloride, pentobarbitone,

phenobarbitone, prochlorperazine mesylate, protein hydrolysate, sulphafurazole, suxamethonium, tetracycline hydrochloride, thiopentone sodium, and solutions of vitamins B and C.

Ampicillin sodium may be added to most intravenous fluids but should not be mixed with blood products or other proteinaceous fluids. In intravenous injections of sodium chloride containing 1% of ampicillin sodium, 90% of the potency may be expected to be retained for 24 hours at 25°. In 5% dextrose infusion ampicillin is much less stable; the solution should be infused within one hour of preparation or the drug may be added by bolus injection into the infusion tubing.

FURTHER INFORMATION. Pharmaceutics of the semisynthetic penicillins—B. Lynn, *Chemist Drugg.*, 1967, **187**, 157, *J. Hosp. Pharm.*, 1970, **28**, 71, and *J. hosp. Pharm.*, 1971, **29**, 183; incompatibilities in intravenous solutions—B. B. Riley, *J. Hosp. Pharm.*, 1970, **28**, 228 and B. Flouvat and P. Lechat, *Thérapie*, 1974, **29**, 337.

Hygroscopicity. It is deliquescent, substantial amounts of moisture being absorbed even at low relative humidities.

Labelling. If the material is not intended for parenteral administration, the label on the container should state that the contents are not to be injected.

Storage. It should be stored in airtight containers at a temperature not exceeding 25°. If it is intended for parenteral administration the containers should be sterile and should be sealed to exclude micro-organisms.

Identification. TESTS. It complies with the tests described for Ampicillin.

MELTING-POINT. About 205°, with decomposition.

Determination in body fluids; Metabolism. See under Ampicillin.

Actions and uses. Ampicillin sodium has the actions described under Ampicillin and on account of its solubility it is used for the preparation of injections; 1.06 grams of ampicillin sodium is approximately equivalent to 1 gram of ampicillin.

It may be administered as a solution in water for injections by intramuscular or intravenous injection.

Solutions for intramuscular injection may be prepared by dissolving the equivalent of 100 milligrams of ampicillin in 0.5 millilitre of water for injections or 250 to 500 milligrams in 2.5 millilitres. Larger doses are painful when given by intramuscular injection and should preferably be given by slow intravenous injection of a solution of 500 milligrams in 10 millilitres of water for injections.

The usual dose by injection is the equivalent of 1 to 3 grams of ampicillin daily in divided doses. Children under 1 year may be given one quarter, and children aged 1 to 10 years half of the adult dose. The usual dose by intrathecal injection is the equivalent of 10 to 40 milligrams of ampicillin daily for adults and 3 to 5 milligrams daily for children.

Undesirable effects; Precautions. As for Ampicillin.

Veterinary uses. Ampicillin sodium is used in the treatment of infections by susceptible organisms. The usual dosage for all species by subcutaneous or intramuscular injection is the equivalent of 2 to 7 milligrams of ampicillin per kilogram body-weight.

Preparations

AMPICILLIN INJECTION: a sterile solution of ampicillin sodium in water for injections. It is prepared by dissolving the contents of a sealed container in water for injections shortly before use. Available as a powder in vials containing ampicillin sodium equivalent to 0.1, 0.25, 0.5, and 1 g of ampicillin.

A standard for this injection is given in the British Pharmacopoeia Addendum 1978

Containers: see the entry on Injections for general information on containers.

Labelling: see the entry on Injections for general information on labelling. In addition, the label on the container should state the amount of the medicament as the equivalent amount of ampicillin.

Storage: the sealed container should be stored at a temperature not exceeding 25°. The injection contains no bactericide and should be used as soon as possible after preparation, but dilute solutions of ampicillin sodium may be stored for up to 1 week without appreciable loss of potency provided they are stored at 2° to 10°.

OTHER PREPARATIONS available include an INJECTION reconstituted from vials of powder containing ampicillin sodium equivalent to 50 mg of ampicillin with cloxacillin sodium equivalent to 25 mg of cloxacillin, an injection reconstituted from vials of powder containing ampicillin sodium equivalent to 250 mg of ampicillin with cloxacillin sodium equivalent to cloxacillin 250 mg, a veterinary intramammary injection containing ampicillin sodium equivalent to 75 mg of ampicillin with cloxacillin sodium equivalent to 200 mg of cloxacillin in 3 g, and an injection reconstituted from vials of powder containing ampicillin sodium equivalent to 250 mg of ampicillin with flucloxacillin sodium equivalent to 250 mg of flucloxacillin.

Ampicillin Trihydrate

(6R)-6-(α-D-Phenylglycylamino)penicillanic acid trihydrate

$C_{16}H_{19}N_3O_4S, 3H_2O = 403.5$

OTHER NAMES: *Penbritin®*; *Pentrexyl®*; *Vidopen®* *Ampiclox®* (with cloxacillin sodium); *Magnapen®* (with flucloxacillin sodium)

A standard is given in the British Pharmacopoeia Addendum 1978

Description. A white microcrystalline odourless powder with a bitter taste.

Solubility. Soluble, at 20°, in 150 parts of water; very slightly soluble in alcohol, in ether, in chloroform, in acetone, and in fixed oils.

Acidity. A 0.25% solution has a pH of 3.5 to 5.5.

Moisture content. 12 to 15%, determined by Fischer titration.

Specific rotation. +280° to +305°, determined on a 0.25% solution.

Hygroscopicity. It absorbs insignificant amounts of moisture at 25° at relative humidities up to about 80% but under damper conditions it absorbs significant amounts.

Storage. It should be stored in airtight containers at a temperature not exceeding 25°.

Identification. TESTS. It complies with the tests described for Ampicillin.

Determination in body fluids; Metabolism. See under Ampicillin.

Actions and uses. Ampicillin trihydrate has the actions described under Ampicillin and is used for the same purposes; 1.15 grams of ampicillin trihydrate is approximately equivalent to 1 gram of ampicillin. It is administered by mouth. The usual dose is the equivalent of 1 to 6 grams of ampicillin daily in divided doses.

Undesirable effects; Precautions. As for Ampicillin.

Veterinary uses. As for Ampicillin.

Preparations

AMPICILLIN CAPSULES: see above under Ampicillin.

AMPICILLIN MIXTURE: see above under Ampicillin.

AMPICILLIN ORAL POWDER: consisting of a mixture of ampicillin trihydrate and lactose or other suitable diluent. Available as a powder containing ampicillin trihydrate equivalent to 10% of ampicillin.

A standard for this powder is given in the British Pharmacopoeia (Veterinary)

Containers and *Storage:* see the entry on Powders for general information on containers and storage. The powder should be stored at a temperature not exceeding 20°.

Labelling: the label on the container should state the amount of the medicament as the equivalent amount of ampicillin. The label also states the date after which the powder is not intended to be used, and the conditions under which it should be stored.

AMPICILLIN TABLETS: available as tablets containing ampicillin trihydrate equivalent to 400 mg of ampicillin.

A standard for these tablets is given in the British Pharmacopoeia (Veterinary)

Containers and *Storage:* see the entry on Tablets for general information on containers and storage. Containers should be airtight. The tablets should be stored at a temperature not exceeding 20°.

Labelling: the label on the container should state the amount of the medicament as the equivalent amount of ampicillin. The label also states the date after which the tablets are not intended to be used, and the conditions under which they should be stored.

PAEDIATRIC AMPICILLIN TABLETS: see above under Ampicillin.

OTHER PREPARATIONS available include CAPSULES containing ampicillin trihydrate equivalent to ampicillin 250 mg with flucloxacillin sodium equivalent to flucloxacillin 250 mg; a MIXTURE containing ampicillin trihydrate equivalent to 125 mg of ampicillin in 1.25 ml when reconstituted, a mixture containing ampicillin trihydrate equivalent to 60 mg of ampicillin with cloxacillin sodium equivalent to 30 mg of cloxacillin in 0.6 ml when reconstituted, and a mixture containing ampicillin trihydrate equivalent to 125 mg of ampicillin with flucloxacillin sodium equivalent to 125 mg of flucloxacillin in 5 ml when reconstituted.

Amprolium Hydrochloride

1-(4-Amino-2-propylpyrimidin-5-ylmethyl)-2-methyl-pyridinium chloride hydrochloride

$C_{14}H_{20}Cl_2N_4 = 315.3$

OTHER NAMES: *Amprol*® (with ethopabate); *Pancoxin*® (with ethopabate and sulphaquinoxaline); *Supacox*® (with ethopabate, sulphaquinoxaline, and pyrimethamine)

A standard is given in the British Pharmacopoeia (Veterinary)

Description. A white odourless powder.

Solubility. Soluble, at 20°, in 2 parts of water and in 170 parts of alcohol; very slightly soluble in ether; practically insoluble in chloroform.

Moisture content. Not more than 1%, determined by drying at 100° *in vacuo.*

Identification. TEST. Dissolve 2.5 mg of naphthalene-2,7-diol in 90 ml of methyl alcohol, add 10 mg of potassium ferricyanide and 50 mg of potassium cyanide dissolved in 10 ml of water, allow to stand for 30 minutes, and add 100 ml of 0.02N sodium hydroxide. To 5 ml of this solution add 1 mg of sample; a deep violet colour is produced.

MELTING-POINT. About 247°, with decomposition.

ULTRAVIOLET ABSORPTION. In 0.1N hydrochloric acid, maxima at 246 nm (E1%, 1cm = 420) and 262 nm (E1%, 1cm = 400).

Veterinary uses. Amprolium hydrochloride is a thiamine antagonist which is used for the prevention of coccidiosis in chickens and turkeys. It is administered in the feed in a concentration of 125 parts per million. It is also used in the treatment of coccidiosis in calves and lambs, the usual dosage being 10 to 20 milligrams per kilogram body-weight daily for 4 to 5 days.

Preparations

AMPROLIUM AND ETHOPABATE PREMIX: consisting of amprolium hydrochloride and ethopabate mixed with a suitable diluent. It must be diluted before administration by mixing thoroughly with the feed.
Available as a premix containing 25% of amprolium hydrochloride and 1.6% of ethopabate.
A standard for this premix is given in the British Pharmacopoeia (Veterinary)
Containers and *Storage:* see the entry on Premixes for general information on containers and storage.

AMPROLIUM, ETHOPABATE, AND SULPHAQUINOXALINE PREMIX: consisting of amprolium hydrochloride, ethopabate, and sulphaquinoxaline, mixed with a suitable diluent. It must be diluted before administration by mixing thoroughly with the feed.
Available as a premix containing 20% of amprolium hydrochloride, 1% of ethopabate, and 12% of sulphaquinoxaline.
A standard for this premix is given in the British Pharmacopoeia (Veterinary)
Containers and *Storage:* see the entry on Premixes for general information on containers and storage.

AMPROLIUM, ETHOPABATE, SULPHAQUINOXALINE, AND PYRIMETHAMINE PREMIX: consisting of amprolium hydrochloride, ethopabate, sulphaquinoxaline, and pyrimethamine, mixed with a suitable diluent. It must be diluted before administration by mixing thoroughly with the feed.
Available as a premix containing 20% of amprolium hydrochloride, 1% of ethopabate, 12% of sulphaquinoxaline, and 1% of pyrimethamine.
A standard for this premix is given in the British Pharmacopoeia (Veterinary)
Containers and *Storage:* see the entry on Premixes for general information on containers and storage.

OTHER PREPARATIONS available include a SOLUTION containing amprolium hydrochloride 7.68% with ethopabate 0.49%.

Amyl Nitrite

A liquid consisting of the nitrites of 3-methylbutan-1-ol, $(CH_3)_2CH.CH_2.CH_2OH$, and 2-methylbutan-1-ol, $CH_3.CH_2.CH(CH_3).CH_2OH$, with other nitrites of the homologous series.

A standard is given in the British Pharmaceutical Codex 1973
CAUTION. *Amyl nitrite forms an explosive mixture with air or oxygen. It is very inflammable and must not be used where it may be ignited.*

Description. A clear, yellow, volatile, inflammable liquid with a fragrant odour.

Solubility. Practically insoluble in water; miscible with alcohol and with ether.

Weight per ml. At 20°, 0.868 to 0.878 g.

Boiling-point. 90° to 100°.

Refractive index. 1.387.

Stability. Amyl nitrite is liable to decompose with evolution of nitrogen, particularly if it has become acid in reaction.
In the preparation of vitrellae, amyl nitrite should pass the following test before filling: shake 5 ml with 9 ml of water, 1 ml of 1N sodium hydroxide, and 1 drop of *phenolphthalein solution,* and allow to stand for 1 minute; the aqueous layer remains alkaline.

Incompatibility. It is incompatible with alcohol, alkali carbonates, caustic alkalis, bromides, iodides, ferrous salts, and phenazone.

Storage. It should be stored in airtight containers, in a cool place, protected from light.

Identification. TESTS. 1. To 4 drops add a mixture of 2 ml of *ferrous sulphate solution* and 5 ml of *dilute hydrochloric acid;* a greenish-brown colour is produced.
2. To 4 drops add 0.5 ml of aniline and 5 ml of glacial acetic acid; a deep-orange red colour is produced.
3. To 2 drops add 2 drops of water and 2 ml of sulphuric acid and dilute to 10 ml with water; the odour of amyl valerate is produced.

Metabolism. ABSORPTION. Absorbed through mucous membranes and absorption through the lungs is rapid.

METABOLIC REACTIONS. Rapidly hydrolysed to form amyl alcohol and nitrite; it is hydrolysed in the gastro-intestinal tract when administered orally and is therefore inactive by this route.

Actions and uses. Amyl nitrite, when inhaled, has actions similar to those described under Glyceryl Trinitrate. After inhalation it is rapidly absorbed, so that the onset of its effect is immediate; its actions last for 4 to 8 minutes.

The chief use of amyl nitrite is in the treatment of an attack of angina of effort; it is contra-indicated, however, in coronary thrombosis. The usual dose by inhalation is 0.12 to 0.3 millilitre. It is also used for the relief of renal and gall-bladder colic.

It is employed in the immediate treatment of cyanide poisoning to induce the formation of methaemoglobin, which combines with the cyanide to form the non-toxic cyanmethaemoglobin.

Poisoning. As for Glyceryl Trinitrate.

Preparation

AMYL NITRITE VITRELLAE: consisting of amyl nitrite enclosed in crushable glass capsules, as described in the entry on Vitrellae. In preparing the vitrellae, the precautions given under Stability (above) should be observed. Available as vitrellae containing 0.2 and 0.3 ml of amyl nitrite.

A standard for these vitrellae is given in the British Pharmaceutical Codex 1973

Containers: they should be supplied in shallow paperboard, metal, or plastic boxes.

Storage: they should be stored in a cool place, as decomposition of the contents may occur at higher temperatures, resulting in the loss of activity and development of high pressure.

Advice for patients: the vitrellae should be crushed between the finger and thumb and the vapour inhaled. They should not be used near a naked flame.

Amylobarbitone

5-Ethyl-5-isopentylbarbituric acid

$C_{11}H_{18}N_2O_3 = 226.3$

OTHER NAMES: Amobarbital; Amylobarb.; *Amytal®* *Drinamyl®* (with dexamphetamine sulphate); *Amylomet®* (with emetine hydrochloride); *Cardiacap A®* (with pentaerythritol tetranitrate); *Hypertane Compound®* (with rauwolfia alkaloids); *Amylozine®* (with trifluoperazine hydrochloride)

A standard is given in the British Pharmacopoeia 1973

Description. A white crystalline odourless powder with a slightly bitter taste.

Solubility. Very slightly soluble in water; soluble, at 20°, in 5 parts of alcohol, in 6 parts of ether, and in 20 parts of chloroform; soluble in solutions of alkali hydroxides and carbonates.

Dissociation constant. pK_a 8.0 (25°).

Hygroscopicity. It absorbs insignificant amounts of moisture at 25° at relative humidities up to about 90%.

Identification. TESTS. It complies with general tests 1 and 3 described under Barbiturates.

MELTING-POINT. About 156°.

ULTRAVIOLET ABSORPTION. In 0.1N sodium hydroxide, maxima at 220 nm (E1%, 1cm = 954) and 244 nm (E1%, 1cm = 365). See also under Barbiturates.

INFRA-RED ABSORPTION. Major peaks at 1319, 1354, 1431, 1696, 1725, and 1758 cm^{-1} (see Appendix 2a: Infra-red Spectra).

THIN-LAYER CHROMATOGRAPHY. See under Thin-layer Chromatography, System 5.

Determination in body fluids. See under Barbiturates.

Metabolism (see also under Barbiturates). ABSORPTION. Readily absorbed after oral administration.

BLOOD CONCENTRATION. After an oral dose of 200 mg of the sodium salt, a plasma concentration of 2 μg/ml is attained after 4 hours and this drops to about 1 μg/ml after 24 hours; in the elderly the 4-hour concentration varies over a wide range and the 24-hour concentration is raised.

HALF-LIFE. Serum half-life, 16 to 24 hours in adults and about 40 hours in the newborn.

DISTRIBUTION. Amylobarbitone crosses the placenta, is secreted in the milk, and is secreted in the saliva in concentrations which parallel those in the serum; the 3'-hydroxy metabolite accumulates in renal function impairment; volume of distribution, about 70 litres; *protein binding,* 40 to 60% bound to plasma proteins.

METABOLIC REACTIONS. Hydroxylation, to form the major metabolite 3'-hydroxyamylobarbitone, the extent of which is decreased in neonates and the elderly; N-hydroxylation also occurs but to a lesser extent; an additional metabolite, 5-(3'-carboxybutyl)-5-ethylbarbituric acid, formed by side-chain oxidation has also been identified.

EXCRETION. In 6 days, 80 to 90% of a dose is excreted in the urine and 4 to 5% is excreted in the faeces; of the excreted material, 30 to 50% is 3'-hydroxyamylobarbitone and 10 to 30% appears to be N-hydroxyamylobarbitone; less than 1% is excreted as unchanged drug in the urine.

FURTHER INFORMATION. 5-(3'-Carboxybutyl)-5-ethylbarbituric acid: a metabolite of amylobarbitone—W. Baldeo *et al., J. Pharm. Pharmac.,* 1977, **29**, 254; elimination of amylobarbitone in mothers and their newborn infants—B. Krauer *et al., Clin. Pharmac. Ther.,* 1973, **14**, 442 and G. H. Draffan *et al., Clin. Pharmac. Ther.,* 1976, **19**, 271; salivary excretion of amylobarbitone—T. Inaba and W. Kalow, *Clin. Pharmac. Ther.,* 1975, **18**, 558; some aspects of the fate of amylobarbitone in man—T. Inaba *et al., Clin. Pharmac. Ther.,* 1976, **20**, 439; N-hydroxyamobarbital: a major metabolite of amobarbital in man—B. K. Tang *et al., Drug Met. Disp.,* 1975, **3**, 479.

Actions and uses. Amylobarbitone is an intermediate-acting barbiturate, the actions and uses of which are described under Barbiturates.

It is given by mouth in a single dose of 100 to 200 milligrams as a hypnotic. Up to 400 milligrams may be given daily in divided doses as a sedative, the usual dose, however, being 30 to 60 milligrams daily.

Undesirable effects; Precautions; Contra-indications; Dependence. See under Barbiturates.

Poisoning. As for Barbiturates, but haemodialysis is not effective.

Preparations

AMYLOBARBITONE TABLETS (*Syn.* Amobarbital Tablets): available as tablets containing 15, 30, 50, 100, and 200 mg of amylobarbitone.

A standard for these tablets is given in the British Pharmacopoeia 1973

Containers and *Storage:* see the entry on Tablets for general information on containers and storage. Containers should be airtight.

Advice for patients: hypnotic doses should be taken half to 1 hour before bedtime. The tablets may cause drowsiness on the following day; persons affected should not drive or operate machinery. Alcohol should be avoided.

OTHER PREPARATIONS available include CAPSULES containing amylobarbitone 65 mg with dexamphetamine sulphate 10 mg in a slow-release formulation, capsules containing amylobarbitone 97 mg with dexamphetamine sulphate 15 mg in a slow-release formulation, capsules containing amylobarbitone 50 mg with pentaerythritol tetranitrate 30 mg in a slow-release formulation, capsules containing amylobarbitone 65 mg with trifluoperazine hydrochloride equivalent to 2 mg of trifluoperazine in a slow-release formulation; TABLETS containing amylobarbitone 32 mg with dexamphetamine sulphate 5 mg, tablets containing amylobarbitone 30 mg with emetine hydrochloride 200 micrograms, tablets containing amylobarbitone 100 mg with emetine hydrochloride 600 micrograms and tablets containing amylobarbitone 15 mg with rauwolfia alkaloids 2 mg.

Amylobarbitone Sodium

Sodium 5-ethyl-5-isopentylbarbiturate

$C_{11}H_{17}N_2NaO_3 = 248.3$

OTHER NAMES: Amobarbital Sodium; Amobarbitalum Natricum; Amylobarb. Sod.; *Sodium Amytal®*; Soluble Amylobarbitone
Tuinal® (with quinalbarbitone sodium)

A standard is given in the European Pharmacopoeia Vol. II

Description. A white, granular, hygroscopic, odourless powder with a bitter taste.

Solubility. Soluble, at 20°, in less than ½ part of water and in 2 parts of alcohol; practically insoluble in ether and in chloroform.

Alkalinity. A 10% solution has a pH of not more than 11.

Moisture content. Not more than 5%, determined by drying at 130°.

Stability; Incompatibility. See under Barbiturates.

Sterilisation. Sterile solutions of amylobarbitone sodium are prepared from sterile powder, immediately before use, by means of an aseptic technique, with water free from carbon dioxide. See also under Barbiturates.

Storage. It should be stored in airtight containers.

Identification. TESTS. 1. Dissolve about 100 mg in 10 ml of water, add 10 ml of *dilute acetic acid*, filter, wash the filter with water and dry the residue at 105°. The residue complies with general tests 1 and 3 described under Barbiturates.

MELTING-POINT. The residue obtained in Test 1, above, melts at about 156°.

Determination in body fluids. See under Barbiturates.

Metabolism. See under Amylobarbitone and also under Barbiturates.

Actions and uses. Amylobarbitone sodium is an intermediate-acting barbiturate, the actions and uses of which are described under Barbiturates and the oral dosage of which is described under Amylobarbitone; 1.1 grams of amylobarbitone sodium is approximately equivalent to 1 gram of amylobarbitone.

It is valuable as a pre-operative sedative when given the night before an operation and it can be used as a basal anaesthetic.

As it may sometimes cause restlessness it is no longer given to patients in labour.

Amylobarbitone sodium may be given by intravenous injection; the dose is 0.3 to 1 gram, adjusted according to the response; usually 500 milligrams is given slowly and this dose is repeated if necessary.

Undesirable effects; Precautions; Contra-indications; Dependence. See Barbiturates.

Poisoning. As for Barbiturates, but haemodialysis is not effective.

Preparations

AMYLOBARBITONE INJECTION: a sterile solution of amylobarbitone sodium in water for injections free from carbon dioxide. It is prepared, immediately before use, by dissolving the contents of a sealed container in water for injections free from carbon dioxide. Available as a powder in ampoules containing 0.125, 0.25, 0.5, and 1 g of amylobarbitone sodium.

A standard for this injection is given in the British Pharmacopoeia 1973

Containers and *Labelling:* see the entry on Injections for general information on containers and labelling.

Storage: the injection decomposes on storage and should be used immediately after preparation.

AMYLOBARBITONE SODIUM CAPSULES (*Syn.* Amobarbital Sodium Capsules; Soluble Amylobarbitone Capsules): consisting of amylobarbitone sodium, in powder, which may be mixed with a suitable inert diluent, enclosed in a hard capsule. The capsule shells may be coloured. Available as capsules containing 60 and 200 mg of amylobarbitone sodium.

A standard for these capsules is given in the British Pharmacopoeia 1973

Containers and *Storage:* see the entry on Capsules for general information on containers and storage.

Advice for patients: hypnotic doses should be taken 15 to 30 minutes before bedtime. The capsules may cause drowsiness on the following day; persons affected should not drive or operate machinery. Alcohol should be avoided.

AMYLOBARBITONE SODIUM TABLETS (*Syn.* Amobarbital Sodium Tablets; Soluble Amylobarbitone Tablets): available as tablets containing 60 and 200 mg of amylobarbitone sodium.

A standard for these tablets is given in the British Pharmacopoeia 1973

Containers and *Storage:* see the entry on Tablets for general information on containers and storage. Containers should be airtight.

Advice for patients: hypnotic doses should be taken 15 to 30 minutes before bedtime. The tablets may cause drowsiness on the following day; persons affected should not drive or operate machinery. Alcohol should be avoided.

OTHER PREPARATIONS available include CAPSULES containing amylobarbitone sodium 50 mg with quinalbarbitone sodium 50 mg, and capsules containing amylobarbitone sodium 100 mg with quinalbarbitone sodium 100 mg.

Anaemia

A condition of the blood in which there is reduction in the concentration of haemoglobin. There may be alteration of the character of the red cells. Symptoms are due to the reduced oxygen carrying capacity of the blood. Anaemia is characterised by weakness, fatigability, drowsiness, pallor, tachycardia, and dyspnoea on exertion. There may also be menstrual disturbances, oedema, a high pulse pressure, palpitations, or heart failure. Angina may occur in patients with coronary insufficiency. It may occur in any condition in which there is haemorrhage, iron loss, poor absorption, low iron intake, a decreased rate of erythropoiesis, or an accelerated destruction of red cells.

Iron-deficiency anaemia is due to inadequate intake of iron or to loss of iron by haemorrhage. Usually the red cells are small (microcytic) and contain less than the normal amount of haemoglobin (hypochromic). This type of anaemia may be treated by the administration of iron compounds as described under Ferrous Sulphate; ferrous and ferric salts are used.

Vitamin B_{12} and folic acid deficiency anaemia (megaloblastic anaemia) is anaemia in which the erythrocytes fail to mature normally because there is a deficiency of either vitamin B_{12} or folic acid. There are fewer red cells but they are larger than normal (macrocytic) and contain the usual quantity of haemoglobin (normochromic). The megaloblastic anaemia is associated with leucopenia, thrombocytopenia, and glossitis. Both folic acid deficiency and vitamin B_{12} deficiency may give rise to gastro-intestinal disturbances including diarrhoea. In addition, untreated vitamin B_{12} deficiency may give rise to neurological disturbances, resulting in myelin degeneration of the posterior and pyramidal tracts of the spinal cord (subacute combined degeneration of the spinal cord). Since other manifestations of vitamin B_{12} deficiency may respond to folic acid, correct diagnosis and treatment is important. Hydroxocobalamin may be used as a source of vitamin B_{12}.

Megaloblastic anaemia due to folic acid deficiency may occur in the elderly, in alcoholics, during pregnancy, in the malabsorption syndrome due to any cause, after continuous administration of large doses of folic acid antagonists such as pyrimethamine or methotrexate, or in epileptics on continuous anticonvulsant treatment. In this last condition the folic acid deficiency may lead to mental deterioration, which can be prevented by giving folic acid and vitamin B_{12} (hydroxocobalamin).

Megaloblastic anaemia due to vitamin B_{12} deficiency occurs in vegetarians who do not eat any animal foodstuffs. It also occurs when there is absence of the intrinsic factor produced by the stomach, which is necessary for the absorption of vitamin B_{12}. Cyanocobalamin labelled with cobalt-57 or -58 is used in the diagnosis of this condition. Absence of intrinsic factor is characteristic of Addisonian pernicious anaemia and also occurs after total gastrectomy.

Haemolytic anaemia is a condition in which there is increased destruction of red cells. The red cells present are usually of normal size and contain the normal quantity of haemoglobin. It may be accompanied by hyperbilirubinaemia, jaundice, splenomegaly, or hepatomegaly. If the haemolysis is intravascular there may also be haemoglobinuria and oliguria. Haemolytic anaemia may be hereditary or due to a reaction to incompatible blood transfusion, chemicals, drugs, infection, autoimmune processes, or other systemic diseases. It is treated by the elimination of the haemolytic agent and the maintenance of fluid balance and renal function.

Aplastic anaemia is a condition in which there is inadequate cell formation as a result of degeneration of the bone marrow. The red cells present are usually of normal size and contain the normal quantity of haemoglobin. If severe, it may be accompanied by thrombocytopenia. It may be idiopathic or due to exposure to certain chemicals such as inorganic arsenic, antineoplastic agents, or ionizing radiation, or as an idiosyncratic reaction to drugs such as chloramphenicol, phenylbutazone, mepacrine, or methoin.

Aplastic anaemia is treated by the removal of the offending substance where possible and transfusion of whole blood until the bone marrow resumes function. Androgens and corticosteroids may be tried to stimulate the bone marrow. The condition has a high mortality.

Anaesthesia

The term anaesthesia is usually applied to the induction of controlled sensory loss sufficient to permit surgical operations. A general anaesthetic is a drug capable of causing loss of sensation together with loss of consciousness and a local anaesthetic is a drug that will induce sensory impairment in a restricted area of the body but without loss of consciousness.

General anaesthesia. Patients undergoing general anaesthesia are usually subjected to three interdependent procedures: premedication following physical examination, the induction of reversible unconsciousness, with analgesics and muscular relaxants as required, and appropriate post-operative care.

PREMEDICATION. Given before surgery, premedicant drugs ideally provide the following three effects: a degree of sedation or tranquillity for the anxious patient and some degree of amnesia subsequently, a reduction in bronchial and salivary secretion, bradycardia, and post-operative vomiting by parasympathetic inhibition, and analgesia to minimise central stimulation during operation in addition to reducing post-operative pain.

The choice of premedicant drugs depends on many factors, including the age and medical history of the patient, the nature of the disease in question, and the nature of the operative procedure and anaesthetic agents to be used. It is becoming increasingly the practice to use oral premedicants, especially the benzodiazepine sedatives on both the night before and the morning of the operation. The oral route is more pleasant for patients and the drugs used are less likely to cause respiratory depression. However, a mixture of analgesic and parasympatholytic drugs administered subcutaneously remains the most widely used premedication. Such mixtures include morphine, papaveretum, or pethidine with hyoscine, atropine, or a phenothiazine derivative.

GENERAL ANAESTHESIA DURING SURGERY. General anaesthetics are given by inhalation or intravenously, these routes permitting some control of the blood levels of the agents used. Anaesthesia is commonly induced by the intravenous administration of a short-acting barbiturate such as methohexitone or thiopentone, or by propanidid and maintained thereafter by means of an inhalational agent, for example, chloroform, cyclopropane, ether, halothane, methoxyflurane, nitrous oxide, trichloroethylene or vinyl ether; these substances also possess analgesic properties. Additional analgesia may be provided during anaesthesia by the intravenous administration of pethidine.

Muscular relaxation is commonly required during general anaesthesia and may be provided by neuromuscular blocking drugs of the depolarising (suxamethonium) type generally used for short procedures and longer-acting non-depolarising (gallamine and tubocurarine) type neuromuscular blocking agents to maintain relaxation for prolonged periods. Neuromuscular paralysis caused by non-depolarising agents is reversed by anticholinesterases (neostigmine and pyridostigmine) which do not reverse the action of depolarising relaxants. Relaxation can also be induced by increasing the concentration of inhalational anaesthetic or by nerve block with a local anaesthetic.

POST-OPERATIVE TREATMENT. The central depressant effects of morphine-like analgesics and the myorelaxant effects of neuromuscular blockers must be reversed if they persist when recovery of consciousness is required. The patient must never be left unattended in the absence of protective reflexes and circulatory stability. Treatment of post-operative pain and vomiting is commonly required.

Local anaesthesia. Local anaesthetics, such as amethocaine, benzocaine, bupivacaine, cinchocaine, cocaine, cyclomethycaine, lignocaine, prilocaine, and procaine, are drugs which block nerve conduction and although they are used for their action on sensory nerve activity they can affect neurone bodies as well as fibres to prevent the genesis or propagation of impulses. Apart from nerves, other conductile tissues like cardiac muscle are affected by local anaesthetics, a property utilised in the treatment of myocardial dysrhythmias with lignocaine or procainamide.

The ease with which fibres in nerve trunks are affected is inversely related to their diameter, the finer sensory nerves being blocked first.

Local anaesthetics are used in several ways. *Surface anaesthesia* is produced by topical application on skin or mucous membranes. *Infiltration anaesthesia* or paralysis of small cutaneous nerves in a localised area is produced by injection into the tissues around the part to be anaesthetised. *Regional anaesthesia* is sensory paralysis produced by local anaesthetic injection around an appropriate nerve or nerve plexus. Such nerve block may also affect motor fibres and cause muscular relaxation. Epidural (injection in epidural space), caudal, paravertebral, and spinal anaesthesia are all varieties of regional anaesthesia. Spinal anaesthetics are given by intrathecal injection, and solutions of greater density than the cerebrospinal fluid fall to the part of the spinal column affecting the lower limbs, while solutions of lower density than cerebrospinal fluid affect the thoracic region and solutions with the same density as cerebrospinal fluid affect the nerves at the level where the injection is made. Vasoconstrictor drugs like noradrenaline and adrenaline help to limit the spread of a local anaesthetic from its sites of injection, and thereby prolong its effect.

Ancylostomiasis

A bowel infection caused by the hookworms *Ancylostoma duodenale* and *Necator americanus*.

Ova develop in warm, moist soil and infect man through the skin of the feet where they may cause a local dermatitis ("ground itch"). The larvae pass by way of the bloodstream to the lungs where they ascend the trachea and pass down the oesophagus to the small intestine and develop into adult worms. Here they may live for many years producing ova which are passed out in the faeces. The worms feed upon blood, and if present in sufficient numbers, cause iron-deficiency anaemia accompanied by abdominal discomfort, poor nutrition, and lassitude. Hypoalbuminaemia may also occur.

Sanitation is most important in the prophylaxis of hookworm infection.

Substances used in the treatment of hookworm infection include bephenium, hexylresorcinol, and tetrachloroethylene. In severe infections, the patient's general condition may require treatment before the hookworms. Various animal hookworms may invade man. They burrow in the skin at a rate of about 10 mm per day giving rise to intense pruritus ("creeping eruption"). They may be treated with thiabendazole.

Angina Pectoris

A condition in which there is anoxia of cardiac muscle resulting from coronary artery insufficiency.

Attacks may be precipitated by exertion or emotion and are most likely to occur in patients whose coronary arteries are partially occluded by arteriosclerotic lesions. The condition is characterised by paroxysmal pain in the chest which may extend to the shoulder, arms, neck, and jaw.

Patients should regulate the amount of exercise taken so as to minimise the occurrence of attacks, and emotional disturbances and overwork should be avoided. β-Adrenoceptor blocking agents, such as oxprenolol or propranolol, that reduce the oxygen requirement of the heart or vasodilators, such as amyl nitrite, glyceryl trinitrate, or pentaerythritol tetranitrate, that reduce cardiac work and may also increase the myocardial blood supply may be employed to prevent or relieve attacks. When these measures are not successful surgery may be required.

Anise Oil

Obtained by distillation from the dried fruits of star anise, *Illicium verum* Hook. f. (Fam. Illiciaceae), a tree indigenous to south-western China, or from anise, the dried fruits of *Pimpinella anisum* L. (Fam. Umbelliferae), an annual plant cultivated chiefly in Spain, southern Russia, and Bulgaria.

OTHER NAMES: Aniseed Oil; Oleum Anisi

A standard is given in the British Pharmacopoeia 1973

Constituents. Anise oil contains about 80 to 90% of anethole. It contains, in addition, chavicol methyl ether, also known as estragol, an isomer of anethole, which it resembles in odour but not in taste, and *p*-methoxyphenylacetone (anise ketone).

Description. A colourless or pale yellow highly refractive liquid with the characteristic odour of the crushed fruit. When cooled it solidifies at about 15° to a white crystalline mass, but it can be cooled considerably below this temperature without becoming solid provided it is undisturbed; the supercooled liquid immediately solidifies if slightly agitated or if a crystal of anethole is introduced. The crystalline mass melts at about 17°.

Solubility. Soluble, at 20°, in 3 parts of alcohol (90%), sometimes with a slight opalescence.

Weight per ml. At 20°, 0.978 to 0.992 g.

Refractive Index. 1.553 to 1.560.

Optical rotation. $-2°$ to $+1°$.

Stability. Exposure to air causes polymerisaton and some oxidation also takes place with the formation of p-methoxybenzaldehyde (anisaldehyde) and anisic acid.

Storage. It should be stored in well-filled containers, in a cool place, protected from light. If it has solidified, it should be completely melted and mixed before use.

Actions and uses. Anise oil is a carminative and mild expectorant. It is used in mixtures and cough lozenges, often in conjunction with liquorice. The usual dose is 0.05 to 0.2 millilitre.

Preparation

CONCENTRATED ANISE WATER:

Anise oil	20 ml
Alcohol (90%)	700 ml
Water for preparations	to 1000 ml

Dissolve the anise oil in the alcohol and add sufficient of the water, in successive small portions, to produce 1000 ml, shaking vigorously after each addition; add 50 g of sterilised purified talc or other suitable filtering aid, shake occasionally during a few hours, and filter.
A standard for this concentrated water is given in the British Pharmaceutical Codex 1973
Dose: 0.3 to 1 millilitre.

Anise Water is prepared by diluting concentrated anise water with 39 times its volume of water for preparations.

Ankylosing Spondylitis

A chronic arthritis of spinal articulations and the sacro-iliac joints occurring mainly in men aged 20 to 40 years. It is characterised by an inflammatory arthropathy with the formation of granulation tissue leading to erosive changes in the joints. It is often accompanied by a raised erythrocyte sedimentation rate but serological tests for rheumatoid factor are negative.

The disease starts as a low backache together with morning stiffness which gradually progresses upwards. Iritis occurs in about 20% of cases and may be treated by the local application of eye-drops of atropine and corticosteroids. Rare complications include cardiac conduction defects and aortic incompetence. Deformity may become permanent owing to ossification of the joints unless appropriate exercises are provided to maintain the spinal musculature and joint mobility. The disease process may be arrested in the early stages by radiotherapy but this treatment increases the risk of leukaemia. Non-steroidal anti-inflammatory drugs are used to relieve symptoms.

Antazoline Hydrochloride

N-Benzyl-N-(2-imidazolin-2-ylmethyl)aniline hydrochloride

$C_{17}H_{20}ClN_3 = 301.8$

A standard is given in the British Pharmacopoeia 1973

Description. A white crystalline odourless powder with a bitter taste.

Solubility. Soluble, at 20°, in 50 parts of water and in 16 parts of alcohol; very slightly soluble in chloroform and in ether.

Acidity. A 1% solution has a pH of 5 to 6.5.

Dissociation constant. pK_a 10.0 (25°).

Sterilisation. Solutions are sterilised by heating in an autoclave or by filtration.

Storage. It should be stored in airtight containers, protected from light.

Identification. TEST. Dissolve about 50 mg in 5 ml of water and add 0.5 ml of nitric acid; a red colour is produced which quickly changes to dark green.

MELTING-POINT. About 240°, with decomposition.

ULTRAVIOLET ABSORPTION. In 0.1N hydrochloric acid, maxima at 241 nm (E1%, 1cm = 500) and 291 nm (E1%, 1cm = 65).

Determination in body fluids. COLORIMETRY. In urine: interference from metabolites is stated to be avoided—N. Wahba, *et al.*, *Pharmazie*, 1974, **29**, 790.

Metabolism. ABSORPTION. Readily absorbed after oral or parenteral administration.

EXCRETION. About 1.5% of an oral dose is excreted unchanged in the urine in 24 hours.

Actions and uses. Antazoline has the actions, uses, and undesirable effects of the antihistamine drugs, as described under Promethazine Hydrochloride; it is one of the weakest of these compounds. It is about 15 times less active than promethazine hydrochloride and the duration of action is shorter.

Antazoline hydrochloride is administered by mouth; it is also applied as a 0.5% solution to the skin and to the mucous membrane of the eye and nose. A 2% cream or ointment is used as an antipruritic, but it is less effective than preparations containing corticosteroids and it may give rise to skin sensitisation.

The usual dose is 100 to 300 milligrams daily in divided doses.

Poisoning. As for Promethazine Hydrochloride.

Antazoline Mesylate

N-Benzyl-N-(2-imidazolin-2-ylmethyl)aniline methanesulphonate

$C_{17}H_{19}N_3, CH_3SO_3H = 361.5$

OTHER NAME: Antazoline Methanesulphonate

A standard is given in the British Pharmaceutical Codex 1973

Description. A white odourless powder.

Solubility. Soluble, at 20°, in 6 parts of water, in 7 parts of alcohol, and in 12 parts of chloroform; practically insoluble in ether.

Acidity. A 1% solution has a pH of 4 to 6.5.

Moisture content. Not more than 2.5%, determined by drying over phosphorus pentoxide *in vacuo*.

Hygroscopicity. It is slightly hygroscopic, significant amounts of moisture being absorbed at 20° at relative humidities above about 70%.

Sterilisation. Solutions are sterilised by heating in an autoclave in sealed containers in which the air has been replaced by nitrogen or other suitable gas, or by filtration.

Storage. It should be stored in airtight containers, protected from light.

Identification. TESTS. 1. Dissolve about 500 mg in 30 ml of water, add 1 ml of *sodium hydroxide solution*, extract with 20 ml of chloroform, wash the extract with 5 ml of water, and evaporate off the chloroform; the residue, after drying over phosphorus pentoxide *in vacuo*, melts at about 121°.
2. Dissolve about 50 mg in 5 ml of water and add 0.5 ml of nitric acid; a red colour is produced which rapidly becomes green.

MELTING-POINT. About 166°.

ULTRAVIOLET ABSORPTION. In 0.1N hydrochloric acid, maximum at 243 nm (E1%, 1cm = 398).

INFRA-RED ABSORPTION. Major peaks at 700, 750, 1042, 1164, 1508, and 1599 cm^{-1} (see Appendix 2a: Infra-red Spectra).

THIN-LAYER CHROMATOGRAPHY. See under Thin-layer Chromatography, System 4.

Determination in body fluids; Metabolism. See under Antazoline Hydrochloride.

Actions and uses. Antazoline mesylate has the actions and uses, described under Antazoline Hydrochloride. It is usually given by injection in a solution containing 50 milligrams in 1 millilitre. The usual dose is 50 to 100 milligrams by intramuscular or slow intravenous injection.

Poisoning. As for Promethazine Hydrochloride.

Antibiotics

see under ANTIMICROBIALS

Anticoagulant and Preservative Solutions for Blood

Sterile pyrogen-free solutions of sodium citrate or sodium acid citrate and dextrose in water for injections. They may contain appropriate quantities of citric acid or sodium acid phosphate as buffering agents. Suitable solutions may be prepared according to the following formulae.

Acid Citrate Dextrose Solution (ACD)

Formula A: sodium citrate 22 g, citric acid monohydrate 8 g (*or* anhydrous citric acid 7.3 g), dextrose monohydrate for parenteral use 24.5 g (*or* anhydrous dextrose 22.4 g), water for injections to 1000 ml. Volume for the collection of 100 ml of blood: 15 ml.

Formula B: sodium citrate 13.2 g, citric acid monohydrate 4.8 g (*or* anhydrous citric acid 4.4 g), dextrose monohydrate for parenteral use 14.7 g (*or* anhydrous dextrose 13.4 g), water for injections to 1000 ml. Volume for the collection of 100 ml of blood: 25 ml.

Formula C: sodium acid citrate 29 to 40 g, dextrose monohydrate for parenteral use 25 g (*or* anhydrous dextrose 22.9 g), water for injections to 1000 ml. Volume for the collection of 100 ml of blood: 15 ml.

Formula D: sodium acid citrate 20 to 25 g, dextrose monohydrate for parenteral use 30 g (*or* anhydrous dextrose 27.4 g), water for injections to 1000 ml. Volume for the collection of 100 ml of blood: 28.6 ml.

Citrate Phosphate Dextrose Solution

Sodium citrate 26.3 g, citric acid monohydrate 3.27 g (*or* anhydrous citric acid 2.99 g), dextrose monohydrate for parenteral use 25.5 g (*or* anhydrous dextrose 23.2 g), sodium acid phosphate 2.51 g, water for injections to 1000 ml. Volume for the collection of 100 ml of blood: 14 ml.

A standard for the above solutions is given in the British Pharmacopoeia Addendum 1978

Preparation of Solutions. Dissolve the ingredients of the required formulation in the water for injections, add sufficient of the water for injections to produce the required volume, and clarify by filtration. Immediately distribute the solution into the final containers, seal, and sterilise by heating in an autoclave without delay.

Containers. See the entry on Solutions for general information on containers.

Labelling. See the entry on Solutions for general information on labelling. The direction that the label on the sealed container states that the solution is not to be used for injection does not apply to this preparation. In addition, the label on the container should state the composition and volume of the solution, the date after which the solution is not intended to be used, and the conditions under which it should be stored.

Storage. The solutions should be protected from light.

Uses. The solutions are used to prevent the coagulation of blood which is collected for transfusion or for the preparation of other blood products. The acidity of the solutions minimises caramelisation during sterilisation and the dextrose delays haemolysis of the red blood corpuscles.

Antihaemophilic Fraction, Human, Dried

Dried human antihaemophilic fraction is prepared from human plasma; it is rich in clotting factor VIII.

A standard is given in the British Pharmacopoeia Addendum 1978

The human plasma is obtained from blood from human subjects who comply with the requirements for donors given under Blood, Whole Human. The blood is withdrawn aseptically into a suitable anticoagulant solution. During withdrawal there should be no interruption in the flow from the donor and the container should be gently agitated.

Immediately after withdrawal is complete the blood is cooled to 4° and the plasma is separated from cellular components by centrifugation as soon as possible and not later than 18 hours after collection. Fractionation is begun without delay or, if this is not possible, the plasma is immediately frozen and stored at $-30°$ or below until fractionated.

Human antihaemophilic fraction may be prepared from human plasma so obtained by precipitation under controlled conditions of pH, ionic strength, and temperature, with organic solvents or by freezing and thawing. The precipitate may be washed by extraction with suitable solvents dissolved in sodium citrate solution adjusted to pH 6.8 to 7.2, which may also contain sodium chloride.

The solution is sterilised by filtration through a membrane filter and immediately frozen and dried. No preservative is added.

It is a white powder or friable solid which, when dissolved in a volume of water equal to the volume of water for injections stated on the label, yields a solution which contains not less than 3 units per ml, not less than 0.1 unit per mg of protein of which not more than 80% is fibrinogen, not more than 200 millimoles of sodium ions per litre, and not more than 55 millimoles of citrate ions per litre.

Storage. It should be stored in an atmosphere of nitrogen or *in vacuo*, in sterile containers sealed to exclude micro-organisms and moisture, at a temperature below 6°, and protected from light.

The reconstituted solution should be used immediately after preparation and should be discarded if not used within 3 hours.

Actions and uses. Dried human antihaemophilic fraction is used specifically to control bleeding in haemophiliacs who have a deficiency of coagulation factor VIII. The amount transfused depends upon the circumstances, particularly the immediate cause of the bleeding and the severity of the haemophilia. The object of treatment is to raise the concentration of plasma antihaemophilic globulin to at least 30% of normal and to maintain it at this level until bleeding has ceased. For further information see the entry on Haemophilia.

The use of dried human antihaemophilic fraction carries a risk of transmitting hepatitis, as explained in the entry on Blood Products. A filter should be incorporated in the apparatus used for administration of the reconstituted product.

Antimicrobials

Antimicrobials are substances that are capable even in high dilution of killing or inhibiting the growth of micro-organisms. They may be subdivided into **antibiotics** which are derived from the growth of micro-organisms and **chemotherapeutic substances** which are synthetic agents not occurring naturally. It should be noted that some antibiotics have little or no antimicrobial activity but exhibit a cytotoxic effect on mammalian cells especially tumour cells.

Antibiotics may be classified according to their chemical constitution or on the basis of their activity against various groups of micro-organisms.

Chemical Classification of Antibiotics

Aminoglycosides which contain in their structure glycosides and amino-sugars include framycetin, gentamicin, kanamycin, neomycin, streptomycin, and tobramycin.

Spectinomycin is related chemically, but as it contains no amino-sugar moiety it is classified as an *aminocyclitol*, not an aminoglycoside.

Cephalosporins have a ring structure (5-thia-1-azabicyclo[4.2.0]octane) chemically related to that of the penicillins. The main characteristics of the cephalosporins are described under Cephaloridine but some modification of activity occurs on changing the side-chains in positions 3 and 7. Some of the cephalosporins are suitable for administration by mouth and some by injection. They include cephalexin, cephaloridine, cephalothin, cephazolin, and cephradine.

Macrolides contain in their structure a large lactone ring. They include erythromycin and rifampicin. This group also includes oleandomycin and spiramycin.

Penicillins are based on an unstable ring structure known as the beta-lactam structure with various side-chains mainly in position 6. The ring structure may be defined as 4-thia-1-azabicyclo[3.2.0]heptane or azeto[2,1-b]thiazole. The beta-lactam structure also occurs in the cephalosporins.

The main properties of the penicillins are described under Benzylpenicillin. By changing the side-chain at position 6 penicillins with a variety of properties are obtained; some are acid stable and may be administered by mouth, some are resistant to staphylococcal penicillinase, and some are effective against bacteria that are resistant to benzylpenicillin. Sparingly soluble salts of penicillin such as the benethamine, benzathine, and procaine salts of benzylpenicillin are used in the formulation of sustained-release preparations. Penicillins include amoxycillin, ampicillin, benzylpenicillin, carbenicillin, cloxacillin, flucloxacillin, methicillin, phenethicillin, phenoxymethylpenicillin, and propicillin. This group also includes carfecillin, mecillinam, and talampicillin.

Polyenes contain in their structure a number (4, 5, 6, or 7) of conjugated double bonds. The best known polyenes have antifungal properties; they include amphotericin and nystatin. This group includes candicidin.

Polypeptide antibiotics contain in their structure a number of peptide-linked amino-acid residues. They include bacitracin, capreomycin, colistin, and polymyxin B. This group also includes bleomycin.

Tetracyclines include a number of variations on the basic 1,11-dioxonaphthacene-2-carboxamide structure of tetracycline. The main properties of this group are described under Tetracycline Hydrochloride. They include chlortetracycline, demeclocycline, doxycycline, lymecycline, methacycline, minocycline, oxytetracycline, and tetracycline. The antitumour agents daunorubicin and doxorubicin have a related structure.

Miscellaneous antibiotics. A number of antibiotics are not related to any recognised group and are usually considered individually. They include chloramphenicol, clindamycin, cycloserine, fusidic acid, griseofulvin, lincomycin, novobiocin, vancomycin, and viomycin. This group also includes the antitumour agents actinomycin C and actinomycin D.

Chemotherapeutic substances

Certain synthetic chemical substances are used for a similar purpose to antibiotics. They include clotrimazole, ethambutol, flucytosine, isoniazid, metronidazole, miconazole, nalidixic acid, nitrofurantoin, pyrazinamide, sodium aminosalicylate, sulphonamides, and trimethoprim.

Classification According to Antimicrobial Spectrum

Bacteria may be divided into Gram-positive and Gram-negative types and may be coccal or rod shaped.

Gram-positive genera include *Bacillus, Clostridium, Corynebacterium, Micrococcus,* and *Streptococcus.* Gram-negative genera include *Brucella, Escherichia, Haemophilus, Klebsiella, Neisseria, Pasteurella, Proteus, Pseudomonas, Salmonella, Serratia, Shigella,* and *Vibrio.*

A classification of antimicrobials according to the spectrum of activity is given below.

Active against Gram-positive bacteria and Gram-negative cocci: clindamycin and lincomycin (not for *Neisseria*), erythromycin, fusidic acid, standard penicillins (benzylpenicillin, phenoxymethylpenicillin), antistaphylococcal penicillins (cloxacillin, flucloxacillin, methicillin), rifampicin (mainly used for tuberculosis), and spectinomycin (used in the treatment of penicillin-resistant gonococci).

Active against Gram-negative bacilli (this group includes some penicillins that are also effective against Gram-positive organisms and some aminoglycosides that are effective against staphylococci).

FOR SYSTEMIC USE:

Aminoglycosides (gentamicin, kanamycin, streptomycin, and tobramycin; some of the foregoing are used also for tuberculosis).

Penicillins (amoxycillin, ampicillin, carbenicillin, carfecillin, mecillinam, and talampicillin).

Polypeptides (bacitracin, colistin, and polymyxin B).

FOR URINARY INFECTIONS ONLY:

Nalidixic acid and nitrofurantoin. This group also includes hexamine and hexamine mandelate.

FOR TOPICAL USE:

Neomycin.

BROAD-SPECTRUM ANTIMICROBIALS:

Cephalosporins (cephalexin, cephaloridine, cephalothin, cephazoline and cephradine).

Chloramphenicol.

Sulphonamides (sulphadiazine, sulphadimidine, sulphafurazole, etc.; also co-trimoxazole).

Tetracyclines (chlortetracycline, doxycycline, lymecycline, methacycline, minocycline, oxytetracycline, and tetracycline).

Used for specific infections

Anaerobic organisms—lincomycin and metronidazole.

Tuberculosis—capreomycin, cycloserine, ethambutol, isoniazid, pyrazinamide, rifampicin, sodium aminosalicylate, streptomycin and other aminoglycosides, and viomycin.

Antifungals—amphotericin, candicidin, clotrimazole, flucytosine, griseofulvin, miconazole, and nystatin.

Antivirals—amantadine, cytarabine, idoxuridine, and methisazone.

Administration

Antibiotics and other antimicrobials should be selected and used in a manner that will minimise the spread of resistant organisms, as described in the entry on Resistance to Antibiotics.

Antibiotics used systemically for the treatment of acute infections are usually prescribed in short courses lasting up to a week or 10 days. The doses should be administered at regular intervals so as to maintain adequate blood levels and a prescribed course of treatment should be completed even though the symptoms have subsided. Many antibiotics, especially penicillins, are not well absorbed when given by mouth but absorption is improved if they are taken on an empty stomach; the absorption of others, notably fusidic acid and griseofulvin, is improved by the presence of fatty food and bile in the gut and they should be taken with or after meals.

Antimony Potassium Tartrate

$C_4H_4KO_7Sb = 324.9$

OTHER NAMES: Antim. Pot. Tart.; Potassium Antimonyltartrate; Tartar Emetic

A standard is given in the British Pharmaceutical Codex 1973

Description. Odourless colourless transparent crystals or white granular powder with a sweet taste.

Solubility. Soluble, at 20°, in 13 parts of water and in 20 parts of glycerol; soluble in 3 parts of boiling water; practically insoluble in alcohol.

Acidity. Solutions in water are acid to litmus.

Moisture content. It may occur as the hemihydrate with about 2.7% of moisture, but the salt effloresces in dry air, and the commercial material rarely contains more than 1% of moisture. The salt becomes anhydrous at 100° and does not readily rehydrate on exposure to the atmosphere.

Stability. A solution prepared for injection, after sterilisation, may be expected to show no increase in toxicity when stored at temperatures ranging from 4° to 40° for 1 year.

FURTHER INFORMATION. Effects of sterilisation and storage on toxicity of injections—G. F. Somers and T. D. Whittet, *Pharm. J.*, ii/1958, 494.

Incompatibility. It is incompatible with acids and alkalis, salts of heavy metals, albumin, soap, and tannins.

Sterilisation. Solutions for injection are sterilised by heating in an autoclave or by filtration.

Storage. It should be stored in airtight containers.

Actions and uses. Antimony potassium tartrate has the actions, uses, and undesirable effects described under Antimony Sodium Tartrate and is used in similar dosage. It is less soluble and more irritant than the sodium salt, which is therefore more suitable for intravenous injection.

It was formerly used as an emetic in a dose of 30 to 60 milligrams but has been superseded by safer drugs.

Precautions; Poisoning. As for Antimony Sodium Tartrate.

Antimony Sodium Tartrate

$C_4H_4NaO_7Sb = 308.8$

OTHER NAMES: Antim. Sod. Tart.; Sodium Antimonyltartrate

A standard is given in the British Pharmacopoeia 1973

Description. Colourless or whitish, odourless, hygroscopic scales or powder, with a sweetish taste.

Solubility. Soluble, at 20°, in 1.5 parts of water; practically insoluble in alcohol.

Acidity. Solutions in water are acid to litmus.

Moisture content. Not more than 6%, determined by drying at 105°.

Stability. The solution for injection, after sterilisation, shows no increase in toxicity when stored at temperatures ranging from 4° to 40° for 1 year.

FURTHER INFORMATION. Effects of sterilisation and storage on toxicity of injections—G. F. Somers and T. D. Whittet, *Pharm. J.*, ii/1958, 494.

Incompatibility. It is incompatible with acids and alkalis, salts of heavy metals, albumin, soap, and tannins.

Sterilisation. Solutions for injection are sterilised by heating in an autoclave or by filtration.

Storage. It should be stored in airtight containers.

BLOOD CONCENTRATION. Blood concentrations of antimony are variable but in untreated subjects they are about 3 ng/ml and in treated subjects during the 6 months after treatment, up to about 33 ng/ml.

DISTRIBUTION. Antimony accumulates in the body and may persist in elevated concentrations for over a year after treatment.

EXCRETION. Slowly excreted in bile and urine.

FURTHER INFORMATION. M. M. Mansour et al., Nature Lond., 1967, **214**, 819.

Actions and uses. Antimony sodium tartrate has an irritant action on mucous membranes and when given by mouth causes nausea and vomiting. It is used in the treatment of schistosomiasis.

The initial dose is 30 milligrams given by slow intravenous injection, care being taken to avoid leakage into the surrounding tissues. On the second day 60 milligrams is given; on the third day 90 milligrams; and on the fourth day 120 milligrams; thereafter a dose of 120 milligrams is given on every other day until a total of 1.2 to 2.4 grams has been administered. A total dose of 1.8 grams usually suffices for the treatment of Schistosoma haematobium infection but for S. mansoni and S. japonicum infections a total dose of 1.8 to 2.4 grams may be needed. The course may be repeated after an interval of 2 months. The dose for children is initially 500 micrograms per kilogram body-weight and the maximum total dose 30 to 35 milligrams per kilogram body-weight.

Antimony sodium tartrate is also used for the treatment of mucocutaneous leishmaniasis for which the dose is 100 milligrams given by slow intravenous injection on alternate days. The total dose is up to 1.5 grams. The single dose for children is 1.5 milligrams per kilogram body-weight, with a total dose of 20 milligrams per kilogram.

Undesirable effects. Undesirable effects frequently occur and include cough, anorexia, nausea, vomiting, diarrhoea, and abdominal, thoracic, muscle, and joint pains. Acute vascular collapse resembling an anaphylactic response sometimes occurs.

Changes in the electrocardiogram are usually observed during treatment, the most common being flattening or inversion of the T-wave. This effect is a property of all organic trivalent antimony derivatives.

Precautions. Antimony sodium tartrate should never be given by intramuscular or subcutaneous injection because it causes severe pain and tissue necrosis; great care should be taken not to inject solutions outside the vein. Antimony sodium tartrate should only be given under skilled supervision with the patient at complete bed-rest. It should not be given to patients with liver, kidney, or serious circulatory and heart disease, severe anaemia, or tuberculosis.

Poisoning. In antimony poisoning persistent vomiting and diarrhoea occur, followed by muscular weakness, suppression of urine, collapse, and convulsions.

Treatment should be designed to remove the poison; if the drug has been taken by mouth and vomiting has not occurred, the stomach should be washed out. Calcium hydroxide, or magnesium oxide may be given to precipitate the antimony in the stomach.

In poisoning caused by intravenous injection of antimony salts, the heart is frequently affected and artificial cardiac stimulation may be required for a while; the patient must be kept warm and a high fluid intake ensured. Injections of dimercaprol should be given.

Preparation

ANTIMONY SODIUM TARTRATE INJECTION (Syn. Sodium Antimonyltartrate Injection): a sterile solution of antimony sodium tartrate in water for injections. It is sterilised by heating in an autoclave or by filtration. Available as an injection containing 60 mg of antimony sodium tartrate per ml.

A standard for this injection is given in the British Pharmacopoeia 1973

Containers and Labelling: see the entry on Injections for general information on containers and labelling.

Antisera

OTHER NAME: Immunosera

Antisera are preparations from native sera containing substances that have a specific prophylactic or therapeutic action when injected into persons exposed to or suffering from a disease due to a specific micro-organism. In preparing antisera, preparations from cultures of the specific organisms or their products are injected into horses or other animals so as to produce immunity, a condition which is manifested by the formation of **antibodies** in the animals' blood. Antibodies are associated with the globulin fraction of plasma or serum.

The general term **antigen** is used to describe any substance which, when injected into the body, will elicit the formation of antibodies, substances which are antagonistic to or otherwise reactive with the antigen. The antigens in common use include toxins, toxoids, and bacterial and viral vaccines.

Antisera are usually concentrated; leptospira antiserum and snake venom antiserum are exceptions. In the case of antitoxic sera, the globulins or their derivatives are obtained by treatment with a proteolytic enzyme; pepsin-treated antitoxic sera are usually termed refined antitoxins. It is desirable to use purified products whenever possible so as to avoid the injection of excessive amounts of foreign proteins which may give rise to reactions. The injection of animal protein may be avoided by the use of the appropriate human immunoglobulin (if available) in place of antiserum.

Antitoxic sera. In preparing antitoxic sera, the antigen used is either the specific toxin, or, more usually, the toxoid. Toxins are poisonous substances which are excreted into the substrate when certain pathogenic bacteria are grown in artificial culture media and they can be demonstrated in the media after the organisms have been removed by filtration; they are sometimes referred to as soluble toxins or **exotoxins.** These exotoxins can be rendered non-toxic or harmless by adding formaldehyde solution and incubating for some days or weeks, usually at 37°; filtrates detoxicated in this way are known as **toxoids** or **formol toxoids.**

Non-lethal amounts of toxin, or the corresponding toxoid, are injected in gradually increasing doses into animals, usually horses. Specific antitoxins develop in the plasma and the animals become actively immune. When the examination of small samples of blood shows that a satisfactory degree of immunity has been produced, larger volumes of blood are withdrawn from the jugular vein and the plasma or serum is processed.

Antibacterial sera are prepared against certain bacteria which do not produce exotoxins. When graded doses of suspensions of living or dead bacteria, or preparations from these suspensions, are injected into horses or other animals, antibodies develop that can combine with the antigens of the organisms and render them susceptible to phagocytosis or lysis by the action of complement. When the blood contains a sufficient amount of antibody it is collected and processed.

Antiviral sera are not usually obtained from animals injected with specific viruses. The immune globulins are usually obtained from the plasma or serum of human patients who have recovered from certain virus diseases, of adults who have had the disease in the past, or of persons who have been artificially immunised. Human immunoglobulin, prepared from pools of adult human plasma and containing the antibodies of normal adults, is used in the prophylaxis of certain virus diseases. Rabies antiserum may be obtained from animals, usually horses, by injecting gradually increasing doses of a rabies vaccine. It is customary first to use a killed vaccine and then, when some immunity is established, to use living virus as an antigen. When a sufficient virus-neutralising titre is reached the blood is collected and may be processed.

Antisera issued in liquid form are distributed under aseptic conditions into sterile containers which are then sealed to exclude micro-organisms. A suitable antibacterial substance, in a concentration sufficient to prevent the growth of micro-organisms, is usually added; this is essential when antisera are issued in multiple-dose containers.

For native antisera, solutions of globulins, and liquid preparations obtained by simple fractionation with salts, the rate of deterioration during storage at 0° is negligible for 5 years and at 5° does not exceed in each year 5% of the previous year's activity. At higher temperatures the annual rate of deterioration is greater; at 15° it may be about 10%, at 20° it may approach 20%, and at 37° preparations may lose 25 to 50% of their activity in a year. With enzyme-treated antisera the rate of deterioration is usually less; they are most stable at pH 5.0 to 6.5, when the rate of deterioration at 0° to 5° is negligible; up to 15° it does not exceed 3%, and at 20°, 5%; at 37° preparations may lose 10 to 20% of their activity in a year.

Storage. Antisera should be protected from light and stored at 2° to 10°; they should not be allowed to freeze. The amount of antiserum placed in each container must be sufficient to ensure that, when stored under these conditions, the number of units stated on the label is still present at the end of the period during which the preparation is intended to be used.

Actions and uses. When antitoxins and other antibodies developed in the blood of one individual are transferred to a second individual by injecting a suitable quantity of the blood or serum containing the antibodies, passive immunity is conferred. This type of immunity is relatively quickly established, the rapidity depending upon the route of injection; antibodies do not remain in the blood of the second individual for longer than a few weeks, owing to the elimination of the foreign protein by the body. The rate of elimination is much slower, however, when homologous serum is used. Individuals who have received foreign protein in serum on a previous occasion may eliminate this protein subsequently with extreme rapidity. It is important, therefore, to follow the conferment of passive immunity, which is largely an emergency procedure, by the injection of suitable antigens to produce active immunity.

Antitoxic sera have the specific power of neutralising the toxins formed by micro-organisms and rendering them harmless to susceptible animals.

Antibacterial sera appear to act by rendering the micro-organisms susceptible to phagocytosis.

Antiviral sera are believed to act mainly by preventing the specific virus from entering the tissue cells and, as they cannot repair the harmfull cell damage, their chief value is prophylactic rather than therapeutic.

Serum reactions. These are liable to occur after the injection of any serum of animal origin. The more serious general reactions are: (1) *Serum anaphylaxis,* a condition of severe shock appearing within a few minutes of the injection, or with less intensity up to two hours afterwards. (2) *Serum sickness,* a syndrome of rashes, pyrexia, and joint-pains occurring typically seven to twelve days, or less commonly three to four days, after the injection; the accelerated reaction is seen in persons who have previously received serum. (3) *Thermal reaction,* a sudden pyrexia accompanied by rigor occurring after the intravenous injection of certain batches of serum; it is not due to serum sensitivity, but is probably caused by pyrogenic substances produced during processing.

The use of enzyme-treated serum has considerably diminished the incidence of serum sickness and the symptoms are usually mild and transient. Serum anaphylaxis, although very rare, may still occur and may prove dangerous in susceptible subjects.

Intradermal, conjunctival, and scratch tests for the detection of serum sensitivity are unreliable and are not recommended.

Before injecting serum, information should be obtained as to whether previous injections of serum have been received and whether the patient is subject to allergic diseases, especially asthma and infantile eczema. If there is no history of previous serum injection or of allergic reaction, the dose of serum may be given intramuscularly; if there is time, however, or if injections of serum have been given previously, a trial dose of 0.2 millilitre of the serum should be given subcutaneously; if no *general* reaction develops within 30 minutes, the main dose of serum is given intramuscularly.

If the patient is subject to allergic diseases, the first trial dose should be 0.2 millilitre of a 1 in 10 dilution of the serum, given subcutaneously; if no *general* reaction develops during an interval of 30 minutes, a subcutaneous injection of 0.2 millilitre of undiluted serum is given and, if a further 30 minutes elapses without incident, the main dose is given intramuscularly.

Whenever serum is to be injected, by whatever route, the patient must be kept under observation for at least 30 minutes after the injection and adrenaline injection and corticosteroids kept in readiness for emergency use. Serum should never be given by the intravenous route unless a preliminary intramuscular injection, given at least 30 minutes beforehand, has been tolerated. For intravenous use the serum should be at room temperature, the injection should be given very slowly, and the patient should be recumbent during the injection and for at least an hour afterwards.

Antoxidants

Many pharmaceutical preparations deteriorate on storage because of oxidation of one or more of the ingredients on exposure to atmospheric oxygen. Such autoxidation reactions are chain reactions which are often initiated by ultraviolet radiation in the presence of a trace of oxygen and which involve the formation of highly active free radicals; these reactions are often catalysed by traces of cupric, ferric, and other heavy-metal ions.

Pharmaceutical substances that are especially susceptible to oxidation include unsaturated oils and fats, compounds with aldehyde groups (paraldehyde and vanillin), and compounds with phenolic groups (adrenaline and morphine); plastics and rubber, used in containers and closures, also tend to oxidise on storage.

Autoxidation reactions can be inhibited by the addition of small amounts of substances known as antioxidants. These substances can be classified into three groups: true antioxidants or "anti-oxygens", reducing agents, and antioxidant synergists.

True antioxidants are substances which probably inhibit oxidation by reacting with free radicals to block the chain reaction. Such substances are not effective against oxidising agents. Examples of true antioxidants are ascorbyl palmitate, butylated hydroxyanisole, butylated hydroxytoluene, dodecyl gallate, ethyl gallate, nordihydroguaiaretic acid, octyl gallate, propyl gallate, thymol, and α-tocopherol.

Reducing agents are substances which have a lower redox potential than the drug that they are intended to protect; they are, therefore, more readily oxidised than the drug and are effective against oxidising agents. In many medicines reducing agents probably react also with free radicals to block chain reactions. Examples of reducing agents are ascorbic acid, sodium metabisulphite, and sodium sulphite. Isoascorbic acid and sodium formaldehyde sulphoxylate have also been used as reducing agents.

Antioxidant synergists are substances that probably have little antioxidant effect if used alone but enhance appreciably the action of true antioxidants by reacting with those heavy-metal ions that catalyse autoxidation. Examples of antioxidant synergists are citric acid, disodium edetate, lecithin, phosphoric acid, and tartaric acid. Monoisopropyl citrate has also been used as an antioxidant synergist. Mixtures of true antioxidants and of true antioxidants with reducing agents sometimes show synergism.

The ideal antioxidant for a pharmaceutical preparation is effective in low concentration under the expected conditions of storage and use, soluble in the vehicle, stable, harmless, non-irritant, unlikely to cause allergies, odourless, tasteless, and compatible with other ingredients and the materials used in the container and closure.

In practice, the choice of an antioxidant depends upon the route of administration and the physical and chemical nature of the medicine. For emulsions, the antioxidant should usually be preferentially soluble in the oily phase. Because of the complexity of free-radical reactions, it is rarely possible to predict the effectiveness of various antioxidants in a particular preparation. Stability tests should be carried out to determine the relative effectiveness of various concentrations of different antioxidants.

In Great Britain, the antioxidants which may be added to foods are controlled by The Antioxidant in Food Regulations, 1974 (SI 1974: No. 1120) and the Antioxidants in Food (Scotland) Regulations, 1974 [SI 1974: No. 1339 (S. 117)].

Antioxidants permitted in foods include ascorbic acid, calcium and sodium ascorbate, ascorbyl palmitate, extracts of natural origin rich in tocopherols, and synthetic α-, γ-, and δ-tocopherols.

The regulations control the antioxidants which can be added to various foods and which should not be added to food intended mainly for babies or young children.

The Seventeenth and Twentieth Reports of the Joint FAO/WHO Expert Committee on Food Additives give information on estimated acceptable daily intake for permitted substances of various kinds and this is indicated in some of the examples below.

ALPHA TOCOPHERYL ACETATE.* True antioxidant; up to 10 parts per million of tocopherol may be added to liquid paraffin.

ASCORBIC ACID.* Reducing agent.

ASCORBYL PALMITATE. True antioxidant; estimated acceptable daily intake, up to 1.25 mg per kg body-weight; used as an antioxidant in food.

BUTYLATED HYDROXYANISOLE.* True antioxidant; temporary estimated acceptable daily intake, up to 500 micrograms per kg body-weight alone and may be mixed with butylated hydroxytoluene provided that combination does not exceed this figure; this antioxidant, or mixture with butylated hydroxytoluene, may be used in combination with dodecyl, octyl, or propyl gallate provided each is within the limits and the total does not exceed 1000 parts per million in the case of essential oils.

BUTYLATED HYDROXYTOLUENE.* True antioxidant; see butylated hydroxyanisole (above); up to 10 parts per million of butylated hydroxytoluene may be added to liquid paraffin (as an alternative to tocopherol).

CITRIC ACID.* Synergist; no limit is indicated for citric acid and its calcium, potassium, and sodium salts in food.

DILAURYL THIODIPROPIONATE. True antioxidant; estimated acceptable daily intake (as thiodipropionic acid), up to 3 mg per kg body-weight; used as an antioxidant synergist for fats.

DISODIUM EDETATE.* Synergist; estimated acceptable daily intake, up to 2.5 mg per kg body-weight; up to 25 mg of disodium edetate per litre is permitted as an additive to brandy.

DISTEARYL THIODIPROPIONATE. True antioxidant; properties similar to those of dilauryl thiodipropionate (above).

DODECYL GALLATE.* True antioxidant; this substance may be used alone or in any admixture with octyl or propyl gallates in a total concentration of up to 100 parts per million in edible oils and fats, and up to 1000 parts per million for essential oils (see also above under butylated hydroxyanisole); temporary estimated acceptable daily intake, up to 200 micrograms per kg body-weight as total concentration of dodecyl gallate or any admixture with octyl or propyl gallate.

ETHYL GALLATE.* True antioxidant; properties similar to those of dodecyl gallate (above).

ISOASCORBIC ACID. Reducing agent; estimated acceptable daily intake, up to 5 mg per kg body-weight; used as an antioxidant in emulsions of fats and oils; it has no vitamin-C activity.

LECITHIN. Synergist; an oil-soluble phosphate with chelating properties used in oils and fats; usually effective in a concentration of 0.02 to 0.2%; also used as an emulsifying agent; main commercially available varieties are egg lecithin and vegetable lecithin.

MONOISOPROPYL CITRATE. Synergist.

NORDIHYDROGUAIARETIC ACID. True antioxidant; used in oils and fats; usually effective in a concentration of 0.001

to 0.01%; its effectiveness can be enhanced by the addition of an antioxidant synergist such as citric acid or lecithin.

OCTYL GALLATE.* True antioxidant; temporary acceptable daily intake up to 200 micrograms per kg body-weight; should not be used in beverages because of its skin sensitising potential; see dodecyl gallate (above).

PHOSPHORIC ACID.* Synergist; estimated acceptable total daily dietary phosphorus load up to 70 mg per kg body-weight, attention being given to the reverse relationship with calcium intake.

PROPYL GALLATE.* True antioxidant; temporary estimated acceptable daily intake up to 200 micrograms per kg body-weight; see dodecyl gallate (above).

SODIUM FORMALDEHYDE SULPHOXYLATE. Reducing agent; used as a preservative and antioxidant.

SODIUM METABISULPHITE.* Reducing agent; estimated acceptable daily intake (as SO_2), up to 700 micrograms per kg body-weight.

SODIUM SULPHITE.* Reducing agent; estimated acceptable daily intake as for sodium metabisulphite (above).

SULPHUR DIOXIDE. Reducing agent; see sodium metabisulphite (above).

TARTARIC ACID.* Synergist; estimated acceptable daily intake up to 30 mg per kg body-weight.

THIOGLYCEROL (monothioglycerol). Reducing agent.

THIOSORBITOL. True antioxidant.

THIOUREA. True antioxidant.

THYMOL.* True antioxidant.

FURTHER INFORMATION. The factors that affect the autoxidation of organic materials and the mechanism of action of various antioxidants—G. Scott, *Atmospheric Oxidation and Antioxidants*, London, Elsevier, 1966; the measurement and prevention of oxidative decomposition in cosmetics and pharmaceuticals—J. P. Ostendorf, *J. Soc. cosmet. Chem.*, 1965, **16**, 203; the use and rationale of antioxidants and chelating agents in liquid dosage-forms—L. Lachman, *Drug Cosmet. Ind.*, 1968, **102** No. 1, 36; a review of the technological efficacy of some antioxidants and synergists—*WHO Food Additive Series*, No. 3, Geneva, World Health Organisation, 1972.

See also the entry under this title.

Anxiety

Anxiety is an unpleasant mood of tension, apprehension, and fear arising either spontaneously or in response to anticipated troubles which may be real or imagined. It can only be considered abnormal when it is excessive, inappropriate, or without obvious cause. The condition may be induced in susceptible individuals by stress or psychological conflict, or it may be constitutional. It is often associated with depression.

The inner changes of tension and apprehension in anxiety may be accompanied by signs and symptoms of overactivity of the autonomic nervous system including tachycardia, hypertension, increased perspiration, dilated pupils, and decreased salivary and gastric secretion. Anxiety attacks may be single episodes occurring in response to some acute threat or they may be periods of exacerbation of a chronic disturbance of mood (anxiety state).

Anxiety may be treated by psychotherapy in conjunction with sedatives such as the benzodiazepines. Sedatives such as the barbiturates have also been used but are now largely replaced by the benzodiazepines which are more

effective, safer in excessive dosage, and less likely to induce dependence. Some specific somatic symptoms respond to treatment with beta-adrenoceptor blocking agents.

Apomorphine Hydrochloride

The hemihydrate of the hydrochloride of apomorphine, an alkaloid which may be obtained from morphine by the abstraction of the elements of a molecule of water.

$C_{17}H_{18}ClNO_2, \frac{1}{2}H_2O = 312.8$

OTHER NAMES: Apomorph. Hydrochlor.; Apomorphini Hydrochloridum

A standard is given in the European Pharmacopoeia Vol. III

Description. A colourless or greyish-white, glistening, microcrystalline, odourless powder which becomes green on exposure to air and light.

Solubility. Soluble, at 20°, in 50 parts of water and in 50 parts of alcohol; very slightly soluble in chloroform and in ether.

Acidity. A 1% solution has a pH of 4.5 to 5.5.

Moisture content. 2.5 to 4%, determined by drying at 105°.

Specific rotation. −48.5° to −52°, determined on a 1% solution in 0.02N hydrochloric acid.

Dissociation constant. pK_a 7.2 (20°).

Stability. In aqueous solution, apomorphine is oxidised to various derivatives of quinolinedione, which are devoid of emetic properties. Oxidised solutions are emerald green, but the depth of colour is not a reliable indication of the extent of oxidation. The rate of oxidation can be retarded by the addition of dilute hydrochloric acid, to adjust the pH of the solution to 3 to 4, and sodium metabisulphite; the solution should be free from dissolved oxygen.

Apomorphine hydrochloride should not be used if it at once gives an emerald-green solution when 1 part is shaken with 100 parts of water. In addition, apomorphine hydrochloride should not be used if a solution so prepared is deeper in colour than a 0.005% solution of the sample treated as follows: dilute 1 ml with 6 ml of water, add 1 ml of *sodium bicarbonate solution* and 0.5 ml of 0.1N iodine, allow to stand for 30 seconds, add 0.5 ml of 0.1N sodium thiosulphate, and dilute to 10 ml with water.

FURTHER INFORMATION. Loss of biological activity in apomorphine solutions—A. M. Burkman, *J. Pharm. Pharmac.*, 1963, **15**, 461; kinetics of degradation of apomorphine—A. M. Burkman, *J. pharm. Sci.*, 1965, **54**, 325; stability of apomorphine in aqueous solution—P. Lundgren and L. Landersjo, *Acta pharm. suec.*, 1970, **7**, 133.

Incompatibility. It is incompatible with alkaline substances, iodides, tannin, iron salts, and oxidising agents.

Sterilisation. Solutions for injection are sterilised by heating in an autoclave in sealed containers in which the air has been replaced by nitrogen or other suitable gas.

Storage. It should be stored in airtight containers, protected from light.

Identification. TESTS. 1. An aqueous solution is colourless when freshly prepared, but rapidly becomes green on exposure to light and air; it is more stable if it is acidified with hydrochloric acid.
2. Dissolve about 10 mg in 1 ml of water and add *sodium bicarbonate solution*; a precipitate is produced which is colourless at first but rapidly becomes green. The precipitate is soluble in ether to give a purple solution, in chloroform to give a blue solution, and in alcohol to give a green solution.
3. Dissolve about 10 mg in 1 ml of water, add *sodium bicarbonate solution*, followed by 3 drops of *iodine solution*, and shake; an emerald-green colour is produced. Add 5 ml of ether, shake, and allow to separate; the ether layer is deep ruby red and the aqueous layer remains green.
4. Dissolve a few crystals in nitric acid; a dark purple solution is produced.

MELTING-POINT. About 230° with decomposition.

ULTRAVIOLET ABSORPTION. In 0.1N hydrochloric acid, maximum at 273 nm (E1%, 1cm = 550).

Determination in body fluids. ULTRAVIOLET SPECTRO-PHOTOMETRY. In urine—P. N. Kaul *et al.*, *J. pharm. Sci.*, 1961, **50**, 244.

GAS CHROMATOGRAPHY. In plasma—D. M. Baaske *et al.*, *J. Chromat*, 1977, **140**, 57.

Metabolism. DISTRIBUTION. In rats, a large amount of apomorphine is localised in the liver, mainly as the glucuronide.

METABOLIC REACTIONS. In rats, rabbits, and horses, apomorphine is extensively metabolised by conjugation with glucuronic acid; in rabbits, the glucuronide metabolites have been identified as the O^8- and O^4-β-glucuronides; in mice, apomorphine appears to induce its own metabolism.

EXCRETION. In rabbits and horses, it is excreted in the urine as glucuronides; in the rat, most of a dose is excreted as conjugates with about 4% as unchanged drug; in rats, the excretion of unchanged drug appears to be pH-dependent and is increased in acid urine.

FURTHER INFORMATION. Induction and inhibition of glucuronidation of apomorphine in mice—P. N. Kaul and M. W. Conway, *J. pharm. Sci.*, 1971, **60**, 94; isolation and characterisation of "bound" apomorphine —P. N. Kaul *et al.*, *J. pharm. Sci.*, 1961, **50**, 244, 248, and 840.

Actions and uses. Apomorphine hydrochloride is a dopaminergic agent which causes vomiting as a result of central stimulation. A dose of 2 to 8 milligrams by subcutaneous or intramuscular injection can produce vomiting in a few minutes, but the same dose taken by mouth may act merely as an expectorant.
The dose for children is a quarter to three-quarters that for adults. Following its emetic action, it commonly induces sleep. Apomorphine is used in aversion therapy. The effectiveness of apomorphine is reduced by drugs which depress the vomiting centre.

Precautions. Apomorphine should not be given to unconscious patients, to patients with corrosive poisoning, or to patients with respiratory or central nervous system depression because of the danger of vomit being inhaled.

Poisoning. Overdosage may cause excessive vomiting, depression of the central nervous system, respiratory difficulty, a fall in blood pressure, and collapse. Excessive vomiting may be treated with 25 to 50 milligrams of chlorpromazine hydrochloride by intramuscular injection.

Veterinary uses. Apomorphine hydrochloride is administered to dogs as an emetic by subcutaneous injection in doses of 300 to 600 micrograms per kilogram body-weight.

Preparation

APOMORPHINE INJECTION (*Syn.* Apomorphine Hydrochloride Injection): a sterile solution of apomorphine hydrochloride, with 0.1% of sodium metabisulphite, in water for injections free from dissolved air. It is distributed into ampoules, the air in the ampoules being replaced by nitrogen or other suitable gas, and the ampoules are immediately sealed and sterilised by heating in an autoclave. The usual strength is 3 mg of apomorphine hydrochloride per ml.
A standard for this injection is given in the British Pharmacopoeia 1973
Containers and *Labelling:* see the entry on Injections for general information on containers and labelling.

Applications

Applications are liquid or semi-liquid preparations for application to the skin.

Containers. Applications should preferably be dispensed in coloured fluted bottles but other suitable containers may be used provided that such containers are clearly distinguishable from types normally used for medicinal products taken internally.

Labelling. The container should be labelled "For external use only"

Arachis Oil

The refined fixed oil obtained from the seeds of *Arachis hypogaea* L. (Fam. Leguminosae), a plant indigenous to Brazil and widely cultivated in Africa, the Indian subcontinent, China, and America.

OTHER NAMES: Groundnut Oil; Oleum Arachis; Peanut Oil

A standard is given in the British Pharmacopoeia 1973

Constituents. Arachis oil consists of glycerides, the fatty acid constituents of which are chiefly oleic and linoleic acids with smaller amounts of palmitic, arachidic, lignoceric, and stearic acids. The proportion of arachidic and lignoceric acids taken together is usually about 5% and their low solubility in alcohol (70%) is used in testing for arachis oil.
The unrefined oil may sometimes contain toxic substances. For example, the seeds may be affected by fungal attacks producing aflatoxin which becomes a contaminant of the crude oil. These toxic substances are removed by the refining process.

Description. A pale yellow oil with a faint odour.

Solubility. Very slightly soluble in alcohol; miscible with ether, with chloroform, and with light petroleum.

Weight per ml. At 20°, 0.911 to 0.915 g.

Refractive index. 1.468 to 1.472.

Adulterants and substitutes. Other vegetable oils, including cottonseed oil and sesame oil.

Reflux 1 g with 5 ml of *alcoholic potassium hydroxide*, warm with a mixture containing 1.5 ml of acetic acid with 50 ml of alcohol (70%) until the solution is clear, and allow to cool slowly; the development of turbidity only at temperatures below 37° indicates the presence of other vegetable oils.

The presence of cottonseed or sesame oil is indicated by the following test. Mix 2.5 ml with 2.5 ml each of amyl alcohol and a 1% solution of precipitated sulphur in carbon disulphide and heat the mixture in a closed tube by immersing to one-third its depth in boiling water; the development of a pink or red colour within 30 minutes indicates the presence of cottonseed oil. Shake 2 ml with 1 ml of a 1% solution of sucrose in hydrochloric acid; the development of a pink colour in the acid layer on allowing to stand for 5 minutes indicates the presence of sesame oil, if the colour produced is deeper than that produced by repeating the test without the sucrose.

Stability. On exposure to air it thickens very slowly and may become rancid.

Sterilisation. It is sterilised by dry heat.

FURTHER INFORMATION. A study of sterilising conditions for injectable oils—D. Pasquale *et al.*, *Bull. parent. Drug Ass.*, 1964, **18**, No. 3, 1.

Storage. It should be stored in well-filled airtight containers. It becomes cloudy at about 3° and partly solidifies at lower temperatures. If it has solidified it should be completely remelted and mixed before use.

Actions and uses. Arachis oil has properties similar to those of olive oil and is used for the same purposes. Emulsions containing 10% of arachis oil and 40% of dextrose have been used by intragastric drip as a nitrogen-free diet.

Arrowroot

Consists of the starch granules of the rhizome *Maranta arundinacea* L. (Fam. Marantaceae). The plant is indigenous to central America; it is cultivated in tropical and subtropical countries, chiefly in the West Indies, and is imported mainly from St. Vincent.

OTHER NAME: Maranta

A standard is given in the British Pharmaceutical Codex 1973

Varieties. Several grades of St. Vincent or West Indian arrowroot are found in commerce and are usually sold on the basis of their general appearance. The mucilages formed from these varieties differ slightly in viscosity, which may form an additional criterion of quality.

Constituents. Arrowroot consists chiefly of amylose and amylopectin and contains about 14 to 17% of moisture. Incineration of the drug may yield up to 0.3% of ash.

Description. *Macroscopical characters:* a white powder, much of which may cohere to form small irregular masses up to about 8 mm in length; it crepitates slightly when pressed.
It is odourless and tasteless.

Microscopical characters: the diagnostic characters are: starch granules ovoid or ellipsoid, simple, frequently with small local enlargements or tuberosities; hilum well marked, generally situated near the broader end of the granules, usually in the form of a 2-rayed cleft; striations concentric, clearly marked but very fine; granules ranging from 7 to **30** to **50** to 75 μm in their greatest dimension and exhibiting a well-marked cross when viewed between crossed polars.

Adulterants and substitutes. Many starches have been described as arrowroots and are sometimes substituted for arrowroot; the most important of these substitutes are the following.

The starch of the potato, *Solanum tuberosum* L. ("English" arrowroot), which is described under Starch. It is rapidly gelatinised when a sample is treated as described under identification, test 2 (below).

Manihot (Manioc) starch ("Brazilian" or "Rio" arrowroot), often known as cassava or tapioca starch, obtained from *Manihot esculenta* Crantz (Fam. Euphorbiaceae), has subspherical and muller-shaped granules, the smaller ones being about 5 to **12** to 25 μm and the larger ones about 25 to 35 μm in diameter.

Sweet potato starch ("Brazilian" arrowroot), obtained from *Ipomoea batatas* (L.) Poir. (Fam. Convolvulaceae), has rounded, polyhedral, and muller-shaped granules, the smaller ones being about 15 to 22 μm and the larger ones about 25 to **50** to 55 μm in diameter.

"Queensland" arrowroot or "tous-les-mois" starch, from *Canna edulis* Edwards (Fam. Cannaceae), has flattened ovoid granules about 30 to **70** to **100** to 130 μm in diameter.

Sago starch, from *Metroxylon rumphii* Mart., *M. sagu* Rottb., and *M. laeve* Mart. (Fam. Palmae), has ovoid, subspherical, and muller-shaped granules, the smaller ones being about 10 to 20 μm and the larger ones about 50 to **60** to 80 μm in diameter.

"Indian" or "Bombay" arrowroot, from *Curcuma angustifolia* Roxb. and "East Indian" arrowroot, from *C. leucorrhiza* Roxb. (Fam. Zingiberaceae), have scitamineous granules, about 30 to **60** to 140 μm long, 25 to 35 μm wide, and 7 to 8 μm thick.

Identification. TESTS. 1. Boil 1 g with 15 ml of water and cool; a translucent whitish gelatinous mass is formed. Add 0.2 ml of *iodine solution*; a deep blue colour is produced which disappears on warming and reappears on cooling.

2. Add to a sample on a microscope slide 0.2 ml of a 0.9% solution of potassium hydroxide in water, apply a coverglass, and examine under a 4-mm objective; the granules are not gelatinised.

Actions and uses. Arrowroot has the general properties of starch and is used as a gruel in the treatment of diarrhoea. It has been employed as a suspending agent in the preparation of barium meals and is sometimes preferred to starch for use in tablet-making.

Arsanilic Acid

4-Aminophenylarsonic acid

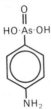

$C_6H_8AsNO_3 = 217.1$

OTHER NAMES: Aminoarsonic Acid; *Pro-Gen*®

A standard is given in the British Pharmacopoeia (Veterinary)

Description. A white or creamy-white, granular, almost odourless powder.

Solubility. Soluble, at 20°, in 200 parts of water and in 40 parts of alcohol; practically insoluble in ether and in chloroform; soluble in solutions of alkalis.

Moisture content. Not more than 2%, determined by drying at 105°.

Identification. TESTS. 1. Dissolve about 50 mg in 10 ml of water, add 100 mg of sodium dithionite dissolved in 2 ml of water, and warm on a water-bath; a yellow precipitate is produced.
2. Fuse about 30 mg with 1 g of sodium carbonate, cool, and extract with 10 ml of water. To 5 ml of the solution add sufficient acetic acid to make it just acid to litmus paper and add 2 ml of *silver nitrate solution*; a chocolate-brown precipitate is produced. To a further 5 ml add sufficient hydrochloric acid to make it just acid to litmus paper, boil, cool, make just alkaline with *dilute ammonia solution*, and add 3 ml of *magnesium-ammonium chloride solution*; a white granular precipitate is produced.

ULTRAVIOLET ABSORPTION. In water, maximum at 250 nm (E1%, 1cm = 725).

Veterinary uses. Arsanilic acid is used for the prevention and treatment of enteric infections.
It has been given in the feed at a rate of 100 parts per million continuously as a growth promoter. For enteric infections up to 250 parts per million may be given in the feed for 3 weeks for pigs or 5 days for poultry.

Preparation
ARSANILIC ACID PREMIX: consisting of arsanilic acid mixed with powdered maize or other suitable diluent. It may contain an antistatic agent.
This preparation is stable to hot pelleting processes. It must be diluted before administration by mixing thoroughly with the feed. Available as a premix containing 22% of arsanilic acid.
A standard for this premix is given in the British Pharmacopoeia (Veterinary)
Containers and *Storage:* see the entry on Premixes for general information on containers and storage.
Labelling: the label on the container should state:
(1) that the preparation should be withdrawn from the feed not less than 10 days before slaughter for human consumption;
(2) that arsanilic acid must not be fed at levels in excess of 100 parts per million to birds producing eggs for human consumption;
(3) that the preparation must not be given to pigs or poultry that are already receiving an arsenical compound in feed or water;
(4) that floor litter from poultry houses must not be fed to livestock; and
(5) that operators should wash hands and exposed skin before meals and after work.

Arteriosclerosis

Arteriosclerosis is a disease in which rigidity and thickening of arteries occurs as a result of the replacement of muscle and elastic tissues in the intimal layer by fibrous tissue.

Atherosclerosis is a common form of arteriosclerosis in which yellowish plaques of atheroma containing cholesterol and other lipid material are formed within the intima and inner media of large and medium sized arteries. It most commonly affects the coronary arteries, cerebral arteries, and peripheral arteries of the lower limb. It is a progressive disease and becomes increasingly common as age advances.
Atheroma causes narrowing and ultimately occlusion of the vessels involved and results in chronic ischaemia of the structures which the vessels supply. Atheroma also provides a surface on which thrombosis can occur and if this happens acute ischaemia and infarction result. The symptoms of ischaemia depend upon the organ supplied by the vessel and upon whether occlusion is acute or chronic. Chronic occlusion may be offset by the development of a collateral circulation.
Atherosclerosis can give rise to angina pectoris, myocardial infarction, and arrhythmias, if occurring in coronary vessels; forgetfulness, confusion, personality changes, or a stroke, if occurring in cerebral vessels; or intermittent claudication of calves and gangrene of toes, if occurring in the arteries of the leg.
Atherosclerosis may cause hypertension either because of the increased peripheral resistance of the narrowed vessels or because of stenosis of the renal artery. Long standing atheroma may extend into the media with weakening of the wall. Aneurysms are formed when rupture of the intima and media allow blood to collect beneath the adventitia which becomes grossly distended. They produce symptoms by pressure on surrounding structures or by rupturing.
Factors which predispose to the development of atherosclerosis include a raised serum lipid level, decreased glucose tolerance, raised blood pressure, obesity, lack of exercise, and cigarette smoking. Control of these factors is the most important element of both prevention and control of atherosclerosis. The patency of severely narrowed vessels may sometimes be restored by surgery. Blood lipid levels may be lowered by control of diet and also by clofibrate and cholestyramine.

Arteriolosclerosis is a form of arteriosclerosis characterised by hardening and thickening of the walls of the arterioles.

Arteritis, Temporal

see GIANT-CELL ARTERITIS

Ascariasis

Ascariasis is one of the commonest helminth infections of the human gastro-intestinal tract and is caused by *Ascaris lumbricoides*, a large roundworm 150–250 mm long. It is transmitted by the faecal-oral route. Swallowed ova hatch in the intestine, and the larvae pass into the bloodstream and travel to the lungs from where they migrate up the trachea and down the oesophagus to mature in the small intestine. Larvae which die on the way set up a foreign-tissue reaction resulting in fever, cough, expectoration, and dyspnoea, with patchy shadowing on the X-ray and eosinophilia. Intestinal infection is usually symptomless, although heavy infection may cause intestinal obstruction.

Drugs used in the treatment of ascariasis include bephenium and piperazine.

Ascorbic Acid

The enolic form of 3-oxo-L-gulofuranolactone.

CH$_2$OH
|
H—C—OH

HO

HO   O

$C_6H_8O_6 = 176.1$

OTHER NAMES: Acidum Ascorbicum; *Ascorbef®*; *Redoxon®*; Vitamin C
Parentrovite® (with vitamins of the B group)

A standard is given in the European Pharmacopoeia Vol. I

Ascorbic acid may be prepared synthetically or obtained by extraction from various vegetable sources. It is a constituent of rose hips, black currants, the juice of citrus fruits, and the ripe fruit of *Capsicum annuum* L. (Fam. Solanaceae).

Description. Almost odourless colourless crystals or a white or very pale yellow crystalline powder with an acidic taste.

Solubility. Soluble, at 20°, in 3.5 parts of water, in 25 parts of alcohol, and in 10 parts of methyl alcohol; practically insoluble in ether and in light petroleum.

Acidity. A 5% solution has a pH of 2.2 to 2.5.

Specific rotation. +20.5° to +21.5°, determined on a 10% solution in water.

Dissociation constants. pK$_a$ 4.2 and 11.6 (25°).

Stability. In the form of crystals or powder, ascorbic acid darkens slowly on exposure to air and light. In aqueous solution ascorbic acid degrades under anaerobic and aerobic conditions; the rate of degradation is increased by light and by ions of heavy metals.
The principal product of oxidation is dehydroascorbic acid; this acid hydrolyses to 2,3-diketogulonic acid which then oxidises to threonic acid and oxalic acid. The rate of oxidation in acidic solution is at a maximum at about pH 4 and a minimum near pH 5.6; oxidation is rapid in alkaline solution. The first stage of oxidation from ascorbic acid to dehydroascorbic acid is reversible.
The stability of ascorbic acid in aqueous solutions improves with increasing concentrations of sodium chloride, the improvement generally being associated with a lower concentration of dissolved oxygen. Propylene glycol has a stabilising effect.
When ascorbic acid solutions are autoclaved, stability is markedly increased if N-hydroxyethylethylenediamine-triacetic acid or diethylenetriaminepenta-acetic acid

(pentetic acid) is present. Improvement is also obtained by use of disodium edetate and, to a lesser extent, by propyl gallate. The stabilising effect results from the chelation of the heavy metal ions which cause decomposition of the ascorbic acid. There are optimal concentrations of chelating agent dependent upon the amounts of heavy metal ions present.

FURTHER INFORMATION. Kinetics of aerobic oxidation of ascorbic acid—S. M. Blaug and B. Hajratwala, *J. pharm. Sci.*, 1972, **61**, 556 and 1974, **63**, 1240; rate of anaerobic degradation in aqueous solution—P. Finholt *et al.*, *J. pharm. Sci.*, 1963, **52**, 948 and 1966, **55**, 1435; studies on stability of injectable solutions—M. A. Kassem *et al.*, *Pharm. Acta Helv.*, 1969, **44**, 611 and 667; stability problems—T. J. Macek, *Am. J. Pharm.*, 1960, **132**, 433; effect of pH on aerobic degradation of solutions—A. R. Rogers and J. A. Yacomeni, *J. Pharm. Pharmac.*, 1971, **23**, 218S; stability in tablets—S. H. Rubin *et al.*, *J. pharm. Sci.*, 1976, **65**, 963; stability in aqueous and fruit-juice vehicles at elevated temperature—M. C. Uprety *et al.*, *J. pharm. Sci.*, 1963, **52**, 1001.

Incompatibility. It is incompatible with ferric salts, oxidising agents, and salts of copper, zinc, and manganese.

Sterilisation. Solutions of the sodium salt for injection are sterilised by heating with a bactericide in sealed containers in which the air has been replaced by nitrogen, or other suitable gas, or by filtration.

Storage. It should be stored in airtight containers free from contact with metal, protected from light.

Identification. TESTS. 1. Dissolve about 50 mg in 1 ml of water, add 1 drop of a freshly prepared 5% solution of sodium nitroprusside and 2 ml of *dilute sodium hydroxide solution*, followed by 0.6 to 0.7 ml of hydrochloric acid, dropwise, and stir; the yellow colour turns blue.
2. Dissolve about 50 mg in 2 ml of water, add 4 drops of *methylene blue solution*, and warm to 40°; the deep blue colour gradually becomes lighter and the solution becomes colourless within 3 minutes.
3. Dissolve about 15 mg in 15 ml of a 5% solution of trichloroacetic acid, add 0.2 g of activated charcoal, shake for 1 minute, and filter until the filtrate is clear; to 5 ml of the filtrate add 1 drop of pyrrole, shake, and heat to 50°; a blue colour is produced.

MELTING-POINT. About 190°, with decomposition.

ULTRAVIOLET ABSORPTION. In 0.01N hydrochloric acid, maximum at 244 nm (E1%, 1cm = 560).

INFRA-RED ABSORPTION. Major peaks at 990, 1031, 1111, 1136, 1316, and 1667 cm^{-1} (see Appendix 2b: Infra-red Spectra).

Determination in body fluids. COLORIMETRY. In urine: after cation exchange resin purification—R. E. Hughes, *Analyst, Lond.*, 1964, **89**, 618.

ULTRAVIOLET SPECTROPHOTOMETRY. In plasma—V. Zannoni *et al.*, *Biochem. Med.*, 1974, **11**, 41.

HIGH-PRESSURE LIQUID CHROMATOGRAPHY. In urine or serum—L. A. Pachla and P. T. Kissinger, *Analyt. Chem.*, 1976, **48**, 364.

Metabolism. ABSORPTION. Well absorbed after oral administration but the proportion of a dose absorbed decreases as the dose is increased; it is absorbed in the mouth, stomach, and intestine; the extent of absorption is reduced in gastro-intestinal disorders; absorption from the intestine appears to be an active saturable process; sustained-release preparations are more completely absorbed than conventional capsules or tablets.

BLOOD CONCENTRATION. Normal concentrations in plasma and in leucocytes are about 5 to 12 $\mu g/ml$ and 250 $\mu g/ml$ of packed cells respectively; after a dose of 2 g, given during a cold when normal concentrations are depleted, plasma concentrations of about 20 $\mu g/ml$ are attained in 2 to 4 hours and concentrations in the leucocytes are increased 2- to 3-fold; after an oral dose of 1 g, peak blood concentrations of 5 to 10 $\mu g/ml$ are attained in 1 to 5 hours; after a similar dose of a sustained-release preparation, peak blood concentrations of 8 to 14 $\mu g/ml$ are attained in 3 to 8 hours; uptake by leucocytes appears to be greater in females than males; normal concentrations of ascorbic acid exhibit circadian and seasonal rhythms and are decreased in the elderly.

HALF-LIFE. Ascorbate concentrations in whole blood decline with a half-life of about 34 hours; other figures have been reported of 11 to 15 hours.

DISTRIBUTION. Widely distributed throughout the body with large amounts present in white blood cells and platelets; after daily doses of 1 g, tissue saturation occurs within 7 days resulting in distinct changes in ascorbic acid pharmacokinetics; volume of distribution, about 80 litres; *protein binding*, 8 to 36% bound to plasma proteins.

METABOLIC REACTIONS. Rapidly metabolised to dehydroascorbic acid, 2,3-diketogulonic acid, oxalate, and carbon dioxide; some sulphate conjugation occurs to form the 3-sulphate; the metabolic turnover of ascorbic acid appears to be greater in females than in males.

EXCRETION. Large doses are rapidly excreted in the urine when in excess of the requirements of the body and after an intravenous dose, about 40% is excreted in 8 hours which is increased to about 70% after tissue saturation; urinary metabolites include diketogulonic acid, oxalate, and small amounts as the sulphate conjugate; the amount of unchanged drug excreted is dose-dependent; in women the excretion of ascorbic acid appears to vary with the stage of the menstrual cycle and it is decreased when taking oral contraceptives.

FURTHER INFORMATION. Quantitative aspects of ascorbic acid metabolism in man—G. L. Atkins *et al.*, *J. biol. Chem.*, 1964, **239**, 2975; metabolism in human scurvy—E. M. Baker *et al.*, *Am. J. clin. Nutr.*, 1971, **24**, 444; factors influencing the metabolic availability of ascorbic acid—H. S. Loh *et al.*, *Clin. Pharmac. Ther.*, 1974, **16**, 390; urinary oxalic acid excretion following ingestion of large amounts of ascorbic acid—H. Takiguchi *et al.*, *J. Vitaminol.*, 1966, **12**, 307; pharmacokinetic implications of ascorbic acid absorption—M. Mayersohn, *Eur. J. Pharmac.*, 1972, **19**, 140; tissue saturation, metabolism, and desaturation of ascorbic acid—C. W. M. Wilson, *Practitioner*, 1974, **212**, 481; ascorbic acid metabolism and the common cold—C. W. M. Wilson and H. S. Loh, *Eur. J. clin. Pharmac.*, 1974, **7**, 421 and C. W. M. Wilson *et al.*, *J. clin. Pharmac.*, 1976, **16**, 19; pharmacokinetics of ascorbic acid in man—G. Zetler *et al.*, *Eur. J. clin. Pharmac.*, 1976, **10**, 273.

Actions and uses. Ascorbic acid is essential for the formation of collagen and intercellular material, and hence for the development of cartilage, bone, and teeth, and for the healing of wounds. It is also essential for the conversion of folic acid to folinic acid. It facilitates the absorption of iron from the gut, 5 milligrams of ascorbic acid being required for each milligram of iron. It also influences the formation of haemoglobin and erythrocyte maturation.

The minimum daily requirement of ascorbic acid is probably about 20 milligrams; this requirement is increased during pregnancy and lactation, in adolescence, in hyperthyroidism, during infections, and after surgery.

Ascorbic acid is used primarily for the prophylaxis and treatment of scurvy. Although this condition is now seldom seen, it may occur in the undernourished and in bottle-fed infants. To prevent infantile scurvy, bottle-fed infants should have their feed supplemented by 2.5 to 5 milligrams of ascorbic acid daily. It is also used in adults in a dosage of 25 to 75 milligrams daily to prevent scurvy in patients on restricted diets and in alcoholics. Supplements of the vitamin may also be necessary to promote healing of wounds and fractures and in those conditions where vomiting, diarrhoea, or diuresis are likely to interfere with its absorption and utilisation. Some types of hypochromic anaemia respond to treatment with ascorbic acid and iron, as ascorbic acid facilitates the absorption of ferrous iron.

Large doses of ascorbic acid are often administered therapeutically, but there is little evidence to show that a daily intake of more than 30 to 50 milligrams has any beneficial effect except in the treatment of methaemoglobinaemia, for which 200 milligrams is given thrice daily; in this dosage ascorbic acid has a diuretic action.

The use of ascorbic acid for the prevention and treatment of the common cold is controversial.

Ascorbic acid is usually administered by mouth; it may also be given parenterally, but since it is absorbed efficiently when taken by mouth parenteral administration is necessary only when absorption from the gastrointestinal tract is unsatisfactory.

Ascorbic acid is used as a reducing agent in ferrous sulphate mixtures and other medicines that are susceptible to autoxidation; a concentration of 0.1 to 0.5% is usually effective. Its effectiveness can be increased by the addition of an oil-soluble antoxidant synergist such as lecithin. A disadvantage of ascorbic acid as a reducing agent is that some of its degradation products are coloured.

Preparations

ASCORBIC ACID INJECTION:

Ascorbic acid	..	..	..	..	10.0 g
Sodium bicarbonate	..	..	..	..	4.8 g
Water for injections	..	..	..		to 100.0 ml

Dissolve, and sterilise the solution by filtration; distribute by means of an aseptic technique, into sterile ampoules, replace the air by sterile nitrogen or other suitable gas, and seal.

A standard for this injection is given in the British Pharmaceutical Codex 1973

Containers: see the entry on Injections for general information on containers. The injection should be supplied in single-dose ampoules.

Labelling: see the entry on Injections for general information on labelling.

Storage: it should be protected from light.

ASCORBIC ACID TABLETS (*Syn.* Vitamin C Tablets): available as tablets containing 25, 50, 100, 200, and 500 mg of ascorbic acid. When prepared by moist granulation and compression as described in the entry on Tablets, the drying of the granules should be carried out at a temperature not exceeding 40° if a drying oven is used.

A standard for these tablets is given in the British Pharmacopoeia 1973

Containers and *Storage:* see the entry on Tablets for general information on containers and storage. Containers should be airtight and light resistant and the tablets should not be in contact with metal.

VITAMINS B AND C INJECTION: a sterile solution of thiamine hydrochloride, pyridoxine hydrochloride, riboflavine or the equivalent amount of riboflavine phosphate (sodium salt), nicotinamide, and ascorbic acid (as the sodium salt), with anhydrous dextrose for the intravenous injection, or benzyl alcohol for the intramuscular injection, in water for injections. Stability during storage is achieved by dividing the ingredients between a pair of ampoules, one (number 1) containing the thiamine hydrochloride, the pyridoxine hydrochloride, the riboflavine and, in the intramuscular injections, the benzyl alcohol, and the other (number 2) containing the ascorbic acid, the nicotinamide, and, in the intravenous injection, the anhydrous dextrose. The air in the number 2 ampoule is replaced by nitrogen or other suitable gas.

The number 1 ampoules and the number 2 ampoules for intravenous injection are sterilised by heating in an autoclave. The number 2 ampoules for intramuscular injection are sterilised by heating with a bactericide; 0.2% chlorocresol is suitable. Alternatively, the solutions are sterilised by filtration.

The injection is prepared by mixing, immediately before use, the contents of a pair of ampoules.

When *Strong Vitamins B and C Injection for intravenous use* is ordered or prescribed, a pair of ampoules, one containing 250 mg of thiamine hydrochloride, 50 mg of pyridoxine hydrochloride, and 4 mg of riboflavine or the equivalent amount of riboflavine phosphate (sodium salt) in 5 ml, the other containing 500 mg of ascorbic acid (as the sodium salt), 160 mg of nicotinamide, and 1 g of anhydrous dextrose in 5 ml, is supplied.

When *Strong Vitamins B and C Injection for intramuscular use* is ordered or prescribed, a pair of ampoules, one containing 250 mg of thiamine hydrochloride, 50 mg of pyridoxine hydrochloride, 4 mg of riboflavine or the equivalent amount of riboflavine phosphate (sodium salt), and 0.14 ml of benzyl alcohol in 5ml, the other containing 500 mg of ascorbic acid (as the sodium salt) and 160 mg of nicotinamide in 2 ml, is supplied.

When *Weak Vitamins B and C Injection for intramuscular use* is ordered or prescribed, a pair of ampoules, one containing 100 mg of thiamine hydrochloride, 50 mg of pyridoxine hydrochloride, 4 mg of riboflavine or the equivalent amount of riboflavine phosphate (sodium salt), and 0.08 ml of benzyl alcohol in 2 ml, the other containing 500 mg of ascorbic acid (as the sodium salt) and 160 mg of nicotinamide in 2 ml, is supplied.

A standard for this injection is given in the British Pharmaceutical Codex 1973

Containers: see the entry on Injections for general information on containers.

Labelling: see the entry on Injections for general information on labelling. In addition, the label on the container should state whether the injection is for intravenous or intramuscular use.

Storage: it should be stored in a cool place, protected from light.

VITAMINS CAPSULES: for each capsule take:

Vitamin D	300 units
Vitamin-A activity	2500 units
Riboflavine	0.5 mg
Thiamine hydrochloride	1.0 mg
Nicotinamide	7.5 mg
Ascorbic acid	15.0 mg

Mix the ingredients, with a suitable fixed vegetable oil

if necessary, and enclose in a soft capsule. The capsule shells may be coloured.

A standard for these capsules is given in the British Pharmaceutical Codex 1973

Containers and *Storage:* see the entry on Capsules for general information on containers and storage. Containers should be light resistant.

Dose: prophylactic, 1 daily; therapeutic, 2 daily.

Advice for patients: the capsules should not be taken for prolonged periods without medical advice.

OTHER PREPARATIONS available include TABLETS containing ascorbic acid 1 g in an effervescent basis.

Ascorbic acid is an ingredient of numerous multiple-vitamin preparations.

Aspirin

2-Acetoxybenzoic acid

$C_9H_8O_4 = 180.2$

OTHER NAMES: Acetylsal. Acid; Acetylsalicylic Acid; Acidum Acetylsalicylicum

The general use of the title "aspirin" is limited, and in any country in which the word "aspirin" is a trade mark it may be used only when applied to the product made by the owners of the trade mark.

A standard is given in the European Pharmacopoeia Vol. I

Description. Odourless colourless crystals or white crystalline powder with a slightly acid taste.

Solubility. Soluble, at 20°, in 300 parts of water, in 7 parts of alcohol, in 20 parts of ether, and in 17 parts of chloroform; soluble in solutions of acetates and citrates and, with decomposition, in solutions of alkali hydroxides and carbonates.

Dissociation constant. pK_a 3.5 (25°).

Stability. In the form of crystals or powder, aspirin is stable in dry air but in contact with moisture it degrades by hydrolysis to acetic acid and salicylic acid. Hydrolysis is catalysed by hydrogen ions and by hydroxide ions. Sodium ions may also catalyse hydrolysis.

In aqueous solutions, the pH of maximum stability is 2 to 3. Aqueous suspensions show appreciable decomposition after storing for only a few days.

Degradation in tablets is increased in the presence of stearates used as lubricants.

FURTHER INFORMATION. Stability in aqueous solution —L. J. Edwards, *Trans. Faraday Soc.*, 1950, **46**, 723, and 1952, **48**, 696, and E. R. Garrett, *J. Am. chem. Soc.*, 1957, **79**, 3401; stability in suspension—K. C. James, *J. Pharm. Pharmac.*, 1958, **10**, 363; stability in tablets— S. S. Kornblum and M. A. Zoglio, *J. pharm. Sci.*, 1967, **56**, 1569, and H. V. Maulding *et al.*, *J. pharm. Sci.*, 1969, **58**, 1359; B. K. Martin, Some chemical and physical properties of aspirin, *Advances in Pharmaceutical Sciences*, H. S. Bean *et al.* (Eds), Vol. 3, London, Academic Press, 1971, page 109.

Storage. It should be stored in airtight containers.

Identification. TESTS. 1. To 200 mg add 4 ml of *dilute sodium hydroxide solution*, boil for 3 minutes, cool, add

5 ml of *dilute sulphuric acid*, and filter; the residue, after washing with water and drying at 105°, melts at about 158°. Dissolve a portion of the residue in water and add *ferric chloride solution;* a purple colour is produced.
2. Heat the filtrate obtained in Test 1 with 2 ml of alcohol and 2 ml of sulphuric acid; the odour of ethyl acetate is produced.
3. Dissolve 1 mg in 2 ml of water to which a few drops of acetone has been added, add 2 drops of a 5% solution of copper sulphate in 10% acetic acid, followed by a few crystals of sodium nitrite; shake, heat to boiling, and boil for 5 minutes; a red colour is produced.

MELTING-POINT. About 142°.

ULTRAVIOLET ABSORPTION. In 0.1N hydrochloric acid, maxima at 229 nm (E1%, 1cm = 434) and 278 nm (E1%, 1cm = 65); in alcohol (95%), maxima at 226 nm (E1%, 1cm = 411) and 278 nm (E1%, 1cm = 58).

INFRA-RED ABSORPTION. Major peaks at 914, 1186, 1220, 1300, 1678, and 1754 cm^{-1} (see Appendix 2a: Infra-red Spectra).

THIN-LAYER CHROMATOGRAPHY. See under Thin-layer Chromatography, System 3.

Determination in body fluids. ULTRAVIOLET SPECTROPHOTOMETRY. In whole blood, plasma, or urine: determined as salicylic acid—G. W. Stevenson, *Analyt. Chem.*, 1960, **32**, 1522; P. Trinder, *Biochem. J.*, 1954, **57**, 301.

GAS CHROMATOGRAPHY. In plasma: simultaneous determination of aspirin and salicylic acid—L. J. Walter *et al.*, *J. pharm. Sci.*, 1974, **63**, 1754.

SPECTROFLUORIMETRY. In whole blood—S. L. Kanter and W. R. Horbaly, *J. pharm. Sci.*, 1971, **60**, 1898.

Metabolism. ABSORPTION. Rapidly absorbed after oral administration but delayed by food; absorption from suppositories is slow and erratic; absorption appears to be impaired in patients with migraine attacks, in patients with achlorhydria, and following administration of polysorbates; in those also taking antacids, absorption takes place more rapidly; some hydrolysis to salicylate occurs before absorption.

BLOOD CONCENTRATION. After an oral dose of 650 mg, peak plasma salicylate concentrations of about 45 µg/ml are attained in 1 to 2 hours; after oral doses of 3 g daily, plasma salicylate concentrations stabilise at about 270 µg/ml; after oral doses of 975 mg thrice daily of a sustained-release preparation, stable salicylate concentrations of about 95 µg/ml are attained; after an oral dose of about 2 g, peak plasma concentrations of aspirin of about 15 µg/ml are attained in about 1 hour and peak plasma concentrations of salicylate of about 130 µg/ml are attained in 2 to 4 hours; saliva concentrations parallel plasma concentrations; ascorbic acid may increase the concentration of salicylate in blood after aspirin administration.

HALF-LIFE. Plasma half-life for aspirin, about 17 minutes and for salicylate, 2 to 4 hours for low doses and up to 19 hours for high doses.

DISTRIBUTION. Rapidly distributed throughout the body; volume of distribution, about 150 ml/kg body-weight; both aspirin and salicylate appear in the milk and cross the placenta; concentrations in synovial fluid are less than those in blood; *protein binding*, salicylate is extensively bound to plasma proteins and will displace uric acid and a number of drugs; aspirin itself is bound to a small extent.

METABOLIC REACTIONS. Rapid hydrolysis to salicylic acid, occurring mainly in the blood, along with glucuronic acid and glycine conjugation to form acyl and ether glucuronides and salicyluronic acid; a small fraction is oxidised to form gentisic acid, 2,3,5-trihydroxybenzoic acid, and 2,3-dihydroxybenzoic acid; serum esterase concentrations may be lower in females than in males and this may account for the higher incidence of gastric ulceration in women.

EXCRETION. Completely excreted in the urine with about 80% of a dose excreted as salicyluronic acid, 10% as salicyl *O*-glucuronide, 5% as salicyl ester glucuronide, and 5 to 10% as free salicylic acid; small amounts may additionally be excreted as gentisic acid or as unchanged drug; salicylates are reabsorbed by the renal tubules in acid urine and thus alkaline diuresis will increase the rate of salicylate excretion. In alkaline urine about 85% of a dose is excreted as free salicylate whilst, in acid urine, about 5% is excreted in this form.

FURTHER INFORMATION. Foetal acquisition and neonatal elimination—L. K. Garrettson *et al.*, *Clin. Pharmac. Ther.*, 1975, **17**, 98; salivary excretion—G. Graham and M. Rowland, *J. pharm. Sci.*, 1972, **61**, 1219; gastro-intestinal blood-loss—J. R. Leonards and G. Levy, *Clin. Pharmac. Ther.*, 1973, **14**, 62; decreased serum salicylate in children with rheumatic fever treated with antacid—G. Levy *et al.*, *New Engl. J. Med.*, 1975, **293**, 323; sex-linked difference in aspirin metabolism—R. Menguy *et al.*, *Nature Lond.*, 1972, **239**, 102; pharmacokinetics of aspirin after intravenous administration—M. Rowland and S. J. Riegelman, *J. pharm. Sci.*, 1968, **57**, 1313; plasma concentrations and bioavailability—V. H. Saggers *et al.*, *Clin. Trials J.*, 1972, **9**, No. 3, 36; effects of food and exercise on absorption—G. N. Volans, *Br. J. clin. Pharmac.*, 1974, **1**, 137; absorption during migraine—G. N. Volans, *Br. med. J.*, iv/1974, 265; plasma salicylate concentrations—E. H. Wiseman, *Curr. ther. Res.*, 1969, **11**, 681.

Bioavailability. The rate of absorption of aspirin is affected by particle size, the small particles being more readily absorbed. Formulations of aspirin containing ascorbic acid appear to be better absorbed. Differences in dissolution rates have been identified between two commercial preparations of aspirin but the reasons for the discrepancy have not been resolved. Aspirin exists in 2 polymorphic forms each having different dissolution rates. Aspirin suppositories are poorly absorbed and show bioavailability variations.
Bioavailability variations are particularly apparent with enteric-coated tablets.

FURTHER INFORMATION. Bioavailability from aspirin tablets—D. F. Biggs *et al.*, *Can. J. pharm. Sci.*, 1977, **12**, 23; bioavailability from suppositories—M. Gibaldi and B. Grundhofer, *J. pharm. Sci.*, 1975, **64**, 1064; bioavailability of aspirin—M. Mayersohn, *J. Am. pharm. Ass.*, 1977, **17**, 107; dissolution of aspirin and aspirin tablets—A. G. Mitchell and D. J. Saville, *J. Pharm. Pharmac.*, 1967, **19**, 729; the polymorphism of aspirin—M. P. Summers *et al.*, *J. Pharm. Pharmac.*, 1970, **22**, 615; gastro-intestinal absorption of two polymorphic forms of aspirin—R. Tawashi, *J. Pharm. Pharmac.*, 1969, **21**, 701.

Actions and uses. Aspirin has analgesic, anti-inflammatory, and antipyretic actions and inhibits prostaglandin synthetase. It is rapidly absorbed from the upper gastro-intestinal tract and its effects are apparent within a few minutes. It is eliminated by the kidneys, excretion beginning shortly after it is administered. Aspirin is given by mouth in a dose of 300 to 900 milligrams for the relief of minor pain and symptoms of inflammation. Up to 3.6 grams may be given daily in divided doses.

Aspirin is also used in the treatment of acute and chronic rheumatic states. For acute episodes, 3.6 to 7.2 grams is given daily in divided doses; for the control of chronic rheumatic disease, 300 to 900 milligrams is administered every 4 hours over long periods.

Aspirin is relatively ineffective for most pains of visceral origin.

Mixtures of aspirin with other analgesics have not been shown to be superior in analgesic effect to the use of only one drug and some of the mixtures have been shown to induce dependence.

Aspirin should not be given to children under one year of age except under medical supervision. The usual dosage as an analgesic for a child from 1 to 2 years is 75 to 150 milligrams not more than 4 times daily, from 3 to 5 years 225 to 300 milligrams not more than 3 times daily, and from 6 to 12 years 300 milligrams not more than 4 times daily. These doses should not be given for more than 2 days except under medical supervision.

The use of aqueous preparations of aspirin, such as mixtures, should be avoided because they decompose rapidly with the liberation of acetic and salicylic acids. Symptoms of gastric irritation may be reduced by taking aspirin after food or with plenty of fluid.

Undesirable effects. Small and occasional doses of aspirin rarely produce serious gastric irritation, but some patients are unable to tolerate it even in low dosage. After large or repeated doses haemorrhage may occur and blood may be present in the stools, although usually in small amounts.

Aspirin produces reactions in hypersensitive patients; skin eruptions and swelling of the mucous membranes of the nose and throat with an asthma-like attack are the most common symptoms. It may give rise to angioneurotic oedema, urticaria, and myocarditis. It decreases platelet adhesiveness and increases the coagulation time of the blood, and infants of mothers who have taken large doses regularly during pregnancy or while breast feeding may have impaired platelet function.

Precautions. The use of aspirin in conjunction with anticoagulant drugs should be avoided as it may increase the risk of haemorrhage. Aspirin may increase the toxic effects of methotrexate and reduce the uricosuric activity of probenecid.

Poisoning. Aspiration and lavage should be carried out even if there is a delay of several hours before treatment is started. The stomach should be washed out with water. Forced alkaline diuresis or haemodialysis may be needed in severe cases. Intravenous injections of sodium chloride with sodium bicarbonate may be required to correct dehydration and metabolic disturbances.

Veterinary uses. Aspirin is an analgesic and antipyretic. The usual dose by mouth is 30 to 100 milligrams per kilogram body-weight. Its use should be avoided in cats as they are unable to metabolise aspirin as effectively as other species and are more susceptible to its toxic effects.

Preparations

ASPIRIN AND CAFFEINE TABLETS (*Syn.* Acetylsalicylic Acid and Caffeine Tablets): for each tablet take:

Aspirin	350 mg
Caffeine	30 mg

A standard for these tablets is given in the British Pharmacopoeia Addendum 1975

Containers and *Storage:* see the entry on Tablets for general information on containers and storage. Containers should be airtight.

Dose: 1 to 2 tablets.

Advice for patients: the tablets should preferably be taken after meals. Treatment should not be continued for longer than 2 days without medical advice.

ASPIRIN AND CODEINE TABLETS (*Syn.* Acetylsalicylic Acid and Codeine Tablets): for each tablet take:

Aspirin	400 mg
Codeine phosphate	8 mg

A standard for these tablets is given in the British Pharmacopoeia Addendum 1975

Containers and *Storage:* see the entry on Tablets for general information on containers and storage. Containers should be airtight and light resistant.

Dose: 1 or 2 tablets.

Advice for patients: the tablets should preferably be taken after meals. Treatment should not be continued for longer than 2 days without medical advice.

ASPIRIN, PARACETAMOL, AND CODEINE TABLETS: for each tablet take:

Aspirin	250.0 mg
Paracetamol..	250.0 mg
Codeine phosphate	9.58 mg

Containers and *Storage:* see the entry on Tablets for general information on containers and storage. Containers should be airtight and light resistant.

Dose: ADULTS: 1 or 2 tablets up to 4 times daily as necessary.

CHILD: 6 to 12 years, half a tablet up to 4 times daily as necessary.

Advice for patients: the tablets should preferably be taken after meals. Treatment should not be continued for longer than 2 days without medical advice.

ASPIRIN, PHENACETIN, AND CODEINE TABLETS (*Syn.* Compound Codeine Tablets): for each tablet take:

Aspirin	250 mg
Phenacetin	250 mg
Codeine phosphate	8 mg

A standard for these tablets is given in the British Pharmacopoeia 1973

Containers and *Storage:* see the entry on Tablets for general information on containers and storage. Containers should be airtight and light resistant.

Dose: 1 or 2 tablets up to 4 times daily as necessary.

Advice for patients: the tablets should preferably be taken after meals. Use for prolonged periods should be avoided.

ASPIRIN TABLETS (*Syn.* Acetylsalicylic Acid Tablets): available as tablets containing 150, 300, 450, 500, and 600 mg of aspirin.

A standard for these tablets is given in the British Pharmacopoeia 1973

Containers and *Storage:* see the entry on Tablets for general information on containers and storage. Containers should be airtight.

Advice for patients: the tablets should preferably be taken after meals. Aspirin should not be used for longer than 2 days or given to children under one year without medical advice.

PAEDIATRIC SOLUBLE ASPIRIN TABLETS (*Syn.* Soluble Tablets of Acetylsalicylic Acid, Paediatric): for each tablet take:

Aspirin, in fine powder	75.0 mg
Saccharin sodium	0.75 mg
Anhydrous citric acid	7.5 mg
Calcium carbonate	25.0 mg

Mix, and prepare by preliminary compression or moist granulation using a non-aqueous liquid excipient, followed by compression as described in the entry on Tablets.

A standard for these tablets is given in the British Pharmaceutical Codex 1973

Containers and *Storage:* see the entry on Tablets for general information on containers and storage. Containers should be airtight.

Dose: CHILD: 1 to 2 years, 1 to 2 tablets not more than 4 times daily; 3 to 5 years, 3 to 4 tablets not more than 3 times daily; 6 to 12 years, 4 tablets not more than 3 or 4 times daily.

Advice for patients: the tablets should be taken dissolved in water, preferably after meals. Aspirin should not be used for longer than 2 days or given to children under one year without medical advice.

SOLUBLE ASPIRIN AND CODEINE TABLETS (*Syn.* Soluble Acetylsalicylic Acid and Codeine Tablets): for each tablet take:

Aspirin, in fine powder	400 mg
Codeine phosphate	8 mg
Saccharin sodium	4 mg
Anhydrous citric acid	40 mg
Calcium carbonate	130 mg

A standard for these tablets is given in the British Pharmacopoeia Addendum 1975

Containers and *Storage:* see the entry on Tablets for general information on containers and storage. Containers should be airtight and light resistant.

Dose: 1 or 2 tablets.

Advice for patients: the tablets should be taken dissolved in water preferably after meals. Treatment should not be continued for longer than 2 days without medical advice.

SOLUBLE ASPIRIN, PHENACETIN, AND CODEINE TABLETS (*Syn.* Soluble Compound Codeine Tablets): for each tablet take:

Aspirin, in fine powder	250 mg
Phenacetin	250 mg
Codeine phosphate	8 mg
Saccharin sodium	5 mg
Anhydrous citric acid	26 mg
Calcium carbonate	80 mg

A standard for these tablets is given in the British Pharmacopoeia 1973

Containers and *Storage:* see the entry on Tablets for general information on containers and storage. Containers should be airtight and light resistant.

Dose: 1 or 2 tablets up to 4 times daily as necessary.

Advice for patients: the tablets should be dissolved in water and taken preferably after meals.

SOLUBLE ASPIRIN TABLETS (*Syn.* Soluble Acetylsalicylic Acid Tablets): for each tablet take:

Aspirin, in fine powder	300 mg
Saccharin sodium	3 mg
Anhydrous citric acid	30 mg
Calcium carbonate	100 mg

When Calcium Aspirin Tablets are prescribed or demanded, Soluble Aspirin Tablets are supplied.

A standard for these tablets is given in the British Pharmacopoeia 1973

Containers and *Storage:* see the entry on Tablets for general information on containers and storage. Containers should be airtight.

Advice for patients: the tablets should be dissolved in water and taken preferably after meals. Aspirin should not be used for longer than 2 days without medical advice.

OTHER PREPARATIONS available include a large number of single and multiple-ingredient preparations containing aspirin many of which are slight variations of the above formulae.

Asthma

Asthma is characterised by wheezing and difficulty in breathing owing to an increased resistance to air flow in the small airways. This increase in resistance is caused by spasm of bronchial smooth muscle, swelling and oedema of bronchial mucous membrane, and blockage of the small airways with viscid sputum. The condition may have well documented triggering factors and be allergic in origin (*extrinsic asthma*); in older subjects with no obvious allergic tendency it is called *intrinsic asthma*. The basic cause of asthma is still unknown, but individual attacks may be precipitated by stress, exercise, bacterial infection, exposure to allergen, etc.

In asthma of the allergic type, the frequency of attacks may be reduced by avoiding contact with known allergens and here measures to control house-dust mites may be particularly effective. In the case of allergy to grass pollens, desensitisation may be effective, and, in addition, prophylaxis with sodium cromoglycate may be of value. Where infection is a precipitating factor, suitable antibiotics should be used.

In general, three groups of drugs are used in the treatment of asthma—bronchodilators, sodium cromoglycate, and corticosteroids. Treatment may be given either in the acute attack or chronically. The aim of chronic treatment is to prevent the development of attacks by the prevention of mediator release or by neutralisation of the mediators before they can produce effects in the lung. Bronchodilators, such as aminophylline, choline theophyllinate, ephedrine, isoprenaline, orciprenaline, pseudoephedrine, salbutamol, and terbutaline, and corticosteroids can be used in the treatment of acute attacks and can also be given chronically. Sodium cromoglycate is ineffective in the acute attack and must be taken continuously prophylactically when the patient is well. The acute attack may be relieved by bronchodilator drugs given as aerosol inhalations, sprays, or injections. In severe acute asthma, large doses of corticosteroids should be started quickly, and a soluble preparation of hydrocortisone should be given intravenously for at least 24 hours at a rate equivalent to 4 milligrams of hydrocortisone per kilogram body-weight every 2 to 3 hours. Bronchodilators should be continued and may be given intravenously or as an aerosol. Administration of oxygen is essential and physiotherapy of great importance.

Chronic treatment may involve oral or aerosol bronchodilators, sodium cromoglycate, oral corticosteroids, or in selected patients aerosol corticosteroids.

There is much controversy about the role of emotional tension and the use of sedatives in the treatment of asthma. Sedatives should never be used in the treatment of a severe acute attack of asthma unless the patient is under close observation and facilities for ventilation are immediately to hand. In chronic management, where stress becomes of greater importance than the asthma itself, the judicious use of sedatives may then be indicated.

Athlete's Foot

see under TINEA INFECTIONS

Atomic Weights of Elements

see under WEIGHTS AND MEASURES

Atrioventricular Block

see under CARDIAC ARRHYTHMIAS

Atropine

(1R,3r,5S)-Tropan-3-yl (±)-tropate, or (±)-hyoscyamine, prepared by racemisation of (−)-hyoscyamine, an alkaloid extracted from *Duboisia* species, *Hyoscyamus muticus* L., and other solanaceous plants, or by synthesis.

$C_{17}H_{23}NO_3 = 289.4$

A standard is given in the British Pharmaceutical Codex 1973

Description. Odourless colourless crystals or a white crystalline powder.

Solubility. Soluble, at 20°, in 400 parts of water, in 3 parts of alcohol, in 60 parts of ether, and in 1 part of chloroform.

Optical rotation. Atropine is optically inactive but it often contains a small proportion of laevorotatory hyoscyamine.

Dissociation constant. pK_a 9.9 (20°).

Stability; Incompatibility. See under Atropine Sulphate.

Identification. TESTS. 1. Dissolve a few crystals in 5 ml of water containing 1 drop of hydrochloric acid and add 5 ml of *gold chloride solution*; a lemon-yellow precipitate is produced which rapidly crystallises. After recrystallisation from 3 ml of boiling water containing 1 drop of hydrochloric acid the precipitate has a minutely crystalline character, is dull and pulverent when dry, and has a melting-point of about 136° (distinction from hyoscyamine).
2. Add a few crystals to 4 drops of fuming nitric acid and evaporate to dryness on a water-bath; a yellow residue is obtained. To the cooled residue add 2 ml of acetone and 4 drops of a 3% solution of potassium hydroxide in methyl alcohol; a deep violet colour is produced. (Hyoscyamine and hyoscine produce the same colour as atropine; the presence of other alkaloids masks the reaction.)
3. To about 10 mg in a porcelain basin add 1.5 ml of a 2% solution of mercuric chloride in alcohol (60%); a yellow colour is produced which changes to red on gently warming (distinction from most other alkaloids except homatropine and hyoscyamine).

MELTING-POINT. About 116°.

ULTRAVIOLET ABSORPTION. In 0.1N sulphuric acid, maxima at 252 nm (E1%, 1cm = 5), 258 nm (E1%, 1cm = 6), and 264 nm (E1%, 1cm = 5).

Metabolism. ABSORPTION. Readily absorbed from mucous membranes, skin, and the gastro-intestinal tract but not from the stomach; after oral administration it is completely absorbed.

DISTRIBUTION. Small amounts are secreted in milk; *protein binding*, about 50% bound to plasma proteins.

METABOLIC REACTIONS. In man, about 50% of a dose is metabolised but the pathways involved are not elucidated; traces of tropic acid and tropine, formed as a result of hydrolysis, are detectable in the urine. The guinea-pig, as demonstrated by experiments *in vitro*, metabolises atropine via N-oxidation and demethylation.

EXCRETION. In 24 hours, 85 to 88% of a dose is excreted in the urine and a trace is excreted in the faeces; in the urine, 50% of the dose is excreted unchanged, less than 2% is excreted as tropic acid, and about 30% is excreted as unknown metabolites.

FURTHER INFORMATION. Metabolism in man—S. C. Kalser and P. L. McLain, *Clin. Pharmac. Ther.*, 1970, **11**, 214 and S. C. Kalser, *Ann. N.Y. Acad. Sci.*, 1971, **179**, 667; metabolic N-oxidation—J. D. Phillipson *et al.*, *J. Pharm. Pharmac.*, 1976, **28**, 687.

Actions and uses. Atropine has central and peripheral actions. It may initially stimulate the central nervous system, causing excitement and restlessness, and in larger doses it produces depression with drowsiness, delirium, and later, coma. It also acts on the lower motor centres and diminishes the muscular rigidity and salivation of parkinsonism. It antagonises the muscarinic actions of acetylcholine and of similarly acting drugs. It diminishes the secretions of the salivary and sweat glands and of the bronchial and gastro-intestinal tract. It also relaxes spasmodic contraction of involuntary muscle, increases the heart rate, and produces vasodilatation. It dilates the pupil, paralyses the muscles of accommodation, and increases intra-ocular pressure. When given by mouth, atropine, administered as the sulphate or methonitrate, is slowly absorbed and takes effect after about three-quarters of an hour; after subcutaneous injection, its effect is maximal within about half an hour.

Atropine is given before the administration of a volatile anaesthetic to prevent excessive bronchial secretion, but hyoscine is often preferred for this purpose. It is also used in the treatment of renal and biliary colic and of asthma to prevent or relieve spasm of involuntary muscle; this action may also explain some of the beneficial effects which follow its use in the treatment of incontinence of urine in children.

Small doses of atropine are sometimes used to prevent excessive peristalsis and colicky pains produced by irritant purgatives.

As it diminishes gastric and intestinal motility it is used in conjunction with other measures in the treatment of gastric and duodenal ulcer. It is, however, more liable to cause undesirable effects than drugs such as propantheline which have a less marked action on the central nervous system.

In the treatment of postencephalitic parkinsonism large

doses of atropine salts are used, although this treatment has been largely replaced by the use of other para-sympatholytics such as benzhexol; the dryness of the mouth which is often associated with these large doses may be relieved by the oral administration of pilocarpine nitrate.

In the treatment of severe anticholinesterase poisoning by, for example, organophosphorus compounds, atropine sulphate may be given intramuscularly in doses of 2 milligrams at intervals of 10 to 30 minutes.

In ophthalmology, atropine has been used to dilate the pupil prior to retinoscopy, but homatropine is to be preferred for this purpose because of its shorter duration of action and the fact that its effect is reversed by physostigmine. Mydriasis due to atropine may be reversed by demecarium but treatment must be continued for several weeks or until all atropine has been cleared as otherwise mydriasis returns as the effect of the demecarium diminishes. Atropine is also applied locally to the conjunctiva to immobilise the ciliary muscle and iris; for this purpose atropine sulphate may be used as 1% aqueous eye-drops or eye ointment; an oily solution of atropine is also used as eye-drops.

The disadvantage of atropine in ophthalmology is that its effect is very persistent and may last for several days and the rise in intra-ocular pressure may precipitate a case of latent glaucoma into an acute attack. In general, it is not used in cases of increased intra-ocular tension, and in the treatment of adults, homatropine is usually preferred. In hypersensitive individuals, atropine gives rise to irritation of the conjunctiva; for these patients, lachesine chloride may be a suitable alternative.

Precautions and contra-indications. Atropine should not be used in patients with glaucoma because it increases intra-ocular tension. It should be used with caution in patients with urinary retention and it should not be used by nursing mothers as atropine will diminish milk flow.

Poisoning. Poisoning by atropine is characterised in the early stages by marked excitement, delirium, dilated pupils, a rapid pulse, and a hot, flushed, dry skin. Belladonna fruits are sometimes a cause of poisoning in children, and gastric lavage with water should be employed.

When atropine or belladonna fruit has been taken by mouth, the stage of excitement should be treated by administration of diazepam when necessary. In the later stages of central depression, artificial respiration may be necessary.

Atropine Methonitrate

(1*R*,3*r*,5*S*)-8-Methyl-3-(±)-tropoyloxytropanium nitrate, the methonitrate of the alkaloid atropine.

$C_{18}H_{26}N_2O_6 = 366.4$

OTHER NAMES: Atrop. Methonit.; *Eumydrin*®; Methyl-atropine Nitrate; Methylatropini Nitras

A standard is given in the European Pharmacopoeia Vol. III

Description. Colourless odourless crystals.

Solubility. Soluble, at 20°, in less than 1 part of water, and in 13 parts of alcohol; practically insoluble in ether and in chloroform.

Acidity or alkalinity. A 10% solution has a pH of 6 to 7.5.

Stability. Aqueous solutions are unstable; stability is enhanced in acid solutions of pH below 6. Alcoholic solutions are stable for 12 months but such solutions should be kept in airtight containers to prevent concentration of the solution by partial evaporation of the solvent.

Sterilisation. Solutions are sterilised by filtration.

Identification. TESTS. 1. To 5 ml of a 1% solution add 0.5 ml of hydrochloric acid and 2.5 ml of *gold chloride solution*; a precipitate is formed which, after recrystallisation from boiling water acidified with hydrochloric acid, melts at about 205° (distinction from atropine and hyoscyamine).
2. To a solution in water add *sodium hydroxide solution*; the alkaloidal base is not precipitated.
3. Add 1 drop of a 1% solution to 4 drops of a 1% solution of diphenylamine in nitrogen-free sulphuric acid; an intense blue colour is produced.
4. It complies with Test 2 described under Atropine.

MELTING-POINT. About 167°.

ULTRAVIOLET ABSORPTION. In 0.1N hydrochloric acid, maxima at 254 nm (E1%, 1cm = 6), 258 nm (E1%, 1cm = 6), and 266 nm.

INFRA-RED ABSORPTION. Major peaks at 1045, 1162, 1176, 1370, 1457, and 1728 cm^{-1} (see Appendix 2a: Infra-red Spectra).

THIN-LAYER CHROMATOGRAPHY. See under Thin-layer Chromatography, System 8.

Metabolism. See under Atropine.

Actions and uses. Atropine methonitrate has the actions described under Atropine. It has less effect on the central nervous system and is less toxic than atropine.

It is used mainly in the treatment of congenital hypertrophic pyloric stenosis; 200 micrograms, or 2 millilitres of a freshly prepared 0.01% aqueous solution, or a solution of similar strength prepared by dilution of a 0.6% alcoholic solution with water, is given by mouth half an hour before food, 7 times during 24 hours. Thereafter the dose is increased by 100 micrograms (1 millilitre) daily to a maximum of 600 micrograms (6 millilitres) per dose and treatment is continued until 10 days after vomiting has ceased. If the patient is in a dehydrated condition it is important to correct this before treatment.

When atropine methonitrate is given as an alcoholic solution the danger of concentration by evaporation should be guarded against; it has been given in this form in the treatment of whooping-cough in infants.

Atropine methonitrate is an ingredient of compound spray solutions used in the treatment of asthma and hay fever.

Precautions and contra-indications. As for Atropine.

Poisoning. As for Atropine.

Preparations

COMPOUND ADRENALINE AND ATROPINE SPRAY:

Adrenaline acid tartrate	.. 8 g
Atropine methonitrate	.. 1 g
Papaverine hydrochloride	.. 8 g
Sodium metabisulphite	.. 1 g
Chlorbutol	.. 5 g
Propylene glycol	50 ml
Purified water, freshly boiled and cooled	to 1000 ml

Adrenaline and atropine compound spray contains the equivalent of about 1 in 225 (4.5 mg in 1 ml) of adrenaline.

A standard for this spray is given in the British Pharmaceutical Codex 1973

Containers: see the entry on Sprays for general information on containers.

Storage: it should be stored in well-filled airtight containers, protected from light.

Advice for patients: the spray solution should be used with an atomiser and inhaled through the mouth. Excessive use of the spray should be avoided.

OTHER PREPARATIONS available include a SOLUTION containing atropine methonitrate 6 mg per ml in alcohol; dilution is not recommended.

Atropine Sulphate

(1R,3r,5S)-3-(±)-Tropoyloxytropanium sulphate monohydrate, the sulphate of the alkaloid atropine.
$(C_{17}H_{23}NO_3)_2,H_2SO_4,H_2O = 694.8$

OTHER NAMES: Atrop. Sulph.; Atropini Sulfas

A standard is given in the European Pharmacopoeia Vol. II

Description. Odourless colourless crystals or white crystalline powder. It effloresces in dry air.

Solubility. Soluble, at 20°, in less than 1 part of water and in 4 parts of alcohol; practically insoluble in ether and in chloroform.

Acidity. A 2% solution has a pH of 4.5 to 6.2.

Moisture content. 2.5 to 4%, determined by drying at 120°.

Stability. In aqueous solution, atropine hydrolyses to tropine and tropic acid but decomposition at room temperature occurs very slowly. Hydrolysis of atropine is catalysed by hydrogen ions and hydroxide ions. At 25°, the rate of hydrolysis is a minimum at pH 3.8. Dehydration of atropine to apoatropine may also occur; apoatropine hydrolyses to tropine and atropic acid.

FURTHER INFORMATION. Stability in aqueous solution —P. Zvirblis *et al., J. Am. pharm. Ass., scient. Edn,* 1956, **45**, 450 and A. A. Kondritzer and P. Zvirblis, *J. Am. pharm. Ass., scient. Edn,* 1957, **46**, 531; chemistry of degradation—E. Bjerkelund *et al., Pharm. Acta Helv.,* 1969, **44**, 744.

Incompatibility. Atropine salts are incompatible with bromides, iodides, alkalis, tannic acid, quinine, and salts of mercury.

Sterilisation. Solutions are sterilised by heating in an autoclave, by heating with a bactericide, or by filtration.

Identification. TESTS. 1. To a 2% solution add *dilute sodium hydroxide solution;* a white precipitate is produced which, after washing and drying, melts at about 116°.

2. It complies with Test 2 described under Atropine.

MELTING-POINT. About 190°, with decomposition, after drying at 135° for 15 minutes.

ULTRAVIOLET ABSORPTION. In 0.1N hydrochloric acid, maxima at 254 nm (E1%, 1cm = 5), 258 nm (E1%, 1cm = 5), and 266 nm.

INFRA-RED ABSORPTION. Major peaks at 1026, 1062, 1081, 1127, 1170, and 1728 cm⁻¹ (see Appendix 2a: Infrared Spectra).

THIN-LAYER CHROMATOGRAPHY. See under Thin-layer Chromatography, System 8.

Metabolism. See under Atropine.

Actions and uses. Atropine sulphate has the actions and uses described under Atropine. The usual dose is 0.25 to 2 milligrams daily in single or divided doses by mouth; alternatively 0.25 to 2 milligrams may be given by subcutaneous, intramuscular, or intravenous injection. The usual dose by subcutaneous, intramuscular, or intravenous injection for children up to 1 year is 250 micrograms, 1 to 5 years 250 to 500 micrograms, and 6 to 12 years 0.5 to 1 milligram.

Precautions and contra-indications. As for Atropine.

Poisoning. As for Atropine.

Veterinary uses. Atropine sulphate is a parasympatholytic, mydriatic, and partial antidote in organophosphorus poisoning.

The usual dose as a parasympatholytic is for horses and cattle 30 to 60 micrograms per kilogram body-weight, pigs 20 to 40 micrograms per kilogram body-weight, sheep 80 to 160 micrograms per kilogram body-weight, dogs and cats 30 to 100 micrograms per kilogram body-weight; these doses are given by subcutaneous injection.

As a partial antidote to organophosphorus poisoning atropine sulphate may be given to all species by intramuscular or intravenous injection in doses of 1 milligram per kilogram body-weight, repeated as necessary.

Preparations

ATROPINE EYE-DROPS (*Syn.* Atropine Sulphate Eye-drops): a sterile solution containing up to 2% of atropine sulphate, with 0.002% of phenylmercuric acetate or nitrate or 0.02% v/v of benzalkonium chloride solution (0.01% w/v of benzalkonium chloride), in purified water. It is prepared by method A, B, or C described in the entry on Eye-drops.

A standard for these eye-drops is given in the British Pharmacopoeia Addendum 1977

Containers: see the entry on Eye-drops for general information on containers. This solution is adversely affected by alkali.

Labelling: see the entry on Eye-drops for general information on labelling.

Advice for patients: see the entry on Eye-drops for general information on the use of eye-drops. Blurring of vision and sensitivity to light may occur for several days after instillation of the drops.

ATROPINE EYE OINTMENT (*Syn.* Oculent. Atrop.): prepared by incorporating atropine sulphate in eye ointment basis, or any other suitable basis, by method A described in the entry on Eye Ointments.

A standard for this eye ointment is given in the British Pharmacopoeia 1973

Containers and *Labelling:* see the entry on Eye Ointments for general information on containers and labelling.

Advice for patients: see the entry on Eye Ointments for general information on the use of eye ointments. Blurring of vision and sensitivity to light may occur for several days after application of the eye ointment.

ATROPINE SULPHATE INJECTION: a sterile solution of atropine sulphate in water for injections. The acidity of the solution is adjusted to pH 3 by the addition of dilute sulphuric acid. The solution is sterilised by heating in an autoclave or by filtration. The usual strength is 1 mg of atropine sulphate per ml. Also available in 1-ml ampoules containing 400 micrograms of atropine sulphate, and in 1-ml ampoules and 25-ml vials containing 600 micrograms of atropine sulphate per ml.
A standard for this injection is given in the British Pharmacopoeia 1973
Containers and *Labelling:* see the entry on Injections for general information on containers and labelling.

ATROPINE SULPHATE TABLETS: available as tablets containing 500 and 600 micrograms of atropine sulphate.
A standard for these tablets is given in the British Pharmacopoeia 1973
Containers and *Storage:* see the entry on Tablets for general information on containers and storage. Containers should be airtight.
Advice for patients: when used as an ulcer suppressant the tablets should be taken half an hour before meals.

Attapulgite, Activated

A purified native aluminium magnesium silicate belonging to the palygorskite-sepiolite group of mineral clays, heated to increase the adsorptive capacity.

OTHER NAMES: *Attasorb®*; *Pharmasorb®*
Atasorb-N® (with neomycin sulphate)

A standard is given in the British Pharmacopoeia Addendum 1977 and the British Pharmacopoeia (Veterinary)

Description. A pale cream or buff very fine powder.

Solubility. Practically insoluble in water and in solutions of alkali hydroxides.

Alkalinity. A 5% suspension in water has a pH of 7.5 to 9.

Actions and uses. Activated attapulgite is an adsorbent which is used similarly to light kaolin, but it has a greater adsorption capacity. The usual dose in the treatment of diarrhoea is 3 grams administered as a 10% suspension 3 or 4 times daily.

Veterinary uses. Activated attapulgite is an adsorbent used in the treatment of diarrhoea, the usual dose for all species being 10 to 150 milligrams per kilogram body-weight.

Preparations

Preparations available include a MIXTURE containing activated attapulgite 3 g and colloidal activated attapulgite 900 mg with neomycin sulphate 321 mg in 30 ml, diluent water, shelf-life of diluted mixture 14 days.

Azaperone

4′ - Fluoro - 4 - [4 - (pyrid - 2 - yl)piperazin - 1 - yl]butyrophenone

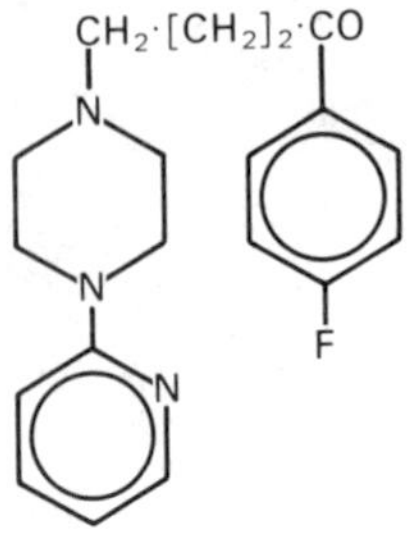

$C_{19}H_{22}FN_3O = 327.4$

OTHER NAMES: *Stresnil®*; *Suicalm®*

A standard is given in the British Pharmacopoeia (Veterinary)

Description. A white to yellowish-white microcrystalline powder.

Solubility. Practically insoluble in water; soluble, at 20°, in 29 parts of alcohol, in 4 parts of chloroform, and in 31 parts of ether.

Sterilisation. Solutions for injection are sterilised by filtration.

Storage. It should be stored in airtight containers, protected from light.

Identification. MELTING-POINT. About 92°.

ULTRAVIOLET ABSORPTION. In a mixture containing 10 volumes of 0.1N hydrochloric acid and 90 volumes of alcohol (95%), maxima at 244 nm (E1%, 1cm = 800) and 310 nm (E1%, 1cm = 187).

Veterinary uses. Azaperone is a tranquilliser used in pigs to reduce stress and control fighting. The usual dose is 0.5 to 2 mg per kilogram body-weight by intramuscular injection, the dose being adjusted in accordance with the response of the animal.

Preparation

AZAPERONE INJECTION: a sterile solution of azaperone, with suitable solubilising and stabilising agents, in water for injections. It is sterilised by filtration. Available in 20-ml bottles containing 40 mg of azaperone per ml.
A standard for this injection is given in the British Pharmacopoeia (Veterinary)
Containers and *Labelling:* see the entry on Injections for general information on containers and labelling.
Storage: it should be protected from light.

Azathioprine

6-(1-Methyl-4-nitroimidazol-5-ylthio)purine

$C_9H_7N_7O_2S = 277.3$

OTHER NAME: *Imuran®*

A standard is given in the British Pharmacopoeia 1973

Description. A pale yellow odourless powder.

Solubility. Practically insoluble in water; very slightly soluble in alcohol and in chloroform; soluble in dilute mineral acids; soluble in dilute solutions of alkali hydroxides but decomposes in stronger solutions.

Moisture content. Not more than 1%, determined by drying at 105° *in vacuo.*

Storage. It should be protected from light.

Identification. TEST. Mix about 20 mg with 100 ml of water, heat, and filter; to 5 ml of the filtrate add 1 ml of hydrochloric acid and 10 mg of zinc powder and allow to stand for 5 minutes; the solution becomes yellow. Filter the solution, cool the filtrate in ice, add 2 drops of a 10% solution of sodium nitrite and 100 mg of sulphamic acid, shake until the bubbles disappear and then add 1 ml of *2-naphthol solution*; a pale pink precipitate is produced.

MELTING-POINT. About 238°, with decomposition.

ULTRAVIOLET ABSORPTION. In 0.1N hydrochloric acid, maximum at 280 nm (E1%, 1cm = 600).

INFRA-RED ABSORPTION. Major peaks at 832, 1237, 1306, 1500, 1531, and 1580 cm⁻¹ (see Appendix 2a: Infra-red Spectra).

Determination in body fluids. ULTRAVIOLET SPECTRO-PHOTOMETRY. In urine—A. H. Chalmers, *Biochem. Med.*, 1975, **12**, 234.

Metabolism. ABSORPTION. Absorbed after oral administration.

DISTRIBUTION. Widely distributed throughout the body.

METABOLIC REACTIONS. Readily converted, mainly in the liver, to its active metabolite, 6-mercaptopurine; it is metabolised along with its active metabolite by xanthine oxidase. The methylnitroimidazole moiety of azathioprine is conjugated with glutathione.

EXCRETION. About 50% of a dose is excreted in the urine in 24 hours, about 10% as unchanged drug.

Actions and uses. Azathioprine is a cytotoxic and im-munosuppressive agent. Its actions partly depend upon its steady conversion into another cytotoxic drug, mer-captopurine, thus providing a prolonged therapeutic effect unobtainable by the use of mercaptopurine itself. The effects of azathioprine appear within 2 to 4 days of administration and about half the dose is excreted in the urine in the first day either as unchanged drug or as its metabolites.

Azathioprine is used as a cytotoxic drug in the treatment of acute leukaemia in a dose of 1.5 to 4 milligrams per kilogram body-weight daily.

As an immunosuppressive agent in organ transplanta-tion to suppress the homograft reaction, 2 to 5 milligrams per kilogram body-weight may be given daily. This is reduced to half as a maintenance dose. In organ trans-plantation, azathioprine is often used with other im-munosuppressive drugs such as corticosteroids and other cytostatic drugs such as actinomycin. In organ trans-plantation, the dose of azathioprine may be temporarily increased and another immunosuppressive agent added if the graft shows signs of rejection.

Azathioprine has also been used for the treatment of some diseases thought to have an immunological mech-anism, such as lupus erythematosus and polyarteritis nodosa, and to reduce the dose of corticosteroids in patients with very severe rheumatoid arthritis, ulcerative colitis, Crohn's disease, and various kinds of nephritis. It is occasionally used in the treatment of severe psoriasis.

Undesirable effects. Azathioprine causes hypoplasia of the bone marrow, the blood cell mainly affected being the granulocyte. Haematological control is therefore essential when the drug is being administered.

Other toxic effects are anorexia, nausea, and malaise; hepatotoxicity has also been observed. It may cause foetal damage. The toxicity of azathioprine is dose de-pendent and may be enhanced if it is given concurrently with allopurinol.

Preparations

AZATHIOPRINE TABLETS: available as tablets containing 50 mg of azathioprine.

A standard for these tablets is given in the British Pharmacopoeia 1973

Containers and *Storage:* see the entry on Tablets for general information on containers and storage. Con-tainers should be airtight and light resistant.

OTHER PREPARATIONS available include an INJECTION consisting of vials of powder containing azathioprine sodium equivalent to 50 mg of azathioprine.

Bacillus Calmette–Guérin Vaccine

A freeze-dried preparation containing live bacteria ob-tained from a strain derived from the bacillus of Calmette and Guérin and known to protect man against tubercu-losis. It is reconstituted immediately before use with an appropriate volume of a suitable sterile liquid.

OTHER NAMES: BCG Vaccine; Dried Tub/Vac/BCG; Freeze-dried BCG Vaccine; Vaccinum Tuberculosis (BCG) Cryodesiccatum

A standard is given in the European Pharmacopoeia Vol. II

Storage. It should be stored as described under Vac-cines. Under these conditions it may be expected to retain its potency for 2 years. The reconstituted vaccine should be used immediately after preparation.

Actions and uses. Bacillus Calmette–Guérin vaccine is used for active immunisation against tuberculosis, prin-cipally for the vaccination of selected groups of the population and of persons likely to be exposed to infec-tion. It is given only to persons who give a negative tuberculin reaction, as described under Old Tuberculin.

A suitable schedule for the immunisation of children is given in the entry on Vaccines.

The vaccine is generally administered intracutaneously over the insertion of the deltoid muscle. The usual dose is 0.1 millilitre by intracutaneous injection.

Bacillus Calmette–Guérin Vaccine, Percutaneous

A suspension of living cells of an authentic strain of the bacillus of Calmette and Guérin with a higher viable bacterial count than Bacillus Calmette–Guérin Vaccine. It is prepared immediately before use by reconstituting the dried vaccine with an appropriate volume of a suitable sterile liquid.

OTHER NAMES: Percut. BCG Vaccine; Tub/Vac/BCG(Perc)

A standard is given in the British Pharmacopoeia 1973

Storage. It should be stored as described under Vaccines. Under these conditions it may be expected to retain its potency for 2 years. The reconstituted vaccine should be used immediately after preparation.

Actions and uses. Percutaneous Bacillus Calmette–Guérin vaccine has the actions and uses described under Bacillus Calmette–Guérin Vaccine, but it is administered by the percutaneous route with the aid of a suitable instrument. On account of its higher viable bacterial count it is not suitable for intracutaneous administration.

Bacitracin Zinc

A zinc salt of bacitracin, one or more of the antimicrobial polypeptides produced by certain strains of *Bacillus licheniformis* and by *B. subtilis* var. *Tracy* and yielding on hydrolysis the amino-acids L-cysteine, D-glutamic acid, L-histidine, L-isoleucine, L-leucine, L-lysine, D-ornithine, D-phenylalanine, and DL-aspartic acid.

OTHER NAMES: *Neobacrin®* (with neomycin sulphate); *Polyfax®* (with polymyxin B sulphate)

A standard is given in the British Pharmacopoeia 1973

Description. A white or pale buff, odourless, hygroscopic powder with a bitter taste.

Solubility. Soluble, at 20°, in 900 parts of water and in 500 parts of alcohol; very slightly soluble in ether; practically insoluble in chloroform.

Moisture content. Not more than 5%, determined by drying at 60° *in vacuo.*

Storage. It should be stored in airtight containers.

Identification. TESTS. 1. Dissolve about 3 mg in 1 ml of water, add 1 ml of a 0.2% solution of ninhydrin in n-butyl alcohol and 0.5 ml of pyridine, and heat at 100° for 5 minutes; a deep purple colour is produced.

2. Ignite, dissolve the residue in *dilute sulphuric acid*, and add 1 drop of a 0.1% solution of copper sulphate and 2 ml of *ammonium mercurithiocyanate solution*; a violet precipitate is produced.

Actions and uses. Bacitracin is an antibiotic which is active against a wide range of Gram-positive organisms and against spirochaetes and some Gram-positive cocci. It is used in the form of its zinc salt in lozenges, ointments, dusting-powders, and aerosol sprays, often in conjunction with other antibiotics such as neomycin or polymyxins, or with hydrocortisone, in the treatment of local infections by susceptible organisms.

In dentistry it may be used as an ingredient of preparations for treating infections of the root canal.

Undesirable effects. Absorption from open wounds or the use of aerosol sprays over the site of an abdominal operation may give rise to signs of renal toxicity.

Preparations

NEOMYCIN AND BACITRACIN OINTMENT:

Neomycin sulphate	..	..	..	..	5 g
Bacitracin zinc	..	..	..	500 000 units
Liquid paraffin	..	..	..	..	100 g
White soft paraffin	..	..	..	to 1000 g

Melt the white soft paraffin, incorporate the liquid paraffin, and stir until cold. Triturate the neomycin sulphate and the bacitracin zinc with a portion of the basis and gradually incorporate the remainder of the basis. The ointment may be expected to retain its potency for 2 years provided that the moisture content of the ointment does not exceed 0.2%. When materials complying with B.P.C. 1973 requirements are used, the moisture content may be expected to be below this figure.

A standard for this ointment is given in the British Pharmaceutical Codex 1973

Containers and *Storage:* see the entry on Ointments for general information on containers and storage. Containers should be airtight.

Advice for patients: the ointment should be applied sparingly to the affected area.

POLYMYXIN AND BACITRACIN EYE OINTMENT: prepared by incorporating polymyxin B sulphate and bacitracin zinc in eye ointment basis, or any other suitable basis, by method B described in the entry on Eye Ointments. Available as an ointment containing 10 000 units of polymyxin B sulphate and 500 units of bacitracin zinc per g.

Containers and *Labelling:* see the entry on Eye Ointments for general information on containers and labelling.

Storage: it should be stored in a cool place.

Advice for patients: see the entry on Eye Ointments for general information on the use of eye ointments. The prescribed course should be completed.

OTHER PREPARATIONS available include an EYE OINTMENT containing neomycin sulphate and bacitracin zinc in the same concentrations as in neomycin and bacitracin ointment; and an OINTMENT containing polymyxin B sulphate and bacitracin zinc in the same concentrations as in polymyxin and bacitracin eye ointment.

Backache

Backache is a common symptom with a large number of different causes.

Mechanical defects of the back due to injury or to structural inadequacy or abnormality produce pain; low back pain (lumbago) due to displacement of an intervertebral disk may be accompanied by sciatica.

Pain in the back may be due to disease of the vertebrae, for example ankylosing spondylitis, infection, or metastatic foci in the vertebrae, or post-menopausal bone thinning as in osteoporosis.

Diseases or conditions in places other than the spine may also produce backache, for example menstruation, pregnancy, rectal disorders, renal disease, pancreatic disease, retroperitoneal tumours, etc.

Backache may also be a symptom of depressive illness.

Treatment should be aimed at the underlying disorder. Pain due to local disorders of the back may be alleviated by reducing the load on the back, by correcting structural weakness, and by analgesics such as salicylates.

Baclofen

4-Amino-3-(4-chlorophenyl)butyric acid

$$NH_2 \cdot CH_2 \cdot CH \cdot CH_2 \cdot COOH$$

$C_{10}H_{12}ClNO_2 = 213.7$

OTHER NAME: *Lioresal*®

Identification. MELTING-POINT. About 207°.

ULTRAVIOLET ABSORPTION. In 0.1N hydrochloric acid, maxima at 220 nm (E1%, 1cm = 473) and 267 nm (E1%, 1cm = 12); in alcohol (95%), maxima at 223 nm (E1%, 1cm = 467) and 268 nm (E1%, 1cm = 12).

INFRA-RED ABSORPTION. Major peaks at 836, 1384, 1396, 1402, 1529, and 1574 cm^{-1} (see Appendix 2a: Infra-red Spectra).

THIN-LAYER CHROMATOGRAPHY. See under Thin-layer Chromatography, System 3.

Determination in body fluids. GAS CHROMATOGRAPHY. In plasma or urine—P. H. Degen and W. Reiss, *J. Chromat.*, 1976, **117**, 399.

Metabolism. ABSORPTION. Readily absorbed after oral administration.

BLOOD CONCENTRATION. After an oral dose of 40 mg, peak plasma concentrations of about 0.6 μg/ml are attained within 2 hours.

HALF-LIFE. Serum half-life, 3 to 4 hours.

DISTRIBUTION. *Protein binding*, about 30% bound to plasma proteins.

METABOLIC REACTIONS. Limited metabolism, mainly deamination.

EXCRETION. About 85% of a dose is excreted unchanged in urine and faeces together with 15% as the deaminated metabolite; 70 to 80% of the recoverable drug and its metabolites is excreted in the urine.

FURTHER INFORMATION. A preliminary report of the pharmacological properties and therapeutic efficacy of baclofen—R. N. Brogden *et al.*, *Drugs*, 1974, **8**, 1.

Actions and uses. Baclofen reduces spasm of voluntary muscle by its action on the motor neurones of the spinal cord. It is used in the treatment of spasticity occurring in multiple sclerosis and other spinal lesions.

It is administered by mouth, starting with a small dose, such as 5 milligrams 3 times a day, and gradually increasing until the spasticity is controlled; doses up to 60 milligrams daily are sufficient in most cases and larger doses up to 100 milligrams daily require careful supervision.

Undesirable effects. Nausea, vomiting, drowsiness, confusion, fatigue, and muscle weakness may occur; these effects are usually dose-dependent.

Precautions and contra-indications. It should be used with caution in psychiatric states, in patients with a history of gastric ulceration, and in those being treated with antihypertensive drugs. It is contra-indicated in patients with a history of epilepsy.

Poisoning. A high fluid intake should be maintained and diuretics administered if necessary to eliminate the substance through the kidneys. Controlled respiration is required when the respiratory muscles are affected.

Preparations

Preparations available include TABLETS containing baclofen 10 mg.

Bang's Disease

see BRUCELLOSIS

Barbiturates

The barbiturates are derivatives of barbituric acid (malonyl urea: 2,4,6-trioxohexahydropyrimidine) in which both of the hydrogen atoms at position 5 are replaced by alkenyl, alkyl, alkynyl, aryl, arylalkyl, or alicyclic groups; the nitrogen atom at position 1 may be methylated. Substitution of sulphur for oxygen at position 2 gives the thiobarbiturates. An enolic form exists in equilibrium with the trioxo form and because of this the barbiturates act as weak acids and form stable sodium and calcium salts.

Stability. Barbiturates can be divided into two groups—the free barbituric acids which have a low solubility in water, and their sodium (or other metal) salts which are more soluble.

The free barbituric acids are generally stable compounds and no special storage requirements are necessary. Stable aqueous solutions may be prepared by incorporating a suitable solubilising agent such as alcohol in the formulation. Because alcohol potentiates the sedative action of barbiturates, alternatives such as glycerol and propylene glycol are used. In some cases combinations of two or three such adjuvants are employed.

The sodium or other alkali or alkaline earth metal salts (sometimes referred to as "soluble barbiturates") are generally hygroscopic. When exposed to air they absorb carbon dioxide and the free barbituric acid is liberated. Storage in airtight containers is therefore essential.

Aqueous solutions of the soluble barbiturates decompose, the rate of decomposition increasing with rise in temperature. For example, amylobarbitone sodium, barbitone sodium, and phenobarbitone sodium have been reported to show the following decomposition in 10% solutions in water at 20°: after 15 days, 3 to 4%; after 30 days, 6 to 8%; after 90 days, about 15%. The rate of decomposition of soluble barbiturates may be increased in the presence of other substances such as sodium chloride or dextrose. The addition of propylene glycol, macrogol 400, alcohol, and glycerol to aqueous solutions of amylobarbitone sodium, barbitone sodium, pentobarbitone sodium, and phenobarbitone sodium, has a stabilising effect. Glycerol has relatively little stabilising action compared with the other adjuvants. Propylene glycol, macrogol 400, and alcohol confer approximately equal degrees of stabilisation. Solutions of the soluble barbiturates in propylene glycol or in macrogol 400 are stable to heating at 100° for 24 hours and can be stored without deterioration for one year at 20°.

Incompatibility. Solutions of sodium salts are incompatible with acidic substances (including carbon dioxide and ammonium chloride) owing to precipitation of the free barbituric acids. As the sodium salts of barbituric acids are alkaline in solution they decompose certain vitamins such as ascorbic acid and thiamine hydrochloride. Ammonia is evolved on mixing the alkaline solution with solutions of ammonium salts, and chloral is decomposed to produce chloroform.

Formation of complexes of low solubility may occur between barbiturates and weak bases, as for example, when solutions of phenobarbitone sodium are mixed with those of calcium chloride, magnesium sulphate, diphenhydramine hydrochloride, and codeine phosphate. Hence precipitation may occur even though the barbiturate is normally soluble at the pH of the medium. Phenobarbitone is reported to form a complex of reduced solubility with macrogol 4000, and the latter should therefore not be included in tablet formulations.

Sterilisation. Barbiturates are decomposed on heating and sterile solutions are therefore usually prepared by dissolving the sterile dry barbiturate in water for injections or other suitable solvent. Solutions are generally prepared immediately before use, and if the solvent is water, it should be free from carbon dioxide.

Aqueous solutions of soluble barbiturates containing a high proportion of propylene glycol are stable and can be sterilised by heating with a bactericide at 98° to 100° for 30 minutes. The presence of propylene glycol also allows a portion of the soluble barbiturate to be replaced by the corresponding acid if a pH adjustment is necessary. These stabilised solutions must be well diluted with water for injections or other suitable injection solution before administration.

Identification. GENERAL TESTS. 1. Place on a filter paper a few mg of the powdered substance or a portion of powdered tablets, or, if stated in the individual monograph, of the precipitated material; add a few drops of acetone, allow to dry, brush any loose powder off the paper, add 1 drop of *cobalt nitrate solution* to the spot on the filter paper, allow to dry, and expose the spot to ammonia vapour; a bright purple colour is produced.
2. To a solution in sulphuric acid add a trace of sodium nitrite and warm; an orange-yellow solution with a brownish sheen is given by barbiturates having a phenyl substituent.
3. The melting-point of the 4-nitrobenzyl derivative may be used as an aid to the identification of certain barbiturates: triturate about 600 mg with 150 mg of anhydrous sodium carbonate and 5 ml of water, add 450 mg of 4-nitrobenzyl chloride dissolved in 10 ml of alcohol (95%), heat for 30 minutes on a water-bath, and allow to stand for 1 hour. Filter, wash the filter with 10 ml of 1N sodium hydroxide and then with water and recrystallise the residue from alcohol (95%). The derivatives have the following melting-points:

150° (or 168°) Amylobarbitone
150° Butobarbitone
155° Secbutobarbitone
156° Quinalbarbitone
168° (or 150°) Amylobarbitone
182° Phenobarbitone

MELTING-POINT. The melting-points given below are those of the free barbituric acids; the method for separating the free acid is given, where appropriate, in the individual monographs.

94° Methohexitone	160° Thiopentone
96° Quinalbarbitone	166° Secbutobarbitone
124° Butobarbitone	172° Cyclobarbitone
128° Pentobarbitone	176° Phenobarbitone
156° Amylobarbitone	

ULTRAVIOLET ABSORPTION. The 5,5-disubstituted barbiturates exhibit ultraviolet absorption only in strongly alkaline solution, due to ionisation which takes place in two stages. At the first stage, at about pH 10, an absorption maximum occurs at about 240 nm; at the second stage at about pH 13, the maximum shifts to about 255 nm. In the case of 1,5,5-trisubstituted barbiturates, the ionisation does not proceed beyond the first stage. None of these compounds exhibits any significant absorption below about pH 8.6. The thiobarbiturates exhibit absorption maxima in both alkaline and acid solutions.

These absorption characteristics may be used to distinguish the various types of barbiturates: to 5 ml of a suitable aqueous solution of the sample add 1 drop of 2N ammonia (to bring the solution to about pH 10) and immediately record the ultraviolet absorption spectrum. Add 1 drop of 2N sulphuric acid (to bring the solution to about pH 2) and again record the ultraviolet absorption spectrum. Finally, add 1 drop of 4N sodium hydroxide solution (to bring the solution to about pH 13) and record the spectrum. Details of the absorption maxima are given in the following table:

	absorption maxima (nm)		
	(approximate)		
barbiturate	pH 10	pH 2	pH 13
5,5-disubstituted barbiturates	240	—	255
1,5,5-trisubstituted barbiturates	240	—	240
thiobarbiturates	255, 305	239, 290	305
methohexitone	250	228	250

Details of the ultraviolet absorption of individual barbiturates are given in the appropriate monographs.

INFRA-RED ABSORPTION. Details of the infra-red absorption of individual barbiturates are given in the appropriate monographs.

THIN-LAYER CHROMATOGRAPHY. See under Thin-layer Chromatography, System 5.

Determination in body fluids. DITHIZONE TITRATION. In blood: quick screening method—A. S. Curry, *Br. med. J.*, i/1964, 354; W. M. Clow and A. C. A. Smith, *Scott. med. J.*, 1967, **12**, 307.

ULTRAVIOLET SPECTROPHOTOMETRY. In blood: 5,5-disubstituted barbiturates—P. M. G. Broughton, *Biochem. J.*, 1956, **63**, 207; G. W. Stevenson, *Analyt. Chem.*, 1961, **33**, 1374. In blood: low concentrations—H. M. Stone and C. R. Henwood, *J. forens. Sci. Soc.*, 1967, **7**, 51.

GAS CHROMATOGRAPHY. In plasma—R. J. Flanagan and G. Withers, *J. clin. Path.*, 1972, **25**, 899. In plasma or urine—D. J. Berry, *J. Chromat.*, 1973, **86**, 89. In whole blood—R. G. Cooper *et al.*, *Clin. Chem.*, 1972, **18**, 1343.

RADIOIMMUNOASSAY. In biological tissues and fluids—S. Spector and E. J. Flynn, *Science*, 1971, **174**, 1036.

REVIEW of methods for determining barbiturates in body fluids—J. Bogan and H. Smith, *J. forens. Sci. Soc.*, 1967, 7, 37.

Metabolism. The barbiturates all have pK_a values within the range 7.2 to 8.1 and are, therefore, partly in the non-ionised state at pH values within the physiological range.

Since the non-ionised forms are lipid soluble to varying extents, their passage through biological membranes by passive diffusion will also vary. These variations in lipid solubility and membrane transfer result in different rates of uptake and release from the tissues and it is this variation that accounts for the differences in the duration of action within the barbiturate group of drugs.

ABSORPTION. The very short-acting barbiturates are usually administered intravenously as the calcium or sodium salts. The other barbiturates are sometimes administered by this route as salts but usually they are administered orally either as salts or as free acids. The barbiturates are readily absorbed after oral administration. The salts appear to be more rapidly absorbed than the corresponding acids.

DISTRIBUTION. The very short-acting barbiturates are rapidly taken up by those tissues which have high blood flows and high membrane permeabilities, including the brain (*see* the section on blood flow-rate in the entry on Metabolism of Drugs). There is also uptake by other tissues such as the liver, heart, and kidney, and ultimately they accumulate in the body fat from which they are slowly released. The intermediate- and long-acting barbiturates are not taken up by the tissues as rapidly and do not accumulate in body fat. Hence their concentration in the blood remains higher for longer periods.

All the barbiturates are protein bound to some extent, with the range between barbitone, which is about 5% bound, and thiopentone, which is about 75% bound. The extent of protein binding corresponds with lipid solubility.

All the barbiturates diffuse across the placenta and they are also found in the milk of lactating mothers.

METABOLIC REACTIONS. The very short-acting barbiturates are metabolised completely but slowly, the intermediate group is also metabolised extensively, but the long-acting barbiturates are only metabolised to a very small extent. The barbiturates are metabolised mainly in the liver.

There are four principal routes of metabolism: oxidation of C_5-substituents, N-dealkylation, replacement of thio-groups at C_2 by oxo-groups, and ring fission.

Oxidation of C_5-substituents. This is the major route of metabolism in which one or both of the side-chains are hydroxylated and possibly further oxidised. This usually occurs on the largest substituent group, whether it is aromatic, alicyclic, or aliphatic.

Aromatic substituents are hydroxylated primarily at the 4'-position and, possibly, to a minor extent, at the 2'-position. Cyclohexyl substituents are hydroxylated and may be further oxidised at the 3'-position. For aliphatic substituents, oxidation of the longest side-chain occurs at the terminal (ω) or penultimate ($\omega-1$) atom. The ω-position may be further oxidised to the carboxylic acid, and the ($\omega-1$)-position to the ketone.

When the initial hydroxylation forms an asymmetric centre, both this reaction and later oxidation may be stereoselective where only one form may be further oxidised. The metabolites derived from oxidation may be conjugated, usually as glucuronides but sometimes as sulphates.

N-Dealkylation. This reaction removes alkyl groups from the 1-position, and the rate of dealkylation decreases with increasing chain length of the N-substituent.

Sulphur replacement. The sulphur of the 2-thiobarbiturates is replaced by oxygen to form the corresponding oxybarbiturate. The extent of this reaction is not known but it is not a major metabolic route.

Ring fission. This reaction, occurring between positions 1 and 6, produces substituted malonylureas, which may be further metabolised to release urea or, if the original compound is a thiobarbiturate, thiourea. This reaction occurs to a very minor extent in man.

ENZYME INDUCTION AND INHIBITION. The activities of the hepatic enzymes responsible for the metabolism of the barbiturates are stimulated by many drugs, pesticides, and food additives, resulting in enhanced barbiturate metabolism (see "Activities of the drug metabolising enzymes" in Metabolism of Drugs).

In animals, some of the drugs that stimulate barbiturate metabolism are the barbiturates themselves, glutethimide, meprobamate, chlorpromazine, and phenytoin. Morphine and certain related compounds inhibit the action of these hepatic enzymes.

Some drugs initially inhibit barbiturate metabolism by competing with the barbiturates for these enzymes, but after a period of 10 to 12 hours, the enzyme activities are increased due to enzyme induction. Some steroids such as spironolactone and testosterone fall within this category. The barbiturates themselves will enhance the metabolism of many other drugs and their induction abilities are possibly related to their plasma half-lives. The fact that the barbiturates can stimulate their own metabolism contributes to the development of tolerance to their activity.

EXCRETION. The barbiturates and their metabolites are excreted mainly in the urine and very little is found in the faeces. In general, the unchanged barbiturates are slowly excreted since they are reabsorbed from the kidney tubules. The rates of excretion of the long-acting barbiturates (those which are poorly soluble in lipid) are increased by an increase in urine flow, and an increase in pH value of the urine will increase the rate of excretion of phenobarbitone.

Actions and uses. Barbiturates have a hypnotic action, but in therapeutic doses they have little or no effect on the medullary centres, so that blood pressure and respiration are not influenced. They may, however, have serious effects, even in hypnotic doses, in patients with chronic bronchitis. They were formerly used as hypnotics and sedatives but as they are especially dangerous in excessive dosage and owing to the danger of developing dependence, safer drugs such as benzodiazepines and chloral derivatives are now preferred. Certain barbiturates are however still used as anticonvulsants and for producing anaesthesia.

There is considerable variation in the duration of action of the barbiturates and they may be roughly classified in the following groups, each of which has its special therapeutic indications:

LONG-ACTING BARBITURATES: these include barbitone and phenobarbitone. Because of its depressant effect on the motor cortex phenobarbitone is used alone or with other anticonvulsants in the treatment of epilepsy. It is also used as a sedative in the treatment of disorders when anxiety and stress are present.

INTERMEDIATE-ACTING BARBITURATES: these include amylobarbitone, butobarbitone, cyclobarbitone, pentobarbitone, quinalbarbitone, and secbutobarbitone.

They are used as soporifics, their action ending not more than 8 hours after administration. They may also be used for pre-operative medication to induce a quiet and restful condition in the patient.

VERY SHORT-ACTING BARBITURATES: these include methohexitone and thiopentone. They are used mainly as rapid-acting intravenous anaesthetics, either alone or, more usually, as a preliminary to inhalation anaesthesia.

Undesirable effects. Patients vary in their response to the barbiturates and the hypnotic state is occasionally preceded by excitement and delirium and by confusion in the elderly. Prolonged administration may lead to tolerance and the dosage may need to be increased to obtain the desired soporific effect.

Increased dosage is liable to produce toxic effects, which may be either acute or chronic. The acute symptoms depend on the nature and dose of the barbiturate used; short-acting barbiturates give rise to respiratory and circulatory failure and the long-acting group to deep unconsciousness, which is followed by congestion of the lungs and "barbiturate pneumonia".

Symptoms of chronic poisoning include nystagmus, tremor, mild changes in the patient's mental condition, such as loss of memory, inability to concentrate, giddiness, depression, and dullness of mental perception, and also skin rashes of various types. It may precipitate acute porphyria.

Haemorrhagic bullae frequently accompany poisoning by long-acting barbiturates.

Precautions. Barbiturates may increase the rate of metabolism of other drugs as described above under Enzyme Induction and Inhibition, and caution should therefore be exercised in giving barbiturates with other drugs that are metabolised by the liver, such as folic acid, griseofulvin, pethidine, phenylbutazone, phenytoin, and anticoagulants of the coumarin type.

Barbiturates should be used with caution in late pregnancy since they cross the placenta and may cause respiratory depression in the offspring. They should be used with caution in nursing mothers since they diminish milk flow and the small amounts present in the milk may cause enzyme induction in infants.

Contra-indications. The majority of the barbiturates are detoxicated by the liver and are therefore contra-indicated where there is extensive liver damage; phenobarbitone is, however, mainly excreted unchanged in the urine.

Dependence. Barbiturates may give rise to dependence of the barbiturate-alcohol type as described under Drug Dependence.

Poisoning. The aims in treating barbiturate poisoning are to maintain respiration and to eliminate the drug. If the drug has been taken by mouth, the stomach should be washed out with warm water and filled with a dilute sodium sulphate solution to promote peristalsis.

Fluid may also be given by intravenous infusion, usually as sodium chloride and dextrose injection, but care must be taken not to give too much as it may increase the risk of bronchopneumonia due to oedema of the lungs.

The most important aspects of the treatment of barbiturate poisoning are careful nursing and the administration of oxygen if necessary. In cases which do not respond to these measures, haemodialysis may be used in addition.

FURTHER INFORMATION. M. T. Bush and D. Sanders, Metabolic fate of drugs: barbiturates and closely related compounds, *Annual Review of Pharmacology*, 1967, **7**,

57; L. C. Mark, Pharmacokinetics of the barbiturates, *Acute Barbiturate Poisoning*, H. Matthew (Ed.), Excerpta Medica, Amsterdam, 1971, p. 75; D. V. Park, Biochemistry of the barbiturates, *Acute Barbiturate Poisoning*, H. Matthew (Ed.), Excerpta Medica, Amsterdam, 1971, p. 7.

Barium Sulphate

$BaSO_4 = 233.4$

OTHER NAMES: Barii Sulfas; *Baritop®*; *Barosperse®*; *Micropaque®*; *Microtrast®*; *Steripaque®*

A standard is given in the European Pharmacopoeia Vol. I

Description. A fine, heavy, white, odourless powder.

Solubility. Practically insoluble in water; very slightly soluble in hydrochloric acid, in nitric acid, and in solutions of many salts.

Stability. Suspensions of barium sulphate are liable to be affected on storage by sulphate-splitting micro-organisms, especially in the presence of small amounts of alcohol and saccharin.

Actions and uses. Barium sulphate is used as a contrast medium for the X-ray examination of the gastro-intestinal tract. It is administered as a suspension and is not absorbed.

Preparations

BARIUM SULPHATE MIXTURE (*Syn.* Barium Sulphate Suspension): containing not less than 75% w/v of barium sulphate in an aqueous vehicle. It may contain suitable colouring, flavouring, and preservative agents and a suitable dispersing agent. Available as a mixture and a sterile mixture containing 100% w/v of barium sulphate.

A standard for this mixture is given in the British Pharmacopoeia Addendum 1978

Containers and *Labelling:* see the entry on Mixtures for general information on containers and labelling.

BARIUM SULPHATE POWDER FOR MIXTURE (*Syn.* Barium Sulphate for Suspension): consisting of barium sulphate together with suitable colouring, flavouring, and preservative agents. It contains not less than 85% w/v of barium sulphate and may contain a suitable dispersing agent. A powder for mixture containing 92% of barium sulphate is available.

A standard for this powder for mixture is given in the British Pharmacopoeia Addendum 1978

Labelling: see the entry on Mixtures for general information on labelling.

OTHER PREPARATIONS available include MIXTURES (sterile) containing barium sulphate 30 and 50% w/v and a PASTE containing barium sulphate 70% w/w.

Beclomethasone Dipropionate

9α-Chloro-11β,17α,21-trihydroxy-16β-methylpregna-1,4-diene-3,20-dione 17,21-dipropionate

$C_{28}H_{37}ClO_7 = 521.0$

OTHER NAMES: *Beconase*®; *Becotide*®; *Propaderm*®

A standard is given in the British Pharmacopoeia 1973

Description. A white to creamy-white odourless powder.

Solubility. Practically insoluble in water; soluble, at 20°, in 60 parts of alcohol and in 8 parts of chloroform.

Specific rotation. +88° to +94°, determined on a 1% solution in dioxan.

Storage. It should be protected from light.

Identification. TEST. It complies with Test 3 described under Cortisone Acetate (presence of acetyl groups).

MELTING-POINT. About 212° with decomposition.

ULTRAVIOLET ABSORPTION. In dehydrated alcohol, maximum at 238 nm (E1%, 1cm = 292).

INFRA-RED ABSORPTION. Major peaks at 890, 1190, 1608, 1650, 1730, and 1755 cm^{-1} (see Appendix 2a: Infra-red Spectra).

THIN-LAYER CHROMATOGRAPHY. See under Thin-layer Chromatography, System 10.

Metabolism. ABSORPTION. After an oral dose, administered as capsules or microfine suspension, 61 to 76% and about 90% is absorbed respectively; after inhalation, 20 to 25% reaches the lungs, the remainder being swallowed.

BLOOD CONCENTRATION. After an oral dose of 4 mg of the dipropionate, administered as capsules or as a microfine suspension, peak plasma concentrations of 9 to 15 ng/ml and about 20 ng/ml are attained in 3 to 5 hours respectively.

METABOLIC REACTIONS. Hydrolysis and conjugation.

EXCRETION. 10 to 15% of a dose is excreted in the urine as unidentified conjugates and free steroid; 36 to 67% is excreted in the faeces, mainly via the bile as dipropionate, propionate, and free base.

FURTHER INFORMATION. Absorption and metabolism—L. E. Martin *et al.*, *Clin. Pharmac. Ther.*, 1974, **15**, 267; pharmacological properties and therapeutic efficacy of beclomethasone dipropionate corticosteroid inhaler—J. B. Wilcox and G. S. Avery, *Drugs*, 1973, **6**, 84.

Actions and uses. Beclomethasone dipropionate is a corticosteroid for topical application with an action that is more potent than that of hydrocortisone. It has marked vasoconstrictor and anti-inflammatory activity.

It is suitable for use when local corticosteroid treatment is required and is applied as a lotion or ointment containing up to 0.025% or as a cream containing up to 0.5%. Its effectiveness is increased by dissolving it in propylene glycol before incorporation in an ointment basis.

Beclomethasone dipropionate applications may be used with or without conventional dressings, or under an occlusive dressing such as polythene when a more intensive effect is required, as in chronic psoriasis. However, if large areas are treated under occlusive dressings, sufficient of the drug may be absorbed to give rise to systemic effects.

Beclomethasone dipropionate may also be administered as an aerosol inhalation in the treatment of asthma, the usual dosage being 100 micrograms 3 or 4 times a day. It is also used as a nasal spray for the treatment of allergic rhinitis, the usual dose being 50 micrograms into each nostril 4 times a day.

Precautions. It should not be used on infected skin without the simultaneous application of a suitable anti-bacterial agent.

Preparations

BECLOMETHASONE AEROSOL INHALATION: a suspension of beclomethasone dipropionate, in powder of suitable particle size, in a suitable mixture of aerosol propellents, which may contain a surface-active agent, stabilising agents, and other adjuvants. It is packed in a pressurised container fitted with a special metering valve and either an oral or a nasal adaptor.

Available as an aerosol inhalation in two forms, one for nasal application and one for oral application, each delivering 50 micrograms of beclomethasone dipropionate to the patient each time the valve is actuated. The prescriber should state which form of preparation is to be supplied. The preparation for nasal application is entitled beclomethasone insufflation in the British National Formulary 1976–78.

Containers, Labelling, and *Storage:* see the entry on Aerosol Inhalations for general information on containers, labelling, and storage.

Advice for patients: see the entry on Aerosol Inhalations for general information on the use of aerosol inhalations. The patient should be advised verbally to read the instructions on the leaflet enclosed with the product.

When used in conjunction with salbutamol or another bronchodilator the bronchodilator should be given first and beclomethasone aerosol inhalation used 5 minutes later. When initiating treatment there may be a time lag of up to 3 weeks before a full therapeutic response is obtained. Treatment should not be discontinued without the advice of the prescriber.

BECLOMETHASONE CREAM: a dispersion of beclomethasone dipropionate, in very fine powder, in a suitable cream basis. Available as creams containing 0.025 and 0.5% of beclomethasone dipropionate.

When a strength less than that available from the manufacturer is prescribed, the stronger cream may be diluted, taking hygienic precautions, with cetomacrogol cream (formula A). The diluted cream must be freshly prepared.

A standard for this cream is given in the British Pharmacopoeia Addendum 1975

Containers and *Labelling:* see the entry on Creams for general information on containers and labelling.

Storage: see the entry on Creams for general information on storage. It should be stored at a temperature not exceeding 25°, protected from light.

Advice for patients: the cream should be applied sparingly to the affected area.

BECLOMETHASONE OINTMENT: a solution of beclomethasone dipropionate in propylene glycol incorporated in a paraffin ointment basis. Available as an ointment containing 0.025% of beclomethasone dipropionate.

When a strength less than that available from the manufacturer is prescribed, the 0.025% ointment may be diluted with white soft paraffin.

A standard for this ointment is given in the British Pharmacopoeia Addendum 1975

Containers and *Labelling:* see the entry on Ointments for general information on containers and labelling.

Storage: it should be stored at a temperature not exceeding 25°, protected from light.

Advice for patients: the ointment should be applied sparingly to the affected area.

OTHER PREPARATIONS available include a CREAM containing beclomethasone dipropionate 0.025% with clioquinol 3%, diluent cetomacrogol cream (formula A); a LOTION containing beclomethasone dipropionate 0.025%, not to be diluted; an OINTMENT containing beclomethasone dipropionate 0.025% with chlortetracycline hydrochloride 3%, diluent white soft paraffin; and an ointment containing beclomethasone dipropionate 0.025% with clioquinol 3%, diluent white soft paraffin.

Beeswax, White

Obtained by bleaching yellow beeswax. The bleaching may be effected by exposure of the wax in thin layers to the action of air, sunlight, and moisture, or by treatment with chemicals such as potassium dichromate and sulphuric acid.

OTHER NAME: Cera Alba

A standard is given in the British Pharmacopoeia 1973

Constituents. See Beeswax, Yellow.

Description. A yellowish-white solid with a faint characteristic odour; in thin layers it is translucent. It has a melting-point of about 63°.

Solubility. Practically insoluble in water; slightly soluble in alcohol; soluble in warm ether, in chloroform, and in fixed and volatile oils.

Adulterants and substitutes. Stearic acid, Japan wax, hard paraffin, and tallow have been reported as adulterants (see Beeswax, Yellow).

Uses. White beeswax is used chiefly to stiffen ointments and occasionally to adjust the melting-point of suppositories. It has been used, often in conjunction with borax or spermaceti, in the preparation of water-in-oil creams.

Beeswax, Yellow

A secretion formed by the hive bee, *Apis mellifera* L., and possibly other species of *Apis* (Fam. Apidae), used by the insect to form the cells of the honeycomb. After extraction of the honey, the wax is melted with water, separated, and strained.

OTHER NAME: Cera Flava

A standard is given in the British Pharmaceutical Codex 1973

Constituents. Yellow beeswax contains about 70% of esters of straight-chain monohydric alcohols with even-number carbon chains from C_{24} to C_{36} esterified with straight-chain acids which also have even numbers of carbon atoms up to C_{36} together with some C_{18}-hydroxy acids. The chief ester is myricyl palmitate (melissyl palmitate; triacontanol hexadecanoate).

Hydrocarbons having odd-numbered straight carbon chains from C_{21} to C_{33} are also present to the extent of about 20%. In addition, up to about 6% of unidentified pollen pigment compounds, free wax acids, lactones, and cholesteryl esters, are present.

Description. A yellowish-brown solid, somewhat brittle when cold, but becoming plastic when warm; fracture dull and granular. It has an agreeable and honey-like odour. It has a melting-point of about 63°.

Solubility. Practically insoluble in water; slightly soluble in alcohol; soluble in warm ether, in chloroform, and in fixed and volatile oils.

Adulterants and substitutes. Colophony, hard paraffin, various fats and waxes, stearic acid, soap, and foreign colouring matters have been reported as adulterants.

Boil 5 g with 80 ml of a 10% solution of sodium hydroxide, replace the water lost by evaporation, cool, filter through glass wool or asbestos, and acidify to litmus paper with hydrochloric acid; the development of a turbidity indicates the presence of fats, fatty acids, Japan wax, or resin.

Gently reflux 3 g with 30 ml of *potassium hydroxide solution in aldehyde-free alcohol* for 2 hours, place in a bath of water at 80°, and allow to cool, swirling the flask continuously; the development of cloudiness or globule formation before the temperature reaches 65° indicates the presence of ceresin, paraffin, or certain other waxes.

Sterilisation. Horsley's wax (see Uses) is sterilised by dry heat.

Uses. Yellow beeswax is used in the preparation of ointments in which the yellow colour is not objectionable.

A preparation of 10% of phenol in a mixture of olive oil and yellow beeswax is known as Horsley's wax (bone wax) and is used to control haemorrhage in bone in cranial surgery.

Belladonna Herb

The dried leaves, or leaves and other aerial parts, of *Atropa belladonna* L. (Fam. Solanaceae) collected when the plants are in flower. The plant is a tall branching herbaceous perennial, indigenous to and cultivated in Europe.

OTHER NAMES: Bellad. Leaf; Belladonna Leaf; Belladonnae Folium

When Belladonna Herb, Belladonna Leaf, Belladonnae Folium, Powdered Belladonna Herb, or Belladonnae Herbae Pulvis is prescribed, Prepared Belladonna Herb is dispensed.

A standard is given in the European Pharmacopoeia Vol. I

Constituents. Belladonna herb contains the alkaloid (−)-hyoscyamine (the laevo isomer of atropine), the total quantity of alkaloid present in dried herb of good quality being about 0.15 to 0.6%. The herb also contains β-methylaesculetin, which gives a blue fluorescence in ultraviolet light, and small quantities of hyoscine, belladonnine, and other alkaloids.

Other constituents are variable amounts of volatile bases, including pyridine, *N*-methylpyrroline and *N*-methylpyrrolidine.

Up to 3% of stem with a diameter greater than 5 mm may be present. It yields up to 4% of acid-insoluble ash.

Description. UNGROUND DRUG. *Macroscopical characters:* leaves thin, brittle, yellowish-green, alternate but arranged in pairs on upper stems, each pair consisting of a larger and a smaller leaf, simple; petiole up to

40 mm long; lamina broadly ovate, usually from 50 to
250 mm long and 30 to 120 mm broad, margin entire,
apex acuminate, base somewhat decurrent down the
petiole, venation pinnate, secondary veins leaving midrib
at angle of about 60° and anastomosing near the margin;
surface slightly hairy.

Flowers borne singly upon short drooping pedicels
arising in axils of paired leaves; calyx gamosepalous,
forming a cup about 5 mm deep and bearing 5 triangular
lobes about 12.5 mm long; corolla campanulate, livid
purple, about 20 mm long and 15 mm wide, with 5 small
reflexed lobes; stamens 5, epipetalous; ovary superior,
bilocular, ovules numerous, placentation axile.

Fruit, a berry; when ripe, purplish black, up to about
12 mm in diameter, bearing persistent inferior calyx
with widely spreading lobes; seeds numerous, brown,
reticulate.

It has a slight odour and a bitter unpleasant taste.

Microscopical characters: the diagnostic characters are:
Leaf: *epidermal cells* with slightly sinuous anticlinal
walls, *cuticle* striated; *stomata* anisocytic, occurring on
both surfaces, stomatal index (abaxial surface) 20 to **22**
to 23; *trichomes* (a) *non-glandular*, occasional, uniseriate, (b) *glandular*, either short, clavate, with multicellular heads, or less frequently long, with uniseriate stalks
and unicellular heads; *mesophyll*, with one layer of
palisade parenchyma, the palisade ratio varying from 5
to 7 (mean of 20 observations); *idioblasts* containing
microsphenoidal *crystals* of calcium oxalate present in
mesophyll; *phloem* intraxylary in midrib and petiole
vascular bundles.
Stem: *fibres* present in pericycle and xylem; *phloem*
intraxylary; *xylem* with wide vessels; microsphenoidal
crystals of calcium oxalate present in idioblasts of
parenchyma.
Pollen grains: subspherical, 37 to 50 μm in diameter,
containing minute starch granules and droplets of oil,
extine marked with rows of fine pits radiating from the
poles to the equator where they number about 84, 3 *pores*
about 8 μm in diameter, 3 *germinal furrows* extending
nearly to the poles.

POWDERED DRUG: Powdered Belladonna Herb. A green
powder possessing the diagnostic microscopical characters, odour, and taste of the unground drug.

Adulterants and substitutes. Indian belladonna, from
A. acuminata Royle ex Lindley, has leaves which are
usually brownish-green, oblong-elliptical, tapering both
at the apex and the base of the lamina; the flowers have
a yellowish-brown corolla. The microscopical characters
are similar to those of belladonna herb, but the stomatal
index is 16.5 to **17.5** to 19.0. (−)-Hyoscyamine and
hyoscine may be present.
The leaves of *Phytolacca americana* L. (*P. decandra* L.)
and other species of *Phytolacca* (Fam. Phytolaccaceae),
of *Scopolia carniolica* Jacq. and *Solanum nigrum* L.
(Fam. Solanaceae), and of *Ailanthus altissima* (Mill.)
Swingle (Fam. Simarubaceae), occur at times as substitutes for belladonna herb. They are best distinguished
by their microscopical features: phytolacca leaves contain idioblasts with acicular raphides of calcium oxalate;
scopolia leaves possess stomata on the under surface
only and the palisade ratio varies from 3 to 5, occasionally 6, while the fruit, a nearly spherical pyxis, is
usually present; ailanthus leaves have cluster crystals of
calcium oxalate near the veins and unicellular thick-
walled trichomes; leaves of *S. nigrum* have a palisade
ratio varying from 2 to 4.
Scopolia carniolica leaves contain 0.5% of (−)-hyo-

scyamine and hyoscine. *S. nigrum* contains alkaloids
based on solanidine and tomatidine.

Storage. It should be stored in a cool dry place, protected from light.

Identification. TEST. Shake 1 g, in powder, for 2 minutes
with 10 ml of 0.1N sulphuric acid, filter, and to the
filtrate add 2 ml of *dilute ammonia solution* and 5 ml of
water; extract with 15 ml of solvent ether, cautiously, to
avoid emulsion formation, separate, dry the ether layer
over anhydrous sodium sulphate, and filter; evaporate
off the ether in a porcelain dish, add 10 drops of fuming
nitric acid and evaporate to dryness over a small flame,
add 10 ml of acetone and, dropwise, a 3% solution of
potassium hydroxide in alcohol (95%); a deep violet
colour develops.

Actions and uses. The actions of preparations of belladonna herb are chiefly due to the hyoscyamine or
atropine they contain.
Belladonna is used to decrease secretions of the sweat,
salivary, and gastric glands. It acts as a powerful
spasmolytic in intestinal colic and, given with purgatives,
allays griping. It is also used for the relief of spasm
associated with biliary and renal colic.

Precautions and contra-indications. As for Atropine.

Poisoning. In cases of poisoning by belladonna herb or
its alkaloids, the procedure described under Atropine
should be adopted.

Preparations

ALUMINIUM HYDROXIDE AND BELLADONNA MIXTURE:

Belladonna tincture	100 ml
Chloroform spirit	50 ml
Aluminium hydroxide gel	to 1000 ml

It must be freshly prepared.
Containers: see the entry on Mixtures for general
information on containers. It should be supplied in
wide-mouthed containers.
Labelling: see the entry on Mixtures for general information on labelling.
Dose: 5 millilitres suitably diluted.
Advice for patients: the mixture may be taken alone, or
with water or other fluid between meals. The mixture
should not be used for longer than a few days without
medical advice.

BELLADONNA DRY EXTRACT: *Small-scale preparation:*

Belladonna herb, in moderately coarse powder	1000 g
Belladonna herb, in fine powder, dried at 80°	a sufficient quantity
Alcohol (70%)	a sufficient quantity

Percolate the belladonna herb in moderately coarse
powder with the alcohol until 4000 ml of percolate has
been obtained. Determine the proportion of total solids
in the percolate by evaporating 20 ml, drying the residue
at 80°, and weighing. Determine also the proportion of
alkaloids in the percolate by the assay for belladonna
tincture, using 50 ml, and the proportion of alkaloids
present in the belladonna herb in fine powder.
From the results of the three determinations, calculate
the amount of belladonna herb in fine powder that must
be added to the percolate to produce a dry extract containing 1% of alkaloids, calculated as hyoscyamine.
Add to the percolate a somewhat smaller amount of
belladonna herb in fine powder than calculation has
shown to be necessary, remove the alcohol by evaporating to dryness under reduced pressure at a temperature
not exceeding 60°, and dry in a current of air at 80°.

Powder the residue, add the final necessary amount of belladonna herb in fine powder, and triturate in a dry, slightly warmed mortar until thoroughly mixed. Pass the powdered extract through a No. 710 sieve and mix.

Manufacture: prepare the extract by the above method, appropriately scaled up.

In making this preparation, the alcohol (70%) may be replaced by industrial methylated spirit diluted so as to be of equivalent alcoholic strength, provided that the law and the statutory regulations governing the use of industrial methylated spirit are observed.

Belladonna dry extract contains, in 60 mg, 600 micrograms of total alkaloids, calculated as hyoscyamine.

A standard for this extract is given in the British Pharmacopoeia 1973

Storage: it should be stored in small, wide-mouthed, airtight containers, in a cool place.

Dose: 15 to 60 milligrams.

BELLADONNA TINCTURE:

Belladonna herb, in moderately coarse powder	100 g
Alcohol (70%) .. .. .. a sufficient quantity	

Prepare about 900 ml of a tincture by the percolation process. Determine the proportion of alkaloids in this tincture by the assay for belladonna tincture and add, if necessary, sufficient alcohol (70%) to produce a belladonna tincture of the required strength.

Belladonna tincture contains, in 2 ml, 600 micrograms of total alkaloids, calculated as hyoscyamine.

A standard for this tincture is given in the British Pharmacopoeia 1973

Dose: 0.5 to 2 ml.

CASCARA AND BELLADONNA MIXTURE (*Syn.* Compound Cascara Mixture):

Cascara elixir	200 ml
Belladonna tincture	50 ml
Chloroform water, double-strength	500 ml
Water for preparations	to 1000 ml

It must be freshly prepared.

Containers and *Labelling:* see the entry on Mixtures for general information on containers and labelling.

Dose: 10 to 20 millilitres.

Advice for patients: the mixture should not be used for longer than a few days without medical advice. It may colour the urine red or yellow.

MAGNESIUM TRISILICATE AND BELLADONNA MIXTURE:

Belladonna tincture	50 ml
Magnesium trisilicate mixture	to 1000 ml

It must be freshly prepared.

Containers and *Labelling:* see the entry on Mixtures for general information on containers and labelling.

Dose: 10 to 20 millilitres.

Advice for patients: the mixture may be taken alone or with water or other fluid between meals. It should not be used for longer than a few days without medical advice.

PAEDIATRIC BELLADONNA AND EPHEDRINE MIXTURE:

Belladonna tincture	30.0 ml
Ephedrine hydrochloride	1.5 g
Potassium iodide	10.0 g
Concentrated anise water	20.0 ml
Benzoic acid solution	20.0 ml
Liquorice liquid extract	30.0 ml
Syrup..	100.0 ml
Water for preparations	to 1000.0 ml

It should be recently prepared.

A standard for this mixture is given in the British Pharmaceutical Codex 1973

Containers and *Labelling:* see the entry on Mixtures for general information on containers and labelling.

Dose: CHILD: up to 1 year, 5 millilitres; 1 to 5 years, 10 millilitres.

Advice for patients: the mixture should not be used for longer than a few days without medical advice.

PAEDIATRIC   BELLADONNA   AND   IPECACUANHA MIXTURE:

Belladonna tincture	30 ml
Ipecacuanha tincture	20 ml
Sodium bicarbonate	20 g
Tolu syrup	200 ml
Chloroform water, double-strength	500 ml
Water for preparations	to 1000 ml

It must be freshly prepared.

Containers and *Labelling:* see the entry on Mixtures for general information on containers and labelling.

Dose: CHILD: up to 1 year, 5 millilitres; 1 to 5 years, 10 millilitres.

Advice for patients: the mixture should not be used for longer than a few days without medical advice.

PAEDIATRIC BELLADONNA MIXTURE:

Belladonna tincture	30 ml
Compound orange spirit	2 ml
Benzoic acid solution	20 ml
Glycerol	100 ml
Syrup..	200 ml
Water for preparations	to 1000 ml

It should be recently prepared.

A standard for this mixture is given in the British Pharmaceutical Codex 1973

Containers and *Labelling:* see the entry on Mixtures for general information on containers and labelling.

Dose: CHILD: up to 1 year, 5 millilitres; 1 to 5 years, 10 millilitres.

Advice for patients: when used in the treatment of colic, the dose should be taken half an hour before meals. The mixture should not be taken for longer than a few days without medical advice.

PREPARED BELLADONNA HERB (*Syn.* Belladonnae Pulvis Normatus; Prep. Bellad.; Prepared Belladonna): obtained by reducing belladonna herb to a fine powder and adjusting, if necessary, to the required alkaloidal content. When adjustment is necessary, powdered lactose or powdered belladonna herb of lower alkaloidal content is added.

It is a fine greyish-green powder with a slightly nauseous odour and a slightly bitter taste. It possesses the diagnostic microscopical characters of powdered belladonna herb. If the material contains lactose, crystals may be observed when a sample is mounted in glycerol.

Prepared belladonna herb contains 0.3% of alkaloids, calculated as hyoscyamine, $C_{17}H_{23}NO_3$.

A standard for this powder is given in the European Pharmacopoeia Vol. I

Storage: it should be stored in airtight containers, in a cool place, protected from light.

Dose: 30 to 200 milligrams.

OTHER PREPARATIONS available include numerous multiple-ingredient preparations, containing belladonna in the form of an extract or tincture.

Belladonna Root

The dried root, or root and rootstock, of *Atropa bella-donna* L. (Fam. Solanaceae), entire or longitudinally divided. The plant is a tall branching herbaceous perennial, indigenous to and cultivated in Europe.

OTHER NAME: Bellad. Root

A standard is given in the British Pharmaceutical Codex 1973

Constituents. Belladonna root contains the alkaloid (−)-hyoscyamine (the laevo isomer of atropine), and traces of hyoscine. The drug also contains β-methylaesculetin, which gives a blue fluorescence in ultraviolet light. The total amount of alkaloid in the root varies from about 0.3 to 0.8%. Up to 2% of foreign organic matter may also be present. It yields up to 2% of acid-insoluble ash.

Description. UNGROUND DRUG. *Macroscopical characters:* root simple or occasionally branched, subcylindrical, occurring entire or split longitudinally, the pieces being about 100 to 300 mm long and up to about 40 mm wide at the crown; external covering of cork, thin pale greyish-brown, longitudinally wrinkled; fracture short; smoothed, transversely cut surface whitish to brownish showing dark cambium line separating the narrow bark, devoid of fibres, from the mainly parenchymatous xylem containing scattered groups of vessels; vessels most numerous and inconspicuously radiate just to inner side of cambium; root crown exhibiting a central pith, a markedly radiate xylem, and a bark with a few phloem fibres.
It has a slight odour and a faintly bitter starchy taste.

Microscopical characters: the diagnostic characters are: Root: *cork* cells in several layers; *phloem fibres* and *sclereids* absent; *parenchyma* abundant, containing *starch* as simple or occasional 2- to 5- compound granules, individual granules 3 to **8** to **16** to 30 μm in diameter; *idioblasts* containing microsphenoidal *crystals* of calcium oxalate, about 1 to 7 μm; *vessels* about 20 to **60** to **120** to 180 μm in diameter, individual elements about 50 to **145** to **175** to 410 μm long, their walls with closely arranged bordered pits; *xylem fibres* thin-walled; *intraxylary phloem* in small, scattered groups; primary xylem and a little secondary xylem forming a compact diarch or occasionally triarch strand.
Rootstock: similar in most particulars to the root, except for presence of occasional *phloem fibres*, lignified *xylem parenchyma*, and occasional *fibres* in intraxylary phloem.

POWDERED DRUG: Powdered Belladonna Root. A grey to light-brown powder possessing the diagnostic microscopical characters, odour, and taste of the unground drug.

Adulterants and substitutes. Indian belladonna root, derived from *A. acuminata* Royle ex Lindley, closely resembles belladonna root; the secondary xylem is yellowish in colour and is arranged in 1 to 4 concentric cylinders separated by narrow cylinders of parenchyma and sieve-tissue, the whole being traversed radially by numerous medullary rays; the rootstock has a similarly constructed xylem. It contains 0.45 to 0.47% of non-volatile alkaloids and volatile bases. (−)-Hyoscyamine and hyoscine may be present.
Phytolacca, or poke root, from *Phytolacca americana* L. (*P. decandra* L.) (Fam. Phytolaccaceae), is sometimes substituted for belladonna and may be detected by the presence of concentric cylinders of separate vascular bundles alternating with cylinders of parenchyma, and, in powder, by the presence of acicular crystals of calcium oxalate.
Scopolia, the dried rhizome of *Scopolia carniolica* Jacq. (Fam. Solanaceae), has also occurred as a substitute and can be recognised by its yellowish-brown colour, the numerous cup-shaped stem-scars on the upper surface, the horny central pith, and microscopically by the preponderance of reticulate vessels. It contains 0.5% of (−)-hyoscyamine and hyoscine.

Storage. It should be stored in a cool dry place.

Identification. See under Belladonna Herb.

Actions and uses. Belladonna root has actions similar to those described under Belladonna Herb. It is used chiefly in preparations for external application, but there is no reliable evidence that belladonna, when applied externally, is absorbed in sufficient amount to produce systemic effects.
Liniments containing belladonna are sometimes used as counter-irritants but the efficacy of these preparations is not due to belladonna.
Although there is little evidence that belladonna has any analgesic action, belladonna glycerin and belladonna plaster have been used locally to allay pain. Belladonna suppositories have been used to relieve the painful spasm of anal fistula.

Poisoning. The procedure as described under Atropine should be adopted.

Preparation

BELLADONNA LIQUID EXTRACT: *Small-scale preparation:*

Belladonna root, in
  moderately coarse powder .. .. .. 1000 g
Alcohol (80%) .. .. .. a sufficient quantity
Exhaust the belladonna root with the alcohol by percolation and evaporate the percolate under reduced pressure to the consistency of a soft extract. Determine the proportion of total alkaloids in the soft extract and dissolve it in sufficient of the alcohol to produce an extract of the required strength; allow the extract to stand for not less than 12 hours and filter if necessary.
Manufacture: prepare the extract by the above method, appropriately scaled up.
Belladonna liquid extract contains 7.5 mg per ml of total alkaloids, calculated as hyoscyamine.
A standard for this liquid extract is given in the British Pharmaceutical Codex 1973

Bendrofluazide

3-Benzyl-3,4-dihydro-6-trifluoromethyl-2*H*-benzo-1,2,4-thiadiazine-7-sulphonamide 1,1-dioxide

$C_{15}H_{14}F_3N_3O_4S_2 = 421.4$

OTHER NAMES: *Aprinox*®; Bendroflumethiazide; *Berko-zide*®; *Neo-NaClex*®
Tenavoid® (with meprobamate); *Centyl K*® and *Neo-NaClex K*® (both with potassium chloride)

A standard is given in the British Pharmacopoeia 1973

Description. A white, crystalline, odourless, tasteless powder.

Solubility. Very slightly soluble in water; soluble, at 20°, in 17 parts of alcohol, in 500 parts of ether, and in 1.5 parts of acetone; practically insoluble in chloroform.

Dissociation constant. pK_a 8.5 (25°).

Identification. TESTS. 1. Mix about 20 mg with a strong solution of potassium permanganate acidified with sulphuric acid, and warm; the odour of benzaldehyde is produced (distinction from hydroflumethiazide).
2. Mix about 20 mg with a mixture of 2.5 ml of hydrochloric acid and 2.5 ml of water, boil, cool in ice, and add successively 0.5 ml of a 0.1% solution of sodium nitrite, 0.5 ml of a 0.5% solution of ammonium sulphamate, and 0.5 ml of a 0.1% solution of N-(1-naphthyl)-ethylenediamine; a deep red colour is produced.

ULTRAVIOLET ABSORPTION. In 0.01N sodium hydroxide, maxima at 273 nm (E1%, 1cm = 415) and 329 nm (E1%, 1cm = 80); in alcohol (95%), maxima at 275 nm (E1%, 1cm = 580) and 327 nm (E1%, 1cm = 103).

INFRA-RED ABSORPTION. Major peaks at 1145, 1155, 1170, 1338, 1518, and 1621 cm^{-1} (see Appendix 2a: Infra-red Spectra).

THIN-LAYER CHROMATOGRAPHY. See under Thin-layer Chromatography, System 6.

Metabolism. ABSORPTION. Readily absorbed after oral administration.

BLOOD CONCENTRATION. After an oral dose of 10 mg, peak plasma concentrations of 50 to 100 ng/ml are attained in 2 to 2.5 hours.

HALF-LIFE. Plasma half-life, during the period 4 to 10 hours following oral administration, about 2.7 hours.

DISTRIBUTION. *Protein binding*, about 95% bound to plasma proteins in dogs.

METABOLIC REACTIONS. Not significantly metabolised.

EXCRETION. 45 to 77% of a dose is excreted unchanged in the urine of dogs in 24 hours.

FURTHER INFORMATION. Plasma levels in man—B. Beermann *et al.*, *Eur. J. clin. Pharmac.*, 1976, **10**, 293; pharmacology of bendrofluazide—J. J. Piala *et al.*, *J. Pharmac. exp. Ther.*, 1961, **134**, 273.

Actions and uses. Bendrofluazide is a thiazide diuretic which has actions and uses similar to those described under Chlorothiazide; it is effective in smaller doses than chlorothiazide and produces a more prolonged diuresis, which continues for about 18 hours.
The initial dosage is 5 to 20 milligrams by mouth once a day and this may be reduced to 2.5 to 10 milligrams daily or on alternate days for maintenance.

Undesirable effects; Precautions. As for Chlorothiazide.
Bendrofluazide inhibits lactation and should be avoided in nursing mothers.

Veterinary uses. Bendrofluazide is a diuretic used in dogs in doses of up to 500 micrograms per kilogram body-weight and in cats in doses of 150 micrograms per kilogram body-weight daily. Potassium supplements may be given to reduce the risk of hypokalaemia.

Preparations

BENDROFLUAZIDE TABLETS: available as tablets containing 2.5 and 5 mg of bendrofluazide.
A standard for these tablets is given in the British Pharmacopoeia 1973

Containers and *Storage:* see the entry on Tablets for general information on containers and storage. Containers should be airtight.
Advice for patients: daily doses should preferably be taken in the morning. Treatment should not be discontinued without the advice of the prescriber.

OTHER PREPARATIONS available include TABLETS containing bendrofluazide 3 mg with meprobamate 200 mg, tablets containing bendrofluazide 2.5 mg with potassium chloride 573 mg (7.7 mmol K$^+$) in a slow-release formulation and tablets containing bendrofluazide 2.5 mg with potassium chloride 630 mg (8.4 mmol K$^+$) in a slow-release formulation.

Benethamine Penicillin

The N-benzylphenethylamine salt of benzylpenicillin.

$C_{15}H_{17}N, C_{16}H_{18}N_2O_4S = 545.7$

OTHER NAMES: Beneth. Penicil.
Propen® (with procaine penicillin); *Triplopen*® (with benzylpenicillin and procaine penicillin)

A standard is given in the British Pharmaceutical Codex 1973

One mega-unit of penicillin is contained in approximately 1 gram of benethamine penicillin.

Description. A white odourless crystalline powder.

Solubility. Soluble, at 20°, in 1500 parts of water, in 50 parts of chloroform, in 100 parts of acetone (50%), and in 50 parts of methyl alcohol (75%).

Acidity. A 1.5% suspension has a pH of 5.5 to 7.

Specific rotation. +120° to +125°, determined on a 1% solution in chloroform.

Labelling. If the material is intended for the preparation of injections, the label should state "Benethamine Penicillin for Injection".

Storage. It should be stored in airtight containers in a cool place. If it is intended for parenteral administration the containers should be sterile and sealed to exclude micro-organisms.

Identification. TEST. Mix about 1 g with 5 ml of *dilute sodium hydroxide solution*, shake for 2 minutes, extract with two successive 10-ml portions of solvent ether, evaporate the combined extracts to dryness, dissolve the residue in 5 ml of alcohol (95%), warm with 5 ml of a saturated solution of picrolonic acid in alcohol (95%), and cool; a precipitate is formed which, after recrystallisation from alcohol (95%) and drying, melts at about 230°.

INFRA-RED ABSORPTION. Major peaks at 755, 1258, 1336, 1562, 1663, and 1773 cm^{-1} (see Appendix 2a: Infra-red Spectra).

Actions and uses. Benethamine penicillin has antibacterial actions similar to those described under Benzylpenicillin.
As it is only slightly soluble in water, it releases penicillin slowly into the circulation after intramuscular injection; a single dose of 300 to 600 milligrams (approximately 300 000 to 600 000 units of penicillin) will maintain an

effective concentration of penicillin in the blood for 3 or 4 days.

Like benzathine penicillin it can be added to preparations containing benzylpenicillin and procaine penicillin to give an injection producing immediate and prolonged antibacterial effect.

Undesirable effects; Precautions. As for Benzylpenicillin.

Preparations

FORTIFIED BENETHAMINE PENICILLIN INJECTION (*Syn.* Benethamine Penicillin with Benzylpenicillin Sodium and Procaine Penicillin Injection; Triple Penicillin Injection): a sterile suspension of benethamine penicillin and procaine penicillin, with appropriate pharmaceutical adjuvants, in a solution of benzylpenicillin sodium in water for injections. It is prepared by adding water for injections to the contents of a sealed container shortly before use.

Available as a powder in vials containing 475 mg (500 000 units) of benethamine penicillin, 300 mg (500 000 units) of benzylpenicillin (sodium salt), and 250 mg (250 000 units) of procaine penicillin.

A standard for this injection is given in the British Pharmaceutical Codex 1973

Containers: see the entry on Injections for general information on containers.

Labelling: see the entry on Injections for general information on labelling. In addition, the name on the label should be "Fortified Benethamine Penicillin for Injection" and the label on the sealed container should state that the contents are to be used for intramuscular injection only.

Storage: the sealed containers should be stored in a cool place.

The injection contains no bactericide and should be used as soon as possible after preparation, but the injection may be expected to retain its potency for 14 days when stored at 2° to 10°.

OTHER PREPARATIONS available include a veterinary INJECTION containing benethamine penicillin 141.5 mg (150 000 units) with procaine penicillin 150 mg (150 000 units) per ml in 30- and 100-ml vials.

Benorylate

4-Acetamidophenyl 2-acetoxybenzoate

$C_{17}H_{15}NO_5 = 313.3$

OTHER NAME: *Benoral*®

Description. An odourless, tasteless, white, crystalline powder.

Solubility. Practically insoluble in water; soluble in 88 parts of alcohol, in 18 parts of chloroform, in 900 parts of ether, in 22 parts of acetone, and in 66 parts of methyl alcohol.

Identification. MELTING-POINT. About 177°.

ULTRAVIOLET ABSORPTION. In alcohol (95%), maximum at 242 nm (E1%, 1 cm = 746).

INFRA-RED ABSORPTION. Major peaks at 1053, 1183, 1202, 1260, 1668, and 1740 cm^{-1} (see Appendix 2a: Infrared Spectra).

THIN-LAYER CHROMATOGRAPHY. See under Thin-layer Chromatography, System 3.

Metabolism. ABSORPTION. Readily absorbed after oral administration; not significantly hydrolysed prior to absorption.

BLOOD CONCENTRATION. After an oral dose of 4 g as a 40% suspension, peak plasma concentrations for unchanged drug of about 2 μg/ml are attained by 30 minutes and peak plasma concentrations of salicylate of about 120 μg/ml are attained by about 3 hours.

DISTRIBUTION. Enters synovial fluid and tissues.

METABOLIC REACTIONS. Rapidly hydrolysed in blood to paracetamol and acetylsalicylic acid.

EXCRETION. In 3 days, about 80% of a dose is excreted as salicylate metabolites and 70% as paracetamol metabolites; 13 to 15% of a dose is excreted in the faeces.

FURTHER INFORMATION. Absorption and metabolism in man—A. Robertson *et al.*, *Xenobiotica*, 1972, **2**, 339; a symposium on benorylate, *Scand. J. Rheumatol.*, 1975, Suppl. 13.

Actions and uses. Benorylate is an analgesic, antipyretic, and anti-inflammatory substance. When administered by mouth it is slowly absorbed and in the blood stream and liver it is hydrolysed with the formation of paracetamol and acetylsalicylic acid.

It is used for the relief of pain and inflammation in rheumatic disease and as an antipyretic in influenza and other febrile conditions.

The usual dose as an antipyretic and for the relief of moderate pain is 1 gram repeated up to 4 times daily as required. For the symptomatic treatment of rheumatoid arthritis and other painful conditions, 4 to 8 grams may be given daily in divided doses. For the relief of pain in children, the usual dose daily in divided doses is: 3 months to 1 year, 100 milligrams per kilogram bodyweight; 1 to 5 years, 1 to 1.5 grams; and 6 to 12 years, up to 2 grams. Larger doses, up to 1 gram 3 or 4 times daily may be given for rheumatoid arthritis in children over one year.

Undesirable effects. Nausea, constipation, drowsiness, rashes, dizziness, and tinnitus may occur.

Precautions and contra-indications. The use of benorylate in conjunction with anticoagulant drugs should be avoided as it may increase the risk of haemorrhage. It is contra-indicated in patients who are sensitive to aspirin.

It should be administered with caution in renal or hepatic insufficiency and in patients with a history of peptic ulceration.

Poisoning. As for Aspirin and Paracetamol.

Preparations

Preparations available include a MIXTURE containing 2 g of benorylate in 5 ml, diluent syrup, shelf-life of diluted mixture 14 days; and TABLETS containing benorylate 750 mg.

Benserazide Hydrochloride

2-Amino-3-hydroxy-2'-(2,3,4-trihydroxybenzyl)propionohydrazide hydrochloride

$C_{10}H_{16}ClN_3O_5 = 293.7$

OTHER NAME: *Madopar*® (with levodopa)

Description. A crystalline solid.

Identification. MELTING-POINT. About 95°.

Metabolism. ABSORPTION. Rapidly absorbed after oral administration.

DISTRIBUTION. In rats, benserazide is distributed almost completely outside the brain and will therefore block extracerebral decarboxylase whilst leaving intracerebral decarboxylase activity intact.

METABOLIC REACTIONS. Appears to be rapidly metabolised.

EXCRETION. In 7 days about 60% of an oral dose and 90% of an intravenous dose is excreted in the urine, most of this being excreted in the first 12 hours. About 10% and 30% of the respective doses are excreted in the faeces in the 7-day period.

FURTHER INFORMATION. Excretion in man and distribution in rat—D. E. Schwartz *et al.*, *Eur. J. clin. Pharmac.*, 1974, **7**, 39.

Actions and uses. Benserazide hydrochloride inhibits the action of the enzyme dopa decarboxylase in the extracerebral tissues. It is used in conjunction with levodopa in the treatment of parkinsonism; competitive inhibition of dopa decarboxylase decreases the metabolism of levodopa in the peripheral tissues thereby increasing the amount of levodopa available to pass into the brain. Because of this, control of parkinsonism may be obtained without the severe side-effects obtained when levodopa is used alone.

When levodopa is given in conjunction with benserazide, dosage should be reduced to about one quarter of the amount required when levodopa is given alone. The usual dosage of benserazide is the equivalent of 25 to 500 milligrams of benserazide base daily, in the ratio of 1 to 4 with levodopa; 1.1 grams of benserazide hydrochloride is approximately equivalent to 1 gram of benserazide.

Undesirable effects. Benserazide enhances the undesirable effects of levodopa, but to a somewhat lesser extent than it enhances its action against parkinsonism.

Preparation

LEVODOPA AND BENSERAZIDE CAPSULES: consisting of levodopa and benserazide hydrochloride, which may be mixed with a suitable inert diluent, enclosed in a hard capsule. The capsule shells may be coloured.

Available as capsules containing 100 mg of levodopa and benserazide hydrochloride equivalent to 25 mg of benserazide, and as capsules containing 200 mg of levodopa and benserazide hydrochloride equivalent to 50 mg of benserazide.

Containers and *Storage:* see the entry on Capsules for general information on containers and storage. Containers should be light resistant.

Advice for patients: the capsules should be taken after meals. Treatment should not be discontinued without the advice of the prescriber. The capsules may affect mental concentration in the first few days of treatment and the urine may darken in colour.

Bentonite

A native colloidal hydrated aluminium silicate, the principal constituent being montmorillonite, $Al_2O_3,4SiO_2,H_2O$.

OTHER NAME: Bentonitum

A standard is given in the European Pharmacopoeia Vol. III

Materials suitable for pharmaceutical purposes are generally obtained from Wyoming; African and Italian bentonites are used for packing and other non-pharmaceutical purposes.

Description. *Macroscopical characters:* a very fine homogeneous, greyish-white, odourless powder with a yellowish tint and a slightly earthy taste.

Microscopical characters: bentonite consists of particles about 50 to 150 μm and numerous smaller particles about 1 to 2 μm; the larger particles have rounded corners and an uneven surface with frequent cracks; mounted in *safranine solution* or *alcoholic methylene blue solution*, the particles are strongly stained red or blue respectively; mounted in alcohol (95%) and irrigated with water, the larger fragments, as they come in contact with the water, rapidly swell to give a jelly-like matrix in which numerous minute particles are embedded; mounted in cresol, it becomes nearly invisible but shines brightly on a dark field between crossed polars.

Solubility. Practically insoluble in water, but swells into a homogeneous mass; practically insoluble in organic solvents.

Alkalinity. A 2% suspension has a pH of 9 to 10.5.

Moisture content. 5 to 12%, determined by drying at 105°.

Sterilisation. It is sterilised by dry heat, after previously drying at 100°; aqueous suspensions are sterilised by heating in an autoclave.

Storage. It should be stored in airtight containers.

Uses. Bentonite absorbs water readily to form either sols or gels, depending upon its concentration, a preparation containing about 7% of bentonite being just pourable. The sols are suitable for suspending powders in aqueous preparations such as calamine lotion, and the gels for ointment and cream bases; these preparations have a pH of about 9.

The gelling property of bentonite is much reduced in the presence of acid and increased by the addition of such alkaline substances as magnesium oxide. In aqueous sols and gels, bentonite particles are negatively charged and flocculation occurs when electrolytes or positively charged suspensions are added. Because of this property, bentonite is sometimes used in clarifying turbid liquids.

Sols and gels may conveniently be prepared by sprinkling

the bentonite on the surface of hot water and allowing to stand for about 24 hours, stirring occasionally when the bentonite has become thoroughly wetted. Water should not be added to bentonite alone, but a satisfactory dispersal in water may be effected if the bentonite is first triturated with glycerol or if it is intimately mixed with powders such as calamine or zinc oxide.

For suspending powders in aqueous preparations and for the preparation of cream bases containing suitable proportions of oil-in-water emulsifying agents such as emulsifying wax and self-emulsifying monostearin, 2% of bentonite is adequate. A preparation containing 10 to 20% of bentonite and 10% of glycerol is also suitable as a basis. A sol containing 5% is convenient for dispensing purposes.

Bentonite should be sterilised before it is used for preparations intended for application to open wounds.

Benzaldehyde

$C_6H_5 . CHO = 106.1$

A standard is given in the British Pharmaceutical Codex 1973

Description. A clear colourless liquid with an odour characteristic of bitter almonds and a burning aromatic taste. The colour becomes yellowish on storage. It oxidises in air to benzoic acid and is volatile with steam.

Solubility. Soluble, at 20°, in 350 parts of water; miscible with alcohol and with ether.

Weight per ml. At 20°, 1.043 to 1.049 g.

Refractive index. At 20°, 1.544 to 1.546.

Boiling-point. About 179°.

Storage. It should be stored in well-filled airtight containers, in a cool place, protected from light.

Uses. Benzaldehyde is used as a flavouring agent. A syrup containing 0.2% v/v of benzaldehyde spirit may be used as an alternative to wild cherry syrup.

Preparation

BENZALDEHYDE SPIRIT:

Benzaldehyde	..	..	..	..	10 ml
Alcohol (90%)	..	..	..	..	800 ml
Purified water	..	..	..	..	to 1000 ml

Dissolve the benzaldehyde in the alcohol and add sufficient of the water to produce the required volume.
A standard for this spirit is given in the British Pharmaceutical Codex 1973
Storage: it should be stored in well-filled airtight containers, in a cool place, protected from light.

Benzalkonium Chloride Solution

An aqueous solution containing a mixture of alkyl-benzyldimethylammonium chlorides, equivalent to 50% of $C_6H_5 . CH_2 . N(CH_3)_2(C_{13}H_{27}) . Cl$. The alkyl groups contain 8 to 18 carbon atoms.

OTHER NAMES: *Agriclens®*; *BTC 50®*; *Capitol®*; *Cycloton B50®*; *Empigen BAC®*; *Hyamine 3500®*; *Marinol Blue®*; *Morpan BC®*; *Roccal®*; *Silquat B10* and *B50®*; *Vantoc CL®*
Benzets® (with benzocaine); *Drapolene®* (with cetrimide); *Stomobar®*, *Stomogel®*, and *Stomosol®* (with chlorhexidine gluconate); *Sporostacin®* (with chlordantoin)

A standard is given in the British Pharmacopoeia 1973

Description. A clear colourless to pale yellow syrupy liquid with an aromatic odour, and a very bitter taste.

Solubility. Miscible with water and with alcohol.

Incompatibility. It is incompatible with soaps and similar anionic compounds, and alkali hydroxides.
It may also be incompatible with ingredients of some commercial rubber mixes.
Incompatibilities have been reported with other substances including aluminium salts, fluorescein sodium, hydrogen peroxide, kaolin, hydrous wool fat, and some sulphonamides.

Sterilisation. Solutions are sterilised by heating in an autoclave or by filtration.

Preparation and storage of solutions. See the statement on aqueous solutions of antiseptics in the entry on Solutions.

Identification. TESTS. 1. Mix 4 drops with 10 ml of water and divide the solution into two portions. To the first portion add 1.5 ml of *dilute nitric acid*; a white precipitate is produced which is soluble in alcohol (95%). To the second portion add 1.5 ml of *mercuric chloride test-solution*; a white precipitate is produced which is soluble in alcohol (95%).
2. Evaporate 0.5 ml to dryness on a water-bath, dissolve the residue in 1 ml of sulphuric acid, add 100 mg of potassium nitrate, and heat on a water-bath for 5 minutes; cool, dilute to 10 ml with water, add 500 mg of zinc powder, and again heat on a water-bath for 5 minutes; to 2 ml of the clear supernatant liquid add 0.5 ml of *sodium nitrite solution*, cool in ice, and add 3 ml of *2-naphthol solution*; an orange-red colour is produced.
3. Dilute with water; the solution is neutral or slightly alkaline to *litmus solution* and foams strongly on shaking.

ULTRAVIOLET ABSORPTION. In water, maxima at 256 nm (E1%, 1cm = 4.9), at 262 nm (E1%, 1cm = 5.8), and at 268 nm (E1%, 1cm = 4.6); inflexion at 252 nm.

Actions and uses. Benzalkonium chloride has the actions and uses of the quaternary ammonium compounds, as described under Cetrimide. Benzalkonium chloride solution may be used, in a dilution of 1 in 500, for the pre-operative preparation of unbroken skin, but for application to mucous membranes and denuded skin the dilution should not be stronger than 1 in 1000. In obstetrics and for application to wounds and burns, dilutions of 1 in 500 to 1 in 1000 may be used. Dilutions of 1 in 10000 are employed for irrigation of the bladder, urethra, and vagina, and a concentration not exceeding 1 in 20000 for retention lavage.
Rubber articles should not be stored in benzalkonium solutions.
Benzalkonium lozenges are used to relieve painful infections of the mouth and throat.
Benzalkonium chloride solution is widely used as a preservative for eye-drops. For this purpose it is usually employed in a 0.02% v/v dilution and may be used in this concentration in the process of sterilisation by heating with a bactericide. Enhancement of antibacterial effect by inclusion of disodium edetate in solutions containing benzalkonium chloride has been reported. It is not suitable for eye-drops containing local anaesthetics because it accelerates the dehydrating effect of the local anaesthetic on the cornea.

Precautions. Benzalkonium chloride should not be applied repeatedly and wet dressings should not be left in contact with the skin, as hypersensitivity may develop.

Preparations

BENZALKONIUM LOZENGES (*Syn.* Benzalkonium Chloride Lozenges): for each lozenge take:

Benzalkonium chloride solution	0.001 ml
Menthol	0.6 mg
Thymol	0.6 mg
Eucalyptus oil	0.002 ml
Lemon oil	0.002 ml

Prepare by moist granulation and compression, as described in the entry on Lozenges. Each lozenge weighs about 1 gram.

A standard for these lozenges is given in the British Pharmaceutical Codex 1973
Containers: see the entry on Lozenges for general information on containers.
Advice for patients: the lozenges should be allowed to dissolve slowly in the mouth.

OTHER PREPARATIONS available include a veterinary APPLICATION (with F.D.&C. blue no. 1 as marker) containing benzalkonium chloride 3.3% in an aerosol pack; a CREAM containing benzalkonium chloride 0.01% with cetrimide 0.2%, a cream containing benzalkonium chloride 10% with chlordantoin 1%, a cream containing benzalkonium chloride 0.5% with chlorhexidine gluconate 0.09%; a GEL containing benzalkonium chloride 0.5%, a gel containing benzalkonium chloride 1% with chlorhexidine gluconate 0.1%; LOZENGES containing benzalkonium chloride 500 micrograms with benzocaine 1 mg; a SOLUTION containing benzalkonium chloride 1%, a solution and a veterinary solution containing benzalkonium chloride 10%, and a solution containing benzalkonium chloride 10% with chlorhexidine gluconate 1%.

Benzathine Penicillin

The *NN'*-dibenzylethylenediamine salt of benzylpenicillin; it contains a variable amount of water of crystallisation.

$$C_{16}H_{20}N_2,(C_{16}H_{18}N_2O_4S)_2 = 909.1$$

OTHER NAMES: Benzathine Penicillin G; Benzylpenicillinum Benzathinum; *Penidural*® *Duphaphen LA*®, *Ethacillin PA*®, *Ilcocillin LA*®, and *Lentrax*® (all with procaine penicillin); *Penidural AP*® (with benzylpenicillin potassium and procaine penicillin)

A standard is given in the European Pharmacopoeia Vol. III

1.2 mega units of penicillin is contained in approximately 900 milligrams of benzathine penicillin.

Description. A white hygroscopic odourless powder.

Solubility. Very slightly soluble in water, in alcohol, in ether, and in chloroform; soluble, at 20°, in 10 parts of formamide and in 7 parts of dimethylformamide.

Moisture content. 5 to 8%, determined by Fischer titration.

Stability. When stored protected from moisture at room temperature, the dry material retains its potency for up to 5 years. Aqueous suspensions of benzathine penicillin have a maximum stability when buffered to pH 6 to 7 and

stored at a low temperature. Degradation follows zero order kinetics as only material in solution degrades. Buffered aqueous suspensions containing 25 to 50 mg of benzathine penicillin per ml may be expected to retain their potency for 2 years when stored at a temperature not exceeding 25°.

Hygroscopicity. At a relative humidity of 80% it absorbs significant amounts of moisture at 25°. It absorbs 4% of moisture after 1 hour rising to a maximum of 8% after 4 hours.

Labelling. If the material is not intended for parenteral administration the label on the container states that the contents are not to be injected.

Storage. It should be stored in airtight containers at a temperature not exceeding 25°, protected from light. If it is intended for parenteral administration the containers should be sterile and sealed to exclude micro-organisms.

Identification. TESTS. 1. It complies with Test 1 described under Benzylpenicillin.
2. Shake about 100 mg with 1 ml of 1N sodium hydroxide for 2 minutes, extract with two 3-ml portions of solvent ether, evaporate the extracts to dryness, dissolve a small portion of the residue in 2 ml of glacial acetic acid and add 1 ml of *potassium dichromate solution*; a golden-yellow precipitate is produced.
3. Dissolve the remainder of the residue obtained in Test 2 in 1 ml of alcohol (50%), add 5 ml of *trinitrophenol solution*, heat at 90° for 5 minutes, and allow to cool slowly; a precipitate is produced which, after recrystallisation from hot alcohol (25%) containing a small quantity of trinitrophenol, melts at about 214°.

MELTING-POINT. About 131°, with decomposition.

ULTRAVIOLET ABSORPTION. In methyl alcohol, maxima at 251 nm (E1%, 1cm = 9), 257 nm (E1%, 1cm = 9), 263 nm (E1%, 1cm = 6), 266 nm (E1%, 1cm = 4), and 320 nm.

Actions and uses. Benzathine penicillin is a benzylpenicillin derivative of low solubility, the action of which is due to release of benzylpenicillin. When given by mouth it is hydrolysed in the gut with the formation of benzylpenicillin which is absorbed. The maximum concentration of penicillin in the blood is obtained less rapidly than after a comparable dose of a soluble salt of benzylpenicillin by injection but the level is maintained for a longer period, and therapeutic doses usually give an effective concentration for 6 hours; absorption of the penicillin from the gastro-intestinal tract is not affected by the food intake.
The usual dose by mouth for adults is 450 milligrams 3 or 4 times daily, and for a child 150 to 300 milligrams or 15 milligrams per kilogram body-weight 3 or 4 times daily.
Intramuscular injections of benzathine penicillin are used to provide a prolonged effect and avoid the need for repeated injections after an initial dose of benzylpenicillin, especially in infants and children with acute streptococcal infections or when oral therapy is unreliable because of a lack of parental cooperation. A dose of 900 milligrams provides therapeutic blood levels (at least 0.03 microgram per ml) for 2 to 3 weeks. Fortnightly injections may be used to prevent relapses of rheumatic fever in patients who cannot be relied upon to take the drug regularly by mouth.

Undesirable effects; Precautions. As for Benzylpenicillin.

Veterinary uses. Benzathine penicillin is a slow-release form of penicillin used in all species by intramuscular injection in a dosage of 5 milligrams per kilogram body-weight every 2 weeks.

Preparations

FORTIFIED BENZATHINE PENICILLIN INJECTION (*Syn.* Benzathine Penicillin with Benzylpenicillin Potassium and Procaine Penicillin Injection): a sterile suspension of benzathine penicillin and procaine penicillin, with appropriate pharmaceutical adjuvants, in a solution of benzylpenicillin potassium in water for injections.

It is prepared by adding water for injections to the contents of a sealed container shortly before use.

Available as a powder in vials containing 600000 units (450 mg) of benzathine penicillin, 300000 units (190 mg) of benzylpenicillin potassium, and 300000 units (300 mg) of procaine penicillin.

A standard for this injection is given in the British Pharmaceutical Codex 1973

Containers: see the entry on Injections for general information on containers.

Labelling: see the entry on Injections for general information on labelling. In addition, the label on the sealed container should state "Fortified Benzathine Penicillin for Injection", and that the contents are to be used for intramuscular injection only.

Storage: the injection contains no bactericide and should be used as soon as possible after preparation but the injection may be expected to retain its potency for up to 7 days provided that it is stored at 2° to 4°.

OTHER PREPARATIONS available include an INJECTION containing benzathine penicillin 300000 units (225 mg) per ml in 10-ml vials, a veterinary injection containing benzathine penicillin 150000 units (112.5 mg) with procaine penicillin 150000 units (150 mg) per ml in 50-, 90-, and 100-ml vials; a MIXTURE containing benzathine penicillin 300000 units (225 mg) in 5 ml, diluent syrup, shelf-life of diluted mixture 14 days, and a mixture containing benzathine penicillin 150000 units (112.5 mg) per ml.

Benzhexol Hydrochloride

1-(3-Cyclohexyl-3-hydroxy-3-phenylpropyl)piperidinium chloride

$C_{20}H_{32}ClNO = 337.9$

OTHER NAMES: *Artane*®; Trihexyphenidyl Hydrochloride

A standard is given in the British Pharmacopoeia 1973

Description. A white or creamy-white, crystalline, almost odourless powder with a bitter taste followed by tingling and numbness.

Solubility. Soluble, at 20°, in 100 parts of water, in 22 parts of alcohol, in 15 parts of chloroform, and in 10 parts of methyl alcohol.

Acidity. A saturated solution has a pH of 5 to 6.

Identification. TESTS. 1. Dissolve 500 mg in 5 ml of warm methanol and make the solution just alkaline to litmus paper with *sodium hydroxide solution*; a precipitate is produced which, after recrystallisation from methanol, melts at about 114°.

MELTING-POINT. About 250°, with decomposition.

ULTRAVIOLET ABSORPTION. In 0.1N hydrochloric acid, maxima at 254 nm, 258 nm (E1%, 1cm = 5.6), and 266 nm; in alcohol (95%), maxima at 254 nm (E1%, 1cm = 5), 259 nm (E1%, 1cm = 5.5), and 266 nm.

INFRA-RED ABSORPTION. Major peaks at 702, 756, 973, 1196, 1206, and 1447 cm^{-1} (see Appendix 2a: Infra-red Spectra).

THIN-LAYER CHROMATOGRAPHY. See under Thin-layer Chromatography, System 8.

Actions and uses. Benzhexol antagonises some of the actions of acetylcholine in a manner similar to that described under Atropine, although it is less active; it diminishes salivation, increases the heart rate, dilates the pupil, and reduces the spasm of involuntary muscle, particularly of the intestine. In small doses it depresses the central nervous system, but larger doses cause cerebral excitement.

Benzhexol is used in the treatment of post-encephalitic, arteriosclerotic, and idiopathic types of parkinsonism. In all types of parkinsonism, benzhexol usually increases mobility and decreases rigidity, but it has only a limited effect on the tremors; the frequency and duration of oculogyric crises are also diminished.

Treatment is usually begun with a dosage of 1 to 2 milligrams of benzhexol hydrochloride by mouth 3 times daily and this is gradually increased to 20 milligrams daily in divided doses. Post-encephalitic patients as a rule tolerate and require higher doses, sometimes as much as 100 milligrams daily.

Benzhexol is sometimes given in conjunction with solanaceous alkaloids or other drugs used for the relief of parkinsonism.

Undesirable effects. Giddiness, dryness of the mouth, nausea, vomiting, and blurred vision occur occasionally but readily disappear when the dose is reduced.

Precautions and contra-indications. As for Atropine.

Preparations

BENZHEXOL TABLETS: available as tablets containing 2 and 5 mg of benzhexol hydrochloride.

A standard for these tablets is given in the British Pharmacopoeia 1973

Containers and *Storage:* see the entry on Tablets for general information on containers and storage. Containers should be airtight.

Advice for patients: the tablets should be taken before meals if the patient is inconvenienced by dryness of the mouth or after meals if there are gastro-intestinal disturbances. Treatment should not be discontinued without the advice of the prescriber.

OTHER PREPARATIONS available include CAPSULES containing benzhexol hydrochloride 5 mg in a slow-release formulation.

Benzocaine

Ethyl 4-aminobenzoate

$C_9H_{11}NO_2 = 165.2$

OTHER NAMES: Benzocainum; Ethyl Aminobenzoate
AAA® (with cetalkonium chloride); *Hibitane*® (with
chlorhexidine hydrochloride); *Auraltone*® (with phenazone); *Intralgin*® (with salicylamide); *Tyrozets*® (with
tyrothricin)

*A standard is given in the European Pharmacopoeia
Vol. I*

Description. Colourless crystals or a white crystalline
powder, with a bitter taste followed by local anaesthesia
of the tongue.

Solubility. Very slightly soluble in water; soluble, at 20°,
in 8 parts of alcohol, in 4 parts of ether, in 2 parts of
chloroform, and in 50 parts of fixed oils.

Dissociation constant. pK_a 2.5 (20°).

Storage. It should be stored in airtight containers, protected from light.

Identification. TESTS. 1. Dissolve about 100 mg in 2 ml
of *dilute hydrochloric acid* with the aid of heat if
necessary, cool in ice, add 4 ml of a 1% solution of
sodium nitrite, and pour the mixture into 2 ml of *2-
naphthol solution* containing 1 g of sodium acetate; an
orange-red precipitate is produced.
2. Mix about 50 mg with 2 drops of acetic acid and 5 drops
of sulphuric acid, and heat; the odour of ethyl acetate
is produced.
3. A 2% solution in water, made with the addition of
sufficient hydrochloric acid, gives a precipitate with
iodine solution but not with *potassium mercuri-iodide
solution* (distinction from procaine).

MELTING-POINT. About 90°.

ULTRAVIOLET ABSORPTION. In 0.1N hydrochloric acid,
maximum at 226 nm (E1%, 1cm = 654); in 0.1N sodium
hydroxide, maxima at 220 nm (E1%, 1cm = 740) and
264 nm (E1%, 1cm = 857); in alcohol (95%), maxima
at 221 nm (E1%, 1cm = 519) and 291 nm (E1%,
1cm = 1142).

INFRA-RED ABSORPTION. Major peaks at 1128, 1175,
1282, 1314, 1599, and 1681 cm⁻¹ (see Appendix 2a: Infra-
red Spectra).

THIN-LAYER CHROMATOGRAPHY. See under Thin-layer
Chromatography, System 2.

Metabolism. METABOLIC REACTIONS. Hydrolysis to
4-aminobenzoic acid.

FURTHER INFORMATION. Absorption and distribution
after absorption from suppositories in rats—J. W. Ayres
et al., J. pharm. Sci., 1976, **65**, 832.

Actions and uses. Benzocaine is a sparingly soluble
local anaesthetic with a toxicity about one-tenth that of
cocaine. It may be given by mouth to relieve the pain
of gastric carcinoma and is used, as an insufflation or as
a 2% solution in equal parts of alcohol and water, in
the symptomatic treatment of tuberculous laryngitis.
Benzocaine has been given by injection into the sub-

mucous and subcutaneous tissues in the treatment of
pruritus ani and anal fissure.
Benzocaine lozenges and compound benzocaine lozenges, allowed to dissolve slowly in the mouth, produce
a local anaesthetic effect and are used to prevent nausea
and vomiting during such procedures as the taking of
impressions for or the fitting of dentures and the passing
of instruments for laryngoscopy, bronchoscopy, or gastroscopy. These lozenges may also be used to relieve the
pain arising from lacerations of the tongue or cheek,
acute pharyngitis, tonsillectomy, or carcinoma of the
mouth.
Compound benzocaine ointment may be applied to burns
and cancerous ulcerations and is of value for the relief
of intractable pruritus.
Benzocaine has also been used in suppositories and
pessaries containing 500 milligrams and in the form of
a dusting-powder containing 10%.

Poisoning. As for Procaine Hydrochloride.

Preparations

BENZOCAINE LOZENGES: for each lozenge take:

Benzocaine .. .. 10 mg

Prepare by the method for compressed lozenges, as
described in the entry on Lozenges. Each lozenge weighs
about 1 gram.
Containers: see the entry on Lozenges for general information on containers.
Advice for patients: the lozenges should be allowed to
dissolve slowly in the mouth.

COMPOUND BENZOCAINE LOZENGES: for each lozenge
take:

Benzocaine .. .. 100 mg
Menthol .. .. 3 mg

Prepare by the method for compressed lozenges, as
described in the entry on Lozenges, adding the menthol
dissolved in a little alcohol (95%) to the dried granules.
Each lozenge weighs about 1 gram.
*A standard for these lozenges is given in the British
Pharmaceutical Codex 1973*
Containers: see the entry on Lozenges for general in-
formation on containers.
Advice for patients: the lozenges should be allowed to
dissolve slowly in the mouth.

OTHER PREPARATIONS available include EAR-DROPS containing benzocaine 1% with phenazone 5%; a GEL containing benzocaine 2% with salicylamide 5%; LOZENGES
containing benzocaine 2 mg with chlorhexidine hydrochloride 5 mg, lozenges containing benzocaine 5 mg with
tyrothricin 1 mg; and a SPRAY containing benzocaine
1.5% with cetalkonium chloride 0.0413% in an aerosol
pack delivering benzocaine 1.5 mg and cetalkonium
chloride 40 micrograms each time the valve is actuated.

Benzoic Acid

$C_6H_5.CO_2H = 122.1$

A standard is given in the British Pharmacopoeia 1973

Description. Colourless light feathery plates or needles
or a white powder with a slight characteristic odour.

Solubility. Soluble, at 20°, in 350 parts of water and in
3 parts of alcohol; readily soluble in ether, in chloroform,
and in fixed and volatile oils.

Dissociation constant. pK_a 4.2 (20°).

Identification. TEST. Mix 200 mg with 20 ml of water and

1 ml of 1N sodium hydroxide, gently warm the mixture, filter, and to the filtrate add *ferric chloride test-solution*; a buff-coloured precipitate is produced.

MELTING-POINT. About 122°, forming a feathery sublimate.

INFRA-RED ABSORPTION. Major peaks at 709, 1296, 1329, 1427, 1459, and 1689 cm^{-1} (see Appendix 2a: Infra-red Spectra).

Metabolism. METABOLIC REACTIONS. Conjugated with glycine to form hippuric acid; there are species differences and, in animals, metabolites include the glucuronide and hydroxylated forms.

EXCRETION. An oral dose of 1 mg/kg is completely excreted in the urine as hippuric acid in 12 hours; 97% may be excreted in the first 4 hours.

FURTHER INFORMATION. Fate of benzoic acid in various species—J. W. Bridges *et al.*, *Biochem. J.*, 1970, **118**, 47; renal contribution to conversion of benzoic acid to hippuric acid—S. H. Wan and S. Riegelman, *J. pharm. Sci.*, 1972, **61**, 1278.

Actions and uses. Benzoic acid has antibacterial and antifungal properties. In a concentration of 0.1% it is a moderately effective preservative provided that the pH of the preparation is not above 5.0. It is used as a preservative in certain acid food products.
Compound benzoic acid ointment is used in the treatment of fungal infections of the skin.

Preparations

BENZOIC ACID SOLUTION:

Benzoic acid	50 g
Propylene glycol	750 ml
Purified water, freshly boiled and cooled	to 1000 ml

Dissolve the benzoic acid in the propylene glycol and add sufficient water, in small quantities and with constant stirring, to produce the required volume.
A standard for this solution is given in the British Pharmaceutical Codex 1973

COMPOUND BENZOIC ACID OINTMENT (*Syn.* Whitfield's Ointment):

Benzoic acid, in fine powder	60 g
Salicylic acid, in fine powder	30 g
Emulsifying ointment	910 g

Triturate the benzoic acid and the salicylic acid with a portion of the emulsifying ointment until smooth and gradually incorporate the remainder of the ointment.
A standard for this ointment is given in the British Pharmaceutical Codex 1973
Containers: see the entry on Ointments for general information on containers.
Advice for patients: the ointment should be applied sparingly to the affected area. It should not be applied to broken or inflamed skin. Prolonged use should be avoided and its use should be discontinued if excessive dryness or irritation of the skin occurs.

Benzoin

A balsamic resin obtained from the incised stem of *Styrax benzoin* Dryand. and of *S. paralleloneurus* Perkins (Fam. Styracaceae) and known in commerce as Sumatra benzoin.

A standard is given in the British Pharmaceutical Codex 1973

Constituents. Benzoin contains various resinous esters of benzoic and cinnamic acids, together with free benzoic, cinnamic, siaresinolic (19-hydroxyoleanolic acid) and sumaresinolic (6-hydroxyoleanolic acid) acids. The proportion of total cinnamic acid is usually about twice that of total benzoic acid.

Description. Hard brittle masses consisting of whitish tears embedded in a greyish-brown to reddish-brown translucent matrix and known in commerce as block benzoin; it also occurs in the form of tears with cream-coloured surfaces and, when broken, exhibiting surfaces having a milky-white colour.
It has an agreeable and balsamic odour.

Adulterants and substitutes. Siam benzoin from *Styrax tonkinensis* (Pierre) Craib ex Hartwich (Fam. Styracaceae) exported from Thailand and Vietnam. A standard for Siam benzoin is given in the European Pharmacopoeia Vol. III. It occurs in tears having a slight odour of vanillin; the surface is brownish-red with a varnished appearance; the tears are milky-white internally. Siam benzoin is not found in block form, although the lowest grade of Vietnamese material, comprising powdery and small granular material, is usually found to be caked giving an appearance of being in block form in the 2-kg bags or packets in which it is exported. The major constituent is coniferyl benzoate together with benzoic acid, triterpenoid acids, and vanillin. When warmed with *potassium permanganate solution* it yields no odour of benzaldehyde.
Penang or "glassy" Penang benzoin, having a greyish vitreous appearance with no aromatic odour, and Palembang benzoin, consisting of a reddish resinous mass in which are embedded a few scattered tears with a slight odour, both from Sumatra, have been substituted for benzoin.

Storage. It should be stored in a cool place.

Identification. TESTS. 1. Heat 0.5 g gently in a dry test-tube; it melts and evolves white fumes, which form a white crystalline sublimate.
2. Warm gently 1 g, in powder, with 5 ml of *potassium permanganate solution*; a distinct odour of benzaldehyde is produced (distinction from Siam benzoin).
3. Triturate 100 mg, in powder, with 5 ml of alcohol (95%), filter, and to the filtrate add 0.5 ml of a 5% solution of ferric chloride in alcohol (95%); no bright green colour is produced (distinction from Siam benzoin).

Actions and uses. Benzoin is an ingredient of inhalations which are used, by adding 5 millilitres of the inhalation to 500 millilitres of hot water (or 1 teaspoonful to a pint) and inhaling the vapour, in the treatment of catarrh of the upper respiratory tract.

Preparations

BENZOIN INHALATION:

Benzoin, crushed	100 g
Prepared storax	50 g
Alcohol (95%)	to 1000 ml

Macerate the benzoin and the prepared storax with 750 ml of the alcohol for 24 hours. Filter and pass sufficient of the alcohol through the filter to produce the required volume.
In making this preparation, the alcohol (95%) may be replaced by industrial methylated spirit, provided that the law and the statutory regulations governing the use of industrial methylated spirit are observed.
A standard for this inhalation is given in the British Pharmaceutical Codex 1973

Containers: see the entry on Inhalations for general information on containers.

Advice for patients: see the entry on Inhalations for general information on the use of inhalations.

BENZOIN TINCTURE (*Syn.* Simple Tincture of Benzoin):

Benzoin, crushed	100 g
Alcohol (90%)	to 1000 ml

Macerate the benzoin with 800 ml of the alcohol for 1 hour, with frequent agitation; filter and pass sufficient alcohol through the filter to produce the required volume.

A standard for this tincture is given in the British Pharmaceutical Codex 1973

Dose: 2.5 to 5 millilitres.

COMPOUND BENZOIN TINCTURE (*Syn.* Friars' Balsam):

Benzoin, crushed	100 g
Aloes	20 g
Tolu balsam	25 g
Prepared storax	75 g
Alcohol (90%)	to 1000 ml

Macerate the materials with 800 ml of the alcohol in a closed vessel for not less than 2 days, shaking occasionally; filter and pass sufficient of the alcohol through the filter to produce the required volume.

A standard for this tincture is given in the British Pharmaceutical Codex 1973

Advice for patients: see the entry on Inhalations for general information on its use as an inhalation. For the treatment of cuts and grazes, it should be applied undiluted to the skin.

MENTHOL AND BENZOIN INHALATION:

Menthol	20 g
Benzoin Inhalation	to 1000 ml

A standard for this inhalation is given in the British Pharmaceutical Codex 1973

Containers: see the entry on Inhalations for general information on containers.

Advice for patients: see the entry on Inhalations for general information on the use of inhalations.

Benztropine Mesylate

(1*R*,3*r*,5*S*)-3-Benzhydryloxytropanium methane-sulphonate

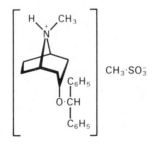

$C_{22}H_{29}NO_4S = 403.5$

OTHER NAMES: Benztropine methanesulphonate; *Cogentin*®

A standard is given in the British Pharmacopoeia 1973

Description. A white crystalline odourless powder with a bitter taste.

Solubility. Soluble, at 20°, in less than 1 part of water and in 1.5 parts of alcohol; practically insoluble in ether.

Moisture content. Not more than 5%, determined by drying at 105°.

Dissociation constant. pK_a 10.0 (20°).

Sterilisation. Solutions for injection are sterilised by heating in an autoclave or by filtration.

Storage. It should be stored in airtight containers.

Identification. TESTS. 1. Add about 1 mg to 4 drops of fuming nitric acid; a reddish-yellow colour is produced. Evaporate the mixture to dryness; a brownish-yellow oily residue is obtained which becomes yellow on the addition of 2 ml of acetone and gives a brownish-red precipitate on the addition of 4 drops of a 3% solution of potassium hydroxide in methanol.

2. Dissolve about 10 mg in 10 ml of sulphuric acid; an orange solution is produced. To 5 ml of the solution add 0.2 ml of *potassium dichromate solution*, warm, and allow to stand; the colour slowly changes from red to brown. Pour the remainder of the original solution into about 10 ml of water; a colourless opalescent solution is produced.

3. Dissolve about 10 mg in 2 ml of water and pour into 5 ml of hot *trinitrophenol solution*; the precipitate, after drying at 105°, melts at about 185°.

MELTING-POINT. About 143°.

ULTRAVIOLET ABSORPTION. In 0.1N sulphuric acid, maxima at 253 nm (E1%, 1cm = 11) and 259 nm (E1%, 1cm = 12); in water, maxima at 253 nm (E1%, 1cm = 9.6) and 258 nm (E1%, 1cm = 11).

INFRA-RED ABSORPTION. Major peaks at 700, 710, 740, 1050, 1192, and 1228 cm^{-1} (see Appendix 2a: Infra-red Spectra).

THIN-LAYER CHROMATOGRAPHY. See under Thin-layer Chromatography, System 8.

Actions and uses. Benztropine antagonises some of the actions of acetylcholine in a manner similar to that described under Atropine. It depresses the motor cortex and also has an antihistamine-like effect. It reduces spasm and tremor of voluntary muscle and is used in the treatment of parkinsonism, usually in conjunction with other drugs.

The initial daily dosage is 500 micrograms of benztropine mesylate by mouth, gradually increased according to the response of the patient; the effective dosage is usually from 2 to 6 milligrams daily in divided doses. Similar doses may be given by intramuscular or intravenous injection.

Undesirable effects. As for Benzhexol Hydrochloride.

Precautions and contra-indications. As for Atropine.

Preparations

BENZTROPINE INJECTION: a sterile solution of benztropine mesylate. It is sterilised by heating in an autoclave or by filtration. Available in 2-ml ampoules containing 1 mg of benztropine mesylate per ml.

Containers and *Labelling:* see the entry on Injections for general information on containers and labelling.

Storage: it should be stored in a cool place, protected from light. It should not be allowed to freeze.

BENZTROPINE TABLETS: available as tablets containing 2 mg of benztropine mesylate.

A standard for these tablets is given in the British Pharmacopoeia 1973

Containers and *Storage:* see the entry on Tablets for general information on containers and storage. Containers should be airtight.

Advice for patients: daily doses should preferably be

taken at bedtime. The tablets should be taken before meals if the patient is inconvenienced by dryness of the mouth, or after meals if there are gastro-intestinal disturbances. Treatment should not be discontinued without the advice of the prescriber. The tablets may cause drowsiness; persons affected should not drive or operate machinery. Alcohol should be avoided.

Benzyl Alcohol

$C_6H_5 \cdot CH_2OH = 108.1$

A standard is given in the British Pharmacopoeia 1973

Description. A colourless, almost odourless liquid with a sharp and burning taste.

Solubility. Soluble, at 20°, in 25 parts of water; miscible with alcohol, with ether, and with chloroform.

Weight per ml. At 20°, 1.043 to 1.046 g.

Boiling-point. About 205°.

Refractive index. 1.538 to 1.541.

Sterilisation. Solutions for injection are sterilised by heating in an autoclave or by filtration.

Identification. TEST. Add 2 drops to a strong solution of potassium permanganate acidified with sulphuric acid; the odour of benzaldehyde is produced.

Actions and uses. Benzyl alcohol is a weak local anaesthetic with antiseptic properties. It is therefore included as a preservative in some injections, at a strength of 1%, and is an effective bactericide up to pH 6. Benzyl alcohol is almost non-toxic and non-irritant, but strong solutions may cause oedema and pain when injected.

Benzyl Benzoate

$C_{14}H_{12}O_2 = 212.2$ $\quad C_6H_5 \cdot CO \cdot O \cdot CH_2 \cdot C_6H_5$

OTHER NAME: *Ascabiol*®

A standard is given in the British Pharmacopoeia 1973

Description. Colourless crystals or oily liquid with a faintly aromatic odour and a sharp burning taste.

Solubility. Practically insoluble in water and in glycerol; soluble in alcohol, in chloroform, and in ether.

Weight per ml. At 20°, 1.116 to 1.120 g.

Refractive index. At 20°, 1.568 to 1.570.

Boiling-point. About 320°.

Incompatibility. It is incompatible with alkalis.

Identification. TESTS. 1. Mix 2 g with 25 ml of *alcoholic potassium hydroxide solution* and boil for 2 hours under a reflux condenser; evaporate the alcohol on a water-bath, add 50 ml of water, and distil until the liquid distilling is no longer turbid. Reserve the distillate. Acidify the liquid remaining in the flask with *dilute hydrochloric acid*; a white crystalline precipitate of benzoic acid is produced.
2. To the distillate reserved in Test 1 add 2.5 g of potassium permanganate and 2 ml of *sodium hydroxide solution*, boil for 15 minutes under a reflux condenser, cool, filter, and acidify the filtrate with *dilute hydrochloric acid*; a white crystalline precipitate of benzoic acid is produced.

ULTRAVIOLET ABSORPTION. In alcohol (95%), maximum at 230 nm (E1%, 1cm = 843).

Metabolism. METABOLIC REACTIONS. Rapidly hydrolysed to benzoic acid and benzyl alcohol; benzyl alcohol is oxidised to the acid, which is conjugated with glycine to form hippuric acid.

EXCRETION. Excreted in the urine mainly as hippuric acid.

Actions and uses. Benzyl benzoate is an acaricide used in the treatment of scabies. The patient is scrubbed with soft soap in a hot bath to open up the burrows and, immediately after drying, benzyl benzoate application is applied over the whole body surface below the neck and is allowed to dry. A second application is made the following day in the same way after a hot bath. Bedding and clothing should be disinfected, preferably by sterilisation. Close contacts should also be treated.
Although more than one course of treatment may be necessary, benzyl benzoate is more efficient, cleaner, and easier to use than sulphur preparations but it may not be effective in some cases of Norwegian scabies.
Benzyl benzoate is also used in the treatment of pediculosis but as resistance to its action is commonly encountered, it has been largely replaced by carbaryl or malathion. When applied to the scalp, the eyes, ears, and lips should be protected.

Preparation

BENZYL BENZOATE APPLICATION:

Benzyl benzoate	..	..	..	..	250 g
Emulsifying wax	..	..	..	..	20 g
Purified water, freshly boiled and cooled	..	..	..	..	to 1000 ml

Mix the benzyl benzoate with the emulsifying wax, previously melted at a low temperature; pour the warm mixture into most of the water, previously warmed to the same temperature, stir thoroughly, add sufficient water to produce the required volume, and mix.
A standard for this application is given in the British Pharmacopoeia 1973
Containers and *Labelling:* see the entry on Applications for general information on containers and labelling.
Advice for patients: for the treatment of scabies a hot bath should be taken and the body thoroughly dried. The preparation should be applied to the body with the aid of a suitable brush and allowed to dry, but it should not be applied to the head and face.
For the treatment of pediculosis the affected area should be thoroughly washed and dried before application. The preparation should be applied to the affected and adjacent areas and should not be washed off for the next 24 hours. The application should not be applied to broken or inflamed skin; contact with the eyes, ears, and lips should be avoided.

Benzyl Hydroxybenzoate

Benzyl 4-hydroxybenzoate

$$CO \cdot O \cdot CH_2 \cdot C_6H_5$$

OH

$C_{14}H_{12}O_3 = 228.3$

OTHER NAMES: Benzylparaben; *Nipabenzyl®*

A standard is given in the British Pharmacopoeia Addendum 1978

Description. An odourless, white to creamy-white, crystalline powder.

Solubility. Practically insoluble in water; soluble, at 20°, in 2.5 parts of alcohol and in 6 parts of ether; soluble in solutions of alkali hydroxides.

Identification. TEST. It complies with the test described under Methyl Hydroxybenzoate.

MELTING-POINT. About 112°.

ULTRAVIOLET ABSORPTION. In alcohol (95%), maximum at 260 nm (E1%, 1cm = 760).

Uses. Benzyl hydroxybenzoate has preservative properties, as described under Methyl Hydroxybenzoate.
It is used in a concentration of 0.01% in conjunction with other hydroxybenzoates as a preservative in aqueous preparations.

Benzylpenicillin

The potassium or the sodium salt of (6R)-6-phenylacetamidopenicillanic acid, an antimicrobial acid produced by growing certain strains of *Penicillium notatum* or related organisms under appropriate conditions in a suitable culture medium. One mega unit of penicillin is contained in approximately 600 milligrams of benzylpenicillin.

$C_{16}H_{17}KN_2O_4S = 372.5$
$C_{16}H_{17}N_2NaO_4S = 356.4$

OTHER NAMES: Benzylpenicillin Potassium; Benzylpenicillin Sodium; Benzylpenicillinum Kalicum; Benzylpenicillinum Natricum; Crystalline Penicillin G; *Crystapen®*; Penicillin; Penicillin G
Strypen Forte® (with dihydrostreptomycin sulphate); *Crystamycin®* (with streptomycin sulphate)

A standard is given in the European Pharmacopoeia Vol. II

Description. Both salts are white, finely crystalline, hygroscopic powders with a faint characteristic odour.

Solubility. Very soluble in water; practically insoluble in fixed oils and in liquid paraffin.

Acidity or alkalinity. A 10% solution has a pH of 5.5 to 7.5.

Moisture content. Not more than 1%, determined by Fischer titration.

Specific rotation. Potassium salt, not less than +270°, sodium salt not less than +282°, both determined on a 2% solution.

Dissociation constant. pK_a 2.7 (25°).

Stability. The stability of benzylpenicillin depends mainly on its moisture content; provided that it contains less than 0.5%, it can be stored at room temperature for 2 to 3 years without significant loss of potency.
For maximum stability, aqueous solutions of benzyl-

penicillin should be buffered at pH 6 to 7 and kept at a low temperature. Dilute solutions are more stable than concentrated ones, probably because less penicilloic acid is produced on hydrolysis with the lower concentration.

Incompatibility. In addition to acids, alkalis, and penicillinase, numerous other substances inactivate benzylpenicillin at varying rates. Traces of heavy metals (copper, lead, zinc, or mercury) have a deleterious action on penicillin solutions.
Although high concentrations of ethyl alcohol should be avoided, rigorous exclusion of alcohol from preparations is unnecessary and it can be used to wipe caps of bottles containing either the dry powder or its solutions for injection.
Low concentrations of glycerol (say 10%) have little effect on the deterioration of aqueous solutions of benzylpenicillin, but high concentrations increase the loss of activity; impurities in the glycerol may be responsible for some of the inactivation. Similar effects occur with propylene glycol.
Benzylpenicillin in slightly alkaline solution is rapidly inactivated by cysteine and other aminothiol compounds.
Benzylpenicillin salts are incompatible with sympathomimetic amines and hydrochlorides of the tetracyclines, the degree of incompatibility being dependent on concentrations, pH of vehicles, and time.
Other substances with an adverse effect on benzylpenicillin include compounds leached from vulcanised rubber, oxidising agents (especially in the presence of trace metals), organic peroxides, thiomersal, wool alcohols, cetostearyl alcohol, paraffins, macrogols, cocoa butter, and many ionic and non-ionic surface-active agents.
Benzylpenicillin should not be given by intravenous infusion in dextrose injection because the acidity of the solution will bring about rapid decomposition, up to half of the activity being lost in a few hours; this loss is likely to be increased if sodium bicarbonate is added in an attempt to neutralise the acidity; it may, however, be safely injected into the drip tubing after being well diluted with sodium chloride injection, normal doses being administered over 1 to 2 minutes and larger doses more slowly.

Hygroscopicity. Both salts are hygroscopic, but the potassium salt is less so. At relative humidities up to 55%, they absorb insignificant amounts of moisture at 25°; at relative humidities between 55 and 80%, the amounts absorbed by the potassium salt are larger but still small (about 0.4% in 12 days at a relative humidity of 70%), but with the sodium salt significant amounts are absorbed at relative humidities between 55 and 70%; under damper conditions, both salts absorb substantial amounts of moisture.

Labelling. The label on the container states whether the contents are the sodium or the potassium salt. If the material is not intended for parenteral administration, the label also states that the contents are not to be injected.

Storage. It should be stored in airtight containers at a temperature not exceeding 30°. If it is intended for parenteral administration, the containers must be sterile and sealed to exclude micro-organisms.

Identification. TEST. Mix 2 mg with 2 mg of chromotropic acid sodium salt and 2 ml of sulphuric acid and immerse in a suitable liquid at 150° for 4 minutes; the solution becomes a pale yellowish colour before it finally chars (distinction from certain other penicillins).

ULTRAVIOLET ABSORPTION. Potassium salt, in water, maximum at 264 nm (E1%, 1cm = 4.7). Sodium salt, in water, maximum at 264 nm (E1%, 1cm = 4.9); in 0.1N sodium hydroxide, maxima at 252 nm (E1%, 1cm = 6) and 258 nm (E1%, 1cm = 6).

INFRA-RED ABSORPTION. Major peaks at 1310, 1420, 1500, 1620, 1700, and 1777 cm^{-1} (see Appendix 2a: Infra-red Spectra).

Metabolism. ABSORPTION. 20 to 30% of a dose administered as a water-soluble salt is absorbed in active form after oral administration. The remainder is inactivated by organisms in the gastro-intestinal tract and by gastric juice; the inactivation may be decreased by the administration of buffers or antacids but excess buffer will also destroy the drug and antacids will adsorb the drug and delay its absorption; oral administration to infants under 6 months of age results in almost complete absorption; parenteral administration results in rapid absorption.

BLOOD CONCENTRATION. After an oral dose of 60 to 600 mg, peak serum concentrations of 1 to 12 µg/ml are attained in 3 to 6 hours; after an intramuscular dose of 180 mg as a water-soluble salt, peak serum concentrations of about 20 µg/ml are attained in 20 to 30 minutes; minimum effective concentration, 0.006 to 2 µg/ml.

HALF-LIFE. Serum half-life, 30 to 160 minutes. Administration of probenecid or phenylbutazone increases the half-life significantly.

DISTRIBUTION. Enters most tissues, lesions, and serous cavities; small amounts enter bone marrow, abscesses, pleural fluid, and cerebrospinal fluid; the amount in the cerebrospinal fluid may be increased if the meninges are inflamed; benzylpenicillin crosses the placenta and small amounts are secreted in the milk; *protein binding*, 20 to 65% bound to plasma proteins.

EXCRETION. After oral administration, 15 to 25% is excreted in the urine and after intramuscular injection about 60% appears in the urine in 1 hour and about 95% in 4 hours; urinary excretion may be delayed by probenecid or phenylbutazone; up to half the urinary excreted material may be excreted in active form; small amounts are excreted in the bile but little or no active drug is detectable in the faeces. Urinary excretion is reduced in neonates.

FURTHER INFORMATION. Effects of age and other drugs on benzylpenicillin half-life—J. Kampmann et al., Clin. Pharmac. Ther., 1972, **13**, 516; protein binding—C. M. Kunin, Clin. Pharmac. Ther., 1968, **7**, 180; pharmacokinetics after intravenous injection in normal subjects and those with renal function impairment—M. E. Plant et al., J. lab. clin. Med., 1969, **74**, 412; excretion—H. D. Riley, J. clin. Pharmac., 1967, **7**, 312.

Actions and uses. Benzylpenicillin is a highly potent antibiotic from which a group of semisynthetic penicillins have been derived for special clinical purposes. These penicillins share the following characteristics and many of them release benzylpenicillin in the tissues and share the same mode of excretion.

The penicillins act mainly by interfering with the synthesis of the bacterial cell membrane and are therefore more effective when the bacterial cell is growing. They may give rise to cell-wall-free variants of certain species of bacteria. The mammalian cell membrane is only affected at high dose levels exceeding 12 grams (20 mega units) daily which may cause haemolysis. The penicillins have additional bactericidal effects within the bacterial cell which occur at high dose levels and may affect dormant bacteria.

The penicillins are readily absorbed through the intestinal mucosa into the blood stream and diffuse into all body fluids but varying proportions are carried bound to protein. Only free penicillin is active but the protein-bound material acts as a reservoir which replaces the free material as the latter is excreted. The cerebrospinal fluid contains a relatively low concentration of total penicillin in the normal patient because it contains only the free component. When there is inflammation of the meninges and a proteinaceous exudate the levels are the same as in blood.

Free penicillin is rapidly excreted but its half-life can be prolonged by the administration of probenecid, 500 milligrams 3 or 4 times daily by mouth, which blocks the tubular component of the excretion. Most of the penicillin is excreted active and unchanged but some is degraded in the liver and kidneys through various pathways and excreted in inactive forms.

Benzylpenicillin is mainly used to treat infections by the Gram-positive pyogenic organisms, species of Neisseria and Actinomyces, Bacillus anthracis, species of Clostridium, Corynebacterium, and Erysipelothrix, and Spirillum minus and the spirochaetes. However, it would probably be effective against many of the Gram-negative bacteria as well as the "resistant" staphylococci were it not for strains and species which produce a variety of penicillinases. These are enzymes which are excreted by the bacteria and destroy the penicillin by opening the β-lactam ring. The production of these enzymes is an inherited characteristic which seldom (if ever) results from mutation. The spread of "resistant" strains particularly of staphylococci through the community is largely a result of replacement of sensitive by naturally resistant strains.

As benzylpenicillin is largely destroyed by the acid in the gastric juice it is administered parenterally; for oral use phenoxymethylpenicillin is preferred.

For the treatment of most acute illnesses due to penicillin-sensitive organisms a dose of 150 to 600 milligrams (250 000 to 1 000 000 units) of benzylpenicillin is given, usually by intramuscular injection, 2 to 4 times daily. Much larger amounts and more frequent administration may be needed for the treatment of subacute bacterial endocarditis and fulminating infections. As much as 24 grams (40 mega units) daily may be given by continuous intravenous infusion.

Benzylpenicillin may also be given by intravenous, intrathecal, subconjunctival, and intra-ocular injection. The parenteral dose for children corresponding to an adult dose of 300 milligrams is up to 1 year 75 milligrams, 1 to 5 years 150 milligrams, and 6 to 12 years 300 milligrams.

The intrathecal dose for adults is 6 to 12 milligrams dissolved in 10 millilitres of water for injections or withdrawn cerebrospinal fluid. The corresponding dose for newborn infants is 1.5 to 3 milligrams and for children aged 4 to 14 years 3 to 6 milligrams.

Benzylpenicillin may be applied to the eye in concentrations of 1.5 to 12 milligrams per millilitre. A solution containing 1.5 milligrams (2500 units) per millilitre is used in the treatment of ophthalmia neonatorum. It may be prepared by dissolving the contents of a vial containing 12 milligrams (20 000 units) in 8 millilitres of a sterile vehicle and transferring the solution to previously sterilised eye-drop bottles, aseptic precautions being taken throughout. A suitable vehicle is a solution containing 0.5% of sodium citrate and 0.85% of sodium chloride with 0.002% of phenylmercuric nitrate in freshly distilled water. This vehicle is sterilised by heating in an autoclave and is stable for 1 year. When used to prepare a solution of benzylpenicillin as directed above, the resultant buffered isotonic solution is stable for 14 days when stored at 2° to 10° or for 4 days at temperatures approaching 20°. When vials containing 12 milligrams of benzylpenicillin are not available any other strength may be used, appropriate adjustments being made in respect of quantity of vehicle used. Unbuffered solutions may also be used but are less stable.

Benzylpenicillin may be injected subconjunctivally in concentrations of 150 to 600 milligrams in 0.5 millilitre of lignocaine and adrenaline injection or intra-ocularly in concentrations of 0.6 to 1.2 milligrams in 0.1 millilitre of water for injections.

For intramuscular injection doses up to 300 milligrams (500 000 units) of benzylpenicillin may be dissolved in 1 millilitre of water for injections, and larger doses in 2 millilitres. As all except the weakest solutions are hypertonic, sodium chloride injection should not be used as the solvent. When a high dose is needed as may be the case in many cases of subacute bacterial endocarditis due to *Streptococcus viridans* or *S. faecalis* a continuous intravenous infusion in dextrose injection (5%) may be preferred to avoid the painful sites caused by large volumes of hypertonic injections. When such infusions are given over long periods there may be a danger of fungal infections occurring at the injection site.

The effect of intramuscular doses of benzylpenicillin may be prolonged by the use of procaine penicillin suspensions from which penicillin is released for up to 12 hours. They are not suitable for high dosage levels. Benzylpenicillin may be used with streptomycin or other bactericidal drugs in the treatment of bacterial endocarditis but synergy with other antibiotics is believed not to occur and many consider that the synchronous use of a bacteriostatic agent is of no advantage.

Undesirable effects. A cell-wall-damaging effect in high concentrations limits the intrathecal dose to a maximum of 12 milligrams (20 000 units) of benzylpenicillin in an adult.

All penicillins carry a risk of hypersensitivity which develops most readily as a result of topical application. It is possible that pure penicillin is not the cause of the allergy in many cases but that degradation products appearing during manufacture or storage or during metabolism of the penicillins in the body are responsible. Some but not all of the allergic responses may be avoided by using specially purified preparations.

These allergies are common to the whole group and penicillins should be avoided or used with great caution in patients with a history of allergy to any form of penicillin. The reaction usually develops during the second week of the first course of treatment and consists of an urticarial rash and fever. Subsequent administration can lead to more serious reactions of the serum sickness type and deaths have occasionally resulted from anaphylaxis.

Encephalopathy may occasionally follow the intravenous administration of high doses of benzylpenicillin in patients with renal failure.

Precautions. As with all antibiotics, penicillin should not be used either prophylactically or for an established infection unless there is a positive indication that it is necessary. Otherwise penicillin will become less useful because of replacement of bacterial flora by resistant strains and the presence in the community of many individuals allergic to this group of drugs.

Benzylpenicillin should only be given to patients thought to be allergic to it if there is no satisfactory alternative and the infection is life-threatening. Preparations should be made to deal with anaphylactic shock before the first dose is given.

Small amounts of benzylpenicillin may be secreted in the milk of nursing mothers and may provoke allergic reactions in infants that are allergic to penicillins.

Benzylpenicillin should not be used topically either on the skin or mucous membranes. When high doses are given the effect of the associated sodium or potassium ions should be taken into account and the appropriate salt or mixture of salts should be used.

Veterinary uses. Benzylpenicillin is an antibacterial agent used in all species by intramuscular injection in a dosage of 3 to 6 milligrams per kilogram body-weight up to 6 times a day. It is given to cattle by intramammary injection in doses of 60 milligrams into each infected quarter, repeated daily if necessary for 2 or 3 days.

Preparations

BENZYLPENICILLIN INJECTION (*Syn.* Penicillin Injection): a sterile solution of benzylpenicillin in water for injections. It may contain a suitable buffering agent. It is prepared by dissolving the contents of a sealed container in water for injections shortly before use. Available as a powder in vials containing 12 mg (20 000 units), 300 mg (500 000 units), and 600 mg (1 mega unit) of benzylpenicillin, and in bottles containing 3 g (5 mega units) and 6 g (10 mega units). The powder in the bottles also contains 4.5% of sodium citrate.

A standard for this injection is given in the British Pharmacopoeia 1973

Containers: see the entry on Injections for general information on containers.

Labelling: see the entry on Injections for general information on labelling. In addition, the label on the sealed container should state whether the contents are benzylpenicillin (potassium salt) or benzylpenicillin (sodium salt).

Storage: the sealed container should be stored at a temperature not exceeding 30°. The injection contains no bactericide and should be used as soon as possible after preparation, but solutions of benzylpenicillin may be expected to retain their potency for up to 7 days after preparation, or for up to 14 days if a buffering agent is present, provided they are stored at 2° to 10°.

BENZYLPENICILLIN TABLETS (*Syn.* Penicillin Tablets): available as tablets containing 250 mg (400 000 units) of benzylpenicillin. They may be coated with sugar or other suitable material.

A standard for these tablets is given in the British Pharmacopoeia 1973

Containers and *Storage:* see the entry on Tablets for general information on containers and storage. Containers should be airtight.

The tablets should be stored at a temperature not exceeding 30°.

Advice for patients: the tablets should be taken at regular intervals, preferably half to 1 hour before meals. The prescribed course should be completed.

OTHER PREPARATIONS available include ELIXIRS containing benzylpenicillin 125 mg (200 000 units) and 250 mg (400 000 units) in 5 ml when reconstituted, diluent syrup, shelf-life of diluted elixir 7 days at room temperature or 14 days at 2° to 10°; an INTRAMAMMARY INJECTION containing benzylpenicillin potassium 300 mg (500 000 units) with dihydrostreptomycin sulphate equivalent to 250 mg of dihydrostreptomycin in 5-ml tubes; and an INJECTION reconstituted from vials of powder containing benzylpenicillin sodium 300 mg (500 000 units) with streptomycin sulphate equivalent to 500 mg of streptomycin.

Benzylpenicillin is an ingredient of fortified benethamine penicillin injection, fortified benzathine penicillin injection, and fortified procaine penicillin injection.

Bephenium Hydroxynaphthoate

Benzyldimethyl-2-phenoxyethylammonium 3-hydroxy-naphthalene-2-carboxylate

$C_{28}H_{29}NO_4 = 443.5$

OTHER NAMES: *Alcopar®*; *Frantin®*

A standard is given in the British Pharmacopoeia Addendum 1977 and the British Pharmacopoeia (Veterinary)

Description. A yellow crystalline odourless powder.

Solubility. Practically insoluble in water; soluble in 50 parts of alcohol.

Moisture content. Not more than 1%, determined by drying at 105°.

Identification. TESTS. 1. Examine under screened ultra-violet radiation; a green fluorescence is produced.
2. Dissolve 200 mg in 10 ml of warm dehydrated alcohol, add 15 ml of *trinitrophenol solution*, and allow to stand; a precipitate is produced which, after washing with alcohol (95%) and then with water, and drying at 105°, melts at about 134°, with decomposition.

MELTING-POINT. About 170°, with decomposition.

INFRA-RED ABSORPTION. Major peaks at 768, 1233, 1359, 1370, 1391, and 1452 cm^{-1} (see Appendix 2a: Infra-red Spectra).

Actions and uses. Bephenium hydroxynaphthoate is an anthelmintic which is effective against a wide variety of intestinal nematodes. It is sparingly soluble, and only a small fraction of the dose given by mouth is absorbed from the gastro-intestinal tract.

Bephenium hydroxynaphthoate in a single dose of 5 grams by mouth is usually effective in removing hookworms of the species *Ancylostoma duodenale* and roundworms (*Ascaris*). Children under 2 years or less than 10 kilograms body-weight may be given 2.5 grams, and older children the adult dose. 1 gram of bephenium hydroxynaphthoate is approximately equivalent to 600 milligrams of bephenium. The dose should be given on an empty stomach and food withheld for one hour afterwards. In severely infected cases treatment may be repeated on 3 consecutive days or at intervals of 7 to 10 days. Since no purge is necessary and bephenium hydroxynaphthoate is relatively non-toxic it is particularly suitable for use by patients with anaemia or diarrhoea.

Bephenium hydroxynaphthoate is less effective against *Necator americanus* and single doses on several successive days may be needed to remove all the worms. It is also effective against intestinal trichostrongyliasis and has a slight effect against whipworms (*Trichuris*).

Undesirable effects. It may occasionally cause transient diarrhoea and the bitter taste may cause nausea and sometimes vomiting.

Veterinary uses. Bephenium hydroxynaphthoate is an anthelmintic used mainly in the control of parasitic gastro-enteritis caused by *Nematodirus* infections in lambs of 4 weeks of age and older. It is administered by mouth as a single dose of 200 milligrams per kilogram body-weight repeated every 3 weeks during periods of risk. The minimum period between completion of treatment and slaughter for human consumption should be 7 days.

Preparations

BEPHENIUM DISPERSIBLE POWDER (*Syn.* Bephenium Hydroxynaphthoate Dispersible Powder): consisting of bephenium hydroxynaphthoate mixed with suitable non-toxic wetting and suspending agents. It contains 90% of bephenium hydroxynaphthoate.
A standard for this dispersible powder is given in the British Pharmacopoeia (Veterinary)
Containers and *Storage:* see the entry on Powders for general information on containers and storage.
Labelling: the label on the container should state the method of using the preparation.

BEPHENIUM GRANULES: consisting of bephenium hydroxynaphthoate with starch and other suitable pharmaceutical adjuvants. Available as sachets containing 5 g of granules equivalent to 2.5 g of bephenium.
A standard for these granules is given in the British Pharmaceutical Codex 1973
Storage: they should be stored in well-filled airtight containers, in a cool place.
Advice for patients: the granules should be taken mixed with milk or a sweet drink. They should be taken on an empty stomach and food withheld for 1 hour afterwards.

BEPHENIUM ORAL PASTE (*Syn.* Bephenium Hydroxynaphthoate Oral Paste): consisting of bephenium hydroxynaphthoate mixed with suitable edible diluents. Available as a paste containing 56% w/w of bephenium hydroxynaphthoate.
A standard for this oral paste is given in the British Pharmacopoeia (Veterinary)
Containers and *Labelling:* see the entry on Oral Pastes for general information on containers and labelling.

Beri-beri

Beri-beri is due to a deficiency of thiamine (vitamin B$_1$) in the diet. It occurs mainly in famine conditions and is sometimes precipitated by high carbohydrate intake following starvation. Early symptoms include anorexia, vomiting, and apathy. Enlargement of the heart gives rise to high output failure and severe oedema. Changes in the nervous system may occur giving rise to weakness, paraesthesiae, tenderness in the calf of the leg, paralysis of lower motor neurones, diminution of tendon reflexes, and encephalopathy.

Treatment is described under Thiamine Hydrochloride.

Betamethasone

9α - Fluoro - 11β,17α,21 - trihydroxy - 16β - methylpregna-1,4-diene-3,20-dione

$C_{22}H_{29}FO_5 = 392.5$

OTHER NAMES: Betameth.; Betamethasonum; *Betnelan®*; *Betsolan®*

A standard is given in the European Pharmacopoeia Vol. II

Description. A white to creamy-white odourless powder.

Solubility. Very slightly soluble in water; soluble, at 20°, in 75 parts of alcohol and in 1100 parts of chloroform.

Specific rotation. +114° to +122°, determined on a 0.5% solution in dioxan.

Preparation of solid dosage forms. In order to achieve a satisfactory rate of dissolution betamethasone in the form of an ultra-fine powder should be used.

Storage. It should be protected from light.

Identification. TESTS. 1. To a warm 1% solution in alcohol add an equal volume of *potassium cupri-tartrate solution*; a red precipitate is produced.
2. Heat 0.5 ml of *chromic-sulphuric acid mixture* in a small test-tube in a water-bath for 5 minutes; the solution wets the sides of the tube and there is no greasiness. Add about 2 mg of the sample and again heat in a water-bath for 5 minutes; the solution does not wet the sides of the tube and does not pour readily from the tube.

MELTING-POINT. About 240°, with decomposition.

ULTRAVIOLET ABSORPTION. In alcohol (95%), maximum at 240 nm (E1%, 1cm = 385).

INFRA-RED ABSORPTION. Major peaks at 1046, 1056, 1606, 1617, 1660, and 1710 cm^{-1} (see Appendix 2a: Infra-red Spectra).

THIN-LAYER CHROMATOGRAPHY. See under Thin-layer Chromatography, System 10.

Metabolism. ABSORPTION. Betamethasone and its phosphate ester are absorbed after oral administration but the valerate is not absorbed; after topical application small amounts of the valerate may be absorbed systemically during prolonged usage.

DISTRIBUTION. *Protein binding*, 60 to 65% bound to plasma proteins.

Actions and uses. Betamethasone has actions and uses similar to those of prednisolone and is effective in much lower dosage; 1 milligram of betamethasone is approximately equivalent in glucocorticoid activity to 5 milligrams of prednisolone.
It may be used in the treatment of all conditions for which cortisone acetate is indicated except adrenocortical deficiency states for which its lack of sodium retaining properties makes it less suitable than cortisone.
In rheumatoid arthritis, 0.5 to 2 milligrams daily may be given by mouth in divided doses, the dosage being modified according to the response; as Cushing's syndrome may occur after a few weeks at the full dosage level it is usual to give the lowest dose that controls symptoms adequately, preferably not more than 1 milligram daily. In disseminated disorders of connective tissue, such as polyarteritis nodosa and systemic lupus erythematosus, much larger doses are often necessary. In the treatment of asthma 1 to 5 milligrams may be given daily in divided doses.

Undesirable effects; Precautions and contra-indications. As for Cortisone Acetate.

Veterinary uses. Betamethasone is a glucocorticoid used to reduce pain, oedema, and self-inflicted injury associated with inflammation, especially of the skin, tendons, and joints. The usual dose for dogs and cats is 20 micrograms per kilogram body-weight in divided doses. Betamethasone is administered to cattle in doses of 20 to 30 milligrams by intramuscular injection to induce parturition.

Preparations

BETAMETHASONE TABLETS: available as tablets containing 250 and 500 micrograms of betamethasone.
A standard for these tablets is given in the British Pharmacopoeia 1973
Containers and *Storage:* see the entry on Tablets for general information on containers and storage. Containers should be airtight and light resistant.
Advice for patients: in long-term use, treatment should not be discontinued without the advice of the prescriber. Patients may carry an identification card giving details of their treatment and the name of the prescriber who should be contacted in the event of accident, feverish illness, diarrhoea, vomiting, or alimentary disturbances. In short-term treatment, the prescribed course should be completed.

OTHER PREPARATIONS available include a veterinary INJECTION containing betamethasone 2 mg per ml in 20- and 50-ml vials.

Betamethasone Sodium Phosphate

9α - Fluoro - 11β,17α,21 - trihydroxy - 16β - methylpregna-1,4-diene-3,20-dione 21-(disodium phosphate), the disodium salt of the 21-phosphate ester of betamethasone.

$C_{22}H_{28}FNa_2O_8P = 516.4$

OTHER NAMES: Betameth. Sod. Phos.; *Betnesol®*; *Betsolan®*
Betsovet® (with betamethasone 21-adamantoate)

A standard is given in the British Pharmacopoeia 1973

Description. A white hygroscopic odourless powder with a bitter taste.

Solubility. Soluble, at 20°, in 2 parts of water and in 350 parts of dehydrated alcohol; practically insoluble in chloroform.

Moisture content. Not more than 8%, determined by Fischer titration.

Specific rotation. +98° to +104°, determined on a 1% solution.

Stability. Aqueous solutions having a pH of about 8 are stable if protected from light. Particular care must be taken to prevent microbial contamination of the solutions so as to avoid hydrolysis of the ester by phosphatase which is a common product of microbial metabolism.

Sterilisation. Solutions are sterilised by filtration.

Storage. It should be stored in airtight containers, protected from light.

Identification. TESTS. 1. It complies with Test 2 described under Betamethasone.
2. Dissolve about 2 mg in 2 ml of sulphuric acid and allow to stand for 5 minutes; no red colour is produced (distinction from prednisolone sodium phosphate).

ULTRAVIOLET ABSORPTION. In water, maximum at 241 nm (E1%, 1cm = 297).

THIN-LAYER CHROMATOGRAPHY. See under Thin-layer Chromatography, System 10.

Metabolism. See under Betamethasone.

Actions and uses. Betamethasone sodium phosphate has the actions and uses described under Betamethasone; 1.3 grams of betamethasone sodium phosphate is equivalent to 1 gram of betamethasone. It is soluble in water, and is used as an anti-inflammatory agent in preparations for local application to the ear and eye.
The usual dose by mouth is the equivalent of 0.5 to 5 milligrams of betamethasone daily in divided doses.
It is also given in doses equivalent to up to 8 milligrams of betamethasone by intra-articular or intra-bursal injection in rheumatoid arthritis to relieve local pain and swelling in affected joints, and by intramuscular or intravenous injection for systemic effect, the usual dose being the equivalent of 4 to 20 milligrams of betamethasone.

Undesirable effects; Precautions and contra-indications. As for Cortisone Acetate.

Veterinary uses. Betamethasone sodium phosphate is a soluble glucocorticoid used to reduce allergic and inflammatory reactions. It is used in dermatitis, tendonitis, and arthritis.
The usual dose by intramuscular injection for all species is the equivalent of 20 to 50 micrograms of betamethasone per kilogram body-weight, and by intra-articular injection in horses the equivalent of 2 to 10 milligrams of betamethasone repeated at long intervals in accordance with the response of the animal.
Betamethasone sodium phosphate is also administered by intravenous injection in doses up to the equivalent of 20 micrograms of betamethasone per kilogram body-weight in shock, and by intramuscular injection in doses equivalent to 20 to 30 milligrams of betamethasone for the induction of parturition in cattle in the last 20 days of pregnancy. Betamethasone sodium phosphate is also applied topically as a cream containing 0.1% with neomycin sulphate 0.5% in dermatitis.

Preparations

BETAMETHASONE EYE-DROPS (*Syn.* Betamethasone Sodium Phosphate Eye-drops): consisting of a sterile solution containing betamethasone sodium phosphate, with a suitable preservative and stabilising agent, in purified water. It is prepared by method B described in the entry on Eye-drops. Available as eye-drops containing 0.1% of betamethasone sodium phosphate in 5- and 10-ml bottles.
A standard for these eye-drops is given in the British Pharmaceutical Codex 1973
Containers and *Labelling:* see the entry on Eye-drops for general information on containers and labelling.
Storage: it should be stored in a cool place, protected from light. It should not be allowed to freeze. The eye-drops should preferably be used within 4 weeks of first opening the container.
Advice for patients: see the entry on Eye-drops for general information on the use of eye-drops.

BETAMETHASONE SODIUM PHOSPHATE INJECTION: a sterile solution of betamethasone sodium phosphate, with suitable stabilising agents, in water for injections. It is sterilised by filtration. Available in 1-ml ampoules containing betamethasone sodium phosphate equivalent to 4 mg of betamethasone per ml and, for veterinary use, in 20- and 50-ml vials containing betamethasone sodium phosphate equivalent to 2 mg of betamethasone per ml.
A standard for this injection is given in the British Pharmacopoeia 1973
Containers: see the entry on Injections for general information on containers.
Labelling: see the entry on Injections for general information on labelling. In addition, the label on the container should state the amount of the medicament as the equivalent amount of betamethasone in a suitable dose-volume.
Storage: it should be stored at a temperature not exceeding 30°, protected from light. It should not be allowed to freeze.

BETAMETHASONE SODIUM PHOSPHATE TABLETS: available as tablets containing betamethasone sodium phosphate equivalent to 500 micrograms of betamethasone; they may be coloured.
A standard for these tablets is given in the British Pharmacopoeia 1973
Containers and *Storage:* see the entry on Tablets for general information on containers and storage. Containers should be airtight and light resistant. The tablets are hygroscopic and should not be handled. Discoloration and failure to produce a clear solution when dissolved in water indicate degradation.
Labelling: the label on the container should state the amount of the medicament as the equivalent amount of betamethasone.
Advice for patients: the tablets should preferably be dissolved in water. In long-term use, treatment should not be discontinued without the advice of the prescriber. Patients may carry an identification card giving details of their treatment and the name of the prescriber who should be contacted in the event of accident, feverish illness, diarrhoea, vomiting, or alimentary disturbances. In short-term treatment, the prescribed course should be completed.

OTHER PREPARATIONS available include a CREAM and a veterinary cream containing betamethasone sodium phosphate 0.1% with neomycin sulphate 0.5%; EYE-DROPS and veterinary eye-drops containing betamethasone sodium phosphate 0.1%, with neomycin sulphate 0.5%; an EYE OINTMENT containing betamethasone sodium phosphate 0.1%, an eye ointment containing betamethasone sodium phosphate 0.1% with neomycin sulphate 0.5%; and a veterinary INJECTION containing betamethasone sodium phosphate equivalent to 1 mg of betamethasone with betamethasone adamantoate 20 mg per ml in 5-ml vials.

Betamethasone Valerate

9α - Fluoro - 11β,17α,21 - trihydroxy - 16β - methylpregna-1,4-diene-3,20-dione 17-valerate.

$C_{27}H_{37}FO_6 = 476.6$

OTHER NAMES: Betameth. Valerate; *Betnovate*®; *Bextasol*®
Betnovate-A, *-C*, *-N*® (with chlortetracycline hydrochloride, clioquinol, and neomycin sulphate, respectively); *Vetsovate*® (with neomycin sulphate)

A standard is given in the British Pharmacopoeia 1973

Description. A white to creamy-white odourless powder.

Solubility. Very slightly soluble in water and in light petroleum; soluble, at 20°, in 12 parts of alcohol and in 2 parts of chloroform.

Specific rotation. +75° to +81°, determined in a 1% solution in dioxan.

Stability. Aqueous solutions have their maximum stability at pH 5.0. In neutral and alkaline solutions the substance is converted to betamethasone 21-valerate which has only about one-tenth of the clinical activity of the 17-valerate.

Incompatibility. It is inactivated by coal tar, salicylic acid, and many other substances.

Storage. It should be protected from light.

Identification. TESTS. 1. It complies with Test 2 described under Betamethasone.
2. Mix about 50 mg with 2 ml of 0.5N alcoholic potassium hydroxide, heat on a water-bath for 5 minutes, cool, add 2 ml of sulphuric acid (50% v/v), and boil gently for 1 minute; the odour of ethyl valerate is produced.

MELTING-POINT. About 190°, with decomposition.

ULTRAVIOLET ABSORPTION. In dehydrated alcohol, maximum at 240 nm (E1%, 1cm = 325).

INFRA-RED ABSORPTION. Major peaks at 1060, 1181, 1603, 1616, 1658, and 1731 cm^{-1} (see Appendix 2a: Infra-red Spectra).

THIN-LAYER CHROMATOGRAPHY. See under Thin-layer Chromatography, System 10.

Metabolism. See under Betamethasone.

Actions and uses. Betamethasone valerate is a corticosteroid for topical application and is applied as an ointment, cream, or lotion. The affected area of skin is treated once or twice daily. The anti-inflammatory effect is enhanced by covering with an occlusive dressing, but if large areas are treated in this way sufficient of the drug may be absorbed to give rise to systemic effects.
Betamethasone valerate is also used as an aerosol inhalation for the prophylaxis of asthma and seasonal rhinitis, up to 800 micrograms being administered daily in divided doses.
Betamethasone valerate is an ingredient of ointments and suppositories for the relief of pain and inflammation due to haemorrhoids.

Undesirable effects. Sensitisation occurs occasionally.

Precautions. It should not be used on infected skin without the simultaneous application of a suitable antibacterial agent.

Preparations

BETAMETHASONE AEROSOL INHALATION: a suspension of betamethasone valerate in a suitable mixture of aerosol propellents, which may contain a surface-active agent, stabilising agents, and other adjuvants. It is packed in a pressurised container fitted with a special metering valve and an oral adapter.
Available as an aerosol inhalation delivering 100 micrograms of betamethasone valerate to the patient each time the valve is actuated.
Containers, Labelling, and *Storage:* see the entry on Aerosol Inhalations for general information on containers, labelling, and storage.
Advice for patients: see the entry on Aerosol Inhalations for general information on the use of aerosol inhalations. The patient should be advised verbally to read the instructions on the leaflet enclosed with the product. When used in conjunction with salbutamol or another bronchodilator, the bronchodilator should be given first and betamethasone aerosol inhalation used 5 minutes later. When initiating treatment, there may be a time lag of up to 3 weeks before a full therapeutic response is obtained. Treatment should not be discontinued without the advice of the prescriber.

BETAMETHASONE VALERATE CREAM (*Syn.* Betamethasone Cream): a dispersion of betamethasone valerate in a suitable water-miscible basis containing a buffering agent and chlorocresol as the preservative.
When a strength less than that available from the manufacturer is prescribed, the stronger cream may be diluted, taking hygienic precautions, with cetomacrogol cream (formula A). The diluted cream must be freshly prepared. Diluents or medicaments which have an alkaline pH accelerate conversion of the active ingredient to the less active betamethasone 21-valerate. Coal tar preparations are examples of medicaments which are strongly alkaline and tar (that is, wood tar), which has an acid pH, is more suitable for mixing with betamethasone valerate cream.
Available as a cream containing betamethasone valerate equivalent to 0.1% of betamethasone.
A standard for this cream is given in the British Pharmaceutical Codex 1973
Containers, Labelling, and *Storage:* see the entry on Creams for general information on containers, labelling, and storage.
Advice for patients: the cream should be applied sparingly to the affected area.

BETAMETHASONE VALERATE LOTION (*Syn.* Betamethasone Lotion): a dispersion of betamethasone valerate in a suitable lotion basis. It may contain a preservative.
The lotion should neither be diluted nor mixed with any other preparation.
Available as a lotion containing betamethasone valerate equivalent to 0.1% of betamethasone.
A standard for this lotion is given in the British Pharmaceutical Codex 1973
Containers and *Labelling:* see the entry on Lotions for general information on containers and labelling.
The recommendation under Labelling concerning dilution of lotions does not apply to this preparation.
Storage: it should be stored in airtight containers at a temperature not exceeding 30°.

Advice for patients: the lotion should be applied sparingly to the affected area.

BETAMETHASONE VALERATE OINTMENT (*Syn.* Betamethasone Ointment): a dispersion of betamethasone valerate in a suitable anhydrous greasy basis.

When a strength less than that available from the manufacturer is prescribed, the stronger ointment may be diluted with white soft paraffin. Admixture with other materials may promote degradation of the active ingredient, especially if water is present.

Available as an ointment containing betamethasone valerate equivalent to 0.1% of betamethasone.

A standard for this ointment is given in the British Pharmaceutical Codex 1973

Containers and *Labelling:* see the entry on Ointments for general information on containers and labelling.

Advice for patients: the ointment should be applied sparingly to the affected area.

BETAMETHASONE VALERATE SCALP APPLICATION (*Syn.* Betamethasone Application; Betamethasone Scalp Application; Betamethasone Valerate Application): a solution of betamethasone valerate in aqueous isopropyl alcohol. It may contain a suitable thickening agent to render the preparation slightly viscous.

The application should neither be diluted nor mixed with any other preparation.

Available as a solution containing betamethasone valerate equivalent to 0.1% w/w of betamethasone.

A standard for this application is given in the British Pharmaceutical Codex 1973

Containers: see the entry on Applications for general information on containers.

Labelling: see the entry on Applications for general information on labelling. In addition, the container should be labelled "Caution. This preparation is inflammable. Keep away from a naked flame." A warning should be given to keep the preparation away from the eyes.

Storage: it should be stored in a cool place, protected from light.

Advice for patients: the preparation should be applied sparingly to the scalp.

BETAMETHASONE VALERATE WITH CHLORTETRACYCLINE OINTMENT (*Syn.* Betamethasone with Chlortetracycline Ointment): a dispersion of betamethasone valerate and chlortetracycline hydrochloride in a suitable anhydrous greasy basis. It contains betamethasone valerate equivalent to 0.1% of betamethasone and 3% of chlortetracycline hydrochloride.

When an ointment containing a lower proportion of betamethasone valerate and chlortetracycline hydrochloride than that available from the manufacturer is prescribed, the stronger ointment may be diluted with white soft paraffin. When an ointment containing a lower proportion of betamethasone valerate but the same proportion of chlortetracycline hydrochloride is prescribed, the ointment may be diluted with chlortetracycline ointment. Admixture of the ointment with other materials may promote degradation of the active ingredients, especially if water is present.

A standard for this ointment is given in the British Pharmaceutical Codex 1973

Containers and *Labelling:* see the entry on Ointments for general information on containers and labelling.

Advice for patients: it should be applied sparingly to the affected area. The ointment stains the skin, hair, and fabric; a dressing may be applied.

OTHER PREPARATIONS available include a CREAM and a veterinary cream containing betamethasone valerate equivalent to betamethasone 0.1% with clioquinol 3%, a cream containing betamethasone valerate equivalent to betamethasone 0.1% with neomycin sulphate 0.5%; a LOTION containing betamethasone valerate equivalent to betamethasone 0.1% with neomycin sulphate 0.5%; an OINTMENT containing betamethasone valerate equivalent to betamethasone 0.1% with clioquinol 3% and an ointment containing betamethasone valerate equivalent to betamethasone 0.1% with neomycin sulphate 0.5%.

Bethanidine Sulphate

1-Benzyl-2,3-dimethylguanidine sulphate

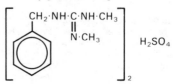

$C_{20}H_{32}N_6O_4S = 452.6$

OTHER NAME: *Esbatal*®

A standard is given in the British Pharmacopoeia 1973

Description. A white odourless powder with a bitter taste.

Solubility. Soluble, at 20°, in 1 part of water and in 30 parts of alcohol; practically insoluble in ether.

Moisture content. Not more than 1%, determined by drying at 105°.

Dissociation constant. pK_a about 12.

Identification. TESTS. 1. Dissolve about 25 mg in 5 ml of water, add 1.5 ml of *sodium hydroxide solution*, 1 ml of *1-naphthol solution*, and dropwise with shaking, 0.5 ml of *dilute sodium hypochlorite solution*; a deep violet colour is produced which darkens on standing.
2. Dissolve about 100 mg in 10 ml of water and add 20 ml of *trinitrophenol solution*; a precipitate is produced which, after washing with water, melts at about 148°.

MELTING-POINT. About 280°.

ULTRAVIOLET ABSORPTION. In water, maxima at 251 nm (E1%, 1cm = 7), 257 nm (E1%, 1cm = 9), and 263 nm (E1%, 1cm = 7).

INFRA-RED ABSORPTION. Major peaks at 701, 1111, 1174, 1192, 1483, and 1630 cm^{-1} (see Appendix 2a: Infra-red Spectra).

Determination in body fluids. ULTRAVIOLET SPECTROPHOTOMETRY. In urine—A. McCoubrey, *J. Pharm. Pharmac.*, 1962, **14**, 798.

SPECTROFLUORIMETRY. In plasma—C. N. Corder *et al.*, *J. pharm. Sci.*, 1975, **64**, 785.

Metabolism. ABSORPTION. Readily absorbed after oral administration.

BLOOD CONCENTRATION. After an oral dose of 10 mg of the hemisulphate, peak plasma concentrations of about 50 to 300 ng/ml are attained in 2 to 4 hours; after an intravenous dose of 25 mg of the hemisulphate, a plasma concentration of about 400 ng/ml is attained soon after dosing, which falls to about 100 ng/ml after 2 hours.

HALF-LIFE. Plasma half-life, 7 to 11 hours.

DISTRIBUTION. Volume of distribution, about 400 litres (determined in 1 subject only); *protein binding*, less than 8% bound to plasma albumin *in vitro*.

METABOLIC REACTIONS. No metabolites have been detected in man; in rats, the desmethyl, didesmethyl, and glucuronic acid-conjugate derivatives have been isolated, and in dogs, hippuric acid has also been found as a metabolite.

EXCRETION. After an intravenous dose about 90% is excreted unchanged in 3 to 4 days and after an oral dose 70 to 85% is excreted in the urine and 3 to 25% in the faeces.

FURTHER INFORMATION. Blood concentration and excretion—A. N. Chremos *et al.*, *J. pharm. Sci.*, 1976, **65**, 140; blood concentration—C. N. Corder *et al.*, *J. pharm. Sci.*, 1975, **64**, 785; pharmacokinetics and excretion—D. Shen *et al.*, *Clin. Pharmac. Ther.*, 1975, 17, 363.

Actions and uses. Bethanidine is a hypotensive agent which reduces blood pressure by selectively blocking transmission at the post-ganglionic adrenergic nerve endings. In tissue concentrations reached with oral therapeutic doses it prevents release of noradrenaline at the nerve ending without producing noradrenaline depletion, but in higher concentrations depletion may occur. Parenteral administration causes an initial increase in blood pressure, probably due to release of noradrenaline from adrenergic nerve endings.

Bethanidine is used to control hypertension. It causes a greater fall in blood pressure in the erect than in the supine position. The effect of a single oral dose reaches a maximum in 4 hours and is complete within 12 hours. Treatment is started with an oral dosage of 5 to 10 milligrams of bethanidine sulphate twice daily, increasing to 4 times daily and then by increments of 10 to 20 milligrams daily in divided doses until the optimum dosage is reached.

Up to 200 milligrams may be given daily in divided doses. After bethanidine is discontinued, pretreatment levels of blood pressure are reached in 24 hours. Tolerance to bethanidine may occur, making necessary a progressive increase in dose. A thiazide diuretic may be given with bethanidine to enhance the antihypertensive effect.

The antihypertensive effect of bethanidine is prevented or reversed by simultaneous treatment with antidepressant drugs of the imipramine and amitriptyline (tricyclic) type which block the neuronal uptake of bethanidine.

Bethanidine potentiates the pressor action of directly-acting sympathomimetic amines (see under Sympathomimetics).

Undesirable effects. Severe postural hypotension and interference with sexual function in the male may occur. Diarrhoea occurs more rarely than when similar drugs are used.

Precautions and contra-indications. Since bethanidine may enhance the effects of circulating catecholamines, it is contra-indicated in phaeochromocytoma. It should be used with caution in patients with renal failure.

Preparation

BETHANIDINE TABLETS: available as tablets containing 10 and 50 mg of bethanidine sulphate; they may be coloured.
A standard for these tablets is given in the British Pharmacopoeia 1973
Containers and *Storage:* see the entry on Tablets for general information on containers and storage. Containers should be airtight.
Advice for patients: the tablets should be taken at regular intervals preferably after meals. Treatment should not be discontinued without the advice of the prescriber.

Bilharziasis

see SCHISTOSOMIASIS

Bioavailability

The term "bioavailability" has been used to describe a number of concepts associated with the effect of administration of a drug preparation, including the extent of absorption of the drug into the blood stream, the availability of the drug at receptor sites, and the therapeutic effectiveness of the preparation. However, the term is used here to describe the biological availability of a drug from a preparation, this availability being quantified in terms of the amount and rate of appearance of the drug in an appropriate body fluid, such as blood, urine, or saliva, after the administration of the preparation. Such measurements may be used as a means of comparing the bioavailability of a drug in alternative formulations—*see* Assessment of Bioavailability, below. The therapeutic action of a drug is dependent on an adequate concentration of the drug reaching the site of action and this concentration is dependent on the passage of the drug across biological membranes. The rate and extent of absorption of a drug by the body is influenced by a number of biological and physiological factors (*see* the entry on Metabolism of Drugs), but it may also be affected by the rate at which the drug dissolves in the body fluid at or before the site of absorption. Frequently, this dissolution is the rate-limiting factor in the absorption process.

Effective dispersal of the drug particles in the body fluid and the solubility of the drug in that fluid may both affect the rate of dissolution and these factors, in turn, may be dependent on the physico-chemical characteristics of the drug itself and on other materials and manufacturing processes used in the preparation of the dosage form. Thus it is possible for an unsuitable formulation to interfere seriously with the effectiveness of the drug being administered.

Factors Affecting Absorption from Drug Preparations

Drug Characteristics

SOLUBILITY. The solubility of a drug substance in body fluids will depend on the nature of the substance, whether it is acidic, neutral, or basic, and on the pH conditions existing at the absorption site (*see* the entry on Metabolism of Drugs). The solubility of a drug substance may sometimes be modified for particular purposes by the formation of derivatives, such as esters, which break down to the drug substance before absorption.

PARTICLE SIZE. An increase in total surface area, brought about by decreasing the size of the particles of the drug, may increase the rate of dissolution and so increase the rate and amount of absorption. This is especially important for poorly soluble drugs and for certain preparations such as suspensions and aerosol inhalations. Powders having an exceptionally small particle size, however, may be difficult to wet, with a consequent reduction in the solution rate.

POLYMORPHISM. A chemical substance may exist in more than one crystalline form (polymorph), each of which may have a different rate of dissolution. In addition, there may be differences in solution rate between an amorphous and a crystalline form of a substance, the amorphous form often having the faster dissolution rate. Certain drugs, for instance novobiocin, are unstable in the amorphous form and revert to a crystalline form when suspended in an aqueous medium, with a consequent reduction in dissolution rate. Chloramphenicol palmitate, an ester which is used as a source of chloramphenicol in oral preparations, exists in three crystalline forms and one amorphous form. Only one of the polymorphs is hydrolysed rapidly in the gut with the formation of chloramphenicol; the remainder are inactive.

SOLVATION. If a drug exists in both a solvated and a non-solvated form, especially a hydrated and an anhydrous form, the different solvates may vary in solubility or in solution rate, and thus the absorption rates of the two forms may differ.

Formulation

Factors associated with formulation and processing which may affect the dispersion and rate of dissolution of the drug vary according to the type of preparation.

AEROSOL INHALATIONS. The active substance is usually dispersed or dissolved in the propellent system and the particle size of the drug and the size of the droplets produced by the spray mechanism are of particular importance in procuring efficient distribution of the drug in the respiratory tract. A proportion of the drug may be trapped in both the mouthpiece of the aerosol and in the mouth and upper airways of the patient and careful design of the valve and mouthpiece are essential.

CAPSULES. Release of the contents is effected by solution of the capsule shell in the gastro-intestinal fluid. The shell material must be easily soluble and must not interact with the drug. When the drug substance is incorporated in a solution or suspension, usually in a flexible capsule shell, there are unlikely to be problems with drug absorption. When the drug substance is present as a solid or a semi-solid, which may be a powder, granules, or a paste, usually in a hard capsule shell, the rate and degree of dispersion after release from the capsule shell, and hence the absorption of the drug, may be affected by the particle size and the degree of compaction. When adjuvants such as binders, diluents, lubricants, or surface-active agents are incorporated they must be carefully selected in order to ensure that there is no interaction with the drug or inhibition of absorption.

CREAMS AND OINTMENTS. The mechanism of absorption through the skin is not fully understood but the degree of skin penetration by a drug substance is determined primarily by the physico-chemical characteristics of the substance itself. The vehicle in which the substance is incorporated may either assist or impede the absorption process. In order to obtain the best skin penetration, the drug substance should be dissolved in a vehicle which favours its passage into the lipid phase and the study of the oil/water partition coefficient of the drug, or of derivatives of the drug, is of value when the formulation of topical preparations is under consideration. If the drug is poorly soluble and is suspended in the vehicle, then the particle size is especially important. For further information see the entry on Creams.

ENEMAS. These are either solutions or suspensions and hence usually provide good absorption characteristics for those drugs which are administered in this way. However, special formulation techniques are required in order to ensure that the preparation is retained for a sufficient length of time for absorption of the drug to take place.

EYE PREPARATIONS. Not all drugs which are applied to the eye are absorbed but where absorption does occur it may be affected by the pH of the vehicle and by the presence of additives such as thickening agents and surface-active agents. When the drug is incorporated in an ointment basis the hydrophilic or lipophilic character of the basis may affect absorption.

SOLUTIONS. Administration of a drug in solution is usually the best way to achieve rapid absorption. However, there may be practical limitations such as solubility, taste, stability, and convenience of administration.

SUPPOSITORIES. The partition coefficient of the drug in the selected basis should ensure that there is effective release of the drug into body fluids. Absorption may also be affected by other characteristics such as the melting-point of the basis and the viscosity of the melted basis and also the particle size of the drug and the manner in which it has been incorporated, that is, as a solution, an emulsion, or a suspension.

SUSPENSIONS. A suspension will usually provide more rapid dispersion and dissolution of the drug than either tablets or capsules, provided that the drug is in appropriate particle size, can be redispersed easily, and does not settle excessively or "cake" on storage. Growth of the primary particles due to the action of surfactants, emulsifiers, or other adjuvants which may have been used in the formulation may be a problem.

TABLETS. Because tablets are compressed, quick dispersion and dissolution of the drug are more difficult to achieve. Efficient disintegration is an important requirement but it does not necessarily ensure good dispersion and dissolution of the drug because the size and nature of the particles which are produced are also controlling factors. The most important factor is the rate of dissolution of the drug from the disintegrating particles and this may be affected by the granulation or other mixing procedure, the degree of compression, and the presence of fillers, binders, or surface-active agents.

The formulation of tablets may be varied in numerous ways in order to provide a rate of absorption appropriate to the particular drug, for example, rapid absorption, sustained absorption over a short period, prolonged absorption ("slow" tablets), or absorption in a specific part of the intestine (enteric-coated tablets). When tablets are coated, the thickness and nature of the coating may affect the absorption characteristics.

Assessment of Bioavailability

It is necessary to have some means whereby drug formulations can be assessed in terms of the extent to which they make the drug available to the body. Ideally, this assessment would involve measurement of the amount of drug available at the site of action at suitable periods of time after administration. In practice, this is not generally possible because either the precise site of action is not known or, in the few cases where it can be identified (for example, heart disease, bronchial asthma, and thyrotoxicosis), it is impracticable to determine the drug concentrations attained. However, it is possible to determine the concentrations of the drug in a selected body fluid over a period of time after administration of the preparation and hence obtain an indication of the amount and rate of absorption of the drug from the preparation. In the context of the determination of the concentration of a drug in body fluids, the word "drug" should be interpreted to include metabolites, where appropriate, for the particular drug substance and the analytical method being used.

These measurements form the basis of a test *in vivo* for the comparative bioavailability of alternative formulations of a drug. The body fluid used in such measurements is frequently blood, but may be some other fluid such as urine or saliva. The most commonly used method involves the construction of plasma concentration/time curves.

Plasma Concentration/Time Curves

Serial samples of plasma are withdrawn from the subject and are examined for drug content at specified periods of time after administration of the preparation. If the drug concentrations are plotted against time, a curve is obtained which usually shows a fairly steep rise to a peak concentration followed by a slow reduction in concentration over a longer period of time (FIG. 1).

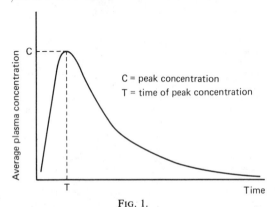

C = peak concentration
T = time of peak concentration

FIG. 1.

The shape of the curve is dependent on a number of factors. Elimination of the drug begins as soon as it appears in the blood and absorption, distribution, and elimination (metabolism and excretion) will all modify the shape of the curve.

There are three important parameters which can be derived from this curve, namely, the peak concentration, the time of the peak concentration, and the area under the curve.

PEAK CONCENTRATION. This represents the highest concentration of the drug achieved in the blood. It is reached when the rate of appearance of the drug in the blood no longer exceeds its rate of removal by distribution, metabolism, and excretion.

TIME OF PEAK CONCENTRATION. This is related to the rate of absorption and can be used to assess that rate.

AREA UNDER THE CURVE. This is related to the total amount of drug absorbed from the dose although, as noted above, the shape of the curve (and hence the area under it) will be modified by the kinetics of distribution, metabolism, and excretion.

The values obtained for these parameters may or may not be related to the therapeutic activity, and if there is a relationship it may not be linear. Nevertheless, the plasma concentration/time curve can be used as a basis for the comparison of alternative formulations.

Urinary Excretion

Measurement of the urinary excretion of a drug or of the drug and its metabolites can also be used in studies on comparative bioavailability. It has the advantage that samples are more easily obtained and it is less unpleasant for the subject than the method using blood samples. In addition, the concentration of the drug in the urine is usually greater than that in the blood and less sensitive analytical methods can often be used.

The measurement of urinary excretion is usually only applicable to those drugs of which a significant amount is excreted unchanged and can only be used as a routine method if it has been shown that, in the same subject, the urinary excretion of the drug is proportional to the plasma concentrations. Where the distribution and excretion is more complex, the information gained from urinary measurements can only be used as a supplement to that gained from blood measurements.

The important parameters in urinary measurements are the cumulative amount excreted and the rate at which this excretion takes place (FIG. 2). When measurements of urinary excretion of a drug are used, it may be necessary to control the pH of the urine for those drugs which are partially ionised at physiological pH values and where there is a significant difference in solubility between the ionised and the non-ionised form (see the section on renal excretion in the entry on Metabolism of Drugs).

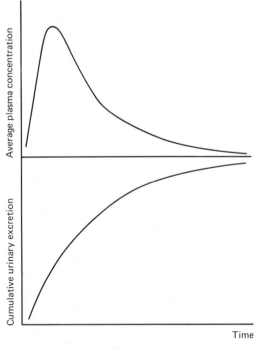

FIG. 2.

Salivary Excretion

During the processes of distribution and elimination, certain drugs are secreted in the saliva. It has been demonstrated for a number of drugs that the concentrations of drug in saliva samples over a period of time after administration follow a similar course to the plasma concentrations. The concentrations found in saliva often differ from those found in the blood but the concentration/time profiles have been shown to be directly related for some drugs and hence it may be possible to predict plasma concentrations from saliva concentrations.

The method has been used in comparative bioavailability studies and has the advantages that samples are more easily obtainable than with blood and results may be more useful than those obtained from urine studies because the pH of the saliva usually remains more constant than that of urine. A disadvantage of the method is that measurements of drug secreted in the saliva may be distorted by the retention of the drug in the mouth after oral administration.

Drugs which have been studied by this method include digoxin, isoniazid, lignocaine, lithium salts, mexiletine, phenazone, and salicylates.

Comparative Bioavailability and Bioequivalence

The measurement of plasma concentrations has been the most usual method used for comparative bioavailability studies. For the purpose of comparing formulations of a drug, plasma concentration/time curves are constructed for equivalent doses of the sample and for a standard preparation. The standard preparation may be one which is already recognised as being acceptable, as for instance an original product for which the therapeutic dose range is known and which has been used satisfactorily in clinical situations for some time, or the standard preparation can be an aqueous solution of the drug taken orally, or an intravenous injection where this is appropriate to the particular drug. These tests are carried out in normal healthy subjects and with randomised crossover designs to compensate for differences between test subjects.

If the plasma concentration/time curve of the test formulation is essentially the same as that of the standard, the two products are said to be " bioequivalent " and the clinical effect of the two products can be expected to be the same. However, if the curves are significantly different, a number of possibilities arise.

A significant difference in the plasma concentration/time curve of two products does not necessarily indicate that there will be a significant difference in therapeutic effect. The curves in FIG. 3 illustrate that if a drug is clinically effective over a wide range of concentrations and if the minimum toxic dose is well above the peak concentration, the fact that different formulations are not demonstrably bioequivalent may not be of importance. In this example the areas under the curves are similar, indicating similar total absorption, but the rate of absorption from Formulation X is much faster than that of Formulation Y and this may or may not be significant, depending on the particular drug and the use for which it is required. For instance, if a rapid response is desired, Formulation X would be chosen.

When there is a narrow range between the minimum therapeutic concentration and the minimum toxic concentration, especially when it is necessary for a patient to be standardised on an accurate dose regimen, the concept of bioequivalence is of fundamental importance. In FIG. 4, it can be seen that Formulation X is likely to produce toxic effects, whilst FIG. 5 shows the reverse situation where Formulation Y is likely to be ineffective due to poor absorption.

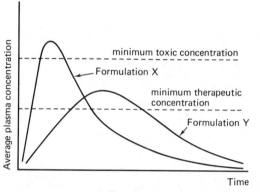

FIG. 4.

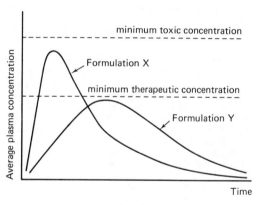

FIG. 5.

The availability of a drug from a formulation, when compared with a standard can be expressed as a percentage:

$$\frac{\text{area under curve for test formulation}}{\text{area under curve for standard}} \times 100$$

The figure obtained will have validity only if, for the drug being examined, the kinetics of absorption and distribution are not dependent on the dose.

The minimum effective concentration and the minimum toxic concentration for the drug will vary from person to person. The decision on what are acceptable values for total availability, and for the other parameters, is a matter of judgement based on a consideration of the absorption profiles obtained in the test and of the known clinical characteristics and therapeutic use of the drug being tested. When a new drug formulation is shown to provide a significantly greater availability than did a previous formulation, then it may be necessary to devise a new dose schedule.

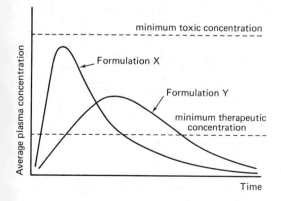

FIG. 3.

Dissolution Tests

The investigation of bioequivalence by means of determinations in biological fluids presents difficulties because it is time-consuming, it requires the use of human subjects, it is affected by a number of variables, and it cannot be applied for routine testing. It would be desirable to have a test *in vitro* for use in these studies but it would be necessary to show a correlation between the test *in vitro* and the test *in vivo*. Certain tests can be carried out on the materials used in manufacture in order to ensure that they have the correct physico-chemical characteristics such as particle size or polymorphic form, but no test *in vitro* has been devised which can predict with confidence the bioequivalence of drug preparations. However, a test which can be considered in this context is the dissolution test for tablets.

Tablets are normally subjected to the disintegration test which indicates the time taken for the tablet to break down into its constituent particles when subjected to conditions similar to those in the gut. The dissolution test shows the rate at which the drug passes into solution from the tablet, and this is an important factor in controlling the availability of the drug. Such a test can, under certain circumstances, provide a means of comparing a new formulation with one that is known to be therapeutically effective, but the test must be treated with caution because the results have not always been found to correlate with absorption *in vivo*. Where such correlation can be demonstrated, the test can be used as a screening test. The test can also be used to monitor commercial production of an established product.

Initiation of Bioequivalence Studies

Difficulties associated with the biological non-equivalence of multiple formulations of the same drug have been reported for only a small proportion of the drugs in general use. Evidence of the non-equivalence of two or more formulations has sometimes been obtained from observations of clinical failures or of toxic reactions. However, this is an unreliable method for the detection of such problems because changes in clinical effect after administration of alternative preparations may be due to other factors such as variations in patient response, changes in the disease process, or failure of the patient to carry out the instructions. In addition, the observation of clinical response is of limited sensitivity, except for a few drugs whose action can be determined easily and accurately by some measurable effect. For instance, blood-sugar concentrations can be determined as a means of measuring the effect of hypoglycaemic drugs, whereas there is no method for quantifying the effects of antidepressant drugs.

Bioequivalence studies may need to be initiated when (a) a number of different formulations are available from several manufacturers, (b) the therapeutic dose of the drug is close to its toxic dose, (c) the drug substance is relatively insoluble, or may become insoluble, in gastro-intestinal fluids, (d) the drug has been shown to be incompletely absorbed from the gastro-intestinal tract, and (e) reports have indicated the possibility of non-equivalence between formulations.

Studies of bioavailability will also be necessary for those drugs for which the kinetics of absorption, distribution, and elimination are dependent on the dose (for instance, phenytoin and salicylates) and also for those drugs for which the metabolism is dependent on the rate of absorption and which have therapeutically active or toxic metabolites.

Bioavailability must always be considered when new formulations or manufacturing techniques are under investigation.

Biperiden

1-(Bicyclo[2.2.1]hept-5-en-2-yl)-1-phenyl-3-piperid-inopropan-1-ol

$C_{21}H_{29}NO = 311.5$

OTHER NAME: *Akineton®*

A standard is given in the British Pharmacopoeia Addendum 1975

Description. A white crystalline odourless powder.

Solubility. Very slightly soluble in water; soluble, at 20°, in 75 parts of alcohol, in 14 parts of ether, and in 2 parts of chloroform.

Sterilisation. Solutions of the lactate salt are sterilised by heating in an autoclave or by filtration.

Storage. It should be protected from light.

Identification. TESTS. 1. Add about 50 mg to 5 ml of phosphoric acid and allow to stand; a green colour is produced.
2. Dissolve about 10 mg in a mixture of 5 ml of water and 2 ml of *dilute sulphuric acid* and then add 0.1N potassium permanganate dropwise; the colour of the permanganate is discharged.

MELTING-POINT. About 114°.

INFRA-RED ABSORPTION. Major peaks at 704, 735, 758, 1000, 1124, and 1149 cm^{-1} (see Appendix 2b: Infra-red Spectra).

Actions and uses. Biperiden antagonises some of the actions of acetylcholine in a manner similar to that described under Atropine and is used in the treatment of idiopathic, encephalitic, and arteriosclerotic types of parkinsonism or of extra-pyramidal disorders induced by treatment with drugs such as reserpine or the phenothiazines.

Biperiden hydrochloride is administered by mouth in a dosage of 1 to 6 milligrams daily in divided doses. Biperiden lactate is administered by intramuscular or slow intravenous injection to obtain rapid control in severe cases or when oral treatment has not been successful. It is used in the treatment of dystonic reactions which may include oculogyric and lingual crises. The usual dosage is 5 to 20 milligrams daily in divided doses. 1.1 grams of biperiden hydrochloride or 1.3 grams of biperiden lactate is equivalent to 1 gram of biperiden.

Undesirable effects. As for Benzhexol Hydrochloride.

Precautions and contra-indications. As for Atropine.

Preparations

BIPERIDEN LACTATE INJECTION (*Syn.* Biperiden Injection): a sterile solution of biperiden lactate, prepared by the interaction of biperiden with lactic acid, with a suitable buffering agent, in water for injections. It is sterilised by heating in an autoclave or by filtration. Available in 1-ml ampoules containing 5 mg of biperiden lactate.

A standard for this injection is given in the British Pharmacopoeia Addendum 1975

Containers and *Labelling:* see the entry on Injections for general information on containers and labelling.

Storage: it should be protected from light.

OTHER PREPARATIONS available include TABLETS containing biperiden hydrochloride 2 mg.

Bisacodyl

4,4'-(Pyrid-2-ylmethylene)bis(phenyl acetate)

$C_{22}H_{19}NO_4 = 361.4$

OTHER NAMES: *Dulcolax*®
Dulcodos® (with dioctyl sodium sulphosuccinate)

A standard is given in the British Pharmacopoeia 1973

CAUTION. *Inhalation of the powder and contact with the eyes, skin and mucous membranes should be avoided.*

Description. An odourless tasteless white crystalline powder.

Solubility. Very slightly soluble in water; soluble, at 20°, in 100 parts of alcohol, in 170 parts of ether, and in 35 parts of chloroform.

Stability. Degradation by hydrolysis may occur yielding the mono- and bis-hydroxy compounds. The rate of hydrolysis in solution is dependent upon pH and increases with rise in temperature. Under optimum moisture-free conditions in solid dosage forms, the rate of hydrolysis is negligible.

Storage. It should be stored in airtight containers, protected from light.

Identification. MELTING-POINT. About 134°.

ULTRAVIOLET ABSORPTION. In 0.1N sulphuric acid, maximum at 264 nm (E1%, 1cm = 266); in 0.1N methanolic potassium hydroxide, maximum at 248 nm (E1%, 1cm = 650).

Metabolism. ABSORPTION. Poorly absorbed after oral administration.

METABOLIC REACTIONS. Hydrolysis to form bis(4-hydroxyphenyl)pyrid-2-ylmethane and conjugation with glucuronic acid.

EXCRETION. Excreted in the bile and urine as the glucuronic acid conjugate of the hydrolysis product; most of the dose is recovered in the faeces as the unconjugated hydrolysis product.

FURTHER INFORMATION. Metabolism and excretion—R. Jauch *et al.*, *Arzneimittel-Forsch.*, 1975, **25**, 1796.

Actions and uses. Bisacodyl is a laxative used for the treatment of constipation, for evacuation of the colon before radiological examination of the abdomen, or endoscopy, and before or after surgical operations. It has little or no action on the small intestine.

Doses of 5 to 10 milligrams may be given by mouth and act within 6 to 12 hours. Suppositories of 10 milligrams given by rectum act within one hour. Children under 10 years may be given 5 milligrams by mouth or by rectum.

Undesirable effects. Occasionally severe abdominal cramps may occur. Suppositories sometimes cause local rectal irritation.

Preparations

BISACODYL SUPPOSITORIES: prepared as described in the entry on Suppositories by incorporating bisacodyl in a suitable basis. Available as suppositories containing 5 and 10 mg of bisacodyl.

A standard for these suppositories is given in the British Pharmacopoeia 1973

Containers and *Storage:* see the entry on Suppositories for general information on containers and storage.

Advice for patients: see the entry on Suppositories for general information on the use of suppositories. They should not be used for longer than a few days without medical advice.

BISACODYL TABLETS: available as tablets containing 5 mg of bisacodyl; they are enteric coated and sugar coated; the coat may be coloured.

A standard for these tablets is given in the British Pharmacopoeia 1973

Containers and *Storage:* see the entry on Tablets for general information on containers and storage. Containers should be airtight.

Advice for patients: the tablets should be taken after meals; they should be swallowed whole and milk or antacids should not be taken within 1 hour. They should not be used for longer than a few days without medical advice.

OTHER PREPARATIONS available include a SOLUTION, for rectal administration, containing bisacodyl 2.74 mg per ml with a suitable macrogol and buffering agents; and TABLETS containing bisacodyl 5 mg with dioctyl sodium sulphosuccinate 100 mg.

Bismuth Carbonate

A basic carbonate the composition of which varies with the conditions under which it is precipitated. It corresponds approximately to the formula $(BiO)_2CO_3,\frac{1}{2}H_2O$. The bulk density also varies considerably, depending upon the conditions of precipitation.

OTHER NAMES: Bism. Carb.; Bismuth Subcarbonate; Bismuthi Subcarbonas; *Lac Bismuth*®

A standard is given in the European Pharmacopoeia Vol. II

Description. An odourless tasteless white or creamy-white powder.

Solubility. Practically insoluble in water and in neutral organic solvents; completely soluble with effervescence in mineral acids.

Moisture content. Not more than 1%, determined by drying at 105°.

Storage. It should be protected from light.

Actions and uses. Bismuth carbonate is a very weak antacid which has been used in doses of 0.6 to 2 grams to treat dyspepsia. There is little justification for its use as it has only weak antacid properties.

Preparations

Preparations available include a MIXTURE containing bismuth carbonate 650 mg in 5 ml.

Bismuth Subgallate

OTHER NAMES: Basic Bismuth Gallate; Bism. Subgall.; Bismuth Oxygallate

A standard is given in the British Pharmaceutical Codex 1973

Description. An odourless tasteless citron-yellow powder.

Solubility. Practically insoluble in water, in alcohol, and in ether; readily soluble in hot mineral acids, with decomposition, and in solutions of alkali hydroxides, forming clear yellow solutions which rapidly become dark red.

Moisture content. Not more than 7%, determined by drying at 105°.

Incompatibility. It is incompatible with alkaline sulphur compounds and iron salts.

Storage. It should be stored in airtight containers, protected from light.

Actions and uses. Bismuth subgallate is used in the form of suppositories for the treatment of haemorrhoids and as an ingredient of dusting-powders.

Preparations

BISMUTH SUBGALLATE SUPPOSITORIES: prepared as described in the entry on Suppositories by incorporating bismuth subgallate in theobroma oil or other suitable basis. Approximately 3 g of bismuth subgallate displaces 1 g of theobroma oil.
A standard for these suppositories is given in the British Pharmaceutical Codex 1973
Containers and *Storage:* see the entry on Suppositories for general information on containers and storage.
Advice for patients: see the entry on Suppositories for general information on the use of suppositories. They should be used night and morning and after defaecation unless otherwise directed.

COMPOUND BISMUTH SUBGALLATE SUPPOSITORIES (*Syn.* Compound Bismuth and Resorcin Suppositories): for each suppository take:

Bismuth subgallate	200 mg
Resorcinol	60 mg
Zinc oxide	120 mg
Castor oil	60 mg
Theobroma oil, or other suitable basis	sufficient to fill a 1-g mould

Powder the bismuth subgallate and the resorcinol, mix with the zinc oxide and the castor oil, and make into a smooth paste with part of the melted basis; gradually incorporate the remainder of the melted basis and pour into the mould. The following quantities displace approximately 1 g of theobroma oil: bismuth subgallate 2.7 g; zinc oxide 4.7 g; castor oil 1 g; resorcinol 1.5 g.
A standard for these suppositories is given in the British Pharmaceutical Codex 1973
Containers and *Storage:* see the entry on Suppositories for general information on containers and storage.
Advice for patients: see the entry on Suppositories for

general information on the use of suppositories. They should be used night and morning and after defaecation unless otherwise directed.

Bismuth Subnitrate

A basic salt which corresponds approximately in composition to the formula $6Bi_2O_3,5N_2O_5,9H_2O$.

OTHER NAMES: Bism. Subnit.; Bismuth Oxynitrate *Forgastrin*® (with animal charcoal)

A standard is given in the British Pharmaceutical Codex 1973

Description. An odourless, tasteless, white, micro-crystalline powder.

Solubility. Practically insoluble in water and in alcohol; readily soluble in dilute nitric acid and in dilute hydrochloric acid.

Moisture content. Not more than 2%, determined by drying at 105°.

Incompatibility. It is incompatible with carbonates and bicarbonates, iodides, tannin, and sulphur.

Storage. It should be protected from light.

Actions and uses. Bismuth subnitrate has been used with iodoform in the preparation of an antiseptic paste. It has been given internally for the same purposes as bismuth carbonate but its continued use may cause methaemoglobinaemia.

Preparations

Preparations available include a veterinary POWDER containing bismuth subnitrate 2.5% with animal charcoal 27%.
Bismuth subnitrate is an ingredient of compound resorcinol ointment—see under Resorcinol.

Bites

see INSECT BITES AND STINGS

Black Currant

The fresh ripe fruits of *Ribes nigrum* L. (Fam. Grossulariaceae), together with their pedicels and rachides. The plant is cultivated in temperate regions, especially in Europe, Australia and Canada.

OTHER NAME: Ribes Nigrum

A standard is given in the British Pharmaceutical Codex 1973

Constituents. Black currant contains invert sugar (about 6 to 8%), citric, malic, and ascorbic acids (giving an acidity equivalent to about 3% of citric acid), pectin, and colouring matter. The ascorbic acid content of the fruit varies from 100 to 300 mg per 100 g.

Description. *Macroscopical characters:* berries globose, ranging in diameter from about 7 to 15 mm, occurring in pendulous racemes; epicarp shiny black externally, enclosing a yellowish-green translucent pulp containing numerous flattened ovoid seeds, about 2.5 mm long, 1.25 mm wide, and 1 mm thick; berry crowned with withered remains of 5-cleft calyx; pedicels thin, up to about 10 mm long, attached to a rachis of varying length.

It has a strong characteristic odour and a pleasantly acidic taste.

Microscopical characters: the diagnostic characters are: epicarp: *glands* yellow, disk-shaped, roughly circular or broadly elliptical, varying in diameter from about 140 to 240 μm, each consisting of a single layer of cells attached in the centre to the epicarp by means of a short multiseriate stalk.
Calyx: *trichomes* unicellular, blunt-ended, with thin, crooked walls, about 10 to 14 mm wide and averaging about 350 μm in length.
Seed: testa with *pigment layer* composed of small cells with horse-shoe-shaped wall thickenings as seen in cross section, each cell containing 1 or 2 prismatic *crystals* of calcium oxalate; *endosperm* cells with irregularly thickened walls.

Uses. Black currant is rich in ascorbic acid and is used in the form of a syrup as a dietary supplement, particularly for children. The syrup is also used as a flavouring agent in cough mixtures.

Preparation

BLACK CURRANT SYRUP (*Syn.* Syrupus Ribis Nigri): prepared from black currant or, alternatively, from the concentrated black currant juice of commerce.
To obtain the clarified juice, pulp a sufficient quantity of black currant, stir in sufficient pectinase of commerce to destroy the pectin, allow to stand for 24 hours, press, clarify the juice, and, if necessary, adjust the weight per ml at 20° to not less than 1.045 g by the addition of water.
To prepare the syrup add 700 g of sucrose to 560 ml of the clarified juice or to a suitable quantity of concentrated juice diluted with water to the same weight per ml at 20°, stir until dissolved, and add sufficient benzoic acid to produce a final content of not more than 800 parts per million, or sufficient sulphurous acid or sodium metabisulphite to produce a final content of not more than 350 parts per million w/w of sulphur dioxide.
A dye, or a mixture of dyes, may be added, provided that any dye used is of food grade of commerce and that its use for colouring food is permitted in the country concerned.
Black currant syrup contains in 10 ml about 7.5 mg of ascorbic acid.
A standard for this syrup is given in the British Pharmaceutical Codex 1973
Storage: it should be stored in well-filled airtight containers, in a cool place, protected from light.
Dose: 5 to 10 millilitres.

Black Disease Vaccine

see CLOSTRIDIUM OEDEMATIENS TYPE B VACCINE

Blackleg Vaccine

see CLOSTRIDIUM CHAUVOEI VACCINE

Blepharitis

Blepharitis is an inflammation of the eyelids in which there may be secondary infection with staphylococci; in the ulcerative form there is widespread staphylococcal infection of the eyelash follicles.
Treatment is similar to that for styes, together with improvement in hygiene where necessary to prevent reinfection.

Blood Corpuscles, Concentrated Human Red

Whole human blood from which part of the plasma and anticoagulant solution has been removed.

OTHER NAME: Concentrate of Human Red Blood Cells

The concentrate is usually prepared within 24 to 48 hours of the blood being collected, with equipment consisting of sterilised plastic containers linked by tubing so that the inner surface of the system is continuous and sterile. The containers and associated tubing are centrifuged or allowed to stand and a quantity of the supernatant liquid equivalent to not less than 40% of the volume of the whole human blood is removed from the sedimented red cells.
The concentrate may also be prepared, not more than 12 hours before use, from whole human blood, not more than 14 days old, collected in glass containers. After sedimentation the plasma is removed by siphoning through sterile tubing; aseptic precautions must be observed throughout the preparation.
It is a dark red fluid which may separate on standing into a sediment of red blood corpuscles and a supernatant layer of yellow plasma.
It has a haemoglobin concentration of not less than 15.5% w/v.

A standard is given in the British Pharmacopoeia 1973

Storage. It should be stored in sterile containers sealed to exclude micro-organisms at 4° to 6°. When prepared in plastic equipment it may be used up to 21 days from the date of collection of the blood. When prepared from blood collected in glass containers it should be used within 12 hours of its preparation.
It should not be used if there is any visible evidence of deterioration.

Actions and uses. Transfusions of concentrated human red blood corpuscles are given for the treatment of various forms of anaemia; the haemoglobin concentration of the blood of the average adult is raised by about 2 grams per 100 millilitres by the concentrated human red blood corpuscles obtained from 1080 millilitres of whole human blood.
The use of concentrated human red blood corpuscles carries a risk of transmitting hepatitis, as explained in the entry on Blood Products.

Blood Pressure

see HYPERTENSION, ARTERIAL

Blood Products

Preparations of human blood are available from commercial sources in some countries but they are not prepared commercially in the United Kingdom. In England and Wales, they are provided by the Department of Health and Social Security. Human immunoglobulin for the prevention of infectious diseases is available from the Public Health Laboratory Service, and for treating hypogammaglobulinaemia or immune deficiency states from the Division of Immunology, Clinical Research Centre, Harrow, Middlesex, or the Regional Immunology Laboratory, East Birmingham General Hospital, Bordesley, Birmingham. Human fibrin foam and human thrombin are available from the Blood Products Laboratory, Lister Institute of Preventive Medicine,

Elstree, and the other preparations are available from Regional Transfusion Centres.

In Scotland, preparations of human blood are available from the centres of the Scottish National Blood Transfusion Association, and in Northern Ireland through the Regional Transfusion Centre.

Post-transfusion hepatitis

Transfusion of blood containing hepatitis-B surface antigen is associated with the occurrence of hepatitis in recipients; hepatitis may however follow transfusion of blood in which the antigen cannot be detected by screening methods at present used. Thus the exclusion of donors whose blood contains the antigen diminishes but does not necessarily eliminate the risk of transmitting hepatitis. Forms of hepatitis other than hepatitis B may apparently also be transmitted by blood and blood products.

Whole human blood, concentrated red blood corpuscles, human antihaemophilic fraction, dried human fibrinogen, dried human fibrinogen for isotopic labelling, dried human plasma, dried human serum, and dried human thrombin therefore carry a risk of transmitting serum hepatitis.

Preparations of albumin that have been heated for 10 hours at 60° and preparations of immunoglobulin made by ethanol fractionation, do not transmit hepatitis.

Manipulation of blood products. All the apparatus and materials brought into contact with preparations of human blood should be free from pyrogens. Water for injections should be used to prepare all aqueous solutions and apparatus should be thoroughly rinsed with it before sterilisation. A suitable filter should be included in transfusion apparatus.

Blood preparations are described in the following entries:

Albumin Fraction (Saline), Human
Albumin Fraction (Saline), Human, Dried
Albumin, Human
Albumin, Human Dried
Antihaemophilic Fraction, Human, Dried
Blood, Whole Human
Blood Corpuscles, Concentrated Human Red
Factor IX Fraction, Dried Human
Fibrin Foam, Human
Fibrinogen, Dried Human
Fibrinogen, Dried Human, for Isotopic Labelling
Immunoglobulin Injection, Anti-D (Rh$_0$)
Immunoglobulin Injection, Human Normal
Immunoglobulin Injection, Human Rabies
Immunoglobulin Injection, Human Tetanus
Immunoglobulin Injection, Human Vaccinia
Plasma, Dried Human
Serum, Dried Human
Thrombin, Dried Human
See also Anticoagulant and Preservative Solutions for Blood.

Blood, Whole Human

Blood withdrawn from adult human beings and mixed with an anticoagulant solution.

OTHER NAMES: Human Blood; Sanguis Humanus

Blood donors must be healthy adults who are, as far as can be ascertained by a registered medical practitioner after inspection or simple clinical examination and consideration of their medical history, free from diseases transmissible by blood transfusion. The donor's blood must have been tested with negative results for evidence of syphilitic infection and presence of hepatitis-B surface antigen. The haemoglobin content of the blood must not be less than 12.5% w/v (female donors) or 13.2% w/v (male donors). Not more than 420 to 440 ml of blood is drawn on one occasion and a donor should preferably not be called upon to give blood more often than once in 6 months.

The blood is withdrawn aseptically through a closed system of sterile tubing which leads into the sterile final container in which the anticoagulant solution has been placed before sterilisation. During collection the container should be gently agitated to mix the blood and anticoagulant solution.

The blood remaining in the tubing after collection is used for grouping the blood and for the tests for freedom from syphilis and from hepatitis-B surface antigen; the ABO group is determined by examination of both cells and serum, and the Rh group by examination of the cells.

Immediately after collection, the container is sealed and cooled to 4° to 6° and thereafter is opened only for administering the blood; a separate sample of the blood mixed with anticoagulant should be provided for compatibility testing.

Anticoagulant solutions are described in the entry on Anticoagulant and Preservative Solutions for Blood.

Whole human blood prepared with a suitable solution may be used up to 21 days after collection.

Whole human blood is a dark red fluid which separates on standing into a sediment of red blood corpuscles and a yellow supernatant plasma free from visible products of haemolysis; the line of demarcation is sharp, but a continuous or interrupted greyish layer of leucocytes may form on the surface of the red blood corpuscles. The plasma may be clear, or turbid due to the presence of fat, which may form a white layer on the surface of the plasma.

It has a haemoglobin concentration of not less than 9.7% w/v.

A standard is given in the European Pharmacopoeia Vol. III

Storage. It should be stored, in sterile containers sealed to exclude micro-organisms, at 4° to 6° until needed for use, except during any periods necessary for its examination and transport at higher temperatures; such periods should not exceed 30 minutes, after which the blood should immediately be cooled again to 4° to 6°.

During storage, certain elements in the blood diminish in amount or disappear; leucocytes disintegrate in a few hours, most of the platelets and certain clotting factors, particularly factor VIII, disappear in a few days, and prothrombin and complement gradually decrease.

Stored whole human blood is a potentially dangerous fluid, the maintenance of the sterility of which depends entirely upon meticulous attention to cleanliness, faultless asepsis, and accurate and constant refrigeration from collection until use.

The fitness of whole human blood for transfusion can be judged only by its appearance. During storage, haemolysis of the red blood corpuscles occurs, and a red colour, which obscures the line of demarcation between the plasma and the sediment of corpuscles, may develop in the plasma immediately above the corpuscular layer. Whole human blood which shows these signs of haemolysis should not be used.

Haemolysis also results if blood is frozen or heated and if it becomes infected; infection usually causes rapid and total haemolysis, but certain Gram-negative organisms may flourish at 4° to 6° without causing any visible haemolysis.

Actions and uses. Whole human blood is used for transfusion, either to replace red blood corpuscles, clotting factors, or other normal constituents partly or completely missing from the patient's blood, or to restore blood volume.

The amount of whole human blood transfused and the rate at which it is given depend upon the patient's age and general condition, and on the state of his circulatory system, and upon the indication for transfusion. The haemoglobin concentration of the blood of the average adult is raised by about 1 gram per 100 millilitres by the transfusion of 540 millilitres of whole human blood.

Whole human blood should not be transfused, except in grave emergency, unless the ABO and Rh groups of the patient's and the donor's blood have been verified and a compatibility check made between the patient's serum and the donor's red cells.

The Rh group of a recipient should always be determined, as at least 50% of Rh-negative recipients may develop Rh antibodies if transfused with Rh-positive blood. A proportion of Rh-negative mothers may become immunised to the Rh factor during pregnancy by bearing Rh-positive foetuses which have inherited the Rh factor from their fathers.

Any of these immunised persons, if subsequently transfused with Rh-positive blood, may suffer a haemolytic reaction which may be fatal. Moreover, a transfusion of Rh-positive blood may sensitise an Rh-negative female, so that subsequent Rh-positive children may be affected with haemolytic disease of the newborn. Ideally all patients should be transfused with blood of homologous Rh group.

In grave emergencies, group O Rh-negative blood, plasma, human albumin fraction (saline), or plasma substitute, may be given while the patient's group is determined and a compatibility test is done; there are, however, few occasions on which there is not time to do these tests before transfusion.

The use of whole human blood carries a risk of transmitting hepatitis, as explained in the entry on Blood Products.

Bluetongue Vaccine, Living

A freeze-dried preparation containing a mixture of several antigenically distinct modified strains of bluetongue virus. It is reconstituted immediately before use with an appropriate volume of a suitable sterile liquid.

A standard is given in the British Pharmacopoeia (Veterinary)

Storage. The dried vaccine should be protected from light and stored at 2° to 8° when it may be expected to retain its potency for at least 12 months. It should be used immediately after reconstitution.

Veterinary uses. It is administered to sheep by subcutaneous injection for the prevention of bluetongue.

Boils

Boils or furuncles form a painful red swelling with a central pustule the slough or core of which separates before healing occurs. They arise from staphylococcal infection of the hair follicles.

Treatment consists in cleansing the skin with a suitable antiseptic and the application of an antibacterial cream preferably containing an antibiotic to which the infecting organism is sensitive. The external nares and perianal skin, which are possible reservoirs of infecting organisms, should also be treated. Boils may be dressed with magnesium sulphate paste for a limited period.

Furunculosis, or recurrent boils, may require systemic treatment with antibiotics.

Carbuncles are similar to boils but more extensive. They may be formed by the spread of perifollicular necrosis in the subcutaneous tissues or by the confluence of several infected follicles. Carbuncles suppurate to the skin and later separate as a slough.

Borax

$Na_2B_4O_7,10H_2O = 381.4$

OTHER NAMES: Sodium Borate; Sodium Tetraborate

A standard is given in the European Pharmacopoeia Vol. I

Description. Odourless colourless crystals or white powder, with a saline and alkaline taste.

Solubility. Soluble, at 20°, in 20 parts of water and in 1 part of glycerol; soluble in less than 1 part of boiling water; practically insoluble in alcohol.

Alkalinity. A 5% solution has a pH of 9 to 9.6.

Stability. It effloresces on exposure to air and on ignition it loses its water of crystallisation.

Incompatibility. It precipitates many alkaloids, including cocaine, from solutions of their salts. It is incompatible with mercuric chloride, zinc sulphate, and other metallic salts.

Sterilisation. Solutions are sterilised by heating in an autoclave or by filtration.

Storage. It should be stored in airtight containers, in a cool place.

Actions and uses. Borax has a feeble antibacterial action similar to that of boric acid. It has been used in a lotion in the treatment of inflammatory conditions of the eye, and in gargles and mouth-washes. Lozenges of borax have been used for their astringent action.

Undesirable effects. Excessive use of preparations containing borax may lead to toxic effects due to absorption, as described under Boric Acid, and they should therefore be used sparingly.

Poisoning. The procedure described under Boric Acid should be adopted.

Preparation

Borax is an ingredient of compound thymol glycerin.

Boric Acid

$H_3BO_3 = 61.83$

OTHER NAMES: Acidum Boricum; Boracic Acid

A standard is given in the European Pharmacopoeia Vol. I

Boric acid is a weak acid, and its alkali salts, which are hydrolysed, particularly in dilute solution, are alkaline. It volatilises in steam. When heated to 100°, it loses water and is slowly converted into metaboric acid, HBO_2; at 140° tetraboric acid, $H_2B_4O_7$, is formed and at higher temperatures, boron trioxide, B_2O_3.

Description. Odourless, white, unctuous, shining scales, crystals, or powder with a slightly acid and bitter taste and a sweetish after-taste.

Solubility. Soluble, at 20°, in 20 parts of water, in 16 parts of alcohol, and in 4 parts of glycerol; soluble in 3 parts of boiling water.

Acidity. A 3% solution has a pH of 3.8 to 4.8.

Dissociation constant. pK_a 9.2 (25°).

Sterilisation. Solutions are sterilised by heating in an autoclave or by filtration.

Metabolism. ABSORPTION. Absorbed after oral administration but does not readily penetrate intact skin, although it may be absorbed through denuded skin, serous or mucous membranes, or granulating tissue.

EXCRETION. About 50% of the amount absorbed is excreted in the urine in 12 hours, the remainder probably being excreted during the following 3 to 7 days.

Actions and uses. Boric acid has feeble antibacterial and antifungal properties. Aqueous solutions have been used as mouth-washes, eye lotions, and skin lotions, and as douches for irrigating the bladder and vagina and hot fomentations for ulcers, whitlows, boils, and carbuncles. Its value for these purposes is doubtful; there are more effective and safer antibacterial and antifungal agents.

Undesirable effects. Because boric acid is excreted very slowly, repeated doses, by whatever route they are given, have a cumulative effect. When ingested it causes gastro-intestinal irritation with loss of appetite and a toxic action on the kidneys.

Toxic effects may result from absorption and fatal cases of poisoning have been recorded in infants following the application of strong ointments of boric acid to extensive raw areas; deaths have also occurred from the absorption arising from the lavage of body cavities with solutions of boric acid.

Poisoning. If the boric acid has been ingested, gastric lavage or an emetic should be employed and a purgative dose of magnesium sulphate given. The patient should be kept warm and treated for shock. Convulsions may be controlled by diazepam.

Preparations

CHLORINATED LIME AND BORIC ACID SOLUTION (*Syn.* Eusol):

Chlorinated lime	..	..	..	..	12.5 g
Boric acid, in powder	..	..	..	12.5 g
Water for preparations	..	..	..	to 1000.0 ml

Reduce the chlorinated lime to fine powder, triturate it with sufficient of the water to form a paste, and add a further portion of the water; add the boric acid, shake well, add sufficient water to produce the required volume, allow to stand, and filter. It must be freshly prepared.

Alternatively, mix each ingredient with a separate portion of water and store in well-filled airtight containers; when required, mix together appropriate quantities of the two liquids, shake well, allow to stand, and filter if necessary.

The preparation may also be made from the mixed dry ingredients, known as "Eupad", a slight modification of the first method being used.

A standard for this solution is given in the British Pharmaceutical Codex 1973

Labelling: the label on the container should state the date after which the solution is not intended to be used.

Storage: it should be stored in well-filled airtight bottles, in a cool place, protected from light. It deteriorates on storage and should be used within 2 weeks of its preparation.

Advice for patients: for use as an antiseptic wound dressing and cleansing agent. It has a bleaching action and will destroy most dyes.

OTHER PREPARATION: boric acid is an ingredient of surgical chlorinated soda solution.

Botulinum Antitoxin

A preparation containing antitoxic globulins that have the specific power of neutralising the toxins formed by *Clostridium botulinum* type A, type B, or type E, or any mixture of types A, B, and E.

OTHER NAMES: Bot/Ser; Immunoserum Antibotulinicum

A standard is given in the European Pharmacopoeia Vol. II

When Mixed Botulinum Antitoxin is ordered or Botulinum Antitoxin is ordered the types to be present not being stated, antitoxin prepared from types A, B, and E is supplied.

Storage. It should be stored as described under Antisera.

Actions and uses. Botulism is a condition of acute toxaemia characterised by paralysis of muscles caused by toxin present in infected food at the time it is consumed. Botulinum toxin is an extremely powerful poison acting peripherally by interfering with the release of acetylcholine at the neuromuscular junction. The earliest symptoms of its action are blurred or double vision, giddiness, ptosis, vomiting, diarrhoea, and difficulty in swallowing and speaking.

Botulinum antitoxin has been successfully used in the treatment of intoxication due to type E, the antitoxin neutralising circulating toxin. Similar considerations apply to intoxications with type B but treatment with antitoxin is probably less effective against the more powerful and rapidly acting type A toxin. However, since no alternative treatment is known, it is advisable to give the antitoxin.

Antitoxin should be given as early as possible in the course of the disease, but since type B and type E toxins may persist for some time in the circulation, late administration may be of some help. The usual dose is not less than 50 000 units each of type A and type B and not less than 5000 units of type E by intramuscular or intravenous injection. Since the type of toxin is seldom known, the polyvalent antitoxin is usually given.

In cases of suspected infection, prophylactic doses of not less than 10 000 units each of type A and type B and not less than 1000 units of type E may be given by subcutaneous or intramuscular injection.

Serum reactions. See under Antisera.

Botulinum Vaccine

see CLOSTRIDIUM BOTULINUM VACCINE

Bradycardia

see under CARDIAC ARRHYTHMIAS

Braxy Vaccine

see CLOSTRIDIUM SEPTICUM VACCINE

Bretylium Tosylate

2-Bromobenzyl-*N*-ethyldimethylammonium toluene-4-sulphonate

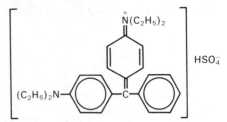

$C_{18}H_{24}BrNO_3S = 414.4$

OTHER NAME: *Bretylate®*

Description. A white crystalline powder.

Solubility. Soluble in 1 part of water and in less than 1 part of alcohol; practically insoluble in ether.

Identification. MELTING-POINT. About 85°.

INFRA-RED ABSORPTION. Major peaks at 680, 820, 1010, 1031, 1124, and 1190 cm^{-1} (see Appendix 2b: Infra-red Spectra).

Determination in body fluids. ULTRAVIOLET SPECTRO-PHOTOMETRY. In blood or urine—C. D. Johnson and J. P. Revill, *Acta pharmac. tox.*, 1965, **22**, 112.

Metabolism. ABSORPTION. Incompletely and irregularly absorbed after oral administration; the extent of absorption is increased after fasting.

BLOOD CONCENTRATION. After an intramuscular dose of 300 mg, the plasma concentration declines from about 1.3 μg/ml after 30 minutes to 0.6 μg/ml after 16 hours.

HALF-LIFE. The decline in plasma concentration after an intramuscular dose is multiphasic.

METABOLIC REACTIONS. Bretylium tosylate does not appear to be metabolised in the body.

EXCRETION. Up to 75% of a dose is excreted in the urine as bretylium in 24 hours and about 85% in 96 hours; the proportion of the dose excreted is dose-dependent, about 10% of a 5-g dose being excreted in 24 hours and 30% of a 200-mg dose being excreted in the same period; urinary excretion is delayed by renal function impairment.

FURTHER INFORMATION. Disposition of bretylium in man and rat—R. Kuntzman *et al.*, *Clin. Pharmac. Ther.*, 1970, **11**, 829.

Actions and uses. Bretylium tosylate has adrenergic neurone blocking actions and is used in the treatment of ventricular dysrhythmias. Since the effect of bretylium does not become apparent until up to 2 hours after administration it is usual to employ anti-dysrhythmic drugs such as lignocaine, procainamide, or quinidine, and to resort to bretylium when other drugs are not effective or if dysrhythmias recur, when bretylium may restore the sinus rhythm.

The usual dose of bretylium tosylate given by intramuscular injection is 5 milligrams per kilogram body-weight which may be repeated at intervals of 6 to 8 hours.

Bretylium tosylate has been administered by mouth for the treatment of hypertension but absorption from the gastro-intestinal tract is incomplete and unreliable and it is no longer used for this purpose.

Precautions. Bretylium should be used only where adequate facilities for monitoring its effects on the heart are available. Since it causes a reduction in blood pressure, patients should remain recumbent during treatment. The use of pressor amines in conjunction with bretylium is not recommended.

Poisoning. Overdosage with bretylium should be treated by supportive measures and careful administration of noradrenaline or phenylephrine.

Preparations

Preparations available include an INJECTION containing bretylium tosylate 50 mg per ml in 2-ml ampoules.

Brilliant Green

Diethyl 4-(4-diethylaminobenzhydrylidene)cyclohexa-2,5-dien-1-ylideneammonium hydrogen sulphate (Colour Index No. 42040)

$C_{27}H_{34}N_2O_4S = 482.6$

OTHER NAME: Viride Nitens

A standard is given in the British Pharmacopoeia 1973

Description. Small glistening golden crystals.

Solubility. Soluble, at 20°, in 5 parts of water and in 12 parts of alcohol.

Dissociation constant. pK$_a$ 7.9 (25°).

Incompatibility. It is incompatible with anionic, oxidising, and reducing substances.

Identification. TESTS. 1. To 10 ml of a 0.05% solution add a few drops of hydrochloric acid; the green colour changes to reddish-yellow.
2. To 10 ml of a 0.05% solution add 1 ml of hydrochloric acid and a few drops of *sodium hydroxide solution*; a pale green precipitate is produced.
3. To 10 ml of a 0.05% solution add 200 mg of zinc powder and warm; the solution becomes colourless and the colour is not restored immediately on exposure to air.

Actions and uses. Brilliant green is an antiseptic which is used in the treatment of infected wounds and burns. It is applied as a 0.05 to 0.1% solution in water or hypertonic saline. A solution containing 0.5% each of brilliant green and crystal violet has been used for disinfecting the skin.

A paint containing 0.5% each of brilliant green and mercuric chloride in industrial methylated spirit is used for the treatment of paronychia.

Preparation

BRILLIANT GREEN AND CRYSTAL VIOLET PAINT (*Syn.* Liquor Tinctorium; Pigmentum Caeruleum; Pigmentum Tinctorium; Solution of Brilliant Green and Crystal Violet):

Brilliant green	..	..	..	..	..	.. 5 g
Crystal violet	..	..	..	..	..	.. 5 g
Alcohol (90%)	..	..	..	..	..	500 ml
Water for preparations	..		..	..	..	to 1000 ml

Dissolve the brilliant green and the crystal violet in the alcohol and add sufficient water to produce the required volume.

In making this preparation the alcohol (90%) may be replaced by industrial methylated spirit diluted so as to be of equivalent alcoholic strength, provided that the law and the statutory regulations governing the use of industrial methylated spirit are observed.

A standard for this paint is given in the British Pharmaceutical Codex 1973

Containers, Labelling, and *Storage:* see the entry on Paints for general information on containers, labelling, and storage.

Advice for patients: the paint should be applied undiluted to the affected area. It stains the hair, skin, and fabric.

Bromhexine Hydrochloride

2-Amino-3,5-dibromobenzyl(cyclohexyl)methylammonium chloride

$C_{14}H_{21}Br_2ClN_2 = 412.6$

OTHER NAMES: *Bisolvon®*; *Broncholin®*
Alupent Expectorant® (with orciprenaline sulphate); *Bisolvomycin®* (with oxytetracycline hydrochloride)

Description. A white crystalline powder.

Solubility. Soluble in 250 parts of water; soluble in hot alcohol and in glacial acetic acid; practically insoluble in chloroform.

Incompatibility. It is incompatible with solutions of sodium chloride.

Identification. MELTING-POINT. About 235°.

Metabolism. ABSORPTION. Well absorbed after oral administration.

BLOOD CONCENTRATION. Peak plasma concentrations are attained within about 1 hour.

DISTRIBUTION. Rapidly distributed.

METABOLIC REACTIONS. Sulphate and glucuronic acid conjugation; other routes are not yet elucidated.

EXCRETION. After an oral dose, about 70% is excreted in the urine in 24 hours and, in 5 days, about 90% is excreted in urine and 4% in the faeces. After an intravenous dose, about 50% is excreted in urine in 24 hours and, in 5 days, about 80% is excreted in urine and 5% in faeces.

FURTHER INFORMATION. Absorption, distribution, and excretion—R. Jauch and R. Hankwitz, *Arzneimittel-Forsch.*, 1975, **25**, 1954.

Actions and uses. Bromhexine hydrochloride is a mucolytic agent which changes the structure of bronchial secretions by rarefication and fragmentation of the mucopolysaccharide fibres, leading to a reduction in the viscosity of the sputum.

It is used in the treatment of conditions of the respiratory tract associated with retention of mucoid secretions, such as bronchitis and asthma.

The usual dose by mouth for adults is 8 to 16 milligrams 4 times daily, for children under 1 year 2 milligrams twice daily, 1 to 5 years 4 milligrams twice daily, and 6 to 12 years 4 milligrams 4 times daily. The dose by slow intravenous injection, intravenous infusion, or intramuscular injection for children and adults over 12 years is 16 to 48 milligrams daily.

Undesirable effects. Bromhexine may give rise to gastro-intestinal disturbances and increased serum transaminase levels.

Precautions. It should be administered with caution to patients with gastric ulceration.

Preparations

Preparations available include CAPSULES containing bromhexine hydrochloride 8 mg with oxytetracycline hydrochloride 250 mg; an ELIXIR containing bromhexine hydrochloride 4 mg with chloroform 17.5 mg in 5 ml, diluent water or sorbitol solution, shelf-life of diluted elixir 14 days; an INJECTION containing bromhexine hydrochloride 2 mg per ml in 2-ml ampoules; a veterinary injection containing bromhexine hydrochloride 3 mg per ml in 50-ml bottles; a MIXTURE containing bromhexine hydrochloride 4 mg with orciprenaline sulphate 10 mg in 5 ml, diluent sorbitol solution or syrup, life of diluted mixture 14 days; a veterinary POWDER containing bromhexine hydrochloride approximately 1%; and TABLETS containing bromhexine hydrochloride 8 mg.

Bromocriptine

see under HYPOTHALAMIC RELEASING FACTORS

Bronchitis

Bronchitis, or inflammation of the trachea and bronchi, is characterised by an initially unproductive cough with a feeling of tightness in the chest and sometimes wheezing respiration.

Acute bronchitis is caused by infection with pyogenic organisms such as *Streptococcus pneumoniae*, often precipitated by infection such as a cold, influenza, measles, or whooping cough.

Chronic bronchitis usually develops as a result of long-term irritation of the bronchial mucosa by dust, tobacco smoke, and other irritants. This disorder usually originates in later adult life and is aggravated by damp, fog, and changes in temperature.

Infections with *Haemophilus influenzae* or *Str. pneumoniae* are common in chronic bronchitis and should be treated with appropriate antibacterial agents and, if necessary, occupation or environment should be changed to avoid contact with irritants.

Brucella Abortus (Strain 19) Vaccine, Living

A fluid or freeze-dried preparation of a culture of a strain of *Brucella abortus* of low virulence known as United States Department of Agriculture Strain 19. The freeze-dried preparation is reconstituted immediately before use with an appropriate volume of a suitable sterile liquid.

OTHER NAME: Contagious Abortion (Strain 19) Vaccine, Living

A standard is given in the British Pharmacopoeia (Veterinary)

Storage. The freeze-dried vaccine and the fluid vaccine should be protected from light and stored at 2° to 8°; the fluid vaccine should not be allowed to freeze. The freeze-dried vaccine may be expected to retain its potency for at least 2 years and the fluid vaccine for at least 3 months. The dried vaccine should be used immediately after reconstitution.

Veterinary uses. It is administered by subcutaneous injection to female cattle for prophylaxis of infection by *Brucella abortus*. In the United Kingdom, usage is restricted to the vaccination of female calves from the 91st to the 180th day of life.

Brucella Abortus (Strain 45/20) Vaccine, Inactivated

A water-in-oil emulsion of a culture of *Brucella abortus* derived from strain 45/20 (McEwen), inactivated in such a manner that immunogenic activity is retained.

A standard is given in the British Pharmacopoeia (Veterinary)

Storage. The vaccine should be protected from light and stored at 2° to 8° when it may be expected to retain its potency for at least 2 years. It should not be allowed to freeze.

Veterinary uses. It is administered by subcutaneous or intramuscular injection to female cattle for the prophylaxis or treatment of infection by *Brucella abortus*. It may be used in the United Kingdom only under licence in eradication areas; in non-eradication areas the vaccine may be used privately by the owner whose herd is not participating in an official brucellosis scheme.

Brucellosis

Brucellosis (Undulant fever; Bang's disease; Malta fever) is an infectious disease caused by organisms of the genus *Brucella*. It is a disease of animals but may infect man by direct contact with secretions, excretions, or meat or by the consumption of untreated milk or milk products from infected animals. *Br. abortus* is acquired from cattle, *Br. suis* from pigs, and *Br. melitensis* from goats.

The inoculation period is usually about 2 weeks, although it may be up to several months. Onset of the disease is gradual with mild fever, malaise, headache, generalised muscle pains, and mild gastro-intestinal disturbances. Brucellosis then follows a chronic course with exacerbations interspersed by relatively asymptomatic intermissions.

Exacerbations are characterised by the sudden onset of pyrexia, sometimes with rigor, and with an increased severity of symptoms. There may also be insomnia, depression, and considerable debility. Brucellosis may give rise to granulomatous nodules in the bone marrow, spleen, liver, kidneys, and other organs. The liver and spleen become enlarged and tender and may be palpable once the disease is established.

Brucellosis may be treated with tetracyclines or alternatively streptomycin or sulphadiazine. These anti-microbials may be used alone or, more commonly, combination therapy is used. Prolonged treatment may be required to eliminate the disease. In the severely ill patient corticosteroids may be required during the first few days of antibiotic treatment to prevent excessive immunological reactions due to the large amounts of antigenic material that may be released.

Bumetanide

3-Butylamino-4-phenoxy-5-sulphamoylbenzoic acid

$C_{17}H_{20}N_2O_5S = 364.4$

OTHER NAME: *Burinex®*
Burinex-K® (with potassium chloride)

Description. An odourless white crystalline powder with a slightly bitter taste.

Identification. MELTING-POINT. About 230°.

INFRA-RED ABSORPTION. Major peaks at 1149, 1205, 1220, 1333, 1587, and 1695 cm⁻¹ (see Appendix 2b: Infra-red Spectra).

Determination in body fluids. GAS CHROMATOGRAPHY. In serum or urine—D. L. Davies *et al.*, *Clin. Pharmac. Ther.*, 1974, **15**, 141.

Metabolism. ABSORPTION. Rapidly absorbed after oral administration.

BLOOD CONCENTRATION. After an oral dose of 1 mg, peak serum concentrations of about 40 ng/ml are achieved in 30 minutes.

DISTRIBUTION. Apparent volume of distribution 12 litres. *Protein binding*, 95 to 97% bound to plasma proteins.

EXCRETION. About 35% of an oral dose of 1 mg is excreted unchanged in the urine in 6 hours.

FURTHER INFORMATION. Renal action, therapeutic use, and pharmacokinetics—D. L. Davies *et al.*, *Clin. Pharmac. Ther.*, 1974, **15**, 141.

Actions and uses. Bumetanide is a diuretic with actions and uses similar to those of frusemide but has a slightly more rapid onset of action after oral administration. Diuresis begins within 30 minutes and the maximum effect is obtained within 1 to 2 hours. After intravenous injection diuresis occurs within a few minutes and is complete after about 2 hours. Bumetanide may sometimes be effective when tolerance to frusemide has developed.

The usual daily dose by mouth is 1 to 2 milligrams in single or divided doses. In refractory cases the dose may, in exceptional circumstances, be increased to 40 milligrams daily but careful biochemical control is necessary.

Bumetanide may be given by intramuscular or intravenous injection of a solution of the sodium derivative usually in doses of 0.5 to 1 milligram when a rapid response is required in cardiac or pulmonary oedema. It may also be given by infusion in dextrose injection (5%), sodium chloride injection, or sodium chloride and dextrose injection in a dose of 2 to 5 milligrams in

500 millilitres of infusion fluid over a period of 30 to 60 minutes.

Undesirable effects. As for Frusemide. In addition it may cause gastro-intestinal disturbances, rashes, and muscle cramps.

Precautions; Contra-indications. As for Frusemide.

Preparations

Preparations available include an INJECTION containing bumetanide 250 micrograms per ml in 4- and 25-ml ampoules; TABLETS containing bumetanide 1 and 5 mg, and tablets containing bumetanide 500 micrograms with potassium chloride 573 mg (K$^+$ 7.7 mmol) in a slow-release formulation.

Bunamidine Hydrochloride

NN-Dibutyl-4-hexyloxy-1-naphthamidine hydrochloride

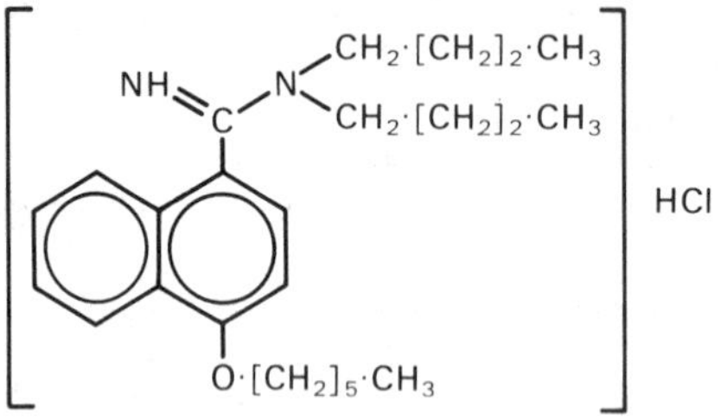

$C_{25}H_{39}ClN_2O = 419.1$

OTHER NAME: *Scolaban*®

A standard is given in the British Pharmacopoeia (Veterinary)

CAUTION. *Bunamidine hydrochloride is irritant, especially to the eyes, and should be handled cautiously. It is administered in coated tablets which should not be broken.*

Description. A white crystalline almost odourless powder.

Solubility. Soluble, at 20°, in 200 parts of water, in 2 parts of alcohol, and in 2 parts of chloroform; practically insoluble in ether.

Moisture content. Not more than 1%, determined by drying at 105°.

Identification. ULTRAVIOLET ABSORPTION. In 0.1N hydrochloric acid, maximum at 298 nm (E1%, 1cm = 220).

Veterinary uses. Bunamidine hydrochloride is used to eliminate tapeworms (*Taenia, Dipylidium,* and *Echinococcus* species) in dogs and cats.
The usual dose is the equivalent of 20 to 50 milligrams of bunamidine per kilogram body-weight as a single dose. Care should be taken in assessing dosage in animals under 2 kilograms body-weight.
Unweaned puppies and kittens should not be treated

Preparation

BUNAMIDINE TABLETS (*Syn.* Bunamidine Hydrochloride Tablets): available as tablets containing bunamidine hydrochloride equivalent to 100 and 200 mg of bunamidine; they are compression coated.
A standard for these tablets is given in the British Pharmacopoeia (Veterinary)
Containers and *Storage:* see the entry on Tablets for

general information on containers and storage. Containers should be airtight.
Labelling: the label on the container should state the amount of the medicament as the equivalent amount of bunamidine. In addition, the label should state that the tablets should be administered whole, and not broken, crushed, mixed with food, or dissolved in liquid, and that care should be taken to avoid transferring particles of the tablets to the eye.

Bupivacaine Hydrochloride

(±) - 1 - Butyl - *N* - 2,6 - xylylpiperidine - 2 - carboxamide hydrochloride monohydrate

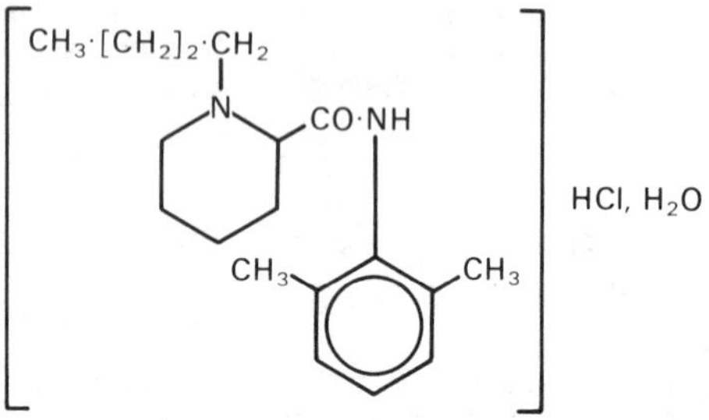

$C_{18}H_{29}ClN_2O,H_2O = 342.9$

OTHER NAME: *Marcain*®

A standard is given in the British Pharmacopoeia 1973

Description. A white crystalline odourless powder with a bitter taste.

Solubility. Soluble, at 20°, in 25 parts of water and in 8 parts of alcohol; very slightly soluble in ether and in chloroform.

Moisture content. 4.5 to 6%, determined by drying at 105°.

Acidity. A 1% solution has a pH of 4.5 to 6.

Sterilisation. Solutions are sterilised by heating in an autoclave or by filtration.

Storage. It should be stored in airtight containers.

Identification. TEST. Dissolve about 150 mg in 10 ml of water and add 15 ml of *trinitrophenol solution*; a precipitate is produced which, after rapidly washing with a little water followed by successive 2-ml portions of methanol and finally with ether, melts at about 194°.

MELTING-POINT. About 250°.

ULTRAVIOLET ABSORPTION. In 0.01N hydrochloric acid, maxima at 263 nm (E1%, 1cm = 14), and at 271 nm (E1%, 1cm = 11).

INFRA-RED ABSORPTION. Major peaks at 1282, 1389, 1429, 1471, 1515, and 1667 cm^{-1} (see Appendix 2b: Infra-red Spectra).

Determination in body fluids. GAS CHROMATOGRAPHY. In blood or plasma—G. T. Tucker, *Anesthesiology,* 1970, **32,** 255; in blood—A. Berlin *et al., J. Pharm. Pharmac.,* 1973, **25,** 466.

Metabolism. BLOOD CONCENTRATION. After an intravenous dose of 50 mg, plasma concentrations of 1.2 μg/ml are obtained after 10 minutes, dropping to 0.1 μg/ml after 2 hours; after a peridural dose of 150 to 225 mg, peak plasma concentrations of 1 to 2.3 μg/ml are attained within 20 minutes and cerebrospinal fluid concentrations of 30 μg/ml are obtained within 30 minutes.

HALF-LIFE. The decline in plasma concentration is biphasic, the half-life of the initial phase being 7 minutes and the half-life of the second about 75 minutes; other reports give a half-life for the second phase of 2 to 2.5 hours.

DISTRIBUTION. The distribution of bupivacaine fits a 2-compartment open model; volume of distribution, about 34 litres; bupivacaine crosses the placenta and enters the cerebrospinal fluid; *protein binding*, 80 to 90% bound to plasma proteins of which 30 to 35% is bound to plasma albumin.

EXCRETION. Less than 10% of a dose is excreted in the urine unchanged; urinary excretion is complete in 24 hours.

FURTHER INFORMATION. Blood concentration, protein binding, and excretion—L. E. Mather *et al., Clin. Pharmac. Ther.*, 1971, **12**, 935; blood concentrations—D. C. Moore *et al., Anesthesiology*, 1976, **45**, 39; protein binding and placental transfer—J. Thomas *et al., Clin. Pharmac. Ther.*, 1976, **19**, 426.

Actions and uses. Bupivacaine is a local anaesthetic with an action similar to lignocaine but of longer duration. Its laevo-isomer has an even more prolonged action than bupivacaine.

Bupivacaine is used in local and spinal anaesthesia and may also be used to produce surface anaesthesia. It is usually administered as a solution containing 0.5% of bupivacaine hydrochloride with adrenaline 1 in 200 000 or 0.25% with adrenaline 1 in 400 000. Local anaesthesia lasting up to 7 hours may be obtained with these solutions, but the total quantity administered over a period of 4 hours should not contain more than 2 milligrams of bupivacaine hydrochloride per kilogram body-weight; this is approximately equivalent to 40 to 60 millilitres of the 0.25% solution or 20 to 30 millilitres of the 0.5% solution for an adult.

Like other local anaesthetics, bupivacaine may have a quinidine-like action on the heart, but it is not used as an antiarrhythmic agent.

Undesirable effects. The toxic effects of bupivacaine are similar to those of other local anaesthetics. Hypotension, muscular twitching, respiratory depression, and convulsions may occur with overdosage.

Precautions. Special care, including the recording of the foetal heart rate, should be taken when using bupivacaine to produce paracervical block in labour, as serious foetal bradycardia may be produced; if this condition occurs the intravenous administration of atropine sulphate may be required.

Preparations

Preparations available include an INJECTION containing bupivacaine hydrochloride 0.25 and 0.5% in 10-ml ampoules, an injection containing bupivacaine hydrochloride 0.25% with adrenaline 1 in 400 000 in 10-ml ampoules, and an injection containing bupivacaine hydrochloride 0.5% with adrenaline 1 in 200 000 in 10-ml ampoules.

Burkitt's Lymphoma

see under LYMPHOPROLIFERATIVE DISEASES

Bursal Disease Vaccine

see INFECTIOUS BURSAL DISEASE VACCINE

Busulphan

Tetramethylenebis(methanesulphonate)

$$CH_3 \cdot SO_2 \cdot O \cdot [CH_2]_4 \cdot O \cdot SO_2 \cdot CH_3$$

$C_6H_{14}O_6S_2 = 246.3$

OTHER NAME: *Myleran®*

A standard is given in the British Pharmacopoeia 1973

CAUTION. *Busulphan is irritant and contact with the skin or inhalation of dust should be avoided.*

Description. A white crystalline odourless powder.

Solubility. Soluble, at 20°, in 750 parts of water (in which it is slowly hydrolysed) and in 25 parts of acetone; very slightly soluble in alcohol.

Moisture content. Not more than 2%, determined by drying at 60° *in vacuo*.

Storage. It should be stored in airtight containers, protected from light.

Identification. TESTS. 1. Mix 100 mg with 100 mg of potassium nitrate and 250 mg of potassium hydroxide, fuse, allow to cool, dissolve the residue in water, acidify the solution with *dilute hydrochloric acid*, and add a few drops of *barium chloride solution*; a white precipitate is produced.

2. Dissolve about 100 mg, with the aid of heat, in a mixture of 15 ml of water and 1 ml of *sodium hydroxide solution*; an intense, characteristic, pyridine-like odour is produced. Reserve one half of the solution and to the other half add one drop of *potassium permanganate solution*; the purple colour changes to violet, then to blue, and finally to emerald-green. Acidify the reserved solution with *dilute sulphuric acid* and add one drop of *potassium permanganate solution*; the colour of the permanganate is not discharged.

MELTING-POINT. About 116°.

INFRA-RED ABSORPTION. Major peaks at 861, 934, 980, 1178, 1336, and 1356 cm^{-1} (see Appendix 2a: Infra-red Spectra).

Metabolism. ABSORPTION. Readily absorbed after oral administration.

BLOOD CONCENTRATION. Busulphan is rapidly cleared from the plasma.

DISTRIBUTION. Taken up by the tissues, especially tumour cells in which small amounts bind to cellular proteins and nucleic acids.

METABOLIC REACTIONS. Metabolites are formed by cyclic alkylation of thiol groups in the cells, probably via glutathione.

EXCRETION. Up to about 50% of a dose is excreted in the urine as sulphur-containing metabolites; no unchanged drug is present in urine.

FURTHER INFORMATION. General review on antineoplastic agents—A. H. Chalmers *et al., Drugs*, 1972, **3**, 227; metabolism and excretion—H. Vodopick *et al., J. Lab. clin. Med.*, 1969, **73**, 266.

Actions and uses. Busulphan is a cytotoxic agent. Its effects are caused by inhibition of cell division. This cytotoxic action is, when therapeutic doses are given, mainly exerted on the bone marrow and especially on the production of granulocytes. Platelet production is very liable to be depressed, with resultant thrombocytopenia. Busulphan is given by mouth in the treatment of chronic myeloid leukaemia. In most cases it produces early symptomatic relief and reduction in the size of the spleen. A dosage of 2 to 4 milligrams daily for several weeks will usually produce a prolonged remission.

Busulphan may also be used for maintenance therapy, the usual daily dosage being 0.5 to 2 milligrams.

In exceptional circumstances, doses of 6 milligrams or more daily may be given for short periods; this, however, increases the risk of irreversible bone-marrow damage. After large doses of busulphan, a rapid fall in the granulocyte count occurs, but with small repeated doses this may not commence for several weeks. A rise in the haemoglobin level and in the red-cell count is associated with a favourable response.

Busulphan is also useful in the treatment of polycythaemia vera and myelosclerosis.

Undesirable effects. Prolonged therapy with busulphan can cause fibrosing alveolitis. Other undesirable effects are hyperpigmentation and amenorrhoea.

Precautions. Weekly examinations of the blood are necessary during busulphan therapy; the platelet count reaches a minimum several weeks after the granulocyte count has reached a stable level.

Preparation

BUSULPHAN TABLETS: available as tablets containing 0.5 and 2 mg of busulphan; they are compression coated or sugar coated. The method of preparation should be such that water does not come into contact with materials used to make the tablets at any stage.

A standard for these tablets is given in the British Pharmacopoeia 1973

Containers and *Storage:* see the entry on Tablets for general information on containers and storage. Containers should be airtight.

Butobarbitone

5-Butyl-5-ethylbarbituric acid

$C_{10}H_{16}N_2O_3 = 212.2$

OTHER NAMES: Butethal; Butobarb.; Butobarbital; Butobarbitalum; *Soneryl®*
Butomet® (with emetine hydrochloride); *Sonergan®* (with promethazine hydrochloride)

A standard is given in the European Pharmacopoeia Vol. II

Description. Colourless crystals or white crystalline powder with a very slight odour and a slightly bitter taste.

Solubility. Soluble, at 20°, in 250 parts of water, in 1 part of alcohol, in 10 parts of ether, and in 3 parts of chloroform; readily soluble in solutions of alkali hydroxides and carbonates.

Dissociation constant. pK_a 8.0 (25°).

Hygroscopicity. It absorbs insignificant amounts of moisture at 25° at relative humidities up to about 90%.

Identification. TESTS. It complies with general tests 1 and 3 described under Barbiturates.

MELTING-POINT. About 124°.

ULTRAVIOLET ABSORPTION. In 0.1N sodium hydroxide, maximum at 243 nm (E1%, 1cm = 351).

INFRA-RED ABSORPTION. Major peaks at 1323, 1337, 1435, 1696, 1727, and 1760 cm⁻¹ (see Appendix 2a: Infrared Spectra).

THIN-LAYER CHROMATOGRAPHY. See under Thin-layer Chromatography, System 5.

Determination in body fluids. See under Barbiturates.

Metabolism (see also under Barbiturates).

HALF-LIFE. Plasma half-life, about 55 hours.

DISTRIBUTION. *Protein binding,* about 26% bound to plasma proteins.

METABOLIC REACTIONS. Side-chain oxidation at the (ω-1)-position to form hydroxy- or oxo-metabolites and at the ω-position to form the carboxy-metabolite.

EXCRETION. After an oral dose of 200 mg, 5 to 9% is excreted in the urine unchanged, 22 to 28% is excreted as 3'-hydroxybutobarbitone, 14 to 18% as 3'-oxobutobarbitone, and 4 to 8% as 5-(3'-carboxypropyl)-5-ethylbarbituric acid; about 54% of a dose is excreted in the urine in about 8 days.

FURTHER INFORMATION. Butobarbitone and its metabolites in man—J. Grove *et al., J. Pharm. Pharmac.,* 1974, **26**, 175, J. N. T. Gilbert *et al., J. Pharm. Pharmac.,* 1974, **26**, Suppl. 16P, and J. N. T. Gilbert and J. W. Powell, *Biomed. mass Spectrom.,* 1974, **1**, 142.

Actions and uses. Butobarbitone is an intermediate-acting barbiturate, the actions and uses of which are described under Barbiturates.

When given by mouth in doses of 100 to 200 milligrams it induces sleep in about half an hour. It has also been given by rectum in suppositories in doses of 200 to 300 milligrams.

Undesirable effects; Precautions; Contra-indications; Dependence; Poisoning. As for Barbiturates.

Preparations

BUTOBARBITONE TABLETS: available as tablets containing 100 mg of butobarbitone; they may be coloured.

A standard for these tablets is given in the British Pharmacopoeia 1973

Containers and *Storage:* see the entry on Tablets for general information on containers and storage. Containers should be airtight.

Advice for patients: hypnotic doses should be taken half an hour before bedtime. The tablets may cause drowsiness on the following day; persons affected should not drive or operate machinery. Alcohol should be avoided.

OTHER PREPARATIONS available include TABLETS containing butobarbitone 100 mg with emetine hydrochloride 600 micrograms, and tablets containing butobarbitone 75 mg with promethazine hydrochloride 15 mg.

Butyl Aminobenzoate

Butyl 4-aminobenzoate

$C_{11}H_{15}NO_2 = 193.2$

OTHER NAME: Butamben

A standard is given in the British Pharmacopoeia (Veterinary)

Description. A white crystalline odourless powder.

Solubility. Very slightly soluble in water; soluble, at 20°, in 3 parts of alcohol, in 2 parts of ether, and in 1 part of chloroform; soluble in dilute mineral acids.

Storage. It should be protected from light.

Identification. TESTS. 1. Dissolve about 1 g in 10 ml of 1N hydrochloric acid and add 90 ml of water; a white precipitate is produced (distinction from benzocaine). Filter and to 1 ml of the filtrate add 4 drops of *iodine solution*; a dark brown precipitate is produced which changes to large reddish-brown prisms on prolonged standing (distinction from benzocaine). To a further portion of the filtrate add *methyl red solution* and then add 0.1N sodium hydroxide until the indicator just changes to yellow; a white crystalline precipitate is produced (distinction from procaine).
2. Dissolve 100 mg in 2 ml of *dilute hydrochloric acid*, cool in ice, add 4 ml of a 1% solution of sodium nitrite, and pour the mixture into 2 ml of *2-naphthol solution* containing 1 g of sodium acetate; a red precipitate is produced (test for primary aromatic amines).

MELTING-POINT. About 58°.

ULTRAVIOLET ABSORPTION. In alcohol (95%), maximum at 294 nm (E1%, 1cm = 1050).

Veterinary uses. Butyl aminobenzoate has local anaesthetic properties and is used in skin applications to reduce irritation.

Preparation

Butyl aminobenzoate is an ingredient of piperonyl butoxide application.

Butyl Hydroxybenzoate

Butyl 4-hydroxybenzoate

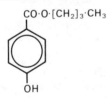

$C_{11}H_{14}O_3 = 194.2$

OTHER NAMES: Butylparaben; *Nipabutyl®*

A standard is given in the British Pharmacopoeia Addendum 1978

Description. A white crystalline odourless powder.

Solubility. Soluble, at 20°, in 5000 parts of water, in 1 part of alcohol, and in 250 parts of glycerol; soluble in solutions of alkali hydroxides.

Identification. TEST. It complies with the test described under Methyl Hydroxybenzoate.

MELTING-POINT. About 70°.

ULTRAVIOLET ABSORPTION. In alcohol (95%), maximum at 259 nm (E1%, 1cm = 840).

Uses. Butyl hydroxybenzoate has preservative properties as described under Methyl Hydroxybenzoate. It is used in a concentration of 0.02% in conjunction with other hydroxybenzoates as a preservative in aqueous preparations.

Butylated Hydroxyanisole

2-*tert*-Butyl-4-methoxyphenol containing a variable amount of 3-*tert*-butyl-4-methoxyphenol.

$C_{11}H_{16}O_2 = 180.2$

OTHER NAMES: BHA; *Embanox BHA®*; *Nipantiox 1-F®*; *Tenox BHA®*
Embanox 7® (with dodecyl gallate)

A standard is given in the British Pharmacopoeia Addendum 1975

Description. A white crystalline powder or a yellowish-white waxy solid with an aromatic odour.

Solubility. Practically insoluble in water; soluble, at 20°, in 4 parts of alcohol, in 2 parts of propylene glycol, in 3 parts of arachis oil, in 100 parts of liquid paraffin, and in 4 parts of lard; soluble in solutions of alkali hydroxides.

Storage. It should be protected from light.

Identification. TESTS. 1. Dissolve a few crystals in 10 ml of alcohol (95%), add 0.5 ml of a 0.2% solution of potassium ferricyanide and 0.5 ml of a 0.5% solution of ferric ammonium sulphate in 1N sulphuric acid; a green to blue colour is produced.
2. Dissolve about 100 mg in 10 ml of alcohol (95%), add 2 ml of a 2% solution of borax and a few crystals of dichloroquinonechloroimine; a blue colour is produced (distinction from butylated hydroxytoluene).

MELTING-POINT. About 63°.

INFRA-RED ABSORPTION. Major peaks at 805, 1050, 1185, 1202, 1222, and 1425 cm^{-1} (see Appendix 2a: Infra-red Spectra).

Metabolism. ABSORPTION. Absorbed after oral administration.

DISTRIBUTION. Stored in body fat.

EXCRETION. Less than 1% is excreted unchanged and 27 to 77% is excreted as the glucuronic acid conjugate in the urine in 24 hours.

Uses. Butylated hydroxyanisole is used as an antioxidant for preserving oils and fats. It may be used either alone or with propyl, octyl, or dodecyl gallate; an antioxidant synergist such as citric acid or phosphoric acid is sometimes added. A mixture consisting of butylated hydroxyanisole 20%, propyl gallate 6%, and citric acid 4% in propylene glycol is commonly used in foods and cosmetics.
Butylated hydroxyanisole may be dissolved in many oils at room temperature, or by warming slightly; it dissolves readily in molten fats. Care should be taken not to incorporate air in the oil or fat while dissolving the antioxidant.
Up to 200 parts per million of butylated hydroxyanisole or butylated hydroxytoluene, or a mixture of these, may be used in pharmaceutical practice for the preservation of fixed oils, fats, or vitamin oil concentrates; in the United Kingdom, up to 1000 parts per million may be added to essential oils used in foods, but inclusion of antioxidants is not usually permitted in essential oils for pharmaceutical use.

Butylated Hydroxytoluene

2,6-Di-*tert*-butyl-*p*-cresol

$C_{15}H_{24}O = 220.4$

OTHER NAMES: *Anullex BHT®*; BHT; *Embanox BHT®*; *Tenox BHT®*; *Topanol OC®*

A standard is given in the British Pharmacopoeia 1973

Description. Odourless colourless crystals or white crystalline powder.

Solubility. Practically insoluble in water, in glycerol, and in propylene glycol; soluble, at 20°, in 4 parts of alcohol, in 0.5 part of ether, in 3 parts of fixed oils, and in 5 parts of liquid paraffin; very slightly soluble in solutions of alkali hydroxides.

Identification. TESTS. 1. It complies with Test 1 described under Butylated Hydroxyanisole.
2. Carry out Test 2 described under Butylated Hydroxyanisole; not more than a faint blue colour is produced (distinction from butylated hydroxyanisole).

MELTING-POINT. About 69°.

ULTRAVIOLET ABSORPTION. In dehydrated alcohol, maximum at 278 nm (E1%, 1cm = 85).

Metabolism. ABSORPTION. Readily absorbed after oral administration.

METABOLIC REACTIONS. Oxidation of the methyl group to a carboxyl group, oxidation of one *tert*-butyl group to a methylpropionic acid group, possibly oxidation of the other *tert*-butyl group to a methyl propionaldehyde group, and glucuronic acid conjugation.

EXCRETION. About 50% of a dose is excreted in urine as metabolites in 24 hours.

FURTHER INFORMATION. Metabolism and excretion—G. M. Holder et al., *J. Pharm. Pharmac.*, 1970, 22, 375.

Uses. Butylated hydroxytoluene is used in the same proportions and for the same purposes as butylated hydroxyanisole.

Cachets

Cachets consist of a dry powder enclosed in a shell and form a convenient method of administering a medicament having an unpleasant taste. The shells are usually prepared from a mixture of rice flour and water by moulding into a suitable shape and drying. The shells thus made are available in two forms: the slip-over or dry-closing type, and the flanged type which is closed by moistening the edges and pressing the two halves together in a machine. Cachets are available in various sizes holding from 0.2 to 1.5 grams of a powder of medium density.
A medicament having a dose of less than 60 milligrams should be triturated with sufficient lactose to produce about 200 milligrams before filling into a cachet. Hygroscopic medicaments should not be enclosed in cachets.

Administration. Cachets are immersed in water for a few seconds, placed on the tongue, and swallowed with a draught of water.

Containers and storage. Cachets should be stored and supplied in containers which provide adequate protection against moisture and crushing.
They should preferably be supplied in wide-mouthed glass or plastic containers, or aluminium containers internally coated with a suitable lacquer or lined with paper; lacquered or lined screw-cap closures or plastic caps should be used.

Cade Oil

Obtained by the destructive distillation of the branches and wood of *Juniperus oxycedrus* L. (Fam. Cupressaceae), a tree common in the Mediterranean areas of North Africa, France, and Spain.

OTHER NAMES: Juniper Tar Oil; Oleum Cadinum

A standard is given in the British Pharmaceutical Codex 1973

Constituents. Cade oil contains guaiacol, together with ethylguaiacol, creosol, the sesquiterpene cadinene, and a varying amount of non-volatile material.

Description. It is a dark reddish-brown or almost black oily liquid with an empyreumatic odour.

Solubility. Very slightly soluble in water; partly soluble in cold alcohol (90%); almost entirely soluble in hot alcohol (90%); soluble, at 20°, in 3 parts of ether; soluble in chloroform.

Weight per ml. At 20°, 0.970 to 1.010 g.

Refractive index. 1.510 to 1.530.

Adulterants and substitutes. Pine tar oil, obtained as a tarry fraction in the destructive distillation of the wood of various species of *Pinus*, *Larix*, and *Abies*.
Shake 1 ml with 15 ml of light petroleum (boiling-range, 40° to 60°) and filter; shake 10 ml of the filtrate with 10 ml of *strong copper acetate solution*, allow to separate, and to 10 ml of the upper layer add 20 ml of solvent ether; the production of a green colour or a brown colour which is deeper than a pale brown indicates the presence of pine tar oil.

Identification. TESTS. 1. To 5 ml add 0.2 ml of a 0.1% solution of ferric chloride in water; a red colour is produced.
2. Boil 5 ml with 2 ml of *potassium cupri-tartrate solution*; a red precipitate is formed.

Actions and uses. Cade oil has been used in local applications for the treatment of psoriasis but has now been almost completely replaced by coal tar preparations.

Preparation

Cade oil is an ingredient of compound resorcinol ointment.

Caffeine

7-Methyltheophylline

$C_8H_{10}N_4O_2 = 194.2$

OTHER NAMES: Anhydrous Caffeine; Coffeinum

A standard is given in the European Pharmacopoeia Vol. II

Caffeine is obtained chiefly from tea waste or coffee or from the dried leaves of *Camellia sinensis* (L.) O. Kuntze; it may also be prepared synthetically. When crystallised from water, caffeine contains one molecule of water of crystallisation, but it is anhydrous when crystallised from alcohol, chloroform, or ether.

Description. Odourless white silky crystals or white crystalline powder with a bitter taste.

Solubility. Soluble, at 20°, in 60 parts of water and in 130 parts of alcohol; very slightly soluble in ether; soluble in chloroform.

Stability. Caffeine is a very weak base and is decomposed by strong solutions of caustic alkalis; its salts are decomposed by water.

Storage. It should be stored in airtight containers.

Identification. TESTS. 1. It complies with Test 2 described under Aminophylline.
2. To 5 drops of a saturated solution add 1 ml of a 5% solution of tannic acid; a precipitate is produced which redissolves on addition of a further 4 ml of the reagent.
3. To a saturated solution add a few drops of *iodine solution*; the solution remains clear. Add a few drops of *dilute hydrochloric acid*; a brown precipitate is produced. Neutralise with *dilute sodium hydroxide solution*; the precipitate redissolves.

MELTING-POINT. About 236°.

ULTRAVIOLET ABSORPTION. In 0.1N hydrochloric acid, maximum at 275 nm (E1%, 1cm = 490); similar figures are obtained in alkaline solution and in alcoholic solution.

INFRA-RED ABSORPTION. Major peaks at 747, 1454, 1480, 1548, 1658, and 1698 cm^{-1} (see Appendix 2a: Infra-red Spectra).

THIN-LAYER CHROMATOGRAPHY. See under Thin-layer Chromatography, System 12.

Determination in body fluids. ULTRAVIOLET SPECTROPHOTOMETRY. In serum or urine—J. I. Routh *et al.*, *Clin. Chem.*, 1969, **15**, 661.

GAS CHROMATOGRAPHY. In plasma: also contains a review of previous methods—F. L. Grab and J. A. Reinstein, *J. pharm. Sci.*, 1968, **57**, 1703.

Metabolism. ABSORPTION. Rapidly but irregularly absorbed after oral administration; the absorption of caffeine is pH-related, an increase in pH increasing its absorption.

BLOOD CONCENTRATION. After an oral dose of 100 mg of caffeine, peak plasma concentrations of 1.5 to 2 μg/ml are attained within 1 to 2 hours.

HALF-LIFE. Plasma half-life, 4 to 10 hours.

DISTRIBUTION. Rapidly distributed throughout the body-water but it does not appear to accumulate in any particular tissues; the uptake of caffeine by the brain is increased if meprobamate or isoniazid is administered concurrently; caffeine is secreted in milk and concentrations of caffeine in saliva are approximately equal to those in plasma; *protein binding*, about 15% bound to plasma proteins.

METABOLIC REACTIONS. *N*-Demethylation and oxidation, and ring cleavage. The drug metabolising enzymes of the liver are stimulated following the ingestion of large amounts of caffeine.

EXCRETION. In 48 hours, 45% of a dose is excreted in the urine as 1-methylxanthine and 1-methyluric acid; other metabolites excreted in the urine include theophylline, 1,7-dimethylxanthine, 7-methylxanthine, and 1,3-dimethyluric acid, together with unchanged caffeine; after an intravenous dose of 500 mg, about 1% is excreted unchanged in the urine.

FURTHER INFORMATION. Blood concentration, half-life, saliva concentration—C. E. Cook *et al.*, *J. Pharmac. exp. Ther.*, 1976, **199**, 679; metabolism—H. H. Cornish and A. A. Christman, *J. biol. Chem.*, 1957, **228**, 315; blood concentration—F. L. Grab and J. A. Reinstein, *J. pharm. Sci.*, 1968, **57**, 1703; metabolism in rats—K. L. Khanna *et al.*, *Toxic. appl. Pharmac.*, 1972, **23**, 720; metabolism—R. N. Warren, *J. Chromat.*, 1969, **40**, 468.

Actions and uses. Caffeine has a stimulating effect on the central nervous system and a weak diuretic action. It may increase renal blood flow or the proportion of functioning glomeruli, but its main action is due to reduction of the normal tubular resorption. The usual dose is 100 to 300 milligrams.
Caffeine is less effective as a diuretic than theobromine, but it has more central stimulant effect. Moderate doses cause insomnia. Caffeine is frequently included in compound analgesic preparations with aspirin or codeine, and is often administered with ergotamine tartrate in migraine preparations.

Preparations

ASPIRIN AND CAFFEINE TABLETS (*Syn.* Acetylsalicylic Acid and Caffeine Tablets): for each tablet take:

Aspirin	350 mg
Caffeine	30 mg

A standard for these tablets is given in the British Pharmacopoeia Addendum 1975
Containers and *Storage:* see the entry on Tablets for general information on containers and storage. Containers should be airtight.
Dose: 1 or 2 tablets.
Advice for patients: the tablets should preferably be taken after meals. Treatment should not be continued for longer than 2 days without medical advice.

CAFFEINE IODIDE ELIXIR:

Caffeine	30 g
Sodium iodide	90 g
Chloroform	2 ml
Liquorice liquid extract	60 ml
Decoction prepared from a sufficient quantity of recently ground roasted coffee of commerce and water for preparations to	1000 ml

To make the decoction, add 100 g of the recently ground roasted coffee to 1000 ml of the boiling water, boil for 1 minute, strain, and pour sufficient water over the contents of the strainer to produce 1000 ml when cold. Dissolve the caffeine and the sodium iodide in 500 ml of the decoction, add the liquorice liquid extract, the chloroform, and sufficient of the decoction to produce the required volume, and mix.
A standard for this elixir is given in the British Pharmaceutical Codex 1973
Containers: see the entry on Elixirs for general information on containers.
Dose: 5 millilitres.
Advice for patients: the elixir should not be used for longer than a few days or given to children without medical advice.

Caffeine Hydrate

7-Methyltheophylline monohydrate
$C_8H_{10}N_4O_2,H_2O = 212.2$

OTHER NAMES: Caffeine Monohydrate; Coffeinum Monohydricum

A standard is given in the European Pharmacopoeia Vol. II

Description. Odourless white silky crystals or white crystalline powder with a bitter taste.

Solubility. Soluble, at 20°, in 60 parts of water and in 110 parts of alcohol; very slightly soluble in ether; soluble in chloroform with separation of water.

Moisture content. 5 to 9%, determined by drying at 105°.

Stability. It effloresces on exposure to dry air and loses its water of crystallisation when heated, becoming anhydrous at 100°.

Storage. It should be stored in airtight containers.

Identification. TESTS. It complies with the tests described under Caffeine.

MELTING-POINT. About 236°.

Determination in body fluids. See under Caffeine.

Metabolism. See under Caffeine.

Actions and uses. Caffeine hydrate has the actions and uses described under Caffeine. The usual dose is 100 to 300 milligrams.

Cajuput Oil

Obtained from the fresh leaves and twigs of certain species of *Melaleuca*, such as *M. cajuputi* Powell and *M. leucadendron* (L.) L. (Fam. Myrtaceae), trees indigenous to Northern Australia and the Malay Archipelago. The oil is distilled mainly in the Molucca Islands and rectified by steam distillation.

OTHER NAME: Oleum Cajuputi

A standard is given in the British Pharmaceutical Codex 1973

Constituents. The chief constituents of cajuput oil are cineole, terpineol (both free and esterified), terpenes, and sesquiterpenes.

Description. It is a colourless, yellow, or green liquid with an agreeable camphoraceous odour.

Solubility. Soluble, at 20°, in 2 parts of alcohol (80%), becoming less soluble with age; miscible with alcohol (90%).

Weight per ml. At 20°, 0.910 to 0.923 g.

Refractive index. 1.464 to 1.472.

Optical rotation. +1° to −4°.

Storage. It should be stored in well-filled airtight containers, in a cool place, protected from light.

Actions and uses. Cajuput oil is a mild counter-irritant and is a constituent of some ointments and liniments.

Preparation

Cajuput oil is an ingredient of compound methyl salicylate ointment.

Calamine

A basic zinc carbonate suitably coloured with ferric oxide.

OTHER NAME: Prepared Calamine

A standard is given in the British Pharmacopoeia 1973

Description. An amorphous, impalpable, pink or reddish-brown powder, the shade depending upon the variety and amount of ferric oxide present and the process by which it is incorporated.

Solubility. Practically insoluble in water; almost completely soluble in hydrochloric acid, with effervescence.

Actions and uses. Calamine has a mild astringent action on the skin and is used in dusting-powders, lotions, and ointments to relieve the discomfort of dermatitis.

Calamine lotion cools the skin by evaporation and is useful for allaying the pain and swelling of sunburn.

Oily calamine lotion is a soothing application for the treatment of eczema. A formula for this preparation was included in the British Pharmaceutical Codex 1973. It consisted of calamine 50 g, wool fat 10 g, oleic acid 5 ml, arachis oil 500 ml, and calcium hydroxide solution to 1000 ml, and was prepared by triturating the calamine with the wool fat, the arachis oil, and the oleic acid, previously melted together, adding the calcium hydroxide solution, and shaking vigorously. This preparation has been criticised because the emulsion sometimes separates and may be difficult to re-emulsify. The lotion is not preserved, and cannot be adequately preserved without fundamentally changing the formulation.

Preparations

AQUEOUS CALAMINE CREAM (*Syn.* Calamine Cream):

Calamine	..	..	..	..	..	40 g
Zinc oxide	..	..	..	..	..	30 g
Emulsifying wax	..	..	..	..	..	60 g
Arachis oil	..	..	..	..	..	300 g
Purified water, freshly boiled and cooled			..	570 g

Melt the emulsifying wax with the aid of gentle heat, add the arachis oil, and warm; add 400 g of the water at the same temperature and stir until cold. Triturate the calamine and the zinc oxide with the remainder of the water and incorporate in the cream.

A standard for this cream is given in the British Pharmaceutical Codex 1973

Containers, Labelling, and Storage: see the entry on Creams for general information on containers, labelling, and storage.

CALAMINE AND COAL TAR OINTMENT (*Syn.* Compound Calamine Ointment; Unguentum Sedativum):

Calamine, finely sifted	..	..	..	125 g
Strong coal tar solution	..	..	..	25 g
Zinc oxide, finely sifted	..	..	..	125 g
Hydrous wool fat	..	..	..	250 g
White soft paraffin	..	..	..	475 g

Melt together the hydrous wool fat and the white soft paraffin, incorporate the calamine, the zinc oxide, and the strong coal tar solution, and stir until cold.

A standard for this ointment is given in the British Pharmaceutical Codex 1973

Containers and Labelling: see the entry on Ointments for general information on containers and labelling. Containers should prevent evaporation.

Advice for patients: the ointment should not be applied

to broken or inflamed skin or near the eyes. It stains the skin, hair, and fabric.

CALAMINE LOTION:

Calamine	..	..	..	..	..	150 g
Zinc oxide	..	..	..	..	..	50 g
Sodium citrate	..	..	..	..	.. 5 g
Bentonite	..	..	..	..	..	30 g
Liquefied phenol	..	..	..	..	..	5 ml
Glycerol	..	..	..	..	..	50 ml

Purified water, freshly boiled and
  cooled   ..   ..   to 1000 ml

Triturate the calamine, the zinc oxide, and the bentonite with a solution consisting of the sodium citrate dissolved in about 700 ml of the water; add the liquefied phenol, the glycerol, and sufficient water to produce the required volume and mix.

A standard for this lotion is given in the British Pharmacopoeia 1973
Containers and *Labelling:* see the entry on Lotions for general information on containers and labelling.
Advice for patients: the lotion should be applied to the skin as required and allowed to dry.

CALAMINE OINTMENT:

Calamine, finely sifted	..	..	..	150 g
White soft paraffin	..	..	..	850 g

Triturate the calamine with a portion of the white soft paraffin until smooth and gradually incorporate the remainder of the paraffin.

A standard for this ointment is given in the British Pharmaceutical Codex 1973
Containers and *Labelling:* see the entry on Ointments for general information on containers and labelling.

COMPOUND CALAMINE APPLICATION (*Syn.* Compound Calamine Cream; Compound Calamine Liniment):

Calamine, finely sifted	..	..	..	100 g
Zinc oxide, finely sifted	..	..	..	50 g
Wool fat	..	..	..	..	25 g
Zinc stearate	..	..	..	..	25 g
Yellow soft paraffin	..	..	..	250 g
Liquid paraffin	..	..	..	..	550 g

Triturate the calamine and the zinc oxide to a smooth paste with a portion of the liquid paraffin. Melt together the zinc stearate, the wool fat, and the yellow soft paraffin at a low temperature and mix with more of the liquid paraffin; incorporate this mixture with the calamine and zinc oxide paste, add the remainder of the liquid paraffin, and mix.

A standard for this application is given in the British Pharmaceutical Codex 1973
Containers and *Labelling:* see the entry on Applications for general information on containers and labelling.
Advice for patients: the preparation should be applied to the skin as required and allowed to dry.

Calciferol

9,10-Secoergosta-5,7,10(19),22-tetraen-3β-ol

$C_{28}H_{44}O = 396.7$

OTHER NAMES: Ergocalciferol; Ergocalciferolum; *Sterogyl-15®*; Vitamin D_2
Calcinate® and *Chocovite®* (both with calcium gluconate)

A standard is given in the European Pharmacopoeia Vol. II Supplement

Description. Odourless, tasteless, colourless or slightly yellow crystals or white or slightly yellow powder.

Solubility. Practically insoluble in water; soluble, at 20°, in 2 parts of alcohol, in 2 parts of ether, in less than 1 part of chloroform, in 10 parts of acetone, and in 50 to 100 parts of fixed oils.

Specific rotation. +103° to +107°, determined on a 4% solution in dehydrated alcohol.

Stability. It rapidly develops a brown colour in the presence of oxygen. Free iodine and traces of metals such as copper promote rapid degradation of calciferol.

Sterilisation. Solutions in ethyl oleate for injection are sterilised by filtration.

Storage. It should be stored in hermetically sealed glass containers in which the air has been replaced by an inert gas, in a cool place, protected from light.

Identification. TESTS. 1. Dissolve about 10 mg in 5 ml of chloroform and add 2 ml of acetic anhydride and 5 drops of sulphuric acid; a red colour develops immediately, quickly turning through violet to blue and finally green.
2. Dissolve about 1 mg in 1 ml of chloroform and add 4 ml of *antimony trichloride solution*; a yellowish-orange colour develops.

MELTING-POINT. About 115°.

ULTRAVIOLET ABSORPTION. In alcohol (95%), maximum at 265 nm (E1%, 1cm = 475).

Determination in body fluids. GAS CHROMATOGRAPHY. In serum: initial thin-layer chromatographic separation—J. R. Evans, *Clinica chim. Acta*, 1972, **42**, 343.

Metabolism. ABSORPTION. Well absorbed after oral administration but decreased absorption may occur with impaired liver and biliary function.

BLOOD CONCENTRATION. During therapy with monthly doses of 100 000 units intramuscularly, serum concentrations of 10 to 30 ng/ml of the 25-hydroxylated metabolite are obtained.

HALF-LIFE. About 960 hours.

DISTRIBUTION. Stored in liver; secreted in milk; *protein binding*, in the blood, bound to α- and β-lipoproteins.

METABOLIC REACTIONS. 25-Hydroxylation in the liver followed by hydroxylation at positions 1α or 24 by the kidney; rate of kidney metabolism controlled by para-thyroid hormone; possible conjugation with sulphate or glucuronic acid.

EXCRETION. Excreted mainly in the bile along with small amounts in the urine; no unchanged calciferol is excreted in the urine.

FURTHER INFORMATION. See under Cholecalciferol.

Actions and uses. Calciferol has the actions and uses of naturally occurring vitamin D, which is necessary for the absorption of calcium and phosphorus and for bone formation.

Deficiency of vitamin D results in rickets in children and osteomalacia in adults and is one of the causes of reduction in bone density leading to fractures in the elderly. Children and infants require relatively more vitamin D than adults, their daily requirements being about 400 units (10 micrograms) but it is important that infants should not be given more than 800 units daily because of the danger of causing hypercalcaemia. The daily requirement of the mother in pregnancy and lactation is also of the order of 400 units (10 micro-grams).

Vitamin D is inactivated, probably through enzyme systems, by the continuous administration of anticon-vulsants, such as phenytoin. Vitamin D deficiency may therefore occur in epileptics under treatment.

In the treatment of vitamin-D-deficiency rickets the mini-mum daily dose is 1000 units (25 micrograms) but 3000 to 4000 units (75 to 100 micrograms) may be given for rapid healing; cases of vitamin-D-resistant rickets may require as much as 20 000 units (500 micrograms) daily or even more (500 000 to 1 000 000 units has been given).

Calciferol is given with calcium for the treatment of infantile tetany. It may also be administered in conditions associated with poor absorption of vitamin D such as steatorrhoea, biliary obstruction, and diarrhoea. Large doses of calciferol (50 000 to 100 000 units daily) may be used instead of dihydrotachysterol for the control of hypoparathyroidism. Massive doses of calciferol should no longer be used for the treatment of arthritis owing to the danger of toxic effects.

Vitamin D_3 (cholecalciferol) is obtained by the ultraviolet irradiation of 7-dehydrocholesterol. Some vitamin D_3 is formed in the body during irradiation with sunlight. It occurs in various fish-liver oils and it is responsible for the antirachitic action of cod- and other fish-liver oils. Hence it is sometimes described as "natural" vitamin D. Its chemical structure and physiological action are similar to those of calciferol, although there is some evidence of a difference in antirachitic activity in man.

Undesirable effects. Excessive doses, that is, 150 000 units (3.75 milligrams) or more daily given over pro-longed periods, may give rise to anorexia, nausea, vomiting, diarrhoea, loss of weight, headache, polyuria, thirst, vertigo, and eventually a raised blood urea. The urinary excretion of calcium is raised and metastatic calcification may occur, particularly in the arteries and kidneys.

Treatment of overdosage consists in withdrawing the calciferol, reducing the dietary calcium intake, and promptly correcting dehydration and electrolyte distur-bances. Hydrocortisone is administered in a dose of 40 milligrams every 8 hours to lower the hypercalcaemia

of hypervitaminosis D. If this fails calcitonin may be administered by injection. Phosphate infusions should not be administered in this situation owing to the dangers of metastatic calcification. The absorption of calcium can be reduced by giving sodium sulphate by mouth and magnesium sulphate by injection.

Precautions. There is danger of overdosage of calciferol in infants and in patients with chronic renal failure. Liquid preparations for infants and children should be particularly carefully measured. Calciferol should be used with caution during pregnancy and lactation as excessive doses may give rise to hypercalcaemia in the offspring.

Calciferol appears to take slightly longer to act and slightly longer to cease acting than dihydrotachysterol and it is therefore even more important to avoid over-dosage with calciferol than with dihydrotachysterol.

Veterinary uses. Calciferol has been used for the pre-vention of hypocalcaemia (milk fever) in cattle, the usual dose being 15 to 30 mega-units (375 to 750 milligrams) daily by injection beginning 4 days before the expected date of parturition and continuing for a day or 2 but not more than 1 week afterwards. Calciferol has been largely replaced by 1α-hydroxycholecalciferol for this purpose.

Preparations

CALCIFEROL INJECTION:

Calciferol or cholecalciferol	..	..	.. 750 mg
Ethyl oleate, peroxide-free	..	..	.. to 100 ml

Unless the injection is prepared without the aid of heat the ethyl oleate used should not require more than 0.15 ml of 0.01N sodium thiosulphate when subjected to the B.P. limit test for peroxides in ethyl oleate. In addition, it should not darken in colour significantly when heated at 150° for 1 hour.

Dissolve, and sterilise the solution by filtration. Alterna-tively, sterilise sufficient of the ethyl oleate by dry heat and allow to cool; by means of an aseptic technique, dissolve the calciferol in the bulk of the cold sterile ethyl oleate and add sufficient of the ethyl oleate to produce the required volume. By means of an aseptic technique, distribute the sterile solution into sterile ampoules, re-place the air in the ampoules with sterile nitrogen or other suitable gas, and seal. Calciferol injection contains, in 1 ml, 300 000 units of antirachitic activity (vitamin D).

A standard for this injection is given in the British Pharmaceutical Codex 1973

Containers: see the entry on Injections for general infor-mation on containers. The injection should be supplied in single-dose ampoules.

Labelling: see the entry on Injections for general in-formation on labelling.

Storage: it should be stored in a cool place, protected from light.

CALCIFEROL SOLUTION (*Syn.* Vitamin D_2 Solution): a solution of calciferol in a suitable vegetable oil. It may be prepared by warming to 40° a 1% suspension of calciferol in a suitable vegetable oil such as arachis oil. To facilitate solution, carbon dioxide is bubbled through the preparation and sufficient oil is added to produce a solution containing, in 1 ml, 75 micrograms of calciferol (3000 units of antirachitic activity, vitamin D).

A standard for this solution is given in the British Pharmacopoeia 1973

Containers and *Storage:* it should be stored in well-filled airtight containers, in a cool place, protected from light.

Labelling: the label on the container should state the number of units of antirachitic activity (vitamin D) in 1 ml.

Advice for patients: the dose should be carefully measured.

CALCIUM WITH VITAMIN D TABLETS: for each tablet take:

Calcium sodium lactate	450.0 mg
Calcium phosphate	150.0 mg
Calciferol	0.0125 mg

Mix the calcium sodium lactate with the calcium phosphate and granulate by moist granulation as described in the entry on Tablets; dry the granules, add the calciferol, either dissolved in a suitable quantity of a fixed oil, as a pre-granulated dispersion, or as a triturate with calcium phosphate, and prepare by compression.

In making this preparation, the calcium sodium lactate may be replaced by calcium lactate, using 300 mg of calcium lactate for each 450 mg of calcium sodium lactate. Alternatively, a suitable mixture of calcium sodium lactate with calcium lactate may be used.

Each tablet contains 500 units of antirachitic activity (vitamin D).

A standard for these tablets is given in the British Pharmaceutical Codex 1973

Containers and *Storage:* see the entry on Tablets for general information on containers and storage. Containers should be airtight. The tablets should be stored in a cool place.

Labelling: a direction to crush the tablets before administration should be given on the label.

Dose: 1 tablet.

Advice for patients: the tablets should preferably be taken after meals. They should not be taken for prolonged periods without medical advice.

STRONG CALCIFEROL TABLETS (*Syn.* Strong Vitamin D$_2$ Tablets): may be prepared by mixing a solution of calciferol in a suitable fixed oil with granules of chocolate basis or other appropriate diluent such that each tablet contains 1.25 mg of calciferol (50 000 units of antirachitic activity, vitamin D); they are sugar coated.

When Calciferol Tablets are prescribed or demanded, Strong Calciferol Tablets should not be dispensed or supplied unless it is confirmed that the strong tablets are intended.

A standard for these tablets is given in the British Pharmacopoeia 1973

Containers and *Storage:* see the entry on Tablets for general information on containers and storage. Containers should be airtight. The tablets should be stored in a cool place.

Labelling: the label on the container should state the amount of the medicament as 1.25 mg of calciferol, equivalent to 50 000 units of antirachitic activity (vitamin D).

Advice for patients: the tablets should be taken only under medical supervision.

OTHER PREPARATIONS available include a SOLUTION containing calciferol 15 mg (600 000 units of antirachitic activity, vitamin D) in 1.5 ml; TABLETS containing calciferol 12.5 micrograms (500 units of antirachitic activity, vitamin D) with calcium gluconate 300 mg, and tablets containing calciferol 15 micrograms (600 units of antirachitic activity, vitamin D) with calcium gluconate 500 mg.

Calcined Magnesite

Consists chiefly of magnesium oxide and may be prepared by igniting naturally-occurring magnesite (magnesium carbonate). It contains not less than 85% of MgO.

A standard is given in the British Pharmacopoeia (Veterinary)

Description. An odourless white or sand-coloured powder or granules.

Solubility. Very slightly soluble in water; incompletely soluble in dilute mineral acids.

Veterinary uses. Calcined magnesite is used to prevent hypomagnesaemia in animals with an inadequate dietary intake. The usual dosage for cattle is 60 grams daily and for calves and sheep 15 grams daily.

Calcitonin (Pork)

A polypeptide hormone of ultimobranchial origin which lowers the calcium concentration in the plasma of mammals by diminishing the rate of bone resorption. It is prepared from dried pork thyroid by extraction with dilute acid or organic solvents and purified by precipitation.

OTHER NAME: *Calcitare®*

A standard is given in the British Pharmacopoeia Addendum 1975

Description. A white powder.

Solubility. Soluble in water; practically insoluble in acetone, in alcohol, in chloroform, and in ether; soluble in solutions of alkali hydroxides; very slightly soluble in solutions of mineral acids.

Moisture content. Not more than 6% determined by drying over phosphorus pentoxide *in vacuo*.

Storage. It should be stored at a temperature not exceeding 25°, protected from light. Under these conditions it may be expected to retain its potency for at least 2 years from the date of manufacture.

Identification. ULTRAVIOLET ABSORPTION. In 0.01N hydrochloric acid, maximum at 278 nm (E1%, 1cm = 12 to 20).

Metabolism. METABOLIC REACTIONS. Degraded in the kidneys and liver.

FURTHER INFORMATION. Plasma clearance of synthetic human calcitonin—R. Ardaillon *et al., J. clin. Invest.,* 1970, **49**, 2345.

Actions and uses. Calcitonin reduces the plasma calcium level and protects the skeleton from calcium loss by inhibiting resorption of calcium from the bones.

In the treatment of Paget's disease a dose of 160 units may be given daily by intramuscular or subcutaneous injection to reduce the excessive resorption of bone. After treatment for 1 or 2 months the serum alkaline phosphatase and urinary hydroxyproline concentrations may be expected to fall towards normal levels and determinations made at intervals may be used to monitor the course of treatment and establish a suitable maintenance dose.

Calcitonin is also used in the management of hypercalcaemia due to immobilisation, thyrotoxicosis, vitamin-D intoxication, hyperparathyroidism or malignancy, or of unknown origin. Dosage is adjusted according to the severity of the condition and the hypocalcaemic response of the patient.

The unit is identical with the international unit of calcitonin, porcine (1974) and is contained in 4.74 mg of the standard preparation.

Undesirable effects. Transient nausea may occur, particularly when calcitonin is administered by intravenous injection.

Precautions. It should be used with caution in patients with a history of allergy.

Preparation

CALCITONIN (PORK) INJECTION: a sterile solution of calcitonin (pork) with a suitable bactericide and either gelatin or appropriate quantities of sodium chloride and acetate ions in water for injections. It is prepared by dissolving the contents of a sealed container in the solvent shortly before use. The bactericide is present in the solvent.

Available as a powder in vials containing 50 units of calcitonin (pork) for reconstitution with saline-acetate diluent for intravenous injection and as a powder in vials containing 160 units of calcitonin (pork) for reconstitution with a diluent containing gelatin for subcutaneous or intramuscular injection.

A standard for this injection is given in the British Pharmacopoeia Addendum 1978

Containers and *Labelling:* see the entry on Injections for general information on containers and labelling.

Storage: the sealed container should be stored at a temperature not exceeding 25°, protected from light. Under these conditions it may be expected to retain its potency for at least 2 years from the date of manufacture. The injection should be used as soon as possible after preparation but solutions may be expected to retain their potency for up to 7 days provided they are stored at 2° to 10°.

Calcium Acetate

$(CH_3.CO_2)_2Ca = 158.2$

A standard is given in the British Pharmaceutical Codex 1973

Description. An odourless white hygroscopic powder.

Solubility. Soluble, at 20°, in 3 parts of water; very slightly soluble in alcohol.

Alkalinity. A 5% solution in water has a pH of 7.2 to 8.2.

Moisture content. Not more than 8%, determined by Fischer titration.

Storage. It should be stored in airtight containers.

Uses. Calcium acetate is a source of calcium ions and may be used to adjust the calcium content of solutions for haemodialysis.

Calcium Alginate

OTHER NAME: *Calgitex®* (with sodium alginate)

Consists chiefly of the calcium salt of alginic acid. It may contain a small proportion of sodium alginate in order to give a product which, although insoluble in water, is more easily absorbed by the body tissues.

A standard is given in the British Pharmaceutical Codex 1973

Description. An odourless white to pale yellowish-brown powder or fibres.

Solubility. Practically insoluble in water and in organic solvents; soluble in solutions of sodium citrate.

Moisture content. Not more than 22%, determined by drying at 105°.

Sterilisation. Solutions are sterilised as described under Alginic Acid.

Identification. TESTS. 1. It complies with Test 1 described under Alginic Acid.
2. Boil 100 mg with 5 ml of water; the sample does not dissolve. Add 2 ml of *sodium carbonate solution* and boil for 1 minute; a white precipitate is formed. Centrifuge and acidify the clear solution; a gelatinous precipitate is produced.

Uses. Calcium alginate is used as an absorbable haemostatic. Fibres of calcium alginate are prepared in a form resembling gauze or wool and this is used to cover lacerated wounds or burns.

Calcium alginate dressings, frequently soaked in sodium alginate solution, are used to pack sinuses, fistulas, and bleeding tooth sockets; the dressings are also used similarly to cover surgical incisions and sites from which skin grafts have been removed.

Calcium alginate is also used as a tablet disintegrant.

Calcium Carbonate

$CaCO_3 = 100.1$

OTHER NAMES: Calc. Carb.; Calcii Carbonas; Precipitated Calcium Carbonate; Precipitated Chalk

A standard is given in the European Pharmacopoeia Vol. I

Description. A white odourless powder.

Solubility. Very slightly soluble in water; the solubility is increased by the presence of carbon dioxide in the water.

Moisture content. Not more than 2%, determined by drying at 200°.

Hygroscopicity. It absorbs insignificant amounts of moisture at 25° at relative humidities up to about 90%.

Sterilisation. It is sterilised by heating in a closed container at a temperature not lower than 160° for sufficient time to ensure that the whole of the powder is maintained at this temperature for 1 hour.

Actions and uses. Calcium carbonate is a very effective antacid which tends to cause constipation. It is usually given with other antacid substances in mixtures, powders, and tablets in doses of 1 to 5 grams, repeated in accordance with the needs of the patient.

Calcium carbonate is also used as a basis for dentifrices.

Undesirable effects. Continued use may cause hypercalcaemia and alkalosis.

Preparations

COMPOUND CALCIUM CARBONATE POWDER:

Calcium carbonate	..	..	..	..	375 g
Light kaolin or light kaolin (natural) ..		..	125 g
Heavy magnesium carbonate	..	..	..	125 g
Sodium bicarbonate	..	..	..	..	375 g

Mix, as described in the entry on Powders.

A standard for this powder is given in the British Pharmaceutical Codex 1973

Containers and *Storage:* see the entry on Powders for general information on containers and storage.

Dose: 1 to 5 grams.

Advice for patients: the powder should be taken, mixed with a little water or other fluid, between meals. Treatment should not be continued for longer than a few days without medical advice.

Calcium carbonate is an ingredient of compound magnesium carbonate powder.

Calcium Chloride

$CaCl_2,2H_2O = 147.0$

OTHER NAMES: Calc. Chlor.; Calcii Chloridum; Calcium Chloride Dihydrate

NOTE. The name Calcium Chloride has also been applied to the hexahydrate, $CaCl_2,6H_2O = 219.1$, and to the anhydrous salt, $CaCl_2 = 111.0$.

A standard is given in the European Pharmacopoeia Vol. I

Description. A white, crystalline, odourless, deliquescent powder with a slightly bitter taste.

Solubility. Soluble, at 20°, in less than 1 part of water and of alcohol.

Incompatibility. It is incompatible with soluble carbonates, phosphates, sulphates, and tartrates.

Sterilisation. Solutions are sterilised by heating in an autoclave or by filtration.

Storage. It should be stored in airtight containers at a temperature not exceeding 25°.

Actions and uses. Calcium chloride has the actions of soluble calcium salts, as described under Calcium Gluconate, and is used in the preparation of solutions for injection, although calcium gluconate is now usually preferred for this purpose.

It is irritant when given by intramuscular or subcutaneous injection and rapid intravenous injection is liable to cause thrombosis; it should therefore be administered by slow intravenous injection, from 6 to 10 millilitres of a 5 to 10% solution (340 to 680 millimoles or 680 to 1360 milliequivalents of Ca^{2+} per litre) being given. A solution containing 10% of the anhydrous salt, equivalent to about 13% of the dihydrate is given in a dose of 10 millilitres by direct intravenous injection in the treatment of cardiac arrest.

Preparation

Calcium chloride is an ingredient of compound sodium lactate injection.

Calcium Copperedetate

The dihydrate of the copper chelate of the calcium salt of ethylenediamine-*NNN'N'*-tetra-acetic acid

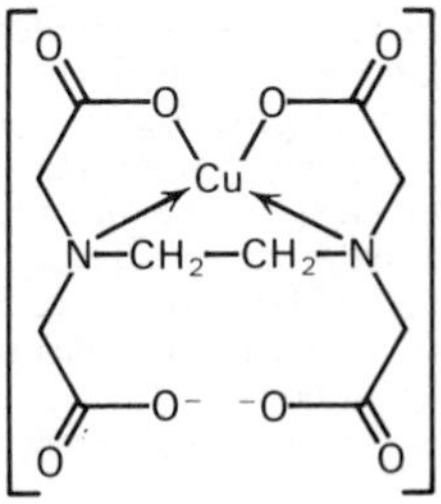

$C_{10}H_{12}CaCuN_2O_8,2H_2O = 427.6$

OTHER NAME: *Coprin*®

A standard is given in the British Pharmacopoeia (Veterinary)

Description. A blue, crystalline, almost odourless powder.

Solubility. Soluble in 7 parts of water, the solution gradually precipitating the tetrahydrate; practically insoluble in alcohol.

Moisture content. Not more than 2%, determined by drying at 105°.

Storage. It should be stored in airtight containers.

Identification. TESTS. 1. Dissolve about 200 mg in 5 ml of water and add 1 ml of acetic acid (33% w/w) and 2 ml of *potassium iodide solution*; the solution remains clear and deep blue.

2. Ignite about 200 mg, dissolve the residue in 3 ml of *dilute hydrochloric acid*, neutralise the solution to litmus paper by the addition of *dilute ammonia solution*, and add 1 ml of acetic acid (33% w/w) and 2 ml of *potassium iodide solution*; a white precipitate is formed and iodine is liberated, colouring the supernatant liquid brown.

3. Ignite about 200 mg, dissolve the residue in 10 ml of *dilute hydrochloric acid*, and pass hydrogen sulphide through the solution; a black precipitate is produced. Filter, boil the filtrate to remove hydrogen sulphide and neutralise to litmus paper by the addition of *dilute ammonia solution*; the solution gives the reactions of calcium.

Veterinary uses. Calcium copperedetate is used in the prevention and treatment of copper deficiency in ruminants.

It is administered by subcutaneous injection to cattle in a dosage of the equivalent of 200 micrograms of copper per kilogram body-weight as a single dose. Pregnant ewes may be given the equivalent of 0.1 to 1 milligram of copper per kilogram body-weight by subcutaneous injection as a single dose for the prevention of swayback in lambs. The dose should be adjusted for the presence of copper in the diet and in other medicines.

Preparation

CALCIUM COPPEREDETATE INJECTION: a sterile suspension of calcium copperedetate with suitable dispersing and stabilising agents in an oil-in-water emulsion. Available in pre-filled syringes containing calcium copperedetate equivalent to 100 mg of copper per ml and as an injection containing calcium copperedetate equivalent to 50 mg of copper per ml.

A standard for this injection is given in the British Pharmacopoeia (Veterinary)

Containers: see the entry on Injections for general information on containers.

Labelling: see the entry on Injections for general information on labelling. In addition, the label on the container should state the amount of the medicament as the equivalent amount of copper in a suitable dose-volume.

Calcium Gluconate

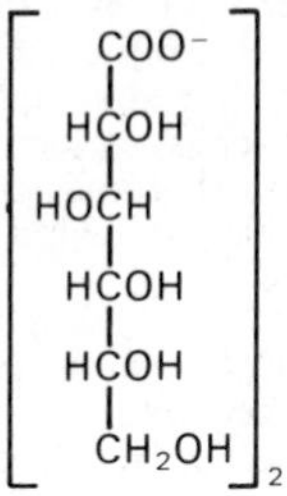

$C_{12}H_{22}CaO_{14},H_2O = 448.4$

OTHER NAMES: Calc. Glucon.; Calcii Gluconas

Calcibor® (with boric acid and in some preparations also with magnesium hypophosphite); *Calcinate*® and *Chocovite*® (both with calciferol)

A standard is given in the European Pharmacopoeia Vol. II

Description. An odourless, tasteless, white, crystalline powder or granules.

Solubility. Slowly soluble, at 20°, in 30 parts of water; soluble in 5 parts of boiling water; practically insoluble in dehydrated alcohol, in ether, and in chloroform.

Incompatibility. It is incompatible with oxidising agents, citrates, and soluble carbonates, phosphates, and sulphates.

Sterilisation. Solutions for injection are sterilised by heating in an autoclave.

Actions and uses. Calcium is an essential element of the tissues and of the blood, which contains approximately 10 milligrams per 100 millilitres (2.5 millimoles per litre); of this, about 7 milligrams is in ionised form and the remainder is in colloidal form united with proteins. The average daily requirement of calcium is 500 milligrams, but larger amounts are necessary during periods of growth, pregnancy, and lactation.

Inadequate calcium intake or absorption in infancy leads to rickets, which is characterised by malformation and imperfect calcification of bones and teeth; the demand by the infant upon the mother during pregnancy and lactation may cause depletion of calcium from the maternal bones, resulting in osteomalacia. These deficiencies are more often caused by lack of vitamin D in the diet than by lack of calcium, but both calcium salts and vitamin D should be employed in their treatment.

Calcium balance is influenced by the parathyroid hormone, excess of which mobilises calcium from the bones, increases the calcium level and the proportion of ionic, compared with bound, calcium in the blood, and increases the excretion of this ion. Deficiency of parathyroid hormone reverses these effects. An abnormally low level of ionic calcium in the blood causes increased excitability of muscle and nerve tissues and may produce tetany or even convulsions; conversely, a high level of ionic calcium decreases muscular and nervous excitability. Calcium gluconate by mouth or by intravenous injection, or calcium chloride by intravenous injection, is therefore used in the treatment of tetany arising in association with parathyroid deficiency, rickets, chronic renal disease, uraemia, and coeliac disease in children, and to check hypocalcaemic convulsions in children.

A high-calcium diet has been used in the treatment of lead poisoning, in which it causes the deposition of lead in bone in the form of an insoluble double salt. In the treatment of lead colic, calcium gluconate intravenously gives prompt relief from the acute pain. Conversely, a low-calcium diet, together with the administration of ammonium chloride, accelerates the excretion of lead, but caution is necessary because the rapid mobilisation of the lead may provoke severe symptoms of plumbism. Calcium gluconate, being tasteless and non-irritant to the stomach, is a more acceptable salt for oral administration than the chloride or lactate.

A dose of 1 to 6 grams (2.23 to 13.4 millimoles, or 4.5 to 27 milliequivalents, of Ca^{2+}) may be given by mouth and repeated in accordance with the needs of the patient. Children may be given half of the dose for an adult. Calcium gluconate is also given by intramuscular injection as a 10% solution the usual dose being 1 gram. In urgent cases, 1 to 2 grams (2.23 to 4.46 millimoles, or 4.5 to 8.9 milliequivalents of Ca^{2+}) may be given by intravenous injection. The usual dose for children by intravenous administration of the diluted solution is up to 1 year 300 milligrams (0.67 millimole or 1.34 milliequivalents of Ca^{2+}), 1 to 5 years 300 to 600 milligrams (0.67 to 1.34 millimoles or 1.34 to 2.68 milliequivalents of Ca^{2+}), and 6 to 12 years 0.6 to 1 gram (1.34 to 2.23 millimoles or 2.68 to 4.46 milliequivalents). Injections of calcium salts should not be given during digitalis therapy.

Calcium gluconate is also administered in suppositories containing 1 gram.

Veterinary uses. Calcium gluconate is administered to animals in the form of calcium borogluconate injection for the treatment of hypocalcaemia. The usual dose in all species is 85 to 250 milligrams (equivalent to approximately 7.5 to 22.5 milligrams of calcium) per kilogram body-weight by subcutaneous or intravenous injection. It may also be given by mouth to dogs and cats in a dosage of 100 to 300 milligrams per kilogram body-weight.

Preparations

CALCIUM BOROGLUCONATE INJECTION: a sterile solution of calcium gluconate with boric acid in water for injections. It may contain up to 0.2% of chlorocresol. The content of boric acid is not more than 2.3 times the content of calcium. It is sterilised by filtration, but it may be sterilised by heating in an autoclave or by heating with a bactericide provided that precautions are taken to ensure that a precipitate does not form during sterilisation or storage.

The general instruction that intravenous injections having a single-dose volume greater than 15 millilitres must not contain an added bactericide does not apply to this preparation.

Available in 400-ml packs containing the equivalent of approximately 1.5, 2.25, and 3% of calcium.

A standard for this injection is given in the British Pharmacopoeia (Veterinary)

Containers: see the entry on Injections for general information on containers.

Labelling: see the entry on Injections for general information on labelling. In addition, the label on the container should state the amount of the medicament as the equivalent amount of calcium in a suitable dose-volume. The label should also state the proportion of boric acid present.

Storage: it should be stored at a temperature not exceeding 20°, protected from light.

CALCIUM GLUCONATE INJECTION: a sterile solution of calcium gluconate, up to 5% of which may be replaced by calcium D-saccharate or other suitable harmless calcium salt as stabilising agent, in water for injections. It is distributed into ampoules, and the ampoules are sealed and sterilised by heating in an autoclave. Available as a solution containing 10% of calcium gluconate, equivalent to 0.89% of calcium (225 millimoles or 450 milliequivalents of Ca^{2+} per litre).

A standard for this injection is given in the British Pharmacopoeia 1973

Containers: see the entry on Injections for general information on containers.

Labelling: see the entry on Injections for general information on labelling. In addition, the label on the container should state the amount of the medicament as the percentage w/v of calcium gluconate equivalent to the total amount of calcium present.

Storage: as the injection is a supersaturated solution, it must be completely free from solid particles. If such particles are present, separation of crystals may occur.

A solution which contains any solid material is unsuitable for use.

CALCIUM GLUCONATE TABLETS: for each tablet take:

Calcium gluconate..	600.0 mg
Vanillin	0.5 mg
Prepared theobroma	150.0 mg
Sucrose	450.0 mg

Mix, and prepare by moist granulation and compression as described in the entry on Tablets.

A standard for these tablets is given in the British Pharmaceutical Codex 1973

Containers and *Storage:* see the entry on Tablets for general information on containers and storage. Containers should be airtight.

Labelling: a direction to chew the tablets before they are swallowed should be given on the label.

Advice for patients: the tablets should not be taken for prolonged periods without medical advice.

EFFERVESCENT CALCIUM GLUCONATE TABLETS: for each tablet take:

Calcium gluconate..	1 g
Saccharin sodium	1 mg
Anhydrous citric acid	150 mg
Tartaric acid	300 mg
Sodium bicarbonate	375 mg

Mix, and prepare by moist granulation, using a non-aqueous liquid excipient, and compression as described in the entry on Tablets.

A standard for these tablets is given in the British Pharmaceutical Codex 1973

Containers and *Storage:* see the entry on Tablets for general information on containers and storage. Containers should be well filled and airtight. The tablets should be stored in a cool place.

Labelling: a direction to dissolve the tablets in water and take the solution as soon as the tablets have dissolved should be given on the label.

Advice for patients: the tablets should not be taken for prolonged periods without medical advice.

OTHER PREPARATIONS available include veterinary INJECTIONS containing calcium borogluconate 20, 30, and 40%, each with magnesium hypophosphite 3% in 400-ml packs.

Calcium Hydrogen Phosphate

$CaHPO_4,2H_2O = 172.1$

OTHER NAMES: Calcii Hydrogenophosphas; Dibasic Calcium Phosphate; Dicalcium Phosphate; *Emcompress*®

A standard is given in the European Pharmacopoeia Vol. III

Description. An odourless, tasteless, white, crystalline powder. It may lose water on exposure to air.

Solubility. Practically insoluble in cold water and partly decomposes in hot water; practically insoluble in alcohol; soluble in dilute hydrochloric and nitric acids.

Storage. It should be stored in airtight containers.

Uses. Calcium hydrogen phosphate has been used as a source of calcium and phosphorus when inadequate amounts are present in the diet. Suitable forms of calcium hydrogen phosphate are used as an aid to the preparation of tablets by direct compression.

Calcium Hydroxide

$Ca(OH)_2 = 74.09$

A standard is given in the British Pharmacopoeia 1973

Description. A soft white powder with an alkaline and slightly bitter taste.

Solubility. Almost completely soluble in 600 parts of water; less soluble in hot water; more soluble in aqueous solutions of glycerol and of sugars. It dissolves in solutions of sucrose with the formation of calcium saccharosates. A solution in water is alkaline and readily absorbs carbon dioxide.

Sterilisation. It is sterilised by heating at a temperature not lower than 160° for sufficient time to ensure that the whole of the powder is maintained at this temperature for 1 hour.

Storage. It should be stored in airtight containers.

Actions and uses. Calcium hydroxide is an antacid and astringent. It has been given by mouth as the solution, which, when added to milk, prevents the formation of large clots of curd in the stomach.

Preparation

CALCIUM HYDROXIDE SOLUTION (*Syn.* Lime Water):

Calcium hydroxide	10 g
Purified water, freshly boiled and cooled	1000 ml

Shake together thoroughly and repeatedly; allow to stand until clear. The clear solution may be drawn off with a siphon, as required. It contains about 0.16% of calcium hydroxide.

A standard for this solution is given in the British Pharmaceutical Codex 1973

Storage: it should be stored in well-filled airtight containers.

Calcium Lactate

The calcium salt of (*RS*)-2-hydroxypropionic acid or mixtures of (*R*)-, (*S*)-, and (*RS*)-2-hydroxypropionic acids. It contains a variable amount (approximately 4 to 5 molecules) of water of crystallisation.

$(C_3H_5O_3)_2Ca = 218.2$

OTHER NAME: Calcii Lactas

A standard is given in the European Pharmacopoeia Vol. III

Description. A white crystalline or granular powder which is odourless or has a slight but not unpleasant odour. It effloresces on exposure to air and becomes anhydrous when heated at 100°.

Solubility. Soluble, at 25°, in 20 parts of water; readily soluble in hot water; very slightly soluble in alcohol; practically insoluble in ether.

Moisture content. 24 to 30%, determined by drying at 125°.

Storage. It should be stored in airtight containers.

Actions and uses. Calcium lactate has the actions of soluble calcium salts as described under Calcium Gluconate.

The usual dose is 5 grams, repeated in accordance with the needs of the patient.

Veterinary uses. Calcium lactate is used in the treatment of calcium deficiency in dogs and cats, the usual dose being 20 to 100 milligrams per kilogram body-weight.

Preparations

CALCIUM LACTATE TABLETS: available as tablets containing 300 and 600 mg of calcium lactate.
A standard for these tablets is given in the British Pharmacopoeia 1973
Containers and *Storage:* see the entry on Tablets for general information on containers and storage. Containers should be airtight.
Advice for patients: the tablets should preferably be taken after meals. They should not be taken for prolonged periods without medical advice.

CALCIUM WITH VITAMIN D TABLETS: see under Calcium Sodium Lactate.
These tablets may be made with calcium lactate, calcium sodium lactate, or a mixture of calcium lactate and calcium sodium lactate.

Calcium Phosphate

Consists chiefly of tricalcium diorthophosphate $Ca_3(PO_4)_2$, together with calcium phosphates of more acidic or basic character. Calcium phosphate is sometimes supplied as "tribasic calcium phosphate", but the pure compound, $Ca_3(PO_4)_2$, has not been obtained.

A standard is given in the British Pharmaceutical Codex 1973

Description. A white, odourless, tasteless, amorphous powder.

Solubility. Very slightly soluble in water; soluble in dilute hydrochloric and nitric acids.

Hygroscopicity. At relative humidities between about 15 and 65%, the equilibrium moisture contents at 25° are about 2%, but at relative humidities above about 75%, it absorbs small amounts of moisture.

Uses. Calcium phosphate is a useful non-hygroscopic diluent for powders and vegetable extracts, but it should not be used as a diluent or excipient in calciferol preparations because it may considerably modify the results of the administration of high doses of the vitamin.
It is not a satisfactory source of calcium or of phosphorus for therapeutic use owing to its insolubility and limited absorption.

Calcium Sodium Lactate

$2C_3H_5NaO_3,(C_3H_5O_3)_2Ca,4H_2O = 514.4$

OTHER NAME: Calc. Sod. Lact.

A standard is given in the British Pharmacopoeia Addendum 1977 and the British Pharmacopoeia (Veterinary)

Description. White deliquescent powder or granules with a slight and characteristic odour and a bitter and slightly acid taste. It melts when heated above 100° and loses water of crystallisation on further heating.

Solubility. Soluble, at 20°, in 14 parts of water; soluble in 25 parts of boiling alcohol; practically insoluble in ether.

Storage. It should be stored in airtight containers.

Actions and uses. Calcium sodium lactate has the actions of soluble calcium salts, as described under Calcium Gluconate. Each gram of calcium sodium lactate is approximately equivalent to 1.15 grams of calcium gluconate or 0.6 gram of calcium lactate. It is usually given by mouth in doses of 0.3 to 2 grams.

Veterinary uses. Calcium sodium lactate is used in the treatment of calcium deficiency in dogs and cats. The usual dose is 50 to 100 milligrams per kilogram body-weight.

Preparation

CALCIUM WITH VITAMIN D TABLETS: for each tablet take:

Calcium sodium lactate	450.0 mg
Calcium phosphate	150.0 mg
Calciferol	0.0125 mg

Mix the calcium sodium lactate with the calcium phosphate and granulate by moist granulation as described in the entry on Tablets; dry the granules, add the calciferol, either dissolved in a suitable quantity of a fixed oil, as a pre-granulated dispersion, or as a triturate with calcium phosphate, and prepare by compression.
In making this preparation, the calcium sodium lactate may be replaced by calcium lactate, 300 mg of calcium lactate being used for each 450 mg of calcium sodium lactate. Alternatively, a suitable mixture of calcium sodium lactate with calcium lactate may be used. Each tablet contains 500 units of antirachitic activity (vitamin D).
A standard for these tablets is given in the British Pharmaceutical Codex 1973
Containers and *Storage:* see the entry on Tablets for general information on containers and storage. Containers should be airtight. The tablets should be stored in a cool place.
Labelling: a direction to crush the tablets before administration should be given on the label.
Dose: 1 tablet.
Advice for patients: the tablets should preferably be taken after meals. They should not be taken for prolonged periods without medical advice.

Calcium Sulphate, Dried

$CaSO_4,\frac{1}{2}H_2O = 145.1$

A powdered gypsum, $CaSO_4,2H_2O$, which has been heated at about 150° until three-quarters of the water of crystallisation has been lost.

OTHER NAMES: Calcined Gypsum; Exsiccated Calcium Sulphate; Plaster of Paris
A standard is given in the British Pharmaceutical Codex 1973

Description. An odourless white hygroscopic powder.

Solubility. Very slightly soluble in water; more soluble in dilute mineral acids; practically insoluble in alcohol.

Setting properties. When it is mixed with a little water it forms a smooth paste which rapidly sets to a hard mass, but if completely dehydrated or heated above 200°, or if much atmospheric moisture has been absorbed, it loses this property. The setting-time is retarded by adding a colloid such as dextrin, acacia, glue, methylcellulose, or any substance which will decrease the solubility, such as alcohol or a citrate; it is accelerated by adding substances such as gypsum, sodium chloride, alum, or potassium sulphate.
It rapidly deteriorates in the presence of moisture. Deterioration is indicated either by too rapid setting or by very slow setting, the set mass being more or less weakened and friable according to the degree of deterioration.

Storage. It should be stored in airtight containers.

Uses. Dried calcium sulphate, consisting of a mixture of amorphous and crystalline forms, is used in the preparation of plaster of Paris bandage.

Bandages may be prepared extemporaneously by applying dried calcium sulphate thickly to a material such as check muslin or book muslin before rolling; after rolling, the bandage is thoroughly wetted and wound round the limb.

Alternatively, the dried calcium sulphate may be mixed to a thin cream in a basin and the unrolled bandaging material passed through the cream immediately before applying to the limb; 1½ to 2 parts of water to 1 part of dried calcium sulphate is a suitable proportion for the cream; a 5% solution of dextrin may be used in place of water.

The plaster will set and a splint form in 15 to 20 minutes. The bulk of the mass increases slightly as the plaster sets; interstices are thus filled and close application obtained.

Dried calcium sulphate is also employed in dental practice for making plaster casts.

Camphor

Bornan-2-one

$C_{10}H_{16}O = 152.2$

A crystalline ketonic substance obtained from the wood of *Cinnamomum camphora* (L.) T. F. Nees and Eberm. (Fam. Lauraceae), a tree growing abundantly in Taiwan, Japan, and China. The wood, in small pieces, is subjected to a process of steam distillation; the crude natural camphor obtained contains a variable quantity of camphor oil and is purified by sublimation. Camphor may also be prepared by synthesis.

A standard is given in the British Pharmacopoeia 1973

Description. A colourless crystalline solid with a characteristic penetrating odour and a taste which is pungent and aromatic, followed by a sensation of cold. According to the manner of condensation, it is obtained as "bells" or "flowers" of camphor; "blocks" and "tablets" are obtained by compression of the powder or by sublimation. It may readily be powdered by trituration with a few drops of alcohol or other volatile organic solvent.

Camphor burns readily with a bright, smoky flame, and volatilises at ordinary temperatures.

Solubility. Soluble, at 20°, in 700 parts of water, in 1 part of alcohol, and in less than 1 part of chloroform; very soluble in ether and in fixed oils.

Melting-point. About 177°.

Specific rotation. Natural camphor: +40° to +43°, determined on a 10% solution in alcohol (95%). Synthetic camphor is optically inactive.

Storage. It should be stored in airtight containers, in a cool place.

Metabolism. ABSORPTION. Absorbed through mucous membranes and from the tissues after injection.

METABOLIC REACTIONS. Mainly hydroxylation to yield hydroxycamphor metabolites which are conjugated with glucuronic acid; some oxidation to yield a carboxylic acid also occurs; the keto-group remains unchanged.

EXCRETION. Excreted in the urine as glucuronides.

FURTHER INFORMATION. Metabolism: reduction and hydroxylation of camphor—K. C. Leibman and E. Ortiz, *Drug Met. Disp.*, 1973, **1**, 543.

Actions and uses. Applied externally, camphor is a mild analgesic and rubefacient and is used in liniments, such as camphor liniment, as a counter-irritant in the treatment of fibrositis and neuralgia.

Poisoning. Poisoning has occurred through the accidental administration of camphor liniment to young children in mistake for castor oil. The symptoms are nausea, vomiting, colic, disturbed vision, delirium, and epileptic convulsions. Recovery is the rule, but in rare cases death may occur from respiratory failure.

The stomach should be evacuated by stomach tube or by emesis and the delirium and convulsions controlled by diazepam, given intravenously if necessary.

Preparations

CAMPHOR LINIMENT (*Syn.* Camphorated Oil):

Camphor	200 g
Arachis oil	800 g

Dissolve the camphor in the arachis oil in a closed vessel.

A standard for this liniment is given in the British Pharmacopoeia 1973

Containers and *Labelling:* see the entry on Liniments for general information on containers and labelling.

Storage: it should be stored in airtight containers in a cool place.

Advice for patients: the liniment should be applied to the skin with considerable friction. It should not be applied to broken or inflamed skin or near to the eyes or mucous membranes.

CAMPHORATED OPIUM TINCTURE (*Syn.* Paregoric):

Opium tincture	50 ml
Camphor	.. 3 g
Benzoic acid	.. 5 g
Anise oil	3 ml
Alcohol (60%)	to 1000 ml

Dissolve the benzoic acid, the camphor, and the anise oil in 900 ml of the alcohol, add the opium tincture and sufficient alcohol to produce the required volume, mix, and filter if necessary. It contains, in 10 ml, 5 mg of morphine, calculated as anhydrous morphine.

A standard for this tincture is given in the British Pharmacopoeia 1973

Dose: 2 to 10 millilitres.

CONCENTRATED CAMPHOR WATER:

Camphor	40 g
Alcohol (90%)	600 ml
Water for preparations	to 1000 ml

Dissolve the camphor in the alcohol and add sufficient water in successive small portions to produce the required volume, shaking vigorously after each addition.

A standard for this concentrated water is given in the British Pharmaceutical Codex 1973

Dose: 0.3 to 1 millilitre.

Camphor Water is prepared by diluting concentrated camphor water with 39 times its volume of water for preparations. The concentrated camphor water should be added in small portions to the bulk of the vehicle, shaking vigorously after each addition.

CONCENTRATED CAMPHORATED OPIUM TINCTURE (*Syn.* Liquor Opii Camphoratus Concentratus):

Opium tincture	400 ml
Camphor	24 g
Benzoic acid	40 g
Anise oil	24 ml
Alcohol (95%)	400 ml
Water for preparations	to 1000 ml

Dissolve the benzoic acid, the camphor, and the anise oil in the alcohol, add the opium tincture and sufficient water to produce the required volume, mix, and filter if necessary. It is approximately 8 times as strong as camphorated opium tincture.

A standard for this tincture is given in the British Pharmaceutical Codex 1973
Dose: 0.25 to 1.25 millilitres.

SOAP LINIMENT (*Syn.* Linimentum Saponis):

Camphor	40 g
Oleic acid	40 g
Rosemary oil	15 ml
Potassium hydroxide solution	140 ml
Alcohol (90%)	700 ml
Purified water, freshly boiled and cooled	to 1000 ml

Dissolve the oleic acid in 500 ml of the alcohol and add, with stirring, the potassium hydroxide solution. Dissolve the camphor and the rosemary oil in the remainder of the alcohol, mix the two solutions, add sufficient of the water to produce the required volume, mix, allow to stand for not less than 7 days, and filter.

In making this preparation the alcohol (90%) may be replaced by industrial methylated spirit diluted so as to be of equivalent alcoholic strength, provided that the law and the statutory regulations governing the use of industrial methylated spirit are observed.

A standard for this liniment is given in the British Pharmaceutical Codex 1973
Containers and *Labelling:* see the entry on Liniments for general information on containers and labelling.
Advice for patients: the liniment should be applied to the skin with considerable friction. It should not be applied to broken or inflamed skin or near to the eyes or mucous membranes.

Cancer

see NEOPLASTIC DISEASE

Candicidin

A mixture of antifungal heptaenes produced by the growth of *Streptomyces griseus* and other species of *Streptomyces*.

OTHER NAME: *Candeptin*®

A standard is given in the British Pharmacopoeia Addendum 1975

Description. A yellow powder with a faint acrid odour.

Solubility. Very slightly soluble in water, in alcohol, in acetone, and in n-butyl alcohol; soluble, at 20°, in 7 parts of dimethyl sulphoxide and in 15 parts of a mixture containing 9 volumes of tetrahydrofuran and 1 volume of water.

Alkalinity. A 1% suspension in water has a pH of 8 to 10.

Moisture content. Not more than 3.5%, determined by drying at 60° *in vacuo.*

Storage. It should be stored in airtight containers, protected from light.

Identification. TEST. To 1 ml of a 0.001% solution in dimethyl sulphoxide add 5 ml of phosphoric acid to form a lower layer; a blue ring is immediately formed at the interface. Mix the liquids; the mixture becomes intensely blue. Add 15 ml of water and mix; the solution becomes pale straw-coloured.

Actions and uses. Candicidin is an antibiotic with antifungal activity. It is especially active against species of *Candida*. It is not well absorbed when given by mouth but is used mainly as a local application in the treatment of susceptible infections.

In the treatment of vaginal candidiasis an ointment containing 0.06% or a vaginal tablet containing 3 milligrams is applied twice daily for 14 days. An ointment containing 0.5 to 1.0% was formerly used for the treatment of skin infections including resistant paronychia.

Undesirable effects. Slight local irritation may rarely occur.

Preparations

CANDICIDIN OINTMENT: a dispersion of candicidin in a suitable anhydrous greasy basis. Available as an ointment containing 0.06% w/w of candicidin.
Containers and *Labelling:* see the entry on Ointments for general information on containers and labelling.
Advice for patients: for the treatment of vaginal candidiasis the ointment should be applied high into the vagina with a suitable applicator, preferably at night. The prescribed course should be completed. For topical use the ointment should be applied sparingly to the affected area.

OTHER PREPARATIONS available include TABLETS, for intravaginal use, containing candicidin 3 mg.

Candidiasis

Candidiasis, also known as moniliasis or thrush, is an acute or chronic fungal infection of skin or mucous membranes caused by the yeast-like organism *Candida albicans*. There is frequently a predisposing condition such as diabetes, pregnancy, or the use of antibiotics, oral contraceptives, or corticosteroids.

Candidiasis of the mucous membranes of the oral cavity, vagina, or rectum is characterised by a fiery red and painful mucosa with multiple creamy patches of exudate. There may be a thick white discharge from the vagina, accompanied by pruritus. Candidiasis of the skin is characterised by reddening and maceration of the skin, especially in the skin folds, together with moist white scales.

Candida may occasionally invade local tissue directly or spread haematogenously to give rise to septicaemia, meningitis, or endocarditis; this is a rare but severe disease and is usually fatal.

Treatment. Local candidiasis responds to good skin hygiene and local applications of nystatin or amphotericin. Treatment of systemic candidiasis may be attempted with systemic antimycotics but is not always successful.

Canine Contagious Hepatitis Vaccine, Inactivated

A preparation of infective tissue or liquid containing canine contagious hepatitis virus which has been inactivated by physical or chemical means.

OTHER NAME: Canine Infectious Hepatitis Vaccine, Inactivated

A standard is given in the British Pharmacopoeia (Veterinary)

Storage. The vaccine should be protected from light and stored at 2° to 8° when it may be expected to retain its potency for at least 12 months.

Veterinary uses. It is administered by subcutaneous injection to dogs for prophylaxis of canine contagious hepatitis.

Canine Contagious Hepatitis Vaccine, Living

A freeze-dried preparation of cell-culture liquid containing canine contagious hepatitis virus which has been modified by serial passage in cell culture. It is reconstituted immediately before use with an appropriate volume of a suitable sterile liquid.

OTHER NAMES: Canine Infectious Hepatitis Vaccine, Living; Freeze-dried Canine Contagious Hepatitis Live Vaccine; Vaccinum Vivum Hepatitidis Canis Contagiosae Cryodesiccatum

A standard is given in the European Pharmacopoeia Vol. III Supplement

Storage. The dried vaccine should be protected from light and stored at 2° to 8° when it may be expected to retain its potency for at least 12 months. It should be used immediately after reconstitution.

Veterinary uses. It is administered by subcutaneous or intramuscular injection to dogs for prophylaxis of canine contagious hepatitis.

Capreomycin Sulphate

A mixture of the sulphates of the antimicrobial substances produced by certain strains of *Streptomyces capreolus*.

OTHER NAME: *Capastat*®

A standard is given in the British Pharmacopoeia 1973

Description. A white odourless solid.

Solubility. Soluble, at 20°, in 1 part of water; very slightly soluble in alcohol; practically insoluble in ether and in chloroform.

Acidity. A 3% solution has a pH of 4.5 to 7.5.

Optical rotation. A solution is laevorotatory.

Labelling. If the material is not intended for parenteral administration, the label on the container states that the contents are not to be injected.

Storage. It should be stored in airtight containers, in a cool place. If it is intended for parenteral administration, the containers should be sterile and sealed to exclude micro-organisms.

Identification. ULTRAVIOLET ABSORPTION. In 0.1N hydrochloric acid, maximum at 268 nm (E1%, 1cm=300); in 0.1N sodium hydroxide, maximum at 287 nm (E1%, 1cm = 200).

Metabolism. ABSORPTION. Not absorbed after oral administration.

BLOOD CONCENTRATION. After an intramuscular dose of 1 g, peak serum concentrations of about 30 μg/ml are attained in 1 to 2 hours and after 8 hours the serum concentration falls to about 5 μg/ml; only traces are found in the serum after 24 hours in patients with normal kidney function.

EXCRETION. About 50% of a dose is excreted in the urine in 12 hours.

Actions and uses. Capreomycin is an antibiotic which is effective against *Mycobacterium tuberculosis*. It is tuberculostatic but, like other members of the aminoglycoside group of antibiotics, it should not be used alone because of the rapid emergence of drug resistance. Capreomycin is used in treatment of tuberculosis as a second-line or reserve drug for patients who cannot tolerate certain other drugs or whose tuberculous infection is not susceptible to them. It is less effective, even in conjunction with other drugs, than streptomycin, rifampicin, ethambutol, or prothionamide, and should be used together with at least one of these substances, the choice depending on bacterial sensitivity and the patient's tolerance. It is preferable to kanamycin because the incidence of serious undesirable effects at effective dosage is lower.

Capreomycin sulphate is administered by intramuscular injection as it is not absorbed from the gastro-intestinal tract. The usual dose is 1 mega unit, equivalent to approximately 1 gram of capreomycin daily. It shows marked cross-resistance to kanamycin, neomycin, and viomycin but not to streptomycin, and no allergy is shared with streptomycin.

Undesirable effects. Progressive renal damage, nitrogen retention, and disturbances of calcium and potassium metabolism may occur. Vertigo, tinnitus, and sometimes deafness occur as a result of a selective toxic action similar to but independent of the action of streptomycin and kanamycin, and these changes may be irreversible. Allergic skin rashes rarely occur.

Precautions and contra-indications. Capreomycin should not be given to patients with impaired renal function and it should be withdrawn if tinnitus or hearing defects occur.

Drug interactions. As for Streptomycin Sulphate.

Preparation

CAPREOMYCIN INJECTION: a sterile solution of capreomycin sulphate in water for injections. It is prepared by dissolving the contents of a sealed container in water for injections shortly before use. Available as a powder in vials containing 1 mega unit of capreomycin sulphate equivalent to approximately 1 g of capreomycin.
A standard for this injection is given in the British Pharmacopoeia 1973
Containers: see the entry on Injections for general information on containers.
Labelling: see the entry on Injections for general information on labelling. In addition, the label on the container states the number of units per mg.
Storage: the sealed container should be stored in a cool place. The injection contains no bactericide and should be used as soon as possible after preparation but solutions of capreomycin sulphate may be expected to retain their potency for up to 14 days provided they are stored at 2° to 10°.

Capsicum

The dried ripe fruits of *Capsicum annuum* var. *minimum* (Miller) Heiser and small-fruited varieties of *C. frutescens* L. (Fam. Solanaceae), small erect shrubs cultivated in central and east Africa and in other tropical countries. In commerce, all small-fruited varieties are referred to as chillies and the larger less pungent varieties as capsicums.

OTHER NAME: Chillies

A standard is given in the British Pharmaceutical Codex 1973

Varieties. Numerous varieties of chillies occur in commerce. Mombasa chillies, grown and collected in Uganda and on the mainland of Tanzania, are dull in colour; the pods are broad and short, and the stalk is present. Zanzibar chillies are more attractive in appearance. Central African chillies (Zambian chillies), with somewhat slender pods, are brighter in colour and almost free from stalk.

Constituents. Capsicum contains about 0.5 to 0.9% of the colourless crystalline pungent principle capsaicin (8-methyl-N-vanillylnon-6-enamide), which melts at about 65° and is volatile at higher temperatures, the vapour being extremely irritating. The carotenoid pigments, capsanthin, capsorubin, zeaxanthin, cryptoxanthin, lutein, and carotene are also present, together with thiamine and ascorbic acid.

Capsicum also contains a fatty oil (about 4 to 16%) and protein. It yields to alcohol (60%) from 20 to 30% of extractive and to acetone about 10%. Up to 3% of calyces and pedicels and up to 1% of foreign organic matter may be present. It yields up to 8% of ash.

Description. UNGROUND DRUG. *Macroscopical characters:* Fruit dull orange-red or red, oblong conical with an obtuse apex, 2-celled, length about 12 to 25 mm, diameter up to 7 mm at widest part, occasionally attached to a 5-toothed inferior calyx and a straight pedicel about 1 mm thick; calyx and pedicel together measuring about 20 to 30 mm.

Pericarp somewhat shrivelled, glabrous and translucent, enclosing about 10 to 20 flat reniform seeds.

Seeds 3 to 4 mm long, either loose or attached to a reddish dissepiment.

It has a characteristic but not powerful odour and an extremely pungent taste.

The pungency is not destroyed by boiling with a 2% solution of sodium hydroxide in water (distinction from ginger) but is destroyed by *potassium permanganate solution.*

Microscopical characters: the diagnostic characters are: Pericarp: *outer epidermis* with cells often arranged in rows of 5 to 7, anticlinal walls straight, moderately and evenly thickened, *cuticle* uniformly striated; parenchymatous cells frequently containing droplets of *red oil,* occasionally containing microsphenoidal *crystals* of calcium oxalate; *inner epidermis* with characteristic island groups of *sclerenchymatous cells* having somewhat wavy, moderately thick, pitted and lignified anticlinal walls, groups separated by thin-walled parenchyma.

Seeds: *epidermis* composed of large, sinuous cells with thin outer walls but strongly thickened, pitted, radial and inner walls; *endosperm* parenchymatous, cells with drops of *fixed oil* and *aleurone grains* 3 to 6 μm in diameter.

Calyx: *outer epidermis* with anisocytic *stomata, inner epidermis* with many trichomes but no stomata; *trichomes* glandular, with uniseriate stalks and multi-cellular heads; mesophyll with many idioblasts containing microsphenoidal *crystals* of calcium oxalate.

Pedicel: *epidermis* of somewhat axially elongated subrectangular cells, with numerous *stomata* and scattered glandular *trichomes; cortex* of 7 to 8 layers of thin-walled cellulosic parenchyma with occasional idioblasts containing microsphenoidal *crystals* of calcium oxalate; *fibres* in isolated groups 2 to 3 cells wide and 1 cell thick, to outer side of narrow cylinder of phloem; *intraxylary phloem,* with *fibres* to inner side; *pith* parenchymatous, with large central cavity.

POWDERED DRUG. Powdered Capsicum. An orange to brownish-red powder possessing the diagnostic microscopical characters, odour, and taste of the unground drug; strongly sternutatory.

Adulterants and substitutes. Japanese chillies possess about one-quarter of the pungency of the African varieties, but are valued for their bright colour. They are derived from an unnamed species of *Capsicum;* they are free from stalk and are distinguished by their somewhat larger size and very bright reddish colour; the cells of the epidermis of the pericarp have a smooth cuticle, strongly thickened anticlinal walls, and a radiate lumen; the cells of the single-layered hypoderm have somewhat thick pitted cuticularised walls.

Paprika is extensively grown and used in central and southern Europe and is derived from mild races of *C. annuum;* the fruits are large and more or less tetrahedral and have a conspicuous green calyx.

Other varieties commonly occurring in commerce include East African capsicums, originating from Malawi and Tanzania, Ethiopian capsicums, Nigerian chillies, and Chinese chillies and capsicums. Varieties occasionally seen include chillies from Thailand, Indonesia, Sierra Leone, Natal, and India.

Ground Cayenne pepper of commerce is normally a blend of any of the varieties mentioned.

Storage. It should be stored in a cool dry place, protected from light.

Actions and uses. Capsicum has a carminative action but it is now rarely used medicinally. It has been applied externally in the form of an ointment as a rubefacient in the treatment of rheumatism.

Preparation

CAPSICUM OINTMENT:

Capsicum oleoresin	..	..	..	..	15 g
Emulsifying wax	..	..	..	..	50 g
Simple ointment	..	..	..	..	935 g

Melt together the simple ointment and the emulsifying wax, incorporate the capsicum oleoresin, and stir until cold.

Capsicum oleoresin may be prepared by the following method:

Exhaust capsicum, previously crushed, by percolation with acetone, or with alcohol (90%) in an apparatus for the continuous extraction of drugs. Evaporate off the solvent and extract the residue with successive quantities of the cold alcohol until the insoluble material is free from pungency. Mix the alcoholic solutions and evaporate off the alcohol.

In making capsicum oleoresin the alcohol (90%) may be replaced by industrial methylated spirit diluted so as to be of equivalent alcoholic strength, provided that the law and statutory regulations governing the use of industrial methylated spirit are observed.

CAUTION. *Capsicum oleoresin is a powerful irritant and even a minute quantity produces an intense burning sensation in contact with the eyes and tender parts of the skin. A dilute solution of potassium permanganate may be used to allay skin irritation and cocaine eye-drops may be required to relieve pain in the eyes.*

The oleoresin is soluble in alcohol, in acetone, in chloroform and in essential oils, and soluble, with opalescence in fixed oils. It should be stored in airtight containers. If separation occurs, the oleoresin should be warmed and mixed before use.

Standards for the ointment and the oleoresin are given in the British Pharmaceutical Codex 1973

Containers and *Labelling:* see the entry on Ointments for general information on containers and labelling.

Advice for patients: the ointment should be rubbed lightly on the affected area. It should not be applied to broken or inflamed skin or near the eyes or mucous membranes.

Capsules

A capsule is a dose of one or more medicinal substances enclosed in a hard or soft (flexible) gelatin shell. Capsules are convenient for the oral administration of many solid or liquid substances, especially those that have an unpleasant taste or odour.

A standard is given in the British Pharmacopoeia 1973

Shells. Hard capsule shells are cylindrical with hemispherical ends and consist of a body with an overfitting cap; after filling, the two components may be more effectively joined by fusion or by means of an additional sealing band or a locking device.

Hard shells are most commonly made from gelatin of a high gel strength; they may contain preservatives such as benzoic acid, hydroxybenzoate esters, or sulphur dioxide, and opacifying agents such as titanium dioxide. Coloured shells are permitted for some capsules. The moisture content of hard shells varies between 12 and 15%, and to prevent undesirable physical changes exposure to extremes of humidity should be avoided. Sizes of hard capsules range from 000, the largest, which will hold about 900 mg of a medium density powder, to 5, the smallest, which will hold up to 100 mg.

In soft or flexible capsules the medicament is enclosed within a single continuous shell, which may be spherical, ovoid, cylindrical with hemispherical ends, or pearshaped. A suitable grade of gelatin, dissolved in water, together with glycerol, sorbitol, or propylene glycol as plasticiser, is used to form shells of suitable hardness or flexibility; preservatives, opacifying agents and, when permitted, colorants may also be included.

Soft capsules are usually manufactured on a large scale. Forming and filling are carried out concurrently by a continuous mechanical process.

Contents. Medicaments in the form of dry powder or granules are usually presented in hard capsules. An advantage of hard capsules is that, usually, fewer additives are required than for tablets although lubricants, glidants, and disintegrants may still be necessary. Hard capsules may also be convenient for extemporaneous dispensing or for small-scale production. It may be possible to separate incompatible ingredients by enclosing a smaller capsule containing one substance within a larger capsule containing the other substances, or by the use of coated granules.

In both hard and soft capsules unpleasant tastes or odours can be masked and the medicament is given reasonable protection from air and moisture, and can be protected from light if necessary.

Soft capsules are generally used for non-aqueous liquids such as vitamin-containing oils and oily solutions of anthelmintics or hormones. Solid medicaments are mainly incorporated as solutions or dispersions in vegetable oils, alone or with surface-active agents; low-molecular weight macrogols have also been used as vehicles.

Substances which contain an appreciable amount of water or other solvent of gelatin are not suitable for filling directly into soft capsules. Alcohols and volatile organic compounds can diffuse through the capsule shell, while aldehydes and alkalis have a tanning effect on the gelatin.

Diluents. It is customary to issue capsules almost completely filled. An inert diluent is usually necessary when the dose of the medicament is less than 100 mg and also for larger doses if the capsules are filled by machine. The choice of diluent is governed in part by the method of filling adopted.

For hard capsules the powdered medicament and diluent must be compatible and the mixture should maintain homogeneity during processing; if filled mechanically, the flow characteristics or cohesiveness should be appropriate to the type of filling machinery used. Suitable diluents for both large- and small-scale processing include lactose, magnesium carbonate, magnesium oxide, calcium carbonate, starch, mannitol, and kaolin.

Manufacturing. Most hard capsule shells are made on automatic machines in which the shells are moulded on steel pins then dried, stripped, trimmed, and assembled. Empty shells can be filled either on high-speed equipment used in the pharmaceutical industry or on semi-automatic or hand-operated fillers for small-scale production.

Soft capsules are usually formed and filled in one operation on large-scale equipment. Machines which utilise rotary or reciprocating dies to form capsules are available for liquids and a rotary machine has also been developed to form and fill powdered or granular materials.

Small-scale preparation. Hand filling of hard capsules can be achieved either by pressing the inverted capsule body into a layer of the powdered medicament or by pressing the powder into the body when held on its side. These methods are slow and the handling which is entailed increases the risk of deterioration of the capsule shell. Small numbers of capsules are more easily filled using a simple apparatus in which the capsules are held in holes and filled by means of a funnel suitably supported.

Small-scale or extemporaneous production of soft capsules is rarely feasible.

Absorption rates. Absorption from hard capsules is closely related to formulation and preparation. Unlike tablets, the contents of hard capsules are not usually heavily compressed and, provided that the gastric or intestinal fluids can easily penetrate the contents after the shell has ruptured, absorption of a medicament from a capsule may be more rapid than from a tablet.

However, several factors affect absorption rates; among these are the particle size distribution, crystal form and habit of sparingly soluble medicaments, the presence of wetting agents, and the physicochemical characteristics of diluents, fillers, and lubricants. (See the entry on Bioavailability for further information.)

Enteric coating. Enteric-coated capsules are treated or coated so that the capsule passes unchanged through the stomach but the contents are released in the intestinal fluid. Capsules resistant to gastric juice may be indicated for medicaments which are gastric irritants, or for medicaments which are destroyed by gastric juice or which are required to be released in the small intestine. Shells treated with formaldehyde, keratin, shellac, or salol have been used but enteric film coatings are now employed, including cellacephate (cellulose acetate phthalate), vinyl polymers and copolymers with maleic anhydride, and a range of acrylic resins.

Enteric coatings are sometimes applied to the capsule contents instead of to the shells.

Sustained release. Capsules may be formulated to release the medicament at such a rate that an effective initial blood level is achieved and an adequate level is subsequently maintained over a period of several hours. In one form of sustained release capsule a hard capsule contains the medicament incorporated into large numbers of small sucrose or sucrose and starch pellets. Uncoated pellets provide the medicament for immediate absorption while pellets coated to varying thicknesses with a slowly-permeable covering disintegrate at different rates to release the medicament over a sustained period. The coating materials usually comprise waxes or lipids blended with water-dispersible stearates, alcohols or esters of high molecular weight.

A similar coating procedure is followed for other types of sustained release capsules in which the starting material is the medicament either in crystal form or as granules.

Other products in capsule shells. Eye ointments, and medicaments for administration by rectum or vagina may be enclosed in capsule shells, and shells and contents may be modified to suit the mode of administration. Inhalation cartridges are also prepared in capsule shells; they are intended for insufflation from a device that pierces the shells and releases the contents for inhalation.

Microencapsulation. Solid particles, liquid droplets, or dispersions in sizes from a few micrometres upwards can be individually coated by microencapsulation techniques.

Microencapsulation is of value to protect volatile or unstable medicaments, to separate incompatible substances, to mask unpleasant tastes or odours, and to achieve controlled release of medicaments. Among the wide range of coating materials used are gelatin, acacia, starches and water-soluble celluloses, water-soluble polymers, waxes, lipids, and resins.

For pharmaceutical substances the most common microencapsulation processes are: spray coating of solid particles suspended in air; coacervation, deposition and fixing from immiscible colloidal phases; mechanical envelopment using centrifugal force; and spray-drying or spray-congealing of high-melting-point coatings. Although the nature of the original coating materials influences the physicochemical characteristics of the microencapsulated product, in many instances dry free-flowing powders can be produced.

Administration of capsules. Capsules are intended to be swallowed whole.

Containers for capsules. Since capsule shells are permeable to water vapour and their physical properties can be affected by humidity changes, containers for both filled and unfilled capsules should provide adequate protection from moisture and also from crushing. Bottles, jars or vials should preferably be of amber coloured glass or plastic and fitted with suitably lined metal or plastic screw caps or close-fitting caps of other types. Cylindrical aluminium containers should be suitably lined and fitted with an aluminium screw cap or a close-fitting plastic cap.

Strip-packed or blister-packed capsules may be dispensed in cartons or wallets of paperboard.

Storage. Capsules should be stored at temperatures not exceeding 25°, unless a lower temperature is specified for a particular preparation.

Further information. Hard gelatin capsules—B. E. Jones and T. D. Turner, *Pharm. J.*, ii/1974, 614. Pharmacopoeial requirements—B. E. Jones and J.-F. V. Törnblum, *Pharm. Acta Helv.*, 1975, **50**, 33. Release of drugs from gelatin capsules—J. M. Newton, *Pharm. Weekbl. Ned.*, 1972, **107**, 485; J. M. Newton *et al.*, *J. Pharm. Pharmac.*, 1971, **23**, 452 and 156S; J. M. Newton and G. Rawley, *J. Pharm. Pharmac.*, 1970, **22**, 163S. Enteric coating—B. E. Jones, *Manuf. Chem. and Aerosol News*, 1970, **41** (5), 53; L. C. Lappas and W. McKeehan, *J. pharm. Sci.*, 1967, **56**, 1257; K. Lehmann, *Manuf. Chem. and Aerosol News*, 1973, **44** (5), 36 and **44** (6), 39. Microencapsulation—E. Doelker and P. Buri, *Pharm. Acta Helv.*, 1975, **50**, 73; M. Gutcho, *Capsule Technology and Microencapsulation*, Noyes Data Corporation, New Jersey, U.S.A., 1972. Capsule-filling machines—K. Ridgway and J. A. B. Callow, *Pharm. J.*, ii/1973, 281.

Caramel

A preparation made by heating a suitable water-soluble carbohydrate with a suitable accelerator until a black viscid mass is formed, which is then adjusted to the required standard by the addition of water, and strained.

OTHER NAMES: Burnt Sugar; Saccharum Ustum

A standard is given in the British Pharmaceutical Codex 1973

Description. A thick but free-flowing dark brown liquid with a slight odour.

Solubility. Miscible with water, with dilute alcohols (up to about 60% v/v), with dilute mineral acids, and with *sodium hydroxide solution*; immiscible with chloroform and with ether; it is precipitated by strong alcohol.

Weight per ml. A 10% solution has a weight per ml of 1.023 to 1.025 g.

Acidity. A 10% solution has a pH of 3 to 5.5.

Uses. Caramel is used as a colouring agent and is capable of producing a range of colours from a pale straw to dark brown. It is usually employed as a 50% solution in chloroform water, 2 millilitres of which is sufficient to colour 100 millilitres of most liquid preparations. The 50% solution should be recently prepared as it is liable to mould growth.

Caramel has no calorific value.

Caraway

The dried ripe fruits of *Carum carvi* L. (Fam. Umbelliferae), an erect biennial herb indigenous to and cultivated in central and northern Europe, chiefly in Holland. The plant is cut when the fruit is ripe and the fruits are obtained by threshing.

OTHER NAMES: Caraway Fruit; Caraway Seed; Carum

A standard is given in the British Pharmacopoeia 1973

Constituents. Caraway contains 2.5 to 6% of volatile oil, containing about 55% of carvone; it also contains fixed oil and about 20% of protein. It yields to cold water from 20 to 26% of non-volatile extractive. Up to 2% of foreign organic matter may also be present. It yields up to 1.5% of acid-insoluble ash.

Description. UNGROUND DRUG. *Macroscopical characters:* cremocarp oblong-ellipsoidal, laterally compressed; mericarps glabrous, brown, usually detached from pedicel and carpophores, up to about 7 mm long and 1 to 2 mm broad, tapered to curved ends, with 5 narrow, slightly yellow primary ridges; pericarp thin; endosperm oily, not grooved on commissural surface.
It has a characteristic aromatic odour and taste.

Microscopical characters: the diagnostic characters are: *epidermis* of polygonal cells with outer walls thickened, *cuticle* striated, *stomata* anomocytic; *vittae* 4 dorsal and 2 commissural; *vascular strands* 1 in each ridge, with narrow vessels and a sclerenchyma cap of *fibres* and *sclereids; parenchyma* of mesocarp without reticulate wall thickening, endosperm cells with thick cellulose walls, cells containing much *oil* and numerous *aleurone grains* up to 10 μm in diameter containing minute rosette *crystals* of calcium oxalate.

POWDERED DRUG. Powdered Caraway. A fawn to brown powder possessing the diagnostic microscopical characters, odour, and taste of the unground drug.

Adulterants and substitutes. Fruits from which the volatile oil has been partially removed are sometimes offered; they may be recognised by their dark colour, shrivelled appearance, lack of aroma, and low yield of aqueous extractive (less than 15%).
Levant or Mogador caraway is light brown, the mericarps usually united, about 5 to 6 mm long, the pedicels often being present; the odour and taste are similar to those of caraway; it yields about 1.5% of volatile oil.
Indian dill, a variety of *Anethum graveolens* L. (*A. sowa* Roxb. ex Flem.) (Fam. Umbelliferae), has been substituted for caraway; it consists usually of entire cremocarps which often have the pedicel attached; they are oval, dorsally compressed, pale brown with narrow yellowish wings; each mericarp is straight with three yellowish dorsal ridges and is about 4 to 6 mm long, 2 mm wide, and 1 mm thick, the ratio of length to breadth being about 2.5 to 1.

Storage. It should be stored in a cool dry place.
Powdered caraway should be stored in airtight containers, in a cool place.

Actions and uses. Caraway is a carminative and a flavouring agent.

Caraway Oil

Obtained by distillation from freshly crushed caraway.

OTHER NAMES: Oleum Cari; Oleum Carui

A standard is given in the British Pharmacopoeia Addendum 1978

Constituents. Caraway oil contains about 60% w/w of (+)-carvone; it also contains (+)-limonene.

Description. It is a colourless or pale yellow liquid with a characteristic odour.

Solubility. Soluble, at 20°, in 7 volumes of alcohol (80%).

Weight per ml. At 20°, 0.902 to 0.912 g.

Refractive index. 1.485 to 1.492.

Optical rotation. +74° to +80°.

Storage. It should be stored in well-filled airtight containers, at a temperature not exceeding 25°, protected from light.

Actions and uses. Caraway oil is a carminative and a flavouring agent.
Caraway water is used in the treatment of flatulence and is a suitable vehicle for children's medicines. The usual dose of caraway oil is 0.05 to 0.2 millilitre.

Preparation

CONCENTRATED CARAWAY WATER:

Caraway oil	20 ml
Alcohol (90%)	600 ml
Water for preparations	to 1000 ml

Dissolve the caraway oil in the alcohol and add sufficient water in successive small portions to produce the required volume, shaking vigorously after each addition; add 50 g of sterilised purified talc or other suitable filtering aid, shake occasionally during a few hours, and filter.
A standard for this concentrated water is given in the British Pharmaceutical Codex 1973
Dose: 0.3 to 1 millilitre.

Caraway Water is prepared by diluting concentrated caraway water with 39 times its volume of water for preparations.

Carbachol

(2-Carbamoyloxyethyl)trimethylammonium chloride

$$\left[NH_2 \cdot CO \cdot O \cdot [CH_2]_2 \cdot \overset{+}{N}(CH_3)_3 \right] \ Cl^-$$

$C_6H_{15}ClN_2O_2 = 182.6$

A standard is given in the British Pharmacopoeia 1973

Description. Very hygroscopic, colourless, prismatic crystals or white crystalline powder with a faint fishy odour resembling that of an aliphatic amine.

Solubility. Very soluble in water; soluble, at 20°, in 55 parts of alcohol; very slightly soluble in dehydrated alcohol, in ether, and in acetone.

Moisture content. Not more than 1%, determined by drying at 105°.

Stability. In aqueous solution carbachol degrades by hydrolysis to choline. Hydrolysis is catalysed by hydrogen ions and hydroxide ions. Solutions are most stable at about pH 3.5; even at pH 5 to 6, less than 3% hydrolysis occurs in solutions during sterilisation by heating in an autoclave. The pH of unbuffered solutions is about 7 and may rise to 8 during autoclaving and storage; at pH 8, about 5% hydrolysis occurs in solutions kept for 1 year at 25°.

FURTHER INFORMATION. Stability in aqueous solution —P. Lundgren, *Acta pharm. suec.*, 1969, **6**, 299.

Sterilisation. Solutions are sterilised by heating in an autoclave or by filtration. In addition, eye-drops may be sterilised by heating with a bactericide.

Storage. It should be stored in airtight containers.

Identification. TESTS. 1. Mix about 200 mg with 3 ml of *sodium hydroxide solution* and boil; ammonia is first evolved and, on further boiling, trimethylamine, recognisable by its odour, is evolved.
2. To a 10% solution add a small excess of a 10% solution of gold chloride; a precipitate is produced which, after recrystallisation from hot water, gives shimmering, thin, flat, prismatic crystals which melt at about 184°.

MELTING-POINT. About 210° with decomposition.

Actions and uses. Carbachol has the muscarinic and nicotinic actions of acetylcholine, as described under Physostigmine Salicylate. Whereas acetylcholine is rapidly inactivated by cholinesterase enzymes, carbachol is not and its action is therefore more prolonged. Since it is also resistant to the action of the digestive enzymes, it is effective when administered by mouth in a dose of 2 to 4 milligrams. It is, however, not readily absorbed after oral administration and is usually given by subcutaneous injection.

Carbachol may be used where the effects of parasympathetic stimulation are required. It is of value in the treatment of post-operative intestinal atony and post-operative retention of urine, for which it is given by subcutaneous injection in a dose of 250 micrograms; this dose may be repeated 2 or 3 times at intervals of 30 minutes. It is also used to stop paroxysmal tachycardia when all other measures have failed, but methacholine is usually preferred.

Carbachol has a miotic action and a 0.8% aqueous solution has been used to lower intra-ocular pressure in glaucoma, sometimes in conjunction with other miotics such as physostigmine.

Undesirable effects. Sweating, nausea, faintness, and abdominal pain occur; these are seldom serious and, if necessary, may be readily controlled or prevented by injection of atropine.

Contra-indications. Carbachol is contra-indicated in patients with acute cardiac failure.

Preparations

CARBACHOL EYE-DROPS: consisting of a sterile solution containing up to 3% of carbachol, with 0.02% v/v of benzalkonium chloride solution, in purified water. It is prepared by method A, B, or C described in the entry on Eye-drops.
A standard for these eye-drops is given in the British Pharmaceutical Codex 1973
Containers: see the entry on Eye-drops for general information on containers. This solution is adversely affected by alkali.
Labelling: see the entry on Eye-drops for general information on labelling.
Advice for patients: see the entry on Eye-drops for general information on the use of eye-drops. Treatment should not be discontinued without the advice of the prescriber. Blurring of vision may occur in the first few days of treatment.

CARBACHOL INJECTION: a sterile solution of carbachol, with 5% of anhydrous dextrose, in water for injections. It is sterilised by heating in an autoclave or by filtration. Available in 1-ml ampoules containing 250 micrograms of carbachol.
A standard for this injection is given in the British Pharmacopoeia 1973
Containers and Labelling: see the entry on Injections for general information on containers and labelling.

Carbamazepine

Dibenz[b,f]azepine-5-carboxamide

$C_{15}H_{12}N_2O = 236.3$

OTHER NAME: *Tegretol®*

A standard is given in the British Pharmacopoeia 1973

Description. A white or yellowish-white, crystalline, almost odourless powder; tasteless or with a slightly bitter taste.

Solubility. Very slightly soluble in water and in ether; soluble, at 20°, in 10 parts of alcohol and in 10 parts of chloroform.

Identification. TESTS. 1. It exhibits an intense blue fluorescence under ultraviolet radiation at 366 nm.
2. Mix 100 mg with 2 ml of nitric acid and heat in a water-bath for 3 minutes; an orange-red colour is produced.

MELTING-POINT. About 191°.

ULTRAVIOLET ABSORPTION. In 0.1N sulphuric acid, maximum at 283 nm (E1%, 1cm = 147) and an inflexion at 255 nm; in alcohol (95%), maximum at 285 nm (E1%, 1cm = 490).

Determination in body fluids. GAS CHROMATOGRAPHY. In plasma or urine—A. Gérardin et al., J. pharm. Sci. 1975, **64**, 1940; in plasma—R. J. Perchalski and B. J. Wilder, Clin. Chem., 1974, **20**, 492; in plasma: simultaneous determination of other anticonvulsants (phenobarbitone, methoin, primidone, phenytoin)—J.-C. Roger et al., Clin. Chem., 1973, **19**, 590; in whole blood —M. Sheehan and R. E. Beam, J. pharm. Sci., 1975, **64**, 2004.

HIGH PRESSURE LIQUID CHROMATOGRAPHY. In plasma carbamazepine and its 10,11-epoxide metabolite—M. Eichelbaum and L. Bertilson, J. Chromat., 1975, **103**, 135; in plasma—H. G. M. Westenberg and R. A. de Zeeuw, J. Chromat., 1976, **118**, 217; in blood or plasma —P. M. Kabra and L. J. Marton, Clin. Chem., 1976, **22**, 1070.

REFLECTANCE SPECTROPHOTOMETRY. In serum—U. Breyer, J. Chromat., 1975, **108**, 370; in serum: carbamazepine and its 10,11-epoxide and 10,11-dihydroxy metabolites—H. K. L. Hundt and E. C. Clarke, J. Chromat., 1975, **107**, 149.

Metabolism. ABSORPTION. Readily absorbed after oral administration; the presence of food may slightly increase absorption.

BLOOD CONCENTRATION. After an oral dose of 6 mg/kg as tablets or as a solution in propylene glycol, peak serum concentrations are, respectively, about 4 µg/ml at 2 hours and 6.5 µg/ml at 3 hours; during therapy with about 12.5 mg/kg daily for 6 months, mean plasma concentrations for carbamazepine and its 10,11-epoxide metabolite are about 5 and 1 µg/ml respectively; therapeutic concentrations are in the range 3 to 6 µg/ml; side-effects are suffered by 50% of subjects with blood concentrations in the range of 8.5 to 10 µg/ml.

HALF-LIFE. Plasma half-life, 21 to 53 hours; in infants the half-life is reduced to 8 to 27 hours. After chronic treatment the plasma half-life is significantly reduced.

DISTRIBUTION. Carbamazepine enters the cerebrospinal fluid, crosses the placenta, and is secreted in milk; in blood it is taken up by red blood cells; *protein binding*, 70 to 80% bound to plasma protein and the epoxide metabolite is about 50% bound.

METABOLIC REACTIONS. Hydroxylation to form 10,11-dihydro-10,11-dihydroxy-5*H*-dibenz[*b*,*f*]azepine-5-carboxamide, epoxidation to form the 10,11-epoxide, and glucuronic acid conjugation; appears to induce its own metabolism in rats, and in man it may increase the metabolism of warfarin and phenytoin.

EXCRETION. Less than 1% of a dose is excreted unchanged in the urine; about 25% is excreted in the urine as the 10,11-dihydroxy metabolite.

FURTHER INFORMATION. Salivary concentrations of carbamazepine—R. E. Chambers *et al.*, *Lancet*, i/1977, 656; plasma kinetics and plasma levels of carbamazepine and its 10,11-epoxide—M. Eichelbaum *et al.*, *Eur. J. clin Pharmac.*, 1975, **8**, 337 and 1976, **9**, 417; the 10,11-epoxide of carbamazepine isolated from human urine—A. Frigerio *et al.*, *J. pharm. Sci.*, 1972, **61**, 1144; pharmacokinetics in man—A. P. Gérardin *et al.*, *J. Pharmacokinet. Biopharm.*, 1976, **4**, 521 and R. H. Levy *et al.*, *Clin. Pharmac. Ther.*, 1975, **17**, 657; CSF concentrations and serum protein binding of carbamazepine and its 10,11-epoxide—S. I. Johannsen *et al.*, *Br. J. clin. Pharmac.*, 1976, **3**, 575; kinetics of carbamazepine and its 10,11-epoxide in children—A. Rane *et al.*, *Clin. Pharmac. Ther.*, 1976, **19**, 276.

Actions and uses. Carbamazepine has marked anticonvulsant properties. It is used, particularly in conjunction with other drugs, in the treatment of grand mal epilepsy with temporal lobe features and of temporal lobe epilepsy, the usual dosage being 200 milligrams daily in divided doses, increasing to 1.2 grams daily in divided doses.

Carbamazepine is sometimes effective in the treatment of trigeminal neuralgia, for which purpose an initial dose of 100 milligrams daily may be given and gradually increased until a suitable response is obtained; the average dosage required is 200 milligrams 3 or 4 times a day.

Undesirable effects. Dizziness, dryness of the mouth, diarrhoea, nausea, diplopia, and rashes may occur and, rarely, aplastic anaemia and jaundice.

Precautions and contra-indications. Carbamazepine should not be given to patients who are being treated with a monoamine-oxidase inhibitor, such as isocarboxazid, nialamide, phenelzine, or tranylcypromine, or within about 2 weeks of the discontinuation of such treatment. It should not be administered during the first 3 months of pregnancy unless specifically indicated.

As it is secreted in the milk it should be administered with caution to nursing mothers.

Preparations

CARBAMAZEPINE TABLETS: available as tablets containing 100 and 200 mg of carbamazepine.
A standard for these tablets is given in the British Pharmacopoeia 1973
Containers and *Storage:* see the entry on Tablets for general information on containers and storage. Containers should be airtight.
Advice for patients: treatment should not be discontinued without the advice of the prescriber. The tablets may cause drowsiness; persons affected should not drive or operate machinery. Alcohol should be avoided.

OTHER PREPARATIONS available include a MIXTURE containing carbamazepine 100 mg in 5 ml, diluent tragacanth mucilage, dilution below half strength not advised, shelf-life of diluted mixture 14 days.

Carbenicillin Sodium

The disodium salt of (6*R*)-6-(2-carboxy-2-phenylacetamido)penicillanic acid.

$C_{17}H_{16}N_2Na_2O_6S = 422.4$

OTHER NAMES: Carbenicillin Disodium; *Pyopen*®

A standard is given in the British Pharmacopoeia Addendum 1978

Description. A white hygroscopic odourless powder with a bitter taste.

Solubility. Soluble, at 20°, in 1.2 parts of water and in 25 parts of alcohol; practically insoluble in ether and in chloroform.

Acidity or alkalinity. A 10% solution has a pH of 6 to 8.

Moisture content. 2.5 to 5.5%, determined by Fischer titration.

Specific rotation. +182° to +196°, determined on a 1% solution.

Stability. In a moist atmosphere, carbenicillin sodium, in the form of powder, degrades slowly by decarboxylation to benzylpenicillin; the reaction is retarded by storage at 5°.
In aqueous solution, carbenicillin degrades by hydrolysis. Degradation is catalysed by hydrogen ions and by hydroxide ions. Degradation is also catalysed by monohydrogen or dihydrogen phosphate ions and by monohydrogen citrate ions. At 35°, solutions are most stable at about pH 6.5. In intravenous infusions of dextrose containing 1 to 2% of carbenicillin sodium, 90% of the potency may be expected to be retained at 25°, 24 hours after preparation.

FURTHER INFORMATION. Stability in aqueous solution—H. Zia *et al.*, *Can. J. pharm. Sci.*, 1974, **9**, 112; stability in intravenous infusions—B. Lynn, *J. hosp. Pharm.*, 1970, **28**, 71 and *Eur. J. Cancer*, 1973, **9**, 425; J. Jacobs *et al.*, *Drug Intell. and clin. Pharm.*, 1970, **4**, 204; E. D. Zost and V. A. Yanchick, *Am. J. hosp. Pharm.*, 1972, **29**, 135.

Storage. It should be stored in sterile containers, sealed to exclude micro-organisms and as far as possible moisture, at a temperature not exceeding 5°, protected from light.

Identification. TESTS. 1. Mix 2 mg with 2 mg of chromotropic acid sodium salt and 2 ml of sulphuric acid and immerse in a suitable liquid at 150° for 4 minutes; the colour of the solution changes through yellowish-brown to greenish-brown and finally to dark brown (distinction from certain other penicillins).
2. Heat about 0.5 g in a small sealed container in a water-bath for 3 minutes, remove the seal and immediately replace by a cork fitted with a platinum loop carrying 1 drop of a freshly prepared mixture of 1 ml of

0.5% sodium carbonate, 1 ml of *phenophthalein solution* and 10 ml of water; the reagent is decolorised within 2 minutes.

Metabolism. ABSORPTION. Carbenicillin is acid-labile and rapidly destroyed in the gastro-intestinal tract and is therefore administered by injection.

BLOOD CONCENTRATION. After an intramuscular dose of 1 g, peak serum concentrations of about 25 μg/ml are attained in 1 hour which fall to about 4 μg/ml after 6 hours; after an intravenous dose of 1 g, concentrations of 140 μg/ml are attained in 15 minutes falling to 20 μg/ml in 2 hours; after an intravenous infusion of 12 to 30 g of the sodium salt administered together with probenecid, plasma concentrations of up to 400 μg/ml are obtained.

HALF-LIFE. Serum half-life, about 30 minutes to 1 hour which is increased to 2, 16, and 23 hours in liver disease, renal disease, and liver disease with oliguria, respectively.

DISTRIBUTION. Distributed throughout the body but does not penetrate the cerebrospinal fluid; volume of distribution, about 12 litres; *protein binding*, 47% bound to plasma proteins.

METABOLIC REACTIONS. Glucuronic acid conjugation.

EXCRETION. 65 to 98% of a dose is excreted in the urine, partly as the glucuronide, and up to 15% is excreted in the bile in 6 to 8 hours; urinary excretion is delayed by probenecid.

FURTHER INFORMATION. Human pharmacology and clinical evaluation—J. L. Bran *et al.*, *Clin. Pharmac. Ther.*, 1971, **12**, 525; pharmacokinetics—T. A. Hoffman *et al.*, *Ann. intern. Med.* 1970, **73**, 173 and R. D. Libke *et al.*, *Clin. Pharmac. Ther.*, 1975, **17**, 441.

Actions and uses. Carbenicillin is a semi-synthetic penicillin which resembles ampicillin. It is, however, not absorbed orally and is therefore administered parenterally. It is destroyed by staphylococcal penicillinase. Activity is demonstrable against *Pseudomonas* species and some ampicillin-resistant strains of *Proteus*, and carbenicillin is therefore used primarily for the treatment of infections caused by these organisms. To prevent the development of resistance by these species, for which at present there are few effective drugs, the use of carbenicillin should be limited to serious generalised infections by these organisms. Blood levels may be raised by blocking tubular excretion and high levels must usually be attained if treatment is to succeed. Carbenicillin is sometimes given in conjunction with aminoglycosides for synergistic antibacterial activity and to retard the development of resistance during treatment. Blood levels of 100 micrograms per millilitre may be maintained by slow intravenous administration; levels of over 25 micrograms per millilitre are needed to inactivate most strains of *Pseudomonas aeruginosa*. High concentrations are reached in the bile, but none diffuses into the cerebrospinal fluid.

The dose of carbenicillin sodium for urinary tract infections is 1 to 2 grams intramuscularly every 6 hours or 5 grams intravenously every 4 to 8 hours, given for 5 to 10 days. The corresponding dose for children is 50 to 100 milligrams per kilogram body-weight by intramuscular injection. For the treatment of severe infections and septicaemia 15 to 30 grams daily is given by repeated slow intravenous injection every 4 hours or by infusion over a period of 30 to 40 minutes. The corresponding daily dose for children is 250 to 400 milligrams per kilogram body-weight, increased to 500 milligrams per kilogram body-weight if necessary.

Carbenicillin sodium may be given intrathecally in a dose of 40 milligrams daily. The usual daily dose for children under 2 years is 5 to 10 milligrams and for those over 2 years, 10 to 20 milligrams.

Undesirable effects. Pain may occur at the site of intramuscular injection. Carbenicillin may also give rise to hypersensitivity as described under Benzylpenicillin. High doses of carbenicillin may lead to abnormal bleeding caused by interference with platelet function.

Precautions. The precautions against allergy described under Benzylpenicillin should be observed. Carbenicillin should not be used topically or for infections that would respond to other more active penicillins. Large doses of carbenicillin sodium contain appreciable amounts of sodium and care is needed when it is given to patients on sodium-restricted diets.

Preparation

CARBENICILLIN INJECTION: a sterile solution of carbenicillin sodium in water for injections. It is prepared by dissolving the contents of a sealed container in water for injections immediately before use. Available as a powder in vials containing carbenicillin sodium equivalent to 1 and 5 g of carbenicillin and in infusion bottles containing carbenicillin sodium equivalent to 5 g of carbenicillin. *A standard for this injection is given in the British Pharmacopoeia Addendum 1978*
Containers: see the entry on Injections for general information on containers.
Labelling: see the entry on Injections for general information on labelling. In addition, the label on the container should state the amount of the medicament as the equivalent amount of carbenicillin.
Storage: the sealed container should be stored at a temperature not exceeding 5°, protected from light. The injection decomposes on storage and should be used immediately after preparation.

Carbenoxolone Sodium

The disodium salt of 3β-(3-carboxypropionyloxy)-11-oxo-olean-12-en-30-oic acid

$C_{34}H_{48}Na_2O_7 = 614.7$

OTHER NAMES: *Biogastrone®*; *Bioral®*; *Duogastrone®*

A standard is given in the British Pharmacopoeia 1973

Description. A white or pale cream-coloured hygroscopic powder with a slightly sweet taste followed by a persistent soapy aftertaste.

Solubility. Soluble in 6 parts of water and in 30 parts of alcohol; very slightly soluble in chloroform and in ether.

Alkalinity. A 10% solution has a pH of 7.9 to 8.7.

Moisture content. Not more than 4%, determined by Fischer titration.

Specific rotation. +132° to +140°, determined on a 1%

solution in a mixture of equal volumes of methyl alcohol and 0.04N sodium carbonate.

Storage. It should be stored in airtight containers.

Identification. TEST. Mix 5 mg with 50 mg of resorcinol and 2 ml of sulphuric acid (80% v/v), heat at 200° for 10 minutes, cool, pour into 200 ml of water, and make the mixture just alkaline by the addition of *sodium hydroxide solution*; an intense green fluorescence is produced.

ULTRAVIOLET ABSORPTION. In a mixture of equal volumes of methyl alcohol and 0.04N sodium carbonate, maximum at 256 nm (E1%, 1cm = 200).

Determination in body fluids. GAS CHROMATOGRAPHY. In serum—C. Rhodes and P. A. Wright, *J. Pharm. Pharmac.*, 1974, **26**, 894.

Metabolism. ABSORPTION. Rapidly and almost completely absorbed after oral administration; food delays and decreases absorption; positioned-release capsules, which burst in the region of the pylorus, are readily absorbed.

BLOOD CONCENTRATION. After an oral dose of 100 mg, peak plasma concentrations of about 15 μg/ml are attained in 2 hours; after a single dose of 50 mg as a positioned-release capsule, a peak concentration of 8 to 12 μg/ml is attained at 8 hours; after doses of 300 mg daily as tablets or of 200 mg daily as positioned-release capsules, steady-state plasma concentrations of over 30 and 25 μg/ml, respectively, are attained after 6 to 8 days; following an oral dose two plasma peaks may be observed, one at 1 hour and the other at 4 hours; these are possibly a consequence of enterohepatic circulation but this has been disputed.

HALF-LIFE. Plasma half-life, 13 to 16 hours, and may be subject to wider individual variation; in the elderly the half-life increases to about 26 hours.

DISTRIBUTION. Volume of distribution, 100 ml/kg; almost entirely located in blood, liver, and the gastro-intestinal tract; carbenoxolone may be secreted in the gastro-intestinal tract from the blood; *protein binding*, almost 100% bound to plasma proteins, 80% to albumin, and 20% to globulin which may be reduced in the elderly.

METABOLIC REACTIONS. Conjugation with glucuronic acid or sulphate; gastro-intestinal hydrolysis to glycyrrhetinic acid and succinate also occurs, the succinate being metabolised subsequently to carbon dioxide.

EXCRETION. Excreted almost entirely in the bile with less than 1% in the urine and 12 to 20% exhaled as carbon dioxide; the major biliary metabolite is the 3-glucuronide.

FURTHER INFORMATION. Absorption in the rat—J. W. Bridges *et al.*, *J. Pharm. Pharmac.*, 1976, **28**, 117; review of metabolism—R. M. Pinder *et al.*, *Drugs*, 1976, **11**, 245.

Actions and uses. Carbenoxolone sodium increases the rate of healing of benign gastric ulcers. This is most marked in ambulant patients, but patients who are treated with bed rest do not seem to gain any further obvious benefit from the use of the drug. Its mechanism of action is unknown, and its therapeutic effects on duodenal ulcer have not been proved.

Carbenoxolone also has aldosterone-like actions, giving rise to weight gain, sodium and chloride retention, and hypokalaemia and anti-inflammatory activity in animals, which is reduced by adrenalectomy.

Treatment is started with 50 milligrams of carbenoxolone sodium by mouth 3 times daily after food, increasing to 100 milligrams 3 times daily if required, and is continued for 4 to 6 weeks. A thiazide diuretic with potassium supplements may be given to reduce signs of fluid retention, but spironolactone should not be used as it antagonises the healing properties as well as the unwanted effects of carbenoxolone.

Carbenoxolone is used in the form of a gel or lozenges for the treatment of ulcers in the mouth.

Undesirable effects. Weight gain frequently occurs, with hypertension, and the associated sodium and water retention may precipitate cardiac failure in patients with heart disease. Hypokalaemic paresis may occur rarely and severe muscle damage with myoglobinuria has been described. Marked increases in hepatocellular enzymes are common; they return to normal after stopping treatment.

Precautions. It should be used with care in patients with heart disease or hypertension and treatment should not be continued for more than 4 to 6 weeks. A potassium supplement is usually required.

Preparations

CARBENOXOLONE TABLETS: available as tablets containing 50 mg of carbenoxolone sodium with peppermint oil as flavouring agent.
A standard for these tablets is given in the British Pharmacopoeia 1973
Containers and *Storage:* see the entry on Tablets for general information on containers and storage. Containers should be airtight.
Advice for patients: for the treatment of gastric ulcer the tablets should be taken after meals. The prescribed course should be completed.

OTHER PREPARATIONS available include CAPSULES containing carbenoxolone sodium 50 mg, a GEL containing carbenoxolone sodium 2%, and LOZENGES containing carbenoxolone sodium 5 mg.

Carbidopa

(*S*)-2-(3,4-Dihydroxybenzyl)-2-hydrazinopropionic acid monohydrate

$C_{10}H_{14}N_2O_4, H_2O = 244.2$

OTHER NAME: *Sinemet*® (with levodopa)

Description. A crystalline solid.

Identification. MELTING POINT. About 210°, with decomposition.

INFRA-RED ABSORPTION. Major peaks at 1121, 1260, 1370, 1400, 1455, and 1625 cm^{-1} (see Appendix 2a: Infra-red Spectra).

Determination in body fluids. SPECTROFLUORIMETRY. In plasma: levodopa and dopamine stated not to interfere —S. Vickers and E. K. Stuart, *J. pharm. Sci.*, 1973, **62**, 1550.

Actions and uses. Carbidopa inhibits the action of the enzyme aromatic amino-acid decarboxylase in the extracerebral tissues but enzyme activity in the brain is not affected as the drug does not penetrate the cerebral tissues.

Carbidopa is used in conjunction with levodopa to diminish its conversion to dopamine in the peripheral tissues thus permitting lower doses to be used effectively for the treatment of parkinsonism and reducing the relative incidence of side-effects. The usual dose of carbidopa is between 10 and 200 milligrams daily.

Undesirable effects. It enhances the undesirable effects of levodopa but to a lesser extent than it enhances its action against parkinsonism.

Preparation

LEVODOPA AND CARBIDOPA TABLETS: available as tablets containing 100 mg of levodopa and carbidopa monohydrate equivalent to 10 mg of carbidopa, and as tablets containing 250 mg of levodopa and carbidopa monohydrate equivalent to 25 mg of carbidopa; they may be coloured.

Containers and *Storage:* see the entry on Tablets for general information on containers and storage. Containers should be airtight and light resistant.

Advice for patients: the tablets should be taken after meals. Treatment should not be discontinued without the advice of the prescriber. The tablets may affect mental concentration in the first few days of treatment and may darken the urine.

Carbimazole

Ethyl 3-methyl-2-thioxo-4-imidazoline-1-carboxylate

$C_7H_{10}N_2O_2S = 186.2$

OTHER NAME: *Neo-Mercazole*®

A standard is given in the British Pharmacopoeia 1973

Description. A white or creamy-white crystalline powder with a characteristic odour; tasteless at first followed by a bitter taste.

Solubility. Soluble, at 20°, in 500 parts of water, in 50 parts of alcohol, in 330 parts of ether, in 3 parts of chloroform, and in 17 parts of acetone.

Storage. It should be stored in airtight containers.

Identification. TESTS. 1. To a small quantity add 1 drop of *dilute potassium iodobismuthate solution*; a scarlet colour is produced.

2. Mix 200 mg with 5 ml of *dilute hydrochloric acid*, heat on a water-bath for 1 hour, cool, and extract with three 5-ml portions of chloroform; wash the combined extracts with 0.5 ml of water, filter through a dry filter paper, and evaporate the filtrate to dryness; the residue, after recrystallisation from alcohol (95%), melts at about 140°.

MELTING-POINT. About 123°.

INFRA-RED ABSORPTION. Major peaks at 740, 1150, 1246, 1275, 1463, and 1574 cm⁻¹ (see Appendix 2c: Infra-red Spectra).

Determination in body fluids. HIGH PRESSURE LIQUID CHROMATOGRAPHY. In plasma: determination of the metabolite methimazole—G. F. Skellern *et al.*, *Br. J. clin. Pharmac.*, 1974, **1**, 265.

Metabolism. ABSORPTION. Rapidly absorbed after oral administration.

BLOOD CONCENTRATION. After an oral dose of 60 mg of carbimazole, peak concentrations of the metabolite methimazole of 0.2 to 0.9 μg/ml were attained at 30 to 60 minutes in one group of patients, and in another group at 2 to 3 hours with concentrations of 0.4 to 1.2 μg/ml; the differences in peak concentrations between the groups may be due to variations in the rate of absorption or to variations in the rate of metabolism.

HALF-LIFE. Apparent plasma half-life for methimazole, 3 to 4 hours following an oral dose of carbimazole and 6 to 9 hours following an oral dose of methimazole; the half-life is decreased in hyperthyroid and increased in hypothyroid subjects.

DISTRIBUTION. The metabolite, methimazole, is widely distributed throughout the body and its volume of distribution is about 34 litres; methimazole crosses the placenta and is secreted in milk; *protein binding*, methimazole is 40% bound to plasma proteins.

METABOLIC REACTIONS. Rapidly hydrolysed and decarboxylated to form methimazole in the blood; sulphate conjugation and possibly glucuronic acid conjugation.

EXCRETION. Almost completely excreted in the urine in 24 hours as methimazole and its conjugates; about 3% of a dose is excreted in the faeces; in rats, 10% is excreted in bile as the glucuronide, most of which is reabsorbed after hydrolysis and excreted in the urine.

FURTHER INFORMATION. Metabolism in man—W. D Alexander *et al.*, *Br. med. J*, ii/1969, 290; absorption and excretion of methimazole—J. A. Pittman *et al.*, *J. clin Endocr. Metab.*, 1971, **33**, 182; plasma concentrations of methimazole—G. G. Skellern *et al.*, *Br. J. clin. Pharmac.*, 1974, **1**, 265; altered half-life of methimazole in thyroid dysfunction—E. S. Vessell *et al.*, *Clin. Pharmac. Ther.*, 1975, **17**, 48.

Actions and uses. Carbimazole is an antithyroid substance that depresses the formation of thyroid hormone and so lowers the basal metabolic rate. Its main effect is on the synthesis of iodotyrosines and thyroid hormones. A secondary effect is the reduction of the uptake and concentration of inorganic iodine by the thyroid. I has no antagonistic action to the thyroid hormones which have already formed.

Carbimazole is used to control hyperthyroidism. It is usually given by mouth in a dosage of 30 to 60 milligrams daily in divided doses every 8 hours, according to the severity of the disorder. The dosage is then gradually reduced to the smallest amount that will control the disease, usually 5 to 20 milligrams daily. An alternative method of treatment is to maintain the carbimazole at a higher level in order to block thyroid hormone synthesis and give replacement doses of thyroxine. Marked thyroid enlargement is an indication of excessive dosage; occasionally eye signs worsen as the condition comes under control. After prolonged administration of carbimazole for many months or years, the disorder may abate spontaneously, but it may recur and signs of hyperthyroidism may reappear within some weeks or months of withdrawal of the drug.

Carbimazole is also used in the preparation of patient for thyroidectomy. Under the influence of this therapy the patient is rendered euthyroid and the metabolic rate returns to normal. The drug is usually then discontinued and iodine or iodides substituted for 10 or 12 days before operation to render the gland firmer and less vascular. The dosage for the treatment of neonatal hyperthyroidism is 2.5 milligrams every 8 hours. This treatment may be continued for about 2 months. The dosage of carbimazole for hyperthyroidism in childhood is 10 milligrams, every 8 hours for 1 month, reducing thereafter to 2.5 to 10 milligrams daily according to the clinical response.

Carbimazole does not act quickly enough to be of immediate use in the treatment of thyroid crises or for the rapid control of severe fulminating cases, for which iodine or iodide should be given in order to prevent the release of further thyroid hormone.

Undesirable effects. Granulocytopenia and swelling of the joints rarely occur; rashes may occasionally occur.

Precautions. Patients should be told to report sore throats, fever, or rashes, as these may precede by several days abnormal findings in the circulating blood. Carbimazole may be given during pregnancy to a thyrotoxic patient, but care should be taken lest overdosage adversely affects the foetus and breast feeding should not be undertaken by lactating patients. In thyrotoxic heart failure, carbimazole therapy should be supplemented by treatment with digitalis and diuretics.

Carbimazole should be given with the utmost caution, or not at all, if there is any degree of tracheal obstruction, as high dosage may produce thyroid enlargement and obstructive symptoms may become marked.

Preparation

CARBIMAZOLE TABLETS: available as tablets containing 5 mg of carbimazole; they are compression coated; the coat may be coloured.

A standard for these tablets is given in the British Pharmacopoeia 1973

Containers and *Storage:* see the entry on Tablets for general information on containers and storage. Containers should be airtight.

Advice for patients: the tablets should be taken at regular intervals. Treatment should not be discontinued without the advice of the prescriber.

Carbomer

A synthetic high-molecular-weight polymer of acrylic acid cross-linked with allylsucrose.

OTHER NAME: *Carbopol 934®*

A standard is given in the British Pharmacopoeia Addendum 1975

Description. A white fluffy hygroscopic powder with a slight characteristic odour.

Solubility. Dispersible in water; soluble, after neutralisation with alkali hydroxides or amines, in water, in alcohol, and in glycerol, with the formation of a viscous gel.

Acidity. A 1% dispersion in water has a pH of about 3.

Moisture content. Not more than 2%, determined by drying at 80°.

Incompatibility. Gels are incompatible with benzoic acid, phenol, and sodium benzoate.

Hygroscopicity. It absorbs about 8% of moisture at 25° at a relative humidity of 50%.

Sterilisation. Aqueous gels are sterilised by heating in an autoclave.

Storage. It should be stored in airtight containers.

Uses. Carbomer disperses in water to form an acidic colloidal solution of low viscosity which when neutralised produces a highly viscous gel. The powder is dispersed in water with the aid of a high-speed stirrer, care being taken to avoid the formation of indispersible lumps. The solution is then neutralised, usually with a solution of sodium hydroxide, but other bases such as triethanolamine, ammonia, and di-isopropylamine are sometimes used; each gram of carbomer requires 400 milligrams of sodium hydroxide for neutralisation. During preparation of the gel, the solutions should be agitated slowly with a broad paddle-like stirrer, care being taken to avoid the introduction of air bubbles.

Carbomer gels are most viscous between pH 6 and 11. The viscosity is much reduced if the pH is less than 3 or greater than 12; strong electrolytes also reduce the viscosity.

Suitable antimicrobial preservatives for carbomer gels include chlorocresol 0.1% and thiomersal 0.01%; higher concentrations of these substances may reduce the viscosity of the gels. Benzoic acid is not a suitable preservative since it markedly reduces the viscosity.

Carbomer is used in the form of a neutralised gel as a suspending agent in preparations for internal and external use. The proportion depends upon the required flow properties of the preparation, the other ingredients, and the pH; 0.1 to 0.4% of carbomer is usually sufficient. Gels containing 0.5 to 5% are used as aqueous ointment bases.

Carbomer is used as a binding agent in tablets and in the formulation of sustained-release tablets.

Carbomer is also employed as an emulsifying agent in the preparation of oil-in-water emulsions for external use; for this purpose it is neutralised partly with sodium hydroxide and partly with a long-chain amine such as stearylamine.

Carbon Dioxide

$CO_2 = 44.01$

OTHER NAME: Carbonei Dioxidum

A standard is given in the European Pharmacopoeia Vol. II

Carbon dioxide may be obtained from naturally occurring carbonates, particularly the carbonates of calcium and magnesium, by treatment with an acid, but is more commonly obtained as a by-product of alcoholic fermentation; it is also obtained by the combustion of fuels. It does not support combustion and is about 1.5 times as heavy as air. A solution in water has weakly acidic properties and reddens blue litmus. Carbon dioxide can be liquefied by pressure at a temperature of 31° or lower; at 31° a pressure of 72 atmospheres is required. It is supplied liquefied in metal cylinders.

LIQUID CARBON DIOXIDE is a limpid colourless liquid, which is immiscible with water but readily dissolves in alcohol, ether, and volatile oils; at atmospheric pressure it boils at about −78°.

SOLID CARBON DIOXIDE, "dry ice", is obtainable commercially and is widely used in refrigeration; owing to its low thermal conductivity it is more stable than liquid carbon dioxide. It has a temperature of −80°. A less compact form, "carbon dioxide snow", may be obtained by suddenly releasing liquid carbon dioxide from a cylinder fitted with an internal tube.

Description. A colourless gas.

Solubility. One volume, measured at normal temperature and pressure, dissolves, at 20°, in 1.2 volumes of water.

Storage, labelling, and colour markings. Carbon dioxide for inhalation should be stored in metal cylinders designed to hold compressed gases. Cylinders should be stored in a special room free from materials of an inflammable nature. The room should ideally be cool but in any case the temperature should not exceed 31°.
The whole of the cylinder should be painted grey and the name of the gas or the chemical symbol "CO_2" should be stencilled in paint on the shoulder of the cylinder.
The name or chemical symbol should be clearly and indelibly stamped on the cylinder valve.
Carbon dioxide for "snow"-making should be stored under similar conditions, but in metal cylinders with an internal tube.
Mixtures of carbon dioxide with oxygen are stored and supplied in cylinders painted in the colours described under Oxygen.

Actions and uses. Carbon dioxide, when given by mouth in solution or as carbonates or bicarbonates, promotes the absorption of liquids by the mucous membranes. For this reason aerated waters rapidly relieve thirst, hasten the action of alcohol, and soon cause diuresis. Carbon dioxide in the stomach increases the secretion of gastric juice, particularly its hydrochloric acid. Effervescing waters are useful for masking the unpleasant taste of saline aperients.
Carbon dioxide is important for regulating the acid-base balance of the blood and tissues. Increased metabolic activity results in a corresponding increase in the proportion of carbon dioxide in the tissues and a decrease in the proportion of oxygen.
As carbon dioxide is a natural direct stimulant of the respiratory centre, an increase in the proportion of carbon dioxide inhaled will cause deeper and more frequent respiration. Air normally contains about 0.04% of carbon dioxide; if this concentration is increased to 3% the depth of respiration in the normal subject is doubled; if it is increased to 5%, the depth is almost trebled and the rate of respiration may increase; if it is further raised to 7%, the rate and depth of respiration may be further increased. Higher concentrations cause dyspnoea, raised blood pressure, headache, mental confusion, and eventually (with 10% or more) unconsciousness.
Withdrawal of carbon dioxide after prolonged inhalation commonly produces pallor, lowered blood pressure, severe headache, and nausea or vomiting.
For therapeutic purposes a mixture of 5 or 7% of carbon dioxide in oxygen may be administered. The mixtures are usually available in cylinders or may be prepared by mixing the gases from separate cylinders. They have been used to induce or improve respiration in newborn infants, in drowning persons, and in the treatment of poisoning by carbon monoxide, morphine, hypnotics, and other depressants. For these purposes oxygen in conjunction with artificial respiration is now usually preferred as it is considered that the disadvantages of using respiratory stimulants outweigh any advantages and carbon dioxide may in some circumstances be dangerous.
Mixtures of oxygen and carbon dioxide may be used to accelerate excretion of inhalation anaesthetics by the lungs and so to reduce the risk of bronchitis and vomiting. Carbon dioxide inhalations may relieve persistent hiccup.
Solid carbon dioxide has a destructive action on tissues

and is used to destroy warts and naevi, being applied with light pressure for 5 or 6 seconds. The application is almost painless, but the surrounding tissues should be covered with soft paraffin and the solid shaped, by compressing in a mould or trimming to a point, to suit the part to be treated. A wheal is afterwards formed, followed by a vesicle, but very little scarring occurs. If a second application is necessary, the inflammation from the first must be allowed to subside.

Carbon Tetrachloride

Tetrachloromethane

$CCl_4 = 153.8$

A standard is given in the British Pharmacopoeia (Veterinary)

Description. A clear colourless volatile liquid with a characteristic odour and a burning taste.
It is non-corrosive and non-flammable, but in contact with flame it decomposes with the production of highly toxic products, which have an acrid odour.

Solubility. Very slightly soluble in water; miscible with dehydrated alcohol and with ether.

Weight per ml. At 20°, 1.592 to 1.595 g.

Boiling-point. About 76°.

Refractive index. 1.460 to 1.461.

Storage. It should be stored in airtight containers, protected from light.

Identification. TEST. When heated on a copper wire it imparts a green colour to a colourless flame.

Metabolism. ABSORPTION. Readily absorbed after inhalation and also absorbed after oral administration or through the skin.

DISTRIBUTION. In rabbits, maximum concentrations of both carbon tetrachloride and hexachloroethane, are found in fat.

METABOLIC REACTIONS. In rabbits and dogs, reduction to chloroform and dimerisation to hexachloroethane.

EXCRETION. Excreted slowly via lungs, urine, and faeces.

FURTHER INFORMATION. Metabolic reactions in dogs —T. C. Butler, *J. Pharmac. exp. Ther.*, 1961, **134**, 311 distribution in rabbits—J. S. L. Fowler, *Br. J. Pharmac.*, 1969, **36**, 181P.

Uses. Carbon tetrachloride is used as an industrial solvent but owing to its toxicity it is no longer used in human medicine. Care should be taken to avoid inhaling the vapour or allowing the liquid to be absorbed through the skin.

Veterinary uses. Carbon tetrachloride is used in the treatment of liver fluke infections in sheep. The usual dose is 1 to 3 millilitres by mouth; similar doses have been given by intramuscular injection but administration by this route may lead to severe tissue damage. It should not be used near tupping or lambing time or in obese animals. Because of the possibility of toxic effects, a test dose should be given to some representative animals before carrying out mass treatment of a flock.

Preparations

CARBON TETRACHLORIDE CAPSULES: consisting of carbon tetrachloride enclosed in a soft capsule. Available as capsules containing 0.6, 1, 2, and 5 ml of carbon tetrachloride.

A standard for these capsules is given in the British Pharmacopoeia (Veterinary)
Containers and *Storage:* see the entry on Capsules for general information on containers and storage. Containers should be light resistant.

CARBON TETRACHLORIDE MIXTURE (*Syn.* Carbon Tetrachloride Drench): a solution of carbon tetrachloride in liquid paraffin or other suitable mineral oil. Available as mixtures containing 19.9, 22.5, and 29% v/v of carbon tetrachloride.
A standard for this mixture is given in the British Pharmacopoeia (Veterinary)
Storage: it should be stored in a dark glass or suitable opaque plastic or metal container at a temperature not exceeding 25°.

Carbromal

(2-Bromo-2-ethylbutyryl)urea

$$CH_3 \cdot CH_2 \cdot \overset{\overset{\displaystyle Br}{|}}{\underset{\underset{\displaystyle C_2H_5}{|}}{C}} \cdot CO \cdot NH \cdot CO \cdot NH_2$$

$C_7H_{13}BrN_2O_2 = 237.1$

A standard is given in the British Pharmacopoeia 1973

Description. A white, crystalline, odourless, tasteless powder.

Solubility. Very slightly soluble in water; soluble, at 20°, in 18 parts of alcohol, in 25 parts of ether, and in 2 parts of chloroform.

Identification. TESTS. Heat about 200 mg with 5 ml of 1N sodium hydroxide; ammonia is evolved. The solution gives the reactions characteristic of bromides.

MELTING-POINT. About 118°.

INFRA-RED ABSORPTION. Major peaks at 660, 1370, 1385, 1478, 1600, and 1694 cm^{-1} (see Appendix 2a: Infra-red Spectra).

Determination in body fluids. ULTRAVIOLET SPECTROPHOTOMETRY. Whole blood: determined as free bromide —H. V. Street, *Clinica chim. Acta*, 1960, **5**, 938.

GAS CHROMATOGRAPHY. Whole blood: determined as free bromide—A. W. Archer, *Analyst, Lond.*, 1972, **97**, 428.

Metabolism. ABSORPTION. Readily absorbed following oral administration.

METABOLIC REACTIONS. Debromination to 2-ethylbutyrylurea and hydroxylation to 2-ethyl-2-hydroxybutyric acid.

EXCRETION. Excreted in the urine partly as 2-ethyl-2-hydroxybutyric acid; very little unchanged drug is excreted in the urine.

Actions and uses. Carbromal has sedative and hypnotic properties. It is given as a hypnotic by mouth in doses of 0.3 to 1 gram, or in doses of 250 milligrams together with an intermediate-acting barbiturate.

Undesirable effects. Rashes may occur. Carbromal may release sufficient bromide ions to affect persons hypersensitive to bromides.

Carbuncles

Carbuncles are similar to boils but more extensive. They may be formed by the spread of perifollicular necrosis in the subcutaneous tissues or by the confluence of several infected follicles. Carbuncles suppurate to the skin and later separate as a slough. They may occur as a result of uncontrolled diabetes, nephritis, and reduced immunity to disease.
See also the entry on Boils.

Carcinoma

see NEOPLASTIC DISEASE

Cardamom Fruit

The dried, nearly ripe fruits of *Elettaria cardamomum* Maton var. *minuscula* Burkill (Fam. Zingiberaceae), a plant growing in southern India and produced on the Malabar coast, in Sri Lanka, in Guatemala, and in Tanzania.

OTHER NAME: Cardamomi Fructus

A standard is given in the British Pharmacopoeia 1973

Varieties. Alleppey cardamoms are elongated ovoid in shape, three-sided, varying from about 8 to 20 mm in length and 4 to 10 mm in breadth, green to pale buff in colour, and strongly striated longitudinally.
Mangalore cardamoms, both full-bleached and half-bleached, are about 20 mm long and 15 mm wide, somewhat globular, and with a roughish, somewhat scurfy surface.
"Ceylon greens" resemble Alleppey fruits, but are generally greener, larger, and more elongated.
Guatemalan cardamoms resemble Alleppey cardamoms but are usually greener in colour. The Tanzanian variety resembles Alleppey cardamoms in shape but is pale to dark buff in colour and more strongly striated longitudinally. Ripe split fruits are frequently present.

Constituents. The active constituents are contained in the seeds which yield from about 3 to 8% of a volatile oil; much starch is also present. They yield to alcohol (45%) about 7% of extractive.
Up to 3% of foreign organic matter may be present. It yields up to 3.5% of acid-insoluble ash and up to 6% of ash.

Description. *Macroscopical characters:* Fruit: a trilocular inferior capsule, up to about 20 mm long, ovoid or oblong, dull green to pale buff, plump or slightly shrunken, obtusely triangular in section, nearly smooth or longitudinally striated; apex with beak formed by flower remains, base rounded or with remains of the stalk.
Seeds: in 2 rows in each loculus, forming an adherent mass attached to the axile placenta; seeds pale to dark reddish-brown, about 4 mm long and 3 mm broad, irregularly angular, hard, transversely rugose with 6 to 8 rugae, raphe contained in longitudinal channel, each seed enveloped by a colourless, membranous aril; transversely cut surface of seed showing a brown testa, white starchy perisperm grooved on one side, yellowish endosperm, and a paler embryo.
It has a strongly aromatic agreeable odour and taste.

Microscopical characters: the diagnostic characters are: seed: *aril* composed of flattened, thin-walled, parenchymatous cells; *outer epidermis* of the testa composed of thick-walled, narrow, axially elongated cells, followed by one layer of collapsed parenchyma and one layer (2 to 3 layers near raphe) of large, thin-walled rectangular cells containing *volatile oil*; the layer of conspicuously dark-brown *stegmata*, each cell about 35 or 40 μm long and about 20 μm wide, lumina narrow, bowl-shaped, each containing a warty *silica-body*; inner epidermis consisting of flattened cells; *vessels* few, narrow, with spiral wall thickening; *perisperm* cells thin-walled, containing numerous starch granules in adherent polyhedral masses; individual granules up to 6 μm in diameter; each starch mass with 1 to 7 prismatic *crystals* of calcium oxalate embedded in it.

Substitutes. Ceylon fruits, known as Long Wild Natives, derived from *E. cardamomum* var. *major* Thwaites, are an article of commerce and are readily distinguished by their elongated shape, shrivelled appearance, and rather dark greyish-brown colour; the seeds have about 4 rugae only in their length.

Cluster cardamoms, derived from *Amomum kepulaga* Sprague and Burkill (Fam. Zingiberaceae), have seeds with a camphoraceous taste and with about 14 interrupted rugae in the length of the seed.

The seeds, imported loose, are less aromatic than those freshly removed from the fruit; they are often more fully ripe and hence contain more fixed oil.

Storage. It should be stored in a cool dry place; the seeds should not be stored after removal from the fruit.

Actions and uses. Cardamom is a carminative and a flavouring agent.

In making preparations of cardamom, only the seed is used. The seeds are removed from the capsules, immediately powdered or bruised, and used without delay.

Cardamom Oil

Obtained by distillation from crushed cardamom fruit.

A standard is given in the British Pharmacopoeia Addendum 1978

Constituents. Cardamom oil contains cineole, terpineol, mainly as the acetic ester, and limonene.

Description. It is a colourless or pale yellow liquid with a pungent aromatic odour.

Solubility. Soluble, at 20°, in 6 parts of alcohol (70%).

Weight per ml. At 20°, 0.917 to 0.940 g.

Refractive index. 1.461 to 1.467.

Optical rotation. +20° to +44°.

Storage. It should be stored in well-filled airtight containers, at a temperature not exceeding 25°, protected from light.

Actions and uses. Cardamom oil has carminative properties. It is sometimes used as a flavouring agent.

Preparations

AROMATIC CARDAMOM TINCTURE (*Syn.* Tinctura Carminativa):

Cardamom oil	3 ml
Caraway oil	10 ml
Cinnamon oil	10 ml
Clove oil	10 ml
Strong ginger tincture	60 ml
Alcohol (90%)	to 1000 ml

Mix.
A standard for this tincture is given in the British Pharmaceutical Codex 1973
Dose: 0.12 to 0.6 millilitre.

COMPOUND CARDAMOM TINCTURE:

Cardamom oil	0.45 ml
Cochineal, in moderately coarse powder	7 g
Cinnamon oil	0.225 ml
Caraway oil	0.4 ml
Glycerol	50.0 ml
Alcohol (60%)	to 1000.0 ml

Moisten the cochineal with a sufficient quantity of the alcohol and prepare 900 ml of tincture by the percolation process as described in the entry on Tinctures; add the cardamom oil, the cinnamon oil, the caraway oil, and the glycerol, and sufficient of the alcohol to produce the required volume. Mix, and filter if necessary.
A standard for this tincture is given in the British Pharmacopoeia 1973
Dose: 2 to 5 ml.

Cardiac Arrhythmias

The cardiac arrhythmias (Dysrhythmias) are a group of conditions in which the normal rate or rhythm of the heart is altered. This may be due to interference with the conduction mechanisms in the heart or the generation of impulses which may be associated with disorders of autonomic control.

Tachycardia. In tachycardia the heart rate is abnormally rapid, usually because of diminished vagal tone or sympathetic stimulation. It often occurs in heart failure where it may either assist in maintaining cardiac output or, more commonly, make failure worse by reducing the efficiency of the myocardium. It may be caused by excessive consumption of coffee, alcohol, or tobacco, or by drugs such as atropine and other drugs having an anticholinergic effect that affect the autonomic nervous system, reducing vagal tone. It is usually symptomless and requires no treatment.
Paroxysmal atrial tachycardia is characterised by sudden onset and termination of periods of tachycardia. It may be associated with various forms of heart disease. Attacks may be terminated by massage of the carotid sinus or the use of defibrillant drugs such as quinidine or verapamil, cardiotonic drugs such as digitalis, or beta-adrenergic blocking drugs such as propranolol.

Bradycardia. Bradycardia is an unusually slow heart rate resulting from increased vagal tone or diminished sympathetic tone. It may occur during convalescence from certain infections and is also observed in some normal subjects such as well-trained athletes. Bradycardia also occurs after myocardial infarction and in raised intracranial pressure. Cardiotonic drugs such as digitalis, beta-adrenergic blocking drugs, analgesics of the morphine type, and some antihypertensive drugs, such as clonidine, also slow the heart rate leading to bradycardia.

Ectopic beats. Ectopic beats are cardiac contractions which arise earlier than expected in the cardiac cycle. They are caused by impulse formation at some abnormal focus of electrical activity which may be in either the atria or the ventricles. Most ectopic beats are followed by a diastolic pause, as the ectopic beat renders the cardiac muscle refractory to the effects of the next normal impulse. Thus there is coupling of heart beats followed by a long pause. The premature contraction will produce only a small pulse at the wrist, since there will have been only a short time for cardiac filling.

Ectopic beats may occasionally be observed in people with normal hearts, especially those who consume large quantities of tea, coffee, tobacco, or alcohol. Ectopic beats may also be associated with rheumatic heart disease, ischaemic heart disease, acute myocardial infarction, and hypertension. They may be induced by overdosage with cardiotonic drugs such as digitalis.

Ectopic beats may be symptomless, but if palpitations occur in the absence of organic heart disease patients should be advised to avoid extensive consumption of tea, coffee, alcohol, or tobacco.

Atrial fibrillation. Atrial fibrillation is a common and important cardiac arrhythmia. Integrated atrial contraction disappears and is replaced by irregular rapid fibrillary twitching of the atrial muscle. This leads to irregular rapid ventricular contractions. Thus the pulse in atrial fibrillation is irregular in time and force. The weaker beats may not reach the wrist, so there is a " pulse deficit "—the pulse rate counted at the wrist being lower than that counted at the heart. Some patients may be unaware of any irregular heart action, but many experience palpitations. Attacks of atrial fibrillation may be accompanied by dizziness, syncope, and ischaemic pain. Atrial fibrillation is usually associated with organic heart disease, such as rheumatic heart disease, mitral stenosis, and ischaemic heart disease. Other causative factors include thyrotoxicosis, especially in the elderly, and hypertension. Less commonly carcinoma of the bronchus, other neoplasms, chest disease, congenital heart disease, and bacterial endocarditis and pericarditis may be involved. In the presence of other serious heart disease, the onset of atrial fibrillation may lead to heart failure. Systemic emboli are common complications when atrial fibrillation is due to valvular disease. Onset of atrial fibrillation may be precipitated by alcohol and physical or mental stress.

Any underlying cause should be treated. When there is tachycardia or any evidence of congestive heart failure, cardiotonic drugs such as digitalis are used to reduce the rapid ventricular rate. If there is no evidence of serious organic disease, atrial fibrillation may be converted to normal rhythm by defibrillants such as quinidine or by direct current shock.

Atrial flutter is a condition similar to atrial fibrillation in which there is coordinated but rapid atrial muscle action, slower than in atrial fibrillation but more rapid than in paroxysmal atrial tachycardia. Paroxysms of atrial flutter last much longer than those of paroxysmal atrial tachycardia. Atrial flutter is almost always associated with organic heart disease and readily progresses to the more commonly encountered atrial fibrillation. Symptoms and treatment are similar to those of atrial fibrillation.

Heart block (Atrioventricular block). In heart block there is a defective conduction of the cardiac impulse from the atria to the ventricles. This may be due to a defect in either the atrioventricular node or the bundle of His. In partial heart block the cardiac impulse may be delayed in its conduction from the atria to the ventricles, or intermittent failure of atrioventricular conduction may cause beats to be dropped. In complete heart block there may be complete atrioventricular dissociation so that the ventricles beat at their intrinsic rate of about 30 to 40 beats per minute. This rate is completely dissociated from and unaffected by external stimuli. However, because of the slow rate, there is increased ventricular filling which may maintain a normal cardiac output.

Heart block is usually due either to anatomical lesions of the conducting system, or to coronary artery disease. It may also be a result of overdosage with cardiotonic drugs. In complete heart block there may be no symptoms but attacks of sudden syncope commonly occur (Stokes-Adams syndrome). The loss of consciousness is sudden with no preceding aura, and is associated with extreme bradycardia (10–20 beats per minute). Consciousness returns when the ventricular rate increases. Adrenergic drugs such as isoprenaline may be given by intravenous infusion or by mouth to increase the heart rate and prevent Stokes-Adams attacks, but intolerable palpitations or ventricular extrasystoles may prevent their continued use. Corticosteroids may increase the pulse rate or restore sinus rhythm. However, in established heart block artificial pacemaking of the heart is indicated.

Bundle branch block. This is a condition in which the cardiac impulses reaching the ventricles are incoordinated leading to asynchronous contraction. Treatment for the underlying heart disease may be required.

Ventricular tachycardia. This is a condition in which the ventricles beat rapidly due to an abnormal focus of excitation within the ventricles themselves. It is usually due to coronary atherosclerosis or myocardial infarction, or to overdosage with cardiotonic drugs such as digitalis or sympathomimetic amines. Acute cardiac failure, ventricular fibrillation and death follow if the condition is not treated with direct current shock or antidysrhythmic drugs such as lignocaine, procainamide, phenytoin, quinidine, or intramuscular bretylium.

Ventricular fibrillation. This is a serious condition in which the ventricles fail to contract effectively and cardiac output falls so that perfusion of vital organs such as the brain ceases. Death rapidly follows if the condition is not reversed with antidysrhythmic drugs such as lignocaine, procainamide, or quinidine, or by direct current shock. Its causes are those of ventricular tachycardia.

Cardiac Infarction

see under MYOCARDIAL INFARCTION

Carmine

The aluminium lake of the colouring matter of cochineal, the dried female insect *Dactylopius coccus* Costa. It contains about 50% of carminic acid and may be prepared by treating an aqueous infusion of cochineal with alum.

A standard is given in the British Pharmaceutical Codex 1973

Carmine may be infected with salmonellae and it must be pasteurised or treated in some other appropriate manner to ensure the destruction of any viable salmonella organisms present.

Description. Light bright-red pieces, readily reducible to powder.

Solubility. Practically insoluble in water and in dilute acids; readily soluble in dilute ammonia solution and in other dilute alkaline solutions, forming a dark purplish-red solution.

Moisture content. 10 to 21%, determined by drying at 105°.

Sterilisation. It may be sterilised by heating in an autoclave; if necessary, it should be subsequently dried at 80°.

Storage. It should be stored in airtight containers.

Uses. Carmine is used for colouring ointments, tooth powders, mouth-washes, dusting-powders, medicines, and other preparations. If it is used in solid form, prolonged trituration with a powder is necessary to obtain a good colour and an even distribution. To obtain the maximum colour, carmine should be dissolved in a small quantity of strong ammonia solution before triturating with the powder. The colouring matter is precipitated in acid solution.

Carmine passes unchanged through the gastro-intestinal tract and is used as a "marker" in metabolism experiments in a dose of 200 to 500 milligrams, administered in a cachet or gelatin capsule.

Cascara

The dried bark of *Rhamnus purshiana* DC. (Fam. Rhamnaceae), a small tree growing in North California, Oregon, Washington, and British Columbia.

OTHER NAMES: Casc.; Cascara Sagrada; Rhamni Purshianae Cortex

A standard is given in the European Pharmacopoeia Vol. II

The bark is collected in the spring and early summer and dried. It was formerly available as quilled, channelled, or nearly flat pieces, known commercially as "natural" cascara, but all supplies of the drug are now processed into small, nearly flat, uniform fragments known commercially as "evenised", "processed", or "compact" cascara bark.

Constituents. Cascara contains about 6 to 9% of anthraquinone glycosides; the most important are cascarosides A and B [glucosides of barbaloin, a 10-glucopyranosyl derivative of aloe-emodin anthrone (10-glucopyranosyl-9,10-dihydro-1,8-dihydroxy-3-hydroxymethyl-9-oxoanthracene)] and cascarosides C and D [glucosides of chrysaloin (11-deoxybarbaloin, 10-glucopyranosyl-9,10-dihydro-1,8-dihydroxy-3-methyl-9-oxoanthracene)]. Several glycosides of emodin (9,10-dihydro-1,6,8-trihydroxy-3-methyl-9,10-dioxoanthracene), of emodin oxanthrone (9,10-dihydro-1,6,8,10-tetrahydroxy-3-methyl-9-oxoanthracene), of aloe-emodin (9,10-dihydro-1,8-dihydroxy-3-hydroxymethyl-9,10-dioxoanthracene), and of chrysophanol (9,10-dihydro-1,8-dihydroxy-3-methyl-9,10-dioxoanthracene) are also present. Small quantities of breakdown products from these glycosides occur, including barbaloin, chrysaloin, aloe-emodin, chrysophanol, and emodin. The cascarosides are almost tasteless, but barbaloin and chrysaloin are extremely bitter.

Up to 1% of foreign organic matter may be present. It yields up to 6% of sulphated ash.

The bark yields to water from 23 to 28% of extractive.

Description. UNGROUND DRUG. *Macroscopical characters:* quilled, channelled, or nearly flat pieces from 1 to 4 mm thick, varying greatly in length and breadth, usually broken into small, nearly flat, uniform fragments; outer surface nearly smooth, cork dark purplish-brown and bearing scattered lenticels; usually more or less completely covered by a whitish coat of lichens and some pieces of bark with many small mosses and foliaceous liverworts growing epiphytically on the outer surface; mussel-scale insects also often present; inner surface yellow to reddish-brown or nearly black, with longitudinal striations and faint transverse corrugations; fracture short; somewhat fibrous near inner surface; smoothed transversely cut surface exhibiting a narrow, purplish cork, a yellowish-grey cortex with darker translucent groups of sclerenchymatous cells, and a brownish-yellow phloem traversed by slightly wavy medullary rays.

It has a characteristic nauseous odour and a persistently bitter taste.

Microscopical characters: the diagnostic characters are: *sclereids* in groups in cortex and phloem; *phloem fibres* slender, in bundles accompanied by *crystal sheaths* with prisms of calcium oxalate; *sieve tubes* thin-walled, with well-defined sieve plates on the oblique end walls; *cluster crystals* of calcium oxalate scattered throughout the parenchyma, the cells of which contain a yellow substance; when bryophytic epiphytes are present the powder may contain either the leaves of liverworts, entire or in fragments, exhibiting a lamina one cell thick, composed of isodiametric cells and having no midrib, or the leaves of mosses, having a lamina one cell thick composed of somewhat elongated cells and possessing a midrib several cells thick, or both.

POWDERED DRUG. Powdered Cascara. A light yellowish-brown to olive-brown powder possessing the diagnostic microscopical characters, odour, and taste of the unground drug.

Adulterants and substitutes. The bark of *R. californica* Eschscholz is occasionally substituted for the official drug.

The bark of *R. cathartica* L. is glossy, reddish-brown and has very distinct lenticels.

Frangula bark, the young bark of *Frangula alnus* Mill. (Fam. Rhamnaceae), occurs as single or double quills, about 10 to 20 mm wide, with an outer surface of smooth dark-purplish cork bearing numerous transversely elongated whitish lenticels; when gently scraped, the deep crimson colour of the inner layers of cork becomes evident; fracture short in the cork and cortex and fibrous in the phloem; the older bark is rougher externally, thicker, usually occurring in single quills or channelled pieces; taste sweetish or slightly bitter. The microscopical characters resemble those of cascara, from which it is distinguished by the absence of groups of sclereids.

Storage. It should be stored in a cool place. Powdered cascara should be stored in airtight containers, in a cool place.

Identification. TESTS. 1. Place a small quantity of the drug, in powder, on a microscope slide, add one drop of *sodium hydroxide solution*, and examine. The yellow substance present in the cells of the parenchyma is coloured violet.

2. Heat about 100 mg with 50 ml of water for 15 minutes on a water-bath, cool, filter, and to 10 ml of the filtrate add 20 ml of hydrochloric acid, heat for 15 minutes on a water-bath, cool, transfer to a separating funnel, extract with three 20-ml portions of ether, combine the ether extracts and reserve the aqueous layer. Shake the ethereal solution with 10 ml of *dilute ammonia solution*; a reddish-purple colour is produced in the ammoniacal layer.

3. To the aqueous layer, reserved in Test 2, add 5 g of ferric chloride, heat for 30 minutes on a water-bath, cool, extract with 15 ml of chloroform, wash the chloroform layer with 10 ml of water, discard the water, and shake the chloroform layer with 5 ml of *dilute ammonia solution*; a rose-pink to cherry-red colour is produced in the ammoniacal layer.

Actions and uses. Cascara is an anthraquinone purgative with actions and uses similar to those of senna fruit. It is used as the dry extract in tablets, or as the liquid extract, or as the more pleasant tasting elixir.
The glycosides of cascara are excreted in the milk and may increase bowel activity in breast-fed infants.

Preparations

CASCARA AND BELLADONNA MIXTURE (*Syn.* Compound Cascara Mixture):

Cascara elixir	200 ml
Belladonna tincture	50 ml
Chloroform water, double-strength	500 ml
Water for preparations	to 1000 ml

It must be freshly prepared.
Dose: 10 to 20 millilitres.
Containers and *Labelling:* see the entry on Mixtures for general information on containers and labelling.
Advice for patients: the mixture should not be used for longer than a few days without medical advice. It may colour the urine red or yellow.

CASCARA DRY EXTRACT: may be prepared by exhausting cascara, in coarse powder, with hot purified water by percolation and evaporating the percolate to dryness. It contains at least 13% of total hydroxyanthracene derivatives of which not less than 40% consists of cascarosides; both quantities are calculated as cascaroside A.
A standard for this dry extract is given in the British Pharmacopoeia 1973
Labelling: the label should state the percentage content of total hydroxyanthracene derivatives.
Storage: it should be stored in airtight containers.

CASCARA ELIXIR:

Cascara, in coarse powder	1000.0 g
Saccharin sodium	1.0 g
Light magnesium oxide	50.0 g
Liquorice, unpeeled, in coarse powder	125.0 g
Coriander oil	0.15 ml
Anise oil	0.2 ml
Alcohol (90%)	12.5 ml
Glycerol	300.0 ml
Water for preparations	to 1000.0 ml

Mix the cascara, the liquorice, and the light magnesium oxide and moisten with 1250 ml of boiling water, stirring thoroughly. Macerate for 24 hours in a well-covered vessel, pack moderately tightly in a percolator, and percolate with boiling water until exhausted.
Evaporate the percolate to about 650 ml on a water-bath. Dissolve the saccharin sodium in 12 ml of water and the coriander oil and the anise oil in the alcohol. Mix both solutions with the glycerol and add the concentrated percolate and sufficient water to produce 1000 ml.
Shake thoroughly and allow to stand for not less than 12 hours; filter, if necessary.
A standard for this elixir is given in the British Pharmaceutical Codex 1973
Dose: 2 to 5 millilitres.
Advice for patients: the elixir should not be used for longer than a few days without medical advice. It may colour the urine red or yellow.

CASCARA LIQUID EXTRACT:

Cascara, in coarse powder	1000 g
Alcohol (90%)	250 ml
Purified water	to 1000 ml

Exhaust the cascara with the water by percolation and evaporate the percolate to about 600 ml; add the alcohol, previously mixed with 150 ml of the water and, if necessary, sufficient of the water to produce 1000 ml. Allow to stand for not less than 4 weeks and filter.
A standard for this liquid extract is given in the British Pharmacopoeia 1973
Dose: 2 to 5 millilitres.

CASCARA TABLETS: containing cascara dry extract; they may be sugar-coated. Each tablet contains 17 to 23 mg of total hydroxyanthracene derivatives of which not less than 40% consists of cascarosides; both quantities are calculated as cascaroside A.
A standard for these tablets is given in the British Pharmacopoeia 1973
Containers and *Storage:* see the entry on Tablets for general information on containers and storage. Containers should be airtight.
Dose: 1 or 2 tablets.
Advice for patients: the tablets should not be used for longer than a few days without medical advice. They may colour the urine red or yellow.

OTHER PREPARATION: cascara elixir is an ingredient of compound figs syrup.

Castor Oil

The fixed oil obtained by cold expression from the seeds of *Ricinus communis* L. (Fam. Euphorbiaceae). The expressed oil is steamed to coagulate proteins and, after filtration, is usually bleached by exposure to the sun or by chemical means.

OTHER NAME: Oleum Ricini

A standard is given in the European Pharmacopoeia Vol. III

Constituents. Castor oil consists chiefly of the triglyceride of ricinoleic acid (12-hydroxyoleic acid), which is present to the extent of about 80%. It also contains small amounts of other glycerides, the fatty acid constituents of which include oleic, linoleic, stearic, and 9,10-dihydroxystearic acids.

Description. It is a nearly colourless or faintly yellow viscous oil with a slight odour. On cooling to 0° it remains bright, but on cooling to $-18°$ it congeals to a yellowish mass.
The most distinctive features of the oil are its high density, the highest of any natural fatty oil, its behaviour with light petroleum (see below), its solubility in alcohol (90%), its high acetyl value, and its high viscosity.

Solubility. Soluble, at 20°, in 2.5 parts of alcohol (90%); miscible with dehydrated alcohol, with ether, and with glacial acetic acid.

Weight per ml. At 20°, 0.953 to 0.965 g.

Refractive index. 1.477 to 1.481.

Optical rotation. Not less than $+3.5°$.

Sterilisation. It is sterilised by dry heat.

Storage. It should be stored in well-filled airtight containers.

Identification. TEST. It gives a clear solution with half its volume of light petroleum (boiling-range, 40° to 60°); it is only partially soluble in 2 volumes.

Actions and uses. Castor oil is a purgative, its action being exerted in 4 to 8 hours. The usual dose is 5 to

20 millilitres. It is best administered in milk or fruit juice. It stimulates both the small and the large intestines. Castor oil has been largely replaced by more pleasant and less drastic purgatives unless prompt and thorough evacuation of the bowel is required. It should be used with caution during pregnancy and menstruation.

Castor oil is emollient and is used in preparations such as zinc and castor oil ointment. Sterilised castor oil is a soothing application when dropped into the eye after removal of foreign bodies; it is used as an oily vehicle for eye-drops.

Preparation

ZINC AND CASTOR OIL OINTMENT (*Syn.* Zinc and Castor Oil Cream; Zinc and Castor Oil):

Zinc oxide, finely sifted	75 g
Castor oil	500 g
Cetostearyl alcohol	20 g
White beeswax	100 g
Arachis oil	305 g

Triturate the zinc oxide with a portion of the castor oil until smooth and add the mixture to the remainder of the ingredients previously melted together; stir until the temperature is about 40°.

A standard for this ointment is given in the British Pharmacopoeia 1973
Containers and *Labelling:* see the entry on Ointments for general information on containers and labelling.

Catechu

A dried aqueous extract prepared from the leaves and young shoots of *Uncaria gambir* (Hunter) Roxb. (Fam. Rubiaceae), a climbing shrub indigenous to and cultivated in the Malay Archipelago.

OTHER NAMES: Pale Catechu; Gambir

A standard is given in the British Pharmacopoeia Addendum 1977 and in the British Pharmacopoeia (Veterinary)

Constituents. Catechu contains about 7 to 33% of (+)-catechin, which may be obtained as a tetrahydrate consisting of white silky needles having a melting-point of about 95°.

On drying over sulphuric acid catechin forms a monohydrate having a melting-point of 175°; on drying at 100° it becomes anhydrous and melts at about 177°. It is sparingly soluble in cold water (1 in 1100 to 1200), but more soluble in boiling water and in alcohol, and produces with ferric salts a deep green colour.

Other constituents are 22 to 50% of catechutannic acid, which is coloured dirty green by ferric salts, and small amounts of (+)-epicatechin, quercetin, wax, fixed oil, catechu red, and a fluorescent substance, gambier-fluorescein, and traces of indole alkaloids such as gambirine, gambirtannine, dihydrogambirtannine, and oxogambirtannine. Catechu also contains mineral matter (about 3 to 5%) and vegetable debris.

Catechu contains up to 33% of water-insoluble matter, up to 34% of alcohol (95%)-insoluble matter and up to 15% of moisture.

Description. UNGROUND DRUG. *Macroscopical characters:* cubes, usually irregular and agglutinated and mixed with fragments of broken cubes; friable and porous, measuring about 25 mm in each direction, larger cubes and brick-shaped pieces up to 50 mm long, sometimes broken into angular fragments; external surface light brown to black, freshly broken surface pale cinnamon brown, occasionally showing darker streaks.

It is odourless with a taste which at first is bitter and very astringent but subsequently sweetish.

Microscopical characters: the diagnostic characters are: *crystals,* acicular, numerous in abundant yellowish-brown masses, composed of catechin and soluble in hot water; varying amounts of fragments from the leaves and shoots of the plant also present, including: *trichomes,* unicellular, non-glandular, occurring singly or in groups attached to pieces of epidermis, mostly about 250 to 540 μm long, lignified, with 1 or 2 thin, transverse septa, base pitted, also a few smaller, about 25 to 45 μm long, conical, with unlignified, warty walls; *epidermis of leaves,* cells thin-walled, slightly sinuous and polygonal, *cuticle* finely striated, *stomata* paracytic, on abaxial surface only; *epidermis of corolla* reddish-brown, with numerous non-glandular *trichomes,* these sometimes broken off leaving characteristic pitted and lignified *cicatrices; parenchymatous cells* containing cluster and microsphenoidal crystals of calcium oxalate; *cork* present as occasional fragments; *pollen grains* sub-spherical, about 11 to 18 μm in diameter with 3 pores and 3 furrows, extine covered with minute scattered pits.

POWDERED DRUG: Powdered Catechu. A pale brown, odourless powder possessing the diagnostic microscopical characters and taste of the unground drug.

Adulterants and substitutes. Black catechu (cutch) is the dried aqueous extract prepared from the heartwood of *Acacia catechu* Willd. and possibly other species of *Acacia* (Fam. Leguminosae). It occurs in irregular dark brown to almost black masses, frequently having pieces of brownish-buff leaves attached to them; it contains acacatechin, which is an optically inactive form of catechin, 25 to 50% of catechutannic acid, quercetin, and catechu red.

Incompatibility. It is incompatible with iron salts and with gelatin.

Identification. TEST. Warm 0.3 g with 2 ml of alcohol (95%), cool, and filter; to the filtrate add 2 ml of *sodium hydroxide solution,* shake, add 2 ml of light petroleum (boiling-range, 40° to 60°), shake, and allow to separate; a brilliant greenish fluorescence is produced in the upper layer (distinction from black catechu).

Actions and uses. Catechu is an astringent and is used in conjunction with other astringents in the symptomatic treatment of diarrhoea.

Preparations

CATECHU TINCTURE:

Catechu, crushed	200 g
Cinnamon, bruised	50 g
Alcohol (45%)	1000 ml

Prepare by the maceration process as described in the entry on Tinctures.
A standard for this tincture is given in the British Pharmaceutical Codex 1973
Dose: 2.5 to 5 millilitres.

OTHER PREPARATION: catechu tincture is an ingredient of aromatic chalk with opium mixture.

Cellacephate

Cellulose in which about half of the hydroxyl groups are acetylated and about one-quarter are esterified with one of the two acid groups of phthalic acid.

OTHER NAMES: Cellulose Acetate Phthalate; Cellulosi Acetas Phthalas

A standard is given in the European Pharmacopoeia Vol. III

Description. A white, hygroscopic, tasteless, free-flowing powder or colourless flakes; odourless or with a faint odour of acetic acid.

Solubility. Practically insoluble in water; soluble, at 20°, in 6 parts of a mixture of equal volumes of ethyl acetate and isopropyl alcohol and in 4 parts of acetone containing 0.4% v/v of water (the solution may be slightly turbid if less water is present); soluble in diethylene glycol and in dioxan; very slightly soluble in alcohol and in chloroform.

Moisture content. Not more than 5%, determined by Fischer titration.

Stability. Cellacephate hydrolyses fairly rapidly if its moisture content is above about 6%.

Hygroscopicity. Its equilibrium moisture content, at room temperature and a relative humidity of 50%, is about 5% and, at a relative humidity of 75%, about 9%.

Storage. It should be stored in airtight containers.

Identification. TESTS. 1. Mix about 10 mg with 0.5 ml of alcohol (95%) and 0.5 ml of sulphuric acid; the odour of ethyl acetate is produced.
2. Mix about 50 mg with 2 ml of *dilute sodium hydroxide solution* and 2 ml of water, warm to dissolve, boil to form a gel, and cool; add 3 ml of *dilute hydrochloric acid*, extract with 5 ml of solvent ether, allow to separate, and evaporate the ether layer to dryness. Heat the residue with 10 mg of resorcinol and 0.5 ml of sulphuric acid, allow the reaction to subside, cool, dilute the greenish-brown mixture with 10 ml of water, and make alkaline with *strong ammonia solution*; a reddish-brown solution is produced which, on dilution, has an intense green fluorescence.
3. Dissolve 100 mg in 1 ml of acetone and allow to evaporate in a glass dish; a clear glossy film is produced.

Uses. Cellacephate is used in the form of a solution in a suitable solvent, such as acetone or a mixture of ethyl acetate and isopropyl alcohol, for the enteric coating of tablets and capsules. It is generally used in conjunction with plasticisers, such as diethyl phthalate, castor oil, or triacetin, and waxes such as carnauba wax are often incorporated to retard the penetration of water from acid media.

Cellulose, Microcrystalline

Partially depolymerised cellulose prepared by acid hydrolysis of purified wood cellulose. It has a molecular weight of about 36000.

OTHER NAME: *Avicel*®

A standard is given in the British Pharmaceutical Codex 1973

There are two pharmaceutical grades of microcrystalline cellulose commercially available, one being a colloidal water-dispersible powder having a much smaller average particle size than the other non-dispersible powder. The colloidal type may contain a small percentage of sodium carboxymethylcellulose to aid its dispersion.

Description. A fine, white, odourless powder.

Microscopical characters: mounted in lactophenol the non-dispersible type exhibits particles of various sizes and irregular shapes, many pieces about 100 to 150 μm long and 20 to 30 μm wide showing numerous cracks and a rather irregular outline and also many minute particles about 10 to 50 μm in width or length and marked with short irregular lines.
The particles of the colloidal type are similar in appearance but smaller, most being about 12 to 15 μm or occasionally up to 18 μm, and some rather square, about 40 μm, or somewhat elongated, about 50 μm by 10 to 20 μm.
Between crossed polars on a dark field the material shines brightly.
Crystalline structures are absent.

Solubility. Both types of powder are practically insoluble in water, but the colloidal type is dispersible, forming colloidal suspensions at low concentrations and thixotropic gels at higher concentrations. Both types are partially soluble in dilute alkalis with swelling; practically insoluble in acids and in most organic solvents.

Loss on drying. Not more than 5%, determined by drying at 105°.

Sterilisation. Gels prepared from the colloidal grade are sterilised by heating in an autoclave.

Labelling. The label on the container indicates whether the material is intended for use in tabletting or as a suspending agent.

Identification. TESTS. 1. To about 1 mg add 1 ml of phosphoric acid, heat on a water-bath for 30 minutes, add 4 ml of a 0.2% solution of catechol in phosphoric acid, and heat for a further 30 minutes; a red colour is produced.
2. Soak in *iodine water* for a few minutes and remove the excess of reagent with the aid of a filter paper; it is not stained blue (distinction from starch). Add one or two drops of sulphuric acid (66% v/v); it is stained blue (distinction from certain other cellulose derivatives).
3. Treat with *phloroglucinol solution* followed by hydrochloric acid; no red colour is produced.

Uses. The non-dispersible type of microcrystalline cellulose is used as a binder, filler, disintegrant, and lubricant in tablets. Water-soluble active ingredients can be adsorbed on to the material before compression. The colloidal type of powder is used to produce gels and to act, in conjunction with other materials, as a suspending agent. Although particle size is small, disaggregation in water by high shear produces particles of sub-micron size which interact as a network to form thixotropic gels when the concentration exceeds 1%. The degree of shear-mixing required to produce a gel varies with the grade used and the rheology of a particular grade depends on the intensity of mixing. Gel rheology does not vary greatly with temperature, permitting sterilisation by autoclaving.
The function of sodium carboxymethylcellulose, or other agents used to aid dispersion, is to act as a protective colloid. Unlike some naturally occurring suspending agents, microcrystalline cellulose is free from serious microbiological contamination.
Microcrystalline cellulose is widely used either alone or in conjunction with other cellulose derivatives such as sodium carboxymethylcellulose and hypromellose and clays such as bentonite, which modify susceptibility to

flocculation, thixotropy, and other properties of the gel, as a "bodying" agent, suspending agent, and emulsion stabiliser. By varying the concentrations of components, most insoluble materials can be permanently suspended at a gel consistency which permits pouring.

Cephalexin

(7R)-3-Methyl-7-(α- D-phenylglycylamino)ceph-3-em-4-carboxylic acid monohydrate

$C_{16}H_{17}N_3O_4S,H_2O = 365.4$

OTHER NAMES: Cefalexin; *Ceporex®*; *Keflex®*

A standard is given in the British Pharmacopoeia 1973

Description. A white to cream-coloured crystalline powder with a characteristic odour.

Solubility. Soluble, at 20°, in 100 parts of water and in 30 parts of diluted hydrochloric acid (0.2% w/v); very slightly soluble in alcohol, in ether, in chloroform, and in acetone.

Acidity. A 0.5% solution has a pH of 3.5 to 5.5.

Moisture content. 4 to 8%, determined by Fischer titration.

Dissociation constants. pK_a 5.2 (carboxyl), 7.3 (amine).

Stability. Aqueous solutions and suspensions degrade rapidly in neutral or alkaline systems; in acid conditions they are stable for several days if refrigerated. Stability is optimum at pH 4.5.

FURTHER INFORMATION. Stability and other aspects of formulation—C. M. Bond *et al.*, *Pharm. J.*, ii/1970, 210; H. Bundegaard, *Arch. Pharm. Chemi, scient. Edn*, 1976, **4**, 25; stability and other properties of cephalexin, *Analytical Profiles of Drug Substances*, K. Florey (Ed.), Vol. 4, London, Academic Press, 1975, p. 21; T. Yamana and A. Tsuji, *J. pharm. Sci.*, 1976, **65**, 1563.

Hygroscopicity. It absorbs insignificant amounts of moisture at 20° at relative humidities up to about 20% but under damper conditions it absorbs substantial amounts.

Storage. It should be stored in airtight containers, at a temperature not exceeding 30°, protected from light.

Identification. TESTS. 1. Mix about 20 mg with a few drops of sulphuric acid (80% v/v) containing 1% v/v of nitric acid; a yellow colour is produced.
2. Mix about 20 mg with 5 drops of a 1% v/v solution of glacial acetic acid and add 2 drops of a 1% solution of copper sulphate and 1 drop of 2N sodium hydroxide; an olive-green colour is produced.

ULTRAVIOLET ABSORPTION. In water, maximum at 260 nm (E1%, 1cm = 232).

INFRA-RED ABSORPTION. Major peaks at 1266, 1351, 1389, 1587, 1695, and 1754 cm^{-1} (see Appendix 2b: Infra-red Spectra).

Metabolism. ABSORPTION. Cephalexin is acid stable and is readily absorbed after oral administration; food may delay absorption; intramuscular doses of the lysine salt are well absorbed.

BLOOD CONCENTRATION. After an oral dose of 500 mg, peak serum concentrations of about 20 µg/ml are attained in 1 hour; after intramuscular and intravenous doses of 1 g, serum concentrations of about 20 µg/ml in 1 hour and about 50 µg/ml in 15 minutes are attained respectively; peak concentrations are subject to wide individual variation.

HALF-LIFE. Serum half-life, about 0.5 to 2 hours in patients with normal renal function; in the newborn, it is 2.5 to 5 hours and in patients with severe renal failure, about 20 hours.

DISTRIBUTION. Widely distributed throughout the body, maximum concentrations being reached in the liver and kidneys; cephalexin does not accumulate following multiple doses; it does not enter the cerebrospinal fluid unless the meninges are inflamed but it does cross the placenta and it is secreted in the milk; volume of distribution, about 24 litres; *protein binding*, 6 to 15% bound to plasma proteins.

METABOLIC REACTIONS. Cephalexin is not metabolised in the body.

EXCRETION. 60 to 100% is excreted unchanged in the urine in 8 hours; small amounts are excreted in the bile; probenecid delays renal excretion.

FURTHER INFORMATION. Review of metabolism and pharmacokinetics of cephalosporins—C. H. Nightingale *et al.*, *J. pharm. Sci.*, 1975, **64**, 1899; review of metabolism and pharmacokinetics of cephalexin—T. M. Speight *et al.*, *Drugs*, 1972, **3**, 9.

Actions and uses. Cephalexin is one of the cephalosporin antibiotics and has the same mode of action, antigenicity, and spectrum of activity as cephaloridine. Cephalexin is not affected by Gram-negative penicillinases and this is sometimes of clinical importance but, in general, organisms resistant to other cephalosporins will not respond to cephalexin. Blood levels may be increased by blocking tubular excretion with probenecid.

Cephalexin is well absorbed after oral administration and adequate blood levels can usually be maintained by a dose of 500 milligrams every 6 hours. The usual dose for children is 25 to 50 milligrams per kilogram body-weight daily in divided doses.

Undesirable effects. Cephalexin may cause abdominal discomfort and diarrhoea in some patients but otherwise its side-effects are similar to those described under Cephaloridine.

Precautions. It should be used with caution in allergic patients, especially when there is a history of penicillin allergy.

Preparations

CEPHALEXIN CAPSULES: containing cephalexin, in powder, which may be mixed with a suitable inert diluent, enclosed in a hard capsule. The capsule shells may be coloured. Available as capsules containing 250 and 500 mg of cephalexin.

A standard is given in the British Pharmacopoeia 1973
Containers and *Storage:* see the entry on Capsules for general information on containers and storage.
Labelling: the label on the container should state the directions for storage and the date after which the capsules are not intended to be used.
Advice for patients: the capsules should be taken at

regular intervals. The prescribed course should be completed.

CEPHALEXIN MIXTURE: a suspension of cephalexin in a suitable flavoured vehicle which may be coloured. It is prepared freshly by dispersing granules consisting of the dry mixed ingredients in the specified volume of water for preparations.

When a dose less than or not a multiple of 5 ml is prescribed, the mixture may be diluted, as described in the entry on Mixtures, with a suitable diluent. *Ceporex®* may be diluted with water and *Keflex®* may be diluted with syrup.

Available as mixtures containing, when reconstituted, 125, 250, and 500 mg in 5 ml.

A standard for this mixture is given in the British Pharmaceutical Codex 1973

Containers: see the entry on Mixtures for general information on containers.

Labelling: see the entry on Mixtures for general information on labelling. The name on the label of the container of the dry granules should be "Granules for Cephalexin Mixture".

Storage: the mixture and the diluted mixture should be stored in a cool place and used within the period stated on the label.

Advice for patients: the mixture should be taken at regular intervals. The prescribed course should be completed.

CEPHALEXIN TABLETS: available as tablets containing 250 and 500 mg of cephalexin. They may be coloured; they may be film coated and the coat may be coloured.

A standard for these tablets is given in the British Pharmacopoeia 1973

Containers and *Storage:* see the entry on Tablets for general information on containers and storage. Containers should be airtight.

Labelling: the label on the container should state the directions for storage and the date after which the tablets are not intended to be used.

Advice for patients: the tablets should be taken at regular intervals. The prescribed course should be completed.

OTHER PREPARATIONS available include a MIXTURE containing, when reconstituted, 125 mg of cephalexin in 1.25 ml; and a mixture containing 125 and 250 mg of cephalexin in 5 ml (ready prepared).

Cephaloridine

(7R)-3-(1-Pyridiniomethyl)-7-[(thien-2-yl)acetamido]-ceph-3-em-4-carboxylate (α-form or δ-form)

$C_{19}H_{17}N_3O_4S_2 = 415.5$

OTHER NAMES: Cefaloridinum; *Ceporin®*

A standard is given in the European Pharmacopoeia Vol. III

Description. A white crystalline powder with a bitter taste; odourless or with a slight odour of pyridine. It discolours on exposure to light.

Solubility. Soluble, at 20°, in 5 parts of water and in 1000 parts of alcohol; very slightly soluble in ether and in chloroform.

Acidity. A 10% solution, prepared by dissolving at 30° and cooling to 20°, has a pH of 4 to 6.

Moisture content. Not more than 0.5% (α-form) or not more than 3% (δ-form), determined by Fischer titration.

Specific rotation. +46° to +50°, determined on a 1% solution.

Stability. Solutions containing 1 gram in 500 ml of compound sodium chloride injection, compound sodium lactate injection, Darrow's solution, sodium chloride and dextrose injection, calcium gluconate injection, or dextran injections, may be expected to retain their activity when stored for 24 hours at room temperature.

Incompatibility. Cephaloridine is unstable in solutions which contain both dextrose and sodium bicarbonate.

Labelling. The label on the container states whether the contents are the α-form or the δ-form.

Storage. It should be stored in sterile airtight containers, sealed to exclude micro-organisms, in a cool place, protected from light.

Identification. TESTS. 1. Mix about 20 mg with a few drops of sulphuric acid (80% v/v) containing 1% v/v of nitric acid; a permanent bluish-green colour is produced.
2. To a 0.5% aqueous solution add 1 ml of *chloramine solution* and 2 ml of 0.1N sodium hydroxide; a dull red colour is produced which persists for 1 minute.

ULTRAVIOLET ABSORPTION. In water, maximum at 240 nm (E1%, 1cm = 377).

INFRA-RED ABSORPTION. Major peaks at 1351, 1389, 1471, 1613, 1667, and 1754 cm^{-1} (see Appendix 2b: Infra-red Spectra).

Determination in body fluids. HIGH PRESSURE LIQUID CHROMATOGRAPHY. In serum—J. S. Wold and S. A. Turnipseed, *J. Chromat.*, 1977, **136**, 170.

Metabolism. ABSORPTION. Cephaloridine is acid labile and only about 5% of a dose is absorbed after oral administration; it is therefore administered by injection. Intramuscular doses are readily absorbed.

BLOOD CONCENTRATION. After an intramuscular dose of 0.5 g, peak serum concentrations of 10 to 30 μg/ml are attained within 30 to 60 minutes; after an intravenous dose of 1 g, serum concentrations of about 140 μg/ml are obtained within 10 minutes of administration.

HALF-LIFE. Serum half-life, 1 to 1.5 hours which is increased to about 23 hours in renal function impairment.

DISTRIBUTION. Widely distributed throughout the body but little appears in the cerebrospinal fluid unless the meninges are inflamed; it penetrates inflamed muscle, is secreted in milk, and crosses the placenta; accumulation may occur when renal function is impaired; volume of distribution, about 16 litres; *protein binding*, 20 to 35% bound to plasma proteins.

EXCRETION. 60 to 90% of intramuscular or intravenous doses is excreted unchanged in the urine in 24 hours mainly by glomerular filtration; urinary excretion is unaffected by probenecid. Urinary excretion increases with increasing urinary pH values.

FURTHER INFORMATION. Blood concentration and excretion—M. M. Cahn *et al.*, *J. clin. Pharmac.*, 1974, **14**, 61; P. De Scheppe *et al.*, *J. clin. Pharmac.*, 1973, **13**, 83; half-life in subjects undergoing haemodialysis—J. R. Curtis and M. J. Marshall, *Br. med. J.*, ii/1970, 149; review of metabolism and pharmacokinetics of cephalosporins—C. H. Nightingale *et al.*, *J. pharm. Sci.*, 1975,

64, 1899; availability from different injection sites—D. S. Reeves *et al., Lancet*, ii/1974, 1421.

Actions and uses. Cephaloridine is one of the cephalosporin antibiotics which have chemical structures related to penicillin. Their mode of action on the bacterial cell wall is similar to that of penicillin and like penicillin they are bactericidal. These antibiotics tend to promote allergy especially in patients already allergic to penicillin. They have a broader spectrum than benzylpenicillin, being relatively resistant to staphylococcal penicillinase and to some of the penicillinases produced by *Proteus mirabilis* and other coliform species. Therefore, although the cephalosporin antibiotics have a wide spectrum, resistance may occur in many bacterial species and successful use is dependent upon careful bacteriological assessment.

Cephaloridine is more susceptible to staphylococcal penicillinase than the other cephalosporins.

Cephaloridine is given by intramuscular injection, the usual dose being 0.5 to 1 gram every 8 to 12 hours for an adult or 20 to 40 milligrams per kilogram body-weight daily in divided doses for children. Up to 4 grams daily in divided doses may be given to adults. The dose should be reduced in patients with poor renal function. The administration of probenecid does not significantly increase the blood level of cephaloridine.

It is not absorbed when given by mouth and it diffuses poorly into the cerebrospinal fluid. It may be given intrathecally, the usual adult dose being 50 milligrams daily in 2 to 10 millilitres of sodium chloride injection or of the patient's own cerebrospinal fluid; for children, the usual dose is 500 micrograms per kilogram body-weight daily. Larger doses cause meningism.

Cephaloridine may be given by subconjunctival injection in a dose of 50 milligrams dissolved in 0.5 millilitre of water for injections.

Undesirable effects. High concentrations of cephaloridine in the blood may give rise to renal damage, convulsions, and an auto-immune type of haemolytic anaemia. At lower blood levels the development of a positive Coombs test may interfere with cross-matching procedures. Neutropenia may occur. Allergic rashes may also occur, especially in patients hypersensitive to penicillin.

Precautions. It should be used with care in patients with an allergic diathesis, especially those already sensitised to penicillin. The dose should be reduced in patients with poor renal function, as otherwise further increases in blood urea and tubular damage may occur.

Drug interactions. Cephaloridine may be nephrotoxic when used in conjunction with phenylbutazone. The use of cephaloridine with oral anticoagulants prolongs the prothrombin time. The concurrent use of cephaloridine and aminoglycoside antibiotics or potent diuretics such as frusemide is dangerous because they enhance the renal toxicity of cephaloridine.

Preparation

CEPHALORIDINE INJECTION: a sterile solution of cephaloridine in water for injections. It is prepared by dissolving the contents of a sealed container in water for injections shortly before use. Available as a powder in vials containing 0.1, 0.25, 0.5, and 1 g of cephaloridine as the δ-form.

A standard for this injection is given in the European Pharmacopoeia Vol. III

Containers: see the entry on Injections for general information on containers.

Labelling: see the entry on Injections for general information on labelling. In addition the label on the container should state whether the contents are cephaloridine (α-form) or cephaloridine (δ-form).

Storage: the sealed container should be stored in a cool place, protected from light. The injection contains no bactericide and should be used as soon as possible after preparation but solutions of cephaloridine may be expected to retain their potency for up to 4 days, provided they are stored at 2° to 10°. It should be noted that stored solutions, even if clear, may be supersaturated and should be warmed and thoroughly shaken before use to avoid possible crystallisation in the syringe.

Cephalothin Sodium

Sodium (7R)-7-(thien-2-ylacetamido)cephalosporanate

$C_{16}H_{15}N_2NaO_6S_2 = 418.4$

OTHER NAMES: Cefalotin Sodium; *Keflin®*

A standard is given in the British Pharmacopoeia 1973

Description. A white, crystalline, almost odourless powder.

Solubility. Soluble, at 20°, in 3.5 parts of water and in 700 parts of alcohol; practically insoluble in ether and in chloroform.

Acidity. A 10% solution has a pH of 4.5 to 7.

Stability. Aqueous solutions may be expected to retain their potency for 2 days when stored at 2° to 10° or for at least 6 hours at room temperature.

For intravenous infusion, cephalothin sodium may be administered in solution in dextrose injection (5%), sodium chloride injection, sodium chloride and dextrose injection, sodium lactate injection, and compound sodium lactate injection.

FURTHER INFORMATION. Stability of cephalothin sodium —T. Yamana and A. Tsuji, *J. pharm. Sci.*, 1976, **65**, 1563.

Labelling. If the material is not intended for parenteral administration, the label on the container states that the contents are not to be injected.

Storage. It should be stored in airtight containers, at a temperature not exceeding 25°, protected from light. If it is intended for parenteral administration, the containers should be sterile and sealed to exclude micro-organisms.

Identification. TEST. Mix about 20 mg with a few drops of sulphuric acid (80% v/v) containing 1% v/v of nitric acid; an olive-green colour is produced changing to reddish-brown.

ULTRAVIOLET ABSORPTION. In water, maximum at 237 nm (E1%, 1cm = 337).

INFRA-RED ABSORPTION. Major peaks at 1235, 1333, 1515, 1613, 1639, and 1695 cm^{-1} (see Appendix 2b: Infra-red Spectra).

Metabolism. ABSORPTION. Cephalothin is acid labile and only about 2% of a dose is absorbed after oral administration; it is therefore administered by injection. Intramuscular doses are well absorbed.

BLOOD CONCENTRATION. After an intravenous dose of 0.5 g, serum concentrations of 20 to 40 μg/ml are obtained and after an intramuscular dose of 0.5 g, peak serum concentrations of 6 to 20 μg/ml are attained in about 30 minutes.

HALF-LIFE. Serum half-life, 30 to 85 minutes which may be increased to about 5 to 17 hours in renal disease.

DISTRIBUTION. Widely distributed throughout the body; very little appears in the cerebrospinal fluid even when the meninges are inflamed; it crosses the placenta; small amounts are secreted in milk; *protein binding*, 50 to 80% bound to plasma proteins.

METABOLIC REACTIONS. Deacetylated in the liver to *O*-desacetylcephalothin. In rats, additional metabolites include thienylacetylglycine and thiopheneacetic acid.

EXCRETION. 60 to 90% of a dose is excreted in the urine in 6 hours; of the excreted material, about 75% is unchanged and about 25% is the deacetylated metabolite. Urinary excretion is delayed by probenecid. Cephalothin is excreted to some extent in the bile.

FURTHER INFORMATION. Excretion in patients with renal impairment—C. M. Kunin and N. Atuk, *New Engl. J. Med.*, 1966, **274**, 654; review of metabolism and pharmacokinetics of cephalosporins—C. H. Nightingale *et al.*, *J. pharm. Sci.*, 1975, **64**, 1899.

Actions and uses. Cephalothin is an antibiotic with actions and uses similar to those described under Cephaloridine, but it is less likely to cause renal damage and may therefore be preferred for the treatment of patients with renal failure or those being dialysed.

The principal use of cephalothin is in the treatment of serious infections due to organisms that have become resistant to benzylpenicillin and ampicillin. It does not cross the blood-brain barrier in effective quantities even in purulent meningitis. It is the most active of the cephalosporins against staphylococci.

Cephalothin sodium may be administered in a dosage equivalent to 2 to 6 grams of cephalothin daily, in divided doses, preferably by intravenous injection or by intravenous infusion since intramuscular injection is painful; in life-threatening infections, doses of up to 12 grams may be administered daily in divided doses.

The usual dose for children is the equivalent of 100 milligrams of cephalothin per kilogram body-weight daily and the dose should not generally exceed the equivalent of 160 milligrams per kilogram body-weight daily.

Undesirable effects. As for Cephaloridine.

Precautions. As for Cephaloridine.

To prevent renal damage during prolonged periods of use, as in the treatment of bacterial endocarditis, the glomerular filtration rate should be estimated regularly and the dose varied accordingly. Solutions for intravenous administration should be suitably diluted as concentrated solutions may cause thrombophlebitis.

Drug interactions. As for Cephaloridine.

Preparation

CEPHALOTHIN INJECTION: a sterile solution of cephalothin sodium in water for injections. It is prepared by dissolving the contents of a sealed container in water for injections shortly before use. Available as a powder in ampoules containing cephalothin sodium equivalent to 1 and 4 g of cephalothin.

A standard for this injection is given in the British Pharmacopoeia 1973

Containers: see the entry on Injections for general information on containers.

Labelling: see the entry on Injections for general information on labelling. In addition, the label on the container should state the amount of the medicament as the equivalent amount of cephalothin.

Storage: the sealed container should be stored at a temperature not exceeding 25°, protected from light. The injection contains no bactericide and should be used as soon as possible after preparation but solutions of cephalothin sodium may be expected to retain their potency for up to 48 hours after preparation, provided they are stored at 2° to 10°. If a precipitate forms, it should be redissolved by warming. Concentrated solutions darken in colour.

Cephradine

(7*R*)-7-(α-D-Cyclohexa-1,4-dienylglycylamino)-3-methylceph-3-em-4-carboxylic acid

$C_{16}H_{19}N_3O_4S = 349.4$

OTHER NAMES: Cefradine; *Velosef*®

Description. A white crystalline powder with a characteristic odour.

Solubility. Soluble in 50 parts of water at pH 6 but less soluble at acid or neutral pH; soluble in propylene glycol; very slightly soluble in alcohol and in acetone; practically insoluble in ether and in chloroform.

INFRA-RED ABSORPTION. Major peaks at 1266, 1333, 1389, 1587, 1667, and 1754 cm^{-1} (see Appendix 2b: Infra-red Spectra).

Metabolism. ABSORPTION. Cephradine is acid stable and is rapidly and almost completely absorbed after oral or intramuscular administration; gastro-intestinal absorption may be delayed by the presence of food; after intramuscular administration there appears to be a sex-linked difference in absorption and also a difference dependent upon the injection site used.

BLOOD CONCENTRATION. After 500-mg and 2-g oral doses after fasting, peak serum concentrations of 17 and 42 μg/ml respectively are attained in about 1 hour; after an oral dose of 500 mg to non-fasting subjects, peak concentrations fall to about 8.5 μg/ml and appear about 1.5 hours later; a 1-g dose of probenecid almost doubles the peak concentration in subjects who have fasted; after an intramuscular dose of 1 g of cephradine, peak concentrations of about 13 μg/ml are attained in about 1 hour.

HALF-LIFE. Serum half-life, 0.7 to 1 hour.

DISTRIBUTION. Widely distributed throughout the body and may accumulate if renal function is impaired; small amounts appear in the cerebrospinal fluid when the meninges are inflamed; it crosses the placenta in significant concentrations and is secreted in milk; volume of distribution, about 20 litres; *protein binding*, 6 to 15% bound to plasma proteins.

METABOLIC REACTIONS. Not metabolised in man.

EXCRETION. Up to 100% of a dose is excreted unchanged in the urine with about 30% being excreted in the first

3 hours after oral administration; small amounts may be excreted in the bile; urinary excretion is delayed by probenecid; urinary excretion appears to be less in bedridden than in ambulant patients.

FURTHER INFORMATION. Absorption and excretion—C. Harvengt et al., J. clin. Pharmac., 1973, **13**, 36 and F. L. Minn et al., J. clin. Pharmac., 1976, **16**, 171; influence of probenecid and food on bioavailability of cephradine —T. W. Mischler et al., J. clin. Pharmac., 1974, **14**, 602; review of metabolism and pharmacokinetics of cephalosporins—C. H. Nightingale et al., J. pharm. Sci., 1975, **64**, 1899; sex differences in intramuscular absorption and bioavailability of cephradine—R. A. Vukovich et al., Clin. Pharmac. Ther., 1975, **18**, 215.

Actions and uses. Cephradine is a cephalosporin antibiotic which has the mode of action, antigenicity, and spectrum of activity of cephalexin but its antibiotic activity in vitro is less than that of other parenteral cephalosporins.

Cephradine may be administered by mouth or by intramuscular or intravenous injection. The usual dosage is 250 milligrams every 6 hours for infections of the respiratory tract and 500 milligrams every 6 hours for infections of the gastro-intestinal and urinary tracts. Up to 1 gram may be given every 6 hours in severe or chronic infections.

Children may be given 25 to 50 milligrams per kilogram body-weight daily divided into 4 doses; larger doses may be given to children for severe or chronic infections but the total daily dose should not exceed 4 grams.

Undesirable effects. As for Cephalexin.

Precautions. As for Cephalexin.
The dose should be reduced in patients with poor renal function, as otherwise an increase in blood urea and tubular damage may occur.

Preparations

Preparations available include CAPSULES containing cephradine 250 and 500 mg; an ELIXIR containing cephradine 125 and 250 mg in 5 ml when reconstituted, diluent syrup, life of diluted elixir 7 days; and an INJECTION reconstituted from vials of powder containing cephradine 0.25, 0.5, and 1 g with anhydrous sodium carbonate equivalent to 6 mmol of Na+ per g of cephradine.

Cetomacrogol 1000

A macrogol ether which may be represented by the formula $CH_3.[CH_2]_m.[O.CH_2CH_2]_n.OH$, where m is 15 or 17 and n is 20 to 24. It may be prepared by condensing cetyl or cetostearyl alcohol with ethylene oxide under controlled conditions.

OTHER NAMES: Cyclogol 1000®; Ethylan CET®; Polyethylene Glycol 1000 Monocetyl Ether; Texofor A1P®; Volpo C20®
Collone N1®, Crodex N®, and Cyclogol Wax N1® (all with cetostearyl alcohol)

A standard is given in the British Pharmacopoeia 1973

Description. An almost odourless, cream-coloured, waxy, unctuous mass which melts when heated to a clear brownish-yellow liquid.

Solubility. Soluble in water, in alcohol, and in acetone; practically insoluble in light petroleum.

Incompatibility. It is incompatible with phenols and it reduces the antibacterial activity of quaternary ammonium compounds.

When solutions are added to strong solutions of electrolytes, the cetomacrogol may separate.

Sterilisation. It is sterilised by dry heat.

Storage. It should be stored in airtight containers.

Uses. Cetomacrogol 1000 is a non-ionic emulsifying agent and is used in the preparation of cetomacrogol emulsifying wax, which can be employed as an emulsifying agent for producing oil-in-water creams that are stable over a wide pH range and suitable for the incorporation of many anionic, cationic, and non-ionic medicaments.

Cetomacrogol 1000 is used to disperse volatile oils in water, producing transparent sols; a proportion of 10 parts of cetomacrogol 1000 to 1 part of volatile oil is suitable in most cases.

Preparations

CETOMACROGOL CREAM: may be prepared according to one of the following formulae for use as a diluent as specified in the relevant entries:

Formula A

Cetomacrogol emulsifying ointment	..	..	300 g
Chlorocresol	.. ..		1 g
Purified water, freshly boiled and cooled	.. ..		699 g

Formula B

Cetomacrogol emulsifying ointment	..	..	300.0 g
Propyl hydroxybenzoate..	.. .. ..		0.8 g
Methyl hydroxybenzoate	.. .. ..		1.5 g
Benzyl alcohol	.. ..		15.0 g
Purified water, freshly boiled and cooled	.. ..		682.7 g

Dissolve the preservatives in the water with the aid of gentle heat; melt the cetomacrogol emulsifying ointment on a water-bath, add the solution containing the preservatives at the same temperature, and stir until cold. To help to prevent production of a granular preparation, the temperature of the melted ingredients should not exceed 65°, and in the preparation of a cream according to formula A, the chlorocresol should be dissolved in not less than 50 ml of warm water before adding to the melted emulsifying basis.

An improved product may also be obtained if, instead of using cetomacrogol emulsifying ointment, the appropriate quantities of white soft paraffin, cetomacrogol emulsifying wax, and liquid paraffin are melted together. In view of the difficulty of achieving the highest hygienic standard, it is recommended that the cream should be freshly prepared, unless facilities are available for assessing the microbiological quality of the product.

A standard for this cream is given in the British Pharmaceutical Codex 1973

Containers and Storage: see the entry on Creams for general information on containers and storage. In addition, if the cream is not freshly prepared, it should preferably be packed in small collapsible tubes. A readily breakable seal should cover the closure or the tube may be enclosed in a sealed plastic envelope or sealed carton. Alternatively, the cream may be supplied in jars.

Labelling: see the entry on Creams for general information on labelling.

CETOMACROGOL EMULSIFYING OINTMENT:

Cetomacrogol emulsifying wax	..	..	300 g
Liquid paraffin	.. ..		200 g
White soft paraffin	.. ..		500 g

Melt together, and stir until cold.

Containers and *Storage:* see the entry on Ointments for general information on containers and storage.

CETOMACROGOL EMULSIFYING WAX (*Syn.* Non-ionic Emulsifying Wax):

Cetomacrogol 1000	200 g
Cetostearyl Alcohol	800 g

Melt together, and stir until cold.

A standard for this emulsifying wax is given in the British Pharmacopoeia 1973

Cetostearyl Alcohol

A mixture of solid aliphatic alcohols consisting chiefly of stearyl alcohol, $CH_3.[CH_2]_{16}.CH_2OH$, and cetyl alcohol, $CH_3.[CH_2]_{14}.CH_2OH$, with small amounts of other alcohols, mainly myristyl alcohol, $CH_3.[CH_2]_{12}.CH_2OH$.

OTHER NAME: *Laurex CS*®

A standard is given in the British Pharmacopoeia 1973

It usually consists of about 50 to 70% of stearyl alcohol and about 20 to 35% of cetyl alcohol, but the proportions may vary considerably. Material which is known in commerce as "cetyl alcohol", unless specified as pure, is a cetostearyl alcohol usually containing about 60 to 70% of cetyl alcohol and 20 to 30% of stearyl alcohol. Pure cetyl alcohol, containing not less than 98% of $CH_3.[CH_2]_{14}.CH_2OH$, is also available.

Description. A white or cream-coloured unctuous mass or almost white flakes or granules with a faint characteristic odour and a bland taste.

Solubility. Practically insoluble in water; soluble in ether; less soluble in alcohol and in light petroleum.

Uses. Cetostearyl alcohol is strongly hydrophobic and when used alone has little value as an emulsifying agent. Oil-in-water emulsions produced by hydrophilic substances, such as sulphated fatty alcohols or cetomacrogol, are stabilised over a wide pH range when cetostearyl alcohol is included.

It may be used to increase the viscosity of oil-in-water and water-in-oil emulsions, thereby improving their stability, and may be added to paraffin ointments to improve their emollient properties.

Preparations

AQUEOUS CREAM (*Syn.* Hydrous Emulsifying Ointment):

Emulsifying ointment	300 g
Chlorocresol	1 g
Purified water, freshly boiled and cooled	699 g

Dissolve the chlorocresol in the water with the aid of gentle heat; melt the emulsifying ointment, add the chlorocresol solution at the same temperature, and stir gently until cold.

Containers, Labelling, and *Storage:* see the entry on Creams for general information on containers, labelling, and storage.

BUFFERED CREAM (*Syn.* Cremor Normalis):

Citric acid monohydrate..	5 g
Sodium phosphate..	25 g
Chlorocresol	1 g
Emulsifying ointment	300 g
Purified water, freshly boiled and cooled	669 g

Dissolve the chlorocresol, the citric acid, and the sodium phosphate in the water with the aid of gentle heat; melt the emulsifying ointment and add the solution containing the preservative and the buffers at the same temperature, and stir gently until cold.

A standard for this cream is given in the British Pharmaceutical Codex 1973

Containers, Labelling, and *Storage:* see the entry on Creams for general information on containers, labelling, and storage. When aluminium tubes are used, they should be coated internally with a suitable lacquer.

EMULSIFYING OINTMENT (*Syn.* Ung. Emulsif.):

Emulsifying wax	300 g
White soft paraffin	500 g
Liquid paraffin	200 g

Melt together and stir until cold.

Containers and *Labelling:* see the entry on Ointments for general information on containers and labelling.

EMULSIFYING WAX (*Syn.* Anionic Emulsifying Wax): containing cetostearyl alcohol and sodium lauryl sulphate or similar sodium salts of sulphated higher primary aliphatic alcohols. A satisfactory preparation may be prepared according to the following formula:

Sodium lauryl sulphate	10 g
Cetostearyl alcohol	90 g
Purified water	4 ml

Melt the cetostearyl alcohol and heat to about 95°, add the sodium lauryl sulphate, mix, and add the water; heat to 115° and maintain at this temperature, stirring vigorously, until frothing ceases and the product is translucent, and cool rapidly.

A standard for this emulsifying wax is given in the British Pharmacopoeia 1973

OTHER PREPARATIONS: cetostearyl alcohol is an ingredient of cetomacrogol cream, cetomacrogol emulsifying ointment, cetomacrogol emulsifying wax, and cetrimide emulsifying ointment.

Cetrimide

Consists chiefly of tetradecyltrimethylammonium bromide, together with smaller amounts of dodecyl- and hexadecyl-trimethylammonium bromide.

OTHER NAMES: *Cetaped*®; *Cetavlex*®; *Cetavlon*®; *Cetricream*®; Cetrimidum; Cetrimonium Bromide; *Comulin*®; *Cycloton V*®; *Morpan CHSA*®; *Silquat C100*®; *Vesagex*®.

Drapolene® (with benzalkonium chloride); *Collone QA*®, *Crodex C*®, and *Cycloton A*® (all with cetostearyl alcohol); *Seboderm*® (with cetyl alcohol); *Gomaxine*® (with chlorocresol); *Medi-Sache*®, *Savlodil*®, and *Savlon*® (all with chlorhexidine gluconate); *Siopel*® (with dimethicone).

A standard is given in the European Pharmacopoeia Vol. II

Description. A white to creamy-white, voluminous, free-flowing powder with a faint characteristic odour and a soapy bitter taste.

Solubility. Soluble, at 20°, in 2 parts of water; soluble in alcohol.

Moisture content. Not more than 2%, determined by drying at 105°.

Stability. At ambient temperatures cetrimide is chemically stable in the dry state and in aqueous solution.

Concentrated solutions may be diluted with water or alcohol.

Incompatibility. It is incompatible with soaps and similar anionic compounds, with iodine, and with alkali hydroxides.

Hygroscopicity. At 20°, at relative humidities of 40 to 50%, it absorbs sufficient moisture to cause caking of the powder.

Sterilisation. Solutions are sterilised by heating in an autoclave or by filtration.

Preparation and storage of solutions. See statement on aqueous solutions of antiseptics in the entry on Solutions.
Stock solutions containing up to 40% of cetrimide may be stored and subsequently diluted; as a precaution against contamination with *Pseudomonas* species they should contain at least 7% v/v of ethyl alcohol or 4% v/v of isopropyl alcohol.

Identification. TESTS. 1. A solution in water foams on shaking.
2. To 5 ml of a 2% solution add 2 ml of *potassium ferricyanide solution*; a yellow precipitate is produced.
3. To 5 ml of a 2% solution add 5 ml of *dilute nitric acid*, filter if necessary, add 5 ml of *silver nitrate solution*, and allow to stand for 30 minutes protected from light; a faint yellow precipitate is produced.
4. Mix 5 ml of water, 1 ml of *dilute sulphuric acid*, 2 ml of chloroform, and 1 drop of *methyl orange solution*, and shake; the chloroform layer is colourless. Add to the mixture about 20 mg of the sample, shake, and allow to separate; the chloroform layer is coloured yellow.

MELTING-POINT. In the range 232° to 247°.

Actions and uses. Cetrimide is a quaternary ammonium compound. It is a relatively non-toxic antiseptic with detergent properties. Like other quaternary ammonium compounds it is active against Gram-positive organisms but it is less effective against Gram-negative organisms (especially *Pseudomonas*) and is inactive against acid-fast bacilli and bacterial spores.
Aqueous solutions and creams containing 0.1 to 1% have been used for the treatment of wounds and burns, for pre-operative cleansing of the skin, and for the removal of scabs and crusts in skin diseases. Solutions containing 1 to 3% are used in seborrhoea of the scalp.
For the cleansing and disinfection of utensils, vessels, and apparatus, solutions containing 0.5 to 1% may be used; rubber articles are adversely affected by prolonged or repeated immersion, and polythene tubing and catheters and articles made of plastic should not remain immersed for more than 30 minutes.
To prevent corrosion, 0.4% of sodium nitrite should be added to solutions of cetrimide used for the storage of instruments. Such solutions should be changed at weekly intervals. Syringes and needles which have been stored in cetrimide solutions should be rinsed in water for injections before use. Instruments with cemented glass components should not be allowed to come into contact with cetrimide solutions.
The activity of quaternary compounds is greatly reduced in the presence of organic matter, soap, and anionic compounds.
Cetrimide is used in the preparation of cetrimide emulsifying wax, which can be used as an emulsifying agent for producing oil-in-water creams, suitable for the incorporation of cationic and non-ionic medicaments. For anionic medicaments, emulsifying wax and cetomacrogol emulsifying wax should be used.

Aqueous solutions of cetrimide are used as preservatives in pharmaceutical and cosmetic preparations.

Precautions. Cetrimide should not be applied repeatedly to skin, and wet dressings should not be left in contact with the skin as hypersensitivity may occur.

Preparations

CETRIMIDE CREAM: a solution of cetrimide in a suitable water-miscible basis. A suitable cream may be prepared according to the following formula:

Cetrimide	5 g, or a sufficient quantity
Cetostearyl alcohol	50 g
Liquid paraffin	500 g
Purified water, freshly boiled and cooled	to 1000 g

Melt the cetostearyl alcohol with the aid of gentle heat, add the liquid paraffin, and warm; dissolve the cetrimide in the water at the same temperature and add to the warm mixture, stirring gently until cold. A phosphate buffer may be included. Available as creams containing 0.5, 1, and 2% of cetrimide.
A standard for this cream is given in the British Pharmacopoeia Addendum 1977 and the British Pharmacopoeia (Veterinary)
Containers, Labelling, and *Storage:* see the entry on Creams for general information on containers, labelling, and storage.
Advice for patients: the cream should not be applied repeatedly. Wet dressings should not be applied.

CETRIMIDE EMULSIFYING OINTMENT:

Cetrimide	30 g
Cetostearyl alcohol	270 g
White soft paraffin	500 g
Liquid paraffin	200 g

Melt together the white soft paraffin, the cetostearyl alcohol, and the liquid paraffin, add the cetrimide, and stir until cold.
A standard for this ointment is given in the British Pharmacopoeia 1973
Containers and *Labelling:* see the entry on Ointments for general information on containers and labelling.

CETRIMIDE EMULSIFYING WAX (*Syn.* Cationic Emulsifying Wax):

Cetrimide	100 g
Cetostearyl alcohol	900 g

Melt the cetostearyl alcohol on a water-bath, add the cetrimide, and stir until cold.
A standard for this emulsifying wax is given in the British Pharmaceutical Codex 1973

CETRIMIDE SOLUTION:

Strong cetrimide solution	25 ml
Purified water, freshly boiled and cooled	to 1000 ml

It must be freshly prepared unless it is issued as sterile in sealed containers.
A standard for this solution is given in the British Pharmaceutical Codex 1973
Sterilisation: the solution may be sterilised by heating in an autoclave or by filtration.
Containers: should be thoroughly cleansed before being filled. Closures should be such that the solution does not come into contact with cork. In addition, if the solution is issued as sterile, the directions given in the entry on Solutions should be followed.

Labelling: the label on the container of a non-sterilised solution should state that the solution should not be used later than one week after issue for use.

The label on the sealed container of a solution issued as sterile should state:

(1) the name of the solution as "Sterile Cetrimide Solution",

(2) the words "Not for Injection", and

(3) that the solution should not be used later than one week after the container is first opened.

Advice for patients: excessive use of the solution should be avoided.

STRONG CETRIMIDE SOLUTION: a 40% aqueous solution of cetrimide, containing 7.5% v/v of alcohol (95%) and 0.0075% of tartrazine (food grade of commerce). It may be perfumed.

In making this preparation the alcohol (95%) may be replaced by industrial methylated spirit, provided that the law and the statutory regulations governing the use of industrial methylated spirit are observed.

A standard for this solution is given in the British Pharmaceutical Codex 1973 and in the British Pharmacopoeia (Veterinary)

Containers: should be thoroughly cleansed before being filled. Closures should be such that the solution does not come into contact with cork.

OTHER PREPARATIONS available include a veterinary APPLICATION containing cetrimide 10% in an aerosol pack, an application containing cetrimide 17.5%, a veterinary application containing cetrimide 20% in an aerosol pack; a CREAM containing cetrimide 0.2% with benzalkonium chloride 0.01%, a cream and a veterinary cream containing cetrimide 0.3% with dimethicone 10%, a cream containing cetrimide 0.5% with chlorocresol 0.05%, a cream containing cetrimide 15.6% with cetyl alcohol 15.6%; an OINTMENT containing cetrimide 1%; a SOLUTION containing cetrimide 0.15% with chlorhexidine gluconate 0.015%, a solution, and a veterinary solution containing cetrimide 15% with chlorhexidine gluconate 1.5%.

Cetylpyridinium Chloride

1-Hexadecylpyridinium chloride monohydrate

$C_{21}H_{38}ClN,H_2O = 358.0$

OTHER NAME: *Merocet*®

A standard is given in the British Pharmacopoeia 1973

Description. A white powder with a slight characteristic odour.

Solubility. Soluble, at 20°, in 20 parts of water.

Acidity. A 1% solution has a pH of 5.0 to 5.4.

Moisture content. 4.5 to 5.5%, determined by Fischer titration.

Incompatibility. It is incompatible with soaps and similar anionic compounds.

Storage. It should be stored in airtight containers.

Preparation and storage of solutions. See statement on aqueous solutions of antiseptics in the entry on Solutions.

Identification. TESTS. 1. Heat a small quantity until it melts and a brown colour develops; the odour of pyridine is produced.

2. Dissolve about 20 mg in 10 ml of water and add 3 ml of *potassium ferricyanide solution;* a yellow precipitate is produced.

3. Dissolve about 2 mg in 1 ml of water and add 1 ml of a saturated solution of potassium thiocyanate; a white gelatinous precipitate is produced.

MELTING-POINT. About 81°.

ULTRAVIOLET ABSORPTION. In water, maximum at 258 nm (E1%, 1cm = 120).

Actions and uses. Cetylpyridinium chloride has actions similar to those of Cetrimide.

It is used as a 0.1% solution for minor wounds and burns and as a 1% solution for pre-operative cleansing of the skin. More dilute solutions (0.01 to 0.02%) should be used for application to mucous membranes or to large areas of exposed tissue. Its activity is greatly reduced by the presence of soap or serum.

Lozenges containing cetylpyridinium chloride are used for the treatment of superficial infections of the mouth and throat.

Preparations

Preparations available include LOZENGES containing cetylpyridinium chloride 1.45 mg and a MOUTH-WASH containing cetylpyridinium chloride 0.05% with alcohol 14%.

Chagas' Disease

see under TRYPANOSOMIASIS

Chalk

Native calcium carbonate freed from most of its impurities by elutriation and dried.
$CaCO_3 = 100.1$

OTHER NAMES: Creta; Creta Praeparata; Prepared Chalk

A standard is given in the British Pharmacopoeia 1973

Description. *Macroscopical characters:* odourless, white or greyish-white, amorphous, earthy, friable masses or powder, soft to the touch.

Microscopical characters: chalk consists of the shells of cretaceous fossil foraminifera belonging to several genera, including *Globigerina*, about 35 to 80 μm in diameter, and *Textularia*, about 50 to 180 μm long by 40 to 100 μm across the base, accompanied by large numbers of fossil remains of small algae belonging to the Coccolithophoridaceae and having the appearance of small disks or rings, about 1 to 2 μm in diameter; small amounts of detritus of echinoderms and of molluscs are also present; when mounted in alcohol and irrigated with acetic acid, it dissolves with effervescence.

Solubility. Practically insoluble in water; very slightly soluble in water containing carbon dioxide; soluble in mineral acids with effervescence.

Actions and uses. Chalk is absorbent and antacid, and is an ingredient of mixtures and powders used in the treatment of diarrhoea.

A dose of 1 to 5 grams is given and repeated in accordance with the needs of the patient.

Undesirable effects. Continued use may cause hypercalcaemia and alkalosis.

Veterinary uses. Chalk is an antacid. The usual dose for all species is 300 to 500 milligrams per kilogram body-weight.

Preparations

AROMATIC CHALK POWDER (*Syn.* Pulvis Cretae Aromaticus):

Chalk, in powder	250 g
Cardamom seed, freshly removed from the fruit, powdered, and used at once ..	30 g
Clove, in powder	40 g
Nutmeg, in powder	80 g
Cinnamon, in powder	100 g
Sucrose, in powder	500 g

Mix, as described in the entry on Powders.
A standard for this powder is given in the British Pharmaceutical Codex 1973
Containers and *Storage:* see the entry on Powders for general information on containers and storage. Containers should be airtight.
Dose: 0.5 to 5 grams.
Advice for patients: the powder should be taken mixed with a little water or other fluid. It should not be used for longer than a few days without medical advice.

AROMATIC CHALK WITH OPIUM MIXTURE (*Syn.* Chalk and Opium Mixture; Mistura Cretae Aromatica cum Opio):

Aromatic chalk powder	130 g
Tragacanth, in powder	2 g
Opium tincture	50 ml
Aromatic ammonia solution	50 ml
Compound cardamom tincture	50 ml
Catechu tincture	50 ml
Chloroform water, double-strength	500 ml
Water for preparations	to 1000 ml

It should be recently prepared.
A standard for this mixture is given in the British Pharmaceutical Codex 1973
Containers and *Labelling:* see the entry on Mixtures for general information on containers and labelling.
Dose: ADULT: 10 to 20 millilitres.
CHILD: Up to 1 year, 1 millilitre; 1 to 5 years, 2 to 5 millilitres.
Advice for patients: the mixture should not be used for longer than a few days without medical advice.

AROMATIC CHALK WITH OPIUM POWDER (*Syn.* Pulvis Cretae Aromaticus cum Opio):

Aromatic chalk powder	975 g
Powdered opium	25 g

Mix, as described in the entry on Powders.
A standard for this powder is given in the British Pharmaceutical Codex 1973
Containers and *Storage:* see the entry on Powders for general information on containers and storage. Containers should be airtight.
Dose: 0.5 to 5 grams.
Advice for patients: the powder should be taken mixed with a little water or other fluid. It should not be used for longer than a few days without medical advice.

PAEDIATRIC CHALK MIXTURE (*Syn.* Mistura Cretae pro Infantibus):

Chalk	20 g
Tragacanth, in powder	2 g
Concentrated cinnamon water	4 ml
Syrup	100 ml
Chloroform water, double-strength	500 ml
Water for preparations	to 1000 ml

It should be recently prepared.
A standard for this mixture is given in the British Pharmaceutical Codex 1973
Containers and *Labelling:* see the entry on Mixtures for general information on containers and labelling.
Dose: CHILD: Up to 1 year, 5 millilitres; 1 to 5 years, 10 millilitres.
Advice for patients: the mixture should not be used for longer than a few days without medical advice.

OTHER PREPARATION: chalk is an ingredient of compound magnesium trisilicate powder.

Charcoal

OTHER NAMES: Activated Charcoal; Carbo; Carbo Activatus; *Darco G-60*®; Medicinal Charcoal; *Medicoal*®

A standard is given in the European Pharmacopoeia Vol. III Supplement

Charcoal may be prepared from vegetable matter such as sawdust, peat, cellulose residues, and coconut shells. The raw material is carbonised and subsequently activated at a high temperature, with or without the addition of inorganic salts, in a stream of activating gases such as steam and carbon dioxide.

Alternatively, raw vegetable matter may be treated with a chemical activating agent such as phosphoric acid, zinc chloride, or potassium thiocyanate, the mixture carbonised at a suitable temperature, and the chemical agent removed by washing.

A combination of both processes may also be employed to improve the purity of the finished product.

Commercial varieties of charcoal differ widely in their characteristics, depending largely upon the method of manufacture.

The adsorptive power of charcoal depends upon the total available surface area, which may include external and internal surfaces. Charcoals showing high adsorptive power for gases may be relatively inactive in liquid-phase systems, and charcoals showing high adsorptive power in liquid media may be relatively inactive for gases.

Technical grades of activated charcoal are widely used as purifying and decolorising agents, for the removal of residual gases in low-pressure apparatus, and in respirators as a protection against toxic gases.

Description. A black, very fine, odourless, tasteless powder.

Solubility. Practically insoluble in water and in alcohol.

Moisture content. Not more than 15%, determined by drying at 120°.

Storage. It should be stored in airtight containers.

Actions and uses. Charcoal will adsorb certain substances from solution and when dry is an efficient adsorbent of gases.

It is sometimes given by mouth in doses of 4 to 8 grams to adsorb gases in the treatment of flatulence and intestinal distension, but it is doubtful if it is of much value in these circumstances. It may also be used as a thick suspension containing up to 50 grams in water in the first-aid treatment of poisoning by alkaloids and similar drugs. Charcoal is used to indicate the passage of intestinal contents.

Charcoal is administered in powder, granules, and tablets, sometimes with light kaolin.

Chemotherapeutic Agents

see under ANTIMICROBIALS

Chicken-pox

Chicken-pox (Varicella) is a highly infectious viral disease occurring mainly between the ages of 5 and 15 years; it may however occur in adults in which case the disease is usually more severe. In patients on long-term therapy with corticosteroids or cytotoxic drugs the condition may be severe or even fatal. The causal organism is also responsible for attacks of shingles or herpes zoster which usually occur in patients with partial immunity against varicella. The incubation period is between 11 and 21 days.

In children the appearance of the rash is usually the first sign of the disease but in adults there may be a period of general constitutional upset. The rash appears in crops which change from a macule to a papule to a vesicle to a pustule within 24 hours, and scabbing occurs thereafter. The rash is at first confined to the face and trunk and is almost always present in the axillae; it later extends towards the extremities although there are usually fewer spots on the limbs than on the trunk. Lesions are usually present in all stages of evolution simultaneously. Small lesions also occur in the mouth and these tend to rupture readily. The patient is infective from one day before the appearance of the rash until the last crust has separated.

The patient should be confined to bed only if necessary. If itching is troublesome, soothing or antipruritic lotions (such as calamine or crotamiton) or sterile dusting-powders may be applied, and bathing in potassium permanganate solution (0.02%) is sometimes helpful. Antihistamines may also be administered by mouth. The commonest complication is bacterial infection of the pustules which may occur especially if the patient scratches, and antibacterial treatment may be required. Rarer complications include encephalitis and a widespread varicella pneumonia which can develop in all ages and is sometimes fatal.

Children at particular risk from chicken-pox, for example those with oncological disease receiving treatment with cytotoxic drugs, may be given zoster immune globulin as a prophylactic measure.

Chilblains

Chilblains are local erythematous swellings which occur in cold weather. They may appear on the fingers, toes, ears, or nose and are accompanied by tenderness and itching. They may sometimes blister and ulcerate.

Chilblains may be prevented by wearing thick clothing in cold weather and by adequate indoor heating. When these measures have not been effective, peripheral vasodilators and alpha-adrenoceptor blocking agents have been used. There is no specific treatment for chilblains.

Chloral Hydrate

2,2,2-Trichloroethane-1,1-diol

$$CCl_3 \cdot CH(OH)_2$$

$C_2H_3Cl_3O_2 = 165.4$

OTHER NAMES: Chlorali Hydras; *Noctec*®

A standard is given in the European Pharmacopoeia Vol. II

Description. Colourless transparent crystals with a pungent but not acrid odour and a slightly bitter and caustic taste.

Solubility. Soluble, at 20°, in less than 1 part of water, of alcohol, and of ether, and in 3 parts of chloroform; soluble in fixed and volatile oils.

Stability. It volatilises slowly in air as chloral and water, reverting on condensation to chloral hydrate. In an airtight container volatilisation ceases as soon as the vapour pressure has reached equilibrium.

In the presence of excess free oxygen, chloral hydrate degrades, after a considerable lag-phase, to form phosgene, carbon dioxide, and hydrochloric acid. A solid polymer, thought to be metachloral, is also formed. In neutral aqueous solution, chloral hydrate degrades by an oxidation-reduction process to form dichloroacetaldehyde, trichloroacetic acid, and hydrochloric acid. Traces of water may therefore result in some degradation of this type which is greatly accelerated in the presence of light. The application of heat to neutral or slightly acid solutions also produces this form of degradation.

Strong sulphuric acid causes polymerisation of chloral to form α- and β-parachlorals and in more dilute sulphuric acid amorphous metachloral is produced. In alkaline solution chloral hydrate degrades to chloroform and formate ions.

Provided oxygen is absent, chloral hydrate does not degrade significantly in the presence of sunlight.

Incompatibility. It is incompatible with alkalis, alkaline earths, alkali carbonates, and soluble barbiturates.

It forms a range of molecular complexes or adducts with acetone, alcohols, caffeine, diazepam, dextrose, ether, oxytetracycline, phenacetin, tetracycline, and urea.

It forms a liquid mixture when triturated with many organic compounds such as camphor, menthol, thymol, phenol, and phenazone.

FURTHER INFORMATION. See J. E. Fairbrother, Chloral hydrate, *Analytical Profiles of Drug Substances*, K. Florey (Ed.), Vol. II, London, Academic Press, 1973, p. 85.

Storage. It should be stored in airtight containers.

Identification. TESTS. 1. The addition of *sodium hydroxide solution* produces a cloudy solution with the odour of chloroform.

2. The addition of *sodium sulphide solution* gives a yellow colour which changes to red; on standing, a red precipitate may be formed.

3. Mix 1 ml of *sodium hydroxide solution* and 1 ml of pyridine, shake, and heat in a water-bath for 2 minutes; the reagent remains colourless. The appearance of a pink colour indicates contamination with chloroform or certain other chloro-compounds and the reagent should be discarded. To the colourless reagent obtained above add 1 ml of an aqueous solution of the sample and heat in a water-bath; pink or red colour appears in the pyridine layer. A positive result in this test is also given by chlorbutol, chloroform, trichloroethane, trichloroethanol and trichloroethylene.

MELTING-POINT. When heated, it liquefies between 50° and 58°.

ULTRAVIOLET ABSORPTION. No significant absorption is exhibited in the range 230 to 360 nm.

INFRA-RED ABSORPTION. Major peaks at 820, 971, 1087, and 1299 cm^{-1} (see Appendix 2b: Infra-red Spectra).

Determination in body fluids. GAS CHROMATOGRAPHY. In blood or urine: chloral hydrate and the metabolites trichloroethanol and trichloroacetic acid—D. D. Breimer et al., *J. Chromat.*, 1974, **88**, 55; in blood or urine—J. Wells and G. Cimbura, *J. forens. Sci.*, 1972, **17**, 674.

Metabolism. ABSORPTION. Rapidly absorbed following oral administration.

BLOOD CONCENTRATION. Concentrations of chloral are not detectable in the blood after an oral dose of 1 g; after an oral dose of 15 mg of chloral hydrate, the plasma concentration of trichloroethanol reaches a peak of about 8 μg/ml; plasma levels of trichloroethanol are prolonged and levels of trichloroacetic acid are decreased when alcohol is taken.

HALF-LIFE. The plasma half-life of trichloroethanol and of trichloroacetic acid are 8 and 67 hours respectively.

DISTRIBUTION. Chloral and trichloroethanol pass into the cerebrospinal fluid, into the milk, and cross the placenta; *protein binding*, trichloroethanol 35 % and trichloroacetic acid 94 % bound to plasma albumin; trichloroacetic acid will displace warfarin from plasma proteins.

METABOLIC REACTIONS. Rapid reduction to trichloroethanol which is further conjugated with glucuronic acid, and oxidation to trichloroacetic acid which is the major metabolite.

Trichloroethanol, which is an active metabolite, will competitively inhibit the metabolism of alcohol.

EXCRETION. Trichloroacetic acid is slowly excreted over 24 to 48 hours; about 10 to 30% of a dose of chloral hydrate may be excreted as trichloroethanol glucuronide and about 5% as trichloroethanol in 24 hours; a small amount of trichloroethanol glucuronide may be excreted in the bile.

FURTHER INFORMATION. Metabolism, blood concentration, half-life, protein binding, excretion—E. M. Sellers et al., *Clin. Pharmac. Ther.*, 1973, **14**, 147.

Actions and uses. Chloral hydrate is a hypnotic which is particularly useful for children and elderly patients. When given by mouth, it is rapidly absorbed and acts within half an hour, the effect lasting for about 8 hours. The usual dose for adults is 0.8 to 2 grams. Children may be given 30 to 50 milligrams per kilogram body-weight up to a maximum single dose of 1 gram.

Undesirable effects. Flatulence, abdominal distension, nausea, headache, giddiness, rashes, and blood dyscrasias may occur.

Precautions and contra-indications. Chloral hydrate is a gastric irritant and must be well diluted before administration. It is contra-indicated in patients with severe cardiac disease or marked hepatic or renal dysfunction. Large doses should be avoided during pregnancy as they may give rise to foetal death.

Dependence. It may give rise to dependence of the barbiturate-alcohol type as described under Drug Dependence and it may also enhance the effects of alcohol.

Veterinary uses. Chloral hydrate is used as a hypnotic and sedative for large animals. The usual dose for horses

and cattle is 60 to 100 milligrams per kilogram body-weight. It is also used in doses of 120 to 180 milligrams per kilogram body-weight by intravenous injection as an anaesthetic in horses and cattle.

Preparations

CHLORAL MIXTURE (*Syn.* Chloral Hydrate Mixture):

Chloral hydrate	100 g
Syrup..	200 ml
Water for preparations	to 1000 ml

It should be recently prepared.

When a dose less than or not a multiple of 5 ml is prescribed, the mixture may be diluted, as described in the entry on Mixtures, with a mixture of one volume of syrup and 4 volumes of water for preparations. The diluted mixture must be freshly prepared.

A standard for this mixture is given in the British Pharmaceutical Codex 1973

Containers and *Labelling:* see the entry on Mixtures for general information on containers and labelling.

Dose: ADULT: 5 to 20 millilitres, well diluted with water. CHILD: hypnotic dose, well diluted with water: 1 to 5 years, 2.5 to 5 millilitres; 6 to 12 years, 5 to 10 millilitres.

Advice for patients: the mixture should be taken well diluted. Hypnotic doses should be taken half an hour before bedtime. The mixture may cause drowsiness on the following day; persons affected should not drive or operate machinery. Alcohol should be avoided. The mixture should not be spilled on the skin.

PAEDIATRIC CHLORAL ELIXIR:

Chloral hydrate	40 g
Water for preparations	20 ml
Black currant syrup	200 ml
Syrup..	to 1000 ml

Dissolve the chloral hydrate in the water, add the black currant syrup and sufficient syrup to produce the required volume, and mix. It should be recently prepared.

When a dose less than or not a multiple of 5 ml is prescribed, the elixir may be diluted, as described in the entry on Elixirs, with syrup. The diluted elixir must be freshly prepared.

A standard for this elixir is given in the British Pharmaceutical Codex 1973

Containers and *Labelling:* see the entry on Elixirs for general information on containers and labelling.

Dose: CHILD: Up to 1 year, 5 millilitres.

Advice for patients: the elixir should be taken well diluted. Hypnotic doses should be taken half an hour before bedtime. The elixir should not be spilled on the skin.

STRONG CHLORAL SOLUTION: a solution of chloral hydrate in purified water. It contains 110% (100 micrograms in 90 microlitres) of chloral hydrate.

A standard for this solution is given in the British Pharmacopoeia (Veterinary)

Labelling: the label on the container should state that the solution is not suitable for injection and that it should be well diluted with water before oral administration.

Storage: it should be stored in airtight containers, protected from light.

Dose: HORSES and CATTLE, by mouth, 55 to 90 microlitres per kilogram body-weight.

OTHER PREPARATIONS available include CAPSULES containing chloral hydrate 500 mg.

Chlorambucil

4-[4-Bis(2-chloroethyl)aminophenyl]butyric acid

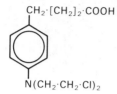

$CH_2 \cdot [CH_2]_2 \cdot COOH$

$N(CH_2 \cdot CH_2 \cdot Cl)_2$

$C_{14}H_{19}Cl_2NO_2 = 304.2$

OTHER NAME: *Leukeran®*

A standard is given in the British Pharmacopoeia 1973

CAUTION: *Care should be taken to avoid inhalation of particles or contact with the skin.*

Description. A white crystalline powder with a slight odour.

Solubility. Practically insoluble in water; soluble, at 20°, in 1.5 parts of alcohol, in 2.5 parts of chloroform, and in 2 parts of acetone.

Storage. It should be stored in airtight containers.

Identification. TESTS. 1. Mix about 400 mg with 10 ml of *dilute hydrochloric acid*, allow to stand for 30 minutes with occasional shaking, and filter; wash the residue with two 10-ml portions of water and reserve the mixed filtrate and washings; the residue after drying over phosphorus pentoxide *in vacuo* for 3 hours, melts at about 146°.
2. To 10 ml of the solution reserved in Test 1 add 0.5 ml of *potassium mercuri-iodide solution*; a buff-coloured precipitate is produced. To a further 10 ml add 0.5 ml of *potassium permanganate solution*; the purple colour is discharged.
3. Mix 600 mg with 4 drops of phenylhydrazine, heat in a water-bath for 10 minutes with occasional stirring, add 2 ml of dehydrated alcohol, heat for 20 seconds, filter immediately, and allow the filtrate to stand for 30 minutes; crystals of phenylhydrazine hydrochloride are formed which, after washing with two 1-ml portions of dehydrated alcohol and drying at 105°, melt at about 245° with decomposition.

MELTING-POINT. About 65°.

INFRA-RED ABSORPTION. Major peaks at 1174, 1228, 1270, 1352, 1505, and 1686 cm⁻¹ (see Appendix 2a: Infra-red Spectra).

Metabolism. ABSORPTION. Readily absorbed after oral administration.

DISTRIBUTION. Strongly adsorbed onto erythrocytes; after a subcutaneous dose to rats, chlorambucil is rapidly distributed with maximum concentrations appearing in the liver and kidneys.

EXCRETION. 60% of a subcutaneous dose to rats is excreted in 24 hours.

FURTHER INFORMATION. Absorption, distribution, and excretion in rats—B. T. Hill and P. G. Riches, *Br. J. Cancer*, 1971, **25**, 831.

Actions and uses. Chlorambucil is a cytotoxic agent which damages cells by fragmentation of nuclear chromosomes.

In the normal dosage, chlorambucil acts mainly on the lymphocytes and to a lesser extent on neutrophils and platelets. Large doses given over prolonged periods can, however, produce severe neutropenia and thrombo-cytopenia and irreversible damage to the bone marrow, with subsequent failure of haemopoiesis.

The best results have been obtained in the treatment of those conditions associated with proliferation of white blood cells, particularly lymphocytes, and in the treatment of follicular lymphoma, lymphocytic lymphoma with or without leukaemia, and some cases of Hodgkin's disease and reticulum-cell sarcoma. It is also effective in the treatment of lymphosarcoma, carcinoma of the breast and ovary, chronic lymphocytic and chronic myelocytic leukaemias, and the macroglobulinaemia of Waldenström.

Chlorambucil is also occasionally used for the treatment of rheumatoid arthritis and systemic lupus erythematosus.

Chlorambucil is better tolerated than mustine or tretamine and, if the dosage is kept low, repeated courses can be given without depression of haemopoiesis.

Chlorambucil is administered by mouth, the usual dosage being 200 micrograms per kilogram body-weight, which corresponds to 10 to 12 milligrams for the average patient, given as a single dose daily for 3 to 6 weeks. This dose should be halved if there is lymphocytic infiltration of the bone marrow or if the bone marrow is hypoplastic, as in cases of long standing and in patients who have undergone extensive treatment. Absorption is more consistent than with tretamine and is not related to food intake, whilst the effect on the bone marrow is more easily controlled.

In general, chlorambucil should not be used within a month of therapeutic irradiation or chemotherapy, as these may have caused some bone-marrow damage. If, however, low doses of radiation have been given to parts remote from the bone marrow and the neutrophil and platelet-cell counts are not depressed, treatment with chlorambucil is permissible. If these cell counts are depressed, they should be allowed to reach normal levels before chlorambucil therapy is begun.

Improvement, if it occurs, is usually apparent by the third week of treatment. If the drug is well tolerated and the blood picture is satisfactory, a daily maintenance dose of 30 to 100 micrograms per kilogram body-weight, which corresponds to about 2 to 5 milligrams for the average adult patient, may be given. Alternatively, short interrupted courses of treatment may be given.

During treatment, total and differential white-cell counts and haemoglobin estimations should be made weekly and skin and mucous membranes examined for signs of haemorrhage.

Undesirable effects. A slowly progressive leucopenia may develop during treatment, but this is reversible on withdrawing the drug.

A fall in the neutrophil count may continue for 10 days after the last dose of chlorambucil. As the total dose of drug approaches 6.5 milligrams per kilogram body-weight (about 400 to 450 milligrams) there is grave risk of irreversible bone-marrow damage.

Preparation

CHLORAMBUCIL TABLETS: available as tablets containing 2 and 5 mg of chlorambucil; they are compression coated or sugar coated and the coat may be coloured.

A standard for these tablets is given in the British Pharmacopoeia 1973

Containers and *Storage:* see the entry on Tablets for general information on containers and storage.

Chloramine

Sodium *N*-chlorotoluene-4-sulphonimidate trihydrate

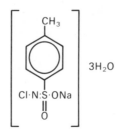

$C_7H_7ClNNaO_2S,3H_2O = 281.7$

OTHER NAMES: Chloraminum; Chloramine-T; *Rendell Foam®*; *Santronex®*

A standard is given in the European Pharmacopoeia Vol. III

Description. A white or slightly yellow efflorescent crystalline powder with the odour of chlorine, and a bitter taste.

Solubility. Soluble, at 20°, in 7 parts of water and in 12 parts of alcohol, with slow decomposition; soluble in 2 parts of boiling water; practically insoluble in ether and in chloroform.

Alkalinity. A 5% solution has a pH of 8 to 10.

Storage. It should be stored in airtight containers, in a cool place, protected from light.

Identification. TESTS. 1. A solution in water turns red litmus paper blue and then bleaches it.
2. Dissolve 500 mg in 10 ml of water and add 10 ml of *dilute hydrogen peroxide solution*; a white precipitate is produced which dissolves on heating the solution. Filter the hot solution and allow to cool; a white crystalline precipitate is produced which, after washing with water and drying at 105°, melts at about 137°.
3. Ignite; sudden decomposition occurs and the residue gives the reactions of sodium and of sulphates.

Actions and uses. Chloramine is a bactericide and in aqueous solution is almost neutral and non-irritant. A 2% solution may be used in the irrigation of wounds.
The stability of solutions may be improved by buffering at pH 9.

Preparations

Preparations available include TABLETS, for vaginal use, containing chloramine 1.1%.

Chloramphenicol

2,2-Dichloro-*N*-[(α*R*,β*R*)-β-hydroxy-α-hydroxymethyl-4-nitrophenethyl]acetamide produced by the growth of *Streptomyces venezuelae*, or prepared synthetically. There are four possible stereoisomers but only the α*R*, β*R* (or D-*threo*) form is active.

$C_{11}H_{12}Cl_2N_2O_5 = 323.1$

OTHER NAMES: *Animycetin®*; Chloramphen.; Chloramphenicolum; *Chloromycetin®*; *Ertilen®*; *Intramycetin®*; *Leukamycin®*; *Kemicetine®*; *Oroject C®*; *Salophen®*
Optocol® (with amethocaine hydrochloride); *Furaphen®* (with furazolidone); *Tanderil Chloramphenicol®* (with oxyphenbutazone); *Otopred®* (with prednisolone)

A standard is given in the European Pharmacopoeia Vol. II

Description. A fine white to greyish-white or yellowish-white crystalline powder or crystals, needles, or elongated plates, with a very bitter taste.

Solubility. Soluble, at 20°, in 400 parts of water, in 2.5 parts of alcohol, and in 7 parts of propylene glycol; soluble in acetone and in ethyl acetate; very slightly soluble in ether.

Acidity. A 0.5% suspension has a pH of 5 to 7.5.

Specific rotation. +18.5° to +21.5°, determined on a 5% solution in alcohol (95%). A solution in ethyl acetate is laevorotatory.

Stability. In aqueous solution, chloramphenicol degrades mainly by hydrolysis to 1-*p*-nitrophenylpropan-1,3-diol-2-amine and dichloroacetic acid; this acid then hydrolyses with the release of chloride ions. Chloramphenicol may also degrade by a photolytic reaction to *p*-nitrobenzaldehyde and other products. Hydrolysis is independent of pH in the range 2 to 7 but it is catalysed by monohydrogen phosphate ions, mono- and dihydrogen citrate ions, and undissociated acetic acid.

FURTHER INFORMATION. Stability in aqueous solution —T. Higuchi and C. D. Bias, *J. Am. pharm. Ass., scient. Edn*, 1953, **42**, 707; T. Higuchi *et al.*, *J. Am. pharm. Ass., scient. Edn*, 1954, **43**, 129; K. C. James and R. H. Leach, *J. Pharm. Pharmac.*, 1970, **22**, 607 and 612 and *Pharm. J.*, i/1970, 477; M. Heward *et al.*, *Pharm. J.*, i/1970, 386; photodegradation—I. K. Shih, *J. pharm. Sci.*, 1971, **60**, 1889; Stability and other properties of chloramphenicol, *Analytical Profiles of Drug Substances*, K. Florey (Ed.), Vol. 4, London, Academic Press, p. 47.

Sterilisation. Solutions in propylene glycol are sterilised by filtration.
Buffered aqueous solutions for use as eye-drops are sterilised by filtration or by heating with a bactericide.

Storage. It should be protected from light.

Identification. TESTS. 1. Dissolve about 10 mg in 1 ml of alcohol (50%), add 3 ml of a 1% solution of calcium chloride and 50 mg of zinc powder, heat on a water-bath for 10 minutes, cool, and filter; to the filtrate add 100 mg of anhydrous sodium acetate and 2 drops of benzoyl chloride, shake for 1 minute, and then add 0.5 ml of *ferric chloride solution* and 3 ml of *dilute hydrochloric acid* and mix; a reddish-violet or purple colour is produced. No such colour is produced when the test is repeated without the zinc powder.

2. To 5 ml of a 0.1% solution add a few drops of *silver nitrate solution*; no precipitate is produced. Heat about 50 mg with 2 ml of *alcoholic potassium hydroxide solution* on a water-bath for 15 minutes, add a small quantity of decolorising charcoal, shake, filter, and to the filtrate add *silver nitrate solution*; a white precipitate is produced which is insoluble in nitric acid but soluble, after washing with water, in *dilute ammonia solution*.

3. Dissolve about 10 mg in 2 ml of alcohol (50%), add 4.5 ml of *dilute sulphuric acid* and about 50 mg of zinc powder, allow to stand for 10 minutes, and decant the supernatant liquid; cool the supernatant liquid in ice, add 0.5 ml of *sodium nitrite solution*, allow to stand for 2 minutes, and then add 1 g of urea followed by 1 ml of *2-naphthol solution* and 2 ml of *sodium hydroxide solution*; a red colour is produced.

MELTING-POINT. About 151°.

ULTRAVIOLET ABSORPTION. In water, maximum at 278 nm (E1%, 1cm = 297).

INFRA-RED ABSORPTION. Major peaks at 820, 847, 1075, 1515, 1562, and 1695 cm^{-1} (see Appendix 2b: Infra-red Spectra).

Determination in body fluids. GAS CHROMATOGRAPHY.
In urine—T. Nakagawa *et al.*, *J. Chromat.*, 1975, **111**, 355.

Bioavailability.
Chloramphenicol has a low solubility in water and thus the method of formulation may have a considerable effect on its rate of absorption. Studies on bioavailability show significant variations in both the peak concentrations in blood and the times at which these occur. These variations may be related to disintegration or dissolution rates or to particle sizes.

Chloramphenicol palmitate has several polymorphic forms each having different absorption characteristics.

FURTHER INFORMATION. Physical and pharmaceutical factors influencing absorption—A. J. Aguiar, *Drug Inform. Bull.*, 1969, **3**, 17, H. Andersgaard *et al.*, *Acta pharm. suec.*, 1971, **8**, 403, and A. J. Glazko *et al.*, *Clin. Pharmac. Ther.*, 1968, **9**, 472.

Metabolism. ABSORPTION.
Well absorbed after oral administration; chloramphenicol esters are hydrolysed in the gastro-intestinal tract prior to absorption; the mono- and di-succinate esters are rapidly absorbed after intramuscular injection but are less effective than when given intravenously.

BLOOD CONCENTRATION. After an oral dose of 500 mg, a peak serum concentration of 8 to 13 μg/ml is attained in 1 to 3 hours; steady-state concentrations of about 4 to 6 μg/ml are attained during a dosage regimen of 500 mg every 6 hours; blood concentrations appear to be higher in females than in males.

HALF-LIFE. Serum half-life in adults after oral administration, 2 to 5 hours which is increased in hepatic function impairment; in the newborn it is 24 to 28 hours.

DISTRIBUTION. Widely distributed throughout the body and appears in the cerebrospinal fluid even in the absence of inflamed meninges; highest tissue concentrations appear in the liver and kidneys; chloramphenicol crosses the placenta and is secreted in the saliva, semen, and milk and in pleural ascitic fluids; *protein binding*, 45 to 60% bound to plasma proteins.

METABOLIC REACTIONS. Extensively metabolised mainly by glucuronic acid conjugation and by deacetylation; prior to absorption it may be acetylated by bacteria in the intestine and then deacetylated by body esterases; conjugation of chloramphenicol is reduced in the new-born; in rats, the metabolism of chloramphenicol is stimulated by phenobarbitone and chloramphenicol itself inhibits the metabolism of dicoumarol, phenytoin, and tolbutamide.

EXCRETION. 70 to 90% of a dose is excreted in the urine in 24 hours; 5 to 10% is excreted unchanged and the rest is excreted mainly as the glucuronide; small amounts are excreted in the bile and faeces.

FURTHER INFORMATION. Absorption—H. Andersgaard *et al.*, *Acta pharm. suec.*, 1971, **8**, 403; elimination in patients with cirrhosis—F. Azzolini, *Int. J. clin. Pharmac.*, 1972, **6**, 130; absorption and dissolution characteristics of oral preparations—H. Bell *et al.*, *Pharmacology*, 1971, **5**, 108 and A. J. Glazko *et al.*, *Clin. Pharmac. Ther.*, 1968, **9**, 472; concentrations in urine and blood in relation to renal function—A. A. Lindberg *et al.*, *Br. med. J.*, ii/1966, 724.

Actions and uses.
Chloramphenicol is an antibiotic with a bacteriostatic action which has a wide range of antimicrobial activity similar to that described under Tetracycline Hydrochloride but including also *Salmonella typhi* and *S. paratyphi*. It is active when administered by mouth, being rapidly absorbed from the gastro-intestinal tract. It enters the bile, cerebrospinal fluid, and urine and passes the placental barrier in therapeutically effective amounts.

It is used in the treatment of typhoid and paratyphoid fevers, but it does not eliminate the typhoid carrier state. Cases resistant to chloramphenicol may be treated with ampicillin or co-trimoxazole; chloramphenicol used in conjunction with ampicillin may be more effective than either drug used alone.

Chloramphenicol is also used in the treatment of *Haemophilus influenzae* meningitis, chronic infections of the urinary tract with a sensitive strain of *Proteus vulgaris* that is resistant to other antibiotics, and rickettsial infections which do not respond to treatment with other drugs.

Chloramphenicol is usually administered by mouth in a dosage of 500 milligrams every 6 hours. A higher initial dosage, with the object of obtaining rapidly a high concentration in the blood, should not be given in the treatment of typhoid fever because of the release of endotoxins from the infecting organisms.

Treatment should be continued for 2 or 3 days after the patient's temperature has returned to normal so as to minimise the risk of relapse, but it is inadvisable to continue the course for more than 10 days or to exceed a total dose of 26 grams.

For a child, the usual daily dosage is 25 to 50 milligrams per kilogram body-weight, given in divided doses at intervals of 6 hours; it should not be given to premature or newborn infants as the Gray syndrome or agranulocytosis may result.

Chloramphenicol is usually administered in capsules; patients unable to swallow the capsules may be given the antibiotic by mouth as a suspension of the palmitate.

Chloramphenicol may be given to seriously ill patients by injection of aqueous solutions of chloramphenicol sodium succinate.

Chloramphenicol is of value when applied to the skin and mucous membranes in the treatment of infections due to sensitive organisms. Ear-drops containing 5 or 10% are used in chronic otorrhoea and are often effective even when such organisms as *Proteus vulgaris* and *Pseudomonas aeruginosa*, which are resistant to many antibacterial agents, are present.

Chloramphenicol is used in the treatment of a wide variety of infections of the eye, and for treatment of superficial infections of the skin such as impetigo, sycosis barbae, and furunculosis.

Undesirable effects. The most serious toxic effect caused by chloramphenicol is that occasionally exerted on the haemopoietic system, resulting in agranulocytosis, thrombocytopenic purpura, or aplastic anaemia. Fatal cases of aplastic anaemia following the administration of chloramphenicol have occurred, and other antibiotics, such as the tetracyclines, are preferred whenever the infecting organism is sensitive to them. Other serious effects may include renal toxicity, optic neuritis, jaundice, and the Stevens-Johnson syndrome. Topical or systemic use of chloramphenicol may give rise to allergic skin rashes and more serious allergic reactions may occur in sensitised patients.

Other toxic reactions, which may occur in a small proportion of patients, include dryness of the mouth, nausea, vomiting, diarrhoea, and urticarial skin rashes. Disturbance of the normal bacterial flora of the mouth and gastro-intestinal tract produced by chloramphenicol may be followed by excessive growth of *Candida albicans* and other fungi on the mucous membrane, producing stomatitis, sore tongue, rectal or vaginal irritation, and, rarely, pneumonia.

The occurrence of the more serious toxic effects is usually associated with high dosage or prolonged administration or with repeated courses of treatment, but blood dyscrasias have also occurred with relatively low dosage. Several months may elapse between the completion of treatment and the onset of aplastic anaemia, and although frequent blood counts are advisable they cannot be relied upon to give adequate warning.

Precautions and contra-indications. Chloramphenicol should not be used for its systemic effect in the treatment of any infection which can be treated with a less toxic antibiotic or a sulphonamide. Its use by mouth is therefore virtually limited to the treatment of typhoid and paratyphoid fevers.

It should preferably be avoided in pregnancy and in nursing mothers.

Drug interactions. Chloramphenicol enhances the effects of phenytoin and hypoglycaemic sulphonylureas.

Veterinary uses. Chloramphenicol is used for the treatment of infections by organisms known to be susceptible to its action and for which safer antibacterial agents are not effective, for example systemic salmonellosis in cattle, respiratory infections in calves, and feline panleucopenia.

The usual dose by mouth for all species is 50 milligrams per kilogram body-weight daily in divided doses but it should not be given by mouth to adult ruminants.

The usual dosage by intramuscular injection for all species is 10 milligrams per kilogram body-weight daily. The usual dose by intrauterine administration in mares and cows is 0.5 to 1 gram and for ewes and sows 250 to 500 milligrams daily.

Preparations

CHLORAMPHENICOL CAPSULES: consisting of chloramphenicol, in powder, which may be mixed with a suitable inert diluent, enclosed in a hard capsule. The capsule shells may be coloured. Available as capsules containing 250 mg of chloramphenicol.

A standard for these capsules is given in the British Pharmacopoeia 1973

Containers and *Storage:* see the entry on Capsules for general information on containers and storage.

Labelling: the label on the container should state the directions for storage and the date after which the capsules are not intended to be used.

Advice for patients: the capsules should be taken at regular intervals. The prescribed course should be completed.

CHLORAMPHENICOL EAR-DROPS: consisting of a solution of chloramphenicol in propylene glycol. Usually a solution containing 5% of chloramphenicol is used but a solution containing 10% is also available.

A standard for these ear-drops is given in the British Pharmaceutical Codex 1973

Containers and *Labelling:* see the entry on Ear-drops for general information on containers and labelling.

Storage: it should be protected from light.

Advice for patients: the prescribed course should be completed.

CHLORAMPHENICOL EYE-DROPS:

Chloramphenicol	0.5 g
Phenylmercuric acetate or nitrate	0.002 g
Borax	0.3 g
Boric acid	1.5 g
Purified water	to 100 ml

Dissolve the boric acid, the borax, and the phenylmercuric salt in 90 ml of the purified water with the aid of heat; adjust the temperature of the solution to 60°, add the chloramphenicol, and maintain the temperature at 60° until the chloramphenicol is dissolved. Cool the solution, add sufficient purified water to produce the required volume, and mix. Then, either (i) sterilise the solution by filtration, and transfer by means of an aseptic technique to sterile containers, which are then closed so as to exclude micro-organisms (method B) or (ii) clarify the solution by filtration, transfer it to the final containers, which are then closed to exclude micro-organisms, and sterilise it by maintaining at 98° to 100° for 30 minutes (method C).

The eye-drops should not be issued for use later than 3 months from the date of preparation, when stored at room temperature in an unopened container.

The preparation is more stable at lower temperatures and provided that it is kept in an unopened container and maintained at a temperature of 2° to 8°, it may be issued for use for up to 17 months from the date of preparation. These storage times assume that the eye-drops will not usually be used for more than 4 weeks after the date of issue for use, so that the total times do not exceed those specified in the storage statement below.

Alternatively, using an aseptic technique, dissolve a sterile dry powder, consisting of the chloramphenicol, the boric acid, the borax, and the phenylmercuric salt, in sterile purified water in the final sterile container. The eye-drops must be freshly prepared when this alternative method is used.

A standard for these eye-drops is given in the British Pharmaceutical Codex 1973

Containers: see the entry on Eye-drops for general information on containers.

Labelling: the label on the container of the eye-drops, except a container issued for an individual patient for domiciliary use should state:
(1) the name of the eye-drops,
(2) the directions for storage, and
(3) the date of preparation.

The label on the container of dry powder used for the preparation of the eye-drops by the alternative method given above should state:
(1) the name of the powder, indicating that it is for the preparation of chloramphenicol eye-drops, and

(2) the weight of chloramphenicol in the container or the volume of eye-drops prepared according to the manufacturer's instructions.

The label on the container or the label on the carton or the package leaflet should state:

(3) the directions for preparing the eye-drops.

The label on a multiple-dose container issued for an individual patient for domiciliary use should state:

(1) that the eye-drops should be kept in a cool place,

(2) if the eye-drops have been prepared by the alternative method given above, "The contents to be discarded if not used before..." [a date 2 weeks after the date of preparation], and

(3) if the eye-drops have been prepared by the other methods given above, the date after which the eye-drops should not be used.

Storage: it should be protected from light. When stored at a temperature of 2° to 8°, it may be expected to retain its potency for 18 months from the date of preparation. When stored at a temperature not exceeding 25°, it may be expected to retain its potency for 4 months from the date of preparation.

Advice for patients: see the entry on Eye-drops for general information on the use of eye-drops. The prescribed course should be completed.

CHLORAMPHENICOL EYE OINTMENT: prepared by incorporating chloramphenicol in eye ointment basis, or any other suitable basis, by method B described in the entry on Eye Ointments. An eye ointment containing 1% of chloramphenicol is available.

A standard for this eye ointment is given in the British Pharmaceutical Codex 1973

Containers and *Labelling:* see the entry on Eye Ointments for general information on containers and labelling.

Advice for patients: see the entry on Eye Ointments for general information on the use of eye ointments. The prescribed course should be completed.

CHLORAMPHENICOL INJECTION: a sterile suspension of chloramphenicol in water for injections. It may contain suitable suspending and stabilising agents. It is prepared by means of an aseptic technique. Available as a suspension containing 150 mg of chloramphenicol per ml in 30, 50, 75, and 100-ml vials.

A standard for this injection is given in the British Pharmacopoeia (Veterinary)

Containers: see the entry on Injections for general information on containers.

Labelling: see the entry on Injections for general information on labelling. In addition, the label on the container should state the amount of the medicament as the amount of chloramphenicol in 1 millilitre, and that the injection is for intramuscular administration only.

Storage: it should be stored in a cool place, protected from light. It should not be allowed to freeze. Under these conditions it may be expected to retain its potency for 2 years.

OTHER PREPARATIONS available include a CREAM containing chloramphenicol 1%, EAR-DROPS containing chloramphenicol 1% with prednisolone 0.25%, an EYE OINTMENT containing chloramphenicol 1% with hydrocortisone acetate 0.5%, an eye ointment containing chloramphenicol 1% with oxyphenbutazone 10%; a veterinary INJECTION containing chloramphenicol (in solution) 150 mg per ml in 50- and 100-ml vials, a veterinary injection containing chloramphenicol (in solution) 200 mg per ml in 50-ml vials, a veterinary injection containing chloramphenicol 250 mg (in solution) per ml in 100-ml vials; a veterinary POWDER (for ophthalmic use) containing chloramphenicol 0.5% with amethocaine

hydrochloride 0.1%; a veterinary (oral) SOLUTION containing chloramphenicol 70 mg per ml; veterinary TABLETS containing chloramphenicol 50 mg, veterinary tablets containing chloramphenicol 500 mg, and tablets containing chloramphenicol 500 mg with furazolidone 250 mg.

Chloramphenicol Palmitate

(2R,3R)-2-(2,2-Dichloroacetamido)-3-hydroxy-3-(4-nitrophenyl)propyl palmitate, the 3-palmitic ester of chloramphenicol.

$C_{27}H_{42}Cl_2N_2O_6 = 561.6$

OTHER NAMES: Chloramphen. Palm.; *Chloromycetin*®

A standard is given in the British Pharmaceutical Codex 1973

Chloramphenicol palmitate exists in three crystalline forms and one amorphous form but only one polymorph, known as polymorph B, is active. In making preparations which contain chloramphenicol palmitate in solid form, any polymorph may be used, but the manufacturing process must be such as to ensure that the final product contains the desired polymorph B.

Description. An almost tasteless, fine, white, unctuous powder with a faint odour.

Solubility. Practically insoluble in water; soluble, at 20°, in 45 parts of alcohol, in 14 parts of ether, and in 6 parts of chloroform.

Specific rotation. +22.5° to +25.5°, determined on a 5% solution in dehydrated alcohol.

Storage. It should be protected from light.

Identification. TEST. Mix about 50 mg with 2 ml of *alcoholic potassium hydroxide solution*, heat on a water-bath for 15 minutes, and add *silver nitrate solution*; a white precipitate is produced which is insoluble in nitric acid but dissolves in *dilute ammonia solution*.

MELTING-POINT. About 89°.

ULTRAVIOLET ABSORPTION. In dehydrated alcohol, maximum at 271 nm (E1%, 1cm = 178).

Determination in body fluids. See under Chloramphenicol.

Metabolism. See under Chloramphenicol.

Actions and uses. Chloramphenicol palmitate has the actions, uses, and undesirable effects described under Chloramphenicol, to which it is hydrolysed in the gastrointestinal tract. Because it is insoluble in water it is almost tasteless and is therefore preferred to chloramphenicol for oral administration to children and to adults when capsules cannot be swallowed; 174 milligrams of chloramphenicol palmitate is equivalent to 100 milligrams of chloramphenicol.

For an adult, the equivalent of 1.5 to 3 grams of chloramphenicol is given daily in divided doses; for a child, the equivalent of 25 to 50 milligrams of chloramphenicol per kilogram body-weight is given daily in divided doses.

Precautions and contra-indications. As for Chloramphenicol.

Preparation

CHLORAMPHENICOL MIXTURE (*Syn.* Chloramphenicol Palmitate Suspension): a suspension of chloramphenicol palmitate in a suitable flavoured vehicle.
The method of manufacture is such that the content of the biologically inactive chloramphenicol palmitate polymorph A is within the prescribed limit in the final product.
Available as a mixture containing chloramphenicol palmitate equivalent to 125 mg of chloramphenicol in 5 ml. When a dose less than or not a multiple of 5 ml is prescribed, the mixture may be diluted, as described in the entry on Mixtures, with syrup. The diluted mixture must be freshly prepared.
A standard for this mixture is given in the British Pharmaceutical Codex 1973
Containers and *Labelling:* see the entry on Mixtures for general information on containers and labelling.
Storage: it should be protected from light.
Advice for patients: the mixture should be taken at regular intervals. The prescribed course should be completed.

Chloramphenicol Sodium Succinate

Sodium (2*R*,3*R*)-2-(2,2-dichloroacetamido)-3-hydroxy-3-(4-nitrophenyl)propyl succinate

$$CH_2 \cdot O \cdot CO \cdot [CH_2]_2 \cdot COONa$$
$$H---C---NH \cdot CO \cdot CHCl_2$$
$$HO---C---H$$

$$NO_2$$

$C_{15}H_{15}Cl_2N_2NaO_8 = 445.2$

OTHER NAMES: Chloramphen. Sod. Succ.; *Chloromycetin*®; *Kemicetine*®

A standard is given in the British Pharmacopoeia Addendum 1977 and the British Pharmacopoeia (Veterinary)

Description. An odourless, hygroscopic, white or yellowish-white powder.

Solubility. Soluble, at 20°, in less than 1 part of water and in 1 part of alcohol; practically insoluble in ether and in chloroform.

Acidity. A 25% solution has a pH of 6 to 7.

Moisture content. Not more than 2%, determined by Fischer titration.

Specific rotation. +5° to +8°, determined on a 5% solution.

Stability. See under Chloramphenicol.

Storage. It should be stored in airtight containers, protected from light.

Identification. TESTS. 1. To about 50 mg add 5 ml of pyridine and 5 ml of *sodium hydroxide solution*, mix well, and heat on a water-bath for a few minutes; a deep red colour develops in the pyridine layer.
2. To about 100 mg add 200 mg of resorcinol and 4 drops of sulphuric acid, heat gently until a deep red solution is produced, and then pour the solution carefully into a large volume of water; an orange-yellow solution with an intense green fluorescence is produced.
3. It complies with Test 2 described under Chloramphenicol.

ULTRAVIOLET ABSORPTION. In ethyl acetate, maximum at 320 nm; in water, maximum at 276 nm (E1%, 1cm = 216).

Determination in body fluids. See under Chloramphenicol.

Metabolism. See under Chloramphenicol.

Actions and uses. Chloramphenicol sodium succinate has the actions, uses, and undesirable effects described under Chloramphenicol, but being soluble in water it is suitable for administration by injection. Solutions containing 10% are administered by intravenous injection. The usual dose for adults is the equivalent of 1 gram of chloramphenicol every 6 to 8 hours; 1.4 grams of chloramphenicol sodium succinate is approximately equivalent to 1 gram of chloramphenicol. Larger doses may be necessary in the treatment of meningitis.
For children aged 6 months to 5 years the usual dose is the equivalent of 50 to 100 milligrams of chloramphenicol per kilogram body-weight daily in divided doses. Premature infants should not be given more than 25 milligrams per kilogram body-weight daily.

Precautions and contra-indications. As for Chloramphenicol.

Veterinary uses. Chloramphenicol sodium succinate is used when a soluble form of chloramphenicol is required for injection. The usual dosage by subcutaneous, intramuscular, or intravenous injection for horses and cattle is the equivalent of 2 to 4 milligrams of chloramphenicol per kilogram body-weight and for foals, calves, dogs, and cats the equivalent of 10 milligrams of chloramphenicol per kilogram body-weight twice daily.

Preparation

CHLORAMPHENICOL SODIUM SUCCINATE INJECTION: a sterile solution of chloramphenicol sodium succinate in dextrose injection (5%), in sodium chloride injection, or in water for injections. It is prepared by dissolving the contents of a sealed container in the vehicle shortly before use. Available as a powder in vials containing chloramphenicol sodium succinate equivalent to 1 and 1.2 g of chloramphenicol.
A standard for this injection is given in the British Pharmacopoeia Addendum 1977 and in the British Pharmacopoeia (Veterinary)
Containers: see the entry on Injections for general information on containers.
Labelling: see the entry on Injections for general information on labelling. In addition, the label on the container should state the amount of the medicament as the equivalent amount of chloramphenicol.
Storage: the sealed container should be protected from light.
The injection contains no bactericide and should be used as soon as possible after preparation, but solutions of chloramphenicol sodium succinate may be expected to retain their potency for up to 24 hours after preparation, provided they are stored at 2° to 10°.

Chlorbutol

2,2,2-Trichloro-1,1-dimethylethanol hemihydrate

$$CCl_3 \cdot C(CH_3)_2 \cdot OH, \tfrac{1}{2}H_2O$$

$C_4H_7Cl_3O, \tfrac{1}{2}H_2O = 186.5$

OTHER NAMES: Chlorbutanol; Chlorobutanol; Chlorobutanolum

A standard is given in the European Pharmacopoeia Vol. III

Description. Colourless crystals with a characteristic musty and somewhat camphoraceous odour and taste. It is volatile at ordinary temperatures.

Solubility. Soluble, at 20°, in 130 parts of water, in less than 1 part of alcohol, and in 8 parts of glycerol; soluble in ether, in chloroform, and in volatile oils.

Acidity or alkalinity. A freshly prepared solution in water is neutral to litmus.

Storage. It should be stored in airtight containers.

Identification. TESTS. 1. To 5 ml of a freshly prepared 0.5% solution add 1 ml of 1N sodium hydroxide followed by 2 ml of *iodine solution*, added slowly; the odour of iodoform develops and a yellow precipitate is produced.
2. Shake 100 mg with 5 ml of 1N sodium hydroxide, add one drop of aniline, and warm; the odour of phenyl isocyanide is produced.
3. Mix about 20 mg with 2 ml of 10N sodium hydroxide and 1 ml of pyridine, heat on a water-bath, and shake; the pyridine layer becomes red.

MELTING-POINT. About 79°.

Actions and uses. Chlorbutol is a mild sedative and local analgesic. Its sedative action resembles that of chloral hydrate but it is less hypnotic and less irritant to mucous membranes. It has been used in the treatment of motion-sickness, but it is less effective for this purpose than hyoscine and the antihistamine drugs. The usual dose is 0.3 to 1.2 grams.
Chlorbutol has antibacterial and antifungal properties. It is used at a concentration of 0.5% as a preservative in eye-drops and injections. At this concentration it is close to its solubility limit at low temperatures and crystallisation from solutions may occur.
Chlorbutol is unstable in alkaline solution and although it is more stable in acid solution at room temperatures, it decomposes appreciably on steaming or autoclaving. It may also be lost from aqueous solutions by volatilisation.

Chlorcyclizine Hydrochloride

(±)-1-(4-Chlorobenzhydryl)-4-methylpiperazine hydrochloride

$C_{18}H_{22}Cl_2N_2 = 337.3$

OTHER NAME: *Histofax*® (with calamine)

A standard is given in the British Pharmacopoeia 1973

Description. A white odourless crystalline powder with a bitter taste.

Solubility. Soluble, at 20°, in 2 parts of water, in 11 parts of alcohol, and in 4 parts of chloroform; very slightly soluble in ether.

Acidity. A 1% solution has a pH of 4.8 to 5.5.

Moisture content. Not more than 2.5%, determined by drying at 120°.

Dissociation constants. pK_a 2.4, 7.8 (25°).

Identification. TESTS. 1. Dissolve 200 mg in 10 ml of water, add 15 ml of *trinitrophenol solution*, filter, and wash the filter with 5 ml of water; the residue, after recrystallisation from alcohol (70%), washing with cold alcohol (70%), and drying at 105° for 30 minutes, melts at about 246°, with decomposition.
2. To about 10 mg add 2 ml of sulphuric acid; a bright yellow colour is produced which disappears when the solution is diluted with water.

MELTING-POINT. About 225°, with decomposition.

ULTRAVIOLET ABSORPTION. In alcohol (95%), maximum at 230 nm (E1%, 1cm = 440).

INFRA-RED ABSORPTION. Major peaks at 704, 725, 758, 870, 990, and 1087 cm^{-1} (see Appendix 2b: Infra-red Spectra).

Determination in body fluids. COLORIMETRY. Tissues —R. Kuntzman *et al.*, *J. Pharmac. exp. Ther.*, 1965, **149**, 29.

Metabolism. ABSORPTION. Readily absorbed after oral administration.

BLOOD CONCENTRATION. After the oral administration of 50 mg 3 times a day for 6 days, plasma concentrations of the metabolite, norchlorcyclizine, of 50 to 115 ng/ml are attained on the first day after cessation of treatment and plasma concentrations of 20 to 40 ng/ml are attained on the tenth day after cessation of treatment; after a single oral dose of 2 mg/kg, plasma concentrations of about 50 ng/ml and 34 ng/ml are attained in 5 hours for unchanged drug and its demethylated metabolite respectively.

HALF-LIFE. Plasma half-life for the demethylated metabolite, 6 to 9 days.

DISTRIBUTION. Widely distributed throughout the body and high concentrations are found in the liver, lungs, kidneys, and spleen; in the rat, both the unchanged drug and its demethylated metabolite cross the placenta; *protein binding*, in dogs, chlorcyclizine is 96% and nor-chlorcyclizine 94% bound to plasma proteins.

METABOLIC REACTIONS. Demethylation to form nor-chlorcyclizine and N-oxidation to form chlorcyclizine N-oxide; ring fission occurs in the rat to form N-(p-chlorobenzhydryl)ethylenediamine; demethylation occurs at a faster rate in male rats than in female rats and it is also increased as a result of enzyme induction by phenobarbitone.

EXCRETION. Slowly excreted in the urine; about 0.5% of a dose is excreted in the urine as the N-oxide in man, in rats about 42% is excreted in the urine as the N-oxide.

FURTHER INFORMATION. Physiological distribution and metabolic inactivation—R. Kuntzman *et al.*, *J. Pharmac. exp. Ther.*, 1965, **149**, 29 and 1967, **155**, 337 and *Ann. N.Y. Acad. Sci.*, 1973, **226**, 131; effects of chronic administration to rats—H. J. Gaertner, *J. Pharmac. exp. Ther.*, 1973, **185**, 195; distribution in pregnant mice —W. J. Waddell, *Drug Met. Disp.*, 1973, **1**, 598.

Actions and uses. Chlorcyclizine hydrochloride has the actions and undesirable effects of the antihistamine drugs, as described under Promethazine Hydrochloride. It has a prolonged action and the usual dosage by mouth for adults is 50 to 100 milligrams once or twice daily.

Poisoning. As for Promethazine Hydrochloride.

Preparations

CHLORCYCLIZINE TABLETS: available as tablets containing 50 mg of chlorcyclizine hydrochloride; they may be sugar coated.

A standard for these tablets is given in the British Pharmacopoeia 1973

Containers and *Storage:* see the entry on Tablets for general information on containers and storage. Containers should be airtight.

Advice for patients: the tablets may cause drowsiness; persons affected should not drive or operate machinery. Alcohol should be avoided.

OTHER PREPARATIONS available include a CREAM containing chlorcyclizine hydrochloride 2% with calamine 8%.

Chlordiazepoxide Hydrochloride

7-Chloro-2-methylamino-5-phenyl-3H-1,4-benzodiazepine 4-oxide hydrochloride

$C_{16}H_{15}Cl_2N_3O = 336.2$

OTHER NAMES: *Calmoden®*; Chlordiazepoxidi Hydrochloridum; *Librium®*; *Tropium®*

A standard is given in the European Pharmacopoeia Vol. III

Description. A white crystalline powder with a slight odour and a very bitter taste.

Solubility. Soluble, at 20°, in 10 parts of water and in 40 parts of alcohol; very slightly soluble in chloroform and in ether.

Acidity. A 10% solution has a pH of 2 to 3.

Dissociation constant. pK_a 4.6 (20°).

Stability. Chlordiazepoxide undergoes hydrolysis to demoxepam by loss of the methylamino group. Demoxepam is further degraded by rupture of the 4,5-azomethine linkage to form an intermediate compound which is subsequently converted to 2-amino-5-chlorobenzophenone. This constitutes the principal degradation route, but the demoxepam also forms a second intermediate, by hydrolysis of the 1,2-amide bond, which subsequently gives rise to a glycine derivative.

FURTHER INFORMATION. Kinetics and mechanisms of hydrolysis of 1,4-benzodiazepines—W. W. Han *et al.*, *J. pharm. Sci.*, 1976, **65**, 1198.

Storage. It should be stored in airtight containers, protected from light.

Identification. TESTS. 1. To about 20 mg add 5 ml of hydrochloric acid and 10 ml of water, heat to boiling,

cool, add 2 ml of 0.1% sodium nitrite solution, allow to stand for 1 minute, add 1 ml of 0.5% ammonium sulphamate solution, allow to stand for 1 minute and add 1 ml of 0.1% of N-1-naphthylethylenediamine dihydrochloride solution; a reddish-violet colour is produced.

2. Dissolve about 200 mg in 4 ml of hot *dilute hydrochloric acid*, boil for 10 minutes, cool, and filter; the filtrate gives the reactions of primary aromatic amines, producing a bright pinkish-red precipitate.

3. Dissolve about 200 mg in 30 ml of water, add 5 ml of *dilute sodium hydroxide solution*, shake, filter, and wash the filter with water; the residue, after drying *in vacuo*, melts at about 240°.

MELTING-POINT. About 215°, with decomposition.

ULTRAVIOLET ABSORPTION. In 0.1N hydrochloric acid, maxima at 246 nm (E1%, 1cm = 1000) and 308 nm (E1%, 1cm = 293); in 0.1N sodium hydroxide, maxima at 246 nm and 262 nm (E1%, 1cm = 1030); in alcohol (95%), maxima at 247 nm (E1%, 1 cm = 891) and 266 nm (E1%, 1cm = 988).

INFRA-RED ABSORPTION. Major peaks at 845, 1146, 1222, 1394, 1425, and 1650 cm^{-1} (see Appendix 2a: Infra-red Spectra).

Determination in body fluids. GAS CHROMATOGRAPHY. Benzodiazepines in blood or plasma—J. A. de Silva *et al.*, *Analyt. Chem.*, 1976, **48**, 10.

REVIEWS OF METHODS FOR BENZODIAZEPINES. J. M. Clifford and W. F. Smythe, *Analyst, Lond.*, 1974, **99**, 241.

Metabolism. ABSORPTION. Readily absorbed after oral administration; the rate of absorption is reduced when antacids are administered concurrently but the extent of absorption is not altered; intramuscular doses are more slowly absorbed than oral doses and suppositories are poorly absorbed.

BLOOD CONCENTRATIONS. After oral doses of 20 to 50 mg of the hydrochloride, peak plasma concentrations of 0.7 to 2 μg/ml are attained in 1 to 6 hours; after similar doses intramuscularly, slightly lower peak concentrations are attained in 2 to 12 hours; desmethylchlordiazepoxide is detectable in plasma after 2 hours, following an oral dose of 20 mg, and reaches concentrations of up to 0.5 μg/ml; demoxepam is not detectable in plasma after administration of a single dose of chlordiazepoxide. During therapy with 30 mg of the hydrochloride daily, steady-state plasma concentrations of 0.7 μg/ml, 0.5 μg/ml, and 0.5 μg/ml are attained for chlordiazepoxide, desmethylchlordiazepoxide, and demoxepam respectively.

HALF-LIFE. Plasma half-life, 6 to 28 hours; following intravenous administration, plasma concentrations exhibit a biphasic decline and the half-lives are about 4 to 15 minutes for the α-phase and 9 to 14 hours for the β-phase.

DISTRIBUTION. Rapidly and widely distributed throughout the body; chlordiazepoxide crosses the placenta and is secreted in milk; volume of distribution, about 25 litres; *protein binding*, about 94% bound to plasma proteins.

METABOLIC REACTIONS. N-Demethylation to form desmethylchlordiazepoxide which is converted to the lactam, demoxepam, which is further cleaved to ring-opened metabolites and further metabolised by reduction to desmethyldiazepam followed by hydroxylation to form oxazepam; conjugation with glucuronic acid; aromatic hydroxylation occurs in rats but not in man;

demoxepam, desmethylchlordiazepoxide, desmethyldiazepam, and oxazepam are active metabolites.

EXCRETION. 60% is excreted in the urine and 10 to 20% in the faeces; less than 2% of a dose is excreted in the urine unchanged and the major urinary metabolites appear to be ring-opened derivatives; in rats, 25% is excreted in the urine as free demoxepam, 15% as glucuronides, mainly of oxazepam, 3.5% as the ring-opened lactam, and small amounts of the 5-p-hydroxy-phenyl- and 7-hydroxy-metabolites.

FURTHER INFORMATION. Pharmacokinetics after administration by various routes and after multiple oral doses—H. G. Boxenbaum *et al.*, *J. Pharmacokinet. Biopharm.*, 1977, **5**, 3 and 25.

Actions and uses. Chlordiazepoxide is a tranquillising drug which relieves nervous tension and anxiety states. It has slight muscle-relaxant properties similar to those of mephenesin.

Dosage depends on the clinical conditions and response of the patient, varying from 15 milligrams of chlordiazepoxide hydrochloride daily in divided doses for mild anxiety states to 60 milligrams daily in divided doses in severe conditions. The daily dosage is reduced to 5 to 20 milligrams in children and elderly and debilitated patients.

Chlordiazepoxide may be given by intramuscular injection for the rapid relief of acute conditions; it must not be given intravenously. Patients receiving injections should be kept under observation, preferably in bed.

Undesirable effects. Drowsiness and ataxia occur, especially with high dosage. Treatment with chlordiazepoxide in the severely disturbed patient sometimes results in paradoxical reactions, provoking excitement instead of sedation.

Chlordiazepoxide may add to the effects of alcohol and reduce ability to drive motor cars and operate moving machinery.

Rashes, blood dyscrasias, and hepatic dysfunction have occasionally been reported.

Precautions. Caution should be exercised in using chlordiazepoxide in conjunction with other drugs that act on the central nervous system.

Dependence. It may give rise to dependence of the barbiturate-alcohol type as described under Drug Dependence.

Preparations

CHLORDIAZEPOXIDE CAPSULES: consisting of chlordiazepoxide hydrochloride, in powder, which may be mixed with a suitable inert diluent, enclosed in a hard capsule; the capsule shells may be coloured. Available as capsules containing 5 and 10 mg of chlordiazepoxide hydrochloride.

A standard for these capsules is given in the British Pharmacopoeia 1973

Containers and *Storage:* see the entry on Capsules for general information on containers and storage. Containers should be light resistant.

Advice for patients: the capsules may cause drowsiness; persons affected should not drive or operate machinery. Alcohol should be avoided.

OTHER PREPARATIONS available include an INJECTION containing chlordiazepoxide hydrochloride equivalent to 100 mg of chlordiazepoxide as a powder in ampoules for reconstitution with 2 ml of solvent; TABLETS containing chlordiazepoxide hydrochloride 5 and 10 mg and tablets containing chlordiazepoxide 5, 10, and 25 mg.

Chlorhexidine Acetate

1,1'-Hexamethylenebis[5-(4-chlorophenyl)biguanide] diacetate

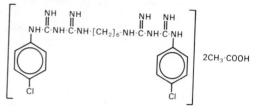

$C_{26}H_{38}Cl_2N_{10}O_4 = 625.6$

OTHER NAMES: *Hibitane*®
Medi-Sache® (with cetrimide)

A standard is given in the British Pharmaceutical Codex 1973

Description. A white to pale cream, odourless, microcrystalline powder.

Solubility. Soluble, at 20°, in 55 parts of water and in 15 parts of alcohol; very slightly soluble in glycerol and in propylene glycol.

Moisture content. Not more than 3.5%, determined by drying at 105°.

Stability. In the form of powder, chlorhexidine acetate is stable at ordinary temperatures but when heated it degrades to 4-chloroaniline; chlorhexidine hydrochloride is less readily degraded by heat than the acetate and can be heated at 115° for one hour without appreciable production of 4-chloroaniline.

In aqueous solution, salts of chlorhexidine degrade by hydrolysis to 4-chloroaniline. Solutions are most stable at pH 5 to 6.

Sterilisation at 100° for 30 minutes has very little effect on chlorhexidine; the concentration of 4-chloroaniline remains within the limit of 500 parts per million. A concentration of 4-chloroaniline of about 3000 parts per million may be produced after sterilisation by heating in an autoclave, but such solutions are unlikely to be toxic.

FURTHER INFORMATION. Stability in aqueous solution —R. R. Goodall *et al.*, *Pharm. J.*, i/1968, 33, F. Jaminet *et al.*, *Pharm. Acta Helv.*, 1970, **45**, 60, and J. Dolby *et al.*, *Pharm. Acta Helv.*, 1972, **47**, 615; toxicity of 4-chloroaniline—A. I. Scott and E. Eccleston, *Proc. Eur. Soc. Stud. Drug Tox.*, 1966, **8**, 195.

Incompatibility. It is incompatible with soaps and similar anionic compounds.

Hygroscopicity. It absorbs insignificant amounts of moisture at temperatures up to 37° at relative humidities up to about 80%.

Sterilisation. Solutions are sterilised by heating in an autoclave at 115° for 30 minutes. The solutions should not be alkaline or contain other ingredients that affect the stability of chlorhexidine. If glass containers are used they should be of neutral glass.

Storage. It should be stored in airtight containers, protected from light.

Preparation and storage of solutions. See the entry on Chlorhexidine Gluconate Solution.

Identification. TESTS. 1. Dissolve about 100 mg in 5 ml of a 20% solution of cetrimide by gently warming and add 1 ml of bromine and 1 ml of *sodium hydroxide solution*; a deep red colour is produced.

2. Dissolve about 100 mg in 10 ml of water and add, while shaking, 0.1 to 0.2 ml of *ammoniacal copper chloride solution*; a purple precipitate is produced immediately which changes to blue on the addition of a further 0.5 ml of *ammoniacal copper chloride solution*.

MELTING-POINT. About 153°.

ULTRAVIOLET ABSORPTION. In methyl alcohol, maximum at 259 nm (E1%, 1cm = 620).

Actions and uses. Chlorhexidine acetate has the actions and undesirable effects described in the entry on Chlorhexidine Gluconate Solution.

It is used as an antibacterial preservative in eye-drops, usually in a concentration of 0.01%.

Preparations

Preparations available include a SOLUTION containing chlorhexidine acetate 0.015% with cetrimide 0.15%.

Chlorhexidine Gluconate Solution

A 20% aqueous solution of 1,1'-hexamethylenebis[5-(4-chlorophenyl)biguanide] digluconate.

$C_{22}H_{30}Cl_2N_{10}.2C_6H_{12}O_7 = 897.8$

OTHER NAMES: *Corsodyl®*; *Dispray®*; *Hibiscrub®*; *Hibitane®*; *Rotersept®*
Eludril® (with amethocaine hydrochloride); *Savlodil®* and *Savlon®* (both with cetrimide)

A standard is given in the British Pharmacopoeia 1973

Description. An almost colourless to pale straw coloured odourless liquid with a bitter taste.

Solubility. Miscible with water, with up to 5 parts of alcohol, and with up to 3 parts of acetone.

Weight per ml. At 20°, 1.06 to 1.07 g.

Acidity. A 5% solution has a pH of 5.5 to 7.

Stability; Incompatibility; Sterilisation. See under Chlorhexidine Acetate.

Storage. It should be stored at a temperature not exceeding 25°, protected from light.

Preparation and storage of solutions. See statement on aqueous solutions of antiseptics in the entry on Solutions.

As a precaution against contamination with *Pseudomonas* species, stock solutions should contain at least 7% v/v of ethyl alcohol or 4% v/v of isopropyl alcohol.

Identification. TESTS. 1. It complies with Test 1 described under Chlorhexidine Acetate, 1 drop of the sample being used.

2. Mix 0.5 ml with 10 ml of water and 0.5 ml of *ferric chloride solution* and heat gently to boiling; a deep orange colour is produced. Add 1 ml of hydrochloric acid; the colour changes to yellow.

3. Mix 0.5 ml with 10 ml of water and add 0.5 ml of *copper sulphate solution*; a white precipitate is produced. Boil the solution; the precipitate flocculates and becomes lilac-coloured.

4. Mix 1 ml with 40 ml of water, cool in ice, and continue as in Test 2 described under Chlorhexidine Hydrochloride.

Actions and uses. Chlorhexidine is an antiseptic which is relatively non-toxic and is active against Gram-positive and Gram-negative organisms. Species of *Proteus* and *Pseudomonas* are relatively less susceptible, and it is inactive against acid-fast bacilli and bacterial spores and fungi.

Solutions containing 0.02 to 0.05% are used for treatment

of wounds and burns, and solutions containing 0.05 to 0.5% for the disinfection of the hands. A 0.02% solution is used for irrigation of the bladder and serous surfaces. A 0.5% solution in alcohol (70%) may be used for preoperative disinfection of the skin. A 0.2% solution in alcohol (7%) is used as a mouth-wash to inhibit the formation of bacterial plaque on the teeth.

To prevent corrosion, 0.1% of sodium nitrite should be added to solutions of chlorhexidine gluconate used for the storage of instruments. Such solutions should be changed at weekly intervals.

Cetrimide and other cationic detergents may be added to chlorhexidine solutions when additional detergent action is required.

Undesirable effects. Strong solutions may cause irritation of the conjunctiva and other sensitive tissues.

Preparations

CHLORHEXIDINE CREAM: containing chlorhexidine gluconate in a suitable water-miscible basis. A suitable cream may be prepared according to the following formula:

Chlorhexidine gluconate solution	..	.. 50 ml, or a sufficient quantity
Cetomacrogol emulsifying wax	..	.. 250 g
Liquid paraffin ..	.. .. ..	.. 100 g
Purified water, freshly boiled and cooled		to 1000 g

Melt the cetomacrogol emulsifying wax in the liquid paraffin at 60° and add, with rapid stirring, to the chlorhexidine gluconate solution, previously diluted to 500 ml with some of the water, at the same temperature; cool, add sufficient of the water to produce the required weight, and mix. Available as a cream containing 50 ml of chlorhexidine gluconate solution in each 1000 g of cream (1% of chlorhexidine gluconate).

A standard for this cream is given in the British Pharmacopoeia Addendum 1977 and in the British Pharmacopoeia (Veterinary)

Containers, Labelling, and *Storage:* see the entry on Creams for general information on containers, labelling, and storage.

Advice for patients: the cream may be applied liberally to the affected area as required. Fabric which has been in contact with chlorhexidine may subsequently stain if washed in solutions containing hypochlorite but solutions containing perborate may be used in laundering.

CHLORHEXIDINE MOUTH-WASH: a 0.2% aqueous solution of chlorhexidine gluconate, containing 7% v/v of alcohol (95%). It may contain suitable colouring and flavouring agents. The mouth-wash should be used undiluted.

Containers and *Labelling:* see the entry on Mouth-washes for general information on containers and labelling.

Advice for patients: the solution should be rinsed around the mouth 3 or 4 times daily as required, avoiding swallowing the preparation. If necessary the teeth should be brushed immediately before using the mouth-wash. Fabric which has been in contact with chlorhexidine may subsequently stain if washed in solutions containing hypochlorite but solutions containing perborate may be used in laundering.

DILUTE CHLORHEXIDINE SOLUTION (*Syn.* Alcoholic Chlorhexidine Solution):

Chlorhexidine gluconate solution	..	..	25 ml
Carmoisine, food grade of commerce		..	0.5 g
Alcohol (95%) ..	.. ..	.. ..	700 ml
Purified water, freshly boiled and cooled	.. ..	..	to 1000 ml

In making this preparation, the alcohol (95%) may be replaced by industrial methylated spirit, provided that the law and the statutory regulations governing the use of industrial methylated spirit are observed; alternatively, if specified by the prescriber, the alcohol (95%) may be replaced by isopropyl alcohol.

When prepared with alcohol (95%) or industrial methylated spirit the solution should be used within 1 year and when prepared with isopropyl alcohol the solution should be used within 3 years of the date of preparation.

A standard for this solution is given in the British Pharmaceutical Codex 1973

Containers: should be thoroughly cleansed before being filled. Closures should be such that the solution does not come into contact with cork.

OTHER PREPARATIONS available include an APPLICATION containing chlorhexidine gluconate 0.02% in an aerosol pack, an application containing chlorhexidine gluconate 0.2% in an aerosol pack, an application containing chlorhexidine gluconate 0.5% in an aerosol pack; a GEL containing chlorhexidine gluconate 1%; a SOLUTION containing chlorhexidine gluconate 4%, a solution containing chlorhexidine gluconate 5%, a solution containing chlorhexidine gluconate 0.015% with cetrimide 0.15%, a solution and a veterinary solution containing chlorhexidine gluconate 1.5% with cetrimide 15%; and a SPRAY containing chlorhexidine gluconate 0.05% with amethocaine hydrochloride 0.015% in an aerosol pack.

Chlorhexidine Hydrochloride

1,1'-Hexamethylenebis[5-(4-chlorophenyl)biguanide] dihydrochloride
$C_{22}H_{32}Cl_4N_{10} = 578.4$

OTHER NAMES: *Hibitane*®
Naseptin® (with neomycin sulphate)

A standard is given in the British Pharmacopoeia 1973

Description. A white crystalline odourless powder with a bitter taste.

Solubility. Soluble at 20°, in 1700 parts of water, in 450 parts of alcohol, and in 50 parts of propylene glycol.

Loss on drying. Not more than 2%, determined by drying at 130°.

Stability; Incompatibility; Hygroscopicity. See the entry on Chlorhexidine Acetate.

Sterilisation. It is sterilised by dry heat.

Storage. It should be stored in airtight containers, protected from light.

Preparation and storage of solutions. See the entry on Chlorhexidine Gluconate Solution.

Identification. TESTS. 1. It complies with Test 1 described under Chlorhexidine Acetate.
2. Dissolve 300 mg in 10 ml of a mixture of equal parts of hydrochloric acid and water, add 40 ml of water, filter, cool the filtrate in ice, add *sodium hydroxide solution* dropwise with stirring until the solution is slightly alkaline to titan yellow paper, add 1 ml in excess, filter, and wash the precipitate with water until free from alkali; the residue, after recrystallisation from alcohol (70%) and drying at 105°, melts at about 132°.

MELTING-POINT. About 255°, with decomposition.

Actions and uses. Chlorhexidine hydrochloride has the actions of chlorhexidine, as described under Chlorhexidine Gluconate Solution. As the hydrochloride is

sparingly soluble in water, it is used when a prolonged action is required. It is used in dusting-powders, creams, and ointments containing 0.1 to 1%, in lozenges containing 5 mg, and as an antiseptic in surgical dressings.

Chlorhexidine and neomycin cream is used for the treatment of nasal carriers of staphylococci.

Preparations

CHLORHEXIDINE AND NEOMYCIN CREAM: containing 0.1% w/w of chlorhexidine hydrochloride with 0.5% w/w of neomycin sulphate in a suitable water-miscible basis. This cream should not be diluted.

Containers and *Labelling:* see the entry on Creams for general information on containers and labelling.

Storage: it should be stored at a temperature not exceeding 25°.

Advice for patients: a small quantity of cream should be placed on the tip of the finger and applied to the inside of each nostril; the cream may be spread further inward by squeezing the nares. For prophylaxis, application should not be discontinued without the advice of the prescriber. For therapy the prescribed course should be completed. Contact with the eyes and ears should be avoided. Fabric which has been in contact with chlorhexidine may subsequently stain if washed in solutions containing hypochlorite but solutions containing perborate may be used in laundering.

CHLORHEXIDINE DUSTING-POWDER:

Chlorhexidine hydrochloride	5 g
Sterilisable maize starch	995 g

Prepare as described in the entry on Powders. Distribute, in quantities of not more than 30 g, into suitable glass containers with reclosable perforated lids or into other suitable containers, and heat for a sufficient length of time to ensure that the whole of the powder is maintained at 150° to 155° for 1 hour.

A standard for this dusting-powder is given in the British Pharmaceutical Codex 1973

Labelling: see the entry on Dusting-powders for general information on labelling.

Advice for patients: the dusting-powder should be dusted lightly on the affected area when required. It should not be applied to open wounds or raw surfaces of a large area. Fabric which has been in contact with chlorhexidine may subsequently stain if washed in solutions containing hypochlorite but solutions containing perborate may be used in laundering.

OTHER PREPARATIONS available include LOZENGES containing chlorhexidine hydrochloride 5 mg with benzocaine 2 mg.

Chlorinated Lime

Slaked lime which has been exposed to chlorine until absorption ceases.

OTHER NAMES: Calx Chlorinata; Chloride of Lime

A standard is given in the British Pharmaceutical Codex 1973

Description. A dull white powder with a characteristic odour.

Solubility. Partly soluble in water and in alcohol.

Stability. On exposure to air it becomes moist and gradually decomposes, carbon dioxide being absorbed and chlorine evolved. It is decomposed by hydrochloric acid with evolution of "available chlorine", upon which its value depends.

The stability of chlorinated lime in tropical climates is increased by admixture with quicklime.

Storage. It should be stored in airtight containers.

Actions and uses. Chlorinated lime is a powerful rapidly acting bactericide and deodorant. Its action is brief because the available chlorine is soon exhausted by combination with organic material. It is used to disinfect faeces, urine, and other infected organic material and as a cleansing agent for closets, drains, and effluents. It is a powerful bleaching agent and will decolorise most dyes.

Chlorinated lime is also used to disinfect swimming baths; it should be added in such an amount that the free chlorine, after combining with any organic matter in the water, is left in a concentration of 0.25 to 1 part per million parts of water.

A concentration of 1 part of free chlorine per million parts of water, maintained for 30 minutes, is an efficient disinfectant for drinking water; the taste of chlorine can be removed by adding a small crystal of sodium thiosulphate to a tumblerful of water.

Hypochlorite solutions have been advocated for the irrigation of wounds and burns and for removing dead tissue and preparing an area for skin grafting. Chlorinated lime and boric acid solution may be applied as a lotion or on gauze as a wet dressing, either alone or diluted with sodium chloride solution (0.9%). Infected wounds treated by the Carrel-Dakin method of continuous or frequent irrigation with surgical chlorinated soda solution containing 0.5% of available chlorine are rapidly cleansed and disinfected, but the solution must be renewed at least every 2 hours. The solution is irritating to the surrounding skin, which should be protected by smearing with soft paraffin. Electrolytically prepared solutions are used similarly, but at the same pH they are no more stable than surgical chlorinated soda solution, although the salt concentration is usually lower.

Surgical chlorinated soda solution is also a valuable cleansing antiseptic for superficial infected wounds and burns, when applied as a lotion or on gauze as a wet dressing. Diluted with 3 or 4 parts of water, it may be used as a gargle for the treatment of tonsillitis and, with 20 to 40 parts of water or normal saline, as an irrigation solution for infections of the bladder and vagina; it is also used as a foot-bath for the prophylaxis of fungal infections of the feet.

Preparations

CHLORINATED LIME AND BORIC ACID SOLUTION (Syn. Eusol):

Chlorinated lime	..	..	..	..	12.5 g
Boric acid, in powder	..	..	..	..	12.5 g
Water for preparations	..	..	..	to 1000 ml

Reduce the chlorinated lime to fine powder, triturate it with sufficient of the water to form a paste, and add a further portion of the water; add the boric acid, shake well, add sufficient water to produce the required volume, allow to stand, and filter. It must be freshly prepared.

Alternatively it may be prepared from stock liquids as described on page 110.

The preparation may also be made from the mixed dry ingredients, known as "Eupad", a slight modification of the first method being used.

A standard for this solution is given in the British Pharmaceutical Codex 1973

Labelling: the label on the container should state the date after which the solution is not intended to be used.

Storage: it should be stored in well-filled airtight bottles, in a cool place, protected from light. It deteriorates on storage and should be used within 2 weeks of its preparation.

Advice for patients: for use as an antiseptic wound dressing and cleansing agent. It has a bleaching action and will destroy most dyes.

SURGICAL CHLORINATED SODA SOLUTION (Syn. Dakin's Solution):

Boric acid	..	..	..	a sufficient quantity
Chlorinated lime	..	..	..	a sufficient quantity
Sodium carbonate	..	..	..	a sufficient quantity
Water for preparations	..	..	..	1000 ml

Determine the proportion of available chlorine in the chlorinated lime by the following method: triturate about 4 g, accurately weighed, with small portions of water, dilute the combined triturates to 1000 ml with water, shake well, and to 100 ml of the suspension add 3 g of potassium iodide in 100 ml of water and 5 ml of acetic acid, and titrate the liberated iodine with 0.1N sodium thiosulphate, each ml of which is equivalent to 0.003545 g of Cl. Prepare the solution by the following method, using the quantities of ingredient indicated in the table.

Available Chlorine in Chlorinated Lime % w/w	Chlorinated Lime g	Sodium Carbonate g	Boric Acid g
30	18.8	37.6	4.00
31	18.2	36.4	3.87
32	17.6	35.2	3.75
33	17.1	34.2	3.64
34	16.6	33.2	3.53
35	16.1	32.2	3.43
36	15.7	31.4	3.33
37	15.3	30.6	3.24
38	14.9	29.8	3.16
39	14.5	29.0	3.08
40	14.1	28.2	3.00

Dissolve the sodium carbonate in the water and add the solution, gradually and with constant trituration, to the chlorinated lime, previously powdered; shake occasionally during 20 minutes, allow to stand for a further 10 minutes, decant, and filter through a bleached filter; dissolve the boric acid in the filtrate.

It should be recently prepared.

A standard for this solution is given in the British Pharmaceutical Codex 1973

Storage: it should be stored in well-filled airtight bottles, in a cool place, protected from light.

Advice for patients: it has a bleaching action and will destroy most dyes.

Chlormerodrin (^{197}Hg) Injection

A sterile solution of 3-chloromercuri-2-methoxypropyl-urea (^{197}Hg) made isotonic with blood by the addition of sodium chloride.

OTHER NAMES: Chlormerodrin (^{197}Hg) Inj.; Chlormerodrini (^{197}Hg) Solutio Iniectabilis

A standard is given in the European Pharmacopoeia Vol. III Supplement

CAUTION. *This material is radioactive and any regulations in force must be complied with.*

Mercury-197 is a radioactive isotope of mercury which decays by electron capture with emission of γ-radiation. The most prominent photon has an energy of 0.069 MeV corresponding to the K X-ray of gold. It has a half-life of 64.4 hours. It may be prepared by neutron irradiation of mercury isotopically enriched in mercury-196.

Description. A clear colourless solution.

Acidity or alkalinity. pH 5 to 8

Sterilisation. It is sterilised by filtration.

Storage. It should be stored in an area assigned for the purpose. The storage conditions should be such that the maximum radiation-dose-rate to which persons may be exposed is reduced to an acceptable level.

Labelling. The label on the container should state:
(1) the content of mercury-197 expressed in millicuries at a given date and hour,
(2) the volume,
(3) the amount of chlormerodrin in the stated volume,
(4) that the injection is radioactive, and
(5) either that the injection does not contain a bactericide or the name and proportion of any added bactericide.

Metabolism. ABSORPTION. Absorbed after oral administration.

DISTRIBUTION. Taken up by tubule cells in the kidney and by brain tumours; *protein binding*, bound to some extent to plasma proteins particularly to albumin.

EXCRETION. Excreted to some extent in the urine.

FURTHER INFORMATION. Protein binding—Y. Cohen and N. Jullien-Saint Guily, *Annls pharm. Fr.*, 1973, **31**, 123.

Actions and uses. Chlormerodrin (^{197}Hg) is used for renal scintigraphy. After intravenous injection, radioactive chlormerodrin is concentrated in the renal tubular cells, the amount reaching a maximum from 1 to 6 hours after administration, the rate of accumulation depending upon the renal blood flow, and the efficiency with which the tubules concentrate the substance; the presence of viable renal tissue may then be shown by scanning the area of the kidneys with a radiation detector. The usual dose for this purpose is 100 microcuries.
Chlormerodrin (^{197}Hg) is discharged slowly from the kidneys and is therefore preferred to sodium iodohippurate (^{131}I), which is discharged too quickly to allow satisfactory scanning.
Chlormerodrin (^{197}Hg) is also used for localisation of the kidneys for biopsy and other purposes. It is also administered by intravenous injection in doses of about 3 millicuries for the localisation of brain tumours in scanning procedures but sodium pertechnetate (^{99m}Tc) injection is generally preferred for this purpose.

Chlormethiazole Edisylate

5-(2-Chloroethyl)-4-methylthiazole ethane-1,2-disulphonate

$C_{14}H_{22}Cl_2N_2O_6S_4 = 513.5$

OTHER NAMES: Chlormethiazole Ethanedisulphonate; Clomethiazole Edisylate; *Heminevrin*®

Description. A white crystalline powder with a characteristic odour which becomes more distinct and unpleasant when the substance is heated.

Solubility. Soluble in water and in warm alcohol; practically insoluble in ether.

Identification. MELTING-POINT. About 127°.

ULTRAVIOLET ABSORPTION. In 0.1N sulphuric acid, maximum at 257 nm (E1%, 1cm = 77).

INFRA-RED ABSORPTION. Major peaks at 781, 826, 1031, 1042, 1205, 1235 cm^{-1} (see Appendix 2b: Infra-red Spectra).

Metabolism. ABSORPTION. Absorbed after oral administration.

BLOOD CONCENTRATION. After an oral dose of 640 mg of the base in capsules, peak plasma concentrations of about 2 μg/ml are attained in 15 to 45 minutes; when the same dose is administered with arachis oil, peak plasma concentrations of about 3.5 μg/ml are attained in 30 minutes; after an oral dose of 1 g of the edisylate as tablets, peak plasma concentrations of about 1 μg/ml are attained within 1 hour; when administered as a 5% mixture with sorbitol at a dose of 500 mg of the edisylate, peak concentrations of about 4 μg/ml are attained in 15 minutes; following an intravenous infusion of 1.2 g, plasma concentrations of 4 to 10 μg/ml are attained within 1 hour after the infusion is stopped.

HALF-LIFE. The decline in plasma concentration after infusion is biphasic, the half-life of the α-phase being 0.5 hours and that of the β-phase, about 4 hours.

DISTRIBUTION. Widely distributed throughout body tissues and crosses the placenta; volume of distribution, about 5.5 litres/kg.

METABOLIC REACTIONS. Appears to be extensively metabolised, probably by first pass metabolism in the liver.

EXCRETION. Less than 5% of a dose is excreted unchanged in the urine.

FURTHER INFORMATION. Plasma concentrations after oral administration—M. Fischler *et al.*, *Acta pharm. suec.*, 1973, **10**, 483; pharmacokinetics in man—R. G. Moore *et al.*, *Eur. J. clin. Pharmac.*, 1975, **8**, 353.

Bioavailability. A 5% mixture of chlormethiazole edisylate with sorbitol is better absorbed than either capsules or tablets. Capsules containing arachis oil along with the base are much better absorbed than capsules containing the base alone.

FURTHER INFORMATION. M. Fischler *et al.*, *Acta pharm. suec.*, 1973, **10**, 483.

Actions and uses. Chlormethiazole edisylate has sedative, hypnotic, and anticonvulsant actions. It is used in the treatment of acute alcoholic and drug withdrawal symptoms, agitated states, and insomnia. It is also used in the treatment of pre-eclamptic toxaemia and certain convulsive conditions.
The usual dose given by mouth in the treatment of alcoholic and drug withdrawal symptoms is 1.5 grams 4 times daily for 2 days, followed by 1 gram 4 times daily for 3 days and then 500 milligrams 4 times daily for 4 days; treatment should not be given for more than 9 days. In the treatment of agitated states, 500 milligrams may be given 3 times daily, and in insomnia, 1 gram may be administered at night.
Chlormethiazole edisylate is administered by slow intravenous infusion in the management of status epilepticus, the usual dosage being in the range 300 to 800 milligrams administered as a 0.8% solution.

Doses of 200 to 400 milligrams may be given by slow intravenous infusion in the treatment of pre-eclamptic toxaemia, subsequent doses being adjusted according to the patient's response.

Undesirable effects. Sneezing, conjunctival irritation, and gastro-intestinal disturbances such as nausea, vomiting, and dyspepsia may occur.

Precautions. Patients should be continuously observed when chlormethiazole edisylate is given by slow intravenous infusion and the rate of administration adjusted to prevent the patient becoming unconscious. It should be administered with caution to patients with obstructive pulmonary disease. It should not be administered to children.

Drug interactions. The action of chlormethiazole edisylate is potentiated by phenothiazines and butyrophenones such as haloperidol.

Preparations

Preparations available include CAPSULES containing chlormethiazole 192 mg, equivalent to 500 mg of chlormethiazole edisylate; an ELIXIR containing chlormethiazole edisylate 250 mg in 5 ml, diluent water, life of diluted elixir 14 days; an INJECTION containing chlormethiazole edisylate 8 mg per ml in 500-ml bottles; and TABLETS containing chlormethiazole edisylate 500 mg.

Chlorocresol

4-Chloro-3-methylphenol

$C_7H_7ClO = 142.6$

OTHER NAMES: Parachlorometacresol; *Wright's Vaporizing Fluid*®

A standard is given in the British Pharmacopoeia 1973

Description. Colourless or faintly coloured crystals with a characteristic phenolic odour. It is volatile in steam.

Solubility. Soluble, at 20°, in 260 parts of water and in less than one part of alcohol; soluble in ether, in terpenes, in fixed oils, and in solutions of alkali hydroxides.

Dissociation constant. pK_a 9.2.

Preparation and storage of solutions. See statement on aqueous solutions of antiseptics in the entry on Solutions.

Identification. TESTS. 1. To a saturated solution in water add 1 drop of *ferric chloride test-solution*; a bluish colour is produced.
2. Mix about 50 mg with 0.5 g of anhydrous sodium bicarbonate, ignite, cool, boil with 5 ml of water, filter, acidify the filtrate with nitric acid, and add a few drops of *silver nitrate solution*; a white precipitate is produced.

MELTING-POINT. About 65°.

Metabolism. METABOLIC REACTIONS. Conjugation with glucuronic acid and sulphate.

EXCRETION. Excreted in the urine mainly as conjugate with very little being excreted unchanged.

Actions and uses. Chlorocresol is a powerful bactericide and fungicide of low toxicity which exerts its action in acid solution and, to a lesser degree, in alkaline solution.

It is used in a concentration of 0.2% in the process of sterilisation by heating with a bactericide for aqueous solutions and suspensions provided they are not intended for ophthalmic use, and in a concentration of 0.1% as a bacteriostat.

It should not be used in solutions intended for intrathecal, intracisternal, or peridural injection, since it may damage delicate tissues; neither should it be used in solutions for intravenous injection where the dose exceeds 15 millilitres.

For use in eye-drops a concentration of 0.05% of chlorocresol may be used as a preservative subject to normal compatibility considerations and provided the drops are not used in conjunction with any surgical procedures on the eye.

It is used as a preservative in creams and other preparations for external use which contain water, but its effectiveness is reduced if oils, fats, or non-ionic surface-active agents are present.

Preparations

Preparations available include a SOLUTION containing chlorocresol 10%.

Chloroform

Trichloromethane to which 1 to 2% v/v of dehydrated alcohol has been added.
$CHCl_3 = 119.4$

A standard is given in the British Pharmacopoeia 1973

Description. A colourless, heavy, volatile liquid with a characteristic odour and a sweet burning taste.

It is non-inflammable, but the strongly heated vapour may be ignited and burns with a green flame with production of noxious vapours.

Solubility. Soluble, at 20°, in 200 parts of water; miscible with dehydrated alcohol, with ether, with most other organic solvents, and with fixed and volatile oils.

Weight per ml. At 20°, 1.474 to 1.479 g.

Stability. On exposure to air and light, trichloromethane is gradually oxidised, becoming contaminated with the very poisonous carbonyl chloride (phosgene) and with chlorine. The decomposition is greatly retarded by the addition of the small percentage of alcohol, which serves also to decompose any carbonyl chloride that may have been formed.

Storage. It should be stored in airtight containers, with glass stoppers or other suitable closures, protected from light.

Identification. TESTS. 1. Mix a few drops with a small amount of resorcinol dissolved in 2N sodium hydroxide, and heat; a red colour is produced.
2. Repeat Test 1, replacing the resorcinol with 2-naphthol; a blue colour is produced.

BOILING-POINT. About 61°.

Determination in body fluids. INFRA-RED SPECTROPHOTOMETRY. In blood—M. Feldstein, *J. forens. Sci.*, 1965, **10**, 207.

GAS CHROMATOGRAPHY. In expired air, blood, or urine—B. J. Fry *et al.*, *Archs int. Pharmacodyn. Thér.*, 1972, **196**, 98.

Metabolism. ABSORPTION. Almost completely absorbed after oral administration and rapidly absorbed after inhalation.

BLOOD CONCENTRATION. After an oral dose of 500 mg in 1 ml of olive oil held in a gelatin capsule, a peak blood concentration of about 0.5 μg/ml is attained in 1 hour and small amounts are detectable for up to 8 hours; adequate anaesthesia occurs at arterial blood concentrations of about 160 μg/ml.

HALF-LIFE. The blood concentration of chloroform declines biphasically after oral administration with a half-life for the α-phase of 9 to 21 minutes and a half-life for the β-phase of about 90 minutes.

DISTRIBUTION. Rapidly distributed throughout the body, taken up in fatty tissues, and rapidly crosses the placenta; volume of distribution, 2 to 3 litres/kg body-weight.

METABOLIC REACTIONS. Metabolised to carbon dioxide; subject to "first pass metabolism" in the liver and lungs.

EXCRETION. Up to 70% of a dose is exhaled unchanged in 8 hours and up to 51% as carbon dioxide in the same period; up to 4% is exhaled in the following 8 hours; less than 0.01% of a dose is excreted in the urine.

FURTHER INFORMATION. Pharmacokinetics—W. L. Chiou, *J. Pharmacokinet. Biopharm.*, 1975, **3**, 193; pulmonary elimination—B. J. Fry *et al.*, *Archs int. Pharmacodyn. Thér.*, 1972, **196**, 98.

Actions and uses. Chloroform is a volatile anaesthetic with a pleasant odour. It is one of the most potent but also one of the most toxic anaesthetics. The vapour is non-inflammable and relatively non-irritant, although the liquid is irritant to both skin and mucous membranes and may cause burns if spilt on them.

Chloroform sensitises the heart to adrenaline and is liable to lead to ventricular fibrillation with sudden cardiac arrest; this is more likely to occur in patients who are excited, and it may be avoided by adequate premedication.

During anaesthesia with chloroform the blood pressure falls, the respiratory centre is depressed, and severe anoxia may occur; this is more likely to occur in exhausted, dehydrated, semi-starved, or toxic patients.

Chloroform is used as an emergency anaesthetic for major first-aid field surgery and for the symptomatic control of convulsions. A concentration of 2 to 3% of the vapour is adequate for induction and 1 to 2% for maintenance of anaesthesia. It is usually administered by open mask or by the semi-closed method, but the use of chloroform in major surgery has been largely discontinued in favour of less toxic drugs.

When taken by mouth, chloroform has an agreeable taste and causes a sensation of warmth. It is used as a carminative and as a flavouring agent in pharmaceutical mixtures and other preparations. It is given in a dosage of 0.06 to 0.3 millilitre.

Externally, chloroform has a rubefacient action and is used as a counter-irritant. It is also used as a solvent for resins, alkaloids, fats, fixed and volatile oils, and rubber.

Chloroform in a concentration of 0.25% is a useful preservative for pharmaceutical mixtures and aqueous extracts of vegetable and animal tissues. However, losses occur because of the volatility of chloroform, especially when containers are opened at intervals for the removal of doses, and mixtures which have lost a proportion of their chloroform content may increase in bacterial content. For further information see the entry on Mixtures.

The administration of chloroform in large doses given in an oily vehicle over a period of time has been shown to give rise to renal tumours in a certain strain of rat. The significance of this finding in relation to human medicine is a matter of dispute but in certain countries there are restrictions on the use of chloroform in medicines.

Possible restrictions on the use of chloroform in the United Kingdom are under consideration; if a decision is made in time a note will be included elsewhere in the text (see Index).

Undesirable effects. Delayed chloroform poisoning occurs from 6 to 24 hours after the administration of the anaesthetic and is characterised by abdominal pain, vomiting and, at a later stage, jaundice. The prolonged use of preparations such as chloroform and morphine tincture which contain substantial amounts of chloroform may give rise to liver damage, especially in children.

Contra-indications. Chloroform should not be administered to patients with renal, hepatic, or cardiovascular disease.

Poisoning. The patient should be kept warm and artificial respiration applied. Where poisoning occurs from swallowing chloroform, gastric lavage should be used.

Preparations

CHLOROFORM AND MORPHINE TINCTURE (*Syn.* Chlorodyne; Tinct. Chlorof. et Morph., B.P. '85):

Chloroform	125 ml
Morphine hydrochloride	2.29 g
Peppermint oil	1 ml
Anaesthetic ether	30 ml
Water for preparations	50 ml
Alcohol (90%)	125 ml
Liquorice liquid extract	125 ml
Treacle, of commerce	125 ml
Syrup	to 1000 ml

Dissolve the peppermint oil in the alcohol, add the water, dissolve the morphine hydrochloride in the mixture, and add the chloroform and the anaesthetic ether. Mix the liquorice extract and the treacle with 400 ml of the syrup, add to the previously formed solution, mix thoroughly, add sufficient syrup to produce the required volume, and mix.

A standard for this tincture is given in the British Pharmacopoeia 1977 and in the British Pharmacopoeia (Veterinary)
Labelling: a direction to shake the bottle well before use should be given on the label.
Storage: it should be stored in airtight containers.
Dose: 0.3 to 0.6 millilitre.

CHLOROFORM SPIRIT:

Chloroform	50 ml
Alcohol (90%)	to 1000 ml

Mix.
A standard for this spirit is given in the British Pharmacopoeia 1973
Dose: 0.25 to 2 ml.

CHLOROFORM WATER (*Syn.* Aq. Chlorof.):

Chloroform	2.5 ml
Purified water, freshly boiled and cooled	to 1000 ml

Shake frequently until solution is effected.
Dose: 10 to 30 millilitres.

CHLOROFORM WATER DOUBLE-STRENGTH:

Chloroform	5 ml
Purified water, freshly boiled and cooled	to 1000 ml

Shake frequently until solution is effected.
Dose: 5 to 15 millilitres.

Chloroquine Phosphate

7-Chloro-4-(4-diethylamino-1-methylbutylamino)quinoline diphosphate

$$2H_3PO_4$$

$$NH \cdot CH \cdot [CH_2]_3 \cdot N(C_2H_5)_2$$
$$CH_3$$

$C_{18}H_{32}ClN_3O_8P_2 = 515.9$

OTHER NAMES: *Aralen®*; *Avloclor®*; *Malarivon®*; *Resochin®*

A standard is given in the British Pharmacopoeia 1973

Description. An odourless white powder with a bitter taste. It discolours on exposure to light.

Solubility. Soluble, at 20°, in 4 parts of water; very slightly soluble in alcohol, in ether, and in chloroform.

Acidity. A 10% solution has a pH of 3.5 to 4.5.

Moisture content. Not more than 1.5%, determined by drying at 105°.

Dissociation constants. pK$_a$ 8.4, 10.8 (20°).

Stability. Solutions of pH 4 to 6 are stable when heated but sensitive to light.

Hygroscopicity. It absorbs insignificant amounts of moisture at temperatures up to 37° at relative humidities up to about 80%.

Sterilisation. Solutions for injection are sterilised by heating in an autoclave or by filtration.

Storage. It should be protected from light.

Identification. TEST. Dissolve about 25 mg in 20 ml of water and add 8 ml of *trinitrophenol solution*; a precipitate is produced which, after washing successively with water, alcohol (95%), and solvent ether, melts at about 207°.

MELTING-POINT. Chloroquine phosphate occurs in two polymorphic forms, one of which melts at about 194° and the other at about 216°.

ULTRAVIOLET ABSORPTION. In 0.1N hydrochloric acid, maxima at 257 nm (E1%, 1cm = 340), 331 nm (E1%, 1cm = 330), and 345 nm (E1%, 1cm = 360).

Determination in body fluids. ULTRAVIOLET SPECTRO-PHOTOMETRY. In blood—V. Waarst, *Arch. Pharm. Chemi*, 1964, **71**, 116.

GAS CHROMATOGRAPHY. In urine—A. Viala *et al., J. Chromat.*, 1975, **111**, 299.

Metabolism. ABSORPTION. Rapidly absorbed after oral administration of the phosphate or sulphate salts; chloroquine delays gastric emptying.

BLOOD CONCENTRATION. During the oral administration of 310 mg of chloroquine as the phosphate daily, plasma concentrations reach a plateau at 10 days with a concentration of about 120 ng/ml; after a 500-mg dose, concentrations of about 700 ng/ml are attained in haemolysed blood in 4 hours and after single oral doses of 400 to 500 mg, peak plasma concentrations of 35 to 220 ng/ml are attained in 2 to 6 hours; chloroquine may be detectable in the blood for as long as 5 years after discontinuation of long-term therapy.

HALF-LIFE. Plasma half-life, about 3 days after single or weekly doses and 6 to 7 days after a treatment period of 14 days with 310 mg daily.

DISTRIBUTION. Widely distributed throughout the body and present in high concentration in the liver, kidneys, lungs, spleen, bone, skin, and melanin-containing tissues such as the eye; in the blood large amounts are taken up by red cells; in mice chloroquine crosses the placenta; *protein binding*, 55% bound to plasma proteins.

METABOLIC REACTIONS. Mainly oxidative *N*-dealkylation and oxidative deamination and also conjugation, possibly with glucuronic acid, of the carboxylic acid metabolites derived from dealkylation and deamination; the metabolites include mono- and bisdesethylchloroquine, 4-(7-chloroquinol-4-ylamino)pentan-1-ol, and 4-(7-chloroquinol-4-ylamino)pentanoic acid and its conjugate.

EXCRETION. Excreted slowly; about 55% is excreted in the urine and about 10% in the faeces by 90 days following therapy with 310 mg of the phosphate for 14 days; the urinary excretion of the unchanged drug is dependent upon urinary pH and larger amounts are excreted in acid urine than in alkaline urine; of the material excreted in the urine, about 70% is unchanged, 23% is desethylchloroquine, 1 to 2% is bisdesethylchloroquine and an unidentified metabolite, and 1 to 2% is excreted as carboxylic acid metabolites in conjugated form.

FURTHER INFORMATION. Affinity of chloroquine for bone—V. W. Fischer and C. D. Fitch, *J. Pharm. Pharmac.*, 1975, **27**, 527; metabolism—E. W. McChesney *et al., J. Pharmac. exp. Ther.*, 1966, **151**, 482 and 1967, **158**, 323; concentrations in the skin—A. Olatunde, *Br. J. Pharmac.*, 1971, **43**, 335; distribution after fatal poisoning—A. E. Robinson *et al., J. Pharm. Pharmac.*, 1970, **22**, 700.

Actions and uses. Chloroquine kills malaria schizonts at all stages of development. It does not affect the sporozoites inoculated by the mosquito or the forms of the parasite that develop in the cells of the human liver. Chloroquine therefore prevents or terminates the clinical symptoms of malaria by suppressing erythrocytic parasites; it does not necessarily eliminate the infection, and overt malaria may develop when the drug is withdrawn. Most patients become completely afebrile within 1 or 2 days after being given therapeutic doses. As a rule it completely eliminates falciparum malaria.

Chloroquine is more active and more rapid in action than mepacrine; it causes fewer toxic side-effects and does not stain the skin yellow.

Chloroquine is used for the suppression and treatment of malaria but it has no true prophylactic action. A total dose equivalent to 1.5 grams of chloroquine base by mouth is usually sufficient to terminate an acute attack of malaria caused by Plasmodium vivax, P. falciparum, or P. malariae; 1 gram of chloroquine phosphate is approximately equivalent to 600 milligrams of chloroquine base. An initial oral dose equivalent to 600 milligrams of the base is followed by the equivalent of 300 milligrams of the base after 6 to 8 hours, and a further dose equivalent to 300 milligrams of the base is given on each of the two following days. Alternatively, the equivalent of 200 to 300 milligrams of chloroquine base may be given daily by intravenous or intramuscular injection.

A single dose equivalent to 450 milligrams of the base is usually sufficient to terminate an attack in a partially immune patient.

For the treatment of cerebral malaria in an adult, a condition in which the patient is unable to swallow, chloroquine may be given in a dose equivalent to 200 to 300 milligrams of the base by intramuscular or intravenous injection as the phosphate or sulphate and repeated if necessary on 2 or 3 occasions at intervals of 4 to 12 hours.

For children suffering from severe malaria, with or without cerebral manifestations, chloroquine may be given intravenously. It is best diluted in 250 ml or more of sodium chloride injection or sodium chloride and dextrose injection and given slowly, each dose being run into a vein over a period of not less than 30 minutes. A single dose of 5 milligrams of chloroquine base per kilogram body-weight is usually given and this dose may be repeated after 6 to 8 hours, if necessary.

For the suppression or so-called prophylaxis of malaria, the equivalent of 300 milligrams of chloroquine base is given regularly by mouth once a week during exposure to the risk and for 4 weeks after leaving a malarious area. This dosage will in most cases suppress all species of the malaria parasite and will cure malaria due to *P. falciparum*. The antimalarial dose for children under one year is one-eighth, 1 to 4 years one-quarter, 5 to 8 years half of the adult dose; older children may be given the same dose as adults.

Chloroquine may be given together with primaquine, pyrimethamine, or proguanil.

Chloroquine has no action on malarial sporozoites or on the tissue forms of *P. vivax*, *P. ovale*, and *P. malariae*. Recrudescences may therefore occur in infections due to these species during the year following the cessation of treatment; to prevent these recrudescences, a single dose equivalent to 600 milligrams of chloroquine base is given by mouth to kill erythrocytic parasites and this is followed by a course of treatment with primaquine.

Malarial infections that are resistant to chloroquine should be treated with quinine, pyrimethamine, proguanil, or chlorproguanil, or with pyrimethamine together with a sulphonamide or sulphone.

Chloroquine is of value in the treatment of hepatic amoebiasis, but it has no effect in intestinal amoebiasis. For the treatment of hepatic amoebiasis and liver abscess, the equivalent of 300 milligrams of chloroquine base (500 milligrams of chloroquine phosphate) is given by mouth twice a day for 2 days or longer and then once a day for a further 2 or 3 weeks.

Chloroquine is also used for the treatment of giardiasis, but mepacrine is more effective. For this purpose, the equivalent of 150 milligrams of chloroquine base (250 milligrams of chloroquine phosphate) is given daily by mouth.

Chloroquine is of value in the treatment of systemic lupus erythematosus, particularly when the skin is involved, and of discoid lupus erythematosus and rheumatoid arthritis. Dosage in these conditions lies within a range equivalent to 150 to 900 milligrams of the base daily. For lupus erythematosus, treatment is usually begun with the equivalent of 300 to 450 milligrams of the base daily by mouth, and this is subsequently reduced to the equivalent of 150 milligrams daily. In the treatment of rheumatoid arthritis, remission of symptoms has been obtained after 2 or 3 months by giving the equivalent of 75 to 300 milligrams of chloroquine base daily by mouth.

Undesirable effects. Chloroquine is well tolerated and toxic effects from antimalarial doses are rare. Pruritus is the most common side-effect; occasionally headache and visual or gastro-intestinal disturbances have been observed. None of these effects is serious and they disappear when administration of the drug is discontinued.

Administration of large doses for periods exceeding 1 to 2 years or, occasionally, shorter periods may produce permanent retinal degeneration and corneal opacities; depigmentation of the skin and hair, wasting of muscle, and acute psychoses may also occur. For this reason, the daily dose for long-term therapy should not exceed 300 milligrams.

Precautions. Chloroquine should not be given to patients who are being treated with a monoamineoxidase inhibitor, such as isocarboxazid, nialamide, phenelzine, or tranylcypromine, or within about 2 weeks of the discontinuation of such treatment. Patients receiving chloroquine over a long period should have an ophthalmic examination every 2 or 3 months. Chloroquine should preferably not be given in pregnancy unless the benefits outweigh the possible risks.

Preparations

CHLOROQUINE PHOSPHATE INJECTION: a sterile solution of chloroquine phosphate in water for injections. It is sterilised by heating in an autoclave or by filtration. The usual strength is the equivalent of 40 mg of chloroquine per ml; 40 mg of chloroquine is approximately equivalent to 64.5 mg of chloroquine phosphate.

A standard for this injection is given in the British Pharmacopoeia 1973

Containers: see the entry on Injections for general information on containers.

Labelling: see the entry on Injections for general information on labelling. In addition, the label should state the amount of the medicament as the equivalent amount of chloroquine.

Storage: it should be protected from light.

CHLOROQUINE PHOSPHATE TABLETS: available as tablets containing 250 mg of chloroquine phosphate; they may be sugar coated; 250 mg of chloroquine phosphate is approximately equivalent to 150 mg of chloroquine.

A standard for these tablets is given in the British Pharmacopoeia 1973

Containers and *Storage:* see the entry on Tablets for general information on containers and storage. Containers should be airtight.

Advice for patients: the tablets should be taken at regular intervals, preferably after meals. For the suppression (prophylaxis) of malaria, doses should be taken during the period at risk and for 4 weeks thereafter. For therapy, the prescribed course should be completed. For the treatment of chronic disease, use of the tablets should not be discontinued without the advice of the prescriber.

OTHER PREPARATIONS available include an ELIXIR containing chloroquine phosphate 80 mg in 5 ml.

Chloroquine Sulphate

7-Chloro-4-(4-diethylamino-1-methylbutylamino)quinoline sulphate monohydrate
$C_{18}H_{28}ClN_3O_4S,H_2O = 436.0$

OTHER NAMES: *Nivaquine®*
Nivembin® (with di-iodohydroxyquinoline)

A standard is given in the British Pharmacopoeia 1973

Description. An odourless white crystalline powder with a bitter taste.

Solubility. Soluble, at 20°, in 3 parts of water; very slightly soluble in alcohol, in ether, and in chloroform.

Acidity. A 10% solution has a pH of 4 to 5.

Moisture content. 3 to 5%, determined by drying at 100° *in vacuo.*

Sterilisation. Solutions for injection are sterilised by heating in an autoclave or by filtration.

Identification. TEST. It complies with the test described under Chloroquine Phosphate.

ULTRAVIOLET ABSORPTION. In 0.01N hydrochloric acid, maxima at 257 nm (E1%, 1cm = 390), 329 nm (E1%, 1cm = 440), and 343 nm (E1%, 1cm = 460).

Determination in body fluids; Metabolism. See under Chloroquine Phosphate.

Actions and uses. Chloroquine sulphate has the actions, uses, and undesirable effects described under Chloroquine Phosphate; 1 gram of chloroquine sulphate is approximately equivalent to 750 milligrams of chloroquine base.
For the suppression of malaria, 400 milligrams of chloroquine sulphate is given regularly by mouth once a week during exposure to the risk and for 4 weeks after leaving a malarious area. To terminate an acute attack of malaria an initial dose of 800 milligrams of chloroquine sulphate is given with subsequent doses of 400 milligrams daily. Alternatively, the equivalent of 200 to 300 milligrams of chloroquine base may be given by intravenous or intramuscular injection daily. For the treatment of hepatic amoebiasis, 400 to 800 milligrams is given daily and for giardiasis 200 milligrams daily.

Precautions. As for Chloroquine Phosphate.

Preparations

CHLOROQUINE SULPHATE INJECTION: a sterile solution of chloroquine sulphate in water for injections. It is sterilised by heating in an autoclave or by filtration. Available in 5-ml ampoules containing chloroquine sulphate equivalent to 40 mg of chloroquine per ml; 40 mg of chloroquine is approximately equivalent to 55 mg of chloroquine sulphate.
A standard for this injection is given in the British Pharmacopoeia 1973
Containers: see the entry on Injections for general information on containers.
Labelling: see the entry on Injections for general information on labelling. In addition, the label on the container should state the amount of the medicament as the equivalent amount of chloroquine.

CHLOROQUINE SULPHATE TABLETS: available as tablets containing 200 mg of chloroquine sulphate; they may be compression coated; 200 mg of chloroquine sulphate is approximately equivalent to 146 mg of chloroquine.
A standard for these tablets is given in the British Pharmacopoeia 1973
Containers and *Storage:* see the entry on Tablets for general information on containers and storage. Containers should be airtight.
Advice for patients: the tablets should be taken at regular intervals, preferably after meals. For the suppression (prophylaxis) of malaria, doses should be taken during the period at risk and for 4 weeks thereafter. For therapy, the prescribed course should be completed. For the treatment of chronic diseases, use of the tablets should not be discontinued without the advice of the prescriber.

OTHER PREPARATIONS available include an ELIXIR containing chloroquine sulphate equivalent to 50 mg of chloroquine in 5 ml, diluent syrup, shelf-life of diluted elixir 14 days; and TABLETS containing chloroquine sulphate 65 mg with di-iodohydroxyquinoline 300 mg.

Chlorothiazide

6-Chloro-2*H*-benzo-1,2,4-thiadiazine-7-sulphonamide 1,1-dioxide

$C_7H_6ClN_3O_4S_2 = 295.7$

OTHER NAME: *Saluric*®

A standard is given in the British Pharmacopoeia 1973

Description. A white crystalline odourless powder with a slightly bitter taste.

Solubility. Very slightly soluble in water; soluble, at 20°, in 650 parts of alcohol and in 100 parts of acetone; practically insoluble in ether and in chloroform.

Moisture content. Not more than 1%, determined by drying at 105°.

Dissociation constants. pK_a 6.8, 9.4.

Storage. It should be stored in airtight containers.

Identification. MELTING-POINT. About 342°, with decomposition.

ULTRAVIOLET ABSORPTION. In 0.1N hydrochloric acid, maxima at 230 nm (E1%, 1cm = 972) and 281 nm (E1%, 1cm = 394); in 0.1N sodium hydroxide, maxima at 230 nm (E1%, 1cm = 741) and 295 nm (E1%, 1cm = 443); in alcohol (95%), maxima at 284 nm (E1%, 1cm = 268) and 297 nm (E1%, 1cm = 269).

INFRA-RED ABSORPTION. Major peaks at 1090, 1125, 1162, 1307, 1385, and 1595 cm⁻¹ (see Appendix 2a: Infra-red Spectra).

THIN-LAYER CHROMATOGRAPHY. See under Thin-layer Chromatography, System 6.

Metabolism. ABSORPTION. Variably absorbed after oral administration.

DISTRIBUTION. Distributed throughout extracellular spaces but does not accumulate in the tissues except the kidney; chlorothiazide crosses the placenta and small amounts are secreted in the milk; *protein binding,* in rats, about 90% bound to plasma proteins which may be reduced by about 10% after the administration of probenecid.

METABOLIC REACTIONS. Not significantly metabolised in man or in dogs and rats.

EXCRETION. After intravenous injection, the whole dose is rapidly excreted in the urine in about 4.5 hours; after oral administration, 13 to 70% is excreted in the urine in 24 hours; urinary excretion may be delayed by the administration of probenecid; in dogs, up to 60% may be excreted in the faeces.

FURTHER INFORMATION. Absorption and excretion— R. E. Kauffman and D. L. Azarnoff, *Clin. Pharmac. Ther.*, 1973, **14**, 886.

Actions and uses. Chlorothiazide is a thiazide diuretic which reduces the resorption of electrolytes by the proximal part of the distal tubules, thereby increasing the excretion of sodium, potassium, and chloride ions, and consequently of water. It also has a minor inhibitory effect on carbonic anhydrase activity but this effect is small and does not appreciably alter the acid-base balance. This effect is not shared by other thiazide diuretics with the exception of hydrochlorothiazide.

Chlorothiazide is rapidly absorbed when given by mouth and produces a response in about 2 hours; the diuresis is maintained for 6 to 12 hours. Tolerance does not develop and the therapeutic efficacy of chlorothiazide is maintained when administered over long periods, but patients may not respond if their glomerular filtration rate is markedly reduced.

The usual initial dosage is 1 to 2 grams each morning for 2 to 3 days, followed by 1 gram daily for a further 2 days. Thereafter, continuous therapy is unnecessary and undesirable; the maintenance dose is adjusted to keep the patient free from oedema, the usual practice being to give the drug every second, third, or fourth day.

Chlorothiazide is used for the treatment of oedema and of the toxaemias of pregnancy. It enhances the effect of antihypertensive agents and is used, usually in doses of 250 to 500 milligrams, alone or in conjunction with hypotensive drugs in the treatment of hypertension.

Undesirable effects. Toxic effects such as hypochloraemic alkalosis, acute pancreatitis, and blood dyscrasias such as agranulocytosis and thrombocytopenia, are rare; allergies, epigastric pain, and nausea occur occasionally and acute episodes may be precipitated in gouty subjects. Chlorothiazide may precipitate hepatic coma in patients with impaired liver function and should be used with great caution when there is renal or hepatic dysfunction. It may aggravate existing diabetes or precipitate the condition from a prediabetic state. It may increase blood uric acid levels and precipitate gout.

Precautions. Prolonged regular administration of chlorothiazide may produce hypokalaemia. This intensifies the effect of digitalis on cardiac muscle and administration of digitalis or its glycosides may have to be temporarily suspended.

Supplements of potassium in the form of chloride, citrate, or gluconate should be given. Some patients also show a chloride deficiency and should preferably receive their potassium supplement in the form of potassium chloride. Supplements should be given after meals several hours after the drug or preferably on the days when chlorothiazide is not given, as otherwise much of the potassium is rapidly excreted under the influence of the drug; the usual amount required is 40 to 80 millimoles, or 3 to 6 grams of potassium chloride, daily in divided doses.

Preparation

CHLOROTHIAZIDE TABLETS: available as tablets containing 500 mg of chlorothiazide.

A standard for these tablets is given in the British Pharmacopoeia 1973

Containers and *Storage:* see the entry on Tablets for general information on containers and storage. Containers should be airtight.

Advice for patients: daily doses should preferably be taken in the morning. Treatment should not be discontinued without the advice of the prescriber.

Chlorotrianisene

Chlorotris(4-methoxyphenyl)ethylene

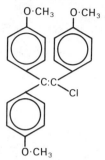

$C_{23}H_{21}ClO_3 = 380.9$

OTHER NAMES: *Tace®*; Tri-*p*-anisylchloroethylene

A standard is given in the British Pharmacopoeia 1973

CAUTION. *Chlorotrianisene is a powerful oestrogen. Contact with the skin or inhalation of the dust should be avoided. Rubber gloves should be worn when handling the powder and, if the powder is dry, a face mask should also be worn.*

Description. Odourless small white crystals or crystalline powder.

Solubility. Very slightly soluble in water; soluble, at 20°, in 360 parts of alcohol, in 28 parts of ether, in 1.5 parts of chloroform, in 7 parts of acetone, and in 100 parts of fixed oils.

Moisture content. Not more than 1%, determined by drying at 80°.

Identification. TESTS. 1. Dissolve about 10 mg in 2 ml of sulphuric acid; a very dark purple colour is produced which, on the addition of 5 ml of water, changes rapidly to pink and, finally, a turbid solution is produced. Add 2 ml of sulphuric acid to form a lower layer; a purple to pink layer is produced at the interface. Shake; a pink solution is produced (distinction from certain other oestrogens).

2. Dissolve about 10 mg in 2 ml of nitric acid; an intense purple colour is produced which, on the addition of 5 ml of water, changes to yellow and a precipitate is produced. Add 5 ml of a 50% solution of sodium hydroxide; an intense yellow colour is produced, the precipitate dissolves, and the odour of benzaldehyde is produced.

3. Dissolve a few crystals in 4 drops of glacial acetic acid, add 1 ml of phosphoric acid, and heat on a water-bath for 3 minutes; a deep pink colour is produced which disappears on the addition of 3 ml of glacial acetic acid (distinction from dienoestrol and stilboestrol).

MELTING-POINT. About 118°.

ULTRAVIOLET ABSORPTION. In alcohol (95%), maxima at 247 nm (E1%, 1cm = 635) and 307 nm (E1%, 1cm = 410).

INFRA-RED ABSORPTION. Major peaks at 813, 1174, 1184, 1250, 1510, and 1606 cm^{-1} (see Appendix 2a: Infra-red Spectra).

THIN-LAYER CHROMATOGRAPHY. See under Thin-layer Chromatography, System 10.

Metabolism. DISTRIBUTION. Stored in body fat from which it is slowly released.

METABOLIC REACTIONS. Slowly converted to an active oestrogenic metabolite.

Actions and uses. Chlorotrianisene is a synthetic oestrogen which has the general actions of the oestrogens, as described under Oestradiol Benzoate.

Chlorotrianisene is given by mouth for the treatment of menopausal disturbances in a dosage of 12 to 24 milligrams daily, for relief in prostatic carcinoma in a dosage of 24 milligrams daily, and for suppression of lactation in a dosage of 48 milligrams daily for 7 days.

Undesirable effects. As for Oestradiol Benzoate. Withdrawal bleeding, nausea, and vomiting are rare.

Preparations

CHLOROTRIANISENE CAPSULES: consisting of a solution of chlorotrianisene in maize oil, enclosed in a soft capsule. The capsule shells may be coloured. Available as capsules containing 12 mg of chlorotrianisene.
A standard for these capsules is given in the British Pharmacopoeia 1973
Containers and *Storage:* see the entry on Capsules for general information on containers and storage.
Advice for patients: the prescribed course should be completed or, where applicable, treatment should not be discontinued without the advice of the prescriber.

CHLOROTRIANISENE TABLETS: available as tablets containing 24 mg of chlorotrianisene.
A standard for these tablets is given in the British Pharmacopoeia 1973
Containers and *Storage:* see the entry on Tablets for general information on containers and storage. Containers should be airtight.
Advice for patients: the prescribed course should be completed or, where applicable, treatment should not be discontinued without the advice of the prescriber.

Chloroxylenol

4-Chloro-3,5-xylenol

$C_8H_9ClO = 156.6$

OTHER NAMES: *Dettol*®; Parachlorometaxylenol

A standard is given in the British Pharmacopoeia Addendum 1977 and the British Pharmacopoeia (Veterinary)

Description. White or creamy-white crystals or crystalline powder with a characteristic odour. It is volatile in steam.

Solubility. Soluble, at 20°, in 3000 parts of water and in 1 part of alcohol; soluble in ether, in terpenes, in fixed oils, and in solutions of alkali hydroxides.

Preparation and storage of solutions. See statement on aqueous solutions of antiseptics in the entry on Solutions.

Identification. TESTS. 1. Dissolve 100 mg in 5 ml of chloroform and add 10 drops of a filtered 1% solution of ferric chloride in chloroform and 2 drops of pyridine; a blue colour is produced.
2. To 5 ml of a saturated solution in water add 0.5 ml of *ferric chloride test-solution*; no bluish colour is produced (distinction from chlorocresol).

3. Mix a small quantity with anhydrous sodium carbonate, ignite strongly, cool, boil with water, acidify with nitric acid, filter, and add *silver nitrate solution*; a white precipitate is produced.

MELTING-POINT. About 115°.

ULTRAVIOLET ABSORPTION. In 0.1N hydrochloric acid, maximum at 279 nm (E1%, 1cm = 83); in 0.1N sodium hydroxide, maximum at 296 nm (E1%, 1cm = 161).

Metabolism. METABOLIC REACTIONS. Conjugation with glucuronic acid and sulphate.

EXCRETION. After an injected dose of 5 g, 14% is excreted in the urine as the glucuronide, 17% as the sulphate, and traces as the unchanged drug; in alkaline urine the excretion of unchanged drug is increased.

Actions and uses. Chloroxylenol is a relatively non-toxic and non-irritant antiseptic. Because it is only slightly soluble in water it is used chiefly as chloroxylenol solution, in which its solubility is increased by the presence of soap and which contains other substances such as terpineol and alcohol.

Chloroxylenol solution is active against Gram-positive and Gram-negative organisms, but species of *Staphylococcus* and *Pseudomonas*, particularly the latter, are relatively less susceptible; it is inactive against bacterial spores.

Chloroxylenol solution is used as an antiseptic for the skin in surgical and obstetrical practice, and also for cuts, wounds, and abrasions. For general purposes a 5% v/v dilution is used, but twice this concentration should be used in adverse conditions or when excessive amounts of blood, serum, or pus are present, as, in common with all bactericides, its activity is reduced by organic matter.

Precautions. Solutions should not be applied repeatedly to and wet dressings should not be left in contact with the skin, as hypersensitivity may occur.

Veterinary uses. Chloroxylenol is used as an antiseptic as described above under Actions and uses.

Preparations

CHLOROXYLENOL SOLUTION (*Syn.* Roxenol):

Chloroxylenol	50 g
Potassium hydroxide	13.6 g
Oleic acid	7.5 ml
Castor oil	63 g
Terpineol	100 ml
Alcohol (95%)	200 ml
Purified water, freshly boiled and cooled	to 1000 ml

Dissolve the potassium hydroxide in 15 ml of the water, add a solution of the castor oil in 63 ml of the alcohol, mix, allow to stand for 1 hour or until a small portion of the mixture remains clear when diluted with 19 times its volume of purified water, and then add the oleic acid. Mix the terpineol with a solution of the chloroxylenol in the remainder of the alcohol, pour into the soap solution, and add sufficient of the water to produce the required volume.

In making this preparation the alcohol (95%) may be replaced by industrial methylated spirit, provided that the law and the statutory regulations governing the use of industrial methylated spirit are observed.

A standard for this solution is given in the British Pharmacopoeia Addendum 1977 and in the British Pharmacopoeia (Veterinary)
Containers: should be thoroughly cleansed before being filled. Closures should be such that the solution does not come into contact with cork.

Advice for patients: the solution should be diluted before use. Wet dressings should not be left in contact with the skin.

OTHER PREPARATIONS available include a CREAM containing chloroxylenol 1.3% with edetic acid 0.2%; a MOUTH-WASH containing chloroxylenol 1.02%; a SOLUTION containing chloroxylenol 4.8%, a solution containing chloroxylenol 6.25%, and a solution containing chloroxylenol 1.44% with terpineol 1.8%.

Chlorphenesin

3-(4-Chlorophenoxy)propane-1,2-diol

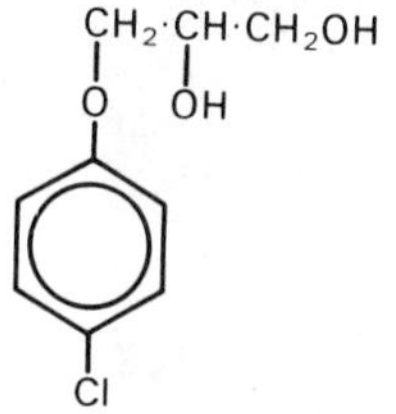

$C_9H_{11}ClO_3 = 202.6$

OTHER NAME: *Mycil*®

A standard is given in the British Pharmacopoeia 1973

Description. White or pale cream-coloured crystals or crystalline aggregates with a slightly phenolic odour and a persistent bitter taste.

Solubility. Soluble, at 20°, in 200 parts of water and in 5 parts of alcohol; soluble in ether; very slightly soluble in fixed oils.

Moisture content. Not more than 1%, determined by drying over phosphorus pentoxide *in vacuo.*

Identification. TESTS. 1. Mix 1 g with 2 ml of methyl carbonate and a few drops of a solution containing 500 mg of sodium in 10 ml of dehydrated alcohol, heat on a water-bath until a gelatinous residue remains, and remove the last traces of solvent by warming under reduced pressure; dissolve the residue as completely as possible in 10 ml of dehydrated alcohol with the aid of heat, filter, and allow to cool; a crystalline precipitate is produced which, after drying in a current of air, melts at about 95°.

2. Mix 500 mg with 1 ml of *sodium hydroxide solution* in a small crucible and boil vigorously until completely dry, taking care to avoid charring; add 4 ml of water, boil to dissolve, cool, slowly add 2 ml of nitric acid, keeping the mixture cool, and add a few drops of *silver nitrate solution;* a white precipitate is produced.

MELTING-POINT. About 80°.

ULTRAVIOLET ABSORPTION. In water, maximum at 280 nm (E1%, 1cm = 65).

INFRA-RED ABSORPTION. Major peaks at 710, 818, 1043, 1109, 1232, and 1488 cm^{-1} (see Appendix 2a: Infra-red Spectra).

Determination in body fluids. GAS CHROMATOGRAPHY. In plasma—J. F. Douglas *et al., J. pharm. Sci.,* 1970, 59, 107.

Actions and uses. Chlorphenesin has antibacterial, antifungal, and trichomonacidal properties and is used for the prophylaxis and treatment of fungal infections of the skin.

Preparations

CHLORPHENESIN CREAM:

Chlorphenesin	5 g
Sodium lauryl sulphate	9 g
Cetostearyl alcohol	81 g
White soft paraffin	150 g
Purified water, freshly boiled and cooled	755 g

Warm the cetostearyl alcohol and the white soft paraffin to 50° and mix. Add, with constant stirring, the sodium lauryl sulphate and the chlorphenesin dissolved in the water at the same temperature and stir until cold.

A standard for this cream is given in the British Pharmaceutical Codex 1973

Containers, Labelling, and *Storage:* see the entry on Creams for general information on containers, labelling, and storage.

Advice for patients: the cream should be rubbed lightly on the affected area. When used in conjunction with chlorphenesin dusting-powder, the cream should be used first and the dusting-powder afterwards. Treatment should be continued for one week after symptoms have disappeared.

CHLORPHENESIN DUSTING-POWDER:

Chlorphenesin	10 g
Zinc oxide	250 g
Purified talc, sterilised	180 g
Starch	560 g

Prepare as described in the entry on Powders.

A standard for this dusting-powder is given in the British Pharmaceutical Codex 1973

Containers and *Labelling:* see the entry on Dusting-powders for general information on containers and labelling.

Advice for patients: the dusting-powder should be dusted lightly onto the affected area after application of chlorphenesin cream. Treatment should be continued for one week after symptoms have disappeared.

Chlorpheniramine Maleate

3-(4-Chlorophenyl)-3-(pyrid-2-yl)-*NN*-dimethylpropyl-amine hydrogen maleate

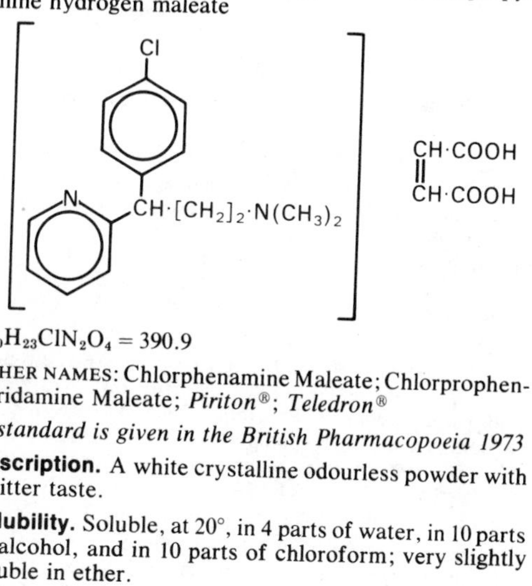

$C_{20}H_{23}ClN_2O_4 = 390.9$

OTHER NAMES: Chlorphenamine Maleate; Chlorprophen-pyridamine Maleate; *Piriton*®; *Teledron*®

A standard is given in the British Pharmacopoeia 1973

Description. A white crystalline odourless powder with a bitter taste.

Solubility. Soluble, at 20°, in 4 parts of water, in 10 parts of alcohol, and in 10 parts of chloroform; very slightly soluble in ether.

Acidity. A 1% solution has a pH of about 4.5.

Dissociation constant. pK$_a$ 9.1 (25°).

Sterilisation. Solutions for injection are sterilised by heating in an autoclave in an atmosphere of nitrogen or other suitable gas.

Storage. It should be protected from light.

Identification. TEST. Dissolve about 500 mg in 5 ml of water, add 2 ml of *strong ammonia solution*, and extract with three 5-ml portions of chloroform; evaporate the aqueous solution to dryness, dissolve the residue in 5 ml of water containing 4 drops of *dilute sulphuric acid*, extract with four 25-ml portions of solvent ether, and evaporate the ether extracts to dryness; the residue melts at about 130°.

ULTRAVIOLET ABSORPTION. In 0.1N sulphuric acid, maximum at 265 nm (E1%, 1cm = 212); in 0.1N sodium hydroxide, maxima at 222 nm (E1%, 1cm = 818) and 263 nm (E1%, 1cm = 142).

INFRA-RED ABSORPTION. Major peaks at 865, 1092, 1356, 1433, 1473, and 1586 cm^{-1} (see Appendix 2a: Infra-red Spectra).

THIN-LAYER CHROMATOGRAPHY. See under Thin-layer Chromatography, System 4.

Determination in body fluids. GAS CHROMATOGRAPHY. In plasma—S. Hanna and A. Tang, *J. pharm. Sci.*, 1974, **63**, 1954.

Metabolism. ABSORPTION. Readily absorbed after oral administration.

BLOOD CONCENTRATION. After an oral dose, peak concentrations appear within 2 to 3 hours; the peak concentration after doses of up to 12 mg has been variously reported as between 20 ng/ml and about 200 ng/ml.

HALF-LIFE. Plasma half-life, after oral administration, has been reported as 12 to 15 hours and about 2 hours; after intravenous administration, the decline in plasma concentration appears to be biphasic with the α-phase having a half-life of 15 minutes and the β-phase a half-life of 28 hours.

DISTRIBUTION. Widely distributed throughout the body tissues and appears to be subject to enterohepatic circulation; *protein binding*, about 70% bound to plasma proteins.

METABOLIC REACTIONS. Extensively metabolised to form polar and non-polar metabolites; 2 metabolites have been identified as a result of N-demethylation and these are monodesmethylchlorpheniramine and didesmethylchlorpheniramine.

EXCRETION. About 35% of a dose is excreted in the urine in 48 hours; the excretion of unchanged drug accounts for about 3 to 10% of the dose but it is increased by an increase in urinary pH and urinary flow; more non-polar metabolites appear to be excreted after intravenous than after oral administration; both demethylated metabolites are excreted in urine; less than 1% of a dose is excreted in the faeces.

FURTHER INFORMATION. Influence of urine pH and flow rate on renal excretion—A. H. Beckett and G. R. Wilkinson, *J. Pharm. Pharmac.*, 1965, **17**, 256; plasma concentrations—S. Hanna and A. Tang, *J. pharm. Sci.*, 1974, **63**, 1954; urinary excretion—P. Kabasakalian *et al.*, *J. pharm. Sci.*, 1968, **57**, 856; metabolism—E. A. Peets *et al.*, *J. Pharmac. exp. Ther.*, 1972, **180**, 464.

Actions and uses. Chlorpheniramine has the actions, uses and undesirable effects of the antihistamine drugs as described under Promethazine Hydrochloride and is effective in smaller doses but it has no marked anti-emetic effect.

The usual dose for an adult is 12 milligrams by mouth daily in divided doses. The usual doses for children are: up to one year 3 milligrams daily in divided doses; 1 to 5 years 6 milligrams daily in divided doses; 6 to 12 years 6 to 12 milligrams daily in divided doses.

In severe allergies, it may be given by intramuscular, subcutaneous, or slow intravenous injection in doses of 10 to 20 milligrams; the total dose given by injection in 24 hours should not normally exceed 40 milligrams.

Poisoning. As for Promethazine Hydrochloride.

Preparations

CHLORPHENIRAMINE ELIXIR (*Syn*. Chlorpheniramine Syrup): a solution of chlorpheniramine maleate in a suitable coloured flavoured vehicle.

When a dose less than or not a multiple of 5 ml is prescribed, the elixir may be diluted, as described in the entry on Elixirs, with syrup. The diluted elixir must be freshly prepared.

Available as an elixir containing 2 mg of chlorpheniramine maleate in 5 ml.

A standard for this elixir is given in the British Pharmaceutical Codex 1973

Containers and *Labelling:* see the entry on Elixirs for general information on containers and labelling.

Storage: it should be stored in a cool place, protected from light.

Advice for patients: the elixir may cause drowsiness; persons affected should not drive or operate machinery. Alcohol should be avoided.

CHLORPHENIRAMINE INJECTION: a sterile solution of chlorpheniramine maleate in water for injections free from dissolved air. It is distributed into the final containers, the air being replaced by nitrogen or other suitable gas, and the containers are sealed and sterilised by heating in an autoclave. Available in 1-ml ampoules containing 10 mg of chlorpheniramine maleate.

A standard for this injection is given in the British Pharmacopoeia 1973

Containers and *Labelling:* see the entry on Injections for general information on containers and labelling.

Storage: it should be protected from light.

CHLORPHENIRAMINE TABLETS: available as tablets containing 4 mg of chlorpheniramine maleate; they may be coloured.

A standard for these tablets is given in the British Pharmacopoeia 1973

Containers and *Storage:* see the entry on Tablets for general information on containers and storage. Containers should be airtight.

Advice for patients: the tablets may cause drowsiness; persons affected should not drive or operate machinery. Alcohol should be avoided.

OTHER PREPARATIONS available include veterinary CAPSULES containing chlorpheniramine maleate 8 mg in a slow-release formulation; and TABLETS containing chlorpheniramine maleate 8 and 12 mg in slow-release formulations.

Chlorproguanil Hydrochloride

1-(3,4-Dichlorophenyl)-5-isopropylbiguanide hydrochloride

$C_{11}H_{16}Cl_3N_5 = 324.6$

OTHER NAME: *Lapudrine*®

A standard is given in the British Pharmacopoeia 1973

Description. A white crystalline odourless powder with a bitter taste.

Solubility. Soluble, at 20°, in 140 parts of water and in 50 parts of alcohol; practically insoluble in ether and in chloroform.

Identification. TESTS. 1. To 10 ml of a saturated solution add 5 drops of *potassium ferrocyanide solution*; a white precipitate is produced which dissolves on the addition of a few drops of *dilute nitric acid*.
2. To 10 ml of a saturated solution add one drop of *copper sulphate solution* and 2.5 ml of *dilute ammonia solution*, shake well, add 5 ml of toluene, and again shake; the toluene layer is coloured purplish-red.
3. To 15 ml of a saturated solution add 2 ml of *sodium hydroxide solution*, extract with 20 ml of solvent ether, wash the extract with water, and evaporate to dryness; the residue, after drying at 105°, melts at about 123°.
4. It complies with Test 1 described under Chlorhexidine Acetate.

ULTRAVIOLET ABSORPTION. In 0.1N sulphuric acid, maximum at 250 nm (E1%, 1cm = 347).

INFRA-RED ABSORPTION. Major peaks at 1407, 1470, 1520, 1562, 1600, and 1620 cm⁻¹ (see Appendix 2a: Infra-red Spectra).

Actions and uses. Chlorproguanil is an antimalarial drug with a mode of action similar to that described under Proguanil Hydrochloride. It is more active than proguanil and has a longer duration of action.
For the causal prophylaxis and suppression of malaria 20 milligrams of chlorproguanil hydrochloride is given by mouth at weekly or fortnightly intervals and administration should be continued for 1 month after leaving a malarious area. It may be given together with chloroquine.
Children under 5 years may be given 10 milligrams at weekly or fortnightly intervals and older children may be given the adult dose.

Undesirable effects. These very rarely occur during the administration of prophylactic doses.

Preparations

CHLORPROGUANIL TABLETS: available as tablets containing 20 mg of chlorproguanil hydrochloride.
A standard for these tablets is given in the British Pharmacopoeia 1973
Containers and *Storage:* see the entry on Tablets for general information on containers and storage. Containers should be airtight.

Advice for patients: doses should be taken at regular intervals, preferably after meals, during the period at risk and for 1 month thereafter.

Chlorpromazine

2-Chloro-10-(3-dimethylaminopropyl)phenothiazine
$C_{17}H_{19}ClN_2S = 318.9$

OTHER NAME: *Largactil*®

A standard is given in the British Pharmaceutical Codex 1973

CAUTION. *Chlorpromazine may cause severe dermatitis in sensitised persons, and pharmacists, nurses, and others who handle the drug frequently should wear masks and rubber gloves.*

Description. An odourless white or creamy-white powder or waxy solid.

Solubility. Practically insoluble in water; soluble, at 20°, in 2 parts of alcohol, in 1 part of ether, and in less than 1 part of chloroform.

Dissociation constant. pK_a 9.3 (20°).

Stability. See under Chlorpromazine Hydrochloride.

Storage. It should be protected from light.

Identification. TESTS. 1. It complies with Test 1 described under Chlorpromazine Hydrochloride.
2. Dissolve about 2 mg in 1 ml of water containing 2 drops of *dilute hydrochloric acid* and add 0.5 ml of a mixture containing 1 volume of nitric acid and 2 volumes of water; a red colour is produced.

MELTING-POINT. About 57°.

ULTRAVIOLET ABSORPTION. In 0.1N hydrochloric acid, maxima at 256 nm (E1%, 1cm = 1035) and 306 nm (E1%, 1cm = 135).

INFRA-RED ABSORPTION. As for Chlorpromazine Hydrochloride.

Determination in body fluids. See under Chlorpromazine Hydrochloride.

Metabolism. See under Chlorpromazine Hydrochloride.

Actions and uses. The actions, uses, and undesirable effects of chlorpromazine are described under Chlorpromazine Hydrochloride.
Chlorpromazine is used in the preparation of suppositories. The usual dose per rectum is 100 milligrams repeated every 6 to 8 hours if necessary.

Precautions and contra-indications. As for Chlorpromazine Hydrochloride.

Preparation

CHLORPROMAZINE SUPPOSITORIES: prepared, as described in the entry on Suppositories, by incorporating chlorpromazine in a hydrogenated vegetable oil or other suitable basis. Available as suppositories containing 100 mg of chlorpromazine.
A standard for these suppositories is given in the British Pharmaceutical Codex 1973
Containers and *Storage:* see the entry on Suppositories for general information on containers and storage. Containers should be light resistant.
Advice for patients: see the entry on Suppositories for general information on the use of suppositories. Daily doses should preferably be taken at night. The sup-

positories may cause drowsiness; persons affected should not drive or operate machinery. Alcohol should be avoided. Chlorpromazine may colour the urine pink.

Chlorpromazine Hydrochloride

2 - Chloro - 10 - (3 - dimethylaminopropyl) phenothiazine hydrochloride

$$CH_2 \cdot [CH_2]_2 \cdot N(CH_3)_2$$

HCl

$C_{17}H_{20}Cl_2N_2S = 355.3$

OTHER NAMES: *Chloractil®*; Chlorpromazini Hydrochloridum; *Largactil®*

A standard is given in the European Pharmacopoeia Vol. III

CAUTION. *Chlorpromazine may cause severe dermatitis in sensitised persons, and pharmacists, nurses, and others who handle the drug frequently should wear masks and rubber gloves.*

Description. A white or cream-coloured powder with a slight odour. It decomposes on exposure to light becoming yellow, pink, and finally violet.

Solubility. Soluble, at 20°, in less than 1 part of water, in 1.3 parts of alcohol, and in 1 part of chloroform; practically insoluble in ether.

Acidity. A 10% solution has a pH of 4 to 5.

Stability. In the form of powder or in aqueous solution, chlorpromazine degrades by photochemical oxidation to chlorpromazine-5-oxide and various phenolic compounds; degraded solutions become brown. Degradation is rapid in alkaline solution.

FURTHER INFORMATION. Stability in aqueous solution —L. J. Ravin *et al.*, *J. Am. pharm. Ass., scient. Edn*, 1958, **47**, 760, A. Felmeister and C. A. Discher., *J. pharm. Sci.*, 1964, **53**, 756, A. Felmeister *et al.*, *J. pharm. Sci.*, 1965, **54**, 1589, and C. L. Huang and F. L. Sands, *J. Chromat.*, 1964, **13**, 246 and *J. pharm. Sci.*, 1967, **56**, 259.

Incompatibility. It is incompatible in aqueous solution with pentobarbitone sodium and phenobarbitone sodium.

Sterilisation. Solutions for injection are sterilised by heating in an autoclave in an atmosphere of nitrogen or other suitable gas.

Storage. It should be protected from light.

Identification. TESTS. 1. Dissolve about 5 mg in 2 ml of sulphuric acid and allow to stand for 5 minutes; a red colour is produced.
2. To 5 ml of a 1% solution add 2 ml of nitric acid; a dark red colour develops which becomes yellowish.

MELTING-POINT. About 196°.

ULTRAVIOLET ABSORPTION. In 0.1N hydrochloric acid, maxima at 256 nm (E1%, 1cm = 920) and 306 nm; in alcohol, maxima at 257 nm (E1%, 1cm = 886) and 313 nm (E1%, 1cm = 123).

INFRA-RED ABSORPTION. Major peaks at 748, 800, 1230, 1246, 1406, and 1450 cm^{-1} (see Appendix 2a: Infra-red Spectra).

THIN-LAYER CHROMATOGRAPHY. See under Thin-layer Chromatography, System 9.

Determination in body fluids. THIN-LAYER CHROMATOGRAPHY. In blood and urine: investigation of metabolites—P. Turano *et al.*, *J. Chromat.*, 1973, **75**, 277. In urine: chlorpromazine and metabolites, colorimetric determination—D. E. Johnson *et al.*, *Psychopharmac. Bull.*, 1970, **6**, 44. In serum and urine: chlorpromazine and metabolites by direct scan spectrodensitometry—T. L. Chan and S. Gershon, *Mikrochim. Acta*, 1973, **3**, 435.

ULTRAVIOLET SPECTROPHOTOMETRY. In blood, serum, or urine; general method for phenothiazine derivatives—J. E. Wallace and J. D. Biggs, *J. pharm. Sci.*, 1971, **16**, 1346.

GAS CHROMATOGRAPHY. In serum—G. W. Christoph *et al.*, *Clinica chim. Acta*, 1972, **38**, 265.

POLAROGRAPHY. In plasma and urine: N-oxide, N-oxide sulphoxide, and sulphoxide metabolites—A. H. Beckett *et al.*, *J. Pharm. Pharmac.*, 1974, **26**, 399.

BIBLIOGRAPHY. For an extensive bibliography of references relating to the determination of phenothiazines and their metabolites see D. E. Johnson *et al.*, *Psychopharmac. Bull.*, 1970, **6**, 44.

Bioavailability. Studies of different proprietary formulations of chlorpromazine have not shown any bioavailability variation except those between liquid and solid oral forms.

FURTHER INFORMATION. Bioavailability—V. F. Smolen *et al.*, *J. clin. Pharmac.*, 1975, **15**, 734.

Metabolism. ABSORPTION. Readily absorbed after oral administration but the extent of absorption may be reduced by the presence of food or by the use of anticholinergic drugs.

BLOOD CONCENTRATION. Plasma concentrations are subject to considerable variation between individual subjects; after an oral dose of 75 to 600 mg daily, plasma concentrations range from 4 to 470 ng/ml with considerable overlap between dose levels; after a single oral dose, there is a tenfold variation in plasma concentrations between individual subjects, the peak being reached in 2 to 3 hours.

HALF-LIFE. Plasma half-life, about 6 hours; in whole blood, about 3 to 4 hours. A plasma half-life of 1.3 days has also been reported.

DISTRIBUTION. Widely distributed throughout the body and readily crosses the placenta; concentrations in the brain may reach 4 to 7 times that in the blood and high concentrations are also detectable in melanin-containing tissues; the desmethyl-, 7-hydroxy-, and sulphoxide-metabolites are taken up by red cells along with traces of the parent drug and its N-oxide; chlorpromazine and its metabolites appear to be subject to enterohepatic circulation; *protein binding*, 90 to 95% bound to plasma proteins.

METABOLIC REACTIONS. Extensively metabolised by sulphoxidation, demethylation, hydroxylation, N-oxidation, glucuronic acid conjugation, and possibly ring fission; these reactions may occur in a number of combinations resulting in the formation of a large number of metabolites; some of the metabolites are active, particularly 7-hydroxychlorpromazine, although less so than the parent drug.
Chlorpromazine may stimulate the drug metabolising enzymes of the liver and may therefore stimulate its own metabolism.

EXCRETION. 20 to 70% of an oral dose is excreted in the urine as phenothiazine metabolites; the majority of the urinary metabolites are conjugated, 5% is excreted as the sulphoxide, and very little is excreted unchanged; about 5% of a dose is excreted in the faeces as phenothiazine metabolites; urinary metabolites are still detectable some 2 to 6 weeks after dosing.

FURTHER INFORMATION. Metabolites in red blood cells —A. H. Beckett and E. E. Essien, *J. Pharm. Pharmac.*, 1973, **25**, 188; S. H. Curry, Action and metabolism of chlorpromazine, *Biological Effects of Drugs in Relation to Their Plasma Concentrations*, A British Pharmacological Society Symposium, D. S. Davies and B. N. C. Prichard (Eds), London, Macmillan, 1973, p. 201; metabolism—I. S. Forrest *et al.*, *J. forens. Sci.*, 1972, **17**, 592; blood concentrations—P. N. Kaul *et al.*, *J. pharm. Sci.*, 1976, **65**, 694; bioequivalency of generic and brand-named chlorpromazine—G. M. Simpson *et al.*, *Clin. Pharmac. Ther.*, 1974, **15**, 631.

Actions and uses. Chlorpromazine is a depressant which blocks dopamine receptors in the central nervous system. It is closely related chemically to promethazine, but it has a much weaker antihistamine action and a stronger local anaesthetic action.

Chlorpromazine reduces the efficiency of the heat-regulating centre so that the patient tends to acquire the temperature of his environment. It produces vasodilatation and a fall in blood pressure, but does not reduce cardiac output. It may induce tachycardia. It reduces salivary and gastric secretions and has a transient anti-adrenaline effect. It causes the skin to become warm, dry, and pale, and it may relieve itching.

Chlorpromazine enhances the action of other central nervous depressants, especially barbiturates and analgesics.

In psychiatry, chlorpromazine is used successfully in the treatment of severe psychomotor excitement and psychotic states. The usual dose by mouth or by subcutaneous or intramuscular injection is 75 to 800 milligrams daily in divided doses. Patients previously aggressive and confused become quiet and co-operative. Within an hour of an oral dose of chlorpromazine and half an hour or less after subcutaneous or intramuscular injection, the patient becomes drowsy, apathetic, less anxious, and occasionally euphoric. A very high proportion of manic depressives in the manic phase have benefited from chlorpromazine.

Chlorpromazine is not excreted in the milk in significant amounts. It should be used with care in elderly and debilitated patients, and withdrawn if the depression deepens. It has proved useful in the treatment of addiction to alcohol, barbiturates, morphine, and pethidine.

Chlorpromazine is a valuable adjunct in the treatment of advanced malignant disease; it may be used to reduce the dose of analgesic required and to delay the need to increase the dose, and it may permit the use of a less potent and less dangerous analgesic. It relieves the nausea and vomiting associated with malignant disease or with the therapy used in its treatment. It not only spares the patient much discomfort, but also helps to maintain his nutrition. It also improves the mental outlook beyond what can be expected from the relief of pain and vomiting. The usual dosage is 25 to 50 milligrams of chlorpromazine hydrochloride by mouth 3 times a day or about half this amount by subcutaneous or intramuscular injection. The dosage may need to be increased as tolerance develops.

In anaesthesia, a mixture of 50 milligrams each of chlorpromazine hydrochloride and promethazine hydrochloride and 100 milligrams of pethidine hydrochloride is sometimes given to render the patient tranquil, free from pain, and easily anaesthetised.

Chlorpromazine is effective in the relief of hiccup and of vomiting provoked by morphine and apomorphine. It also reduces the incidence of post-anaesthetic vomiting, but is less effective than certain antihistamines in the control of motion-sickness.

Chlorpromazine hydrochloride has been used in doses of 50 to 100 milligrams 4 times daily in conjunction with antitoxin in the treatment of tetanus.

Undesirable effects. Pallor, postural hypotension, tachycardia, arrhythmias, hypotonia of voluntary muscle, drowsiness, indifference, dryness of the mouth, nightmares, insomnia, depression, and, rarely, agitation may occur but rarely necessitate discontinuation of treatment.

Chlorpromazine may also give rise to amenorrhoea, galactorrhoea, gynaecomastia, blurred vision, corneal and lens opacity, and pigmentation of the cornea, conjunctiva, skin, and retina. High doses may cause the body temperature to fall but sometimes there may be a rise in temperature; cholestatic hepatitis, blood dyscrasias, contact skin sensitisation, rashes, photosensitivity, and megacolon may occur. It crosses the placenta and may give rise to respiratory depression in the offspring.

Chlorpromazine may cause symptoms resembling parkinsonism and occasionally tardive dyskinesia. Like other phenothiazine derivatives chlorpromazine may precipitate convulsions, especially in overdosage.

Precautions and contra-indications. It is contra-indicated in coma due to direct central nervous depressants such as alcohol, barbiturates, or opiates, and in patients with liver dysfunction or a low leucocyte count. It should not be used in conjunction with drugs, such as thiouracil derivatives, amidopyrine, and phenylbutazone, that depress leucopoiesis.

Caution should be exercised when treating epileptics and those with tachycardia or cardiac insufficiency or being treated with drugs that may give rise to hypotension. Patients on prolonged therapy should be examined for abnormal skin pigmentation on exposed areas of the body and for ocular changes and if necessary the drug should be withdrawn.

Poisoning. In acute poisoning the stomach should be washed out. If there is acute hypotension the patient should be placed in the prone position with the feet raised. Central nervous system depression should be allowed to recover naturally. The body temperature should be allowed to return to normal without active warming, unless the temperature approaches levels at which cardiac arrhythmias may be feared.

Veterinary uses. Chlorpromazine hydrochloride is used as a tranquilliser and for anaesthetic premedication. The usual dose by mouth for dogs is 5 milligrams per kilogram body-weight; by deep intramuscular injection for horses and cattle 0.1 to 1 milligram per kilogram body-weight and for pigs and dogs 1 to 2 milligrams per kilogram body-weight by intramuscular or intravenous injection. Chlorpromazine is generally considered to be unsuitable for cats because of the uncertainty of its action.

Preparations

CHLORPROMAZINE ELIXIR (*Syn.* Chlorpromazine Syrup): a solution of chlorpromazine hydrochloride in a suitable coloured flavoured vehicle.

When a dose less than or not a multiple of 5 ml is

prescribed, the elixir may be diluted, as described in the entry on Elixirs, with syrup. The diluted elixir must be freshly prepared.

Available as an elixir containing 25 mg of chlorpromazine hydrochloride in 5 ml.

A standard for this elixir is given in the British Pharmaceutical Codex 1973

Containers and *Labelling:* see the entry on Elixirs for general information on containers and labelling.

Storage: it should be protected from light.

Advice for patients: daily doses should preferably be taken at night. The elixir may cause drowsiness; persons affected should not drive or operate machinery. Alcohol should be avoided. Chlorpromazine may colour the urine pink. The elixir should not be spilled on the skin.

CHLORPROMAZINE INJECTION: a sterile solution of chlorpromazine hydrochloride, with suitable buffering and stabilising agents, in water for injections free from dissolved air. It is distributed into the final containers, the air being replaced by nitrogen or other suitable gas, and the containers are sealed and sterilised by heating in an autoclave. Available in 5-ml ampoules containing 10 mg of chlorpromazine hydrochloride per ml, in 1- and 2-ml ampoules containing 25 mg of chlorpromazine hydrochloride per ml, and in 5-ml ampoules containing 50 mg of chlorpromazine hydrochloride per ml (for veterinary use).

A standard for this injection is given in the British Pharmacopoeia 1973

Containers and *Labelling:* see the entry on Injections for general information on containers and labelling.

Storage: it should be protected from light.

CHLORPROMAZINE TABLETS: available as tablets containing 10, 25, 50, and 100 mg of chlorpromazine hydrochloride; they are film coated or sugar coated.

A standard for these tablets is given in the British Pharmacopoeia 1973

Containers and *Storage:* see the entry on Tablets for general information on containers and storage. Containers should be airtight.

Advice for patients: daily doses should preferably be taken at night. The tablets may cause drowsiness; persons affected should not drive or operate machinery. Alcohol should be avoided. Chlorpromazine may colour the urine pink.

Chlorpropamide

1-(4-Chlorobenzenesulphonyl)-3-propylurea

SO₂·NH·CO·NH·[CH₂]₂·CH₃

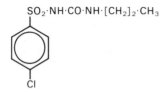

Cl

$C_{10}H_{13}ClN_2O_3S = 276.7$

OTHER NAMES: *Diabinese®*; *Melitase®*

A standard is given in the British Pharmacopoeia 1973

Description. A white, crystalline, odourless, tasteless powder.

Solubility. Practically insoluble in water; soluble, at 20°, in 12 parts of alcohol, in 200 parts of ether, in 9 parts of chloroform, and in 5 parts of acetone; soluble in solutions of alkali hydroxides.

Moisture content. Not more than 1.5%, determined by drying at 105°.

Identification. TESTS. 1. Boil about 100 mg with 8 ml of sulphuric acid (50% w/w) under a reflux condenser for 30 minutes, cool, filter, and reserve the filtrate; the residue, after recrystallisation from water, melts at about 143°.

2. Make the reserved filtrate from Test 1 alkaline with *sodium hydroxide solution* and heat; an ammoniacal odour is produced.

3. Ignite with anhydrous sodium carbonate, cool, extract with water, filter, acidify the filtrate with *dilute nitric acid*, and add *silver nitrate solution*; a white precipitate is produced.

MELTING-POINT. About 128°.

ULTRAVIOLET ABSORPTION. In 0.01N hydrochloric acid (solution prepared by initially dissolving in methyl alcohol and then diluting with 0.01N hydrochloric acid), maximum at 232 nm (E1%, 1cm = 600).

Determination in body fluids. GAS CHROMATOGRAPHY. In serum—W. E. Braselton *et al., Analyt. Lett.,* 1975, **8**, 301. In plasma or blood—S. B. Matin and M. Rowland, *J. Pharm. Pharmac.,* 1973, **25**, 186. In plasma—K. K. Midha *et al., J. Pharm. Sci.,* 1976, **65**, 576.

Metabolism. ABSORPTION. Rapidly and completely absorbed after oral administration.

BLOOD CONCENTRATION. After an oral dose of 250 mg to fasting subjects, peak plasma concentrations of 25 to 36 µg/ml are attained in 1 to 7 hours; after oral doses of 250 mg and 500 mg daily, plasma concentrations of up to 75 and 245 µg/ml respectively are attained 2 hours after dosing; at 2 hours about 95% of the drug in the blood is unchanged.

HALF-LIFE. Plasma half-life, 25 to 42 hours, which may be increased by administration of chloramphenicol, allopurinol, probenecid, dicoumarol, or clofibrate and increased in renal function impairment.

DISTRIBUTION. *Protein binding,* 60 to 88% bound to plasma proteins but chlorpropamide may be displaced by several drugs such as salicylate, aspirin, and phenylbutazone.

METABOLIC REACTIONS. Hydroxylation at the 2- and 3-position of the propyl substituent in the side chain, *N*-dealkylation thus removing the propyl group, and hydrolysis to form the sulphonamide metabolite.

EXCRETION. About 80% of a single oral dose is excreted in the urine in 7 days; of the material excreted in 36 hours, about 40% is unchanged (CPA), 10% is 4-chlorobenzenesulphonamide (CBS), 8% is 4-chlorobenzenesulphonylurea (CBSU), 40% is 1-(4-chlorobenzenesulphonyl)-3-(2-hydroxypropyl)urea (2-hydroxy-CPA), and 2% is 1-(4-chlorobenzenesulphonyl)-3-(3-hydroxypropyl)urea (3-hydroxy-CPA); during long-term therapy, up to 100% is excreted in the urine in 24 hours; of the dose, 18% is unchanged, 2% is CBS, 21% is CBSU, 55% is 2-hydroxy-CPA, and 2% is 3-hydroxy-CPA.

DISEASE STATES. In renal insufficiency the plasma half-life in severe cases may rise to about 200 hours.

FURTHER INFORMATION. Pharmacokinetics and biotransformation—J. A. Taylor, *Clin. Pharmac. Ther.,* 1972, **13**, 710 and T. Taylor *et al., Eur. J. clin. Pharmac.,* 1977, **11**, 207; metabolic fate—R. C. Thomas and R. W. Judy, *J. mednl Chem.,* 1972, **15**, 964.

Actions and uses. Chlorpropamide is a hypoglycaemic agent which is effective when given by mouth. It probably acts by stimulating the release of insulin from the beta cells of the pancreatic islets. Its only advantage over insulin is that it may be given by mouth; it is not a substitute for insulin, as it is effective only in the presence of functioning islet tissue. It is excreted slowly, the effect of a single dose lasting for 24 hours, and the higher blood concentrations which can be maintained with chlorpropamide may make it effective in patients whose blood-sugar levels cannot be controlled adequately with tolbutamide. Hypoglycaemic attacks may, however, be provoked, and may cause prolonged disorientation, especially in elderly patients.

Chlorpropamide is used in the treatment of mild diabetes; it is unsuitable for the treatment of diabetics with more than a trace of ketonuria or with diabetic ketosis.

The initial daily dosage is 100 to 250 milligrams by mouth. The dose should be adjusted to a suitable maintenance level as soon as the diabetic condition allows, otherwise hypoglycaemic attacks with such undesirable effects as vertigo, headache, and confusion may occur.

The maximum effect of chlorpropamide may not be evident for 4 to 7 days and adequate control may not be achieved for several weeks. In cases inadequately controlled with chlorpropamide, metformin may be administered in addition. Chlorpropamide should not be used in obese patients until it has been shown that weight reduction alone fails to control diabetes. Even then it tends to promote obesity and drugs such as metformin may be preferred. The daily dosage should not normally exceed 375 milligrams but up to 500 milligrams has been used.

If the patient is taking less than 20 units of insulin daily it may be possible to change to oral treatment with chlorpropamide without admission to hospital. After some weeks chlorpropamide may fail to control some diabetics, who then require insulin therapy. During periods of stress such as pregnancy, infection, or operation, insulin therapy may be necessary for a time.

Chlorpropamide is also useful in the treatment of many adult patients suffering from mild to moderate diabetes insipidus. The usual daily dosage is 100 milligrams gradually increased if necessary to 500 milligrams.

Undesirable effects. Skin sensitisation, gastro-intestinal disturbances, leucopenia, intolerance to alcohol, and jaundice may occur. Such effects are comparatively rare with a daily dosage of less than 500 milligrams.

In the event of sore throat or fever, repeated white-cell counts should be carried out because abnormalities in the circulating blood may not appear for several days.

Precautions. Caution should be exercised in giving chlorpropamide in conjunction with monoamine-oxidase inhibitors, oral anticoagulants, oxyphenbutazone, phenylbutazone, salicylates, and sulphonamides, which may increase its activity. The activity of chlorpropamide is also enhanced by hepatic or renal failure and by excessive alcohol intake.

Preparation

CHLORPROPAMIDE TABLETS: available as tablets containing 100 and 250 mg of chlorpropamide.
A standard for these tablets is given in the British Pharmacopoeia 1973
Containers and *Storage:* see the entry on Tablets for general information on containers and storage. Containers should be airtight.
Advice for patients: the tablets should be taken at regular intervals, preferably after meals. Treatment should not be discontinued without the advice of the prescriber. Intolerance to alcohol may occur.

Chlortetracycline Hydrochloride

7-Chlorotetracycline hydrochloride, an antimicrobial substance produced by *Streptomyces aureofaciens.*

$C_{22}H_{24}Cl_2N_2O_8 = 515.3$

OTHER NAMES: *Aureomycin®; Aurofac®;* Chlortetracyclini Hydrochloridum
Betnovate A® (with betamethasone valerate); *Propaderm-A®* (with beclomethasone dipropionate); *Aureocort®* (with triamcinolone acetonide)

A standard is given in the European Pharmacopoeia Vol. II

Description. Yellow odourless crystals with a bitter taste.

Solubility. Soluble, at 20°, in 110 parts of water and in 250 parts of alcohol; practically insoluble in propylene glycol.

Acidity. A 1% solution has a pH of 2.3 to 3.3.

Moisture content. Not more than 2%, determined by drying at 60° over phosphorus pentoxide *in vacuo.*

Specific rotation. $-235°$ to $-250°$, determined on a 0.5% solution in 0.1N hydrochloric acid, kept in the dark 30 minutes before measurement.

Dissociation constants. pK_a 3.3, 7.4, 9.3 (25°).

Storage. It should be stored in airtight containers protected from light.

Identification. TESTS. 1. Mix about 500 μg with 2 ml of sulphuric acid; a deep blue colour is produced, changing to bluish-green. Add 1 ml of water; a brownish colour is produced.
2. Prepare a 0.1% solution in *solution of standard pH 7.6* and heat at 100° for 1 minute; the solution exhibits a strong blue fluorescence under ultraviolet radiation.

MELTING-POINT. About 210°, with decomposition.

INFRA-RED ABSORPTION. Major peaks at 1311, 1362, 1447, 1580, 1622, and 1666 cm^{-1} (see Appendix 2a: Infrared Spectra).

Determination in body fluids. ULTRAVIOLET ABSORPTION. In blood or urine—T. Sakaguchi and K. Taguchi, *Pharm. Bull., Tokyo,* 1955, **3**, 303.

Metabolism. ABSORPTION. Readily though not completely absorbed after oral administration. Formulations containing the base are more readily absorbed than those containing the hydrochloride; chlortetracycline exists in two polymorphic forms one being more readily absorbed than the other. The difference appears to be a consequence of differences in solubility.

BLOOD CONCENTRATION. After the oral administration of 250 mg as the base or the hydrochloride, serum concentrations of 0.2 to 1.8 and 0.15 to 1.1 μg/ml are attained 2 to 3 and 6 hours after administration respectively; on average, serum concentrations obtained after administration of the base are higher than those obtained with the hydrochloride.

HALF-LIFE. Plasma half-life, 5 to 6 hours.

DISTRIBUTION. Rapidly distributed throughout the body and enters the cerebrospinal fluid even when the meninges are not inflamed; chlortetracycline is deposited in bones and teeth, it crosses the placenta, and it is secreted in the milk in concentrations about 30% of those in the blood; *protein binding*, 45 to 75% bound to plasma proteins.

EXCRETION. Excreted mainly in the bile and faeces; 10 to 25% of a dose is excreted unchanged in the urine in 10 hours.

FURTHER INFORMATION. Effect of polymorphism on dissolution and absorption—S. Miyazaki *et al.*, *Chem. pharm. Bull.*, *Tokyo*, 1974, **22**, 638; bioavailability—S. Miyazaki *et al.*, *Chem. pharm. Bull.*, *Tokyo*, 1975, **23**, 2151; blood concentrations—H. Welch *et al.*, *Antibiotic Med. clin. Ther.*, 1957, **4**, 414.

Actions and uses. Chlortetracycline hydrochloride has the actions and uses described under Tetracycline Hydrochloride and is given in similar dosage. The usual oral dose for an adult is 250 to 500 milligrams every 6 hours, but up to 3 grams daily may be given in more severe infections.

In general, tetracyclines should not be given to children, but when considered essential the usual dose is 2.5 to 7.5 milligrams per kilogram body-weight every 6 hours. Salts of aluminium, calcium, iron, and magnesium, and antacids and milk, which may decrease the absorption of the tetracyclines, should not be given with chlortetracycline.

Undesirable effects; Precautions and contraindications; Drug interactions. As for Tetracycline Hydrochloride.

Veterinary uses. Chlortetracycline hydrochloride is an antibacterial. The usual dosage by mouth for horses, calves, and pigs is 10 to 20 milligrams per kilogram body-weight daily in divided doses and for dogs and cats 20 to 50 milligrams per kilogram body-weight daily in divided doses. It may be administered to pigs and poultry in a concentration of 130 milligrams per litre of drinking water. The usual dosage by intra-uterine insertion in mares and cows is up to 1 gram and ewes and sows up to 500 milligrams. The usual dosage by intramammary injection in cattle is up to 500 milligrams in each infected quarter daily.

Preparations

BETAMETHASONE VALERATE WITH CHLORTETRACYCLINE OINTMENT (*Syn.* Betamethasone with Chlortetracycline Ointment): a dispersion of betamethasone valerate and chlortetracycline hydrochloride in a suitable anhydrous greasy basis. It contains betamethasone valerate equivalent to 0.1% of betamethasone and 3% of chlortetracycline hydrochloride.

When an ointment containing a lower proportion of betamethasone valerate and chlortetracycline hydrochloride than that available from the manufacturer is prescribed, the stronger ointment may be diluted with white soft paraffin. When an ointment containing a lower proportion of betamethasone valerate but the same proportion of chlortetracycline hydrochloride is prescribed, the ointment may be diluted with chlortetracycline ointment. Admixture of the ointment with other materials may promote degradation of the active ingredients, especially if water is present.

A standard for this ointment is given in the British Pharmaceutical Codex 1973

Containers and *Labelling:* see the entry on Ointments for general information on containers and labelling.

Advice for patients: it should be applied sparingly to the affected area. The ointment stains the skin, hair, and fabric; a dressing may be applied.

CHLORTETRACYCLINE CAPSULES: consisting of chlortetracycline hydrochloride, in powder, which may be mixed with a suitable inert diluent enclosed in a hard capsule. Available as capsules containing 250 mg of chlortetracycline hydrochloride.

A standard for these capsules is given in the British Pharmacopoeia 1973

Containers and *Storage:* see the entry on Capsules for general information on containers and storage.

Labelling: the label on the container should state the date after which the capsules are not intended to be used, and the conditions under which they should be stored.

Advice for patients: the capsules should be taken at regular intervals and salts of aluminium, calcium, iron, and magnesium and antacids and milk should not be taken within 1 hour. The prescribed course should be completed.

CHLORTETRACYCLINE EYE OINTMENT: prepared by incorporating chlortetracycline hydrochloride in eye ointment basis, or any other suitable basis, by method B described in the entry on Eye Ointments. Available as an eye ointment containing 1% of chlortetracycline hydrochloride.

A standard for this eye ointment is given in the British Pharmaceutical Codex 1973

Containers and *Labelling:* see the entry on Eye Ointments for general information on containers and labelling.

Storage: it should be protected from light.

Advice for patients: see the entry on Eye Ointments for general information on the use of eye ointments. The prescribed course should be completed.

CHLORTETRACYCLINE OINTMENT: a dispersion containing up to 3% of chlortetracycline hydrochloride, with 10% of wool fat, in yellow soft paraffin. It is prepared by melting together the wool fat and the yellow soft paraffin, stirring until cold, and incorporating the chlortetracycline hydrochloride in the cold basis.

Chlortetracycline ointment may be prepared with any other suitable basis.

Available as an ointment containing 3% of chlortetracycline hydrochloride.

When a strength less than that available from a manufacturer is prescribed, the 3% ointment may be diluted with a basis consisting of 1 part of wool fat and 9 parts of yellow soft paraffin.

A standard for this ointment is given in the British Pharmaceutical Codex 1973

Containers and *Labelling:* see the entry on Ointments for general information on containers and labelling.

Advice for patients: it should be applied sparingly to the affected area. The ointment stains skin, hair, and fabric; a dressing may be applied.

CHLORTETRACYCLINE SOLUBLE POWDER: consisting of chlortetracycline hydrochloride in a water-soluble diluent consisting of lactose, or other suitable basis, and a suitable green dye. Available as a soluble powder containing 5.5% of chlortetracycline hydrochloride.

A standard for this soluble powder is given in the British Pharmacopoeia (Veterinary)

Containers and *Storage:* see the entry on Powders for general information on containers and storage. Containers should be airtight. The powder should be stored in a cool place.

Labelling: the label on the container should state the amount of the medicament in terms of the concentration of chlortetracycline hydrochloride, the date after which the powder is not intended to be used, and the conditions under which it should be stored.

CHLORTETRACYCLINE TABLETS: available as tablets containing 500 mg of chlortetracycline hydrochloride.
A standard for these tablets is given in the British Pharmacopoeia (Veterinary)
Containers and *Storage:* see the entry on Tablets for general information on containers and storage. Containers should be airtight.
Labelling: the label on the container should state the date after which the tablets are not intended to be used and the conditions under which they should be stored.

OTHER PREPARATIONS available include an APPLICATION containing chlortetracycline hydrochloride 2% with crystal violet 0.5% in an aerosol pack, an application containing chlortetracycline hydrochloride 1% with triamcinolone acetonide 0.025% in an aerosol pack; CAPSULES containing chlortetracycline hydrochloride 250 mg; a CREAM containing chlortetracycline hydrochloride 3%, a cream containing chlortetracycline hydrochloride 3% with triamcinolone acetonide 0.1%, which should not be diluted; an OINTMENT containing chlortetracycline hydrochloride 3% with beclomethasone dipropionate 0.025% which should not be diluted, and an ointment containing chlortetracycline hydrochloride 3% with triamcinolone acetonide 0.1%, which should not be diluted.

OTHER VETERINARY PREPARATIONS available include an APPLICATION (with crystal violet 0.5% as marker) containing chlortetracycline hydrochloride 2% in an aerosol pack; a DUSTING-POWDER containing chlortetracycline hydrochloride 2% with benzocaine 1%; an INTRAMAMMARY INJECTION containing chlortetracycline hydrochloride 71 mg with hydrocortisone 330 micrograms per ml in 6-ml disposable syringes; a PREMIX containing chlortetracycline hydrochloride 10%, and a premix containing chlortetracycline hydrochloride 20%.

Chlorthalidone

3-(4-Chloro-3-sulphamoylphenyl)-3-hydroxyisoindolin-1-one

$C_{14}H_{11}ClN_2O_4S = 338.8$

OTHER NAMES: *Hygroton®*
Hygroton K® (with potassium chloride)

A standard is given in the British Pharmacopoeia 1973

Description. A white or creamy-white, crystalline, odourless, tasteless powder.

Solubility. Very slightly soluble in water; soluble, at 20°, in 150 parts of alcohol, in 650 parts of chloroform, and in 25 parts of methanol; very slightly soluble in ether; soluble in solutions of alkali hydroxides.

Identification. TEST. A solution in sulphuric acid has an intense yellow colour.

MELTING-POINT. About 220°, with decomposition.

ULTRAVIOLET ABSORPTION. In alcohol (95%), maxima at 275 nm (E1%, 1cm = 60) and 284 nm (E1%, 1cm = 45).

INFRA-RED ABSORPTION. Major peaks at 845, 1033, 1160, 1340, 1378, and 1685 cm^{-1} (see Appendix 2c: Infra-red Spectra).

Determination in body fluids. ULTRAVIOLET SPECTROPHOTOMETRY. In plasma, serum or urine: no interference reported from digitalis, chlorpropamide, benzodiazepines, phenobarbitone, aspirin, allopurinol, or methyldopa—M. G. Tweeddale and R. I. Ogilvie, *J. pharm. Sci.*, 1974, **63**, 1065.

GAS CHROMATOGRAPHY. In plasma—M. Ervik and K. Gustavii, *Analyt. Chem.*, 1974, **46**, 39.

Metabolism. ABSORPTION. Well absorbed after oral administration.

BLOOD CONCENTRATION. After an oral dose of 50 mg, peak plasma concentrations of 30 to 200 ng/ml are attained in 2 to 4 hours and after an oral dose of 200 mg peak plasma concentrations of 3 μg/ml are attained in 6 hours; during therapy with 50 mg daily, steady-state concentrations of 210 to 1140 ng/ml are attained and during therapy with 200 mg daily, plasma concentrations of up to 34 μg/ml may be obtained; most of the drug in the blood is bound to red cells and the concentration in red cells may reach 8 to 10 times that in the plasma.

HALF-LIFE. The decline in plasma concentration is biphasic with a half-life for the β-phase in the range 50 to 90 hours.

DISTRIBUTION. Most of the drug is bound to red cells in blood and this binding is maximal after 8 hours; chlorthalidone appears to be localised in renal tissue; volume of distribution, 3 to 12 litres/kg body-weight; the red cell binding of chlorthalidone appears to be reduced significantly by the administration of acetazolamide; *protein binding*, about 50 to 75% of the drug not bound to red cells is bound to plasma proteins.

METABOLIC REACTIONS. Not significantly metabolised in man but metabolites have been detected in rats and rabbits.

EXCRETION. After a single dose, about 30% is excreted in the urine unchanged in 24 hours; during daily therapy, about 50% of the daily dose is excreted in the urine in 24 hours; chlorthalidone appears to be excreted in the bile and about 25% of a dose is recovered in the faeces.

FURTHER INFORMATION. Binding-site interaction of chlorthalidone and acetazolamide—B. Beerman *et al.*, *Clin. Pharmac. Ther.*, 1975, **17**, 424; chlorthalidone concentrations in plasma and red cells—P. Collste *et al.*, *Eur. J. clin. Pharmac.*, 1976, **9**, 319; improved method of estimation in body fluids—M. G. Tweeddale and R. I. Ogilvie, *J. pharm. Sci.*, 1974, **63**, 1065.

Actions and uses. Chlorthalidone is a diuretic which has the actions and uses described under Chlorothiazide. It is effective in smaller doses than chlorothiazide and, as it is more slowly absorbed from the gastro-intestinal tract, its diuretic effect is much more prolonged. It produces diuresis in about 2 hours and this may continue for up to 48 hours.
The usual dosage is 100 to 200 milligrams by mouth on

alternate days, but for severe cases the initial dose may be 400 milligrams.

Undesirable effects; Precautions. As for Chlorothiazide.

Preparations

CHLORTHALIDONE TABLETS: available as tablets containing 50 and 100 mg of chlorthalidone.

A standard for these tablets is given in the British Pharmacopoeia 1973

Containers and *Storage:* see the entry on Tablets for general information on containers and storage. Containers should be airtight.

Advice for patients: daily doses should preferably be taken in the morning. Treatment should not be discontinued without the advice of the prescriber.

OTHER PREPARATIONS available include TABLETS containing chlorthalidone 25 mg with potassium chloride 500 mg (6.7 mmol K^+).

Cholecalciferol

9,10-Secocholesta-5,7,10(19)-trien-3β-ol

$C_{27}H_{44}O = 384.6$

OTHER NAMES: *Super-Suntax®*; Vitamin D_3

A standard is given in the British Pharmacopoeia Addendum 1977 and the British Pharmacopoeia (Veterinary)

Description. White odourless crystals.

Solubility. Practically insoluble in water; soluble in alcohol, in chloroform, in ether, and in acetone; soluble in fixed oils.

Specific rotation. +105° to +112°, determined on a freshly prepared 0.8% solution in aldehyde-free alcohol (95%).

Storage. It should be stored in hermetically sealed containers in which the air has been replaced by an inert gas, in a cool place, protected from light.

Identification. TESTS. 1. Dissolve about 1 mg in 1 ml of ethylene chloride and add 4 ml of *antimony trichloride solution*; a yellowish-orange colour is produced.

2. To a 10% solution in chloroform add 6 drops of acetic anhydride and 2 drops of sulphuric acid; a bright red colour is produced which changes to violet and then to blue-green.

MELTING-POINT. About 84°, determined without powdering or drying.

ULTRAVIOLET ABSORPTION. In aldehyde-free alcohol (95%), maximum at 265 nm (E1%, 1cm = 480).

INFRA-RED ABSORPTION. Major peaks at 893, 971, 1053, 1351, 1370, and 1449 cm^{-1} (see Appendix 2b: Infra-red Spectra).

Metabolism. ABSORPTION. Absorption after oral administration may be decreased in subjects after gastrectomy or with conditions where bile secretion is impaired.

BLOOD CONCENTRATION. Normal serum concentrations of the major metabolite, 25-hydroxycholecalciferol (25-OHD$_3$), are about 15 to 40 ng/ml. Since these concentrations are controlled by dietary intake and exposure to the sun, which aids the formation of cholecalciferol (D$_3$) from its provitamin in the skin, significant individual, geographical, and seasonal variations in concentrations may be expected. Serum concentrations of 25-OHD$_3$ are decreased in epileptics undergoing therapy with anticonvulsants, in subjects with hyperthyroidism, in pregnancy, and in the elderly.

HALF-LIFE. Plasma half-life, about 20 to 30 hours. After an intravenous dose, serum concentrations show a biphasic decline with the half-life of the α-phase being about 2 days and the half-life of the β-phase being about 18 days.

DISTRIBUTION. Secreted in milk; *protein binding*, cholecalciferol and its metabolites are bound to some extent to globulins and to lipoproteins.

METABOLIC REACTIONS. Cholecalciferol is metabolised to active metabolites by hydroxylation. These metabolites are inactivated by conjugation with sulphate or glucuronic acid. The major metabolite is 25-OHD$_3$ which is formed in the liver. The 25-hydroxylated metabolite may be further hydroxylated at positions 1 or 24 principally by the kidneys. The 1α,25-dihydroxy form is preferentially formed but in cases where the 1-hydroxylation reaction is saturated or deficient, the 24,25-dihydroxylated metabolite is produced. The production of the 1α,25-dihydroxy metabolite is controlled by feedback mechanisms linked to the serum concentrations of calcium and phosphorus and to parathyroid hormone. The 1α,24,25-trihydroxylated metabolite is also produced. In pigs, 26-hydroxylation also occurs.

EXCRETION. Most of a dose is excreted in the faeces via the bile. About 25% of the excreted material is excreted as conjugates. No unchanged cholecalciferol is excreted in the urine.

FURTHER INFORMATION. Metabolism and blood concentration of cholecalciferol—M. H. Briggs and M. Briggs, *Med. J. Aust.*, 1974, **1**, 838 and 891; metabolism of calciferol and cholecalciferol—H. F. De Luca and H. K. Schnoes, *A. Rev. Biochem.*, 1976, **45**, 631; metabolism of cholecalciferol in normals and anephrics—R. W. Gray *et al.*, *J. clin. Endocr. Metab.*, 1974, **39**, 1045; blood concentration and metabolism of calciferol and cholecalciferol—J. G. Haddad and T. J. Hahn, *Nature*, 1973, **244**, 515; metabolism of cholecalciferol—G. B. Kolata, *Science*, 1975, **187**, 635; blood concentrations of 25-hydroxy metabolites of calciferol and cholecalciferol in the elderly—E. Lester *et al.*, *Lancet*, i/1977, 979; blood concentration and metabolism of cholecalciferol—E. B. Mawer *et al.*, *Clin. Sci. & mol. Med.*, 1975, **48**, 349; blood concentration of 25-hydroxy metabolite in hyperthyroidism—L. Mosekilde *et al.*, *Lancet*, i/1977, 806; blood concentration of 25-hydroxy metabolite in chronic renal failure—H. E. Nielson *et al.*, *Lancet*, i/1977, 754; blood concentration of 25-hydroxyergocalciferol—R. K. Skinner *et al.*, *Lancet*, i/1977, 720; blood concentration of 25-hydroxy metabolites in pregnancy—C. W. G. Turton *et al.*, *Lancet*, i/1977, 222.

Actions and uses. Cholecalciferol has the actions and uses described under Calciferol and is given in similar dosage. Patients with conditions that have become resistant to calciferol may still respond to cholecalciferol.

Undesirable effects; Precautions. As for Calciferol.

Veterinary uses. Cholecalciferol is used as an antirachitic for poultry by incorporation of 25 to 50 parts per million in the feed. It is used for the prevention of milk fever in cattle, the usual dose being 10 mega units (250 milligrams) as a single-dose 2 to 8 days before the expected data of parturition, but it has been largely superseded for this purpose by 1α-hydroxycholecalciferol.

Preparations

CALCIFEROL INJECTION: see under Calciferol. Preparations available include an INJECTION (veterinary) containing cholecalciferol 6.25 mg (250 000 units of antirachitic activity, vitamin D) per ml in 100-ml vials.

Cholera

Cholera is an acute infectious epidemic disease due to infection with *Vibrio cholerae* (including the El Tor biotype). The organisms are transmitted by the faecal-oral route, water being an important source of infection and the spread of disease being enhanced by poverty and poor sanitation. The incubation period is up to 5 days and cases may be asymptomatic or vary in severity from mild diarrhoea to severe dehydration which may be rapidly fatal.

In the severe form, the condition is characterised by uncontrollable diarrhoea leading to watery, mucoid, odourless, isotonic stools ("rice water stool"), which may be accompanied by sudden vomiting of a similar opalescent fluid. Both the stools and the vomit are highly infective. The total fluid loss may be up to 15 to 20 litres per day and results in marked dehydration and electrolyte imbalance, leading to tissue shrinkage, extreme thirst, low urine output, haemoconcentration, fall in blood pressure, muscle cramps, and general weakness. Treatment consists in replacing the water and electrolyte losses rapidly by the oral or intravenous route (see under Diarrhoea). Large volumes of fluid may be required and the most important ions that require replacement are sodium, potassium, chloride, and bicarbonate. Once rehydration is complete, fluid intake should equal that lost from vomit and stools. Antibacterial drugs such as tetracycline, given intravenously initially, are administered to hasten the elimination of the vibrios. Complications occurring during convalescence include abdominal pains, dizziness, deafness, and, occasionally, acute renal failure. These should be treated symptomatically; they usually resolve spontaneously.

Preventive measures include good sanitation and avoidance of contamination of water and food supplies. A temporary immunity may be produced by vaccination (see Cholera Vaccine).

A full account of the treatment of cholera is included in Principles and Practice of Cholera Control: *Public Health Papers, No. 40*, Geneva, World Health Organization, 1970.

Cholera Vaccine

A sterile suspension of suitable strains of the cholera vibrio, *Vibrio cholerae.*

OTHER NAMES: Cho/Vac; Vaccinum Cholerae

A standard is given in the European Pharmacopoeia Vol. II

Cholera vaccine contains not less than 8000 million vibrios per millilitre prepared from the two main serotypes (Inaba and Ogawa) of the classical biotype and may contain in addition Inaba and Ogawa serotypes of the El Tor biotype.

Storage. It should be stored as described under Vaccines. Under these conditions it may be expected to retain its potency for 18 months.

Actions and uses. Cholera vaccine is used for active immunisation against cholera but the immunity conferred is short-lived. A primary prophylactic course of two injections is recommended, preferably with an interval of 4 weeks between the injections, and this may confer immunity for 5 to 6 months.

The vaccine is administered by subcutaneous or intramuscular injection of the volume stated on the label as the dose, usually the first dose being 0.5 millilitre and the second being 1 millilitre. Further doses of 1 millilitre should be given at intervals of 6 months. Reactions to this vaccine are usually mild.

Choline Salicylate

The choline salt of salicylic acid.

$$HO \cdot [CH_2]_2 \cdot \overset{+}{N}(CH_3)_3 \qquad \left[\begin{array}{c} COO^- \\ OH \end{array} \right]$$

$C_{12}H_{19}NO_4 = 241.3$

OTHER NAMES: *Audax®*; *Bonjela®*; *Teejel®*

Description. An odourless, white, very hygroscopic, crystalline powder.

Solubility. Soluble in water, in alcohol, and in acetone; practically insoluble in ether.

Acidity. A 10% solution has a pH of 6.5.

Melting-point. About 50°.

Storage. It should be stored in airtight containers.

Actions and uses. Choline salicylate is applied topically for the relief of pain and inflammation in local conditions. Ear-drops containing 20% are used in painful conditions of the ear and a paste or gel containing 8.7% is applied to lesions of the mouth.

Precautions and contra-indications. It should not be used in patients who are sensitive to salicylates. The paste should not be used in infants under 4 months and should be used with caution in infants up to 1 year of age.

Preparations

CHOLINE SALICYLATE DENTAL PASTE: a solution of choline salicylate, with a suitable preservative and flavouring agent, in an adhesive gelatinous paste for application to oral surfaces. It contains 8.7% of choline salicylate.

Containers and *Storage:* see the entry on Pastes for general information on containers and storage. It may be packed in small collapsible tubes.

Advice for patients: it should be rubbed gently into the lesions before meals and at night. It should not be used for prolonged periods without medical advice.

OTHER PREPARATIONS available include EAR-DROPS containing choline salicylate 200 mg with ethylene oxide-polyoxypropylene glycol condensate 12.5 mg per ml.

Choline Theophyllinate

The choline salt of theophylline.

HO·[CH$_2$]$_2$·$\overset{+}{N}$(CH$_3$)$_3$

$C_{12}H_{21}N_5O_3 = 283.3$

OTHER NAME: *Choledyl*®

A standard is given in the British Pharmacopoeia 1973

Description. A white crystalline powder which is odourless or has a faint amine-like odour and a slightly saline taste.

Solubility. Soluble, at 20°, in less than 1 part of water and in 10 parts of alcohol; very slightly soluble in ether and in chloroform.

Storage. It should be stored in airtight containers, at a temperature not exceeding 25°, protected from light.

Identification. TESTS. 1. Dissolve 500 mg in 2 ml of water, add 3 ml of *sodium hydroxide solution*, and heat to boiling; the odour of trimethylamine is produced.
2. Dissolve about 10 mg in 1 ml of hydrochloric acid, add 0.1 g of potassium chlorate, and evaporate to dryness in a dish; a reddish residue remains, which becomes purple on exposure to ammonia vapour.

MELTING-POINT. About 189°.

ULTRAVIOLET ABSORPTION. In 0.1N sodium hydroxide, maximum at 275 nm (E1%, 1cm = 420).

INFRA-RED ABSORPTION. Major peaks at 756, 1095, 1412, 1525, 1632, and 1677 cm^{-1} (see Appendix 2a: Infra-red Spectra).

THIN-LAYER CHROMATOGRAPHY. See under Thin-layer Chromatography, System 12.

Metabolism (see also the section on metabolism under Theophylline). ABSORPTION. Rapidly absorbed after oral administration and gives earlier and higher blood concentrations of theophylline than aminophylline.

BLOOD CONCENTRATION. After an oral dose of 600 mg as compression-coated tablets, peak plasma concentrations of about 10 μg/ml are attained in 2 hours; after an oral dose of 314 mg as capsules and as an alcoholic syrup, plasma concentrations of 2.8 to 7 μg/ml and 4 to 10 μg/ml are attained at 4 hours, respectively.

FURTHER INFORMATION. Blood concentrations—K. B. Bulow *et al.*, *Eur. J. clin. Pharmac.*, 1975, **8**, 115.

Actions and uses. Choline theophyllinate has the pharmacological actions of theophylline and is administered by mouth for its bronchodilator effect in the treatment of bronchial asthma and pulmonary emphysema.
The usual adult dosage is 200 milligrams 2 or 3 times a day and for children from 3 to 5 years 60 to 125 milligrams or 6 to 12 years 100 milligrams 3 times a day.
When given by mouth in therapeutically effective doses, choline theophyllinate causes substantially less gastric irritation or nausea than aminophylline.

Preparations

CHOLINE THEOPHYLLINATE ELIXIR: a solution of choline theophyllinate in a suitable coloured flavoured vehicle. Dilution of this elixir is not recommended. Available as an elixir containing 62.5 mg of choline theophyllinate in 5 ml.
Containers and *Labelling*: see the entry on Elixirs for general information on containers and labelling.
Storage: it should be stored at a temperature not exceeding 25°, protected from light.
Advice for patients: the elixir should preferably be taken after meals.

CHOLINE THEOPHYLLINATE TABLETS: available as tablets containing 100 and 200 mg of choline theophyllinate; they are compression coated; the coat may be coloured.
A standard for these tablets is given in the British Pharmacopoeia 1973
Containers and *Storage*: see the entry on Tablets for general information on containers and storage. Containers should be airtight and light resistant. The tablets should be stored at a temperature not exceeding 25°.
Advice for patients: the tablets should preferably be taken after meals.

Chondrocalcinosis

see PYROPHOSPHATE ARTHROPATHY

Choriocarcinoma

Choriocarcinoma is a malignant tumour of the trophoblast. It occurs as the end stage of a degenerating pregnancy which does not spontaneously abort. The trophoblastic epithelium may continue to proliferate, resulting in a hydatidiform mole. This is a benign tumour and is sometimes expelled spontaneously. However, in approximately 10% of women who have had benign trophoblastic disease, choriocarcinoma develops. Careful follow-up of all patients expelling a hydatidiform mole is therefore essential.
Choriocarcinoma causes persistent uterine bleeding following pregnancy or an apparently complete abortion. It may metastasize to the vaginal wall, the lungs, or the brain.
Choriocarcinoma is life threatening but early treatment with cytotoxic drugs, used in conjunction with surgery, reduces the mortality rate to about 10%.
Cytotoxic drugs used in the treatment of choriocarcinoma include mercaptopurine, methotrexate, and vinblastine.

Christmas Disease

see HAEMOPHILIA B under HAEMOPHILIA

Chromatography

see GAS CHROMATOGRAPHY, THIN-LAYER CHROMATOGRAPHY, HIGH PRESSURE LIQUID CHROMATOGRAPHY, and PAPER CHROMATOGRAPHY

Cimetidine

1-Cyano-2-methyl-3-[2-(5-methylimidazol-4-ylmethyl-thio)ethyl]guanidine

$C_{10}H_{16}N_6S = 252.3$

OTHER NAME: *Tagamet*®

Description. A crystalline powder.

Solubility. Soluble in 88 parts of water.

Melting-point. About 142°.

Determination in body fluids. HIGH PRESSURE LIQUID CHROMATOGRAPHY. In blood or urine—W. C. Randolph *et al.*, *J. pharm. Sci.*, 1977, **66**, 148.

Metabolism. ABSORPTION. Rapidly absorbed after oral administration.

BLOOD CONCENTRATION. After an oral dose of 200 mg, peak concentrations, in whole blood, of 0.3 to 1.0 $\mu g/ml$ are attained in 45 to 75 minutes. A concentration of about 0.5 $\mu g/ml$ is required to produce a 50% inhibition of the output of gastric juice stimulated by histamine or pentagastrin.

HALF-LIFE. After intravenous administration, about 2 hours.

DISTRIBUTION. Widely distributed throughout the tissues from which it is rapidly eliminated except from the liver, kidneys, and adrenal cortex; *protein binding*, about 18 to 26% bound to plasma proteins.

METABOLIC REACTIONS. Sulphoxidation. Not all the metabolites have been identified. No differences in metabolism appear to occur after oral or intravenous administration.

EXCRETION. After an intravenous dose, about 60% is excreted in the urine in 2.5 hours and 80 to 100% in 24 hours; after an oral dose, 13 to 35% is excreted in the urine in 2 hours and 60 to 95% in the urine in 24 hours. Of the excreted material, 40 to 70% is unchanged, about 20% is the major metabolite (the sulphoxide), and the remainder is unidentified.

FURTHER INFORMATION. R. W. Brimblecombe *et al.*, *J. int. med. Res.*, 1975, **3**, 86; W. L. Burland *et al.*, *Br. J. clin. Pharmac.*, 1975, **2**, 481; W. C. Randolph *et al.*, *J. pharm. Sci.*, 1977, **66**, 1149; D. C. Taylor *et al.*, *Drug Met. Disp.*, 1978, **6**, 21.

Actions and uses. Cimetidine is an H_2-receptor antagonist which is used to antagonise the effects of histamine on the acid-secreting cells in the gastric mucosa as described under Histamine Receptors. It is used to reduce gastric acid secretion in conditions associated with hyperacidity such as duodenal and peptic ulceration.

The usual oral dose of cimetidine is 200 milligrams, increasing to 400 milligrams when necessary, 3 times a day, and 400 milligrams at night. Treatment should be continued for at least 4 weeks. After the initial course, a maintenance dose of 400 milligrams at night may be given to prevent relapse.

Cimetidine may be administered by intravenous injection in a dosage of 200 milligrams every 4 to 6 hours. The usual dose by intravenous infusion is 100 milligrams, increasing if necessary to 150 milligrams (or 2 milligrams per kilogram body-weight), hourly for 2 hours, repeated at intervals of 4 to 6 hours. If cimetidine is administered by continuous intravenous infusion the hourly rate of infusion should not exceed 75 milligrams. The use of cimetidine in children has not been fully evaluated. A suggested dose is 20 to 40 milligrams per kilogram body-weight daily in divided doses.

Undesirable effects. Diarrhoea, muscle pain, and rashes may occasionally occur and, rarely, increases in serum creatinine values and gynaecomastia.

Precautions. The oral and parenteral dose of cimetidine should not exceed 2 grams daily. Dosage should be reduced in patients with impaired renal function; usually, the dose required in severe renal impairment does not exceed 400 milligrams daily in divided doses.

The effects of prolonged cimetidine treatment have not been fully evaluated. Serum creatinine concentrations should be measured each month during treatment.

Cimetidine should not be withdrawn abruptly but by gradual reduction in dose to avoid rebound acidity and its complications.

Preparations

Preparations available include an ELIXIR containing cimetidine hydrochloride equivalent to 200 mg of cimetidine in 5 ml, diluent syrup, life of diluted elixir 4 weeks; an INJECTION containing cimetidine 100 mg per ml in 2-ml ampoules; and TABLETS containing cimetidine 200 mg.

Cinchocaine

2-Butoxy-*N*-(2-diethylaminoethyl)quinoline-4-carboxamide

$C_{20}H_{29}N_3O_2 = 343.5$

OTHER NAMES: *Dermacaine*®; Dibucaine

A standard is given in the British Pharmaceutical Codex 1973

Description. A white odourless powder.

Solubility. Very slightly soluble in water; soluble in ether.

Moisture content. Not more than 1%, determined by drying over phosphorus pentoxide *in vacuo*.

Dissociation constant. pK_a 7.5 (20°).

Identification. TEST. Dissolve 250 mg in 8 ml of 0.1N hydrochloric acid and add 10 ml of a saturated solution of potassium perchlorate; a precipitate is produced which, after recrystallisation from water and drying, melts at about 132°.

MELTING-POINT. About 64°.

INFRA-RED ABSORPTION. Major peaks at 766, 1340, 1400, 1540, 1598, and 1643 cm^{-1} (see Appendix 2a: Infra-red Spectra).

Actions and uses. Cinchocaine has the local anaesthetic properties described under Cinchocaine Hydrochloride and, because of its solubility in oils, it is employed in the preparation of ointments and oily solutions.

It is used as a 1% ointment for the treatment of irritant and painful conditions of the skin and mucous membranes. A similar preparation has been incorporated in paraffin gauze dressings and used for dressing burns and raw or granulating surfaces.

An oily solution containing 0.5% of cinchocaine is employed in the injection treatment of haemorrhoids, anal fissures, and pruritus ani and for relieving spasm of the anal sphincter. The prolonged analgesia produced by such a solution is especially valuable in the relief of pain following operations on the anus and rectum.

Oily solutions for injection are prepared by an aseptic technique with a suitable oil which has been previously sterilised by heating at 150° for 1 hour.

Poisoning. The procedure as described under Cocaine should be adopted.

Preparations

Preparations available include a CREAM containing cinchocaine 2%.

Cinchocaine Hydrochloride

2-Butoxy-N-(2-diethylaminoethyl)quinoline-4-carbox-amide hydrochloride
$C_{20}H_{30}ClN_3O_2 = 379.9$

OTHER NAMES: Dibucaine Hydrochloride; *Nuper-cainal*®; *Nupercaine*®

A standard is given in the British Pharmacopoeia 1973

Description. Fine, white, hygroscopic, odourless crystals with a slightly bitter taste.

Solubility. Soluble, at 20°, in less than 1 part of water; soluble in alcohol, in chloroform, and in acetone; practically insoluble in ether and in oils.

Acidity. A 2% solution has a pH of 5 to 6.

Moisture content. Not more than 2.5%, determined by drying at 70° *in vacuo*.

Sterilisation. Solutions for injection are sterilised by heating in an autoclave or by filtration.

Storage. It should be stored in airtight containers.

Identification. TEST. 5 ml of a 5% solution complies with the test described under Cinchocaine.

MELTING-POINT. About 98°.

ULTRAVIOLET ABSORPTION. In 1N hydrochloric acid, maxima at 247 nm (E1%, 1cm = 650) and 319 nm (E1%, 1cm = 235).

THIN-LAYER CHROMATOGRAPHY. See under Thin-layer Chromatography, System 2.

Actions and uses. Cinchocaine is a local anaesthetic which is suitable for infiltration, surface, or spinal anaesthesia. Although it is several times more toxic than procaine by injection or cocaine by surface application, it is relatively safer because its local anaesthetic action is greater and it can therefore be used in lower concentrations than are normally employed with procaine or cocaine; in addition, it does not produce the idiosyncratic reactions that may arise after the administration of cocaine.

The risk of toxic effects may be reduced by the inclusion of adrenaline, which delays absorption. Solutions containing adrenaline should not, however, be used for inducing anaesthesia in digits because the profound ischaemia produced may lead to gangrene.

In infiltration anaesthesia, the action of cinchocaine is more prolonged than that of procaine.

For surface application in otorhinolaryngology, cinchocaine hydrochloride is used as a 0.5 or 2% solution. In

ophthalmology, a 0.1% solution produces an analgesic effect comparable to that produced by a 3% solution of cocaine hydrochloride. Water-soluble jellies containing 1 to 5% have been employed as anaesthetic lubricants for the passage of bronchoscopes and nasal and urethral instruments. Cinchocaine suppositories have been used for the relief of pain in anal fissure and haemorrhoids. Lozenges containing 1 milligram may be used for anaesthetising the larynx and pharynx prior to laryngoscopy, bronchoscopy, or gastroscopy, and a 0.1% solution may be injected into the intact urethra before passing a catheter or cystoscope. The onset of analgesia may be preceded by irritation.

For infiltration anaesthesia a 0.03 to 0.1% solution may be used.

For spinal anaesthesia, cinchocaine hydrochloride is usually administered as a 0.1 to 0.5% solution having a higher density than that of cerebrospinal fluid; this solution is prepared by dissolving the requisite dose in dextrose injection (6%). For techniques in which a solution of relatively low density is required, a suitable preparation is a 0.066% solution of cinchocaine hydrochloride in water for injections containing 0.5% of sodium chloride.

Poisoning. The procedure as described under Cocaine should be adopted.

Preparations

Preparations available include a CREAM containing cinchocaine hydrochloride 1.1%, an INJECTION containing cinchocaine hydrochloride 0.5% with dextrose 6%, and an OINTMENT containing cinchocaine hydrochloride 1.1%.

Cineole

The anhydride of *p*-menthane-1,8-diol. It may be obtained from eucalyptus oil, cajuput oil, and other oils.

$C_{10}H_{18}O = 154.3$

OTHER NAME: Eucalyptol

A standard is given in the British Pharmaceutical Codex 1973

Description. A colourless liquid with an aromatic and camphoraceous odour.

Solubility. Miscible with alcohol and with light liquid paraffin.

Weight per ml. At 20°, 0.922 to 0.924 g.

Refractive index. At 20°, 1.456 to 1.460.

Optical rotation. −1° to +1°.

Storage. It should be stored in airtight containers, in a cool place, protected from light.

Actions and uses. Cineole has the actions and uses described under Eucalyptus Oil but it is less irritating to mucous membranes.

It is used with other counter-irritants in some ointments. It is also used as an antiseptic (0.25%) in dentifrices and as a softening agent to adapt gutta percha fillings and cones to cavities and root canals of teeth.

Cineole has been used as an ingredient of oily nasal drops and throat sprays, but oily solutions are unsuitable for these purposes because they inhibit ciliary action and may cause lipoid pneumonia.

Preparation

Cineole is an ingredient of compound methyl salicylate ointment.

Cinnamic Acid

E-β-Phenylacrylic acid

$C_9H_8O_2 = 148.2$

A standard is given in the British Pharmaceutical Codex 1973

Description. Colourless crystals with a faint balsamic odour.

Solubility. Very slightly soluble in water; soluble, at 20°, in 6 parts of alcohol and in 15 parts of ether and of chloroform.

Identification. TEST. Warm 100 mg with 100 mg of potassium permanganate and 5 ml of *dilute sulphuric acid*; the odour of benzaldehyde is produced.

MELTING-POINT. About 133°.

Uses. Cinnamic acid has antibacterial and antifungal properties similar to those of benzoic acid. It is used with benzoic acid as an ingredient of opiate squill pastilles to simulate the flavour of tolu.

Cinnamon

The dried inner bark of the shoots of coppiced trees of *Cinnamomum zeylanicum* Blume (Fam. Lauraceae), a small tree indigenous to and cultivated in Sri Lanka. It is known in commerce as Ceylon cinnamon.

OTHER NAMES: Cinnamomi Cortex; Cinnamon Bark

A standard is given in the British Pharmacopoeia 1973

The trees are cut down to form stools, from which adventitious shoots arise; these are cut off when about 1 or 2 metres in length, the bark is stripped, and the epidermis and cortex removed by scraping; the strips are then packed, the smaller within the larger, and dried to form compound quills.

Varieties. "Quillings" consist of pieces of broken quills obtained during the manipulation of the quills; they yield about 0.9 to 1.3% of volatile oil.

Constituents. Cinnamon contains about 1 to 2% of volatile oil, with tannin and mucilage. It yields to alcohol (90%) about 14 to 16% of extractive and gives 26 to 36% of crude fibre. Up to 2% of foreign organic matter may be present. It yields up to 2% of acid-insoluble ash.

Description. UNGROUND DRUG. *Macroscopical characters:* single or double, closely packed compound quills, up to about 1 m or more in length and about 10 mm in diameter; outer surface dull yellowish-brown, marked with pale longitudinal lines and often with small scars or holes, cork patches rare; inner surface darker and striated longitudinally; bark about 0.5 mm thick, brittle, fracture splintery.

It has a fragrant odour and a warm, sweet, and aromatic taste.

Microscopical characters: the diagnostic characters are: *sclereids* present in the outer phloem, mostly isodiametric, but sometimes slightly elongated tangentially, usually with the inner and radial walls thicker than the outer walls; some sclereids containing starch granules; inner phloem narrow, mainly consisting of tangential bands of sieve tissue alternating with parenchyma, but containing some axially elongated cells filled with *volatile oil* or *mucilage*; *fibres* thick-walled, up to 30 μm in diameter, solitary or in short tangential rows; total length of fibres per gram 230 to **265** to 290 m; *medullary rays* mostly 2 cells wide, consisting of isodiametric cells; simple 2- to 4-compound *starch* granules mostly 4 to 8 and rarely more than 10 μm in diameter; minute acicular *crystals* of calcium oxalate also present in some parenchymatous cells.

POWDERED DRUG. Powdered Cinnamon. A dull yellowish-brown powder possessing the diagnostic microscopical characters, odour, and taste of the unground drug.

Adulterants and substitutes. Jungle cinnamon is obtained from wild plants; the bark is darker, coarser, less carefully trimmed, and less aromatic than the cultivated bark.

Cinnamon chips consist of small pieces of untrimmed bark; they can be distinguished by their lower yield to alcohol (90%) and, microscopically, by the abundance of cork. A similar material to "chips", but of a better quality, is known as "featherings".

Saigon cinnamon is referred to *C. loureirii* Nees; the quills are thicker than those of Ceylon cinnamon and of a greyish-brown colour with lighter patches, warty and ridged externally, and have a sweeter taste.

Java cinnamon is obtained from *C. burmanni* Blume. It may be distinguished by its low yield of extractive to alcohol (90%) and, microscopically, by the presence in the medullary rays of small tabular crystals of calcium oxalate. The odour is less delicate than that of Ceylon cinnamon. The oil contains 75% of cinnamic aldehyde.

Seychelles cinnamon, which is inferior in aroma and flavour, is obtained from plants of *C. zeylanicum* introduced into the Seychelles, where they have become wild. It occurs in broken pieces or as rolled quills.

Cassia bark is known as Chinese cinnamon; it is the dried bark of *C. cassia* Blume, a tree indigenous to Indo-China and southern China. It occurs in single quills or channelled pieces, 50 to 400 mm long, 12 to 18 mm in diameter, and 1 to 3 mm thick; colour dark earthy brown, except where patches of thin greyish cork persist; fracture short and granular in the outer part, but slightly fibrous in the inner part; odour resembling that of cinnamon, but less delicate; taste more mucilaginous and astringent. The chief microscopical characters which distinguish it are the presence of cork in alternating layers of thick- and thin-walled cells, the phloem fibres up to about 40 μm in width, the somewhat larger starch granules, often more than 10 μm in diameter. Cassia bark contains about 1 to 2% of volatile oil. The oil rarely contains less than 85% of cinnamic aldehyde and no eugenol. The total length of fibres present is characteristic, being 27 to **40** to 55 m per gram.

Cayenne cinnamon is *C. zeylanicum* from French Guiana, Brazil, and West Indies.

Oliver or black sassafras bark is *C. oliveri* from Queensland. It contains 1 to 2.4% of volatile oil.

Storage. It should be stored in a cool dry place. Powdered cinnamon should be stored in airtight containers in a cool place.

Actions and uses. Cinnamon is a carminative and is slightly astringent.

Preparation

Powdered cinnamon is an ingredient of aromatic chalk powder.

Cinnamon Oil

Obtained by distillation from cinnamon.

OTHER NAME: Oleum Cinnamomi

A standard is given in the British Pharmacopoeia Addendum 1978

Constituents. Cinnamon oil contains about 70% w/w of cinnamic aldehyde, together with eugenol, phellandrene, and other terpenes.

Description. It is a yellow liquid when freshly distilled, gradually becoming reddish-brown with age; it has a characteristic odour.

Weight per ml. At 20°, 1.000 to 1.035 g.

Refractive index. 1.573 to 1.595.

Optical rotation. 0° to −2°.

Adulterants and substitutes. Cassia oil is obtained from the leaves and twigs of *Cinnamomum cassia* Blume (Fam. Lauraceae); it has a much less delicate odour and taste than cinnamon oil and has a cinnamic aldehyde content of 80% or more, a higher weight per ml, and a higher refractive index.
Cinnamon-leaf oil contains about 80% of eugenol and has a weight per ml intermediate between that of cassia oil and cinnamon oil. The refractive index is lower than that for cinnamon oil. Adulteration with cassia oil or cinnamic aldehyde increases the weight per ml and the cinnamic aldehyde content. Adulteration with cinnamon-leaf oil diminishes the cinnamic aldehyde content and increases the eugenol content and may be detected by the blue-green colour produced on the addition of 0.25 ml of a 5% alcoholic solution of ferric chloride to 10 ml of a 20% alcoholic solution of the oil.

Storage. It should be stored in well-filled airtight containers at a temperature not exceeding 25°, protected from light.

Actions and uses. Cinnamon oil is a carminative and is used largely as a flavouring agent. It has sometimes been used as a preservative because the predominant constituent, cinnamic aldehyde is an effective anti-mould agent for syrups in a concentration of 0.01%.

Preparation

CONCENTRATED CINNAMON WATER:

Cinnamon oil	..	..	..	..	..	20 ml
Alcohol (90%)	..	..	..	..	600 ml
Water for preparations	..	..	..	to 1000 ml

Dissolve the cinnamon oil in the alcohol and add sufficient of the water, in successive small portions, to produce the required volume, shaking vigorously after each addition; add 50 g of sterilised purified talc or other suitable filtering aid, shake occasionally during a few hours, and filter.
A standard for this concentrated water is given in the British Pharmaceutical Codex 1973

Dose: 0.3 to 1 millilitre.
Cinnamon Water is prepared by diluting concentrated cinnamon water with 39 times its volume of water for preparations.

Circulatory Failure, Acute

Acute circulatory failure, or lack of circulation of an adequate blood supply to the tissues and organs, results from arterial hypotension caused by a substantial uncompensated reduction in cardiac output. In transient form this gives rise to syncope, and in more prolonged form to shock.

Syncope (often referred to as a "faint") is a transient reversible loss of consciousness caused by cerebral ischaemia resulting from acute circulatory failure. Reduction in cardiac output may be the result of insufficient venous return to the heart caused by peripheral vasodilatation occurring, for example, in hot weather or by venous pooling below the heart, for example, after prolonged standing. It may also be due to instability of vasomotor control, for example, postural hypotension caused by ganglion-blocking agents or bilateral sympathectomy. Cardiogenic syncope may occur owing to transient failure of the diseased heart to provide sufficient cardiac output. Psychic factors, especially emotional situations, may also precipitate syncope through vagal overactivity.
Syncope is usually preceded by feelings of faintness and by pallor, sweating, and tachypnoea. The hypotensive episode may be accompanied by bradycardia, particularly if due to vagal overactivity. Unconsciousness is brief and recovery may be hastened by laying the patient flat. Syncope which is the result of heart disease, such as myocardial infarction may be followed by shock.

Shock is a condition of acute circulatory failure due to derangement of circulatory control or loss of circulating fluid resulting in severe reduction in cardiac output. Intense sympathetic vasoconstriction maintains the arterial perfusion pressure to the head and other vital organs although at subnormal levels. There is a depression of all vital activities causing weakness, subnormal temperature, sweating, and apathy. Consciousness is generally maintained although syncope may occur if the patient stands up. The skin is pale and cold and the arterial pulse is weak and rapid. There is a reduction in renal blood flow which results in fluid and electrolyte retention.
Shock may be caused by massive loss of body fluids, for example, by external trauma such as haemorrhage, crushing, and burning, or by diarrhoea and vomiting. It may be the result of the release into the circulation of endotoxins or tissue breakdown products, which result in vasodilatation and increased capillary permeability, as in peritonitis, septicaemia, and pancreatitis. Conditions such as pulmonary embolism cause shock by producing a massive disturbance in the normal circulation. Damage to the heart itself, for example, by myocardial infarction, is especially likely to cause shock by reducing cardiac output.
The incidence and severity of shock may be minimised by gentle handling of injuries, protection from cold, treatment of pain, and prevention of losses of blood and electrolytes.
Treatment should be instituted as soon as possible and consists in removing the immediate cause such as haemorrhage, treatment of infection, and replacement of lost fluid by transfusion of blood or plasma as appropriate,

or by other blood volume expanders such as dextran. The patient should be kept warm and pain relieved with analgesics such as parenteral morphine or diamorphine. Care should be taken, however, as large doses may increase circulatory collapse. Where hypotension is marked, sympathomimetic amines may be used to raise blood pressure. Care must however be taken since such drugs may further increase renal vasoconstriction with the danger of renal tubular necrosis. The use of α-adrenoceptor blocking drugs together with transfusion fluids to maintain blood volume has been advocated to increase blood flow to and perfusion of the renal and splanchnic areas.

Cirrhosis of the Liver

Cirrhosis of the liver is a group of chronic diseases of the liver of multiple aetiology characterised by destruction of parenchymal cells and loss of their normal lobular structure with fibrosis and regeneration of the remaining cells to form nodules.

The disease may have a long latent period and in some cases it may be far advanced before symptoms occur. The disturbance of liver architecture may result in a blockage of venous outflow with associated portal hypertension. This gives rise to ascites with abdominal distension and pain, oesophageal varices resulting in haematemesis, and enlargement of the spleen. The disturbed liver structure may also lead to biliary obstruction with associated jaundice and pruritus.

The loss of liver cells and an inefficient blood supply to the regenerated cells results in liver cell failure; metabolism of ingested substances will be particularly affected and toxic products of protein metabolism may cause hepatic encephalopathy leading to coma. The toxic effects of drugs are increased and prolonged.

Other metabolic consequences of liver-cell failure include jaundice, oedema, impairment of synthesis of albumin and of various clotting factors, and delay in breakdown of certain hormones such as hydrocortisone and oestrogens. These excess hormones may result in the formation of spider naevi (vascular abnormalities in the skin produced by arteriolar dilatation), erythema of palms and soles, and, in the male, gynaecomastia and atrophy of the testes. In up to a fifth of patients with cirrhosis the regenerative activity in the hepatic nodule becomes neoplastic, resulting in hepatoma.

Since the disease process cannot be reversed, treatment is designed to prevent further fibrosis and limit the development of fluid retention and encephalopathy. A diet rich in energy and protein should be given unless encephalopathy is present, when protein intake should be limited.

Hepatic coma is prevented or treated by reducing the absorption of toxic nitrogenous substances from the intestine. This is achieved by a reduction in protein intake and reduction of the bacterial population of the gut by antibacterials such as neomycin. Salt intake should be restricted when ascites or oedema are present and diuretics administered if required; in severe ascites, abdominal paracentesis may be required. Surgery may be required where cirrhosis is due to obstruction of the bile ducts. Pruritus, which is most commonly associated with cirrhosis due to biliary obstruction, may be relieved by the use of antihistamines and cholestyramine. Corticosteroids may relieve symptoms and prolong life when used in the active phases of the disease if there is evidence of progressive active hepatitis.

Cirrhosis of the liver accompanied by degenerative changes in the brain may be due to **Wilson's disease**, a recessively inherited disease of copper metabolism in which copper is deposited in the tissues. It manifests itself in the second or third decade of life as tremor, incoordination, and dysarthria, together with cirrhosis of the liver. Treatment aims to decrease total body copper by chelation with penicillamine.

Deposition of iron in the liver as in haemochromatosis may also cause cirrhosis. It is due to an excess intake of iron from multiple blood transfusions or from increased absorption from the gut. It is treated by the removal of iron from the body by phlebotomy or chelation of iron with desferrioxamine.

Citric Acid

2-Hydroxypropane-1,2,3-tricarboxylic acid

$$HOOC \cdot CH_2 \cdot \underset{\underset{OH}{|}}{\overset{\overset{COOH}{|}}{C}} \cdot CH_2 \cdot COOH$$

$C_6H_8O_7 = 192.1$

OTHER NAMES: Acidum Citricum; Anhydrous Citric Acid

A standard is given in the European Pharmacopoeia Vol. III

Description. Colourless odourless crystals or white powder with a strongly acid taste. It is slightly hygroscopic in moist air.

Solubility. Soluble, at 20°, in less than 1 part of water and in 1.5 parts of alcohol; very slightly soluble in ether.

Hygroscopicity. At relative humidities between about 25 and 50% it absorbs insignificant amounts of moisture at 25°; at relative humidities between 50 and 75% it absorbs significant amounts, the monohydrate being formed at relative humidities in the upper part of this range; under damper conditions it absorbs substantial amounts of moisture.

Storage. It should be stored in airtight containers.

Metabolism. See under Citric Acid Monohydrate.

Actions and uses. Citric acid has the actions described under Citric Acid Monohydrate. It is used for the preparation of effervescent tablets.

Citric Acid Monohydrate

2-Hydroxypropane-1,2,3-tricarboxylic acid monohydrate
$C_6H_8O_7, H_2O = 210.1$

OTHER NAME: Acidum Citricum Monohydricum

A standard is given in the European Pharmacopoeia Vol. III

Description. Odourless colourless prismatic crystals or white powder with a strongly acid taste. It is slightly hygroscopic in moist air and slightly efflorescent in warm dry air.

Solubility. Soluble, at 20°, in less than 1 part of water, in 1.5 parts of alcohol, and in 2 parts of glycerol; very slightly soluble in ether.

Stability. At 75° it begins to lose water, at 135° it becomes anhydrous, at about 153° it fuses, and at about 175° it is decomposed into water and aconitic acid.

Hygroscopicity. At relative humidities lower than about 65% it effloresces at 25°, the anhydrous acid being formed at relative humidities lower than about 40%; at relative humidities between about 65 and 75% it absorbs insignificant amounts of moisture, but under damper conditions it absorbs substantial amounts.

Storage. It should be stored in airtight containers.

Metabolism. ABSORPTION. Absorbed after oral administration.

DISTRIBUTION. Citric acid is found naturally in the body and is widely distributed; about 70% of the citric acid in the body is in hard bone and this accounts for 1.5% of bone content.

METABOLIC REACTIONS. It is an important intermediate in carbohydrate metabolism and its major role is in the tricarboxylic acid cycle (Krebs citric acid cycle); it is metabolised to carbon dioxide and water.

EXCRETION. Citric acid is normally excreted in the urine in amounts ranging from 0.4 to 1.5 g daily and this amount is not increased unless very large doses are administered; the urinary excretion of citric acid is increased by the administration of oestrogens, decreased by the administration of androgens, and increased in alkaline urine.

Actions and uses. Citric acid monohydrate and alkali citrates increase the secretion of urine and render it less acidic.

Citric acid monohydrate is used in the preparation of effervescent granules. Effervescent draughts may be prepared with citric acid monohydrate and carbonates or bicarbonates; they are more agreeable if they contain a slight excess of acid.

The following substances form approximately neutral solutions when mixed in the proportions stated with 10 parts of citric acid monohydrate: ammonium bicarbonate 7½ parts, magnesium carbonate 7 parts, potassium bicarbonate 14½ parts, and sodium bicarbonate 12 parts.

A 7% solution of citric acid is approximately equal in acidity to lemon juice.

Citric acid monohydrate is also used as an antoxidant synergist. It is usually effective in a concentration of 0.05 to 0.5%.

Sucrose may crystallise on storage from preparations containing a high proportion of syrup when citric acid is present. The inclusion of invert syrup in the formulation retards crystallisation.

Preparations

PAEDIATRIC SIMPLE LINCTUS:

Simple linctus	250 ml
Syrup..	to 1000 ml

When a dose less than or not a multiple of 5 ml is prescribed, the linctus may be diluted, as described in the entry on Linctuses, with syrup.

A standard for this linctus is given in the British Pharmaceutical Codex 1973

Containers: see the entry on Linctuses for general information on containers.

Storage: it should be stored in a cool place.

Dose: CHILD: 5 to 10 millilitres.

Advice for patients: the linctus should be sipped and swallowed slowly. Treatment should not be continued for longer than a few days without medical advice.

SIMPLE LINCTUS:

Citric acid monohydrate	25 g
Concentrated anise water	10 ml
Amaranth solution	15 ml
Chloroform spirit	60 ml
Syrup..	to 1000 ml

When a dose less than or not a multiple of 5 ml is prescribed, the linctus may be diluted, as described in the entry on Linctuses, with syrup.

A standard for this linctus is given in the British Pharmaceutical Codex 1973

Containers: see the entry on Linctuses for general information on containers.

Storage: it should be stored in a cool place.

Dose: 5 millilitres.

Advice for patients: the linctus should be sipped and swallowed slowly. Treatment should not be continued for longer than a few days without medical advice.

Citronella Oil

Obtained by distillation from *Cymbopogon nardus* Rendle or *C. winterianus* Jowitt (Fam. Graminae) or from varietal or hybrid forms of these species; producing countries include Sri Lanka, Indonesia, Taiwan, and other tropical countries.

OTHER NAME: Oleum Citronellae

A standard is given in the British Pharmaceutical Codex 1973

There are two main types of citronella oil in commerce which differ in odour and composition and are known as Ceylon oil and Java oil; Formosa oil closely resembles the latter.

Constituents. The chief constituents of citronella oil are citronellal and geraniol. Java oil contains about 35% of citronellal and 21% of geraniol and Ceylon oil contains about 10% of citronellal and 18% of geraniol.

Description. A pale to deep yellow oil with a pleasant characteristic odour.

Weight per ml. At 20°, 0.895 to 0.905 g.

Refractive index. Ceylon oil, 1.408 to 1.485; Java oil, 1.468 to 1.473.

Optical rotation. Ceylon oil, −9° to −18°; Java oil, −5° to +2°.

Storage. It should be stored in well-filled airtight containers, in a cool place, protected from light.

Uses. Citronella oil is used as a perfume for soaps and brilliantines.

Clindamycin Hydrochloride

Methyl 7-chloro-6,7,8-trideoxy-6-[(2S,4R)-1-methyl-4-propylprolylamino]-1-thio-β-L-*threo*-D-*galacto*-octopyranoside hydrochloride

$C_{18}H_{34}Cl_2N_2O_5S = 461.4$

OTHER NAME: *Dalacin C*®

Description. A white crystalline powder which is

odourless or has a faint mercaptan-like odour and has a bitter taste.

Solubility. Soluble in 1.3 parts of water, in 1000 parts of chloroform, and in 6 parts of methyl alcohol.

Optical rotation. Solutions are dextrorotatory.

Dissociation constant. pK_a 7.7 (25°).

Determination in body fluids. GAS CHROMATOGRAPHY. In serum—T. F. Brodasky and F. F. Sun, *J. pharm. Sci.*, 1974, **63**, 360.

RADIOIMMUNOASSAY. In serum—T. J. Gilbertson and R. P. Stryd, *Clin. Chem.*, 1976, **22**, 828.

Metabolism. ABSORPTION. Absorption is rapid after oral administration and is delayed by the presence of food; the palmitate is hydrolysed in the gastro-intestinal tract and absorbed as the base; intramuscular absorption of the phosphate is slower than oral absorption and this appears to be due to slower hydrolysis.

BLOOD CONCENTRATION. Peak serum concentrations are attained in 45 minutes to 1 hour; after an oral dose of 500 mg as the base or hydrochloride, serum concentrations of 2.6 to 7.9 μg/ml and 2.8 to 7.1 μg/ml are attained in 1 and 2 hours respectively; after a dose of 300 mg of the phosphate every 8 hours, mean serum concentrations of about 7 μg/ml are attained; steady-state levels are attained after 4 to 5 doses.

HALF-LIFE. Serum half-life, 2 to 3 hours in adults but may be shorter in children and longer in patients with renal disease.

DISTRIBUTION. Well distributed throughout the body but relatively small amounts appear in muscle and saliva; therapeutic concentrations appear in bone, lungs, and synovial fluid but no detectable concentrations are found in the cerebrospinal fluid; clindamycin crosses the placenta and is secreted in the milk; *protein binding*, 25% bound to plasma proteins.

METABOLIC REACTIONS. In rats, the major reactions are N-demethylation and sulphoxidation and, in dogs, the major reactions are sulphoxidation and glucuronic acid conjugation with some N-demethylation.

EXCRETION. 5 to 25% of a dose is excreted unchanged in the urine and 3% is excreted in the faeces; clindamycin is excreted in the bile; in liver disease elimination is increased 2- to 5-fold.

FURTHER INFORMATION. Serum clearance in patients with uraemia—A. M. Joshi and R. M. Stein, *J. clin. Pharmac.*, 1974, **14**, 140; absorption and excretion—R. E. Kauffman *et al.*, *Clin. Pharmac. Ther.*, 1972, **13**, 704; urinary excretion in rat and dog—F. F. Sun, *J. pharm. Sci.*, 1973, **62**, 1657.

Actions and uses. Clindamycin is a semi-synthetic derivative of lincomycin. Its antibacterial spectrum is similar to that of lincomycin and it is active against staphylococci, pneumococci, and bacteroides. It is ineffective against species of *Neisseria*, *Haemophilus*, and *Streptococcus faecalis*. Clindamycin shows cross-resistance with lincomycin.

When given by mouth clindamycin is rapidly absorbed, peak blood levels about twice those obtained after an equal dose of lincomycin being obtained in half to one hour.

Clindamycin is used in the treatment of infections by susceptible organisms, especially severe *Bacteroides* infections, staphylococcal septicaemia, and osteomyelitis. It may be used in patients who are hypersensitive to penicillin.

The usual dose is 150 to 300 milligrams increased in severe infections to 450 milligrams, every 6 hours. Children may be given 3 milligrams per kilogram body-weight, increased in severe infections to 6 milligrams per kilogram body-weight, every 6 hours.

For serious infections clindamycin may be given by injection as the phosphate. The usual dose by intramuscular injection or intravenous infusion is the equivalent of 0.6 to 1.2 grams of clindamycin daily in divided doses, which may be increased in life-threatening infections to 4.8 grams daily. Children over 1 month may be given the equivalent of 15 to 25 (increasing to 40) milligrams of clindamycin per kilogram body-weight daily in divided doses, but in severe infections not less than 300 milligrams should be given daily.

Undesirable effects. Rashes, nausea, vomiting, and diarrhoea may occur.

Precautions. As for Lincomycin Hydrochloride. If diarrhoea occurs treatment should be discontinued as it may indicate the onset of pseudomembranous colitis, a very serious complication.

Preparations

CLINDAMYCIN CAPSULES: consisting of clindamycin hydrochloride, in powder, which may be mixed with a suitable inert diluent, enclosed in a hard capsule. The capsule shells may be coloured. Available as capsules containing clindamycin hydrochloride equivalent to 75 and 150 mg of clindamycin.

Containers and *Storage:* see the entry on Capsules for general information on containers and storage.

Advice for patients: the capsules should be taken at regular intervals. The prescribed course should be completed.

PAEDIATRIC CLINDAMYCIN MIXTURE: a suspension of clindamycin palmitate hydrochloride in a suitable coloured flavoured vehicle. It is prepared freshly by dispersing granules consisting of the dry mixed ingredients in the specified volume of water for preparations.

When a dose less than or not a multiple of 5 ml is prescribed, the mixture may be diluted, as described in the entry on Mixtures, with freshly boiled and cooled purified water. The diluted mixture must be freshly prepared.

Available as a mixture containing clindamycin palmitate hydrochloride equivalent to 75 mg of clindamycin in 5 ml when reconstituted.

Containers: see the entry on Mixtures for general information on containers.

Labelling: see the entry on Mixtures for general information on labelling; the name on the label of the container of the dry granules should be "Granules for Clindamycin Mixture".

Storage: when stored at room temperature the dry granules may be expected to retain their potency for at least 2 years from the date of manufacture. The mixture and the diluted mixture should be used within 2 weeks of preparation.

Advice for patients: the mixture should be taken at regular intervals. The prescribed course should be completed.

Clinical Trials

Clinical trials are experimental procedures for the evaluation of the effects of drugs in human subjects.

Preliminary work. Since clinical trials involve some inconvenience and possible risk to human patients they are only undertaken when there has been adequate preparation and when it is likely that a particular drug will have value in medical practice. The purity of the medicinal substances, excipients, and other adjuncts must be known and there should be adequate information on physical characteristics, formulation, stability, and impurities. Studies of bioavailability, metabolism, pharmacology, toxicology, teratology, and carcinogenicity are usually carried out in more than one animal species. In some countries, including the United Kingdom, a certificate must be obtained from the registration authority before a clinical trial can be carried out.

Design of clinical trials. A trial should be designed to evaluate the effects of the drug under specified conditions, usually by comparing it with a control consisting of a similar preparation or a placebo. It may be of one of the following types.

Controlled trials are designed to compensate for effects such as natural recovery and the psychological effects of taking medicines by comparing the effects of a drug with an established drug of the same type or a placebo, the dosage forms administered being indistinguishable in appearance, taste, etc. In another type of controlled trial the effects of a drug are compared with the natural recovery of untreated patients. Controlled trials may be divided into two types, between-patient trials and cross-over trials.

BETWEEN-PATIENT TRIALS. One group of patients is used as a control while another group receives the preparation under examination. This method is suitable for conditions of limited duration but is subject to error on account of variability between patients.

CROSS-OVER TRIALS. Each patient receives the drug under examination for one period and the control drug or placebo for another period. This method is suitable only for chronic conditions but has the advantage that each patient acts as his own control. Errors may, however, be introduced by a "carry-over" effect or by fluctuations in the patient's condition.

Uncontrolled trials. Controls may be dispensed with when treating conditions that are rapidly fatal and for which there is no standard treatment.

Selection of patients. To eliminate bias patients should be randomly allocated to control and treatment groups. Patients in the two groups should be matched for age, sex, and severity of disease. The consent of patients should be sought after the conditions of the trial have been explained to them and they must be withdrawn from a trial if it appears to be in their best interest to do so.

Double-blind operation. It is usually desirable to make the appearance, taste, and other characteristics of the medicinal product under trial indistinguishable from that of the control drug or placebo and not to reveal to the patients or investigators which patient is receiving each type of treatment. This will eliminate bias in favour of an expected activity.

Arrangement of trial. A *fixed sample* trial is carried out with a previously arranged number of patients and analysis of results is carried out when all treatment is completed. Alternatively, a *sequential* method may be used, in which patients are treated and their numbers added to from time to time, the results being analysed as the trial proceeds until a predetermined statistical significance is reached.

A fixed *dose* may be used throughout the trial but generally the results will be of limited value and it is preferable for a variable dose scheme to be used when possible. It is desirable to obtain evidence that patients are actually taking the drugs according to the schedule by, for example, simple tests on the urine, and to exclude from the trial those patients that are found not to be taking their medicines.

Interpretation of results. In assessing the value of new drugs, it is frequently necessary to read reports of clinical trials and to make a critical appraisal of them. In general, it is desirable that clinical trials should be designed and carried out so as to eliminate bias; the status of the investigators and the institution where the trial was carried out may be taken into account in assessing this aspect of the trial. Before a drug is regarded as acceptable it should be shown to have significant practical advantages over a standard treatment if one is available. It is also desirable that there should be sufficient evidence to establish that the drug does not give rise to important undesirable effects in an undue proportion of patients.

Clioquinol

5-Chloro-7-iodoquinolin-8-ol

$C_9H_5ClINO = 305.5$

OTHER NAMES: Chinoform; *Entero-Valodon®*; *Entero-Vioform®*; Iodochlorhydroxyquin; *Vioform® Oralcer®* (with ascorbic acid)

A standard is given in the British Pharmacopoeia 1973

Description. A yellowish-white to brownish-yellow, voluminous, tasteless powder with a faint characteristic odour.

Solubility. Very slightly soluble in water and in alcohol; soluble in dimethylformamide and in pyridine.

Storage. It should be protected from light.

Identification. MELTING-POINT. About 180°, with decomposition.

INFRA-RED ABSORPTION. Major peaks at 952, 1205, 1333, 1370, 1389, and 1493 cm^{-1} (see Appendix 2b: Infra-red Spectra).

Determination in body fluids. GAS CHROMATOGRAPHY. In plasma—D. B. Jack and W. Riess, *J. pharm. Sci.*, 1973, **62**, 1929; in plasma or urine—P. Hartwig and C. Fagerlund, *J. Chromat.*, 1977, **140**, 170.

HIGH-PRESSURE LIQUID CHROMATOGRAPHY. In urine: conjugates of clioquinol—C-T. Chen *et al.*, *Chem. pharm. Bull.*, Tokyo, 1975, **23**, 2173.

Metabolism. ABSORPTION. Poorly absorbed after oral administration.

BLOOD CONCENTRATION. After oral doses of 250, 750, and 1500 mg peak plasma concentrations of 5, 7 to 23, and 14 to 33 µg/ml are attained respectively at 4 hours.

HALF-LIFE. Plasma half-life after oral administration, 11 to 14 hours.

DISTRIBUTION. Clioquinol does not accumulate in the body nor does it have any special tissue affinity; in animals, highest concentrations are found in the blood, kidneys, and liver.

METABOLIC REACTIONS. Conjugation with glucuronic acid and sulphate.

EXCRETION. 25% of a dose of 750 mg is excreted in the urine in 24 hours; 12.6% of a dose is excreted as the glucuronide in 10 hours; in dogs, 22% of a dose is excreted in the urine and 66% in the faeces in 72 hours with significant amounts appearing in the bile.

FURTHER INFORMATION. Absence of neurotoxicity in animals—R. Hess et al., Lancet, ii/1972, 424; pharmacokinetics—D. B. Jack and W. Riess, J. pharm. Sci., 1973, **62**, 1929; distribution and excretion in animals—K. Schmid et al., Arzneimittel-Forsch., 1973, **23**, 1560.

Actions and uses. Clioquinol is an antiseptic and amoebicide. It is used in the treatment of intestinal amoebiasis and bacillary dysentery, the usual dose being 0.75 to 1.5 grams daily in divided doses. The dose for children is 12 to 25 milligrams per kilogram body-weight daily. For intestinal amoebiasis, treatment should initially be given for 10 days and the course repeated after an interval of 7 to 10 days.

Clioquinol has also been used as a suppository (250 milligrams) or cream or insufflation for the treatment of intestinal trichomoniasis.

For the treatment of skin infections, clioquinol is available in lotions, creams, and ointments, usually in a concentration of 3%.

Undesirable effects. Clioquinol stains skin, clothing, and linen yellow. It occasionally causes hypersensitivity. It has been reported to cause subacute myelo-optic neuropathy.

Precautions. Clioquinol should not be given to patients with liver damage, hyperthyroidism, or iodine sensitivity. Treatment should not exceed the time limits given above under Actions and uses.

Preparations

CLIOQUINOL CREAM:

Clioquinol, in very fine powder	30 g
Chlorocresol	.. 1 g
Cetomacrogol emulsifying ointment	300 g
Purified water, freshly boiled and cooled	669 g

Dissolve the chlorocresol in the water with the aid of gentle heat; melt the cetomacrogol emulsifying ointment on a water-bath, add the chlorocresol solution at the same temperature, stir until cold, and incorporate the clioquinol.

Clioquinol cream may be prepared using any other suitable basis.

A standard for this cream is given in the British Pharmaceutical Codex 1973

Containers and Labelling: see the entry on Creams for general information on containers and labelling. When collapsible tubes are used they should preferably be made of plastic material. If made of aluminium, the inner surface of the tubes should be lacquered.

Storage: it should be protected from light.

Advice for patients: the cream should be applied sparingly to the affected area. It stains skin, hair, and fabric; a dressing may be applied.

HYDROCORTISONE AND CLIOQUINOL OINTMENT:

Hydrocortisone, or hydrocortisone acetate, in ultra-fine powder	10 g
Clioquinol, in very fine powder	30 g
Wool fat	100 g
White soft paraffin	860 g

Melt together the wool fat and white soft paraffin and stir until cold. Incorporate the clioquinol and the hydrocortisone, or hydrocortisone acetate, in the cold basis.

The ointment may be prepared with any other suitable basis.

A standard for this ointment is given in the British Pharmaceutical Codex 1973

Containers and Labelling: see the entry on Ointments for general information on containers and labelling. The ointment should be protected from light. When collapsible tubes are used they should preferably be made of plastic material. If made of aluminium, the inner surface of the tubes should be lacquered.

Advice for patients: the ointment should be applied sparingly to the affected area. It stains skin, hair, and fabric; a dressing may be applied.

OTHER PREPARATIONS available include LOZENGES containing clioquinol 35 mg with ascorbic acid 6 mg; and TABLETS containing clioquinol 250 mg.

Clioquinol, in addition to being an ingredient of hydrocortisone and clioquinol ointment, is included in many preparations for topical application in conjunction with various corticosteroids; it is usually present in a concentration of 30 mg per g with an appropriate quantity of corticosteroid.

Clofazimine

3 - (4 - Chloroanilino) - 10 - (4 - chlorophenyl) - 2,10 - dihydro - 2 - phenazin - 2 - ylideneisopropylamine

$C_{27}H_{22}Cl_2N_4 = 473.4$

OTHER NAME: Lamprene®

Description. Dark red crystals or an orange-red microcrystalline powder.

Solubility. Practically insoluble in water; very slightly soluble in alcohol and in glycols; soluble in dimethylformamide and in macrogol 400.

Identification. MELTING-POINT. About 215°.

ULTRAVIOLET ABSORPTION. In 0.1N sulphuric acid, maximum at 284 nm (E1%, 1cm = 302); in methyl alcohol, maximum at 283 nm (E1%, 1cm = 1520).

Actions and uses. Clofazimine has antibacterial actions against species of Mycobacterium and certain other species such as Actinomyces, Streptomyces, and Nocardia. It is used in the treatment of leprosy, especially when resistance to dapsone has been encountered. In the long-term treatment of lepromatous leprosy of recent onset, the dose is adjusted according to body-weight and severity of the disease. The usual weekly dose for a patient who weighs 40 to 60 kilograms is 100 milligrams, increasing to 600 milligrams weekly if active leprosy or sulphone-resistant bacilli are present. In the treatment of erythema nodosum leprosum and in reactions in non-lepromatous leprosy, 200 milligrams is given daily for 3 weeks. This may be increased or decreased by not more than 100 milligrams per week according to the response of the patient. This dose is decreased by 50 milligrams daily to the smallest dose which will control symptoms; treatment should be continued for at least 6 months. Up to 1.2 grams daily has been given.

Undesirable effects. Gastro-intestinal disturbances may occur. The skin and urine may be temporarily discoloured.

Precautions. Clofazimine should be given with caution to patients with renal or hepatic disease. Doses exceeding 400 milligrams should not be given in the treatment of reactions to non-lepromatous leprosy without continuous observation.

Contra-indications. It is contra-indicated in the first trimester of pregnancy.

Preparation

CLOFAZIMINE CAPSULES: consisting of clofazimine enclosed in a soft capsule. Available as capsules containing 100 mg of clofazimine.
Containers and *Storage:* see the entry on Capsules for general information on containers and storage.
Advice for patients: the capsules should preferably be taken after meals. Treatment should not be discontinued without the advice of the prescriber. A red or reddish-violet colour may be imparted to the skin, particularly around the lesions. The urine may also be discoloured.

Clofibrate

Ethyl 2-(4-chlorophenoxy)-2-methylpropionate

$$O \cdot \underset{\underset{CH_3}{|}}{\overset{\overset{CH_3}{|}}{C}} \cdot CO \cdot O \cdot CH_2 \cdot CH_3$$

$C_{12}H_{15}ClO_3 = 242.7$

OTHER NAMES: *Atromid-S®*; *Liprinal®*

A standard is given in the British Pharmacopoeia 1973

Description. A clear almost colourless liquid with a characteristic faintly acrid odour and a taste acrid at first, becoming sweet.

Solubility. Very slightly soluble in water; miscible with alcohol, with ether, and with chloroform.

Weight per ml. At 20°, 1.138 to 1.144 g.

Refractive index. 1.500 to 1.505.

Identification. TEST. To 1 drop of a 10% solution in solvent ether add 1 drop of a saturated solution of hydroxylammonium chloride in alcohol (95%) and 1 drop of a saturated solution of potassium hydroxide in alcohol (95%), heat for 2 minutes on a water-bath, cool, acidify with 0.5N hydrochloric acid, and add 1 drop of a 1% solution of ferric chloride; a violet colour is produced.

ULTRAVIOLET ABSORPTION. In dehydrated alcohol, maxima at 226 nm (E1%, 1cm = 455), 280 nm (E1%, 1cm = 44), and 288 nm (E1%, 1cm = 31).

INFRA-RED ABSORPTION. Major peaks at 1140, 1175, 1238, 1282, 1486, and 1735 cm^{-1} (see Appendix 2a: Infra-red Spectra).

Determination in body fluids. GAS CHROMATOGRAPHY. In serum—A. Karmen and H. Haut, *Biochem. Med.*, 1975, **12**, 154. In plasma—R. Gugler and C. Jensen, *J. Chromat.*, 1976, **117**, 175.

HIGH PRESSURE LIQUID CHROMATOGRAPHY. In plasma; determination of the metabolite clofibric acid—R. N. Woodhouse *et al.*, *J. Chromat.*, 1977, **137**, 218.

Metabolism. ABSORPTION. Readily absorbed after oral administration.

BLOOD CONCENTRATIONS. After an oral dose of 1 g, peak plasma concentrations of the de-esterified acid, clofibric acid [2-(4-chlorophenoxy)-2-methylpropionic acid], of 43 to 79 µg/ml are attained in 2 to 8 hours and, after doses of 2 g, plasma concentrations of about 200 µg/ml are attained in 1 to 3 hours. During therapy with 1 g twice daily for 10 days, steady-state plasma concentrations of the acid of about 116 µg/ml are attained by 10 days.

HALF-LIFE. Plasma half-life, 12 to 17 hours which may be decreased when free fatty acid concentrations are high; longer half-lives have been reported, especially after repeated doses.

DISTRIBUTION. Clofibrate does not appear to be localised in any tissues; minimal amounts are secreted in the milk; *protein binding*, clofibric acid is about 98% bound to plasma proteins but this may be reduced in the presence of high free fatty acid concentrations.

METABOLISM. Hydrolysed by serum enzymes to the acid, α-*p*-chlorophenoxy-α-methylpropionic acid, which is conjugated with glucuronic acid.

EXCRETION. 85% of a dose is excreted in the urine, 92 to 98% of which is the conjugate.

FURTHER INFORMATION. Plasma concentrations and bioavailability—L. F. Chasseaud *et al.*, *J. clin. Pharmac.*, 1974, **14**, 382; pharmacokinetics—W. G. Crouthamel and R. J. Cenedella, *Pharmacology*, 1975, **13**, 465.

Actions and uses. Clofibrate reduces elevated plasma cholesterol, triglyceride, and phospholipid concentrations, reduces platelet stickiness and fibrinogen concentrations, and increases fibrinolysis. The mechanism of action is not known.
Clofibrate is used in hyperlipidaemia, hypercholesterolaemia, hypertriglyceridaemia, tuberous xanthomatosis, and diabetic exudative lipaemic retinopathy in doses of 1.5 to 2 grams daily.

Undesirable effects. Transient nausea and diarrhoea may occur. In patients with low serum albumin levels, as in the nephrotic syndrome, high concentrations of unbound clofibrate in the plasma may give rise to muscle pain.

Precautions. Clofibrate prolongs the prothrombin time when anticoagulants are being given and careful control of anticoagulant dosage is therefore necessary.

Preparation

CLOFIBRATE CAPSULES: consisting of clofibrate enclosed in a soft capsule. Available as capsules containing 500 mg of clofibrate.
A standard for these capsules is given in the British Pharmacopoeia 1973

Containers and *Storage:* see the entry on Capsules for general information on containers and storage.

Advice for patients: the capsules should preferably be taken after meals. Treatment should not be discontinued without the advice of the prescriber.

Clomiphene Citrate

A mixture of the *cis* and *trans* isomers of 2-[4-(2-chloro-1,2-diphenylvinyl)phenoxy]triethylammonium citrate.

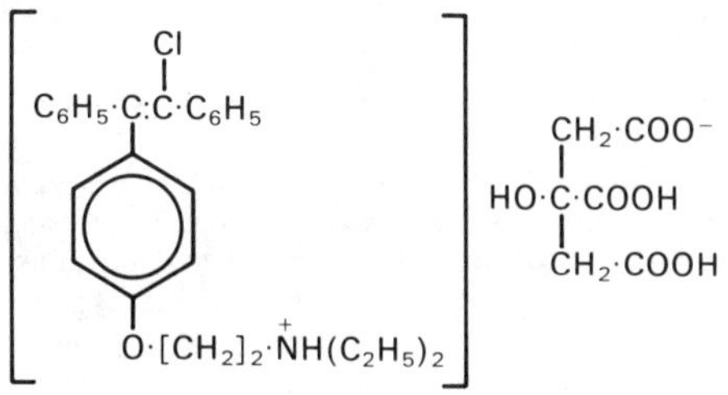

$C_{32}H_{36}ClNO_8 = 598.1$

OTHER NAME: *Clomid*®

A standard is given in the British Pharmacopoeia 1973

Description. A white to pale yellow odourless powder.

Solubility. Soluble, at 20°, in 900 parts of water, in 40 parts of alcohol, and in 800 parts of chloroform; practically insoluble in ether.

Storage. It should be protected from light.

Identification. TEST. Dissolve about 5 mg in 5 ml of a mixture of 1 volume of acetic anhydride and 5 volumes of pyridine and heat on a water-bath; a deep wine-red colour is produced.

MELTING-POINT. About 145°, with decomposition.

ULTRAVIOLET ABSORPTION. In 0.1N hydrochloric acid, maxima at 235 nm (E1%, 1cm = 316) and 292 nm (E1%, 1cm = 176).

Metabolism. ABSORPTION. Readily absorbed after oral administration.

HALF-LIFE. Biological half-life, 5 to 7 days.

DISTRIBUTION. Taken up by oestrogenic-responsive tissues and appears to be subject to enterohepatic circulation.

EXCRETION. Slowly excreted mainly in the faeces via biliary excretion.

Actions and uses. Clomiphene stimulates the production of pituitary gonadotrophins. It is used to induce fertility by the stimulation of ovulation in anovulatory patients. For this purpose, doses of 50 to 200 milligrams of clomiphene citrate are given daily in 2 divided doses for 5 days. Treatment may begin on either the first or the fifth day of the menstrual cycle. In patients with amenorrhoea, treatment can be started at any time. If pregnancy has not occurred after 6 courses of treatment it is unlikely to do so after further courses and treatment should be discontinued.

Clomiphene has also been used in daily doses of 50 to 200 milligrams for the stimulation of spermatogenesis, but its value for this purpose has not been established.

Undesirable effects. Hot flushes, abdominal disturbances, ovarian enlargement, and visual blurring may occur.

Precautions and contra-indications. Clomiphene should not be given to patients with ovarian cysts or endometrial carcinoma or during pregnancy and it is inadvisable to continue treatment for prolonged periods. Patients should be advised of the possible occurrence of multiple pregnancy.

Preparation

CLOMIPHENE TABLETS: available as tablets containing 50 mg of clomiphene citrate.

A standard for these tablets is given in the British Pharmacopoeia 1973

Containers and *Storage:* see the entry on Tablets for general information on containers and storage. Containers should be airtight and light resistant. The tablets should be stored at a temperature not exceeding 25°.

Advice for patients: the prescribed course should be completed.

Clonazepam

5-(2-Chlorophenyl)-1,3-dihydro-7-nitro-2*H*-1,4-benzodiazepin-2-one

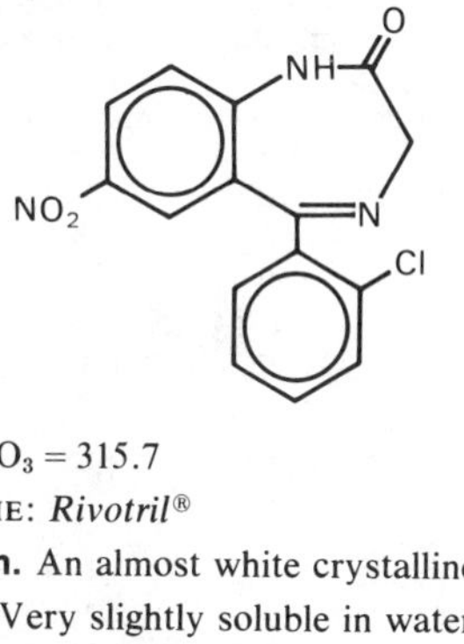

$C_{15}H_{10}ClN_3O_3 = 315.7$

OTHER NAME: *Rivotril*®

Description. An almost white crystalline powder.

Solubility. Very slightly soluble in water.

Dissociation constants. pK_a 1.5, 10.5.

Identification. MELTING-POINT. About 237°.

INFRA-RED ABSORPTION. Major peaks at 748, 1255, 1310, 1333, 1610, and 1685 cm⁻¹ (see Appendix 2a: Infra-red Spectra).

Determination in body fluids. GAS CHROMATOGRAPHY. In plasma—M. Gerna and P. L. Morselli, *J. Chromat.*, 1976, **116**, 445; H. J. Knop *et al.*, *Pharm. Weekbl.*, 1975, **110**, 297. In plasma or serum—E. B. Sollow and C. P. Kenfield, *J. analyt. Toxicol.*, 1977, **1**, 155.

RADIOIMMUNOASSAY. In plasma—W. R. Dixon *et al.*, *J. pharm. Sci.*, 1977, **66**, 235.

Metabolism. ABSORPTION. Rapidly absorbed after oral administration.

BLOOD CONCENTRATION. After an oral dose of 2 mg, peak plasma concentrations of 6 to 24 ng/ml are attained in 1 to 4 hours; during therapy with 2 mg orally thrice daily over 4 months, concentrations of 20 to 49 ng/ml are attained, whilst during therapy with 0.5 mg twice daily, steady-state concentrations of 7 to 13 ng/ml are attained; following an intravenous dose of 2 mg, concentrations in plasma of up to 36 ng/ml are attained within 10 minutes.

HALF-LIFE. The decline in plasma concentration is biphasic with the α-phase lasting 8 to 10 hours and the β-phase having a half-life of 18 to 60 hours.

DISTRIBUTION. Volume of distribution, 1.8 to 4 litres/kg body-weight.

METABOLIC REACTIONS. Reduction of the nitro-group to an amine which is acetylated, and hydroxylation at position 3, the hydroxyl group so formed being conjugated with glucuronic acid or sulphate.

EXCRETION. Less than 0.5% of a dose is excreted unchanged in the urine in 24 hours.

FURTHER INFORMATION. Metabolic and pharmacokinetic studies—A. Berlin and H. Dahlström, *Eur. J. clin. Pharmac.*, 1975, **9**, 155, E. Eschenhof, *Arzneimittel-Forsch.*, 1973, **23**, 390, S. A. Kaplan *et al.*, *J. pharm. Sci.*, 1974, **63**, 527, and J. A. F. de Silva *et al.*, *J. pharm. Sci.*, 1974, **63**, 520.

Actions and uses. Clonazepam has anticonvulsant and weak muscle relaxant actions similar to those described under Diazepam. It is used in the treatment of all types of epilepsy, especially typical and atypical petit mal and myoclonic epilepsies.

Treatment is started with low doses which are increased gradually over 2 to 4 weeks, according to the response of the patient, to a maintenance dosage. The usual daily maintenance dosage given in 3 or 4 divided doses by mouth for adults is 4 to 8 milligrams, for children aged up to 1 year, 0.5 to 1 milligram, for children aged 1 to 5 years, 1 to 3 milligrams and for children aged 6 to 12 years, 3 to 6 milligrams.

In status epilepticus in adults 1 milligram may be administered by slow intravenous injection or infusion and repeated if necessary. Infants and children may be given 500 micrograms by slow intravenous injection or infusion, repeated if necessary.

Undesirable effects. As for Diazepam. Excessive secretion by the salivary glands and bronchi may also occur in infants and children.

Precautions and contra-indications. As for Diazepam.

Preparations

Preparations available include an INJECTION containing clonazepam 1 mg per ml in 1-ml ampoules (supplied with 1-ml ampoules of diluent); and TABLETS containing clonazepam 0.5 and 2 mg.

Clonidine Hydrochloride

N-(2,6-Dichlorophenyl)-2-imidazolin-2-amine hydrochloride

$C_9H_{10}Cl_3N_3 = 266.6$

OTHER NAMES: *Catapres*®; *Dixarit*®

Description. A white powder.

Solubility. Soluble in 15 parts of water, in 27 parts of alcohol, in 38 parts of dehydrated alcohol, and in 270 parts of chloroform; practically insoluble in ether.

Identification. MELTING-POINT. About 313°.

INFRA-RED ABSORPTION. Major peaks at 775, 790, 1435, 1445, 1605, and 1650 cm⁻¹ (see Appendix 2a: Infra-red Spectra).

Determination in body fluids. GAS CHROMATOGRAPHY–MASS SPECTROMETRY. In plasma—C. T. Dollery *et al.*, *Clin. Pharmac. Ther.*, 1976, **19**, 11.

Metabolism. ABSORPTION. Well absorbed after oral administration.

BLOOD CONCENTRATION. After an oral dose of 300 μg, peak plasma concentrations of 1 to 1.5 ng/ml are attained at 1.5 hours.

HALF-LIFE. After oral administration, the plasma half-life is 6 to 23 hours; after intravenous administration, the plasma concentration follows a biphasic decline with a half-life for the α-phase of 2 to 11 minutes and a half-life for the β-phase of 6 to 9 hours.

DISTRIBUTION. Volume of distribution, 2 to 6 litres/kg body-weight.

METABOLIC REACTIONS. In the rat, hydroxylation to form 4-hydroxyclonidine followed by conjugation and also dealkylation to form 2,6-dichlorophenylguanidine.

EXCRETION. About 65% of a dose is excreted in the urine and about 22% in the faeces; about 50% of the amount excreted in the urine is unchanged drug.

FURTHER INFORMATION. Pharmacokinetics and clinical pharmacology—D. S. Davies *et al.*, *Br. J. clin. Pharmac.*, 1976, **3**, 348P, C. T. Dollery *et al.*, *Clin Pharmac. Ther.*, 1976, **19**, 11, and D. Rehbinder and W. Deckers, *Arzneimittel-Forsch.*, 1969, **19**, 169; 2,6-dichlorophenyl-guanidine: a metabolite of clonidine—P. Hodges, *J. Pharm. Pharmac.*, 1976, **28**, 61.

Actions and uses. Clonidine hydrochloride is an antihypertensive agent and has central and peripheral actions. During initial treatment, it causes reduction in blood pressure with a decrease in central sympathetic activity and increased vagal tone. In long-term treatment, it causes the peripheral blood vessels to become less responsive to vasoconstrictor and vasodilator substances and also to sympathetic nerve stimulation.

Clonidine hydrochloride is used in the treatment of hypertension. The initial dose is 50 to 100 micrograms by mouth 3 times daily and is gradually increased until adequate control of the blood pressure is obtained. The usual maintenance dose is 0.3 to 1.2 milligrams daily in divided doses but some patients may require 1.8 milligrams or more daily.

Clonidine hydrochloride may be used in conjunction with other antihypertensive agents.

In hypertensive crises, 150 to 300 micrograms is administered by slow intravenous injection; up to 750 micrograms may be given over a period of 24 hours.

Clonidine hydrochloride is also used for the prophylaxis of migraine or recurrent vascular headache and in the treatment of flushing associated with the menopause. The usual dose is 50 micrograms twice daily increasing after 2 weeks to 75 micrograms twice daily if no response has been obtained.

Undesirable effects. Sedation, dry mouth, and fluid retention may occur during initial treatment. Dizziness, headache, nausea, constipation, euphoria, sleep disturbances, symptoms of Raynaud's disease, and rarely impotence may occur. Facial pallor may occur after intravenous injection and agitation on withdrawal of treatment.

Precautions. It should be administered with caution to patients who are depressed and in Raynaud's disease and thromboangiitis obliterans. Long-term treatment should be withdrawn gradually to prevent rebound hypertension.

The concurrent administration of tricyclic antidepressants decreases the therapeutic action of clonidine.

Preparations

CLONIDINE TABLETS: available as tablets containing 25, 100, and 300 micrograms of clonidine hydrochloride; they may be sugar coated and the coat may be coloured. *Containers* and *Storage:* see the entry on Tablets for general information on containers and storage. Containers should be airtight and light resistant.
Advice for patients: when used in the treatment of hypertension, treatment should not be discontinued without the advice of the prescriber. The tablets may cause drowsiness; persons affected should not drive or operate machinery. Alcohol should be avoided.

OTHER PREPARATIONS available include an INJECTION containing clonidine hydrochloride 150 micrograms per ml in 1-ml ampoules.

Cloprostenol Sodium

The sodium salt of $(\pm)(5Z)$-7-{(1R,2R,3R,5S)-2-[(1E, 3R) - 4 - (3 - chlorophenoxy) - 3 - hydroxybut - 1 - enyl] - 3,5-dihydroxycyclopentyl}hept-5-enoic acid.

$C_{22}H_{28}ClNaO_6 = 446.9$

OTHER NAME: *Estrumate®*

A standard is given in the British Pharmacopoeia (Veterinary)

CAUTION. *Cloprostenol sodium is extremely potent and extraordinary care should be taken in any procedure in which it is used.*

Description. A white amorphous hygroscopic powder.

Solubility. Soluble in water, in alcohol, and in methyl alcohol; practically insoluble in acetone.

Sterilisation. Solutions for injection are sterilised by heating in an autoclave or by filtration.

Storage. It should be stored in airtight containers, in a dry atmosphere, protected from light.

Veterinary uses. Cloprostenol sodium is a luteolytic prostaglandin used in cattle to control dates of oestrus and ovulation in planned breeding programmes. It is also used in cattle to correct certain forms of infertility.
The usual dose is the equivalent of 1 microgram of cloprostenol per kilogram body-weight by intramuscular injection followed after 11 days by a second similar dose; 1.1 grams of cloprostenol sodium is equivalent to 1 gram of cloprostenol.

Preparation

CLOPROSTENOL INJECTION: a sterile solution of cloprostenol sodium in water for injections. It may contain suitable buffering agents. It is sterilised by heating in an autoclave or by filtration. Available in 10- and 20-ml vials containing cloprostenol sodium equivalent to 250 micrograms of cloprostenol per ml.

A standard for this injection is given in the British Pharmacopoeia (Veterinary)
Containers: see the entry on Injections for general information on containers.
Labelling: see the entry on Injections for general information on labelling. In addition, the label on the container should state the amount of the medicament as the equivalent amount of cloprostenol in a suitable dose-volume.
Storage: it should be protected from light.

Clostridium Botulinum Vaccine

A culture in a liquid medium, a filtrate of such a culture, or materials derived therefrom, of *Clostridium botulinum* type C or type D, or a mixture of these types, which has been inactivated in such a manner that immunogenic activity is retained.

OTHER NAME: Botulinum Vaccine

A standard is given in the British Pharmacopoeia (Veterinary)

Storage. The vaccine should be protected from light and stored at 2° to 8°.

Veterinary uses. It is administered to domestic animals by subcutaneous injection for prophylaxis against botulism caused by *Clostridium botulinum* types C and D either singly or in combination.
When Clostridium Botulinum Vaccine is prescribed and the types to be present are not stated, Clostridium Botulinum Vaccine prepared from types C and D is dispensed or supplied.

Clostridium Chauvoei Vaccine

A culture in a liquid medium of a suitable strain or strains of *Clostridium chauvoei* inactivated in such a manner that immunogenic activity is retained.

OTHER NAME: Blackleg Vaccine

A standard is given in the British Pharmacopoeia (Veterinary)

Storage. The vaccine should be protected from light and stored at 2° to 8°.

Veterinary uses. It is administered by subcutaneous injection to cattle and sheep for prophylaxis against infection by *Clostridium chauvoei*.

Clostridium Oedematiens Alpha Antitoxin

The serum of horses or of other suitable animals, immunised with antigens of *Clostridium oedematiens* type B, or a preparation from serum containing the antitoxic globulins that have the specific power of neutralising the alpha toxin formed by *Cl. oedematiens*.

OTHER NAME: Black Disease Antiserum

A standard is given in the British Pharmacopoeia (Veterinary)

Storage. It should be protected from light and stored at 2° to 8°. It should not be allowed to freeze.

Veterinary uses. It is administered to give temporary protection against infective necrotic hepatitis (black disease) in cattle and sheep and *Cl. oedematiens* infections in horses and cattle. It is also used occasionally in the treatment of infected animals.

The usual prophylactic dose by subcutaneous injection for horses and cattle is 15 000 units and for sheep 3000 units.

The usual therapeutic dose by intravenous injection for horses and cattle is 45 000 to 75 000 units and for sheep 9000 to 15 000 units.

Clostridium Oedematiens Type B Vaccine

A culture in a liquid medium, or a filtrate of such a culture, or materials derived therefrom, of *Clostridium oedematiens* type B, inactivated in such a manner that immunogenic activity is retained.

OTHER NAME: Black Disease Vaccine

A standard is given in the British Pharmacopoeia (Veterinary)

Storage. The vaccine should be protected from light and stored at 2° to 8°.

Veterinary uses. It is administered by subcutaneous injection to cattle and sheep for prophylaxis against necrotic hepatitis (black disease) and swelled head in rams.

Clostridium Perfringens Type B Antitoxin

The serum of horses or other suitable animals, immunised with antigens of *Clostridium perfringens* type B, or a preparation of the serum, containing the antitoxic globulins that have the specific power of neutralising the beta and epsilon toxins of *Clostridium perfringens* type B.

OTHER NAMES: Clostridium Welchii Type B Antitoxin; Lamb Dysentery Antiserum

A standard is given in the British Pharmacopoeia (Veterinary)

Storage. It should be protected from light and stored at 2° to 8°. It should not be allowed to freeze.

Veterinary uses. It is used for the prevention of lamb dysentery due to *Clostridium perfringens* type B. The usual dose by subcutaneous injection for sheep is 15 000 units and for lambs 6000 units.

Clostridium Perfringens Type D Antitoxin

The serum of horses or other suitable animals immunised with antigens of *Clostridium perfringens* type D, or a preparation from the serum, containing the antitoxic globulins that have the specific power of neutralising the epsilon toxin of *Clostridium perfringens* type D.

OTHER NAMES: Clostridium Welchii Type D Antitoxin; Enterotoxaemia Antiserum; Pulpy Kidney Antiserum

A standard is given in the British Pharmacopoeia (Veterinary)

Storage. It should be protected from light and stored at 2° to 8°. It should not be allowed to freeze.

Veterinary uses. It is used for the prevention of enterotoxaemia due to *Clostridium perfringens* type D (pulpy kidney disease) in lambs and sheep. The usual dose by subcutaneous injection for sheep is 1500 units and for lambs 600 units.

Clostridium Perfringens Vaccines

Cultures in a liquid medium, or filtrates of such cultures, or materials derived therefrom, of *Clostridium perfringens* type B, type C, or type D, as listed below, or any combination of these types, inactivated in such a manner that immunogenic activity is retained.

Clostridium Perfringens Type B Vaccine

OTHER NAMES: Clostridium Welchii Type B Vaccine; Lamb Dysentery Vaccine

Clostridium Perfringens Type C Vaccine

OTHER NAMES: Clostridium Welchii Type C Vaccine; Struck Vaccine

Clostridium Perfringens Type D Vaccine

OTHER NAMES: Clostridium Welchii Type D Vaccine; Enterotoxaemia Vaccine; Pulpy Kidney Vaccine

Standards are given in the British Pharmacopoeia (Veterinary)

Storage. The vaccines should be protected from light and stored at 2° to 8°. They should not be allowed to freeze.

Veterinary uses. The vaccines are administered by subcutaneous injection to sheep and lambs for prophylaxis of lamb dysentery caused by *Clostridium perfringens* type B, enterotoxaemia caused by *Clostridium perfringens* type C (struck), and enterotoxaemia and pulpy kidney disease caused by *Clostridium perfringens* type D.

The vaccines may also be administered in a similar manner to pregnant horses, cattle, pigs, and goats, for prophylaxis of necrotic toxaemia in such animals and their young.

Clostridium Septicum Vaccine

A preparation in a liquid medium, or a filtrate of such a culture, or materials derived therefrom, of a suitable strain or strains of *Clostridium septicum* inactivated in such a manner that immunogenic activity is retained.

OTHER NAMES: Braxy Vaccine; Malignant Oedema Vaccine

A standard is given in the British Pharmacopoeia (Veterinary)

Storage. It should be protected from light and stored at 2° to 8°. It should not be allowed to freeze.

Veterinary uses. It is administered by subcutaneous injection for prophylaxis of braxy in sheep and lambs; it is also administered to ewes to provide an active immunity through the colostrum to the lamb to prevent navel infection with *Clostridium septicum*.

Clostridium Tetani Antitoxin

The serum of horses or of other suitable animals, or a preparation from the serum, containing the antitoxic globulins that have the specific power of neutralising the toxin formed by *Clostridium tetani*.

OTHER NAME: Tetanus Antitoxin (Veterinary)

A standard is given in the British Pharmacopoeia (Veterinary)

Storage. It should be protected from light and stored at 2° to 8°. It should not be allowed to freeze.

Veterinary uses. It is administered to animals prophylactically following the infliction of wounds and as a pre-operative precaution.

The usual prophylactic dose by subcutaneous injection for horses and cattle is not less than 3000 units, for pigs, sheep, and calves not less than 500 units, and for piglets, lambs, and dogs not less than 250 units.

The usual therapeutic dose by intravenous injection for horses and cattle is not less than 150 000 units; for pigs, calves, and sheep not less than 25 000 units, and for piglets, lambs and dogs not less than 12 500 units.

Clostridium Tetani Vaccine

A preparation containing a filtrate of a culture in a liquid medium, or materials derived therefrom, of a suitable strain or strains of *Clostridium tetani*, inactivated in such a manner that immunogenic activity is retained.

OTHER NAME: Tetanus Toxoid (Veterinary)

A standard is given in the British Pharmacopoeia (Veterinary)

Storage. The vaccine should be protected from light and stored at 2° to 8°. It should not be allowed to freeze.

Veterinary uses. It is administered by subcutaneous injection to animals other than horses, donkeys, and mules for prophylaxis against tetanus.

Clostridium Tetani Vaccine for Equidae

A preparation containing a filtrate of a culture in a liquid medium, or materials derived therefrom, of a suitable strain or strains of *Clostridium tetani*, inactivated in such a manner that immunogenic activity is retained.

OTHER NAME: Tetanus Toxoid for Equidae

A standard is given in the British Pharmacopoeia (Veterinary)

Storage. The vaccine should be protected from light and stored at 2° to 8°. It should not be allowed to freeze.

Veterinary uses. It is administered by deep intramuscular injection to horses, donkeys, and mules, for prophylaxis against tetanus.

Clotrimazole

1-(α-2-Chlorophenylbenzhydryl)imidazole

$C_{22}H_{17}ClN_2 = 344.8$

OTHER NAME: *Canesten*®

Description. A colourless crystalline powder.

Solubility. Practically insoluble in water; soluble in chloroform and in acetone; very slightly soluble in ether.

Identification. INFRA-RED ABSORPTION. Major peaks at 709, 741, 752, 763, 1075, and 1205 cm^{-1} (see Appendix 2b: Infra-red Spectra).

Metabolism. ABSORPTION. Well absorbed after oral administration; after topical application to the skin it rapidly penetrates the epidermis and deeper layers of the skin but less than 0.5% of the dose is absorbed systemically; about 3% of a dose administered as a vaginal pessary is absorbed systemically.

BLOOD CONCENTRATION. Large individual variations occur in serum concentrations after oral administration; after a single oral dose of 1 g, peak serum concentrations of about 15 μg/ml are attained in 3 hours which drop to about 0.3 μg/ml after 36 hours; serum concentrations after doses of 1 g given twice daily for 3 days rise to about 25 μg/ml after 3 days and with a similar daily dosage for 16 days rise to about 70 μg/ml by the last day; in the newborn, peak serum concentrations appear later and are more prolonged than those in adults.

DISTRIBUTION. Widely distributed throughout the body, including the skin, after oral administration; it is secreted in the saliva; on continued therapy it may accumulate in the body; *protein binding*, about 98% bound to plasma proteins.

METABOLIC REACTIONS. Mainly metabolised in the liver to form triphenylmethane or triphenylmethanol derivatives which may be further hydroxylated and conjugated. Clotrimazole stimulates the drug metabolising enzymes of the liver in the rat; it appears to stimulate the *O*-demethylation of mestranol in the same animal.

EXCRETION. About 10% of an oral dose is excreted in the urine in 24 hours and about 25% is excreted in 6 days; very little unchanged drug is excreted in the urine and the major metabolite is α-2-chlorophenyl-α-4-hydroxyphenyl-α-phenylmethane together with its conjugate and the conjugate of α-2-chlorophenyl-αα-diphenylmethane.

FURTHER INFORMATION. Pharmacokinetics—B. Duhm *et al.*, *Postgrad. med. J.*, 1974, **50**, Suppl. 1, 13.

Actions and uses. Clotrimazole is a broad spectrum antifungal and trichomonacidal agent. It is applied topically as a cream or solution containing 1% in the treatment of dermatomycoses due to moulds and yeasts and dermatophytes such as species of *Candida*.

Pessaries containing 100 milligrams are used in the treatment of leucorrhoea and vaginitis caused by infections with *Candida* and *Trichomonas* species. A pessary is inserted daily for 6 days or in severe infections twice daily for up to 12 days.

Clotrimazole cream may be applied intravaginally in vulvo-vaginal candidiasis.

Undesirable effects. Mild irritation and occasionally sensitisation may occur at the site of application.

Preparations

CLOTRIMAZOLE CREAM: a dispersion of clotrimazole in a suitable water-miscible basis. Available as a cream containing 1% of clotrimazole.

Containers, Labelling, and *Storage:* see the entry on Creams for general information on containers, labelling, and storage.

Advice for patients: the cream should be rubbed lightly on the affected area. Treatment should be continued for 2 weeks after symptoms have disappeared.

CLOTRIMAZOLE PESSARIES: available as pessaries containing 100 mg of clotrimazole.

Containers and *Storage:* see the entry on Tablets for general information on containers and storage.

Advice for patients: the pessaries should be inserted high into the vagina with a suitable applicator, preferably at night. The prescribed course should be completed.

OTHER PREPARATIONS available include a SOLUTION containing clotrimazole 1%; a combination pack consisting of cream and pessaries is also available.

Clove

The dried flower-buds of *Syzygium aromaticum* (L.) Merrill and Perry (Fam. Myrtaceae), an evergreen tree indigenous to Amboyna and other Moluccan islands, but now cultivated chiefly in Zanzibar and Pemba, Malagasy, and Penang.

OTHER NAMES: Caryophyllum; Cloves

A standard is given in the British Pharmaceutical Codex 1973

The flower-buds are white when young, becoming green and then crimson during ripening; they are collected when ripe and dried in the sun.

Varieties. The bulk of the supplies of clove comes from Zanzibar and Malagasy; these cloves are somewhat shrunken and are smaller, darker in colour, and less fragrant than Penang cloves which are plump and bright reddish-brown in colour.

Constituents. Clove contains about 15 to 20% of volatile oil of which about 85 to 92% consists of eugenol. It also contains about 13% of tannins, up to 10% of fatty oil, resin, vanillin, eugenin (a chromone), and a crystalline substance, caryophyllin, which is the pentacyclic triterpene oleanolic acid, which is odourless.

Clove yields about 6 to 10% of crude fibre. Up to 1% of foreign organic matter and up to 5% of stalks may also be present. It yields up to 1% of acid-insoluble ash and up to 7% of ash.

Description. UNGROUND DRUG. *Macroscopical characters:* from 10 to 17.5 mm long, reddish-brown, heavier than water; lower portion consisting of a slightly flattened 4-sided hypanthium containing in its upper part 2 loculi with numerous ovules on axile placentae; calyx with 4 thick, acute, divergent sepals surrounding a dome-shaped head consisting of 4 paler, unexpanded, membranous, imbricate petals enclosing numerous incurved stamens and a single stiff erect style; indentation of the hypanthium with the finger-nail causes oil to exude. It has a strong, aromatic, and spicy odour and a pungent taste.

Microscopical characters: the diagnostic characters are: *epidermis* of hypanthium and calyx teeth composed of straight-walled cells about 8 to 10 to 15 to 25 μm, with thick cuticle; *stomata* anomocytic, circular, 30 to 35 μm in diameter; *glands* ovoid, schizolysigenous, up to 200 μm long, found in all parts; phloem *fibres* occasional, isolated; spongy tissue of the hypanthium; *stamens* each with an oil gland in the apex of the connective; anther walls with a *fibrous layer; pollen grains* triangularly lenticular, 15 to 20 μm in diameter; cluster *crystals* of calcium oxalate, 6 to 20 μm in diameter; *starch* absent. A small number of *sclereids* and prismatic *crystals* of calcium oxalate from the stalk.

POWDERED DRUG: Powdered Clove. A brown powder possessing the diagnostic microscopical characters, odour, and taste of the unground drug.

Adulterants and substitutes. "Blown" cloves are the expanded flowers from which the petals and stamens have become detached. Clove "dust" often consists largely of broken stamens, petals, etc.

Clove stalks are up to about 35 mm in length with opposite and decussate branching, the ultimate branches being about 3 mm thick; they are brownish and woody and break with a short fracture; they contain about 5 to 7% of volatile oil, which is less aromatic and somewhat different from that of clove. Clove stalks are said to be used for adulterating powdered clove, in which their presence is easily detected by means of the isodiametric sclereids, by the higher proportion of ash, and by the prisms of calcium oxalate; they yield about 13.6 to 18.7% of crude fibre.

The nearly ripe fruits are also exported under the name "mother cloves" (anthophylli); they contain very little volatile oil and their presence may be detected in powdered clove by the large starch granules which the seeds contain.

Exhausted cloves, from which the oil has been removed by distillation, yield no oil when indented with the finger-nail; they are sometimes artificially coloured.

Storage. It should be stored in a cool dry place.

Powdered clove should be stored in airtight containers, in a cool place.

Actions and uses. Clove is a carminative and a flavouring agent. Infusions of clove have been used as vehicles for mixtures.

Preparation

Powdered clove is an ingredient of aromatic chalk powder.

Clove Oil

Obtained by distillation from clove. It is prepared in Great Britain and also imported from Zanzibar.

OTHER NAME: Oleum Caryophylli

A standard is given in the British Pharmacopoeia 1973

Constituents. The chief constituent of clove oil is eugenol (about 85 to 90% v/v). It also contains the sesquiterpene caryophyllene, furfural, which is probably the cause of the oil darkening on storage, methyl pentyl ketone, which gives the much valued fruity odour to the oil, vanillin, methyl salicylate, and up to about 10% of acetyleugenol.

Description. When freshly distilled it is a colourless or pale yellow liquid with a characteristic odour.

Solubility. Soluble, at 20°, in 2 parts of alcohol (70%); miscible with alcohol (90%) and with ether.

Weight per ml. At 20°, 1.041 to 1.054 g.

Refractive index. At 20°, 1.528 to 1.537.

Optical rotation. 0° to −1.5°.

Adulterants and substitutes. The oils, containing 90% or more of eugenol, distilled from clove stems are less fragrant and are used chiefly as a source of eugenol.

Stability. It darkens with age or on exposure to air, becoming reddish-brown in colour.

Storage. It should be stored in well-filled airtight containers, in a cool place, protected from light; contact with iron or zinc should be avoided.

Actions and uses. Taken by mouth in a dose of 0.05 to 0.2 millilitre, clove oil is carminative. Applied externally to skin and mucous membranes, it is irritant, rubefacient, and slightly analgesic.

Clove oil is used to flavour dentifrices, to which it imparts feebly antiseptic properties. It is used as a local analgesic for hypersensitive dentine, carious cavities, or exposed tooth pulps, but should be used with caution as repeated application may damage the gingival tissues. A mixture of clove oil with zinc oxide is used as a temporary analgesic filling for deep cavities, but eugenol is often preferred to clove oil for this purpose.

There is little evidence of the efficacy of clove oil as a preservative.

Cloxacillin Benzathine

NN' - Dibenzylethylenediammonium bis{(6*R*)-6-[3-(2-chlorophenyl)-5-methylisoxazole-4-carboxamido]penicillanate}

$C_{54}H_{56}Cl_2N_8O_{10}S_2 = 1112.1$

OTHER NAME: *Orbenin Dry Cow*®

A standard is given in the British Pharmacopoeia (Veterinary)

Description. A white odourless powder.

Solubility. Very slightly soluble in water; soluble, at 20°, in 110 parts of alcohol, in 18 parts of chloroform, in 80 parts of acetone, in 170 parts of isopropyl alcohol, and in 3 parts of methyl alcohol; practically insoluble in carbon tetrachloride and light petroleum.

Moisture content. Not more than 5%, determined by Fischer titration.

Storage. It should be protected as far as possible from moisture and stored at a temperature not exceeding 25°. If it is intended for parenteral administration or for intramammary injection, the containers should be sterile and sealed to exclude micro-organisms.

Identification. TESTS. 1. Shake about 100 mg with 1 ml of 1N sodium hydroxide for 2 minutes, add 2 ml of ether, shake for 1 minute, allow to separate, and evaporate 1 ml of the ethereal layer to dryness; dissolve the residue in 2 ml of glacial acetic acid and add 1 ml of *potassium dichromate solution*; a golden yellow precipitate is produced.

2. Mix about 2 mg with 2 mg of chromotropic acid sodium salt and 2 ml of sulphuric acid and immerse in a suitable liquid at 150°; after heating for 1 minute an olive-green colour is produced which changes to purple after heating for a further 2 minutes.

Veterinary uses. Cloxacillin benzathine is used in intramammary injections from which cloxacillin is gradually released. It is used in dry cows to reduce existing bacterial infection, the equivalent of 500 milligrams of cloxacillin being injected into each quarter as a single dose.

Preparation

CLOXACILLIN INTRAMAMMARY INJECTION (SLOW RELEASE) (*Syn.* Cloxacillin Benzathine Intramammary

Injection (Slow Release)): a sterile suspension of cloxacillin benzathine, with suitable suspending agents, in an oily basis. It contains no added colour. Available as an intramammary injection containing cloxacillin benzathine equivalent to 500 mg of cloxacillin in tubes or syringes, for use on 1 occasion only, containing 3 g of suspension.

A standard for this intramammary injection is given in the British Pharmacopoeia (Veterinary)

Containers: see the entry on Intramammary Injections for general information on containers.

Labelling: see the entry on Intramammary Injections for general information on labelling. In addition, the label on the container should state the amount of the medicament as the equivalent amount of cloxacillin.

Cloxacillin Sodium

Sodium (6*R*)-6-[3-(2-chlorophenyl)-5-methylisoxazole-4-carboxamido]penicillanate monohydrate

$C_{19}H_{17}ClN_3NaO_5S,H_2O = 475.9$

OTHER NAMES: Cloxacillinum Natricum; *Orbenin*® *Ampiclox*® (with ampicillin sodium)

A standard is given in the British Pharmacopoeia 1973

Description. A white, crystalline, odourless, hygroscopic powder with an intensely bitter taste.

Solubility. Soluble, at 20°, in 2.5 parts of water, in 30 parts of alcohol, and in 500 parts of chloroform.

Acidity. A 10% solution has a pH of 5 to 7.

Moisture content. Not more than 4.5%, determined by Fischer titration.

Specific rotation. +163° to +172°, determined on a 1% solution.

Dissociation constant. pK$_a$ 2.7 (25°).

Stability. In aqueous solution, cloxacillin sodium degrades by hydrolysis. Degradation is catalysed by hydrogen ions and by hydroxide ions. At 25°, solutions are most stable at pH 6.3; such solutions may be expected to lose 10% of their potency after 12 days. Degradation is considerably accelerated by lactate ions.

Unbuffered solutions containing 2.5 to 20% of cloxacillin sodium may be expected to lose about 5% of their potency when stored for 7 days at 5°. At 25°, losses of up to 15% may be expected after 4 days.

FURTHER INFORMATION. Stability in aqueous solution and in intravenous infusions—B. Lynn, *Chemist Drugg.*, 1967, **187**, 134 and 157, and *J. hosp. Pharm.*, 1970, **28**, 71, H. Bundgaard and K. Ilver, *Dansk Tidsskr. Farm.*, 1970, **44**, 365, and L. Landersjö *et al.*, *Acta pharm. suec.*, 1974, **11**, 563; stability and other aspects of cloxacillin—*Analytical Profiles of Drug Substances*, K. Florey (Ed.), Vol. 4., London, Academic Press, 1975, p. 113.

Labelling. If the material is not intended for parenteral administration, the label on the container states that the contents are not to be injected.

Storage. It should be stored in airtight containers at a temperature not exceeding 25°. If it is intended for parenteral administration the containers should be sterile and sealed to exclude micro-organisms.

Identification. TEST. Mix 2 mg with 2 mg of chromotropic acid sodium salt and 2 ml of sulphuric acid and immerse in a suitable liquid at 150° for 4 minutes; the colour of the solution changes through greenish-yellow to green and finally to purple (distinction from certain other penicillins).

MELTING-POINT. About 170°, with decomposition.

ULTRAVIOLET ABSORPTION. In 0.1N hydrochloric acid, maximum at 352 nm (E1%, 1cm = 67).

INFRA-RED ABSORPTION. Major peaks at 1336, 1495, 1598, 1620, 1659, and 1765 cm^{-1} (see Appendix 2a: Infra-red Spectra).

Metabolism. ABSORPTION. Cloxacillin is acid stable and variably absorbed after oral administration; after an oral dose of 2 g of the sodium salt, 30 to 50% is absorbed.

BLOOD CONCENTRATION. After an oral dose of 500 mg of the sodium salt, a peak plasma concentration of 5 to 12 μg/ml is attained within 30 to 60 minutes; effective concentrations are maintained for 4 to 6 hours after a single dose; after oral doses of 500 mg given to children every 6 hours for 2 days, serum concentrations of about 7 μg/ml are attained 2 hours after the last dose.

HALF-LIFE. Plasma half-life, 30 minutes to 1 hour, which is increased in renal function impairment.

DISTRIBUTION. Well distributed throughout the tissues and does not enter the cerebrospinal fluid; concentrations in synovial fluid reach about half that in the serum during multiple dosing; *protein binding*, 80 to 95% bound to plasma proteins.

EXCRETION. About 60% of a dose is excreted unchanged in the urine; small amounts are excreted in the bile; probenecid delays urinary excretion.

FURTHER INFORMATION. Effect of protein binding on levels of cloxacillin in synovial fluid—A. Howell *et al.*, *Clin. Pharmac. Ther.*, 1972, **13**, 724; pharmacokinetics —E. H. Nauta and H. Mattie, *Br. J. clin. Pharmac.*, 1975, **2**, 111; cloxacillin levels in synovial fluid—J. H. Newman, *Br. med. J.*, iii/1974, 472.

Actions and uses. Cloxacillin is a semisynthetic penicillin which is not decomposed by staphylococcal penicillinase but which has a considerably reduced antibiotic potency compared with benzylpenicillin. It is destroyed by other penicillinases produced by Gram-negative bacteria.

Cloxacillin is mainly of value in the treatment of penicillinase-producing staphylococcal infections. The usual adult dose is the equivalent of 250 milligrams of cloxacillin, dissolved in 1.5 millilitres of water for injections, by intramuscular injection every 4 to 6 hours or the equivalent of 500 milligrams of cloxacillin by mouth, taken before meals to ensure maximum absorption, every 6 hours. In serious infections this can be increased to the equivalent of 2 grams by injection every 4 hours.

The usual oral dose for children, given every 6 hours, is: under 1 year, the equivalent of 62.5 to 125 milligrams of cloxacillin and 1 to 5 years, the equivalent of 125 to 250 milligrams. The usual dose by intramuscular or slow intravenous injection given every 6 hours, is: under 1 year, the equivalent of 62.5 milligrams of cloxacillin, 1 to 5 years, the equivalent of 62.5 to 125 milligrams, and 6 to 12 years, the equivalent of 125 to 250 milligrams. The usual intrathecal dose for adults is the equivalent

of 10 milligrams of cloxacillin and for children the equivalent of 5 to 10 milligrams.

Undesirable effects. Allergic reactions as described under Benzylpenicillin may occur.

Precautions. The same precautions against allergic reactions should be taken as for benzylpenicillin. It should not be used topically or locally in the eye.

Veterinary uses. Cloxacillin sodium is used in intra-mammary injections for the treatment of mastitis in lactating cattle. The usual dose is the equivalent of 200 milligrams of cloxacillin in each infected quarter; 3 doses may be given, at intervals of 24 or 48 hours, according to the release-rate of the basis used.

Preparations

CLOXACILLIN CAPSULES: consisting of cloxacillin sodium, in powder, which may be mixed with a suitable inert diluent, enclosed in a hard capsule. The capsule shells may be coloured. Available as capsules containing cloxacillin sodium equivalent to 250 and 500 mg of cloxacillin.

A standard for these capsules is given in the British Pharmacopoeia 1973

Containers and *Storage:* see the entry on Capsules for general information on containers and storage.

Labelling: the label on the container should state the amount of the medicament as the equivalent amount of cloxacillin. In addition, the label should state the directions for storage and the date after which the capsules are not intended to be used.

Advice for patients: the capsules should be taken at regular intervals, preferably half to 1 hour before meals. The prescribed course should be completed.

CLOXACILLIN ELIXIR (*Syn.* Cloxacillin Syrup): a solution of cloxacillin sodium in a suitable coloured flavoured vehicle. It is prepared freshly by dissolving a powder consisting of the dry mixed ingredients in the specified volume of water for preparations. When a dose less than or not a multiple of 5 ml is prescribed, the elixir may be diluted, as described in the entry on Elixirs, with syrup.

Available as an elixir containing cloxacillin sodium equivalent to 125 mg of cloxacillin in 5 ml when reconstituted.

A standard for this elixir is given in the British Pharmaceutical Codex 1973

Containers and *Labelling:* see the entry on Elixirs for general information on containers and labelling. The name on the label of the container of the dry powder should be "Powder for Cloxacillin Elixir".

Storage: the elixir and the diluted elixir should be stored in a cool place and used within 1 week of preparation.

Advice for patients: the elixir should be taken at regular intervals, preferably half to 1 hour before meals. The prescribed course should be completed.

CLOXACILLIN INJECTION: a sterile solution of cloxacillin sodium in water for injections. It is prepared by dissolving the contents of a sealed container in water for injections shortly before use. Available as a powder in vials containing cloxacillin sodium equivalent to 250 and 500 mg of cloxacillin.

A standard for this injection is given in the British Pharmacopoeia 1973

Containers: see the entry on Injections for general information on containers.

Labelling: see the entry of Injections for general information on labelling. In addition, the label on the container should state the amount of the medicament as the equivalent amount of cloxacillin.

Storage: the sealed container should be stored at a temperature not exceeding 25°. The injection contains no bactericide and should be used as soon as possible after preparation but solutions of cloxacillin sodium may be expected to retain their potency for up to 4 days after preparation, provided they are stored at 2° to 10°.

CLOXACILLIN INTRAMAMMARY INJECTION: a sterile suspension of cloxacillin sodium in an oily basis which may contain suitable suspending and dispersing agents. It contains no added colours. It may be prepared as described in the entry on Intramammary Injections. Available as an injection containing cloxacillin sodium equivalent to 200 mg of cloxacillin (for cattle).
A standard for this intramammary injection is given in the British Pharmacopoeia (Veterinary)
Containers: see the entry on Intramammary Injections for general information on containers.
Labelling: see the entry on Intramammary Injections for general information on labelling. In addition, the label on the container should state the amount of the medicament as the equivalent amount of cloxacillin.

OTHER PREPARATIONS available include an INJECTION reconstituted from vials of powder containing cloxacillin sodium equivalent to 25 mg of cloxacillin with ampicillin sodium equivalent to 50 mg of ampicillin, an injection reconstituted from vials of powder containing cloxacillin sodium equivalent to 250 mg of cloxacillin with ampicillin sodium equivalent to 250 mg of ampicillin; and a MIXTURE containing cloxacillin sodium equivalent to 30 mg of cloxacillin with ampicillin trihydrate equivalent to 60 mg of ampicillin in 0.6 ml when reconstituted.

Coal Tar

see TAR, COAL

Cobalt Oxide

Tricobalt tetraoxide containing a small proportion of dicobalt trioxide.
$Co_3O_4 = 240.8$

OTHER NAME: *Permaco®*

A standard is given in the British Pharmacopoeia (Veterinary)

Description. A black odourless powder.

Solubility. Practically insoluble in water; soluble in mineral acids and in solutions of alkali hydroxides.

Moisture content. Not more than 1%, determined by igniting at 600°.

Veterinary uses. Cobalt oxide is used in the prevention of cobalt deficiency in ruminants. It is administered in depot-tablets ("bullets") from which cobalt is gradually released over a period of several weeks. One depot-tablet is administered to each animal, depot-tablets containing the equivalent of 12 grams of cobalt being suitable for cattle and those containing 4 grams being suitable for sheep.

Preparation

COBALT DEPOT-TABLETS (*Syn.* Cobalt Oxide Depot-tablets): containing approximately 57% of cobalt oxide, 40% of powdered iron, and 3% of sodium silicate. They are extremely hard tablets prepared from a suitable powder by moist granulation and compression, followed

by heating at about 570° for 15 minutes. Available as depot-tablets containing 4 and 12 g of cobalt.
A standard for these depot-tablets is given in the British Pharmacopoeia (Veterinary)
Labelling: the label on the container should state the amount of cobalt contained in each depot-tablet.

Cocaine

Methyl (1*R*,2*R*,3*S*,5*S*)-3-benzoyloxytropane-2-carboxylate *or* methyl benzoylecgonine, an alkaloid occurring in coca together with variable proportions of other alkaloids of closely related structure.

$C_{17}H_{21}NO_4 = 303.4$

A standard is given in the British Pharmacopoeia 1973

Coca consists of the dried leaves of *Erythroxylum coca* Lam. (Bolivian or Huanuco leaf) or of *E. truxillense* Rusby (Peruvian or Truxillo leaf) (Fam. Erythroxylaceae).
The mixed alkaloids of coca are extracted from the powdered leaves by mixing with lime and percolating with naphtha or other similar solvent. Cocaine is either obtained directly from the crude mixture of alkaloids by suitable methods of purification or the mixed alkaloids may be hydrolysed with acid to yield ecgonine, from which, after purification, cocaine may be synthesised.

Description. Odourless colourless crystals or white crystalline powder. It is slightly volatile.

Solubility. Very slightly soluble in water; soluble, at 20°, in 7 parts of alcohol, in 4 parts of ether, in less than 1 part of chloroform, in 30 parts of arachis oil, and in 120 parts of liquid paraffin; practically insoluble in glycerol.

Specific rotation. −79° to −81°, determined on a 2.4% solution in 0.1N hydrochloric acid.

Dissociation constant. pK_a 8.6 (20°).

Sterilisation. Sterile oily solutions are prepared by an aseptic technique.

Identification. TESTS. 1. Mix 100 mg with 1 ml of sulphuric acid, heat at 100° for 5 minutes, cool, and cautiously mix with 2 ml of water; the aromatic odour of methyl benzoate is perceptible and, when the solution is cooled and allowed to stand for several hours, crystals of benzoic acid separate.
2. Dissolve 50 mg in 1.65 ml of 0.1N hydrochloric acid, add 8.5 ml of *alum solution* and 5 ml of *potassium permanganate solution*, and stir briskly for several seconds; characteristic violet plates are produced.

MELTING-POINT. About 97°.

ULTRAVIOLET ABSORPTION. In 0.1N sulphuric acid, maxima at 233 nm (E1%, 1cm = 470) and 275 nm (E1%, 1cm = 38).

INFRA-RED ABSORPTION. Major peaks at 712, 1037, 1110, 1275, 1710, and 1738 cm⁻¹ (see Appendix 2c: Infra-red Spectra).

Determination in body fluids. COLORIMETRY. In plasma

or urine: the metabolites benzoylecgonine and ecgonine are stated not to interfere—L. A. Woods *et al.*, *J. Pharmac. exp. Ther.*, 1951, **101**, 188.

GAS CHROMATOGRAPHY. In plasma or urine: cocaine and metabolites—J. I. Javaid *et al.*, *J. Chromat.*, 1975, **110**, 141; in urine: the metabolite benzoylecgonine—S. Koontz *et al.*, *J. Chromat.*, 1973, **85**, 75; in blood or plasma— B. H. Dvorchik *et al.*, *J. Chromat.*, 1977, **135**, 141.

THIN-LAYER CHROMATOGRAPHY. In urine: identification of metabolites—M. L. Bastos *et al.*, *J. Chromat.*, 1974, **89**, 335.

RADIOIMMUNOASSAY. In urine: metabolites—B. Kaul *et al.*, *J. Pharmac. exp. Ther.*, 1976, **199**, 171.

EVALUATION OF SELECTED METHODS. In urine—J. E. Wallace *et al.*, *J. analyt. Toxicol.*, 1977, **1**, 20.

Metabolism. ABSORPTION. Slowly absorbed as it produces vasoconstriction.

METABOLIC REACTIONS. Hydrolysis to yield benzoyl-ecgonine and ecgonine.

EXCRETION. 1 to 9% of a daily intravenous dose of 120 mg of cocaine is excreted unchanged in the urine and 35 to 55% is excreted as benzoylecgonine; the excretion of unchanged drug is increased when the urine is acid; small amounts of ecgonine are also present in the urine; no unchanged drug is excreted in the faeces.

FURTHER INFORMATION. Excretion—F. Fish and W. D. C. Wilson, *J. Pharm. Pharmac.*, 1969, **21**, 1355; disposition and metabolism in dogs—A. L. Misra *et al.*, *Xenobiotica*, 1976, **6**, 531.

Actions and uses. Cocaine is the oldest local anaesthetic, but because of systemic toxic effects and the danger of causing dependence, its use is now almost entirely restricted to local administration in ophthalmic and ear, nose, and throat surgery.

In low concentrations cocaine affects the nerve fibres and endings concerned with touch and pain more readily than those serving the senses of temperature and pressure, and sensory paralysis may be produced while motor fibres are still active. It should never be applied in an unnecessarily high concentration, as, in addition to risks following absorption, it may produce lasting local damage.

When a suitable concentration of cocaine hydrochloride is applied to the mucous membrane, surface anaesthesia develops in 5 to 10 minutes and persists for 20 to 30 minutes or longer, depending on the concentration used and the vascularity of the tissue.

Cocaine differs from other local anaesthetics in that it behaves as a vasoconstrictor, so that adrenaline need not be added to the solution to intensify and prolong its actions.

When instilled into the eye, cocaine blanches the conjunctiva and dilates the pupil.

Cocaine is used chiefly as the hydrochloride, but the alkaloid is more convenient for the preparation of oily solutions, suppositories, and ointments. A 5 to 10% spray solution may be used for anaesthetising the nose and throat; concentrations up to 20% may be used for the larynx.

Cocaine may be applied to the urethra as a 0.5% solution before cystoscopy, but even this concentration may prove dangerous if there is any lesion in the urethra.

When taken by mouth, cocaine causes a sensation of exhilaration and well-being, due to stimulation of the cerebral cortex. There is also an increased power to work and overcome fatigue, but large doses cause rest-lessness, tremors, and hallucinations. The general action of cocaine is used in its administration with morphine or diamorphine for the relief of pain in patients suffering from advanced malignant disease.

Undesirable effects. Some people have a distinct cocaine idiosyncrasy and may become dangerously ill after quite small doses; the symptoms are headache, faintness, and collapse, and these may occur with alarming rapidity and terminate fatally. The toxic effects of cocaine are more persistent than is usual with other local anaesthetics, as cocaine is less readily broken down and excreted. Cocaine eye-drops may cause loosening of the corneal epithelium and corneal erosion if frequently administered.

Precautions. Cocaine solutions should never be administered by injection for local or regional anaesthesia; other local anaethetics are equally effective and much safer for such use. In particular, cocaine is much too dangerous for administration as a spinal anaesthetic.

Dependence. The repeated use of cocaine may lead to dependence of the cocaine type as described under Drug Dependence. Cocaine addicts inject it subcutaneously or use it in the form of a snuff. The addict suffers from extreme stimulation, loss of memory, and an intolerable craving for the drug; loss of weight is usually marked and there is mental deterioration.

Poisoning. In acute cocaine poisoning, convulsions should be treated with diazepam and respiratory depression may necessitate the use of artificial respiration.

Cocaine Hydrochloride

$(1R,2R,3S,5S)$ - 3 - Benzoyloxy - 2 - methoxycarbonyltro-panium chloride, the hydrochloride of the alkaloid cocaine.

$C_{17}H_{22}ClNO_4 = 339.8$

OTHER NAME: Cocaini Hydrochloridum

A standard is given in the European Pharmacopoeia Vol. II

Description. Odourless hygroscopic colourless crystals or white crystalline powder, with a bitter, sharp taste followed by anaesthesia of the tongue.

Solubility. Soluble, at 20°, in less than 1 part of water, in 4.5 parts of alcohol, in 18 parts of chloroform, and in 3 parts of glycerol; very slightly soluble in ether; practically insoluble in fixed oils.

Specific rotation. −70° to −73°, determined on a 2.5% solution.

Incompatibility. It is incompatible with borax, but a clear aqueous solution may be made by dissolving equal weights of borax and boric acid and adding the cocaine salt in solution. It is also incompatible with alkali hydroxides and carbonates, mercuric chloride, phenol, tannic acid, and soluble silver salts.

Sterilisation. Solutions are sterilised by heating with a bactericide or by filtration.

Storage. It should be stored in airtight containers.

Identification TESTS. It complies with Tests 1 and 2 described under Cocaine.

MELTING-POINT. About 197°, with decomposition.

Determination in body fluids. See under Cocaine.

Metabolism. See under Cocaine.

Actions and uses. Cocaine hydrochloride has the

actions described under Cocaine and is used for the administration of cocaine in aqueous solution. The usual dose in conjunction with an analgesic in terminal illness is 8 to 16 milligrams.

For ophthalmic use, cocaine hydrochloride is employed in solutions containing 1 to 4%, alone or with homatropine hydrobromide. The use of eye-drops containing concentrations of cocaine hydrochloride higher than 5% should be avoided, as it may cause desiccation of the cornea.

Pastilles and lozenges containing 1.5 to 10 milligrams are used to relieve throat irritation and hoarseness.

Solutions containing 2 to 20% of cocaine hydrochloride are applied locally to mucous surfaces prior to operation. These solutions are liable to develop fungoid growth and should therefore contain a preservative such as chlorbutol or chlorocresol.

Undesirable effects; Precautions; Dependence. These are as described under Cocaine.

Poisoning. The procedure as described under Cocaine should be adopted.

Preparations

COCAINE AND HOMATROPINE EYE-DROPS: consisting of a sterile solution containing 2% of cocaine hydrochloride and 2% of homatropine hydrobromide, with 0.01% of chlorhexidine acetate, in purified water. It is prepared by method B or C described in the entry on Eye-drops.

A standard for these eye-drops is given in the British Pharmaceutical Codex 1973

Containers: see the entry on Eye-drops for general information on containers. This solution is adversely affected by alkali.

Labelling: see the entry on Eye-drops for general information on labelling.

COCAINE EYE-DROPS: consisting of a sterile solution containing up to 5% of cocaine hydrochloride, the usual strength being 4%, in purified water. The solution also contains 0.002% of phenylmercuric acetate or nitrate or 0.01% of chlorhexidine acetate. It is prepared by method B or C described in the entry on Eye-drops.

A standard for these eye-drops is given in the British Pharmaceutical Codex 1973

Containers: see the entry on Eye-drops for general information on containers. The solution is adversely affected by alkali.

Labelling: see the entry on Eye-drops for general information on labelling.

DIAMORPHINE AND COCAINE ELIXIR:

Diamorphine hydrochloride .. .. 1 g
Cocaine hydrochloride .. .. 1 g
Alcohol (90%) .. .. 125 ml
Syrup.. .. .. 250 ml
Chloroform water .. .. to 1000 ml

It must be freshly prepared.

When *Diamorphine and Cocaine Elixir* is prescribed without qualification an elixir prepared in accordance with the formula above is supplied.

When *Morphine and Cocaine Elixir* is prescribed without qualification an elixir prepared in accordance with the formula above but containing 1 g of morphine hydrochloride instead of 1 g of diamorphine hydrochloride is supplied. It should be recently prepared.

When *Morphine, Cocaine, and Chlorpromazine Elixir* or *Diamorphine, Cocaine, and Chlorpromazine Elixir* is prescribed, the syrup in the above formula is replaced by chlorpromazine elixir. These preparations should be protected from light.

When specified by the prescriber, the proportion of diamorphine hydrochloride or morphine hydrochloride in the above formulae may be altered.

Dose: the elixir contains in 10 millilitres, 10 milligrams of cocaine hydrochloride and, unless otherwise specified, 10 milligrams of diamorphine hydrochloride or of morphine hydrochloride. The dose-volume (and the proportion of diamorphine hydrochloride or morphine hydrochloride) is determined by the physician in accordance with the needs of the patient.

Cochineal

The dried female insect, *Dactylopius coccus* Costa (Fam. Coccidae), containing eggs and larvae.

OTHER NAMES: Coccus; Coccus Cacti

A standard is given in the British Pharmacopoeia 1973

The insects are indigenous to central America and Mexico, but the drug is now chiefly obtained from Peru and also from the Canary Islands, where the insects are reared upon the branches of various species of *Nopalea* (Fam. Cactaceae). After fecundation the insects increase in size and develop an abundance of red colouring matter. They are then brushed off the plant, killed by the fumes of burning sulphur or charcoal, or by heat, and dried in the sun.

Varieties. "Black-brilliant" cochineal is uniformly purplish-black and consists of insects of which the waxy secretion has been melted by the heat applied during preparation for the market. "Silver-grey" cochineal is greyish-white and retains some or all of the waxy covering in its original condition.

Constituents. Cochineal contains about 10% of the anthraquinone compound 6-D-glucopyranosyl-9,10-dihydro-2,5,7,8-tetrahydroxy-4-methyl-9,10-dioxoanthracene-1-carboxylic acid (carminic acid), which occurs as small red prismatic crystals, soluble in water, in alcohol, and in alkaline solutions.

About 10% of fat and 2% of wax are also present, as well as albuminoids and inorganic matter. The fat consists almost entirely of free oleic, linoleic, and myristic acids. Up to 2% of foreign organic matter may also be present. It yields up to 7% of ash.

Description. *Macroscopical characters:* purplish-black or purplish-grey in colour, about 3.5 to 5.5 mm long and 3 to 4.5 mm broad, oval in outline; dorsal surface convex, transversely wrinkled, and showing about 11 segments; ventral surface flat or slightly concave, whole insects carrying upon anterior part two 7-jointed straight antennae, about 0.3 mm long, 3 pairs of short legs, each about 1 mm long, terminating in a single claw, and a mouth from which projects the remains of a filiform proboscis; drug readily reduced to red or puce-coloured powder.

It has a characteristic odour and taste.

Microscopical characters: the diagnostic characters are: numerous short tubular *wax glands* scattered over the dermis, either singly or in groups; the insect has 2 *eyes*, each composed of a single lens; numerous *larvae*, usually about 150, present in each insect; each larva about 0.75 mm long with *proboscides* appearing as 2 circular coils, one in each side of head; *muscle fibre* abundant.

Adulterants and substitutes. Cochineal has been artificially weighted with inorganic matter. In the case of the "silver-grey" variety, barium or lead carbonate or sulphate has been used, while the "black-brilliant" variety has been "faced" with graphite, ivory black, or manganese dioxide, and has been mixed with very dark grains of magnetic sand containing iron.

Storage. It should be stored in a dry place.

Uses. Cochineal in the form of a tincture or solution is used as a colouring agent but its colouring properties are modified in acid solution.

Cocillana

The dried bark from *Guarea rusbyi* (Britton) Rusby and closely related species (Fam. Meliaceae). It is obtained from Bolivia and Haiti.

OTHER NAMES: Grape Bark; Guapi Bark

A standard is given in the British Pharmaceutical Codex 1973

Constituents. Cocillana contains about 2.3% of resins, about 2.5% of fixed oil, and tannin; traces of an alkaloid and possibly a glycoside are also present. The bark yields about 7.5% of ash.

Description. UNGROUND DRUG. *Macroscopical characters:* large flattish or curved pieces up to about 600 mm long and 150 mm wide and from 5 to 20 mm in thickness; outer surface showing shallow or deep longitudinal fissures according to age; colour grey-brown or orange-brown where cork has been removed, and often bearing whitish patches of lichens; inner surface longitudinally striated with straight or slightly wavy striae and easily detachable fibre strands; fracture short and granular in outer part, coarsely splintery, fibrous, and soft in the much thicker inner part; transversely cut surface showing a narrow outer corky region and wide inner region with dark-coloured, narrow, wavy medullary rays.
It has a slight characteristic odour and a slightly astringent, slightly nauseous taste.

Microscopical characters: the diagnostic characters are: *cork* cells in layers alternating with parenchyma containing yellowish *screleids*, angular or irregular in shape and up to 150 μm long; *fibres* straight, in numerous tangentially elongated groups alternating with tangential bands of dark-coloured *parenchyma* and *sieve tubes*, each fibre group surrounded by a *crystal sheath* with prisms of calcium oxalate from 10 to 25 μm long; *medullary rays* 1 to 3 cells wide; cells of medullary rays and parenchyma with red-brown contents and single sphaeroidal 2- to 4-compound *starch* granules, individual granules 5 to 20 μm in diameter.

POWDERED DRUG: Powdered Cocillana. A greyish-brown powder possessing the diagnostic microscopical characters, odour, and taste of the unground drug.

Adulterants and substitutes. The barks of *G. bangii* Rusby and of species of *Nectandra* (Fam. Lauraceae) have been reported as adulterants.
The bark of *G. bangii* is roughly striate and peels in long thin fibrous strips; it has a more reddish cork; its fracture is tougher and more fibrous, the fibres projecting throughout the inner bark; the screleids are smaller and the crystals less numerous; the powdered bark is light chocolate-brown.
Bark of *Nectandra* species contains oil cells and has a camphoraceous odour.

Actions and uses. Cocillana is an expectorant and, in large doses, an emetic. It has been used as an alternative to ipecacuanha in the treatment of coughs.
It is administered, usually in conjunction with other expectorants, as a 1 in 1 liquid extract prepared with alcohol (60%) by a reserved percolation process; the usual dose of the liquid extract is 0.5 to 1 millilitre, equivalent to 0.5 to 1 gram of cocillana.
The dose for children is one-quarter to three-quarters of the dose for adults.

Coconut Oil

The oil obtained by expression from the dried solid part of the endosperm of *Cocos nucifera* L. (Fam. Palmae), a tree cultivated throughout the tropics.

A standard is given in the British Pharmaceutical Codex 1973

Constituents. Coconut oil contains triglycerides, the fatty acid constituents of which are mainly lauric and myristic acids with smaller proportions of capric, caproic, caprylic, oleic, palmitic, and stearic acids.

Description. It is a white or pearl-white unctuous mass. It is either odourless or has an odour characteristic of coconut. It has a melting-point of about 24°.

Solubility. Soluble, at 60°, in 2 parts of alcohol, less soluble at lower temperatures; soluble in ether and in chloroform.

Refractive index. At 40°, 1.448 to 1.450.

Stability. On exposure to the air, the oil readily becomes rancid, acquiring an unpleasant odour and a strong acid taste.

Storage. It should be stored in well-filled airtight containers, in a cool place, protected from light.

Uses. Coconut oil is used as an ointment basis, particularly in preparations intended for application to the scalp. It is also used to prepare soaps with a high solubility in water.
Coconut oil is used as a source of medium chain-length triglycerides in dietary preparations for patients with fat malabsorption syndromes. The medium chain-length triglycerides are more readily absorbed from the gastro-intestinal tract than long-chain triglycerides and are not dependent on biliary and pancreatic secretions for their absorption.

Preparation

Coconut oil is an ingredient of coal tar and salicylic acid ointment.

Coconut Oil, Fractionated

Coconut oil that has been refined by hydrolysis, followed by fractionation of the liberated fatty acids and re-esterification.

OTHER NAMES: *Alembicol D*®; *MCT Oil*®; *Miglyols*®; Thin Vegetable Oil

A standard is given in the British Pharmacopoeia 1973

Constituents. It consists of a mixture of triglycerides containing only short- and medium-chain saturated fatty acids, mainly octanoic (caprylic) and decanoic (capric) acids.

Description. It is a clear, pale yellow, odourless or almost odourless liquid. It solidifies at about 0° and has a low viscosity even at temperatures near its solidification point.

Solubility. Almost insoluble in water; miscible with alcohol, with ether and with chloroform.

Weight per ml. At 20°, 0.940 to 0.950 g.

Refractive index. 1.450 to 1.453.

Storage. It should be stored in well-filled containers, in a cool place, protected from light.

Uses. Fractionated coconut oil is used as a non-aqueous vehicle for oral preparations, for example, calciferol solution.

Because of its oily nature, the addition of suitable colouring presents difficulties. Permitted oil-soluble colours may be used and the lakes of suitable water-soluble food dyes may be dispersed in the oil; sweetening agents such as saccharin may be added in a similar manner.

Codeine Phosphate

3-O-Methylmorphine phosphate hemihydrate
A sesquihydrate also exists (mol. wt. = 424.4).

$$C_{18}H_{24}NO_7P, \tfrac{1}{2}H_2O = 406.4$$

OTHER NAMES: Codeinii Phosphas
Codis® (with aspirin); Kaodene® (with light kaolin);
Neurodyne®, Panadeine Co®, Paracodol®, Parake® (all with paracetamol); Veganin® (with aspirin and paracetamol)

A standard is given in the European Pharmacopoeia Vol. I

Description. Odourless small colourless crystals or white crystalline powder, with a bitter taste.

Acidity. A 4% solution has a pH of 4.2 to 5.

Moisture content. Not more than 3%, determined by drying at 105°. The sesquihydrate contains 5 to 7% of moisture.

Specific rotation. −98° to −102°, determined on a 2% solution.

Dissociation constant. pK_a 8.2 (20°).

Sterilisation. Solutions for injection are sterilised by heating in an autoclave or by filtration.

Storage. It should be stored in airtight containers, protected from light.

Identification. TESTS. 1. Dissolve a few mg in water and add 1 ml of *potassium iodobismuthate solution*; an orange or orange-red precipitate is produced.
2. Mix about 10 mg with 1 ml of sulphuric acid and 1 drop of *ferric chloride solution*; a blue colour is produced which turns red on the addition of 1 drop of nitric acid (also given by morphine and ethylmorphine).
3. Place a few mg on the surface of a drop of nitric acid; a yellow but no red colour is produced (distinction from morphine).
4. Mix about 1 mg, in a white dish, with 1 drop of sulphuric acid containing 5 mg/ml of selenious acid; a green colour is immediately produced which rapidly

changes to blue, then slowly to dark olive-green (morphine gives an immediate blue colour changing to green).

ULTRAVIOLET ABSORPTION. In 0.1N sulphuric acid, maximum at 285 nm (E1%, 1cm = 42).

THIN-LAYER CHROMATOGRAPHY. See under Thin-layer Chromatography, System 7.

Determination in body fluids. GAS CHROMATOGRAPHY. In serum—W. J. Serfontein et al., J. Pharm. Pharmac., 1975, **27**, 937; in plasma—R. A. Zweidinger et al., J. pharm. Sci., 1976, **65**, 427.

Metabolism. ABSORPTION. Well absorbed after oral administration and after injection.

BLOOD CONCENTRATION. After an oral dose of 15 mg, peak plasma concentrations of 30 ng/ml are attained within 2 hours.

DISTRIBUTION. Widely distributed throughout the body and crosses the placenta.

METABOLIC REACTIONS. Metabolised in the liver by O-demethylation to form morphine, N-demethylation to form norcodeine, and conjugation to form glucuronides and sulphates of both unchanged drug and its metabolites.

EXCRETION. After an oral dose, about 86% is excreted in the urine in 24 hours; of the excreted material, 40 to 70% is free or conjugated codeine, 5 to 15% is free or conjugated morphine, 10 to 20% is free or conjugated norcodeine, and trace amounts may be free or conjugated normorphine; some of the dose is excreted in the bile and trace amounts are found in the faeces; unchanged drug accounts for 6 to 8% of the dose in urine in 24 hours which may be increased to about 10% when the urinary pH is decreased; after an intramuscular dose, 15 to 20% is excreted unchanged in acid urine in 24 hours.

FURTHER INFORMATION. Excretion in urine—W. O. R. Ebbighausen et al., J. pharm. Sci., 1973, **62**, 146, D. P. Vaughan and A. H. Beckett, J. Pharm. Pharmac., 1973, **25**, 104P, and H. W. Elliott et al., Clin. Pharmac. Ther., 1967, **8**, 78; protein binding—J. Judis, J. pharm. Sci., 1977, **66**, 802; in serum and urine—E. Schmerzler et al., J. pharm Sci., 1966, **55**, 155; metabolism of codeine—M. D. Solomon, Clin. Toxicol., 1974, **7**, 255; the fate of morphine and its surrogates—E. L. Way and T. K. Adler, Pharmac. Rev., 1960, **12**, 383.

Actions and uses. Codeine has moderate analgesic and weak cough-suppressant effects. It is also used to check diarrhoea. It is less depressant to the respiratory centre and causes much less nausea and vomiting than morphine. The usual dose is 10 to 60 milligrams.

Undesirable effects. Constipation commonly occurs.

Poisoning. The procedure described under Morphine Hydrochloride should be adopted.

Preparations

ASPIRIN AND CODEINE TABLETS (*Syn.* Acetylsalicylic Acid and Codeine Tablets): for each tablet take:

Aspirin	..	..	..	..	..	400 mg
Codeine phosphate		..	..	..	..	8 mg

A standard for these tablets is given in the British Pharmacopoeia Addendum 1975
Containers and *Storage*: see the entry on Tablets for general information on containers and storage. Containers should be airtight and light resistant.
Dose: 1 or 2 tablets.
Advice for patients: the tablets should preferably be

taken after meals. Treatment should not be continued for longer than 2 days without medical advice.

ASPIRIN, PARACETAMOL, AND CODEINE TABLETS: for each tablet take:

Aspirin	250 mg
Paracetamol..	250 mg
Codeine phosphate	9.58 mg

Containers and *Storage:* see the entry on Tablets for general information on containers and storage. Containers should be airtight and light resistant.
Dose: ADULT: 1 or 2 tablets up to 4 times daily as necessary.
CHILD: 6 to 12 years, half a tablet up to 4 times daily as necessary.
Advice for patients: the tablets should preferably be taken after meals. Treatment should not be continued for longer than 2 days without medical advice.

ASPIRIN, PHENACETIN, AND CODEINE TABLETS (*Syn.* Compound Codeine Tablets): for each tablet take:

Aspirin	250 mg
Phenacetin	250 mg
Codeine phosphate	8 mg

A standard for these tablets is given in the British Pharmacopoeia 1973
Containers and *Storage:* see the entry on Tablets for general information on containers and storage. Containers should be airtight and light resistant.
Dose: 1 or 2 tablets up to 4 times daily as necessary.
Advice for patients: the tablets should preferably be taken after meals. Use for prolonged periods should be avoided.

CODEINE AND PARACETAMOL TABLETS: for each tablet take:

Codeine phosphate	8 mg
Paracetamol..	500 mg

Containers and *Storage:* see the entry on Tablets for general information on containers and storage. Containers should be airtight and light resistant.
Dose: 2 tablets up to 4 times daily as necessary.
Advice for patients: the tablets should not be used for longer than 2 days without medical advice.

CODEINE LINCTUS:

Codeine phosphate	3 g
Compound tartrazine solution	10 ml
Benzoic acid solution	20 ml
Chloroform spirit	20 ml
Water for preparations	20 ml
Lemon syrup	200 ml
Syrup..	to 1000 ml

Dissolve the codeine phosphate in the water, add 500 ml of the syrup, and mix; add the compound tartrazine solution, the benzoic acid solution, the chloroform spirit, the lemon syrup, and sufficient of the syrup to produce the required volume, and mix.
When a dose less than or not a multiple of 5 ml is prescribed, the linctus may be diluted, as described in the entry on Linctuses, with syrup.
Codeine linctus contains, in 5 ml, 15 mg of codeine phosphate.
A standard for this linctus is given in the British Pharmaceutical Codex 1973
Containers: see the entry on Linctuses for general information on containers.
Storage: it should be protected from light.
Dose: 5 millilitres.

Advice for patients: the linctus should be sipped and swallowed slowly. It should not be used for the suppression of productive cough. Treatment should not be continued for longer than a few days without medical advice.

CODEINE PHOSPHATE SYRUP (*Syn.* Codeine Syrup):

Codeine phosphate	5 g
Water for preparations	15 ml
Chloroform spirit	25 ml
Syrup..	to 1000 ml

Dissolve the codeine phosphate in the water, add 750 ml of the syrup, and mix; add the chloroform spirit and sufficient of the syrup to produce the required volume, and mix.
Codeine phosphate syrup contains, in 10 ml, 50 mg of codeine phosphate.
A standard for this syrup is given in the British Pharmaceutical Codex 1973
Storage: it should be protected from light.
Dose: 2.5 to 10 millilitres.
Advice for patients: it should not be used for the suppression of productive cough. Treatment should not be continued for longer than a few days without medical advice.

CODEINE PHOSPHATE TABLETS: available as tablets containing 15, 30, and 60 mg of codeine phosphate.
A standard for these tablets is given in the British Pharmacopoeia 1973
Containers and *Storage:* see the entry on Tablets for general information on containers and storage. Containers should be airtight and light resistant.
Advice for patients: the tablets may cause drowsiness; persons affected should not drive or operate machinery. Alcohol should be avoided.

DIABETIC CODEINE LINCTUS:

Codeine phosphate	3 g
Citric acid monohydrate	5 g
Lemon spirit	1 ml
Compound tartrazine solution	10 ml
Benzoic acid solution	20 ml
Chloroform spirit	20 ml
Water for preparations	20 ml
Sorbitol solution, non-crystallising grade	to 1000 ml

Dissolve the codeine phosphate and the citric acid in the water, add 750 ml of the sorbitol solution, and mix; add the lemon spirit, the compound tartrazine solution, the benzoic acid solution, the chloroform spirit, and sufficient of the sorbitol solution to produce the required volume, and mix. It has a weight per ml at 20° of about 1.27 g.
When a dose less than or not a multiple of 5 ml is prescribed, the linctus may be diluted, as described in the entry on Linctuses, with chloroform water.
Diabetic codeine linctus contains, in 5 ml, 15 mg of codeine phosphate. Each 5 ml contains about 4.2 g of carbohydrate and provides about 16 kilocalories (67 kilojoules).
A standard for this linctus is given in the British Pharmaceutical Codex 1973
Containers: see the entry on Linctuses for general information on containers.
Storage: it should be protected from light.
Dose: 5 millilitres.
Advice for patients: the linctus should be sipped and swallowed slowly. It should not be used for the suppression of productive cough. Treatment should not be

continued for longer than a few days or given to children under 1 year without medical advice.

PAEDIATRIC CODEINE LINCTUS (*Syn.* Codeine Mixture, Paediatric):

Codeine linctus	200 ml
Syrup..	to 1000 ml

When a dose less than or not a multiple of 5 ml is prescribed, the linctus may be diluted, as described in the entry on Linctuses, with syrup.

Paediatric codeine linctus contains, in 5 ml, 3 mg of codeine phosphate.

A standard for this linctus is given in the British Pharmaceutical Codex 1973

Containers: see the entry on Linctuses for general information on containers.

Storage: it should be protected from light.

Dose: CHILD: Up to 1 year, 5 millilitres; 1 to 5 years, 10 millilitres.

Advice for patients: the linctus should be sipped and swallowed slowly. It should not be used for the suppression of productive cough. Treatment should not be continued for longer than a few days or given to children under 1 year without medical advice.

SOLUBLE ASPIRIN AND CODEINE TABLETS (*Syn.* Soluble Acetylsalicylic Acid and Codeine Tablets): for each tablet take:

Aspirin, in fine powder	400 mg
Codeine phosphate	8 mg
Saccharin sodium	4 mg
Citric acid (anhydrous)	40 mg
Calcium carbonate	130 mg

A standard for these tablets is given in the British Pharmacopoeia Addendum 1975

Containers and *Storage:* see the entry on Tablets for general information on containers and storage. Containers should be airtight and light resistant.

Dose: 1 or 2 tablets.

Advice for patients: the tablets should be taken dissolved in water, preferably after meals. Treatment should not be continued for longer than 2 days without medical advice.

SOLUBLE ASPIRIN, PHENACETIN, AND CODEINE TABLETS (*Syn.* Soluble Compound Codeine Tablets): for each tablet take:

Aspirin, in fine powder	250 mg
Phenacetin	250 mg
Codeine phosphate	8 mg
Saccharin sodium	5 mg
Citric acid (anhydrous)	26 mg
Calcium carbonate	80 mg

A standard for these tablets is given in the British Pharmacopoeia 1973

Containers and *Storage:* see the entry on Tablets for general information on containers and storage. Containers should be airtight and light resistant.

Dose: 1 or 2 tablets up to 4 times daily as necessary.

Advice for patients: the tablets should be taken dissolved in water, preferably after meals. Use for prolonged periods should be avoided.

Cod-liver Oil

The fixed oil obtained from the fresh liver of the cod, *Gadus morrhua* (= *G. callarius* L.) (Fam. Gadidae), and other species of *Gadus*, by the application of low-pressure steam at a temperature not exceeding 85°. The oil is cooled to about 0° and filtered to remove the separated fat.

OTHER NAMES: Oleum Jecoris Aselli; Oleum Morrhuae

A standard is given in the British Pharmacopoeia 1973

Constituents. The vitamin-A activity varies very widely in different samples, but an average sample contains about 1000 units per g. The vitamin-D content varies from about 50 to 250 units of antirachitic activity (vitamin D) per g, the average being about 100 units.

The fatty acid constituents of the glycerides of cod-liver oil are largely unsaturated and consist chiefly of docosahexenoic acid and a highly unsaturated acid containing 18 to 22 carbon atoms; glycerides of oleic acid are probably absent, but those of palmitic and stearic acids occur in small quantities.

The unsaponifiable matter consists chiefly of cholesterol with small amounts of batyl alcohol, squalene, and the vitamins A and D.

Cod-liver oil may contain a trace of iodine.

Description. It is a pale yellow liquid with a slightly fishy but not rancid odour. It may contain up to 100 parts per million of dodecyl gallate, or propyl gallate, or any mixture of these substances, as an antoxidant.

When maintained at 0° for 3 hours, it remains bright (limit of stearin).

Solubility. Very slightly soluble in alcohol; miscible with ether, with chloroform, and with light petroleum.

Weight per ml. At 20°, 0.917 to 0.924 g.

Refractive index. 1.478 to 1.482.

Adulterants and substitutes. Other liver oils such as those of the seal (*Phoca* species), haddock (*Melanogrammus aeglefinus*), shark (*Carcharias* species), and coal fish (*Pollachius carbonarius*).

Stability. If properly stored, cod-liver oil retains its potency and characters for many years. Inferior or old oils are liable to be dark in colour, acrid or bitter, unduly acid, and somewhat rancid.

On exposing the oil to sunlight the vitamin A is rapidly destroyed; on exposure to air the oil absorbs oxygen and becomes thicker, but does not dry to a hard varnish.

Storage. It should be stored in well-filled airtight containers, in a cool place, protected from light.

Actions and uses. Cod-liver oil is a valuable source of vitamins A and D and of readily digestible fat. Because of its vitamin-D content, cod-liver oil promotes absorption of calcium and phosphorus from the gut and prevents rickets. Cod-liver oil also contains several unsaturated fatty acids which are essential food factors. These are absent from vitamin A and D concentrates, which are often given in place of cod-liver oil.

The antirachitic activity of cod-liver oil is believed to be due to vitamin D_3 (cholecalciferol), which occurs in various fish-liver oils and may be obtained by the ultra-violet irradiation of 7-dehydrocholesterol; there is some evidence that vitamin D_2 (calciferol) differs from vitamin D_3 in antirachitic activity in man.

Cod-liver oil is used as a dietary supplement for infants and children to prevent the occurrence of rickets and to improve nutrition and calcification of bones in undernourished children and in patients with rickets. It is administered alone, in capsules, and in malt extract with cod-liver oil.

The usual dose for prophylaxis of rickets is not more than 10 millilitres daily, but the continuous daily intake of vitamin D should not exceed 400 units, including vitamin D obtained from other sources.

Cod-liver oil has been advocated for use externally as an application to promote healing in burns, ulcers, and wounds, but there is no evidence to suggest that it is superior to other more acceptable oily preparations.

Veterinary uses. Cod-liver oil is used in animal nutrition as a source of vitamins A and D. The usual dose for horses, cattle, pigs, and sheep is 0.1 millilitre per kilogram body-weight and for dogs and cats 0.2 millilitre per kilogram body-weight.

Preparation

MALT EXTRACT WITH COD-LIVER OIL (*Syn.* Extractum Malti cum Oleo Morrhuae):

Malt Extract	..	..	..	..	900 g
Cod-liver oil	..	..	..	..	100 g

Mix thoroughly with the aid of gentle heat. The extract may be flavoured.

Malt extract with cod-liver oil contains in 30 ml about 4.5 ml of cod-liver oil.

A standard for this extract is given in the British Pharmaceutical Codex 1973

Storage: it should be stored in well-filled airtight containers, in a cool place, protected from light.

Dose: 10 to 30 millilitres daily.

Advice for patients: it should not be taken for prolonged periods without medical advice.

Coeliac Disease

Coeliac disease (Idiopathic steatorrhoea; Gluten enteropathy) is a chronic disorder of the small intestine in which there is an unusual sensitivity to gluten. It is characterised by abnormalities of the jejunal mucosa, malabsorption, and fatty diarrhoea (steatorrhoea). There may also be secondary lactose intolerance. The malabsorption leads to weight loss and deficiency of minerals and vitamins.

Coeliac disease may occur in children or adults and is sometimes familial. In most cases avoidance of foods containing gluten, such as those prepared from wheat, rye, barley, and oats, results in normal intestinal function, but the disease returns if gluten is again ingested. Certain medicines, such as tablets prepared with wheat starch, contain gluten and may affect patients with coeliac disease.

Colchicine

N-[(7*S*)-5,6,7,9-Tetrahydro-1,2,3,10-tetramethoxy-9-oxobenz[*a*]heptalen-7-yl]acetamide, an alkaloid obtained from colchicum corm and seeds.

$C_{22}H_{25}NO_6 = 399.4$

OTHER NAME: *Colbenemid*® (with probenecid)

A standard is given in the British Pharmacopoeia 1973

Description. Pale yellow odourless crystals, amorphous scales, or powder. It has a hay-like odour when damped and warmed, and darkens on exposure to light.

Solubility. Soluble in water, in alcohol, and in chloroform; soluble, at 15.5°, in 160 parts of ether; practically insoluble in light petroleum.

Moderately concentrated aqueous solutions may deposit crystals of a sesquihydrate which is practically insoluble in cold water.

Moisture content. Not more than 2%, determined by drying over phosphorus pentoxide *in vacuo*.

Specific rotation. −425° to −450°, determined on a 1% solution.

Dissociation constant. pK_a 1.7 (20°).

Stability. It darkens on exposure to light. In acidic solution, colchicine is slowly hydrolysed to colchiceine but unbuffered solutions are stable at 20° for at least 6 months. On exposure to ultraviolet radiation, isomers known as "lumicolchicines" are formed; these products may be deposited as crystals.

FURTHER INFORMATION. Stability of colchicine injection —G. Smith *et al.*, *J. Pharm. Pharmac.*, 1963, **15**, 92T.

Sterilisation. Solutions for injection are sterilised by heating in an autoclave or by filtration.

Storage. It should be stored in airtight containers, protected from light.

Identification. TESTS. 1. Dissolve about 50 mg in 1.5 ml of water; a yellow solution is produced, the colour of which is intensified by the addition of a mineral acid.
2. Mix 1 mg with a few drops of sulphuric acid in a white dish; a lemon yellow colour is produced. Add one drop of nitric acid; the colour changes to greenish-blue and then rapidly becomes reddish and finally yellow or almost colourless. Add excess of *sodium hydroxide solution*; a red colour is produced.
3. Mix 30 mg with 1 ml of alcohol (95%) and add 1 drop of *ferric chloride test-solution*; an immediate red colour is produced.

MELTING-POINT. About 154°.

ULTRAVIOLET ABSORPTION. In alcohol (95%), maxima at 243 nm (E1%, 1cm = 730) and 350 nm (E1%, 1cm = 420).

INFRA-RED ABSORPTION. Major peaks at 1090, 1250, 1485, 1550, 1578, and 1610 cm^{-1} (see Appendix 2a: Infra-red Spectra).

Metabolism. ABSORPTION. Readily absorbed after oral administration.

BLOOD CONCENTRATION. After an intravenous infusion of 2 mg, plasma concentrations of 4 to 33 ng/ml are attained in about 15 minutes.

HALF-LIFE. Biological half-life, about 10 to 30 minutes, which is increased in renal function impairment and decreased in hepatic function impairment.

DISTRIBUTION. Colchicine does not appear to be specifically localised in any tissues except the liver and kidneys; it may undergo enterohepatic circulation.

METABOLIC REACTIONS. Demethylation to desmethylcolchicine.

EXCRETION. 5 to 50% of a dose is excreted in the urine in 48 hours; unchanged drug appears to be excreted in both urine and faeces; colchicine may be excreted in the bile and secreted from the blood into the gastro-intestinal tract.

FURTHER INFORMATION. Biliary excretion—A. L. Hunter and C. D. Klaassen, *J. Pharmac. exp. Ther.*, 1975,

192, 605; excretion—E. J. Walaszek *et al.*, *Archs int. Pharmacodyn. Thér.*, 1960, **125**, 371; plasma concentrations—S. L. Wallace *et al.*, *Am. J. Med.*, 1970, **48**, 443.

Actions and uses. Colchicine is used for the relief of pain in acute gout.

For the treatment of acute episodes, it is administered by mouth in a dosage of 1 milligram initially, followed by 500 micrograms every 2 hours until relief is obtained or gastro-intestinal symptoms such as vomiting and diarrhoea make its further use undesirable; the total amount given during a course of treatment should not exceed 10 milligrams. The course should not be repeated within 3 days.

For the prevention of acute episodes, colchicine may be given for long periods in smaller doses, such as 500 micrograms twice daily.

Colchicine has also been given by intravenous injection of 2 to 4 milligrams in sodium chloride injection but this is never justified.

Undesirable effects. In large doses, after a latent period of 1 to 3 hours, colchicine has a marked action on involuntary muscle, especially that of the intestine, and causes severe diarrhoea. Liver damage may occur.

Precautions. As colchicine has antimitotic activity, it should be used with caution in pregnancy and lactation.

Preparations

COLCHICINE TABLETS: available as tablets containing 250 and 500 micrograms of colchicine.

A standard for these tablets is given in the British Pharmacopoeia 1973

Containers and *Storage:* see the entry on Tablets for general information on containers and storage. Containers should be airtight and light resistant.

Advice for patients: when used for the relief of pain in acute gout, not more than 10 milligrams of colchicine should be taken in each course of treatment. The course should not be repeated within 3 days.

OTHER PREPARATIONS available include TABLETS containing colchicine 500 micrograms with probenecid 500 mg.

Colchicum Corm

The corm of the meadow saffron, *Colchicum autumnale* L. (Fam. Liliaceae), a plant widely distributed over central and southern Europe and common in parts of England.

A standard is given in the British Pharmacopoeia 1973

Colchicum corm is collected in early summer after the leaves have died down, and is prepared by removing the scale leaves, slicing transversely, and drying at a temperature not higher than 65°.

Constituents. Colchicum corm contains about 0.08 to 0.15% of the alkaloid colchicine, together with closely related alkaloids; it also contains starch, gum, sugar, tannin, colouring matter, and fat. It may also contain up to 2% of foreign organic matter. It yields about 4% of ash and up to 0.5% of acid-insoluble ash.

Description. UNGROUND DRUG. *Macroscopical characters:* slices, about 2 to 5 mm thick, subreniform or ovate in outline, a few subconical or plano-convex, edges yellowish-brown; fracture short, mealy; transversely cut surfaces white and starchy with numerous scattered vascular bundles showing as small greyish points; cut surface immediately coloured yellow by hydrochloric acid or sulphuric acid (20% v/v).
It is odourless with a bitter and acrid taste.

Microscopical characters: the diagnostic characters are: *epidermal cells* brown, rectangular to polygonal, 40 to **60** to 90 μm wide, anticlinal walls slightly wavy and indistinctly pitted; *stomata* anomocytic, occasional; *ground tissue* of very thin-walled, polygonal, parenchymatous cells about 50 to 100 μm in diameter; cells pitted, containing simple or usually 2- to 3-compound *starch* granules, individual granules spherical, polyhedral, or muller-shaped, about 3 to **12** to **16** to 30 μm in diameter, usually with a triangular or stellate central hilum; numerous slender *vascular bundles* with *vessels* up to 30 μm wide, wall thickening spiral or annular; *crystals* of calcium oxalate absent.

POWDERED DRUG: Powdered Colchicum Corm. A pale buff powder possessing the diagnostic microscopical characters, odour, and taste of the unground drug.

Adulterants and substitutes. Indian colchicum corm consists of the corms of *C. luteum* Baker; they are small, usually entire, and often semi-translucent owing to gelatinisation of the starch. It contains only traces of colchicine.

Colchicum seeds are subspherical, about 2 to 3 mm in diameter, with a projection at the hilum and a strophiole extending along about one-quarter of the circumference; testa reddish-brown, dull, somewhat rough; endosperm hard, oily, and yellowish; embryo straight, about 0.5 mm long, placed radially; odourless; taste unpleasant and bitter; they contain about 0.3 to 0.6% of alkaloids, calculated as colchicine.

Actions and uses. Preparations of colchicum corm relieve the pain and inflammation of acute gout but their use for long periods is not recommended. They may cause considerable gastro-intestinal irritation with vomiting and purging.

Colds

see CORYZA, ACUTE

Colistin Sulphate

A mixture of the sulphates of the antimicrobial substances produced by the growth of a selected strain of *Bacillus polymyxa* var. *colistinus*.

OTHER NAME: *Colomycin*®

A standard is given in the British Pharmacopoeia 1973

Description. A white to cream-coloured powder with a faint odour and a bitter taste.

Solubility. Soluble, at 20°, in less than 2 parts of water and in 300 parts of alcohol; practically insoluble in ether, in chloroform, in acetone, and in propylene glycol.

Acidity. A 1% solution has a pH of 4 to 5.8.

Moisture content. Not more than 3.5%, determined by drying at 60° *in vacuo*.

Specific rotation. −65° to −74°, determined on a 5% solution.

Stability. Aqueous solutions may be expected to retain their potency for 4 weeks when stored at room temperature and for 8 weeks when stored at 2° to 4°.
For use as a dusting-powder colistin sulphate may be diluted with lactose.

The following may be used as cream and ointment bases for colistin sulphate to provide preparations that are stable for 4 weeks at room temperature: aqueous cream alone or mixed in the proportions of 90 parts by weight of aqueous cream with 10 parts by weight of hydrous wool fat; oily cream; and macrogol ointment.

The following may be used as vehicles for colistin sulphate to provide eye-drops or ear-drops that are stable for 4 weeks at room temperature: sterile purified water, which may contain up to 0.9% of sodium chloride for eye-drops; water for preparations, for ear-drops; 0.002% of phenylmercuric nitrate is a suitable preservative.

Storage. It should be stored in airtight containers, protected from light.

Metabolism. ABSORPTION. Poorly absorbed after oral administration of both the sulphate and sulphomethate sodium salts.

BLOOD CONCENTRATION. After an intramuscular dose of 2 mg/kg as the sodium sulphomethate, serum concentrations of 6 to 15 μg/ml are attained in 2 to 3 hours; therapeutic concentrations are in the range 3 to 6 μg/ml.

HALF-LIFE. Serum half-life, 2 to 8 hours after intramuscular injection. The half-life is increased in renal function impairment.

DISTRIBUTION. Well distributed throughout the body, crosses the placenta, and enters the cerebrospinal fluid when the meninges are inflamed; colistin is secreted in the milk; *protein binding*, 50% bound to plasma proteins.

EXCRETION. 40 to 80% of intramuscular doses of the sulphomethate is excreted in the urine mainly as the unchanged drug; the drug is excreted in the urine mainly by glomerular filtration and the rate of excretion is reduced in the aged; colistin is also excreted in the bile. Colistin impairs renal function and may delay the excretion of other drugs.

FURTHER INFORMATION. Serum and urine concentrations—J. Froman *et al.*, *J. Urol.*, 1970, **103**, 210; placental transmission—M. A. MacAulay *et al.*, *Clin. Pharmac. Ther.*, 1967, **8**, 578.

Actions and uses. Colistin is an antibiotic with a range of activity similar to polymyxin B, being active against a wide variety of Gram-negative bacteria, with the exception of strains of *Proteus*. It is poorly absorbed from the gastro-intestinal tract and so when given by mouth it is of no value in systemic infections, but may be useful when antibiotic treatment of gastro-enteritis is thought necessary. Overgrowth of non-susceptible organisms, particularly species of *Proteus*, may occur.

Colistin is usually given in a dosage of 9 to 18 mega units daily in divided doses. The doses for children are as follows: up to 1 year 0.75 to 1.5 mega units daily, 1 to 5 years 1.5 to 2.5 mega units daily, and 6 to 12 years 2.5 to 5 mega units daily. These doses should be given in three divided doses and may be doubled for the treatment of severe infections.

Undesirable effects. The effects described under Colistin Sulphomethate Sodium and in addition rashes, nausea, vomiting, and diarrhoea may occur.

Preparations

COLISTIN TABLETS: available as tablets containing 1.5 mega units of colistin sulphate.
A standard for these tablets is given in the British Pharmacopoeia 1973
Containers and *Storage:* see the entry on Tablets for general information on containers and storage. Containers should be airtight and light resistant.

Advice for patients: the tablets should be taken at regular intervals. The prescribed course should be completed.

OTHER PREPARATIONS available include an ELIXIR containing colistin sulphate 250 000 units in 5 ml when reconstituted, diluent syrup, life of diluted elixir 14 days; and a POWDER (sterile) in vials containing colistin sulphate 1 and 5 g.

Colistin Sulphomethate Sodium

A compound of colistin which may be prepared from colistin sulphate by the action of formaldehyde and sodium bisulphite, whereby amino-groups are sulphomethylated.

OTHER NAMES: Colistimethate Sodium; *Colomycin*®

A standard is given in the British Pharmacopoeia 1973

Description. A cream-coloured powder with a faint odour and a bitter taste.

Solubility. Soluble, at 20°, in less than 2 parts of water and in 500 parts of alcohol; practically insoluble in dehydrated alcohol, in ether, in chloroform, in acetone, and in propylene glycol.

Acidity or alkalinity. A 1% solution has a pH of 6.2 to 7.5.

Moisture content. Not more than 1.5%, determined by drying at 60° *in vacuo*.

Specific rotation. −45° to −49°, determined on a 5% solution.

Stability. Aqueous solutions containing 0.5 or 1% may be expected to retain their potency for 1 week when stored at room temperature or for 8 weeks in the frozen state.

Compatibility. Suitable vehicles for intravenous infusion are dextran 40 injection, dextrose injection (5%), laevulose injection (5%), Ringer's solution for injection, and sodium chloride injection. Infusion should be completed within 6 hours. Colistin sulphomethate injection is compatible with phenylmercuric nitrate, and with acetylcysteine.

Storage. It should be stored in airtight containers, protected from light. If it is intended for parenteral administration, the containers should be sterile and sealed to exclude micro-organisms.

Metabolism. See under Colistin Sulphate.

Actions and uses. Colistin sulphomethate sodium is a compound of colistin which is suitable for administration by injection. It has a range of activity similar to polymyxin B and is used in the treatment of Gram-negative infections, particularly those due to species of *Pseudomonas* and *Klebsiella*, that have failed to respond to other antibiotics. It is administered by intramuscular injection for the treatment of septicaemia and urinary tract infections and by intrathecal injection for meningitis.

The usual dosage for an adult is 3 to 9 mega units daily by intravenous infusion or by intramuscular injection in divided doses.

The usual dose for children up to 1 year is 75 000 to 150 000 units, 1 to 5 years 150 000 to 200 000 units, and 6 to 12 years 300 000 to 500 000 units; these doses may be repeated every 8 hours. Doses of 500 to 1000 units per kilogram body-weight may be given daily by intrathecal injection.

A 0.5% solution is used for subconjunctival injection to treat *Pseudomonas aeruginosa* infections of the eye. Colistin sulphomethate sodium is also used as a solution containing 0.1 to 1% for topical application.

Undesirable effects. Allergy may develop and the drug should not be used again in patients showing allergy to it. If the stated dose is exceeded or the excretion delayed by renal insufficiency, vertigo, perioral paraesthesia, and migraine-like syndromes may develop.
Colistin sulphomethate sodium may also give rise to renal toxicity, hypokalaemia, neuromuscular block, and neurotoxic reactions such as ataxia and apnoea.

Preparation

COLISTIN SULPHOMETHATE INJECTION: a sterile solution of colistin sulphomethate sodium in sodium chloride injection. It is prepared by dissolving the contents of a sealed container in sodium chloride injection shortly before use. Available as a powder in vials containing 0.5 or 1 mega unit of colistin sulphomethate sodium.
A standard for this injection is given in the British Pharmacopoeia 1973
Containers: see the entry on Injections for general information on containers.
Labelling: see the entry on Injections for general information on labelling. In addition, the label on the sealed container should state the amount of the medicament as the number of units contained in it.
Storage: the sealed container should be stored in a cool place, protected from light. The injection contains no bactericide and should be used as soon as possible after preparation but solutions of colistin sulphomethate sodium may be expected to retain their potency for up to 48 hours after preparation, provided they are stored at 2° to 10°.

Collagen Disease

see CONNECTIVE TISSUE DISEASE

Collodions

Collodions are liquid preparations consisting of a solution of pyroxylin in a mixture of organic solvents, usually ether and alcohol. They are intended for local external application and are applied by painting on the skin and allowing to dry. A flexible cellulose film is formed, covering the site of application.
Collodions may be used to seal off minor cuts and wounds or as a means of holding a dissolved medicament in contact with the skin for long periods.
See the entry on Pyroxylin for information on flexible collodion.

Colophony

The residue left after removal, by distillation, of oil of turpentine from the crude oleoresin obtained from various species of *Pinus* (Fam. Pinaceae), including *P. palustris* Mill., *P. elliottii* Engelm., and *P. caribaea* Mor. in North America and *P. pinaster* Ait. in southern Europe.

OTHER NAME: Resin

A standard is given in the British Pharmacopoeia 1973

Constituents. Colophony contains about 90% of resin acids, of which about one-third is abietic acid. The remaining 10% of the resin consists principally of esters of oleic acid, of other fatty acids, and of resin acids. The resin acids appear to undergo change when exposed to air.
The composition of colophony varies according to its source, age, and method of storage.

Solubility. Practically insoluble in water; soluble in alcohol, in ether, in carbon disulphide, and in many fixed and volatile oils; partly soluble in light petroleum.

Description. It occurs as translucent, pale yellow or brownish-yellow, angular, brittle, glassy masses which are readily fusible and have a faint terebinthinate odour and taste.

Adulterants and substitutes. An opaque resin results when water is not entirely removed during the preparation of colophony.
Black resin is the resin obtained from the later runnings from the incisions into the trees, or it may result from long-continued application of heat to the amber-coloured colophony.

Storage. It should be stored in the unground condition.

Identification. TEST. Dissolve 100 mg in 10 ml of acetic anhydride by means of gentle heat, cool, and add 1 drop of sulphuric acid; a bright purplish-red colour, rapidly changing to violet, is produced.

Uses. Colophony is an ingredient of certain plaster-masses and collodions.

Colouring Agents

Colouring agents may be added to medicines to mask an unpleasant appearance or to increase the acceptability of medicines to patients. In manufacturing practice, colouring may be used to prepare products of consistent appearance from raw materials of variable colour.
The usual proportion of dye required to colour a liquid medicine is from 0.0001 to 0.001%. It is usual to employ a colour appropriate to the flavour of the medicine, for example, red with cherry, strawberry, or raspberry, orange or yellow with citrus fruit, and green with mint flavours.

Selection of an appropriate colouring matter. Dyes should be non-toxic and compatible with the ingredients of the medicine. The dyes selected must be permitted for use in medicines in the country concerned. In the United Kingdom, it is proposed that after an interim period only dyes permitted for use in food may be used in medicines, and in approving a permitted list account will be taken of a European Economic Council Directive on food colours (as amended), which lists the following:

Aluminium	Erythrosine
Amaranth	Gold
Anthocyanins	Green S
Beetroot red (betanin)	(acid brilliant green S)
Brilliant black BN	Indigo Carmine
(black PN)	Iron oxides and
Calcium carbonate	hydroxides
Caramel	Patent blue V
Carmoisine (azorubine)	Ponceau 4R
Carotenoids, various	(cochineal red A)
Charcoal	Quinoline yellow
Chlorophylls	Riboflavine
Chlorophylls, copper	Silver
complexes	Sunset yellow FCF
Chlorophyllins, copper	(orange yellow S)
complexes	Tartrazine
Cochineal	Titanium dioxide
Curcumin	Xanthophylls, various

The use in medicines of brilliant blue FCF and red 2G is under consideration, together with the use of other dyes in medicines for external use.

Conjunctivitis

Conjunctivitis is an inflammation of the conjunctiva and may be due to infection or allergic reaction. Infection may be due to staphylococci, streptococci, haemophili, other bacteria, or viruses.

The usual treatment is local application of broad-spectrum antimicrobial agents such as chloramphenicol or neomycin. Treatment should be continued for sufficient time to ensure elimination of the infection as otherwise the condition will recur.

Conjunctivitis of allergic origin may be treated by application of corticosteroids, antihistamines, or sympathomimetics such as adrenaline acid tartrate.

Corticosteroids should not be used in conjunctivitis due to herpes simplex infection because they allow the infection to progress more rapidly. Conjunctivitis due to herpes simplex may be treated with antiviral agents such as idoxuridine; vidarabine may be used in idoxuridine-resistant cases.

Infectious conjunctivitis may be spread by common use of face towels and precautions should be taken to prevent the transfer of infection in crowded situations.

Connective Tissue Diseases

The connective tissue diseases (Collagen diseases) are a group of diseases, most of unknown aetiology, characterised by widespread inflammatory changes in connective tissues and blood vessels. Any system of the body may be involved and symptoms may include arthritis, endocarditis, pericarditis, pleurisy, uveitis, or renal failure.

Diseases in this group include rheumatoid arthritis, polyarteritis nodosa, systemic lupus erythematosus, systemic sclerosis, dermatomyositis, and polymyalgia rheumatica.

Conn's Syndrome

see under HYPERALDOSTERONISM

Constipation

Constipation, or unusually difficult or infrequent evacuation of the bowel, may be caused by lack of dietary roughage, poor bowel training, mechanical obstruction of the bowel by impacted faeces or tumours, disruption of normal habits such as occurs when intercurrent illness or operation confines a patient to bed, adoption of an unsuitable posture for defaecation, or muscular weakness. Some medicines may cause constipation as a side-effect.

Most cases of constipation can be treated by dietary measures. Long-continued constipation should be treated by increasing the bulk of intestinal contents by the use of a high-fibre diet or, failing this, by artificial means using bulk laxatives. If these measures are not successful suitable purgatives which act by lubrication, by osmotic action, or by irritation of intestinal mucosa thereby increasing peristalsis may be used. In paralytic ileus anticholinesterases such as neostigmine may be of value. Emollient laxatives (faecal softeners) include dioctyl sodium sulphosuccinate and liquid paraffin.

Bulk-forming laxatives include ispaghula husk, methylcellulose, and sterculia.

Saline purgatives include magnesium sulphate, potassium acid tartrate, sodium potassium tartrate, sodium sulphate, and tartaric acid.

Stimulant purgatives include aloes, aloin, bisacodyl, cascara, castor oil, danthron, phenolphthalein, rhubarb, and senna.

Anticholinesterases include neostigmine bromide and neostigmine methylsulphate.

Contact Lenses and Contact Lens Solutions

The corneal contact lens is an optical device designed to correct distorted vision and to obviate the wearing of spectacles. Contact lenses can be used in cases of myopia and astigmatism and in clinical conditions where a protective effect is required. Their use is contra-indicated in the presence of active intra-ocular or corneal pathological conditions, in clinical conditions such as herpes simplex, and in circumstances where lachrymal secretion is markedly deficient.

Conventional contact lenses are made of plastic materials and are designated "hard" or "soft" according to their physical characteristics. Hard lenses are generally made from polymerised esters of acrylic acid, polymethylmethacrylate (PMMA) being the most frequently used.

Soft contact lenses can be divided into two categories, namely, "hydrophilic" and "hydrophobic".

Hydrophilic lenses are based on a hydrophilic polymer such as hydroxyethylmethacrylate cross-linked with substances such as hydroxyethyldimethacrylate and polyvinylpyrrolidone. There are many variations which can be made in using these components. Hydrophilic lenses swell to varying degrees when immersed in water; generally the greater the degree of cross-linking the less the amount of water absorbed by the lens. The water of hydrophilic lenses may range from 3% to 85%.

The hydrophobic category of soft lenses is exemplified by those developed from cross-linked dimethylpolysiloxane. About 40% silica is mixed with the siloxane polymer and the whole is heated under pressure to achieve further polymerisation and cross-linking. Hydrophobic hard and soft lens surfaces are not readily wetted by lachrymal fluid and therefore need to be artificially wetted with appropriate fluids before they are applied to the cornea.

Hard contact lenses are misfitted by a calculated amount to permit precorneal tear flow and gaseous exchange. Soft lenses can be closely fitted provided the plastics permit good gaseous exchange.

Routine care of contact lenses of whatever type demands a high standard of hygiene to minimise the possibility of infection of the eye due to lens insertion. Specially formulated solutions have been developed to assist contact lens wearers and to cover the physical aspects of hydration, wetting, and cleansing of the lenses as well as their disinfection.

Care should be exercised in attempting to remove stains from contact lenses and the use of stain removers and neutralising solutions should not be attempted by the wearer. Often the stain is caused by a change in the polymer itself which no chemical treatment will remove.

Different solutions are required for use with hard and soft contact lenses.

The use of eye-drops by patients wearing hydrophilic lenses should be carefully controlled. Preservatives may be absorbed and concentrated in the lenses and subsequently released causing intense irritation in the eye. The usual preservatives used in eye-drops are unsuitable but thiomersal 0.005% may sometimes be used.

Solutions for Use in Association with Hard Contact Lenses

At least two types of solution are needed for adequate care of hard contact lenses. One type is needed for use as an antimicrobial, cleansing, storage, and soaking solution in which lenses can be immersed when they are not being worn and the other solution is required to wet the surface of the lens before application to the cornea and to provide a comfortable cushioning effect for the wearer.

Since the functions of these two types of solution are different the practice of providing combination or all-purpose solutions should be discouraged unless it can be shown that the total solution is free from irritant and toxic effects when introduced into the eye in association with the contact lens. Single-purpose solutions are also used but the solutions commonly available are one, or a combination, of the following solutions.

Soaking and cleansing solutions. Their function is to remove debris and adherent matter from the lens surface after wear without causing damage to the lens. Common contaminants include proteins and lipids derived from the eye tissues, cosmetics, and foreign bodies such as dust particles.

Non-ionic surfactants are used to aid the cleansing effect and some solutions contain enzymes to assist in the removal of organic matter. If not designed specifically to act also as a disinfecting solution, the formulation of a soaking and cleansing solution should include chemical antimicrobial agents in a bacteriostatic concentration.

Storage and disinfecting solutions. Solutions intended for storage of lenses when not in use are generally formulated to provide efficient disinfection. For chemical disinfection benzalkonium chloride is the antimicrobial agent employed in many formulations and it is either used alone or in combination with disodium edetate or in combination with another antimicrobial substance such as chlorhexidine. Thiomersal, also widely used in contact lens solutions, suffers the disadvantage that it is rapidly absorbed from solution by certain types of plastic containers and although often presented in a preparation containing disodium edetate it is incompatible with this substance when the pH is below 7.2.

Potential eye pathogens must be killed by this category of solution and therefore risk of reducing antimicrobial activity should be avoided.

Dry storage of hard contact lenses has been proposed as an alternative to wet storage. The latter is recommended because contamination may survive dry storage whilst immersion in an effective solution will disinfect the lens. Also it ensures the small degree of hydration (about 1.5%) necessary for the proper wetting of the hard lens by tear secretion and solutions and it serves to prevent dimensional changes in the lens, to reduce corneal abrasion, and promote comfort in wear.

Wetting and cushioning solutions. The function of the wetting solution is to enable the lachrymal fluid to rapidly wet the contact lens surface and so permit comfortable wear. A wetting solution must therefore be suitable for direct instillation into the eye without causing irritation. Polyvinyl alcohol and polysorbate 80 are commonly used as wetting agents but the latter has the disadvantage that concentrations of 0.5% or greater are incompatible with benzalkonium and chlorhexidine.

Viscolising agents such as cellulose derivatives are included to provide a cushioning and lubricating effect, an acceptable viscosity lying within the range of 15 to 25 centistokes (0.000015 to 0.000025 $m^2 s^{-1}$). Care must be taken to ensure that the preservative is not incompatible with the viscolising agent.

Wetting solutions also require the inclusion of effective antimicrobial agents to protect them against accidental contamination but because of the prolonged contact of the solution trapped between the inner surface of the contact lens and the cornea, concentrations of antimicrobial substances which are acceptable in eye-drops may be too irritant when used in wetting solutions. By using combinations of certain antimicrobial agents it may be possible to select those which at lower than normal effective concentration together produce equivalent or enhanced activity to the individual agents used at higher concentration. It may be possible, therefore, to avoid irritancy without impairment of antimicrobial activity but the absorbent properties of the particular contact lens material for the proposed antimicrobial agents should first be established as being satisfactorily small.

Saliva has been widely used as a wetting agent for hard contact lens and whilst the physiological components of this material make it an efficient wetting agent, its high bacterial content makes the habit unacceptable. Since lenses are inserted using a finger-tip, scrupulous hand hygiene is also required of the contact lens wearer.

Solutions for Hydrophilic Soft Lenses

Hydrophilic lenses offer the advantages to the patient of easier adaptability and longer uninterrupted wear than hard lenses but the requirements of solutions needed for their care are different since they will permeate the lens.

Two solutions are desirable to meet the requirements for soft lenses, one being a hydrating and preserving solution which should be acceptable for long-term use in the eye. The second solution provides a cleansing and hydrating system after removal of the lens from the eye. Both solutions require the addition of a minimum concentration of bactericide sufficient to protect against accidental contamination during use and which will not be absorbed by the hydrophilic lenses immersed in the solutions to the extent that irritancy is produced by release of bactericide into the eye when the lens is worn. The cold chemical sterilisation of hydrophilic contact lenses by means of specially formulated solutions is still in the stage of development and a combination of cleansing by using an appropriate solution and sterilisation by boiling in a physiological saline solution is recommended by most manufacturers.

Claims have been made for the efficacy of hydrogen peroxide, povidone-iodine, and esters of p-hydroxybenzoic acid in a water-soluble polymer complex as sterilising agents for certain types of hydrophilic lenses.

Antimicrobial Standards for Contact Lens Solutions

In the absence of published standards for the effectiveness of antimicrobial substances included in contact lens solutions onus rests on the manufacturer to demonstrate by adequate testing procedures that the preparation can efficiently combat a level of contamination and within a period of time which is consistent with contact lens practice.

Lens Containers (Storage Kits)

Containers for storage and immersion of contact lenses in the different types of solutions for lens care should be made of materials which are free from substances which will leach out harmful chemicals or absorb essential materials from the contact lens solutions.

The kit should be easy to clean and should have separate labelled compartments for the left and right lens. Sponge materials which are ideal receptacles for micro-organisms and abrasive particulate matter should be avoided. The lens receptacles should be sufficient size not only to cover the lenses but also to permit diffusion into solution of all contaminants on the lens. A minimum of 5 millilitres per lens has been recommended.

Preferably, a disposable case should be supplied with each bottle of disinfecting storage solution and contact lens wearers should be advised to wash and disinfect the lens-case regularly. If cases are to be used for longer periods they should be made of heat-resistant materials to permit regular washing and sterilisation by boiling.

Further Information

Contact lenses—*Drug & Ther. Bull.*, 1974, **12**, 25; cleansing and disinfection of contact lenses—J. Dallos and W. H. Hughes, *Br. J. Ophthal.*, 1972, **56**, 114, D. J. G. Davies and D. A. Norton, *J. Pharm. Pharmac.*, 1975, **27**, 383, R. J. McBride and M. A. L. Mackie, *J. Pharm. Pharmac.*, 1974, **26**, 841, and N. E. Richardson *et al.*, *J. Pharm. Pharmac.*, 1977, **29**, 717; general references and reviews—J. Z. Krezanoski, *J. Am. pharm. Ass.*, 1970, **10**, 13, R. M. E. Richards, *Pharm. J.*, ii/1972, 314, and A. J. Phillips, *Ophthal. Optic.*, 1968, **8**, 1058 and 1969, **9**, 19.

Contagious Bovine Pleuropneumonia Vaccine, Living

A fluid or dried preparation of a culture usually derived from a suitably modified strain of *Mycoplasma mycoides* such as T1 or KH3J. The dried preparation is reconstituted immediately before use with an appropriate volume of a suitable sterile liquid.

A standard is given in the British Pharmacopoeia (Veterinary)

Storage. The fluid vaccine should be protected from light and stored at 2° to 8°; it should not be allowed to freeze. Vaccines prepared from strains T1 or KH3J, but not other suitable strains of *Mycoplasma mycoides*, may be expected to retain their potency for not longer than 1 month.

The dried vaccine should be protected from light and stored between −20° and −30°; under these conditions it may be expected to retain its potency for 12 months. It should be used immediately after reconstitution.

Veterinary uses. It is administered by subcutaneous injection to cattle and buffaloes for prophylaxis of infection with *Mycoplasma mycoides*.

Contagious Pustular Dermatitis Vaccine, Living

A suspension of living contagious pustular dermatitis virus of reduced virulence either obtained from vesico-pustular lesions produced on the skin of healthy lambs or prepared in a suitable cell culture system.

OTHER NAME: Orf Vaccine

A standard is given in the British Pharmacopoeia (Veterinary)

Storage. The vaccine should be protected from light. When stored at a temperature not above −20° it may be expected to retain its potency for 12 months. When stored between −20° and 4°, it may retain its potency for less than 12 months, the actual time depending in part on the mode of preparation.

Veterinary uses. It is administered to sheep, by scarification, for prophylaxis against contagious pustular dermatitis.

Contraception

Unwanted conception may be prevented by a number of methods. The method of choice in any particular case depends on the convenience, the cost, and the views of the person, including any moral or religious prohibitions. The common methods depend upon the prevention of fertilisation of an ovum by a spermatozoon. This can be achieved by avoidance of coitus at the time of ovulation, by suppressing ovulation, by the use of mechanical barriers, or by the use of spermicides. Other methods include the use of loops and other devices placed in the uterus; it is possible that they prevent implantation of the foetus but the mechanism of their action is not established.

Safe period or rhythm methods. Coitus is avoided around the time of ovulation which is estimated by calendar or by observations of changes in body temperature or by a combination of these methods. This method is not entirely reliable but may be regarded as a means of spacing out births rather than as a complete method of contraception.

Mechanical barriers. Condoms or male sheaths provide a fair degree of protection provided that they are of sound quality, free from leakage, are correctly applied, and kept in position throughout coitus. Diaphragms, caps, or vaults are used in the vagina. Medical advice is required regarding size and fitting. These devices provide a reasonable degree of protection provided that they remain in position during coitus and for at least 6 hours thereafter. The efficiency of all mechanical barriers is much increased by using them in conjunction with a spermicide.

Spermicides. Spermicidal drugs are applied to the vagina in the form of pessaries, gels, creams, pastes, soluble tablets, effervescent ("foaming") tablets, and aerosols. They are applied before coitus, and when used alone their efficiency is comparatively low; they may, however, also be used in conjunction with mechanical barriers to provide an effective method.

Suppression of ovulation. Ovulation may be suppressed by the administration of progestogens or oestrogens. They are usually given in combination in order to provide better control of the menstrual cycle and to reduce the dose of oestrogen required. Progestogen-oestrogen treatment increases the risk of thrombo-embolic disease; the risk is usually low when the dose of oestrogen does not exceed 50 micrograms but is increased in patients over 35 years of age, in those who smoke, in those who have taken the tablets for more than 5 years, and in those with hypertension or hyperlipidaemia.

Contraceptive tablets of the progestogen-oestrogen type are taken daily for 21 days, beginning on the fifth day of the menstrual cycle, followed by an interval of 7 days without treatment before the course is repeated. This method is not suitable for patients with arterial hypertension, severe migraine, epilepsy, or where there is a tendency to venous thrombosis, and gynaecological examination is desirable before the method is used and annually while its use is continued. Side-effects may be troublesome and should be minimised by selecting the most suitable of the available commercial products by a process of trial and error if necessary.

Contraceptive tablets of the progestogen-only type (that is, without oestrogen) are administered daily without any interval. Side-effects may be less troublesome, but the menstrual cycle does not usually achieve such regularity as with the progestogen-oestrogen type.

Contraceptive tablets are an efficient method of contraception provided that the doses are regularly administered and that absorption is not reduced by vomiting or diarrhoea.

Certain drugs when given concurrently may reduce the effectiveness of oral contraceptives; these drugs include barbiturates, rifampicin, and anti-epileptics. In general progestogen-only tablets are less effective than progestogen-oestrogen preparations, especially if any doses are omitted.

If any doses of a course of an oral contraceptive have been omitted there is an increased risk of ovulation occurring and it may be desirable to use an additional method of contraception.

Progestogens and oestrogens used in oral contraceptives include ethinyloestradiol, ethynodiol diacetate, lynoestrenol, mestranol, norethisterone, norethynodrel, and norgestrel.

Intra-uterine devices. Coils, loops, spirals, or other shapes, usually made of plastics, inserted into the uterus under medical supervision, provide an efficient method of contraception. The devices may cause pelvic pain on or immediately after insertion, and may sometimes cause excessive periodic pain and blood loss. Means should be provided for verifying that the device is still in position. This type of contraceptive is best accepted by multiparous patients.

Copper Sulphate

Cupric sulphate pentahydrate
$CuSO_4,5H_2O = 249.7$

A standard is given in the British Pharmaceutical Codex 1973 and the British Pharmacopoeia (Veterinary)

Description. Blue triclinic prisms or a blue crystalline powder, slowly efflorescent in air; odourless.

Solubility. Soluble, at 20°, in 3 parts of water and of glycerol; very slightly soluble in alcohol.

Actions and uses. Copper sulphate and other soluble salts of copper have an astringent action on mucous surfaces and in strong solutions are corrosive. Concentrated solutions irritate the gastro-intestinal tract and give rise to violent vomiting and purging.

Traces of copper sulphate are sometimes administered in conjunction with iron in the treatment of microcytic anaemias, but do not significantly enhance the absorption or utilisation of iron.

Copper sulphate is used in copper and zinc sulphate lotion for the treatment of impetigo. Solutions of 0.25 to 0.5% are suitable for ophthalmic use as an astringent.

Copper sulphate is a potent fungicide; in a concentration of 0.5 to 1 part per million it prevents the growth of algae in reservoirs; 5 parts per million will kill the fresh-water snails which act as intermediate hosts in the life-cycle of the parasite causing schistosomiasis.

Veterinary uses. Copper sulphate is used in the treatment of copper deficiency in ruminants, the usual dose being 20 milligrams per kilogram body-weight. Doses of 30 milligrams per kilogram body-weight are administered to ewes for the prevention of swayback in lambs. Copper sulphate has been added to the diet in a proportion of 800 parts per million as a growth promoter for pigs.

Poisoning. In cases of poisoning by salts of copper, white of egg, milk, or magnesia should be given. An emetic is not usually required. Morphine may be given to allay the pain. Penicillamine or sodium calciumedetate can be used to chelate the copper.

Preparations

COPPER AND ZINC SULPHATES LOTION (*Syn.* Copper and Zinc Lotion; Dalibour Water):

Copper sulphate	10 g
Zinc sulphate	15 g
Concentrated camphor water	25 ml
Water for preparations	to 1000 ml

Dissolve the copper sulphate and the zinc sulphate in 900 ml of the water, add the concentrated camphor water in small quantities, shaking vigorously after each addition, and add sufficient water to produce the required volume.

A standard for this lotion is given in the British Pharmaceutical Codex 1973

Containers and *Labelling:* see the entry on Lotions for general information on containers and labelling.

Advice for patients: the lotion may be applied on gauze as a wet dressing.

OTHER PREPARATION: copper sulphate is an ingredient of compound ferrous sulphate tablets.

Cor Pulmonale

see under HYPERTENSION, PULMONARY

Coriander

The dried, nearly ripe fruits of *Coriandrum sativum* L. (Fam. Umbelliferae). The plant is an erect herbaceous annual, indigenous to southern Europe and naturalised throughout temperate Europe. It is cultivated chiefly in Russia, central Europe, England, and north Africa.

A standard is given in the British Pharmacopoeia 1973

Varieties. English fruits average 100 fruits per gram, are a uniform brownish-buff colour, are frequently split into separate mericarps, and contain 0.3 to 0.8% of volatile oil.

Moroccan fruits are larger, averaging less than 75 fruits per gram, are marked with purplish patches, are rarely split, and contain 0.3 to 0.6% of volatile oil.

Russian fruits are smaller, averaging more than 130 fruits per gram, are purplish-brown in colour, are usually whole cremocarps, and contain 0.8 to 1.2% of volatile oil.

Argentine fruits are rather smaller than English, deep brownish-buff in colour, include some split fruits, and contain 0.3 to 0.6% of volatile oil.

Constituents. Coriander contains about 0.3 to 1.2% of volatile oil and about 13% of fixed oil; proteins are also present. Up to 1.5% of acid-insoluble ash and up to 2% of foreign organic matter may be present.

Description. UNGROUND DRUG. *Macroscopical characters:* cremocarp glabrous, sub-globular, about 2 to 4 mm in diameter; primary ridges 10, wavy and less prominent than the 8 straight secondary ridges; mericarps usually remaining united at their margins, generally brown, brownish-yellow, or purplish-brown in colour, apex with a small stylopod and remains of sepals; transversely cut surface showing sclerenchyma in a continuous band in the dorsal part of the pericarp and 2, or rarely more, large vittae on the commissure; endosperm oily, concave on the commissural side.
It has an aromatic odour and an agreeable and spicy taste.

Microscopical characters: the diagnostic characters are: pericarp: *epidermal cells,* if present, composed of thin-walled cells, frequently containing a small prismatic *crystal* of calcium oxalate; mesocarp differentiated into outer, middle, and inner zone; outer zone parenchymatous, containing *degenerate vittae;* 2, or rarely more, *normal vittae* containing *volatile oil* also present on commissural side of each mericarp; middle zone sclerenchymatous, composed of sinuous rows of pitted *fusiform cells* often crossing one another at right angles and forming definite longitudinal strands in the secondary ridges; inner mesocarp partially composed of thin-walled hexagonal *sclereids; inner epidermis* consisting of thin-walled cells with parquetry arrangement.
Endosperm parenchymatous, with thickened cellulose walls, cells containing *fixed oil* and numerous *aleurone* grains, about 4 to 8 μm in diameter, with minute rosette *crystals* of calcium oxalate.

POWDERED DRUG: Powdered Coriander. A fawn to brown powder possessing the diagnostic microscopical characters, odour, and taste of the unground drug.

Adulterants and substitutes. Indian coriander is said to be derived from a geographical race of *C. sativum;* the cremocarps are yellowish-buff, ellipsoidal in shape, up to 8 mm in length, and contain little volatile oil.

Storage. It should be stored in a cool dry place.
Powdered coriander should be stored in airtight containers in a cool place.

Actions and uses. Coriander is a carminative and a flavouring agent.

Coriander Oil

Obtained by distillation from coriander.

OTHER NAME: Oleum Coriandri

A standard is given in the British Pharmacopoeia 1973

Constituents. Coriander oil contains about 65 to 80% of alcohols, chiefly (+)-linalol, together with terpenes.

Description. It is a colourless or pale yellow liquid with the odour of coriander.

Solubility. Soluble, at 20°, in 3 parts of alcohol (70%) and in less than 1 part of alcohol (90%); soluble in ether and in chloroform.

Weight per ml. At 20°, 0.863 to 0.870 g.

Refractive index. 1.462 to 1.472.

Optical rotation. + 8° to + 12°.

Storage. It should be stored in well-filled airtight containers, in a cool place, protected from light.

Actions and uses. Coriander oil is a carminative and is added to purgative medicines to prevent griping. The usual dose is 0.05 to 0.2 millilitre.

Preparations
Coriander oil is an ingredient of cascara elixir and of compound orange spirit.

Corneal Ulcer

The penetration of infecting organisms through the cornea as a result of injury, lack of lachrymal secretion, or reduced resistance to infection may give rise to corneal ulceration and infection of the anterior chamber of the eye. Since such infections may result in blindness, rapid treatment with appropriate antibiotics topically, systemically, and subconjunctivally is required.
Corneal ulcers due to herpes simplex may be treated by application of idoxuridine preparations or of vidarabine in idoxuridine-resistant cases.

Corticotrophin

A preparation which contains the hormone that increases the rate at which corticoid hormones are secreted by the adrenal gland.

OTHER NAMES: ACTH; *Acthar®; Cortico-Gel®;* Corticotrophinum; *Cortrophin ZN®*

A standard is given in the European Pharmacopoeia Vol. III

Corticotrophin is obtained from the acetone-dried powder of the anterior lobes of the pituitary gland of the pig by extraction with hot glacial acetic acid. Impurities are precipitated from the filtered extract by the addition of acetone, and the active material is then precipitated by the addition of solvent ether. The active material is washed free from acetic acid with acetone and purified by adsorption on oxycellulose or by another suitable method. The purified material may be sterilised by a process of filtration and is dried by a suitable method.

Description. White hygroscopic flakes or powder.

Acidity. A 1% solution has a pH of 3 to 5.

Moisture content. Not more than 7%, determined by drying at 60° *in vacuo.*

Storage. It should be stored in airtight containers, at a temperature not exceeding 25°, protected from light. Under these conditions it may be expected to retain its potency for at least 2 years from the date of manufacture.

Actions and uses. Corticotrophin stimulates the adrenal cortex, producing hyperplasia and increasing the hormonal output of the adrenal gland. When thus stimulated the gland increases in weight, loses ascorbic acid and cholesterol, and undergoes histological change, mainly in the zona fasciculata. The clinical effect is therefore similar to, but not identical with, that of cortisone, the patient showing some signs of Cushing's syndrome on prolonged or intensive treatment, as described under Cortisone Acetate.
After intravenous injection, it is effective within a few minutes, and 20 units of corticotrophin given by intravenous infusion over a period of 6 hours or longer causes as much adrenal cortical stimulation as about 6 times this dose given by intramuscular injection at 4- or 6-hourly intervals. The dose by slow intravenous injection for maximum adrenal stimulation is 45 to 90 units according to the age of the patient; the dose should be administered over a period of 8 to 24 hours.
The effect of corticotrophin ceases within either a few

hours or 1 or 2 days of stopping treatment, depending upon the dosage and route of administration, and the symptoms may recur if the disorder is still active. Treatment with corticotrophin should therefore be withdrawn gradually.

Corticotrophin is used in the treatment of the conditions described under Cortisone Acetate with the exception of adrenocortical states (Addison's disease, adrenalectomy). Its rapid action is particularly useful in severe asthma and allergic states; it has the disadvantage that it cannot be given by mouth.

Some patients who have failed to benefit from oral corticosteroids improve when these drugs are replaced by corticotrophin; the reverse also occurs occasionally.

Long-acting preparations of corticotrophin are available; these include preparations in which corticotrophin is combined with zinc hydroxide, or in which the viscosity is increased by the addition of gelatin. With these preparations a single intramuscular dose daily may be sufficient.

Undesirable effects. Undesirable effects of corticotrophin are similar to those described under Cortisone Acetate, but gastro-intestinal side-effects are less common, whereas hypertension and acne are more common. Allergic reactions may occur, with lessening therapeutic effect. Local reactions to the injections may sometimes occur, and may be a real drawback in bleeding states, such as thrombocytopenic purpura, owing to haematoma formation.

Precautions; Contra-indications. Corticotrophin should not be given to patients with peptic ulceration, with active or doubtfully quiescent tuberculous lesions, or with signs of mental instability or hypertension, although in these last two instances each case must be judged on its merits. Diabetes mellitus is aggravated and insulin needs are increased by corticotrophin therapy, and the signs of infective processes may be masked, as described under Cortisone Acetate.

Preparations

CORTICOTROPHIN GELATIN INJECTION (*Syn.* ACTH Gel. Inj.): a sterile solution of corticotrophin in water for injections containing suitably hydrolysed gelatin. It may be prepared by heating a 16% w/w solution of gelatin in water for injections for sufficient time to produce a solution which is mobile at 25°, cooling, and dissolving in the solution the requisite quantity of corticotrophin. The solution is sterilised by filtration and distributed by means of an aseptic technique into sterile containers which are then sealed.

Available in 5-ml vials containing 20, 40, and 80 units of corticotrophin per ml and in 2-ml vials containing 40 units of corticotrophin per ml.

A standard for this injection is given in the British Pharmacopoeia 1973

Containers: see the entry on Injections for general information on containers.

Labelling: see the entry on Injections for general information on labelling. In addition, the label on the container should state the amount of the medicament as the number of units in 1 ml, the animal source, "For subcutaneous or intramuscular use only", and that if necessary the contents should be warmed before use.

Storage: it should be stored at 2° to 10°, protected from light. Under these conditions it may be expected to retain its potency for at least 18 months.

CORTICOTROPHIN INJECTION (*Syn.* Corticotropini Solutio Iniectabilis; ACTH Injection): a sterile solution of corticotrophin in water for injections. It is prepared by dissolving the contents of a sealed container in water for injections immediately before use. The sealed container may also contain added inert substances.

Available as a powder in vials containing 25 and 40 units of corticotrophin.

A standard for this injection is given in the European Pharmacopoeia Vol. III

Containers: see the entry on Injections for general information on containers.

Labelling: see the entry on Injections for general information on labelling. In addition, the label on the container should state the animal source and either "For intravenous use only" or "For subcutaneous or intramuscular use only".

Storage: the sealed container should exclude micro-organisms and, as far as possible, moisture. It should be stored at a temperature not exceeding 25°, protected from light. Under these conditions it may be expected to retain its potency for 2 years. The injection decomposes on storage and should be used immediately after preparation.

CORTICOTROPHIN ZINC INJECTION (*Syn.* ACTH Zinc Inj.; Corticotrophin Zinc Hydroxide Injection; Corticotropini Zinci Hydroxidi Suspensio Iniectabilis): a sterile aqueous suspension of corticotrophin with zinc hydroxide. It may be prepared by adjusting the alkalinity of a sterile aqueous solution of corticotrophin containing a suitable quantity of zinc chloride to pH 8.0 with a sterile solution of sodium hydroxide. The quantity of zinc chloride is the minimum necessary to precipitate at least 90% of the total protein. The suspension is made isotonic with blood by the addition of glycerol or other suitable substance and sodium phosphate is added as a stabiliser. It is distributed by means of an aseptic technique into sterile containers which are then sealed.

Available in 5-ml vials containing 40 units of corticotrophin per ml.

A standard for this injection is given in the European Pharmacopoeia Vol. III

Containers: see the entry on Injections for general information on containers.

Labelling: see the entry on Injections for general information on labelling. In addition, the label on the container should state the amount of the medicament as the number of units in 1 ml, the animal source, "For subcutaneous or intramuscular use only", and that the container should be gently shaken before a dose is withdrawn.

Storage: it should be stored at 2° to 10°. Under these conditions it may be expected to retain its potency for 2 years. It should not be allowed to freeze.

Cortisone Acetate

17α,21-Dihydroxypregn-4-ene-3,11,20-trione 21-acetate

$C_{23}H_{30}O_6 = 402.5$

OTHER NAMES: *Cortelan*®; Cortisoni Acetas; *Cortistab*®; *Cortisyl*®

A standard is given in the European Pharmacopoeia Vol. II

Description. A white crystalline odourless powder.

Solubility. Very slightly soluble in water; soluble, at 20°, in 300 parts of alcohol and in 4 parts of chloroform; soluble in ether, in acetone, and in methyl alcohol.

Moisture content. Not more than 1%, determined by drying at 105°.

Specific rotation. +209° to +219°, determined on a 1% solution in dioxan.

Preparation of solid dosage forms. In order to achieve a satisfactory rate of dissolution, cortisone acetate in the form of an ultra-fine powder should be used.

Stability. Cortisone acetate exists in several polymorphic forms, and when aqueous suspensions are being prepared, all particles should be converted to the most stable of these forms as otherwise crystal growth will occur.

Storage. It should be protected from light.

Identification. TESTS. 1. It complies with Test 1 described under Betamethasone.
2. Dissolve about 200 μg in 1 ml of alcohol (95%), evaporate to dryness *in vacuo*, add 5 ml of 1N sodium hydroxide, and heat at 70° for 30 minutes; a yellow solution is produced which has a strong absorption at 370 nm (distinction from prednisone).
3. To about 15 mg in a test-tube add 3 drops of phosphoric acid and close the tube with a stopper through which passes a smaller test-tube filled with water and on the outside of which hangs a drop of *lanthanum nitrate solution* and heat in a water-bath for 5 minutes (or if necessary bring slowly to the boil over a flame); mix the drop of lanthanum nitrate solution with 1 drop of 0.02N iodine on a white tile and place at the edge of the mixture 1 drop of *dilute ammonia solution*; a blue colour slowly appears at the junction of the two liquids (presence of acetyl groups).

MELTING-POINT. About 240°, with decomposition.

ULTRAVIOLET ABSORPTION. In alcohol, maximum at 240 nm (E1%, 1cm = 390).

INFRA-RED ABSORPTION. Major peaks at 1235, 1279, 1650, 1675, 1700, and 1753 cm^{-1} (see Appendix 2a: Infra-red Spectra).

THIN-LAYER CHROMATOGRAPHY. See under Thin-layer Chromatography, System 10.

Metabolism. ABSORPTION. Readily absorbed after oral administration; absorption after intramuscular doses is slower than that from the oral route.

BLOOD CONCENTRATION. After an oral dose of 200 mg, peak plasma concentrations of cortisone are attained at 2 hours and reach about 20 μg/ml; after the above dose, 2-hour plasma concentrations for the metabolites, hydrocortisone, tetrahydrocortisol, and tetrahydrocortisone are about 60, 59, and 67 μg/ml respectively; in cirrhosis, the plasma concentrations of hydrocortisone are increased as a result of impaired ring-A reduction.

HALF-LIFE. Plasma half-life, about 30 minutes.

DISTRIBUTION. Widely distributed throughout the body; *protein binding*, highly bound to plasma proteins.

METABOLIC REACTIONS. Readily but not completely converted to its active metabolite, hydrocortisone, which is further metabolised by similar routes to those of cortisone itself; in addition to 11-oxo reduction, to form hydrocortisone, cortisone undergoes reduction of the A-ring to form 5β-hydro-metabolites, reduction of the 3-oxo group to form 3α-hydroxy-metabolites, reduction of the 20-oxo group to form 20α- and 20β-hydroxy-metabolites, and also side-chain cleavage to form androsterone metabolites; most of the metabolites are conjugated with glucuronic acid.

EXCRETION. Excreted rapidly in the urine mainly as conjugated metabolites with less than 1% of a dose as unchanged drug.

FURTHER INFORMATION. K. Fotherby and F. James, Metabolism of steroid hormones, *Advances in Steroid Biochemistry and Pharmacology*, M. H. Briggs and G. A. Christie (Eds), Vol. 3, London, Academic Press, 1972, p. 67; conversion of cortisone to cortisol—J. A. Jenkins and P. A. Sampson, *Br. med. J.*, ii/1967, 205.

Actions and uses. Cortisone acetate has the actions and uses of the naturally occurring adrenocortical hormone, hydrocortisone.

It is used in adrenocortical deficiency states and as an anti-inflammatory agent in a large number of disorders. Its action is transitory and relapse soon occurs when therapy is stopped unless the underlying disease has in the meantime spontaneously abated.

With continued therapy, endogenous pituitary secretion of corticotrophin is depressed and the adrenal cortex undergoes involution with diminution in its secretions. Electrolyte balance is affected to varying degrees in different patients; retention of sodium and water may sometimes be observed early in therapy, usually followed by spontaneous diuresis. The urinary potassium level may rise, and metabolic alkalosis, with symptoms of muscular weakness and electrocardiographic evidence of hypokalaemia, may occasionally occur. Carbohydrate metabolism may also be affected in that the blood sugar rises, and glycosuria may occur. Protein metabolism is affected in many patients, continued administration causing a negative nitrogen balance. Resistance of the patient's tissue to bacterial infection is diminished and, as the inflammatory response to infection is also diminished or absent, diagnostic signs of infection may be completely absent; granulation and fibrous growth may be inhibited, although epithelialisation usually continues normally. The main use of cortisone is therefore in those conditions which are self-limiting and where inflammation may be harmful, as in the eye.

Cortisone is rapidly effective when given by mouth and more slowly effective when given by intramuscular injection. Unlike hydrocortisone acetate, it is ineffective when injected into joints or applied to the skin.

In suppressing inflammation, as in the treatment of asthma and rheumatoid arthritis, and in the treatment of disorders of the blood, it is preferable to use prednisolone or some other corticosteroid that has less sodium- and water-retaining effects. When cortisone is used in these conditions, the correct dosage is the lowest that produces the desired effect; 25 milligrams of cortisone acetate is approximately equivalent in glucocorticoid activity to 5 milligrams of prednisolone. Close watch must always be kept for signs of bacterial infections and the appropriate antibiotic given, because cortisone may mask diagnostic features of such infections.

In adrenocortical deficiency states, such as Addison's disease, a daily dosage of 25 to 50 milligrams by mouth is required for maintenance therapy; in most cases cortisone alone is inadequate and fludrocortisone must be given in addition to increase sodium retention. In

Addisonian crisis, intravenous injection of hydrocortisone sodium succinate is to be preferred. In hypopituitarism with secondary adrenocortical deficiency, smaller doses such as 12.5 to 37.5 milligrams daily are usually adequate.

The diseases of the eye which respond to local application of cortisone and its analogues are inflammatory lesions of the anterior segment such as allergic conjunctivitis, and keratitis, acute iritis, non-specific keratitis, and phlyctenular keratoconjunctivitis; initially, 1 or 2 drops of a 0.5 to 2.5% suspension of cortisone acetate in normal saline are placed in the conjunctival sac every hour during the day, the frequency of dosage being gradually decreased as the condition improves. Alternatively, an ointment containing 1% of cortisone acetate may be applied 3 or 4 times a day.

Cortisone has no antibacterial action, does not control degenerative, as opposed to inflammatory, processes and does not remove organised products of inflammation.

Undesirable effects. In some cases gravitational oedema, ascites, and other signs of congestive heart failure may occur, owing to electrolyte imbalance.

Other toxic effects of therapy include features of Cushing's syndrome, such as rounding of the face, hirsutism, striae over the hips and shoulders, and acne; more serious effects are crush fractures of vertebrae, mental changes in those predisposed, hypertension, and possibly thrombo-embolic episodes.

If withdrawal of the drug be sudden and the disease still active, symptoms and signs return rapidly, sometimes with evidence of adrenal exhaustion—the so-called "withdrawal syndrome". This may sometimes prove fatal, or lead to serious progression and worsening of the disease under treatment.

Precautions and contra-indications. Care should be taken in treating diabetic patients, as insulin requirements are usually increased during administration of cortisone. The risk of peptic ulceration is a real one, and caution is necessary in treating patients with past symptoms of peptic ulceration, as relapse and haemorrhage or perforation may occur.

Cortisone should be used with great care in the presence of active or doubtfully quiescent tuberculosis. It may, however, be used in conjunction with specific anti-tuberculous therapy in certain forms of tuberculosis in an attempt to suppress inflammatory features of the disease and adhesion formation.

When cortisone is used in the eye, infections must be controlled by means of antibiotics, sulphonamides, or other antibacterial agents, as otherwise the infection may progress and cause fibrosis, scarring, and even dissolution of the structures affected; it should never be applied to dendritic ulcers, herpetic lesions, or inflammation suspected to be of viral origin, because of the risk of causing blindness. Cortisone delays regeneration of epithelial tissue and must not be used for treating corneal ulcers.

Cortisone should be used with caution in pregnancy, especially during the first 14 weeks, as it may give rise to foetal damage. It should also be used with caution in nursing mothers.

Preparations

CORTISONE INJECTION (*Syn.* Cortisone Acetate Injection): a sterile suspension of cortisone acetate, in very fine particles, with suitable dispersing agents, in water for injections. It is prepared by means of an aseptic technique. Available in 10-ml vials containing 25 mg of cortisone acetate per ml.

A standard for this injection is given in the British Pharmacopoeia 1973

Containers: see the entry on Injections for general information on containers.

Labelling: see the entry on Injections for general information on labelling. In addition, the label should state "Not to be given by intravenous injection".

Storage: it should be stored at room temperature, protected from light.

CORTISONE TABLETS (*Syn.* Cortisone Acetate Tablets): available as tablets containing 5 and 25 mg of cortisone acetate.

A standard for these tablets is given in the British Pharmacopoeia 1973

Containers and *Storage:* see the entry on Tablets for general information on containers and storage. Containers should be airtight and light resistant.

Advice for patients: in long-term use, treatment should not be discontinued without the advice of the prescriber. Patients may carry an identification card giving details of their treatment and the name of the prescriber, who should be contacted in the event of accident, feverish illness, diarrhoea, vomiting, or alimentary disturbances. In short-term treatment, the prescribed course should be completed.

OTHER PREPARATIONS available include EYE-DROPS containing cortisone acetate 1% and an EYE OINTMENT containing cortisone acetate 1%.

Coryza, Acute

Acute coryza (Common cold) is due to infection of the nose, nasopharynx, and upper respiratory tract by a variety of viruses including adenoviruses, some myxoviruses, and rhinoviruses. It is sometimes followed by secondary bacterial infection.

Infection spreads rapidly under crowded conditions, and immunity is of short duration and specific for each strain of virus, while physical resistance may be lowered in ill health or by environmental changes. The condition is characterised by discomfort in the eyes, nose, and throat, and nasal congestion and discharge ("running nose"). There may be sore throat and cough.

Treatment is symptomatic with analgesic and antipyretic drugs to relieve pain and reduce fever and sympathomimetic drugs or steam inhalations to relieve congestion.

Cough

Coughing results from a reflex mechanism when irritant substances stimulate receptors in the upper respiratory tract. It may serve to remove an accumulation of mucus or it may be unproductive and persistent.

Unproductive cough may be treated with suppressants. Productive cough is commonly treated with expectorants which relieve congestion by decreasing the viscosity of the mucus, but the therapeutic value of many expectorants is equivocal. Treatment of coughs should not be continued for more than a few days without medical advice since there may be a serious underlying condition such as chronic bronchitis, tuberculosis, asthma, pulmonary fibrosis, heart failure, or carcinoma, requiring investigation and treatment.

Creams

The term "cream" should be restricted to preparations intended for external use.

Creams are viscous semi-solids and are usually either oil-in-water emulsions (aqueous creams) or water-in-oil emulsions (oily creams). Certain water-miscible bases which have a complex matrix-like physical structure are also known as "creams"; they are often anhydrous or contain only a small proportion of water and are similar in appearance to traditional emulsion-type cream bases.

Creams are used to apply solutions or dispersions of medicaments to the skin for therapeutic or prophylactic purposes where a highly occlusive effect is not necessary. Bland creams may also be applied for their emollient, cooling, or moistening effects upon the skin.

Percutaneous absorption. In creams applied topically for therapeutic effect, it is desirable that the active substance should be released at the skin surface and should penetrate at a suitable rate in sufficient amounts to maintain an effective concentration at the site of action.

Percutaneous absorption is the term used to describe the penetration of substances through skin into the bloodstream.

Of the three main layers of the skin, the hypodermis, the dermis, and the epidermis, the outermost horny layer of the epidermis or *stratum corneum* provides the principal barrier to medicaments and vehicles. The mechanism of percutaneous absorption through intact skin has not been clearly established. Potential routes of penetration are through sweat glands, hair follicles, and sebaceous glands into the dermis or directly through or between the keratinised cells of the *stratum corneum*. Skin appendages provide an area for absorption which is only a fraction of the total skin surface and therefore it seems probable that for most substances epidermal penetration constitutes the main route.

Factors which affect percutaneous absorption. The factors which influence percutaneous absorption can be considered under three main headings: condition of the skin; physicochemical characteristics of the active substance; and effects due to the vehicle.

CONDITION OF THE SKIN. Intact skin presents a barrier to absorption which can be reduced considerably when the skin is damaged or is in the diseased state. The rate of absorption is also influenced by age and by environmental effects on skin temperatures and surface humidity. In plantar and palmar areas of body surface keratin layers are thick and absorption rates are slow; on the face, and particularly behind the ear, absorption is more rapid.

The keratinised cells of the *stratum corneum* have the ability to hold water, and their degree of hydration, which is also related to the environmental humidity and the extent of perspiration, affects the pliancy of the skin. Absorption of active substances is enhanced as the skin becomes more hydrated; this is the principle involved in the use of occlusive dressings where loss of moisture from the skin is retarded by the application of a film of low permeability.

PHYSICOCHEMICAL CHARACTERISTICS OF THE ACTIVE SUBSTANCE. Molecular modification of active substances can have marked effects on their activity. Changes in functional groups which alter the solubility and the partition coefficient of the substance between the vehicle and the skin barrier may retard or enhance the skin penetration rate. For example, when applied topically, most of the esters of the fluorinated corticosteroids have considerably greater activity than hydrocortisone.

There is some evidence that a partition coefficient which approaches unity aids the direct penetration of the skin barrier which has both hydrophilic and hydrophobic properties.

Both penetration and thermodynamic activity (chemical potential) of an ionic substance are influenced by its ionisation constant and by the pH of the skin and of aqueous vehicles. The lipid-soluble non-ionised species of many substances are more rapidly absorbed than their water-soluble salts.

An increase in the concentration of an active substance in a vehicle usually produces an increase in the amount absorbed percutaneously. Molecules of small size in high concentration tend to penetrate more readily than large molecules. Ideally, where polymorphic forms of a substance occur, the form with physical characteristics most suitable for penetration should be selected. The rates of dissolution and subsequent penetration of a substance of low solubility may be enhanced by particle-size reduction.

EFFECTS DUE TO THE VEHICLE. Although the nature of the vehicle can affect the release of an active substance, the intrinsic activity of the substance and its potential for absorption by the skin are more important factors in percutaneous absorption than the ability of the vehicle to penetrate the skin. For most substances, the slowest or rate-determining step in skin penetration is the diffusion rate of the substance in the horny layer of the skin. There is some evidence that for certain steroids that have a very low solubility in the vehicle, the rate of release of the drug from the vehicle is the rate-determining step.

The nature of the vehicle can influence not only the amount of active substance which is dissolved or suspended in it but also the diffusion coefficient of the substance and its partition coefficient between the vehicle and the skin. Substances which have a high affinity for the vehicle have a low thermodynamic activity and are released slowly; their lipid-water partition coefficients are often low. By reducing the solubility of a substance in the vehicle, conditions more favourable for release can usually be obtained. In some instances, the high affinity of the active substance for the vehicle may be due to complexation or "binding" to constituents of the vehicle.

The state of hydration of the skin can also be affected by the vehicle. Increased hydration is achieved, clinically, by reducing evaporation by means of an occlusive layer. Emulsified creams are less occlusive than oleaginous ointment bases, but the water-in-oil type have some occlusive properties.

Humectants may decrease hydration by extracting moisture from the skin itself. Insoluble powders also decrease hydration by disrupting the continuity of oily films at the skin surfaces and by providing an increased surface area for evaporation.

In systems where a weakly ionised active substance is present in the aqueous phase of an oil-in-water emulsion, adjustment of the pH to values above or below the pK_a value will reduce or increase the degree of ionisation with consequent effect on both activity and release.

The diffusion constant of a drug in a vehicle is inversely proportional to viscosity; thus a reduction in viscosity enhances diffusion. Propylene glycol and alcohol have been included in vehicles as solvents for steroids; if their concentration in such systems is carefully controlled they can favourably influence the lipid-water partition coefficients to aid penetration.

Organic liquids such as dimethyl sulphoxide and, to a lesser extent, dimethyl formamide and dimethyl acetamide have the ability to penetrate the skin barrier rapidly. Rates of penetration of substances have been enhanced when dissolved in these solvents. However, irritant, toxic, and undesirable side-effects have restricted the use of such solvents.

Thus, the main function of a vehicle is to carry and release the active substance. In view of the complexity of the absorption mechanisms, the extent to which a vehicle can penetrate the skin is an unreliable basis on which to attempt to predict the effectiveness of the vehicle in enhancing penetration of the active substance.

Cream bases and raw materials. Aqueous creams are usually oil-in-water emulsions. By the selection of anionic, cationic, or non-ionic emulsifying agents it is possible to formulate aqueous creams which are compatible with most active substances.

The water-in-oil emulsions which form oily creams are more frequently used for their emollient and occlusive properties. Such emulsions are formed by metallic soaps, beeswax, wool fat and its derivatives, and some synthetic non-ionic substances.

Non-emulsified systems which have the appearance and consistency of creams have been used as topical vehicles for corticosteroids; they usually comprise a continuous solubilising phase and a solid phase. The solvent in the solubilising phase may be propylene glycol and the solid phase a mixture of a fatty acid and high molecular-weight macrogols.

Raw materials used in creams and other semi-solids are hydrocarbons (hard, soft, and liquid paraffins), alcohols (cetostearyl, cetyl, stearyl), glycols (glycerol, macrogols, propylene glycol), lanolin and its derivatives, fatty acids (oleic, stearic), beeswax, vegetable oils (almond, arachis, castor, coconut, cottonseed, maize, olive), esters (isopropyl myristate), and emulsifying agents. The properties and uses of these materials are described in more detail in individual entries and in the sections on emulsions and emulsifying agents.

Rheology and stability of creams. As emulsified creams are usually non-Newtonian systems their rheological properties vary with the shear forces applied. Thus, viscosity and flow characteristics may change in accordance with the degree to which the systems are homogenised, or with the amount of shear applied during processing either in mechanical devices or by a spatula. Oil-in-water creams may have a visco-elastic gel network the rigidity of which can be increased by the inclusion of higher concentrations of mixed emulsifying agents such as cetrimide with cetostearyl alcohol. In most emulsified systems, the overall viscosity may be increased by increasing the viscosity of the continuous phase, by increasing the content of a single emulsifying agent, or by reducing the globule size by homogenisation.

Major factors which affect the stability of emulsified creams are temperature, cohesive and gravitational forces, physical and surface properties of the oily constituents, and the relative densities, viscosities, and concentrations of the two phases. In formulating creams, the chemical and physical properties of the active substance must be carefully considered: for instance, anionic substances are incompatible with cationic emulsifying agents; hydrolysis of an active substance may be enhanced if an aqueous base is used instead of an anhydrous base, while electrolytes can react with emulsifying agents or may induce gel-formation.

Preparation of creams. Emulsified creams which contain waxes or fatty solids are prepared by heating to 70–75° the oil-soluble or oil-miscible constituents together with the emulsifying agent, if it is oil-soluble. Water-soluble or water-miscible constituents dissolved in or incorpor-ated with the aqueous phase, are heated to a similar temperature and the two phases are mixed. If the dispersed phase occupies only a small volume, it is usual to add this to the continuous phase, otherwise the order of mixing is of little importance. The important factors are that the two phases should be at similar temperatures and addition should be steady, without splashing or vortexing, in order to avoid the entrapment of air. Subsequent cooling should be slow with stirring which is adequate to ensure homogeneity yet minimise aeration. Sudden cooling or excessive aeration can lead to a granular product. After cooling to 30–40°, the cream can usually be homogenised.

All apparatus used in preparation and the final containers should be thoroughly cleaned before use and rinsed with freshly boiled and cooled purified water before drying. Purified water, freshly boiled and cooled, should also be used for the preparation of creams and the highest hygienic standards should be adopted at all stages during processing and filling into containers.

Microbial contamination of creams. Creams, particularly emulsions of the oil-in-water type, provide suitable substrates for the growth of micro-organisms. Even when a preservative is included in a cream, the efficiency of the system may be impaired due to partitioning of the preservative between the oily and aqueous phases of the emulsion or to its partial inactivation by an emulsifying agent or a hydrophilic colloid. Since increasing the preservative content to a more effective level may introduce undesirable clinical side-effects, the concentration of preservative selected is, of necessity, a compromise.

These limitations of preservatives in creams mean that for the prevention of microbial growth less reliance than usual can be placed on preservatives in such systems, and consequently there is an even greater need for high standards of cleanliness during the preparation and handling of creams. Contamination of corticosteroid creams with *Pseudomonas aeruginosa* and other pathogenic organisms can present a risk to patients because of the reduced resistance to local infection caused by steroids. Heavy contamination may also lead to spoilage of the cream itself.

Dilution of creams. If a cream is prescribed with a content of active substance which is less than that available from the manufacturer it may be diluted with a suitable diluent. Suitable diluents are specified in the appropriate entries where the creams are described. Creams used as diluents and the dilutions themselves should be prepared under hygienic conditions; the stability and the bactericidal properties of the original cream should not be reduced on dilution.

The use of an unsuitable diluent may yield a product of limited bactericidal efficiency because the diluent either does not contain a preservative or contains one which is inactivated or incompatible on admixture. A diluent which differs in pH from the original cream may promote chemical breakdown or inactivation of the active substance. Physical breakdown may occur when a system formed by an anionic emulsifier is mixed with a cationic-based emulsion, or with a system which contains cationic active substances. The extent of release or the release rate of an active substance from a cream could be altered by admixture with a diluent of a different emulsion type, or with a diluent which changed the physical form or the complexation behaviour of the active substance. It is inadvisable therefore, to make dilutions in the absence of information on the suitability of the diluent.

Diluted creams must be freshly prepared without the

application of heat; they are usually given a life of 2 weeks from the date of issue.

Containers for creams. Creams should be supplied in well-closed containers which prevent evaporation and contamination of the contents. The materials of construction should be resistant to sorption or diffusion of the contents. Collapsible tubes of metal (to British Standard 4230: 1967) or flexible plastic tubes may be used.

If aluminium tubes are used, a phosphate buffer such as that provided by a mixture of 0.1% of disodium hydrogen phosphate (anhydrous) and 0.02% of sodium dihydrogen phosphate (dihydrate) may be included, if this is specified in the entry describing the cream. The buffer is intended to inhibit corrosion of the aluminium and to reduce the possibility of hydrogen formation. Alternatively, the internal surface of the tube may be coated with a lacquer of a heat-cured epoxy resin. Collapsible tubes may also be lined near the base with a suitable pressure-sensitive sealing coat. Aluminium tubes are not suitable for creams preserved with organic mercury compounds unless adequately protected by a suitable internal lacquer.

Creams may also be supplied in wide-mouthed glass or plastic jars fitted with plastic screw caps with impermeable liners or with close-fitting slip-on lids. Collapsible tubes reduce the risk of bacterial contamination during use and should be used in preference to wide-mouthed jars.

Storage. Creams should preferably be stored in a cool place.

Labelling. The container should be labelled "For external use only" and bear an instruction that it should be stored in a cool place. The strength of active ingredient should be stated as a percentage by weight or by volume. The label on the container of a diluted cream should also state that the contents should not be used later than 2 weeks after issue, unless otherwise stated in the entry describing the cream.

Further information. Percutaneous absorption—B. Idson, *J. pharm. Sci.*, 1975, **64**, 901. Preservatives in emulsified systems—H. S. Bean *et al.*, *J. Pharm. Pharmac.*, 1969, **21**, 173S; G. H. Konning, *Can. J. pharm. Sci.*, 1974, **9**, 103; A. G. Mitchell and S. J. A. Kazmi, *Can. J. pharm. Sci.*, 1975, **10**, 67; B. W. Barry, Rheology, *Advances in Pharmaceutical Sciences*, H. S. Bean *et al.* (Eds), Vol. 4, London, Academic Press, 1974, p. 1. Sterilisation of topical creams—G. P. Polli *et al.*, *J. pharm. Sci.*, 1972, **61**, 1078.

Cresol

A mixture of *o*-, *m*-, and *p*-cresol, $CH_3.C_6H_4.OH$, in which the *meta*-isomer predominates, and of other phenols obtained from coal tar.

A standard is given in the British Pharmacopoeia 1973

Description. An almost colourless to pale brownish-yellow liquid which becomes darker on keeping or on exposure to light; the odour resembles phenol but is more tarry; an aqueous solution has a pungent taste.

The characters of the constituent isomers are as follows:

o-Cresol is a colourless deliquescent solid with a characteristic odour; it becomes yellow on keeping, melts at about 30°, and boils at about 191°.

m-Cresol is a colourless or yellowish liquid, very slightly soluble in water and soluble in organic solvents; it melts at about 10° and boils at about 202°.

p-Cresol is a crystalline solid, very slightly soluble in water and soluble in alcohol and in ether; it melts at about 36° and boils at about 201°.

Weight per ml. At 20°, 1.029 to 1.044 g.

Boiling range. 188° to 205°.

Storage. It should be stored in airtight containers, protected from light.

Preparation and storage of solutions. See statement on aqueous solutions of antiseptics in the entry on Solutions.

Identification. TESTS. 1. Shake 0.5 ml with 300 ml of water, filter, and to a portion of the filtrate add *ferric chloride test-solution*; a transient bluish colour is produced.
2. To another portion of the filtrate obtained in Test 1 add *bromine solution*; a pale yellow flocculent precipitate is produced.

Metabolism. METABOLIC REACTIONS. In rabbits, hydroxylation to form dihydroxytoluene and oxidation at the methyl group to form *p*-hydroxybenzoic acid followed by glucuronic acid and sulphate conjugation; *p*-hydroxybenzoic acid is only formed from the *p*-cresol isomer.

EXCRETION. In rabbits, 60 to 70% of a dose is excreted as a glucuronide, about 15% as a sulphate, about 10% as *p*-hydroxybenzoic acid in free and conjugated forms, and 3% as dihydroxytoluene.

Actions and uses. Cresol has actions similar to those described under Phenol but it is less caustic and less poisonous than phenol. Most pathogens are killed in 10 minutes by exposure to solutions containing 0.3 to 0.6% of cresol but spores require higher concentrations and longer exposure times.

Cresol may be used in place of phenol in lotions and ointments. It is sometimes added, in a concentration of about 0.3%, as a preservative to solutions for parenteral administration.

Cresol is an ingredient of lysol (a 50% v/v solution of cresol in soap solution) which is used as a general antiseptic but which has been largely replaced by similar preparations such as Printol®, Stericol®, and Sudol®, containing other alkyl phenols. When used on the skin, these solutions may be irritant even when well diluted. Lysol and similar preparations may be used as general disinfectants at the following dilutions: for drains, 1 in 20; for heavily infected linen, 1 in 40; for floors and walls, 1 in 100.

Poisoning. As for Phenol.

Cretinism

see HYPOTHYROIDISM

Crohn's Disease

Crohn's disease is a chronic granulomatous and inflammatory disease of unknown cause affecting the small intestine, especially the terminal ileum, although it may involve the colon. It is characterised by abdominal pain, diarrhoea, fever, nutritional deficiencies, and loss of weight. Fistulae and abscesses commonly occur and may open onto the surface of the abdomen, internally, or in the perianal region. The disease most commonly begins in young adults and relapses and remissions occur during its course.

No specific treatment for Crohn's disease is known. Diarrhoea, anaemia, and lactose intolerance may be treated as described elsewhere. Rest and treatment with corticosteroids may be of value and bacterial agents may be used in case of sepsis. Sulphasalazine may be helpful in suppressing the disease and azathioprine may be useful in patients not responding to sulphasalazine and corticosteroids. Surgery is often required for the complications of obstruction or fistulae.

Crotamiton

N-Ethyl-*N*-*o*-tolylcrotonamide

CH₃·CH:CH·CO·N·C₂H₅

$C_{13}H_{17}NO = 203.3$

OTHER NAMES: *Eurax®*
Teevex® (with halopyramine hydrochloride)
A standard is given in the British Pharmacopoeia 1973

Description. A colourless or pale yellow oily liquid with a faint fishy odour. At low temperatures it may solidify partly or completely.

Solubility. Soluble, at 20°, in 400 parts of water; miscible with alcohol and with ether.

Weight per ml. At 20°, 1.004 to 1.009 g.

Refractive index. 1.540 to 1.542.

Boiling-point. About 154°.

Storage. It should be stored in small containers. If it has solidified, it should be completely melted and mixed before use.

Identification. ULTRAVIOLET ABSORPTION. In cyclohexane, maximum at 242 nm (E1%, 1cm = 315).

Actions and uses. Crotamiton is an antipruritic which is applied as a cream or lotion containing 10%. Its actions last for 6 to 10 hours. It has also been used as an acaricide for the treatment of scabies.

Undesirable effects. Sensitivity to crotamiton is rare, but the drug may produce irritation in the presence of acute vesicular dermatitis.

Precautions. It should not be used near the eyes or in cases of acute exudative or vesicular dermatitis.

Preparations

CROTAMITON CREAM (*Syn.* Crotamiton Ointment): a dispersion of crotamiton in a suitable water-miscible basis. It may be perfumed. Available as a cream containing 10% of crotamiton. It should not be diluted.
Containers, Labelling, and *Storage:* see the entry on Creams for general information on containers, labelling, and storage.
Advice for patients: the cream should be rubbed lightly on the affected area when required. Contact with the eyes should be avoided.

CROTAMITON LOTION: a dispersion of crotamiton in a suitable lotion basis. It may be perfumed. Available as an emulsion containing 10% of crotamiton. It should not be diluted.
Containers and *Labelling:* see the entry on Lotions for general information on containers and labelling.

Storage: it should be stored at room temperature. The lotion may solidify at lower temperatures.
Advice for patients: the lotion should be rubbed lightly on the affected area when required. Contact with the eyes should be avoided.

OTHER PREPARATIONS available include a CREAM containing crotamiton 5% with halopyramine hydrochloride 1%, and a cream containing crotamiton 10% with hydrocortisone 0.25%.

Crystal Violet

4-[4,4'-Bis(dimethylamino)benzhydrylidene]cyclohexa-2,5-dienylidenedimethylammonium chloride (Colour Index No. 42555)

$C_{25}H_{30}ClN_3 = 408.0$

OTHER NAMES: Medicinal Gentian Violet; Viola Crystallina
A standard is given in the British Pharmacopoeia 1973

Description. Greenish-bronze odourless crystals or powder.

Solubility. Soluble, at 20°, in 200 parts of water and in 30 parts of glycerol; soluble in alcohol and in chloroform; practically insoluble in ether.

Moisture content. Not more than 9%, determined by drying at 110°.

Identification. TESTS. 1. Sprinkle about 1 mg on to 1 ml of sulphuric acid; it dissolves to give an orange or brownish-red colour. Carefully dilute with water; the colour changes to brown, then to green, and finally to blue.
2. Dissolve about 20 mg in 10 ml of water and add 5 drops of hydrochloric acid. To 5 ml of this solution add *tannic acid solution* dropwise; a deep blue precipitate is produced.
3. To the remainder of the solution prepared in Test 2 add about 500 mg of zinc powder and warm the mixture; the solution is rapidly decolorised. Place a drop of the decolorised solution next to a drop of *dilute ammonia solution* on a filter paper; the zone of contact assumes a blue colour.

Actions and uses. Crystal violet is an antiseptic with a selective action on Gram-positive organisms. It does not irritate the skin. A 0.5% solution is used in the treatment of burns, boils, carbuncles, and mycotic skin infections. A solution containing 0.5% each of crystal violet and brilliant green has been used for disinfecting the skin.

Preparations

BRILLIANT GREEN AND CRYSTAL VIOLET PAINT (*Syn.* Liquor Tinctorium; Pigmentum Caeruleum; Pigmentum Tinctorium; Solution of Brilliant Green and Crystal Violet):

Brilliant green					.. 5 g
Crystal violet					.. 5 g
Alcohol (90%)					500 ml
Water for preparations	..	..	..		to 1000 ml

Dissolve the brilliant green and the crystal violet in the alcohol and add sufficient water to produce the required volume.

In making this preparation the alcohol (90%) may be replaced by industrial methylated spirit diluted so as to be of equivalent alcoholic strength, provided that the law and the statutory regulations governing the use of industrial methylated spirit are observed.

A standard for this paint is given in the British Pharmaceutical Codex 1973

Containers, Labelling, and *Storage:* see the entry on Paints for general information on containers, labelling, and storage.

Advice for patients: the paint should be applied undiluted to the affected area. It stains skin, hair, and fabric.

CRYSTAL VIOLET PAINT (*Syn.* Gentian Violet Paint):

| Crystal violet | | | | | .. 5 g |
| Water for preparations | .. | .. | .. | | to 1000 ml |

Dissolve.

A standard for this paint is given in the British Pharmaceutical Codex 1973

Containers, Labelling, and *Storage:* see the entry on Paints for general information on containers, labelling and storage.

Advice for patients: the paint should be applied undiluted to the affected area. It stains skin, hair, and fabric.

Cushing's Syndrome

The presence of an excessive amount of corticosteroids in the circulation over a period of time gives rise to Cushing's syndrome. There is excess fat accumulation around the neck and trunk ("buffalo-fat"), the face becomes rounded ("mooned") and plethoric, and the skin is thinned and readily bruised. Hirsutism and menstrual irregularities may occur in women and impotence in men. Hypertension, mild polycythaemia, wasting of muscles, osteoporosis, and a diabetic tendency may also occur.

Cushing's syndrome occurs most commonly in women between the ages of 15 and 35. Most cases are due to bilateral adrenal hyperplasia which is due to excessive secretion of corticotrophin. Cushing's syndrome may also be due to benign or malignant adrenocortical tumours, to the production of corticotrophin by carcinomas, or to excessive administration of corticosteroids. Adrenal hyperplasia may be treated by irradiation of the pituitary by means of X-rays or by implantation of radioactive materials or by total adrenalectomy as appropriate. Tumours of the adrenals may be removed, and iatrogenic Cushing's syndrome may be treated by reducing the dose of corticosteroid. Inoperable adrenal carcinoma may be treated with the antineoplastic agent, mitotane (*o,p′* DDD, an analogue of dicophane). Care should be taken not to precipitate an Addisonian crisis due to acute hypoadrenalism.

Cyanocobalamin

Coα-[α-(5,6- Dimethylbenzimidazolyl)] - *Coβ* - cyanocobamide, a cobalt-containing substance which may be obtained from liver or separated from the products of metabolism of various micro-organisms.
$C_{63}H_{88}CoN_{14}O_{14}P = 1355.4$

OTHER NAMES: *Benvet-B12®*; *C-VetB₁₂®*; Cyanocobalaminum; *Cytacon®*; *Cytamen®*; *Hepacon-B12®* *Ce-Cobalin®* (with ascorbic acid)

A standard is given in the European Pharmacopoeia Vol. II

Description. Dark red, odourless, tasteless, hygroscopic crystals or crystalline powder.

Solubility. Soluble, at 20°, in 80 parts of water; soluble in alcohol; practically insoluble in ether, in chloroform, and in acetone.

Moisture content. Not more than 12%, determined by drying at 105°.

Sterilisation. Solutions for injection are sterilised by heating in an autoclave or by filtration.

Storage. It should be stored in airtight containers, protected from light.

Identification. TESTS. 1. Mix in a porcelain dish about 1 mg with about 10 mg of potassium sulphate and 2 drops of *dilute sulphuric acid*, heat carefully to red heat, allow to cool, dissolve the residue in 2 drops of water, add 10 drops of a saturated solution of ammonium thiocyanate and 0.5 ml of benzyl alcohol and shake; a blue colour is formed which is taken up in the benzyl alcohol layer.

2. Fuse about 1 mg with 50 mg of potassium hydrogen sulphate, cool, break up the mass, add 3 ml of water, and boil until dissolved; add sufficient *sodium hydroxide solution* to make the solution just alkaline to *phenolphthalein solution* and add 500 mg of sodium acetate, 0.5 ml of *dilute acetic acid*, and 0.5 ml of a 0.2% solution of disodium 1-nitroso-2-naphthol-3,6-disulphonate; a red or orange-red colour is immediately produced. Add 0.5 ml of hydrochloric acid and boil for 1 minute; the red colour persists.

Metabolism. ABSORPTION. Large doses are irregularly absorbed after oral administration and absorption is impaired when intrinsic factor is deficient or when gastrointestinal disease is present.

BLOOD CONCENTRATION. Serum concentrations of vitamin B_{12}, in healthy subjects, are 110 to 1700 pg/ml when determined by microbiological assay. The large variation is partly due to differences in laboratory techniques including the type of micro-organism used.

HALF-LIFE. Biological half-life, 123 hours.

DISTRIBUTION. Stored in the liver, undergoes enterohepatic circulation, and crosses the placenta.

EXCRETION. 50% of a dose is excreted in the urine in 48 hours along with significant amounts in bile.

FURTHER INFORMATION. Serum concentrations in smokers, in non-smokers, and in pregnancy—J. M. McGarry and J. Andrews, *Br. med. J.*, ii/1972, 74; absorption, metabolism, and excretion—N. K. Shinton, *Br. med. J.*, i/1972, 556.

Actions and uses. Cyanocobalamin has the actions and uses described under Hydroxocobalamin but it is more rapidly excreted and so has the disadvantage that it does not produce such a high initial serum-vitamin-B₁₂ level as hydroxocobalamin and the serum level is not maintained for so long a period.

Cyanocobalamin should not be given by mouth because of its variable absorption.

In the treatment of pernicious anaemia, 5 intramuscular injections, each of 1 to 2 milligrams of cyanocobalamin, are generally given within the first week, followed by 250 micrograms weekly until the blood count is normal;

the usual maintenance dosage is 250 micrograms every 3 or 4 weeks. In all cases the dosage must be related to the patient's response; in patients with neurological abnormalities, the doses should be doubled.

The initial dose of cyanocobalamin for children is the same as that for adults. Subsequent dosage is determined by the haematological response.

Precautions. Cyanocobalamin should not be given before a diagnosis of pernicious anaemia has been fully established because of its ability to mask symptoms of subacute combined degeneration of the spinal cord.

Preparations

CYANOCOBALAMIN INJECTION: a sterile solution of cyanocobalamin, with sufficient acetic acid or hydrochloric acid to adjust the solution to about pH 4.5, in water for injections. It may contain a suitable buffering agent. It is sterilised by heating in an autoclave or by filtration. Available in 1-ml ampoules containing the equivalent of 50, 100, 250, 500, and 1000 micrograms of cyanocobalamin per ml.

Also available, for veterinary use, in 30- and 50-ml vials containing the equivalent of 250 micrograms of anhydrous cyanocobalamin per ml, and in 20- and 50-ml vials containing the equivalent of 1000 micrograms of anhydrous cyanocobalamin per ml.

A standard for this injection is given in the British Pharmacopoeia 1973

Containers: see the entry on Injections for general information on containers.

Labelling: see the entry on Injections for general information on labelling. In addition the label on the container should state the amount of the medicament as the equivalent amount of anhydrous cyanocobalamin in a suitable dose-volume.

Storage: it should be protected from light.

OTHER PREPARATIONS available include an ELIXIR containing cyanocobalamin 35 micrograms in 5 ml, diluent syrup, life of diluted elixir 14 days; an elixir containing cyanocobalamin 6 micrograms with ascorbic acid 2 mg in 1 ml; and TABLETS containing cyanocobalamin 50 micrograms.

Cyanocobalamin (^{57}Co)

Coα - [α - (5,6 - Dimethylbenzimidazolyl)] - Coβ - cyano-[^{57}Co]cobamide. It may be produced by the growth of certain micro-organisms on a medium containing [^{57}Co] cobaltous ions.

A standard is given in the British Pharmacopoeia 1973

CAUTION. This material is radioactive and any regulations in force must be complied with.

Cobalt-57 is a radioactive isotope of cobalt which decays by electron capture with emission of γ-radiation mainly of energy 0.122 MeV. It has a half-life of 270 days. It may be prepared by irradiation of nickel with protons of suitable energy.

Description. A freeze-dried solid supplied in sealed glass containers.

Stability. It decomposes with an accompanying decrease in radiochemical purity but should be issued in such a form that, when stored as indicated below, the rate of decomposition measured in terms of radiochemical purity does not exceed 2% per month during a period of 3 months from the date stated on the label.

Storage. It should be stored in an area assigned for the purpose, protected from light, at a temperature not exceeding 10°. The storage conditions should be such that the maximum radiation-dose-rate to which persons may be exposed is reduced to an acceptable level.

Labelling. The label on the container should state (1) the form of the preparation, (2) the content of cobalt-57 expressed in microcuries or millicuries at a given date, and (3) that the preparation is radioactive. The label on the package should state the total quantity in the container.

Actions and uses. Cyanocobalamin labelled with radioactive cobalt is used to measure the absorption of orally administered cyanocobalamin in the investigation of megaloblastic anaemias and particularly for the detection of pernicious anaemia. Impaired absorption which can be corrected by the simultaneous oral administration of intrinsic factor occurs in pernicious anaemia or following total gastrectomy; impaired absorption which cannot be corrected by intrinsic factor is usually due to disease of the small bowel.

Cyanocobalamin absorption tests are especially useful in cases where haematological investigations are vitiated by premature treatment or where neurological manifestations of pernicious anaemia precede the development of abnormalities in the marrow. The procedure is also used in subjects with pernicious anaemia to standardise preparations of intrinsic factor.

Various methods of performing cyanocobalamin absorption tests are in use. As the proportion of cyanocobalamin absorbed after oral administration depends upon the quantity administered, a standard dose, for example 1 microgram, should be administered; the labelled material may be diluted if necessary with non-radioactive cyanocobalamin so that the standard dose contains a suitable amount of radioactivity for measurement in the test.

A common procedure is the Schilling test, in which a large dose of non-radioactive cyanocobalamin is given by injection to impede uptake by the liver of the absorbed oral dose; the proportion absorbed may be assessed by measuring the radioactivity of the urine.

Other methods involve (a) measuring the radioactivity of the plasma, (b) using a scintillation counter over the liver, and (c) determining the non-absorbed fraction in the faeces after ashing, using a conventional well-type sodium iodide scintillation counter.

Observations of the radioactivity of the urine following intravenous injection of cyanocobalamin (^{57}Co) have also been used for the determination of the glomerular filtration rate of the kidneys.

Cyanocobalamin labelled with cobalt-57 or cobalt-58 is available and both forms are used for the tests; cyanocobalamin labelled with cobalt-60 should not be used because of the long half-life of this isotope. Cyanocobalamin (^{57}Co) may be stored for a longer period and for a given activity provides a lower dose of radiation to the liver.

Solutions of cyanocobalamin (^{57}Co) of high specific activity are used for the estimation in vitro of plasma vitamin-B$_{12}$ concentrations. The dose by mouth for the investigation of the absorption and metabolism of cyanocobalamin is 0.5 to 2 microcuries.

Cyanocobalamin (^{57}Co) Solution

A solution of cyanocobalamin (^{57}Co). It may contain a suitable stabiliser and bactericide. The method of production of cyanocobalamin (^{57}Co) and radiation data for cobalt-57 are given under Cyanocobalamin (^{57}Co).

OTHER NAME: Cyanocobalamini (^{57}Co) Solutio

A standard is given in the European Pharmacopoeia Vol. III

CAUTION. *This material is radioactive and any regulations in force must be complied with.*

Description. A clear colourless or slightly pink solution.

Acidity. pH 4 to 6.

Stability; Storage. As for Cyanocobalamin (^{57}Co).

Labelling. As for Cyanocobalamin (^{57}Co). In addition, the label on the package should state the name of any added stabilising agent.

Actions and uses. As for Cyanocobalamin (^{57}Co).

Cyanocobalamin (^{58}Co)

Coα - [α - (5,6 - Dimethylbenzimidazolyl)] - Coβ - cyano-[^{58}Co]cobamide. It may be produced by the growth of certain micro-organisms on a medium containing [^{58}Co] cobaltous ions.

A standard is given in the British Pharmacopoeia 1973

CAUTION. *This material is radioactive and any regulations in force must be complied with.*

Cobalt-58 is a radioactive isotope of cobalt which decays by $\beta+$-emission and electron capture with emission of photons mainly of energy 0.511MeV (annihilation energy) and 0.810MeV (γ-radiation). It has a half-life of 71.3 days. It may be prepared by neutron irradiation of nickel.

Description. A freeze-dried solid supplied in sealed glass containers.

Stability. It decomposes with an accompanying decrease in radiochemical purity but should be issued in such a form that when stored as indicated below the rate of decomposition, measured in terms of radiochemical purity, does not exceed 2 per cent per month during a period of 3 months from the date stated on the label.

Labelling. The label on the container should state (1) the form of the preparation, (2) the content of cobalt-58 expressed in microcuries or millicuries at a given date, and (3) that the preparation is radioactive. The label on the package should state the total quantity in the container.

Storage. It should be stored in an area assigned for the purpose, protected from light, at a temperature not exceeding 10°. The storage conditions should be such that the maximum radiation-dose-rate to which persons may be exposed is reduced to an acceptable level.

Actions and uses. Cyanocobalamin (^{58}Co) is used in the investigation of megaloblastic anaemias as described under cyanocobalamin (^{57}Co). The usual dose for the investigation of the absorption and metabolism of cyanocobalamin is 0.5 to 2 microcuries.

Cyanocobalamin (^{58}Co) Solution

A solution of cyanocobalamin (^{58}Co). It may contain a suitable stabiliser and bactericide. The method of production of cyanocobalamin (^{58}Co) and radiation data for cobalt-58 are given under cyanocobalamin (^{58}Co).

OTHER NAME: Cyanocobalamini (^{58}Co) Solutio

A standard is given in the European Pharmacopoeia Vol. III

CAUTION. *This material is radioactive and any regulations in force must be complied with.*

Description. A clear colourless or slightly pink solution.

Acidity. pH 4 to 6.

Stability; Storage. As for Cyanocobalamin (^{58}Co).

Labelling. As for Cyanocobalamin (^{58}Co). In addition, the label on the package should state the name of any added stabilising agent.

Actions and uses. As for Cyanocobalamin (^{58}Co).

Cyclizine Hydrochloride

1-Benzhydryl-4-methylpiperazine hydrochloride

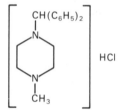

$C_{18}H_{23}ClN_2 = 302.8$

OTHER NAMES: *Marzine$^®$; Valoid$^®$*
Diconal$^®$ (with dipipanone hydrochloride)

A standard is given in the British Pharmacopoeia 1973

Description. A white, crystalline, almost odourless powder with a bitter taste.

Solubility. Soluble, at 20°, in 125 parts of water and in 120 parts of alcohol; practically insoluble in ether.

Dissociation constant. pK$_a$ 8.2 (20°).

Acidity. A 2% solution in a mixture of 2 volumes of alcohol and 3 volumes of water has a pH of about 5.

Moisture content. Not more than 1%, determined by drying at 130°.

Sterilisation. Solutions for injection are sterilised by heating in an autoclave or by filtration.

Identification. TESTS. 1. Mix a few crystals with 1 ml of sulphuric acid; a yellow colour develops in about 1 minute. Pour the solution into 10 ml of cold water; the colour disappears.
2. Dissolve about 500 mg in 10 ml of alcohol (60% v/v) with the aid of heat, cool in ice, and add 1 ml of *sodium hydroxide solution* followed by sufficient water to produce 20 ml; the precipitate, after washing with water and drying at 60° under reduced pressure for 2 hours, melts at about 107°.

MELTING-POINT. About 285°, with decomposition.

ULTRAVIOLET ABSORPTION. In 0.1N hydrochloric acid, maxima at 225 nm (E1%, 1cm = 394), 257 nm (E1%, 1 cm = 24), 262 nm (E1%, 1cm = 25), and 268 nm (E1%, 1cm = 19).

INFRA-RED ABSORPTION. Major peaks at 701, 716, 756, 984, 1449, and 1496 cm⁻¹ (see Appendix 2a: Infra-red Spectra).

THIN-LAYER CHROMATOGRAPHY. See under Thin-layer Chromatography, System 4.

Determination in body fluids. COLORIMETRY. In tissues —R. Kuntzman *et al.*, *J. Pharmac. exp. Ther.*, 1965, **149**, 29.

Metabolism. BLOOD CONCENTRATION. After termination of therapy with oral doses of 50 mg thrice daily for 6 days, plasma concentrations of the major metabolite, norcyclizine, of 4 to 22 ng/ml are attained during day 1 and 3 to 4 ng/ml during day 4.

HALF-LIFE. The plasma half-life of norcyclizine is less than 1 day.

DISTRIBUTION. Norcyclizine is widely distributed throughout the tissues and is localised in the lungs, kidneys, liver, and spleen; *protein binding*, norcyclizine is 60% bound to plasma proteins.

METABOLIC REACTIONS. Extensive *N*-demethylation to form norcyclizine.

EXCRETION. 1 to 1.8 mg of norcyclizine is excreted in the urine in 4 days after a dose of 50 mg thrice daily of cyclizine.

FURTHER INFORMATION. Physiological distribution and metabolic inactivation—R. Kuntzman *et al.*, *J. Pharmac. exp. Ther.*, 1965, **149**, 29; importance of tissue and plasma binding—R. Kuntzman *et al.*, *J. Pharmac. exp. Ther.*, 1967, **158**, 332.

Actions and uses. Cyclizine has the actions, uses, and undesirable effects of the antihistamine drugs, as described under Promethazine Hydrochloride. It is given by mouth for the prevention and relief of motion-sickness; it acts rapidly.

The usual dose for an adult is 50 milligrams of cyclizine hydrochloride 3 times daily, for a child aged 6 to 12 years, 25 milligrams, and for a younger child, 12.5 milligrams. The first dose should be taken 20 minutes before the journey.

Cyclizine has also been used for the relief of the nausea and vomiting of pregnancy and for the symptomatic treatment of vertigo and labyrinthine disorders due to Ménière's disease and other causes.

Poisoning. As for Promethazine Hydrochloride.

Preparations

CYCLIZINE INJECTION: a sterile solution of cyclizine lactate, with sodium metabisulphite, in water for injections. Available in 1-ml ampoules containing 50 mg of cyclizine lactate.

Containers and *Labelling:* see the entry on Injections for general information on containers and labelling.

Storage: it should be stored at room temperature.

Dose: adults and children over 10 years, cyclizine lactate 50 milligrams by intramuscular injection 3 times daily.

CYCLIZINE TABLETS: available as tablets containing 50 mg of cyclizine hydrochloride.

A standard for these tablets is given in the British Pharmacopoeia 1973

Containers and *Storage:* see the entry on Tablets for general information on containers and storage. Containers should be airtight.

Advice for patients: the tablets may cause drowsiness; persons affected should not drive or operate machinery. Alcohol should be avoided.

OTHER PREPARATIONS available include TABLETS containing cyclizine hydrochloride 30 mg with dipipanone hydrochloride 10 mg.

Cyclobarbitone Calcium

Calcium 5-(cyclohex-1-enyl)-5-ethylbarbiturate

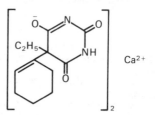

$C_{24}H_{30}CaN_4O_6 = 510.6$

OTHER NAMES: Cyclobarb. Calc.; Cyclobarbital Calcium; Cyclobarbitalum Calcicum; *Phanodorm®*; *Rapidal®* *Cyclomet®* (with emetine hydrochloride)

A standard is given in the European Pharmacopoeia Vol. II

Description. A white or slightly yellowish, odourless, crystalline powder with a bitter persistent taste.

Solubility. Soluble, at 20°, in 100 parts of water; very slightly soluble in alcohol, in ether, and in chloroform.

Moisture content. Not more than 1%, determined by drying at 105°.

Stability; Incompatibility. See under Barbiturates.

Storage. It should be stored in airtight containers.

Identification. TESTS. Dissolve, with the aid of heat, about 400 mg in a mixture of 10 ml of water and 10 ml of acetic acid, and cool; a crystalline precipitate is produced which, after washing with water and drying at 105°, melts at about 172°. The precipitate complies with general Test 1 described under Barbiturates, and, when dissolved in sulphuric acid, gives a yellowish colour which changes to orange on standing.

INFRA-RED ABSORPTION. Major peaks at 1260, 1357, 1389, 1429, 1537, and 1645 cm⁻¹ (see Appendix 2a: Infra-red Spectra).

THIN-LAYER CHROMATOGRAPHY. See under Thin-layer Chromatography, System 5.

Determination in body fluids. See under Barbiturates.

Metabolism (see also under Barbiturates). ABSORPTION. Rapidly absorbed after oral administration; absorption from a solution has been reported to be faster but less complete than absorption from tablets.

BLOOD CONCENTRATION. After an oral dose of 300 mg of the calcium salt, peak plasma concentrations of 7 to 11 μg/ml are attained in 20 to 120 minutes; concentrations over 3 μg/ml are effective in inducing sleep.

HALF-LIFE. Plasma half-life, 8 to 17 hours.

DISTRIBUTION. Volume of distribution, 34 litres.

METABOLIC REACTIONS. Oxidation to ketocyclobarbitone which, in rabbits, is further metabolised.

EXCRETION. 2 to 7% of a dose is excreted unchanged and 18 to 22% is excreted as ketocyclobarbitone; in rabbits about 44% is excreted as ketocyclobarbitone in 1 to 2 days.

FURTHER INFORMATION. Pharmacokinetics and relative

bioavailability—D. D. Breimer and M. A. C. M. Winten, *Eur. J. clin. Pharmac.*, 1976, **9**, 443.

Actions and uses. Cyclobarbitone is an intermediate-acting barbiturate, the actions and uses of which are described under Barbiturates. The usual dose as a hypnotic is 200 to 400 milligrams.

Undesirable effects; Precautions; Contra-indications; Dependence. See under Barbiturates.

Poisoning. As for Barbiturates.

Preparations

CYCLOBARBITONE TABLETS (*Syn.* Cyclobarbital Calcium Tablets): available as tablets containing 200 mg of cyclobarbitone calcium.
A standard for these tablets is given in the British Pharmacopoeia 1973
Containers and *Storage:* see the entry on Tablets for general information on containers and storage. Containers should be airtight.
Advice for patients: hypnotic doses should be taken half an hour before bedtime. The tablets may cause drowsiness on the following day; persons affected should not drive or operate machinery. Alcohol should be avoided.

OTHER PREPARATIONS available include TABLETS containing cyclobarbitone calcium 200 mg with emetine hydrochloride 600 micrograms.

Cyclomethycaine Sulphate

1 - [3 - (4 - Cyclohexyloxybenzoyloxy)propyl] - 2 - methylpiperidinium hydrogen sulphate

$C_{22}H_{35}NO_7S = 457.6$

A standard is given in the British Pharmacopoeia 1973

Description. A white crystalline odourless powder with a bitter taste followed by a sensation of numbness.

Solubility. Soluble, at 20°, in 50 parts of water, in 50 parts of alcohol, and in 227 parts of chloroform; very slightly soluble in dilute mineral acids.

Moisture content. Not more than 1%, determined by drying at 105°.

Sterilisation. Solutions for injection are sterilised by heating in an autoclave or by filtration.

Identification. TEST. Mix 500 mg with 10 ml of alcohol (95%), add 10 ml of *sodium hydroxide solution*, and heat under a reflux condenser for 1 hour; cool and add 7 ml of hydrochloric acid; a precipitate is produced which, after washing with water, drying, and recrystallising from alcohol (60%), melts at about 182°.

MELTING-POINT. About 164°.

ULTRAVIOLET ABSORPTION. In 0.01N hydrochloric acid, maximum at 261 nm (E1%, 1cm = 400).

INFRA-RED ABSORPTION. Major peaks at 775, 1176, 1235, 1250, 1613, and 1724 cm^{-1} (see Appendix 2b: Infra-red Spectra).

Actions and uses. Cyclomethycaine sulphate is a sparingly soluble local anaesthetic which is applied for surface analgesia in cuts and abrasions, skin irritation, burns, pruritus ani and vulvae, haemorrhoids, anal fissures, and cracked nipples. It may be used before cystoscopy, except when injury is present. Analgesia occurs within 5 to 10 minutes and lasts from 4 to 8 hours. Cyclomethycaine is not suitable for otolaryngological or ophthalmic use and should not be used on extensive areas of broken or burnt skin. It does not inactivate sulphonamides.

Undesirable effects. Cyclomethycaine occasionally causes sensitisation reactions.

Poisoning. The procedure as described under Procaine Hydrochloride should be adopted.

Cyclopenthiazide

6-Chloro-3-cyclopentylmethyl - 3,4 - dihydro - 2H - benzo-1,2,4-thiadiazine-7-sulphonamide 1,1-dioxide

$C_{13}H_{18}ClN_3O_4S_2 = 379.9$

OTHER NAMES: *Navidrex* ®
Navidrex-K ® (with potassium chloride)

A standard is given in the British Pharmacopoeia 1973

Description. A white, odourless, almost tasteless powder.

Solubility. Very slightly soluble in water; soluble, at 20°, in 12 parts of alcohol and in 600 parts of chloroform; soluble in ether.

Identification. MELTING-POINT. About 235°, with decomposition.

ULTRAVIOLET ABSORPTION. In 0.1N hydrochloric acid, maxima at 274 nm (E1%, 1cm = 556) and 319 nm (E1%, 1cm = 79).

INFRA-RED ABSORPTION. Major peaks at 1138, 1168, 1181, 1309, 1345, and 1605 cm^{-1} (see Appendix 2a: Infra-red Spectra).

THIN-LAYER CHROMATOGRAPHY. See under Thin-layer Chromatography, System 6.

Determination in body fluids. COLORIMETRY. In urine —H. Sheppard *et al., J. Am. pharm. Ass., scient. Edn,* 1960, **49**, 722.

Actions and uses. Cyclopenthiazide is a thiazide diuretic which has actions and uses similar to those described under Chlorothiazide. The usual dose is 250 to 500 micrograms by mouth, once or twice daily.

Undesirable effects; Precautions. As for Chorothiazide.

Preparations

CYCLOPENTHIAZIDE TABLETS: available as tablets containing 500 micrograms of cyclopenthiazide.
A standard for these tablets is given in the British Pharmacopoeia 1973
Containers and *Storage:* see the entry on Tablets for general information on containers and storage.
Advice for patients: daily doses should preferably be

taken in the morning. Treatment should not be discontinued without the advice of the prescriber.

OTHER PREPARATIONS available include TABLETS containing cyclopenthiazide 250 micrograms with potassium chloride 600 mg (K^+ 8.1 mmol) in a slow-release formulation.

Cyclopentolate Hydrochloride

2-[2-(1-Hydroxycyclopentyl)-2-phenylacetoxy]ethyldimethylammonium chloride

$$\left[\begin{array}{c} \text{C}_6\text{H}_5 \\ | \\ \text{HO} \diagdown \text{CH·CO·O·[CH}_2]_2·\overset{+}{\text{N}}\text{H(CH}_3)_2 \end{array} \right] \text{Cl}^-$$

$C_{17}H_{26}ClNO_3 = 327.9$

OTHER NAME: *Mydrilate*®

A standard is given in the British Pharmacopoeia 1973

Description. A white crystalline powder which is odourless or has a characteristic odour.

Solubility. Soluble, at 20°, in less than 1 part of water and in 5 parts of alcohol; practically insoluble in ether.

Acidity. A 1% solution has a pH of 4.5 to 5.5.

Dissociation constant. pK_a 7.9.

Sterilisation. Solutions are sterilised by filtration.

Identification. TESTS. 1. Dissolve 200 mg in 2 ml of water, add 2 ml of *sodium hydroxide solution*, boil for 1 minute, and add a few drops of nitric acid; an odour resembling that of phenylacetic acid is produced.
2. Dissolve 500 mg in 10 ml of water, add 2 g of potassium carbonate, and extract with two successive 10-ml portions of solvent ether; dry the combined extracts with potassium carbonate, filter, and to the filtrate add 4 drops of dimethyl sulphate and allow to stand for 2 hours; a precipitate is produced which, after recrystallisation from acetone and drying under reduced pressure for 2 hours, melts at about 141° with decomposition. When the residue is mixed with an equal quantity of the original sample, the melting-point of the mixture is not less than 15° lower.

MELTING-POINT. About 136°.

ULTRAVIOLET ABSORPTION. In 0.1N hydrochloric acid, maxima at 254 nm (E1%, 1cm = 5), 258 nm (E1%, 1cm = 5.6), and 266 nm.

INFRA-RED ABSORPTION. Major peaks at 704, 735, 1150, 1200, 1471, and 1735 cm^{-1} (see Appendix 2a: Infra-red Spectra).

THIN-LAYER CHROMATOGRAPHY. See under Thin-layer Chromatography, System 8.

Metabolism. ABSORPTION. The corneal absorption of cyclopentolate is increased when it is applied as a buffered solution with sodium borate; following ophthalmic use, cyclopentolate may be absorbed systemically either by transcorneal absorption, direct topical absorption through the skin, or by absorption from the nasal or nasolachrymal system.

FURTHER INFORMATION. Plasma concentrations—C. R. Bauer *et al.*, *J. Pediat.*, 1973, **92**, 501; corneal absorption —E. S. N. Wang and E. R. Hammarlund, *J. pharm. Sci.*, 1970, **59**, 1559.

Actions and uses. Cyclopentolate has mydriatic and cycloplegic properties similar to those described under Atropine, but it acts more quickly and its effect lasts for a shorter time.

The usual quantity for refraction procedures in adults is 1 drop of a 0.5% solution instilled into the eye; children aged 6 to 16 years usually require 1 drop of a 1% solution and children under 6 years 1 or 2 drops of a 1% solution. As a mydriatic, 1 drop of a 0.5 or 1% solution may be used The mydriatic action may be reversed by pilocarpine.

Cyclopentolate is also used in the treatment of corneal ulceration, iritis, iridocyclitis, keratitis, and choroiditis, 1 or 2 drops of a 0.5 or 1% solution being used as required.

Precautions. Cyclopentolate has relatively little effect on intra-ocular tension in the normal eye, but it should be used with caution in patients with increased intra-ocular pressure.

Preparation

CYCLOPENTOLATE EYE-DROPS: consisting of a sterile solution containing up to 1% w/v of cyclopentolate hydrochloride with 0.02% v/v of benzalkonium chloride solution in purified water. It may also contain boric acid and potassium chloride. Available as eye-drops containing 0.1, 0.5, and 1% of cyclopentolate hydrochloride.

A standard for these eye-drops is given in the British Pharmaceutical Codex 1973

Containers and *Labelling:* see the entry on Eye-drops for general information on containers and labelling.

Storage: it should be stored in a cool place.

Advice for patients: see the entry on Eye-drops for general information on the use of eye-drops. Blurring of vision and sensitivity to light may occur for up to 24 hours after instillation of the drops.

Cyclophosphamide

2-[Bis(2-chloroethyl)amino]perhydro-2H-1,3,2-oxazaphosphorine 2-oxide monohydrate

$$\left[\begin{array}{c} \text{O} \diagup \overset{\displaystyle \text{O}}{\underset{\displaystyle |}{\text{P}}} \diagdown \\ \diagdown \text{N} \diagup ^{\diagdown} \text{N(CH}_2·\text{CH}_2·\text{Cl})_2 \\ \text{NH} \end{array} \right] \text{H}_2\text{O}$$

$C_7H_{15}Cl_2N_2O_2P, H_2O = 279.1$

OTHER NAME: *Endoxana*®

A standard is given in the British Pharmacopoeia 1973

Description. A fine, white, crystalline, odourless powder with a slightly bitter taste.

Solubility. Soluble, at 20°, in 25 parts of water and in 1 part of alcohol; very slightly soluble in ether.

Acidity. A 2% solution has a pH of 4 to 6.

Moisture content. 6 to 7%, determined by Fischer titration.

Stability. It discolours on exposure to light. Aqueous solutions may be kept for a few hours at room temperature but at temperatures above 30° hydrolysis occurs with removal of chlorine atoms.

Storage. It should be stored in airtight containers, protected from light.

Identification. TEST. Dissolve 100 mg in 10 ml of water and add 5 ml of *silver nitrate solution*; no precipitate is produced. Boil; a white precipitate is produced which is insoluble in nitric acid but dissolves on the addition of *dilute ammonia solution* and is reprecipitated by nitric acid.

MELTING-POINT. About 51°.

INFRA-RED ABSORPTION. Major peaks at 945, 975, 1044, 1088, 1128, and 1225 cm^{-1} (see Appendix 2a: Infra-red Spectra).

Determination in body fluids. GAS CHROMATOGRAPHY. In serum or urine—C. Pantarotto *et al.*, *J. pharm. Sci.*, 1974, **63**, 1554.

MASS SPECTROMETRY. In blood—M. Jarman *et al.*, *Clinica chim. Acta*, 1975, **58**, 61.

Metabolism. ABSORPTION. Well absorbed after oral administration.

BLOOD CONCENTRATION. After the intravenous administration of about 9 mg/kg, plasma concentrations of cyclophosphamide of about 26 μg/ml are attained immediately after injection, falling to about 13 μg/ml by 2 hours; after doses of 9 to 12 and 40 to 60 mg/kg, peak concentrations of unbound alkylating metabolites of about 0.3 to 2 and 2 to 13 μg/ml, respectively, are attained in 2 to 3 hours.

HALF-LIFE. Plasma half-life, 3 to 11 hours after intravenous injection.

DISTRIBUTION. Both unchanged drug and its metabolites are found in the lymph, muscles, adipose tissue, skin, cerebrospinal fluid, synovial fluid, saliva, milk, and sweat; in mice, cyclophosphamide crosses the placenta; volume of distribution 21 to 66 litres; *protein binding*, active metabolites are 12 to 56% bound to plasma proteins but cyclophosphamide itself does not appear to be bound.

METABOLIC REACTIONS. Oxidation to 4-hydroxycyclophosphamide which may be further oxidised to 4-keto-cyclophosphamide, or may be metabolised to an aldehyde by ring-fission and N-dealkylation to form the active metabolite, aldophosphamide; aldophosphamide may be oxidised to the carboxylic acid, carboxyphosphamide, or converted to the toxic metabolites, acrolein and phosphoramide mustard.

EXCRETION. 27 to 95% of a dose is excreted in the urine with up to 30% as unchanged drug and 10% as ketocyclophosphamide; small amounts are excreted in the bile and faeces.

FURTHER INFORMATION. Clinical pharmacology—C. M. Bagley *et al.*, *Cancer Res.*, 1973, **33**, 226; pharmacokinetics—J. L. Cohen *et al.*, *Br. J. Pharmac.*, 1971, **43**, 677; metabolic variation in normal subjects—H. T. Mouridsen *et al.*, *Acta pharmac. tox.*, 1974, **35**, 98; A. R. Torkelson *et al.*, Metabolic fate of cyclophosphamide, *Drug Metabolism Reviews*, F. J. Di Carlo (Ed.), Vol. 3, New York, Marcel Dekker, 1974–1975, p. 131.

Actions and uses. Cyclophosphamide is a cytotoxic drug with the actions and uses described under Mustine Hydrochloride. It is broken down, mainly in the liver, probably by phosphoramidases, at the nitrogen-phosphorus linkage, liberating an alkylating agent. Unlike mustine, it has no vesicant action. It may be administered orally, intramuscularly, intravenously, or directly into body cavities.

Cyclophosphamide is used for the treatment of lymphosarcoma, Hodgkin's disease, multiple myeloma, lymphatic leukaemia, ovarian and other carcinomas, tumours of the head and neck, retinoblastoma, and malignant pleural effusions and as an adjuvant in the treatment of inoperable bronchocarcinoma and inoperable carcinoma of the breast.

Cyclophosphamide is occasionally used in the treatment of rheumatoid arthritis and systemic lupus erythematosus.

Cyclophosphamide may also be used to suppress cellular auto-immune reactions in tissue transplantations, such as kidney grafts, in the nephrotic syndrome and nephritis, and for prolonging survival of homografts. It may be used in a dose of up to 3 milligrams per kilogram body-weight daily in the treatment of the nephrotic syndrome in children when treatment with corticosteroids has proved unsuccessful.

The limiting factor in determining dosage and duration of treatment is depression of the white-cell count. If this is kept within the range of 2000 to 5000 white cells per cubic millimetre, treatment can be prolonged. It is started with a daily dosage of 100 milligrams intravenously, increased to 200 to 300 milligrams, or in certain circumstances to 400 milligrams, until a total dose of 6 to 8 grams has been given, the dose depending on the white-cell count. The daily dosage for maintenance therapy is 2.5 to 5 milligrams per kilogram body-weight which should be reduced if the white cell count falls.

For a child, the initial dosage is 5 milligrams per kilogram body-weight daily by intravenous injection; this is repeated until the white-cell count has fallen as far as permissible and then 2 to 5 milligrams per kilogram body-weight daily is given by mouth as a maintenance dose. Treatment can be continued with a maintenance dose for 1 or 2 years if the white-cell count is favourable.

Cyclophosphamide is perhaps one of the safest alkylating agents because depression of the white-cell count from overdosage is readily reversed on withdrawing the drug.

Dosage is expressed in terms of anhydrous cyclophosphamide; 1.1 milligrams of cyclophosphamide is approximately equivalent to 1 milligram of anhydrous cyclophosphamide.

Undesirable effects. Leucopenia (particularly of the neutrophil cells), loss of hair, anorexia, nausea, and vomiting may occur.

Cyclophosphamide may give rise to cystitis but this tendency may be minimised by the administration of large quantities of water. It may also cause sterility in both sexes. Bone-marrow depression occurs less frequently if the drug is given in intermittent large doses.

Preparations

CYCLOPHOSPHAMIDE INJECTION: a sterile solution of cyclophosphamide, with sodium chloride, in water for injections. It is prepared by dissolving the contents of a sealed container, consisting of cyclophosphamide equivalent to 100 parts by weight of anhydrous cyclophosphamide with 45 parts by weight of sodium chloride, in water for injections immediately before use.

Available as a powder in vials containing cyclophosphamide equivalent to 0.1, 0.2, 0.5, and 1 g of anhydrous cyclophosphamide.

A standard for this injection is given in the British Pharmacopoeia 1973

Containers: see the entry on Injections for general information on containers.

Labelling: see the entry on Injections for general information on labelling. In addition, the label on the container should state the amount of the medicament as the equivalent amount of anhydrous cyclophosphamide.

Storage: the sealed container should be protected from light. The injection decomposes on storage and should be used immediately after preparation.

CYCLOPHOSPHAMIDE TABLETS: available as tablets containing cyclophosphamide equivalent to 10 and 50 mg of anhydrous cyclophosphamide; they are compression coated or sugar coated.
A standard for these tablets is given in the British Pharmacopoeia 1973
Containers and *Storage:* see the entry on Tablets for general information on containers and storage. Containers should be airtight and light resistant.

Cyclopropane

$$H_2C \overset{CH_2}{\underset{}{\diagup\diagdown}} CH_2$$

$C_3H_6 = 42.08$

A standard is given in the British Pharmacopoeia 1973

CAUTION. *Cyclopropane is highly inflammable and mixtures of its vapour with oxygen or air at certain concentrations are explosive; it should not be used in the presence of a naked flame or of any electrical apparatus liable to produce a spark. Precautions should be taken against the production of static electrical discharge.*

Description. A colourless inflammable gas with a characteristic odour. It boils at about $-34.5°$ at normal pressure.

Solubility. One volume, measured at normal temperature and pressure, dissolves, at $20°$, in 2.85 volumes of water; soluble in alcohol, in ether, in chloroform, and in fixed oils.

Incompatibility. Cyclopropane is liable to leach some of the material from the walls of rubber or synthetic flexible tubing which may therefore be weakened and result in the development of leaks or sudden bursting of the tubing if it contains gas under pressure. In addition, under certain conditions, admixture of the gas with such materials produces a liquid which, if carried into other parts of the apparatus, may interfere with their function. Appropriate precautions should be taken to minimise these effects.

Storage, labelling, and colour-markings. It should be stored in metal cylinders designed to hold compressed gases. Cylinders should be stored in a special room free from materials of an inflammable nature. The room should be cool. The whole of the cylinder should be painted orange and the name of the gas or chemical symbol "C_3H_6" should be stencilled in paint on the shoulder of the cylinder. The name or chemical symbol of the gas should be clearly and indelibly stamped on the cylinder valve.

Metabolism. ABSORPTION. Readily absorbed after inhalation.

DISTRIBUTION. Localised in adipose tissue and crosses the placenta.

METABOLIC REACTIONS. No evidence of metabolism in man but may be metabolised in the rat.

EXCRETION. Excreted mostly through the lungs as unchanged drug.

FURTHER INFORMATION. Placental transfer—F. Moya and V. Thorndike, *Clin. Pharmac. Ther.*, 1963, **4**, 628.

Actions and uses. Cyclopropane is the most potent of the gaseous anaesthetics.
Its advantages are that it is non-irritant, that induction and recovery are rapid, and that it can be administered with a high percentage of oxygen. It is non-toxic to the liver and kidneys and causes only mild excitement during induction and only slight post-operative vomiting.
Its disadvantages are that it is a respiratory depressant and that it has a tendency to cause cardiac irregularities and increased haemorrhage. It may also cause bronchospasm if surgical stimulation occurs under light anaesthesia, and if it is used in conjunction with thiopentone sodium, laryngospasm may occur.
Because of the risk of explosion, the usual method of administration is by means of a closed circuit. It is usually administered with oxygen; a concentration of 4% of cyclopropane in oxygen produces analgesia, 8% produces light anaesthesia, and 20 to 25% produces surgical anaesthesia.

Precautions. Respiratory depressants in pre-operative medication should be given with caution, and during cyclopropane anaesthesia the pulse must be carefully observed and the use of sympathomimetic drugs, such as adrenaline, should be avoided. A marked fall in systolic blood pressure and varying degrees of lung collapse may be occasional sequelae.

Poisoning. As for Chloroform.

Cycloserine

(R)-4-Aminoisoxazolidin-3-one, an antimicrobial substance produced by the growth of *Streptomyces orchidaceus* or *S. garyphalus*, or obtained by synthesis.

$$H \overset{O}{\underset{NH_2}{\diagup\diagdown}} \overset{NH}{\underset{}{}} O$$

$C_3H_6N_2O_2 = 102.1$

A standard is given in the British Pharmacopoeia 1973

Description. A white or pale yellow, crystalline, hygroscopic, odourless powder with a slightly bitter taste.

Solubility. Soluble, at $20°$, in 10 parts of water and in 50 parts of alcohol; very slightly soluble in ether and in chloroform.

Acidity. A 10% solution has a pH of 5.7 to 6.3.

Specific rotation. $+110°$ to $+114°$, determined on a 5% solution in 2N sodium hydroxide.

Storage. It should be stored in airtight containers at a temperature not exceeding $25°$.

Identification. TEST. To 1 ml of a 0.01% solution in 0.1N sodium hydroxide add 3 ml of *dilute acetic acid* and 1 ml of a freshly prepared mixture of equal parts of a 4% solution of sodium nitroprusside and *sodium hydroxide solution*; a blue colour slowly develops.

MELTING-POINT. About $154°$.

ULTRAVIOLET ABSORPTION. In 0.1N hydrochloric acid, maximum at 219 nm (E1%, 1cm = 344).

Metabolism. ABSORPTION. Well absorbed after oral administration.

BLOOD CONCENTRATION. After a single dose of 250 mg, a peak plasma concentration of 4 μg/ml is attained in 4 hours and, after a dose of 1 g, concentrations of about

15 µg/ml are attained in a similar period; during therapy with 760 mg given every 6 hours for 2 to 3 days, concentrations reach 50 µg/ml or more.

HALF-LIFE. Plasma half-life, 8 to 12 hours.

DISTRIBUTION. Widely distributed and detectable in most body fluids and tissues; cycloserine is found in the cerebrospinal fluid even in the absence of inflamed meninges and it also crosses the placenta and is secreted in the milk; *protein binding*, less than 20% is bound to plasma proteins.

METABOLIC REACTIONS. Converted to β-aminoxyalanine in the rat.

EXCRETION. 66% of a dose is excreted in the urine in about 24 hours, 35% being excreted as unknown metabolites; very little is excreted in the faeces.

Actions and uses. Cycloserine is a water-soluble antibiotic which is active against a wide range of Gram-positive and Gram-negative bacteria, including *Mycobacterium tuberculosis*, streptococci, staphylococci, species of *Klebsiella*, and *Escherichia coli*. Its antibacterial activity is lower than that of other antibiotics available for treating infections due to these micro-organisms and it is therefore used only when the infecting organism has acquired resistance to other agents or when the patient has become hypersensitive to these other agents. It is not active against *Proteus vulgaris*, *Pseudomonas* species, or gonococci.

The main use of cycloserine is in the treatment of pulmonary tuberculosis when an antibiotic of the streptomycin group cannot be used because the organism is resistant or the patient hypersensitive. As with streptomycin, treatment with cycloserine should be combined with other drugs, as described in the entry on Tuberculosis, in order to minimise the emergence of resistant strains.

Cycloserine is given by mouth in an initial dosage of 250 milligrams daily; if no toxic effects are observed in about 2 weeks this dose may be given twice daily, and then 3 times daily if no serious toxic effects have been observed. The usual dosage for children is up to 10 milligrams per kilogram body-weight daily, adjusted in accordance with the blood concentrations observed. Cycloserine is also used in urinary tract infections when other drugs are contra-indicated or ineffective.

Undesirable effects. When the dosage recommended for the treatment of tuberculosis is used, the incidence of side-effects may be as high as 30%; the most common are headache and dizziness, but reflex changes, speech difficulty, convulsions, and coma may also occur. Gastro-intestinal symptoms and changes in serum transaminase may occur, but allergic reactions are uncommon.

Precautions. The blood level of cycloserine should be maintained between 15 and 25 micrograms per millilitre by appropriate adjustment of the dose and the use of lower dosage in patients with renal impairment.

Contra-indications. It should not be given to patients with a history of epilepsy or mental disturbance or with impaired renal function.

Preparations

CYCLOSERINE CAPSULES: consisting of cycloserine, in powder, which may be mixed with a suitable inert diluent, enclosed in a hard capsule. The capsule shells may be coloured. Available as capsules containing 125 and 250 mg of cycloserine.
A standard for these capsules is given in the British Pharmacopoeia 1973

Containers and *Storage:* see the entry on Capsules for general information on containers and storage.
Labelling: the label on the container should state the date after which the capsules are not intended to be used and the conditions under which they should be stored.
Advice for patients: the capsules should be taken at regular intervals. For the treatment of tuberculosis, therapy should not be discontinued without the advice of the prescriber. For the treatment of acute infections, the prescribed course should be completed. The capsules may affect mental concentration; persons affected should not drive or operate machinery. Alcohol should be avoided.

CYCLOSERINE TABLETS: available as tablets containing 250 mg of cycloserine.
A standard for these tablets is given in the British Pharmacopoeia 1973
Containers and *Storage:* see the entry on Tablets for general information on containers and storage. Containers should be airtight.
The tablets should be stored at a temperature not exceeding 25°.
Labelling: the label on the container should state the date after which the tablets are not intended to be used and the conditions under which they should be stored.
Advice for patients: the tablets should be taken at regular intervals. For the treatment of tuberculosis, therapy should not be discontinued without the advice of the prescriber. For the treatment of acute infections, the prescribed course should be completed. The tablets may affect mental concentration; persons affected should not drive or operate machinery. Alcohol should be avoided.

Cyproheptadine Hydrochloride

4-(5*H*-Dibenzo[*a,d*]cyclohepten-5-ylidene)-1-methyl-piperidinium chloride sesquihydrate

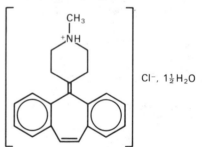

$C_{21}H_{22}ClN,1\frac{1}{2}H_2O = 350.9$

OTHER NAMES: *Periactin*®
Perideca® (with dexamethasone)

A standard is given in the British Pharmacopoeia 1973

Description. A white to slightly yellow, crystalline, almost odourless powder with a slightly bitter taste.

Solubility. Soluble, at 20°, in 275 parts of water, in 35 parts of alcohol, in 16 parts of chloroform, and in 1.5 parts of methyl alcohol; practically insoluble in ether.

Moisture content. 7 to 9%, determined by drying at 100° *in vacuo.*

Storage. It should be stored in airtight containers.

Identification. MELTING-POINT. About 215°, with decomposition.

ULTRAVIOLET ABSORPTION. In 0.1N sulphuric acid, maximum at 286 nm (E1%, 1cm = 312).

INFRA-RED ABSORPTION. Major peaks at 756, 777, 788, 815, 1416, and 1469 cm^{-1} (see Appendix 2a: Infra-red Spectra).

THIN-LAYER CHROMATOGRAPHY. See under Thin-layer Chromatography, System 4.

Metabolism. BLOOD CONCENTRATION. After an oral dose of 5 mg, peak plasma concentrations of drug plus metabolites of 36 to 50 ng/ml are attained at 10 hours; unchanged drug does not appear to be detectable in plasma.

DISTRIBUTION. Drug and metabolites are extensively distributed throughout the tissues; in the rat they are present in high concentrations in the kidneys, liver, and pancreas.

METABOLIC REACTIONS. Aromatic ring hydroxylation, N-demethylation, heterocyclic ring oxidation, and glucuronic acid conjugation; 10,11-epoxidation does not occur in man but is an important additional reaction in the rat.

EXCRETION. 67 to 77% of a dose is excreted in the urine in 6 days, the remainder being excreted in the faeces; the major metabolite in urine is a quaternary ammonium glucuronide conjugate; of the excreted material, 58 to 65% is conjugated with glucuronic acid, 9 to 11% is conjugated with sulphate, 20 to 26% is excreted as polar material not hydrolysable by glucuronidases or sulphatases, and 5 to 6% appears to be unconjugated.

FURTHER INFORMATION. Metabolism—K. L. Hintze *et al.*, *Drug Met. Disp.*, 1975, **3**, 1, C. C. Porter *et al.*, *Drug Met. Disp.*, 1975, **3**, 189, and J. S. Wold and L. J. Fischer, *J. Pharmac. exp. Ther.*, 1972, **183**, 188.

Actions and uses. Cyproheptadine has the actions and uses of the antihistamine drugs as described under Promethazine Hydrochloride and has also been used to stimulate appetite; 1.1 grams of cyproheptadine hydrochloride is approximately equivalent to 1 gram of anhydrous cyproheptadine hydrochloride.

The dose of cyproheptadine hydrochloride is the equivalent of 4 to 20 milligrams of anhydrous cyproheptadine hydrochloride daily in divided doses. The dose for children under 1 year is 1.5 to 3 milligrams daily in divided doses; 1 to 5 years, 6 milligrams daily in divided doses; 6 to 12 years, 12 milligrams daily in divided doses.

Undesirable effects. As for Promethazine Hydrochloride. In addition, cyproheptadine may inhibit lactation.

Poisoning. As for Promethazine Hydrochloride.

Preparations

CYPROHEPTADINE TABLETS: available as tablets containing cyproheptadine hydrochloride equivalent to 4 mg of anhydrous cyproheptadine hydrochloride.

A standard for these tablets is given in the British Pharmacopoeia 1973

Containers and *Storage:* see the entry on Tablets for general information on containers and storage. Containers should be airtight.

Labelling: the label on the container should state the amount of the medicament as the equivalent amount of anhydrous cyproheptadine hydrochloride.

Advice for patients: the tablets may cause drowsiness; persons affected should not drive or operate machinery. Alcohol should be avoided.

OTHER PREPARATIONS available include an ELIXIR containing cyproheptadine hydrochloride equivalent to

anhydrous cyproheptadine hydrochloride 2 mg in 5 ml, diluent syrup, life of the diluted elixir 14 days; and TABLETS containing cyproheptadine hydrochloride equivalent to 4 mg of anhydrous cyproheptadine hydrochloride with dexamethasone 250 micrograms.

Cystitis

see under URINARY TRACT INFECTIONS

Cytarabine

4-Amino-1-β-D-arabinofuranosylpyrimidin-2($1H$)-one *or* 1-β-D-arabinofuranosylcytosine

$C_9H_{13}N_3O_5 = 243.2$

OTHER NAMES: *Cytosar*®; Cytosine Arabinoside

Description. An odourless white crystalline powder.

Solubility. Soluble in 10 parts of water; very slightly soluble in alcohol and in chloroform.

Acidity. A 1% solution has a pH of 4 to 6.

Specific rotation. +154° to +160°, determined on a 1% solution.

Identification. ULTRAVIOLET ABSORPTION. In 0.1N hydrochloric acid, maximum at 281 nm (E1%, 1cm = 563).

INFRA-RED ABSORPTION. Major peaks at 1031, 1075, 1111, 1149, 1176, and 1389 cm^{-1} (see Appendix 2b: Infra-red Spectra).

Metabolism. ABSORPTION. Poorly absorbed after oral administration.

BLOOD CONCENTRATION. Therapeutic plasma concentrations are in the range 100 to 400 ng/ml.

HALF-LIFE. Plasma half-life after intravenous administration, 12 minutes for the α-phase and 111 minutes for the β-phase. Another report gives a half-life of 1 to 2 minutes for the α-phase and 8 to 19 minutes for the β-phase and suggests that the 111-minute value for the β-phase may in fact be a value for a third phase.

DISTRIBUTION. Volume of distribution at steady state, about 20 to 90 litres.

METABOLIC REACTIONS. Deamination in the liver and kidneys to form arabinofuranosyluracil.

EXCRETION. After an intravenous dose, about 70 to 90% is excreted in the urine in 24 hours, mostly as the deamination product along with 5 to 8% as unchanged drug.

FURTHER INFORMATION. Metabolism—R. L. Dedrick *et al.*, *Biochem. Pharmac.*, 1972, **21**, 1; clinical pharmacology—D. H. W. Ho and E. Frei, *Clin. Pharmac.*

Ther., 1971, **12**, 944; pharmacokinetics—R. van Prooijen *et al.*, *Clin. Pharmac. Ther.*, 1977, **21**, 744 and S. H. Wan *et al.*, *Cancer Res.*, 1974, **34**, 392.

Actions and uses. Cytarabine is a cytotoxic antimetabolite that inhibits the synthesis of deoxycytidine and also inhibits the action of cytidylic acid kinase enzymes. It becomes incorporated into nucleic acid and may cause breakages in the chromosomes of human leucocytes.

Cytarabine is used to induce and maintain remissions in acute myeloblastic leukaemias. As it is inactive when given by mouth, it is administered by subcutaneous or intravenous injection or infusion. Lower doses may be more effective when cytarabine is given by slow intravenous infusion than when it is given by intravenous injection.

For the induction of remission, either continuous or intermittent treatment may be used. There are various regimens of continuous treatment. If rapid intravenous injection is used, a starting dose of 2 milligrams per kilogram body-weight may be given daily for children and adults. If the response is not adequate, in the absence of apparent toxicity the dose may be increased to 4 milligrams per kilogram body-weight after 10 days. If slow intravenous infusion is used for continuous treatment, the initial dosage may be 0.5 to 1 milligram per kilogram body-weight over 24 hours for children or adults. This may be increased if necessary after 10 days to 2 milligrams per kilogram body-weight daily, subject to the absence of toxic effects, and this is continued until remission or toxicity occurs.

Alternatively, intermittent treatment may be used to induce remission. The usual daily dose for adults and children is 3 to 5 milligrams per kilogram body-weight, by intravenous infusion or occasionally by intravenous injection, for 5 days. This course may be repeated after an interval of 2 to 9 days. Further courses are given until remission occurs or until signs of toxicity appear. Response to treatment may occur in a week, but may take more than 2 months. For the maintenance of remission 1 milligram per kilogram body-weight may be given by intravenous or subcutaneous injection once or twice weekly.

Undesirable effects. Cytarabine may give rise to bone-marrow suppression with leucopenia, thrombocytopenia, anaemia, and hyperuricaemia. Nausea, vomiting, diarrhoea, abdominal pain, oral ulceration, renal dysfunction, anorexia, sepsis, haemorrhage from mucous membranes, joint and chest pains, and liver damage may also occur.

Precautions. Cytarabine is teratogenic and should be given in pregnancy only when the risks involved can be justified. During treatment with cytarabine, the blood should be monitored for leucocyte and platelet counts and for uric acid to avoid the development of hyperuricaemia. Facilities should be available for the treatment of acute granulocytopenia and infections resulting from it, and for haemorrhage due to thrombocytopenia.

Preparation

CYTARABINE INJECTION: a sterile solution of cytarabine, with 0.9% of benzyl alcohol, in water for injections. It is prepared by dissolving the contents of a sealed container in the solvent shortly before use. The benzyl alcohol is present in the solvent. Available as a powder in vials containing 100 mg of cytarabine. The solvent, 0.9% benzyl alcohol in water for injections, is available in 5-ml ampoules.

Containers and *Labelling:* see the entry on Injections for general information on containers and labelling.

Storage: the injection should be used as soon as possible after preparation but solutions of cytarabine may be expected to retain their potency for up to 48 hours at room temperature.

Danthron

1,8-Dihydroxyanthraquinone

$C_{14}H_8O_4 = 240.2$

OTHER NAMES: *Altan®*; Dihydroxyanthraquinone *Normax®* (with dioctyl sodium sulphosuccinate); *Dorbanex®* (with poloxamer 188); *Normacol-X®* (with sterculia)

A standard is given in the British Pharmacopoeia 1973

Description. An orange, almost odourless, almost tasteless, crystalline powder.

Solubility. Very slightly soluble in water; soluble, at 20°, in 2500 parts of alcohol, in 500 parts of ether, and in 30 parts of chloroform; soluble in solutions of alkali hydroxides.

Identification. TESTS. 1. Dissolve about 50 mg in 10 ml of chloroform, add 5 ml of *dilute ammonia solution*, shake, and allow to separate; the aqueous layer is coloured red.

2. Dissolve about 100 mg in 1 ml of sulphuric acid; a red solution is produced. Dilute with water; a yellow precipitate is produced.

MELTING-POINT. About 195°.

ULTRAVIOLET ABSORPTION. In methyl alcohol, maxima at 224 nm (E1%, 1cm = 1650), 252 nm (E1%, 1cm = 940), and 283 nm (E1%, 1cm = 460); in 0.1N alcoholic sodium hydroxide, maximum at 280 nm (E1%, 1cm = 510).

Actions and uses. Danthron is an anthraquinone purgative which acts by stimulating the muscles of the colon. It may colour the urine pink or red. The usual dose is 25 to 50 milligrams which acts in between 6 and 12 hours.

Veterinary uses. Danthron is used in animals as a purgative. The usual dose in all species is 20 to 50 milligrams per kilogram body-weight as a single dose.

Preparations

Preparations available include CAPSULES containing danthron 25 mg with poloxamer "188" 200 mg, capsules containing danthron 50 mg with dioctyl sodium sulphosuccinate 60 mg; an ELIXIR containing danthron 25 mg with poloxamer "188" 200 mg in 5 ml, diluents syrup or tragacanth mucilage, life of diluted elixir 14 days, and an elixir containing danthron 75 mg with poloxamer "188" 1 g in 5 ml, diluents as above; a PREMIX containing danthron 9.8 %; and TABLETS containing danthron 200 mg in conjunction with granules containing sterculia 62%.

Dapsone

Bis(4-aminophenyl) sulphone

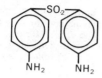

$C_{12}H_{12}N_2O_2S = 248.3$

OTHER NAMES: DADPS; DDS; Diaphenylsulfone

A standard is given in the British Pharmacopoeia 1973

Description. A white or creamy-white, odourless, crystalline powder with a slightly bitter taste.

Solubility. Very slightly soluble in water; soluble, at 20°, in 30 parts of alcohol; soluble in acetone and in dilute mineral acids.

Moisture content. Not more than 1.5%, determined by drying at 105°.

Stability. It becomes discoloured on exposure to light but this is not accompanied by significant decomposition.

Hygroscopicity. It absorbs insignificant amounts of water when stored under ordinary conditions.

Sterilisation. Dapsone is prepared as a sterile powder by the method described under Sulphadimidine. Oily suspensions are sterilised by dry heat.

Identification. MELTING-POINT. About 178°.

ULTRAVIOLET ABSORPTION. In 0.1N hydrochloric acid, maxima at 234 nm (E1%, 1cm = 420) and 288 nm (E1%, 1cm = 350); in methyl alcohol, maxima at 260 nm (E1%, 1cm = 730) and 295 nm (E1%, 1cm = 1200).

Determination in body fluids. COLORIMETRY. In serum —T. N. Higgins and J. D. Taylor, *Clin. Biochem.*, 1973, **6**, 295.

ULTRAVIOLET SPECTROPHOTOMETRY. In urine—J. H. Peters *et al.*, *Int. J. Lepr.*, 1969, **37**, 46.

SPECTROFLUORIMETRY. In plasma or urine—J. H. Peters *et al.*, *J. Lab. clin. Med.*, 1970, **76**, 338.

Metabolism. ABSORPTION. Absorbed slowly but completely after oral administration.

BLOOD CONCENTRATION. After an oral dose of 100 mg, peak serum concentrations of about 2 μg/ml are attained in 3 to 6 hours; after doses of 400 mg twice weekly, peak concentrations of up to 8 μg/ml are attained; blood concentrations are subject to wide variations.

HALF-LIFE. Plasma half-life, 18 to 43 hours.

DISTRIBUTION. Widely distributed throughout the tissues and may persist for several weeks; dapsone is secreted in the milk and is subject to enterohepatic circulation; *protein binding*, 50 to 80% bound to plasma proteins and its monoacetylated metabolite is 97 to 100% bound.

METABOLIC REACTIONS. Acetylation and *N*-oxidation together with glucuronic acid and sulphate conjugation; acetylation exhibits genetic polymorphism similar to the acetylation of isoniazid; acetylated metabolites may be deacetylated; the major *N*-oxidation product is 4-amino-4'-hydroxyaminodiphenylsulphone.

EXCRETION. 70 to 90% of a dose is excreted in the urine with small amounts in the faeces; up to about 20% of a dose is excreted in the urine unchanged together with about 30% as *N*-oxidation products either free (up to 7%)

or conjugated (up to 30%) and the remainder is excreted as glucuronic acid or sulphate conjugates of unchanged drug and its other metabolites.

FURTHER INFORMATION. Absorption and excretion— J. O'D. Alexander *et al.*, *Br. J. Derm.*, 1970, **83**, 620; polymorphic acetylation—R. Gelber *et al.*, *Clin. Pharmac. Ther.*, 1971, **12**, 225; metabolism—Z. H. Israili *et al.*, *J. Pharmac. exp. Ther.*, 1973, **187**, 138 and H. Uehleke and S. Tabarelli, *Archs Pharmac.*, 1973, **278**, 55; genetic factors affecting toxicity—R. J. Cohen *et al.*, *New Engl. J. Med.*, 1968, **279**, 1127.

Actions and uses. Dapsone is an antibacterial substance which, like the sulphonamides, probably acts by preventing the use by certain bacteria of essential metabolites, as its action is antagonised by 4-aminobenzoic acid. Its principal use is in the treatment of leprosy, but it is also of value in unrelated diseases such as dermatitis herpetiformis and mycetoma (maduromycosis). It has a suppressive action on the malaria parasite.

Dapsone is administered by mouth and many dosage schemes have been proposed for the treatment of leprosy. For example, an initial dose of 25 milligrams may be given twice weekly and gradually increased over 3 or 4 months to a maximum of 350 milligrams twice weekly, at which stage the dosage may be changed to 100 milligrams daily if this is more convenient. However, in many cases of leprosy 50 milligrams twice weekly is adequate and gives rise to fewer reactions than higher doses; a dose of 200 milligrams once or twice a week is now rarely exceeded.

The dose corresponding to an adult dose of 50 milligrams is, for children under 1 year 1.25 to 2 milligrams per kilogram body-weight, 1 to 5 years 12.5 to 20 milligrams, and 6 to 12 years 25 milligrams increasing to 50 milligrams.

In certain circumstances, particularly in the treatment of out-patients suffering from leprosy, dapsone may be administered intramuscularly at fortnightly intervals in the form of a suspension of 1.0 to 1.2 grams in 5 millilitres of a sterile vehicle such as arachis oil, chaulmoogra oil, or ethyl esters of hydnocarpus oil, but the injections are liable to cause pain and possibly severe abscess formation.

In tuberculoid leprosy, skin lesions usually disappear in 3 to 9 months and in lepromatous leprosy in 1 to 5 years; in the dimorphous (borderline) form of the disease, lesions disappear in an intermediate period of time. In lepromatous leprosy, acid-fast bacilli can be demonstrated in the skin for months or years after the disappearance of lesions, but these bacilli have undergone characteristic morphological changes, resulting in fragmentation and the appearance of granularity, and, on electron-microscopical examination, appear to be non-viable. However, viable bacilli may persist in the peripheral nervous system, so it is advisable to continue to give maintenance doses of dapsone for 18 months after the disappearance of skin lesions in tuberculoid leprosy and for even longer periods after the disappearance of granular bacilli from the skin in lepromatous leprosy.

In dermatitis herpetiformis the initial dosage is usually 100 milligrams daily, which is gradually reduced to the lowest effective maintenance dose, usually about 25 milligrams on alternate days.

For the suppression of malaria the usual dosage is 100 milligrams of dapsone with 12.5 milligrams of pyrimethamine weekly. The same dosage of dapsone is used in conjunction with other antimalarial drugs in the treatment of chloroquine-resistant *Plasmodium falciparum* infections.

Undesirable effects. Undesirable effects are rare and include anaemia, dermatitis, and hepatitis; psychosis has been reported but has not been proved to be caused by the drug. The anaemia is haemolytic in type and usually disappears when dapsone is withheld. Blood transfusion is required if the anaemia is severe; the administration of a ferrous salt may prove useful by correcting any underlying iron-deficiency anaemia.

Lepra reactions (reactional states), which may complicate the treatment of leprosy, are not toxic effects of dapsone as they can occur during treatment with other unrelated antileprotic drugs, or even when no treatment is being given. Antimalarial drugs, parenteral antimony compounds, and corticosteroids may be of value in the management of these reactions, particularly the type known as erythema nodosum leprosum.

The incidence of untoward effects is greater in coloured races.

Veterinary uses. Dapsone is an antibacterial sulphone used alone or in conjunction with penicillin in the treatment of bovine mastitis. Lactating cows may be given doses of 4 grams daily by intramammary injection in each infected quarter. Dry cows may be given a single dose of 8 to 10 grams by intramammary injection into each quarter for the prophylaxis and treatment of mastitis.

Preparation

DAPSONE TABLETS: the usual strength is 100 mg of dapsone.

A standard for these tablets is given in the British Pharmacopoeia 1973

Containers and *Storage:* see the entry on Tablets for general information on containers and storage. Containers should be airtight.

Advice for patients: when used in the treatment of malaria, doses should be taken at regular intervals and the prescribed course completed.

In leprosy, treatment should not be discontinued without the advice of the prescriber.

Debrisoquine Sulphate

3,4-Dihydroisoquinoline-2(1*H*)-carboxamidine sulphate

$C_{20}H_{28}N_6O_4S = 448.5$

OTHER NAME: *Declinax*®

A standard is given in the British Pharmacopoeia Addendum 1977

Description. A white crystalline odourless powder.

Solubility. Soluble in 40 parts of water; very slightly soluble in alcohol; practically insoluble in chloroform and in ether.

Acidity. A 3% solution has a pH of 5.3 to 6.8.

Storage. It should be stored in airtight containers, protected from light.

Identification. ULTRAVIOLET ABSORPTION. In 0.1N sulphuric acid, maxima at 262 nm (E1%, 1cm = 13.8) and 270 nm (E1%, 1cm = 10.2).

INFRA-RED ABSORPTION. Major peaks at 748, 1045, 1090, 1582, 1612, and 1650 cm⁻¹ (see Appendix 2a: Infra-red Spectra).

Determination in body fluids. GAS CHROMATOGRAPHY. In plasma: debrisoquine and the 4-hydroxy metabolite —S. L. Malcolm and T. R. Marten, *Analyt. Chem.*, 1976, **48**, 807; in blood, plasma, saliva, or urine— M. S. Lennard *et al.*, *J. Chromat.*, 1977, **133**, 161.

Metabolism. ABSORPTION. Rapidly absorbed after oral administration.

BLOOD CONCENTRATION. After an oral dose of 20 mg, peak plasma concentrations of 10 to 50 ng/ml are attained in 2 hours. Peak debrisoquine plasma concentrations following daily administration of 40 mg are between 15 to 180 ng/ml.

HALF-LIFE. The concentration of the unchanged drug in plasma declines biphasically with an α-phase lasting 3.5 to 5.5 hours, followed by a terminal β-phase of 20 to 30 hours.

DISTRIBUTION. Widely distributed in the rat with high concentrations in the kidneys, heart, liver, and lungs.

METABOLIC REACTIONS. Hydroxylation in the 4-position predominates over aromatic hydroxylation at positions 6 and 7. Ring-opened acidic metabolites, produced through hydroxylation at positions 1 and 3 and further oxidation, are also present. There is no evidence of glucuronic acid conjugation in man. 4-Hydroxylation of debrisoquine is polymorphic.

EXCRETION. More than 90% of a dose is excreted within 72 hours of administration, of which 80 to 90% is in the urine. Excretion of unchanged drug in the urine ranges from 8 to 80% of the dose and of the 4-hydroxy metabolite, 0 to 30% of the dose.

FURTHER INFORMATION. Metabolism—J. G. Allen *et al.*, *Drug Met. Disp.*, 1975, **3**, 332 and M. Angelo *et al.*, *Trans. biochem. Soc.*, 1976, **4**, 704; polymorphic hydroxylation in man—A. Mahgoub *et al.*, *Lancet*, ii/1977, 584; plasma concentrations—S. L. Malcolm and T. R. Marten, *Analyt. Chem.*, 1976, **48**, 807; variation in response of hypertensive patients to debrisoquine—J. H. Silas *et al.*, *Br. med. J.*, i/1977, 422.

Actions and uses. Debrisoquine is an antihypertensive agent with actions and uses similar to those of guanethidine sulphate. It lowers blood pressure by selectively blocking transmission at the post-ganglionic adrenergic nerve endings and in tissue concentrations reached with oral therapeutic doses it prevents release of noradrenaline at the nerve endings without producing noradrenaline depletion. Parenteral administration may cause an initial rise in blood pressure, probably due to release of noradrenaline from adrenergic nerve endings.

Debrisoquine is used to control hypertension. It causes a greater fall in blood pressure in the erect than in the supine position. The effect of a single oral dose reaches a maximum within 2 to 3 hours and lasts for about 12 hours in patients with normal renal function.

Debrisoquine is excreted almost entirely through the kidneys and its effects may therefore be increased in patients with renal disease.

In patients with normal renal function treatment is started with an oral dosage of the equivalent of 10 milligrams of debrisoquine twice daily increased by 10 milligrams at intervals of about 3 days until the optimum dosage is reached; maintenance dosage usually lies between the equivalent of 40 and 120 milligrams of debrisoquine daily; 1.3 milligrams of debrisoquine sulphate is equivalent to 1 milligram of debrisoquine.

Tolerance to debrisoquine may occur, making necessary a progressive increase in dose.

A thiazide diuretic may be given with debrisoquine to enhance the antihypertensive effect.

Undesirable effects. Severe postural and effort hypotension, diarrhoea, nasal stuffiness, failure of ejaculation, and fluid retention may occur.

Precautions and contra-indications. Debrisoquine may enhance the effects of circulating catecholamines and may therefore cause a rise in blood pressure. It is contra-indicated in phaeochromocytoma. It should be used with caution in patients with renal insufficiency.

Preparation

DEBRISOQUINE TABLETS: available as tablets containing debrisoquine sulphate equivalent to 10 and 20 mg of debrisoquine base; they may be coloured.

A standard for these tablets is given in the British Pharmacopoeia Addendum 1977.

Containers and *Storage:* see the entry on Tablets for general information on containers and storage. Containers should be airtight.

Advice for patients: the tablets should be taken at regular intervals, preferably after meals. Treatment should not be discontinued without the advice of the prescriber.

Decoquinate

Ethyl 6-decyloxy-7-ethoxy-4-hydroxyquinoline-3-carboxylate

$C_{24}H_{35}NO_5 = 417.5$

OTHER NAME: *Deccox®*

A standard is given in the British Pharmacopoeia (Veterinary)

Description. A cream to buff-coloured, microcrystalline, odourless powder.

Solubility. Practically insoluble in water and in alcohol; very slightly soluble in ether and in chloroform.

Identification. MELTING-POINT. About 242°.

ULTRAVIOLET ABSORPTION. In 0.01N methanolic hydrochloric acid, maximum at 265 nm (E1%, 1cm = 1000).

Veterinary uses. Decoquinate is used to prevent coccidiosis in poultry. It is administered continuously in the feed at a concentration of 40 parts per million. It should not be given to laying birds.

Preparation

DECOQUINATE PREMIX: consisting of decoquinate mixed with powdered cereal or other suitable diluent. This preparation is stable to hot pelleting processes. It must be diluted before administration by mixing thoroughly with the feed. Available as a premix containing 8% of decoquinate.

A standard for this premix is given in the British Pharmacopoeia (Veterinary)

Containers and *Storage:* see the entry on Premixes for general information on containers and storage.

Labelling: the label on the container should state that the preparation should not be given to birds producing eggs for human consumption.

Demeclocycline Hydrochloride

7-Chloro-6-demethyltetracycline hydrochloride, an antimicrobial substance produced by the growth of *Streptomyces aureofaciens.*

$C_{21}H_{22}Cl_2N_2O_8 = 501.3$

OTHER NAMES: Demeclocyclini Hydrochloridum; Demethylchlortetracycline Hydrochloride; *Ledermycin®*

A standard is given in the European Pharmacopoeia Vol. II

Description. A yellow odourless crystalline powder with a bitter taste.

Solubility. Soluble, at 20°, in 30 parts of water and in 45 parts of alcohol; very slightly soluble in acetone, in ether, and in chloroform; soluble in aqueous solutions of alkali hydroxides and carbonates.

Acidity. A 1% solution has a pH of 2 to 3.

Moisture content. Not more than 2%, determined by drying at 60° over phosphorus pentoxide *in vacuo.*

Dissociation constants. pK_a 3.3, 7.2, 9.2 (25°).

Storage. It should be stored in airtight containers, protected from light.

Identification. TESTS. 1. Mix about 500 µg with 2 ml of sulphuric acid; a purple colour is produced. Add 1 ml of water; the colour changes to yellow.

2. Mix about 2 mg with 5 ml of hydrochloric acid and boil for 2 minutes; a yellow colour is produced.

Metabolism. ABSORPTION. Well absorbed after oral administration but absorption may be decreased by divalent and trivalent metal ions, food, and medicaments; demeclocycline is absorbed to a greater extent than tetracycline.

BLOOD CONCENTRATIONS. After an oral dose of 300 mg, a peak serum concentration of about 1.7 µg/ml is attained in 3 to 6 hours; after an intravenous dose of 200 to 500 mg, serum concentrations of 10 to 25 µg/ml are detectable in less than 5 minutes.

HALF-LIFE. Serum half-life, 10 to 15 hours.

DISTRIBUTION. Widely distributed throughout the body and enters the cerebrospinal fluid when the meninges are inflamed; *protein binding,* 36 to 91% bound to plasma proteins.

EXCRETION. 40 to 50% of a dose is excreted in the urine unchanged; large amounts are excreted in the faeces after oral administration but very little is found after intramuscular administration; concentrations reaching 20 to 30 times those in the serum are obtained in the bile but much of this is reabsorbed.

FURTHER INFORMATION. Review of metabolism—M. Finland and L. P. Garrod, *Br. med. J.,* ii/1960, 959.

Actions and uses. Demeclocycline has a range of activity similar to that described under Tetracycline Hydrochloride and is used for similar purposes. As it is excreted more slowly, the concentration in the blood from the same dose is maintained for a longer period.

The usual dosage for an adult is 600 milligrams by mouth daily in 2 to 4 doses. In general tetracyclines should not be given to children but when considered essential the usual dose is 6 to 12 milligrams per kilogram body-weight daily.

Salts of aluminium, calcium, iron, and magnesium, and antacids and milk, which may decrease the absorption of tetracycline from the gut, should not be given with demeclocycline.

Undesirable effects; Precautions and contra-indications. These are described under Tetracycline Hydrochloride; there is the additional hazard of photo-sensitisation which makes it desirable for patients to avoid exposure to sunlight during treatment.

Drug interactions. As for Tetracycline Hydrochloride.

Preparations

DEMECLOCYCLINE CAPSULES (Syn. Demethylchlortetra-cyline Capsules): consisting of demeclocycline hydro-chloride, in powder, which may be mixed with a suitable inert diluent, enclosed in a hard capsule. The capsule shells may be coloured.

Available as capsules containing 150 mg of demeclo-cycline hydrochloride.

A standard for these capsules is given in the British Pharmacopoeia 1973

Containers and *Storage:* see the entry on Capsules for general information on containers and storage. Con-tainers should be light resistant.

Labelling: the label on the container should state the directions for storage and the date after which the cap-sules are not intended to be used.

Advice for patients: the capsules should be taken at regular intervals and salts of aluminium, calcium, iron, and magnesium, and antacids and milk should not be taken within 1 hour. The prescribed course should be completed. Direct exposure to sunlight should be avoided during treatment.

OTHER PREPARATIONS available include TABLETS con-taining demeclocycline hydrochloride 300 mg.

Deoxycortone Acetate

3,20-Dioxopregn-4-en-21-yl acetate

$C_{23}H_{32}O_4 = 372.5$

OTHER NAMES: Deoxycort. Acet.; Desoxycorticosterone Acetate; Desoxycortoni Acetas

A standard is given in the European Pharmacopoeia Vol. II

Description. Odourless colourless crystals or white crystalline powder.

Solubility. Very slightly soluble in water; soluble, at 20°, in 50 parts of alcohol, in 30 parts of acetone, in 170 parts of propylene glycol, in 150 parts of ethyl oleate, in 140 parts of arachis oil, and in other fixed oils.

Specific rotation. +179° to +184°, determined on a 1% solution in alcohol.

Sterilisation. Oily solutions for injection are sterilised by dry heat.

Storage. It should be protected from light.

Identification. TESTS. 1. It complies with Test 1 des-cribed under Betamethasone.

2. It complies with Test 3 described under Cortisone Acetate (presence of acetyl groups).

MELTING-POINT. About 159°.

ULTRAVIOLET ABSORPTION. In alcohol (95%), maximum at 240 nm (E1%, 1cm = 445).

INFRA-RED ABSORPTION. Major peaks at 1244, 1375, 1420, 1667, 1718, and 1745 cm^{-1} (see Appendix 2a: Infra-red Spectra).

THIN-LAYER CHROMATOGRAPHY. See under Thin-layer Chromatography, System 10.

Actions and uses. Deoxycortone is a mineralocorticoid which causes sodium retention and potassium excretion. It is used in conjunction with cortisone or hydrocortisone in the treatment of Addison's disease or after total adren-alectomy in patients in whom cortisone or hydrocor-tisone given alone does not prevent the development of sodium deficiency. For this purpose, however, fludro-cortisone given by mouth is often preferred.

Deoxycortone acetate is given by intramuscular injection in a dosage of 2 to 5 milligrams daily or on alternate days, or as an implant of 100 to 400 milligrams every 4 to 5 months. It may also be given sublingually in a dosage of 2 to 10 milligrams daily in tablets containing 1 milligram.

Undesirable effects. Overdosage causes sodium reten-tion with elevation of blood pressure in both normal and adrenal-deficient subjects, and oedema occasionally occurs.

Preparation

DEOXYCORTONE ACETATE IMPLANTS: consist of sterile cylinders, prepared by heavy compression or fusion, of deoxycortone acetate without the addition of any other substance. The usual strength is 600 mg of deoxycortone acetate.

A standard for these implants is given in the British Pharmacopoeia 1973

Labelling: the label on the container should state the nominal weight.

Storage: they should be protected from light.

Dependence

see DRUG DEPENDENCE

Depression

Depression is an abnormal unpleasant experience of sadness and misery accompanied by loss of interest and a decreased capacity for enjoyment or productive work. It may be accompanied by sleeplessness, dejection, ideas of unworthiness, hypochondriasis, constipation, headache, loss of appetite, or loss of weight. It should be distinguished from the normal response to unhappy events or other environmental stresses which lessens with the passage of time.

Depression may also occur post partum or accompany certain physical illnesses such as hepatitis, Cushing's syndrome, hyperparathyroidism, and brain tumours.

Some individuals respond to environmental stress with excessive depressive reactions in which cases constitutional features must also be involved. Where no environmental stress is apparent the depression is termed endogenous and the patient may suffer in addition from episodes of mania (see Psychoses).

Patients with depression may have difficulty in falling asleep, sleep is fitful and unrefreshing, and the patient may waken early.

Tricyclic antidepressants are usually tried in all forms of depression but are particularly effective in endogenous depression. Monoamine-oxidase inhibitors may be needed in some patients especially those with atypical features of depression. When depression is related to anxiety states, sedatives are used. When depression is related to mania (see Psychoses) major tranquillizers or lithium salts may be required.

Dequalinium Chloride

4, 4' - Diamino - 2, 2' - dimethyl - *NN'* - decamethylenedi - (quinolinium chloride)

$C_{30}H_{40}Cl_2N_4 = 527.6$

OTHER NAMES: *Dequadin®*; *Labosept®*

A standard is given in the British Pharmacopoeia 1973

Description. An odourless creamy-white powder with a bitter taste.

Solubility. Very slightly soluble in water; soluble in 30 parts of boiling water; soluble, at 20°, in 200 parts of propylene glycol.

Moisture content. Not more than 5%, determined by drying at 105° *in vacuo.*

Melting-point. About 315°, with decomposition.

Incompatibility. It is incompatible with soaps and similar anionic compounds, with phenol, and with chlorocresol.

Storage. It should be stored in airtight containers.

Preparation and storage of solutions. See statement on aqueous solutions of antiseptics in the entry on Solutions.

Actions and uses. Dequalinium chloride has antibacterial and antifungal properties. It is active against Gram-positive and Gram-negative bacteria and against *Borrelia vincentii*, *Candida albicans*, and several species of *Trichophyton*. Its action is little affected by the presence of serum.

Dequalinium chloride is used in the treatment of infections of the gums, mouth, and throat, for which it may be administered in lozenges containing 250 micrograms or applied as a paint containing 0.5% in propylene glycol.

Preparations

Preparations available include LOZENGES containing dequalinium chloride 250 micrograms, and PASTILLES containing dequalinium chloride 250 micrograms.

Dermatitis

Inflammation of the skin. Conditions involving dermatitis are described under Eczema.

Dermatomyositis

Dermatomyositis (Polymyositis) is a disorder characterised by inflammatory and degenerative changes in the skin and voluntary muscles. In the skin this results in erythema, scaling, and oedema followed by brownish pigmentation, especially of the skin over affected muscles and joints. In the muscles there is swelling and tenderness accompanied by weakness and sometimes pain which is eventually followed by atrophy and fibrous contractures. When the lesions occur only in the muscles the disease is called polymyositis.

The symptoms of dermatomyositis may be controlled by corticosteroids.

Derris

The dried rhizome and roots of *Derris elliptica* (Roxb.) Benth. and *D. malaccensis* Prain (Fam. Leguminosae) and possibly of other species of *Derris*. The plants are climbers, indigenous to Burma, Thailand, Vietnam, and Malaysia, and have been cultivated in Malaysia, Singapore, Indonesia, the Philippines, Tanzania, and Zaire.

OTHER NAMES: Aker-tuba; Tuba Root

Lonchocarpus may be supplied when derris is demanded; derris may be supplied when lonchocarpus is demanded.

A standard is given in the British Pharmacopoeia (Veterinary)

Varieties. Other species of *Derris*, of which there are over 80, distributed mainly in the tropics of south-east Asia, are known to contain rotenone. Among those that possess insecticidal properties, or contain rotenone, are *D. trifoliata* Lour. (*D. uliginosa* Benth.), *D. philippinensis* Merr., *D. heptaphylla* Merr., *D. polyantha* Perk., *D. thyrsiflora* Benth., *D. robusta* Benth., *D. chinensis* Benth., and *D. amazonica* Killip.

The roots, rhizome, and stem of *D. trifoliata* have been imported, the material consisting mainly of the stem, in pieces 100 to 250 mm long and 8 to 25 mm thick. Portions are commonly found in which two stems have become intertwined. The bark is rusty greyish-brown, very rough, with prominent longitudinal ridges and furrows and numerous reddish-brown warts; it bears the remains of buds protruding at intervals. The outer layer forms grey papery scales, partially detached from the surface. The wood is very tough and hard. The transversely cut surface shows a bark, light-coloured near the outside but darker near the wood; the wood is yellowish to brown, porous and without marked radial structure, and the pith is small. It contains a much smaller proportion of active principle than either *D. elliptica* or *D. malaccensis*.

Constituents. Derris contains a number of toxic crystalline substances, of which (−)-rotenone is the most important. Rotenone ($C_{23}H_{22}O_6$, melting-point about 163°; specific rotation −226°, using a 4% w/v solution in benzene) occurs in amounts of up to about 16%.

Five other related compounds with biological activity have been isolated, these being elliptone and deguelin, together with the hydroxy derivatives, sumatrol, malaccol and toxicarol. Deguelin has not been isolated in its naturally occurring optically active form.

The active constituents are soluble in acetone, in benzene, in chloroform, in ether, and in some other organic solvents, and slightly soluble in alcohol and in mineral oils; they are insoluble in water, in weak acids, and in alkalis. Alkalis, and prolonged boiling with certain solvents, cause a loss of activity due to chemical change or racemisation, or both; pyridine is particularly active in this respect. Carbon tetrachloride gives relatively stable solutions, but rotenone crystallises from such solutions with solvent of crystallisation.

It yields up to 2% of acid-insoluble ash and up to 6% of ash.

Description. UNGROUND DRUG. *Macroscopical characters:* roots, a number sometimes attached to a short piece of rhizome, up to 2 m in length and varying from fine rootlets to roots 8 mm in diameter; very flexible, hard and tough, with a fibrous fracture; externally, greyish-brown to reddish-brown, with numerous fine longitudinal furrows; on thicker pieces, many elongated scars arranged in an irregularly spaced ring formation; the smoothed transversely cut surface showing a brown bark and a wood varying in colour from cream to pale brown, and in larger pieces showing 3 or 4 concentric circles. When viewed in screened ultraviolet radiation, the transversely cut surface and the powder of *D. elliptica* appear grey or yellowish-grey; a filtered ethereal extract (1 in 20) is faintly yellow. *D. malaccenis* treated in the same manner gives an orange colour.

It has a slight but aromatic odour and a taste which is at first slightly bitter but, on chewing, a very persistent sensation of numbness develops in the tongue and gradually extends to the throat.

Microscopical characters: the diagnostic characters are: a 4- or 5-arch primary *xylem* and a wide secondary *xylem* with numerous medullary rays; large xylem *vessels*, usually isolated or rarely in groups of 2 or 3, and about 40 to 220 μm in diameter, also smaller *vessels* in groups of 2 to 6 and about 20 to 40 μm in diameter; *xylem fibres* in groups of 15 to 30; *vessels* and groups of *fibres* embedded in parenchyma which contains *starch* grains, the walls of the cells near the vessels being lignified; *phloem* with tangential bands of *fibres* alternating with parenchyma and sieve-tissue; adjacent to the groups of *fibres*, files of small *parenchymatous cells*, each nearly filled with a *crystal* of calcium oxalate in the form of a prism, about 10 to 20 μm in diameter; *fibres* of both xylem and phloem having only the middle lamellae lignified; *starch* in single or compound grains with 2 to 3 components, single grains rounded or elliptical in outline, components of compound grains, muller-shaped, individual grains about 3 to **6** to **12** to 20 μm in diameter; subrectangular *sclereids* in the phelloderm and pericyclic parenchyma; scattered cells of the parenchyma of the xylem, phloem, and the medullary rays contain rotenone and resin, which appear as a brown mass in the cells.

Incompatibility. Rotenone is readily oxidised in the presence of alkali, and materials of this nature should be avoided in preparing sprays, dips or dusts of derris.

Storage. Derris should be stored in a dry place at a temperature not exceeding 25°.

Veterinary uses. Derris is an insecticide and larvicide. It is chiefly used in the control of ectoparasites of domestic animals.

A dusting-powder or wash containing 1% of derris resins or 0.3% of rotenone, together with sufficient of

a suitable dispersing agent, has been used for the control of warble fly in cattle.

Although it is generally harmless to mammals, derris is extremely toxic to fish, and dip, spray, or wash residues should be allowed to drain into streams or ponds.

Preparations

LONCHOCARPUS DUSTING-POWDER: consisting of powdered lonchocarpus root, powdered derris root, or a mixture of the two, mixed with suitable inert diluents. Available as a dusting-powder containing 1% of rotenone.

When Derris Dusting-powder is demanded, Lonchocarpus Dusting-powder may be supplied.

A standard for this dusting-powder is given in the British Pharmacopoeia (Veterinary)

PREPARED LONCHOCARPUS (Syn. Prepared Lonchocarpus Powder; Lonchocarpus Praeparata): consisting of lonchocarpus or derris, or a mixture of the two, which has been reduced to fine powder and adjusted, if necessary, by the addition of fine powder prepared from lonchocarpus or derris of lower or higher rotenone content, to produce a powder of the required strength. It contains 5% of rotenone.

When Prepared Derris, Prepared Derris Powder, or Derris Praeparata is demanded, Prepared Lonchocarpus may be supplied.

A standard for this powder is given in the British Pharmacopoeia (Veterinary)

Description: a cream to buff powder with a slight odour and a bitter or acrid taste causing a persistent sensation of numbness in the mouth and throat. The diagnostic characters are: *cork cells, sclereids, fibres,* and *parenchymatous cells* described under Derris and Lonchocarpus; if prepared from lonchocarpus only, or from a mixture of lonchocarpus and derris, it contains in addition bordered pitted *vessels* up to 500 μm in diameter, *crystals* of calcium oxalate in the form of prisms up to 30 μm long and *starch granules* up to 25 μm in diameter; if prepared from derris only it contains in addition bordered pitted *vessels* up to 220 μm in diameter, *crystals* of calcium oxalate in the form of prisms up to 20 μm long, and *starch granules* up to 20 μm in diameter.

Incompatibility: rotenone is readily oxidised in the presence of alkali and materials of this nature should be avoided in preparing sprays, dip concentrates, or dusting-powders containing lonchocarpus or derris.

Storage: it should be stored in airtight containers, at a temperature not exceeding 25°, protected from light.

Actions and uses: prepared lonchocarpus depends for its action on the presence of rotenone and other constituents of the drugs and is used as described under Derris.

Desferrioxamine Mesylate

30-Amino-3,14,25-trihydroxy-3,9,14,20,25-penta-azatriacontane-2,10,13,21,24-pentaone methanesulphonate

$$NH_2 \cdot [CH_2]_5 \cdot N \cdot C \cdot [CH_2]_2 \cdot C \cdot NH \cdot [CH_2]_5 \cdot N \cdot C \cdot [CH_2]_2 \cdot C \cdot NH \cdot [CH_2]_5 \cdot N \cdot C \cdot CH_3, \ CH_3 \cdot SO_3H$$

$$C_{26}H_{52}N_6O_{11}S = 656.8$$

OTHER NAMES: Deferoxamine Mesylate; *Desferal*®; Desferrioxamine Methanesulphonate

A standard is given in the British Pharmacopoeia 1973

Description. An odourless white to cream-coloured powder with a bitter taste.

Solubility. Soluble, at 20°, in 5 parts of water and in

20 parts of alcohol; practically insoluble in ether, in chloroform, and in dehydrated alcohol.

Acidity. A 10% solution has a pH of 4.5 to 6.5.

Moisture content. Not more than 2%, determined by Fischer titration.

Storage. It should be stored in airtight containers, at a temperature not exceeding 4°, protected from light.

Metabolism. ABSORPTION. Poorly absorbed after oral administration.

EXCRETION. After an intravenous dose of 154 mg of ^{59}Fe-labelled desferrioxamine, 13 to 65% of the radio-activity is excreted in the urine in 24 hours and a further 1 to 7% after 48 hours.

Actions and uses. Desferrioxamine mesylate is a chelating agent with a specific affinity for iron. It combines with any available iron in the tissues and body fluids and is excreted through the kidneys as ferrioxamine B. Desferrioxamine mesylate is used for the removal of iron in poisoning due to iron. For this purpose it is injected intramuscularly in doses of 2 grams dissolved in 8 to 12 millilitres of water for injections. Gastric lavage should be carried out as quickly as possible with 1% sodium bicarbonate solution. Oral administration of 5 grams of desferrioxamine mesylate in 50 millilitres of fluid should then be used to bind any iron remaining in the stomach and to prevent any further absorption. Intubation may be necessary in comatose patients. Desferrioxamine mesylate may also be administered by continuous intravenous infusion at a rate of not more than 15 milligrams per kilogram body-weight per hour to a maximum dose of 80 milligrams per kilogram body-weight in 24 hours; it may be added to sodium chloride injection or dextrose injection.

Intramuscular injection may be repeated at intervals of 12 hours and if large amounts of iron have been taken it may have to be given to a maximum of 12 grams. The quantity of desferrioxamine given by injection in poisoning should be related to the serum iron level. In suitable cases oral treatment as described above may be given and a decision whether to give injection treatment made when serum iron determinations have been made. Young children with serum levels above 5 milligrams per litre or adults with serum levels of over 8 milligrams per litre require treatment by injection.

Desferrioxamine mesylate is also used in a variety of haemolytic anaemias to remove iron from the body. Dosage is 1 to 1.5 grams daily, given in 1 to 3 intra-muscular injections. Intermittent maintenance treatment may be necessary for several months. It is used in conjunction with venesection in patients with primary haemochromatosis and is the only treatment applicable in secondary haemochromatosis. It has also been used in the treatment of thalassaemia in children.

Eye-drops containing 10% of desferrioxamine mesylate are used for the treatment of ocular siderosis. A suitable vehicle consists of 0.5% of methylcellulose 4000, with 1% of benzyl alcohol, in water for injections. The vehicle is prepared by dispersing the methylcellulose in sufficient of the water, previously heated to 90°, cooling with continuous stirring until the temperature reaches 35°, and adding the benzyl alcohol and sufficient of the water to produce the required volume. The solution is filtered through a number 1 and then a number 2 sintered glass filter, transferred in 5-ml portions to suitable containers (see the entry on Eye-drops), and heated in an autoclave at 110° for 20 minutes. To prepare the eye-drops, 5 ml of the vehicle is transferred aseptically to a vial containing 500 mg of the desferrioxamine mesylate and

shaken, care being taken to ensure that solution is complete, and the solution returned to the eye-drop container. The eye-drops decompose on storage and should be prepared when required for use and discarded not later than 1 week after preparation.

Undesirable effects. Rapid intravenous injection of desferrioxamine mesylate may produce anaphylactic reactions and the rate of injection should never exceed 15 milligrams per kilogram body-weight per hour. There may be pain at the site of intramuscular injection.

Preparation

DESFERRIOXAMINE INJECTION: a sterile solution of desferrioxamine mesylate in water for injections. It is prepared, immediately before use, by dissolving the contents of a sealed container in water for injections. Available as a powder in vials containing 500 mg of desferrioxamine mesylate.

A standard for this injection is given in the British Pharmacopoeia 1973
Containers and *Labelling:* see the entry on Injections for general information on containers and labelling.
Storage: the sealed container should be stored at a temperature not exceeding 4°, protected from light. The injection decomposes on storage and should be used immediately after preparation. Cloudy solutions are unsuitable for use and should be discarded.

Desipramine Hydrochloride

3-(10,11-Dihydro-5*H*-dibenz[*b,f*]azepin-5-yl)-*N*-methyl-propylamine hydrochloride

$C_{18}H_{23}ClN_2 = 302.8$

OTHER NAMES: Desipramini Hydrochloridum; *Pertofran*®

A standard is given in the European Pharmacopoeia Vol. III Supplement

Description. A white crystalline odourless powder with a bitter taste, slightly burning, followed by a sensation of numbness.

Solubility. Soluble, at 20°, in 20 parts of water, in 20 parts of alcohol, and in 4 parts of chloroform; very slightly soluble in ether.

Acidity. A 10% solution has a pH of 4.5 to 5.7.

Dissociation constant. pK_a 9.4.

Sterilisation. Solutions for injection are sterilised by heating in an autoclave or by filtration.

Storage. It should be stored in airtight containers, protected from light.

Identification. TESTS. 1. Dissolve a few mg in 2 ml of nitric acid; an intense blue colour is produced (also given by imipramine).
2. Dissolve about 50 mg in 3 ml of warm water, cool, and add 1 drop of a 2.5% solution of quinhydrone in methyl alcohol; a red colour is gradually produced (distinction from imipramine).
3. Dissolve 500 mg in 20 ml of alcohol, boil, add 5 ml of

a saturated solution of trinitrophenol in alcohol, and allow to cool; the precipitate, after washing with alcohol and drying, melts at about 161°.

MELTING-POINT. About 214°.

ULTRAVIOLET ABSORPTION. In 0.01N hydrochloric acid, maximum at 251 nm (E1%, 1cm = 270) and a shoulder at 270 nm.

INFRA-RED ABSORPTION. Major peaks at 741, 746, 763, 1235, 1449, and 1471 cm⁻¹ (see Appendix 2b: Infra-red Spectra).

Determination in body fluids. GAS CHROMATOGRAPHY. In serum—M. Ervik *et al.*, *Acta pharm. suec.*, 1970, **7**, 625.
Further information may be found under Imipramine Hydrochloride (desipramine is a metabolite of imipramine).

Metabolism. ABSORPTION. Well absorbed after oral administration.

BLOOD CONCENTRATION. During therapy with oral doses of 25 mg thrice daily, plasma concentrations ranged from 8 to 290 ng/ml; therapeutic plasma concentrations are in the range 35 to 100 ng/ml and concentrations above 100 ng/ml may be toxic.

HALF-LIFE. Plasma half-life, 12 hours to 2 days.

DISTRIBUTION. Volume of distribution 15 to 40 litres/kg; in animals, desipramine crosses the placenta; *protein binding*, about 90% bound to plasma proteins.

METABOLIC REACTIONS. Aromatic hydroxylation and possibly hydroxylamine formation. In rats, desipramine inhibits the microsomal oxidation of guanethidine, propranolol, and barbiturates.

EXCRETION. Less than 5% of a dose is excreted in the urine as unchanged drug; the urinary excretion of unchanged drug is pH-dependent and is increased in acid urine.

FURTHER INFORMATION. Metabolism—W. Hammer *et al.*, *Clin. Pharmac. Ther.*, 1969, **10**, 44, A. H. Beckett and S. Al-Sarraj, *J. Pharm. Pharmac.*, 1973, **25**, 335, and C. Von Bahr *et al.*, *Acta pharmac. tox.*, 1974, **34**, 58; serum concentrations—M. Ervik *et al.*, *Acta pharm. suec.*, 1970, **7**, 625; plasma concentrations—W. M. Hammer and B. B. Brodie, *J. Pharmac. exp. Ther.*, 1967, **157**, 503; excretion—F. Sjoqvist *et al.*, *Clin. Pharmac. Ther.*, 1969, **10**, 826.

Actions and uses. Desipramine hydrochloride is a tricyclic antidepressant with actions and uses similar to those described under Amitriptyline Hydrochloride but it has a less tranquillising action.
The usual oral dosage of desipramine hydrochloride is initially 50 to 75 milligrams daily in divided doses, increasing to 150 to 200 milligrams daily over a period of about 5 days. When a satisfactory response has been obtained the drug should be gradually withdrawn, but prolonged maintenance therapy with a daily dosage of 100 to 150 milligrams may be necessary. As desipramine hydrochloride may give rise to insomnia, it should not be administered in the evening.

Undesirable effects; Precautions and contra-indications; Drug interactions. As for Amitriptyline Hydrochloride.

Preparation

DESIPRAMINE TABLETS: available as tablets containing 25 mg of desipramine hydrochloride; they are sugar coated; the coat may be coloured.

A standard for these tablets is given in the British Pharmacopoeia 1973
Containers and *Storage:* see the entry on Tablets for general information on containers and storage. Containers should be airtight.
Advice for patients: when initiating treatment there may be a time-lag of up to 3 weeks before a full therapeutic response is obtained. The tablets may affect mental concentration or occasionally cause drowsiness; persons affected should not drive or operate machinery. Alcohol should be avoided. To avoid possible insomnia, doses should not be taken for several hours before bedtime.

Deslanoside

Deacetyl-lanatoside C, 3-[(*O*-β-D-glucopyranosyl-(1→4)-*O*-2,6-dideoxy-β-D-*ribo*-hexopyranosyl-(1→4)-*O*-2,6-dideoxy-β-D-*ribo*-hexopyranosyl-(1→4)-*O*-2,6-dideoxy-β-D-*ribo*-hexopyranosyl)oxy]-12,14-dihydroxy-3β,5β,12β,14β-card-20(22)-enolide

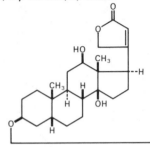

$C_{47}H_{74}O_{19} = 943.1$

OTHER NAME: *Cedilanid®* (this name is also applied to preparations of lanatoside C)

A standard is given in the British Pharmacopoeia Addendum 1977

Description. Odourless hygroscopic white crystals or powder.

Solubility. Very slightly soluble in water, in alcohol, in ether, and in chloroform.

Moisture content. Not more than 7%, determined by drying over phosphorus pentoxide *in vacuo.*

Hygroscopicity. It absorbs about 7% of moisture when exposed to air.

Sterilisation. Solutions for injection are sterilised by heating in an autoclave or by filtration.

Storage. It should be stored in airtight containers, protected from light.

Identification. TESTS. 1. Dissolve about 5 mg in 5 ml of glacial acetic acid, add 2 drops of *ferric chloride test-solution*, mix, and then add carefully 2 ml of sulphuric acid so as to form a lower layer; a brown ring is formed at the interface of the two layers, and the upper layer becomes green, changing to blue on standing. Digitoxin and digoxin also respond to this test.
2. Mix about 500 µg with 0.5 ml of alcohol (60%) and

add 0.25 ml of *dinitrobenzoic acid solution* and 2 drops of *dilute sodium hydroxide solution;* the suspension becomes violet. Digitoxin and digoxin also respond to this test.

MELTING-POINT. It melts indistinctly in the range 220° to 235°.

Metabolism. ABSORPTION. Erratically absorbed after oral administration.

HALF-LIFE. Serum half-life, about 36 hours.

DISTRIBUTION. *Protein binding,* weakly bound to plasma proteins.

METABOLIC REACTIONS. Hydrolysis to form digoxin.

EXCRETION. After a single oral dose, about 80% is excreted in the urine unchanged and about 15% is excreted as digoxin; during maintenance therapy, 30% of the daily dose is excreted in the urine and 3% in the faeces daily, and of the excreted material in the urine, 25% is unchanged and 5% is digoxin.

Actions and uses. Deslanoside has the actions described under Digitalis Leaf. It is derived from lanatoside C but is administered by intravenous or intramuscular injection and is usually reserved for medical emergencies such as pulmonary oedema or left ventricular failure.
The characteristic effects of deslanoside are produced in 10 to 30 minutes, reaching a maximum in 1 to 2 hours, regressing between 16 and 36 hours after administration, and disappearing within 3 to 6 days. The usual digitalising dose is 1 to 1.6 milligrams. When the emergency is past, a suitable oral preparation of a digitalis glycoside should be substituted for maintenance therapy.

Undesirable effects. The undesirable effects described under Digitalis Leaf may occur and may be severe and of rapid onset when deslanoside is given intravenously.

Precautions. As for Digitalis Leaf. The injection should be diluted with sodium chloride injection and injected slowly to minimise toxic effects.

Poisoning. The procedure as described under Digitalis Leaf should be adopted.

Preparation

DESLANOSIDE INJECTION: a sterile solution containing 0.02% of deslanoside, with suitable buffering agents, in water for injections. It is sterilised by heating in an autoclave or by filtration. Available in 2-ml ampoules containing 200 micrograms of deslanoside per ml.
A standard for this injection is given in the British Pharmacopoeia Addendum 1977
Containers and *Labelling:* see the entry on Injections for general information on containers and labelling.
Storage: it should be protected from light.

Dexamethasone

9α - Fluoro - 11β,17α,21 - trihydroxy - 16α - methylpregna-1,4-diene-3,20-dione

$C_{22}H_{29}FO_5 = 392.5$

OTHER NAMES: *Decadron®*; *Dexadreson®*; Dexameth.; Dexamethasonum; *Opticorten®*; *Oradexon®*; *Sisotek®* *Perideca®* (with cyproheptadine hydrochloride); *Maxidex®* (with hypromellose); *Decaspray®* (with neomycin sulphate)

A standard is given in the European Pharmacopoeia Vol. III

Description. A white odourless powder.

Solubility. Very slightly soluble in water; soluble, at 20°, in 42 parts of alcohol and in 165 parts of chloroform.

Specific rotation. +75° to +80°, determined on a 1% solution in dioxan.

Storage. It should be protected from light.

Identification. TESTS. It complies with Tests 1 and 2 described under Betamethasone.

MELTING-POINT. About 253°, with decomposition.

ULTRAVIOLET ABSORPTION. In alcohol (95%), maximum at 240 nm (E1%, 1cm = 385).

INFRA-RED ABSORPTION. Major peaks at 896, 1057, 1071, 1608, 1622, and 1663 cm^{-1} (see Appendix 2a: Infra-red Spectra).

THIN-LAYER CHROMATOGRAPHY. See under Thin-layer Chromatography, System 10.

Determination in body fluids. RADIOIMMUNOASSAY. In plasma or urine—J. English *et al., Eur. J. clin. Pharmac.,* 1975, **9**, 239.

HIGH PRESSURE LIQUID CHROMATOGRAPHY. In plasma— J. C. K. Loo and N. Jordan, *J. Chromat.,* 1977, **143**, 314.

Metabolism. ABSORPTION. Rapidly absorbed after oral administration; intramuscular doses of the acetate are more slowly absorbed than similar doses of the phosphate.

BLOOD CONCENTRATION. After an oral dose of 12 mg, peak plasma concentrations of 100 to 170 ng/ml are attained in 1 to 3 hours; after an oral dose as a solution, peak concentrations may be attained as early as 10 minutes; after a 12-mg dose of a soluble salt intravenously, concentrations of 100 to 200 ng/ml are obtained at 1 hour; the minimum concentrations to give maximal pituitary suppression are 5 to 10 ng/ml.

HALF-LIFE. Plasma half-life, 2 to 5 hours.

DISTRIBUTION. *Protein binding,* about 77% bound to plasma proteins.

METABOLIC REACTIONS. Metabolised to polar metabolites; in rats, two metabolites have been identified as 6-hydroxydexamethasone and 20-dihydrodexamethasone; phenobarbitone and phenytoin may induce dexamethasone metabolism.

EXCRETION. Up to about 65% of a dose is excreted in the urine in 24 hours; urinary excretion of dexamethasone is increased after low dosage following concomitant administration of phenytoin.

FURTHER INFORMATION. Bioavailability—D. E. Duggan *et al., Clin. Pharmac. Ther.,* 1975, **18**, 205 and L. E. Hare *et al., Clin. Pharmac. Ther.,* 1975, **18**, 330; plasma and urine concentrations—J. English *et al., Eur. J. clin. Pharmac.,* 1975, **9**, 239; metabolism: effect of phenytoin —N. Haque *et al., J. clin. Endocr. Metab.,* 1972, **34**, 44 and W. Jubiz *et al., New Engl. J. Med.,* 1970, **283**, 11; absorption and disposal—J. C. Melby and S. L. Dale, *Clin. Pharmac. Ther.,* 1969, **10**, 344.

Actions and uses. Dexamethasone has actions and uses similar to those of prednisolone but is effective in lower dosage; 1 milligram of dexamethasone is approximately equivalent in glucocorticoid activity to 5 milligrams of prednisolone.

Dexamethasone is used in the treatment of all conditions for which cortisone acetate is indicated, except adreno-cortical deficiency states, for which its diminished sodium-retaining properties make it less suitable than cortisone.

It is given by mouth in a dosage of 0.5 to 2 milligrams daily in divided doses, but in potentially fatal conditions, such as leukaemia or pemphigus, up to 12 milligrams daily may be given. Soluble salts such as dexamethasone sodium phosphate may be administered by injection.

Undesirable effects; Precautions and contra-indications. As for Cortisone Acetate.

Veterinary uses. Dexamethasone is a glucocorticoid used in animals to reduce allergic and inflammatory reactions. The usual dose for dogs and cats is 25 to 100 micrograms per kilogram body-weight.

Preparations

DEXAMETHASONE TABLETS: available as tablets containing 0.25, 0.5, 0.75, 2, 5, and 10 mg of dexamethasone; they may be coloured.

A standard for these tablets is given in the British Pharmacopoeia 1973

Containers and *Storage:* see the entry on Tablets for general information on containers and storage. Containers should be airtight and light resistant.

Advice for patients: in long term use treatment should not be discontinued without the advice of the prescriber. Patients may carry an identification card giving details of their treatment and the name of the prescriber, who should be contacted in the event of accident, feverish illness, diarrhoea, vomiting, or alimentary disturbances. In short-term treatment the prescribed course should be completed.

OTHER PREPARATIONS available include an APPLICATION containing dexamethasone 10 mg with neomycin sulphate 50 mg in 90 g, an aerosol pack delivering dexamethasone 75 micrograms with neomycin sulphate 375 micrograms per second when the valve is actuated; EYE-DROPS containing dexamethasone 0.1% and hypromellose 0.5%; and a veterinary INJECTION containing dexamethasone 2 mg per ml in 30-ml vials.

Dexamethasone Sodium Phosphate

9α-Fluoro-11β,17α,21-trihydroxy-16α-methylpregna-1,4-diene-3,20-dione 21-(disodium phosphate)

$C_{22}H_{28}FNa_2O_8P = 516.4$

OTHER NAMES: *Decadron®*; *Dexadreson®*; Dexameth. Sod. Phos.; *Duphacort Q®*; *Oradexon®*

Dupha-Duocort® (with dexamethasone acetate); *Dexafort®* (with dexamethasone phenylpropionate)

A standard is given in the British Pharmacopoeia Addendum 1977 and the British Pharmacopoeia (Veterinary)

Description. A white hygroscopic powder.

Solubility. Soluble in 2 parts of water; soluble in dehydrated alcohol; practically insoluble in chloroform.

Alkalinity. A 1% solution has a pH of 7.5 to 9.5.

Specific rotation. +74° to +79°, determined on a 1% solution.

Sterilisation. Solutions for injection are sterilised by filtration.

Storage. It should be stored in airtight containers, protected from light.

Identification. TESTS. 1. It complies with Test 2 described under Betamethasone.

2. Dissolve about 2 mg in 2 ml of sulphuric acid and allow to stand for 5 minutes; a pale straw colour is produced (distinction from prednisolone sodium phosphate).

Determination in body fluids. See under Dexamethasone.

Metabolism. See under Dexamethasone.

Actions and uses. Dexamethasone sodium phosphate is a water-soluble substance that has the actions and uses described under Dexamethasone; 1.3 milligrams of dexamethasone sodium phosphate is approximately equivalent to 1.2 milligrams of dexamethasone phosphate or 1 milligram of dexamethasone.

Dexamethasone sodium phosphate is administered by intravenous infusion in sodium chloride injection or dextrose injection (5%) in an initial dosage of the equivalent of 0.5 to 20 milligrams of dexamethasone phosphate daily. Subsequently, dosage is adjusted according to the patient's condition and given by intravenous or intramuscular injection.

In states of shock doses equivalent to 2 to 6 milligrams of dexamethasone per kilogram body-weight may be given by intravenous injection or infusion and repeated if necessary after 2 to 6 hours.

Dexamethasone sodium phosphate is of value in relieving cerebral oedema associated with cerebral tumours, cerebro-vascular embolism, or head surgery or injury. The usual initial dose is the equivalent of 10 milligrams of dexamethasone phosphate by intravenous injection, followed by the equivalent of 4 milligrams of dexamethasone phosphate every 6 hours by intramuscular injection.

In the palliative management of inoperable cerebral tumours a smaller maintenance dose of the equivalent of 2 milligrams of dexamethasone phosphate may be used 2 or 3 times a day, and adjusted according to the response of the patient.

Because of its long biological half-life, dexamethasone sodium phosphate is used in diagnostic testing of adreno-cortical hyperfunction by suppressing the secretion of corticotrophin from the pituitary gland.

Dexamethasone sodium phosphate is also used in eye-drops and other preparations for topical treatment of inflammatory or allergic conditions of the eye and skin.

Undesirable effects; Precautions and contra-indications. As for Cortisone Acetate.

Veterinary uses. Dexamethasone sodium phosphate is a soluble glucocorticoid used in animals to reduce allergic and inflammatory reactions, especially in dermatitis, tenosynovitis, and arthritis. It is also used for the induction of premature parturition in cows, mares, and ewes, and in treating ketosis of ruminants. Dexamethasone sodium phosphate may also be given intravenously in the treatment of shock.

The usual dose by intramuscular injection in all species is the equivalent of 20 to 100 micrograms of dexamethasone per kilogram body-weight daily. Similar doses may be given by mouth to dogs and cats. Single doses of the equivalent of 10 milligrams of dexamethasone for horses and 2 milligrams for dogs may be given by intra-articular or periarticular injection.

Preparations

DEXAMETHASONE SODIUM PHOSPHATE INJECTION: a sterile solution of dexamethasone sodium phosphate, with suitable stabilising agents, in water for injections. It is sterilised by filtration.

Available in 50-ml vials containing 2 mg of dexamethasone sodium phosphate per ml, and in 20- and 50-ml vials containing dexamethasone sodium phosphate equivalent to 2 mg of dexamethasone per ml. Also available for human use in 1-ml ampoules containing 5 mg of dexamethasone sodium phosphate per ml, in 2-ml vials containing dexamethasone sodium phosphate equivalent to 4 mg of dexamethasone phosphate (approximately 3.3 mg of dexamethasone) per ml, in 2-ml vials containing dexamethasone sodium phosphate equivalent to 4 mg of dexamethasone per ml, and in 5-ml vials containing dexamethasone sodium phosphate equivalent to 20 mg of dexamethasone per ml.

A standard for this injection is given in the British Pharmacopoeia (Veterinary)

Containers: see the entry on Injections for general information on containers.

Labelling: see the entry on Injections for general information on labelling. In addition, the label on the container should state the amount of the medicament as the equivalent amount of dexamethasone in a suitable dose-volume.

Storage: it should be stored in a cool place, protected from light.

OTHER PREPARATIONS available include a veterinary INJECTION containing dexamethasone sodium phosphate 1 mg with dexamethasone acetate 1 mg per ml in 50-ml vials, and a veterinary injection containing dexamethasone sodium phosphate equivalent to 1 mg of dexamethasone with dexamethasone phenylpropionate equivalent to 2 mg of dexamethasone per ml in 50-ml vials.

Dexamphetamine Sulphate

(S)-α-Methylphenethylammonium sulphate

$$\left[C_6H_5 \cdot CH_2 - \overset{\overset{H}{|}}{\underset{\underset{CH_3}{|}}{C}} - \overset{+}{N}H_3 \right]_2 SO_4^{2-}$$

$C_{18}H_{28}N_2O_4S = 368.5$

OTHER NAMES: *Dexamed®*; Dexamphet. Sulph.; *Dexedrine®*; Dextro Amphetamine Sulphate
Drinamyl® (with amylobarbitone); *Steladex®* (with trifluoperazine hydrochloride)

A standard is given in the British Pharmacopoeia 1973

Description. A white crystalline odourless powder with a saline slightly bitter taste.

Solubility. Soluble, at 20°, in 9 parts of water and in 800 parts of alcohol; practically insoluble in ether.

Acidity. A 5% solution has a pH of 5 to 6.

Dissociation constant. pK_a 9.9.

Specific rotation. +19.5° to +22.0°, determined on an 8% solution.

Identification. TESTS. 1. It complies with Test 1 described under Amphetamine Sulphate; the precipitate melts at about 157°.
2. It complies with Test 2 described under Amphetamine Sulphate.

MELTING-POINT. Above 300°.

Determination in body fluids. GAS CHROMATOGRAPHY. In plasma—D. B. Campbell, *J. Pharm. Pharmac.*, 1969, **21**, 129.

Metabolism. ABSORPTION. Well absorbed after oral administration.

BLOOD CONCENTRATION. After an oral dose of 10 to 15 mg of the sulphate, peak plasma concentrations of 40 to 50 ng/ml are attained in 1 to 1.5 hours falling to 2 ng/ml at 8 to 10 hours.

DISTRIBUTION. Rapidly distributed throughout the body.

METABOLIC REACTIONS. Hydroxylation to form 4-hydroxyamphetamine and 4-hydroxynorephedrine; the (−)-form of amphetamine is not metabolised to 4-hydroxynorephedrine; in rabbits, dexamphetamine is metabolised to phenylacetone which is conjugated with glucuronic acid or glycine; phenylacetone is produced in human tissue *in vitro*.

EXCRETION. The urinary excretion of dexamphetamine is pH-dependent; in acid urine, up to 70% is excreted unchanged in 16 hours and in alkaline urine, about 2 to 9% is excreted.

FURTHER INFORMATION. Excretion—A. M. Asatoor *et al.*, *Br. J. Pharmac.*, 1965, **24**, 293, A. H. Beckett and G. T. Tucker, *J. Pharm. Pharmac.*, 1966, **18**, 72S, and B. Wesley-Hadzija, *J. Pharm. Pharmac.*, 1971, **23**, 366; plasma concentrations—D. B. Campbell, *J. Pharm. Pharmac.* 1969, **21**, 129; metabolism—J. H. Cavanaugh *et al.*, *Clin. Pharmac. Ther.*, 1970, **11**, 656; absorption and excretion—E. Rosen *et al.*, *J. pharm. Sci.*, 1967, **56**, 365.

Actions and uses. Dexamphetamine is a sympathomimetic drug which has the actions and uses described under Amphetamine Sulphate but it is about twice as potent as the racemic compound.

Tolerance occurs after treatment for 2 or 3 weeks during which time psychological dependence may already have been induced.

Dexamphetamine has been used for the treatment of obesity but its use has declined because it is of doubtful value and it carries the risk of producing dependence. It has no effect on the basal metabolic rate or on nitrogen excretion but it makes a restricted food intake more acceptable to the patient, and for this purpose it has been given by mouth in a dosage of 10 milligrams 2 or 3 times a day about half an hour before food. To avoid insomnia the last dose should be taken several hours before bedtime.

Precautions. Dexamphetamine sulphate should not be given to patients who are being treated with a monoamine-oxidase inhibitor, such as isocarboxazid, nialamide, phenelzine, or tranylcypromine, or within about 2 weeks of the discontinuation of such treatment.

Its indiscriminate use in attempts to increase capacity for

work or to overcome fatigue is undesirable, as it is liable to lead to dependence.

Contra-indications. As for Amphetamine Sulphate.

Dependence. It may give rise to dependence of the amphetamine type as described under Drug Dependence.

Poisoning. As for Amphetamine Sulphate.

Preparations

DEXAMPHETAMINE TABLETS: available as tablets containing 5 mg of dexamphetamine sulphate.
A standard for these tablets is given in the British Pharmacopoeia 1973
Containers and *Storage:* see the entry on Tablets for general information on containers and storage. Containers should be airtight.
Advice for patients: the tablets may affect mental concentration; persons so affected should not drive or operate machinery. To avoid insomnia doses should not be taken for several hours before bedtime.

OTHER PREPARATIONS available include CAPSULES containing dexamphetamine sulphate 10 and 15 mg in a slow-release formulation, capsules containing dexamphetamine sulphate 10 mg with amylobarbitone 65 mg in a slow-release formulation, capsules containing dexamphetamine sulphate 15 mg with amylobarbitone 97 mg in a slow-release formulation, capsules containing dexamphetamine sulphate 10 mg with trifluoperazine hydrochloride equivalent to 2 mg of trifluoperazine base, and TABLETS containing dexamphetamine sulphate 5 mg with amylobarbitone 32 mg.

Dextrans

Polymers of glucose in which the linkages between the glucose units are almost entirely of the α-1,6 type. They are produced by the fermentation of sucrose by a strain of *Leuconostoc mesenteroides* (National Collection of Type Cultures No. 10817) followed by hydrolysis and fractionation to give dextrans having different ranges of average molecular weight. Each fraction is designated by a number which, when multiplied by 1000, indicates the weight average molecular weight of that polymer.
The dextran injections are almost colourless, slightly viscous solutions. They are either metabolised as a polysaccharide or excreted; none of them is retained in the body.

Dextran 40 Injection

A sterile 10% solution of dextrans in dextrose injection (5%) or sodium chloride injection. It is sterilised by heating in an autoclave or by filtration. Available in 500-ml containers.

OTHER NAMES: *Gentran 40*®; *Lomodex 40*®; *Rheomacrodex*®

A standard is given in the British Pharmacopoeia 1973

Containers and labelling. See the entry on Injections for general information on containers and labelling.

Storage. It should not be exposed to undue fluctuations in temperature.

Actions and uses. Dextran 40 injection, given intravenously, inhibits the intravascular aggregation of red blood cells, the so-called sludging of blood, which may occur in many pathological conditions associated with local slowing of blood flow. Sludging of the blood may also occur in normal subjects, in whom it is of no path-

ological significance. It is suggested that red blood cell aggregates may plug arterioles and capillaries and so diminish blood flow locally, with the production of tissue anoxia and finally necrosis. However, the clinical implications of intravascular sludging of blood are still uncertain.
As dextran 40 injection inhibits red-cell aggregation and lowers blood viscosity, it may improve local blood supply. It has been recommended for the treatment of a wide variety of clinical conditions where impaired blood flow results in local ischaemia.
In the doses used, dextran 40 injection increases plasma volume for a short time, thereby reducing blood viscosity and increasing blood flow; some of the therapeutic effects claimed for it may be the result of this. Half of a dose is excreted by the kidneys unchanged in 3 hours and most is excreted or metabolised within about 24 hours. It does not interfere with the cross-matching of blood, blood clotting or bleeding mechanisms, or fibrinolysis; it is compatible with heparin.
The initial dose of dextran 40 injection is 500 to 1000 millilitres by intravenous injection, the first 500 millilitres being injected over a period of 30 minutes. This may be followed by 1000 to 2000 millilitres daily by continuous intravenous infusion for 2 days, followed by 500 to 1000 millilitres daily for a further 3 days. In cardiovascular surgery, 20 millilitres per kilogram body-weight may be added to the perfusion fluid. In vascular surgery, 500 millilitres may be given intravenously immediately before and 500 millilitres during the operation, followed post-operatively by 500 millilitres daily for 3 days as a continuous intravenous infusion.
Dextran 40 injection has been recommended for use in vascular and cardiac surgery to reduce the risk of thrombosis, in oligaemic and traumatic shock, severe burns and crush injuries, fat embolism, myocardial and cerebral ischaemia, venous thrombosis, arterial embolism, pancreatitis, and peritonitis, and also in angiography.

Precautions and contra-indications. Dextran 40 injection should be given with caution to patients with congestive heart failure, renal impairment, or polycythaemia, and after blood and electrolyte replacement. It should not be administered at a rate greater than 500 millilitres an hour to dehydrated patients. It is contra-indicated in patients with thrombocytopenia, as it lowers the platelet count, and in severe congestive heart failure and renal failure with anuria.

Dextran 70 Injection

A sterile 6% solution of dextran 70 in dextrose injection (5%) or in sodium chloride injection. It is sterilised by heating in an autoclave or by filtration. Available in 500-ml containers.

OTHER NAMES: *Gentran 70*®; *Lomodex 70*®; *Macrodex*®

A standard is given in the British Pharmacopoeia 1973

Containers and labelling. See the entry on Injections for general information on containers and labelling.

Storage. It should not be exposed to undue fluctuations in temperature.

Actions and uses. Dextran 70 injection has actions and uses similar to those described under Dextran 110 Injection. About 30% is excreted unchanged in the urine in 6 hours.
It is also used in the prevention of post-operative thrombosis, 500 to 1000 millilitres being given over 4 to 6 hours, followed by further doses of 500 millilitres on alternate days.

Precautions and contra-indications. As for Dextran 40 Injection.

Dextran 110 Injection

A sterile 6% solution of dextran 110 in dextrose injection (5%) or sodium chloride injection. It is sterilised by heating in an autoclave or by filtration. Available in 500-ml containers.

OTHER NAME: *Dextraven 110®*

A standard is given in the British Pharmacopoeia 1973

Containers and labelling. See the entry on Injections for general information on containers and labelling.

Storage. It should not be exposed to undue fluctuations in temperature.

Actions and uses. Dextran 110 injection, given intravenously, is an effective temporary plasma substitute, because its osmotic pressure is approximately the same as that of the plasma proteins. When infused, about 40% is excreted unchanged in the urine in 24 hours but a significant proportion is retained in the circulation for 2 or 3 days, a period long enough for the normal physiological replacement of the plasma proteins.

Dextran 110 injection helps to maintain the blood volume and to increase the venous return. It raises a lowered blood pressure.

Dextran 110 injection is used to restore blood volume if this has been reduced by haemorrhage, extravasation of blood or plasma, injury, shock, surgery, or burns. It is also used prophylactically in major surgery to maintain the blood pressure and prevent surgical shock during long operations or those associated with much haemorrhage.

The dose of dextran 110 injection and the rate of infusion depend on the condition being treated or whether it is used prophylactically. After moderate blood loss, 500 millilitres infused rapidly during 15 minutes and a further 500 millilitres given during 30 to 45 minutes may suffice. For the treatment of severe haemorrhage, 1000 millilitres may be infused rapidly with a further 500 millilitres given more slowly later if necessary. In the case of injury and shock, plasma proteins leak into the tissues and draw water osmotically from the blood. These conditions may be treated by infusing 500 millilitres or more, the rate of infusion depending on the degree of shock. Large quantities may be needed in the first few days for the treatment of burns, during which 3000 millilitres may be given; electrolytes are also required.

For prophylaxis during surgical operations associated with blood loss or shock, intravenous drip at the rate of 10 to 20 drops a minute is given as soon as the patient has been anaesthetised, and the rate adjusted to maintain a normal blood pressure during the operation.

Precautions and contra-indications. Blood samples for cross matching should be taken from patients before infusion with dextran 110 injection in case blood or packed cells need to be given later. These may be necessary after infusing large quantities of dextran 110 injection, which is unable to transport oxygen and dilutes the blood-clotting factors. It should not be used for the treatment of haemorrhage associated with hypofibrinogenaemia.

Dextromethorphan Hydrobromide

(+)-3-Methoxy-*N*-methylmorphinan   hydrobromide monohydrate

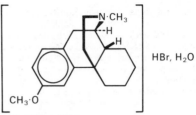

$C_{18}H_{26}BrNO,H_2O = 370.3$

OTHER NAMES: *Cosylan®*
Dexylets® (with phenylephrine hydrochloride)

A standard is given in the British Pharmacopoeia 1973

Description. A white crystalline odourless powder with a bitter taste.

Solubility. Soluble, at 20°, in 60 parts of water and in 10 parts of alcohol; soluble in chloroform with separation of water; practically insoluble in ether.

Acidity. A 2% solution has a pH of 5.2 to 6.5.

Moisture content. 4 to 5.5%, determined by drying at 80° *in vacuo*.

Dissociation constant. pK_a 8.3.

Storage. It should be stored in airtight containers.

Identification. TESTS. 1. Mix about 50 mg with 2 ml of *dilute sulphuric acid* and add 1 ml of a freshly prepared solution made by dissolving 0.7 g of mercuric nitrate in 4 ml of water and adding 0.1 g of sodium nitrite and filtering; no immediate red colour is produced. Heat the solution for 15 minutes; a yellow to red colour develops.
2. Dissolve 5 mg in 1 ml of water, add 1 drop of *dilute hydrochloric acid*, and a mixture of 1 ml of *potassium ferricyanide solution*, 1 drop of *ferric chloride test-solution*, and 4 ml of water; no green or bluish-green colour develops within 15 minutes (distinction from morphine).
3. Add 1 mg to 1 ml of a 1% solution of ammonium molybdate in sulphuric acid; a greenish-yellow colour develops.

MELTING-POINT. About 125°, with decomposition.

ULTRAVIOLET ABSORPTION. In water, maximum at 278 nm (E1%, 1cm = 55).

THIN-LAYER CHROMATOGRAPHY. See under Thin-layer Chromatography, System 7.

Determination in body fluids. GAS CHROMATOGRAPHY. In plasma—A. Noirfalaise, *J. Chromat.*, 1974, **90**, 392.

Metabolism. ABSORPTION. Absorbed after oral administration.

BLOOD CONCENTRATION. After an oral dose of 30 mg of the hydrobromide, 10, 25, and 10% of the dose is detectable in the blood at 1, 2.5, and 6 hours respectively after administration.

METABOLIC REACTIONS. *N*-Demethylation and *O*-demethylation followed by sulphate or glucuronic acid conjugation; the major metabolite is (±)-3-hydroxy-*N*-methylmorphinan and the other metabolites are (+)-3-hydroxymorphinan and possibly (+)-3-methoxymorphinan and their respective conjugates.

EXCRETION. Up to 56% of a dose is excreted in the urine, about 8% being excreted unchanged in 6 hours; in rats, dextromethorphan is excreted in the bile and twice as much may be detectable in the faeces than in the urine.

FURTHER INFORMATION. Micro-method of determining concentrations in blood—W. E. Large *et al.*, *J. pharm. Sci.*, 1968, **57**, 124.

Actions and uses. Dextromethorphan hydrobromide has a depressant action on the cough centre similar to that described under Codeine Phosphate, but it has no analgesic or expectorant effect, no other depressant action on the central nervous system, nor any other established pharmacological action. Its use does not lead to addiction.

The recommended dosage is 15 to 30 milligrams by mouth once to 4 times a day, or half this dose for a child. Much higher doses have been used repeatedly without harm.

Preparations

DEXTROMETHORPHAN TABLETS: available as tablets containing 15 mg of dextromethorphan hydrobromide; they are sugar coated.
A standard for these tablets is given in the British Pharmacopoeia 1973
Containers and *Storage:* see the entry on Tablets for general information on containers and storage. Containers should be airtight.

OTHER PREPARATIONS available include an ELIXIR containing dextromethorphan hydrobromide 13.5 mg in 5 ml, diluent syrup, life of diluted elixir 14 days; LOZENGES containing dextromethorphan hydrobromide 2.5 mg with phenylephrine hydrochloride 500 micrograms.

Dextromoramide Tartrate

(+)-1-(3-Methyl-4-morpholino-2,2-diphenylbutyryl)pyrrolidine hydrogen tartrate.

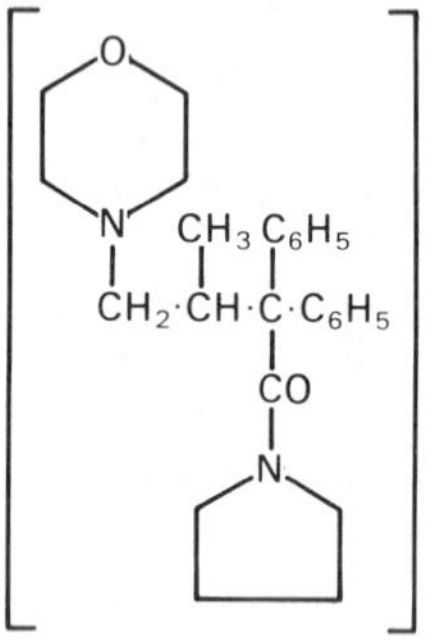

$C_{29}H_{38}N_2O_8 = 542.6$

OTHER NAME: *Palfium®*

A standard is given in the British Pharmacopoeia 1973

Description. An odourless white crystalline powder with a bitter taste.

Solubility. Soluble, at 20°, in 25 parts of water and in 85 parts of alcohol; practically insoluble in chloroform.

Melting-point. About 190°, with slight decomposition.

Specific rotation. +24.5° to +25.7°, determined on a 3% solution.

Sterilisation. Solutions for injection are sterilised by heating in an autoclave or by filtration.

ULTRAVIOLET ABSORPTION. In 1N hydrochloric acid, maxima at 254 nm (E1%, 1cm = 7), 259 nm (E1%, 1cm = 7.7), and 264 nm (E1%, 1cm = 6.7).

Actions and uses. Dextromoramide is a potent analgesic with actions and uses similar to those of methadone hydrochloride. It is used for the alleviation of severe pain.

The usual dose is the equivalent of 5 milligrams of dextromoramide by mouth or by subcutaneous or intramuscular injection, repeated in accordance with the needs of the patient.

Undesirable effects. Nausea, vomiting, dizziness, faintness, and constriction of the pupil may occur. As with morphine, many of these effects occur more often in ambulant than in recumbent patients. When administered in therapeutic doses for prolonged periods, dextromoramide may lead to the development of tolerance, euphoria, and dependence of the morphine type (see under Drug Dependence). Dextromoramide is a powerful respiratory depressant. Cumulation occurs with repeated dosage.

Precautions. It should be used with caution in patients with hepatic insufficiency or hypotension.

Poisoning. The procedure as described under Morphine Hydrochloride should be adopted.

Preparations

DEXTROMORAMIDE INJECTION (*Syn.* Dextromoramide Tartrate Injection): a sterile solution of dextromoramide tartrate, with sodium chloride, in water for injections. It is sterilised by heating in an autoclave or by filtration. Available in 1-ml ampoules as a solution containing dextromoramide tartrate equivalent to 5 and 10 mg of dextromoramide.
A standard for this injection is given in the British Pharmaceutical Codex 1973
Containers and *Labelling:* see the entry on Injections for general information on containers and labelling.

DEXTROMORAMIDE TABLETS: available as tablets containing dextromoramide tartrate equivalent to 5 and 10 mg of dextromoramide.
A standard for these tablets is given in the British Pharmacopoeia 1973
Containers and *Storage:* see the entry on Tablets for general information on containers and storage. Containers should be airtight.
Labelling: the label on the container should state the amount of the medicament as the equivalent amount of dextromoramide.

OTHER PREPARATIONS available include SUPPOSITORIES containing dextromoramide tartrate equivalent to 10 mg of dextromoramide.

Dextropropoxyphene Hydrochloride

(+)-(2S,3R)-4-Dimethylamino-3-methyl-1,2-diphenyl-but-2-yl propionate hydrochloride *or* (+)-dimethyl[(2R, 3S)-2-methyl-3,4-diphenyl-3-propionyloxybutyl]-ammonium chloride

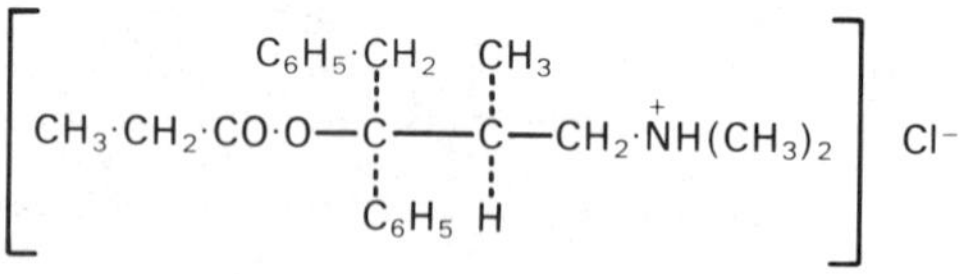

$C_{22}H_{30}ClNO_2 = 375.9$

OTHER NAMES: *Depronal SA®*; Propoxyphene Hydrochloride; *SK 65®*
Distalgesic® (with paracetamol)

A standard is given in the British Pharmacopoeia 1973

Description. A white or slightly yellow odourless powder with a bitter taste.

Solubility. Soluble, at 20°, in 0.3 part of water, in

1.5 parts of alcohol, and in 0.6 part of chloroform; practically insoluble in ether.

Specific rotation. +36° to +40°, determined on a 1% solution.

Sterilisation. Solutions for injection are sterilised by filtration.

Storage. It should be stored in airtight containers.

Identification. MELTING-POINT. About 165°.

THIN-LAYER CHROMATOGRAPHY. See under Thin-layer Chromatography, System 7.

Determination in body fluids. SPECTROPHOTOMETRY. In blood and urine—J. E. Wallace et al., J. forens. Sci., 1972, **17**, 164.

GAS CHROMATOGRAPHY. In plasma: dextropropoxyphene and its metabolite nordextropropoxyphene—K. Verebely and C. E. Inturrisi, J. Chromat., 1973, **75**, 195; in plasma: dextropropoxyphene and major metabolites —J. F. Nash et al., J. pharm. Sci., 1975, **64**, 429 and M. Cleeman, J. Chromat., 1977, **132**, 287; in blood and urine—see J. E. Wallace et al., above.

FLUORIMETRY. In urine: stated to avoid interference from main metabolite—J. C. Valentour et al., Clin. Chem., 1974, **20**, 275.

Metabolism. ABSORPTION. The hydrochloride and napsylate salts of dextropropoxyphene are readily absorbed after oral administration.

BLOOD CONCENTRATION. After an oral dose of 65 mg of the hydrochloride, a peak plasma concentration of 0.02 to 0.15 μg/ml is attained in 1 to 3 hours, and after an equivalent dose of the napsylate (100 mg), a similar peak concentration is attained in 2 to 3 hours; after an intravenous dose of 50 to 65 mg of the hydrochloride, a plasma concentration of 0.17 to 0.49 μg/ml is attained in 15 to 30 minutes, and after a similar intramuscular dose, a peak plasma concentration of 0.02 to 0.18 μg/ml is attained in 2 to 3 hours.

HALF-LIFE. After the oral administration of the napsylate, the plasma half-life is about 11 hours for dextropropoxyphene and about 35 hours for the N-demethylated metabolite (norpropoxyphene); after oral, intramuscular, and intravenous administration of the hydrochloride, plasma half-lives are about 3.5, 3.5, and 2 hours respectively. Other reports of plasma half-life for dextropropoxyphene are in the range 2 to 6 hours.

DISTRIBUTION. Rapidly distributed and concentrated in the brain, lungs, liver, and kidneys, and possibly in the body fat.

METABOLIC REACTIONS. N-Demethylation to norpropoxyphene and to dinorpropoxyphene which may be cyclised. Dextropropoxyphene is subject to substantial first pass metabolism.

EXCRETION. 60 to 70% of a dose is excreted in the urine in 5 days, about 5% as unchanged drug, mainly in the first 24 hours, and the remainder as N-demethyldextropropoxyphene in unconjugated form.

FURTHER INFORMATION. Excretion—R. E. McMahon et al., Toxic. appl. Pharmac., 1971, **19**, 427; plasma concentration—J. F. Nash et al., Toxic. appl. Pharmac., 1971, **19**, 537; plasma concentration of dextropropoxyphene and metabolites—J. F. Nash et al., J. pharm. Sci., 1975, **64**, 429; first pass effect—D. Perrier and M. Gibaldi, J. clin. Pharmac., 1972, **12**, 449; review of bioavailability and of metabolism—R. I. Poust et al., J. Am. pharm. Ass., 1976, **16**, 100; half-life, plasma concentration—K. Verebely and C. E. Inturrisi, Clin.

Pharmac. Ther., 1974, **15**, 302; plasma concentrations of dextropropoxyphene and norpropoxyphene, half-lives —R. L. Wolen et al., Clin. Pharmac. Ther., 1975, **17**, 15.

Actions and uses. Dextropropoxyphene is an analgesic of potency similar to codeine but it is less constipating. It does not have antitussive or anti-inflammatory properties. Unlike most potent analgesics its use does not appear to lead to tolerance and euphoria and it rarely causes dependence.

Up to 260 milligrams of dextropropoxyphene hydrochloride may be taken daily.

Its action as an analgesic develops rapidly; a dose of 65 milligrams of dextropropoxyphene hydrochloride produces its full effect in 1 to 2 hours and lasts for 5 to 6 hours. It is frequently given in conjunction with aspirin or paracetamol.

Undesirable effects. Nausea, vomiting, drowsiness, dizziness, and rashes may occur. Abuse of dextropropoxyphene has been reported and drug dependence of the morphine type may rarely occur.

Poisoning. Large doses depress respiration, and alcohol and barbiturates enhance the toxic effects of dextropropoxyphene.

Where an overdose of a preparation containing both dextropropoxyphene and paracetamol has been taken, the effects of dextropropoxyphene appear rapidly and should be treated first.

Analeptics should not be given as they may provoke convulsions.

Nalorphine, levallorphan, or naloxone should be given and if necessary artificial respiration should be applied.

Preparations

Preparations available include CAPSULES containing dextropropoxyphene hydrochloride 65 mg, capsules containing dextropropoxyphene hydrochloride 150 mg in a slow-release formulation, and TABLETS containing dextropropoxyphene hydrochloride 32.5 mg with paracetamol 325 mg.

Dextropropoxyphene Napsylate

(+)-(2S,3R)-4-Dimethylamino-3-methyl-1,2-diphenylbut-2-yl propionate naphthalene-2-sulphonate monohydrate or (+)-dimethyl[(2R,3S)-2-methyl-3,4-diphenyl-3-propionyloxybutyl]ammonium naphthalene-2-sulphonate monohydrate

$C_{32}H_{37}NO_5S,H_2O = 565.7$

OTHER NAMES: Doloxene®; Propoxyphene Napsylate Distalgesic Soluble® (with paracetamol); Dolosan® and Napsalgesic® (both with aspirin)

A standard is given in the British Pharmacopoeia 1973

Description. A white odourless powder with a bitter taste.

Solubility. Very slightly soluble in water; soluble, at 20°, in 13 parts of alcohol and in 3 parts of chloroform.

Melting-point. About 160°.

Moisture content. 3 to 5%, determined by Fischer titration.

Determination in body fluids; Metabolism. See under Dextropropoxyphene Hydrochloride.

Actions and uses. Dextropropoxyphene napsylate has the actions, uses, and undesirable effects described under Dextropropoxyphene Hydrochloride, but it is less bitter and less irritant to the mucous membranes; 100 milligrams of dextropropoxyphene napsylate is approximately equivalent to 65 milligrams of dextropropoxyphene hydrochloride.

The usual dosage is up to 400 milligrams daily in divided doses.

Poisoning.   As   for   Dextropropoxyphene   Hydrochloride.

Preparations

DEXTROPROPOXYPHENE CAPSULES (*Syn.* Propoxyphene Capsules): consisting of dextropropoxyphene napsylate, in powder, which may be mixed with a suitable inert diluent, enclosed in a hard capsule. The capsule shells may be coloured.

Available as capsules containing dextropropoxyphene napsylate equivalent to 65 mg of dextropropoxyphene hydrochloride.

A standard for these capsules is given in the British Pharmacopoeia 1973

Containers and *Storage:* see the entry on Capsules for general information on containers and storage.

Labelling: the label on the container should state the amount of the medicament as the equivalent amount of dextropropoxyphene hydrochloride.

Advice for patients: the capsules may cause drowsiness; persons affected should not drive or operate machinery. Alcohol should be avoided.

OTHER PREPARATIONS available include TABLETS containing dextropropoxyphene napsylate 50 mg with aspirin 500 mg, tablets containing dextropropoxyphene napsylate 100 mg with aspirin 325 mg, and soluble tablets containing dextropropoxyphene napsylate 50 mg with paracetamol 325 mg.

Dextrose

D-(+)-Glucopyranose monohydrate
$C_6H_{12}O_6,H_2O = 198.2$

OTHER NAMES: Dextrose Monohydrate; Glucose

A standard is given in the British Pharmacopoeia 1973

Description. Odourless colourless crystals or white or cream-coloured crystalline or granular powder with a sweet taste.

Solubility. Soluble, at 20°, in 1 part of water and in 200 parts of alcohol; soluble in glycerol.

Moisture content. 7 to 10%, determined by drying at 105°.

Specific rotation. +52.5° to +53.0°, determined on a solution prepared by dissolving 10 g in 50 ml of water, adding 0.2 ml of *dilute ammonia solution*, diluting to 100 ml, and allowing to stand for 30 minutes.

Identification. TESTS. 1. Heat a small quantity; it melts, swells up, and burns, evolving an odour of burnt sugar. 2. Heat a small quantity with *potassium cupri-tartrate solution;* a copious precipitate of cuprous oxide is produced.

Metabolism. ABSORPTION. Readily absorbed after oral administration by both active and passive mechanisms.

BLOOD CONCENTRATION. Normal concentrations in the blood are about 0.8 mg/ml which may rise to 1.8 mg/ml postprandially; in diabetes, blood concentrations may rise to over 2.5 mg/ml.

HALF-LIFE. Postprandial concentrations fall to fasting concentrations within 2 to 3 hours.

DISTRIBUTION. Widely distributed and utilised throughout the tissues; it is utilised directly or stored in liver and muscle as glycogen; the utilisation of dextrose is hormonally controlled.

METABOLIC REACTIONS. Formed from food carbohydrates by enzymatic hydrolysis in the gastro-intestinal tract; dextrose is an important source of energy and its oxidation results in the formation of stores of energy in high-energy phosphate bonds; dextrose is ultimately metabolised to carbon dioxide and water but may be converted to glycogen for storage or to lactic acid when oxygen is deficient.

EXCRETION. Dextrose is not normally excreted in the urine. However, at blood concentrations greater than 1.8 mg/ml, the renal threshold is exceeded.

Actions and uses. The chief use of dextrose is as a food and it is the substance to which carbohydrates, when given by mouth, are mainly converted. It also has an indirect food value because of the part it plays in the metabolism of fats and proteins. In the absence of sufficient glucose, the amount of fat oxidised is greatly increased and by-products such as hydroxybutyric acid and acetoacetic acid accumulate in the blood giving rise to ketosis.

Dextrose is given in all conditions associated with insufficiency of carbohydrates; it provides a rapidly available source of energy.

Aqueous solutions of dextrose are given by intravenous injection to increase the volume of the circulating blood in shock and to counteract dehydration; when it is desired to replace excessive salt loss, as in persistent vomiting, sodium chloride may be included in the solution.

Hypertonic dextrose solutions (10 to 50%) are given by intravenous injection to provide temporary relief from the symptoms of increased intracranial pressure and for hypoglycaemic coma, but such solutions are liable to cause venous thrombosis at the site of injection.

Dextrose may be administered by mouth in solution or, when necessary, a 5% solution may be given rectally as a retention enema.

Dextrose is given by mouth in a single dose of 50 grams, after overnight fasting, in glucose tolerance tests for the detection of diabetic conditions. Patients should be kept under observation since the test may precipitate ketoacidosis.

When dextrose is required in infant feeding to supplement the carbohydrate content of cows' milk, dextrose (monohydrate) is usually employed.

Undesirable effects. Dextrose injections, and particularly hypertonic dextrose injections, may have a low pH, and such solutions when injected may irritate the venous intima near the site of the injection so causing thrombophlebitis.

Veterinary uses. See under Dextrose, Anhydrous.

Preparation

COMPOUND SODIUM CHLORIDE AND DEXTROSE POWDER (*Syn.* Electrolyte Powder): for each powder take:

Sodium chloride, in powder	0.50 g
Dextrose (monohydrate), in powder	20.00 g
Potassium chloride, in powder	0.75 g
Sodium bicarbonate, in powder	0.75 g

Mix, as described in the entry on Powders, and dispense in airtight single-unit containers or wrap individually using an inner waxed paper or an outer covering of metal foil.

It contains in 1 litre, when reconstituted (see below), 35 mmol of Na$^+$, 20 mmol of K$^+$, 37 mmol of Cl$^-$, 18 mmol of HCO$_3^-$, and 200 mmol of dextrose. The total osmolarity is 310 mosmol per litre.

When Small Size Compound Sodium Chloride and Dextrose Powder is ordered, a powder of identical composition containing 8.8 g in each single-unit container is supplied; the powder is dissolved, as described under Uses, in sufficient water, recently boiled and cooled, to make 200 ml (7 fl. oz.) of solution.

Compound sodium chloride and dextrose powder, and small size compound sodium chloride and dextrose powder, may be flavoured.

A standard for this powder is given in the British Pharmaceutical Codex Supplement 1976

Labelling: directions for using the powder should be stated on the label or in a leaflet or card enclosed with the powders or single-dose units issued to the patient.

Uses: one powder or single-dose unit (22 g) is dissolved in sufficient water, recently boiled and cooled, to make 500 ml (17½ fl. oz.) of solution. Hygienic precautions should be taken throughout the preparation. Any portion of the solution remaining after 24 hours should be discarded.

The solution is administered by mouth as directed for rehydration and electrolyte replacement in the treatment of infantile diarrhoea.

Dextrose, Anhydrous

D-(+)-glucopyranose

$C_6H_{12}O_6 = 180.2$

OTHER NAMES: Anhydrous Dextrose for Parenteral Use; Anhydrous Glucose; Dextrosum Anhydricum ad Usum Parenterale

A standard is given in the European Pharmacopoeia Vol. II

Description. A white crystalline odourless powder with a sweet taste.

Solubility. Soluble, at 20°, in 1 part of water and in 200 parts of alcohol; soluble in glycerol.

Moisture content. Not more than 1%, determined by Fischer titration.

Specific rotation; Identification; Metabolism. See under Dextrose.

Sterilisation. Solutions for injection are sterilised immediately after preparation by heating in an autoclave.

Actions and uses. Anhydrous dextrose is used for the preparation of injections of dextrose, the actions and uses of which are described under Dextrose.

Veterinary uses. Dextrose is used in the treatment of ketosis in ruminants, the usual dose being 200 grams for cattle and 50 grams for sheep, administered by slow intravenous injection. It is also used as a carbohydrate source in feed supplements and in the treatment of hypoglycaemia in piglets, the usual dose being 3 grams

by intra-peritoneal injection, and in dogs, the usual dose being 500 milligrams per kilogram body-weight by slow intravenous injection.

Preparations

DEXTROSE INJECTION: a sterile solution of anhydrous dextrose, or the equivalent amount of dextrose monohydrate for parenteral use, in water for injections. It is sterilised, immediately after preparation, by heating in an autoclave. The usual strength is one containing 5% of anhydrous dextrose but various other strengths are used including a solution containing 50% of anhydrous dextrose described separately below.

A standard for this injection is given in the British Pharmacopoeia 1973

Containers: see the entry on Injections for general information on containers.

Labelling: see the entry on Injections for general information on labelling. In addition, the label on the container should state the amount of the medicament as the amount of anhydrous dextrose in grams per litre.

Storage: it should be stored at a temperature not exceeding 25°.

POTASSIUM CHLORIDE AND DEXTROSE INJECTION: a sterile solution of potassium chloride, with anhydrous dextrose or the equivalent amount of dextrose monohydrate for parenteral use, in water for injections. It is sterilised, immediately after preparation, by heating in an autoclave. The usual strength is 0.3% of potassium chloride (40 millimoles each of K$^+$ and Cl$^-$ per litre) with 5% of anhydrous dextrose.

A standard for this injection is given in the British Pharmacopoeia 1973

Containers: see the entry on Injections for general information on containers.

Labelling: see the entry on Injections for general information on labelling. In addition, the label on the container should state the amounts of the medicaments as the percentages w/v of potassium chloride and anhydrous dextrose.

When the injection is intended for intravenous infusion, the label should also state that rapid infusion may be harmful and the approximate concentrations, in millimoles per litre, of the potassium ions and the chloride ions and the number of grams per litre of anhydrous dextrose.

Storage: it should be stored at a temperature not exceeding 25°.

POTASSIUM CHLORIDE, SODIUM CHLORIDE, AND DEXTROSE INJECTION: a sterile solution of potassium chloride, sodium chloride, and anhydrous dextrose or the equivalent amount of dextrose monohydrate for parenteral use, in water for injections. It is sterilised, immediately after preparation, by heating in an autoclave. It contains 0.18% of sodium chloride (30 mmol of Na$^+$ per litre) and 4% of anhydrous dextrose. The usual strengths of potassium chloride are those that provide between 10 and 40 mmol of K$^+$ per litre. The prescriber should state the strength of potassium chloride required in millimoles per litre.

A standard for this injection is given in the British Pharmacopoeia Addendum 1978

Containers: see the entry on Injections for general information on containers.

Labelling: see the entry on Injections for general information on labelling. In addition, the label on the container should state the amounts of the medicaments as the percentage w/v of potassium chloride, a sodium chloride content of 0.18% w/v, and an anhydrous dextrose content of 4% w/v, the concentration of potassium chloride in grams per litre and the approximate concentration of K^+ in millimoles per litre, a sodium chloride content of 1.8 g per litre equivalent to approximately 30 mmol of Na^+ per litre, the Cl^- content in millimoles per litre, and an anhydrous dextrose content of 40 g per litre.

The label should also state that rapid infusion may be harmful, and that solutions containing visible solid particles must not be used.

Storage: it should be stored at a temperature not exceeding 25°. On storage, separation of small solid particles from glass containers may occur. Solutions containing such particles must not be used.

SODIUM CHLORIDE AND DEXTROSE INJECTION: a sterile solution of sodium chloride, with anhydrous dextrose or the equivalent amount of dextrose monohydrate for parenteral use, in water for injections. It is sterilised, immediately after preparation, by heating in an autoclave. The usual strength is 0.18% of sodium chloride (30 millimoles each of Na^+ and Cl^- per litre) with 4% of anhydrous dextrose.

A standard for this injection is given in the British Pharmacopoeia 1973

Containers: see the entry on Injections for general information on containers.

Labelling: see the entry on Injections for general information on labelling. In addition, the label on the container should state the amounts of the medicaments as the percentages w/v of sodium chloride and anhydrous dextrose. When the injection is intended for intravenous infusion, the label should also state the approximate concentrations, in millimoles per litre, of the sodium ions and the chloride ions and the number of grams per litre of anhydrous dextrose.

Storage: it should be stored at a temperature not exceeding 25°. On storage, the solution may cause separation of small solid particles from glass containers. Solutions containing such particles must not be used.

STRONG DEXTROSE INJECTION:

Anhydrous dextrose	..	..	..	50 g
Water for injections	..	..	..	to 100 ml

Dissolve and clarify by filtration. Sterilise, immediately after preparation, by heating in an autoclave. In making this preparation the anhydrous dextrose may be replaced by the equivalent amount of dextrose monohydrate for parenteral use.

A standard for this injection is given in the British Pharmaceutical Codex 1973

Containers: see the entry on Injections for general information on containers.

Labelling: see the entry on Injections for general information on labelling. In addition, the label on the container should state the amount of the medicament as the amount of anhydrous dextrose in grams per litre.

Storage: it should be stored at a temperature not exceeding 25°.

Dextrose Monohydrate for Parenteral Use

D-(+)-Glucopyranose monohydrate
$C_6H_{12}O_6,H_2O = 198.2$

OTHER NAMES: Dextrosum Monohydricum ad Usum Parenterale; Glucose for Parenteral Use

A standard is given in the European Pharmacopoeia Vol. II

Description; Solubility; Moisture content; Specific rotation. See under Dextrose.

Sterilisation. Solutions for injection are sterilised, immediately after preparation, by heating in an autoclave.

Identification; Metabolism. See under Dextrose.

Uses. Dextrose monohydrate for parenteral use is used for the preparation of injections of dextrose, as described under Dextrose, Anhydrous.

Diabetes Insipidus

Diabetes insipidus is due to a deficiency of antidiuretic hormone or, occasionally, to insensitivity of the renal tubules to the hormone. It is characterised by the passage of large volumes of very dilute urine. The loss of fluid may amount to 10 to 20 litres daily and results in constant thirst, constipation, and dry skin.

The usual treatment is replacement of the antidiuretic hormone by desmopressin, lypressin, or pituitary (posterior lobe), but chlorpropamide, thiazide diuretics, clofibrate, and carbamazepine, which have some antidiuretic effects, may also be used in some cases.

Diabetes Mellitus

Diabetes mellitus is a disease characterised by persistent hyperglycaemia usually with glycosuria, caused by a deficiency of or the diminished effectiveness of insulin. The condition may be of multifactorial origin in which hereditary factors, age, sex, pregnancy, obesity, infections, and stress may have some bearing on the development of the condition or it may be precipitated by hormonal disorders such as acromegaly or Cushing's syndrome or by administration of drugs such as corticosteroids or diuretics.

Juvenile-onset diabetes. This usually develops during the first forty years of life in patients who are of normal or less than normal weight. The onset of symptoms is frequently sudden and acute but can be insidious. Classical symptoms include thirst, polyuria, dehydration, and loss of energy and weight. Blurred vision, paraesthesias in the hands and feet, cramp in the legs at night, and constipation may also occur. Pruritus vulvae and disturbances or cessation of menstruation are common in women and in men there may be decreased libido. The diabetes is said to be insulin-dependent as the administration of insulin is a necessary part of treatment.

The presence of ketones in the urine is an early indication of a progression towards diabetic coma. The ketones occur as a result of abnormal breakdown of fats by the liver. Their accumulation in the blood leads to their excretion in the urine (ketonuria) and in the breath which has a sweet sickly smell. Ketonuria may be associated with a dry furred tongue, cracked lips, rapid pulse, and low blood pressure; mental confusion and apathy may also be present.

The condition should be treated initially with insulin injection (soluble insulin) and fluid replacement. Subsequently, carbohydrate feeds are given at regular intervals together with plenty of fluids.

Where the condition has progressed to diabetic coma it should be treated as described under Insulin Injection.

Maturity-onset diabetes. This usually appears in middle-aged or elderly patients who are often obese. It occurs more frequently in women than in men and is usually mild. Ketosis and other classical symptoms are usually absent, but there may be pruritus vulvae in women. The presence of chronic recurrent sepsis, neuropathy, and retinopathy may be indicative of long-standing diabetes.

In many of these patients the diabetes may be controlled by diet alone, but if this is unsuccessful it may be possible to obtain control by diet together with the administration of sulphonylureas such as chlorpropamide or tolbutamide; if this fails to produce stabilisation the simultaneous administration of sulphonylureas and a biguanide such as metformin may be successful as their effects are additive.

Treatment of diabetes. Treatment should abolish the symptoms of diabetes, reduce blood glucose levels to as near normal as possible, and maintain a suitable body-weight. Carbohydrate restriction is necessary in all diabetics and involves regulation of the amount and timing of food intake, particularly intake of carbohydrates. The patient will require advice on a dietary regimen and this should take into account his energy expenditure. Alcoholic beverages may be included in the diet provided that allowance for their carbohydrate content is made in the diet.

The patient should be educated in the management of his disease so that he is able to adjust therapy to cover alterations in energy expenditure, changes in the timing of meals, and illness. He should be taught to test samples of urine for the presence of glycosuria and the proper timing for the taking of these samples. He should be taught to recognise the onset of hypoglycaemia which may be very rapid; its symptoms and treatment are described under Insulin Injection.

If an attack of hypoglycaemia occurs and no adequate explanation can be found, the patient should be re-examined and a new schedule of treatment established.

Complications of diabetes. Diabetics are more liable than normal people to suffer from infections, particularly staphylococcal skin infections, pulmonary tuberculosis, and urinary tract infections. The following vascular, ocular, renal, nervous and other complications also occur.

VASCULAR. Diabetics are liable to all forms of arterial degeneration including coronary and cerebral artery disease and obliterative arterial disease of the legs. Other complications of vascular disease include renal failure, blindness, hypertension, and congestive heart failure.

OCULAR. There may be blurring of vision resulting from changes in blood-sugar level; when the level is high, some patients become myopic and when low they become hypermetropic. Temporary change is common in early insulin treatment. Cataract occurs rarely in young diabetics with severe disease. Retinopathy occurs fairly commonly and is related to duration rather than severity of the disease.

RENAL. Renal lesions may occur in longstanding diabetes. There is no specific treatment. Diuretics, low protein diet, and blood transfusions may increase the patient's comfort and prolong life.

NERVOUS. Neuropathy may occur, generally affecting the lower limbs. Paraesthesiae of the hands and feet are followed by hyperaesthesiae and loss of perception of heat, pin prick, vibration, and deep pain. Impotence also occurs and is secondary to autonomic neuropathy. Impaired cardiovascular reflexes lead to postural hypotension. No satisfactory treatment is available but strict control of diabetes may lead to recovery.

PREGNANCY. There is a slightly increased maternal mortality in diabetic mothers and foetal loss is increased.

The insulin requirement is increased during the last 6 months of pregnancy. Mothers who have given birth to heavy babies should be examined for diabetes.

Dialysis

The property of a semi-permeable membrane of allowing substances of low molecular weight to pass through but preventing passage of substances of high molecular weight may be used to effect excretion of excess of water and accumulated waste products or other toxic substances normally excreted from the body by the kidney in cases where, due to disease or injury, renal failure has occurred, or to augment the action of the kidney in the treatment of poisoning.

Solutions containing electrolytes and dextrose formulated to simulate an ideal extracellular fluid are placed in contact with one surface of the membrane and the patient's blood in contact with the opposite surface, allowing exchange of ions between the two media. Increasing the osmolarity of solutions by raising the concentrations of dextrose helps to eliminate water from the body, while reducing the concentration of specific electrolytes allows selective removal of electrolytes from the blood to correct imbalances.

Two forms of treatment are used, one being termed haemodialysis and the other intraperitoneal dialysis.

Haemodialysis. An artificial semi-permeable membrane is used. This is enclosed in a machine which is connected via tubing to the patient's circulatory system in a manner such that the patient's blood is diverted through the machine and brought into contact with one surface of the membrane before being returned to the circulation. Meanwhile, the dialysing fluid is pumped to the machine so that it flows over the other surface of the membrane, allowing exchange of ions to take place. It is usual to perform a minor surgical operation to provide access points for connecting the machine into the patient's circulatory system. With training and suitable assistance, the patient may be able to carry out the procedure in his own home.

The solutions required depend on the type of machine used. In one type of machine, the dialysing solution is prepared in a container attached to the machine by dissolving the ingredients in suitable water (usually softened mains water). This arrangement is suitable for the treatment of individual patients undergoing special treatment (for example treatment for poisoning). Other machines require a concentrated solution of standard composition which is diluted with softened mains water by means of a proportioning pump. The diluted solution is passed over the membrane and discarded. Formulae for suitable solutions are given below.

A more recent development is a machine which circulates the dialysis solution over the membrane and then through an adsorbent which removes the products of dialysis; the solution is then recycled. This process uses considerably less solution than the single-pass process and requires a haemodialysis solution of slightly different composition.

Techniques have also been developed for the removal by dialysis of so-called "middle molecules" which are substances of higher molecular weight than the substances usually removed by dialysis.

Intraperitoneal dialysis. The dialysing fluid is introduced into the peritoneum by cannula and exchange is effected across the peritoneal membrane. After a suitable interval the solution is replaced or it may be recycled through an adsorbent chamber. The process requires no special connecting points on the body but it is much less effective than haemodialysis.

Haemodialysis solutions (Syn. Haemodialysis fluids; Dialysing solutions for artificial kidney)

Although there is no necessity for haemodialysis solutions to be sterile, precautions should be taken to prevent heavy bacterial contamination during their preparation and use, as some metabolic products of bacteria can pass through the membrane of the artificial kidney.

A number of concentrated solutions, each differing in composition and in the extent to which they must be diluted, are in use. They usually contain sodium acetate as a source of bicarbonate, because this salt is more soluble in water than sodium bicarbonate.

The quantities of the salts in the concentrated haemodialysis solutions are such that when the solutions are diluted to an appropriate extent, usually 35 or 40 times, the final concentrations of the ions, per litre, are usually in the ranges:

sodium, 130 to 140 mmol; potassium, 0 to 4 mmol; calcium, 1.5 to 2 mmol; magnesium, 0.45 to 0.75 mmol; bicarbonate (or its equivalent as acetate or lactate), 25 to 35 mmol; and chloride, 101 to 112 mmol. The final concentration of dextrose is usually 0.1 to 0.2 per cent.

Suitable concentrated solutions may be prepared according to the following formulae:

CONCENTRATED HAEMODIALYSIS SOLUTION (35×)

Potassium chloride	2.6 g
Dextrose (monohydrate)..	70.0 g
Sodium acetate	166.6 g
Sodium chloride	194.5 g
Purified water, freshly boiled and	
cooled	to 1000 ml

For each 35 litres of haemodialysis solution required in the artificial kidney, dilute 1 litre of concentrated haemodialysis solution (35×) with 34 litres of the appropriate type of water (see below).

The diluted solution, when prepared with purified water, contains in 1 litre the following concentrations of ions: 130 mmol of Na^+, 1.0 mmol of K^+, the equivalent of 35 mmol of HCO_3^-, and 96 mmol of Cl^-.

CONCENTRATED HAEMODIALYSIS SOLUTION (40×)

Potassium chloride	4.0 g
Dextrose (monohydrate)..	80.0 g
Sodium acetate	190.4 g
Sodium chloride	222.4 g
Lactic acid	4 ml
Purified water, freshly boiled and	
cooled	to 1000 ml

For each 40 litres of haemodialysis solution required in the artificial kidney, dilute 1 litre of concentrated haemodialysis solution (40×) with 39 litres of the appropriate type of water (see below).

The diluted solution, when prepared with purified water, contains in 1 litre the following concentrations of ions: 130 mmol of Na^+, 1.3 mmol of K^+, the equivalent of 36 mmol of HCO_3^-, and 96 mmol of Cl^-.

WATER FOR DILUTING CONCENTRATED HAEMODIALYSIS SOLUTIONS. Mains water, mains water softened by base exchange, or purified water is used.

Where purified water is used, the formulae given above are suitable for use without modification in respect of the sodium content of the diluted solution.

In hard water areas, if mains water is to be used, it is usual to pass it first through a base-exchange water softener, but in removing the calcium and magnesium salts responsible for the hardness, equivalent amounts of sodium ions are introduced into the softened water. These amounts vary from 5 to 7 mmol per litre in the London area, but will differ in other places, and, in addition, might be subject to seasonal variation in any given area.

In soft water areas where the natural calcium content of mains water is less than 1.5 mmol per litre, softening may or may not be carried out and the ordinary mains water may be used, allowance again being made, if necessary, for the sodium present. Whichever type of water is used for diluting the concentrate, it should be de-gassed and filtered to remove particles larger than 25 micrometres.

INCLUSION OF CALCIUM AND MAGNESIUM IONS. The calcium and magnesium ions required in the diluted haemodialysis solution may be obtained in some areas simply by using the unsoftened mains water to dilute the concentrate. In other areas, supplementary additions of calcium acetate or calcium chloride and magnesium acetate or magnesium chloride may need to be made. If purified water or softened mains water is used as the diluent, the whole of the required calcium and magnesium ions in the form of the salts must either be added to the dilute artifical kidney solution or included in the concentrated solution.

A standard for the above haemodialysis solutions is given in the British Pharmaceutical Codex 1973

Containers: concentrated haemodialysis solutions are supplied in suitable glass or plastic containers which do not release ions or harmful substances into the solution. Separation of solid particles from the glass containers may occur on storage; solutions containing such particles must not be used.

Labelling: the label on the container of the concentrated solution should state the strength of the solution as a percentage or weight per litre for each ingredient, the quantity of dextrose being expressed in terms of anhydrous dextrose, $C_6H_{12}O_6$, the number of millimoles of each ion present per litre, that the solution must be diluted before use, and the directions for diluting the solution.

The label may state, in addition, the number of milliequivalents of each ion present per litre.

Storage: Concentrated Haemodialysis Solution (40×) should be kept in a warm place as it is liable to deposit crystals on keeping.

Uses: haemodialysis solutions are employed, as described above, in cases of temporary or permanent renal failure, in the artificial kidney to remove the excess of water and accumulated waste products normally excreted from the body by the kidney, and to correct electrolyte imbalance.

In the treatment of poisoning, elimination of poisons of low molecular weight, e.g. aspirin and certain barbiturates, as well as substances of higher molecular weight which diffuse across the dialyser membrane, may be hastened by haemodialysis; elimination may sometimes be assisted by adjustment of the pH of the dialysis solution. Substances that are strongly bound to body protein are not effectively removed by dialysis.

Haemodialysis has been shown to be of value in the treatment of renal failure occurring with *P. falciparum* infections (malignant tertian malaria). In this condition renal damage associated with tubular necrosis may give rise to oliguria or anuria with uraemia. Dialysis may prolong life until the renal lesion has healed and should be considered in all patients with *P. falciparum* infections who have oliguria and a rising blood urea.

In patients with a severe degree of renal damage, dialysis may need to be continued for several weeks and for such patients haemodialysis is the only practicable method. For those with less severe degrees of renal damage intraperitoneal dialysis may be satisfactory.

Cholera, severe dysentery, and gastroenteritis, particularly in infants and young children, may similarly give rise to renal damage necessitating haemodialysis or peritoneal dialysis.

Concentrated Haemodialysis Solution (35×) contains in 1 litre approximately 4500 mmol of Na^+, 35 mmol of K^+, the equivalent of 1225 mmol of HCO_3^-, and 3360 mmol of Cl^-.

Concentrated Haemodialysis Solution (40×) contains in 1 litre approximately 5200 mmol of Na^+, 54 mmol of K^+, the equivalent of 1445 mmol of HCO_3^-, and 3855 mmol of Cl^-.

Intraperitoneal dialysis solutions (*Syn.* Intraperitoneal dialysis fluids; Peritoneal dialysis solutions)

Sterile aqueous solutions of electrolytes and dextrose approximating in composition to a normal extracellular body fluid. They contain sodium ions, calcium ions, and magnesium ions, in association with chloride ions and bicarbonate ions. Either lactate or acetate is used as the source of the bicarbonate ions.

The solutions are rendered slightly hypertonic by the inclusion of dextrose, which is usually present in a concentration of about 1.4%, but when a more rapid removal of water is required, the tonicity is increased by including higher concentrations of dextrose, which can be up to 7%.

Potassium chloride is usually administered separately in accordance with the needs of the patient.

Suitable solutions may be prepared according to the following formulae:

INTRAPERITONEAL DIALYSIS SOLUTION (LACTATE)

Magnesium chloride	0.15 g
Calcium chloride	0.26 g
Lactic acid } equivalent to	
Sodium hydroxide } sodium lactate	5.00 g
Sodium chloride	5.60 g
Anhydrous dextrose	13.60 g
Sodium metabisulphite	0.05 g
Water for injections	to 1000 ml

The quantity of sodium lactate required may be obtained from 3.8 ml of the lactic acid and 1.8 g of the sodium hydroxide and the procedure described under Lactic Acid for the preparation of sodium lactate injection followed; if the sodium lactate is prepared in this way, a small quantity of sodium chloride is formed and consequently the amount of sodium chloride in the recipe should be reduced by an amount corresponding to the volume of hydrochloric acid used in the preparation of the solution.

Dissolve the other ingredients in a portion of the water, mix with the sodium lactate solution, filter, and sterilise by heating in an autoclave; the type of autoclave used should be such that rapid cooling of the solution may be effected, in order to prevent caramelisation of the dextrose.

INTRAPERITONEAL DIALYSIS SOLUTION (ACETATE)

Magnesium chloride	0.152 g
Calcium chloride	0.220 g
Sodium acetate	4.760 g
Sodium chloride	5.560 g
Anhydrous dextrose	17.000 g
Sodium metabisulphite	0.150 g
Water for injections	to 1000 ml

Dissolve, filter, and sterilise by heating in an autoclave; the type of autoclave used should be such that rapid cooling of the solution may be effected, in order to prevent caramelisation of the dextrose.

A standard for the above intraperitoneal dialysis solutions is given in the British Pharmaceutical Codex 1973

Containers: intraperitoneal dialysis solutions are supplied in suitable glass or plastic containers which do not release ions or harmful substances into the solution. Separation of solid particles from the glass containers may occur on storage; solutions containing such particles must not be used.

Labelling: the label on the container should state the strength of the solution, as a percentage or weight per litre for each ingredient, the quantity of dextrose being expressed in terms of anhydrous dextrose, $C_6H_{12}O_6$, the number of millimoles of each ion present per litre, the volume of solution in the container, that the solution is not for intravenous administration, and that any portion of the solution remaining after the contents are first used should be discarded.

The label may state, in addition, the number of milli-equivalents of each ion per litre.

Uses: intraperitoneal dialysis solutions are used for the same purposes as haemodialysis solutions, as described above. They are infused into the peritoneal cavity through a catheter under aseptic conditions, allowed to remain in the body for about 1 hour, and then drained from the cavity through the catheter.

Intraperitoneal dialysis solution (*lactate*) contains in 1 litre approximately 140 mmol of Na^+, 1.8 mmol of Ca^{2+}, 0.75 mmol of Mg^{2+}, 100 mmol of Cl^-, and the equivalent of 45 mmol of HCO_3^- (as lactate).

Intraperitoneal dialysis solution (*acetate*) contains in 1 litre approximately 130 mmol of Na^+, 1.5 mmol of Ca^{2+}, 0.75 mmol of Mg^{2+}, 100 mmol of Cl^-, and the equivalent of 35.0 mmol of HCO_3^- (as acetate).

Diamorphine Hydrochloride

3,6-*O*-Diacetylmorphine hydrochloride monohydrate

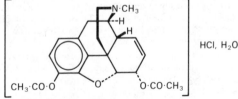

$C_{21}H_{24}ClNO_5,H_2O = 423.9$

OTHER NAME: Heroin Hydrochloride

A standard is given in the British Pharmacopoeia 1973

Description. An almost white, crystalline, odourless powder with a bitter taste.

Solubility. Soluble, at 20°, in 1.6 parts of water, in 12 parts of alcohol, and in 1.6 parts of chloroform; practically insoluble in ether.

Moisture content. Not more than 4.5%, determined by drying at 105°.

Dissociation constant. pK_a 7.6 (23°).

Stability. In aqueous solution, diamorphine hydrolyses to 3-*O*- and 6-*O*-acetylmorphine and then to morphine. Hydrolysis is catalysed by hydrogen ions and hydroxide ions. At 25°, aqueous solutions are most stable at about pH 4; in solutions at pH 4, 10% degradation occurs in about 5 days at 25°, in 5 weeks at 4°, and in 7 weeks at 0°.

FURTHER INFORMATION. Hydrolysis in aqueous solution —E. A. Davey and J. B. Murray, *Pharm. J.*, ii/1969, 737; stability of elixir of diamorphine and cocaine—E. W. Gold, *J. Hosp. Pharm.*, 1973, **31**, 12 and R. G. Twycross, *Pharm. J.*, i/1974, 153.

Incompatibility. It is incompatible with mineral acids and with alkalis. Sodium chloride precipitates diamorphine from solutions and is not suitable for adjusting the tonicity of solutions.

Sterilisation. It is sterilised by dissolving the powder in sterile purified water, filtering the solution through a sterile bacteria-proof filter, and transferring the solution aseptically to suitable previously sterilised containers; the solvent is evaporated off by freeze-drying and the dry sterile product transferred aseptically to the final previously sterilised containers which are then sealed to exclude micro-organisms.

Storage. It should be stored in airtight containers, protected from light.

Identification. TESTS. 1. Moisten a few crystals with nitric acid; a yellow colour is produced which changes to greenish-blue on warming and reverts to yellow on cooling.
2. Dissolve 100 mg in 1 ml of sulphuric acid, warm, cool, add 6 ml of water and a mixture of 0.5 ml of *potassium ferricyanide solution* and 0.025 ml of *ferric chloride test-solution;* a deep blue colour is produced.
3. Dissolve 100 mg in 1 ml of alcohol, add 1 ml of sulphuric acid, and warm; the odour of ethyl acetate is produced.

MELTING-POINT. About 231°.

ULTRAVIOLET ABSORPTION. In water, maximum at 279 nm (E1%, 1cm = 40); in 0.1N sodium hydroxide, maximum at 299 nm due to morphine formed by hydrolysis (E1%, 1cm = 60).

THIN-LAYER CHROMATOGRAPHY. See under Thin-layer Chromatography, System 7.

Determination in body fluids. GAS CHROMATOGRAPHY. In urine: diamorphine and metabolites—S. Y. Yeh and R. L. McQuinn, *J. pharm. Sci.*, 1975, **64**, 1237; in blood: diamorphine and metabolites—D. A. Smith and W. J. Cole, *J. Chromat.*, 1975, **105**, 377.

COLUMN, GAS, AND THIN-LAYER CHROMATOGRAPHY. In urine: identification of metabolites—S. Y. Yeh *et al.*, *J. pharm. Sci.*, 1977, **66**, 201.

SURVEY of screening methods for urine—D. Sohn *et al.*, *Analyt. Chem.*, 1973, **45**, 1498.

Metabolism. ABSORPTION. Rapidly and completely absorbed after oral administration or by injection; absorption from the gastro-intestinal tract may be erratic and availability upon inhalation varies according to the method of inhalation used.

BLOOD CONCENTRATION. In cases of fatal overdose total morphine concentrations of 100 to 900 ng/ml have been detected.

HALF-LIFE. In cases of overdose the serum concentrations decrease biphasically with the α-phase having a half-life of 1.9 to 3.1 hours and the β-phase, a half-life of 10 to 44 hours.

DISTRIBUTION. The diamorphine metabolites, morphine and 6-monoacetylmorphine, rapidly cross the blood-brain barrier; morphine crosses the placenta and is secreted in the milk.

METABOLIC REACTIONS. Rapidly hydrolysed to 6-monoacetylmorphine which is further hydrolysed to morphine; normorphine is also formed; all metabolites may be conjugated with glucuronic acid; morphine may be conjugated at positions 3 or 6.

EXCRETION. Up to 80% of a dose is recovered in the urine in 24 hours, after oral or parenteral administration; most of the dose is recovered as morphine-3-glucuronide with about 5 to 7% as free morphine, 1% as 6-monoacetylmorphine, 0.1% as unchanged drug, and trace amounts of the other metabolites; after inhalation 14 to 20% of the dose appears in the urine; morphine metabolites are excreted in the bile.

FURTHER INFORMATION. Actions and metabolism on continuous intravenous infusion—H. W. Elliott *et al.*, *Clin. Pharmac. Ther.*, 1971, **12**, 806; morphine concentrations and survival periods in acute heroin fatalities—J. C. Garriott and W. Q. Sturner, *New Engl. J. Med.*, 1973, **289**, 1276; assessment of inhalation as a mode of administration by heroin addicts—B. P. Mo and E. L. Way, *J. Pharmac. exp. Ther.*, 1966, **154**, 142; alimentary absorption and urinary excretion—R. G. Twycross *et al.*, *Br. J. clin. Pharmac.*, 1974, **1**, 491; identification of metabolites—S. Y. Yeh *et al.*, *J. pharm. Sci.*, 1977, **66**, 201.

Actions and uses. Diamorphine has actions similar to those described under Morphine Hydrochloride, but it is more potent than morphine. It has less tendency to cause vomiting and constipation and is particularly effective in the relief of cough, for which purpose it is administered in a dose of 1.5 to 6 milligrams as the elixir or linctus.

Diamorphine is given by subcutaneous or intramuscular injection in a dose of 5 to 10 milligrams increasing if necessary for the relief of pain and restlessness in the terminal stages of carcinoma and other fatal illnesses. It is also given by mouth in a similar dosage alone or in conjunction with cocaine for the same purpose. Chlorpromazine may be used at the same time but perphenazine is sometimes preferred as it causes less sedation.

Solutions for injection are prepared immediately before use by an aseptic technique.

Undesirable effects. Diamorphine produces dependence of the morphine type (see under Drug Dependence) more readily than morphine and the effects are worse, greater mental and moral deterioration occurring. Diamorphine crosses the placenta and is secreted in the milk and may cause respiratory depression and dependence in the newborn.

It should be used with great caution and only when less dangerous analgesics and cough suppressants have proved inadequate or unsuitable.

Poisoning. The procedure as described under Morphine Hydrochloride should be adopted.

Preparations

DIAMORPHINE AND COCAINE ELIXIR:

Diamorphine hydrochloride	..	..	..	.. 1 g
Cocaine hydrochloride	..	..	..	.. 1 g
Alcohol (90%)	..	..	..	.. 125 ml
Syrup..	..	..	..	.. 250 ml
Chloroform water ..	..	..	..	to 1000 ml

It must be freshly prepared.

When *Diamorphine and Cocaine Elixir* is prescribed without qualification an elixir prepared in accordance with the formula above is supplied.

When *Morphine and Cocaine Elixir* is prescribed without qualification an elixir prepared in accordance with the formula above but containing 1 g of morphine hydrochloride instead of 1 g of diamorphine hydrochloride is supplied. It should be recently prepared.

When *Morphine, Cocaine, and Chlorpromazine Elixir* or *Diamorphine, Cocaine, and Chlorpromazine Elixir* is prescribed, the syrup in the above formulae is replaced by chlorpromazine elixir. These preparations should be protected from light.

When specified by the prescriber, the proportion of diamorphine hydrochloride or morphine hydrochloride in the above formulae may be altered.

Dose: the elixir contains, in 10 millilitres, 10 milligrams of cocaine hydrochloride and, unless otherwise specified, 10 milligrams of diamorphine hydrochloride or of morphine hydrochloride. The dose volume (and the proportion of diamorphine hydrochloride or morphine hydrochloride) is determined by the physician in accordance with the needs of the patient.

DIAMORPHINE INJECTION: a sterile solution of diamorphine hydrochloride in water for injections. It is prepared by dissolving the contents of a sealed container in water for injections immediately before use. Available as a powder in ampoules containing 5, 10, and 30 mg of diamorphine hydrochloride. Sodium chloride precipitates diamorphine from solutions and is not suitable for adjusting the tonicity of the injection.

A standard for this injection is given in the British Pharmacopoeia 1973

Containers and *Labelling:* see the entry on Injections for general information on containers and labelling.

Storage: the sealed container should be protected from light. The injection decomposes on storage and should be used immediately after preparation.

DIAMORPHINE LINCTUS:

Diamorphine hydrochloride	..	..	..	600 mg
Compound tartrazine solution	..	..	..	12 ml
Glycerol	..	..	..	.. 250 ml
Oxymel	..	..	..	.. 250 ml
Syrup..	..	..	..	to 1000 ml

Dissolve the diamorphine hydrochloride in the compound tartrazine solution, add the oxymel, the glycerol, and sufficient syrup to produce the required volume, and mix. It must be freshly prepared.

When a dose less than or not a multiple of 5 ml is prescribed, the linctus may be diluted, as described in the entry on Linctuses, with syrup.

Diamorphine linctus contains, in 5 ml, 3 mg of diamorphine hydrochloride.

A standard for this linctus is given in the British Pharmaceutical Codex 1973

Dose: 2.5 to 10 millilitres.

Diamphenethide

$\beta\beta'$-Oxydi(aceto-*p*-phenetidide)

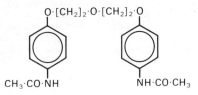

$C_{20}H_{24}N_2O_5 = 372.4$

OTHER NAME: *Coriban*®

A standard is given in the British Pharmacopoeia (Veterinary)

Description. A white to pale buff powder.

Solubility. Practically insoluble in water; soluble in 160 parts of alcohol, in 500 parts of chloroform, and in 150 parts of methyl alcohol; practically insoluble in ether.

Moisture content. Not more than 5%, determined by drying at 100° *in vacuo*.

Veterinary uses. Diamphenethide is a fasciolacide used in the treatment of acute and chronic liver-fluke diseases in sheep. The usual dose is 100 milligrams per kilogram body-weight, repeated at intervals of 5 to 8 weeks as required. Operators administering the preparation should wash splashes from the skin and eyes immediately.

The minimum period between cessation of treatment and slaughter of the animal for human consumption is 7 days.

Preparation

DIAMPHENETHIDE MIXTURE (*Syn.* Diamphenethide Suspension): a suspension of diamphenethide, with suitable suspending and dispersing agents, in an aqueous vehicle. Available as a suspension containing 18% of diamphenethide in 4.5-litre containers.

A standard for this mixture is given in the British Pharmacopoeia (Veterinary)

Labelling: see the entry on Mixtures for general information on labelling.

Storage: it should not be allowed to freeze.

Diarrhoea

Diarrhoea is the frequent passage of stools which are too fluid. The cause may be a disorder of the stomach, biliary system, or small or large bowel, a systemic illness, or the ingestion of drugs, toxins, or poisons. In its acute form it may be caused by food poisoning, by bowel infection, or by ingestion of bacterial toxins as described under gastro-enteritis and typhoid. Chronic diarrhoea may be due to disease such as malabsorption, colitis, or cancer, to infestation with amoebae, *Giardia lamblia*, or occasionally worms, disturbances of intestinal motility (including nervous diarrhoea), and the effects of drugs. Treatment is directed if possible to the underlying cause.

For symptomatic therapy, adsorbent powders or mixtures are used to treat mild diarrhoea, and morphine-like drugs which reduce intestinal movement may be given in the more severe cases.

Bulk-forming laxatives such as methylcellulose may be useful in taking up excess fluid in diarrhoea and also in controlling loose motions in patients with an ileostomy or a colostomy.

In severe diarrhoea, dehydration may occur, especially

in infants, elderly patients, or in cholera, and rehydration should be carried out by means of oral, or, if necessary, intravenous fluids. Oral rehydration fluid contains salts to replace electrolyte loss and dextrose (glucose) to assist absorption. A suitable fluid for infantile diarrhoeas may be prepared from compound sodium chloride and dextrose powder. In adult diarrhoea due to cholera, the pattern of electrolyte loss is different and a fluid prepared from sodium chloride 3.5 grams, dextrose monohydrate 20 grams, potassium chloride 1.5 grams, sodium bicarbonate 2.5 grams, and water to 1000 millilitres may be used.

Faecal impaction is a condition occurring mainly in the elderly which may give rise to "spurious diarrhoea" in which liquid faeces are passed without the original faecal mass being expelled. The condition is treated by evacuation of the rectum by suppositories, by enema, or by manual removal.

Diaveridine

5-Veratrylpyrimidine-2,4-diamine

$C_{13}H_{16}N_4O_2 = 260.3$

OTHER NAME: *Saquadil*® (with sulphaquinoxaline)

A standard is given in the British Pharmacopoeia (Veterinary)

Description. A white or creamy-white, odourless, tasteless powder.

Solubility. Very slightly soluble in water and in alcohol; soluble, at 20°, in 600 parts of chloroform.

Moisture content. Not more than 1%, determined by drying at 105°.

Identification. TEST. Mix 250 mg with 0.5 ml of a mixture of equal volumes of acetic anhydride and glacial acetic acid, heat under a reflux condenser for 10 minutes, cool, add, with constant stirring, 5 ml of water and 2.5 ml of 2N sodium hydroxide, and allow to stand for 20 minutes; a precipitate is produced which, after washing with water and drying at 105°, melts at about 186°.

MELTING-POINT. About 233°.

ULTRAVIOLET ABSORPTION. In 0.1N hydrochloric acid, maximum at 276 nm (E1%, 1cm = 300).

INFRA-RED ABSORPTION. Major peaks at 1250, 1460, 1510, 1600, 1630, and 1645 cm⁻¹ (see Appendix 2c: Infra-red Spectra).

Veterinary uses. Diaveridine is used to prevent coccidiosis in poultry. It is administered continuously in the feed at a concentration of 15 parts per million in conjunction with sulphaquinoxaline 85 parts per million. It may also be administered in a concentration of 45 parts per million in conjunction with sulphaquinoxaline in drinking water for periods of 3 days separated by intervals of 2 days when unmedicated water is given.

Preparation

DIAVERIDINE AND SULPHAQUINOXALINE PREMIX consisting of diaveridine and sulphaquinoxaline mixed with a suitable diluent. It must be diluted before administration by mixing thoroughly with the feed. Available as a premix containing 3.3% of diaveridine and 18.7% of sulphaquinoxaline.

A standard for this premix is given in the British Pharmacopoeia (Veterinary)

Containers and *Storage:* see the entry on Premixes for general information on containers and storage.

OTHER PREPARATIONS available include a solution containing diaveridine 14 mg with sulphaquinoxaline 16 mg per ml.

Diazepam

7-Chloro-1,3-dihydro-1-methyl-5-phenyl-2H-1,4-benzodiazepin-2-one

$C_{16}H_{13}ClN_2O = 284.7$

OTHER NAMES: *Atensine*®; *Tensium*®; *Valium*®

A standard is given in the British Pharmacopoeia 1973

Description. A white crystalline odourless powder.

Solubility. Very slightly soluble in water; soluble in 24 parts of alcohol, in less than 2 parts of chloroform, in 55 parts of ether, in 8 parts of acetone, and in 60 parts of propylene glycol.

Dissociation constant. pK_a 3.3 (20°).

Stability. Diazepam degrades by hydrolysis of the 4,5-azomethine bond to form an intermediate compound which is in turn hydrolysed to produce a glycine derivative and 2-methylamino-5-chlorobenzophenone. In solutions of pH below 3.3 the degradation reaction is not reversible. At pH values above 3.3 the first stage of hydrolysis is reversible.

FURTHER INFORMATION. Kinetics and mechanisms of hydrolysis of benzodiazepines—W. W. Ham *et al.*, *J. pharm. Sci.*, 1977, **66**, 573.

Storage. It should be stored in airtight containers, protected from light.

Identification. TEST. It complies with Test 1 described under Chlordiazepoxide Hydrochloride.

MELTING-POINT. About 132°.

ULTRAVIOLET ABSORPTION. In 0.1N hydrochloric acid, maxima at 243 nm (E1%, 1cm = 964), 287 nm (E1%, 1cm = 490), and 364 nm (E1%, 1cm = 148); in alcohol (95%), maximum at 229 nm (E1%, 1cm = 1082).

INFRA-RED ABSORPTION. Major peaks at 705, 1128, 1315, 1338, 1470, and 1671 cm⁻¹ (see Appendix 2a: Infra-red Spectra).

Determination in body fluids. SPECTROPHOTOMETRY. In blood—J. A. F. de Silva *et al.*, *J. pharm. Sci.*, 1966, **55**, 692.

GAS CHROMATOGRAPHY. In blood and urine: diazepam

and metabolites—J. A. F. de Silva and C. V. Puglisi, *Analyt. Chem.*, 1970, **42**, 1725; in serum and urine: diazepam and metabolites—J. M. Steyn and H. K. L. Hundt, *J. Chromat.*, 1975, **107**, 196; in plasma—D. M. Rutherford, *J. Chromat.*, 1977, **137**, 439.

HIGH PRESSURE LIQUID CHROMATOGRAPHY. In plasma: diazepam and *N*-desmethyldiazepam—R. R. Brodie *et al.*, *J. Chromat.*, 1978, **150**, 361.

REVIEWS. Methods for benzodiazepines—see under Chlordiazepoxide Hydrochloride.

Metabolism. ABSORPTION. Rapidly and completely absorbed after oral administration; following intramuscular injection, the absorption is variable, the major influences being the site and depth of injection.

BLOOD CONCENTRATION. After an oral dose of 10 to 30 mg, peak plasma concentrations of 130 to 500 ng/ml are attained in 0.5 to 4 hours; during therapy with oral doses of 30 to 60 mg daily, steady state concentrations of 0.5 to 2 μg/ml are attained; after intramuscular doses of 20 mg, peak plasma concentrations of 35 to 290 ng/ml are attained in 1 to 1.5 hours; and after an intravenous dose of 20 mg, a concentration of about 1.6 μg/ml is attained within 15 minutes; minimum effective plasma concentrations are about 400 ng/ml; concentrations of diazepam in the blood of alcoholics appear to be reduced.

HALF-LIFE. The decline in plasma concentration appears to be biphasic with a half-life of 1 to 10 hours for the α-phase and a half-life of 2 to 8 days for the β-phase; other estimates of half-life have been recorded in the range 8 to 93 hours; the plasma half-life appears to be increased in the aged, in subjects with renal function impairment, and in cirrhotics; it is increased in premature infants and decreased in children aged 4 to 8 years.

DISTRIBUTION. Extensively distributed and may accumulate following continuous dosage; high concentrations appear in adipose tissue and small amounts are taken up by red blood cells; both diazepam and its major metabolite, desmethyldiazepam, cross the placenta and are secreted in the milk; volume of distribution, 1 to 2 litres per kg body-weight; during long-term therapy, desmethyldiazepam accumulates in the cerebrospinal fluid; *protein binding*, about 97% bound to plasma proteins.

METABOLIC REACTIONS. *N*-demethylation, 3-hydroxylation, and glucuronic acid conjugation; aromatic hydroxylation occurs in the rat but not to any extent in man; the metabolites formed are *N*-desmethyldiazepam which is the major blood metabolite, temazepam, oxazepam, and their glucuronides; the newborn have a limited capacity to hydroxylate diazepam. Diazepam in high doses or on prolonged administration induces the metabolism of itself and of other drugs.

EXCRETION. About 70% is excreted in the urine and 10% in the faeces; the urinary metabolites include 3-hydroxydiazepam and oxazepam and their conjugates; diazepam is excreted to some extent in the bile.

FURTHER INFORMATION. Factors influencing plasma concentrations—R. A. Assaf *et al.*, *Br. J. clin. Pharmac.*, 1974, **1**, 343P; in breast milk—R. Brandt, *Arzneimittel-Forsch.*, 1976, **26**, 454; plasma concentrations—H. H. Dasberg *et al.*, *Clin. Pharmac. Ther.*, 1974, **15**, 473; cumulation of *N*-desmethyl metabolite in cerebrospinal fluid—J. Hendel, *Acta pharmac. tox.*, 1975, **37**, 1 7; metabolism in normal man—L. Hillestad *et al.*, *Clin. Pharmac. Ther.*, 1974, **16**, 479 and 485; pharmacokinetics—S. A. Kaplan *et al.*, *J. pharm. Sci.*, 1973, **62**, 1789 and U. Klotz *et al.*, *J. clin. Invest.*, 1975, **55**, 347; biliary elimination—W. A. Mahon *et al.*, *Clin.*

Pharmac. Ther., 1976, **19**, 443; placental transfer and disposition in newborn—M. Mandelli *et al.*, *Clin. Pharmac. Ther.*, 1975, **17**, 564; metabolism in chronic alcoholic patients—R. Sellman *et al.*, *Acta pharmac. tox.*, 1975, **36**, 25 and 33; induction effect of diazepam on its own metabolism—R. Sellman *et al.*, *Acta pharmac. tox.*, 1975, **37**, 345; pharmacokinetics—E. Van der Kleijn *et al.*, *Acta pharmac. tox.*, 1971, **29**, Suppl. 3, 109; metabolism during chronic medication—I. A. Zingales, *J. Chromat.*, 1973, **75**, 55; pharmacokinetic review—M. Mandelli *et al.*, *Clin. Pharmacokinet.*, 1978, **3**, 72.

Actions and uses. Diazepam has tranquillising properties similar to those described under Chlordiazepoxide Hydrochloride.

It is used in the treatment of psychoneurotic disorders, when anxiety and nervous tension are present; it has also been used to relieve muscle spasm in various conditions, in the treatment of status epilepticus, in acute alcohol withdrawal, and for preoperative medication.

Dosage depends upon the clinical condition and response of the patient, varying from 5 to 30 milligrams daily in divided doses in the treatment of anxiety and nervous tension, this dosage being reduced in elderly and debilitated patients. In anxious children, the daily dose is usually 1 to 5 milligrams.

In status epilepticus and tetanus, a dose of 10 milligrams of diazepam may be given by intramuscular or intravenous injection. Patients should be kept under observation in the supine position in bed for at least one hour after injection.

When given undiluted by the intravenous route the injection should be administered at a rate not exceeding 5 milligrams per minute. When given by intravenous infusion the solution should be diluted to contain not more than 10 milligrams of diazepam in 125 millilitres of infusion solution.

Undesirable effects. Drowsiness, ataxia, dryness of the mouth, and hypotension may occur. In severely disturbed patients, diazepam, like chlordiazepoxide, may sometimes provoke aggressive behaviour rather than sedation. Rashes, blood dyscrasias, and hepatic dysfunction may rarely occur.

Diazepam may reduce the patient's ability to drive motor cars or operate moving machinery.

Precautions and contra-indications. Caution should be exercised in using diazepam in conjunction with alcohol and with other drugs that act on the central nervous system.

When used adjunctively in convulsive disorders, diazepam may increase the frequency and severity of grand mal seizures, necessitating an increased dosage of anticonvulsant drugs. Abrupt withdrawal may be associated with temporary increase in frequency and severity of seizures.

Diazepam should be used with caution in patients with acute narrow-angle glaucoma.

Diazepam should also be used with caution in nursing mothers; it is secreted in the milk and in high dosage may give rise to sedation in breast-fed infants. It crosses the placenta and high doses in late pregnancy may cause lethargy and hypotonia in the offspring.

Dependence. Diazepam may give rise to dependence of the barbiturate-alcohol type as described in the entry on Drug Dependence.

Preparations

DIAZEPAM CAPSULES: consisting of diazepam, which may be mixed with a suitable inert diluent, enclosed in a hard capsule. The capsule shells may be coloured. Available as capsules containing 2 and 5 mg of diazepam.

A standard for these capsules is given in the British Pharmacopoeia 1973

Containers and *Storage:* see the entry on Capsules for general information on containers and storage. Containers should be light resistant.

Advice for patients: the capsules may cause drowsiness; persons affected should not drive or operate machinery. Alcohol should be avoided.

DIAZEPAM ELIXIR: a solution of diazepam in a suitable coloured flavoured vehicle.

When a dose less than or not a multiple of 5 ml is prescribed, the elixir may be diluted, as described in the entry on Elixirs, with syrup or sorbitol solution. The diluted elixir must be freshly prepared and should be well shaken.

Available as a solution containing 2 mg of diazepam in 5 ml.

Containers and *Labelling:* see the entry on Elixirs for general information on containers and labelling.

Storage: it should be stored in a cool place, protected from light.

Advice for patients: the elixir may cause drowsiness; persons affected should not drive or operate machinery. Alcohol should be avoided.

DIAZEPAM INJECTION: a sterile solution of diazepam in propylene glycol. Available in 2- and 5-ml ampoules containing 5 mg of diazepam per ml.

Containers and *Labelling:* see the entry on Injections for general information on containers and labelling.

Storage: it should be protected from light.

DIAZEPAM TABLETS: available as tablets containing 2, 5, and 10 mg of diazepam; they may be coloured.

A standard for these tablets is given in the British Pharmacopoeia 1973

Containers and *Storage:* see the entry on Tablets for general information on containers and storage. Containers should be airtight and light resistant.

Advice for patients: the tablets may cause drowsiness; persons affected should not drive or operate machinery. Alcohol should be avoided.

Diazoxide

7-Chloro-3-methyl-2*H*-benzo-1,2,4-thiadiazine 1,1-dioxide

$C_8H_7ClN_2O_2S = 230.7$

OTHER NAME: *Eudemine®*

A standard is given in the British Pharmacopoeia Addendum 1975

Description. An odourless white crystalline powder.

Solubility. Very slightly soluble in water; soluble, at 20°, in 250 parts of alcohol; very slightly soluble in ether and in chloroform; soluble in solutions of alkali hydroxides.

Sterilisation. Solutions of the sodium salt for injection are sterilised by heating in an autoclave or by filtration.

Identification. MELTING-POINT. About 330°.

ULTRAVIOLET ABSORPTION. In 0.1N sodium hydroxide, maximum at 280 nm (E1%, 1cm = 590); in alcohol, maximum at 270 nm (E1%, 1cm = 455).

INFRA-RED ABSORPTION. Major peaks at 813, 1111, 1136, 1163, 1299, and 1493 cm^{-1} (see Appendix 2b: Infra-red Spectra).

Determination in body fluids. ULTRAVIOLET SPECTRO-PHOTOMETRY. In blood—S. Symchowicz *et al.*, *J. pharm. Sci.*, 1967, **56**, 912.

Metabolism. ABSORPTION. Well absorbed after oral administration. The extent of absorption is related to the dissolution rate of the formulation.

BLOOD CONCENTRATION. After an oral dose of 300 mg, peak plasma concentrations of about 15 μg/ml are attained in about 5 hours; after an intravenous dose of 210 to 300 mg, plasma concentrations of 40 μg/ml are attained within 30 minutes falling to 20 to 30 μg/ml at 1 hour; maintenance doses in children give plasma concentrations of 15 to 50 μg/ml.

HALF-LIFE. Plasma half-life in adults, 20 to 70 hours, and in children, 9 to 24 hours.

DISTRIBUTION. Volume of distribution, 13 to 23 litres which is increased in renal function impairment and decreased in children; diazoxide does not appear to be localised in any particular tissues; it crosses the placenta and also enters the cerebrospinal fluid; *protein binding,* about 90% bound to plasma proteins, which may be reduced in renal function impairment depending upon the reduction in plasma albumin concentration which may occur.

METABOLIC REACTIONS. Oxidation of the methyl group to an alcohol which is conjugated with sulphate or further metabolised to the carboxylic acid.

EXCRETION. Up to 90% of a dose is excreted in the urine in 5 to 6 days; 6 to 50% appears to be excreted unchanged along with the hydroxy and carboxylic acid metabolites which account for 20 to 30% of the excreted material; the amounts of unchanged drug excreted in the urine of hypertensive patients appear to be reduced; this may be a consequence of the antidiuretic activity of diazoxide when administered in large doses; about 2% of a dose is excreted in the faeces.

FURTHER INFORMATION. Metabolism and disposition (a review)—P. G. Dayton *et al.*, *Drug Met. Disp.*, 1975, **3**, 226; decreased plasma protein binding in uraemia—K. O'Malley *et al.*, *Clin. Pharmac. Ther.*, 1975, **18**, 53; pharmacokinetics and response in renal failure—R. M. Pearson, *Clin. Pharmacokinet.*, 1977, **2**, 198 and R. M. Pearson and A. M. Breckenridge, *Br. J. clin. Pharmac.*, 1976, **3**, 169; disposition in children—A. W. Pruitt *et al.*, *Clin. Pharmac. Ther.*, 1973, **14**, 73; metabolism—A. W. Pruitt *et al.*, *J. Pharmac. exp. Ther.*, 1974, **188**, 248; concentrations in urine and plasma—W. Sadee *et al.*, *J. Pharmacokinet. Biopharm.*, 1973, **1**, 195.

Actions and uses. Diazoxide has antihypertensive and antihypoglycaemic actions. Its antihypertensive effect is due to dilatation of peripheral arterioles. Its antihypoglycaemic effect may be due to a direct action on the β-cells of the pancreas, thus reducing the release of stored insulin, to stimulation of catecholamine release, to a direct action on the liver increasing the rate of glucose output, or to a combination of these mechanisms. Diazoxide is used in severe hypertension which has failed to respond to treatment with other drugs; it is also useful for the rapid reduction of blood pressure in hypertensive crises. It may be administered by rapid intravenous injection in a dose of 300 milligrams; further doses of 300 milligrams may be given intravenously at intervals of 2 to 3 hours up to a maximum of 1.2 grams in 24 hours. The usual dose by mouth is 0.4 to 1 gram daily in divided doses.

Diazoxide is also used in the treatment of intractable hypoglycaemia where surgery is impracticable. It is administered orally in an initial dose of 5 milligrams per kilogram body-weight daily in divided doses. The dose may be increased until satisfactory control is obtained. In adults with tumours producing large amounts of insulin, up to 1 gram daily may be necessary. The initial dose for children is 5 milligrams per kilogram body-weight daily in divided doses; in idiopathic hypoglycaemia a dose of 10 to 15 milligrams per kilogram body-weight may be required.

Undesirable effects. In the treatment of hypertension there may be associated hyperglycaemia and when treating hypoglycaemia there may be profound hypotension and pain in the chest. When administered by mouth diazoxide may give rise to hypertrichosis, especially in children, and oedema, anorexia, nausea, and vomiting may occur. Rashes, leucopenia, thrombocytopenia, hyperuricaemia, cardiac arrhythmias, and extrapyramidal side-effects occur rarely.

When administered during pregnancy there is a high incidence of alopecia in the newborn.

Precautions. In long-term therapy regular examination of the blood for changes in white-cell and platelet counts should be undertaken. In children there should be regular assessment of growth, bone, and psychological maturation.

Preparations

DIAZOXIDE INJECTION: a sterile solution of diazoxide sodium, prepared by the interaction of diazoxide with sodium hydroxide, in water for injections. It is sterilised by heating in an autoclave or by filtration. Available as a solution containing diazoxide sodium equivalent to 15 mg of diazoxide per ml in 20-ml ampoules. It should be neither mixed with other drugs nor diluted.

A standard for this injection is given in the British Pharmacopoeia Addendum 1975

Containers and *Labelling:* see the entry on Injections for general information on containers and labelling.

Storage: it should be protected from light.

DIAZOXIDE TABLETS: available as sugar-coated tablets containing 50 mg of diazoxide.

A standard for these tablets is given in the British Pharmacopoeia Addendum 1975

Containers and *Storage:* see the entry on Tablets for general information on containers and storage. Containers should be airtight.

Advice for patients: the tablets should be taken at regular intervals. Treatment should not be discontinued without the advice of the prescriber.

Dibromopropamidine Isethionate

The bis(2-hydroxyethanesulphonate) of 3,3'-dibromo-4,4'-trimethylenedioxydibenzamidine *or* of 4,4'-trimethylenedioxybis(3-bromobenzamidine)

$C_{21}H_{30}Br_2N_4O_{10}S_2 = 722.4$

OTHER NAMES: *Brolene®*; *Brulidine®* *Otamidyl®* (with di(4-amidinophenyl)amine dihydrochloride); *Dibrogan®* and *Phenergan®* (both with promethazine)

A standard is given in the British Pharmacopoeia 1973

Description. An odourless white crystalline powder with a bitter taste.

Solubility. Soluble, at 20°, in 2 parts of water, in 60 parts of alcohol, and in 20 parts of glycerol; practically insoluble in ether, in chloroform, in fixed oils, and in liquid paraffin.

Acidity. A 5% solution has a pH of 5 to 7.

Moisture content. Not more than 2%, determined by drying at 105°.

Sterilisation. Aqueous solutions are sterilised by filtration.

Storage. It should be stored in airtight containers.

Identification. TESTS. 1. Dissolve about 200 mg in 20 ml of water, divide the solution into two portions, and to one portion add 1 ml of *dilute sulphuric acid*; a white precipitate is produced. To the other portion of solution add 4 drops of *sodium hydroxide solution*; a white precipitate is produced (also given by pentamidine isethionate).

2. Dissolve about 5 mg in 10 ml of water, add 1 ml of a 0.1% solution of glyoxal sodium bisulphite and 1 ml of a solution prepared by dissolving 4 g of boric acid in 27 ml of 1N sodium hydroxide diluted to 100 ml with water, and heat on a water-bath for 10 minutes; a magenta colour is produced (also given by pentamidine isethionate).

3. Mix about 100 mg with 500 mg of anhydrous sodium carbonate, ignite, extract the residue with 20 ml of water, filter, neutralise the filtrate to litmus paper with nitric acid, and add *silver nitrate solution*; a yellowish curdy precipitate is produced which is somewhat soluble in *strong ammonia solution* but insoluble in *dilute ammonia solution.*

ULTRAVIOLET ABSORPTION. In 0.01N hydrochloric acid, maximum at 261 nm (E1%, 1cm = 340).

INFRA-RED ABSORPTION. Major peaks at 1047, 1190, 1266, 1456, 1479, and 1654 cm^{-1} (see Appendix 2a: Infra-red Spectra).

Actions and uses. Dibromopropamidine is an antibacterial and fungistatic agent for external use.

It is active against various streptococci and against *Staphylococcus aureus*, including forms resistant to penicillin and other antibiotics, and against certain Gram-negative bacilli, particularly *Escherichia coli*, *Proteus vulgaris*, and some strains of *Pseudomonas aeruginosa*. Its antibacterial action is not inhibited by pus, blood, or 4-aminobenzoic acid.

A cream containing 0.15% of dibromopropamidine isethionate has been used as a first-aid dressing for wounds, abrasions, burns, and scalds.

An eye ointment containing 0.15% is used in acute infections of the conjunctiva and in blepharitis.

Preparations

Preparations available include a CREAM containing dibromopropamidine isethionate 0.15%, a cream containing dibromopropamidine isethionate 0.15% with promethazine 2%, a veterinary cream containing dibromopropamidine isethionate 0.165% with promethazine 2%, EAR-DROPS containing dibromopropamidine isethionate 0.15% with di(4-amidinophenyl)amine dihydrochloride 0.5%, and EYE OINTMENT containing dibromopropamidine isethionate 0.15%.

Dichlofenthion

O-2,4-Dichlorophenyl OO-diethyl phosphorothioate

$C_{10}H_{13}Cl_2O_3PS = 315.1$

A standard is given in the British Pharmacopoeia (Veterinary)

Description. A colourless or pale yellow oily liquid.

Solubility. Immiscible with water; miscible with alcohol, with benzene, and with chloroform.

Weight per ml. At 20°, 1.296 to 1.316 g.

Refractive index. At 25°, 1.530 to 1.533.

Veterinary uses. Dichlofenthion is an insecticide which is used as an ingredient of sheep dips.

Preparation

DICHLOFENTHION AND GAMMA BENZENE HEXACHLORIDE DIP CONCENTRATE: a solution consisting of dichlofenthion and gamma benzene hexachloride mixed with suitable pharmaceutical adjuvants to produce an emulsifiable concentrate. It may contain a suitable preservative.
Available as a concentrate containing 2.5% of dichlofenthion and 2% of gamma benzene hexachloride. It must be diluted before use.
A standard for this dip concentrate is given in the British Pharmacopoeia (Veterinary)
Replenishment of baths: see the entry on Dip Concentrates for general information on the replenishment of baths.

Dichloralphenazone

A complex of chloral hydrate and phenazone.

$[CCl_3 \cdot CH(OH)_2]_2$

$C_{15}H_{18}Cl_6N_2O_5 = 519.0$

OTHER NAMES: *Bonadorm*®; *Dormwell*®; *Welldorm*® *Paedo-Sed*® (with paracetamol)

A standard is given in the British Pharmacopoeia 1973

Description. A white microcrystalline powder with a slight odour characteristic of chloral hydrate and a taste which is saline at first, becoming acrid.

Solubility. Soluble, at 20°, in 10 parts of water, in 1 part of alcohol, and in 2 parts of chloroform; soluble in dilute acids.

Stability. Formation of an insoluble, inactive, 4-substituted condensation product, 2,3-dimethyl-1-phenyl-4-(2,2,2-trichloro-1-hydroxyethyl)pyrazolin-5-one, may occur, especially at elevated temperatures. Chloral hydrate may be lost by volatilisation.
In aqueous solution, dichloralphenazone behaves as a mixture of chloral hydrate and phenazone and will exhibit the stability characteristics of these two substances. For example, in alkaline solution, chloroform is liberated from the chloral hydrate.

Hygroscopicity. It is hygroscopic, although less so than chloral hydrate.

Sterilisation. Solutions are sterilised by filtration.

Storage. It should be stored in airtight containers in a cool place.

Identification. TESTS. 1. Dissolve 100 mg in 10 ml of water containing 100 mg of sodium nitrite and add 1 ml of *dilute sulphuric acid*; a green colour is produced.
2. It complies with Test 3 described under Chloral Hydrate.

MELTING-POINT. About 65°.

Determination in body fluids; Metabolism. After administration, dichloralphenazone acts as a mixture of chloral hydrate and phenazone, and reference should be made to the entries on these substances.

Actions and uses. Dichloralphenazone has the actions of its constituents, chloral and phenazone. It is used as described under Chloral Hydrate but is less likely to cause nausea and vomiting.
A dose of 650 milligrams may be given 2 or 3 times a day as a sedative. In domiciliary midwifery it is an effective sedative in a dose of 1.3 to 2.6 grams.
Dichloralphenazone is particularly suitable for geriatric patients, a suitable dose being 1.3 grams. As a hypnotic, 0.65 to 2 grams may be given as a single dose for an adult; children up to 1 year may be given 90 to 270 milligrams, 1 to 5 years 270 to 540 milligrams, and 6 to 12 years 540 to 675 milligrams. Doses should be taken with fluid since chloral is a gastric irritant.

Undesirable effects. Flatulence, abdominal distension, nausea, rashes, pruritus, headache, and lassitude may rarely occur.

Contra-indications. It is contra-indicated in acute intermittent porphyria since it may precipitate an acute attack.

Dependence. It may give rise to dependence of the barbiturate-alcohol type as described under Drug Dependence and it may also enhance the effects of alcohol.

Drug interactions. It may increase the difficulty in controlling oral anticoagulant therapy.

Preparations

DICHLORALPHENAZONE ELIXIR: a solution of dichloralphenazone in a suitable coloured flavoured vehicle. When a dose less than or not a multiple of 5 ml is prescribed, the elixir may be diluted, as described in the entry on Elixirs, with syrup. The diluted elixir must be freshly prepared.

Available as a solution containing 225 mg of dichloralphenazone in 5 ml.

A standard for this elixir is given in the British Pharmaceutical Codex 1973

Containers and *Labelling:* see the entry on Elixirs for general information on containers and labelling.

Storage: it should be stored in well-filled airtight containers, in a cool place, protected from light.

Advice for patients: the elixir should be taken diluted with water. Hypnotic doses should be taken 20 minutes before bedtime. The elixir may cause drowsiness on the following day; persons affected should not drive or operate machinery. Alcohol should be avoided.

DICHLORALPHENAZONE TABLETS: available as tablets containing 650 mg of dichloralphenazone with peppermint oil as flavouring agent; the tablets may be coated with sugar or other suitable material and the coat may be coloured.

A standard for these tablets is given in the British Pharmacopoeia 1973

Containers and *Storage:* see the entry on Tablets for general information on containers and storage. Containers should be airtight. The tablets should be stored in a cool place.

Advice for patients: the tablets should be swallowed with water. Hypnotic doses should be taken 20 minutes before bedtime. The tablets may cause drowsiness on the following day; persons affected should not drive or operate machinery. Alcohol should be avoided.

OTHER PREPARATIONS available include an ELIXIR containing dichloralphenazone 200 mg with paracetamol 100 mg in 5 ml, diluent syrup, life of diluted elixir 14 days; other diluents such as orange juice or milk may also be used.

Dichlorodifluoromethane

$CCl_2F_2 = 120.9$

OTHER NAMES: *Arcton 12*®; Difluorodichloromethane; *Isceon 12*®; Propellent 12; Refrigerant 12

Dichlorodifluoromethane is gaseous at ordinary temperatures but is liquefied by compression and is supplied in liquid form in suitable containers.

A standard is given in the British Pharmaceutical Codex 1973

Description. A clear, colourless, non-inflammable, very volatile liquid with a faintly ethereal odour.

Solubility. In the liquid state it is immiscible with water and miscible with dehydrated alcohol.

Weight per ml. At 15°, about 1.35 g and, at −35°, about 1.50 g.

Boiling-point. About −29.8°.

Storage. It should be stored in suitable metal containers in a cool place away from any fire risk.

Metabolism. For information on pharmacokinetics in dogs see S. Niazi and W. L. Chiou, *J. pharm. Sci.*, 1977, **66**, 49.

Uses. Dichlorodifluoromethane is used as a refrigerant and as an aerosol propellant, as described in the entry on Propellents. It is gaseous at room temperature and must be handled in a closed system under pressure. It is sometimes used as the sole propellent, particularly if its vapour pressure is likely to be reduced by other constituents of the preparation. More commonly it is mixed with either trichlorofluoromethane or dichlorotetrafluoroethane to form propellent 12/11 or propellent 12/114 mixtures.

Typical aerosol preparations using propellent 12/11 mixtures are spray bandages and analgesic or anaesthetic sprays. Propellent 12/114 mixtures are used mainly in antibronchitic and antiasthmatic sprays and in nasal and dermatological sprays.

Preparations

See under Trichlorofluoromethane.

Dichlorophen

2,2'-Methylenebis(4-chlorophenol) *or* 4,4'-dichloro-2,2'-methylenediphenol

$C_{13}H_{10}Cl_2O_2 = 269.1$

OTHER NAMES: *Anthiphen*®; *Dicestal*®

A standard is given in the British Pharmacopoeia 1973

Description. A white to slightly cream-coloured powder with a very slight phenolic odour and a saline and phenolic taste.

Solubility. Very slightly soluble in water; soluble, at 20°, in 1 part of alcohol and in less than 1 part of ether.

Moisture content. Not more than 1%, determined by drying at 105°.

Identification. TEST. Dissolve 200 mg in a mixture of 5 ml of water and 5 ml of *sodium hydroxide solution*, cool in ice, and add a solution prepared by mixing 1 ml of *sodium nitrite solution* with a cold solution containing 0.15 ml of aniline in a mixture of 4 ml of water and 1 ml of hydrochloric acid; a reddish-brown precipitate is produced.

MELTING-POINT. About 176°.

ULTRAVIOLET ABSORPTION. In 0.1N sodium hydroxide, maxima at 245 nm (E1%, 1cm = 650) and 304 nm (E1%, 1cm = 270).

Actions and uses. Dichlorophen is a taenicide with a direct lethal action on the worm. It is active against all species of tapeworm, including fish tapeworms (*Diphyllobothrium latum*) and dwarf tapeworms (*Hymenolepis nana*).

After the tapeworm has been killed, the segments are partially digested in the intestine and they are therefore largely unrecognisable in the stools, so that it is impossible to be sure whether the scolex has been removed. There is no necessity for preliminary starvation or the administration of a laxative.

Dichlorophen is best given in the morning on an empty stomach, as the dosing is usually followed in 2 to 3 hours by intestinal colic and the passing of a few loose stools. Dichlorophen is administered in a dose of 6 grams for an adult or 2 to 4 grams for a child on the morning of 2 successive days.

Undesirable effects. Vomiting occurs occasionally and there is the possibility that segments or ova regurgitated into the stomach could cause cysticercosis.

Contra-indications. Dichlorophen is contra-indicated in liver or severe cardiovascular disease, in febrile illness, in pregnancy, or when purgation is undesirable.

Veterinary uses. Dichlorophen is used in the treatment of tapeworm infections (*Taenia* and *Dipylidium* spp.) in dogs and cats in a dose of 200 milligrams per kilogram body-weight repeated, if required, after 10 days.
An ointment containing 2% or an aerosol spray is used for the treatment of ringworm.

Preparations

DICHLOROPHEN AEROSOL SPRAY: a solution of dichlorophen in a suitable solvent to which suitable propellents have been added. It may contain a suitable dye to act as a marker. It is packed in a pressurised container fitted with a suitable valve.
Available as aerosol sprays containing 2, 7, 7.5 and 10% w/w of dichlorophen.
A standard for this aerosol spray is given in the British Pharmacopoeia (Veterinary)
Containers and *Storage:* see the entry on Aerosol Inhalations for general information on containers and storage.
Labelling: the label on the container should state the weight of dichlorophen present in the container, the total weight of contents, the name and proportion of any added dye, and directions for using the preparation.

DICHLOROPHEN TABLETS: available as tablets containing 500 mg of dichlorophen.
A standard for these tablets is given in the British Pharmacopoeia 1973
Containers and *Storage:* see the entry on Tablets for general information on containers and storage. Containers should be airtight.
Advice for patients: daily doses should preferably be taken in the morning before breakfast. The prescribed course should be completed.

Dichlorotetrafluoroethane

1,2-Dichloro-1,1,2,2-tetrafluoroethane
$CClF_2 . CClF_2 = 170.9$

OTHER NAMES: *Arcton 114®*; *Isceon 114®*; Propellent 114; Refrigerant 114; Tetrafluorodichloroethane

A standard is given in the British Pharmaceutical Codex 1973

Dichlorotetrafluoroethane is gaseous at ordinary temperatures but is liquefied by compression and is supplied in liquid form in suitable metal containers.

Description. A clear, colourless, non-inflammable, very volatile liquid with a faintly ethereal odour.

Solubility. In the liquid state it is immiscible with water and miscible with dehydrated alcohol.

Weight per ml. At 15°, about 1.49 g and, at −35°, about 1.63 g.

Boiling-point. About 3.5°.

Storage. It should be stored in suitable metal containers, in a cool place away from any fire risk.

Uses. Dichlorotetrafluoroethane is used as a refrigerant and as an aerosol propellant, as described in the entry on Propellents. It is gaseous at room temperature and must be handled either in a closed system under pressure or as a refrigerated liquid in an open system. It is stable in the presence of water and may be used in place of trichlorofluoromethane as a means of controlling the

pressure in aqueous formulations. A range of pressures can be achieved with different mixtures of dichlorotetrafluoroethane and dichlorodifluoromethane.

Dichlorphenamide

4,5-Dichlorobenzene-1,3-disulphonamide

$C_6H_6Cl_2N_2O_4S_2 = 305.2$

OTHER NAMES: *Daranide®*; *Oratrol®*

A standard is given in the British Pharmacopoeia 1973

Description. A white crystalline powder with a slight odour and taste and a bitter after-taste.

Solubility. Very slightly soluble in water and in chloroform; soluble, at 20°, in 30 parts of alcohol; soluble in solutions of alkali hydroxides.

Moisture content. Not more than 1%, determined by drying at 100° *in vacuo.*

Identification. MELTING-POINT. About 240°.

ULTRAVIOLET ABSORPTION. In 0.1N sodium hydroxide, maxima at 285 nm (E1%, 1cm = 42) and 294 nm (E1%, 1cm = 36).

INFRA-RED ABSORPTION. Major peaks at 706, 881, 906, 1163, 1180, and 1333 cm⁻¹ (see Appendix 2a: Infra-red Spectra).

Actions and uses. Dichlorphenamide is a carbonic-anhydrase inhibitor which has an action similar to but more prolonged than that described under Acetazolamide but which also causes an increase in chloride excretion.
Dichlorphenamide is used to effect reduction of the intra-ocular pressure in the treatment of various types of glaucoma, for which the initial dose is 100 to 200 milligrams by mouth, followed by 100 milligrams every 12 hours until the desired result is achieved, after which a maintenance dosage of 25 to 50 milligrams is given 1 to 3 times a day. Its effect begins within 1 hour and reaches a maximum within 2 to 4 hours.

Undesirable effects. Anorexia, nausea and vomiting, numbness and paraesthesia of the extremities, confusion, drowsiness, tremors, ataxia, and tinnitus may occur.

Precautions. The concomitant use of miotics is essential when treating all types of glaucoma with dichlorphenamide. Its use over prolonged periods in chronic cases results in considerable electrolyte depletion and symptoms of potassium deficiency may develop, in which case potassium supplements should be given; such treatment does not interfere with the ocular effects of the drug.

Preparation

DICHLORPHENAMIDE TABLETS: available as tablets containing 50 mg of dichlorphenamide; they may be coloured.
A standard for these tablets is given in the British Pharmacopoeia 1973
Containers and *Storage:* see the entry on Tablets for

general information on containers and storage. Containers should be airtight.

Advice for patients: daily doses should preferably be taken in the morning. When used in glaucoma, treatment should not be discontinued without the advice of the prescriber. The tablets may cause drowsiness; persons affected should not drive or operate machinery. Alcohol should be avoided.

Dicobalt Edetate

Dicobalt ethylenediamine-*NNN'N'*-tetra-acetate

$$\left[\begin{array}{cc} \text{-OOC·CH}_2 & \text{CH}_2\text{·COO}^- \\ & \diagdown \hspace{0.5cm} \diagup \\ & \text{N·CH}_2\text{·CH}_2\text{·N} \\ & \diagup \hspace{0.5cm} \diagdown \\ \text{-OOC·CH}_2 & \text{CH}_2\text{·COO}^- \end{array} \right] 2\text{Co}^{2+}$$

$C_{10}H_{12}Co_2N_2O_8 = 406.1$

OTHER NAMES: Cobalt Edetate; *Kelocyanor*®

Actions and uses. Dicobalt edetate forms a stable complex with cyanide ions and is used in the treatment of cyanide poisoning to render cyanide harmless. Treatment must be started as rapidly as possible.

The usual dose is 40 millilitres of an injection containing a total of 600 milligrams of dicobalt edetate by intravenous injection followed immediately by 50 millilitres of strong dextrose injection. If there is no response, a further 20 millilitres of the dicobalt edetate injection is administered followed by a further 50 millilitres of strong dextrose injection or alternatively treatment with sodium nitrite injection and sodium thiosulphate injection may be given as described under Sodium Nitrite.

Undesirable effects. Injection of dicobalt edetate initially causes a fall in blood pressure, an increased pulse rate, and vomiting, but these effects should last for only about 1 minute.

Precautions. As dicobalt edetate is toxic it should only be given to patients with cyanide poisoning.

Preparations

Preparations available include an INJECTION containing dicobalt edetate 15 mg per ml in 20-ml ampoules.

Dicophane

A mixture consisting chiefly of 1,1,1-trichloro-2,2-bis(4-chlorophenyl)ethane, with variable quantities of an isomer, and the carbinol resulting from condensation of one molecular proportion of chlorobenzene with chloral hydrate.

$C_{14}H_9Cl_5 = 354.5$

OTHER NAMES: Chlorophenothane; DDT
Esoderm® (with gamma benzene hexachloride)

A standard is given in the British Pharmacopoeia 1973

Description. White crystals, powder, flakes, or small granules, which are odourless or have a slight aromatic odour.

Solubility. Very slightly soluble in water; soluble in carbon tetrachloride; soluble, at 20°, in 50 parts of alcohol and in 10 parts of most fixed oils.

Moisture content. Not more than 1%, determined by Fischer titration.

Storage. It should be stored in airtight containers.

Identification. TESTS. 1. Heat a small quantity until it melts and continue heating; decomposition occurs and hydrogen chloride is evolved.
2. Mix a small quantity with a 0.5% solution of hydroquinone in nitrogen-free sulphuric acid and heat; a wine-red colour is produced.

MELTING-POINT. About 109°.

Actions and uses. Dicophane is an insecticide and larvicide. It is active whether ingested by the insect or absorbed through the cuticle and, because of its low volatility, retains its activity for long periods under a variety of conditions. It does not, however, have the immediate lethal effect of derris and pyrethrum. A 0.25% aqueous suspension is used as an insecticidal spray. Dicophane has been applied to the head as a 2% application to kill lice and it has been used as a dusting-powder containing 2 to 10% for the disinfection of clothing.

The development of resistant strains in species of insects which are normally susceptible has been reported.

Undesirable effects. In mammals, dicophane acts mainly as a peripheral nerve poison, but appears also to have an action on the central nervous system. Ingestion of dicophane may be lethal. Occasionally, hepatic insufficiency may develop without premonitory symptoms or associated nervous signs; when this happens, there is a rapid loss in body-weight and anaemia and leucocytosis develop. Kidney damage may also occur. These hepatic and renal conditions appear to be reversible.

Precautions. Protective clothing, including a face mask, should be worn when handling concentrated solutions of dicophane in organic solvents, as the risk of absorption is considerable. Warning of toxicity is usually given by loss of appetite, muscular weakness, and fine tremors; if at this stage further contact with dicophane is avoided, these effects usually disappear spontaneously.

The widespread use of dicophane as a general insecticide is undesirable because of the persistence of toxic residues.

Poisoning. Solutions of dicophane, if swallowed, may produce vomiting, diarrhoea, and collapse; these conditions should be treated symptomatically. Dicophane may also give rise to a prolonged tendency to convulsions, which may require treatment with diazepam.

Preparations

Preparations available include an APPLICATION containing dicophane 1% with gamma benzene hexachloride 1%, in a shampoo basis and a LOTION containing dicophane 1% with gamma benzene hexachloride 1%.

Dicyclomine Hydrochloride

2-[Bi(cyclohexyl)carbonyloxy]triethylammonium chloride

$C_{19}H_{36}ClNO_2 = 346.0$

OTHER NAME: *Merbentyl*®

A standard is given in the British Pharmacopoeia 1973

Description. An odourless white crystalline powder with a bitter taste followed by local numbness.

Solubility. Soluble, at 20°, in 20 parts of water, in 5 parts of alcohol, and in 2 parts of chloroform; practically insoluble in ether.

Acidity. A 1% solution has a pH of 5 to 5.5.

Moisture content. Not more than 1%, determined by drying at 105°.

Identification. TEST. To 3 ml of a 0.1% solution of sodium lauryl sulphate add 5 ml of chloroform and 1 drop of a 0.25% solution of methylene blue, mix gently and allow to separate; the chloroform layer is blue. Dissolve about 20 mg of the sample in 2 ml of water, add to the mixture, shake gently and again allow to separate; the blue colour is transferred to the aqueous layer.

MELTING-POINT. About 173°.

ULTRAVIOLET ABSORPTION. In 0.1N sulphuric acid, there are no maxima in the range 230 nm to 360 nm.

INFRA-RED ABSORPTION. Major peaks at 1136, 1184, 1197, 1214, 1453, and 1714 cm^{-1} (see Appendix 2a: Infrared Spectra).

THIN-LAYER CHROMATOGRAPHY. See under Thin-layer Chromatography, System 8.

Determination in body fluids. GAS CHROMATOGRAPHY. In plasma—P. J. Meffin *et al.*, *Analyt. Chem.*, 1973, **45**, 1964.

Metabolism. ABSORPTION. Rapidly absorbed after oral administration.

BLOOD CONCENTRATION. After oral administration of 20 mg, peak plasma concentrations of about 20 ng/ml are attained in about 1.5 hours.

HALF-LIFE. The plasma half-life of drug plus metabolites is about 5 hours.

EXCRETION. 80% of an oral dose is excreted in the urine and about 10% is excreted in the faeces.

FURTHER INFORMATION. Metabolism—I. E. Danhof *et al.*, *Toxic. appl. Pharmac.*, 1968, **13**, 16; plasma concentrations—P. J. Meffin *et al.*, *Analyt. Chem.*, 1973, **45**, 1964.

Actions and uses. Dicyclomine has peripheral actions similar to but much weaker than those described under Atropine. It has been given by mouth to diminish gastric secretion and to reduce gastric and intestinal motility in the treatment of peptic ulceration and pylorospasm.

The usual dosage of dicyclomine is 30 to 60 milligrams daily in divided doses. Children up to 1 year may be given 5 milligrams before feeds, and children aged 1 to 5 years 5 to 10 milligrams 3 times daily.

Undesirable effects. As for Benzhexol Hydrochloride but less frequent and less severe.

Precautions and contra-indications. As for Atropine.

Preparations

DICYCLOMINE ELIXIR (*Syn.* Dicyclomine Syrup): a solution of dicyclomine hydrochloride in a suitable, coloured, flavoured vehicle. Available as an elixir containing 10 mg of dicyclomine hydrochloride in 5 ml. When a dose less than or not a multiple of 5 ml is prescribed, the elixir may be diluted, as described in the entry on Elixirs, with syrup. The diluted elixir must be freshly prepared.
A standard for this elixir is given in the British Pharmaceutical Codex 1973
Containers and *Labelling:* see the entry on Elixirs for general information on containers and labelling.
Storage: it should be protected from light.

DICYCLOMINE TABLETS: available as tablets containing 10 mg of dicyclomine hydrochloride.
A standard for these tablets is given in the British Pharmacopoeia 1973
Containers and *Storage:* see the entry on Tablets for general information on containers and storage. Containers should be airtight.

Dienoestrol

(Z,Z)-4,4'-[1,2-Bis(ethylidene)ethylene]diphenol

$C_{18}H_{18}O_2 = 266.3$

OTHER NAMES: Dienestrol; Dienoestrolum; *Hormofemin*®

A standard is given in the European Pharmacopoeia Vol. III

CAUTION. *Dienoestrol is a powerful oestrogen. Contact with the skin or inhalation of the dust should be avoided. Rubber gloves should be worn when handling the powder and, if the powder is dry, a face mask should be worn.*

Description. A white crystalline odourless powder.

Solubility. Very slightly soluble in water; soluble, at 20°, in 8 parts of alcohol, in 15 parts of ether, and in 5 parts of acetone; soluble in solutions of alkali hydroxides.

Storage. It should be protected from light.

Identification. TESTS. 1. Dissolve about 1 mg in 5 ml of glacial acetic acid, add 0.2 ml of a 1% v/v solution of bromine in glacial acetic acid, allow to stand for 20 seconds, add 1 drop of *liquefied phenol*, and heat in a water-bath for 2 minutes; an emerald-green colour is produced. Add a few mg of sucrose and continue heating on a water-bath; the green colour changes through deep blue, grey, and yellow to reddish-brown.

2. Dissolve about 1 mg in 5 ml of glacial acetic acid, add 1 ml of a 1% v/v solution of bromine in glacial acetic acid, and heat in a water-bath for 2 minutes; place 0.5 ml of this solution in a dry test-tube, add 0.5 ml of dehydrated

alcohol, mix, and add 10 ml of water; a reddish-violet colour is produced. Add 5 ml of chloroform, shake, and allow to separate; the chloroform layer is coloured deep orange-red and the aqueous layer is almost colourless.
3. Dissolve about 500 µg in 0.2 ml of glacial acetic acid, add 1 ml of phosphoric acid, and heat in a water-bath for 3 minutes; a red-violet colour is produced. Add 3 ml of glacial acetic acid; the colour becomes bluish-violet (distinction from stilboestrol).

MELTING-POINT. About 232°.

ULTRAVIOLET ABSORPTION. In alcohol (95%), maxima at 228 nm (E1%, 1cm = 1200) and 276 nm (E1%, 1cm = 160).

INFRA-RED ABSORPTION. Major peaks at 829, 1174, 1208, 1250, 1335, and 1512 cm^{-1} (see Appendix 2a: Infra-red Spectra).

THIN-LAYER CHROMATOGRAPHY. See under Thin-layer Chromatography, System 10.

Actions and uses. Dienoestrol has oestrogenic properties similar to those of stilboestrol but it is less potent. For menopausal symptoms, 0.5 to 5 milligrams of dienoestrol may be given daily.
For suppression of lactation, 15 milligrams may be given thrice daily for 3 days followed by 15 milligrams daily for 6 days.
The usual dosage for carcinoma of the prostate and mammary carcinoma is 15 to 30 milligrams daily.

Veterinary uses. Dienoestrol has been used in the treatment of infertility in farm animals. The usual dose for horses, cattle, sheep, and pigs is up to 10 micrograms per kilogram body-weight by subcutaneous injection.

Preparations

DIENOESTROL CREAM: a dispersion of dienoestrol in a suitable water-miscible basis. It may contain benzoic acid. Available as a cream containing 0.01% of dienoestrol with 0.2% of benzoic acid and as a cream containing 0.16% of dienoestrol.
Containers, Labelling, and *Storage:* see the entry on Creams for general information on containers, labelling, and storage.
Advice for patients: the cream should be applied high into the vagina with a suitable applicator, preferably at night. The prescribed course should be completed.

DIENOESTROL TABLETS: available as tablets containing 0.3 and 5 mg of dienoestrol.
A standard for these tablets is given in the British Pharmacopoeia 1973
Containers and *Storage:* see the entry on Tablets for general information on containers and storage. Containers should be airtight and light resistant.
Advice for patients: the prescribed course should be completed, or where applicable treatment should not be discontinued without the advice of the prescriber.

Diethyl Phthalate

Ethyl benzene-1,2-dicarboxylate

$C_{12}H_{14}O_4 = 222.2$

OTHER NAME: Ethyl Phthalate

A standard is given in the British Pharmaceutical Codex 1973

Description. A clear, colourless, somewhat viscous liquid with a slight odour.

Solubility. Practically insoluble in water; miscible with alcohol, with ether, and with aromatic hydrocarbons.

Weight per ml. At 20°, 1.115 to 1.119 g.

Refractive index. At 20°, 1.500 to 1.505.

Boiling-point. About 295°.

Identification. TESTS. 1. Mix 1 g with 5 ml of *alcoholic potassium hydroxide solution*, boil gently for 10 minutes, add 5 ml of water, evaporate to half its volume, cool, add 1 ml of hydrochloric acid, and filter; melt the dried residue, add 0.5 g of resorcinol and 1 drop of chloroform, heat at 180° for 3 minutes, cool, add 1 ml of *sodium hydroxide solution*, and pour into water; an intense yellowish-green fluorescence is produced.
2. Boil under a reflux condenser for 2 hours with 0.5N sodium hydroxide; the product gives the reactions characteristic of ethyl alcohol and, on acidification, a white precipitate is formed which, after recrystallisation from water and drying, melts at about 215°.

Uses. Diethyl phthalate is used as a solvent and plasticiser for cellacephate, cellulose acetate, nitrocellulose, and rubber. It is also used as a denaturant of alcohol, for example, in surgical spirit.

Undesirable effects. It is irritant to mucous membranes and when taken in large amounts causes paralysis of the central nervous system.

Diethylcarbamazine Citrate

NN-Diethyl-4-methylpiperazine-1-carboxamide dihydrogen citrate

$C_{16}H_{29}N_3O_8 = 391.4$

OTHER NAMES: *Banocide®*; *Caritrol®*; *Dicarocide®*; Diethylcarbam. Cit.; *Franocide®*; *Hetrazan®*; *Husk®* *Banminth D®* (with morantel tartrate)

A standard is given in the British Pharmacopoeia 1973

Description. An odourless white crystalline powder with a bitter acid taste.

Solubility. Soluble in water; soluble, at 20°, in 35 parts of alcohol; practically insoluble in ether, in chloroform, and in acetone.

Dissociation constant. pK_a 7.7 (25°).

Sterilisation. Solutions for injection are sterilised by heating in an autoclave or by filtration.

Storage. It should be stored in airtight containers.

Identification. TEST. Dissolve about 500 mg in 2 ml of water, make alkaline with *sodium hydroxide solution*, extract with four 5-ml portions of chloroform, wash the combined extracts with water, evaporate to dryness, add to the residue 1 ml of ethyl iodide, and heat gently under a reflux condenser for 5 minutes; cool the solution, separate the viscous yellow oil produced, dissolve it in alcohol (95%), add, with continuous stirring, sufficient solvent ether to precipitate the quaternary ammonium salt, and filter; the residue, after reprecipitation with ether from alcohol (95%) and drying at 105°, melts at about 152°.

MELTING-POINT. About 137°.

Metabolism. ABSORPTION. Readily absorbed after oral administration, reaching peak concentrations in the plasma within 1 to 2 hours.

METABOLIC REACTIONS. N-Dealkylation and N-oxidation.

EXCRETION. About 97% of an oral dose, administered to rats, is excreted in the urine with about 15% as unchanged drug, 23% as the N-dealkylated metabolite, 1-ethylcarbamoyl-4-methylpiperazine, and about 50% as the oxide, 1-diethylcarbamoyl-4-methylpiperazine-4-oxide. Other urinary metabolites in the rat include piperazine, N-methylpiperazine, and diethylcarbamoyl-piperazine.

FURTHER INFORMATION. Metabolism in rats—J. K. Faulkner and K. J. A. Smith, *Xenobiotica*, 1972, **2**, 59; plasma concentrations in man—D. B. A. Hutchinson and B. C. Weatherley, *Trans. R. Soc. trop. Med. Hyg.*, 1977, **71**, 542.

Actions and uses. Diethylcarbamazine is used in the treatment and prophylaxis of filarial infections, and is effective when given by mouth.

In the treatment of *Wuchereria bancrofti* infections the microfilariae are rapidly eliminated from the blood stream. The drug has no direct toxic action upon the larvae and it is thought that it may act by so modifying them that they are trapped by reticulo-endothelial cells in the liver sinusoids. This action upon microfilariae is important in helping to limit the spread of filariasis by the insect vector. The action of diethylcarbamazine upon the adult worms is much less rapid and they may persist for several months, but, after they have been eliminated, microfilariae do not often reappear in the peripheral blood. Local reactions sometimes appear at the sites which commonly harbour adult worms.

In loaiasis both microfilariae and adult worms are killed; in onchocerciasis the microfilariae may be killed, but the adult parasites are less affected.

A suitable course of treatment for *Loa loa* or *W. bancrofti* infections is 6 milligrams of diethylcarbamazine citrate per kilogram body-weight by mouth daily in single or divided doses for 3 or 4 weeks. For mass treatment in endemic areas, 6 milligrams per kilogram body-weight given at weekly or monthly intervals to a total of 9 doses is effective. Larger doses of 20 or 30 milligrams per kilogram body-weight have been given without serious side-effects.

Because reactions are especially prominent in *Brugia malayi* and *Onchocerca volvulus* infections, it is important in the treatment of these diseases to start with small doses; a single dose of not more than 2 milligrams of diethylcarbamazine citrate per kilogram body-weight should be given on the first day and the dosage should be gradually increased until the full course can be given.

In general, the dose for children is the same as that for adults.

Undesirable effects. Anorexia, drowsiness, headache, nausea, and vomiting sometimes occur, but are seldom serious. The release of foreign protein in the tissues by the death of adult worms or larvae often provokes allergic reactions, including fever, tender swelling, muscular pains, and skin rashes.

Precautions and contra-indications. It is unwise to use diethylcarbamazine for mass treatment of populations where onchocerciasis is common, because in this infection the allergic reactions may involve the eyes. In such cases individual treatment after first giving a test dose for 2 days is recommended. If severe allergic reactions occur, treatment should be stopped and an antihistamine drug or corticosteroid administered.

Veterinary uses. Diethylcarbamazine citrate is an anthelmintic. It is used in the treatment of parasitic bronchitis in cattle, sheep, and pigs, the usual dose being 20 milligrams per kilogram body-weight by mouth or by intramuscular injection for 3 successive days.

It is also used in the treatment of filariasis and ascariasis in dogs and cats, the usual dose by mouth being 50 milligrams per kilogram body-weight.

Preparations

DIETHYLCARBAMAZINE INJECTION: a sterile solution of diethylcarbamazine citrate, or of diethylcarbamazine and citric acid, in water for injections. If necessary, the pH is adjusted to about 6.5. It is sterilised by heating in an autoclave or by filtration.

Available in 100-, 200-, 350-, and 400-ml packs containing the equivalent of 400 mg of diethylcarbamazine citrate per ml.

A standard for this injection is given in the British Pharmacopoeia (Veterinary)

Containers and *Labelling:* see the entry on Injections for general information on containers and labelling.

DIETHYLCARBAMAZINE TABLETS: available as tablets containing 50, 100 and 200 mg of diethylcarbamazine citrate.

A standard for these tablets is given in the British Pharmacopoeia 1973

Containers and *Storage:* see the entry on Tablets for general information on containers and storage. Containers should be airtight.

Advice for patients: prophylaxis should not be discontinued without the advice of the prescriber. For treatment of infections the prescribed course should be completed.

OTHER PREPARATIONS available include a veterinary MIXTURE containing diethylcarbamazine citrate 5.09% with morantel tartrate 2%.

Diethylpropion Hydrochloride

1-Benzoyltriethylammonium chloride

$$\left[\begin{array}{c} C_6H_5 \cdot CO \cdot \overset{|}{C}H \cdot \overset{+}{N}H(C_2H_5)_2 \\ CH_3 \end{array} \right] Cl^-$$

$C_{13}H_{20}ClNO = 241.8$

OTHER NAME: *Tenuate*®

Description. A white or off-white crystalline powder with a slight odour and a slightly bitter taste.

Solubility. Soluble in 0.5 part of water, in 3 parts of alcohol, and in 3 parts of chloroform; practically insoluble in ether.

Identification. TEST. Mix about 25 mg with 2 ml of a solution containing 2 g of citric acid monohydrate in 100 ml of acetic anhydride and heat for 15 minutes on a water-bath; a red to purple colour is produced.

MELTING-POINT. About 175°, with decomposition.

INFRA-RED ABSORPTION. Major peaks at 701, 1230, 1287, 1383, 1443, and 1682 cm^{-1} (see Appendix 2a: Infra-red Spectra).

Metabolism. ABSORPTION. Readily absorbed after oral administration.

HALF-LIFE. Determined from urinary excretion, 1.5 to 3 hours in subjects whose urines are acid.

METABOLIC REACTIONS. N-Dealkylation, reduction, de-amination, and N-hydroxylation; ketoreduction is stereoselective resulting in the formation of *threo*-hydroxylated metabolites; glucuronide formation also occurs along with the formation of hippuric and mandelic acids.

EXCRETION. 80 to 90% of a dose is excreted in the urine; the amount excreted in the urine is reduced when the urine is alkaline; of the urinary excreted material, N-ethylaminopropiophenone, norephedrine, and hippuric acid are the main metabolites along with small amounts of unchanged drug, aminopropiophenone, N-diethyl-norephedrine, and N-ethylnorephedrine.

FURTHER INFORMATION. Excretion—F. Banci *et al.*, *Arzneimittel-Forsch.*, 1971, **21**, 1616; metabolism and excretion—E. C. Schrieber *et al.*, *J. Pharmac. exp. Ther.*, 1968, **159**, 372, B. Testa, *Acta pharm. suec.*, 1973, **10**, 441, B. Testa and A. H. Beckett, *J. Pharm. Pharmac.*, 1973, **25**, 119, and B. Testa and A. H. Beckett, *Pharm. Acta Helv.*, 1974, **49**, 21.

Actions and uses. Diethylpropion hydrochloride is a sympathomimetic agent used as an appetite suppressant in the treatment of obesity.

The usual dose given by mouth to adults is 25 milligrams thrice daily or 75 to 150 milligrams daily taken as a sustained-release preparation early in the morning or afternoon.

Undesirable effects. It may give rise to anxiety and insomnia and dependence of the amphetamine type, as described in the entry on Drug Dependence.

Precautions and contra-indications. It should not be given to patients who are being treated with a mono-amine-oxidase inhibitor such as isocarboxazid, nialamide, phenelzine, or tranylcypromine or within about 2 weeks of the discontinuation of such treatment. It is undesirable to administer diethylpropion to children. Diethylpropion may cause a reversal of the effects of antihypertensive drugs.

Preparations
Preparations available include TABLETS containing diethylpropion hydrochloride 25 mg, and tablets containing diethylpropion hydrochloride 75 mg in a slow-release formulation.

Diethylthiambutene Hydrochloride

NN-Diethyl-1-methyl-3,3-di(thien-2-yl)prop-2-enyl-ammonium chloride

$C_{16}H_{22}ClNS_2 = 327.9$

OTHER NAME: *Themalon®*

A standard is given in the British Pharmacopoeia (*Veterinary*)

Description. A white crystalline odourless powder.

Solubility. Soluble, at 20°, in 2 parts of water and in 1 part of alcohol; practically insoluble in ether.

Sterilisation. Diethylthiambutene hydrochloride is usually supplied as a sterile product. Solutions for injection are prepared by dissolving the sterile product, immediately before use, in the required amount of water for injections (see below).

Identification. TESTS. 1. Dissolve about 20 mg in 1 ml of sulphuric acid; a bright red colour is produced. Dilute gradually with water, keeping the mixture well cooled; the colour changes to dark red and then to dark green. 2. Dissolve about 0.2 g in 10 ml of water and to 5 ml of the solution add 4 drops of *potassium mercuri-iodide solution*; a cream-coloured precipitate is produced. To the other 5 ml of solution add 1 ml of *dilute nitric acid*; a white precipitate is produced.

MELTING-POINT. About 152°.

INFRA-RED ABSORPTION. Major peaks at 714, 741, 855, 1250, 1429, and 1471 cm^{-1} (see Appendix 2b: Infra-red Spectra).

Veterinary uses. Diethylthiambutene hydrochloride is a narcotic analgesic used in dogs, the level of anaesthesia depending on the dose and route of administration.

The usual dose by intravenous injection is 1 to 4 milligrams per kilogram body-weight; by intramuscular injection 2.5 to 10 milligrams per kilogram body-weight, and by subcutaneous injection 5 to 20 milligrams per kilogram body-weight; nalorphine is a suitable antagonist.

Preparation

DIETHYLTHIAMBUTENE SOLUTION-TABLETS FOR INJECTION: available as sterile solution-tablets containing 50 mg of diethylthiambutene hydrochloride.
A standard for these solution-tablets is given in the British Pharmacopoeia (Veterinary)
Labelling: the label on the container should state the amount of diethylthiambutene hydrochloride in each tablet and that the solution for injection is prepared by dissolving the solution-tablet in water for injections.

Diethyltoluamide

NN-Diethyl-*m*-toluamide

$C_{12}H_{17}NO = 191.3$

OTHER NAME: *Metadelphene®*

A standard is given in the British Pharmacopoeia Addendum 1975

Description. A colourless or faintly yellow odourless liquid.

Solubility. Very slightly soluble in water and in glycerol; miscible with alcohol, with isopropyl alcohol, with ether, and with chloroform.

Weight per ml. At 20°, 0.997 to 1.000 g.

Refractive index. At 20°, 1.521 to 1.524.

Boiling-point. About 111° at a pressure of 1 mmHg.

Identification. TESTS. 1. Mix 2 ml with 25 ml of 50% v/v hydrochloric acid, heat under a reflux condenser for 1 hour, make the mixture alkaline with *sodium hydroxide solution*, cool, extract with three 30-ml portions of solvent ether, and reserve the aqueous layer; evaporate the mixed ether extracts to dryness, dissolve the residue in 5 ml of *dilute hydrochloric acid*, cool to 5°, add 5 ml of *sodium nitrite solution*, allow to stand for 10 minutes at 5°, add 10 ml of water, and extract with 20 ml of solvent ether; evaporate the ether, add 1 g of phenol to the residue, cool, and add 1 ml of sulphuric acid; an intense green colour is produced which becomes red on pouring into water and green on making alkaline with *dilute sodium hydroxide solution*.

2. Acidify the aqueous layer reserved in Test 1, extract with two 20-ml portions of solvent ether, and evaporate the ether extract to dryness; the residue, after drying at 60°, melts at about 108°.

Actions and uses. Diethyltoluamide is an insect repellent that is effective against mosquitoes, midges, mites, ticks, and fleas. It is applied to exposed skin as a 50 to 75% solution in alcohol or isopropyl alcohol which is effective for several hours. The same solution is used to impregnate clothing made of wool, cotton, or nylon, but certain fibres such as rayon may be adversely affected. Diethyltoluamide is also used as a leech repellent.

Undesirable effects. It may irritate tender areas of the skin. Hypersensitivity has been reported.

Precautions. Solutions should not be applied to broken skin or near the eyes and lips, to mucous surfaces, or to the antecubital or popliteal fossae or the groins.

Digitalis Lanata Leaf

Consists of the dried leaves of *Digitalis lanata* Ehrh. (Fam. Scrophulariaceae). The plant is a biennial, indigenous to Austria and the Balkans, and cultivated in Great Britain and other temperate countries.

The leaves are rapidly dried, as soon as possible after collection, at a temperature not exceeding 60°.

OTHER NAMES: Austrian Digitalis; Austrian Foxglove; Woolly Foxglove Leaf

A standard is given in the British Pharmaceutical Codex 1973

Constituents. Digitalis lanata leaf contains about 1 to 1.4% of a mixture of cardioactive glycosides, of which the most important is digoxin, which may be classified into 5 series, each based on a different steroidal aglycone.

The A series, based on digitoxigenin [3β,14-dihydroxy-5β-card-20(22)-enolide], includes the following glycosides: lanatoside A (acetylpurpurea glycoside A); purpurea glycoside A (deacetyllanatoside A), in which the hydroxyl group in position 3 of the aglycone is substituted by a chain of 3 digitoxose units with a terminal glucose unit and formed from lanatoside A by removal of the acetyl group; acetyldigitoxin, formed from lanatoside A by removal of the terminal glucose unit; and digitoxin, formed from lanatoside A by removal of the acetyl group and the terminal glucose unit.

The B series, based on gitoxigenin (16-hydroxydigitoxigenin), includes the analagous glycosides lanatoside

B, purpurea glycoside B, acetylgitoxin, and gitoxin. Other members of this series which are also present in the leaf are: digitalinum verum (glucodigitalogitoxigenin), formed by the addition of one glucose unit and one digitalose (a deoxy sugar) unit to gitoxigenin; strospeside (digitalogitoxigenin), formed by addition of one digitalose unit to gitoxigenin; and gitorin (glucodigitoxogitoxigenin), formed by the addition of one digitoxose (an α-deoxy sugar) unit and one glucose unit to gitoxigenin.

The C, D, and E series, based respectively on digoxigenin (12-hydroxydigitoxigenin), diginatigenin (12,16-dihydroxydigitoxigenin), and gitaloxigenin (16-formylgitoxigenin), include the following glycosides with structures analogous to those in the A and B series: deacetyllanatoside C, deacetyllanatoside D, and glucogitaloxin; acetyldigoxin, acetyldiginatin, and acetylgitaloxin; and digoxin, diginatin, and gitaloxin.

The secondary glycosides digitoxin, gitoxin, digoxin, diginatin, and gitaloxin all have in position 3 of the aglycone, a chain of 3 digitoxose units; removal of these sugar groups yields the corresponding, almost inactive, aglycones which are present in the leaf in only small amounts. The glycosides diginin and digifolin, which are also present, are not cardioactive.

Up to 2% of foreign organic matter may be present.

Description. UNGROUND DRUG: *Macroscopical characters:* leaves brittle, oblong-lanceolate, 20 to **50** to **150** to 300 mm long and 4 to **20** to 45 mm wide, sessile, margin entire and ciliate in the basal half of the leaf, becoming wavy toothed towards the apex; surface apparently glabrous; midrib strongly marked, and the main secondary veins, about 2 or 3 on each side of the basal third or quarter of the midrib, leaving it at an angle of 10° to 30° and curving towards the acute apex.

It has a slight odour and a characteristic bitter taste.

Microscopical characters: the diagnostic characters are: *epidermal cells* of both surfaces with slightly sinuous and irregularly beaded anticlinal walls; *stomata* numerous, anomocytic, occurring on both surfaces; *water pores* single or in groups of 2 to 4 on the margin at intervals of about 1 to 5 mm; *trichomes:* (a) marginal, uniseriate, non-glandular, 9 to **10** to **14** to 20 cells long, (b) glandular, with bicellular heads and unicellular stalks, on both surfaces, and a few, chiefly on the adaxial surface, with 2- to 10-celled uniseriate stalks and unicellular heads; *mesophyll* with 1 to 3 rows of palisade cells; *phloem fibres* and *crystals* absent.

POWDERED DRUG: Powdered Digitalis Lanata Leaf. A green powder possessing the diagnostic microscopical characters, odour, and taste of the unground drug.

Storage. It should be stored in airtight containers, protected from light.

Uses. Digitalis lanata leaf is a source of digoxin and certain other glycosides.

Poisoning. Withdrawal of the drug is usually sufficient but in very severe cases the administration of potassium salts orally, or even parenterally, may be required.

Digitalis Leaf

The dried leaves of *Digitalis purpurea* L. (Fam. Scrophulariaceae), a biennial herb widely distributed and cultivated throughout Europe and indigenous to and cultivated in England.

The leaves are rapidly dried, as soon as possible after collection, at a temperature not exceeding 60°.

OTHER NAMES: Digitalis; Digitalis Folium; Digitalis Purpureae Folium

When Digitalis Leaf, Digitalis Folium, Digitalis, Powdered Digitalis Leaf, Digitalis Folii Pulvis, or Pulvis Digitalis is prescribed, Prepared Digitalis is dispensed.

A standard is given in the European Pharmacopoeia Vol. III

Constituents. Digitalis leaf contains about 0.2 to 0.45% of a mixture of cardioactive glycosides, the majority of which can be classified into 3 series—the A, B, and E series described under Digitalis Lanata Leaf.
The glycosides of the A series in digitalis leaf are purpurea glycoside A and digitoxin, together with odoroside H, in which the hydroxyl group in position 3 of the aglycone digitoxigenin is substituted by the digitalose unit.
The glycosides of the B series are purpurea glycoside B, gitoxin, digitalinum verum, strospeside, and gitorin, while those of the E series are glucogitaloxin and gitaloxin, together with glucoverodoxin and verodoxin, the 16-formyl esters of digitalinum verum and strospeside respectively.
There is some evidence that the relative proportions of the A and B series vary with the strain of plants. The percentages of individual glycosides in the total glycosidal mixture vary considerably; both primary and secondary glycosides are present, the latter constituting about 10 to 20% of the total.
The steroidal saponins digitonin and gitonin are present in the leaf. Hydrolytic enzymes also occur and, in the presence of moisture, readily break down the primary glycosides to secondary glycosides; it is possible that such breakdowns lead to loss of therapeutic activity.
Digitalis seeds contain glucodigifucoside and glucodigiproside (glycosides of the A series), together with digitalinum verum and other cardiac glycosides, and digitonin and gitonin.
Up to 5% of acid-insoluble ash may be present.

Description. UNGROUND DRUG. *Macroscopical characters:* leaf brittle, greyish-green, about 100 to 400 mm long and 40 to 150 mm wide, ovate-lanceolate to broadly ovate and petiolate; lamina with crenate, serrate, or dentate margin, decurrent base, subacute apex, and pinnate venation; petiole about one-quarter equal in length to the lamina, winged, the lowest veins running down the wings; upper surface hairy, lower surface usually densely pubescent and marked by the reticulation of raised veinlets.
It has a slight odour and a distinctly bitter taste.

Microscopical characters: the diagnostic characters are: *epidermal cells* about 30 to 75 μm wide or long, with wavy anticlinal walls; *stomata* anomocytic, more numerous on abaxial than adaxial surface; *water pores* large, 1, or rarely 2, at the apex of most marginal teeth; *trichomes:* (a) usually 3 to 5 cells long, bluntly pointed, and finely warty, (b) glandular, stalk unicellular or more rarely uniseriate, head unicellular or bicellular; *midrib* strongly projecting on abaxial surface, containing an arc of radiate *xylem* and below this a narrow band of *phloem* and a narrow layer of *collenchyma*; *endodermoid* sheath enclosing midrib bundle, containing starch; *crystals* and *sclerenchyma* absent.

POWDERED DRUG: Powdered Digitalis Leaf. A green powder possessing the diagnostic microscopical characters, odour, and taste of the unground drug.

Adulterants and substitutes. Digitalis has been known to be adulterated with *Verbascum thapsus* L. (Fam. Scrophulariaceae), *Symphytum officinale* L. (Fam. Bora-

ginaceae), *Primula vulgaris* Huds. (Fam. Primulaceae), *Inula conyza* DC. (Fam. Compositae), *Urtica dioica* L. (Fam. Urticaceae), *D. thapsi* L., and *D. lutea* L.

Storage. It should be stored in airtight containers, protected from light.

Identification. TESTS. 1. Boil 1 g in powder with 10 ml of alcohol (70%) for 2 minutes and filter; to 5 ml of the filtrate add 10 ml of water and 5 ml of chloroform, separate the lower layer, and evaporate to dryness; dissolve the cooled residue in 3 ml of glacial acetic acid containing 0.1 ml of *ferric chloride test-solution* and transfer this solution to the surface of 2 ml of sulphuric acid; a reddish-brown layer forms at the interface and the upper layer gradually acquires a bluish-green colour which darkens on standing.
2. Boil 1 g in powder with 20 ml of alcohol (50%) and 10 ml of *lead acetate solution* for 2 minutes, allow to cool, and centrifuge; shake the supernatant solution with 2 portions, each of 15 ml, of chloroform; if necessary, separate the 2 layers by centrifuging; dry the combined chloroform layers over anhydrous sodium sulphate and filter; evaporate 5 ml of the solution to dryness on a water-bath and to the residue add 2 ml of *dinitrobenzoic acid solution* and 1 ml of 1N sodium hydroxide solution; a red-violet colour develops within 5 minutes.
3. Evaporate 5 ml of the chloroform solution, prepared as described in Test 2, to dryness on a water-bath; to the residue add 3 ml of *xanthydrol solution* and heat for 3 minutes on a water-bath; a red colour develops.

Actions and uses. Digitalis acts mainly upon the cardiovascular system, its action being due to the glycosides it contains. It increases excitability of cardiac muscle and produces more forceful contractions. Its effect in congestive heart failure is therefore to increase cardiac output and relieve venous congestion. The consequent improvement of the circulation through the kidneys may result in diuresis and loss of oedema fluid.
Digitalis depresses conduction in the atrioventricular bundle producing a slower ventricular beat, which is valuable in atrial fibrillation.
Digitalis will frequently convert atrial flutter into fibrillation and, upon withdrawal of the drug, normal sinus rhythm may be restored.
The principal glycosides are metabolised slowly, and about 25% of the activity of a dose is still present in the body after 10 days.
The effects of digitalis in congestive heart failure may be produced rapidly or slowly according to the method of administration. If a patient is severely ill and has not recently received treatment with digitalis, rapid digitalisation is necessary and is best achieved by intravenous injection of a soluble preparation such as digoxin. Alternatively, if the patient can take the drug by mouth a total dose of 2 grams of prepared digitalis is given in the first 24 hours. Half the total is given at once, and the other half in divided doses at 6-hourly intervals, but such rapid digitalisation is rarely necessary. The patient may be digitalised more slowly by giving 200 milligrams of prepared digitalis 3 times daily for 2 or 3 days, followed by half or two-thirds of this dosage for a further 2 or 3 days. It is usually necessary to continue digitalis therapy indefinitely. The daily dosage required is usually of the order of 60 to 200 milligrams of prepared digitalis.
The value of digitalis in high-output failure is less evident, and it may even be contra-indicated.

Undesirable effects. Mild toxic effects, such as headache, anorexia, and nausea, are commonly associated with the therapeutic action of the drug.
More severe symptoms, such as vomiting, diarrhoea,

profound bradycardia, ventricular tachycardia, or the development of cardiac irregularities, such as extrasystoles and coupling, and disturbances of colour vision, are indications of overdosage.

Treatment may be temporarily withheld before continuing with a smaller dose.

Precautions. Especial care should be taken in assessing the maintenance dose for elderly patients, particularly when they are receiving intensive diuretic therapy which may give rise to hypokalaemia and precipitate symptoms of digitalis toxicity.

Poisoning. Withdrawal of the drug is usually sufficient but in very severe cases the administration of potassium salts orally or even parenterally may be required. Cardiac monitoring should be carried out to detect arrhythmias. If anti-arrhythmic drugs are required they should be used with caution.

Preparations

PREPARED DIGITALIS (*Syn.* Digitalis Pulverata; Powdered Digitalis; Prep. Digit.): obtained by reducing digitalis leaf to a powder not coarser than a moderately coarse powder, no portion being rejected, and determining its activity by comparison with that of the standard preparation on the hearts of guinea-pigs. Other methods compare the action of the preparations on the hearts of frogs, cats, or pigeons.

When adjustment is necessary, a weaker powdered digitalis leaf or powdered grass is added.

For therapeutic administration, it contains 10 units in 1 gram.

It is a green powder with a slight odour and a distinctly bitter taste.

Microscopical characters: it possesses the diagnostic microscopical characters described under Digitalis Leaf; if powdered grass is present, the histological details vary with the species but for those most likely to occur the following characters are diagnostic: *trichomes* represented by scarce to abundant, long or short, unicellular hairs with thin or thick walls and by prickles with bulbous bases and short barbs; *epidermis* typically consisting of parallel longitudinal files of cells, the cells in many or all of the files being of 2 distinct sizes referred to as "long" and "short" respectively; short-cells commonly solitary or in pairs, many of them containing solitary *silica-bodies*, the shapes of which are diagnostic for the species of grass concerned; short-cells in which no silica-bodies are present usually have suberised walls and are termed cork cells; stomata with characteristic dumb-bell-shaped guard cells, restricted to certain files of cells in the intercostal zones; *crystals* absent; *pollen grains* spherical, each with a single pore.

A standard for this powder is given in the British Pharmacopoeia 1973

Labelling: the label on the container should state the number of units in 1 gram.

Storage: it should be stored in airtight containers, protected from light.

Actions and uses: prepared digitalis has the actions, uses, and undesirable effects described under Digitalis Leaf; the usual initial dose for rapid digitalisation is 1 to 1.5 grams, in divided doses and the maintenance dose is 100 to 200 milligrams daily.

Precautions; Poisoning: as for Digitalis Leaf.

PREPARED DIGITALIS TABLETS (*Syn.* Digitalis Tablets): containing prepared digitalis in fine powder and containing 10 units in 1 g. Available as tablets containing 30, 60, and 100 mg.

A standard for these tablets is given in the British Pharmacopoeia 1973

Containers and *Storage:* see the entry on Tablets for general information on containers and storage. Containers should be airtight.

Advice for patients: the tablets should be taken at regular intervals, preferably before meals. If there are gastrointestinal disturbances, the dose may be taken after meals. Treatment should not be discontinued without the advice of the prescriber.

Digitoxin

3-[(O-2,6-Dideoxy-β-D-*ribo*-hexopyranosyl-(1→4)-O-2,6-dideoxy-β-D-*ribo*-hexopyranosyl-(1→4)-O-2,6-dideoxy-β-D-*ribo*-hexopyranosyl)oxy]-14-hydroxy-3β,5β,14β-card-20(22)-enolide, a crystalline glycoside obtained from suitable species of *Digitalis*.

$C_{41}H_{64}O_{13} = 764.9$

OTHER NAMES: Digitaline Cristallisée; *Digitaline Nativelle*®; Digitoxinum; Digitoxoside

A standard is given in the European Pharmacopoeia Vol. I

Description. A white powder.

Solubility. Practically insoluble in water; soluble, at 20°, in 150 parts of alcohol and in 40 parts of chloroform; very slightly soluble in ether.

Sterilisation. Alcoholic solutions and solutions in propylene glycol are sterilised by heating in an autoclave.

Storage. It should be stored in airtight containers, protected from light.

Identification. TESTS. 1. It complies with Tests 1 and 2 described under Deslanoside.

2. Prepare a solution in a mixture of equal parts of alcohol and chloroform, place 1 drop of the solution on a filter paper (Whatman no. 7) and spray with a 10% solution of antimony pentachloride in chloroform; a yellow colour is produced which changes to purple. Warm the spot in hot air for 5 to 10 minutes; the colour changes to black.

MELTING-POINT. About 256°.

INFRA-RED ABSORPTION. Major peaks at 990, 1010, 1058, 1072, 1125, and 1740 cm^{-1} (see Appendix 2a: Infra-red Spectra).

Determination in body fluids. DOUBLE ISOTOPE DILUTION DERIVATIVE. In plasma or urine—D. S. Lukas and R. E. Peterson, *J. clin. Invest.*, 1966, **45**, 782.

THIN-LAYER CHROMATOGRAPHY. In serum—D. B. Faber et al., *J. Chromat.*, 1977, **143**, 95.

REVIEW. Cardiac glycosides in blood—T. W. Smith and E. Haber, *Am. J. med. Sci.*, 1970, **259**, 301.

Metabolism. ABSORPTION. Rapidly and completely absorbed, mainly in the jejunum and also in the duodenum and stomach, after oral administration.

BLOOD CONCENTRATION. Therapeutic serum concentrations range from 10 to 40 ng/ml and toxic symptoms develop when serum concentrations reach about 45 ng/ml; on a maintenance dosage of 800 μg daily, mean serum concentrations of about 20 ng/ml are obtained.

HALF-LIFE. Serum half-life, 4 to 9 days.

DISTRIBUTION. More widely distributed than digoxin; crosses the placenta; *protein binding*, 95% bound to plasma proteins.

METABOLIC REACTIONS. Highly metabolised, mainly in the liver, via hydroxylation to form digoxin and via hydroxylation and removal of one or two digitoxose molecules to form digoxigenin-bis-digitoxoside and digoxigenin-mono-digitoxoside; epidigitoxigenin and its glucuronic acid conjugate are also formed; the metabolism of digitoxin is enhanced by barbiturates.

EXCRETION. In 3 weeks about 60 to 80% of a dose is excreted in the urine, 10% as unchanged drug; during oral maintenance therapy with 100 to 300 μg daily, about 16 to 30% of the dose is excreted in the urine and about 2 to 17% in the faeces daily; of the urinary excretion, 2% is unchanged drug, 8% is active digoxin, and 22% is inactive metabolites; urinary excretion of digitoxin is unaffected by diuretics but it is reduced in patients with uraemia; digitoxin appears to be extensively excreted in the bile as polar conjugates which may be reabsorbed from the gastro-intestinal tract.

Actions and uses. Digitoxin has the actions, uses, and undesirable effects described under Digitalis Leaf. It is the most potent and most cumulative of the digitalis glycosides. It is completely and readily absorbed when given by mouth, and is equally active when given by injection.

For rapid digitalisation of patients who have not been given cardiac glycosides within the preceding two weeks, 1 to 1.5 milligrams may be given by mouth in divided doses over 1 or 2 days. The maintenance dosage is 50 to 200 micrograms daily. However, digoxin is more suitable for rapid digitalisation as it has a shorter duration of action and its effect is therefore more readily controlled.

When vomiting or other oral conditions prevent oral administration, digitoxin may be given by intramuscular or slow intravenous injection; the usual digitalising dosage is 1.2 milligrams daily in divided doses not exceeding 500 micrograms.

For intravenous injection, the dose is dissolved in a mixture of alcohol, glycerol, and water, and for intramuscular injection it is dissolved in propylene glycol.

If toxic effects arise, further doses of digitoxin should be withheld.

Digitoxin must be carefully distinguished from digitalin (amorphous digitalin), a standardised mixture of glyco-

sides prepared from digitalis seeds, which does not contain digitoxin or gitoxin and is given in much larger doses.

Precautions; Poisoning. As for Digitalis Leaf.

Preparations

DIGITOXIN TABLETS: available as tablets containing 100 micrograms of digitoxin; they may be coloured.

A standard for these tablets is given in the British Pharmacopoeia 1973

Containers and *Storage:* see the entry on Tablets for general information on containers and storage. Containers should be airtight.

Advice for patients: the tablets should be taken at regular intervals, preferably before meals. If there are gastro-intestinal disturbances the dose may be taken after meals. Treatment should not be discontinued without the advice of the prescriber.

OTHER PREPARATIONS available include an INJECTION containing digitoxin 200 micrograms per ml in 1-ml ampoules and a SOLUTION containing digitoxin 1 mg per ml (1 in 1000).

Digoxin

3-[(*O*-2,6-Dideoxy-β-D-*ribo*-hexopyranosyl-(1→4)-*O*-2,6-dideoxy-β-D-*ribo*-hexopyranosyl-(1→4)-*O*-2,6-dideoxy-β-D-*ribo*-hexopyranosyl)oxy]-12,14-dihydroxy-3β, 5β,12β,14β-card-20(22)-enolide, a crystalline glycoside obtained from digitalis lanata leaf.

$C_{41}H_{64}O_{14} = 780.9$

OTHER NAMES: *Diganox®*; Digoxinum; *Lanoxin®*

A standard is given in the European Pharmacopoeia Vol. I

Description. It occurs as colourless crystals or a white powder.

Solubility. Very slightly soluble in water, in dehydrated alcohol, and in chloroform; soluble at 20°, in 122 parts of alcohol (80%) and in 4 parts of pyridine.

Stability. Digoxin is stable in aqueous solution at pH 7 but in acid solution it is hydrolysed directly or through intermediate glycosides to the aglycone digoxigenin. At

37° the half-life of digoxin is 13 minutes at pH 1.0 and 130 minutes at pH 2.0.

FURTHER INFORMATION. Stability in aqueous solution— L. A. Sternson and R. D. Shaffer, *J. pharm. Sci.*, 1978, **67**, 327.

Sterilisation. Alcoholic solutions for injection are sterilised by heating in an autoclave.

Storage. It should be stored in airtight containers, protected from light.

Identification. TESTS. 1. It complies with Tests 1 and 2 described under Deslanoside.
2. It complies with Test 2 described under Digitoxin.

INFRA-RED ABSORPTION. Major peaks at 1000, 1017, 1054, 1073, 1172, and 1720 cm^{-1} (see Appendix 2a: Infra-red Spectra).

Determination in body fluids. GAS CHROMATOGRAPHY. In plasma—E. Watson and S. M. Kalman, *J. Chromat.*, 1971, **56**, 209.

RADIOIMMUNOASSAY. In serum—T. W. Smith *et al.*, *New Engl. J. Med.*, 1969, **281**, 1212; in serum or urine— A. Brock, *Acta pharmac. tox.*, 1974, **34**, 198.

OTHER METHOD. In plasma: inhibition by digitalis glycosides of the transport of ^{86}Rb into erythrocytes— A. Bertler and A. Redfors, *Clin. Pharmac. Ther.*, 1970, **11**, 665.

REVIEW. Cardiac glycosides in blood—T. W. Smith and E. Haber, *Am. J. med. Sci.*, 1970, **259**, 301.

Metabolism. ABSORPTION. The absorption of digoxin after oral administration is variable and subject to bio-availability differences; absorption occurs mainly in the small intestine and in the stomach; in the presence of food, absorption is delayed but not reduced; absorption is decreased following the administration of antacids, metoclopramide, colestipol, or cholestyramine, or in patients with malabsorption syndrome or gastro-intestinal hypermotility; in tablet form, about 50 to 65% of a dose is absorbed and, as a solution, about 80% is absorbed.

BLOOD CONCENTRATION. Therapeutic serum concentrations are in the range 0.5 to 2.5 ng/ml and toxic reactions occur with serum concentrations above 3 ng/ml; after a single dose of 500 μg in tablet form, peak serum concentrations of 1.2 to 4.8 ng/ml are attained in 30 to 90 minutes and after maintenance doses of 125 to 500 μg, mean serum concentrations of 0.5 to 1.5 ng/ml are attained; after an intravenous injection of 250 μg, concentrations of about 6 and 3 ng/ml are attained within 30 and 60 minutes respectively.

HALF-LIFE. Serum half-life, about 35 hours after oral administration and about 33 hours after intravenous administration.

DISTRIBUTION. Digoxin is rapidly distributed throughout the body and less than 20% of the total digoxin in the body is located in the blood; the ratios of myocardial concentrations to blood concentrations are in the range 40 to 150:1; skeletal muscle concentrations are less than that in the myocardium but since the skeletal muscle comprises 43% of the body mass, large amounts of digoxin are stored outside its site of action; myocardial binding of digoxin is influenced by blood concentrations of digoxin itself and by the concentrations of Na$^+$, Ca^{2+}, Mg^{2+}, blood pH values, oxygen tension, and thyroid function; *protein binding*, about 30% bound to plasma protein.

METABOLIC REACTIONS. Stepwise removal of the sugar moieties to form digoxigenin which is further metabolised to inactive metabolites which may be excreted in the free or conjugated form; reduction to dihydrodigoxin followed by hydrolysis may also occur.

EXCRETION. After an intravenous dose, up to 80% is excreted in the urine and the remainder is excreted in the faeces via the bile; of the material excreted in the urine 80 to 90% is unchanged, 10% is in the dihydro-form, and a small amount includes digoxigenin and the mono- and bis-digitoxosides; of the material excreted in the bile, 50% is excreted unchanged, 25% is digoxin bisdigitoxoside, 25% is digoxin monodigitoxoside, and about 1% is digoxigenin.

Bioavailability. The difference between the therapeutic and toxic blood levels of digoxin is very small and it is therefore essential to control the amount of bioavailable digoxin. It has been established that different formulations, and in some cases different batches of the same formulation, of digoxin tablets can vary considerably both in digoxin content and in bioavailability, up to a sevenfold variation in blood levels having been demonstrated between different formulations of the same labelled strength.

The differences in bioavailability have been shown to correspond very closely with variations in the dissolution rate. The British Pharmacopoeia now includes a single-tablet assay to give closer control of the digoxin content, and a standard for rate of dissolution. It requires that not less than 75% of digoxin in a tablet should be dissolved in 1 hour.

It has been suggested that differences in particle size and crystal form are mainly responsible for the variations in dissolution rate.

Actions and uses. Digoxin has the actions and uses described under Digitalis Leaf.

It is excreted more rapidly than other digitalis glycosides and its action is therefore less cumulative. Digoxin is of particular value for rapid digitalisation in the treatment of atrial fibrillation and congestive heart failure. When it is given by mouth, its characteristic effect is produced in about 1 hour and reaches its maximum in about 6 to 7 hours. The usual digitalising dosage is 1 to 1.5 milligrams by mouth in single or divided doses, followed by 250 to 500 micrograms every 6 hours until the desired therapeutic effect is obtained. The usual maintenance dosage is 250 micrograms 1 to 3 times daily.

For rapid digitalisation of patients who have not been given cardiac glycosides within the preceding 2 weeks, or if the patient is unable to swallow, digoxin may be given by slow intravenous injection in a dose of 0.5 to 1 milligram; its action then begins in about 5 to 10 minutes and reaches a maximum in 1 to 2 hours. Care should be taken to prevent any of the solution escaping into the perivenous tissues. The risk of producing toxic effects on the heart is much greater if digoxin is given intravenously.

Digoxin may also be given by intramuscular injection but the injection may be painful.

Undesirable effects. The undesirable effects described under Digitalis Leaf may occur, but as digoxin is excreted more rapidly than most other cardiac glycosides it is less likely to give rise to cumulative effects.

Precautions; Poisoning. As for Digitalis Leaf.

Veterinary uses. Digoxin is used in animals as a myocardial stimulant and in the treatment of atrial fibrillation. The usual initial dose for dogs and cats is 50 to 100 micrograms per kilogram body-weight which is reduced to a maintenance level of 10 to 25 micrograms per kilogram body-weight, adjusted in accordance with the response of the animal over not less than 2 weeks.

Preparations

DIGOXIN INJECTION:

Digoxin	25 mg
Citric acid monohydrate..	75 mg
Sodium phosphate..	450 mg
Alcohol (80%)	12.5 ml
Propylene glycol	40.0 ml
Water for injections	to 100.0 ml

Dissolve the digoxin in the alcohol and add the propylene glycol; dissolve the citric acid and the sodium phosphate in a portion of the water, add to the first solution, and then add sufficient water to produce the required volume. Distribute the solution into ampoules, seal, and sterilise by heating in an autoclave.
Digoxin injection contains, in 4 ml, 1 mg of digoxin.
A standard for this injection is given in the British Pharmacopoeia 1973
Containers and *Labelling:* see the entry on Injections for general information on containers and labelling.
Storage: it should be protected from light.

DIGOXIN TABLETS: available as tablets containing 62.5, 125, and 250 micrograms of digoxin.
A standard for these tablets is given in the British Pharmacopoeia Addendum 1977
Containers and *Storage:* see the entry on Tablets for general information on containers and storage. Containers should be airtight.
Advice for patients: the tablets should be taken at regular intervals, preferably before meals. If there are gastro-intestinal disturbances, the dose may be taken after meals. Treatment should not be discontinued without the advice of the prescriber.

PAEDIATRIC DIGOXIN ELIXIR: a solution containing 0.005% of digoxin, 10% v/v of alcohol, and sodium phosphate, with methyl hydroxybenzoate, or other suitable preservative, in a suitable coloured flavoured vehicle. The solution is adjusted to pH 7. This elixir should not be diluted.
The general direction given in the entry on Elixirs that the preparation should be diluted so that the dose is contained in 5 ml does not apply to this elixir. The dose prescribed should be measured by means of a graduated pipette.
Paediatric digoxin elixir contains in 1 ml 50 micrograms of digoxin.
A standard for this elixir is given in the British Pharmaceutical Codex 1973
Labelling: see the entry on Elixirs for general information on labelling.
Storage: it should be stored in a cool place, protected from light.
Advice for patients: the elixir should be taken at regular intervals, preferably before meals. If there are gastro-intestinal disturbances, the dose may be taken after meals. Treatment should not be discontinued without the advice of the prescriber.

PAEDIATRIC DIGOXIN INJECTION:

Digoxin	10 mg
Citric acid monohydrate..	75 mg
Sodium phosphate..	450 mg
Alcohol (80%)	12.5 ml
Propylene glycol	40.0 ml
Water for injections	to 100.0 ml

Dissolve the digoxin in the alcohol and add the propylene

glycol; dissolve the citric acid and the sodium phosphate in a portion of the water, add to the first solution, and then add sufficient water to produce the required volume. Distribute the solution into ampoules, seal, and sterilise by heating in an autoclave.
Paediatric digoxin injection contains, in 0.25 ml, 25 micrograms, and, in 1 ml, 100 micrograms of digoxin.
A standard for this injection is given in the British Pharmacopoeia Addendum 1975
Containers and *Labelling:* see the entry on Injections for general information on containers and labelling.
Storage: it should be protected from light.

Dihydrocodeine Tartrate

7,8-Dihydro-3-*O*-methylmorphine hydrogen tartrate

$C_{18}H_{23}NO_3,C_4H_6O_6 = 451.5$

OTHER NAMES: *DF 118*®
Onadox-118® (with aspirin); *Paramol-118*® (with paracetamol)

A standard is given in the British Pharmacopoeia 1973

Description. Odourless colourless crystals or white crystalline powder.

Solubility. Soluble, at 20°, in 4.5 parts of water; very slightly soluble in alcohol; practically insoluble in ether.

Dissociation constant. pK_a 8.8 (25°).

Specific rotation. $-71.5°$ to $-73.5°$, determined on a 5% solution.

Acidity. A 10% solution has a pH of 3.2 to 4.2.

Sterilisation. Solutions for injection are sterilised by heating in an autoclave or by filtration.

Storage. It should be protected from light.

Identification. TESTS. 1. Mix a few mg with 1 ml of sulphuric acid containing 1 drop of *formaldehyde solution*; a purple colour is produced (distinction from pholcodine).
2. Mix a few mg with one drop of nitric acid; a yellow, but no red, colour is produced (distinction from morphine).
3. Mix 100 mg with 1 ml of sulphuric acid, add 1 drop of *ferric chloride test-solution*, and warm gently; a brownish-yellow colour is produced. Add 1 drop of *dilute nitric acid*; no red colour is produced (distinction from codeine and morphine).

MELTING-POINT. About 192°.

ULTRAVIOLET ABSORPTION. In water, maximum at 284 nm (E1%, 1cm = 36).

Metabolism. ABSORPTION. Well absorbed after oral administration.

DISTRIBUTION. Crosses the placenta.

EXCRETION. After an oral dose of 52 mg, 20 to 30% is excreted in the urine in 24 hours and after an intramuscular dose of about 43 mg, 40 to 60% is excreted in the urine over the same period; the excretion of the oral dose is increased to about 35% when the urine is acid; 30 to 45% of the urinary excreted material is conjugated.

FURTHER INFORMATION. See D. P. Vaughan and A. H. Beckett, *J. Pharm. Pharmac.*, 1973, **25**, 104P.

Actions and uses. Dihydrocodeine is an analgesic intermediate in potency between codeine and morphine, and with a duration of action of about 3 hours. Sedation and euphoria are less marked than with morphine. Dihydrocodeine is also used as an antitussive and it has been used in conjunction with phenothiazine derivatives to relieve symptoms in terminal carcinoma.
The usual dose of dihydrocodeine tartrate as an analgesic is 30 milligrams and if this does not give relief the dose may be repeated. The response may not be enhanced by increasing the dose. Children may be given 500 micrograms per kilogram body-weight. The usual dose as an antitussive is 10 milligrams.

Undesirable effects. Dihydrocodeine may cause constipation, nausea, and giddiness. It may give rise to dependence of the morphine type, as described in the entry on Drug Dependence, but this is less likely to occur than with morphine.

Precautions. Dihydrocodeine should be used with caution in patients with asthma or impaired liver function.

Preparations

DIHYDROCODEINE AND PARACETAMOL TABLETS: for each tablet take:

Dihydrocodeine tartrate .. .. 10 mg
Paracetamol.. .. .. 500 mg

Containers and *Storage:* see the entry on Tablets for general information on containers and storage. Containers should be airtight.
Dose: 2 tablets up to 4 times daily, as necessary.
Advice for patients: the tablets should preferably be taken after meals.

DIHYDROCODEINE INJECTION: a sterile solution of dihydrocodeine tartrate, with 0.1% of sodium metabisulphite, in water for injections. It is sterilised by heating in an autoclave or by filtration. Available as an injection containing 50 mg of dihydrocodeine tartrate per ml in 1-ml ampoules.
A standard for this injection is given in the British Pharmacopoeia 1973
Containers and *Labelling:* see the entry on Injections for general information on containers and labelling.
Storage: it should be protected from light.

DIHYDROCODEINE TABLETS: available as tablets containing 30 mg of dihydrocodeine tartrate.
A standard for these tablets is given in the British Pharmacopoeia 1973
Containers and *Storage:* see the entry on Tablets for general information on containers and storage. Containers should be airtight and light resistant.
Advice for patients: the tablets should preferably be taken after meals.

OTHER PREPARATIONS available include an ELIXIR containing dihydrocodeine tartrate 10 mg in 5 ml, diluent syrup, life of diluted elixir 14 days; and TABLETS containing dihydrocodeine tartrate 10 mg with soluble aspirin equivalent to 300 mg of aspirin.

Dihydrostreptomycin Sulphate

O-2-Deoxy-2-methylamino-α-L-glucopyranosyl-(1→2)-
O-5-deoxy-3-*C*-hydroxymethyl-α-L-lyxofuranosyl-
(1→4)-N^1N^3-diamidino-D-streptamine sulphate

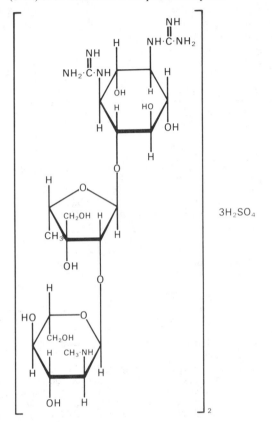

$(C_{21}H_{41}N_7O_{12})_2,3H_2SO_4 = 1461.5$

OTHER NAMES: *Strypen Forte*® (with benzylpenicillin potassium); *Ilcocillin Dry Cow*®, *Ilcocillin PS*®, *Streptocillin*®, *Streptopen*®, *Strypen*®, and *Strypen Forte Rapid*® (all with procaine penicillin); *Dimycin*® and *Ilcocillin S*® (both with streptomycin sulphate)

A standard is given in the British Pharmacopoeia (Veterinary)

Description. A white hygroscopic odourless powder.

Solubility. Soluble in water; practically insoluble in alcohol, in chloroform, and in ether.

Acidity. A 25% solution has a pH of 4.5 to 7.

Moisture content. Not more than 7%, determined by drying at 60° over phosphorus pentoxide *in vacuo*.

Incompatibility. It is incompatible with substances yielding calcium ions in solution, calcium sulphate being precipitated.

Storage. It should be stored in well-closed containers, which as far as possible prevent access of moisture, at a temperature not exceeding 30°. If it is intended for parenteral administration, the containers should be sterile and sealed to exclude micro-organisms.

Identification. TESTS. 1. Dissolve about 100 mg in 2 ml of water and add 1 ml of *1-naphthol solution* and 2 ml of a mixture containing equal volumes of *dilute sodium hypochlorite solution* and water; a red colour is produced.

2. Mix a small quantity with 1N sodium hydroxide, boil for a few minutes, and add a slight excess of hydrochloric acid followed by a few drops of *ferric chloride test-solution*; not more than a faint violet colour is produced (distinction from streptomycin sulphate).

Metabolism. See under Streptomycin Sulphate.

Veterinary uses. Dihydrostreptomycin sulphate is used in animals as an antibacterial agent. It is commonly administered in conjunction with penicillin to obtain a broad spectrum of antibacterial activity. The usual dose by subcutaneous or intramuscular injection for all species except cats is the equivalent of 10 milligrams of dihydrostreptomycin per kilogram body-weight twice daily.

When given by intramammary injection in cattle the usual dose is the equivalent of 100 to 500 milligrams of dihydrostreptomycin into each infected quarter.

Preparations

DIHYDROSTREPTOMYCIN INJECTION: a sterile solution of dihydrostreptomycin sulphate in water for injections. It is prepared by dissolving the contents of a sealed container in water for injections shortly before use.

A standard for this injections is given in the British Pharmacopoeia (Veterinary)

Containers: see the entry on Injections for general information on containers.

Labelling: see the entry on Injections for general information on labelling. In addition, the label on the container should state the amount of the medicament as the equivalent amount of dihydrostreptomycin in mg.

Storage: the sealed container should be stored at a temperature not exceeding 30°. The injection contains no bactericide and should be used as soon as possible after preparation but solutions of dihydrostreptomycin sulphate may be expected to retain their potency for up to 1 month, provided they are stored at a temperature not exceeding 4°.

OTHER VETERINARY PREPARATIONS available include an INJECTION containing dihydrostreptomycin sulphate equivalent to 125 mg of dihydrostreptomycin with streptomycin sulphate equivalent to 125 mg of streptomycin per ml in 100-ml vials, an injection containing dihydrostreptomycin sulphate 250 mg with procaine penicillin 200 mg (200000 units) per ml in 50- and 100-ml vials, an injection containing dihydrostreptomycin sulphate equivalent to 250 mg of dihydrostreptomycin with procaine penicillin 250 mg (250000 units) per ml in 30-, 90-, and 100-ml vials, an injection containing dihydrostreptomycin sulphate equivalent to 500 mg of dihydrostreptomycin with streptomycin sulphate equivalent to 500 mg of streptomycin in 3 ml in 30- and 100-ml vials, an INTRAMAMMARY INJECTION containing dihydrostreptomycin sulphate equivalent to 100 mg of dihydrostreptomycin with procaine penicillin 100 mg (100000 units) in a single dose tube, an intramammary injection containing dihydrostreptomycin sulphate equivalent to 250 mg of dihydrostreptomycin with procaine penicillin 300 mg (300000 units) in a single dose tube, an intramammary injection containing dihydrostreptomycin sulphate equivalent to 250 mg of dihydrostreptomycin with benzylpenicillin potassium 300 mg (300000 units) in a single dose tube, an intramammary injection containing dihydrostreptomycin sulphate equivalent to 500 mg of dihydrostreptomycin with procaine penicillin 1 g (1 mega unit) in a single dose tube in both normal and slow-release

formulations, and an intramammary injection containing dihydrostreptomycin sulphate equivalent to 1 g of dihydrostreptomycin with procaine penicillin 1 g (1 mega unit) in a single dose tube.

Dihydrotachysterol

9,10-Secoergosta-5,7,22-trien-3β-ol

$C_{28}H_{46}O = 398.7$

OTHER NAME: *AT10*®

A standard is given in the British Pharmacopoeia 1973

Description. Odourless colourless crystals or white crystalline powder.

Solubility. Very slightly soluble in water; soluble, at 20°, in 20 parts of alcohol, in less than 1 part of chloroform, in 3 parts of ether, and in 50 parts of arachis oil.

Specific rotation. +100° to +103°, determined on a 2% solution in dehydrated alcohol.

Storage. It should be stored in hermetically sealed glass containers in which the air has been replaced by an inert gas, in a cool place, protected from light.

Identification. TEST. Mix about 5 mg with 2 ml of *antimony trichloride solution* and warm in a water-bath; a red colour is produced.

MELTING-POINT. About 127°; it also occurs in another form which melts at about 113°.

ULTRAVIOLET ABSORPTION. In methyl alcohol, maxima at 242 nm (E1%, 1cm = 870), 251 nm (E1%, 1cm = 1000), and 261 nm (E1%, 1cm = 650).

Actions and uses. The actions of dihydrotachysterol resemble those of calciferol and vitamin D$_3$. It has a powerful antirachitic action in cases of steatorrhoea, chronic renal failure, and hypophosphataemia. It also has some antirachitic effect in cases of classical vitamin-D deficiency, although it is less potent than calciferol in this respect. It promotes the absorption of calcium from the intestine and the mobilisation of calcium from bone as effectively as calciferol.

Dihydrotachysterol acts more rapidly and is more rapidly eliminated than calciferol and its action is therefore more readily controlled; in practice, calciferol is generally used for the treatment of vitamin-D deficiency and dihydrotachysterol for other conditions.

Dihydrotachysterol is effective when given orally for the treatment of all forms of hypoparathyroidism with lowered plasma-calcium. A dosage of 1 to 2 milligrams daily raises the plasma-calcium to normal in 5 to 10 days. In an emergency, 8 milligrams may be given daily for 2 days, followed by 4 milligrams daily for 2 days and

2 milligrams daily thereafter. Dosage should be adjusted in accordance with the plasma and urinary calcium. When this level becomes normal a maintenance dose of 0.5 to 2 milligrams of dihydrotachysterol is given; as dihydrotachysterol is slowly metabolised and excreted, the maintenance dose need be given only every other day. No changes in the normal dietary calcium intake are necessary.

The dose for children is initially the same as for adults, but as dihydrotachysterol is cumulative in action, and the therapeutic dose is often close to the toxic dose, treatment should be carefully controlled by monitoring the serum calcium.

Dihydrotachysterol is administered in cases of vitamin-D-resistant rickets and osteomalacia in the doses mentioned, until the serum-alkaline-phosphatase level returns to normal. The dose is then reduced considerably or even stopped, as the dosage that causes a reasonably rapid cure of the rickets will constitute an overdose if it is continued.

Undesirable effects. The therapeutic dose is close to that producing toxic effects. Overdosage causes decalcification of bone, increased urinary excretion of calcium, hypercalcaemia, metastatic calcification, and eventually a raised blood-urea. The symptoms are anorexia, nausea, vomiting, polyuria, vertigo, thirst, and abdominal cramps.

Treatment consists in withdrawing the dihydrotachysterol, reducing the dietary calcium intake, and increasing the fluid intake.

Precautions. Dosage may need revision in the case of patients who have undergone thyroidectomy or treatment with radioactive iodine or who are receiving a high calcium intake, as in a milk diet.

Dihydrotachysterol should be used with caution during pregnancy and lactation as excessive doses may give rise to hypercalcaemia in the offspring.

Preparations

Preparations available include a SOLUTION containing dihydrotachysterol 250 μg per ml.

Di-iodohydroxyquinoline

5,7-Di-iodoquinolin-8-ol

$C_9H_5I_2NO = 397.0$

OTHER NAMES: Di-iodohydroxyquin; *Diodoquin®*; and *Embequin®* (both available only in certain overseas countries); *Floraquin®*; *Zoaquin®*

A standard is given in the British Pharmacopoeia 1973

Description. An odourless, tasteless, pale yellowish to yellowish-brown, microcrystalline powder.

Solubility. Very slightly soluble in water, in alcohol, and in ether.

Storage. It should be protected from light.

Identification. MELTING-POINT. In the range 200° to 215°, with decomposition.

ULTRAVIOLET ABSORPTION. In a solution prepared by

dissolving 5 mg in 100 ml of dioxan and diluting 5 ml to 100 ml with dehydrated alcohol, maximum at 258 nm (E1%, 1cm = 1060).

Metabolism. ABSORPTION. Poorly and irregularly absorbed after oral administration.

DISTRIBUTION. Iodine released from di-iodohydroxyquinoline is found in the thyroid, spleen, lungs, and muscles.

METABOLIC REACTIONS. Iodine is slowly released; the drug may be conjugated with glucuronic acid or with sulphate.

EXCRETION. About 5% of an oral dose of 300 mg is excreted in the urine as the glucuronic acid conjugate in 10 hours.

FURTHER INFORMATION. Absorption and urinary excretion—L. Berggren and O. Hansson, *Clin. Pharmac. Ther.*, 1968, **9**, 67.

Actions and uses. Di-iodohydroxyquinoline is an amoebicide. When given by mouth, a large proportion of the dose reaches the large intestine, where it is thought to act upon the amoebae living in the lumen or upon the bacteria on which they feed.

Di-iodohydroxyquinoline is used chiefly in the treatment of chronic infections. It is less satisfactory than emetine or metronidazole for the treatment of acute amoebic dysentery, but is frequently used to supplement emetine therapy.

It may be used prophylactically in endemic areas and for the treatment of asymptomatic cyst passers. The drug has been used for the treatment of *Giardia lamblia* and *Balantidium coli* infections and locally for the treatment of trichomoniasis and candidiasis.

Di-iodohydroxyquinoline is given by mouth in a dosage of 300 to 600 milligrams 3 or 4 times daily for 21 days; the dose for cyst passers is 0.6 to 2.1 grams daily and for prophylaxis 300 milligrams 3 times a day. The daily dose for children is 30 milligrams per kilogram body-weight given in divided doses.

Courses of treatment with di-iodohydroxyquinoline are often supplemented by treatment with other amoebicides.

Pessaries of di-iodohydroxyquinoline are used for the treatment of trichomonal and candidal vaginitis.

Undesirable effects. Pruritus ani, furunculosis, abdominal pain with nausea, vomiting, diarrhoea, and headache may occur. Slight enlargement of the thyroid gland is common.

Di-iodohydroxyquinoline may occasionally give rise to optic neuritis especially when dosage is high and prolonged.

Contra-indications. It should not be administered to iodine-sensitive persons or to those with thyroid disease.

Preparations

DI-IODOHYDROXYQUINOLINE PESSARIES: for each pessary take:

Di-iodohydroxyquinoline	..	..	..		100 mg
Phosphoric acid	..	..	..	..	17 mg
Boric acid	..	..	..	..	65 mg
Lactose	..	..	..	..	180 mg
Anhydrous dextrose	..	..	..		300 mg

Mix, and prepare by moist granulation and compression as described in the entry on Tablets.

A standard for these pessaries is given in the British Pharmaceutical Codex 1973

Containers and *Storage:* see the entry on Tablets for general information on containers and storage. Containers should be light resistant.

Advice for patients: the pessaries should be moistened with water and inserted high into the vagina with a suitable applicator, preferably at night. The prescribed course should be completed and should not be interrupted during menstruation.

DI-IODOHYDROXYQUINOLINE TABLETS: available as tablets containing 300 and 650 mg of di-iodohydroxyquinoline, and as veterinary tablets containing 5 g of di-iodohydroxyquinoline.

A standard for these tablets is given in the British Pharmacopoeia 1973
Containers and *Storage:* see the entry on Tablets for general information on containers and storage. Containers should be airtight and light resistant.

Advice for patients: the tablets should be taken at regular intervals preferably after meals. When used for prophylaxis doses should be taken throughout the period at risk. When used for therapy the prescribed course should be completed.

Dill Oil

Obtained by distillation from the dried ripe fruits of *Anethum graveolens* L. (Fam. Umbelliferae). It closely resembles caraway oil, but usually contains less carvone.

OTHER NAME: Oleum Anethi

A standard is given in the British Pharmaceutical Codex 1973

Constituents. Dill oil contains about 50% of carvone, the remainder consisting chiefly of (+)-limonene.

Description. It is a colourless or pale yellow liquid which becomes yellowish-brown on storage. It has an odour characteristic of the crushed fruit.

Solubility. Soluble, at 20°, in 1 part of alcohol (90%) and in 10 parts of alcohol (80%).

Weight per ml. At 20°, 0.895 to 0.910 g.

Refractive index. 1.481 to 1.492.

Optical rotation. +70° to +80°.

Adulterants and substitutes. East Indian dill oil, from *Anethum sowa* Roxb. ex Hem. is distinguished by its higher weight per ml and lower optical rotation, and by its containing dill apiole, which boils at 285° and, having a weight per ml of about 1.15 g, sinks in water. Genuine dill oil contains no constituent boiling at so high a temperature and no portion of the distillate sinks in water.

Storage. It should be stored in well-filled airtight containers, in a cool place, protected from light.

Actions and uses. Dill oil is a carminative and is used as dill water in the treatment of flatulence in infants. Dill water is a useful vehicle for children's medicines. The usual dose of dill oil is 0.05 to 0.2 millilitre.

Preparations

CONCENTRATED DILL WATER (*Syn.* Aqua Anethi Concentrata):

Dill oil	..	..	..	..	..	20 ml
Alcohol (90%)	..	..	..	..	600 ml
Water for preparations	..	..	..	to 1000 ml

Dissolve the dill oil in the alcohol and add sufficient water, in successive small portions, to produce 1000 ml,

shaking vigorously after each addition; add 50 g of sterilised purified talc or other suitable filtering aid, shake occasionally during a few hours, and filter.

A standard for this concentrated water is given in the British Pharmaceutical Codex 1973
Dose: 0.3 to 1 millilitre.

Dill Water is prepared by diluting concentrated dill water with 39 times its volume of water for preparations.

Diloxanide Furoate

4-(*N*-Methyl-2,2-dichloroacetamido)phenyl 2-furoate

$C_{14}H_{11}Cl_2NO_4 = 328.2$

OTHER NAME: *Furamide*® (available only in certain overseas countries)

A standard is given in the British Pharmacopoeia 1973

Description. An odourless, tasteless, white, crystalline powder.

Solubility. Very slightly soluble in water; soluble, at 20°, in 100 parts of alcohol, in 130 parts of ether, and in 2.5 parts of chloroform.

Melting-point. About 115°.

Storage. It should be protected from light.

ULTRAVIOLET ABSORPTION. In alcohol (95%), maximum at 258 nm (E1%, 1cm = 700).

Metabolism. ABSORPTION. Readily absorbed after oral administration as the base. The furoate is hydrolysed prior to absorption and appears to be less well absorbed than diloxanide.

EXCRETION. Diloxanide is excreted in both the urine and the faeces.

Actions and uses. Diloxanide furoate is used in the treatment of amoebiasis. It has a direct effect upon the amoebae in the gut and has no antibacterial action. It is used as an alternative to di-iodohydroxyquinoline or emetine and bismuth iodide in the treatment of acute and chronic intestinal amoebiasis and of asymptomatic carriers. It is also used together with chloroquine in the treatment of amoebic hepatitis.

Doses of 500 milligrams are given 3 times a day for 10 days. For children the usual dose is 20 milligrams per kilogram body-weight daily in divided doses for 10 days.

Preparation

DILOXANIDE FUROATE TABLETS: available as tablets containing 500 mg of diloxanide furoate.

A standard for these tablets is given in the British Pharmacopoeia 1973

Containers and *Storage:* see the entry on Tablets for general information on containers and storage. Containers should be airtight and light resistant.

Advice for patients: the tablets should be taken at regular intervals and the prescribed course should be completed.

Dilution

Formulated or proprietary products may have to be diluted (1) so that the required dose is contained in 5 ml or multiple thereof of elixirs, linctuses, or mixtures, as indicated in the relevant entries, or (2) when a cream, ointment, lotion, or similar preparation, is required in a form more dilute than is usually available.

Liquid internal medicines. Where the full formula is known, the vehicle, that is, all the inert ingredients, can be used as a diluent. Frequently, however, a simpler diluent is specified for ease of working. The composition of proprietary products is not usually completely disclosed, and therefore only a diluent recommended by the manufacturer should be used.

Preparations to be applied externally. Only recommended diluents should be used to avoid incompatibility which may result in phase inversion and separation or lack of preservation. Incompatibility may also lead to changes in the rate of release of the drug from the preparation. Creams liable to contamination should be adequately preserved. The diluent should preferably contain the same preservative at the same strength as that of the product concerned. Lack of preservative in a diluent, or use of an incompatible preservative system, may reduce the concentration of the preservative in the final diluted product to a level at which it may no longer be effective.

Stability. Most dilutions prepared as above are chemically stable and adequately preserved microbiologically but it is not recommended that extemporaneous dilutions should be stored for long periods. It is recommended that the dilutions should be freshly prepared and used within an arbitrary time limit, usually 14 days.

A few liquid medicines for internal use cannot be diluted satisfactorily and in these cases a suitable measure should be provided to measure the dose. In cases where an ointment or cream cannot be satisfactorily diluted the prescriber should be consulted.

Dimenhydrinate

2-Benzhydryloxy-*NN*-dimethylethylamine salt of 8-chlorotheophylline

$C_{24}H_{28}ClN_5O_3 = 470.0$

OTHER NAMES: Diphenhydramine Theoclate; *Dramamine*®; *Gravol*®

A standard is given in the British Pharmacopoeia 1973

Description. An odourless white crystalline powder with a bitter taste followed by local numbness.

Solubility. Soluble, at 20°, in 95 parts of water, in 2 parts of alcohol, and in 2 parts of chloroform; very slightly soluble in ether.

Sterilisation. Solutions for injection are sterilised by heating with a bactericide.

Storage. It should be stored in airtight containers.

Identification. TESTS. 1. Dissolve about 500 mg in 30 ml of alcohol (50%), add 30 ml of water and 4 ml of *strong ammonia solution*, extract with two 20-ml portions of ether, wash the combined extracts with 10 ml of water, add 2 ml of hydrochloric acid, and evaporate almost to dryness; the residue complies with Test 2 described under Diphenhydramine Hydrochloride.

2. Dissolve about 250 mg in 15 ml of alcohol (50%), add 15 ml of water and 2 ml of *dilute sulphuric acid*, and cool in ice for 30 minutes. Dissolve 10 mg of the precipitate obtained in 1 ml of hydrochloric acid, add 100 mg of potassium chlorate, and evaporate to dryness; a reddish residue remains which becomes purple when exposed to the vapour of *dilute ammonia solution*.

MELTING-POINT. About 105°.

Actions and uses. Dimenhydrinate has the actions, uses, and undesirable effects of the antihistamine drugs, as described under Promethazine Hydrochloride, its activity being due to its diphenhydramine content. It is given by mouth for the prevention and relief of motion-sickness.

The usual dose for an adult is 50 milligrams, for a child aged 6 to 12 years 25 milligrams, and for a younger child 12.5 milligrams. The first dose should be taken 30 minutes before a journey and the dose repeated not more than twice in 24 hours. Doses may be given by mouth, by rectum, or by intramuscular or intravenous injection.

Dimenhydrinate is also used for the symptomatic treatment of irradiation sickness and of vertigo and labyrinthine disorders due to Ménière's disease.

Poisoning. As for Promethazine Hydrochloride.

Preparations

DIMENHYDRINATE INJECTION: a sterile solution of dimenhydrinate, with 5% v/v of benzyl alcohol, in a mixture of equal volumes of propylene glycol and water for injections. Available in 1-ml ampoules containing 50 mg of dimenhydrinate.
A standard for this injection is given in the British Pharmacopoeia 1973
Containers and *Labelling:* see the entry on Injections for general information on containers and labelling.

DIMENHYDRINATE TABLETS: available as tablets containing 50 mg of dimenhydrinate; they may be coloured.
A standard for these tablets is given in the British Pharmacopoeia 1973
Containers and *Storage:* see the entry on Tablets for general information on containers and storage. Containers should be airtight.
Advice for patients: the tablets may cause drowsiness; persons affected should not drive or operate machinery. Alcohol should be avoided.

OTHER PREPARATIONS available include SUPPOSITORIES containing dimenhydrinate 50 and 100 mg.

Dimercaprol

2,3-Dimercaptopropan-1-ol

$C_3H_8OS_2 = 124.2$

OTHER NAMES: B.A.L.; British Anti-Lewisite; Dimercaprolum

A standard is given in the European Pharmacopoeia Vol. I

Description. A clear colourless or slightly yellow liquid with an alliaceous odour.

Solubility. Soluble, at 20°, in 20 parts of water and in 18 parts of arachis oil; miscible with alcohol and with benzyl benzoate.

Weight per ml. At 20°, 1.239 to 1.259 g.

Acidity. A saturated solution has a pH of 5 to 6.5.

Refractive index. At 20°, 1.568 to 1.574.

Boiling-point. About 80° at a pressure of 1.9 mmHg.

Sterilisation. Oily solutions for injection are sterilised by dry heat in an atmosphere of nitrogen or other suitable gas.

Storage. It should be stored in small well-filled airtight containers, at a temperature of 2° to 10°, protected from light.

Identification. TESTS. 1. Dissolve 0.1 ml in 4 ml of water and to 2 ml of the solution add *lead acetate solution*; a yellow precipitate is produced.
2. To the remainder of the solution prepared in Test 1 add 1 ml of 0.1N iodine; the colour of the iodine is discharged.

Metabolism. BLOOD CONCENTRATION. After intramuscular injection, peak blood concentrations are attained within 2 hours.

HALF-LIFE. Blood concentrations decrease by 50% after 4 hours.

EXCRETION. Rapidly excreted in the urine, chelated with metal ions; alkaline urine prevents dissociation of the chelate and therefore helps to protect the kidneys.

Actions and uses. Dimercaprol combines in the body with arsenic, mercury, and other heavy metals which inhibit the pyruvate-oxidase system by competing for the sulphydryl groups in proteins. It has a greater affinity than the proteins have for these metals and the resulting compounds are stable and rapidly excreted by the kidneys.

Dimercaprol is used in the treatment of acute poisoning by arsenic, mercury, gold, bismuth, thallium, and antimony; it should not be used in the treatment of iron or cadmium poisoning but it may be used in conjunction with sodium calciumedetate in the treatment of lead poisoning.

The toxic manifestations of arsenic therapy respond to treatment with dimercaprol, the first to disappear being haemorrhagic encephalitis, fever, agranulocytosis, and optic neuritis; exfoliative dermatitis and hyperkeratosis usually clear within 21 days, but aplastic anaemia shows no response. For the treatment of severe symptoms of arsenic poisoning, one scale of dosage consists in giving 3 milligrams of dimercaprol per kilogram body-weight by intramuscular injection every 4 hours for the first 2 days, 4 times on the third day, and twice daily for the next 10 days or until recovery is complete. For milder symptoms, 4 doses of 2.5 milligrams per kilogram body-weight are given daily at intervals of 4 hours for the first 2 days, followed by 2 doses on the third day and 1 or 2 doses daily for the next 10 days or until recovery is complete. Larger doses appear to be necessary for the treatment of mercurial poisoning.

For the treatment of gold poisoning, the dosage scheme is the same as that for the milder symptoms of arsenic poisoning.

Accidental contamination of the eyes with arsenical vesicants is successfully treated by instilling a 5 to 10% solution of dimercaprol in oil into the conjunctival sac; if given within 5 minutes of contamination there is complete recovery.

Local applications have also proved useful in the treatment of chromium dermatitis.

Undesirable effects. In doses of 4 to 5 milligrams per kilogram body-weight, dimercaprol gives rise to malaise, nausea, vomiting, lachrymation, salivation, headache, and burning sensation of the lips, mouth, throat, and eyes, together with a feeling of constriction in the throat and chest and an increase in systolic and diastolic blood pressure; the maximum effect is reached in about 15 to 20 minutes. The dosage usually employed, however, seldom produces reactions severe enough to warrant cessation of treatment. Single doses of up to 8 milligrams per kilogram body-weight have been given; the toxic effects last only a few hours and are completely reversible.

Veterinary uses. Dimercaprol is used in animals in the treatment of poisoning by arsenic or mercury. The usual dose for all species by intramuscular injection is 2.5 to 3 milligrams per kilogram body-weight, repeated as necessary. In severe arsenic poisoning the dose may be repeated every 4 hours for the first 2 days, every 6 hours on the third day, and twice daily for the next 10 days.

Preparation

DIMERCAPROL INJECTION (*Syn.* B.A.L. Injection):

Dimercaprol	..	..	..	..	..	.. 5 g
Benzyl benzoate	..	..	..	..	..	9.6 ml
Arachis oil	..	..	..	..	..	to 100.0 ml

Dissolve the dimercaprol in the benzyl benzoate and add sufficient arachis oil to produce the required volume. Add sufficient 5N alcoholic ammonia to adjust the pH from 6.8 to 7.0; add about 200 mg of decolorising charcoal, stir, allow to stand for not less than 1 hour, and filter. Distribute the solution into ampoules, replace the air in the ampoules with nitrogen or other suitable gas, seal, and sterilise by dry heat.

It contains 800 mg of dimercaprol in 16 ml. Available in 2-ml ampoules.

A standard for this injection is given in the British Pharmacopoeia 1973

Containers: see the entry on Injections for general information on containers.

Labelling: see the entry on Injections for general information on labelling. In addition, the label on the container should state the nature of the solvent and that the preparation is for intramuscular injection only.

Dimethicone

Polydimethylsiloxane

$$CH_3 \left[\begin{array}{c} CH_3 \\ | \\ Si \cdot O \\ | \\ CH_3 \end{array} \right]_n \begin{array}{c} CH_3 \\ | \\ Si \cdot CH_3 \\ | \\ CH_3 \end{array}$$

OTHER NAMES: Dimethyl Silicone Fluid; Dimethylsiloxane; *Dow Corning 360 Medical Fluid*®; *Lancepol Paediatric*®; *Silicone Fluids F 111*®

Asilone® and *Siloxyl*® (with dried aluminium hydroxide gel); *Siopel*® (with cetrimide); *Sprilon*® (with zinc oxide)

Standards for Dimethicones 20, 200, 350, 500, and 1000 are given in the British Pharmaceutical Codex 1973

Dimethicone is prepared by hydrolysing a mixture of dichlorodimethylsilane, $(CH_3)_2SiCl_2$, and chlorotrimethylsilane, $(CH_3)_3SiCl$. The products of hydrolysis contain active silanol groups, (SiOH), through which condensation polymerisation proceeds. By varying the proportion of chlorotrimethylsilane, which acts as a chain terminator, silicones of varying molecular weight are prepared.

As the molecular weight increases, the products become more viscous and fluids are available throughout the viscosity range of 0.65 to 3 000 000 centistokes. The various grades are distinguished by the numbers appended after each name, each number corresponding approximately to the viscosity of the product, in centistokes.

Description. A clear colourless odourless liquid.

Solubility. Soluble in ether, in xylene, in chlorinated hydrocarbons, and in solvent naphtha; dimethicones 20, 200, 350, and 500 are also soluble in amyl acetate, in cyclohexane, in light petroleum, and in kerosene; dimethicones 20, 200, 350, 500, and 1000 are practically insoluble in water, in alcohol, in methyl alcohol, and in acetone.

Weight per ml. At 20°, dimethicone 20, 0.940 to 0.965 g; dimethicones 200, 350, 500, and 1000, 0.965 to 0.980 g.

Actions and uses. The dimethicones are water-repellent liquids which have a low surface tension. They are stable to heat and are resistant to most chemical substances, although they are affected by strong acids.

Dimethicones are used in industrial barrier creams for protecting the skin against irritant substances. Creams, lotions, and ointments containing 10 to 30% of a dimethicone are employed for the prevention of bedsores and to protect the skin against trauma from urine or faecal discharge. Dimethicones are also used in conjunction with antacids to assist the expulsion of flatus prior to radiographic examination of the gastro-intestinal tract.

Dimethicones are used to form a water-repellent film on glass vials. A typical method is to rinse clean dry vials with a 2% solution of dimethicone 1000 in xylene, drain off the excess solution, and dry the vials at 110°; the vials are then heated for three hours at 250° to 275° in order to bond the dimethicone to the glass. Solutions and suspensions can be drained completely from vials which have been so treated.

Repeated use with a dimethicone will make glass apparatus water-repellent, although cleaning with toluene after use will remove most of the polymer.

Solutions of a dimethicone in ether or light petroleum are used as syringe lubricants; for this purpose, however, a methylphenylsiloxane is sometimes preferred because of its better lubricating properties and greater stability at high temperatures.

Dimethicones with added silica are used in the treatment of flatulence and as antifrothing agents in manufacturing processes.

Precautions. Dimethicone preparations should not be applied where free drainage is necessary or to inflamed or abraded skin. They may be irritant to the eye.

Preparations

DIMETHICONE CREAM (*Syn.* Silicone Cream):

Dimethicone 350	..	..	..	..	100 g
Cetrimide	..	..	..	..	.. 5 g
Chlorocresol	..	..	..	..	.. 1 g
Cetostearyl alcohol	..	..	..	..	50 g
Liquid paraffin	..	..	..	..	400 g
Purified water, freshly boiled and cooled	..	..	..	..	444 g

Warm and mix together the dimethicone 350, the liquid paraffin, and the cetostearyl alcohol until homogeneous; add, with mechanical stirring, the cetrimide and the chlorocresol dissolved in the water at the same temperature and stir until cold.

A standard for this cream is given in the British Pharmaceutical Codex 1973

Containers, Labelling, and *Storage:* see the entry on Creams for general information on containers, labelling, and storage.

Advice for patients: the cream should be applied sparingly and massaged well into the skin. It should not be applied to inflamed or broken skin.

OTHER PREPARATIONS available include an APPLICATION containing dimethicone 2% with zinc oxide 24% in an aerosol pack, a CREAM and a veterinary cream containing dimethicone 10% with cetrimide 0.3%, an EMULSION containing dimethicone 20 mg in 0.3 ml, and TABLETS containing dimethicone 250 mg with dried aluminium hydroxide gel 500 mg.

Dimethisterone

17-Hydroxy-6α,21-dimethyl-17α-pregn-4-en-20-yn-3-one monohydrate

$C_{23}H_{32}O_2,H_2O = 358.5$

A standard is given in the British Pharmacopoeia 1973

Description. A white crystalline odourless powder.

Solubility. Practically insoluble in water; soluble, at 20°, in 3 parts of alcohol, in 0.7 part of chloroform, in 1 part of pyridine, and in 80 parts of arachis oil.

Moisture content. 3.5 to 5.5%, determined by Fischer titration.

Storage. It should be protected from light.

Identification. MELTING-POINT. About 100°, with decomposition.

ULTRAVIOLET ABSORPTION. In alcohol (95%), maximum at 240 nm (E1%, 1cm = 423).

INFRA-RED ABSORPTION. Major peaks at 876, 1275, 1364, 1385, 1605, and 1658 cm^{-1} (see Appendix 2a: Infra-red Spectra).

THIN-LAYER CHROMATOGRAPHY. See under Thin-layer Chromatography, System 10.

Actions and uses. Dimethisterone is a synthetic progestogen which has actions and uses similar to those described under Progesterone.

It is active when given by mouth and is approximately as effective by this route as an equal weight of parenterally administered progesterone.

Dimethisterone may be used in a dosage of 15 to 40 milligrams daily in divided doses during the second half of the menstrual cycle for the treatment of functional uterine haemorrhage.

Undesirable effects. In large doses, dimethisterone may give rise to pelvic pain, breast turgidity, and vertigo.

Precautions and contra-indications. As for Progesterone.

Preparation

DIMETHISTERONE TABLETS. The usual strength is 5 mg. *A standard for these tablets is given in the British Pharmacopoeia 1973*
Containers and *Storage:* see the entry on Tablets for general information on containers and storage. Containers should be airtight and light resistant.
Advice for patients: the prescribed course should be completed or, where applicable, treatment should not be discontinued without the advice of the prescriber.

Dimethyl Phthalate

Methyl benzene-1,2-dicarboxylate

CO·O·CH₃
CO·O·CH₃

$C_{10}H_{10}O_4 = 194.2$

OTHER NAMES: DMP; Methyl Phthalate

A standard is given in the British Pharmacopoeia 1973

Description. A colourless or faintly coloured liquid which is odourless or has a faint odour.

Solubility. Soluble, at 20°, in 250 parts of water; miscible with alcohol, with ether, and with most organic solvents.

Weight per ml. At 20°, 1.186 to 1.192 g.

Refractive index. 1.515 to 1.517.

Boiling-point. About 280°, with decomposition.

Storage. Contact with plastic materials should be avoided.

Identification. TEST. It complies with Test 1 described under Diethyl Phthalate.

Actions and uses. Dimethyl phthalate is an insect repellent and is very effective against mosquitoes, midges, mites, ticks, and fleas.
Owing to its low volatility, it is active for 3 to 5 hours when applied to the skin, but profuse sweating greatly reduces the effective repellent time. It is usually applied as a cream or lotion containing at least 40% of dimethyl phthalate; weaker preparations are not effective as insect repellents.
Dimethyl phthalate may be used to impregnate clothing, but dibutyl phthalate is usually preferred.
It should not be allowed to come into contact with garments of rayon or other man-made fibres or with plastic spectacle frames.

Undesirable effects. Dimethyl phthalate has no serious irritant or toxic effects, although it may cause temporary smarting in tender areas of skin; it should not be applied near the eyes or to mucous surfaces.

Dimethyl Sulphoxide

$CH_3 . SO . CH_3 = 78.1$

OTHER NAMES: *Demavet*®
Fluvet DMSO® (with flumethasone)

A standard is given in the British Pharmacopoeia Addendum 1975

Description. A colourless hygroscopic liquid which is odourless or has a slight odour characteristic of dimethyl sulphide.

Solubility. Miscible with water, with alcohol, with ether, and with most organic solvents; immiscible with paraffin hydrocarbons.

Weight per ml. At 20°, 1.099 to 1.101 g.

Refractive index. At 20°, 1.478 to 1.479.

Storage. It should be stored in airtight containers, contact with plastics being avoided, protected from light.

Identification. TEST. Cautiously add 1.5 ml, dropwise, to 2.5 ml of hydriodic acid cooled in ice and filter rapidly; the residue, after drying under reduced pressure, is an unstable deep violet crystalline solid with an unpleasant odour and soluble in chloroform to give a red solution.

Metabolism. ABSORPTION. Readily absorbed after injection or oral or percutaneous administration.

BLOOD CONCENTRATION. After an oral dose of 1 g/kg body-weight, peak serum concentrations of unchanged drug of about 2 to 3 mg/ml are attained in 1.5 to 8 hours; after a percutaneous dose of 1 g/kg, applied over the entire body surface, a peak serum concentration of about 0.5 mg/ml is attained in 4 to 8 hours.

HALF-LIFE. Serum half-life, about 20 hours.

DISTRIBUTION. Widely distributed throughout the body and permeates body water but appears to accumulate primarily in soft tissues with accumulation in hard tissues occurring more slowly; the sulphone appears in the serum after 48 hours and may persist for up to 400 hours.

METABOLIC REACTIONS. Oxidation to dimethyl sulphone; in cats, dimethyl sulphide has been identified as a metabolite.

EXCRETION. After an oral dose, 30 to 68% is excreted in the urine unchanged and 21 to 23% is excreted as the sulphone; after a percutaneous dose, about 13% is excreted unchanged and 5 to 10% is excreted as the sulphone; in cats, about 3% of a dose is excreted through the lungs as dimethyl sulphide.

FURTHER INFORMATION. Respiratory excretion in cats —H. H. Borgstedt and V. Di Stefano, *Toxic. appl. Pharmac.*, 1967, **10**, 523; absorption, excretion, and metabolism in man—H. B. Hucker *et al.*, *J. Pharmac. exp. Ther.*, 1967, **155**, 309.

Uses. Dimethyl sulphoxide is a polar solvent which is aprotic and thus lacks basic and acidic properties. Like dimethylacetamide and dimethylformamide, it possesses exceptional solvent properties. These derive from its capacity to associate with both ionic species and neutral molecules which are either polar or polarisable.
Structural complexes, which dimethyl sulphoxide forms with water, proteins, and lipids give rise to its most important property, namely, its ready penetration and diffusion through biological membranes. It is probable that as dimethyl sulphoxide penetrates the stratum corneum, it displaces bound water and substitutes a looser structure. The permeability of the latter is then typically 10 to 50 times greater to other compounds than untreated skin. The cutaneous penetration of corticosteroids and many other compounds is thus enhanced by its use although the skin normally remains impermeable to drugs of high molecular weight, such as peptides. The pro-

portion of solvent must be greater than 80% before absorption rates are greatly increased.

A 5% solution of idoxuridine in dimethyl sulphoxide is used in the topical treatment of cutaneous herpes zoster eruptions.

Dimethyl sulphoxide has important cryophylactic properties, sharing with glycerol, pyridine-N-oxide, and some glycols marked ability to protect living cells, such as spermatozoa and lymphocytes, against damage during freezing and thawing. It also possesses marked radioprotective characteristics, modifying the damage caused to cells by ionising radiation.

Undesirable effects. It may give rise to a transient burning and stinging sensation and repeated applications may be associated with dermatitis. It imparts a garlic-like odour to the breath. Enhancement of the skin penetration may, with some drugs, give rise to toxic effects.

Precautions. It should not be applied to the eyes and mucous surfaces.

Preparations

Preparations available include an APPLICATION containing dimethyl sulphoxide 90% and an application containing dimethyl sulphoxide 90% with flumethasone 0.005%.

Dimetridazole

1,2-Dimethyl-5-nitroimidazole

$C_5H_7N_3O_2 = 141.1$

OTHER NAME: *Emtryl®*

A standard is given in the British Pharmacopoeia (Veterinary)

CAUTION. *Direct contact with the skin and inhalation of dust should be avoided.*

Description. An almost white to brownish-yellow odourless powder which darkens on exposure to light.

Solubility. Very slightly soluble in water; soluble, at 20°, in 30 parts of alcohol, in 170 parts of ether, and in 5 parts of chloroform.

Moisture content. Not more than 1%, determined by Fischer titration.

Storage. It should be protected from light.

Identification. TEST. Dissolve about 100 mg in 20 ml of anaesthetic ether, add 10 ml of a 1% solution of trinitrophenol in anaesthetic ether, induce crystallisation, and allow to stand; a precipitate is produced which, after washing with anaesthetic ether and drying at 105°, melts at about 160°.

MELTING-POINT. About 139°.

ULTRAVIOLET ABSORPTION. In methyl alcohol, maximum at 309 nm (E1%, 1cm = 650).

Veterinary uses. Dimetridazole is used for the prevention of blackhead in turkeys and for the control of swine dysentery.

The usual dose for poultry is 75 to 250 parts per million in the drinking water or 75 to 500 parts per million in the feed; it should not be fed to laying birds.

The usual dose for pigs is 250 parts per million in the drinking water or 200 to 500 parts per million in the feed.

Preparations

DIMETRIDAZOLE PREMIX: consisting of dimetridazole mixed with a suitable diluent. This preparation is stable to hot pelleting processes. It must be diluted before administration by mixing thoroughly with the feed. Available as a premix containing 22.5% of dimetridazole.

A standard for this premix is given in the British Pharmacopoeia (Veterinary)

Containers and *Storage:* see the entry on Premixes for general information on containers and storage. It should be protected from light.

DIMETRIDAZOLE SOLUBLE POWDER: consisting of dimetridazole in a water-soluble diluent. Available as a soluble powder containing 40% of dimetridazole.

A standard for this soluble powder is given in the British Pharmacopoeia (Veterinary)

Containers and *Storage:* see the entry on Powders for general information on containers and storage. Containers should be light resistant.

Labelling: the label on the container should state the proportion of dimetridazole in the preparation and directions for the medication of drinking water.

DIMETRIDAZOLE TABLETS: available as tablets containing 100 mg of dimetridazole. They may be prepared by moist granulation and compression as described in the entry on Tablets.

A standard for these tablets is given in the British Veterinary Codex Supplement 1970

Containers and *Storage:* see the entry on Tablets for general information on containers and storage. Containers should be light resistant.

Dinitolmide

3,5-Dinitro-*o*-toluamide

$C_8H_7N_3O_5 = 225.1$

OTHER NAME: *Zoalene®*

A standard is given in the British Pharmacopoeia (Veterinary)

Description. A cream to light tan odourless powder.

Solubility. Practically insoluble in water; soluble, at 20°, in 100 parts of alcohol, in 15 parts of acetone, in 650 parts of chloroform, and in 850 parts of ether.

Moisture content. Not more than 1%, determined by drying at 105°.

Identification. TEST. Mix 1 g with 20 ml of sulphuric acid (50% v/v), heat under a reflux condenser for 1 hour, cool, and add 50 ml of water; a precipitate is produced which, after washing with water and drying at 105°, melts at about 205°.

MELTING-POINT. About 179°.

Veterinary uses. Dinitolmide is used as a coccidiostat in poultry in a dosage of 200 parts per million in the feed.

Dinoprost Trometamol Salt

The 2-amino-2-(hydroxymethyl)propane-1,3-diol salt of (1R,2R,3R,5S)-7-{3,5-dihydroxy-2-[(3S)-3-hydroxyoct-1(E)-enyl]cyclopentyl}hept-5(Z)-enoic acid

$C_{20}H_{34}O_5,C_4H_{11}NO_3 = 475.6$

OTHER NAMES: *Lutalyse*®; PGF$_{2\alpha}$ THAM salt; Prostaglandin F$_{2\alpha}$ Trometamol; *Prostin F2 Alpha*®

Description. A white to off-white very hygroscopic crystalline powder.

Solubility. Soluble in 5 parts of water.

Melting-point. About 100°.

Metabolism. BLOOD CONCENTRATION. Venous blood concentrations of less than 75 to 430 pg/ml are sufficient to induce uterine contractions.

DISTRIBUTION. Dinoprost and dinoprostone are the two major natural prostaglandins found in man. They are synthesised in almost all tissues.

METABOLIC REACTIONS. Rapidly metabolised by dehydrogenation of the side chain hydroxyl group, β-oxidation of the carboxyl group, and ω-oxidation of the alkyl side chain to form a large number of metabolites; the major metabolites are the 5β- and 5α- forms of 5,7α-dihydroxy-11-oxotetranorprosta-1,6-dioic acid.

EXCRETION. 90 to 95% of an intravenous dose is excreted in the urine in 5 to 7 hours.

FURTHER INFORMATION. Reviews—P. B. Curtis-Prior, *Prostaglandins: An Introduction to their Biochemistry, Physiology and Pharmacology*, Oxford, North Holland Publishing Company, 1976, and T. O. Osterling *et al.*, *J. pharm. Sci.*, 1972, **61**, 1861.

Actions and uses. Dinoprost trometamol salt is a soluble salt of prostaglandin F$_{2\alpha}$. It may be administered by intravenous infusion, extra-amniotically, or intra-amniotically to stimulate uterine contractions as described under Dinoprostone but it is less potent.
It is administered by intravenous infusion for the induction of labour, for therapeutic termination of pregnancy, for missed abortion or foetal death in utero, and for expulsion of a hydatidiform mole. It is also administered by the extra-amniotic route for the therapeutic termination of pregnancy and by the intra-amniotic route for the therapeutic termination of pregnancy during the second trimester.
For the induction of labour and for foetal death in utero, a solution containing the equivalent of 15 micrograms of dinoprost per millilitre is infused at the rate of 2.5 micrograms per minute for at least 30 minutes and then adjusted as necessary. Larger doses may be required for foetal death in utero, and 5 micrograms per minute may be infused initially and increased at hourly intervals.
For the therapeutic termination of pregnancy, missed abortion, and hydatidiform mole, a solution containing 50 micrograms of dinoprost per millilitre is infused at a rate of 25 micrograms of dinoprost per minute for at least 30 minutes and then increased if necessary to 50 micrograms per minute. For the therapeutic termina-

tion of pregnancy, the initial dose by the extra-amniotic route is the equivalent of 375 micrograms of dinoprost; subsequent doses of 375 to 750 micrograms may be administered at intervals of 2 hours depending on the uterine response. By the intra-amniotic route, the equivalent of 40 milligrams of dinoprost is injected slowly into the amniotic sac as a solution containing 5 milligrams per millilitre.

Undesirable effects; Precautions; Contra-indications. As for Dinoprostone.

Veterinary uses. Dinoprost trometamol salt is a luteolytic prostaglandin used in cattle and horses to control the timing of oestrus and ovulation, to correct certain forms of infertility, and to terminate early pregnancy. It is also used to induce parturition in cattle. It is given as a single intramuscular injection, the usual dose for cattle being the equivalent of 25 to 35 milligrams of dinoprost and for mares the equivalent of 5 milligrams of dinoprost.

Preparations

Preparations available include an INJECTION containing dinoprost trometamol salt equivalent to 5 mg of dinoprost per ml in 1.5- and 5-ml ampoules for intravenous use, 1.5-ml ampoules with diluent for extra-amniotic use, and 4- and 8-ml ampoules for intra-amniotic use.

Dinoprostone

(1R,2R,3R)-7-{3-Hydroxy-2-[(3S)-3-hydroxyoct-1(E)-enyl]-5-oxocyclopentyl}hept-5(Z)-enoic acid *or* (8R,11R,12R,15S)-11,15-dihydroxy-9-oxaprosta-5(Z),13(E)-dienoic acid

$C_{20}H_{32}O_5 = 352.5$

OTHER NAMES: Prostaglandin E$_2$; *Prostin E2*®

Description. A white to off-white crystalline solid.

Solubility. Soluble in 1000 parts of water; soluble in alcohol.

Identification. MELTING-POINT. About 65°.

Stability. Solutions in alcohol or NN-dimethylacetamide are stable for at least 2 years when stored as described below. Aqueous solutions are unstable and should be used within 24 hours when stored at 4°.

Storage. Alcoholic solutions should be stored at 4°. Solutions in NN-dimethylacetamide should be stored below 20° and should not be allowed to come into contact with plastics unless diluted.

Metabolism. DISTRIBUTION. Dinoprostone and dinoprost are the two major natural prostaglandins found in man. They are synthesised in almost all tissues.

METABOLIC REACTIONS. Rapidly metabolised by dehydrogenation of the side chain hydroxyl group, p-oxidation of the carboxyl group and ω-oxidation of the alkyl side chain to form a large number of metabolites; the major metabolites are 7α-hydroxy-5,11-dioxotetranorprosta-1,16-dioic acid in man and 11α,15-dihydroxy-9-oxoprost-5-enoic acid and 11α-hydroxy-9,15-dioxoprost-5-enoic acid in guinea pigs.

EXCRETION. About 50% of an intravenous dose is excreted in the urine in 5 hours.

FURTHER INFORMATION. See under Dinoprost Trometamol Salt.

Actions and uses. Dinoprostone is used to stimulate uterine contractions of labour when there are no foetal or maternal contra-indications. For this purpose it is administered by mouth as an oral solution diluted to contain 100 micrograms per millilitre or as tablets of 500 micrograms.

When administering the oral solution, a test dose of 500 micrograms is given, followed after 30 minutes by a dose of 1 milligram; doses of 1 milligram, 1.5 milligrams, and 2 milligrams are then administered at two-hourly intervals depending on the uterine response.

The initial dose of the tablets is 500 micrograms followed by doses of 500 micrograms every hour increasing to 1 milligram hourly if necessary, the maximum single dose being 1.5 milligrams.

Dinoprostone may be administered by the intravenous route to stimulate uterine contraction in order to expel uterine contents for the induction of labour, and in foetal death in utero, and in a higher dosage for the therapeutic termination of pregnancy, missed abortion, and hydatidiform mole.

For the induction of labour and foetal death in utero the usual dose, by intravenous infusion, is 0.25 microgram per minute as a solution in dextrose injection (5%) or sodium chloride injection containing 1.5 micrograms per millilitre for 30 minutes. This dose is then adjusted according to the patient's response. Foetal death in utero may require higher doses. An initial rate of 0.5 microgram per minute may be used with stepwise increases at intervals of not less than 1 hour.

For the therapeutic termination of pregnancy, missed abortion, and hydatidiform mole, a solution containing 5 micrograms per millilitre may be given by intravenous infusion, at a rate of 2.5 micrograms of dinoprostone per minute for 30 minutes, and continued at this rate or increased to 5 micrograms per minute if necessary for at least 4 hours after which the rate of administration may be further increased if necessary. Alternatively, the extra-amniotic route may be used for the therapeutic termination of pregnancy in an initial dose of 1 millilitre of solution containing 100 micrograms followed by doses of 100 to 200 micrograms every 2 hours depending on the response of the patient.

Dinoprostone has been given intra-amniotically as an initial injection of 1 milligram followed by two further 1-milligram doses at 10-minute intervals. In cases of diminished uterine activity a further dose of 3 milligrams of dinoprostone may be given after 12 hours.

Undesirable effects. Nausea, vomiting, diarrhoea, pyrexia, elevated white blood cell count, and vasovagal symptoms such as flushing, shivering, headache and dizziness may occur.

Precautions. It should be administered with caution to patients with glaucoma, raised intra-ocular pressure, or asthma. Cephalopelvic relationships should be known before administering dinoprostone for the induction of labour. Uterine activity, foetal status, and the progression of cervical dilatation should be monitored during the administration of dinoprostone. In addition it should be used with caution in patients where there is a history of difficult labour or of pelvic infection.

Dinoprostone may potentiate the effect of oxytocin and the use of these drugs concurrently should be monitored.

Contra-indications. Dinoprostone should not be administered to patients who are sensitive to prostaglandins or for whom oxytocic drugs are contra-indicated. The extra-amniotic route should not be used in the presence of cervicitis or vaginal infections.

Preparations

Preparations available include an INJECTION containing dinoprostone 1 mg per ml in 0.75-ml ampoules and 10 mg per ml in 0.5-ml ampoules for intravenous use, an injection containing dinoprostone 10 mg per ml in 0.5-ml ampoules with diluent for extra-amniotic use, a SOLUTION in NN-dimethylacetamide containing dinoprostone 10 mg per ml in 0.5-ml ampoules (for dilution before oral administration), and TABLETS containing dinoprostone 500 micrograms.

Dioctyl Sodium Sulphosuccinate

Sodium 1,4-bis(2-ethylhexyl) sulphosuccinate

$$CO \cdot O \cdot CH_2 \cdot \overset{\displaystyle C_2H_5}{\underset{\displaystyle}{CH}} \cdot [CH_2]_3 \cdot CH_3$$
$$\underset{\displaystyle}{CH_2}$$
$$NaSO_3 \cdot CH$$
$$CO \cdot O \cdot CH_2 \cdot \underset{\displaystyle C_2H_5}{CH} \cdot [CH_2]_3 \cdot CH_3$$

$C_{20}H_{37}NaO_7S = 444.6$

OTHER NAMES: *Aerosol OT*®; *Condanol SB-DO 60%*®; *Dioctyl-Medo*®; *Manoxol OT/P*®; *Molcer*®; *Siponol O*®; *Soliwax*®; *Waxsol*®

Dulcodos® (with bisacodyl); *Normax*® (with danthron); *Audinorm*® (with glycerol)

A standard is given in the British Pharmaceutical Codex 1973

Description. Hygroscopic white waxy masses or flakes with a characteristic odour.

Solubility. Soluble, at 20°, in 70 parts of water, higher concentrations forming a thick gel; soluble in 1 part of chloroform, in 1 part of ether, and in 3 parts of alcohol.

Moisture content. Not more than 3%, determined by drying at 105°.

Stability. It is stable in acid solution but hydrolyses slowly in weak alkaline solutions and rapidly in solution above pH 9.

Storage. It should be stored in airtight containers.

Identification. TEST. To 5 ml of a 0.1% solution add 1 ml of *dilute sulphuric acid*, 10 ml of chloroform, and 0.2 ml of *dimethyl yellow solution*, and shake; the chloroform layer is coloured red. Add 50 mg of cetrimide and shake; the colour of the chloroform layer changes to yellow.

Metabolism. ABSORPTION. Dioctyl sodium sulphosuccinate appears to be absorbed after oral administration.

EXCRETION. After oral administration of 100 to 200 mg of dioctyl sodium sulphosuccinate to patients with indwelling T-tube biliary drainage, biliary concentrations of up to 15 to 20 μg/ml are attained in 2 to 4 hours.

FURTHER INFORMATION. Excretion in bile—C. A. Dujovne *et al.*, *Clin. Pharmac. Ther.*, 1972, **13**, 602.

Actions and uses. Dioctyl sodium sulphosuccinate is an anionic surface-active agent. When taken by mouth exerts a softening effect on the faeces and has a laxative action.

The usual dose for adults is 50 to 100 milligrams on alternate days. The dose for children is one half and for infants one quarter of the dose for adults.

A 0.25% solution is used as an enema for the removal of impacted faeces. A 5% solution has been used for softening wax in the ear.

Dioctyl sodium sulphosuccinate is also used as a tablet disintegrant.

Preparations

Preparations available include CAPSULES containing dioctyl sodium sulphosuccinate 60 mg with danthron 50 mg; EAR-DROPS containing dioctyl sodium sulphosuccinate 5% in both multiple-dose containers and as single-dose forms, ear-drops containing dioctyl sodium sulphosuccinate 5% with glycerol 10%; an ELIXIR containing dioctyl sodium sulphosuccinate 12.5 mg in 5 ml (also for rectal use); a SOLUTION containing dioctyl sodium sulphosuccinate 1%; TABLETS containing dioctyl sodium sulphosuccinate 20 and 100 mg, and tablets containing dioctyl sodium sulphosuccinate 100 mg with bisacodyl 5 mg.

Dioxathion

A technical product consisting mainly of *cis* and *trans* isomers of *SS'*-1,4-dioxane-2,3-diyl bis(*OO*-diethyl phosphorodithioate), the remainder consisting of related materials which are also active.

$C_{12}H_{26}O_6P_2S_4 = 456.5$

OTHER NAMES: *Delnav*®
Tick Dip (Liquid) Cooper® (with gamma benzene hexachloride)

A standard is given in the British Pharmacopoeia (Veterinary)

CAUTION. *Dioxathion is very toxic when inhaled, swallowed, or spilled on the skin. It can be removed from the skin by washing with soap and water. Contaminated material should be immersed in a 2% solution of sodium hydroxide for several hours.*

Description. A dark amber-coloured liquid with an odour characteristic of sulphides.

Solubility. Practically insoluble in water; miscible with alcohol, with acetone, with benzene, and with xylene.

Weight per ml. At 25°, 1.240 to 1.270 g.

Refractive index. 1.540 to 1.550.

Storage. It should be stored in airtight containers at a temperature not exceeding 25°.

Identification. TESTS. 1. Mix about 10 mg with 10 mg of anhydrous sodium acetate, dissolve with the aid of heat in 5 ml of a 10% solution of potassium hydroxide in methyl alcohol, cool, and filter; to the filtrate add 1 ml of a 0.5% solution of dichloroquinonechloroimine in alcohol (95%); a reddish-brown colour is produced which changes to brown on dilution with 20 ml of water.

2. Boil a small quantity with perchloric acid (72%) for a few minutes, cool, and dilute with water; the solution gives the reactions of phosphates.

Veterinary uses. Dioxathion is an insecticide and acaricide used in the control of cattle ticks and of ticks, lice, keds, and blowfly of sheep. The usual strength of cattle dips is 0.05 to 0.1% and of sheep dips 0.025 to 0.1%.

Preparation

DIOXATHION DIP CONCENTRATE: consisting of dioxathion mixed with suitable pharmaceutical adjuvants to produce an emulsifiable concentrate. It may contain a suitable preservative. Available as a concentrate containing 25% w/v of dioxathion. It must be diluted before use to produce an emulsion containing about 0.1% of dioxathion.

A standard for this dip concentrate is given in the British Pharmacopoeia (Veterinary)

Labelling: see the entry on Dip Concentrates for general information on labelling.

Dip Concentrates

Preparations intended for dilution with water to make an insecticidal wash in which animals may be completely immersed in order to kill ectoparasites and, in some cases, to provide protection against reinfestation. Usually, the same preparations may be applied to the animals in the form of sprays, but the effectiveness of spraying depends upon the parasite to be controlled and the species of animal and the length of its coat.

Dip concentrates may take the form of wettable dispersible powders or pastes, emulsion concentrates, or simple solutions of water-soluble insecticides.

Suspension dip concentrates. Wettable dispersible powders or pastes must be of fine particle size in order to avoid rapid sedimentation or fall in concentration in the dipping bath. Mixing with water must be thorough so that an even suspension is formed; a preliminary creaming of the dip concentrate with water may be necessary before adding it to the bath. In the case of sheep-dipping baths, the final mixing can be achieved by thorough agitation with wooden paddles. In large deep cattle-dipping baths, the final mixing, or the resuspension of dip washes which have been standing, may be carried out by dipping 25 to 50 head of cattle which are later dipped again.

Emulsion dip concentrates. May be of the "black fluid", "white fluid", or "miscible oil" types. They may require to be mixed by a creaming process, small quantities of water being added with stirring so as to form a primary emulsion which can then be mixed with the main bulk of water in the dipping bath. Some paste concentrates require the use of hot water in the preparation of the primary emulsion. The resulting emulsions must be stable, as any breakdown of the emulsion may reduce its efficacy and may expose the treated animals to toxic hazards. When "black fluids" are used, hard waters must first be softened by means of washing soda before mixing is attempted.

Replenishment and exhaustion of baths. Sheep dips should normally be used for dipping one flock only and the residue then discarded. Cattle dipping-baths are used at regular intervals and may be kept in use for many months before being emptied and recharged. In both cases, replenishments should be regularly made as dipping proceeds, in order to compensate for the dip-wash retained on the coats of the animals.

Because the amount of insecticide in the wash draining from dipped animals may be less than that in the original wash, there may be a progressive decrease in the concentration of the insecticide in the bath as dipping proceeds, a phenomenon known as "exhaustion". In certain cases, such as some arsenical and lime-sulphur dips, the degree of exhaustion can be determined by bath-side tests. To counteract this exhaustion, it is necessary to replenish the bath frequently with dipping-wash at a higher concentration than was originally used.

Bacterial contamination. When the dip has no bacteriostatic properties, it is advisable to add a suitable substance to the dip concentrate or to the bath in order to prevent the growth of undesirable micro-organisms.

Precautions in using organophosphorus dips. If the active ingredient of a dip is an organophosphorus compound, users should exercise great care when handling the preparation, even when it has been diluted, in order to avoid accidentally splashing themselves with it. All the precautions given on the label or the package leaflet should be strictly observed.

Labelling. The label on the container should state the names and proportions of medicaments, the name and proportion of any added preservative, and the name and quantity of diluent and the method to be employed in preparing the diluted dip concentrate for use.

The label on the container of a preparation containing an organophosphorus compound or the package leaflet should state: (1) that the preparation is an organophosphorus compound; (2) the precautions to be taken in respect of the animals under treatment, namely, (a) the minimum period, if any, which must elapse between cessation of treatment of the animals and slaughter for human consumption, and (b) that the preparation should not be used if the animals are not in a fit state for treatment or during unsuitable weather conditions; (3) the precautions to be taken to protect the operators, namely, that they (c) should wear suitable protective clothing when handling the concentrate or dip wash and freshly dipped animals, (d) should wash the concentrate or dip wash from the eyes or exposed skin immediately if splashed, (e) should wash hands and exposed skin before meals and after work, (f) should avoid working in a spray mist, and (g) should not handle the preparation if they are under medical advice not to work with organophosphorus compounds; and (4) the precautions to be taken to protect wild life and others, namely, (h) that the preparation is toxic to fish, so that residues of the used preparation should not be allowed to drain into ditches, ponds, or waterways, (j) that the container should be stored, securely closed, in a safe place and away from foodstuffs, and (k) that the used container should be thoroughly washed out, safely disposed of, and not left lying about.

Diphenhydramine Hydrochloride

2-Benzhydryloxyethyl-*NN*-dimethylammonium chloride

$$[(C_6H_5)_2 \cdot CH \cdot O \cdot [CH_2]_2 \cdot \overset{+}{N}H(CH_3)_2] \ Cl^-$$

$C_{17}H_{22}ClNO = 291.8$

OTHER NAMES: *Benadryl®*; *Histergan®*
Newmarket Cough Syrup® (with theophylline)

A standard is given in the British Pharmacopoeia 1973

Description. A white crystalline odourless powder with a bitter taste followed by a sensation of numbness.

Solubility. Soluble, at 20°, in 1 part of water, in 2 parts of alcohol, in 2 parts of chloroform, and in 50 parts of acetone; very slightly soluble in ether.

Dissociation constant. pK_a 9.0 (25°).

Sterilisation. Solutions for injection are sterilised by filtration.

Storage. It should be stored in airtight containers, protected from light.

Identification. TESTS. 1. Mix 5 ml of a 2% solution with 3 ml of hydrochloric acid, boil for 3 minutes, and cool in ice; the precipitate, after recrystallisation from water, melts at about 64°.

2. To 10 ml of a hot 1% solution in water add *trinitrophenol solution*, dropwise; the precipitate, after recrystallisation from alcohol, melts at about 130°.

MELTING-POINT. About 170°.

ULTRAVIOLET ABSORPTION. In 0.1N hydrochloric acid, maxima at 254 nm (E1%, 1cm = 13) and 260 nm (E1%, 1cm = 14.5); in alcohol (95%), maxima at 253 nm (E1%, 1cm = 12), 258 nm (E1%, 1cm = 15), and 264 nm (E1%, 1cm = 12).

INFRA-RED ABSORPTION. Major peaks at 713, 754, 1017, 1103, 1180, and 1454 cm^{-1} (see Appendix 2a: Infra-red Spectra).

THIN-LAYER CHROMATOGRAPHY. See under Thin-layer Chromatography, System 4.

Determination in body fluids. GAS CHROMATOGRAPHY. In plasma—K. S. Albert *et al.*, *Res. Commun. chem. Path. Pharmac.*, 1974, **7**, 95 and R. Baugh and R. T. Calvert, *Br. J. clin. Pharmac.*, 1976, **3**, 1062.

ULTRAVIOLET SPECTROPHOTOMETRY. In urine—B. Caddy *et al.*, *Analyst, Lond.*, 1975, **100**, 563.

Metabolism. ABSORPTION. Readily absorbed after oral administration.

BLOOD CONCENTRATION. After an oral dose of 50 mg of the hydrochloride as a solution and as a capsule, plasma concentrations of 50 to 54 ng/ml and 20 to 38 ng/ml are attained at 1 hour respectively; at 2 hours, the respective plasma concentrations are 64 to 70 ng/ml and 45 to 51 ng/ml; after an intravenous infusion of 50 mg of the hydrochloride, plasma concentrations of 179 to 258 ng/ml are attained at 1 hour.

HALF-LIFE. The plasma half-life after an oral dose is 13 to 21 hours and after an intravenous infusion 7 to 10 hours.

DISTRIBUTION. *Protein binding*, 98% bound to plasma proteins.

METABOLIC REACTIONS. Extensively metabolised; about 50% of an oral dose is metabolised in the liver before reaching the general circulation. Reactions include N-dealkylation and deamination.

EXCRETION. In the urine up to 3% of a dose is excreted unchanged, up to 13% as basic amines and up to 65% as diphenylmethane metabolites. The major urinary metabolite appears to be diphenylmethoxyacetic acid in free or conjugated form.

FURTHER INFORMATION. Pharmacokinetics—K. S Albert *et al.*, *J. Pharmacokinet. Biopharm.*, 1975, **3**, 159 metabolic disposition—A. J. Glazko *et al.*, *Clin. Pharmac. Ther.*, 1974, **16**, 1066.

Bioavailability. Absorption from soft gelatin capsules

appears to be better than from sugar-coated tablets—U. Gundert-Remy *et al., Drugs Germ.*, 1975, **18**, 99.

Actions and uses. Diphenhydramine has the actions, uses, and undesirable effects of antihistamine drugs, as described under Promethazine Hydrochloride. It is one of the less active but more sedating of the group and is sometimes used for its sedative properties. It is usually administered by mouth, although it may be given parenterally if necessary.

The usual adult dose is 50 to 200 milligrams by mouth daily in divided doses. The oral dose for children under 1 year is 6.25 to 12.5 milligrams 3 times daily, 2 to 5 years 12.5 to 25 milligrams 3 to 4 times daily, and 6 to 12 years 25 to 50 milligrams 3 or 4 times daily.

Because of its mild spasmolytic properties diphenhydramine is sometimes used as an ingredient of preparations for the relief of cough. It has also been used for the treatment of parkinsonism and for the prevention of motion-sickness.

Poisoning. As for Promethazine Hydrochloride.

Preparations

DIPHENHYDRAMINE CAPSULES: consisting of diphenhydramine hydrochloride, in powder, which may be mixed with a suitable inert diluent, enclosed in a hard capsule. The capsule shells may be coloured. Available as capsules containing 25 mg of diphenhydramine hydrochloride.

A standard for these capsules is given in the British Pharmacopoeia 1973

Containers and *Storage:* see the entry on Capsules for general information on containers and storage.

Advice for patients: the capsules may cause drowsiness; persons affected should not drive or operate machinery. Alcohol should be avoided.

DIPHENHYDRAMINE ELIXIR: a solution of diphenhydramine hydrochloride in a suitable coloured flavoured vehicle.

When a dose less than or not a multiple of 5 ml is prescribed, the elixir may be diluted, as described in the entry on Elixirs, with syrup. The diluted elixir must be freshly prepared, unless a preservative is added to the diluent; 0.2% of methyl hydroxybenzoate is a suitable preservative.

Available as an elixir containing 10 mg of diphenhydramine hydrochloride in 5 ml.

A standard for this elixir is given in the British Pharmaceutical Codex 1973

Containers and *Labelling:* see the entry on Elixirs for general information on containers and labelling.

Storage: it should be protected from light.

Advice for patients: the elixir may cause drowsiness; persons affected should not drive or operate machinery. Alcohol should be avoided.

OTHER PREPARATIONS available include a CREAM containing diphenhydramine hydrochloride 2%; a veterinary MIXTURE containing diphenhydramine hydrochloride 2.6 mg with theophylline 3.5 mg per ml; and TABLETS containing diphenhydramine hydrochloride 25 and 50 mg.

Diphenoxylate Hydrochloride

-(3-Cyano-3,3-diphenylpropyl)-4-ethoxycarbonyl-4-phenylpiperidinium chloride

$C_{30}H_{33}ClN_2O_2 = 489.1$

OTHER NAMES: *Lomotil*® and *Reasec*® (both with atropine sulphate)

A standard is given in the British Pharmacopoeia 1973

Description. A white odourless powder.

Solubility. Very slightly soluble in water; soluble, at 20°, in 50 parts of alcohol, in 2.5 parts of chloroform, and in 40 parts of acetone; practically insoluble in ether.

Acidity. A saturated solution has a pH of about 3.3.

Identification. TEST. Dissolve a few mg in 5 ml of water and add 2 drops of *potassium mercuri-iodide solution*; a cream-coloured precipitate is produced.

MELTING-POINT. About 223°.

ULTRAVIOLET ABSORPTION. In a mixture of 1 volume of 1N hydrochloric acid and 99 volumes of methyl alcohol, maxima at 252 nm (E1%, 1cm = 11), 258 nm (E1%, 1cm = 13), and 264 nm (E1%, 1cm = 10).

Metabolism. ABSORPTION. Rapidly absorbed after oral administration.

BLOOD CONCENTRATION. After an oral dose of 5 mg, peak plasma concentrations of unchanged drug of about 10 ng/ml are attained in 2 hours and peak concentrations of diphenoxylic acid, the major metabolite in blood, of about 40 ng/ml are attained after the same period.

HALF-LIFE. Plasma half-life, about 2.5 hours for unchanged drug and about 4 hours for diphenoxylic acid.

DISTRIBUTION. Widely distributed throughout the body; volume of distribution, about 320 litres.

METABOLIC REACTIONS. Extensively metabolised by hydrolysis, hydroxylation, and conjugation with glucuronic acid.

EXCRETION. About 14% and 50% of a dose is excreted in 96 hours in the urine and faeces respectively; the major urinary metabolites are diphenoxylic acid and hydroxy-diphenoxylic acid both in free and conjugated forms; less than 0.1% of a dose is excreted in the urine unchanged.

FURTHER INFORMATION. Pharmacokinetics and metabolism—A. Karim *et al., Clin. Pharmac. Ther.*, 1972, **13**, 407.

Actions and uses. Diphenoxylate has an inhibitory action on intestinal motility and is used in the symptomatic control of both acute and chronic diarrhoea, however caused. Response to treatment is usually rapid and the prompt control reduces the dehydration associated with diarrhoea.

Diphenoxylate has no antibacterial properties, and its use in controlling the symptoms of diarrhoea does not remove the need for specific therapy when the diarrhoea is caused by bacterial or parasitic infection.

Diphenoxylate is also used in colostomy and ileostomy for reducing the frequency as well as the fluidity of the stools.

It is given in doses of 5 to 10 milligrams 3 or 4 times a

day until the diarrhoea is controlled, when the dose may be reduced according to need to 5 milligrams daily.
The dose for children is from a quarter to three quarters of the adult dose.

Undesirable effects. Although undesirable effects are not frequent, nausea, dizziness, and sedation may occur; other side-effects include rash, pruritus, and insomnia; euphoria and abdominal distension have also been reported.

Precautions and contra-indications. Diphenoxylate is contra-indicated in patients with impaired liver function. The possibility that it may enhance the action of barbiturates should be borne in mind.
Although it has a structural relationship with pethidine, it has no analgesic action, but it appears to be capable of preventing withdrawal symptoms in known narcotic addicts and the addiction liability approximates to that of codeine.
When diphenoxylate is used for short-term administration, the risk of addiction is negligible, and excessive use is discouraged by the addition of a subclinical dose of atropine.

Preparations
Preparations available include an ELIXIR containing diphenoxylate hydrochloride 2.5 mg with atropine sulphate 25 micrograms in 5 ml, diluent glycerol, life of diluted elixir 14 days; and TABLETS containing diphenoxylate hydrochloride 2.5 mg with atropine sulphate 25 micrograms.

Diphenylpyraline Hydrochloride

4-Benzhydryloxy-1-methylpiperidinium chloride

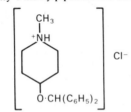

$C_{19}H_{24}ClNO = 317.9$

OTHER NAMES: *Histryl®; Lergoban®*

A standard is given in the British Pharmacopoeia Addendum 1975

Description. An odourless white powder.

Solubility. Soluble, at 20°, in 1 part of water, in 3 parts of alcohol, and in 2 parts of chloroform; practically insoluble in ether.

Moisture content. Not more than 1%, determined by drying at 105°.

Identification. TESTS. 1. Dissolve about 10 mg in 10 ml of sulphuric acid; an orange solution is produced. To 5 ml of the solution add 4 drops of *potassium dichromate solution*, warm, and allow to stand; the colour of the solution slowly changes from red to brown. Pour the remainder of the solution into about 10 ml of water; a colourless, opalescent solution is produced.
2. Dissolve about 100 mg in 10 ml of water, heat the solution and add, dropwise, *trinitrophenol solution* until precipitation is complete; the precipitate, after recrystallisation from alcohol (95%), melts at about 168°.

MELTING-POINT. About 206°.

ULTRAVIOLET ABSORPTION. In 0.1N hydrochloric acid, maxima at 255 nm (E1%, 1cm = 12) and 260 nm (E1%, 1cm = 13.2); in alcohol (95%), maxima at 255 nm (E1%, 1cm = 10.7), 260 nm (E1%, 1cm = 12), and 266 nm (E1%, 1cm = 9.5).

INFRA-RED ABSORPTION. Major peaks at 709, 748, 762, 1051, 1067, and 1450 cm⁻¹ (see Appendix 2a: Infra-red Spectra).

THIN-LAYER CHROMATOGRAPHY. See under Thin-layer Chromatography, System 4.

Determination in body fluids. ULTRAVIOLET SPECTROPHOTOMETRY. In urine: prior separation by thin-layer chromatography—H.-D. Dell *et al., Z. analyt. Chem.*, 1975, **277**, 208.

Metabolism. HALF-LIFE. Based on urinary excretion data, 24 to 40 hours.

EXCRETION. 2 to 9% of a dose is excreted unchanged.

FURTHER INFORMATION. Half-life in man—G. Graham and A. G. Bolt, *J. Pharmacokinet. Biopharm.*, 1974, **2**, 191.

Actions and uses. Diphenylpyraline has the actions, uses, and undesirable effects of the antihistamine drugs, as described under Promethazine Hydrochloride.
The usual dose of diphenylpyraline hydrochloride for the relief of allergic conditions is 3 to 4.5 milligrams 4 times a day or 5 to 10 milligrams of a slow-release preparation twice a day.

Poisoning. As for Promethazine Hydrochloride.

Preparations
Preparations available include CAPSULES containing diphenylpyraline hydrochloride 2.5 and 5 mg in a slow-release formulation; an ELIXIR containing diphenylpyraline hydrochloride 1.5 mg in 5 ml, diluent syrup, life of diluted syrup 14 days; and TABLETS containing diphenylpyraline hydrochloride 5 mg in a slow-release formulation.

Diphtheria and Tetanus Vaccine

A mixture of diphtheria formol toxoid and tetanus formol toxoid.

OTHER NAMES: Diphtheria-Tetanus Prophylactic; DT/Vac/FT

A standard is given in the British Pharmacopoeia 1973

Storage. It should be stored as described under Vaccines.

Actions and uses. Diphtheria and tetanus vaccine is especially useful for reinforcing doses for children at about 3 to 5 years of age or at school or nursery school entry who no longer require immunisation against pertussis. A suitable schedule for the immunisation of children is given under Vaccines.
The vaccine is administered by intramuscular or deep subcutaneous injection of 0.5 or 1 millilitre as stated on the label as the dose.

Diphtheria and Tetanus Vaccine, Adsorbed

Prepared from diphtheria formol toxoid containing no less than 1500 *flocculation equivalents* (1500 Lf) per mg of protein nitrogen, tetanus formol toxoid containing no ess than 500 *flocculation equivalents* (500 Lf) per mg of protein nitrogen, and a mineral carrier which may be aluminium hydroxide, aluminium phosphate, or calcium phosphate. It contains not more than 1.25 mg of Al or 1.3 mg of Ca in the recommended dose.

OTHER NAMES: Adsorbed Diphtheria-Tetanus Prophylactic; DT/Vac/Adsorbed; Vaccinum Diphthericum et Tetanicum Adsorbatum

The antigenic properties of this vaccine are adversely affected by exposure to the action of phenol or cresol; bactericides of this type are not added to the vacine.

A standard is given in the European Pharmacopoeia Vol. III Supplement

Storage. It should be stored as described under Vaccines. Under these conditions it may be expected to retain its potency for 3 years.

Actions and uses. Adsorbed diphtheria and tetanus vaccine is used for both the primary immunisation and reinforcing dose for children in the prophylaxis of diphtheria and tetanus. A suitable schedule for the immunisation of children is given under Vaccines.

The vaccine is administered by intramuscular or deep subcutaneous injection of 0.5 or 1 millilitre as stated on the label as the dose.

Diphtheria Antitoxin

A preparation containing antitoxic globulins that have the specific power of neutralising the toxin formed by *Corynebacterium diphtheriae* and rendering it harmless to susceptible animals.

OTHER NAMES: Dip/Ser; Immunoserum Antidiphthericum

A standard is given in the European Pharmacopoeia Vol. II

Storage. It should be stored as described under Antisera.

Actions and uses. Diphtheria antitoxin neutralises the toxin produced by *C. diphtheriae* locally at the site of infection, but does not affect the pathological changes already induced by the toxin. It can neutralise the toxin present in the circulation, but it is unlikely that it can neutralise that which is fixed in the tissues.

The dose of antitoxin varies according to the severity and stage of the disease, but not with the age of the patient; a child requires at least as large a dose as an adult. As mortality increases rapidly with delay in administering antitoxin, an adequate dose should be given as soon as the disease is diagnosed or suspected without waiting for the results of the culture.

When the attack is mild or of moderate severity, doses of 10 000 to 30 000 units should be given intramuscularly; doses of 40 000 to 100 000 units or even more should be given in severe cases.

Whenever a dose of more than 40 000 units is thought to be necessary, the intravenous route should be used; first a portion of the dose is given intramuscularly, followed half to two hours later by the bulk of the dose intravenously.

It should be appreciated that 24 hours after the intramuscular injection of a dose, the antitoxin titre in the patient's circulation is only about half that attained after the intravenous injection of the same amount. If at any time the amount of antitoxin given is considered to be inadequate, an additional dose should be administered intravenously.

The prophylactic dose is 500 to 2000 units, usually injected intramuscularly. The passive immunity thus conferred usually lasts about 2 weeks. Passive immunisation may be combined with active immunisation, as described under Diphtheria Vaccine.

Serum reactions. See under Antisera.

Diphtheria, Tetanus, and Pertussis Vaccine

A mixture of diphtheria formol toxoid, tetanus formol toxoid, and a suspension of killed *Bordetella pertussis*.

OTHER NAMES: Diphtheria-Tetanus-Whooping-cough Prophylactic; DTPer/Vac

A standard is given in the British Pharmacopoeia 1973

Storage. It should be stored as described under Vaccines.

Actions and uses. Diphtheria, tetanus, and pertussis vaccine is used for primary immunisation against diphtheria, tetanus, and whooping-cough. A suitable schedule for the immunisation of children is given under Vaccines.

The vaccine is administered by intramuscular or deep subcutaneous injection of 0.5 or 1 millilitre as stated on the label as the dose.

A reinforcing dose is desirable at school or nursery-school entry; as it is considered that the risk of whooping-cough is over by then, diphtheria and tetanus vaccine is generally used. Diphtheria and tetanus vaccine is also used when administration of pertussis vaccine is considered undesirable and in these cases, for primary immunisation, adsorbed diphtheria and tetanus vaccine is used.

Diphtheria, Tetanus, and Pertussis Vaccine, Adsorbed

Prepared from diphtheria formol toxoid, containing not less than 1500 *flocculation equivalents* (1500 Lf) per mg of protein nitrogen, tetanus toxoid containing not less than 500 *flocculation equivalents* (500 Lf) per mg of protein nitrogen, a suspension of killed *Bordetella pertussis* containing not more than 20×10^9 bacilli in each human dose, and a mineral carrier which may be aluminium hydroxide, aluminium phosphate, or calcium phosphate. It contains not more than 1.25 mg of Al or 1.3 mg of Ca in the recommended dose.

OTHER NAMES: Adsorbed Diphtheria-Tetanus-Whooping-cough Prophylactic; DTPer/Vac/Adsorbed; Vaccinum Diphthericum, Tetanicum, et Pertussis Adsorbatum

The antigenic properties of this vaccine are adversely affected by exposure to the action of phenol or cresol; bactericides of this type are not added to the vaccine.

A standard is given in the European Pharmacopoeia Vol. III Supplement

Storage. It should be stored as described under Vaccines. Under these conditions it may be expected to retain its potency for 2 years.

Actions and uses. Adsorbed diphtheria, tetanus, and pertussis vaccine is used for primary immunisation against diphtheria, tetanus, and whooping-cough in the same manner as diphtheria, tetanus, and pertussis vaccine (above).

The vaccine is administered by intramuscular or deep subcutaneous injection of 0.5 or 1 millilitres as stated on the label as the dose.

Diphtheria, Tetanus, and Poliomyelitis Vaccine

A mixture of diphtheria formol toxoid, tetanus formol toxoid, and poliomyelitis vaccine (inactivated).

OTHER NAME: DTPol/Vac

A standard is given in the British Pharmacopoeia 1973

Storage. It should be stored as described under Vaccines. Under these conditions it may be expected to retain its potency for 1 year.

Actions and uses. Diphtheria, tetanus, and poliomyelitis vaccine is used to reinforce the immunity of children who have previously been immunised against diphtheria, tetanus, and poliomyelitis, particularly at the time of school or nursery-school entry. A suitable schedule for the immunisation of children is given under Vaccines. The vaccine is administered by intramuscular or deep subcutaneous injection of the volume stated on the label as the dose.

Diphtheria, Tetanus, Pertussis, and Poliomyelitis Vaccine

A mixture of diphtheria formol toxoid, tetanus formol toxoid, a suspension of killed *Bordetella pertussis*, and poliomyelitis vaccine (inactivated).

OTHER NAMES: Diphtheria-Tetanus-Whooping-cough-Poliomyelitis Prophylactic; DTPerPol/Vac

A standard is given in the British Pharmacopoeia 1973

Storage. It should be stored as described under Vaccines. Under these conditions it may be expected to retain its potency for 1 year.

Actions and uses. Diphtheria, tetanus, pertussis, and poliomyelitis vaccine is used for the active immunisation of infants against diphtheria, tetanus, whooping-cough, and poliomyelitis. Primary immunisation should consist of 3 injections, the second following the first after an interval of 6 to 8 weeks, and the third following the second after an interval of 4 to 6 months; immunisation should be initiated at age 3 months and should be completed by the end of the first year of life.

The vaccine is administered by intramuscular or deep subcutaneous injection of 0.5 or 1 millilitre as stated on the label as the dose.

Diphtheria Vaccine

Prepared from diphtheria toxin produced by the growth of *Corynebacterium diphtheriae*. The toxin is converted to diphtheria formol toxoid by treatment with formaldehyde solution. It contains not less than 25 *flocculation equivalents* (25 Lf) in the recommended dose.

OTHER NAMES: Diphtheria Prophylactic; Dip/Vac/FT

A standard is given in the British Pharmacopoeia 1973

Storage. It should be stored as described under Vaccines.

Actions and uses. Diphtheria vaccines are used for active immunisation against diphtheria.

For primary immunisation of infants, the most commonly used preparation is diphtheria, tetanus, and pertussis vaccine. In this vaccine the pertussis component acts as an adjuvant for the diphtheria toxoid. Primary immunisation should consist of 3 injections, the second following the first after an interval of 6 to 8 weeks, and the third following the second after an interval of 4 to 6 months; immunisation should be initiated at age 3 months and should be completed by the end of the first year of life.

For the primary immunisation of children to whom the administration of pertussis vaccine is considered undesirable, adsorbed diphtheria and tetanus vaccine should be used. If primary vaccination against diphtheria only is required, adsorbed diphtheria vaccine must be used; diphtheria vaccine is no longer regarded as adequate for the primary immunisation of children.

At school entry a further reinforcing dose is recommended; for this purpose diphtheria vaccine, adsorbed diphtheria vaccine, or diphtheria, tetanus, and poliomyelitis vaccine may be used.

The vaccine is administered by intramuscular or deep subcutaneous injection using the volume stated on the label as the dose.

Some guide to the liability of patients to suffer undue reactions during immunisation is provided by the response to the control in the Schick test (see under Schick Test Toxin).

Diphtheria Vaccine, Adsorbed

Prepared from diphtheria formol toxoid containing not less than 1500 *flocculation equivalents* (1500 Lf) per mg of protein nitrogen and a mineral carrier which may be aluminium hydroxide, aluminium phosphate, or calcium phosphate. It contains not more than 1.25 mg of Al or 1.3 mg of Ca in the recommended dose.

OTHER NAMES: Adsorbed Diphtheria Prophylactic; Dip/Vac/Adsorbed; Vaccinum Diphthericum Adsorbatum

The antigenic properties of this vaccine are adversely affected by exposure to the action of phenol or cresol; bactericides of this type are not added to the vaccine.

A standard is given in the European Pharmacopoeia Vol. III Supplement

Storage. It should be stored as described under Vaccines. Under these conditions it may be expected to retain its potency for 3 years.

Actions and uses. Adsorbed diphtheria vaccine is used for active immunisation against diphtheria when simultaneous immunisation against tetanus or tetanus and pertussis is not required. Primary immunisation should consist of 3 injections, the second following the first after an interval of 6 to 8 weeks, and the third following the second after an interval of 4 to 6 months; immunisation should be initiated at age 3 months and should be completed by the end of the first year of life. When primary immunisation is required, adsorbed diphtheria vaccine is used. For the reinforcement of primary immunisation, diphtheria vaccine or adsorbed diphtheria vaccine is used.

The vaccine is administered by intramuscular or deep subcutaneous injection using the volume stated on the label as the dose.

Some guide to the liability of patients to suffer undue reactions during immunisation is provided by the response to the control in the Schick test.

Dipipanone Hydrochloride

1-(5-Oxo-4,4-diphenylhept-2-yl)piperidinium chloride monohydrate

$C_{24}H_{32}ClNO,H_2O = 404.0$

OTHER NAMES: Piperidyl Methadone Hydrochloride
Diconal® (with cyclizine hydrochloride)

A standard is given in the British Pharmacopoeia 1973

Description. An almost odourless, white, crystalline powder with a bitter taste followed by a sensation of numbness and burning.

Solubility. Soluble, at 20°, in 40 parts of water, in 1.5 parts of alcohol, and in 6 parts of acetone; practically insoluble in ether.

Acidity. A 2.5% solution has a pH of 4 to 6.

Moisture content. 4 to 5%, determined by Fischer titration.

Dissociation constant. pK_a 8.5 (25°).

Sterilisation. Solutions for injection are sterilised by heating in an autoclave or by filtration.

Identification. TESTS. 1. Dissolve about 200 mg in 10 ml of water and add 1 ml of *potassium mercuri-iodide solution*; a white precipitate is produced.
2. Dissolve about 100 mg in 10 ml of water, add 10 ml of a 1% solution of trinitrophenol and 1 drop of hydrochloric acid, and shake vigorously; a precipitate is produced which, after recrystallisation from alcohol (70%) and drying at 105°, melts at about 141°.

MELTING-POINT. About 125°.

Metabolism. ABSORPTION. Absorbed after oral administration.

METABOLIC REACTIONS. Metabolised in the liver.

EXCRETION. Excreted in the urine and faeces.

Actions and uses. Dipipanone has a strong analgesic action which begins about 15 minutes after an intramuscular injection and persists for 4 to 6 hours.
Dipipanone, like methadone, has relatively little sedative and hypnotic action. It can be used to maintain relief of pain when morphine or pethidine has ceased to be effective, the usual dosage being 25 milligrams of dipipanone hydrochloride, repeated every 6 hours if necessary, by subcutaneous or intramuscular injection.
Dipipanone is also used in conjunction with cyclizine hydrochloride. The usual dose by mouth is 10 milligrams gradually increased to 30 milligrams in conjunction with 3 times its weight of cyclizine hydrochloride as an anti-emetic.

Undesirable effects. Nausea and vomiting may occur.

Precautions. Dipipanone should not be given intravenously as it may produce an alarming fall in blood pressure. Undue respiratory depression may be relieved by giving 5 to 10 milligrams of nalorphine hydrobromide intravenously.
In the presence of severe liver or kidney damage the action of dipipanone may be prolonged and it should be used with special caution in such cases.

Dependence. Prolonged administration of therapeutic doses may lead to the development of dependence of the morphine type, as described under Drug Dependence.

Preparations

DIPIPANONE INJECTION: a sterile solution of dipipanone hydrochloride in water for injections. The acidity of the solution is adjusted to pH 4.5 by the addition of hydrochloric acid. The solution is sterilised by heating in an autoclave or by filtration.
A standard for this injection is given in the British Pharmacopoeia 1973
Containers and *Labelling:* see the entry on Injections for general information on containers and labelling.
Storage: it should be protected from light.

OTHER PREPARATIONS available include TABLETS containing dipipanone hydrochloride 10 mg with cyclizine hydrochloride 30 mg.

Diprenorphine Hydrochloride

N-Cyclopropylmethyl-7,8-dihydro-7α-(1-hydroxy-1-methylethyl)-O^6-methyl-6α,14α-ethanonormorphine hydrochloride

$C_{26}H_{36}ClNO_4 = 462.0$

OTHER NAME: *Revivon*®

A standard is given in the British Pharmacopoeia (Veterinary)

Description. A white crystalline powder.

Solubility. Soluble, at 20°, in 30 parts of water, in 160 parts of alcohol (95%), and in 2500 parts of chloroform; practically insoluble in ether.

Acidity. A 2% solution has a pH of 4.5 to 6.

Moisture content. Not more than 2%, determined by drying at 105°.

Specific rotation. −97° to −107°, determined on a 2% solution in methyl alcohol.

Sterilisation. Solutions for injection are sterilised by heating in an autoclave or by filtration.

Storage. It should be stored in airtight containers, protected from light.

Identification. ULTRAVIOLET ABSORPTION. In 0.1N hydrochloric acid, maximum at 287 nm (E1%, 1cm = 35); in 0.1N sodium hydroxide, maximum at 301 nm (E1%, 1cm = 55).

Veterinary uses. Diprenorphine hydrochloride is a narcotic antagonist which is used to reverse the action of etorphine.
The dose administered by intravenous injection is approximately 30 to 300 micrograms per kilogram body-weight determined in accordance with the response of

the animal and is usually about 1.2 milligrams of diprenorphine for each milligram of etorphine hydrochloride for large animals or 4 milligrams of diprenorphine for each milligram of etorphine hydrochloride for small animals.

Preparation

DIPRENORPHINE INJECTION: a sterile solution of diprenorphine hydrochloride, with methylene blue and chlorocresol, in water for injections. The acidity of the solution is adjusted to pH 4. The solution is sterilised by heating in an autoclave or by filtration.

Available in 20-ml vials containing diprenorphine hydrochloride equivalent to 272 micrograms of diprenorphine per ml with 0.001% of methylene blue and 0.1% of chlorocresol and in 10-ml vials containing diprenorphine hydrochloride equivalent to 3 mg of diprenorphine per ml with 0.001% of methylene blue and 0.1% of chlorocresol.

A standard for this injection is given in the British Pharmacopoeia (Veterinary)

Containers: see the entry on Injections for general information on containers.

Labelling: see the entry on Injections for general information on labelling. In addition, the label on the container should state the amount of the medicament as the equivalent amount of diprenorphine in a suitable dose-volume.

Storage: it should be protected from light.

Dipyridamole

2,6-Bis[bis(2-hydroxyethyl)amino]-4,8-dipiperidinopyrimido[5,4-*d*]pyrimidine

$C_{24}H_{40}N_8O_4 = 504.6$

OTHER NAME: *Persantin*®

Description. An odourless, intensely yellow, crystalline powder with a bitter taste. Solutions have a yellowish-blue fluorescence.

Solubility. Very slightly soluble in water; soluble in chloroform and in methyl alcohol; practically insoluble in ether and in light petroleum; soluble in dilute mineral acids.

Identification. MELTING-POINT. About 163°.

ULTRAVIOLET ABSORPTION. In 0.1N sulphuric acid, maxima at 236 nm (E1%, 1cm = 520) and 282 nm (E1%, 1cm = 533).

INFRA-RED ABSORPTION. Major peaks at 1010, 1214, 1354, 1436, 1464, and 1526 cm^{-1} (see Appendix 2a: Infrared Spectra).

Metabolism. ABSORPTION. Readily absorbed after oral administration.

BLOOD CONCENTRATION. After a single oral dose of 50 mg, peak serum concentrations are attained in about 1.5 hours; after oral doses of 200 mg rising to 400 mg daily by day 3, peak concentrations after the morning dose on day 4 are about 1.2 mg/litre at 1.5 hours.

METABOLIC REACTIONS. Glucuronic acid conjugation.

EXCRETION. Excreted mainly in the faeces; small amounts are excreted as the glucuronide.

FURTHER INFORMATION. Blood concentration—S. M. Rajah *et al.*, *Br. J. clin. Pharmac.*, 1977, **4**, 129.

Actions and uses. Dipyridamole is a coronary vasodilator and reduces platelet adhesiveness by inhibiting adenosine diphosphate induced platelet aggregation. It is used in the treatment of coronary insufficiency and to prevent thrombosis and emboli in patients who have had prosthetic valve surgery.

The usual dose by mouth for adults is 50 milligrams 3 times daily, taken before food; alternatively, 10 to 20 milligrams may be given by slow intravenous injection 2 or 3 times daily.

Undesirable effects. Gastro-intestinal disturbances, headache, faintness and dizziness may occur. The administration of dipyridamole, especially by injection, may cause a reduction in blood pressure, particularly in hypertensive patients.

Contra-indications. Dipyridamole should not be given by injection to patients with myocardial infarction when shock or hypotension is also present.

Preparations

Preparations available include an INJECTION containing dipyridamole 5 mg per ml in 2-ml ampoules and TABLETS containing dipyridamole 25 and 100 mg.

Disodium Edetate

Disodium dihydrogen ethylenediamine-*NNN'N'*-tetraacetate dihydrate

$C_{10}H_{14}N_2Na_2O_8,2H_2O = 372.2$

OTHER NAMES: Disodium Edathamil; Edetate Disodium; *Limclair*®; *Sequestrene NA2*®

A standard is given in the British Pharmacopoeia 1973

Description. A white crystalline odourless powder with a slightly acid taste.

Solubility. Soluble, at 20°, in 11 parts of water; very slightly soluble in alcohol; practically insoluble in ether and in chloroform.

Acidity. A 5% solution has a pH of 4 to 5.5.

Sterilisation. Strong solutions, prepared with the aid of sodium hydroxide to give the trisodium salt, are sterilised by heating in an autoclave.

Actions and uses. Disodium edetate is a chelating substance which has a strong affinity for divalent and tervalent metals. It is poorly absorbed after oral administration and is usually administered by intravenous injection.

It is used as a decalcifying agent in the treatment of hypercalcaemia, as the calcium ion loses its physiological properties when firmly bound in a chelate ring; the complex thus formed is not metabolised in the body and is rapidly excreted by the kidneys.

The usual daily dosage for an adult is up to 70 milligrams per kilogram body-weight and for a child up to 60 milligrams per kilogram body-weight, given as trisodium edetate injection, diluted to about 500 millilitres with sodium chloride injection or dextrose injection (5%), by slow intravenous injection over a period of 2 to 3 hours; 1 gram of disodium edetate (dihydrate) is approximately equivalent to 1 gram of trisodium edetate. Rapid injection may cause a dangerous fall in the serum-calcium level, leading to convulsions and cardiac arrest, and will also damage the vein used for the injection. Treatment is usually given for 5 days, followed by 2 days' rest; the course may be repeated as often as necessary.

Disodium edetate is used for the removal of calcium deposits from lime burns of the eye, a suitable strength of solution being 0.38% with 0.1% of sodium bicarbonate.

For the inactivation of bacterial collagenase as an adjunct to antibiotic treatment of keratopathy caused by *Pseudomonas aeruginosa*, eye-drops containing 0.38% buffered to pH 7.0 may be used.

Damage to the cornea resulting from the presence of epithelial collagenase may be treated with eye-drops containing 1.9 or 3.8% buffered to pH 7.0. A suitable buffer consists of sodium acid phosphate 0.42% and sodium phosphate 1.43%; benzalkonium chloride is a suitable preservative.

Disodium edetate is also used as an antioxidant synergist in aqueous preparations. It acts by removing traces of heavy metals which often catalyse autoxidation reactions; a concentration of 0.01 to 0.05% is usually effective in enhancing stability.

Undesirable effects. Overdosage may lead to renal damage and haemorrhagic manifestations.

Milder undesirable effects such as nausea, diarrhoea, and cramp occur occasionally and reactions on the skin and mucous membranes have been reported; these symptoms subside when treatment is stopped.

Precautions. During treatment, the serum-calcium level should be checked repeatedly; if signs of tetany occur the infusion rate should be reduced or treatment discontinued and, if necessary, a solution of a calcium salt should be injected.

Preparation

TRISODIUM EDETATE INJECTION:

Disodium edetate	20.8 g
Sodium hydroxide..	2.5 g
	or a sufficient quantity
Water for injections	to 100 ml

Suspend the disodium edetate in about 80 ml of the water; prepare an approximately 10% solution of sodium hydroxide in water for injections and add to the suspension, with continuous stirring, until a pH of 7.4 is obtained; add sufficient of the water to produce the required volume, and filter. Distribute the solution into ampoules and sterilise by heating in an autoclave. Trisodium edetate injection contains, in 1 ml, the equivalent of 200 mg of trisodium edetate. Available as an injection in ampoules of 5 ml.

A standard for this injection is given in the British Pharmacopoeia 1973
Containers: see the entry on Injections for general information on containers. They should be made from lead-free glass.
Labelling: see the entry on Injections for general information on labelling. In addition the label on the container should state the amount of the medicament as the equivalent amount of trisodium edetate in a suitable dose-volume, and that the injection should be diluted with sodium chloride injection or dextrose injection before administration.

Dissociation Constants

Most medicinal substances are either weak acids or weak bases and, in aqueous solution, are only partially dissociated. The extent of this dissociation is one of a number of important parameters which affect the absorption, distribution, and metabolism of the drug in the body (see Metabolism of Drugs). In order to obtain a quantitative measure of the extent of this dissociation at a particular temperature the *dissociation constant* is determined—the terms "ionisation constant" and "acidity constant" have also been used to describe this parameter.

For a weak acid dissolved in water, the dissociation is expressed as the equilibrium

$$HA + H_2O \rightleftharpoons H_3O^+ + A^-$$

Similarly, for a weak base dissolved in water, the dissociation is expressed by the equilibrium

$$B + H_2O \rightleftharpoons BH^+ + OH^-$$

However, in order that a base may be treated in a similar way to an acid, advantage is taken of the amphiprotic character of water which undergoes self-ionisation, and the dissociation of a weak base may then be expressed by the equilibrium

$$BH^+ + H_2O \rightleftharpoons H_3O^+ + B$$

This method of expression makes it possible to discuss base strengths in terms of the strength of the conjugate acid and thus express the dissociation of acids and bases on the same scale, just as pH is used for both acidity and alkalinity.

The strength of an acid is governed by its tendency to yield protons, and the quantitative measure of this in water at a particular temperature is given by the expression

$$K_a = \frac{a_{H_3O^+} \cdot a_{A^-}}{a_{HA}}$$

where K_a = the thermodynamic dissociation constant, and $a_{H_3O^+}$, a_{A^-}, and a_{HA} are the thermodynamic activities of the hydrated proton, anion, and undissociated acid respectively.

Similarly, the strength of a base is given by the expression

$$K_a = \frac{a_{H_3O^+} \cdot a_B}{a_{BH^+}}$$

Thermodynamic activities are used in order to allow for the departure from ideality of real solutions, and the thermodynamic dissociation constant is independent of the concentration. If concentrations are used in the above expressions instead of thermodynamic activities, the resulting dissociation constant, sometimes known as the *apparent dissociation constant*, is dependent on the concentration. This figure will differ from the thermodynamic dissociation constant but, for dilute solutions, the difference is small and for many purposes the apparent dissociation constant is an adequate parameter to use in comparative studies on drugs. At infinite dilution the two constants are equal.

pK$_a$ Values

The pK$_a$ value of a drug is the negative logarithm (base 10) of the dissociation constant, i.e. $-\log K_a = pK_a$. Since $-\log a_{H_3O^+} = pH$, by taking logarithms of the expression given above for the thermodynamic dissociation constant of a weak acid in aqueous solution, the following relationship is obtained:

$$pK_a = pH + \log \frac{a_{HA}}{a_{A^-}}$$

and for a weak base:

$$pK_a = pH + \log \frac{a_{BH^+}}{a_B}$$

In both of these relationships, the activity "a" is substituted by the concentration (molality "m") if the apparent dissociation constant is to be determined.

Thus the determination of a pK$_a$ value requires the measurement of the pH and the ratio of the activities (or of the concentrations) of the dissociated and undissociated species present at a particular temperature. This ratio depends only on the pK$_a$ and the pH. If the pH of the aqueous solution is controlled by a buffer, the ratio will vary only with the pK$_a$, that is, with the nature of the acid or base being examined. This applies regardless of whether or not the acid or base has previously been neutralised because salts of weak acids or bases are hydrolysed partly in solution to the parent acids or bases.

Values for pK$_a$ are usually quoted for bases, a practice which has largely superseded the earlier custom of using the dissociation constant K$_b$ and the corresponding pK$_b$. Values of pK$_b$ can be converted to pK$_a$ by the use of the relationship pK$_a$ + pK$_b$ = pK$_w$, where pK$_w$ is the negative logarithm of the ion product of water at the temperature used. For normal purposes this figure can be taken as 14.

Percentage Ionisation

The percentage of an acid or base which is non-ionised depends on the pH and the pK$_a$. As it is only the non-ionised species of drugs which penetrate lipid membranes with any facility (by passive diffusion) it is useful to know the percentage ionisation for a given drug (i.e. for a given pK$_a$ value) at a given pH.

For an acid, percentage $A^- = \dfrac{100}{1 + \text{antilog}(pK_a - pH)}$

For a base, percentage $BH^+ = \dfrac{100}{1 + \text{antilog}(pH - pK_a)}$

The percentage ionisation is extremely sensitive to pH changes, particularly when the pH lies close to the pK$_a$ (see Table).

PERCENTAGE IONISATION

pK$_a$−pH	Percentage Cationic Ionisation	Percentage Anionic Ionisation
+3	99.90	0.0999
+2	99.01	0.990
+1	90.91	9.09
+0.5	75.97	24.03
+0.2	61.32	38.68
0	50	50
−0.2	38.68	61.32
−0.5	24.03	75.97
−1	9.09	90.91
−2	0.990	99.01
−3	0.0999	99.90

Measurement of Dissociation Constants

The three most important methods for the measurement of dissociation constants are the potentiometric, spectrophotometric, and conductimetric methods. Of these, the conductimetric method is normally used only in specialist hands and the potentiometric and spectrophotometric methods are the methods of choice. A number of other methods have been used in special cases, usually when there is some intractable difficulty associated with the use of the above methods.

Potentiometric method. (*i*) *e.m.f. measurements:* e.m.f. measurements may be used to determine the exact thermodynamic dissociation constant.

For an acid (HA), the measurements are made in a cell of the type:

Pt H$_2$(g) $\vdots$ HA(aq)(m_1), KA(aq)(m_2), KCl(aq)(m_3) $\vdots$ AgCl(s) Ag

where m_1, m_2, and m_3 are the stoicheiometric molalities. By means of suitable equations, values of apparent dissociation constant can be determined and extrapolated to zero ionic strength to give the thermodynamic dissociation constant.

An analogous procedure is used for a cationic acid BH$^+$, but in a cell of the type:

Pt H$_2$(g) $\vdots$ BH$^+$Cl$^-$(aq)(m_1), B(aq)(m_2) $\vdots$ AgCl(s) Ag

(*ii*) *pH measurements:* the apparent dissociation of a substance can be determined by the measurement of the pH of a partially neutralised solution of the substance. This follows from the relationship, for example, for a weak acid:

$$pK_a = pH + \log \frac{m_{HA}}{m_{A^-}}$$

The procedure requires the titration of the substance being examined by a strong base (or in the case of a weak base, by a strong acid). After the addition of each increment of titrant, the pH is measured by a potentiometric pH-measuring device incorporating a glass electrode and a reference electrode, which is frequently a calomel electrode. The ratio of the molalities is calculated from the stoicheiometry of the system after the addition of each increment.

The titrant acid or base is generally at least ten times as concentrated as the compound being titrated and carbon dioxide-free nitrogen is bubbled through the solution in order to avoid reaction with the atmosphere. An automatic titrimeter can be used to record, rapidly and accurately, a titration curve in which pH is plotted against volume of titrant. The minimum volume of solution that can be titrated depends mainly on the size of the electrode system and specially designed apparatus can be used for automatic titrimetry on the micro-scale.

At least nine increments of titrant should be added from which nine pK$_a$ values are calculated, so that the observed scatter will give an indication of the precision of the results. It is evident from the relationship, above, that the pK$_a$ is equal to the pH at half-neutralisation (when $m_{HA} = m_{A^-}$). This value can be readily obtained from a titration curve and this is a useful method if an approximate pK$_a$ value is required.

The determination of pK$_a$ by the measurement of pH has the advantage that the exact concentration of the compound being titrated need not be known because it can be calculated from the end-point of the titration.

Values of apparent pK$_a$ determined in this way can have activity corrections applied, if necessary, and this is desirable when concentrations exceed 0.01M.

Spectrophotometric method. If either or both of the dissociated and undissociated species of the substance absorb in the ultraviolet region, and if the spectrum of each form is different, then this property may be used to measure the ratio of the concentrations. If the pH is also measured, then the pK_a may be calculated from the relationships given above under "pK_a Values". The spectrophotometric method is slower and less convenient than the potentiometric titration procedure but it is valuable for compounds whose pK_a values are less than 2 or more than 11 (for which other methods are unsuitable) and in cases where the solubility of the compound is too low for potentiometry.

The compound is dissolved, at equal concentrations, in a series of non-absorbing buffer solutions and the pH of each solution is measured potentiometrically. The two pH values at the extreme ends of the range must be such that the compound exists either wholly in the undissociated form or wholly in the dissociated form. At the intermediate values of pH there will be a mixture of the two forms. It can be seen from the foregoing table of percentage ionisation that the two extreme pH values must lie not less than 2 pH units away from the pK_a value of the compound, when there will be at least 99% of either the dissociated or the undissociated form. The buffer solutions which are used must be virtually transparent at the wavelength used for the measurements and must be capable of being prepared at low ionic strength.

The absorbance of each solution is measured at a wavelength chosen so that there is the greatest difference in absorbance between the dissociated and undissociated forms; the temperature of the solutions is standardised and the measurements are made against an equivalent buffer solution in the reference cell.

A pK_a value for a weak acid can now be calculated from the data obtained for each of the intermediate members of the series of solutions by the use of the relationship:

$$pK_a = pH + \log \frac{E_d - E_{obs}}{E_{obs} - E_n}$$

Similarly, for a weak base:

$$pK_a = pH + \log \frac{E_{obs} - E_n}{E_d - E_{obs}}$$

where,

E_d = extinction of the totally ionised form,
E_n = extinction of the totally non-ionised form,
E_{obs} = extinction of the intermediate buffered solution

It is recommended that measurements are made on seven intermediate solutions, giving seven pK_a values, from which the degree of precision may be ascertained. The pK_a values determined by this method are *apparent* pK_a values in spite of the low concentrations used. This is because of the presence of buffer salts and the measurement of the pH of the solutions by a potentiometric method.

Conductimetric method. The conductimetric method is the classical method of determining dissociation constants of acids but it has been largely displaced by the potentiometric and spectrophotometric methods. The degree of dissociation of an acid is given by the ratio of the molar conductances at a given concentration to the molar conductance at infinite dilution, and hence

$$K_a = \frac{\alpha^2 c}{1 - \alpha}$$

where α is the degree of dissociation at concentration c. Molar conductances of solutions of different concen-

trations are measured in a conductivity cell with platinised electrodes at a carefully controlled temperature. The value of the molar conductance at infinite dilution cannot be determined directly, since the ionisation of water interferes. However, it is calculated from measurements of the conductivity of solutions of the sodium salt of the weak acid.

The use of the conductimetric method is generally restricted to acids with pK_a values below 6 but its advantage is that it can be used at concentrations as low as 10^{-5}M.

Other methods. If the acid is very strong ($K_a > 10^{-1}$) it is necessary to use high concentrations to achieve a suitable ratio of dissociated to undissociated molecule. The usual spectrophotometric procedures are unsuitable at high concentrations but if the acid has a suitable *Raman spectrum* the dissociation constant can be determined.

Nuclear magnetic resonance spectra can also be used to determine the dissociation constants of very weak acids or bases by plotting the chemical shift of a non-exchanging proton, near to the ionising group, against pH for a series of solutions.

Solubility measurements can be used to determine dissociation constants by comparing the total solubility of the dissociated and undissociated forms with the solubility in solutions which are sufficiently acid to repress ionisation. This method is particularly suited to compounds whose solubilities are too low for the potentiometric method to be used.

The measurement of the *partition* of a substance between two phases can also be used.

FURTHER INFORMATION. *The Determination of Ionisation Constants*, 2nd Edn, A. Albert and E. P. Serjeant, London, Chapman and Hall, 1971.

Evaluation of Dissociation Constants

A very large number of dissociation constants have been reported in the literature and these have been determined by a variety of methods and for a variety of purposes. It is, therefore, difficult to assess the reliability of reported figures. However, it is important to consider both the degree of accuracy required for the purpose which the user has in mind, and the degree of accuracy of the reported figure.

1. In the biological sciences, where pK_a values may be used to correlate with some property of a complex living system, very accurate values may not be required. However, if a pK_a value is used to determine the percentages of dissociated and undissociated species in a buffered solution such as a biological fluid, then small changes in the quantity "$pH - pK_a$" produce large changes in the percentage when "$pH - pK_a$" is small. In such cases a greater accuracy may be required.

2. Apparent dissociation constants are usually quoted to one decimal place; thermodynamic dissociation constants are usually quoted to more than one decimal place. Accurate values should be reported with a numerical estimate of both accuracy and precision; where no such estimate is given, values should be treated with caution.

3. The chemical and physical properties of the compound will dictate the method of determination. The simple potentiometric titration procedure is best suited to compounds having sufficient solubility and with pK_a values between 5 and 9. If the values are below 5 or above 9, then hydrogen ion or hydroxyl ion concentrations should be allowed for in the calculations. If the result is recorded as one value calculated at half-neutralisation, than the accuracy of the figure is doubtful.

If the spectrophotometric method is used, there must be

a suitable difference in absorbance between the dissociated and undissociated forms. It should be established that there is no danger of decomposition of the compound in acidic or alkaline solutions.

Conductimetric determinations are likely to suffer from contamination with carbon dioxide from the atmosphere.

Special methods must be used for compounds with pK_a values below 2 or above 11, and these values must be treated with reserve.

4. Ideally, all determinations should be carried out in aqueous solution. Some figures have been reported in other solvents, notably aqueous alcohol, and these figures vary considerably from those determined in water. For instance, acetic acid has a pK_a, at 25°, of 4.76 in water and 5.84 in alcohol (50%), and the anilinium ion has a pK_a, at 25°, of 4.64 in water and 3.92 in alcohol (50%).

5. Dissociation constants vary with temperature. Determinations are usually carried out at 25°, but solubility characteristics or other factors may require the use of other temperatures.

6. The concentration at which the constant is determined should be noted, although for concentrations below 0.01M, corrections for concentration are negligible.

7. If a compound has more than one acidic group or more than one basic group, special calculation procedures may be needed. In the common case of a diacidic base or a dibasic acid, ordinary methods may be used to calculate pK_{a_1} and pK_{a_2} provided that they differ by more than 2.7. If the values differ by less than 2.7, the compound is said to have overlapping pK_a values and special calculations are needed. The method of calculation for reported figures of this type should be studied. If a compound is amphoteric and has both an acidic and a basic group, pK_{a_1} and pK_{a_2} will have the normal values for the groups. However, if an internal salt is formed (zwitterion), when the acidic pK_a is lower than the basic pK_a, the values may be different from those of the simple analogues because of mutual interaction between the ionising groups.

Note. Because of the number of methods that can be used for the determination of dissociation constants, there are often wide differences in the figures given in the scientific literature. The figures given for pK_a values of medicinal substances in this volume have been taken from published data and should be regarded only as approximate.

Disulfiram

Tetraethylthiuram disulphide

$$(C_2H_5)_2 \cdot N \cdot \overset{\overset{\displaystyle S}{\|}}{C} \cdot S \cdot S \cdot \overset{\overset{\displaystyle S}{\|}}{C} \cdot N(C_2H_5)_2$$

$C_{10}H_{20}N_2S_4 = 296.5$

OTHER NAME: *Antabuse*®

A standard is given in the British Pharmacopoeia Addendum 1978

Description. An odourless white powder.

Solubility. Practically insoluble in water; soluble, at 20°, in 65 parts of alcohol, in 20 parts of ether, and in 2 parts of chloroform.

Storage. It should be stored in airtight containers, protected from light.

Identification. TEST. Dissolve about 5 mg in 5 ml of alcohol (95%) and add 1 ml of a 10% solution of potassium cyanide; a yellow colour is produced which changes to green and finally to bluish-green.

MELTING-POINT. About 71°.

INFRA-RED ABSORPTION. Major peaks at 917, 962, 1149, 1190, 1266, and 1515 cm^{-1} (see Appendix 2b: Infra-red Spectra).

Determination in body fluids. COLORIMETRY. In blood or urine—S. L. Tompsett, *Acta pharmac. tox.*, 1964, **21**, 20; in blood, serum, or urine: disulfiram and its metabolites—A. M. Sauter *et al.*, *Arzneimittel-Forsch.*, 1976, **26**, 173.

THIN-LAYER CHROMATOGRAPHY. In urine: detection of the metabolite diethylamine—D. H. Neiderhiser *et al.*, *J. Chromat.*, 1976, **117**, 187.

GAS CHROMATOGRAPHY. In expired air: detection of the metabolite carbon disulphide—J. Wells and E. Koves, *J. Chromat.*, 1974, **92**, 442; in blood—A. M. Sauter and J. P. von Wartburg, *J. Chromat.*, 1977, **133**, 167.

Metabolism. ABSORPTION. Incompletely absorbed after oral administration.

BLOOD CONCENTRATION. After a dose of 200 mg, peak blood concentrations of about 4.5 μg/ml are attained in 12 hours.

EXCRETION. 20% of a dose is excreted unchanged in the faeces and the remainder is slowly excreted as metabolites in the urine; excreted in the lungs as carbon disulphide.

FURTHER INFORMATION. Blood concentrations—M. W. Brown *et al.*, *J. Pharm. Pharmac.*, 1974, **26**, 95P.

Actions and uses. Disulfiram is used as an adjunctive treatment in patients with chronic alcoholism but is only of value in patients who are willing to co-operate.

Disulfiram interferes with the oxidation of alcohol, causing acetaldehyde to accumulate in the body. This evokes an unpleasant reaction as early as 10 minutes after ingestion of alcohol. The reaction includes flushing of the face, throbbing headache, dyspnoea, palpitations, tachycardia, nausea, and vomiting. With large doses of alcohol cardiac arrhythmias, hypotension, and collapse may also occur.

In a typical regimen, the patient is warned not to take any alcohol and is given 800 milligrams of disulfiram on the first day of treatment, 600 milligrams on the second day, 400 milligrams on the third day, 200 milligrams on the fourth and fifth days, and 200 reducing to 100 milligrams thereafter. Treatment may be continued for up to 12 months. On the fifth day of treatment, the patient may be given a challenge dose of 10 to 15 millilitres of alcohol (95%) to evoke a reaction in order to demonstrate its effects to the patient.

Undesirable effects. Drowsiness, fatigue, nausea, constipation, reduced libido, allergic dermatitis, and peripheral neuritis may occur. Psychotic reactions including depressive psychosis, paranoia, schizophrenia, and mania occur rarely.

Precautions. Disulfiram should be administered with caution to patients with renal, hepatic, or respiratory disease, diabetes mellitus, and epilepsy.

Contra-indications. Disulfiram should not be given to patients with cardiac failure, coronary artery disease, and psychotic illness or to patients who are pregnant or addicted to narcotic drugs.

Drug interactions. Disulfiram potentiates the action of

paraldehyde and barbiturates. Caution should be exercised in administering disulfiram in conjunction with any drugs that affect the central nervous system. When given in conjunction with metronidazole acute psychoses and confusional states may occur.

Preparation

DISULFIRAM TABLETS: available as tablets containing 200 mg of disulfiram.
A standard for these tablets is given in the British Pharmacopoeia Addendum 1978
Containers and Storage: see the entry on Tablets for general information on containers and storage. Containers should be airtight and light resistant.
Advice for patients: during treatment, and for 7 days thereafter, foods, medicines, toilet preparations, or any other products containing alcohol must not be used. Patients may carry an identification card giving details of their treatment, to be shown when medical or dental treatment is required.

Dithranol

Anthracene-1,8,9-triol

$C_{14}H_{10}O_3 = 226.2$

OTHER NAMES: Anthralin; Dioxyanthranol; *Dithrocream®*; *Psoradrate®*
Dithrolan® and *Stie-Lasan®* (both with salicylic acid)

A standard is given in the British Pharmacopoeia 1973

CAUTION. *Dithranol is a powerful irritant and should be kept away from the eyes and tender parts of the skin.*

Description. A yellow odourless tasteless powder.

Solubility. Practically insoluble in water; very slightly soluble in alcohol and in ether; soluble in chloroform, in acetone, and in fixed oils.

Moisture content. Not more than 1%, determined by drying at 105°.

Storage. It should be stored in airtight containers, protected from light.

Identification. TEST. Dissolve about 5 mg in 5 ml of 1N sodium hydroxide; a clear fluorescent yellow or orange solution is formed which turns red on exposure to air (distinction from 1,2-dihydroxyanthranol).

MELTING-POINT. About 178°.

ULTRAVIOLET ABSORPTION. In chloroform, maximum at 354 nm (E1%, 1cm = 440).

Actions and uses. Dithranol is used, in a concentration of 0.01 to 1%, in external preparations for the treatment of psoriasis. It also has fungicidal properties and is used for the treatment of ringworm infections and other chronic dermatoses.

Precautions. As some patients are intolerant of the usual concentrations of dithranol, a preliminary test for sensitivity should be carried out with the ointment to guard against an excessive reaction.

Preparations

DITHRANOL OINTMENT (*Syn.* Ung. Dithranol.): prepared by triturating dithranol, in fine powder, with yellow soft paraffin, adding sufficient yellow soft paraffin to produce an ointment of the required strength, and mixing thoroughly. If a more viscous preparation is required, a suitable proportion of hard paraffin may be incorporated in the yellow soft paraffin by melting together at a low temperature and stirring until cold.
A standard for this ointment is given in the British Pharmacopoeia 1973
Containers and Labelling: see the entry on Ointments for general information on containers and labelling. The ointment should be protected from light.
Advice for patients: the ointment should be applied carefully to the lesions; a dressing may be applied. Contact with normal skin should be avoided and it should not be applied to inflamed or broken skin or near the eyes or mucous membranes. The hands should be washed thoroughly after use. The ointment will cause redness and staining of the skin and discolour clothing and fair hair.

DITHRANOL PASTE: consisting of a dispersion containing up to 1% of dithranol in zinc and salicylic acid paste. It is prepared by mixing the dithranol thoroughly with a portion of the zinc and salicylic acid paste until smooth and then gradually incorporating the remainder of the paste.
When Weak Dithranol Paste is ordered or prescribed, a paste containing 0.1% of dithranol is supplied. When Strong Dithranol Paste is ordered or prescribed, a paste containing 1% of dithranol is supplied.
A standard for this paste is given in the British Pharmaceutical Codex 1973
Containers and Storage: see the entry on Pastes for general information on containers and storage. The paste should be protected from light.
Advice for patients: the paste should be applied liberally and carefully to the lesions with a suitable applicator; a dressing may be applied. Contact with normal skin should be avoided and it should not be applied to inflamed or broken skin or near to the eyes or mucous membranes. The hands should be washed thoroughly after use. The paste will cause redness and staining of the skin and discolour clothing and fair hair.

OTHER PREPARATIONS available include a CREAM containing dithranol 0.1%, a cream containing dithranol 0.25%, an OINTMENT containing dithranol 0.4% with salicylic acid 0.4% and an ointment containing dithranol 0.5% with salicylic acid 0.5%.

Diuretics

Diuretics increase the rate of formation of urine by the kidney and so hasten the elimination of water from the body.

Mechanism of action. Diuretics act by increasing the rate of glomerular filtration or by inhibiting tubular resorption. Xanthines increase renal blood flow which leads to an increase in the glomerular filtration rate. Other diuretics inhibit resorption from the tubule. They include the thiazides (acting mainly on the proximal part of the distal tubule), bumetanide, ethacrynic acid, and frusemide (loop diuretics), acting mainly on the loop of Henle, and various potassium-sparing diuretics such as amiloride and triamterene that act mainly on the distal part of the distal tubule. The carbonic anhydrase inhibitor acetazolamide and the aldosterone antagonist spironolactone also reduce resorption from the tubules. Osmotic diuretics increase the osmotic pressure of the glomerular filtrate and thereby decrease its resorption from the tubule.

With many diuretics more than one mechanism may be involved; for example, chlorothiazide, which may inhibit sodium resorption in the proximal part of the distal tubule, also has minor inhibitory activity on carbonic anhydrase.

Thiazide diuretics act mainly by inhibiting resorption from the proximal part of the distal tubule. They cause a moderate diuresis and loss of potassium ions. The action is described in more detail under Chlorothiazide. Thiazide diuretics are derived from 1,2,4-thiadiazine 1,1-dioxide. They include bendrofluazide, chlorothiazide, cyclopenthiazide, hydrochlorothiazide, and hydroflumethiazide. A number of diuretics bearing some chemical resemblance to the thiazides are also available. They act in a similar way but some, such as chlorthalidone, have a more prolonged action.

Loop diuretics act mainly by inhibiting resorption from the tubule, including the ascending loop of Henle. They cause a rapid intense diuresis and may sometimes be effective when thiazides are not. They cause loss of potassium ions. They include bumetanide, ethacrynic acid, and frusemide.

Mercurial diuretics act by inhibiting resorption in the renal tubules and they do not cause marked loss of potassium ions. They may give rise to alkalosis which limits their action and is reduced by preliminary administration of an acidifying agent such as ammonium chloride. As mercurial diuretics must be given by injection, they have been largely replaced by thiazides except in refractory cases. They include mersalyl sodium.

Carbonic anhydrase inhibitors reduce the rate of interaction between water and carbon dioxide so reducing the availability of hydrogen ions and resulting in the excretion of an increased amount of sodium and bicarbonate. The urine becomes alkaline and in continued use of the diuretic a metabolic acidosis develops.

When carbonic anhydrase inhibitors are used for longer than a few days, their action becomes self-limiting and diuresis ceases. This is because metabolic acidosis causes a depletion of bicarbonate ion and an excess of hydrogen ions in the extracellular fluid, which becomes available for exchange and overcomes the effect of a carbonic anhydrase inhibitor. Thus, except in the treatment of glaucoma carbonic anhydrase inhibitors have been replaced by other diuretics. They include acetazolamide.

Aldosterone antagonists and other potassium-sparing diuretics. Aldosterone antagonists inhibit the exchange of sodium and potassium ions in the distal part of the distal tubule by competition with the hormone aldosterone, thus producing a weak diuresis with loss of sodium and retention of potassium. They include spironolactone.

A number of diuretics with an action on the distal part of distal tubular resorption produce a weak diuresis with potassium retention. They are frequently used in conjunction with other diuretics such as the thiazides to produce a strong diuresis while conserving body potassium. When potassium-sparing diuretics such as spironolactone, amiloride, and triamterene are given in conjunction with loop diuretics and thiazide diuretics, the excessive use of potassium supplements should be avoided owing to the risk of hyperkalaemia.

Xanthines increase renal blood flow and the rate of glomerular filtration thereby producing a mild diuresis.

They include aminophylline, caffeine, theobromine, and theophylline.

Osmotic diuretics. Substances that increase the osmotic pressure of the glomerular filtrate increase diuresis. They are used to supplement the action of more powerful diuretics and when there is a risk of acute renal failure, for example, in surgical procedures undertaken in the presence of obstructive jaundice. They include mannitol and urea.

Uses of diuretics. Diuretics are used to remove excess salt and water from the body in the treatment of oedema and to maintain a diuresis in patients at risk from acute renal failure. They are also used in the treatment of hypertension.

Selection of the appropriate diuretic. In congestive heart failure thiazide diuretics will usually remove excess sodium and water without causing profound electrolyte depletion or circulatory collapse. However, they should be used in an intermittent regimen to allow homeostatic mechanisms to function between doses and prevent early onset of potassium depletion. In acute pulmonary oedema, it is essential to remove fluid from the lungs rapidly and for this purpose the fast-acting loop diuretics are suitable.

In renal insufficiency, conventional doses of many diuretics cease to be effective and high doses of loop diuretics are usually necessary.

In hepatic insufficiency, ascites may be associated with a high concentration of circulating aldosterone resulting in reduced body stores of potassium. To prevent further electrolyte imbalance it is desirable to remove excess fluid slowly and to prevent loss of potassium. Spironolactone should therefore be used and, if necessary, its action may be supplemented by the addition of a loop diuretic.

In hypertension, thiazide diuretics may effect some reduction in arterial pressure but other diuretics may also be used. They are usually administered in conjunction with antihypertensive drugs.

For rapid removal of fluid in emergencies or when other diuretics are ineffective, bumetanide, ethacrynic acid, or frusemide may be given.

Dodecyl Gallate

Dodecyl 3,4,5-trihydroxybenzoate

$$CO \cdot O \cdot [CH_2]_{11} \cdot CH_3$$

$C_{19}H_{30}O_5 = 338.4$

OTHER NAME: *Progallin LA®*

A standard is given in the British Pharmacopoeia 1973

Description. A white or creamy-white, odourless, tasteless powder.

Solubility. Practically insoluble in water; soluble, at 20°, in 3.5 parts of alcohol, in 4 parts of ether, in 60 parts of chloroform, in 2 parts of acetone, in 30 parts of arachis oil, in 1.5 parts of methyl alcohol, and in 60 parts of propylene glycol.

Storage. It should be stored in airtight containers, contact with metals being avoided, protected from light.

Identification. TESTS. 1. Dissolve about 10 mg in a mixture of 2.5 ml of acetone and 2.5 ml of water and add 5 ml of *dilute ammonia solution*; a deep pink colour is produced. Allow the mixture to stand for about 20 minutes; the colour becomes orange-brown. Shake the mixture; the pink colour is restored.
2. Dissolve about 5 mg in a mixture of 25 ml of acetone and 25 ml of water and add 1 drop of *ferric chloride solution*; a purplish-blue colour is produced which rapidly becomes bluish-black.

MELTING-POINT. About 97°.

ULTRAVIOLET ABSORPTION. In methyl alcohol, maximum at 275 nm (E1%, 1cm = 300).

Metabolism. METABOLIC REACTIONS. Hydrolysed to gallic acid which is methylated or conjugated with glucuronic acid.

EXCRETION. Excreted as gallic acid, 4-O-methylgallic acid, and a glucuronide.

Uses. Dodecyl gallate is used as an antoxidant for preserving oils and fats; it is also used to inhibit autoxidation of ether, paraldehyde, and similar substances which develop peroxides in the presence of oxygen.
Anhydrous oils and fats may contain up to 0.01% of dodecyl gallate and volatile oils up to 0.1%; dodecyl gallate is dissolved in fixed oils by warming the mixture to 70° to 80° and in solid fats by warming until the fat is just melted.
The formation of peroxides in ether is inhibited by 0.01% of dodecyl gallate and the oxidation of paraldehyde is retarded by 0.05%.

Domiphen Bromide

A mixture of alkyldimethyl-2-phenoxyethylammonium bromides. It consists chiefly of dodecyldimethyl-2-phenoxyethylammonium bromide, $\{C_6H_5.O[CH_2]_2.N-(CH_3)_2(C_{12}H_{25})\}^+Br^-$ ($C_{22}H_{40}BrNO = 414.5$).

OTHER NAME: *Bradosol*®

A standard is given in the British Pharmacopoeia 1973

Description. Colourless or faintly yellow crystalline flakes with a bitter soapy taste.

Solubility. Soluble, at 20°, in less than 2 parts of water and of alcohol and in 30 parts of acetone.

Moisture content. Not more than 1%, determined by drying at 70° *in vacuo*.

Incompatibility. It is incompatible with soaps and similar anionic detergents and with alkali hydroxides.

Storage. It should be stored in airtight containers.

Preparation and storage of solutions. See statement on aqueous solutions of antiseptics in the entry on Solutions.

Identification. TEST. Dissolve about 10 mg in 10 ml of water and add 2 drops of *eosin solution* and 100 ml of water; an intense pink colour is produced.

MELTING-POINT. In the range 106° to 116°.

ULTRAVIOLET ABSORPTION. In water, maxima at 268 nm (E1%, 1cm = 30) and 274 nm (E1%, 1cm = 25).

Actions and uses. Domiphen bromide has the actions and uses of the quaternary ammonium compounds, as described under Cetrimide, in addition to which it has antifungal activity.
The activity of domiphen bromide is enhanced in alkaline media, but reduced in the presence of acid, organic

matter, blood, and pus. Its activity is also reduced in the presence of soap; consequently all traces of soap should be removed from the skin before applying domiphen bromide.
A 0.02% aqueous solution has been used in obstetrics, for application to wounds and burns, and for irrigation of the bladder and urethra.
Lozenges containing 500 micrograms of domiphen bromide are used for the treatment of bacterial and fungal infections of the mouth and throat.
Domiphen bromide is used as an antiseptic in some medicated surgical dressings.

Precautions. Continuous use may bring about defatting of the skin of the hands; protection against this may be provided by the application of a suitable cream, such as hydrous ointment, containing wool alcohols or wool fat.

Preparations
Preparations available include LOZENGES containing domiphen bromide 500 micrograms.

Dopamine

see under HYPOTHALAMIC RELEASING FACTORS

Dothiepin Hydrochloride

3-(6H-Dibenzo[b,e]thiepin-11-ylidene)propyl-NN-dimethylammonium chloride. It consists predominantly of the *trans*-isomer.

$C_{19}H_{22}ClNS = 331.9$

OTHER NAMES: Dosulepin Hydrochloride; *Prothiaden*®

A standard is given in the British Pharmacopoeia Addendum 1975

Description. A white to faintly yellow, crystalline, almost odourless powder.

Solubility. Soluble, at 20°, in 2 parts of water, in 8 parts of alcohol, and in 2 parts of chloroform; very slightly soluble in ether.

Storage. It should be stored in airtight containers, protected from light.

Identification. TEST. Dissolve 1 mg in 5 ml of sulphuric acid; a dark red colour is produced.

MELTING-POINT. About 224°, with decomposition.

ULTRAVIOLET ABSORPTION. In 0.1N hydrochloric acid, maxima at 229 nm (E1%, 1cm = 800) and 303 nm (E1%, 1cm = 108) and an inflexion at 260 nm.

INFRA-RED ABSORPTION. Major peaks at 727, 747, 763, 1252, 1420, and 1467 cm⁻¹ (see Appendix 2a: Infra-red Spectra).

Determination in body fluids. HIGH PRESSURE LIQUID CHROMATOGRAPHY. In plasma or serum—R. R. Brodie et al., *J. int. med. Res.*, 1977, **5**, 387.

Actions and uses. Dothiepin is a tricyclic antidepressant with actions and uses similar to those described under Amitriptyline Hydrochloride. It is used in the treatment of depression and anxiety associated with depression. Dothiepin hydrochloride is given in a dosage of 50 to 150 milligrams daily in divided doses; where insomnia is a problem, a large proportion of the dose should be given at night.

Undesirable effects; Precautions and contra-indications; Drug interactions. As for Amitriptyline Hydrochloride.

Preparations

DOTHIEPIN CAPSULES: consisting of dothiepin hydrochloride, in powder, which may be mixed with a suitable inert diluent, enclosed in a hard capsule. The capsule shells may be coloured. Available as capsules containing 25 mg of dothiepin hydrochloride.

A standard for these capsules is given in the British Pharmacopoeia Addendum 1975

Containers and *Storage:* see the entry on Capsules for general information on containers and storage.

Advice for patients: daily doses should preferably be taken at night. When initiating treatment there may be a time-lag of up to 10 days before a therapeutic response is obtained.

The capsules may cause drowsiness; persons affected should not drive or operate machinery. Alcohol should be avoided.

OTHER PREPARATIONS available include TABLETS containing dothiepin hydrochloride 75 mg.

Doxapram Hydrochloride

1-Ethyl-4-(2-morpholinoethyl)-3,3-diphenyl-2-pyrrolidone hydrochloride monohydrate

$C_{24}H_{31}ClN_2O_2,H_2O = 433.0$

OTHER NAME: *Dopram*®

Description. An odourless, white or off-white, crystalline powder.

Solubility. Soluble in 50 parts of water; soluble in alcohol and in chloroform; practically insoluble in ether.

Acidity. A 1% solution has a pH of 3.5 to 5.

Moisture content. 3 to 4.5%, determined by drying at 105°.

Incompatibility. Solutions are incompatible with alkaline substances and compatible with dextrose injection (5%).

Storage. It should be stored in airtight containers.

Identification. MELTING-POINT. About 220°

INFRA-RED ABSORPTION. Major peaks at 696, 710, 753, 1253, 1423, and 1683 cm^{-1} (see Appendix 2a: Infra-red Spectra).

Determination in body fluids. GAS CHROMATOGRAPHY. In plasma—R. H. Robson and L. F. Prescott, *J. Chromat.*, 1977, **143**, 527.

Metabolism. DISTRIBUTION. In dogs, doxapram metabolites are widely distributed throughout the tissues with high concentrations appearing in fatty tissues, liver, pancreas, and adrenal glands.

METABOLIC REACTIONS. Rapidly metabolised to a number of metabolites; the probable metabolic reactions include oxidation of the morpholine ring to the 2-ketone, N-dealkylation of the ring nitrogen, ring fission of the morpholine group followed by N-dealkylation, deamination, and oxidation of the resultant side-chain; hydroxylation of the phenyl groups does not seem to occur.

EXCRETION. In dogs, 30 to 40% of a dose is excreted in the urine in 24 to 48 hours and 30 to 40% is excreted in the faeces via the bile over a similar period; very little unchanged drug is excreted by either route.

FURTHER INFORMATION. R. B. Bruce *et al.*, *J. mednl Chem.*, 1965, **8**, 157; J. E. Pitts *et al.*, *Xenobiotica*, 1973, **3**, 73.

Actions and uses. Doxapram hydrochloride is a respiratory stimulant with actions and uses similar to those of Nikethamide.

It is used to decrease recovery time after analgesia and to counteract respiratory depression caused by narcotic analgesics or occurring after operations. The usual dosage is 1 to 1.5 milligrams per kilogram body-weight by intravenous injection, repeated at intervals of 1 hour if necessary.

Doxapram hydrochloride may also be given by intravenous infusion in the treatment of respiratory failure. The usual dosage is 0.5 to 4 milligrams per minute, adjusted according to the response of the patient.

In the differential diagnosis of post-operative apnoea, a single dose of 1 to 1.5 milligrams per kilogram body-weight may be given by intravenous injection. Apnoea resulting from depression of the central nervous system responds to this treatment while that due to partial neuromuscular blockade is unaffected.

Undesirable effects. Doxapram may give rise to dizziness, hypertension, and sensation of warmth, especially in the perineum.

Precautions and contra-indications. It should be given with caution to patients who are being treated with a monoamine-oxidase inhibitor, such as isocarboxazid, nialamide, phenelzine, or tranylcypromine, or who have been so treated within the previous 2 weeks. Caution should be observed in administering doxapram to epileptic patients.

It is contra-indicated in severe hypertension, coronary artery disease, thyrotoxicosis, airway obstruction, and cerebrovascular accident.

Preparations

DOXAPRAM INJECTION: a sterile solution of doxapram hydrochloride in water for injections. Available in 5-ml ampoules containing 20 mg of doxapram hydrochloride per ml.

Containers and *Labelling:* see the entry on Injections for general information on containers and labelling.

Storage: it should not be allowed to freeze.

OTHER PREPARATIONS available include an INJECTION containing doxapram hydrochloride 2 mg per ml in dextrose injection (5%) in 500-ml infusion bottles.

Doxepin Hydrochloride

A mixture of the *cis*- and *trans*-isomers of 3-(6H-dibenz[b,e]oxepin-11-ylidene)propyl-NN-dimethylammonium chloride.

$C_{19}H_{22}ClNO = 315.8$

OTHER NAME: *Sinequan*®

A standard is given in the British Pharmacopoeia Addendum 1975

Description. A white crystalline powder with a slight amine-like odour.

Solubility. Soluble, at 20°, in 1.5 parts of water, in 1 part of alcohol, and in 2 parts of chloroform.

Moisture content. Not more than 1%, determined by drying at 105°.

Storage. It should be protected from light.

Identification. TEST. Dissolve about 5 mg in 2 ml of nitric acid; a red colour is produced.

MELTING-POINT. About 188°.

ULTRAVIOLET ABSORPTION. In 0.1N methanolic hydrochloric acid, maximum at 297 nm (E1%, 1cm = 131).

INFRA-RED ABSORPTION. Major peaks at 750, 768, 1006, 1198, 1438, and 1478 cm^{-1} (see Appendix 2a: Infra-red Spectra).

Determination in body fluids. COLORIMETRY. In serum or urine: doxepin and some of its metabolites—A. Devreindt *et al.*, *Arzneimittel-Forsch.*, 1973, **23**, 863.

SPECTROPHOTOMETRY: SPECTROFLUORIMETRY. In serum or urine—see A. Devreindt *et al.*, above.

GAS CHROMATOGRAPHY. In urine—L. J. Dusci and L. P. Hackett, *J. Chromat.*, 1971, **61**, 231; in serum: doxepin and its metabolite monodemethyldoxepin—S. V. Reite *et al.*, *Meddr. norsk farm. Selsk.*, 1975, **37**, 141.

Metabolism. ABSORPTION. Well absorbed after oral administration.

BLOOD CONCENTRATION. During therapy with oral doses of 50 to 300 mg, plasma concentrations of drug plus metabolites of 25 to 140 ng/ml are obtained.

DISTRIBUTION. In rats, doxepin and its metabolites are rapidly distributed throughout the tissues with high concentrations appearing in the liver, kidneys, and lungs; doxepin has an affinity for melanin and crosses the blood/brain and the placental barriers.

METABOLIC REACTIONS. In rats and man, demethylation, N-oxidation, aromatic hydroxylation, and glucuronic acid conjugation. The demethylated metabolite is an active metabolite.

EXCRETION. In man, about 0.4% of a dose is excreted unchanged in the urine in 24 hours; in dogs, 50%, and in rats, 60% of a dose is excreted in the urine.

FURTHER INFORMATION. Doxepin: a review—*Drugs*, 1971, **1**, 194; plasma concentrations—J. E. O'Brien and O. N. Hinsvark, *J. pharm. Sci.*, 1976, **65**, 1068; urinary excretion—L. J. Dusci and L. P. Hackett, *J. Chromat.*, 1971, **61**, 231; a review of pharmacological properties and

therapeutic efficacy—R. M. Pinder *et al.*, *Drugs*, 1977, **13**, 161.

Actions and uses. Doxepin hydrochloride is a tricyclic antidepressant with actions and uses similar to those described under Amitriptyline Hydrochloride.
The usual dose is the equivalent of 50 to 150 milligrams of doxepin daily, in divided doses; 1.1 grams of doxepin hydrochloride is approximately equivalent to 1 gram of doxepin.

Undesirable effects; Precautions and contra-indications; Drug interactions. As for Amitriptyline Hydrochloride.

Preparation

DOXEPIN CAPSULES: consisting of doxepin hydrochloride, which may be mixed with a suitable inert diluent, enclosed in a hard capsule. The capsule shells may be coloured. Available as capsules containing doxepin hydrochloride equivalent to 10, 25, 50, and 75 mg of doxepin.
A standard for these capsules is given in the British Pharmacopoeia Addendum 1975
Containers and *Storage:* see the entry on Capsules for general information on containers and storage.
Advice for patients: daily doses should preferably be taken at night. When initiating treatment there may be a time-lag of up to 2 weeks before a full therapeutic response is obtained. The capsules may cause drowsiness; persons affected should not drive or operate machinery. Alcohol should be avoided.

Doxycycline Hydrochloride

6-Deoxy-5β-hydroxytetracycline hydrochloride hemiethanolate hemihydrate

$C_{22}H_{25}ClN_2O_8,\frac{1}{2}C_2H_5OH,\frac{1}{2}H_2O = 512.9$

OTHER NAMES: Doxycycline Hyclate; *Vibramycin*®

A standard is given in the British Pharmacopoeia 1973

Description. A yellow crystalline powder with a slightly ethanolic odour and a bitter taste.

Solubility. Soluble, at 20°, in 3 parts of water and in 4 parts of methyl alcohol; practically insoluble in chloroform.

Acidity. A 1% solution has a pH of 2 to 3.

Moisture content. 1.4 to 2.8%, determined by Fischer titration. It also contains 4.3 to 6% of ethyl alcohol.

Dissociation constants. pK$_a$ 3.5, 7.7, 9.5 (20°).

Storage. It should be stored in airtight containers, protected from light.

Identification. TEST. To about 500 μg add 2 ml of sulphuric acid; a yellow colour is produced.

ULTRAVIOLET ABSORPTION. In 0.1N hydrochloric acid, maxima at 270 nm (E1%, 1cm = 415) and 348 nm (E1%, 1cm = 257); in alcohol (95%), maxima at 277 nm (E1%, 1cm = 329) and 365 nm (E1%, 1cm = 333); in 0.1N sodium hydroxide, maxima at 239 nm (E1%, 1cm = 375), 282 nm (E1%, 1cm = 286), and 381 nm (E1%, 1cm = 308).

INFRA-RED ABSORPTION. Major peaks at 1220, 1244, 1462, 1580, 1613, and 1660 cm⁻¹ (see Appendix 2a: Infrared Spectra).

Determination in body fluids. MICROBIOLOGICAL ASSAY. In serum or urine—N. H. Steigbigel *et al.*, *Am. J. med. Sci.*, 1968, **255**, 296.

Metabolism. ABSORPTION. Readily absorbed after oral administration; the extent of absorption may be decreased by the presence of aluminium hydroxide gels and by other antacids and by ferrous sulphate; absorption of doxycycline is not much affected by food or by zinc sulphate and it is more completely absorbed than tetracycline.

BLOOD CONCENTRATION. After an oral dose of 200 mg followed by 100 mg daily, blood concentrations are maintained at 1.5 to 4.5 μg/ml with peak concentrations of up to 7.0 μg/ml being attained 2 hours after dosing; after a single oral dose of 500 mg of the hydrochloride, peak serum concentrations of about 15 μg/ml are attained at 4 hours; minimum effective concentrations are about 1 μg/ml and concentrations above this are maintained for up to 4 days following the 500-mg dose.

HALF-LIFE. Plasma half-life, 15 to 23 hours, which may be increased after multiple dosing and decreased following concurrent antiepileptic drug therapy.

DISTRIBUTION. Enters the synovial fluid, seminal fluid, lungs, lymph, and sputum; low concentrations are attained in the cerebrospinal fluid; doxycycline crosses the placenta and is secreted in the milk; it does not accumulate in renal function impairment; *protein binding*, 25 to 93% bound to plasma proteins.

EXCRETION. 25 to 40% of a dose is excreted in the urine in 24 hours and about 80% in 3 days; variable amounts are excreted in the faeces; urinary excretion of doxycycline is increased by about 50% when the urine is alkaline; its excretion is not much influenced by renal disease; it is excreted in the bile in concentrations about 15 times those in the blood.

FURTHER INFORMATION: Serum concentrations—B. K. Adadevoh *et al.*, *Br. med. J.*, i/1976, 880; excretion—J. M. Jaffe *et al.*, *J. pharm. Sci.*, 1974, **63**, 1256; blood concentrations—B. J. Liebowitz *et al.*, *Curr. ther. Res.*, 1972, **14**, 820; absorption and distribution—W. A. Mahon *et al.*, *Can. med. Ass. J.*, 1970, **103**, 1031; interaction with some antiepileptic drugs—O. Penttilä *et al.*, *Br. med. J.*, ii/1974, 470; effect of zinc sulphate on absorption of doxycycline—O. Penttilä *et al.*, *Eur. J. clin. Pharmac.*, 1975, **9**, 131.

Bioavailability. A study of 2 formulations—J. D. Arcilla *et al.*, *Curr. ther. Res.*, 1974, **16**, 1126.

Actions and uses. Doxycycline has the actions and uses described under Tetracycline Hydrochloride but differs from tetracycline in having a high lipid solubility. Higher concentrations are reached in secretions such as those of the bronchi and nasal sinuses than with other tetracyclines.

The usual initial dose is the equivalent of 200 milligrams of doxycycline, followed by 100 milligrams daily, but this may be increased to 200 milligrams daily for the treatment of infections caused by organisms for which the minimum inhibitory concentration is greater than 0.6 microgram per millilitre; the usual dosage for children is 3 milligrams per kilogram body-weight daily; 1.15 grams of doxycycline hydrochloride is approximately equivalent to 1 gram of doxycycline.

Precautions and contra-indications. As for Tetracycline Hydrochloride.

Doxycycline rarely gives rise to increased blood-urea concentrations in renal failure and may therefore be preferable to other tetracyclines in renal insufficiency.

Drug interactions. As for Tetracycline Hydrochloride.

Blood concentrations of doxycycline are reduced by the concurrent administration of anticonvulsants such as barbiturates, carbamazepine, and phenytoin.

Preparation

DOXYCYCLINE CAPSULES: consisting of doxycycline hydrochloride, in powder, which may be mixed with a suitable inert diluent, enclosed in a hard capsule. The capsule shells may be coloured. Available as capsules containing doxycycline hydrochloride equivalent to 100 mg of doxycycline.

A standard for these capsules is given in the British Pharmacopoeia 1973

Containers and *Storage:* see the entry on Capsules for general information on containers and storage.

Labelling: the label on the container should state the amount of the medicament as the equivalent amount of doxycycline, the date after which the capsules are not intended to be used, and the conditions under which they should be stored.

Advice for patients: the capsules should be taken at regular intervals. Salts of aluminium, calcium, iron, and magnesium, and antacids should not be taken within 1 hour. The prescribed course should be completed.

Dracunculiasis

see under FILARIASIS

Driving and Drugs

Certain medicines may temporarily impair a patient's alertness, skill, and judgement and so render him incapable of correctly driving a motor vehicle or operating moving machinery.

Any substance that affects the central nervous system may have an effect on ability to drive, especially substances known to cause drowsiness, dizziness, or distorted perception or judgement.

The medicines that cause drowsiness are tranquillisers and hypnotics and others that have sedative side-effects, such as analgesics, anticonvulsants, antihistamines, motion-sickness remedies, and certain antidepressants. Alcohol has a similar effect and it is therefore particularly dangerous to drive when taking sedative drugs in conjunction with alcohol.

Medicines that may cause giddiness and fainting include insulin and substances that reduce blood pressure such as antihypertensive agents and isoprenaline. Medicines that alter perception and judgement include those substances that allay anxiety, including tranquillisers and antidepressants. Perception may also be distorted by drugs such as cannabis and lysergide.

Ability to drive may also be affected by substances that cause visual disturbances, for example anticholinergics, ethambutol, indomethacin, and nalidixic acid; visual acuity, colour perception, and dark adaptation may be affected.

Driving ability is most likely to be reduced when the drug treatment is being initiated and before tolerance has developed; conversely, in the case of stimulant substances, the greatest effects on driving may occur when drowsiness occurs as the effect of the drug wears off or when it is withdrawn.

Drug Dependence

Drugs that alter mood or behaviour and that are administered repeatedly over a period of time may give rise to drug dependence, that is, a compulsive desire to continue to take the drug. The characteristics of the dependent state vary with the drug used and may be divided into two main types, namely, psychic and physical dependence. Thus, for example, the abuse of amphetamine and cocaine is originated and maintained by the desire to attain maximum euphoria (psychic dependence) but there is no physical dependence. Other drugs, for example, morphine, create psychic dependence which is soon supplemented by physical dependence. Discontinuation of the drug interferes with the normal functioning of the body and withdrawal symptoms occur which can be relieved by further doses of the drug.

Morphine type. Drug dependence of the morphine type is characterised by (i) strong psychic dependence, (ii) an early development of physical dependence, which increases in intensity as the dosage is increased, and (iii) development of tolerance, necessitating increased dosage to obtain the initial effects.

Barbiturate-alcohol type. Drug dependence of the barbiturate-alcohol type is characterised by (i) a strong psychic dependence, (ii) intoxication manifested by sedation, sleep, coma, stupor, impaired cognition and judgement, and ataxia, (iii) development of tolerance, (iv) partial cross tolerance between members of the group, and (v) a dangerous type of physical dependence manifested by anxiety, insomnia, weakness, tremors, abnormalities in the electroencephalogram, convulsions, and delirium on withdrawal.

Cocaine type. Drug dependence of the cocaine type is characterised by (i) strong psychic dependence, (ii) no development of physical dependence and therefore absence of characteristic abstinence syndrome when the drug is withdrawn, (iii) absence of tolerance and sensitisation to the drug's effects in some cases, and (iv) a strong desire for rapid repetition of the dose.

Cannabis type. Drug dependence of the cannabis type is characterised by (i) moderate to strong psychic dependence on account of the desired subjective effects, (ii) absence of physical dependence and therefore of a characteristic abstinence syndrome when the drug is withdrawn, and (iii) lack of tendency to increase the dose and no evidence of tolerance.

Amphetamine type. Drug dependence of the amphetamine type is characterised by (i) strong psychic dependence, (ii) a high degree of tolerance, and (iii) no readily evident physical dependence and consequently no characteristic abstinence syndrome, although withdrawal will be followed by a state of mental and physical depression with electroencephalographic changes as the stimulatory effect of the drug diminishes.

Hallucinogen (lysergide) type. Drug dependence of the hallucinogen type is characterised by (i) mild psychic dependence, (ii) no physical dependence, and (iii) a high degree of tolerance. The chief dangers to the individual arise from the psychological effects of hallucinogenic drugs.

Detection of drug abuse in young persons. The spread of drug abuse in young persons may progress to dependence on the more dangerous drugs with consequent moral and physical impairment. Occasional abuse of drugs is relatively common but sometimes leads to chronic abuse. Parents, teachers, and others, who wish to be aware of drug abuse in its early stages should look for mood changes in young persons, often occurring at the weekend or immediately following it.

Amphetamines give rise to increased activity and the pupil of the eye may be dilated. Irritability and depression follow as the effect of the drug decreases.

Barbiturates and other sedatives may give rise to a "drunken" state, with drowsiness and possibly coma.

Cannabis tends to produce a brief elevation of mood followed by sedation. It is usually detected by reddening of the eyes and the pungent smell after smoking. An unusual thirst may occur after smoking.

Lysergide (LSD). A disorientated or dream-like state may be observed.

Morphine-like compounds cause sedation, facial flushing, and contraction of the pupils. Marks on the skin may be found in persons using diamorphine by injection, and there may be marked withdrawal symptoms in these subjects.

Pharmacists may sometimes receive requests from drug abusers who are seeking substances that may be obtained for this purpose without medical prescription. Caution should therefore be exercised in dealing with requests for volatile solvents such as cleaning fluids, mixtures containing antihistamines, analgesics, and dilutions of morphine-like substances which are sometimes used for this purpose.

Drug Interactions

see INTERACTIONS OF DRUGS

Dusting-powders

Dusting-powders are used externally and are usually mixtures of two or more substances in fine powder free from grittiness. They may be prepared as described in the entry on Powders.

Talc, kaolin, and other natural mineral ingredients are liable to be heavily contaminated with bacteria, including *Clostridium tetani*, *Cl. perfringens* (*Cl. welchii*), and *Bacillus anthracis*. Such ingredients should be sterilised by heating for a sufficient length of time to ensure that the whole of the powder has been maintained at a temperature not lower than 160° for not less than one hour before mixing with the other ingredients. This procedure is not necessary when the final product is subjected to a sterilisation process, as indicated in the individual monograph, but must be carried out in all other cases. Dusting-powders should be dusted lightly on the affected area. They should not be applied to open wounds or to raw surfaces of large area.

Containers. Unless otherwise specified, dusting-powders should be dispensed in suitable coloured glass or plastic jars, preferably fitted with a reclosable perforated lid.

Labelling. The container should be labelled "For external use only". The label on containers of dusting-powders for veterinary use should state, in addition, the names and proportions of the medicaments and whether the contents are sterile.

Dydrogesterone

9β,10α-Pregna-4,6-diene-3,20-dione

$C_{21}H_{28}O_2 = 312.5$

OTHER NAME: *Duphaston*®

A standard is given in the British Pharmacopoeia Addendum 1978

Description. A white crystalline odourless powder.

Solubility. Practically insoluble in water; soluble, at 20°, in 52 parts of alcohol, in 140 parts of ether, in 2 parts of chloroform, in 17 parts of acetone, in 40 parts of methyl alcohol, and in 180 parts of fixed oils.

Specific rotation. −446° to −464°, determined on a 1% solution in dioxan.

Storage. It should be stored in airtight containers, protected from light.

Identification. TEST. Dissolve about 50 mg in 5 ml of dehydrated alcohol, add 50 mg of hydroxylammonium chloride and 50 mg of anhydrous sodium acetate, and heat under a reflux condenser for 2 hours; evaporate the solution to a volume of about 3 ml and add 10 ml of water; a precipitate is produced which, after washing with two 3-ml portions of water and two 3-ml portions of warm methyl alcohol, melts at about 275°, with decomposition.

MELTING-POINT. About 169°.

ULTRAVIOLET ABSORPTION. In alcohol (95%), maximum at 284 nm (E1%, 1cm = 803).

INFRA-RED ABSORPTION. Major peaks at 1197, 1232, 1581, 1622, 1660, and 1697 cm⁻¹ (see Appendix 2a: Infra-red Spectra).

THIN-LAYER CHROMATOGRAPHY. See under Thin-layer Chromatography, System 10.

Metabolism. ABSORPTION. Absorbed after oral administration.

METABOLIC REACTIONS. Ketoreduction to form the 20α- and 20β-hydroxy-metabolites and glucuronic acid conjugation; the 4-en-3-one structure in the A-ring is metabolically stable since it is protected by both the double bond at carbon 6 and by the 9β,10α-retro structure; about 10 unidentified metabolites have been isolated; 17-hydroxylation occurs *in vitro* with placental preparations.

EXCRETION. About 50% of a dose is excreted in the urine as the 20α-hydroxy metabolite along with smaller amounts of the 20β-hydroxy form; the drug or its metabolites are excreted in both urine and bile.

FURTHER INFORMATION. See J. H. H. Thijssen, The metabolism of orally active synthetic progestational compounds, *International Encyclopedia of Pharmacology and Therapeutics*, Section 48, M. Tausk (Ed.), Vol. 2, Oxford, Pergamon Press, 1972, p. 220.

Actions and uses. Dydrogesterone has actions similar to those of progesterone but, being a derivative of retroprogesterone, it does not have androgenic or oestrogenic properties and does not prevent ovulation or suppress pituitary secretion of gonadotrophins. It does not raise body temperature.

Dydrogesterone is used in the differential diagnosis of amenorrhoea. It is used together with oestrogens in the treatment of mild dysfunctional menorrhagia and to prevent metrorrhagia. In doses of 5 milligrams 4 times daily from the fifth day of the menstrual cycle for 20 days, it may relieve pain and spasm in dysmenorrhoea. Treatment for 6 months or more with 10 to 30 milligrams daily in divided doses from day 5 to 25 of the menstrual cycle may be used for the treatment of endometriosis. Dydrogesterone is used to maintain pregnancy in threatened abortion due to progesterone deficiency, but its value is uncertain; it does not lead to virilisation of the foetus. It is of no value as an oral contraceptive.

Undesirable effects. Dydrogesterone occasionally causes nausea and vomiting but this is usually mild. Uterine bleeding may occur during treatment but usually responds to reduction in dose with increased frequency of administration.

Preparation

DYDROGESTERONE TABLETS: available as tablets containing 10 mg of dydrogesterone.

A standard for these tablets is given in the British Pharmacopoeia Addendum 1978

Containers and *Storage:* see the entry on Tablets for general information on containers and storage. Containers should be airtight and light resistant.

Advice for patients: the prescribed course should be completed or, where applicable, treatment should not be discontinued without the advice of the prescriber.

Dysentery

see under SHIGELLA INFECTION

Dysmenorrhoea

Dysmenorrhoea is painful menstruation. The pain may occur before or at the onset of menstrual bleeding or late in menstruation. Uncoordinated uterine contractions due to shedding of endometrium cause pain, lasting for 12 to 24 hours, around the time of the beginning of menstruation. Dysmenorrhoea due to endometriosis or pelvic infection usually starts 2 or more days before menstruation and continues throughout menstruation.

Ear-drops

Ear-drops are solutions or suspensions of medicaments in water, glycerol, diluted alcohol, propylene glycol, or other suitable solvent, for instillation into the ear.

Containers. Ear-drops should be supplied in coloured fluted glass bottles fitted with a plastic screw cap incorporating a glass dropper tube fitted with a rubber teat, or in plastic squeeze bottles fitted with a plastic cap incorporating a dropper device.

Labelling. The container should be labelled "For external use only".

Eclampsia

see under TOXAEMIA OF PREGNANCY

Ecothiopate Iodide

(2-Diethoxyphosphorylthioethyl)trimethylammonium iodide

$$[(CH_3)_3\overset{+}{N}\cdot[CH_2]_2\cdot S\cdot \underset{\underset{O}{\|}}{P}(O\cdot C_2H_5)_2] \quad I^-$$

$C_9H_{23}INO_3PS = 383.2$

OTHER NAME: *Phospholine Iodide®*

A standard is given in the British Pharmacopoeia 1973

Description. A white crystalline hygroscopic powder with an alliaceous odour.

Solubility. Soluble, at 20°, in 1 part of water, in 25 parts of alcohol, and in 3 parts of methyl alcohol; very slightly soluble in other organic solvents.

Acidity. Solutions have a pH of about 4.

Moisture content. Not more than 1%, determined by drying at 50° *in vacuo.*

Storage. It should be stored in airtight containers, at a temperature of 2° to 10°, protected from light. Under these conditions it may be expected to retain its potency for 18 months.

Identification. TEST. Dissolve about 100 mg in 2 ml of water and add 1 ml of nitric acid; a brown precipitate of iodine is formed. To 1 drop of the mixture add 1 ml of carbon tetrachloride and shake; a pink colour develops in the carbon tetrachloride layer. Heat the remainder of the mixture until colourless, cool, and dilute to 10 ml with water; the solution gives the reactions of phosphates.

MELTING-POINT. About 119°, with decomposition.

Actions and uses. Ecothiopate iodide is a powerful long-acting inhibitor of cholinesterase. It is applied locally for the reduction of intra-ocular tension.

In the treatment of glaucoma, 1 drop of a 0.03 or 0.06% solution may be instilled into the conjunctival sac twice daily. Patients who have failed to respond to other miotics used in conjunction with sympathomimetics and carbonic anhydrase inhibitors may sometimes be treated successfully with a higher concentration of ecothiopate iodide, such as 0.125 or 0.25%.

In the treatment of esotropia, 1 drop of a 0.125% solution should be instilled into each eye daily at bedtime and if a satisfactory response is obtained treatment may be continued with 1 drop of a 0.06% solution daily or 1 drop of a 0.125% solution every other day.

Undesirable effects. Systemic absorption of ecothiopate may occur during ocular treatment, and general anticholinesterase effects, including potentiation of muscle relaxants of the depolarising type, may result. Ecothiopate eye-drops may also precipitate iritis.

Preparation

ECOTHIOPATE EYE-DROPS: consisting of a sterile solution of ecothiopate iodide with 0.06% of boric acid, 0.5% of chlorbutol, 1.2% of mannitol, 0.8% of potassium acetate, and 0.026% of anhydrous sodium phosphate in purified water. It is prepared freshly by dissolving, aseptically, a sterile dry powder consisting of the ecothiopate iodide with the potassium acetate in a sterile diluent containing the other ingredients in the final sterile container. Available as a solution containing, when reconstituted, 0.03, 0.06, 0.125, and 0.25% of ecothiopate iodide.

Containers: see the entry on Eye-drops for general information on containers.

Labelling: see the entry on Eye-drops for general information on labelling. The label on the container of the eye-drops, except a container issued for an individual patient for domiciliary use should state: (1) the name of the eye-drops, (2) the directions for storage, and (3) the date of preparation.

The label on the container of dry powder used for the preparation of the eye-drops should state: (1) the name of the powder, indicating that it is for the preparation of ecothiopate eye-drops and (2) the weight of ecothiopate iodide in the container or the volume of eye-drops prepared according to the manufacturer's instructions. The label on the container or the label on the carton or the package leaflet should state (3) the direction for preparing the eye-drops.

The label on a multiple-dose container issued for an individual patient for domiciliary use should state: (1) that the eye-drops should be kept in a refrigerator and (2) the date after which the eye-drops should not be used.

Storage: it should be protected from light. The sterile dry powder should be stored at a temperature of 2° to 10°. Under these conditions it may be expected to retain its potency for 18 months. After preparation, the eye-drops may be expected to retain their potency for 1 month when stored at a temperature not exceeding 25° or, when stored at 2° to 10°, until the expiry date as specified by the manufacturer.

Advice for patients: see the entry on Eye-drops for general information on the use of eye-drops. The eye-drops should preferably be instilled at night. The treatment should not be discontinued without the advice of the prescriber. Headache and disturbances of vision may occur in the first few days of treatment.

Eczema

Eczema is an inflammation of the skin with itching and weeping. It commonly appears as a uniformly distributed pattern of papulovesicles on an erythematous ground. In subacute and chronic eczema there is epidermal thickening and scaliness but vesicles and weeping may be absent. Contact eczema (contact dermatitis) usually occurs in exposed areas and is associated with exposure to an allergen from the patient's occupation, clothing, or treatment with topical preparations. Infantile eczema is often associated with asthma and hay fever. It usually affects the forehead, cheeks, and other areas in infancy; if it persists to adult life the flexures of knees and elbows and wrists and hands are most usually affected.

Contact eczema may be treated by removal of the allergen followed by a short course of treatment with an antihistamine by mouth and if necessary local application of a corticosteroid cream or lotion. Treatment of infantile eczema may require similar measures but often on a long-term basis and it may be necessary to use emulsifying ointment instead of soap.

Endogenous eczema may be treated by bland applications and dressings to protect the lesions while the underlying condition of the patient receives appropriate treatment. Minor tranquillisers may be helpful in some cases. Irritation may be reduced by aqueous creams and lotions which reduce the skin temperature by evaporation. Preparations of tar may be applied topically to treat chronic eczema when the lesions become lichenified.

Weeping eczemas may be treated with wet dressings of potassium permanganate (0.01%), and corticosteroid ointment or creams may be applied if necessary to reduce inflammation.

The topical application of antibiotics is required when infection is present but there is a danger of sensitisation. Systemic treatment with antibiotics and corticosteroids is occasionally required.

Edrophonium Chloride

Ethyl(3-hydroxyphenyl)dimethylammonium chloride

$C_{10}H_{16}ClNO = 201.7$

OTHER NAME: *Tensilon®*

A standard is given in the British Pharmacopoeia 1973

Description. A white crystalline odourless powder with a bitter and saline taste.

Solubility. Soluble, at 20°, in 0.5 part of water and in 5 parts of alcohol; practically insoluble in ether and in chloroform.

Acidity. A 10% solution has a pH of 4 to 5.

Sterilisation. Solutions for injection are sterilised by heating in an autoclave or by filtration.

Storage. It should be stored in airtight containers, protected from light.

Identification. TEST. Dissolve about 50 mg in 2 ml of water and add 1 drop of *ferric chloride test-solution*; a reddish-violet colour is produced.

MELTING-POINT. About 168°, with decomposition.

ULTRAVIOLET ABSORPTION. In 0.1N hydrochloric acid, maximum at 273 nm (E1%, 1cm = 110); in 0.1N sodium hydroxide, maxima at 240 nm (E1%, 1cm = 550) and 294 nm (E1%, 1cm = 170).

Metabolism. HALF-LIFE. In rats, edrophonium is rapidly removed from the circulation and the removal appears to be biphasic.

DISTRIBUTION. In rats, localised in liver and kidneys and 5 minutes after an intravenous injection greater than 50% of the dose can be accounted for in the tissues; in rats, volume of distribution 1.5 litres/kg.

METABOLIC REACTIONS. Glucuronic acid conjugation.

EXCRETION. In rats, about 50% of a parenteral dose is excreted in the urine in 24 hours as unchanged drug and as glucuronic acid conjugate; about 5% is excreted in the bile of rats in 6 hours mostly as the glucuronide.

FURTHER INFORMATION. Excretion, metabolites in bile, and plasma concentrations—D. J. Back and T. N. Calvey, *Br. J. Pharmac.*, 1972, **44**, 534 and 1972, **46**, 355, and T. N. Calvey and D. J. Back, *J. Pharm. Pharmac.*, 1971, **23**, 642.

Actions and uses. Edrophonium chloride is an anticholinesterase drug with actions qualitatively similar to those of neostigmine methylsulphate. Its actions are rapid in onset and of short duration. It is of particular value in the diagnosis of myasthenia gravis.

It is given by intravenous injection in doses of 2 to 10 milligrams; the usual procedure is to inject 2 milli-grams and, if no change in clinical signs occurs within 30 seconds, to continue with the injection of a further 8 milligrams. The dose of edrophonium chloride for a child of up to 35 kilograms body-weight is 1 milligram, given by intravenous injection; 2 milligrams may be given by intramuscular injection when intravenous injection is difficult.

In untreated patients with myasthenia gravis, there is immediate subjective improvement and muscle strength increases. This effect usually lasts only for about 5 minutes, after which time the typical signs and symptoms return; because of its brief action edrophonium chloride is not suitable for the routine treatment of myasthenia gravis or for use as an antagonist to curare-like drugs.

Edrophonium chloride is used in a similar way to determine whether or not a patient with severe symptoms of myasthenia gravis is suffering from the effects of inadequate or excessive treatment with anticholinesterase drugs. If treatment has been inadequate, edrophonium chloride will produce an immediate amelioration of symptoms, whereas in cholinergic crisis due to overtreatment the symptoms will be aggravated or unchanged.

Preparation

EDROPHONIUM INJECTION: a sterile solution of edrophonium chloride in water for injections. It is sterilised by heating in an autoclave or by filtration. Available in 1-ml ampoules containing 10 mg of edrophonium chloride.

A standard for this injection is given in the British Pharmacopoeia 1973

Containers and *Labelling*: see the entry on Injections for general information on containers and labelling.

Storage: it should be protected from light.

Elixirs

Elixirs are clear, pleasantly flavoured, liquid preparations of potent or nauseous medicaments. The vehicle frequently contains a high proportion of alcohol, sugar, glycerol, or propylene glycol together with adjuvants such as colouring matter, other sweetening or flavouring agents, and preservatives.

Stability of elixirs. In general, elixirs are reasonably stable preparations provided they are stored in well-filled containers and are not diluted or mixed with other preparations. Any special precautions which may be necessary are indicated in the relevant monographs.

Some elixirs which cannot be kept for long periods are supplied in the form of granules or powder to which a specified quantity of water is added to prepare the elixir just before issue for use, and an appropriate warning regarding their limited stability is given on the label.

Microbial contamination. Elixirs do not usually support the growth of micro-organisms but, as they are liable to contain a high proportion of syrup, dilution or admixture with other preparations may create a suitable growth medium for micro-organisms.

Dilution of elixirs. When a dose ordered or prescribed is less than or not a multiple of 5 millilitres, the elixir should be diluted with the vehicle recommended under the individual elixir, so that the dose to be measured for the patient is one 5-millilitre spoonful or a multiple thereof.

Diluted elixirs must always be freshly prepared and not

more than 2 weeks' supply should be issued at a time unless otherwise specified in the entry on a particular elixir.

Containers. Elixirs should be dispensed in plain bottles of colourless or amber glass.

Labelling. A. The label on a container of an elixir issued by the manufacturer should state: (1) for elixirs other than those for which a full recipe is given in this volume, the name and concentration of the active ingredient; and (2) directions for storage. If the elixir is one which is to be prepared freshly before issue to the patient, the label on the container of granules or powder should state: (3) the name of the preparation in the form of "Granules (or Powder) for the Elixir", as specified under the individual elixir; (4) the name and concentration of the active ingredient in the elixir when prepared according to the manufacturer's instructions; (5) directions for storage; and (6) the date after which the granules or powder should not be used.

The label on the container, or the package leaflet, or the label on the package states: (1) the directions for preparing the elixir; (2) the directions for storage of the elixir; and (3) the period during which the elixir may be expected to retain its potency when stored under the stated conditions.

B. The label on the container of an elixir issued to the patient on a prescription should state, in addition to the prescriber's directions: (1) any special storage direction as directed in the entry on a particular elixir; and (2) if such a recommendation is made by the manufacturer, the date after which the elixir should not be used; or, if the elixir has been diluted before issue "The contents to be discarded if not taken before. . . [a date 2 weeks, or other period specified by the manufacturer or under the individual elixir, after the date of issue]".

Eltor Vaccine

A suspension of suitable killed strains of the El Tor biotype of *Vibrio cholerae*. It consists of a mixture of equal parts of vaccines prepared from smooth strains of the two main serotypes, Inaba and Ogawa. It contains not less than 8000 vibrios per millilitre.

OTHER NAME: Eltor/Vac

A standard is given in the British Pharmacopoeia 1973

Storage. It should be stored as described under Vaccines.

Actions and uses. Eltor vaccine is used for the same purpose as cholera vaccine, but it is not recognised as complying with the requirements for the international vaccination certificate.

The vaccine is administered as described under Cholera Vaccine by subcutaneous or intramuscular injection of the volume stated on the label as the dose, usually the first dose being 0.5 millilitre and the second being 1 millilitre.

Emetine Hydrochloride

(2S,3R,11bS)-3-Ethyl-2,3,4,6,7,11b-hexahydro-9,10-dimethoxy-2-[(1R)-1,2,3,4-tetrahydro-6,7-dimethoxyisoquinolin-1-yl]-1H-benzo[a]quinolizine dihydrochloride heptahydrate, the hydrochloride of emetine, an alkaloid obtained from ipecacuanha or prepared by methylating cephaëline or by synthesis.

$C_{29}H_{42}Cl_2N_2O_4,7H_2O = 679.7$

OTHER NAME: Emet. Hydrochlor.

A standard is given in the British Pharmacopoeia 1973

Description. A white, crystalline, odourless powder with a bitter taste; it becomes faintly yellow on exposure to light.

Solubility. Soluble in water and in alcohol.

Moisture content. 15 to 19%, determined by drying at 105°.

Specific rotation. +17° to +18.3°, determined on a 6% solution.

Dissociation constants. pK_a 7.4, 8.3 (25°).

Stability. Solutions of emetine hydrochloride are most stable to heating at 120° when buffered to pH 2, but solutions of pH 3.5 are sufficiently stable to be heat sterilised. Stability to heat is improved by removal of oxygen and by the addition of disodium edetate (to remove copper ions). Solutions are affected by radiation of wavelength 254 nm; the pH of maximum stability is 3 to 7 and photochemical stability is unaffected by the presence of oxygen.

FURTHER INFORMATION. Quantitative aspects of emetine degradation—C. Schuyt *et al.*, *Pharm. Weekbl. Ned.*, 1977, **12**, 1125.

Sterilisation. Solutions for injection are sterilised by heating with a bactericide or by filtration.

Storage. It should be stored in airtight containers, protected from light.

Identification. TEST. Mix 5 mg of molybdenum trioxide with 1 ml of sulphuric acid and sprinkle over the surface a small quantity of the sample; a bright green colour is produced.

INFRA-RED ABSORPTION. Major peaks at 1111, 1220, 1235, 1250, 1449, and 1493 cm^{-1} (see Appendix 2b: Infrared Spectra).

Determination in body fluids. SPECTROFLUORIMETRY. In tissues, blood, or urine—B. Davis *et al.*, *J. Pharm. Pharmac.*, 1962, **14**, 249.

Metabolism. ABSORPTION. Rapidly absorbed from parenteral sites.

DISTRIBUTION. Concentrates in the kidneys, lungs, liver, and spleen; continuous therapy leads to accumulation in the body.

METABOLIC REACTIONS. Emetine is not metabolised.

EXCRETION. Excreted unchanged in the urine at a slow rate; it is detectable in the urine some 40 to 60 days after treatment has ended.

Actions and uses. Emetine hydrochloride is an amoebicide. With the exception of chloroquine, it is the only effective agent for the treatment of extra-intestinal amoebiasis.

When injected subcutaneously it rapidly relieves the symptoms of amoebic dysentery, but because it does not eliminate cysts it does not effect a cure, nor does it eliminate the infection from asymptomatic cyst passers who spread the disease. It is, however, of value for the treatment of amoebic hepatitis and amoebic involvement of the lungs, brain, and other tissues.

Owing to the toxicity of emetine, chloroquine is the drug of choice, and emetine is usually reserved for cases of extra-intestinal amoebiasis that do not respond to chloroquine; sometimes the two drugs are used together.

Injections of emetine will not usually eradicate the intestinal infection and it is therefore necessary to give supplementary treatment by mouth with another amoebicide such as emetine and bismuth iodide, diloxanide furoate, or metronidazole. Many schedules of treatment have been devised in which alternating courses and combinations of various amoebicides are given. Amoebic ulcers are always secondarily infected with bacteria and in some patients amoebicidal drugs have little action until the secondary infection is controlled by sulphonamides or by antibiotics.

For the treatment of acute amoebic dysentery, a daily dosage of 60 milligrams of emetine hydrochloride is administered by subcutaneous or intramuscular injection until the symptoms are controlled; 3 or 4 doses are usually sufficient and the total dose should not exceed 750 milligrams. It should not be given intravenously owing to its cardiotoxic action. The usual dose for debilitated and underweight patients is 30 milligrams. Patients should be kept in bed during treatment and for several days thereafter; 6 to 8 weeks should elapse between courses of emetine hydrochloride.

The usual daily doses for children by subcutaneous or intramuscular injection are: up to one year, 1 milligram per kilogram body-weight; 1 to 5 years, 15 to 25 milligrams; and 6 to 12 years, 30 to 45 milligrams.

Undesirable effects. When given by mouth, emetine has an irritant action upon mucous membranes. In small doses it causes increased bronchial secretion and perspiration; larger doses, of about 6 milligrams of emetine hydrochloride, cause vomiting.

Injections of emetine are sometimes painful and may cause local induration or necrosis of tissue. Prolonged administration may produce degenerative changes in the kidney tubules, liver, and muscles, and may give rise to peripheral neuritis. Its effect upon heart muscle causes changes in the electrocardiogram; rarely, acute degenerative myocarditis with cardiac irregularities and failure may occur.

Contra-indications. Emetine is contra-indicated if there is severe cardiac or renal involvement, in elderly or debilitated patients, in pregnancy, and in children, unless other drugs such as metronidazole or chloroquine have failed.

Preparation

EMETINE INJECTION: a sterile solution of emetine hydrochloride in water for injections. The acidity of the solution is adjusted to pH 3 by the addition of dilute hydrochloric acid. The solution is sterilised by heating in an autoclave or by filtration. The usual strength is 60 mg of emetine hydrochloride per ml.

A standard for this injection is given in the British Pharmacopoeia 1973

Containers and *Labelling:* see the entry on Injections for general information on containers and labelling.

Storage: it should be protected from light.

Emulsifying Agents

Emulsifying agents prevent coalescence of the dispersed globules in emulsified systems by forming barriers at the interfaces; they may also facilitate the initial dispersion of globules by reducing interfacial tension.

Characteristics and Mode of Action

An efficient emulsifying agent should have both lipophilic and hydrophilic properties in reasonable balance such that, at the interfaces of the system, the lipophilic non-polar groups of the emulsifying agent, which are attracted to the oil phase, and the hydrophilic polar groups, which are orientated towards the water, form a stable film. The interfacial film may act as a barrier to coalescence by physical or chemical effects due to the adsorbed emulsifying agent, by the repulsive effect of electrically charged groups, or by a combination of the two.

Generally, an emulsifying agent having a hydrophilic group which is large compared with the non-polar lipophilic portion of the molecule favours formation of an oil-in-water emulsion. An emulsifier with a relatively larger lipophilic group tends to produce a water-in-oil emulsion. The degree to which the emulsifying agent is soluble in each phase may give an indication which type of emulsion will be formed although other factors such as viscosity and phase volume ratio will have an influence.

Selection of Emulsifying Agent

The ideal emulsifying agent for pharmaceutical purposes should be stable, inert, and free from toxic and irritant properties; it should be odourless, tasteless, and colourless and low concentrations should produce stable emulsions of the desired type. Although emulsifiers of natural origin are widely used in pharmaceutical emulsions, the number of synthetic emulsifying agents which can be used for emulsions for oral ingestion is relatively small.

More rigid interfacial films can often be achieved by the use of two emulsifying agents. In such a combination, the secondary emulsifying agent usually has more lipophilic properties than the primary emulsifying agent and the two may complex to form highly charged condensed interfacial films. If the secondary emulsifier is added in quantities exceeding those needed to form a complex, the viscosity of the emulsion may be increased with a consequent improvement in stability.

Types of Emulsifying Agent

Emulsifying agents can be broadly classified into three groups, synthetic substances, natural products, and finely divided solids.

Synthetic Substances

The location of their surface activity on dissociation can be used to divide the synthetic emulsifiers into four further groups, anionic, cationic, non-ionic, and ampholytic.

Anionic emulsifying agents. Soaps formed from long chain (C_{12} to C_{18}) fatty acids, sulphated alcohols, and sulphonates comprise many of the anionic emulsifying agents in common use. On dissociation, the long-chain anion imparts surface activity, while the cation is inactive. Soaps and similar anionic agents are unsuitable for emulsions for internal use because of their unpleasant taste and irritant action on the intestinal mucosa. Good oil-in-water emulsions can be prepared from the alkali soaps, but they become unstable below pH 10 and are incompatible with acids and polyvalent inorganic and long-chain organic cations. Calcium, magnesium, zinc, and aluminium soaps are water-insoluble and form water-in-oil emulsions. Amine soaps yield oil-in-water emulsions and are made *in situ* by reaction between amines such as triethanolamine or isopropanolamine and fatty acids; they are less alkaline than alkali soaps (pH about 8) and more resistant to calcium ions or changes in pH. In the case of sulphated alcohols, such as sodium lauryl sulphate or triethanolamine lauryl sulphate, the hydrophilic group is the sulphuric acid ester; they often have strong wetting properties and form oil-in-water emulsions but usually require a secondary emulsifier. Such emulsions have a pH of approximately 7 and are fairly resistant to pH change; they are used in creams and ointments. Dioctyl sodium sulphosuccinate is the sulphonate most commonly used in pharmacy; it is an effective wetting agent and forms oil-in-water emulsions preferentially when supplemented with a secondary emulsifier.

Cationic emulsifying agents. Cationic emulsifying agents dissociate to yield the surface-active cation and the inactive anion. Typical examples are quaternary ammonium compounds such as cetrimide, benzalkonium chloride, and domiphen bromide which, although used as emulsifying agents, have wider application as bactericides. By the use of a secondary emulsifier, oil-in-water emulsions for external application can be prepared which are stable over the pH range 3 to 7.
Emulsions made with cationic emulsifying agents are incompatible with those made with anionic materials.

Non-ionic emulsifying agents. The advantages of non-ionic emulsifying agents, which do not dissociate, are their high resistance to electrolytes, pH changes, and polyvalent inorganic cations; they are also compatible with other surface-active agents. One disadvantage is their tendency, when present in excess, to bind or to inactivate preservatives with phenolic or carboxylic acid groups.
Non-ionic emulsifiers can be made, often by the use of long-chain ethylene oxide polymers, in different physical forms with varying or balanced hydrophilic and lipophilic characteristics. The type of emulsion produced can depend on the hydrophilic-lipophilic balance of the emulsifying agent and this may be defined by the HLB number (see below).
Emulsions suitable for internal use can be made with certain non-ionic emulsifying agents, such as polysorbates and sorbitan esters.
Non-ionic materials constitute the largest group of emulsifying agents and include glyceryl esters, polyoxyethylene glycol esters and ethers, sorbitan esters, and polyoxyethylene sorbitan esters.
Glyceryl monostearate is a typical glyceryl ester, predominantly lipophilic and insoluble in water; it is a poor emulsifier but an effective stabiliser. However, with added soap, as in self-emulsifying monostearin, it can be used as a primary emulsifier for oil-in-water creams or lotions.
Polyoxyethylene glycol (macrogol) esters form emulsions which are less resistant to pH changes than those made with the ethers. Polyoxyethylene glycol (macrogol) ethers have a strong ether linkage and produce very stable emulsions which withstand acids and alkalis.
In sorbitan esters, the lipophilic element is predominant and these oil-soluble emulsifiers produce water-in-oil emulsions. The polysorbates are polyoxyethylene sorbitan mono- and tri-stearates, oleates, laurates, and palmitates; they yield oil-in-water emulsions of good stability which are resistant to pH changes and electrolytes. Polysorbate 80 is used in the preparation of parenteral emulsions and to emulsify dietary oils and fats. Mixtures of two non-ionic emulsifiers of different hydrophilic-lipophilic balance are often used in practice.

Ampholytic emulsifying agents. The surface-active agents are not widely used as emulsifiers; their chief applications are as bactericidal detergents or in shampoos which are non-irritant to the eyes. The ionic characteristics of ampholytic emulsifiers depend on the pH of the system; below a specific acid pH for each agent they are cationic and above a defined alkaline pH they are anionic, while at intermediate pH they behave as zwitterions. The main types of ampholytic substances are available as fatty acid derivatives, amino acids, and long-chain betaines.

Natural Products

Many traditional emulsifying agents are derived from plant or animal sources. Such substances are often complex and of undefined or variable chemical composition; they are thus subject to considerable variation in emulsifying power. In most cases, the mode of action of natural emulsifying agents is more dependent on increasing the viscosity of the aqueous phase than on surface activity at the interface and they are frequently used as stabilising agents in conjunction with a primary emulsifier.
The presence of microbial contamination is a major limitation of many natural emulsifiers and this can lead to rapid spoilage unless adequate preservatives are included. Some vegetable materials hydrolyse on storage with consequent reduction in emulsification power.

Gums and polysaccharides. In this group tragacanth and acacia are the most widely used, particularly in emulsions for internal use. Acacia yields stable emulsions of low viscosity which are often thickened with other gums such as tragacanth or agar. Emulsions of tragacanth alone are less stable and of coarser texture than those of acacia.
Agar is a poor emulsifier but produces viscous mucilages or gels; it is included in concentrations of about 1% as a stabiliser in acacia emulsions. Chondrus or Irish moss is also more effective as a viscolising agent than as a primary emulsifier. Other products from seaweed are salts of alginic acid which are available in a range of viscosity grades of reasonable consistency. They are used at a concentration of about 1% as thickeners and stabilisers, but tend to precipitate at pH values below 5 or in the presence of heavy metal ions.
Pectin has similar properties to tragacanth and is mainly used as a stabiliser.
Saponins are effective primary emulsifiers with marked surface activity which have only limited use in pharmacy in the form of quillaia liquid extract.
Methylcellulose and sodium carboxymethylcellulose are commonly used as emulsifiers and viscolising agents; both are used at concentrations of up to 2% and are available in various viscosity grades. Methylcellulose is non-ionic while sodium carboxymethylcellulose is anionic.

Emulsifying agents from animal sources. Steroidal emulsifying agents derived from animals include wool fat, wool alcohols, beeswax, cholesterol, and the bile salts sodium glycocholate and sodium taurocholate.
Wool fat and wool alcohols are used in topical preparations; they absorb water and form water-in-oil emul-

sions with other oils and fats. Wool alcohol is a more effective emulsifier than wool fat but both substances can be chemically modified to liquid or solid forms with different solvent and surface-active characteristics.

Cholesterol and related sterols are the principal emulsifying agents in lanolin products and beeswax; cholesterol also emulsifies the fatty substances in the human diet in conjunction with the bile salts and pancreatic fluids.

Lecithin, a phosphatide present with cholesterol in egg yolk and also in soya bean, shows surface activity and yields oil-in-water emulsions; it also has antoxidant activity but degrades rapidly in unpreserved systems. In oil-in-water emulsions made with egg yolk the hydrophilic effect of lecithin exceeds the lipophilic affinity of the cholesterol and a high degree of stability is obtained. One egg yolk will emulsify approximately 60 ml of volatile oil or 120 ml of fixed oils; such emulsions must contain a preservative.

Proteins. Gelatin and casein are only of limited value as emulsifiers, particularly in small-scale production; however, oil-in-water emulsions can be produced and improved by homogenisation. If type A (cationic) gelatin is used, acidic emulsions of pH 3 can be prepared, while for emulsions of pH 8 and above, type B gelatin is used.

Finely Divided Solids

A number of colloidal clays and several inorganic substances are effective emulsifiers when in the finely divided state and although the emulsions which result are often of coarse texture they show good stability and are less prone to microbial spoilage than many of those made with natural emulsifiers.

Of the colloidal clays, one of the most widely used in pharmacy is bentonite; others are aluminium magnesium silicate, attapulgite, and laponites. The clays absorb considerable amounts of water to form gels and in concentrations of 2 to 5% usually form oil-in-water emulsions, although bentonite will stabilise emulsion systems of either type.

Insoluble hydroxides and oxides of aluminium and magnesium can be absorbed at oil-water interfaces and are therefore of value as emulsifiers though relatively high concentrations are required. Hydrated aluminium oxide will emulsify oils in a disperse phase containing alcohol and will also stabilise water-in-oil emulsions. Magnesium hydroxide and magnesium oxide will form oil-in-water emulsions which usually require homogenisation.

The HLB System

The balance between the hydrophilic and lipophilic moieties of a surface-active molecule has been used as the basis for a more rational means of selecting and classifying emulsifying agents than the empirical methods traditionally used. In the HLB (hydrophile-lipophile balance) system, which was originally developed for non-ionic emulsifiers, each emulsifying agent is assigned a number between 1 and 20. In the case of non-ionic substances the number is calculated from the hydrocarbon chain length and the number of polar groupings; for other emulsifiers HLB values have been derived from other characteristics such as water solubility, dielectric constant, interfacial tension, and cloud points. As a rough guide, emulsifiers with HLB values of between 3 and 6 are lipophilic and form water-in-oil emulsions, while values of 8 to 18 indicate predominantly hydrophilic characteristics and the formation of oil-in-water emulsions. The relationship between HLB numbers and surfactant properties is as follows:

HLB range	Property
4–6	Emulsifying agents (w/o)
7–9	Wetting agents
8–18	Emulsifying agents (o/w)
13–15	Detergents
10–18	Solubilising agents

Extensive lists of HLB values for emulsifying agents have appeared in the literature. In addition, many oils and waxy materials used in emulsions have been given a "required HLB" value, determined by experiment, to facilitate the selection of the appropriate emulsifier. Examples of "required HLB" values are given below.

"REQUIRED HLB" VALUES FOR
OILS AND WAXES

	Emulsion type	
	o/w	w/o
Beeswax	12	5
Castor oil	14	—
Cetyl alcohol	15	—
Cottonseed oil	9	—
Paraffin, hard	10	4
Paraffin, liquid	12	4
Paraffin, soft	12	4
Stearic acid	16	—

Since HLB values can be added it is possible to calculate the amounts required for a mixture of two emulsifiers, one of low HLB and the other of high HLB value in order to obtain a blend of appropriate HLB for the oil to be emulsified. Greater efficiency is often obtained by using a blend of emulsifiers in this manner instead of a single substance. The following example illustrates the method used to determine the proportions of two emulsifiers:

Polysorbate 80 (HLB = 15) and sorbitan mono-oleate (HLB = 4.3) are to be used as the emulsifiers in the following oil-in-water system:

Liquid paraffin (req. HLB = 12)	30 g
Wool fat (req. HLB = 10)	5 g
Emulsifying agents (polysorbate 80) (sorbitan mono-oleate)	5 g
Water	to 100 g

1. Required HLB for the oily phase

$$= \frac{30}{35} \times 12 + \frac{5}{35} \times 10 = 11.7$$

2. Proportion of emulsifying agents required can then be calculated. If X is the percentage of polysorbate 80 in the blend $100-X$ is the percentage of sorbitan mono-oleate.

$$\text{Required HLB} = 11.7 = \frac{X}{100} \times 15 + \frac{(100-X)}{100} \times 4.3$$

$$X = 69\%$$

Therefore, in the final formulation the content of polysorbate 80 is 3.45 g and of sorbitan mono-oleate is 1.55 g.

The HLB system was originally devised for non-ionic emulsifiers but it has since been extended to include anionic and cationic substances. Some modification has been necessary and in the case of sodium lauryl sulphate which has marked hydrophilic activity an HLB number of 40 has been allocated. Furthermore HLB values may not be precise and several pairs of different emulsifiers with the same HLB numbers may not all produce similar emulsions. It is often necessary to prepare a series of emulsions in order to determine the optimum combination. Moreover, the HLB calculations do not take into account the concentration of emulsifier to be used. As a rough guide, 2% is considered optimum with a maximum of 5%, but again a series of samples may have to be prepared to determine the optimum concentration.

Further Information

For further information on emulsions see P. Becher, *Emulsions, Theory and Practice*, New York, Rheinhold, 1965; J. D. Davies and E. K. Rideal, *Interfacial Phenomena*, 2nd Edn, London, Academic Press, 1963; W. C. Griffin *et al.*, *Drug Cosmet. Ind.*, 1967, **101**, 41; B. Ecanow *et al.*, Emulsion technology, *Dispensing of Medication*, J. E. Hoover (Ed.), 8th Edn, Easton, Mack Publishing, 1971, p. 189; *Emulsions and Emulsion Technology, Part II*, K. Lissant (Ed.), New York, Marcel Dekker, 1974.

Emulsions

An emulsion consists of two immiscible liquid phases, one of which is finely subdivided and uniformly dispersed in the other; the system is stabilised by the presence of an emulsifying agent. The dispersed liquid, or internal phase, usually comprises globules of sizes down to 0.1 micrometre which are distributed within the external or continuous phase. In pharmaceutical emulsions, one phase is usually water while the other is an oil, fat, or waxy substance and systems are referred to as oil-in-water or water-in-oil. Emulsions can be prepared in which the dispersed particles are smaller than 0.1 micrometre; such particles tend to behave as colloids and the micro-emulsions formed may be transparent. Brownian movement of colloidal particles and subsequent collision leads to coalescence into larger globules of reduced mobility.

Emulsions can vary in viscosity from liquid to semi-solid. In pharmaceutical practice, it has been generally accepted that the title "emulsions" is applied to liquid preparations intended for oral administration. Semi-solid emulsions are referred to as creams and this title is usually restricted to preparations for external application.

Emulsions for oral ingestion are almost invariably of the oil-in-water type and are a convenient means for the presentation, in a diluted and possibly flavoured form, of oils and fats or oily solutions of water-insoluble or unpalatable drugs. Sterile oil-in-water emulsions of oily nutrients and vitamins together with carbohydrates have been used for feeding patients intravenously. The oil globules in such emulsions must be mainly about 1 micrometre and not greater than 5 micrometres in diameter and the emulsifying agent must be carefully selected. The intestinal absorption of oil from an oil-in-water emulsion taken orally is usually enhanced when globules have been homogenised to below 1 micrometre in diameter.

Methods of identification of emulsion type. The phase type of an emulsified system may be determined by examining the miscibility of its continuous phase when shaken or stirred with oil or water; care must be taken during dilution as phase inversion may occur. Since a continuous phase which is aqueous will transmit an electric current and one which consists of oil will not, electrical conductance can be used to distinguish between oil-in-water and water-in-oil systems.

When an emulsion is mixed with a water-soluble dye such

as amaranth and examined under a microscope, the continuous phase, if aqueous, should be coloured. If, however, an oil-soluble dye such as Sudan III is incorporated, the oil phase is coloured.

Another microscopic test requires that a drop of the emulsion is exposed to ultraviolet radiation. Because many oils fluoresce under ultraviolet radiation, a water-in-oil emulsion should show continuous fluorescence while in an oil-in-water type only the globules fluoresce.

Stability of emulsions. Although an emulsion can usually be formed from two immiscible liquids by the application of efficient agitation and adequate shearing forces, in most instances the dispersed droplets will rapidly coalesce and the original phases will re-form unless a suitable emulsifying agent is also present. Emulsifying agents of various types are examined in more detail in the entry on this subject.

Coalescence still occurs to some extent even in the presence of an emulsifying agent, especially of globules smaller than 0.5 micrometre, but in a stable emulsion the globules remain uniformly distributed throughout the continuous phase. Physical instability of emulsions can appear in three main forms, as "cracking" or separation, as "creaming" or sedimentation, or as flocculation or coagulation.

In "cracking", the globules of the dispersed phase coalesce due to rupture of the interfacial film. Film breakdown can often arise from chemical incompatibility of the emulsifier with additives or other constituents of the system; it may also be induced by exposure to increased or reduced temperatures. If the amount of the dispersed phase is increased until it approaches or exceeds the theoretical maximum of 74% of the total volume, the emulsion may "invert" (from oil-in-water to water-in-oil or vice versa) or it may completely break down. Inversion may also occur during the cooling of a heated emulsion or when electrolytes are added.

"Creaming" occurs when the dispersed globules move upwards through the continuous phase; in sedimentation the movement is downwards. A "creamed" emulsion can usually be redispersed by shaking as the globules do not coalesce to any great extent. Effecting a reduction in the particle size of the dispersed globules or an increase in the viscosity of the continuous phase are methods by which the rate of "creaming" can be reduced.

When flocculation occurs, the globules aggregate in clumps but the interfacial films do not necessarily break; often the globules can be redispersed by shaking. However, it is usual for flocculation to precede coalescence, though this does not occur in every case.

The chemical stability of components of an emulsion may be influenced by their distribution within the system, and conditions for oxidation or hydrolysis may be enhanced due to the extensive liquid interfaces.

Preparation of emulsions. Before an emulsion is prepared the oil-soluble and water-soluble constituents are separated, dissolved if necessary in the appropriate phase, and a suitable emulsifying agent is selected for the type of emulsion required (water-in-oil or oil-in-water); this also is dissolved in either the aqueous or the oil phase. Ideally, the internal phase volume should be between 40 and 60% of the total volume; lower phase volumes increase the tendency to "cream" or sediment, while higher volumes tend to cause inversion in emulsions of high viscosity. If it is necessary to melt or to heat constituents to maintain a fluid state in either phase, the other phase should be brought to a similar temperature before mixing and emulsification.

Generally, the dispersed phase is gradually added to the

continuous phase and often a more viscous primary concentrated emulsion is formed before the main bulk of the continuous phase is incorporated. Alternatively, the continuous phase may be added gradually to the disperse phase; while the disperse phase is in excess it will constitute the continuous phase of the first emulsion formed but as addition continues the first emulsion should invert to form the required type.

In a less frequently used method, all the emulsifying agent is mixed with a portion of one phase and then a portion of the other phase is incorporated. Successive additions of each phase are made until all have been included.

Emulsions for external application (creams, applications, liniments, and lotions) often include waxy solids which require melting before mixing; in cases such as these the order of mixing is less important. When soaps are included as emulsifiers these can be prepared at the interface by bringing together the fatty acid in the oil phase and the alkali in the aqueous phase.

Equipment. The mortar and pestle is a simple and inexpensive piece of equipment for the extemporaneous preparation of small quantities of emulsions although its efficiency is limited and in some systems globules may exceed 10 micrometres.

Electric mixers can also be used on the small scale though care must be taken to avoid excessive entrapment of air. On the larger scale, more controlled agitation and greater shearing forces can be obtained by using mechanical stirrers although their value may be limited for viscous emulsions. Colloid mills are suitable for continuous processing and produce high rates of shear and globules of very low particle size; the equipment may need cooling during operation.

Homogenisers are made for small-scale and large-scale production and may be used to both mix and emulsify a product or to improve the quality of a coarse emulsion pre-mixed in other equipment. The shearing forces produced can often be adjusted if the emulsion is to be recirculated through the equipment; small particle size ranges are produced.

By using oscillating devices, ultrasonic vibrations can be set up within coarse emulsions to induce cavitation and thus reduce the particle size of globules; equipment of this type is available for large- and small-scale production.

Preservation of emulsions. Micro-organisms can rapidly proliferate in emulsified systems with a high water content, particularly if carbohydrates, proteins, or steroidal materials are also present. Ideally, any preservative included in an emulsion should have both fungicidal and bactericidal activity since spoilage in such systems is often due to moulds and yeasts.

The polymorphic nature of emulsions presents special problems in preservation due to the partitioning of the preservative between the oily and the aqueous phases. To protect the product it is necessary to have an effective bactericidal and fungicidal concentration of preservative in the aqueous phase, but in order to achieve this the total concentration of preservative required may be clinically unacceptable if the preservative has a high partition coefficient between the particular oil and water.

Other problems can arise from interactions between preservatives and constituents of the emulsion. The presence of non-ionic emulsifying agents such as polysorbates or compounds with polyoxyethylene groups can inhibit or inactivate phenolic preservatives while hydroxybenzoate esters can be partially inactivated due to binding with polysorbates, povidone, certain macrogols, methylcellulose, and gelatin. Complexation of methylcellulose with hydroxybenzoates has also been reported.

Further information is given in the entry on Preservatives.

Antoxidants. In an emulsion where air may be incorporated during preparation and there is a large oil-water interface, conditions can be suitable for oxidation of the unsaturated organic compounds present in the vegetable oils, mineral oils, vitamin oils, and steroidal materials which are common constituents of emulsions. Inhibition of the rancidity and spoilage which can result from oxidation can be achieved by the inclusion in the oils of antoxidants such as the alkyl gallates, butylated hydroxyanisole, butylated hydroxytoluene, and tocopherols.

Further information is given in the entry on Antoxidants.

Containers for emulsions. Emulsions for internal use should be supplied in wide-mouthed bottles fitted with plastic screw closures which provide an airtight seal; metal caps should be avoided. Containers should be well filled to minimise evaporation and condensation during storage.

Labelling. A direction to shake the bottle should be given on the label.

FURTHER INFORMATION. Use of fat emulsions in parenteral nutrition—H. C. Meng, *Drug Intell. clin. Pharm.*, 1972, **6**, 321; evaluation of sustained-action parenteral emulsions—J. J. Windheuser *et al.*, *Bull. parent. Drug Ass.*, 1970, **24**, 286. Physical stability: emulsion stabilisation by non-ionic surfactants, experiment and theory (review)—A. T. Florence and J. A. Rogers, *J. Pharm. Pharmac.*, 1971, **23**, 153, 233; stability of oil-in-water emulsions (review)—E. R. Garrett, *J. pharm. Sci.*, 1965, **54**, 1557; J. A. Kitchener and P. R. Musselwhite, *Emulsion Science*, P. Sherman (Ed.), London, Academic Press, 1968. Phase inversion of emulsions (review)—V. B. Sunderland, *Aust. J. pharm. Sci.*, 1974, NS3 (1), 13. Stability testing and prediction: prediction of stability in pharmaceutical preparations: oil-in-water emulsion stability and the analytical ultracentrifuge—E. R. Garrett, *J. pharm. Sci.*, 1962, **51**, 35; accelerated stability testing of emulsions—M. J. Groves, *Pestic. Sci.*, 1970, **1**, 274; accelerated testing of emulsion stability—P. Sherman, *Soap Perfum. Cosm.*, 1971, **44**, 693; physical stability testing of pharmaceuticals—J. E. Tingstad, *J. pharm. Sci.*, 1964, **53**, 955. Emulsion theory: P. Becher, *Emulsions, Theory and Practice*, 2nd Edn, New York, Rheinhold, 1965; C. G. Sumner, *Clayton's Theory of Emulsions and their Technical Treatment*, 5th Edn, London, Churchill, 1954. Small-scale preparation of emulsions—W. C. Griffin *et al.*, *Drug Cosmet. Ind.*, 1967, **101**, 52; C. Gunn and S. J. Carter, *Dispensing for Pharmaceutical Students*, 12th Edn, London, Pitman, 1975; R. F. White, *Spalton's Pharmaceutical Emulsions and Emulsifying Agents*, 4th Edn, London, Chemist and Druggist, 1964. Equipment: small-scale emulsifying machinery—C. W. Ridout, *Manuf. Chem.*, 1961, **32**, 101; pharmaceutical applications of ultrasonics (review)—D. M. Skauen, *J. pharm. Sci.*, 1967, **56**, 1373. Preservation of emulsions against microbial attack—D. L. Wedderburn, *Advances in Pharmaceutical Sciences*, H. S. Bean *et al.* (Eds), Vol. 1, London, Academic Press, 1964.

Endometriosis

Endometriosis is a condition in which functioning endometrial tissue is found in an abnormal location. Common sites for the ectopic endometriosis include the ovary, broad ligament, utero-rectal pouch, rectum, and sigmoid colon. The endometrial tissue forms a cyst which responds to the cyclic changes in oestrogen and progesterone by proliferating and bleeding into the cyst at the time of menstruation. Some of the fluid is absorbed resulting in a tarry cyst which may grow as large as an orange. Rupture of such a cyst may result in multiple adhesions.

The symptoms of endometriosis are very varied, depending upon location, but usually include pain around the time of menstruation and menstrual irregularities.

Remission or cure of endometriosis may be achieved by a course of treatment with progestational steroids with or without oestrogens, or by surgery.

Pregnancy will usually result in cure of endometriosis. Progestogens used in the treatment of endometriosis include ethynodiol, medroxyprogesterone acetate, norethisterone, and norethynodrel.

Enemas

Enemas are aqueous or oily solutions or suspensions for rectal administration. Any solid substances or oils contained in them should be uniformly dispersed.

Enemas are given for their anthelmintic, anti-inflammatory, nutritive, purgative, or sedative effects, or for X-ray examination of the lower bowel.

Retention enemas should preferably be used after defaecation; they should be administered slowly with the patient lying on one side and the patient should then lie prone and retain the enema for at least 30 minutes to allow distribution and absorption of the medicament.

Large-volume enemas should be warmed to body temperature before administration.

Containers. Enemas should be supplied in coloured fluted glass bottles or in single-use plastic packs fitted with a rectal nozzle which should be lubricated before use.

Enterobiasis

Enterobiasis (Oxyuriasis) is a helminth infection caused by the threadworm *Enterobius vermicularis* which is about 10 to 15 mm long. Ova which are swallowed hatch, develop, and copulate in the small intestine. The males die and the females travel to the rectum where they work their way out of the anus and lay their eggs on the perineum causing pruritus ani. Infection and reinfection may be caused by the ova via the faecal-oral route, and by hatched larvae which migrate through the anus. Several members of a family may be affected.

Substances used in the treatment of threadworm infection include piperazine, thiabendazole, and viprynium.

Ephedrine

(−)-(1R,2S)-2-Methylamino-1-phenylpropan-1-ol hemihydrate, an alkaloid obtained from certain species of *Ephedra*, particularly *E. sinica* Stapf and *E. equisetina* Bunge, indigenous to China, and *E. gerardiana* Wall. (Fam. Ephedraceae), indigenous to India. The structure exists in four isomeric forms, *l*-ephedrine and *d*-ephedrine

and *l*- and *d*-pseudoephedrine, but only *l*-ephedrine and *d*-pseudoephedrine occur naturally. Ephedrine may also be prepared synthetically.

$$\left[C_6H_5 - \overset{OH}{\underset{H}{\overset{|}{C}}} - \overset{NH\cdot CH_3}{\underset{H}{\overset{|}{C}}} - CH_3 \right] \tfrac{1}{2}H_2O$$

$C_{10}H_{15}NO, \tfrac{1}{2}H_2O = 174.2$

OTHER NAMES: Ephedrinum; Ephedrinum Hydratum; Hydrated Ephedrine

A standard is given in the European Pharmacopoeia Vol. III

Description. Colourless hexagonal prismatic crystals or a white crystalline powder with a bitter taste; odourless or with a slight aromatic odour.

Solubility. Soluble, at 20°, in 36 parts of water, in less than 1 part of alcohol, and in 20 parts of glycerol; soluble in 25 parts of olive oil and in 100 parts of liquid paraffin with separation of water; soluble in ether and in chloroform with turbidity due to separation of water. The anhydrous alkaloid forms clear solutions in liquid paraffin.

Moisture content. 4.5 to 5.5%, determined by Fischer titration.

Specific rotation. −41° to −43°, determined on a 4.5% solution in *dilute hydrochloric acid.*

Dissociation constant. pK_a 9.6 (25°).

Storage. It should be stored in airtight containers, protected from light.

Identification. TESTS. 1. Dissolve about 10 mg in 1 ml of water and add 4 drops of *strong sodium hydroxide solution* and 4 drops of *copper sulphate solution*; a violet colour is produced. Add 2 ml of ether and shake; the ethereal layer is purple and the aqueous layer is blue.

2. Dissolve 1 g in 20 ml of carbon tetrachloride, add a small quantity of copper turnings and shake frequently; a turbidity appears followed by a copious precipitate. Allow to stand for 15 minutes, remove the copper turnings, and filter; the residue, after washing with three successive 5-ml portions of carbon tetrachloride, recrystallising from a mixture of ether and alcohol (95%), and drying at 105°, melts at about 218°.

MELTING-POINT. About 41°.

ULTRAVIOLET ABSORPTION. In 0.1N hydrochloric acid, maxima at 253 nm (E1%, 1cm = 8.0), 259 nm (E1%, 1cm = 9.4), and 265 nm (E1%, 1cm = 6.9); in alcohol (95%), maxima at 254 nm (E1%, 1cm = 8.6), 259 nm (E1%, 1cm = 9.9), and 265 nm (E1%, 1cm = 7.8).

Determination in body fluids. ULTRAVIOLET SPECTRO-PHOTOMETRY. In serum and urine: phenylpropanolamine and pseudoephedrine are stated to interfere—J. E. Wallace, *J. pharm. Sci.*, 1969, **58**, 1489.

GAS CHROMATOGRAPHY. In urine—A. H. Beckett *et al.*, *J. Pharm. Pharmac.*, 1972, **24**, 65P. In plasma—M. E. Pickup and J. W. Paterson, *J. Pharm. Pharmac.*, 1974, **26**, 561.

Metabolism. ABSORPTION. Readily absorbed after oral or percutaneous administration; gastro-intestinal absorption is increased by antacids but decreased by kaolin.

BLOOD CONCENTRATION. After an oral dose of 22 mg of the hydrochloride, peak plasma concentrations of 40 to 140 ng/ml are attained and, after an oral daily dose of 33 mg of the hydrochloride, peak plasma concentrations of 65 to 120 ng/ml are attained during therapy; effective bronchodilator plasma concentrations are in the range 35 to 80 ng/ml.

HALF-LIFE. Plasma half-life, 3 to 11 hours.

DISTRIBUTION. Accumulates in the liver, lungs, kidneys, spleen, and brain.

METABOLIC REACTIONS. N-Demethylation and oxidative deamination followed by conjugation.

EXCRETION. Up to about 95% of a dose may be excreted in the urine in 24 hours, 55 to 75% as unchanged drug, 8 to 20% as the N-demethylated metabolite, and 4 to 13% as deaminated metabolites such as benzoic acid, hippuric acid, and 1-phenyl-propane-1,2-diol; the rate of urinary excretion of ephedrine is pH-dependent and is increased in acid urine.

FURTHER INFORMATION. Urinary excretion—A. H. Beckett *et al.*, *J. Pharm. Pharmac.*, 1972, **24**, 65P; pharmacokinetics—J. F. Costello, *Br. J. clin. Pharmac.*, 1975, **2**, 180P; bronchodilator effects—C. S. May *et al.*, *Br. J. clin. Pharmac.*, 1975, **2**, 533; metabolism—P. S. Sever *et al.*, *Eur. J. clin. Pharmac.*, 1975, **9**, 193; absorption, metabolism, and excretion—G. R. Wilkinson and A. H. Beckett, *J. Pharmac. exp. Ther.*, 1968, **162**, 139.

Actions and uses. Ephedrine is a sympathomimetic amine with direct and indirect effects on adrenoreceptors. It resembles adrenaline and amphetamine in its actions.

When given by mouth in therapeutic doses as the hydrochloride, ephedrine constricts the peripheral vessels, thus raising the blood pressure. It relaxes the bronchioles and decreases the tone and peristaltic movements of the intestine but contracts the uterus. It contracts the sphincter but relaxes the detrusor muscle of the bladder, dilates the pupil, and stimulates the central nervous system. The prolonged administration of ephedrine has no cumulative effect but tolerance may develop.

Ephedrine hydrochloride has been given by intramuscular injection to combat a fall in blood pressure arising from attacks of syncope or anaphylactic shock. It is given by mouth or by subcutaneous injection to prevent attacks of bronchial spasm; its action is delayed in onset and is only fully established after about 1 hour, but its effect lasts for about 4 hours. Belladonna or atropine is often administered with ephedrine to augment its bronchodilator actions.

It is given by mouth for the treatment or prevention of attacks of bronchospasm in asthma and is widely prescribed in admixture with theophylline and barbiturates, although it is doubtful whether these compound preparations are more effective than ephedrine alone.

Its action on the bladder may be used in controlling nocturnal enuresis in children.

It is applied locally, usually in the form of a solution of a soluble ephedrine salt to relieve congestion of mucous membranes in acute sinusitis, hay fever, urticaria, and serum sickness but excessive use may lead to a worsening of the condition.

It has been used in conjunction with neostigmine to decrease the fatigue of voluntary muscle in myasthenia gravis.

Undesirable effects. A variety of undesirable effects may arise in patients with idiosyncrasy to ephedrine or as a result of overdosage. These effects include anxiety, restlessness, nausea, muscular weakness and tremors, sweating and thirst, and sometimes dermatitis. The insomnia produced in adults by ephedrine may be re-lieved by the administration of a benzodiazepine such as nitrazepam. In patients with prostatic hypertrophy, ephedrine may give rise to retention of urine.

Precautions and contra-indications. Ephedrine should not be given to patients who are being treated with a monoamine-oxidase inhibitor, such as isocarboxazid, nialamide, phenelzine, or tranylcypromine, or within about 2 weeks of the discontinuation of such treatment. Because of its effects on the cardiovascular system, ephedrine is contra-indicated in coronary thrombosis and thyrotoxicosis. It should be used with caution in patients with urinary retention and hypertension.

Ephedrine Hydrochloride

(−)-(1R,2S)-N-(1-Hydroxy-1-phenylprop-2-yl)-N-methylammonium chloride
$C_{10}H_{16}ClNO = 201.7$

OTHER NAMES: Ephed. Hydrochlor.; Ephedrini Hydrochloridum
CAM® (with butethamate citrate); *Argotone®* (with mild silver protein); *Rubelix®* (with pholcodine)

A standard is given in the European Pharmacopoeia Vol. III

Description. Odourless, colourless crystals or white crystalline powder, with a bitter taste.

Solubility. Soluble, at 20°, in 4 parts of water and in 17 parts of alcohol; very slightly soluble in chloroform.

Specific rotation. −33.5° to −35.5°, determined on a 5% solution.

Dissociation constant. See under Ephedrine.

Sterilisation. Solutions for injection are sterilised by heating in an autoclave or by filtration.

Storage. It should be stored in airtight containers, protected from light.

Identification. TESTS. It complies with the tests described under Ephedrine.

MELTING-POINT. About 218°.

ULTRAVIOLET ABSORPTION. See under Ephedrine.

INFRA-RED ABSORPTION. Major peaks at 699, 705, 754, 994, 1049, and 1453 cm⁻¹ (see Appendix 2a: Infra-red Spectra).

Determination in body fluids. See under Ephedrine.

Metabolism. See under Ephedrine.

Actions and uses. Ephedrine hydrochloride has the actions, uses, and undesirable effects described under Ephedrine. It is the form in which ephedrine is usually given by mouth or by injection, although great care is necessary in the parenteral administration of aqueous solutions of the drug.

The usual dose by mouth is 15 to 60 milligrams. Children up to 1 year may be given 7.5 milligrams, 1 to 5 years 15 milligrams, and 6 to 12 years 30 milligrams. These doses may be given 3 times daily.

Aqueous solutions containing 0.5 to 5% are used for application to mucous membranes. The nasal drops may be used to reduce swelling of the turbinate bodies in hay fever and catarrhal infections.

Precautions and contra-indications. As for Ephedrine.

Preparations

EPHEDRINE ELIXIR (*Syn.* Ephedrine Hydrochloride Elixir):

Ephedrine hydrochloride	3.0 g
Lemon spirit	0.2 ml
Compound tartrazine solution	10.0 ml
Chloroform spirit	40.0 ml
Water for preparations	60.0 ml
Alcohol (90%)	100.0 ml
Invert syrup	200.0 ml
Glycerol	200.0 ml
Syrup..	to 1000.0 ml

Dissolve the ephedrine hydrochloride in the water, add the glycerol, the compound tartrazine solution, the alcohol, the chloroform spirit, the lemon spirit, the invert syrup, and sufficient syrup to produce the required volume, and mix.

It contains in 5 ml, 15 mg of ephedrine hydrochloride. When a dose less than or not a multiple of 5 ml is prescribed, the elixir may be diluted, as described in the entry on Elixirs, with syrup. The diluted elixir must be freshly prepared.

A standard for this elixir is given in the British Pharmaceutical Codex 1973

EPHEDRINE HYDROCHLORIDE TABLETS: available as tablets containing 30 and 60 mg of ephedrine hydrochloride.

A standard for these tablets is given in the British Pharmacopoeia 1973

Containers and *Storage:* see the entry on Tablets for general information on containers and storage. Containers should be airtight.

EPHEDRINE NASAL DROPS:

Ephedrine hydrochloride	0.5 g
Chlorbutol	0.5 g
Sodium chloride	0.5 g
Water for preparations	to 100 ml

A standard for these nasal drops is given in the British Pharmaceutical Codex 1973

Containers: see the entry on Nasal Drops for general information on containers.

Advice for patients: prolonged or excessive use of the nasal drops should be avoided.

PAEDIATRIC BELLADONNA AND EPHEDRINE MIXTURE:

Belladonna tincture	30 ml
Ephedrine hydrochloride	1.5 g
Potassium iodide	10.0 g
Concentrated anise water	20 ml
Benzoic acid solution	20 ml
Liquorice liquid extract	30 ml
Syrup..	100 ml
Water for preparations	to 1000 ml

It should be recently prepared.

A standard for this mixture is given in the British Pharmaceutical Codex 1973

Dose: CHILD: up to 1 year, 5 millilitres; 1 to 5 years, 10 millilitres.

Advice for patients: the mixture should not be used for longer than a few days without medical advice.

OTHER PREPARATIONS available include an ELIXIR containing ephedrine hydrochloride 4 mg with butethamate citrate 4 mg in 5 ml, diluent syrup or water, life of diluted elixir 14 days; an elixir containing ephedrine hydrochloride 6 mg with pholcodine 4 mg in 5 ml, diluent syrup, life of diluted elixir 14 days; EYE-DROPS containing ephedrine hydrochloride 5% (in single-dose form); and NASAL DROPS containing ephedrine hydrochloride 0.9% with mild silver protein 1%.

Epilepsy

Epilepsy is characterised by seizures caused by paroxysmal disturbances in the electrical activity of the brain. An epileptic fit may be defined as a transitory disorder of cerebral function usually associated with a disturbance of consciousness and accompanied by sudden excessive electrical changes in the cerebral neurones. It may be idiopathic or may be precipitated by an underlying tumour or the administration of certain drugs such as chlorpromazine.

Generalised seizures are characterised by a loss of consciousness accompanied by generalised symmetrical electrical changes. These include the grand mal and petit mal epilepsies.

Grand mal (major fits). The patient experiences episodes of loss of consciousness and spasm of musculature including the respiratory muscles lasting for about half a minute. A characteristic cry may be made and this is followed by a further half minute in which jerky movements of the tongue and jaw may be observed and there may be tongue biting and incontinence. A comatose state follows, merging into normal sleep.

Phenobarbitone and phenytoin sodium are the drugs principally used in the prevention of grand mal fits but a number of other drugs, including carbamazepine, ethotoin, methoin, primidone, sodium valproate, and sulthiame, are sometimes used.

Petit mal. This form of epilepsy begins in childhood and may persist into adult life. It is characterised by frequent transitory lapses of consciousness. Occasionally there is jerking of the arm or, rarely, akinetic seizure in which the patient falls to the ground.

Medicines commonly used in the treatment of petit mal epilepsy include acetazolamide, clonazepam, ethosuximide, paramethadione, sodium valproate, and troxidone.

Psychomotor seizures are usually caused by disturbance in a localised area of the brain most commonly in the temporal lobe and are therefore sometimes referred to as *temporal lobe epilepsy.* The fits are characterised by a dream-like state and amnesia but consciousness is not usually lost. Hallucinations of colour, taste, and hearing may occur.

The drugs used in the treatment of psychomotor seizures are primidone and sulthiame, and sometimes carbamazepine, diazepam, phenytoin, and sodium valproate.

Myoclonic jerks are manifested as random involuntary movements usually involving the upper limbs, frequently provoked by noise or other sensory stimuli. These seizures are commonly associated with petit mal, less frequently with grand mal epilepsy, and rarely with progressive mental deterioration.

The usual drugs used in treatment are clonazepam, diazepam, and ethosuximide.

Salaam attacks or infantile spasms are sudden repetitive contractions of limbs and trunk beginning in the first year of life and associated with mental retardation. Corticotrophin and nitrazepam are used in the treatment of infantile spasms.

Status epilepticus is a condition in which fits occur in rapid succession without a recovery period and consequently it may have a fatal outcome unless rapidly controlled. It may be precipitated by abrupt withdrawal of anticonvulsant drugs or alcohol. It may be necessary to gag the patient to ensure all airways are clear.

Status epilepticus may be controlled by injection, intravenously if possible, of diazepam, phenobarbitone sodium, or phenytoin sodium; intramuscular injections of paraldehyde are also used.

Epinephrine

see ADRENALINE

Ergometrine Maleate

The hydrogen maleate of ergometrine, (6aR,9R)-4,6,6a,7,8,9-hexahydro-N-[(2S)-1-hydroxyprop-2-yl]-7-methylindolo[4,3-fg]quinoline-9-carboxamide *or* (+)-N-[(2S)-1-hydroxyprop-2-yl]-D-lysergamide, a water-soluble alkaloid obtained from ergot or prepared by partial synthesis.

$C_{23}H_{27}N_3O_6 = 441.5$

OTHER NAMES: Ergometrinii Maleas; Ergonovine Maleate

Syntometrine® (with oxytocin)

A standard is given in the European Pharmacopoeia Vol. I

Description. A white or yellowish, crystalline, odourless powder.

Solubility. Soluble, at 20°, in 40 parts of water, giving a solution with a blue fluorescence, and in 100 parts of alcohol (90%); practically insoluble in ether and in chloroform.

Acidity. A 1% solution has a pH of 3 to 5.

Moisture content. Not more than 2%, determined by drying at 80° *in vacuo*.

Specific rotation. +50° to +56°, determined on a 1% solution.

Dissociation constant. pK_a 6.8 (20°).

Sterilisation. Solutions for injection are sterilised by heating in an autoclave in an atmosphere of nitrogen or other suitable gas.

Storage. It should be stored in an atmosphere of nitrogen, in hermetically sealed containers, in a cool place, protected from light.

Identification. TESTS. 1. To 2 drops of a 1% solution add 10 drops of water; the solution shows a blue fluorescence. Add 1 drop of *iodine solution*; a dark brown flocculent precipitate is produced.

2. To 2 drops of a 1% solution add 1 ml of glacial acetic acid, 1 drop of *ferric chloride solution*, and 1 ml of phosphoric acid, and heat on a water-bath at 80°; after a few minutes a blue or violet colour develops.

3. To 1 drop of a 1% solution add 10 drops of water and 1 ml of *dimethylaminobenzaldehyde solution*; an intense dark blue colour is produced.

MELTING-POINT. About 167°, with decomposition.

Determination in body fluids. THIN-LAYER CHROMATOGRAPHY. In urine: separation and identification—A. S. Curry, *J. Pharm. Pharmac.*, 1959, **11**, 411.

Metabolism. METABOLIC REACTIONS. Hydroxylation and glucuronic acid conjugation and possibly N-demethylation.

EXCRETION. The glucuronides of ergometrine and ergometrinine are excreted in the bile of rats along with the glucuronides of 12-hydroxyergometrine and 12-hydroxyergometrinine following a dose of ergometrine.

FURTHER INFORMATION. Metabolites in rat bile—M. V. Slaytor and S. E. Wright, *J. mednl pharm. Chem.*, 1962, **5**, 483.

Actions and uses. Ergometrine is the alkaloid responsible for the oxytocic activity of aqueous extracts of ergot.

When administered by mouth in solution, ergometrine causes contractions of the uterus, which begin about 8 minutes after administration; after about an hour, the contractions become less frequent.

When ergometrine is administered by intramuscular injection, uterine contractions begin within 2 minutes; when the injection is given intravenously, they begin within 1 minute.

Its action is slower in onset and more prolonged than that of oxytocin.

The usual dose by mouth is 0.5 to 1 milligram, the usual intramuscular dose is 0.2 to 1 milligram, and the intravenous dose is 100 to 500 micrograms.

Ergometrine has little effect on the sympathetic nervous system, and in this respect differs from ergotamine.

Ergometrine is used mainly in the prevention and treatment of post-partum haemorrhage due to uterine atony. It may be given in conjunction with oxytocin. In emergencies, when a rapid response is needed, it may be given intravenously.

Precautions. It should not be given during the first or second stage of labour, as the contraction might cause the death of the foetus or rupture the uterus. Because of its powerful oxytocic action, it is not generally administered before the expulsion of the placenta.

Preparations

ERGOMETRINE AND OXYTOCIN INJECTION: a sterile solution of ergometrine maleate and synthetic oxytocin in water for injections. It may contain suitable stabilising agents. The acidity of the solution is adjusted to pH 3.3 by the addition of maleic acid. The solution is sterilised by filtration, distributed by means of an aseptic technique, into sterile ampoules, the air in the ampoules is replaced with sterile nitrogen or other suitable gas, and the ampoules are immediately sealed. Available as an injection containing 500 micrograms of ergometrine maleate and 5 units (oxytocic) of synthetic oxytocin per ml in 1-ml ampoules.

A standard for this injection is given in the British Pharmacopoeia Addendum 1978

Containers: see the entry on Injections for general information on containers.

Labelling: see the entry on Injections for general information on labelling. In addition, the label on the container should state the amount of the medicament with respect to the oxytocin as the number of units (oxytocic) per ml and the label on the container or the label on the package should also state that the oxytocin is synthetic.

Storage: it should be stored at a temperature not exceeding 25°, protected from light. Under these conditions it may be expected to retain its potency for at least 2 years from the date of manufacture.

ERGOMETRINE INJECTION (*Syn.* Ergonovine Maleate Injection): a sterile solution of ergometrine maleate in water for injections free from dissolved air. It may contain suitable stabilising agents. The acidity of the solution is adjusted to pH3 by the addition of maleic acid. The solution is distributed into ampoules, the air in the ampoules is replaced with nitrogen or other suitable gas, and the ampoules are immediately sealed. It is sterilised by heating in an autoclave. The solution should be protected from light during preparation.
The usual strength is 500 micrograms of ergometrine maleate per ml.
A standard for this injection is given in the British Pharmacopoeia 1973
Containers and *Labelling:* see the entry on Injections for general information on containers and labelling.
Storage: it should be protected from light.

ERGOMETRINE TABLETS (*Syn.* Ergonovine Maleate Tablets): available as tablets containing 250 and 500 micrograms of ergometrine maleate.
A standard for these tablets is given in the British Pharmacopoeia 1973
Containers and *Storage:* see the entry on Tablets for general information on containers and storage. Containers should be airtight and light resistant.

Ergotamine Tartrate

The tartrate of ergotamine, $(-)$-N-{(2R,5S,10aS,10bS)-5-benzyl-10b-hydroxy-2-methyl-3,6-dioxoperhydro-oxazolo[3,2 - a]pyrrolo[2,1-c]pyrazin-2-yl}-D-lysergamide, an alkaloid obtained from certain species of ergot. It may contain 2 molecules of methanol of crystallisation.

$C_{70}H_{76}N_{10}O_{16} = 1313.4$

OTHER NAMES: Ergotamini Tartras; *Femergin*®; *Lingraine*®; *Medihaler Ergotamine*®
Cafergot® and *Effergot*® (both with caffeine)

A standard is given in the European Pharmacopoeia Vol. III

Description. Odourless colourless crystals or white crystalline powder.

Solubility. Soluble in water, the solution possibly becoming turbid, but the turbidity may be removed by adding tartaric acid; soluble, at 20°, in 500 parts of alcohol (90%).

Acidity. A 0.25% suspension has a pH of 4 to 6.

Moisture content. Not more than 6%, determined by drying at 95° *in vacuo*.

Dissociation constant. pK_a 6.3 (25°).

Stability. In aqueous solution, ergotamine degrades by epimerisation to ergotaminine until an equilibrium is attained between the two substances. In acidic solu-

tions, ergotamine and ergotaminine invert to form aci-ergotamine and aci-ergotaminine. Ergotamine also degrades by hydrolysis to lysergic acid amide and isolysergic acid amide, by photolysis to various lumi-compounds, and by oxidation.
The rate of degradation due to reactions other than epimerisation is minimal at pH 3.6.

FURTHER INFORMATION. Stability in aqueous solution —B. Kreilgård and J. Kisbye, *Arch. Pharm. Chemi, scient. Edn*, 1974, **2**, 1 and 38.

Sterilisation. Solutions for injection are sterilised by filtration and immediately sealed into containers the air in which is replaced by nitrogen or other suitable gas.

Storage. It should be stored in an atmosphere of nitrogen, in hermetically sealed containers, in a cool place, protected from light.

Identification. TESTS. 1. It complies with Tests 2 and 3 described under Ergometrine Maleate.
2. Dissolve about 2 mg in 2 ml of *dilute sulphuric acid* with the aid of gentle heat, dissolve a few mg of magnesium powder in the solution, add 25 mg of resorcinol, shake to dissolve, carefully pour 2 ml of sulphuric acid to form a lower layer, and warm gently; a red ring forms at the interface of the two liquids and spreads throughout the lower layer.

MELTING-POINT. It decomposes, without melting, at about 190°.

Determination in body fluids. THIN-LAYER CHROMATOGRAPHY. In plasma—M. Amin and W. Sepp, *J. Chromat.*, 1976, **118**, 225.

Metabolism. Poorly absorbed after oral administration; rapidly metabolised in the body and very little unchanged drug is excreted in the urine.

Actions and uses. Ergotamine stimulates and, in large doses, paralyses the motor terminations of the sympathetic nerves. Prolonged administration produces gangrene due to constriction of the peripheral arterioles with consequent arrest of blood flow. When given by intravenous injection it causes contraction of involuntary muscle, including that of the uterus, and a rise in blood pressure.
Ergotamine is used chiefly in the treatment of migraine. It acts most reliably when given by subcutaneous or intramuscular injection, but it is often given by mouth, preferably sublingually, or in suppositories. The most successful results are obtained when it is given before the symptoms are fully established.
The initial dose of ergotamine tartrate is 1 to 2 milligrams by mouth at the first warning of an attack repeated if necessary at half hour intervals until relief is obtained. The most effective therapeutic results are obtained when the drug is injected subcutaneously or intramuscularly in doses of 250 to 500 micrograms. Ergotamine tartrate may also be given rectally in doses of 2 milligrams repeated at hourly intervals if necessary. The restriction given below under "Precautions and contra-indications" should be observed.
Ergotamine tartrate can be administered by oral inhalation in a dose of 360 micrograms at the beginning of an attack of migraine. This may be repeated after 5 minutes if necessary. Not more than 6 inhalations a day or 15 a week should be taken.

Undesirable effects. Ergotamine, when used in the recommended doses for the treatment of migraine, rarely produces undesirable effects other than headache, nausea, and vomiting; occasionally, however, it produces muscular weakness and pain. In large repeated doses it can produce all the symptoms of ergot poisoning, including gangrene of the extremities and serious mental derangement.

Precautions and contra-indications. It should be used with caution in patients with peripheral vascular and ischaemic heart disease and it should preferably not be given to such patients by injection. It should also be given with caution to patients receiving oral contraceptives. Not more than 6 to 8 milligrams of ergotamine tartrate should be taken orally or rectally for any 1 attack of migraine, and not more than 12 milligrams in any 1 week. Ergotamine tartrate should not be used for the prophylaxis of migraine. It should not be given during preganancy or lactation or in serious liver or kidney disease.

Poisoning. In the event of overdosage the stomach should be washed out and amyl nitrite inhaled.

Preparations

COMPOUND ERGOTAMINE SUPPOSITORIES: containing ergotamine tartrate, caffeine, butalbital, and belladonna alkaloids in a suitable basis. Available as suppositories containing 2 mg of ergotamine tartrate, 100 mg of caffeine, 100 mg of butalbital, and 250 micrograms of belladonna alkaloids.
Containers and Storage: see the entry on Suppositories for general information on containers and storage. The suppositories should be stored in a cool place.
Advice for patients: see the entry on Suppositories for general information on the use of suppositories. The suppositories should be used as indicated by the prescriber at the first warning of an attack and the patient instructed to lie down in a darkened room for 2 hours after initiating treatment. Not more than 3 suppositories of ergotamine tartrate should be used in 24 hours or 5 suppositories in any 1 week.

ERGOTAMINE AEROSOL INHALATION: a suspension of ergotamine tartrate, in sufficiently fine powder to meet the requirements of the standard, in a suitable mixture of aerosol propellents, which may contain a surface-active agent, stabilising agents, and other adjuvants. It is packed in a pressurised container fitted with a special metering valve and an oral adapter.
Available as an aerosol inhalation delivering 360 micrograms of ergotamine tartrate to the patient each time the valve is actuated.
A standard for this aerosol inhalation is given in the British Pharmaceutical Codex 1973
Containers, Labelling, and Storage: see the entry on Aerosol Inhalations for general information on containers, labelling, and storage.
Advice for patients: see the entry on Aerosol Inhalations for general information on the use of aerosol inhalations. The patient should be advised verbally to read the instructions on the leaflet enclosed with the product. The aerosol inhalation should be used as indicated by the prescriber at the first warning of an attack and the patient instructed to lie down in a darkened room for 2 hours after initiating treatment. Not more than 6 inhalations of ergotamine tartrate should be taken in 24 hours or 15 inhalations in any 1 week.

ERGOTAMINE INJECTION: a sterile solution of ergotamine tartrate with alcohol (95%) and glycerol in water for injections. The acidity of the solution is adjusted to pH 3.3 by the addition of tartaric acid. 60% of the total alkaloidal content is present as ergotamine tartrate. The solution is sterilised by filtration and, by means of an aseptic technique, distributed into sterile ampoules, the air in which is replaced by sterile nitrogen or other

suitable gas, and the ampoules are immediately sealed. Available as an injection containing 500 micrograms of ergotamine tartrate per ml in 1-ml ampoules.
A standard for this injection is given in the British Pharmacopoeia Addendum 1977
Containers and Labelling: see the entry on Injections for general information on containers and labelling.
Storage: it should be protected from light.

ERGOTAMINE TABLETS: available as tablets containing 1 and 2 mg of ergotamine tartrate; they are sugar coated.
A standard for these tablets is given in the British Pharmacopoeia 1973
Containers and Storage: see the entry on Tablets for general information on containers and storage. Containers should be airtight.
Advice for patients: the tablets should be taken as indicated by the prescriber at the first warning of an attack and the patient instructed to lie down in a darkened room for 2 hours after initiating treatment. Not more than 6 to 8 milligrams of ergotamine tartrate should be taken in 24 hours or 12 milligrams in any 1 week.

OTHER PREPARATIONS available include TABLETS containing ergotamine tartrate 1 mg with caffeine 100 mg, and tablets containing ergotamine tartrate 2 mg with caffeine 50 mg in an effervescent formulation.

Erythromycin

(2R,3S,4S,5R,6R,8R,10R,11R,12S,13R)-5-(3-Amino-3,4,6-trideoxy-NN-dimethyl-β-L-xylo-hexopyranosyl-oxy)-3-(2,6-dideoxy-3C,3O-dimethyl-α-L-ribo-hexopy-ranosyloxy)-13-ethyl-6,11,12-trihydroxy-2,4,6,8,10,12-hexamethyl-9-oxotridecan-13-olide, an antimicrobial substance produced by certain strains of Streptomyces erythreus Waksman.

$C_{37}H_{67}NO_{13} = 733.9$

OTHER NAMES: Erycen®; Erythrocin®; Erythromid®; Erytrotil®; Erythromycinum; Ilotycin®; Retcin®

A standard is given in the European Pharmacopoeia Vol. II

Description. Odourless, slightly hygroscopic, white or slightly yellow crystals or powder with a bitter taste.

Solubility. Soluble, at 20°, in 1000 parts of water, less soluble in hot water; soluble, at 20°, in 5 parts of alcohol and of ether and in 6 parts of chloroform; soluble in dilute hydrochloric acid.

Alkalinity. A saturated solution has a pH of 8 to 10.5.

Moisture content. Not more than 6.5%, determined by Fischer titration.

Specific rotation. $-71°$ to $-78°$, determined on a 2% solution in alcohol (95%) and measured 30 minutes after preparation of the solution.

Storage. It should be stored in airtight containers, protected from light, at a temperature below 30°.

Identification. TESTS. 1. To about 5 mg add 2 ml of sulphuric acid and shake gently; a reddish-brown colour is produced.

2. Dissolve about 3 mg in 2 ml of acetone and add 2 ml of hydrochloric acid; an orange colour is produced which changes to red and then to a deep purplish-red. Add 2 ml of chloroform and shake; the chloroform layer is coloured purple.

3. To about 5 mg add 5 ml of a 0.02% solution of xanthydrol in a mixture of 1 volume of hydrochloric acid and 99 volumes of acetic acid and heat on a water-bath; a red colour is produced.

MELTING-POINT. About 135°.

Determination in body fluids. SPECTROFLUORIMETRY. In whole blood, plasma, or serum—K. Tserng and J. G. Wagner, *Analyt. Chem.*, 1976, **48**, 348.

Metabolism. ABSORPTION. The base is destroyed by acid and is therefore administered in a resistant coating or as a stable ester; the esters which dissolve more slowly appear to be better absorbed than those which dissolve quickly; the rates of absorption of the base, estolate, and stearate salts are diminished by the presence of food; the stearate is hydrolysed in the intestine and the free erythromycin is absorbed but the estolate is absorbed as an ester and is then hydrolysed.

BLOOD CONCENTRATION. After an oral dose of 500 mg of the base, stearate, or estolate, peak serum concentrations of 0.9 to 1.4, 0.4 to 1.8, and 1.4 to 5.0 $\mu g/ml$ are attained respectively in 1 to 4 hours; after an intravenous dose of 250 mg of the gluceptate, serum concentrations of 3 to 10 $\mu g/ml$ are attained.

HALF-LIFE. Serum half-life for erythromycin, 1.2 to 4 hours, and for the estolate, about 1.6 hours; in subjects with oliguria the half-life is about 5 hours.

DISTRIBUTION. Erythromycin is widely distributed throughout the body; some retention occurs in the liver and spleen and it enters the cerebrospinal fluid when the meninges are inflamed; it crosses the placenta and is secreted in the milk; erythromycin also enters the pleural, synovial, and peritoneal fluids, and the aqueous humour; it may accumulate upon repeated dosage; *protein binding*, erythromycin is reported to be 20 to 70% bound, the stearate being more bound but less so than the estolate which is reported to be about 98% bound to plasma proteins.

METABOLIC REACTIONS. Hydrolysis of the ester forms and demethylation.

EXCRETION. 5 to 15% of a dose of erythromycin is excreted in the urine and large amounts of unchanged drug are excreted in the bile; the estolate is excreted as erythromycin or as the propionate.

FURTHER INFORMATION. Bioavailability—E. Triggs and M. A. Neaverson, *Med. J. Aust.*, 1973, **2**, 344; metabolism—J. Viallier *et al.*, *Thérapie*, 1961, **16**, 878; pharmacokinetics—J. Tréfouël and R. Paul, *Thérapie*, 1959, **14**, 171; protein binding—R. C. Gordon *et al.*, *J. pharm. Sci.*, 1973, **62**, 1074 and R. G. Weigund and A. H. C. Chun, *J. pharm. Sci.*, 1972, **61**, 425.

Actions and uses. Erythromycin is an antibiotic which is bacteriostatic under the conditions of clinical use and is effective in the treatment of infections due to a wide range of organisms. It acts by interfering with ribosomal protein synthesis within the bacterial cell.

When given by mouth it enters all tissues of the body except the meningeal space; it is excreted in the bile and by glomerular filtration but more than half is metabolised in the body so that it does not accumulate very rapidly in renal failure. Therapeutically active blood levels are maintained for 6 hours as erythromycin is largely excreted in the bile and re-absorbed.

Erythromycin is used mainly in the treatment of infections of patients allergic to penicillin and of infections caused by penicillinase-producing staphylococci, but it is also effective against infections due to many strains of leptospirae, of entamoebae, and of *Diplococcus pneumoniae, Streptococcus pyogenes, Streptococcus viridans, Haemophilus influenzae,* and *Bordetella pertussis.*

Its chief disadvantage is the ready induction within the bacterial cell of an alternative enzyme system which renders the drug ineffective and also produces resistance to other macrolide antibiotics and to lincomycin, leading to cross-resistance and interference, especially when these drugs are used in combination. It may also give rise to the dissemination of resistant strains in the community. Erythromycin should therefore be used only when other antibiotics cannot be used and when it has been established that the infecting organism is sensitive to its action.

Erythromycin is used in a dosage of 1 to 2 grams daily in divided doses.

As erythromycin is partially destroyed by acid gastric juice it is administered in enteric-coated tablets. Some erythromycin compounds are better absorbed than the base when given by mouth.

Externally, erythromycin is used as a 1% ointment for pyogenic skin infections and as a 0.5 to 1% ointment for eye infections.

Undesirable effects. Abdominal discomfort or pain and allergic drug eruptions may rarely occur.

Precautions. It should be administered with caution to patients with hepatic insufficiency.

Veterinary uses. Erythromycin is an antibacterial agent used mainly for the control of penicillin-resistant organisms and mycoplasmal infections.

The usual dose by deep intramuscular injection for cattle and sheep is 2 to 4 milligrams per kilogram body-weight, for pigs 2 to 6 milligrams per kilogram body-weight, for dogs and cats 2 to 10 milligrams per kilogram body-weight, and for poultry 10 to 40 milligrams per kilogram body-weight. The usual dose by mouth for dogs and cats is 2 to 10 milligrams per kilogram body-weight twice daily.

For sinusitis in turkeys, 100 milligrams may be injected into each sinus after removing the exudate and repeated if required after 5 to 7 days.

For respiratory mycoplasmosis in poultry, 100 parts per million may be given in the drinking water for 3 days or 100 parts per million in the feed for 5 days.

Preparations

ERYTHROMYCIN INJECTION: a sterile solution of erythromycin, with 2% of butyl aminobenzoate, in a non-aqueous water-miscible vehicle. It is sterilised by heating in an autoclave or by filtration. This preparation must not be mixed with water. Available in 50-ml vials containing 220 mg of erythromycin per ml.

A standard for this injection is given in the British Veterinary Codex Supplement 1970

Containers: see the entry on Injections for general information on containers.

Labelling: see the entry on Injections for general information on labelling. In addition, the label on the container should state that animals should not be slaughtered for human consumption within 48 hours after cessation of treatment, and that milk should not be drawn for human consumption from lactating animals within 48 hours after cessation of treatment.

Storage: it should be stored at a temperature not exceeding 30°, protected from light. It should not be allowed to freeze.

ERYTHROMYCIN SOLUBLE POWDER: consisting of erythromycin mixed with a suitable solubilising agent. It may contain suitable pharmaceutical adjuvants and colouring matter. Available as a soluble powder containing 30% of erythromycin.

A standard for this soluble powder is given in the British Veterinary Codex Supplement 1970

Containers and *Storage:* see the entry on Powders for general information on containers and storage. Containers should be airtight and light resistant.

Labelling: the label on the container should state the proportion of erythromycin in the preparation and directions for the medication of drinking water.

ERYTHROMYCIN TABLETS: available as tablets containing 250 mg of erythromycin; they are enteric coated and either film coated or sugar coated; the coat may be coloured.

A standard for these tablets is given in the British Pharmacopoeia 1973

Containers and *Storage:* see the entry on Tablets for general information on containers and storage. Containers should be airtight.

Labelling: the label on the container should state the date after which the tablets are not intended to be used, and the conditions under which they should be stored.

Advice for patients: the tablets should be taken at regular intervals preferably half to 1 hour before meals. They should be swallowed whole and milk and antacids should not be taken within 1 hour. The prescribed course should be completed.

OTHER VETERINARY PREPARATIONS available include an INTRAMAMMARY INJECTION containing erythromycin 52.5 mg per ml in 6-ml disposable syringes.

Erythromycin Estolate

Erythromycin 2'-propionate dodecyl sulphate
$C_{40}H_{71}NO_{14},C_{12}H_{26}O_4S = 1056.4$

OTHER NAME: *Ilosone®*

A standard is given in the British Pharmacopoeia 1973

Description. A white, crystalline, odourless, tasteless powder.

Solubility. Very slightly soluble in water; soluble, at 20°, in 2 parts of alcohol; soluble in chloroform; practically insoluble in dilute hydrochloric acid.

Moisture content. Not more than 4%, determined by Fischer titration.

Storage. It should be stored in airtight containers, protected from light.

Identification. TEST. Dissolve about 15 mg in 2 ml of acetone and add 2 ml of hydrochloric acid; an orange-red colour is produced which changes to red and then to deep purple. Add 2 ml of chloroform and shake; the chloroform layer is coloured purple.

MELTING-POINT. About 136°.

Determination in body fluids; Metabolism. See under Erythromycin.

Actions and uses. Erythromycin estolate has the antibacterial actions described under Erythromycin.

When given by mouth it is rapidly absorbed and, after therapeutic doses, the concentration of erythromycin in the blood is higher and a therapeutic level is maintained for a longer period than after equivalent doses of erythromycin; 144 milligrams of erythromycin estolate is approximately equivalent to 100 milligrams of erythromycin.

A dose equivalent to 1 to 2 grams of erythromycin may be given daily in divided doses for not more than 10 days. The oral dose for children, given every 6 hours is up to 1 year the equivalent of 80 milligrams of erythromycin, 1 to 5 years the equivalent of 125 milligrams, and 6 to 12 years the equivalent of 200 to 250 milligrams.

Erythromycin estolate is used for the treatment of pneumococcal, streptococcal, and staphylococcal infections in children.

Undesirable effects. Cholestatic jaundice has occasionally been reported after treatment has been continued for more than 10 days.

Contra-indications. It is contra-indicated in patients who develop jaundice in the course of treatment, even after the jaundice has subsided.

Preparations

ERYTHROMYCIN ESTOLATE CAPSULES: consisting of erythromycin estolate, which may be mixed with a suitable inert diluent, enclosed in a hard capsule. The capsule shells may be coloured. Available as capsules containing erythromycin estolate equivalent to 250 mg of erythromycin.

A standard for these capsules is given in the British Pharmacopoeia 1973

Containers and *Storage:* see the entry on Capsules for general information on containers and storage.

Labelling: the label on the container should state the amount of the medicament as the equivalent amount of erythromycin. In addition, the label on the container should state the date after which the capsules are not intended to be used, and the conditions under which they should be stored.

Advice for patients: the capsules should be taken at regular intervals. The prescribed course should be completed.

OTHER PREPARATIONS available include a MIXTURE containing erythromycin estolate equivalent to 125 and 250 mg of erythromycin in 5 ml, diluent syrup, life of diluted mixture 14 days; and TABLETS containing erythromycin estolate equivalent to 500 mg of erythromycin.

Erythromycin Ethylsuccinate

The ethyl succinate ester of erythromycin.
$C_{43}H_{75}NO_{16} = 862.1$

OTHER NAMES: *Erythrocin®; Erythroped®*

Description. A white or slightly yellow, odourless, almost tasteless, crystalline powder.

Solubility. Very slightly soluble in water; soluble in alcohol, in chloroform and in liquid macrogols.

Actions and uses. Erythromycin ethylsuccinate has the actions and uses described under Erythromycin and is administered by mouth or by deep intramuscular injection.

The usual dose for an adult is the equivalent of 1 to 2 grams of erythromycin daily by mouth in divided doses, increasing in severe infections to the equivalent of 4 grams or more daily. The usual dose given by mouth to children is the equivalent of 30 milligrams per kilogram body-weight daily in divided doses, increasing to the equivalent of 50 milligrams per kilogram body-weight daily if necessary.

The usual dose for an adult given by deep intramuscular injection is the equivalent of 100 milligrams of ery-thromycin every 8 to 12 hours, increasing to the equi-valent of 100 milligrams every 4 hours in more severe infections. For children of 15 kilograms body-weight the equivalent of 50 milligrams of erythromycin may be administered by intramuscular injection every 4 to 12 hours and for children of less than 15 kilograms body-weight, provided an adequate muscle mass is present, the equivalent of 3 to 4 milligrams per kilogram body-weight may be administered every 4 to 12 hours.

Undesirable effects; Precautions. As for Erythromycin.

Preparations

Preparations available include an INJECTION containing erythromycin ethylsuccinate equivalent to 50 mg of ery-thromycin per ml (in a macrogol basis) in 2-ml ampoules; and a MIXTURE containing erythromycin ethylsuccinate equivalent to 125, 250, and 500 mg of erythromycin in 5 ml when reconstituted, diluent syrup.

Erythromycin Stearate

The stearate of erythromycin ($C_{37}H_{67}NO_{13},C_{18}H_{36}O_2 = 1018.4$), with stearic acid and sodium stearate.

OTHER NAME: *Erythrocin®*

A standard is given in the British Pharmacopoeia 1973

Description. Almost odourless, colourless or slightly yellow crystals or a white or slightly yellow powder with a slightly bitter taste.

Solubility. Very slightly soluble in water and in acetone; partly soluble in alcohol, in chloroform, in isopropyl alcohol, and in methyl alcohol.

Moisture content. Not more than 4%, determined by Fischer titration.

Storage. It should be stored in airtight containers, pro-tected from light.

Identification. TESTS. 1. It complies with Tests 1 and 2 described under Erythromycin.

2. Mix about 100 mg with 5 ml of *dilute hydrochloric acid* and boil; oily globules appear on the surface of the liquid. Cool, remove the fatty layer, heat with 3 ml of 0.1N sodium hydroxide, and cool; the solution sets to a gel. Add 10 ml of hot water and shake; the solution froths. To 1 ml add *calcium chloride solution*; a granular precipitate which is insoluble in hydrochloric acid is produced.

Determination in body fluids; Metabolism. See under Erythromycin.

Actions and uses. Erythromycin stearate has the actions, uses, and undesirable effects described under Erythromycin, but it is less bitter.

The usual dose by mouth for adults and children in terms of erythromycin base is as given under Erythromycin

Ethylsuccinate; 138 milligrams of erythromycin stearate is approximately equivalent to 100 milligrams of erythromycin.

Preparations

ERYTHROMYCIN MIXTURE (*Syn.* Erythromycin Suspen-sion): a suspension of erythromycin stearate in a suitable coloured flavoured vehicle. It contains erythromycin stearate equivalent to 100 mg of erythromycin in 5 ml. When a dose less than or not a multiple of 5 ml is prescribed, the mixture may be diluted, as described in the entry on Mixtures, with syrup. The diluted mixture must be freshly prepared.

A standard for this mixture is given in the British Pharmaceutical Codex 1973

Containers and *Labelling:* see the entry on Mixtures for general information on containers and labelling.

Storage: the mixture and the diluted mixture should be stored in a cool place.

Advice for patients: the mixture should be taken at regular intervals, preferably after meals. The prescribed course should be completed.

ERYTHROMYCIN STEARATE TABLETS: available as tablets containing erythromycin stearate equivalent to 250 and 500 mg of erythromycin; they are film coated; the coat may be coloured.

A standard for these tablets is given in the British Pharmacopoeia 1973

Containers and *Storage:* see the entry on Tablets for general information on containers and storage. Con-tainers should be airtight and light resistant.

Advice for patients: the tablets should be taken at regular intervals, preferably after meals. The prescribed course should be completed.

Ethacrynic Acid

2,3-Dichloro-4-(2-ethylacryloyl)phenoxyacetic acid

$C_{13}H_{12}Cl_2O_4 = 303.1$

OTHER NAMES: Acidum Etacrynicum; *Edecrin®*; Eta-crynic Acid

A standard is given in the European Pharmacopoeia Vol. III Supplement

CAUTION. *Ethacrynic acid, especially in the form of dust, is irritating to the skin, eyes, and mucous membranes.*

Description. A white crystalline odourless powder.

Solubility. Very slightly soluble in water; soluble at 20°, in 1.6 parts of alcohol, in 3.5 parts of ether, and in 6 parts of chloroform. It forms water-soluble compounds with hydroxides, alkali carbonates, and ammonia.

Stability. Solutions of the sodium salt at pH 7 may be kept at room temperature for short periods, but are less stable at lower pH.

Identification. TESTS. 1. To about 25 mg add 2 ml of 1N sodium hydroxide, heat for 5 minutes in a water-bath, cool, add 5 drops of sulphuric acid (50%, v/v) followed by 0.5 ml of a 10% solution of chromatropic acid sodium salt and, cautiously, 2 ml of sulphuric acid; a deep violet colour is produced.

2. Dissolve about 5 mg in 1 ml of sulphuric acid; a yellow colour with a slight greenish tinge develops.

MELTING-POINT. About 123°.

ULTRAVIOLET ABSORPTION. In a mixture of 1 volume of 1N hydrochloric acid and 99 volumes of methyl alcohol, maximum at 270 nm (E1%, 1cm = 115) and a shoulder at 285 nm.

INFRA-RED ABSORPTION. Major peaks at 1077, 1249, 1279, 1586, 1661, and 1726 cm^{-1} (see Appendix 2a: Infra-red Spectra).

THIN-LAYER CHROMATOGRAPHY. See under Thin-layer Chromatography, System 6.

Metabolism. ABSORPTION. Readily absorbed after oral administration.

HALF-LIFE. Plasma half-life, less than 1 hour.

DISTRIBUTION. Ethacrynic acid is detectable in the liver and kidneys; *protein binding*, significantly bound to plasma proteins.

METABOLIC REACTION. Conjugation to form a cysteine derivative.

EXCRETION. After intravenous administration, 30% is excreted in the bile and 60% in the urine in 24 hours; urinary excretion is pH-dependent and the material excreted in the urine is composed of unchanged drug, a cysteine conjugate, and a third unstable metabolite; mercurial compounds and probenecid delay urinary excretion.

FURTHER INFORMATION. Renotropic characteristics— K. H. Beyer et al., J. Pharmac. exp. Ther., 1965, **147**, 1.

Actions and uses. Ethacrynic acid is a loop diuretic which acts by reducing resorption of sodium and chloride in the proximal renal tubule, in the ascending loop of Henle and, to a lesser extent, in the distal renal tubules; distal tubular potassium secretion is also increased to a variable degree. Urinary pH is decreased, bicarbonate excretion is diminished, ammonium excretion is increased, and serum uric acid levels may be increased. The intense initial enhancement of sodium and chloride excretion may diminish on prolonged use, but potassium and hydrogen-ion losses may be increased.

Ethacrynic acid is rapidly absorbed when given by mouth and produces an intense diuresis beginning in about 30 minutes and reaching a maximum in about 2 hours. The usual dosage is 50 to 200 milligrams daily in divided doses, and a daily dosage of 400 milligrams should not be exceeded. Ethacrynic acid should preferably be given with food. It is of value for the treatment of oedema and for fluid retention.

In the form of its sodium salt, ethacrynic acid may be given by slow intravenous injection, when it produces a rapid and intense natriuresis and diuresis; doses equivalent to 50 to 100 milligrams of ethacrynic acid may be used in the treatment of pulmonary oedema.

When a blood transfusion is administered to a chronically anaemic patient who cannot be treated by more conservative means, a dose equivalent to 12.5 to 50 milligrams of ethacrynic acid may be given separately to prevent pulmonary oedema.

Undesirable effects. Anorexia, nausea, vomiting, diarrhoea, dysphagia, headache, blurred vision, confusion, transient loss of hearing, and rashes may occur. Prolonged use may give rise to a hypochloraemic alkalosis and electrolyte imbalance; hypokalaemia may occur. Ethacrynic acid may increase the blood level of urea

nitrogen. Its use may occasionally precipitate an acute attack of gout or, more rarely thrombocytopenia.

Precautions. During prolonged treatment, potassium supplements should be given, the usual amount required being about 40 to 80 millimoles, or 3 to 6 grams, of potassium chloride daily in divided doses. As ethacrynic acid may cause hypoglycaemia, its use in diabetic patients should be carefully controlled. Breast-feeding should be discontinued during treatment.

Preparations

ETHACRYNIC ACID INJECTION: a sterile solution of ethacrynic acid, in the form of the sodium salt, in dextrose injection (5%) or in sodium chloride injection. It is prepared by dissolving the contents of a sealed container in the solvent shortly before use.

Available as a powder in vials containing ethacrynate sodium equivalent to 50 mg of ethacrynic acid.

Containers: see the entry on Injections for general information on containers.

Labelling: see the entry on Injections for general information on labelling. In addition, the label on the container should state the amount of the medicament as the equivalent amount of ethacrynic acid.

Storage: the injection contains no bactericide and should be used as soon as possible after preparation but solutions of ethacrynate sodium may be expected to retain their potency for up to 24 hours provided they are stored at 2° to 10°.

ETHACRYNIC ACID TABLETS: available as tablets containing 50 mg of ethacrynic acid.

A standard for these tablets is given in the British Pharmacopoeia 1973

Containers and *Storage:* see the entry on Tablets for general information on containers and storage. Containers should be airtight.

Advice for patients: daily doses should preferably be taken after breakfast.

Ethambutol Hydrochloride

(+)-NN'-Bis[(R)-1-hydroxymethylpropyl]ethylenediammonium chloride

$$\left[\begin{array}{c} \underset{\underset{CH_2OH}{|}}{\overset{\overset{H}{|}}{C_2H_5-C-\overset{+}{N}H_2\cdot CH_2\cdot CH_2\cdot \overset{+}{N}H_2-\underset{\underset{H}{|}}{\overset{\overset{CH_2OH}{|}}{C}-C_2H_5}}} \end{array} \right] \ 2Cl^-$$

$C_{10}H_{26}Cl_2N_2O_2 = 277.2$

OTHER NAMES: *Myambutol*®
Mynah® (with isoniazid)

A standard is given in the British Pharmacopoeia 1973

Description. A white crystalline odourless powder.

Solubility. Soluble, at 20°, in 1 part of water, in 30 parts of alcohol, in 850 parts of chloroform, and in 9 parts of methyl alcohol; very slightly soluble in ether.

Specific rotation. +5.8° to +6.6°, determined at 25° on a 10% solution.

Dissociation constants. pK$_a$ 6.3, 9.5 (20°).

Storage. It should be stored in airtight containers.

Identification. TEST. Dissolve about 100 mg in 10 ml of water and add 2 ml of a 1% solution of copper sulphate followed by 1 ml of 1N sodium hydroxide; a distinct blue colour is produced.

MELTING-POINT. About 201°.

Determination in body fluids. GAS CHROMATOGRAPHY. In urine—V. Strind and B. Salvesen, *Meddr norsk farm. Selsk.*, 1974, **36**, 44.

Metabolism. ABSORPTION. Readily absorbed after oral administration.

BLOOD CONCENTRATION. After an oral dose of 25 mg/kg body-weight of the hydrochloride, peak serum concentrations of 2 to 5 μg/ml are attained in 2 to 4 hours; at 24 hours, serum concentrations are negligible; during continuous therapy with 15 to 25 mg/kg body-weight daily of the hydrochloride, serum concentrations of 2 to 5 μg/ml are maintained.

HALF-LIFE. Plasma half-life, about 8 hours.

DISTRIBUTION. Ethambutol does not accumulate in the tissues except in cases of renal failure; it enters the cerebrospinal fluid when the meninges are inflamed and, in the blood, more is found in red cells than in plasma.

METABOLIC REACTIONS. Oxidation to 2,2'-ethylenedi-iminodibutyric acid and to an aldehyde.

EXCRETION. Up to 70% of a dose is excreted in the urine, 50% as unchanged drug and 8 to 15% as metabolites; about 20% is excreted unchanged in the faeces.

FURTHER INFORMATION. Metabolism—E. A. Peets and D. A. Buyske, *Biochem. Pharmac.*, 1964, **13**, 1403; concentrations in cerebrospinal fluid and serum—E. A. Peets *et al.*, *Am. Rev. resp. Dis.*, 1965, **91**, 51; J. A. Pilheu *et al.*, *Tubercle*, 1971, **52**, 117.

Actions and uses. Ethambutol is used in the treatment of mycobacterial infections, particularly tuberculosis. It is active against some strains of *Mycobacterium tuberculosis* that are resistant to other drugs and cross-resistance between ethambutol and other antitubercular drugs does not occur. It should always be given simultaneously with other tuberculostatic agents to delay the development of resistance (see under Tuberculosis). Ethambutol hydrochloride is given to adults and children in a dosage of 15 milligrams per kilogram body-weight daily. When re-treatment is necessary, as in cases of relapse, a daily dosage of 25 milligrams per kilogram body-weight may be given.

Undesirable effects. A serious toxic effect is the insidious onset of visual loss which may be manifested as a restriction of the visual field or as a loss of colour discrimination. This effect may occur on the prolonged administration of doses of 25 milligrams per kilogram body-weight and is associated with progressive depletion of copper and zinc; it may be reversed if treatment with ethambutol is stopped promptly, and in some cases treatment may be resumed at a lower dose level. Allergic rashes and gastro-intestinal disturbances may rarely occur.

Precautions and contra-indications. Dosage should be appropriately reduced in patients with impaired renal function and serum concentrations should not be allowed to exceed 5 micrograms per millilitre. The eyes should be examined periodically and treatment should be terminated if visual defects appear.

Preparations

ETHAMBUTOL TABLETS: available as tablets containing 100 and 400 mg of ethambutol hydrochloride; they may be coated with sugar or other suitable material and the coat may be coloured.
A standard for these tablets is given in the British Pharmacopoeia 1973
Containers and *Storage:* see the entry on Tablets for general information on containers and storage. Containers should be airtight.
Advice for patients: the tablets should be taken at regular intervals. Treatment should not be discontinued without the advice of the prescriber. Visual defects should be reported immediately.

OTHER PREPARATIONS available include a POWDER in bottles containing ethambutol hydrochloride 50 g and TABLETS containing ethambutol hydrochloride 200, 250, 300, and 365 mg each with isoniazid 100 mg.

Ethanolamine

2-Aminoethanol

$$NH_2 \cdot CH_2 \cdot CH_2OH$$

$C_2H_7NO = 61.08$

OTHER NAME: Monoethanolamine

A standard is given in the British Pharmaceutical Codex 1973

Description. A clear colourless or pale yellow liquid with a slight odour.

Solubility. Miscible with water and with alcohol; very slightly soluble in ether and in light petroleum.

Weight per ml. At 20°, 1.014 to 1.023 g.

Refractive index. At 20°, 1.453 to 1.459.

Dissociation constant. pK_a 9.4 (25°).

Sterilisation. Solutions are sterilised by heating in an autoclave.

Identification. TESTS. 1. It is alkaline to *litmus solution.*
2. To 2 drops add 300 mg of trinitrophenol and 1 ml of water and evaporate to dryness on a water-bath; the residue, after crystallising from alcohol (95%) and drying at 105°, melts at about 160°.
3. When freshly distilled and the first half of the distillate rejected, it freezes at about 10°.

Actions and uses. Ethanolamine, combined with oleic acid, is given by intravenous injection as a sclerosing agent in the treatment of varicose veins. If it escapes into the perivenous tissues during injection it causes less sloughing than some other sclerosants and allergic reactions rarely follow its use.
Ethanolamine is administered as the injection, the dose of 2 to 5 millilitres being divided into 3 or 4 portions, which are injected at different sites. The treatment is usually given at intervals of about a week until the varices have been completely occluded.

Contra-indications. It is contra-indicated where there is thrombosis of the deep veins of the leg or acute phlebitis.

Preparation

ETHANOLAMINE OLEATE INJECTION:

Ethanolamine	..	..	..	..	0.91 g
Oleic acid	..	..	..	..	4.23 g
Benzyl alcohol	..	..	..	..	2 ml
Water for injections	..	..	..	to 100 ml

Shake the oleic acid with 50 ml of the water in a closed container and gradually add the ethanolamine, shaking between each addition until combination is complete. Add the benzyl alcohol, shake, and add sufficient of the water to produce the required volume. Sterilise by heating in an autoclave. It is not necessary to add an additional bactericide when the injection is supplied in multiple-dose containers.

A standard for this injection is given in the British Pharmaceutical Codex 1973
Containers: see the entry on Injections for general information on containers.
Labelling: see the entry on Injections for general information on labelling. In addition, the label on the container and the label or wrapper on the package should state that the injection contains about 5% of ethanolamine oleate and that the contents are to be used for intravenous injection only as a sclerosing agent.
Storage: it should be protected from light.

Ethchlorvynol

1-Chloro-3-ethylpent-1-en-4-yn-3-ol

$$\underset{\underset{C_2H_5}{|}}{CH{:}C{\cdot}\overset{\overset{OH}{|}}{C}{\cdot}CH{:}CHCl}$$

$C_7H_9ClO = 144.6$

OTHER NAME: *Serenesil®*

A standard is given in the British Pharmacopoeia 1973

Description. A colourless to yellow liquid with a characteristic and pungent odour and a slightly bitter pungent taste.

Solubility. Practically insoluble in water; miscible with alcohol, with ether, with chloroform, and with acetone.

Weight per ml. At 20°, 1.070 to 1.074 g.

Refractive index. At 20°, 1.4770 to 1.4805.

Storage. It should be stored in airtight containers protected from light. It should not be allowed to come into contact with metal.

Identification. TESTS. 1. Mix 2 drops with a mixture containing 4 ml of water, 3 ml of sulphuric acid, and 8 ml of alcohol (95%), and heat at 40° for 5 minutes; a red colour is produced which turns to dark brown on standing.
2. Add 2 drops to 20 ml of alcohol (95%) containing 2 drops of *bromophenol blue solution,* neutralise the mixture by the addition of a 0.04% solution of sodium hydroxide or of a 0.1% solution of nitric acid, and add *alcoholic silver nitrate solution* which has previously been neutralised in a similar manner; the solution immediately turns yellow.
3. Carefully mix 2 volumes of acetic acid (50% v/v) with 1 volume of a 2% solution of diphenylamine in sulphuric acid, and add 3 ml of this mixture to 2 ml of the test solution; a red colour develops which is stable for several hours. The test is sensitive to about 1 ppm and a test solution can be prepared by shaking 1 drop of the substance with 100 ml of water. The test can also be applied to urine or to gastric washings.

Determination in body fluids. ULTRAVIOLET SPECTROPHOTOMETRY. In serum or urine—J. E. Wallace *et al., Clin. Chem.,* 1974, **20,** 159.

GAS CHROMATOGRAPHY. In blood or urine—P. F. Gibson and N. Wright, *J. pharm. Sci.,* 1972, **61,** 169. In serum—M. A. Evenson and M. A. Poquette, *Clin. Chem.,* 1974, **20,** 212. In blood, urine, or gastric fluid—H. H. McCurdy, *J. analyt. Toxicol.,* 1977, **1,** 164. In plasma or urine—R. J. Flannagan and T. D. Lee, *J. Chromat.,* 1977, **137,** 119.

Metabolism. ABSORPTION. Rapidly absorbed after oral administration.

BLOOD CONCENTRATION. After an oral dose of 500 mg, peak serum concentrations of 4.0 to 6.5 μg/ml are attained in 1 to 3 hours.

HALF-LIFE. Plasma half-life, about 6 hours.

DISTRIBUTION. Highly localised in the tissues especially in adipose tissue.

METABOLIC REACTIONS. Ethchlorvynol is extensively metabolised but the nature of its metabolites is unknown.

EXCRETION. In 24 hours about 0.025% of a dose is excreted in the urine either as unchanged drug or as the sulphate or glucuronide.

FURTHER INFORMATION. Concentrations in serum and urine—L. M. Cummins *et al., J. pharm. Sci.,* 1971, **60,** 261; concentrations in plasma and urine—J. K. Dawborn *et al., Med. J. Aust.,* ii/1972, 702.

Actions and uses. Ethchlorvynol has a hypnotic action resembling that of an intermediate-acting barbiturate, the actions and uses of which are described under Barbiturates. Sleep lasting for 4 to 6 hours is produced within about 20 minutes by oral doses of 0.25 to 1 gram. As a sedative, a dose of 100 to 250 milligrams has been given twice daily.

Undesirable effects. Dizziness, nausea, and vomiting may occur.

Precautions. See under Barbiturates. Exaggerated reactions may occur if it is taken with alcohol.

Dependence. Ethchlorvynol may give rise to dependence of the barbiturate-alcohol type as described under Drug Dependence.

Preparation

ETHCHLORVYNOL CAPSULES: consisting of ethchlorvynol enclosed in a soft capsule. The capsule shells may be coloured. Available as capsules containing 500 mg of ethchlorvynol.
A standard for these capsules is given in the British Pharmacopoeia 1973
Containers and *Storage:* see the entry on Capsules for general information on containers and storage. Containers should be light resistant.
Advice for patients: the capsules should preferably be taken with food 20 minutes before bedtime. They may cause drowsiness on the following day; persons affected should not drive or operate machinery. Alcohol should be avoided.

Ether, Anaesthetic

Diethyl ether which has been purified and contains up to 0.002% w/v of a suitable stabiliser, such as propyl gallate or hydroquinone, to retard the formation of ether peroxides.
$C_2H_5.O.C_2H_5 = 74.12$

OTHER NAMES: Aether Anaestheticus; Ether

A standard is given in the European Pharmacopoeia Vol. III

CAUTION. *Anaesthetic ether is highly inflammable and mixtures of its vapour with oxygen or air at certain concentrations are explosive; it should not be used in the presence of a naked flame or of any electrical apparatus liable to produce a spark. Precautions should be taken against the production of static electrical discharge.*

Description. A clear, colourless, very mobile liquid with a characteristic odour and a sweet burning taste. It is very volatile and inflammable.

Solubility. Soluble, at 20°, in 10 parts of water; miscible with alcohol, with chloroform, and with fixed and volatile oils.

Boiling-point. About 35°. Explosive peroxides are generated by atmospheric oxidation and it is dangerous to distil a sample which contains peroxides.

Storage. It should be stored in dry airtight containers in a cool place, protected from light. If the container is closed by a cork, this should be protected with metal foil. Ether remaining in a partly used container may deteriorate rapidly.

Determination in body fluids. INFRA-RED SPECTRO-PHOTOMETRY. In blood—M. Feldstein, *J. forens. Sci.*, 1965, **10**, 207.

Metabolism. ABSORPTION. Readily absorbed after inhalation.

DISTRIBUTION. Widely distributed throughout the body and crosses the placenta.

METABOLIC REACTIONS. In mice, ether appears to be converted into acetate which is utilised in anabolic processes. Ether, administered in sub-anaesthetic concentrations to rats, appears to stimulate the metabolism of hexobarbitone.

EXCRETION. About 90% of an inhaled dose is exhaled, rapidly at first and then more slowly; some unchanged ether may be excreted in the urine.

Actions and uses. Anaesthetic ether is a volatile anaesthetic. It is much less depressant to the medullary centres than chloroform and causes less fall in blood pressure and less depression of respiration.

Ether does not lead to ventricular fibrillation in the induction stage, nor does prolonged ether anaesthesia produce a direct toxic action on the heart. It causes peripheral vasodilatation, especially of skin vessels, and this is a cause of the increased capillary oozing that may occur when ether is used. The white-cell count may rise 300% after ether anaesthesia.

Although ether produces slight transient toxic effects on the liver and kidneys, it does not give rise to severe delayed poisoning and it has a wide margin of safety.

The chief disadvantage of ether as an anaesthetic is its irritant action on the mucous membrane of the respiratory tract; it stimulates the secretion of saliva and mucus from the bronchial tree. Frequently, atropine, or hyoscine, and morphine are given about one hour before the induction of anaesthesia; the atropine or hyoscine inhibits the bronchial secretion, thus reducing the risk of inhalation pneumonia, while the morphine reduces the amount of anaesthetic required.

Laryngeal spasm is an occasional complication of ether anaesthesia. Prolonged contact with ether spilt on any tissue produces necrosis.

The concentration of ether in the inspired air necessary to produce anaesthesia is normally from 6 to 7% by volume, although it may be desirable to exceed this concentration, especially during induction. It is administered on an open mask or by semi-closed or closed methods. When ether is used alone in this way it requires a long time for the induction of anaesthesia, thus prolonging the stage of excitement. To reduce or obviate this, it is current practice to premedicate the patient and to employ mixtures of ether with other anaesthetics, such as nitrous oxide.

Poisoning. In the event of poisoning by ether, resulting in collapse, the procedure described under Chloroform

should be adopted. Convulsions, which are frequently fatal, occasionally occur in patients under deep ether anaesthesia, especially under hot or humid conditions, but their occurrence does not seem to be related to the presence, as impurities, of peroxides or aldehydes. The evidence seems rather to support the view that patients so affected have a predisposition to convulsions.

If ether convulsions occur, artificial respiration may be required to prevent respiratory failure, and a solution of a soluble barbiturate or diazepam may be given by intravenous injection.

Ether, Solvent

Diethyl ether
$C_2H_5.O.C_2H_5 = 74.12$

A standard is given in the British Pharmacopoeia 1973

CAUTION. *Solvent ether is highly inflammable and mixtures of its vapour with oxygen or air at certain concentrations are explosive; it should not be used in the presence of a naked flame or of any electrical apparatus liable to produce a spark. Precautions should be taken against the production of static electrical discharge.*

Description; Solubility; Boiling-point. As for Ether, Anaesthetic.

Storage. It should be stored in dry airtight containers, in a cool place, protected from light. If the container is closed by a cork, this should be protected with metal foil.

Determination in body fluids; Metabolism. As for Ether, Anaesthetic.

Uses. Solvent ether is used as a solvent for oils, resins, and many other substances. It is also used, with suitable precautions against the risk of fire, for cleaning the skin before surgical operations and for removing adhesive plaster from the skin. Solvent ether may contain aldehydes and other impurities and is unsuitable for use in preparations administered internally.

Ethinyloestradiol

19-Nor-17α-pregna-1,3,5(10)-trien-20-yne-3,17-diol

$C_{20}H_{24}O_2 = 296.4$

OTHER NAMES: Aethinyloestradiolum; Ethinyl Estradiol; Ethinylestradiolum; Ethinyloestr.; *Lynoral*®
Paralut® (with ethisterone); *Conova 30*®, *Demulen 50*®, *Metrulen 50*®, and *Ovulen 50*® (all with ethynodiol diacetate); *Minilyn*® (with lynoestrenol); *Climatone*®, *Declimone*®, *Menolet*®, *Mepilin*®, and *Mixogen*® (all with methyltestosterone); *Brevinor*® and *Ovysmen*® (both with norethisterone); *Anovlar 21*®, *Controvlar*®, *Gynovlar 21*®, *Loestrin 20*®, *Minovlar*®, *Norlestrin*®, and *Orlest 21*® (all with norethisterone acetate); *Eugynon*®, *Microgynon*®, and *Ovran*® (all with norgestrel or D-norgestrel)

A standard is given in the European Pharmacopoeia Vol. II

CAUTION. *Ethinyloestradiol is a powerful oestrogen. Contact with the skin or inhalation of the dust should be avoided. Rubber gloves should be worn when handling the powder and, if the powder is dry, a face mask should also be worn.*

Description. A white or slightly yellowish-white, crystalline, odourless powder.

Solubility. Very slightly soluble in water; soluble, at 20°, in 6 parts of alcohol, in 4 parts of ether, in 20 parts of chloroform, in 5 parts of acetone, and in 4 parts of dioxan; soluble in solutions of alkali hydroxides.

Moisture content. Not more than 1%, determined by drying at 105°.

Specific rotation. A 5% solution in dioxan is slightly dextrorotatory (less than +5°).

Storage. It should be stored in airtight containers, protected from light, in a cool place.

Identification. TESTS. 1. Dissolve 2 mg in 2 ml of sulphuric acid; the solution is orange-red by transmitted light and shows a yellowish-green fluorescence by reflected light.
2. To 1 ml of the solution prepared in Test 1 add 1 drop of *ferric ammonium sulphate solution* and 2 ml of water; a reddish-brown flocculent precipitate is produced.
3. To 1 ml of the solution prepared in Test 1 add 2 ml of water; a rose-red flocculent precipitate is produced.
4. Dissolve about 25 mg in 10 ml of a 5% solution of potassium hydroxide in a glass-stoppered tube and add 100 mg of benzoyl chloride, and shake; a precipitate is produced which, after recrystallisation from methyl alcohol, melts at about 201°.

MELTING-POINT. About 183°. It may also occur in another polymorphic form which melts at about 143°.

INFRA-RED ABSORPTION. Major peaks at 645, 1055, 1259, 1301, 1388, and 1501 cm⁻¹ (see Appendix 2a: Infra-red Spectra).

THIN-LAYER CHROMATOGRAPHY. See under Thin-layer Chromatography, System 10.

Metabolism. ABSORPTION. Well absorbed after oral administration.

BLOOD CONCENTRATION. After an intravenous dose of 50 μg, 5 to 15% of the dose is present in the total plasma volume at 1 hour and 0.3 to 3.5% is present at 24 hours.

HALF-LIFE. The decline in plasma concentration appears to be biphasic with a half-life of 7 hours for the initial phase and of about 50 hours for the second phase; the half-life determined from urinary excretion data is about 25 hours.

DISTRIBUTION. Localised in uterine tissues and also in the ovary and in fatty tissues; 4 to 9% of the dose may be localised in fatty tissues; it is secreted in the milk of rats in small amounts.

METABOLIC REACTIONS. Metabolised to D-homo-oestradiol-17$\alpha\beta$, 2-methoxyethinyloestradiol and 2-hydroxyethinyloestradiol 3-methylether along with glucuronide and sulphate formation.

EXCRETION. 30 to 60% of a dose is excreted in the urine in 5 days; of the excreted material about 40% is glucuronide, 12% is sulphate, and 19% is unconjugated of which about 70% is unchanged; about 30% is excreted in the faeces of which about one third is unchanged drug; ethinyloestradiol is excreted in the bile mainly as sulphate and also as glucuronide.

FURTHER INFORMATION. Metabolism—M. T. Abdel-Aziz and K. I. H. Williams, *Steroids*, 1970, **15**, 695;

secretion in milk of lactating rats—D. I. Cargill *et al.*, *Proc. Soc. exp. Biol. Med.*, 1969, **131**, 1362; metabolism—J. W. Goldzieher and D. C. Kraemer, *Acta Endocr., Copenh.*, 1972, **166**, Suppl. 1, 389, S. Kamyab *et al.*, *Nature*, 1969, **221**, 360, B. D. Kulkarni and J. W. Goldzieher, *Contraception*, 1970, **1**, 47, and M. J. Reed *et al.*, *J. Endocr.*, 1972, **55**, 351; biliary metabolites—B. G. Steinetz *et al.*, *Proc. Soc. exp. Biol. Med.*, 1967, **124**, 1283; plasma concentrations—R. J. Warren and K. Fotherby, *J. Endocr.*, 1973, **59**, 369.

Actions and uses. Ethinyloestradiol has the actions and uses of the oestrogens, as described under Oestradiol Benzoate.

In the treatment of menopausal symptoms, an initial dosage of 10 to 50 micrograms is given by mouth 3 times a day; for maintenance, 10 micrograms once or twice a day may be sufficient. A progestational agent may be required in addition during the second half of the cycle.

For the treatment of primary amenorrhoea, 20 micrograms is given twice daily for 24 days. A progestational agent, for example, norethisterone, should be given in a dosage of 5 milligrams a day for the last 10 days and the cycle repeated once bleeding has ceased.

Functional uterine bleeding may be treated with 500 micrograms once or twice a day, or smaller doses more frequently, until the bleeding is controlled. The dosage is then reduced to 50 micrograms once to 3 times a day for 20 days; 5 milligrams of progesterone is sometimes given daily for the last 5 days.

For the inhibition of lactation, 100 micrograms is given 3 times a day for 3 days, and then 50 micrograms twice daily for 2 days and once daily for 3 more days.

For the palliative treatment of carcinoma of the prostate and of the breast, 1 to 2 milligrams is given daily, the dosage in the former condition being controlled by periodic estimations of the serum acid phosphatase.

Ethinyloestradiol is also used as the oestrogenic component of progestogen-oestrogen oral contraceptive tablets.

Undesirable effects. In addition to the undesirable effects described under Oestradiol Benzoate, headache, dizziness, nausea, and vomiting may occur.

Veterinary uses. Ethinyloestradiol has been used in the treatment of infertility and uterine infections in cattle. The usual dose is 0.5 to 2 milligrams by intra-uterine infusion as a single dose.

Preparations

ETHINYLOESTRADIOL TABLETS: available as tablets containing 10, 20, 50, and 100 micrograms and 1 mg of ethinyloestradiol.

A standard for these tablets is given in the British Pharmacopoeia 1973

Containers and *Storage:* see the entry on Tablets for general information on containers and storage. Containers should be airtight and light resistant.

Advice for patients: the prescribed course should be completed or, where applicable, treatment should not be discontinued without the advice of the prescriber.

OTHER PREPARATIONS available include TABLETS containing ethinyloestradiol 4.4 micrograms with methyltestosterone 3.6 mg; ethinyloestradiol 5 micrograms with methyltestosterone 2.5 and 5 mg; ethinyloestradiol 10 micrograms with methyltestosterone 3 mg; ethinyloestradiol 15 micrograms with methyltestosterone 5 mg; ethinyloestradiol 20 micrograms with norethisterone acetate 1 mg; ethinyloestradiol 30 micrograms with ethynodiol diacetate 2 mg, ethinyloestradiol 30 micrograms with D-norgestrel 150 and 250 micrograms, and with norgestrel 500 micrograms; ethinyloestradiol 35 micrograms with norethisterone 500 micrograms; ethinyloestradiol 50 micrograms with ethisterone 10 mg, with ethynodiol diacetate 500 micrograms and 1 and 2 mg, with lynoestrenol 2.5 mg, with norethisterone acetate 1, 2.5, 3, and 4 mg, with norgestrel 500 micrograms; and ethinyloestradiol 100 micrograms with ethisterone 50 mg.

Ethionamide

2-Ethylpyridine-4-carbothioamide

$C_8H_{10}N_2S = 166.2$

OTHER NAME: *Trescatyl*®

A standard is given in the British Pharmacopoeia 1973

Description. A bright yellow crystalline powder with a slight odour and an unpleasant sulphurous taste.

Solubility. Practically insoluble in water; soluble, at 20°, in 30 parts of alcohol, in 600 parts of ether, and in 350 parts of chloroform.

Moisture content. Not more than 1%, determined by drying at 105°.

Storage. It should be protected from light.

Identification. TESTS. 1. Mix about 100 mg with 5 ml of *sodium hydroxide solution* and heat; the vapours evolved turn red litmus paper blue.
2. Mix about 100 mg with 5 ml of 1N hydrochloric acid and heat; the vapours evolved blacken lead paper.

MELTING-POINT. About 163°.

ULTRAVIOLET ABSORPTION. In 0.1N sulphuric acid, maxima at 230 nm (E1%, 1cm = 638) and 276 nm (E1%, 1cm = 410) and a shoulder at 317 nm; in alcohol (95%), maximum at 290 nm (E1%, 1cm = 415).

INFRA-RED ABSORPTION. Major peaks at 813, 870, 885, 1149, 1282, and 1587 cm^{-1} (see Appendix 2b: Infra-red Spectra).

Metabolism. ABSORPTION. Readily absorbed after oral administration.

BLOOD CONCENTRATION. After an oral dose of 1 g, peak plasma concentrations of up to 20 μg/ml are attained in 3 hours which fall to about 3 μg/ml after 9 hours and to less than 1 μg/ml after 24 hours.

HALF-LIFE. 2 to 4 hours.

DISTRIBUTION. Widely distributed throughout the body and enters the cerebrospinal fluid when the meninges are both normal and inflamed.

METABOLIC REACTIONS. Extensively metabolised to a number of metabolites by N-methylation, sulphoxidation, desulphuration, and deamination.

EXCRETION. 25 to 30% of a dose is excreted in the urine in 8 hours; about 8.5% is excreted unchanged after oral administration and 2.5% is excreted unchanged after rectal administration.

FURTHER INFORMATION. Metabolites of ethionamide —A. Bieder *et al., Annls pharm. Fr.,* 1966, **24**, 493; metabolism—J. P. Johnston *et al., J. Pharm. Pharmac.,* 1967, **19**, 1.

Actions and uses. Ethionamide is a tuberculostatic agent with uses similar to those of sodium aminosalicylate. It is active against some strains of *Mycobacterium tuberculosis* that are resistant to other tuberculostatic drugs, although there may be cross-resistance between ethionamide and the thiosemicarbazones.

Originally sensitive strains of *M. tuberculosis* rapidly become resistant to ethionamide if it is used alone in the treatment of tuberculosis. The simultaneous administration of other tuberculostatic agents delays the development of resistance (see under Tuberculosis).

In the treatment of pulmonary and extrapulmonary tuberculosis, the usual dosage of ethionamide by mouth is 750 to 1000 milligrams daily in divided doses, but 500 milligrams may be sufficient for some patients.

The usual initial dose for children up to 10 years is 12 to 15 milligrams per kilogram body-weight daily in divided doses. This, if tolerance permits, may be gradually increased over a period of 15 days and some patients have received up to 20 milligrams per kilogram body-weight of ethionamide daily in divided doses. A maximum daily dosage of 750 milligrams should not be exceeded. Children over 10 may be given the adult dose.

Undesirable effects. Disturbances of the alimentary tract, including a metallic taste, stomatitis, excessive salivation, nausea, vomiting, and diarrhoea, may occur in patients receiving more than 500 milligrams daily.

Liver damage, hypotension, convulsions, peripheral neuropathy, alopecia, gynaecomastia, impotence, menstrual disturbances, drowsiness, slight deafness, diplopia, headache, insomnia, and skin rashes have been reported. The administration of ethionamide to patients with diabetes mellitus may cause difficulty in controlling the diabetes. When it is given concurrently with other tuberculostatic drugs it may intensify their adverse effects.

Contra-indications. It should not be given in early pregnancy as it may give rise to foetal malformations.

Preparation

ETHIONAMIDE TABLETS: available as tablets containing 125 mg of ethionamide. They may be sugar coated and the coat may be coloured.
A standard for these tablets is given in the British Pharmacopoeia 1973
Containers and *Storage:* see the entry on Tablets for general information on containers and storage. Containers should be airtight.
Advice for patients: the tablets should preferably be taken after meals and daily doses preferably at bedtime. Treatment should not be discontinued without the advice of the prescriber.

Ethisterone

17-Hydroxy-17α-pregn-4-en-20-yn-3-one

$C_{21}H_{28}O_2 = 312.5$

OTHER NAMES: Anhydrohydroxyprogesterone; Ethinyltestosterone; *Gestone-oral*®
Paralut® (with ethinyloestradiol)

A standard is given in the British Pharmacopoeia 1973

Description. A white crystalline odourless powder.

Solubility. Practically insoluble in water; soluble, at 20°, in 1000 parts of alcohol, in 110 parts of chloroform, in 750 parts of acetone, and in 35 parts of pyridine; very slightly soluble in vegetable oils.

Moisture content. Not more than 1%, determined by drying at 105°.

Specific rotation. +29° to +33°, determined on a 1% solution in pyridine.

Storage. It should be stored in airtight containers, protected from light.

Identification. MELTING-POINT. About 274°.

ULTRAVIOLET ABSORPTION. In dehydrated alcohol, maximum at 240 nm (E1%, 1cm = 520).

INFRA-RED ABSORPTION. Major peaks at 1062, 1125, 1235, 1383, 1614, and 1660 cm^{-1} (see Appendix 2a: Infrared Spectra).

THIN-LAYER CHORMATOGRAPHY. See under Thin-layer Chromatography, System 10.

Actions and uses. Ethisterone is a progestational agent that is effective when given by mouth, preferably sublingually, the usual dose being 25 milligrams daily in single or divided doses although up to 100 milligrams daily has been used. It has been largely replaced by other compounds such as norethisterone which have less virilising action.

Ethisterone is also given in conjunction with ethinyl-oestradiol for the treatment of amenorrhoea, the usual dosage being 50 milligrams of ethisterone with 50 micrograms of ethinyloestradiol daily for 3 days.

Precautions and contra-indications. As for Progesterone.

Preparations

ETHISTERONE TABLETS (*Syn.* Ethinyltestosterone Tablets): available as tablets containing 5, 10, and 25 mg of ethisterone.

A standard for these tablets is given in the British Pharmacopoeia 1973

Containers and *Storage:* see the entry on Tablets for general information on containers and storage. Containers should be airtight and light resistant.

Advice for patients: the prescribed course should be completed or, where applicable, treatment should not be discontinued without the advice of the prescriber.

OTHER PREPARATIONS available include TABLETS containing ethisterone 10 mg with ethinyloestradiol 50 micrograms and tablets containing ethisterone 50 mg with ethinyloestradiol 100 micrograms.

Ethopabate

Methyl 4-acetamido-2-ethoxybenzoate

CO·O·CH$_3$

O·C$_2$H$_5$

NH·CO·CH$_3$

C$_{12}$H$_{15}$NO$_4$ = 237.3

OTHER NAMES: *Amprol*® (with amprolium hydrochloride); *Pancoxin*® (with amprolium hydrochloride and sulphaquinoxaline); *Supacox*® (with amprolium hydrochloride, sulphaquinoxaline, and pyrimethamine)

A standard is given in the British Pharmacopoeia (Veterinary)

Description. A white or pinkish-white odourless powder.

Solubility. Soluble, at 20°, in 2000 parts of water, in 30 parts of alcohol, in 10 parts of chloroform, in 600 parts of ether, and in 15 parts of methyl alcohol.

Moisture content. Not more than 1%, determined by drying at 100° *in vacuo.*

Identification. MELTING-POINT. About 148°.

ULTRAVIOLET ABSORPTION. In methyl alcohol, maxima at 268 nm (E1%, 1cm = 812) and 299 nm (E1%, 1cm = 362).

Veterinary uses. Ethopabate is used in conjunction with other coccidiostats in the control of coccidiosis in turkeys and chickens. The usual dose is up to 6 parts per million in the feed.

Preparations

AMPROLIUM AND ETHOPABATE PREMIX: consisting of amprolium hydrochloride and ethopabate mixed with a suitable diluent. It must be diluted before administration by mixing thoroughly with the feed.

Available as a premix containing 25% of amprolium hydrochloride and 1.6% of ethopabate.

A standard for this premix is given in the British Pharmacopoeia (Veterinary)

Containers and *Storage:* see the entry on Premixes for general information on containers and storage.

AMPROLIUM, ETHOPABATE, AND SULPHAQUINOXALINE PREMIX: consisting of amprolium hydrochloride, ethopabate, and sulphaquinoxaline, mixed with a suitable diluent. It must be diluted before administration by mixing thoroughly with the feed.

Available as a premix containing 20% of amprolium hydrochloride, 1% of ethopabate, and 12% of sulphaquinoxaline.

A standard for this premix is given in the British Pharmacopoeia (Veterinary)

Containers and *Storage:* see the entry on Premixes for general information on containers and storage.

AMPROLIUM, ETHOPABATE, SULPHAQUINOXALINE, AND PYRIMETHAMINE PREMIX: consisting of amprolium hydrochloride, ethopabate, sulphaquinoxaline, and pyrimethamine mixed with a suitable diluent. It must be diluted before administration by mixing thoroughly with the feed.

Available as a premix containing 20% of amprolium hydrochloride, 1% of ethopabate, 12% of sulphaquinoxaline, and 1% of pyrimethamine.

A standard for this premix is given in the British Pharmacopoeia (Veterinary)

Containers and *Storage:* see the entry on Premixes for general information on containers and storage.

OTHER PREPARATIONS available include a SOLUTION containing ethopabate 0.49% with amprolium hydrochloride 7.68%.

Ethosuximide

2-Ethyl-2-methylsuccinimide *or* 3-ethyl-3-methylpyrro-lidine-2,5-dione

$C_7H_{11}NO_2 = 141.2$

OTHER NAMES: *Emeside*®; *Zarontin*®

A standard is given in the British Pharmacopoeia 1973

Description. A white odourless powder or waxy solid with a slightly bitter taste.

Solubility. Soluble, at 20°, in 4.5 parts of water and in less than 1 part of alcohol, of ether, and of chloroform.

Dissociation constant. pK_a 9.5.

Identification. TEST. Mix about 100 mg with 200 mg of resorcinol and 2 drops of sulphuric acid, heat at 140° for 5 minutes, add 5 ml of water, make alkaline with *sodium hydroxide solution*, and pour a few drops of the mixture into a large volume of water; a bright green fluorescence is produced.

MELTING-POINT. About 46°.

ULTRAVIOLET ABSORPTION. In alcohol (95%), maximum at 248 nm (E1%, 1cm = 8.5).

INFRA-RED ABSORPTION. Major peaks at 1130, 1208, 1348, 1376, 1700, and 1777 cm^{-1} (see Appendix 2a: Infra-red Spectra).

Determination in body fluids. ULTRAVIOLET SPECTRO-PHOTOMETRY. In serum—S. E. Hansen, *Acta pharmac. tox.*, 1963, **20**, 286.

GAS CHROMATOGRAPHY. In serum—E. B. Solow and J. B. Green, *Clinica chim. Acta*, 1971, **33**, 87; in plasma or urine—E. Van der Kleijn *et al.*, *J. Pharm. Pharmac.*, 1973, **25**, 324.

Metabolism. ABSORPTION. Readily absorbed after oral administration.

BLOOD CONCENTRATION. After oral doses of 10 to 45 mg/kg daily, plasma concentrations of up to 150 μg/ml are attained; after a single dose of about 20 mg/kg, peak plasma concentrations of about 70 μg/ml are attained in about 2 hours; after large daily doses, plasma concentrations steadily increase until the fourth to seventh days; therapeutic plasma concentrations are in the range 40 to 70 μg/ml.

HALF-LIFE. Plasma half-life, 50 to 60 hours in adults and about 30 hours in children.

DISTRIBUTION. Uniformly distributed throughout the body and enters the cerebrospinal fluid; ethosuximide crosses the placenta; *protein binding*, weakly and not significantly bound to plasma proteins.

METABOLIC REACTIONS. Hydroxylation to produce several metabolites including 2-ethyl-3-hydroxy-2-methylsuccinimide and 2-(1-hydroxyethyl)-2-methyl-succinimide; the latter is further oxidised to produce 2-acetyl-2-methylsuccinimide.

EXCRETION. 10 to 20% is excreted in the urine as un-changed drug and metabolites after a single dose.

FURTHER INFORMATION. Absorption and elimination in children—R. A. Buchanan *et al.*, *J. clin. Pharmac.*, 1969, **9**, 393; plasma concentrations—R. A. Buchanan *et al.*, *Clin. Pharmac. Ther.*, 1976, **19**, 143; concentrations

in blood—A. F. Haerer *et al.*, *J. clin. Pharmac.*, 1970, **10**, 370; metabolism in rat and man—M. G. Horning *et al.*, *Drug Met. Disp.*, 1973, **1**, 569 and P. G. Preste *et al.*, *J. pharm. Sci.*, 1974, **63**, 467; concentrations in plasma and urine—E. Van der Kleijn *et al.*, *J. Pharm. Pharmac.*, 1973, **25**, 324.

Actions and uses. Ethosuximide is an anticonvulsant used in the treatment of petit mal. Pure petit mal responds better than mixed petit mal.

Ethosuximide may be administered in combination with other anticonvulsants, such as phenobarbitone, pheny-toin sodium, or primidone, to treat petit mal when it co-exists with grand mal or other forms of epilepsy. Occasionally, the use of this combined treatment may increase the frequency of the grand mal attacks in these cases and the medication used for controlling the major seizures may require adjustment. Patients with petit mal who have proved to be resistant to other anticonvulsants have been treated successfully with ethosuximide.

The initial dosage for patients under 6 years of age is 250 milligrams daily and, for patients 6 years of age and over, 500 milligrams daily in divided doses. Dosage thereafter should be adjusted by small increments, according to the response of the patient, to a maximum of 1 gram for a child of 6 years and of 2 grams for an adult, daily in divided doses.

Undesirable effects. Mild reactions, which are usually transient, may occur initially; these include drowsiness, headache, and gastric upset. Occasionally, skin rashes have occurred.

Haematological reactions, including leucopenia, agran-ulocytosis, and aplastic anaemia, have sometimes occurred with ethosuximide therapy. Administration to patients with temporal lobe seizures may precipitate an acute psychosis.

Preparations

ETHOSUXIMIDE CAPSULES: consisting of ethosuximide, which may be mixed with a suitable inert diluent, en-closed in a soft capsule. The capsule shells may be coloured. Available as capsules containing 250 mg of ethosuximide.

A standard for these capsules is given in the British Pharmacopoeia 1973
Containers and *Storage:* see the entry on Capsules for general information on containers and storage.
Advice for patients: the capsules should be taken at regular intervals, preferably after meals. Treatment should not be discontinued without the advice of the prescriber. The capsules may cause drowsiness; persons affected should not drive or operate machinery. Alcohol should be avoided.

ETHOSUXIMIDE ELIXIR (*Syn.* Ethosuximide Syrup): a solution of ethosuximide in a suitable coloured flavoured vehicle. Available as an elixir containing 250 mg of etho-suximide in 5 ml.

When a dose less than or not a multiple of 5 ml is prescribed, the elixir may be diluted, as described in the entry on Elixirs, with a suitable diluent. The diluted elixir must be freshly prepared. *Emeside*® may be diluted with water for preparations and *Zarontin*® may be diluted with syrup.

A standard for this elixir is given in the British Pharmaceutical Codex 1973
Containers and *Labelling:* see the entry on Elixirs for general information on containers and labelling.
Storage: it should be stored in a cool place.
Advice for patients: the elixir should be taken at regular intervals, preferably after meals. Treatment should not

be discontinued without the advice of the prescriber. The elixir may cause drowsiness; persons affected should not drive or operate machinery. Alcohol should be avoided.

Ethotoin

3-Ethyl-5-phenylimidazolidine-2,4-dione

$C_{11}H_{12}N_2O_2 = 204.2$

OTHER NAME: *Peganone*®

A standard is given in the British Pharmacopoeia 1973

Description. A white, crystalline, almost odourless, almost tasteless powder.

Solubility. Practically insoluble in water; soluble, at 20°, in 4 parts of dehydrated alcohol, in 25 parts of ether, and in 1.5 parts of chloroform.

Melting-point. About 90°.

Moisture content. Not more than 1%, determined by Fischer titration.

Actions and uses. Ethotoin has an anticonvulsant action resembling that described under Phenytoin Sodium but it is much less effective and is less liable to produce undesirable effects. Ethotoin is usually given in conjunction with other anticonvulsant drugs, such as phenobarbitone and phenytoin, in the treatment of grand mal epilepsy. The initial dosage for an adult is 1 gram by mouth daily, gradually increased to 2 or 3 grams daily while the dosage of the other anticonvulsant drugs given at the same time is gradually reduced. The initial daily dosage for a child is 500 milligrams, which may be gradually increased to 2 grams.

Undesirable effects. Ethotoin seldom produces visual disturbances or hyperplasia of the gums, but occasionally skin rashes, nausea, vomiting, dizziness, headache, and drowsiness may occur.

Precautions; Drug interactions. As for Phenytoin Sodium.

Preparation

ETHOTOIN TABLETS: available as tablets containing 500 mg of ethotoin.
A standard for these tablets is given in the British Pharmacopoeia 1973
Containers and *Storage:* see the entry on Tablets for general information on containers and storage. Containers should be airtight.
Advice for patients: the tablets should preferably be taken after meals. When initiating treatment there may be a time-lag of up to 2 weeks before a full therapeutic response is obtained. Treatment should not be discontinued without the advice of the prescriber. The tablets may cause drowsiness; persons affected should not drive or operate machinery. Alcohol should be avoided.

Ethyl Chloride

Chloroethane
$C_2H_5Cl = 64.51$

A standard is given in the British Pharmacopoeia 1973

CAUTION. *Ethyl chloride is highly inflammable and mixtures of the gas with 5 to 15% of air are explosive.*

Ethyl chloride is prepared by the action of hydrogen chloride on ethyl alcohol and may contain a small variable proportion of methyl chloride if industrial methylated spirit is used as the source of alcohol.

Description. It is a gas at ordinary temperatures and pressures but is liquefied by slight compression, forming a colourless, mobile, inflammable, very volatile liquid, in which form it is usually supplied. It has a pleasant ethereal odour and a burning taste. It has a flash-point of $-58°$ F (closed-cup test).

Solubility. Very slightly soluble in water; miscible with alcohol and with ether.

Weight per ml. At 0°, about 0.92 g.

Boiling-point. Under normal pressure, about 12°.

Storage. It should be stored in a cool place, protected from light.

Actions and uses. Ethyl chloride is a volatile anaesthetic which was formerly used for the induction of general anaesthesia but it has been superseded by safer agents. Ethyl chloride has been used as a local anaesthetic, the intense cold produced by the rapid evaporation of the spray rendering the tissues insensitive by freezing, but this procedure is not recommended.

Poisoning. In the event of poisoning, resulting in collapse, the procedure as described under Chloroform should be adopted.

Ethyl Gallate

Ethyl 3,4,5-trihydroxybenzoate

$C_9H_{10}O_5 = 198.2$

OTHER NAME: *Progallin A*®

A standard is given in the British Pharmacopoeia Addendum 1978

Description. A white to creamy-white, odourless, crystalline powder.

Solubility. Soluble, at 20°, in 500 parts of water, in 3 parts of alcohol, in 3 parts of ether, and in 20 000 parts of arachis oil.

Moisture content. Not more than 1%, determined by drying at 105°.

Storage. It should be stored in airtight containers, contact with metals being avoided, protected from light.

Identification. TEST. It complies with Test 2 described under Dodecyl Gallate.

MELTING-POINT. About 152°.

Uses. Ethyl gallate is used as an antioxidant for preserving oils and fats as described under Dodecyl Gallate. Since it is more soluble in water than the higher alkyl gallates, it can be used to inhibit the autoxidation of aqueous preparations.

Ethyl Hydroxybenzoate

Ethyl 4-hydroxybenzoate

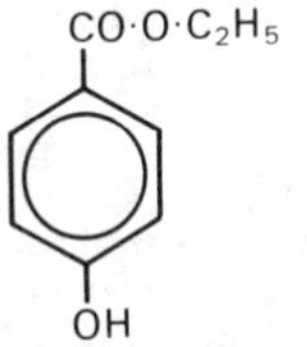

CO·O·C$_2$H$_5$

OH

$C_9H_{10}O_3 = 166.2$

OTHER NAMES: Ethylparaben; *Nipagin A*®

A standard is given in the British Pharmacopoeia Addendum 1978

Description. An odourless white crystalline powder.

Solubility. Soluble, at 20°, in 1500 parts of water, in 2 parts of alcohol, in 3.5 parts of ether, and in 200 parts of glycerol; soluble in solutions of alkali hydroxides.

Identification. TEST. It complies with the test described under Methyl Hydroxybenzoate.

MELTING-POINT. About 117°.

Uses. Ethyl hydroxybenzoate has preservative properties, as described under Methyl Hydroxybenzoate. It is used in a concentration of 0.05% in conjunction with other hydroxybenzoates as a preservative in aqueous preparations.

Ethyl Oleate

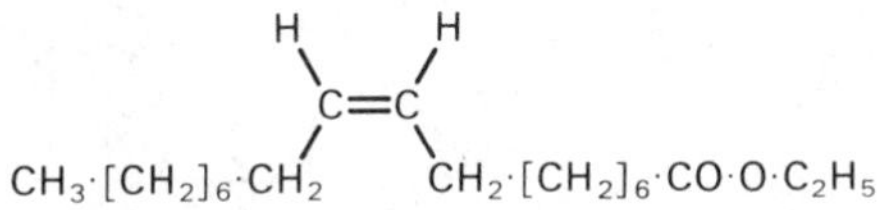

H   H

C=C

CH$_3$·[CH$_2$]$_6$·CH$_2$ CH$_2$·[CH$_2$]$_6$·CO·O·C$_2$H$_5$

$C_{20}H_{38}O_2 = 310.5$

A standard is given in the British Pharmacopoeia 1973

Description. A pale yellow, oily, almost odourless liquid with a taste somewhat resembling that of olive oil.

Solubility. Practically insoluble in water; miscible with alcohol, with ether, with chloroform, and with fixed oils.

Weight per ml. 0.869 to 0.874 g.

Stability. On storage in contact with air it is slowly oxidised. A suitable antoxidant may be added to retard oxidation.

Sterilisation. It is sterilised by dry heat.

Labelling. The label on the container states the name and proportion of any added antoxidant.

Storage. It should be stored in small, well-filled, airtight containers or in an atmosphere of nitrogen, protected from light.

Uses. Ethyl oleate has properties similar to those of certain fixed oils such as almond and arachis oils, except that it is less viscous, is a better solvent, and is more rapidly absorbed by the tissues. It is therefore sometimes used instead of fixed oils as a vehicle for injections.

Ethylenediamine Hydrate

NH$_2$·CH$_2$·CH$_2$·NH$_2$, H$_2$O

$C_2H_8N_2, H_2O = 78.11$

A standard is given in the British Pharmacopoeia 1973

Description. A clear, colourless or slightly yellow, strongly alkaline liquid with an ammoniacal odour.

Solubility. Miscible with water and with alcohol.

Storage. It should be stored in airtight containers, protected from light.

Identification. TEST. Mix 1 ml with 5 ml of water and to 3 drops of the mixture add 2 ml of a 1% solution of copper sulphate and shake; a purplish-blue colour is produced.

Uses. Ethylenediamine hydrate is used in the preparation of aminophylline injection.

Ethylmorphine Hydrochloride

3-O-Ethylmorphine hydrochloride dihydrate

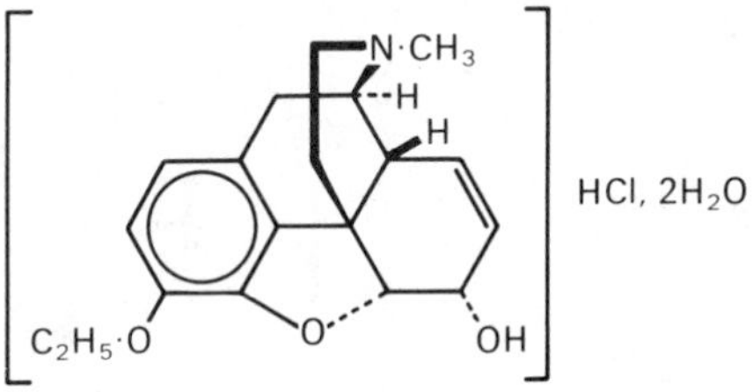

N·CH$_3$

--H

H

HCl, 2H$_2$O

C$_2$H$_5$·O   O   OH

$C_{19}H_{24}ClNO_3, 2H_2O = 385.9$

OTHER NAMES: Aethylmorphini Hydrochloridum; Ethylmorphini Hydrochloridum

A standard is given in the European Pharmacopoeia Vol. III

Description. A white, minutely crystalline, odourless powder with a bitter taste.

Solubility. Soluble, at 20°, in 12 parts of water and in 25 parts of alcohol; soluble in 1 part of warm alcohol; very slightly soluble in chloroform; practically insoluble in ether.

Acidity. A 2% solution has a pH of 4 to 5.4

Loss on drying. 8 to 10%, determined by drying at 105°.

Specific rotation. $-102°$ to $-105°$, determined on a 2% solution.

Dissociation constant. pK_a 8.2 (20°).

Sterilisation. Solutions are sterilised by heating with a bactericide or by filtration.

Storage. It should be protected from light.

Identification. TESTS. 1. Dissolve about 5 mg in 5 ml of water and add 1 ml of *potassium iodobismuthate solution*; an orange or orange-red precipitate is produced. 2. To about 10 mg add 1 ml of sulphuric acid and 1 drop of *ferric chloride test-solution* and warm; a blue colour is produced. Add 1 drop of nitric acid; the colour changes to red. 3. Dissolve about 600 mg in 6 ml of water, add 15 ml of 0.1N sodium hydroxide, and induce crystallisation; a white crystalline precipitate is produced which, after washing with water, recrystallising from water, and drying *in vacuo*, melts at about 85°.

MELTING-POINT. About 123°.

ULTRAVIOLET ABSORPTION. In 0.2N sulphuric acid, maximum at 285 nm (E1%, 1cm = 49).

INFRA-RED ABSORPTION. Major peaks at 952, 1042, 1064,

1136, 1190, and 1266 cm^{-1} (see Appendix 2b: Infra-red Spectra).

THIN-LAYER CHROMATOGRAPHY. See under Thin-layer Chromatography, System 7.

Actions and uses. Ethylmorphine has some of the actions of morphine and codeine but does not depress the respiratory centre to the same extent as morphine. A 1 to 5% solution of ethylmorphine hydrochloride has been used in ophthalmic practice in the treatment of corneal ulceration, iritis, and glaucoma; ethylmorphine increases the blood supply to the tissues and may provoke a sharp burning sensation and some oedema of the conjunctiva, but this soon subsides.

Ethylmorphine has also been used as an ingredient of linctuses to allay cough in bronchitis, bronchial asthma, and whooping-cough. For the relief of cough it is used in doses of 5 to 30 milligrams.

Ethyloestrenol

19-Nor-17α-pregn-4-en-17-ol

$C_{20}H_{32}O = 288.5$

OTHER NAMES: Ethylestrenol; *Orabolin*®

A standard is given in the British Pharmacopoeia Addendum 1975

Description. A white crystalline odourless powder.

Solubility. Very slightly soluble in water; soluble, at 20°, in 9 parts of alcohol, in 6 parts of ether, and in 2 parts of chloroform.

Specific rotation. +29° to +33°, determined on a 1% solution in dioxan.

Storage. It should be stored in a cool place, protected from light.

Identification. MELTING-POINT. About 89°.

ULTRAVIOLET ABSORPTION. In methyl alcohol there is no significant absorption in the range 230 to 350 nm.

INFRA-RED ABSORPTION. Major peaks at 975, 995, 1040, 1302, 1434, and 1450 cm^{-1} (see Appendix 2a: Infra-red Spectra).

THIN-LAYER CHROMATOGRAPHY. See under Thin-layer Chromatography, System 10.

Actions and uses. Ethyloestrenol has actions and uses similar to those described under Methandienone but it is devoid of androgenic effects. In high dosage it has a slight progestational activity.

Ethyloestrenol is used to promote nitrogen and calcium retention and protein synthesis in debility states, in post-operative recovery and convalescence, in the treatment of osteoporosis, and during prolonged treatment with corticosteroids.

The usual dosage for an adult is 2 to 4 milligrams daily in divided doses, but doses of up to 10 milligrams daily have been given. Children usually require about 50 micrograms per kilogram body-weight daily in divided doses.

Undesirable effects. Slight progestational effects may be observed when dosage exceeds the recommended range. Nausea, vomiting, and fluid retention may occur.

Precautions and contra-indications. It should be given with caution in the presence of liver disease. Doses above the recommended range should not be given to women during the first half of the menstrual cycle. It should be used with caution in children because of the possibility of reducing normal growth. It is contra-indicated in pregnancy and in carcinoma of the prostate.

Drug interactions. It prolongs the prothrombin time in patients being treated with oral anticoagulants.

Veterinary uses. Ethyloestrenol is an anabolic steroid which is effective when given by mouth. It is used in the treatment of convalescent and debilitated animals and to promote healing of wounds and fractures. The usual dose for dogs and cats is 50 micrograms per kilogram body-weight daily.

Preparation

ETHYLOESTRENOL TABLETS: available as tablets containing 2 mg of ethyloestrenol.

A standard for these tablets is given in the British Pharmacopoeia Addendum 1975

Containers and *Storage:* see the entry on Tablets for general information on containers and storage. Containers should be airtight and light resistant. The tablets should be stored in a cool place.

Ethynodiol Diacetate

19-Nor-17α-pregn-4-en-20-yne-3β,17-diol diacetate

$C_{24}H_{32}O_4 = 384.5$

OTHER NAMES: *Femulen*®

Demulen 50®, *Metrulen 50*®, *Ovamin 30*®, and *Ovulen 50*® (all with ethinyloestradiol); *Demulen*®, *Metrulen*®, *Metrulen M*®, and *Ovulen 1 mg*® (all with mestranol)

A standard is given in the British Pharmacopoeia 1973

Description. A white crystalline odourless powder.

Solubility. Very slightly soluble in water; soluble, at 20°, in 15 parts of alcohol, in 3.5 parts of ether, and in 1 part of chloroform.

Specific rotation. −70° to −76°, determined on a 1% solution in chloroform.

Storage. It should be stored in airtight containers, protected from light.

Identification. TEST. It complies with Test 3 described under Cortisone Acetate (presence of acetyl groups).

MELTING-POINT. About 128°.

THIN-LAYER CHROMATOGRAPHY. See under Thin-layer Chromatography, System 10.

Determination in body fluids. RADIOIMMUNOASSAY. In plasma—C. Walls *et al.*, *J. Steroid Biochem.*, 1977, **8**, 167.

Metabolism. ABSORPTION. Rapidly absorbed after oral administration.

HALF-LIFE. Plasma half-life for drug plus metabolites, about 25 hours.

DISTRIBUTION. There does not appear to be any selective tissue uptake of ethynodiol diacetate or its metabolites; ethynodiol is secreted in the milk and, in mice, crosses the placenta.

METABOLIC REACTIONS. Hydrolysis, reduction of ring A, formation of a keto-group at carbon 3, aromatisation of ring A, double bond formation at position 6, and hydroxylation to the mono-, di-, and polyhydroxy-metabolites; conjugation also occurs but most of the water-soluble metabolites appear to be unconjugated hydroxylated metabolites; metabolites detected in man *in vivo* include 17α-ethinyl-3β,10β,17β-trihydroxy-5α-oestrane, 17α-ethinyl-17β-hydroxyoestr-4-en-3-one (norethindrone), and 3α- and 3β-hydroxy-5α- and 5β-saturated metabolites and also small amounts of ethinyloestradiol.

EXCRETION. 13 to 67% of a dose is excreted in the urine and 13 to 25% is excreted in the faeces; the major urinary metabolites appear to be polyhydroxylated oestranes.

FURTHER INFORMATION. Metabolism—P. K. Besch *et al.*, *Metabolism*, 1965, **14**, 432, C. E. Cook *et al.*, *J. Pharmac. exp. Ther.*, 1973, **185**, 696, R. I. Freudenthal *et al.*, *J. Pharmac. exp. Ther.*, 1971, **177**, 468 and 1972, **182**, 328, Y. Kishimoto *et al.*, *Xenobiotica*, 1972, **2**, 237, and H. Watanabe *et al.*, *Steroids*, 1968, **11**, 97; excretion in milk—G. Pincus *et al.*, *Nature*, 1966, **212**, 924.

Actions and uses. Ethynodiol diacetate is a synthetic progestational steroid hormone which has an action similar to that of norethisterone. It is active when taken by mouth and is generally used in conjunction with oestrogens.

In the treatment of primary and secondary amenorrhoea and of functional uterine bleeding, it is given daily in a dosage of 1 or 2 milligrams from the fifth day of the menstrual cycle and continuing until the twenty-fourth day; withdrawal bleeding usually occurs 1 to 3 days after discontinuing treatment. For the treatment of endometriosis, doses of 4 milligrams or more are given daily for periods of 9 to 12 months.

Ethynodiol diacetate is used in conjunction with oestrogens as an oral contraceptive to inhibit ovulation. For this purpose doses of 0.5 to 2 milligrams are given daily, with ethinyloestradiol or mestranol, from the fifth to the twenty-fourth day of each menstrual cycle. The course is repeated after an interval of 1 week. Regular administration is essential.

Undesirable effects; Precautions and contra-indications. As for Norethisterone.

Preparations

Preparations available include TABLETS containing ethynodiol diacetate 500 micrograms; tablets containing ethynodiol diacetate 500 micrograms, 1 mg, and 2 mg, each with ethinyloestradiol 50 micrograms; tablets containing ethynodiol diacetate 2 mg with ethinyloestradiol 30 micrograms; and tablets containing ethynodiol diacetate 500 micrograms, 1 mg, and 2 mg, each with mestranol 100 micrograms.

Etorphine Hydrochloride

7,8-Dihydro-7α-[(1R)-1-hydroxy-1-methylbutyl]-O^6-methyl-6α,14α-ethenomorphine hydrochloride

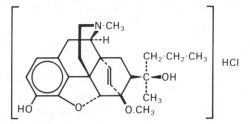

$C_{25}H_{34}ClNO_4 = 448.0$

OTHER NAMES: *Immobilon*® (with acepromazine maleate or methotrimeprazine for large and small animals respectively); M99

A standard is given in the British Pharmacopoeia (Veterinary)

CAUTION. *Etorphine is a powerful analgesic. It should be handled with care and precautions should be taken to avoid inhalation of airborne particles.*

Description. A white microcrystalline powder.

Solubility. Soluble, at 20°, in 40 parts of water, in 30 parts of alcohol, and in 2200 parts of chloroform; practically insoluble in ether.

Acidity. A 2% solution has a pH of 4 to 5.5.

Moisture content. Not more than 4%, determined by drying at 105°.

Specific rotation. −122° to −132°, determined on a 2% solution in methyl alcohol.

Sterilisation. Solutions are sterilised by heating in an autoclave or by filtration.

Storage. It should be stored in airtight containers, protected from light.

Identification. TEST. To about 100 mg add 2 ml of sulphuric acid; a reddish-brown colour is produced.

MELTING-POINT. About 266°.

ULTRAVIOLET ABSORPTION. In 0.1N hydrochloric acid, maximum at 289 nm (E1%, 1cm = 34); in 0.1N sodium hydroxide, maximum at 302 nm (E1%, 1cm = 60).

Veterinary uses. Etorphine hydrochloride is a narcotic analgesic used with tranquillisers to immobilise animals and produce neuroleptanalgesia. Effects should be reversed by a suitable antagonist such as diprenorphine (for animals) and naloxone or nalorphine (for human patients accidentally exposed).

Etorphine is very toxic to man if accidentally injected or absorbed through the skin; suitable precautions should be taken and the appropriate antagonist should be kept available whenever etorphine or its preparations are being handled.

The dose of etorphine hydrochloride in conjunction with acepromazine or methotrimeprazine is as given below for the appropriate preparations.

Preparations

ETORPHINE AND ACEPROMAZINE INJECTION: a sterile solution of etorphine hydrochloride and acepromazine maleate, with sodium chloride and a suitable preservative, in water for injections. The acidity of the solution is adjusted to pH 4. The solution is sterilised by heating in an autoclave or by filtration. It contains 2.45 mg of etorphine hydrochloride and 10 mg of acepromazine maleate per ml. Available in 10-ml vials.

A standard for this injection is given in the British Pharmacopoeia (Veterinary)

Containers and *Labelling:* see the entry on Injections for general information on containers and labelling.

Storage: it should be protected from light.

Dose: horses and cattle, 0.5 millilitre per 50 kilograms body-weight by intravenous or intramuscular injection; sheep, 0.25 millilitre per 50 kilograms body-weight by intramuscular injection; pigs, 0.5 millilitre per 50 kilograms body-weight by intramuscular injection.

ETORPHINE AND METHOTRIMEPRAZINE INJECTION: a sterile solution of etorphine hydrochloride and methotrimeprazine, with suitable stabilising agents, in water for injections. The acidity of the solution is adjusted to pH 4. The solution is sterilised by heating in an autoclave or by filtration. It contains 74 micrograms of etorphine hydrochloride and 18 mg of methotrimeprazine per ml. Available in 20-ml vials.

A standard for this injection is given in the British Pharmacopoeia (Veterinary)

Containers and *Labelling:* see the entry on Injections for general information on containers and labelling.

Storage: it should be protected from light.

Dose: dogs, 0.1 millilitre per kilogram body-weight by intramuscular injection or 0.05 millilitre per kilogram body-weight by intravenous injection.

Eucalyptus Oil

Obtained by rectifying the oil distilled from the fresh leaves and terminal branchlets of species of *Eucalyptus* (Fam. Myrtaceae) which yield oils containing a large proportion of cineole but little phellandrene.

OTHER NAMES: Eucalypti Aetheroleum; Oleum Eucalypti

A standard is given in the European Pharmacopoeia Vol. III

Commercial sources of eucalyptus oil are Spain and Portugal, where the oil is derived from *E. globulus* Labill., and Australia, where several species of *Eucalyptus* are used. Two species yielding oil of suitable quality are *E. fruticetorum* F. von Mueller (*E. polybractea* R. T. Baker) and *E. smithii* R. T. Baker.

Constituents. Contains chiefly cineole, which is also known as eucalyptol. It also contains (+)-α-pinene and other terpenes; phellandrene may also be present in small quantities.

Description. A colourless or pale yellow liquid with an aromatic camphoraceous odour.

Solubility. Soluble, at 20°, in 5 parts of alcohol (70%); miscible with alcohol (90%), with dehydrated alcohol, with oils, with fats, and with paraffins.

Weight per ml. At 20°, 0.904 to 0.924 g.

Refractive index. 1.458 to 1.470.

Optical rotation. 0° to +10°.

Storage. It should be stored in well-filled airtight containers, in a cool place, protected from light.

Actions and uses. Eucalyptus oil has been applied to the skin in ointments and liniments as a counter-irritant. To relieve cough in chronic bronchitis it is inhaled from steam with other volatile compounds such as menthol. It is an ingredient of pastilles for the symptomatic relief of common cold. The usual dose is 0.05 to 0.2 millilitre.

Oily solutions of eucalyptus oil should not be used as nasal drops because the vehicle inhibits ciliary movements and may cause lipoid pneumonia.

Preparation

MENTHOL AND EUCALYPTUS INHALATION:

Menthol	20 g
Eucalyptus oil	100 ml
Light magnesium carbonate	70 g
Water for preparations	to 1000 ml

Dissolve the menthol in the eucalyptus oil and add the light magnesium carbonate and sufficient of the water to produce the required volume.

A standard for this inhalation is given in the British Pharmaceutical Codex 1973

Containers and *Labelling:* see the entry on Inhalations for general information on containers and labelling.

Advice for patients: see the entry on Inhalations for general information on the use of inhalations.

Extracts

Extracts are concentrated products containing the active principles of crude drugs.

Liquid extracts are prepared by maceration or percolation with suitable solvents followed by concentration, and are usually of such a strength that 1 part by volume of the product is equivalent to 1 part by weight of the crude drug. If, however, the active principle is of a potent nature and permits of an assay, the liquid extract is adjusted to a definite strength.

Dry extracts are prepared by evaporating the extractive from the crude drug to dryness, usually under reduced pressure. If the active principle is of a potent nature and permits of an assay, the dried extractive is adjusted to a definite strength by dilution with an inert diluent. The strength of the adjusted dry extract bears no relation to the content of active principle in the crude drug but is determined by the dose, its strength being so adjusted that the maximum dose is not less than 60 milligrams. Lactose and starch are suitable diluents for most dried extractives; if the dried extractive is deliquescent, however, an absorbent diluent, such as calcium phosphate, is used.

Soft extracts are prepared by evaporating the extractive from the crude drug until a soft mass is obtained.

Preparation of extracts. Extracts are prepared on a small scale by the methods described in the entries on appropriate drugs. When an extract is manufactured in larger quantities, the same method, appropriately scaled up, is used; for certain liquid extracts the following alternative method is permitted: the crude powdered drug is exhausted by percolating with a suitable solvent, the solvent is removed by evaporating the percolate to the consistence of a soft extract, and the extractive is subsequently mixed with an appropriate volume of a suitable mixture of alcohol and water to yield a product that complies with the required standard.

Storage. Deliquescent dry and soft extracts should be stored in airtight containers.

Eye-drops

Eye-drops are sterile liquids for instillation into the conjunctival sac; they contain medicaments dissolved or suspended in aqueous or oily vehicles. Eye-drops may be in single-dose forms or in multiple-application containers.

Types of medicament which are dispensed in the form of eye-drops for both therapeutic and diagnostic purposes include antimicrobials, mydriatics, cycloplegics, miotics, local anaesthetics, and anti-inflammatory agents. Some medicaments produce mainly local effects; they may not necessarily penetrate the cornea. Miotics, mydriatics, most anti-inflammatory agents, and some antimicrobials pass through the precorneal film and the cornea by either passive diffusion or active transport processes. Penetration of the cornea appears to be enhanced when the medicament is soluble in both lipids and water or when its molecules are small.

Aqueous eye-drops to be presented in multiple-application containers are prepared in a vehicle which is both bactericidal and fungicidal; for this purpose, solutions containing phenylmercuric acetate or nitrate (0.002%), benzalkonium chloride (0.01%), or chlorhexidine acetate (0.01%) are generally suitable. The choice of antimicrobial substance may be governed in some eye-drops by the compatibility of the medicament with other constituents or by the duration of the period during which the eye-drops are likely to be used. In local anaesthetic eye-drops which reduce the blink reflex of the eye, or in eye-drops for patients with exposure keratitis, benzalkonium chloride is not a suitable preservative because of its surface activity on the precorneal film.

Adjuvants which are used in some eye-drops include buffers, sodium metabisulphite, and disodium edetate. Buffers may be used to maintain the pH of the eye-drops at an optimum to minimise chemical breakdown or to increase comfort for the user. Both sodium metabisulphite and disodium edetate are effective in retarding oxidation reactions and, in some systems, disodium edetate also enhances the bactericidal activity of benzalkonium chloride and chlorhexidine acetate.

Thickening agents such as hypromellose and other cellulose derivatives are included in certain eye-drops. Other substances such as povidone and polyvinyl alcohol are used to decrease the contact angle between the solution and the eye. An increase in the viscosity of eye-drops can enhance the therapeutic effect by extending the contact time of the medicament with the eye surface, or it may enhance comfort, especially in patients with deficient tear secretion. It is not usual to adjust the tonicity of the drops with the exception of those used as "artificial tears", for example, hypromellose eye-drops.

Single-dose forms consist of about 0.5 ml of the eye-drops in a flexible applicator pack enclosed in a sealed outer container; the applicator pack and its contents are sterile. The solution should comply with the formula specified in the relevant monograph except that the preservative is omitted.

It is known that some medicaments can be concentrated in soft hydrophilic contact lenses with consequent modification of the intensity and duration of the therapeutic action; also, concentration of a preservative in the contact lens may lead to eye irritation. Wherever possible, wearers of such lenses should remove them before administration of therapeutic preparations but if this is not practicable the use of a single-dose form may be preferable.

When the eye-drops are dispensed for domiciliary use, the user should be warned of the need to avoid contamination during application. It has been suggested that a suitably worded leaflet be issued to the patient. In general, a container of eye-drops may be used for domiciliary purposes for about 4 weeks after first opening the container.

When the eye-drops are dispensed for use in hospital wards, individual supplies of previously unopened containers should be provided for each patient. When both eyes are being treated, a separate container should be used for each eye. Single-dose forms are required in all circumstances in which the dangers of infection are high. When single-dose forms are specified but are not available, multiple-application containers may be used, provided that the same principle is adhered to, that is, use of a previously unopened container for 1 patient on 1 occasion only.

Fluorescein eye-drops for use in any area in a hospital should only be supplied in single-dose form. Sterile fluorescein strips are available, individually wrapped; these may also be used.

Eye-drops used in hospital wards should be discarded not later than 1 week after first opening the container. When used for treating a patient before an operation on the eye, they should be discarded at the time of the operation and, if treatment with eye-drops is continued after the operation, fresh supplies should be provided. Similarly, at the time of discharge of the patient from the hospital, eye-drops in use should be discarded and, if treatment is to be continued, fresh supplies should be given to the patient.

Eye-drops for use in out-patient departments, except fluorescein eye-drops, may be supplied and used in multiple-application containers. The contents of opened containers should be discarded at the end of each day, but, if an incorporated dropper becomes contaminated, the remaining contents should be discarded immediately. A patient who undergoes out-patient surgery which requires the use of eye-drops should be treated with a separate supply of eye-drops from a previously unopened container and given a further fresh supply, if prescribed, after the operation.

Eye-drops for use in clinics for external eye-diseases and ophthalmic accident and emergency departments should be supplied in single-dose form or, if this is not possible, in multiple-application containers used for 1 application only. This precaution is necessary because of the risk of transferring certain viral infections. A particular danger is that infection could be transferred by handling the outside surface of a multiple-application container. Provided that the normal hand-washing procedure is followed before and after examination of each patient, special precautions for maintaining the outer surface of the container free from contamination, by washing with sterile purified water, for example, are unnecessary.

Eye-drops for use in operating theatres should be supplied in single-dose form or, if this is not possible, in multiple-application containers used for one application only. When possible, the outer surface of containers should be sterile and supplied with a sterile overwrap, or else the outer surface of the packs should, as far as possible, be rendered free from contamination by a suitable method such as washing with sterile purified water or by spraying with an antiseptic solution just before the packs are taken into the operating theatre for use.

Hospital and clinic staff and patients should be made aware of the dangers of misuse of eye-drops and should be given guidance on their correct use.

Eye-drops formulated for use in the conventional manner of instilling 1 or 2 drops into the conjunctival sac are not suitable for introduction into the anterior chamber of the eye during surgical procedures. Solutions for the latter purpose should likewise be sterile but should not contain any preservative.

Preparation of eye-drops. A prime requirement of eye-drops is that they should be sterile and, when dispensed in a multiple-application container, they should be effectively preserved against any accidentally-introduced contamination with micro-organisms. Standards of cleanliness for apparatus, containers and the preparation should be similar to those adopted for injections. Guidance on the cleansing of equipment and components of the containers is given in the entry on Sterilisation.

Rubber teats must be cleansed, impregnated with the selected antimicrobial substance and any other preservative included in the eye-drops, and stored in the impregnating solution, as described for the pretreatment of rubber caps in the entry on Sterilisation. It should be established by preliminary tests that the rubber teats are compatible with the antimicrobial substance to be used; they should not yield a turbidity or precipitate when autoclaved in a solution of the selected antimicrobial substance after they have been subjected to this pretreatment. To minimise particulate contamination, eye-drops should be clarified by filtration, ideally through a microporous membrane.

Except where the only source of supply is a ready-prepared commercially produced pack containing a larger amount, not more than 10 ml of the eye-drops should be supplied in a multiple-application container and if more than 10 ml is dispensed at one time, the total quantity of solution should be supplied in an appropriate number of containers.

Eye-drops may be prepared and sterilised by the following methods:

Method A. The medicament is dissolved in the aqueous vehicle containing one of the prescribed antimicrobial substances and any other preservative specified in the individual monograph; the solution is clarified by filtration, transferred to the final containers, which are then closed so as to exclude micro-organisms, and sterilised by heating in an autoclave.

Method B. The medicament is dissolved in the aqueous vehicle containing one of the prescribed antimicrobial substances and any other preservative specified in the individual monograph; the solution is sterilised by filtration and transferred, by means of an aseptic technique, to sterile containers which are then closed so as to exclude micro-organisms.

Method C. The medicament is dissolved in the aqueous vehicle containing one of the prescribed antimicrobial substances and any other preservative specified in the individual monograph; the solution is clarified by filtration, transferred to the final containers which are then closed to exclude micro-organisms, and sterilised by maintaining at 98° to 100° for 30 minutes.

Eye-drops may be prepared by any other method provided that the final product is identical in appearance, quality, and composition with a product prepared by the appropriate method described above or by the method given for a specific preparation.

Containers for eye-drops. Eye-drops should be dispensed in amber-coloured bottles of neutral or surface-treated glass which comply with British Standard 1679: 1974 Part 5. These containers are fitted with a phenolic plastic screw cap which incorporates a neutral glass dropper tube with a natural or synthetic rubber teat; alternatively, the bottle is closed with a plain screw cap of phenolic plastic fitted with a suitable liner, and a complete sterile dropper assembly supplied separately within a sealed package. Applicator bottles made of a suitable plastic, or of a combination of glass and a suitable plastic, may also be used.

Rubber teats, or bottles made of surface-treated glass, should not be autoclaved more than once. If the eye-drops contain benzalkonium chloride, teats of silicone rubber should be used unless the suitability of other types of rubber has been established (as described under Preparation of eye-drops, above).

When a closure is used which incorporates a silicone rubber teat, storage of the filled container should be limited to 3 months.

This is because silicone rubber is permeable to water vapour and a steady loss of water can occur from containers fitted with teats of this material. Teats made of butyl or natural rubber are usually less permeable to water vapour than those of silicone rubber. If eye-drops for which a silicone rubber teat is appropriate are to be stored for more than 3 months, the complete dropper assembly should be supplied separately as a wrapped sterilised unit, as described above. The dropper assembly is exchanged for the plain phenolic cap and liner used to close the container just before issue for use or the patient is instructed to do this on first opening the container.

The cap is covered with an easily removed seal, or the package or carton may be suitably sealed, to prevent the removal of the contents without the seal being broken. For use in operating theatres, the external surface of the pack should, when possible, be sterile and enclosed in a sterile overwrap.

Labelling of eye-drops. Except when issued to the individual patient for domiciliary use, the label on the container or the label or wrapper on the package should indicate the name of the preparation and the concentration of the active ingredients, and the name and concentration of the antimicrobial substances included in the eye-drops. In addition, the labels on containers of eye-drops prepared for use in hospitals should indicate the expiry date and that the contents are sterile until opened. In the case of single-dose forms, the inner container may bear letters and figures by which the active ingredient and its concentration can be identified; if such letters and figures are used, the outer wrapper or containers should be labelled in accordance with the requirements for multiple-application containers.

The following code is suggested:

Adrenaline Eye-drops, Neutral	..	..	ADN
Amethocaine Eye-drops ..	..	..	..	AME
Atropine Sulphate Eye-drops	..	..	..	ATR
Betamethasone Eye-drops	..	..	..	BET
Carbachol Eye-drops	..	..	..	CAR
Chloramphenicol Eye-drops	..	..	..	CPL
Cocaine Eye-drops	..	..	..	CCN
Cyclopentolate Eye-drops	..	..	..	CYC
Fluorescein Eye-drops ..	..	..	..	FLN
Homatropine Eye-drops ..	..	..	..	HOM
Hydrocortisone Eye-drops	..	..	..	HCOR
Hyoscine Eye-drops	..	..	..	HYO
Hypromellose Eye-drops	..	..	..	HPRM
Lachesine Eye-drops	..	..	..	LAC
Neomycin Eye-drops	..	..	..	NEO
Phenylephrine Eye-drops	..	..	..	PHNL
Physostigmine Eye-drops	..	..	..	ESR
Pilocarpine Eye-drops ..	..	..	..	PIL
Prednisolone Eye-drops ..	..	..	..	PRED
Proxymetacaine Eye-drops	..	..	..	PROX
Sulphacetamide Eye-drops	..	..	..	SULF
Zinc Sulphate Eye-drops	..	..	..	ZSU

The word "SALINE" may also be used as a code on the inner container of single-dose forms and as such indicates that the contents are a sterile 0.9% solution of sodium chloride in purified water.

Colour Codes. Opinion is divided on the desirability of using coloured labels as a rapid means of identifying general types of eye-drops. Some hospitals have already adopted colour codes, and to avoid confusion it is desirable that the system used should be uniform. It is therefore suggested that when colour coding is used mydriatics should be indicated by *red* and miotics by *blue* and that these colours should not be used for other types of eye-drops.

Further information. Eye preparations in hospitals, *Pharm. J.*, i/1975, 278.

Eye Lotions

Sterile aqueous solutions used, usually undiluted, for bathing the eyes. There are two types of eye lotion:
(1) sterile aqueous solutions which contain no bactericide; these are used once only for first-aid or for a period of treatment not longer than 24 hours; and
(2) aqueous solutions (sterile when issued) containing a bactericide for intermittent domiciliary use for up to 7 days.

Preparation of eye lotions. All apparatus and containers used in the preparation and packaging of eye lotions should be thoroughly cleansed. The medicament and bactericide, if included, are dissolved in water and the solution is clarified by filtration before transfer to the final container. After closing the container to exclude micro-organisms, the container is sterilised by heating in an autoclave.

Alternatively, the solution is sterilised by filtration and transferred aseptically to the final sterile containers which are then closed to exclude micro-organisms.

Containers. Eye lotions should preferably be supplied in coloured fluted glass bottles, fitted with screw-cap closures; cork wads should not be used. The complete container should be capable of withstanding heating in an autoclave and the closure should prevent subsequent ingress of micro-organisms. Closures should be covered with a readily breakable seal.

Eye lotions should be dispensed in containers which hold a volume sufficient for one treatment of the patient lasting not more than 24 hours for sterile solutions or 7 days for preserved eye lotions; suitable volumes are 25 ml and 200 ml respectively.

Labelling. For sterile type 1 solutions which do not contain a bactericide, the label on the container should indicate that the contents are sterile until opened, that contamination in use should be avoided as far as possible, and that any unused portion of the contents should be discarded after 24 hours.

For type 2 solutions, the label on the container should state the date after which the contents are not intended to be used and, unless otherwise specified by the manufacturer, that any of the solution that remains 7 days after first opening the container should preferably be discarded.

Uses. Application of eye lotions to the eyes is usually effected by means of a small disposable device, a sterile eye-bath, or, when controlled flow is required, a suitable irrigator.

Because eye lotions are applied in larger volumes than eye-drops, the extent of dilution of the lachrymal fluid is increased, and it is therefore desirable that eye lotions should be made iso-osmotic with tears to ensure comfort for the patient.

Eye lotions containing weak acid or alkali, chelating agents, or specific chemical reagents, have been used in the past mainly for the emergency treatment of burns in the eye caused by particular substances. As such solutions are now thought to be of limited value in emergencies, they have been largely replaced by sterile sodium chloride eye lotion which is useful for first-aid treatment and for the removal of conjunctival discharges. For convenience for first-aid use, commercial plastic packs of sodium chloride injection (0.9%), which is identical in composition with sodium chloride eye lotion, may be used.

Solutions containing sodium bicarbonate, usually in a strength of 2%, have been used in hospitals for the treatment of blepharitis. However, such solutions have only limited stability, as they may cause particles to separate from glass containers or become increasingly alkaline due to loss of carbon dioxide by permeation through plastic containers.

Eye Ointments

Sterile semi-solid preparations for application to the conjunctival sac or to the eyelid margin; they contain medicaments dissolved or dispersed in a suitable non-irritant basis.

In using eye ointments, precautions should be taken to avoid contamination. For domiciliary use, the ointment is best applied directly from the tube or with the aid of a clean glass rod. When used in hospital wards, a single-application pack should be opened, if necessary, with a sterile instrument and the eye ointment applied directly to the eye. When a multiple-application container is used, the eye ointment should be applied to the eye with a sterile applicator. Sterile applicators should preferably be supplied singly in sealed packs and should each be used for one application only.

Eye ointments usually contain substances with antimicrobial, anti-inflammatory, mydriatic, or miotic properties. To maintain stability or to protect the preparation from contamination, antoxidants, stabilisers, or antimicrobial substances may also be included. Insoluble medicaments which are suspended in the basis should be reduced to an extremely fine powder before incorporation to avoid irritation to the eye.

Oleaginous and mainly anhydrous materials have commonly been used as bases for eye ointments. All bases used for eye ointments should be non-irritant to the eye and should permit diffusion of the medicament when in contact with the fluids at the eye surface. More recently, absorption bases, mineral oil gelled with polyethylene, or water-soluble bases containing macrogols, have been introduced as eye ointment bases; however, there is little published information on the bioavailability of medicaments from eye ointment bases, whatever their type.

Preparation of eye ointments. The apparatus used in the preparation of eye ointments must be thoroughly cleansed and sterilised. A suitable basis for eye ointments may be prepared according to the following formula:

EYE OINTMENT BASIS

Liquid paraffin	100 g
Wool fat	100 g
Yellow soft paraffin	800 g

Heat together the wool fat, the yellow soft paraffin, and

the liquid paraffin; filter while hot through a coarse filter paper in a heated funnel. Sterilise by heating for a sufficient time to ensure that the whole of the basis is maintained at a temperature of 150° for one hour, and allow to cool, taking precautions to avoid contamination with micro-organisms, before incorporating the sterile medicament.

For eye ointments intended to be used in tropical or subtropical climates, the proportions of the paraffins may be varied, or hard paraffin may be included, when prevailing high temperatures otherwise make the ointments too soft for convenience.

Eye ointments are prepared, by means of an aseptic technique, by either of the following methods:

Method A. If the medicament is readily soluble in water forming a stable solution, it is dissolved in the minimum quantity of water and the solution is sterilised by autoclaving or by filtration and incorporated gradually in the melted sterile basis, the mixture being stirred continuously until it is cold. The eye ointment is then transferred to the final sterile containers, which are closed to exclude micro-organisms.

Method B. If it is not readily soluble in water or if the aqueous solution is unstable, the sterile medicament (see entry on Sterilisation), reduced to a suitable particle-size range, is thoroughly mixed with a small quantity of the melted sterile basis, and then incorporated with the remainder of the sterile basis. The eye ointment is then transferred to the final sterile containers, which are closed so as to exclude micro-organisms.

Other methods. Methods appropriate to sterilisation by ionising radiation may also be used (see the entry on Sterilisation).

Containers. Eye ointments for multiple application should be packed in small, sterilised, collapsible tubes of suitable metal or plastic; it should be possible to fit a cannula, and the tube must be closed to prevent ingress of micro-organisms. Metal tubes used for eye ointments should comply with British Standard 4230: 1967. All containers should be as free as possible from dirt and particles of the material used in their construction. Screw caps, if fitted, should not contain wads made from cork. Alternatively, eye ointments may be supplied in single-application containers such as soft gelatin capsules with applicator tips.

Unless the eye ointment has been prepared extemporaneously, the screw cap should be covered with a readily breakable seal or, alternatively, the whole container should be sealed in an outer package such as a paperboard carton or pouch of paper, plastic, or cellulose film.

Quantity supplied. Not more than 5 grams should be supplied in each container.

Labelling. Except when an eye ointment is dispensed on a medical prescription for an individual patient, the label on the container, or on the sealed outer package, should indicate that the contents are sterile provided that the container has not been opened.

Note. When Simple Eye Ointment or Non-medicated Eye Ointment is ordered or prescribed, sterile eye ointment basis is supplied.

Factor IX Fraction, Dried Human

Prepared from human plasma; it is rich in clotting factors II, IX, and X and may also contain clotting factor VII.

OTHER NAME: Human Coagulation Factor (II, IX, and X)

A standard is given in the British Pharmacopoeia Addendum 1978

Dried human factor IX fraction is prepared by a suitable fractionation technique from plasma that has been obtained as described under Dried Human Antihaemophilic Fraction or from plasma which has been kept in the liquid state at a temperature not above 6° for not more than 48 hours or not higher than −30° for not more than 12 months. The solution is sterilised by filtration through a membrane filter and immediately frozen and dried. No preservative is added.

It is a white or slightly coloured powder or friable solid which, when dissolved in a volume of water equal to the volume of water for injections stated on the label, yields a solution which contains not less than 20 units of clotting factor IX per ml, not more than 300 millimoles of sodium ions per litre, not more than 60 millimoles of citrate ions per litre, and not more than 50 millimoles of phosphate ions per litre.

Storage. It should be stored *in vacuo* or under nitrogen, in sterile containers sealed to exclude micro-organisms and moisture, at a temperature below 6°, protected from light. The reconstituted solution should be used immediately after preparation and should be discarded if not used within 3 hours.

Actions and uses. Dried human factor IX fraction is used to control bleeding in patients with a rare deficiency of coagulation factor IX (Christmas disease), and the even less common deficiencies of factor II or factor X.

The amount transfused depends upon the circumstances, particularly the immediate cause of the bleeding, and the severity of the haemophilia. The object of treatment is to raise the concentration of plasma antihaemophilic globulin to at least 30% of normal and to maintain it at this level until bleeding has ceased. For further information see the entry on Haemophilia.

The use of dried human factor IX fraction carries a risk of transmitting hepatitis, as explained in the entry on Blood Products.

A filter should be incorporated in the apparatus used for administration of the reconstituted product.

Faintness

see under CIRCULATORY FAILURE

Feline Infectious Enteritis Vaccine, Living

A freeze-dried preparation of cell-culture liquid containing the virus of feline infectious enteritis which has been modified by serial passage in cell culture. It is reconstituted immediately before use with an appropriate volume of a suitable sterile liquid.

OTHER NAME: Feline Panleucopoenia Vaccine, Living

A standard is given in the British Pharmacopoeia (Veterinary)

Storage. The dried vaccine should be protected from light and stored at 2° to 8° when it may be expected to retain its potency for at least 12 months. It should be used immediately after reconstitution.

Veterinary uses. It is administered by subcutaneous or intramuscular injection to cats and other felidae for prophylaxis against feline infectious enteritis.

Fenfluramine Hydrochloride

N-Ethyl-α-methyl-3-trifluoromethylphenethylammonium chloride

$$CH_2 \cdot \overset{\overset{\displaystyle CH_3}{|}}{CH} \cdot \overset{+}{N}H_2 \cdot C_2H_5 \qquad Cl^-$$

(structure with CF_3 substituted benzene ring)

$C_{12}H_{17}ClF_3N = 267.7$

OTHER NAME: *Ponderax®*

A standard is given in the British Pharmacopoeia 1973

Description. A white crystalline odourless powder with a slightly bitter taste.

Solubility. Soluble, at 20°, in 20 parts of water, in 10 parts of alcohol, and in 10 parts of chloroform; very slightly soluble in ether.

Dissociation constant. pK_a 9.1 (25°).

Moisture content. Not more than 1%, determined by drying at 105°.

Identification. MELTING-POINT. About 170°.

ULTRAVIOLET ABSORPTION. In 0.1N sulphuric acid, maxima at 259 nm (E1%, 1cm = 16), 263 nm (E1%, 1cm = 22), and 270 nm (E1%, 1cm = 19.5).

INFRA-RED ABSORPTION. Major peaks at 748, 793, 1070, 1116, 1165, and 1333 cm^{-1} (see Appendix 2a: Infra-red Spectra).

Determination in body fluids. GAS CHROMATOGRAPHY. In urine: fenfluramine and metabolites—A. H. Beckett *et al.*, *J. Pharm. Pharmac.*, 1971, **23**, 950. In plasma or urine: fenfluramine and metabolites—D. B. Campbell, *J. Chromat.*, 1970, **49**, 442.

Metabolism. ABSORPTION. Readily and completely absorbed after oral administration although the rate may vary between individuals; absorption from sugar-coated tablets occurs more slowly than from ordinary tablets during the first hour after administration.

BLOOD CONCENTRATION. After an oral dose of 60 mg of the hydrochloride, peak plasma concentrations of 30 to 70 ng/ml occur within 2 to 3 hours for fenfluramine and about 16 ng/ml within 4 to 6 hours for its metabolite, norfenfluramine; after 6 to 8 hours following the above dose, plasma concentrations of unchanged drug fall to about 10 ng/ml; after a daily dose of 20 mg, plasma concentrations reach a steady state of 40 to 120 ng/ml after 9 to 14 days.

HALF-LIFE. Plasma half-life, 11 to 30 hours, the half-life being shorter when the urine is acid.

DISTRIBUTION. Fenfluramine is widely distributed throughout the body and accumulates in the brain, fat, muscles, liver, and other tissues; in the blood it is taken up by the red cells in concentrations reaching 40% higher than those in the plasma; fenfluramine crosses the placenta in animals and probably does so to a significant extent in man.

METABOLIC REACTIONS. Fenfluramine is subject to extensive first-pass metabolism after oral administration and is metabolised by N-de-ethylation to form the active metabolite, norfenfluramine, followed by de-amination to m-trifluoromethylbenzoic acid which is conjugated with glycine to form m-trifluoromethyl-hippuric acid.

EXCRETION. The rate of excretion of fenfluramine is influenced by urinary pH and urinary flow; 80 to 100% of a dose is excreted in the urine although in cases of overdosage some of the drug may be excreted in the bile and into the stomach; up to 5% of a dose may be excreted in the faeces as unchanged drug and nor-fenfluramine; in acid urine, 6 to 30% of a dose is excreted unchanged, 3 to 22% is de-ethylated, and 66 to 93% is excreted as m-trifluoromethylhippuric acid; in alkaline urine, about 2% is excreted as unchanged drug and norfenfluramine and, in uncontrolled urinary pH conditions, 3 to 10% is unchanged drug and 3 to 14% is norfenfluramine; no free m-trifluoromethylbenzoic acid is present in the urine of man but it is found in that of dogs.

FURTHER INFORMATION. Absorption and urinary excretion—A. H. Beckett and L. G. Brookes, *J. Pharm. Pharmac.*, 1967, **19**, 425; pharmacokinetics of absorption, distribution, and elimination—A. H. Beckett and J. A. Salmon, *J. Pharm. Pharmac.*, 1972, **24**, 108; metabolism—R. B. Bruce and W. R. Maynard, *J. pharm. Sci.*, 1968, **57**, 1173; pharmacological properties—R. M. Pinder *et al.*, *Drugs*, 1975, **10**, 241.

Actions and uses. Fenfluramine is an anorectic agent chemically related to amphetamine. It is used as an aid in the treatment of obesity. Unlike amphetamine, however, fenfluramine may cause drowsiness, especially early in treatment; it does not raise the blood pressure and may increase the antihypertensive effect of beth-anidine, guanethidine, methyldopa, and reserpine, but not that of debrisoquine.

The usual initial dose is 20 milligrams twice daily, increasing if necessary by 20 to 40 milligrams at intervals of 1 week to a maximum of 120 milligrams daily. Doses of up to 40 milligrams daily do not cause marked disturbance of sleep patterns, but this may occur on higher dosage, possibly accompanied by vivid or disturbing dreams.

Undesirable effects. Fenfluramine may give rise to diarrhoea. While its abuse potential appears to be low, the appearance of depressive symptoms some days after cessation of therapy may lead to a desire to recommence taking the drug.

Precautions and contra-indications. Fenfluramine should not be given to patients who are being treated with a monoamine-oxidase inhibitor, such as isocarboxazid, nialamide, phenelzine, or tranylcypromine, or within about 2 weeks of the discontinuation of such treatment. It is probably best avoided in patients with a recent history of depressive illness and during the first 3 months of pregnancy.

Preparations

FENFLURAMINE TABLETS: available as tablets containing 20 mg of fenfluramine hydrochloride. They are film coated or sugar coated and the coat may be coloured.
A standard for these tablets is given in the British Pharmacopoeia 1973
Containers and *Storage:* see the entry on Tablets for general information on containers and storage. Containers should be airtight.
Advice for patients: the tablets should preferably be taken half an hour before meals. They may cause drowsiness; persons affected should not drive or operate machinery. Alcohol should be avoided.

OTHER PREPARATIONS available include CAPSULES containing fenfluramine hydrochloride 60 mg, in a slow-release formulation.

Fennel

Consists of the dried fruits of cultivated plants of *Foeniculum vulgare* Mill. var. *vulgare* (Fam. Umbelliferae). The plant is indigenous to Europe, but commercial supplies come from India and China with small quantities from Egypt.

OTHER NAMES: Fennel Fruit; Foeniculum

A standard is given in the British Pharmaceutical Codex 1973

Varieties. Saxon fennel fruits are about 8 to 10 mm long; they yield about 4% of volatile oil of which over 20% may consist of fenchone.

Russian, Galician, and Rumanian fennels closely resemble one another; they are usually shorter than the Saxon variety and yield a volatile oil containing a slightly smaller proportion of fenchone.

Indian fennel fruits are greenish-brown or yellowish-brown and 6 to 7 mm long; Chinese are slightly darker in colour.

The name bitter fennel is sometimes applied to fennel.

Constituents. Fennel yields 0.8 to 4% of volatile oil, the chief constituents of which are anethole and (+)-fenchone. Up to 1.5% of foreign organic matter may be present. It yields up to 1.5% of acid-insoluble ash.

Description. UNGROUND DRUG. *Macroscopical characters:* fruits usually entire cremocarps with pedicels attached, up to about 10 mm long and 4 mm wide; cremocarp oblong, laterally compressed, greenish-brown or yellowish-brown to brown, glabrous, with short bifid stylopod at apex; mericarps with 5 prominent yellowish primary ridges, transverse section showing in the pericarp 2 commissural vittae and 4 dorsal vittae occurring between the primary ridges, each ridge with a vascular strand; embryo small, embedded in upper end of abundant oily endosperm, commissural surface of endosperm not grooved.

It has an aromatic odour and an aromatic and camphoraceous taste.

Microscopical characters: the diagnostic characters are: *outer epidermis* of pericarp composed of tetrahedral to polyhedral cells; cuticle not striated; *stomata* anomocytic, occasional; mesocarp with lignified and *reticulate parenchyma; inner epidermis* of pericarp with cells frequently showing a parquetry arrangement; *vittae* brown; *endosperm* composed of polyhedral, thick-walled cells containing *fixed oil* and *aleurone grains* with minute rosette *crystals* of calcium oxalate; *trichomes* and *starch* absent.

POWDERED DRUG. Powdered Fennel. A greenish-yellow to yellowish-brown powder possessing the diagnostic microscopical characters, odour, and taste of the unground drug.

Adulterants and substitutes. The French sweet fennel, or Roman fennel [*Foeniculum vulgare* Mill. var. *dulce* (Mill.) Thellung], yields only about 2% of volatile oil, which is practically free from fenchone.

Exhausted or partially exhausted fennel is deficient in oil and therefore deficient in odour.

Storage. It should be stored in a cool dry place. Powdered fennel should be stored in airtight containers in a cool place.

Actions and uses. Fennel is a carminative and a flavouring agent.

Fenoprofen Calcium

Calcium 2-(3-phenoxyphenyl)propionate dihydrate

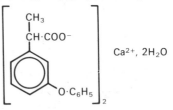

$(C_{15}H_{13}O_3)_2Ca,2H_2O = 558.6$

OTHER NAME: *Fenopron*®

Identification. ULTRAVIOLET ABSORPTION. In 0.1N hydrochloric acid, maximum at 274 nm (E1%, 1cm = 64); in alcohol (95%), maximum at 274 nm (E1%, 1cm = 67).

INFRA-RED ABSORPTION. Major peaks at 696, 1225, 1417, 1443, 1483, and 1562 cm^{-1} (see Appendix 2a: Infra-red Spectra).

THIN-LAYER CHROMATOGRAPHY. See under Thin-layer Chromatography, System 3.

Determination in body fluids. GAS CHROMATOGRAPHY. In plasma—J. F. Nash *et al.*, *J. pharm. Sci.*, 1971, **60**, 1062.

Metabolism. ABSORPTION. Readily absorbed after the oral administration of the calcium or sodium salt; the extent of absorption is decreased by the presence of food but is unaffected by the presence of antacids.

BLOOD CONCENTRATION. After an oral dose of 250 mg of the calcium salt, peak plasma concentrations of about 26 μg/ml are attained within 2 hours; after an intravenous dose of 250 mg of the sodium salt, plasma concentrations of about 56 μg/ml are attained immediately after administration and fall to about 20 μg/ml after 2 hours; blood concentrations of fenoprofen are reduced when aspirin is administered concurrently; this reduction is not due to a reduction in absorption and may be due to competition for plasma protein binding sites thereby exposing more unbound fenoprofen to metabolism.

HALF-LIFE. Plasma half-life, 2 to 3 hours.

DISTRIBUTION. Small amounts are secreted in the milk; *protein binding*, about 99% bound to plasma proteins; fenoprofen may displace warfarin from binding sites to a small extent.

METABOLIC REACTIONS. Almost completely metabolised by hydroxylation at the 4-position and glucuronic acid conjugation.

EXCRETION. 90% of a dose is excreted in the urine and about 2% in the faeces in 24 hours; of the urinary excreted material, about 3% is unchanged, 45% is fenoprofen glucuronide, 42% is 4-hydroxyfenoprofen glucuronide, and about 2% is free 4-hydroxyfenoprofen; the remaining 8% appears to be composed of 2 acid-labile metabolites.

ENZYME INDUCTION. The metabolism of fenoprofen appears to be stimulated by phenobarbitone.

FURTHER INFORMATION. Physiological disposition and gastro-intestinal effects—A. Rubin *et al.*, *Curr. med. Res. Opin.*, 1974, **2**, 529.

Actions and uses. Fenoprofen is an analgesic with anti-inflammatory properties and has the actions and uses described under Ibuprofen but it is more effective and has a greater incidence of gastro-intestinal side-effects.

The usual dosage is the equivalent of 600 milligrams of fenoprofen 3 to 4 times daily. This may be reduced to a lower maintenance dosage in patients who respond well. The daily dosage should not exceed the equivalent of 3 grams of fenoprofen; 1.2 grams of fenoprofen calcium is approximately equivalent to 1 gram of fenoprofen.

Undesirable effects. Mild gastro-intestinal upsets may occur and occasionally rashes.

Precautions. As for Ibuprofen.

Preparations

Preparations available include TABLETS containing fenoprofen calcium equivalent to 300 and 600 mg of fenoprofen.

Fentanyl Citrate

N-(1-Phenethylpiperid-4-yl)propionanilide citrate

$C_{22}H_{28}N_2O,C_6H_8O_7 = 528.6$

OTHER NAMES: *Sublimaze*®
Hypnorm® (with fluanisone); *Thalamonal*® (with droperidol)

A standard is given in the British Pharmacopoeia Addendum 1977 and the British Pharmacopoeia (Veterinary)

CAUTION. *Fentanyl is a powerful analgesic. It should be handled with care and precautions should be taken to avoid the inhalation of airborne particles.*

Description. A white crystalline powder or white granules.

Solubility. Soluble, at 20°, in 40 parts of water, in 140 parts of alcohol, in 350 parts of chloroform, and in 10 parts of methyl alcohol; very slightly soluble in ether.

Sterilisation. Solutions are sterilised by heating in an autoclave or by filtration.

Storage. It should be stored in airtight containers, protected from light.

Identification. MELTING-POINT. About 149°.

ULTRAVIOLET ABSORPTION. In water, maxima at 251 nm (E1%, 1cm = 7.2), at 257 nm (E1%, 1cm = 8.2), and at 262 nm (E1%, 1cm = 6.4).

Actions and uses. Fentanyl citrate is a narcotic analgesic with actions similar to those described under Morphine Hydrochloride. It is a much more potent analgesic and respiratory depressant but has a shorter duration of action. The full analgesic effect develops one minute after intravenous injection and persists for about 30 minutes but a level of analgesia sufficient to relieve post-operative pain may last for about 6 hours.
Fentanyl citrate is used to produce states of surgical analgesia. It is often used in conjunction with a neuroleptic such as droperidol to induce a degree of analgesia with a tranquillising effect ("neuroleptanalgesia") so that the patient, whilst able to co-operate, remains calm and indifferent to the surroundings. In addition, it may be used to produce respiratory depression in patients undergoing surgery where assisted respiration is necessary.
Fentanyl citrate may be given by intramuscular injection as premedication, usually in conjunction with droperidol, in a dosage equivalent to 50 to 100 micrograms of fentanyl for adults and 20 to 75 micrograms for children 15 to 45 minutes pre-operatively.
During surgery, under general anaesthesia, the initial dose for adults is the equivalent of 100 to 200 micrograms of fentanyl by intravenous injection and for children the equivalent of 3 to 5 micrograms of fentanyl per kilogram body-weight. To maintain adequate analgesia in adults, doses of 50 micrograms should be given intravenously every 20 to 30 minutes depending on the degree of pain. Where assisted respiration is necessary during surgery, the initial dose of fentanyl may be increased to 200 to 600 micrograms for adults and 10 to 15 micrograms per kilogram body-weight for children.
Respiratory depression is maintained with the equivalent of 50 to 200 micrograms of fentanyl every 20 to 30 minutes.
Fentanyl citrate is occasionally used to relieve severe pain, as in myocardial infarction.

Undesirable effects; Dependence; Poisoning. As for Morphine Hydrochloride.

Precautions. Fentanyl citrate should not be given to patients who are being treated with a monoamine-oxidase inhibitor such as isocarboxazid, nialamide, phenelzine, or tranylcypromine, or within about 2 weeks of the discontinuation of such treatment.

Veterinary uses. Fentanyl citrate is a narcotic analgesic used with tranquillisers to produce neuroleptanalgesia. The usual dose by intramuscular injection for dogs is 50 to 100 micrograms per kilogram body-weight.

Preparations

Preparations available include an INJECTION containing fentanyl citrate equivalent to 50 micrograms of fentanyl per ml in 2- and 10-ml ampoules, an injection containing fentanyl citrate equivalent to 50 micrograms of fentanyl with droperidol 2.5 mg per ml in 2-ml ampoules, and a veterinary injection containing fentanyl citrate 315 micrograms with fluanisone 10 mg per ml in 10-ml bottles.

Fenthion

OO-Dimethyl *O*-4-methylthio-*m*-tolyl phosphorothioate

$C_{10}H_{15}O_3PS_2 = 278.3$

OTHER NAME: *Tiguvon*®

A standard is given in the British Pharmacopoeia (Veterinary)

Description. A yellowish-brown oily substance.

Solubility. Immiscible with water; miscible with alcohol, with benzene, and with chloroform.

Identification. TEST. Mix 0.15 ml with 3 ml of isopropyl alcohol and 200 mg of potassium hydroxide, heat on a water-bath for 15 minutes, add 5 ml of water, heat for a further 5 minutes, cool, dilute to 50 ml with water, and add 3 ml of *iodine solution*; a green colour is produced which gradually fades.

Veterinary uses. Fenthion is an insecticide. It is applied at a dosage of 5 to 10 milligrams per kilogram body-weight as a 2% solution in liquid paraffin to the backs of cattle to treat louse infections and to prevent the damage that would be caused by the migration of warble fly larvae.

Preparations

Preparations available include a SOLUTION (in liquid paraffin) containing fenthion 2% w/w.

Ferric Ammonium Citrate

A complex ammonium ferric citrate.

OTHER NAMES: Ferr. Ammon. Cit.; Iron and Ammonium Citrate

A standard is given in the British Pharmacopoeia 1973

Description. Deliquescent, dark red, thin, transparent scales or brown, shiny, granular powder with an astringent taste.

Solubility. Soluble, at 20°, in less than 1 part of water; very slightly soluble in alcohol.

Stability. Aqueous solutions of ferric ammonium citrate are particularly liable to grow moulds; chloroform or some other suitable preservative should be added.

Incompatibility. It is incompatible with mineral salts, alkali carbonates, and vegetable astringents.

Storage. It should be stored in airtight containers, protected from light.

Actions and uses. Ferric ammonium citrate has the actions and uses of iron salts, as described under Ferrous Sulphate; 100 milligrams contains approximately 20 milligrams of Fe.
When given by mouth, it is better tolerated than the astringent preparations of iron. Doses of up to 9 grams daily in divided doses may be needed for the treatment of iron-deficiency anaemias. The usual dose for an adult is 2 grams (as 10 millilitres of ferric ammonium citrate mixture) up to 4 times daily. The usual dose for children up to 1 year is 400 milligrams (5 millilitres of paediatric ferric ammonium citrate mixture) up to 4 times daily and for children aged 1 to 5 years 800 milligrams (10 millilitres of paediatric ferric ammonium citrate mixture) up to 4 times daily.

Undesirable effects. Large doses sometimes produce diarrhoea.

Poisoning. As for Ferrous Sulphate.

Preparations

FERRIC AMMONIUM CITRATE MIXTURE (*Syn.* Iron and Ammonium Citrate Mixture):

Ferric ammonium citrate	..	..	..	200 g
Chloroform water, double-strength	..	..	500 ml
Water for preparations	..	..	..	to 1000 ml

It should be recently prepared.
A standard for this mixture is given in the British Pharmaceutical Codex 1973
Containers: see the entry on Mixtures for general information on containers.
Advice for patients: the dose may be taken alone or with water and should be swallowed through a straw to prevent blackening of the teeth. The mixture should preferably be taken before meals; if there are gastro-intestinal disturbances the dose may be taken after meals. Antacids should not be taken within 1 hour. The mixture should not be taken for prolonged periods without medical advice. It may blacken the faeces.

PAEDIATRIC FERRIC AMMONIUM CITRATE MIXTURE (*Syn.* Paediatric Iron and Ammonium Citrate Mixture):

Ferric ammonium citrate	..	..	..	80 g
Compound orange spirit	..	..	..	2 ml
Syrup	..	..	..	..	100 ml
Chloroform water, double-strength	..	..	500 ml
Water for preparations	..	..	..	to 1000 ml

It should be recently prepared.
A standard for this mixture is given in the British Pharmaceutical Codex 1973
Containers: see the entry on Mixtures for general information on containers.
Advice for patients: the dose should be taken well diluted with water and swallowed through a straw to prevent blackening of the teeth. The mixture should preferably be taken before meals; if there are gastro-intestinal disturbances the dose may be taken after meals. Antacids should not be taken within 1 hour.
The mixture should not be taken for prolonged periods without medical advice. It may blacken the faeces.

Ferric Citrate (^{59}Fe) Injection

A sterile solution containing iron-59 in the ferric state, 1% of sodium citrate, and sufficient sodium chloride to make the solution isotonic with blood.

A standard is given in the British Pharmacopoeia 1973

CAUTION. *This material is radioactive and any regulations in force must be complied with.*

Iron-59 is a radioactive isotope of iron which decays by emission of β^--radiation mainly of maximum energy 0.27 and 0.47 MeV and γ-radiation mainly of energy 1.10 and 1.29 MeV. It has a half-life of 44.6 days.
It may be prepared by neutron irradiation of iron-58 sufficiently low in iron-54 to ensure that the final content of iron-55 is not more than 2 per cent of the total activity; cobalt-60 is removed from the irradiated material during preparation.

Description. A clear colourless or faintly orange-brown solution.

Acidity or alkalinity. pH 6 to 8.

Sterilisation. It is sterilised by heating in an autoclave.

Storage. It should be stored in an area assigned for the purpose. The storage conditions should be such that the maximum radiation-dose-rate to which persons may be exposed is reduced to an acceptable level. Glass containers may darken under the effects of radiation.

Labelling. The label on the container should state: (1) the content of iron-59 expressed in microcuries or millicuries at a given date, (2) that the injection is radioactive, and (3) either that it does not contain a bactericide or the name and proportion of any added bactericide.
The label on the package should state (1) the total volume in the container, (2) the content of total iron, and (3) the calculated content of iron-55.

Actions and uses. Ferric citrate (^{59}Fe) injection is used in the investigation of iron metabolism, especially in anaemia and iron-storage disorders. For this purpose it is given by mouth or by intravenous injection. The fraction of the radioactivity absorbed after oral administration with ascorbic acid is assessed by measuring the residue in the faeces or by determining the total body radioactivity immediately after ingestion and again after an interval. A dose of 5 to 20 microcuries is usually administered for these tests.

The rate of fall in the circulating radioactivity of the isotope following an intravenous injection of (^{59}Fe) ferric citrate may be measured to determine the turnover rate of plasma iron and red-cell iron. The incorporation of iron-59 into newly formed red cells can be measured; this may be useful in assessing marrow function in conditions associated with abnormalities of red-cell production, such as anaemias and polycythaemia. The dose usually administered for this purpose is about 5 microcuries. Iron-59 has also been used to measure red-cell life-span. Iron-59 emits high-energy γ-rays which can be detected by a scintillation counter at the body surface. The passage of the isotope through underlying organs, including the liver, spleen, heart, and bone marrow of the lumbar or sacral regions of the vertebral column, can thus be followed. This is of value in detecting abnormalities of iron storage such as occur in primary and secondary haemochromatosis, and it may also be used to assess the distribution of sites of erythropoiesis in myeloid metaplasia.

Ferrous Fumarate

$C_4H_2FeO_4 = 169.9$

OTHER NAMES: *Fersaday*®; *Fersamal*®; *Galfer*® *Co-Ferol*®, *Ferrocap F-350*®, *Folex-350*®, *Galfer FA*®, *Norfer*®, *Pregaday*®, and *Tifol*® (all with folic acid); *Ferrocap*® (with thiamine hydrochloride)

A standard is given in the British Pharmacopoeia 1973

Description. A fine, reddish-orange to reddish-brown, almost odourless powder with a slightly astringent taste.

Solubility. Very slightly soluble in water and in alcohol.

Moisture content. Not more than 1%, determined by drying at 105°.

Actions and uses. Ferrous fumarate has the actions and uses of iron salts, as described under Ferrous Sulphate; 100 milligrams contains approximately 32 milligrams of Fe.
Initially, 400 to 600 milligrams of ferrous fumarate may be given daily in divided doses and reduced to a maintenance dosage of 200 milligrams daily. The usual therapeutic dose for children up to 1 year is 35 milligrams, 1 to 5 years 70 milligrams, and 6 to 12 years 140 milligrams, 3 times daily.

Poisoning. As for Ferrous Sulphate.

Preparations

FERROUS FUMARATE TABLETS: available as tablets containing 200 mg of ferrous fumarate, equivalent to 65 mg of iron.
A standard for these tablets is given in the British Pharmacopoeia 1973

Containers and *Storage:* see the entry on Tablets for general information on containers and storage. Containers should be airtight.

Advice for patients: the tablets should preferably be taken before meals; if there are gastro-intestinal disturbances doses may be taken after meals. Antacids should not be taken within 1 hour.

The tablets should not be taken for prolonged periods without medical advice. They may blacken the faeces.

IRON AND FOLIC ACID TABLETS: available as tablets containing 308 mg of ferrous fumarate equivalent to 100 mg of iron and 350 micrograms of folic acid; they may be coated with sugar or other suitable material and the coat may be coloured.

Containers and *Storage:* see the entry on Tablets for general information on containers and storage. Containers should be airtight.

Advice for patients: the tablets should preferably be taken before meals; if there are gastro-intestinal disturbances doses may be taken after meals. Antacids should not be taken within 1 hour.

The tablets should not be taken for prolonged periods without medical advice. They may blacken the faeces.

OTHER PREPARATIONS available include CAPSULES containing 312 mg of ferrous fumarate, capsules containing ferrous fumarate 300 mg with folic acid 300 micrograms, capsules containing ferrous fumarate 308 mg with folic acid 350 micrograms, capsules containing ferrous fumarate 330 mg with folic acid 350 micrograms, capsules containing ferrous fumarate 330 mg with thiamine hydrochloride 5 mg in a slow-release formulation; a MIXTURE containing ferrous fumarate 140 mg in 5 ml, diluent syrup, life of diluted mixture 14 days; TABLETS (sugar coated) containing ferrous fumarate 308 mg, tablets containing ferrous fumarate 120 mg with folic acid 200 micrograms, and tablets containing ferrous fumarate 200 mg with folic acid 125 mg.

Ferrous Gluconate

$C_{12}H_{22}FeO_{14},2H_2O = 482.2$

OTHER NAMES: Ferrosi Gluconas; *Fergon*® *Sidros*® (with ascorbic acid); *Feravol-F*® (with folic acid); *Dellipsoids D28*® and *Feravol-G*® (with thiamine hydrochloride)

A standard is given in the European Pharmacopoeia Vol. III Supplement

Description. A grey powder or granules with a green or yellow tint, a slight odour resembling that of burnt sugar, and a taste which is saline at first and then slightly chalybeate.

Solubility. Soluble, at 20°, in 8 parts of water; very slightly soluble in alcohol.

Acidity. A 10% solution has a pH of 3.7 to 6.

Moisture content. 5 to 11%, determined by drying at 105°.

Storage. It should be stored in airtight containers, protected from light.

Actions and uses. Ferrous gluconate has the actions and uses of iron salts, as described under Ferrous Sulphate; 100 milligrams contains approximately 12 milligrams of Fe.

Initially, 1.2 to 1.8 grams of ferrous gluconate may be given daily in divided doses and reduced to a maintenance dosage of 600 milligrams daily. The usual therapeutic dose for children aged 6 to 12 years is 300 milligrams 3 times daily.

Poisoning. As for Ferrous Sulphate.

Preparations

FERROUS GLUCONATE TABLETS: available as tablets containing 300 mg of ferrous gluconate; they are sugar coated; the coat may be coloured.
A standard for these tablets is given in the British Pharmacopoeia 1973
Containers and *Storage:* see the entry on Tablets for general information on containers and storage. Containers should be airtight.
Advice for patients: the tablets should preferably be taken before meals; if there are gastro-intestinal disturbances doses may be taken after meals. Antacids should not be taken within 1 hour.
The tablets should not be taken for prolonged periods without medical advice. They may blacken the faeces.

OTHER PREPARATIONS available include an ELIXIR containing ferrous gluconate 300 mg with thiamine hydrochloride 1 mg in 5 ml; TABLETS containing ferrous gluconate 300 mg with ascorbic acid 30 mg, tablets containing ferrous gluconate 300 mg with folic acid 3 mg and 5 mg, and tablets containing ferrous gluconate 200 mg with thiamine hydrochloride 1 mg.

Ferrous Succinate

A basic salt prepared by the interaction of sodium succinate and ferrous sulphate in boiling aqueous solution.

OTHER NAMES: *Ferromyn*®
Ferromyn S® (with succinic acid)

A standard is given in the British Pharmacopoeia 1973

Description. An almost tasteless brownish-yellow to brown amorphous powder with a slight odour.

Solubility. Very slightly soluble in water and in alcohol; soluble in dilute mineral acids.

Moisture content. Not more than 1%, determined by drying at 105°.

Storage. It should be stored in airtight containers, protected from light.

Actions and uses. Ferrous succinate has the actions and uses described under Ferrous Sulphate, but it produces a lower incidence of undesirable gastro-intestinal effects; 100 milligrams of ferrous succinate contains approximately 35 milligrams of iron.

Initially, 400 to 600 milligrams of ferrous succinate may be given daily in divided doses and reduced to a maintenance dosage of 200 milligrams daily. The usual therapeutic dose for children up to 1 year is up to 100 milligrams daily, from 1 to 5 years 100 to 300 milligrams daily, and from 6 to 12 years 300 to 400 milligrams daily in divided doses.

Ferrous succinate should be administered before meals to obtain maximum absorption.

Poisoning. As for Ferrous Sulphate.

Preparations

FERROUS SUCCINATE CAPSULES: consisting of ferrous succinate, in powder, which may be mixed with a suitable inert diluent, enclosed in a hard capsule. The capsule shells may be coloured. The usual strength is 100 mg of ferrous succinate.
A standard for these capsules is given in the British Pharmacopoeia 1973
Containers and *Storage:* see the entry on Capsules for general information on containers and storage. Containers should be light resistant.
Advice for patients: the capsules should preferably be taken before meals; if there are gastro-intestinal disturbances doses may be taken after meals. Antacids should not be taken within 1 hour.
The capsules should not be taken for prolonged periods without medical advice. They may blacken the faeces.

FERROUS SUCCINATE TABLETS: available as tablets containing 100 mg of ferrous succinate; they may be sugar coated and the coat may be coloured.
A standard for these tablets is given in the British Pharmacopoeia 1973
Containers and *Storage:* see the entry on Tablets for general information on containers and storage. Containers should be airtight and light resistant. The tablets should be stored in a cool place.
Advice for patients: the tablets should preferably be taken before meals; if there are gastro-intestinal disturbances doses may be taken after meals. Antacids should not be taken within 1 hour. The tablets should not be taken for prolonged periods without medical advice. They may blacken the faeces.

OTHER PREPARATIONS available include an ELIXIR containing ferrous succinate 106 mg in 5 ml, diluent syrup, life of diluted elixir 14 days; and TABLETS containing ferrous succinate 106 mg with succinic acid 110 mg.

Ferrous Sulphate

$FeSO_4,7H_2O = 278.0$

OTHER NAME: Ferrosi Sulfas

A standard is given in the European Pharmacopoeia Vol. II

Description. A pale green crystalline powder or bluish-green crystals with a metallic astringent taste.

Solubility. Soluble, at 20°, in 1.5 parts of water; practically insoluble in alcohol.

Acidity. A 5% solution has a pH of 3 to 4.

Stability. Ferrous sulphate loses 6 molecules of water of crystallisation at 38°; at higher temperatures basic sulphates are produced. When exposed to moist air it is oxidised and becomes brown in colour.
Granular ferrous sulphate, prepared by precipitation with alcohol from a slightly acidic solution, is less liable to oxidation than crystalline powder.

Storage. It should be stored in airtight containers.

Actions and uses. Iron is essential for the formation of haemoglobin and hence for the oxidative process of living tissues. The amount of iron required daily for the formation of haemoglobin is 2 to 2.5 milligrams but, because of poor absorption, the actual intake to provide this must be greater—up to 20 to 25 milligrams. The daily requirement is raised during pregnancy and after severe or continuous haemorrhage.

Absorption of iron from food, or from iron compounds administered by mouth, takes place in the duodenum and jejunum in amounts ranging from 1 to 50 milligrams daily, depending upon the needs of the body. The presence of free succinic acid and ascorbic acid may aid the absorption of iron salts; it is decreased in the presence of antacids. Iron absorbed from the gastro-intestinal tract combines with protein and is deposited in the intestinal mucosa. Iron liberated by the destruction of red blood cells is stored in the liver and spleen. It is mobilised from these depots when required for haemoglobin formation.

Compounds of iron are used in all forms of iron-deficiency and hypochromic anaemia, anaemia of pregnancy, the nutritional anaemia of infants, anaemia due to excessive or repeated haemorrhage, and anaemia associated with infections and malignant disease. In the treatment of macrocytic anaemia, preparations of iron given alone are of no value, but they may be of value as a supplement to vitamin-B_{12} therapy whenever the reserves of iron are depleted and the increase in haemoglobin does not parallel the rise in the number of blood cells. The soluble ferrous salts are the most satisfactory of the iron preparations for effecting haemoglobin formation; ferric salts are relatively ineffective.

Since only a small and variable proportion of the iron administered by mouth is absorbed, large doses of iron salts are necessary to produce a remission in iron-deficiency anaemia. Full doses of ferrous sulphate should be administered 3 or 4 times a day; 100 milligrams contains approximately 20 milligrams of Fe.

The usual prophylactic and maintenance dose of ferrous sulphate is 300 milligrams daily. The usual therapeutic dosage is 0.9 to 1.8 grams daily in divided doses. The usual therapeutic dose for children under 1 year is 180 milligrams daily, 1 to 5 years 360 milligrams daily, and 6 to 12 years 600 milligrams daily, in divided doses. Large doses often produce gastro-intestinal irritation and vomiting and diarrhoea and should be given after meals to reduce gastric irritation; continued administration may sometimes produce constipation. Patients intolerant of oral administration may be treated with parenteral iron preparations.

When iron compounds are given by mouth for the treatment of anaemia it may take up to 3 months for the haemoglobin to reach normal values and treatment should be continued for 6 months in cases of severe anaemia.

Poisoning. Fatal poisoning has occurred in children after ingestion of ferrous sulphate. The procedure described under Desferrioxamine Mesylate should be followed. Doses of 1 gram or more should be considered toxic in children, and treatment for poisoning started immediately.

If desferrioxamine is not available the patient must be encouraged to vomit without delay and thereafter the stomach should be washed out with a 5% solution of sodium bicarbonate and about 300 millilitres of the solution should be left in the stomach. Gastric lavage should not be done after the first hour, owing to the danger of perforation. A saline cathartic should be given to speed the elimination of the ferrous sulphate. Fluid loss should be replaced by intravenous administration of compound sodium lactate injection or sodium chloride and dextrose injection. In severe cases exchange transfusion may help.

All oral iron preparations are probably equally toxic per unit of soluble iron they contain.

Veterinary uses. Ferrous sulphate is used in the prevention and treatment of iron deficiency anaemias. The usual dose by mouth for piglets is 10 to 30 milligrams per kilogram body-weight.

Preparations

FERROUS SULPHATE MIXTURE:

Ferrous sulphate	30 g
Ascorbic acid	2 g
Orange syrup	50 ml
Chloroform water, double-strength	500 ml
Water for preparations	to 1000 ml

It should be recently prepared. The use of certain types of tap water, particularly those with temporary hardness, may lead to discoloration of this mixture. Freshly boiled and cooled purified water gives a satisfactory colourless or very pale yellow product.

A standard for this mixture is given in the British Pharmaceutical Codex 1973

Containers: see the entry on Mixtures for general information on containers.

Storage: when stored in filled unopened containers at room temperature, it may be expected to have a shelf-life of about 4 weeks. Once the container has been opened the mixture should preferably be used within about 1 week.

Advice for patients: the dose should be taken well diluted with water and swallowed through a straw to prevent blackening of the teeth. The mixture should preferably be taken before meals; if there are gastro-intestinal disturbances doses may be taken after meals. Antacids should not be taken within 1 hour.

The mixture should not be taken for prolonged periods without medical advice. It may blacken the faeces.

PAEDIATRIC FERROUS SULPHATE MIXTURE:

Ferrous sulphate	12 g
Ascorbic acid	2 g
Orange syrup	100 ml
Chloroform water, double-strength	500 ml
Water for preparations	to 1000 ml

It should be recently prepared. The use of certain types of tap water, particularly those with temporary hardness, may lead to discoloration of this mixture. Freshly boiled and cooled purified water gives a satisfactory colourless or very pale yellow product.

A standard for this mixture is given in the British Pharmaceutical Codex 1973

Containers: see the entry on Mixtures for general information on containers.

Storage: when stored in filled unopened containers at room temperature, it may be expected to have a shelf-life of about 4 weeks. Once the container has been opened the mixture should preferably be used within about 1 week.

Advice for patients: as for Ferrous Sulphate Mixture (above).

Ferrous Sulphate, Dried

Ferrous sulphate from which part of the water of crystallisation has been removed by drying at 40°.

OTHER NAMES: Exsiccated Ferrous Sulphate; *Feospan®*; *Ferro-Gradumet®*; *Slow-Fe®*; *Toniron®* *Fefol®*, *Ferrograd-Folic®*, *Folvron®*, *Pregfol®*, and *Slow-Fe Folic®* (all with folic acid); *Ferrograd-C®* (with sodium ascorbate)

A standard is given in the British Pharmacopoeia 1973

Description. A greyish-white powder with a metallic astringent taste.

Solubility. Slowly but almost completely soluble in freshly boiled and cooled water.

Storage. It should be stored in airtight containers.

Actions and uses. Dried ferrous sulphate has the actions and uses of iron salts as described under Ferrous Sulphate; 100 milligrams contains approximately 30 milligrams of Fe.

The usual prophylactic and maintenance dose is 200 milligrams daily and the usual therapeutic dose is 0.6 to 1.2 grams daily in divided doses. The therapeutic dose for children under 1 year is 120 milligrams daily, 1 to 5 years 240 milligrams daily, and 6 to 12 years 400 milligrams daily in divided doses.

Preparations

COMPOUND FERROUS SULPHATE TABLETS: for each tablet take:

Dried ferrous sulphate	a quantity equivalent to 170 mg of $FeSO_4$
Copper sulphate	2.5 mg
Manganese sulphate	2.5 mg

Mix, and prepare by moist granulation and compression as described in the entry on Tablets. The tablets may be coated with sugar or other suitable material and the coat may be coloured.

The manufacturing techniques used in the preparation of these tablets should ensure that increases in the disintegration time on prolonged storage do not exceed the limit. Alternatively, an appropriate expiry date should be specified on the label. Each tablet contains about 60 mg of iron.

A standard for these tablets is given in the British Pharmaceutical Codex 1973

Containers and *Storage:* see the entry on Tablets for general information on containers and storage. Containers should be airtight and light resistant.

Advice for patients: as for Ferrous Sulphate Tablets (below).

FERROUS SULPHATE TABLETS: available as tablets containing 200 and 300 mg of dried ferrous sulphate equivalent to about 60 and 90 mg of iron respectively; they may be film coated or sugar coated and the coat may be coloured. Sugar-coated tablets are supplied unless the contrary is indicated.

A standard for these tablets is given in the British Pharmacopoeia 1973

Containers and *Storage:* see the entry on Tablets for general information on containers and storage. Containers should be airtight.

Advice for patients: the tablets should preferably be taken before meals; if gastro-intestinal disturbances occur the dose may be taken after meals. Antacids should not be taken within 1 hour.

The tablets should not be taken for prolonged periods without medical advice. They may blacken the faeces.

OTHER PREPARATIONS available include CAPSULES containing dried ferrous sulphate 150 mg in a slow-release formulation, capsules containing dried ferrous sulphate 150 mg with folic acid 500 micrograms in a slow-release formulation, capsules containing dried ferrous sulphate 270 mg with folic acid 500 micrograms; TABLETS containing dried ferrous sulphate 160 and 325 mg in slow-release formulations, enteric-coated tablets containing dried ferrous sulphate 200 mg, tablets containing dried ferrous sulphate 160 mg with folic acid 400 micrograms in a slow-release formulation, tablets containing dried ferrous suphate 194 mg with folic acid 1.7 mg, tablets containing dried ferrous sulphate 325 mg with folic acid 350 micrograms in a slow-release formulation, and tablets containing dried ferrous sulphate 325 mg with sodium ascorbate equivalent to 500 mg of ascorbic acid.

Fibrillation

see under CARDIAC ARRHYTHMIAS

Fibrin Foam, Human

A dry artificial sponge of human fibrin.

A standard is given in the British Pharmaceutical Codex 1973

Human fibrin foam is prepared by clotting with human thrombin a foam of a solution of human fibrinogen. The clotted foam is dried from the frozen state, cut into strips, and sterilised by heating at 130° for 3 hours. It is a firm, light, white, spongy material.

Storage. It should be stored in sterile containers sealed to exclude micro-organisms and moisture, at a temperature below 25°, and protected from light.

Actions and uses. Human fibrin foam is used, in conjunction with human thrombin, as a haemostatic agent in surgery in sites in which bleeding cannot easily be controlled by the commoner methods of haemostasis.

A piece of the foam is cut to the required size, saturated with a solution of thrombin in sodium chloride injection, and placed in contact with the bleeding-point. Blood coagulates in contact with the thrombin in the interstices of the foam, which acts as a scaffold for the clot thus formed. Since all the clotting materials are of human origin, they may be left in place when the wound is closed.

Fibrinogen, Dried Human

A sterile dried preparation of the soluble constituent of liquid human plasma which, on the addition of human thrombin, is transformed into fibrin.

A standard is given in the British Pharmacopoeia 1973

Dried human fibrinogen may be prepared from human plasma separated from whole human blood by precipitation with organic solvents such as alcohol under controlled conditions of pH, ionic strength, and temperature. The precipitate is dissolved in a solution of sodium chloride and sodium citrate and dried from the frozen state; no preservative is added.

It is a white powder or friable solid which, when reconstituted with a volume of water equal to the volume of water for injections stated on the label, forms an almost colourless, opalescent solution which clots on the addition of thrombin on standing.

When fibrinogen is so reconstituted the resultant solution contains: (a) 1.0 to 1.5% w/v of fibrinogen, comprising not less than 70% of the total protein present, (b) not more than 200 millimoles of sodium ions per litre, and (c) not more than 25 millimoles of citrate ions per litre.

Storage. It should be stored in an atmosphere of nitrogen, in sterile containers sealed to exclude micro-organisms and moisture, at a temperature below 25°, and protected from light.

Fig   359

Actions and uses. Dried human fibrinogen is used to control haemorrhage associated with the defibrination syndrome which may occur in the presence of certain obstetrical conditions such as premature separation of the placenta or death of the foetus *in utero* or in association with cardiac operations. Haemorrhage does not usually occur until the fibrinogen level, which should be determined before treatment, has fallen below 100 mg per 100 ml of plasma. The transfusion of a solution of 2 to 6 grams of dried fibrinogen will usually control haemorrhage in these conditions.

Fibrinogen is also used to raise the fibrinogen level during operations on patients with the very rare abnormality, congenital afibrinogenaemia.

Dried human fibrinogen is used in conjunction with human thrombin to fix nerve sutures and to improve the adhesion of skin and mucous membrane grafts.

Dried human fibrinogen is reconstituted by adding, using an aseptic technique, a volume of water for injections not greater than the original volume of the fibrinogen solution before drying. The fibrinogen dissolves slowly and the container may be rocked but should not be shaken to aid solution; if shaken, frothing will occur which will impede solution.

Dried human fibrinogen should be used immediately after reconstitution; it must not be used more than 3 hours after reconstitution.

The use of dried human fibrinogen carries a risk of transmitting hepatitis, as explained in the entry on Blood Products.

Fibrinogen, Dried Human, For Isotopic Labelling

A preparation of the soluble constituent of liquid human plasma which, on addition of human thrombin, is transformed into fibrin.

A standard is given in the British Pharmacopoeia 1973

Dried human fibrinogen for isotopic labelling is prepared from liquid human plasma obtained from selected donors by precipitating with organic solvents such as alcohol under controlled conditions of pH, ionic strength, and temperature, dissolving the precipitate in a solution of sodium chloride and sodium citrate, and drying from the frozen state.

It is a white powder or friable solid. When dissolved in a volume of water equal to the volume of water for injections stated on the label not less than 90% of the total protein present is clottable.

Storage. It should be stored in an atmosphere of nitrogen, in sterile containers sealed to exclude micro-organisms and moisture, at 2° to 10°, and protected from light.

Actions and uses. Dried human fibrinogen for isotopic labelling is used mainly in the form of iodine-125 or iodine-131 labelled preparations for the detection of deep venous thrombosis.

The use of dried human fibrinogen for isotopic labelling carries a risk of transmitting hepatitis, as explained in the entry on Blood Products.

Fibrocystic Disease

Fibrocystic disease is an autosomal recessive genetically transmitted disease characterised by a widespread disorder of mucus-secreting glands in which mucus is unduly viscid and results in retention of secretion, secondary infection, and fibrosis. It occurs particularly in the gut, bronchi, pancreas, liver, and sweat glands. It is usually revealed in early infancy when there may be intestinal distension, wasting due to malabsorption, and recurrent chest infections.

Malabsorption is treated with a low-fat, high-protein diet and pancreatic enzyme replacement with meals. Long-term antibiotic therapy may be needed to prevent recurrent chest infections.

Fig

The dried succulent fruit of *Ficus carica* L. (Fam. Moraceae). The tree is indigenous to western Asia and is cultivated in most subtropical and warm climates. When the fruits are ripe, they are collected and dried in the sun.

OTHER NAME: Ficus

A standard is given in the British Pharmaceutical Codex 1973

Varieties. The varieties are known in commerce as "natural", "pulled" or "lacoum", and "layer" figs. "Natural" figs are those which are packed loose and retain to some extent their original shape. "Pulled" figs have been kneaded and pulled to make them supple. "Layer" figs have been cut into halves and closely packed, so that they are compressed and flattened.

Constituents. Fig contains about 50% of sugars, consisting principally of invert sugar with some sucrose. Small quantities of citric, acetic, and malic acids, and a proteolytic enzyme, ficin, are also present.

Description. *Macroscopical characters:* fruit compound, soft, fleshy, brown or yellowish-brown, sometimes covered with a saccharine efflorescence; at the summit a small opening surrounded by scales and at the base a short, stalk-like prolongation; fruit up to about 50 mm in length and breadth, consisting of a hollow receptacle bearing on the inner surface numerous drupelets, each containing a stone about 1.5 to 2 mm long; seed containing endosperm and a curved embryo. It has a pleasantly fruity odour and a sweet taste.

Microscopical characters: the diagnostic characters are: receptacle: *epidermal cells* polyhedral, *stomata* raised, *trichomes* unicellular and uniseriate, thick-walled, of varying length, up to about 300 μm; *hypodermis* composed of rounded polyhedral cells, some containing small rosette *crystals* of calcium oxalate; *aerenchyma* made up of large, irregular cells, forming greater part of the receptacle, containing large rosette *crystals* of calcium oxalate and interspersed with numerous *latex tubes*, about 30 to 50 μm wide, and slender *vascular bundles*.

Pericarp: *epicarp* consisting of radially elongated cells with mucilaginous outer walls; *mesocarp* of delicate often disorganised cells; *endocarp* of radially elongated *sclereids* with pitted walls. Endosperm and embryo: small cells containing *aleurone grains* and *fixed oil*; *starch* absent.

Storage. It should be stored in a dry place.

Actions and uses. Fig has demulcent properties and is used in confections and syrups with senna and other purgatives.

Preparation

COMPOUND FIGS SYRUP (*Syn.* Aromatic Syrup of Figs):

Fig, cut small	320 g
Sucrose	540 g
Cascara elixir	50 ml
Compound rhubarb tincture	50 ml
Senna liquid extract	100 ml
Water for preparations	to 1000 ml

Add the fig to 800 ml of boiling water, digest at a gentle heat for 1 hour, strain, express, and wash the pulp with sufficient warm water to produce 800 ml; evaporate the liquid to one half its volume, dissolve the sucrose in the concentrated liquid, add the compound rhubarb tincture, the senna liquid extract, the cascara elixir, and sufficient water to produce the required volume, and mix.
A standard for this syrup is given in the British Pharmaceutical Codex 1973
Dose: 2.5 to 10 millilitres.

Filariasis

A disease caused by the presence of filarial worms within the body.

Wuchereria bancrofti and *Brugia malayi* are similar filarial worms 40 to 100 mm long which live in lymph vessels and nodes, especially in the region of the pelvis and genitalia, and give rise to lymphatic obstruction and elephantiasis. The fertilised female worm releases microfilariae into the lymph and thence the bloodstream. These microfilariae are held in the pulmonary vessels, but at night they enter the general circulation and may be ingested by night-biting mosquitoes. After further development in the mosquitoes, they may be reinjected into man.
Infection with *Wuchereria bancrofti* or *Brugia malayi* gives rise at first to lymphangitis and lymphadenitis accompanied by fever and malaise. Later there may be lymphatic obstruction due to dead or dying worms, giving rise to lymph varicosities, chronic hydrocele, etc. Long-standing lymphatic blockage results in elephantiasis of a limb.
Diethylcarbamazine acts primarily on the microfilariae but may also destroy the adult worms. The destruction of large numbers of microfilariae may give rise to an acute allergic reaction which may be reduced by antihistamines or corticosteroids.

Loaiasis is a disease caused by the filarial nematode *Loa loa* which is 30 to 70 mm long and transmitted by flies of the genus *Chrysops*.
Infection gives rise to the appearance of transient erythematous swellings (calabar swellings) mainly on the limbs, caused by the migration of the worms through the subcutaneous tissues, resulting in local allergic phenomena. They may also migrate across the eye where they may be seen in the field of view. Microfilariae are released by the female into the blood, where they appear during the daytime and are infective to the insect vector. These microfilariae may result in generalised allergic phenomena.
Loaiasis is treated with diethylcarbamazine; antihistamines or sometimes corticosteroids may be needed to control allergic reaction to treatment.

Onchocerciasis (river blindness) is a filarial disease caused by nematodes of the genus *Onchocerca*, which are transmitted by *Simulium* flies. It is characterised by a persistent irritating skin rash, corneal opacities, skin nodules, and muscular pains.

After the infective larvae are injected into man, they grow in nodules in the tissues. After 10 to 18 months, the females produce a large number of microfilariae which invade the skin producing a low-grade inflammatory reaction. Here they are available to the insect vectors. It is the microfilariae which give rise to disease. When they die they release a foreign protein that provokes a tissue reaction. In the skin this gives rise to a small, persistent, papular, irritating eruption; in the eye it may lead to blindness and in muscles it may cause pain. The microfilariae are destroyed with diethylcarbamazine. Suramin is used to kill the adult parasites.

Dracunculiasis is caused by the guinea-worm *Dracunculus medinensis* which is about 1 metre long and lives in connective tissues. The small crustacean *Cyclops* is its intermediate host and infection is acquired when infected *Cyclops* are ingested in drinking water.
The larvae penetrate the wall of the small intestine and develop in connective tissues. The mature female travels to the legs or arms and bores through to the surface where it secretes a toxic substance which causes a blister to appear. This bursts and the worm releases embryos whenever the limb is immersed in water. Generalised urticaria occurs and there may be aching or intense itching in the affected area. The worm may be visible below the surface of the skin and may sometimes be gradually extracted over a period of several days, but surgery may damage the worm and may give rise to undesirable reactions.
The worms may be killed with suitable anthelmintics such as niridazole or thiabendazole.

Flavouring Agents

Flavouring agents are used to mask unpleasant tastes and make medicines more acceptable to patients, especially children. The type of flavour is usually chosen according to the taste to be disguised or masked. *Fruit flavours* help to disguise acid or sour flavours, *liquorice* and *cinnamon* are effective with saline tastes, and *chocolate* and various *fruit syrups* help to disguise bitter tastes. Emulsions are often flavoured with *benzaldehyde* or *vanillin*. Some improvement in acceptability may be achieved by adjusting the sweetness and viscosity of preparations and by incorporating a colour associated with the flavour used.

Stability of flavouring agents. Flavouring agents may be affected by pH, oxidation, reduction, or hydrolysis. Some synthetic flavours are more stable than the corresponding natural materials.

Fleas

Fleas are small laterally compressed wingless ectoparasitic arthropods with mouth parts adapted to piercing and sucking. Eggs are dropped haphazardly and hatch in 3 to 4 days. Larval or adult fleas may remain dormant in dust for months.
The two major groups of fleas which infect man are the Pulicidae (including *Pulex irritans*, the human flea) and *Xenopsylla* spp. (the rat flea). Flea bites are small, discrete, erythematous, sometimes petechial spots, which are usually irritating especially in individuals already sensitised to them.
Dusting-powders containing insecticides such as gamma benzene hexachloride and dicophane have been used as an aid to the elimination of flea infections.

Fluanisone

4'-Fluoro-4-[4-(2-methoxyphenyl)piperazin-1-yl]butyro-
phenone

$C_{21}H_{25}FN_2O_2 = 356.4$

OTHER NAME: *Hypnorm*®

*A standard is given in the British Pharmacopoeia
(Veterinary)*

Description. Odourless, almost white to buff-coloured
crystals or powder.

Solubility. Practically insoluble in water; soluble, at 20°,
in 12 parts of alcohol, in 22 parts of ether, and in 1 part
of chloroform; soluble in dilute solutions of organic
acids.

Sterilisation. Solutions are sterilised by heating in an
autoclave or by filtration.

Storage. It should be stored in airtight containers,
protected from light.

Identification. TEST. It complies with Test 2 described
under Betamethasone.

MELTING-POINT. About 74°.

ULTRAVIOLET ABSORPTION. In a mixture of 1 volume of
0.1N hydrochloric acid and 9 volumes of isopropyl
alcohol, maximum at 243 nm (E1%, 1cm = 550).

INFRA-RED ABSORPTION. Major peaks at 750, 1155, 1235,
1497, 1600, and 1690 cm^{-1} (see Appendix 2c: Infra-red
Spectra).

Veterinary uses. Fluanisone is a tranquilliser used in
conjunction with a narcotic analgesic (fentanyl) to
produce neuroleptanalgesia. The usual dose by intramuscular injection in dogs is 5 milligrams per kilogram
body-weight.

Preparations

Preparations available include a veterinary INJECTION
containing fluanisone 10 mg with fentanyl citrate
315 micrograms per ml in 10-ml bottles.

Flucloxacillin Sodium

Sodium (6R)-6-[3-(2-chloro-6-fluorophenyl)-5-methyl-
isoxazole-4-carboxamido]penicillanate monohydrate

$C_{19}H_{16}ClFN_3NaO_5S,H_2O = 493.9$

OTHER NAMES: Floxacillin Sodium; *Floxapen*®

Magnapen® (with ampicillin sodium or ampicillin
trihydrate)

Description. A white crystalline powder with a characteristic bitter taste.

Solubility. Soluble in 1 part of water, in 8 parts of
alcohol, and in 8 parts of acetone.

Acidity. A 10% solution has a pH of about 6.

Stability. In aqueous solutions, decomposition occurs
slowly at the pH for maximum stability (approximately
6.5); such solutions lose only a small proportion of their
potency when kept for several days at room temperatures. Solutions in sodium chloride injection or dextrose
injection may be used for 24 hours at room temperature.

FURTHER INFORMATION. Stability in aqueous solution
and in intravenous infusions—B. Lynn, *J. Hosp.
Pharm.*, 1971, **29**, 183.

Storage. It should be stored in airtight containers at a
temperature not exceeding 25°. If it is intended for
parenteral administration, the containers should be
sterile and sealed to exclude micro-organisms.

Identification. ULTRAVIOLET ABSORPTION. In alcohol
(95%), maximum at 270 nm (E1%, 1cm = 24).

INFRA-RED ABSORPTION. Major peaks at 1337, 1495,
1603, 1622, 1660, and 1767 cm^{-1} (see Appendix 2a: Infra-
red Spectra).

Metabolism. ABSORPTION. Well absorbed after oral
administration; it is better absorbed than cloxacillin; it
is less well absorbed if taken after food.

BLOOD CONCENTRATION. After an oral dose of 250 mg,
peak serum concentrations of up to 26 μg/ml are attained
within about 1 hour in fasted subjects; in unfasted subjects, the peak concentration is reduced by 50% and
occurs about 2 hours later.

HALF-LIFE. Plasma half-life, 45 to 50 minutes.

DISTRIBUTION. Volume of distribution, about 8 litres; it
does not enter the cerebrospinal fluid; *protein binding*,
90 to 95% bound to plasma proteins.

EXCRETION. 20 to 50% of an oral dose is excreted in the
urine and up to 90% may be excreted in the urine after
intramuscular doses; the urinary excretion of flucloxacillin is delayed by probenecid.

FURTHER INFORMATION. Serum concentrations and protein binding—G. P. Bodey *et al.*, *Clin. Pharmac. Ther.*,
1972, **13**, 512 and R. Sutherland *et al.*, *Br. med. J.*,
iv/1970, 455; pharmacokinetics—E. H. Nauta and H.
Mattie, *Br. J. clin. Pharmac.*, 1975, **2**, 111.

Actions and uses. Flucloxacillin sodium has the actions
and uses described under Cloxacillin Sodium but when
given by mouth it gives peak blood levels higher than
those obtained with an equivalent dose of cloxacillin
sodium.

The usual adult dose is the equivalent of 250 mg of
flucloxacillin 4 times a day by mouth or by intramuscular
injection and 250 to 500 mg 4 times a day by slow
intravenous or once-daily by intra-articular injection.
Flucloxacillin sodium may also be administered intra-
pleurally in a daily dose equivalent to 250 mg of flucloxacillin and using an aerosol in a dosage equivalent to
125 to 250 mg of flucloxacillin 4 times a day. In severe
infections these doses may be doubled.

The dose for children up to 2 years is one quarter and
from 2 to 10 years one half of the adult dose.

Undesirable effects. Allergic reactions as described
under Benzylpenicillin may occur.

Precautions. The same precautions against allergic reactions should be taken as for Benzylpenicillin. It should not be used topically or locally in the eye.

Preparations

FLUCLOXACILLIN CAPSULES: consisting of flucloxacillin sodium, in powder, which may be mixed with a suitable inert diluent, enclosed in a hard capsule. The capsule shells may be coloured. Available as capsules containing flucloxacillin sodium equivalent to 250 mg of flucloxacillin.

Containers and *Storage:* see the entry on Capsules for general information on containers and storage. The capsules should be stored in a cool place.

Advice for patients: the capsules should be taken at regular intervals, preferably half to 1 hour before meals. The prescribed course should be completed.

FLUCLOXACILLIN INJECTION: a sterile solution of flucloxacillin sodium in water for injections. It is prepared by dissolving the contents of a sealed container in water for injections immediately before use. Available as a powder in vials containing flucloxacillin sodium equivalent to 250 and 500 mg of flucloxacillin.

Containers: see the entry on Injections for general information on containers.

Labelling: see the entry on Injections for general information on labelling. In addition, the label on the container should state the amount of the medicament as the equivalent amount of flucloxacillin.

Storage: the sealed container should be stored in a cool place.

OTHER PREPARATIONS available include CAPSULES containing flucloxacillin sodium equivalent to 250 mg of flucloxacillin with ampicillin trihydrate equivalent to 250 mg of ampicillin; an ELIXIR containing flucloxacillin sodium equivalent to 125 mg of flucloxacillin in 5 ml when reconstituted, diluent syrup, an elixir containing flucloxacillin sodium equivalent to 125 mg of flucloxacillin with ampicillin trihydrate equivalent to 125 mg of ampicillin in 5 ml when reconstituted; and an INJECTION reconstituted from a powder in vials containing flucloxacillin sodium equivalent to 250 mg of flucloxacillin with ampicillin sodium equivalent to 250 mg of ampicillin.

Flucytosine

4-Amino-5-fluoropyrimidin-2(1*H*)-one

$C_4H_4FN_3O = 129.1$

OTHER NAME: *Alcobon*®

Description. An odourless, white or off-white, crystalline powder.

Solubility. Soluble in 67 parts of water; very slightly soluble in alcohol; practically insoluble in chloroform and in ether.

Storage. It should be stored in airtight containers, protected from light.

Identification. MELTING-POINT. About 295°, with decomposition.

ULTRAVIOLET ABSORPTION. In dilute hydrochloric acid, maximum at 285 nm.

Determination in body fluids. GAS CHROMATOGRAPHY. In serum: in the presence of amphotericin—S. A. Harding *et al.*, *Clin. Chem.*, 1976, **22**, 772.

MICROBIOLOGICAL ASSAY. In serum—R. G. Blaker and B. J. Doutt, *Antimicrob. Ag. Chemother.*, 1972, **2**, 502; in serum: in the presence of amphotericin—E. R. Block and J. E. Bennett, *Antimicrob. Ag. Chemother.*, 1972, **1**, 476; in serum or urine—R. J. Holt and R. L. Newman, *J. clin. Path.*, 1973, **26**, 167.

Metabolism. ABSORPTION. Well absorbed after oral administration.

BLOOD CONCENTRATION. During therapy with 100 mg/kg body-weight daily, serum concentrations of 1 to 80 μg/ml are attained; after doses of 8 to 12 g daily concentrations of up to 180 μg/ml are attained; therapeutic concentrations are in the range 30 to 100 μg/ml.

HALF-LIFE. Serum half-life, 2 to 8 hours; the half-life may be doubled in patients with renal function impairment.

DISTRIBUTION. Widely distributed throughout the body and has a volume of distribution of 0.5 to 1.0 litre/kg body-weight; readily enters the cerebrospinal fluid and concentrations in this fluid attain about 80% of those in serum; *protein binding*, about 50% bound to serum proteins.

EXCRETION. 90% of a dose is excreted unchanged in the urine in 24 hours; in patients with impaired renal function, urinary excretion occurs more slowly.

FURTHER INFORMATION. Serum concentrations and urinary excretion—R. R. Davies and D. S. Reeves, *Br. med. J.*, i/1971, 577; pharmacokinetics—J. R. Horn and D. L. Giusti, *Drug Intell. & clin. Pharm.*, 1975, **9**, 180.

Actions and uses. Flucytosine is an antifungal substance used in the treatment of systemic and urinary tract infections by sensitive fungi, especially strains of *Candida albicans*, *Cryptococcus neoformans*, *Torulopsis*, *Aspergillus fumigatus*, and chromomycotic fungi. It is frequently used in conjunction with amphotericin. It is administered by mouth.

In the treatment of severe infections a dose of 200 milligrams per kilogram body-weight is given daily in 4 divided doses to children and adults, but lower doses such as 100 to 150 milligrams per kilogram body-weight daily may be effective if the infecting organism is very sensitive. Smaller doses should be given to patients with renal impairment.

When flucytosine cannot be given by mouth it may be administered in similar dosage by slow intravenous injection or intraperitoneal infusion of a solution suitably diluted with sodium chloride injection or dextrose injection (5%); somewhat lower doses may be effective by these routes.

Flucytosine has also been applied as a 10% ointment.

Undesirable effects. Nausea, vomiting, diarrhoea, rashes, leucopenia, and thrombocytopenia may occur. Liver function may be affected.

Precautions. Blood examinations, liver function tests, and tests for sensitivity of organisms should be carried out at intervals. Blood concentration should be monitored, especially in patients with renal impairment. Flucytosine is teratogenic and should not be given in pregnancy.

Preparations

FLUCYTOSINE TABLETS: available as tablets containing 500 mg of flucytosine.

Containers and *Storage:* see the entry on Tablets for general information on containers and storage. Containers should be airtight and light resistant.

Advice for patients: the tablets should be taken at regular intervals. The dose may be taken over a period of 15 minutes to minimise nausea. The prescribed course should be completed.

OTHER PREPARATIONS available include an INJECTION containing 1% of flucytosine in 250-ml bottles.

Fludrocortisone Acetate

9α - Fluoro - 11β,17α,21 - trihydroxypregn - 4 - ene - 3,20-dione 21-acetate

$C_{23}H_{31}FO_6 = 422.5$

OTHER NAME: *Florinef*®

A standard is given in the British Pharmacopoeia 1973

Description. An odourless, hygroscopic, white, crystalline powder.

Solubility. Very slightly soluble in water; soluble, at 20°, in 50 parts of alcohol, in 250 parts of ether, and in 50 parts of chloroform.

Moisture content. Not more than 1%, determined by drying at 105°.

Specific rotation. +148° to +156°, determined on a 1% solution in dioxan.

Storage. It should be stored in airtight containers, protected from light.

Identification. TESTS. 1. It complies with Tests 1 and 2 described under Betamethasone.
2. It complies with Test 3 described under Cortisone Acetate (presence of acetyl groups).

MELTING-POINT. About 225°. It may also occur in a form which melts at about 209°.

ULTRAVIOLET ABSORPTION. In dehydrated alcohol, maximum at 240 nm (E1%, 1cm = 405).

INFRA-RED ABSORPTION. Major peaks at 1041, 1247, 1273, 1360, 1649, and 1712 cm^{-1} (see Appendix 2a: Infra-red Spectra).

THIN-LAYER CHROMATOGRAPHY. See under Thin-layer Chromatography, System 10.

Metabolism. ABSORPTION. Rapidly and completely absorbed after oral administration; it is absorbed to some extent through the skin since pituitary-adrenal axis suppression occurs following topical application.

BLOOD CONCENTRATION. After an oral dose of 100 μg of the alcohol, peak plasma concentrations of 1.2 to 1.7 ng/ml are attained in 1.5 to 2 hours; after an intravenous dose of 100 μg of the alcohol, initial plasma concentrations of 1.6 to 2.4 ng/ml are attained which fall to about 1 ng/ml after 3 to 4 hours; after administration of the acetate, only the non-esterified alcohol is detectable in the blood.

HALF-LIFE. Plasma half-life for fludrocortisone after intravenous administration, about 30 minutes; following administration of the acetate to dogs, the blood concentration shows a triphasic decline and each phase may represent the elimination of a metabolite.

DISTRIBUTION. Widely distributed throughout the body; *protein binding,* fludrocortisone is 70 to 80% bound to serum proteins, mainly to the globulin fractions.

METABOLIC REACTIONS. Hydrolysis to produce the non-esterified alcohol.

EXCRETION. In rats most of a dose is excreted in the bile, and in dogs and guinea-pigs most of the dose is excreted in the urine.

FURTHER INFORMATION. Pharmacokinetics—A. Garbe and H. Wenzl, *Arzneimittel-Forsch.,* 1971, **21**, 1127, W. Vogt *et al., Arzneimittel-Forsch.,* 1971, **21**, 1133, and H. Wenzl *et al., Arzneimittel-Forsch.,* 1971, **21**, 1110, 1115, 1123.

Actions and uses. Fludrocortisone has powerful glucocorticoid and mineralocorticoid actions. Given alone in adrenocortical deficiency states, its mineralocorticoid action is relatively stronger than its glucocorticoid action, and oedema and other signs of salt and water retention appear within a few days of starting treatment. With a dosage which is just enough to correct sodium loss in Addison's disease or in adrenalectomised subjects, the glucocorticoid action of fludrocortisone is insufficient to maintain the patient in normal health. For this reason fludrocortisone acetate is usually given by mouth in low dosage, such as 100 micrograms every 1 to 5 days, together with the usual maintenance replacement dose of cortisone acetate, to those adrenocortical-deficient patients who become sodium deficient on cortisone alone.

In some patients adrenalectomised for metastatic carcinomatosis, symptoms of sodium deficiency may occur when the malignant process begins to extend again after the regression caused by the operation; in such cases fludrocortisone is of value.

Undesirable effects. Excessive dosage may result not only in Cushingoid features with oedema and electrolyte imbalance but also in marked muscle weakness and in hyperglycaemia.

Preparation

FLUDROCORTISONE TABLETS: available as tablets containing 100 micrograms and 1 mg of fludrocortisone acetate; they may be coloured.

A standard for these tablets is given in the British Pharmacopoeia 1973

Containers and *Storage:* see the entry on Tablets for general information on containers and storage. Containers should be airtight and light resistant.

Advice for patients: in long-term use, treatment should not be discontinued without the advice of the prescriber. Patients may carry an identification card giving details of their treatment and the name of the prescriber, who should be contacted in the event of accident, feverish illness, diarrhoea, vomiting, or alimentary disturbances. In short-term treatment the prescribed course should be completed.

Flufenamic Acid

N-(ααα-Trifluoro-m-tolyl)anthranilic acid

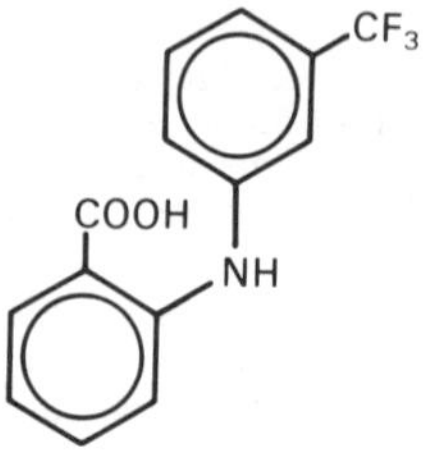

$C_{14}H_{10}F_3NO_2 = 281.2$

OTHER NAME: *Arlef*®

A standard is given in the British Pharmacopoeia Addendum 1975

Description. A pale yellow, crystalline, odourless powder.

Solubility. Very slightly soluble in water; soluble, at 20°, in 4 parts of alcohol, in 3 parts of ether, and in 7 parts of chloroform.

Identification. TESTS. 1. Dissolve about 25 mg in 15 ml of chloroform and examine the solution under ultra-violet radiation; a strong bluish-white fluorescence is observed.
2. Heat 0.5 ml of *chromic-sulphuric acid mixture* in a small test-tube in a water-bath for 5 minutes; the solution wets the sides of the tube and there is no greasiness. Add about 2 mg of the sample and again heat in a water-bath for 5 minutes; the solution does not wet the sides of the tube and does not pour easily from the tube.

MELTING-POINT. About 124°; on further heating it re-solidifies and melts again at about 135°.

ULTRAVIOLET ABSORPTION. In a mixture of 1 volume of 1N hydrochloric acid and 99 volumes of methyl alcohol, maxima at 287 nm (E1%, 1cm = 570) and 344 nm (E1%, 1cm = 295).

INFRA-RED ABSORPTION. Major peaks at 698, 796, 1118, 1166, 1180, and 1661 cm⁻¹ (see Appendix 2a: Infra-red Spectra).

THIN-LAYER CHROMATOGRAPHY. See under Thin-layer Chromatography, System 3.

Determination in body fluids. COLORIMETRY. In urine: determination of fluorine—H.-D. Dell and J. Fiedler, *Z. analyt. Chem.*, 1974, **270**, 278.

SPECTROFLUORIMETRY. In urine—H.-D. Dell and R. Kamp, *Arch. Pharm., Berl.*, 1970, **303**, 785.

Metabolism. ABSORPTION. Well absorbed after oral administration.

BLOOD CONCENTRATION. During therapy with oral doses of 200 mg thrice daily, plasma concentrations of 0.3 to 17 μg/ml are attained; after a single dose of 500 mg, peak concentrations of about 20 μg/ml are attained in about 2 hours.

HALF-LIFE. Plasma half-life, about 3 hours.

DISTRIBUTION. Small amounts are secreted in the milk; *protein binding*, strongly bound to plasma proteins.

METABOLIC REACTIONS. Hydroxylation and glucuronic acid conjugation.

EXCRETION. 20 to 30% of a dose is excreted in the urine and 5% in the faeces; the major urinary metabolite is the glucuronide.

FURTHER INFORMATION. Excretion in breast milk— R. A. Buchanan *et al.*, *Curr. ther. Res.*, 1969, **11**, 533.

Actions and uses. Flufenamic acid is an analgesic with minor anti-inflammatory properties and has the actions and uses described under Ibuprofen. It may be given with caution to patients with peptic ulceration. The usual dosage for adults is 400 to 600 milligrams daily in divided doses.

Undesirable effects. As for Ibuprofen. Flufenamic acid may give rise to diarrhoea and abnormalities in liver function which may necessitate discontinuation of treatment.

Precautions. As for Ibuprofen.

Contra-indications. It is contra-indicated in pregnancy and lactation. Flufenamic acid should not be adminis-tered to children. Its use should be avoided in patients with inflammatory bowel disease, or renal or hepatic disease.

Preparation

FLUFENAMIC ACID CAPSULES: consisting of flufenamic acid, in powder, which may be mixed with a suitable inert diluent, enclosed in a hard capsule. The capsule shells may be coloured. Available as capsules containing 100 mg of flufenamic acid.
A standard for these capsules is given in the British Pharmacopoeia Addendum 1975
Containers and *Storage:* see the entry on Capsules for general information on containers and storage.
Advice for patients: the capsules should preferably be taken after meals.

Fluocinolone Acetonide

6α,9α - Difluoro - 11β,21 - dihydroxy - 16α,17α - isopropyl-idenedioxypregna-1.4-diene-3,20-dione

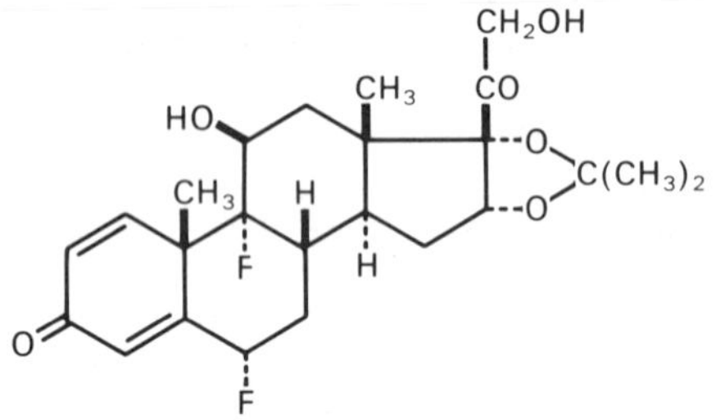

$C_{24}H_{30}F_2O_6 = 452.5$

OTHER NAMES: *Synalar*®; *Synandone*®
Synalar-N® (with neomycin sulphate)

A standard is given in the British Pharmacopoeia 1973

Description. An odourless white crystalline powder.

Solubility. Practically insoluble in water; soluble, at 20°, in 26 parts of dehydrated alcohol, in 15 parts of chloroform, and in 10 parts of acetone; very slightly soluble in light petroleum.

Moisture content. Not more than 1%, determined by drying at 50° *in vacuo.*

Specific rotation. +92° to +96°, determined on a 1% solution in dioxan.

Storage. It should be protected from light.

Identification. TESTS. It complies with Tests 1 and 2 described under Betamethasone.

MELTING-POINT. About 275°, with decomposition.

ULTRAVIOLET ABSORPTION. In dehydrated alcohol, maximum at 240 nm (E1%, 1cm = 360).

INFRA-RED ABSORPTION. Major peaks at 910, 1056, 1074, 1615, 1629, and 1669 cm^{-1} (see Appendix 2a: Infra-red Spectra).

THIN-LAYER CHROMATOGRAPHY. See under Thin-layer Chromatography, System 10.

Metabolism. ABSORPTION. After topical application, fluocinolone acetonide penetrates the skin poorly; the use of occlusive techniques increases penetration.

DISTRIBUTION. After a subcutaneous dose to mice, high concentrations are attained in the liver with lower concentrations appearing in the lungs, kidneys, pituitary and adrenal glands, skeletal muscle, myocardium, and lachrymal glands.

EXCRETION. After a subcutaneous dose to mice, about 80% of the dose is excreted in the faeces via the bile and about 6% is excreted in the urine; after a percutaneous dose to man, about 0.3% is excreted in the urine.

FURTHER INFORMATION. Percutaneous absorption in different vehicles—M. F. Coldman *et al.*, *J. pharm. Sci.*, 1969, **58**, 1098; percutaneous absorption and urinary excretion—H. L. Maibach and R. J. Feldmann, *Clin. Res.*, 1966, **14**, 270; fate of fluocinolone acetonide administered subcutaneously and percutaneously in mice —T. Takahashi *et al.*, *Chem. pharm. Bull.*, *Tokyo*, 1971, **19**, 309.

Actions and uses. Fluocinolone acetonide is a corticosteroid for topical application that is more potent than hydrocortisone; it should not be given by mouth. It is applied as an ointment, lotion, or cream containing up to 0.025%, and is generally used either without dressings or with conventional bandaging, but if the area is covered with a non-porous dressing such as polythene the effect is greatly enhanced. This method of application is suitable for small areas in chronic skin conditions, but if the preparation is used over large areas, sufficient of the drug may be absorbed through the skin to give rise to systemic effects. In certain intractable skin conditions a cream containing 0.2% may be used.

Precautions. It should not be used on infected skin without the simultaneous application of a suitable antibacterial agent.

Preparations

FLUOCINOLONE CREAM (*Syn.* Fluocinolone Acetonide Cream): a dispersion of fluocinolone acetonide in a suitable water-miscible basis containing a mixture of benzyl alcohol, methyl hydroxybenzoate, and propyl hydroxybenzoate as the preservative system. Available as creams containing 0.01, 0.025, and 0.2% of fluocinolone acetonide.
When a strength less than those available from the manufacturer is prescribed, the 0.025% cream may be diluted, with hygienic precautions, with cetomacrogol cream (formula B). The diluted cream must be freshly prepared.
Diluents or medicaments which are strongly alkaline or acid, or which contain oxidising agents, accelerate the decomposition of fluocinolone acetonide. Diluents which contain ionic emulsifying compounds may be incompatible with the basis. Emulsifying ointment and aqueous cream are examples of such diluents.
A standard for this cream is given in the British Pharmaceutical Codex 1973
Containers, Labelling, and *Storage:* see the entry on Creams for general information on containers, labelling, and storage.
Advice for patients: the cream should be applied sparingly to the affected area.

FLUOCINOLONE GEL: containing fluocinolone acetonide in a suitable water-miscible basis. Available as a gel containing 0.025% of fluocinolone acetonide. This preparation should not be diluted.
Advice for patients: the gel should be applied sparingly to the affected area.

FLUOCINOLONE OINTMENT: a dispersion of fluocinolone acetonide in a suitable anhydrous greasy basis. Available as ointments containing 0.01% and 0.025% of fluocinolone acetonide.
When a strength less than those available from the manufacturer is prescribed, the 0.025% ointment may be diluted with white or yellow soft paraffin or with eye ointment basis.
A standard for this ointment is given in the British Pharmaceutical Codex 1973
Containers, Labelling, and *Storage:* see the entry on Ointments for general information on containers, labelling, and storage.
Advice for patients: the ointment should be applied sparingly to the affected area.

OTHER PREPARATIONS available include a CREAM containing fluocinolone acetonide 0.025% with clioquinol 3%, diluents as indicated under Fluocinolone Cream, a cream containing fluocinolone acetonide 0.025% with neomycin sulphate 0.5%; a LOTION containing fluocinolone acetonide 0.025%, diluent cetostearyl alcohol 2.5% and cetomacrogol 1000 0.5% in water, a veterinary lotion containing fluocinolone acetonide 0.025% with neomycin sulphate 0.5%; an OINTMENT containing fluocinolone acetonide 0.025% with clioquinol 3%, diluents as indicated under Fluocinolone Ointment, and an ointment containing fluocinolone acetonide 0.025% with neomycin sulphate 0.5%.

Fluocortolone Hexanoate

6α - Fluoro - 11β,21 - dihydroxy - 16α - methylpregna - 1,4- diene-3,20-dione 21-hexanoate

$C_{28}H_{39}FO_5 = 474.6$

OTHER NAMES: Fluocortolone Caproate
Ficoid® and *Ultralanum*® (both with fluocortolone or fluocortolone pivalate); *Ultradil*® (with fluocortolone pivalate)

A standard is given in the British Pharmacopoeia 1973

Description. An odourless, white or creamy-white, crystalline powder.

Solubility. Practically insoluble in water and in ether; very slightly soluble in alcohol and in methyl alcohol; soluble, at 20°, in 18 parts of chloroform.

Specific rotation. +97° to +103°, determined on a 1% solution in dioxan.

Storage. It should be protected from light.

Identification. TESTS. 1. It complies with Test 2 described under Betamethasone.
2. Mix about 1 mg with 2 ml of a mixture containing 3 volumes of sulphuric acid and 2 volumes of glacial acetic acid and heat for 1 minute on a water-bath; a red colour is produced. Add 5 ml of water; the colour changes to violet-red.
3. Mix about 50 mg with 2 ml of 0.5N alcoholic potassium hydroxide and heat in a water-bath for 5 minutes; add 3 ml of water, evaporate the alcohol, add 2 ml of sulphuric acid (50% v/v), and again heat on a water-bath; the odour of hexanoic acid develops.

MELTING-POINT. About 244°.

ULTRAVIOLET ABSORPTION. In methyl alcohol, maximum at 242 nm (E1%, 1cm = 340).

INFRA-RED ABSORPTION. Major peaks at 1163, 1176, 1622, 1658, 1722, and 1747 cm^{-1} (see Appendix 2a: Infra-red Spectra).

THIN-LAYER CHROMATOGRAPHY. See under Thin-layer Chromatography, System 10.

Actions and uses. Fluocortolone hexanoate is a corticosteroid intended for topical application. It has the powerful anti-inflammatory actions of fluocortolone, and although the onset of action is less rapid than with fluocortolone or fluocortolone pivalate, it is more prolonged.
It is used with fluocortolone as an ointment containing 0.25% of each constituent, or as a cream or lotion with fluocortolone pivalate.
Initially, it may be necessary to apply the ointment 3 times a day, but later a dressing once daily may be adequate. With such dressings, excessive absorption and consequent systemic effects are unlikely except in infants. In psoriasis and other refractory conditions, the ointment should be applied thinly and covered with an occlusive dressing. Large areas of the body should not be occluded in this way because of the increased risk of systemic effects and disturbances of the heat-regulating mechanism.

Precautions. Fluocortolone hexanoate should not be used on infected skin without the simultaneous application of a suitable antibacterial agent.

Preparations

Preparations available include a CREAM containing fluocortolone hexanoate 0.1% with fluocortolone pivalate 0.1%, a cream containing fluocortolone hexanoate 0.25% with fluocortolone pivalate 0.25%, diluent (for both strengths) aqueous cream, life of diluted creams 14 days; a LOTION containing fluocortolone hexanoate 0.25% with fluocortolone pivalate 0.25%, diluent water, life of diluted lotion 14 days; an OINTMENT containing fluocortolone hexanoate 0.1% with fluocortolone pivalate 0.1%, and an ointment containing fluocortolone hexanoate 0.25% with fluocortolone 0.25%, diluent (for both ointments) oily cream, life of diluted ointment 14 days.

Fluocortolone Pivalate

6α - Fluoro - 11β,21 - dihydroxy - 16α - methylpregna - 1,4-diene-3,20-dione 21-pivalate

$C_{27}H_{37}FO_5 = 460.6$

OTHER NAMES: Fluocortolone Trimethylacetate
Ficoid®, *Ultradil*®, and *Ultralanum*® (all with fluocortolone hexanoate)

A standard is given in the British Pharmacopoeia 1973

Description. An odourless, white or creamy-white, crystalline powder.

Solubility. Very slightly soluble in water; soluble, at 20°, in 36 parts of alcohol, in 3 parts of chloroform, and in 18 parts of methyl alcohol.

Specific rotation. +100° to +105°, determined on a 1% solution in dioxan.

Storage. It should be protected from light.

Identification. TESTS. 1. It complies with Test 2 described under Betamethasone.
2. It complies with Test 2 described under Fluocortolone Hexanoate.
3. Mix about 50 mg with 2 ml of 0.5N alcoholic potassium hydroxide and heat in a water-bath for 5 minutes; add 2 ml of water, evaporate the alcohol, add 2 ml of sulphuric acid (50% v/v), extract with 5 ml of solvent ether, and evaporate the ether; the odour of pivalic acid is produced.

MELTING-POINT. About 187°.

ULTRAVIOLET ABSORPTION. In methyl alcohol, maximum at 240 nm (E1%, 1cm = 335).

INFRA-RED ABSORPTION. Major peaks at 1159, 1285, 1605, 1619, 1662, and 1725 cm^{-1} (see Appendix 2a: Infra-red Spectra).

THIN-LAYER CHROMATOGRAPHY. See under Thin-layer Chromatography, System 10.

Actions and uses. Fluocortolone pivalate has the general anti-inflammatory properties of fluocortolone, as described under Fluocortolone Hexanoate.
It is used in conjunction with fluocortolone hexanoate in creams and lotions when the free alcohol would not be suitable owing to its instability.

Precautions. Fluocortolone pivalate should not be used on infected skin without the simultaneous application of a suitable antibacterial agent.

Preparations

Preparations available include a CREAM containing fluocortolone pivalate 0.1% with fluocortolone hexanoate 0.1%, a cream containing fluocortolone pivalate 0.25% with fluocortolone hexanoate 0.25%, diluent (for both strengths) aqueous cream, life of diluted creams 14 days; a LOTION containing fluocortolone pivalate 0.25% with fluocortolone hexanoate 0.25%, diluent water, life of diluted lotion 14 days; and an OINTMENT containing fluocortolone pivalate 0.1% with fluocortolone hexanoate 0.1%, diluent oily cream, life of diluted ointment 14 days.

Fluorescein Sodium

The disodium salt of 2-(6-hydroxy-3-oxo-3*H*-xanthen-9-yl)benzoic acid.

$C_{20}H_{10}Na_2O_5 = 376.3$

OTHER NAMES: *Fluor-Amps®*; Fluoresceinum Natricum; *Fluorets®*; *Fluoro-I-Strip®*; Soluble Fluorescein

A standard is given in the British Pharmacopoeia 1973

Description. An orange-red, hygroscopic, odourless, almost tasteless powder.

Solubility. Soluble, at 20°, in 1.5 parts of water and in 10 parts of alcohol.

Moisture content. Not more than 10%, determined by drying at 105°.

Sterilisation. Solutions are sterilised by heating in an autoclave.

Storage. It should be stored in airtight containers.

Identification. TESTS. 1. A solution is strongly fluorescent, even in extreme dilution. Acidify the solution; the fluorescence disappears. Make the solution alkaline; the fluorescence reappears.

2. Place 1 drop of a 0.05% solution on a filter paper; the paper is coloured yellow. Expose the moist paper to the vapour of bromine for 1 minute and then to the vapour of ammonia; the yellow colour becomes deep pink.

Uses. Fluorescein sodium is used in ophthalmic practice as a diagnostic agent for detecting lesions and foreign bodies; a 2% solution is commonly used for this purpose. When introduced into the eye, it does not stain the normal cornea but ulcers, or parts deprived of epithelium, become green and foreign bodies are seen surrounded by a green ring. Since it is applied to abraded corneas, special care should be taken to avoid bacterial contamination.

Solutions containing 5 to 20% of fluorescein sodium have been administered by intravenous injection for diagnostic purposes, such as the investigation of circulatory disorders and the differentiation of normal and malignant tissues when examined in ultraviolet light.

Preparations

FLUORESCEIN EYE-DROPS: consisting of a sterile solution containing up to 2% of fluorescein sodium in purified water. It is prepared by Method A, B, or C described in the entry on Eye-drops. When prepared by Method C it contains 0.002% of phenylmercuric acetate or nitrate. Available as eye-drops in a single-dose form containing 1% and 2% of fluorescein sodium.

A standard for these eye-drops is given in the British Pharmaceutical Codex 1973

Containers: see the entry on Eye-drops for general information on containers. The eye-drops should preferably be supplied in single-dose containers but if only multiple-dose containers are available they may be used provided they are discarded after use on one occasion.

Labelling: see the entry on Eye-drops for general information on labelling. When supplied in a multiple-dose container a direction should be given that it should be discarded after use on one occasion.

OTHER PREPARATIONS available include an INJECTION containing fluorescein sodium 5, 10, 15, 20, and 25% in 5-ml ampoules; and OPHTHALMIC STRIPS containing fluorescein sodium 1 and 9 mg.

Fluorouracil

5-Fluoropyrimidine-2,4(1*H*,3*H*)-dione

$C_4H_3FN_2O_2 = 130.08$

OTHER NAME: *Efudix®*

CAUTION. *Fluorouracil is irritant and contact with skin and mucous membranes should be avoided.*

Description. A white, almost odourless powder.

Solubility. Soluble in water; very slightly soluble in alcohol; practically insoluble in chloroform and in ether.

Storage. It should be stored in airtight containers, protected from light.

Identification. MELTING-POINT. About 282°, with decomposition.

INFRA-RED ABSORPTION. Major peaks at 820, 1220, 1250, 1429, 1667, and 1724 cm^{-1} (see Appendix 2b: Infra-red Spectra).

Determination in body fluids. GAS CHROMATOGRAPHY. In urine: initial separation by ion-exchange—K. V. Rao *et al.*, *J. pharm. Sci.*, 1974, **63**, 1328.

Actions and uses. Fluorouracil is a cytotoxic agent. It is an analogue of uracil, a component of ribonucleic acid, and is believed to exert its effect in malignant disease by interfering with nucleic acid biosynthesis. It is used alone or in conjunction with radiotherapy in the palliative treatment of cancers of the gastro-intestinal tract, breast, and respiratory tract.

The usual dosage is 15 milligrams per kilogram body-weight daily by intravenous infusion in dextrose injection (5%) but the total daily dose should not exceed 1 gram. Treatment should be continued daily until a total of 12 to 15 grams has been administered or until signs of toxicity occur. An interval of 4 to 6 weeks should then elapse before a further course is given. Alternatively, fluorouracil may be given in courses of 5 days at a dosage of 1 gram daily by intravenous infusion. This is often well tolerated but an interval of 4 to 6 weeks should elapse between courses.

Fluorouracil may also be given by intravenous injection. The usual daily dosage is 12 milligrams per kilogram body-weight up to a maximum of 1 gram for 3 days. If there is no evidence of toxicity, this is followed by three doses each of 6 milligrams per kilogram body-weight on alternate days and a maintenance dosage of 5 to 15 milligrams per kilogram body-weight weekly.

Fluorouracil may be administered intra-arterially for regional perfusion in a dosage of 5 to 7 milligrams per kilogram body-weight daily.

It may be applied as a 5% cream or ointment or as a 1 to 5% solution in propylene glycol in the treatment of solar keratoses and other malignant conditions of the skin.

Undesirable effects. Nausea, vomiting, diarrhoea, alopecia, dermatitis, leucopenia, and bone-marrow depression may occur.

Precautions and contra-indications. Regular examinations of the blood should be made during treatment and the initial dosage should be reduced in patients who are debilitated, have poor renal or hepatic function, or have undergone major surgery. It should not be given in pregnancy.

Preparations

FLUOROURACIL INJECTION: a sterile solution of the trometamol salt of fluorouracil in water for injections. Available as an injection containing the equivalent of 50 mg of fluorouracil per ml in 5-ml ampoules. The solution is further diluted before use with dextrose injection (5%) or water for injections for parenteral administration or with fruit juice or other suitable beverage for oral administration.

Containers and *Labelling:* see the entry on Injections for general information on containers and labelling.

Storage: it should be stored at room temperature, protected from light.

OTHER PREPARATIONS available include a CREAM containing fluorouracil 5%.

In the female it is given in doses of 20 milligrams in the treatment of inoperable breast cancer and in a dosage of 1 to 5 milligrams daily in functional uterine bleeding and dysmenorrhoea.

In the male it is given in the treatment of hypogonadism and eunuchoidism in a dosage of 5 to 10 milligrams daily.

It is administered for its anabolic effect in the treatment of osteoporosis in a dosage of 2 to 10 milligrams daily.

Precautions and contra-indications. The precautions described under Testosterone should be observed; increased erythropoiesis and hypercalcaemia are rare. Salt retention and oedema may be corrected by salt restriction and administration of diuretics.

Fluoxymesterone is contra-indicated in patients with impaired liver function or prostatic carcinoma.

Preparation

FLUOXYMESTERONE TABLETS: available as tablets containing 5 mg of fluoxymesterone.

A standard for these tablets is given in the British Pharmacopoeia 1973

Containers and *Storage:* see the entry on Tablets for general information on containers and storage. Containers should be airtight and light resistant.

Advice for patients: treatment should not be discontinued without the advice of the prescriber.

Fluoxymesterone

9α-Fluoro-11β,17β-dihydroxy- 17α-methylandrost-4-en-3-one

$C_{20}H_{29}FO_3 = 336.4$

OTHER NAME: *Ultandren*®

A standard is given in the British Pharmacopoeia 1973

Description. An odourless, white or creamy-white, crystalline powder.

Solubility. Very slightly soluble in water; soluble, at 20°, in 70 parts of alcohol and in 200 parts of chloroform.

Moisture content. Not more than 1%, determined by drying over phosphorus pentoxide *in vacuo.*

Specific rotation. +102° to +112°, determined on a 1% solution in alcohol (95%).

Storage. It should be stored in airtight containers, protected from light.

Identification. TEST. It complies with Test 2 described under Betamethasone.

MELTING-POINT. About 278°.

ULTRAVIOLET ABSORPTION. In dehydrated alcohol, maximum at 240 nm (E1%, 1cm = 495).

INFRA-RED ABSORPTION. Major peaks at 867, 1036, 1247, 1350, 1627, and 1654 cm⁻¹ (see Appendix 2a: Infra-red Spectra).

THIN-LAYER CHROMATOGRAPHY. See under Thin-layer Chromatography, System 10.

Actions and uses. Fluoxymesterone is an androgenic hormone which has the actions and uses described under Testosterone. It is effective when given by mouth.

Fluphenazine Decanoate

2-{4-[3-(2-Trifluoromethylphenothiazin-10-yl)propyl]-piperazin-1-yl}ethyl decanoate

$C_{32}H_{44}F_3N_3O_2S = 591.8$

OTHER NAME: *Modecate*®

A standard is given in the British Pharmacopoeia Addendum 1975

Description. A pale yellow viscous liquid or a yellow crystalline oily solid with a faint and ester-like odour.

Solubility. Practically insoluble in water; miscible with dehydrated alcohol, with ether, and with chloroform; soluble in fixed oils.

Moisture content. Not more than 1%, determined by drying at 60° *in vacuo.*

Sterilisation. Oily solutions for injection are sterilised by filtration.

Storage. It should be protected from light.

Identification. TEST. Dissolve about 5 mg in 2 ml of sulphuric acid and allow to stand for 5 minutes; a reddish-brown colour is produced.

ULTRAVIOLET ABSORPTION. In dehydrated alcohol, maxima at 261 nm (E1%, 1cm = 600) and at 310 nm.

Determination in body fluids; Metabolism. See under Fluphenazine Hydrochloride.

Actions and uses. Fluphenazine decanoate has actions and uses similar to those described under Fluphenazine Hydrochloride, but it is administered as an oily solution with a prolonged action.

It is usual to administer an initial dose of 12.5 milligrams of fluphenazine decanoate by deep intramuscular injection; this dose, which may be expected to control psychotic symptoms for 4 to 7 days, enables an assessment to be made of the extrapyramidal effects of the drug. Subsequently, doses of 25 milligrams may be administered and the dose adjusted and repeated at intervals of 14 to 35 days as necessary to maintain the response. Children under 12 years and adults over 60 years may be given half the adult dose.

1.2 milligrams of fluphenazine decanoate is approximately equivalent to 1 milligram of fluphenazine hydrochloride.

Undesirable effects; Contra-indications; Poisoning. As for Fluphenazine Hydrochloride.

Preparation

FLUPHENAZINE DECANOATE INJECTION: a sterile solution of fluphenazine decanoate in sesame oil. It is sterilised by filtration. Available as an injection containing 25 mg of fluphenazine decanoate per ml in 0.5-, 1-, and 2-ml ampoules, 1- and 2-ml disposable syringes, and 10-ml vials.

A standard for this injection is given in the British Pharmacopoeia Addendum 1975

Containers: see the entry on Injections for general information on containers.

Labelling: see the entry on Injections for general information on labelling. In addition the label on the container should state the name of the solvent and that the injection is for intramuscular injection only.

Storage: it should be protected from light.

Fluphenazine Enanthate

2-{4-[3-(2-Trifluoromethylphenothiazin-10-yl)propyl]-piperazin-1-yl}ethyl heptanoate

CH₂·CH₂·CH₂—N⟩ ⟨N—CH₂·CH₂·O·CO·[CH₂]₅·CH₃

$C_{29}H_{38}F_3N_3O_2S = 549.7$

OTHER NAME: *Moditen Enanthate®*

A standard is given in the British Pharmacopoeia Addendum 1975

Description. A pale yellow viscous liquid or a yellow crystalline oily solid with a faint ester-like odour.

Solubility. Practically insoluble in water; miscible with dehydrated alcohol, with ether, and with chloroform; soluble in fixed oils.

Moisture content. Not more than 1%, determined by drying at 60° *in vacuo.*

Sterilisation. Oily solutions are sterilised by filtration.

Storage. It should be protected from light.

Identification. TEST. Dissolve about 5 mg in 2 ml of sulphuric acid and allow to stand for 5 minutes; a reddish-brown colour is produced.

ULTRAVIOLET ABSORPTION. In dehydrated alcohol, maxima at 261 nm (E1%, 1cm = 640) and 310 nm.

Determination in body fluids; Metabolism. See under Fluphenazine Hydrochloride.

Actions and uses. Fluphenazine enanthate has actions and uses similar to those described under Fluphenazine Decanoate, but its action is less prolonged.

An initial dose of 12.5 milligrams of fluphenazine enanthate is given by deep intramuscular injection as described under Fluphenazine Decanoate. Subsequently, a dose of 25 milligrams may be expected to control psychotic symptoms for 10 to 28 days.

Children under 12 years and adults over 60 years may be given half of the adult dose.

1.1 milligrams of fluphenazine enanthate is approximately equivalent to 1 milligram of fluphenazine hydrochloride.

Undesirable effects; Contra-indications; Poisoning. As for Fluphenazine Hydrochloride.

Preparation

FLUPHENAZINE ENANTHATE INJECTION: a sterile solution of fluphenazine enanthate in sesame oil. It is sterilised by filtration. Available as an injection containing 25 mg of fluphenazine enanthate per ml in 1-ml ampoules and 10-ml vials.

A standard for this injection is given in the British Pharmacopoeia Addendum 1975

Containers: see the entry on Injections for general information on containers.

Labelling: see the entry on Injections for general information on labelling. In addition, the label on the container should state the name of the solvent and that the injection is for intramuscular injection only.

Storage: it should be protected from light.

Fluphenazine Hydrochloride

2-{4-[3-(2-Trifluoromethylphenothiazin-10-yl)propyl]-piperazin-1-yl}ethanol dihydrochloride

$C_{22}H_{28}Cl_2F_3N_3OS = 510.4$

OTHER NAMES: *Moditen®*
Motipress® and *Motival®* (both with nortriptyline hydrochloride)

A standard is given in the British Pharmacopoeia 1973

Description. An odourless white crystalline powder with a bitter taste.

Solubility. Soluble, at 20°, in 10 parts of water; very slightly soluble in alcohol and in ether.

Acidity. A 5% solution has a pH of 1.9 to 2.3.

Moisture content. Not more than 1%, determined by drying at 105°.

Dissociation constant. pK_a 8.1 (20°).

Storage. It should be stored in airtight containers, protected from light.

Identification. TEST. Dissolve about 5 mg in 2 ml of sulphuric acid and allow to stand for 5 minutes; an orange colour is produced.

ULTRAVIOLET ABSORPTION. In 0.1N hydrochloric acid, maxima at 257 nm (E1%, 1cm = 576) and 308 nm (E1%, 1cm = 68); in alcohol (95%), maxima at 262 nm (E1%, 1cm = 667) and 312 nm (E1%, 1cm = 72).

INFRA-RED ABSORPTION. Major peaks at 767, 1116, 1144, 1245, 1338, and 1422 cm⁻¹ (see Appendix 2a: Infra-red Spectra).

THIN-LAYER CHROMATOGRAPHY. See under Thin-layer Chromatography, System 9.

Determination in body fluids. SPECTROFLUORIMETRY. In serum—S. L. Tompsett, *Acta pharmac. tox.*, 1968, **26**, 298.

GAS CHROMATOGRAPHY. In urine: fluphenazine and its sulphoxide—M. I. Kelsey *et al.*, *J. Chromat.*, 1973, **75**, 294.

Metabolism. ABSORPTION. The hydrochloride is well absorbed after oral administration; the decanoate and enanthate are slowly absorbed from sites of injection.

BLOOD CONCENTRATION. During therapy with daily doses of 150 mg of the dihydrochloride, plasma concentrations of unchanged drug reach 100 to 250 ng/ml at 1 hour following the first morning dose; concentrations of the sulphoxide metabolite are of a similar order.

DISTRIBUTION. The base, enanthate, and the sulphoxide metabolite penetrate many tissues but only the base can cross the blood/brain barrier.

METABOLIC REACTIONS. Sulphoxidation and conjugation with glucuronic acid or sulphate.

EXCRETION. After an oral dose of the hydrochloride, 60% is excreted in the urine and 20% in the faeces in 7 days; after an intramuscular dose of the enanthate, 26% is excreted in the faeces and 14% in the urine in 14 days; after an intramuscular dose of the decanoate, 17% is excreted in the faeces and 6% in the urine in 30 days; after an oral dose, 0.3 to 0.6% is excreted in the urine unchanged in 24 hours and 0.3 to 0.7% is excreted as the sulphoxide in a similar period; 6 to 25% of an oral dose is excreted in the faeces in 24 hours mostly as unchanged drug; the major urinary metabolite in dogs appears to be 7-hydroxyfluphenazine in the free or conjugated form.

FURTHER INFORMATION. Distribution and metabolism —A. G. Ebert and S. M. Hess, *J. Pharmac. exp. Ther.*, 1965, **148**, 412; biological disposition and metabolic fate, excretion, and transformation—J. Dreyfuss *et al.*, *J. pharm. Sci.*, 1971, **60**, 821, 829; metabolic study—A. Viala *et al.*, *Annls pharm. Fr.*, 1969, **27**, 511.

Actions and uses. Fluphenazine hydrochloride is a tranquilliser with actions similar to those of Trifluoperazine Hydrochloride. It has anti-emetic properties, but little sedative and hypotensive action, and it produces less tachycardia than chlorpromazine.

It is used mainly in the treatment of schizophrenia and paranoid states and is also of value in severe anxiety disorders and for senile confusion.

For anxiety states fluphenazine hydrochloride is given in a dosage of 1 to 2 milligrams daily in single or divided doses and in the treatment of schizophrenia a dosage of up to 15 milligrams daily in divided doses may be given.

Undesirable effects. Extrapyramidal syndromes are particularly likely to occur. Dystonic reactions and akathisia are common and may not be recognised when they do not resemble classical parkinsonism; dyskinesias may become irreversible. Occasionally galactorrhoea, augmentation of epilepsy, epigastric pain, or jaundice may occur.

Contra-indications. It is contra-indicated in patients with renal, hepatic, or cardiac insufficiency, phaeochromocytoma, or sensitivity to phenothiazine derivatives.

Poisoning. Heat loss should be prevented and blood pressure maintained by changing posture. Drugs such as benzhexol may be required for any dystonic effects.

Preparations

FLUPHENAZINE TABLETS: available as tablets containing 1, 2.5, and 5 mg of fluphenazine hydrochloride; they are sugar coated and the coat may be coloured.

A standard for these tablets is given in the British Pharmacopoeia 1973

Containers and *Storage:* see the entry on Tablets for general information on containers and storage. Containers should be airtight.

Advice for patients: daily doses should preferably be taken in the morning. The tablets may cause drowsiness; persons affected should not drive or operate machinery. Alcohol should be avoided.

OTHER PREPARATIONS available include an ELIXIR containing fluphenazine hydrochloride 2.5 mg in 5 ml, diluent syrup, life of diluted elixir 1 month; TABLETS containing fluphenazine hydrochloride 500 micrograms with nortriptyline hydrochloride equivalent to 10 mg of nortriptyline, and tablets containing fluphenazine hydrochloride 1.5 mg with nortriptyline hydrochloride equivalent to 30 mg of nortriptyline.

Fluprostenol Sodium

Sodium (±)-7-{(1R,2R,3R,5S)-3,5-dihydroxy-2-[(3R)-3-hydroxy-4-(3-trifluoromethylphenoxy)but-1(E)-enyl]-cyclopent-1-yl}hept-5(Z)-enoate

$C_{23}H_{28}F_3NaO_6 = 480.5$

OTHER NAME: *Equimate*®

A standard is given in the British Pharmacopoeia (Veterinary)

CAUTION. *Fluprostenol sodium is extremely potent and extraordinary care should be taken in any procedure in which it is used.*

Description. A white amorphous hygroscopic powder.

Solubility. Soluble in water, in alcohol, and in methyl alcohol; practically insoluble in acetone.

Storage. It should be stored in airtight containers, protected from light.

Veterinary uses. Fluprostenol sodium is a luteolytic prostaglandin used in mares to control dates of oestrus and ovulation in planned breeding programmes. It is also used to correct certain forms of infertility.

The usual dose is the equivalent of 0.5 microgram of fluprostenol per kilogram body-weight by intramuscular injection as a single dose.

Preparation

FLUPROSTENOL INJECTION: a sterile solution of fluprostenol sodium in water for injections. It may contain suitable buffering agents. It is sterilised by heating in an autoclave or by filtration. Available in 5-ml disposable syringes containing fluprostenol sodium equivalent to 50 micrograms of fluprostenol per ml.

A standard for this injection is given in the British Pharmacopoeia (Veterinary)

Containers: see the entry on Injections for general information on containers.

Labelling: see the entry on Injections for general information on labelling. In addition, the label on the container should state the amount of the medicament as the equivalent amount of fluprostenol in a suitable dose-volume.

Storage: it should be protected from light.

Folic Acid

N-4-(2-Amino-4-hydroxypterid-6-ylmethylamino)ben-zoyl-L-glutamic acid

$C_{19}H_{19}N_7O_6 = 441.4$

OTHER NAMES: Pteroylglutamic Acid
Co-Ferol®, Ferrocap F-350®, Folex-350®, Galfer FA®, Norfer®, Pregaday®, and *Tifol®* (all with ferrous fum-arate); *Feravol-F®* (with ferrous gluconate); *Kelfolate®* (with ferrous glycine sulphate); *Fefol®, Ferrograd-Folic®, Folvron®, Pregfol®,* and *Slow-Fe Folic®* (all with dried ferrous sulphate)

A standard is given in the British Pharmacopoeia 1973

Folic acid is identical with the liver *Lactobacillus casei* factor, and is present, either free or combined with several L(+)-glutamic acid moieties in peptide linkages, in liver, yeast, and certain other natural products.

Description. An orange-yellow, microcrystalline, almost odourless, tasteless powder.

Solubility. Practically insoluble in cold water and in alcohol; soluble in 5000 parts of boiling water; soluble in dilute sodium hydroxide solution, yielding a clear orange-brown solution.

Moisture content. 5 to 8.5%, determined by drying at 100° *in vacuo.*

Specific rotation. About +20°, determined on a 0.5% solution in 0.1N sodium hydroxide.

Stability. Solutions in purified water adjusted to pH 8.0 may be kept for 6 weeks at room temperatures. Decomposition occurs more rapidly at higher temperatures or in the presence of thiamine, riboflavine, or heavy metal ions.

Incompatibility. It is incompatible with oxidising and reducing agents and heavy metal ions.

Sterilisation. Solutions of the sodium salt for injection are sterilised by filtration.

Storage. It should be stored in airtight containers, protected from light.

Identification. ULTRAVIOLET ABSORPTION. In 0.1N sodium hydroxide, maxima at 256 nm (E1%, 1cm = 550), 283 nm (E1%, 1cm = 550), and at 365 nm (E1%, 1cm = 185).

INFRA-RED ABSORPTION. Major peaks at 1191, 1335, 1480, 1602, 1636, and 1686 cm^{-1} (see Appendix 2a: Infra-red Spectra).

Metabolism. ABSORPTION. Rapidly absorbed after oral administration, mainly from the proximal part of the small intestine; absorption is greatly reduced in coeliac disease; anticonvulsants may inhibit the absorption of folate.

BLOOD CONCENTRATION. Physiological blood concentrations are about 350 ng/ml.

HALF-LIFE. Biological half-life, about 0.7 hours.

DISTRIBUTION. Widely and rapidly distributed throughout the body and large amounts are stored in the liver, mainly as methylated folate; normal body stores are of the order 5 to 10 mg, 50% of which is found in the liver; *protein binding,* about 66% bound to plasma proteins.

METABOLIC REACTIONS. Metabolised by reduction and methylation to 5-methyltetrahydrofolate and by oxidation to folinic acid.

EXCRETION. 20 to 90% of an ingested dose is excreted in the urine in 24 hours; the percentage of a dose excreted appears to be dose-dependent as after a 5-mg dose 50% is excreted in 24 hours and after a 15-mg dose about 90% is excreted in 24 hours; urinary excretion products include folinic acid; excretion is increased after the administration of methotrexate.

Actions and uses. Folic acid is present in many foods, partly as free folic acid but mainly in the conjugated form with several glutamic acid residues. The best sources are green leafy vegetables, meat, offal, and cereals.

Without folic acid, the living cell cannot divide but is halted in metaphase; this property underlies the use of folic acid antagonists in the treatment of neoplastic disease. Folic acid is necessary for the normal production of red blood cells, including maturation of megaloblasts into normoblasts.

Folic acid is absorbed mainly from the proximal part of the small intestine. It is enzymically reduced in the body to tetrahydrofolic acid, a coenzyme that is involved in purine and pyrimidine nucleotide synthesis and some amino-acid conversion. The human requirement is from about 50 micrograms daily in infancy to about 100 micro-grams daily in the adult, the actual amount being determined by metabolic and cell-turnover rates. The total body folic acid stores are 5 to 10 milligrams.

Symptoms of deficiency in man include megaloblastic haematopoiesis, glossitis, diarrhoea, loss of weight, and neurological manifestations. A deficiency may occur in pregnancy, in the malabsorption syndrome, after continuous administration of large doses of pyrimethamine and co-trimoxazole, and in epileptics on continuous anti-convulsive treatment. In this last condition the folic acid deficiency may lead to mental deterioration, which can be prevented by giving folic acid and vitamin B$_{12}$. Minor variations of folic acid metabolism may occur in patients with cardiac failure and rheumatoid arthritis. Folate deficiency may occur in women taking oral contraceptives.

Folic acid produces a haematopoietic response in pernicious anaemia (but see precautions and contra-indications), nutritional macrocytic anaemia, megaloblastic anaemia of infancy and pregnancy, pellagra, sprue, idiopathic steatorrhoea, coeliac disease, and following gastrectomy. Folic acid is administered for the treatment of megaloblastic anaemia due to these conditions, to the malabsorption syndrome, and to the continuous use of anticonvulsants, particularly primidone and phenytoin. It is of no value in the treatment of other forms of anaemia.

Folic acid may be given by mouth in an initial dosage of 10 to 20 milligrams daily for 14 days or until a haematopoietic response has been obtained; the daily maintenance dosage is 2.5 to 10 milligrams.

Children aged up to 1 year may be given a maintenance dose of 250 micrograms per kilogram body-weight daily, 1 to 5 years 2.5 milligrams daily, and 6 to 12 years 5 milligrams daily. An initial dosage of twice the maintenance dose may be given for 2 days. During pregnancy and lactation a daily intake of up to 800 micrograms may be required. Folic acid may also be administered by intramuscular injection as the sodium salt.

Precautions and contra-indications. Folic acid should never be given in the treatment of pernicious anaemia because it fails to prevent the onset of subacute combined degeneration of the cord; the therapy of choice in pernicious anaemia is hydroxocobalamin or cyanocobalamin.

Large and continuous doses of folic acid may lower the blood level of vitamin B_{12}.

Preparations

FOLIC ACID TABLETS: the usual strength is 5 mg of folic acid.

A standard for these tablets is given in the British Pharmacopoeia 1973

Containers and *Storage:* see the entry on Tablets for general information on containers and storage. Containers should be airtight and light resistant.

IRON AND FOLIC ACID TABLETS: they contain 308 mg of ferrous fumarate equivalent to 100 mg of iron and 350 micrograms of folic acid; they may be coated with sugar or other suitable material and the coat may be coloured.

Containers and *Storage:* see the entry on Tablets for general information on containers and storage. Containers should be airtight.

Advice for patients: the tablets should preferably be taken before meals; if there are gastro-intestinal disturbances doses may be taken after meals. Antacids should not be taken within 1 hour.

The tablets should not be taken for prolonged periods without medical advice. They may blacken the faeces.

OTHER PREPARATIONS available include CAPSULES containing folic acid 300 micrograms with ferrous fumarate 300 mg, capsules containing folic acid 350 micrograms with ferrous fumarate 308 mg, capsules containing folic acid 350 micrograms with ferrous fumarate 330 mg, capsules containing folic acid 500 micrograms with dried ferrous sulphate 150 mg in a slow-release formulation, capsules containing folic acid 500 micrograms with dried ferrous sulphate 270 mg; TABLETS containing folic acid 125 micrograms with ferrous fumarate 200 mg, tablets containing folic acid 150 micrograms with ferrous glycine sulphate 225 mg, tablets containing folic acid 200 micrograms with ferrous fumarate 120 mg, tablets containing folic acid 3 mg with ferrous gluconate 300 mg, tablets containing folic acid 5 mg with ferrous gluconate 300 mg, tablets containing folic acid 350 micrograms with dried ferrous sulphate 325 mg in a slow-release formulation, tablets containing folic acid 400 micrograms with dried ferrous sulphate 160 mg in a slow-release formulation, and tablets containing folic acid 1.7 mg with dried ferrous sulphate 194 mg.

Foot and Mouth Disease Vaccine

A liquid preparation containing one or more types or sub-types of foot and mouth disease virus which have been inactivated in such a manner that immunogenic activity is retained. An adjuvant is incorporated.

A standard is given in the British Pharmacopoeia (Veterinary)

Storage. The vaccine should be protected from light and stored at 2° to 8° when it may be expected to retain its potency for 12 months. Vaccines containing aluminium hydroxide should not be allowed to freeze.

Veterinary uses. The vaccine is administered by subcutaneous injection to cattle, sheep, and pigs for prophylaxis of foot and mouth disease. In many countries, it may be used only when authorised. The type of vaccine chosen is dependent on the strains of virus which are present in or expected to enter the country in which the vaccine is to be used.

Formaldehyde Solution

An aqueous solution containing about 36% w/w of formaldehyde, H.CHO, with methyl alcohol to delay polymerisation of the formaldehyde to solid paraformaldehyde, $(CH_2O)_n$.

OTHER NAMES: *Emoform®*; Formalin; *Veracur®*

NOTE: *the general use of the name "formalin" is limited, and in any country in which the word "formalin" is a trade mark it may be used only when applied to the product made by the owners of the trade mark.*

A standard is given in the British Pharmacopoeia 1973

Description. A colourless liquid with a characteristic irritating odour and a burning taste.

Solubility. Miscible with water and with alcohol.

Stability. A white deposit may form on storage; its formation occurs more rapidly if the solution is kept in a cold place.

Incompatibility. It is incompatible with ammonia, with gelatin, and with oxidising agents.

Storage. It should be stored in airtight containers in a moderately warm place.

Actions and uses. Formaldehyde solution is a powerful antiseptic, but is very irritant to mucous membranes. It reacts with and precipitates proteins, and when applied undiluted hardens the skin. It is used in antiseptic mouthwashes and gargles. It has been used mixed with thymol, cresol, glycerol, and zinc oxide as a mummifying agent for residual dental pulp tissue and with equal parts of cresol or creosote as a dressing for septic root canals. It is used to remove the specific toxicity of bacterial toxins in the preparation of toxoids.

For the disinfection of rooms, formaldehyde solution may be used as a spray, or the gas may be liberated by heat. When fumigation is effected by spraying, an equal volume of industrial methylated spirit must be added to the solution in order to prevent polymerisation in the droplets and on surfaces after deposition. When vaporisation is effected by heat, 500 millilitres of formaldehyde solution added to 1 litre of water is boiled in a stainless steel vessel over an electric hot-plate; this volume is sufficient for 1000 cubic feet (25 m³) of air space. Alternatively, 170 grams of potassium permanganate added to 500 millilitres of undiluted formaldehyde solution will cause violent boiling within ten seconds and the production of sufficient moist formaldehyde gas to disinfect the same cubic capacity. During fumigation, the room must be effectively sealed and maintained at a temperature above 18°; contact with the vapour must continue for more than 4 hours, and preferably overnight.

For the disinfection of bedding and similar objects, larger quantities of formaldehyde solution must be vaporised to allow for the absorption of formaldehyde by the materials. Formaldehyde solution does not damage metals or fabrics, but it should not be used for disinfection when other more reliable methods are possible.

Formaldehyde solution has also been used for the disinfection of membranes used in renal dialysis.

Diluted to 10 volumes with saline solution it is used as a preservative for pathological specimens; it is not suitable for preserving urine for subsequent examination.

Undesirable effects. The vapour of formaldehyde may cause lachrymation and, if inhaled, irritation of the respiratory tract.

Poisoning. Formaldehyde poisoning is characterised by severe abdominal pain, which may be followed by collapse and death; in less severe cases, acute nephritis with oliguria may result. Gastric lavage should be carried out or an emetic administered; diluted aromatic ammonia spirit may be given by mouth.

Preparations

FORMALDEHYDE LOTION:

Formaldehyde solution	30 ml
Water for preparations	to 1000 ml

It must be freshly prepared.

Containers: it should be dispensed in coloured fluted bottles; plastic containers are generally unsuitable for this preparation.

Labelling: the container should be labelled "For external use only".

Storage: it should be stored in a moderately warm place.

OTHER PREPARATIONS available include a GEL containing formaldehyde solution 1.5% v/v; and a (tooth) PASTE containing formaldehyde solution 1.3% v/v.

Fowl-pox Vaccine, Living

A freeze-dried preparation derived from cell cultures or eggs infected with pigeon-pox virus, modified fowl-pox virus, or modified turkey-pox virus. It is reconstituted immediately before use with an appropriate volume of a suitable sterile liquid.

A standard is given in the British Pharmacopoeia (Veterinary)

Storage. The dried vaccine should be protected from light and stored at 2° to 8° when it may be expected to retain its potency for 12 months. It should be used immediately after reconstitution.

Veterinary uses. It is administered to turkeys and chickens, either by piercing the non-vascular membranous triangle of skin above the elbow joint with a needle dipped in the vaccine or by application to the feather follicles for prophylaxis of fowl pox.

Framycetin Sulphate

The sulphate of 2-deoxy-4-O-(2,6-diamino-2,6-dideoxy-α-D-glucopyranosyl)-5-O-[3-O-(2,6-diamino-2,6-dideoxy-α-L-idopyranosyl)-β-D-ribofuranosyl]streptamine (neomycin B), an antimicrobial base produced by certain strains of *Streptomyces fradiae* or *Streptomyces decaris*.

$C_{23}H_{46}N_6O_{13},3H_2SO_4 = 908.9$

OTHER NAMES: *Framomycin®*; *Framygen®*; *Soframycin®* *Enterfram®* (with light kaolin); *Framycort®* (with hydrocortisone acetate)

A standard is given in the British Pharmacopoeia 1973

Description. A white or yellowish-white, odourless, tasteless, hygroscopic powder.

Solubility. Soluble, at 20°, in 1 part of water; practically insoluble in alcohol, in ether, and in chloroform.

Moisture content. Not more than 5%, determined by Fischer titration.

Acidity. A 1% solution has a pH of 6 to 7.

Specific rotation. +52° to +56.5°, determined on a 10% solution.

Storage. It should be stored in airtight containers, protected from light, at a temperature not exceeding 30°.

Metabolism. Very little is absorbed after oral administration and most of a dose is recovered unchanged from the faeces. It may accumulate in the body in renal function impairment.

Actions and uses. Framycetin sulphate is an aminoglycoside antibiotic with actions and uses similar to those of neomycin sulphate. It shares the same spectrum of activity and cross resistance with neomycin and some other members of the same group. It is too toxic for parenteral administration. It has been used for the prevention and treatment of infections of the skin, eyes, and large bowel, as described under Neomycin Sulphate. The dose for bacillary dysentery and gastro-enteritis for adults is 1 to 3 grams daily in divided doses at intervals of 6 hours. The dose for infants is 250 to 375 milligrams daily and for children 375 to 750 milligrams (approximately 30 to 60 milligrams per kilogram body-weight) daily in divided doses for 5 days. Treatment should not be continued for more than 8 days.

For bowel preparation, 1 gram is administered every 6 hours for 2 to 3 days before surgery. Alternatively, 750 milligrams may be given twice daily before and after surgery for a total period not exceeding 8 days.

Sterile solutions of framycetin sulphate have been used as instillations into body cavities such as the chest and bladder but some absorption may occur resulting in toxicity to the kidneys and eighth cranial nerve. The maximum daily dosage should not exceed 500 milligrams. In bladder irrigations up to 500 milligrams has been used daily in 100 to 150 millilitres of sterile water.

Precautions. As for Neomycin Sulphate.

Veterinary uses. Framycetin sulphate is an antibacterial used mainly in the control of enteritis due to *Escherichia coli.*

The usual dose by mouth for all species is 10 milligrams per kilogram body-weight daily but it should not be administered by mouth to adult ruminants. The usual dosage by intramuscular injection for all species is 10 milligrams per kilogram body-weight daily.

Preparations

FRAMYCETIN EAR-DROPS: a solution of framycetin sulphate in a suitable aqueous vehicle. Available as ear-drops containing 0.5% of framycetin sulphate.

Containers and *Labelling:* see the entry on Ear-drops for general information on containers and labelling.

Storage: it should be stored in a cool place; it should not be allowed to freeze.

Advice for patients: the prescribed course should be completed.

FRAMYCETIN EYE-DROPS: a sterile solution of framycetin sulphate in a suitable aqueous vehicle. Available as eye-drops containing 0.5% of framycetin sulphate.

Containers and *Labelling:* see the entry on Eye-drops for general information on containers and labelling.

Storage: it should be stored in a cool place; it should not be allowed to freeze.

Advice for patients: see the entry on Eye-drops for general information on the use of eye-drops. The prescribed course should be completed.

FRAMYCETIN EYE OINTMENT: prepared by incorporating framycetin sulphate in eye ointment basis or any other suitable basis by method B described in the entry on Eye Ointments. Available as an eye ointment containing 0.5% of framycetin sulphate.

Containers and *Labelling:* see the entry on Eye Ointments for general information on containers and labelling.

Storage: it should be stored in a cool place.

Advice for patients: see the entry on Eye Ointments for general information on the use of eye ointments. The prescribed course should be completed.

OTHER PREPARATIONS available include a CREAM containing framycetin sulphate 0.5%, a cream containing framycetin sulphate 1.5% with gramicidin 0.005%; EAR-DROPS containing framycetin sulphate 0.5% with hydro-cortisone acetate 0.5%; EYE-DROPS containing framycetin sulphate 0.5% with hydrocortisone acetate 0.5%; an EYE OINTMENT containing framycetin sulphate 0.5% with hydrocortisone acetate 0.5%; a MIXTURE containing framycetin sulphate 300 mg with light kaolin 6 g in 30 ml, diluent water, diluted mixture to be used immediately; an OINTMENT containing framycetin sulphate 0.5% with hydrocortisone acetate 0.5%, an ointment containing framycetin sulphate 1.5% with gramicidin 0.005%; and TABLETS containing framycetin sulphate 250 mg.

OTHER VETERINARY PREPARATIONS available include an INJECTION containing framycetin sulphate 50 mg per ml in 50-ml vials, an injection containing framycetin sulphate 100 mg per ml in 50-ml vials, an injection containing framycetin sulphate 150 mg per ml in 100-ml vials; an ORAL PASTE containing framycetin sulphate 100 mg per dose in 10-dose disposable syringe applicators; a soluble POWDER containing framycetin sulphate 250 mg per g; and a PREMIX containing framycetin sulphate 10%.

Fructosaemia

Fructosaemia (inherited fructose intolerance) is an autosomal inborn error of metabolism due to lack of fructose diphosphate aldolase B and consequent inability to metabolise fructose. Fructose or sucrose may give rise to vomiting, hypoglycaemia, failure to gain weight, anorexia, hepatomegaly, and later renal damage. Fructosaemia is treated by the exclusion of cane sugar, honey and fruit, particularly dried fruit, from the diet.

Sorbitol, which is a common ingredient of fruit squashes, should also be avoided as it is converted to fructose.

Frusemide

4-Chloro-N-furfuryl-5-sulphamoylanthranilic acid

$C_{12}H_{11}ClN_2O_5S = 330.7$

OTHER NAMES: *Dryptal®*; *Frusid®*; Furosemide; Furosemidum; *Lasix®*

Diumide® and *Lasikal®* (both with potassium chloride)

A standard is given in the European Pharmacopoeia Vol. III Supplement

Description. A white, crystalline, odourless, almost tasteless powder.

Solubility. Very slightly soluble in water and in chloroform; soluble, at 20°, in 75 parts of alcohol and in 850 parts of ether; soluble in solutions of alkali hydroxides.

Dissociation constant. pK_a 3.9.

Identification. TESTS. 1. Dissolve about 25 mg in 2.5 ml of alcohol (95%) and add 2 ml of *dimethylaminobenzaldehyde solution*; a green colour is produced which becomes deep red.

2. Dissolve about 12 mg in 5 ml of alcohol (95%) and add 10 ml of water. Mix 4 drops of this solution with 10 ml of *dilute hydrochloric acid*, heat under a reflux condenser

for 15 minutes, cool, add 18 ml of 1N sodium hydroxide and 1 ml of a 0.5% solution of sodium nitrite, and allow to stand for 3 minutes; add 2 ml of a 2.5% solution of sulphamic acid, mix, and add 1 ml of a 0.5% solution of N-(1-naphthyl)ethylenediamine dihydrochloride; a red-violet colour is produced.

MELTING-POINT. About 206°, with decomposition.

ULTRAVIOLET ABSORPTION. In 0.1N sodium hydroxide, maxima at 226 nm (E1%, 1cm = 1147), 273 nm (E1%, 1cm = 557), and 336 nm (E1%, 1cm = 133); in alcohol (95%), maxima at 228 nm (E1%, 1cm = 945), 276 nm (E1%, 1cm = 588), and 336 nm (E1%, 1cm = 144).

INFRA-RED ABSORPTION. Major peaks at 1143, 1241, 1323, 1561, 1590, and 1669 cm^{-1} (see Appendix 2a: Infra-red Spectra).

Determination in body fluids. SPECTROFLUORIMETRY. In serum or urine—A. W. Forrey et al., Clin. Chem., 1974, **20**, 152.

GAS CHROMATOGRAPHY. In plasma—B. Lindstroem and M. Molander, J. Chromat., 1974, **101**, 219.

HIGH PRESSURE LIQUID CHROMATOGRAPHY. In serum or urine—A. D. Blair et al., J. pharm. Sci., 1975, **64**, 1334.

Metabolism. ABSORPTION. Rapidly absorbed after oral administration; the rate of absorption is decreased by food.

BLOOD CONCENTRATION. After an oral dose of 80 mg to fasting subjects, peak plasma concentrations of about 22 μg/ml are attained in about 1 hour.

HALF-LIFE. Plasma half-life after intravenous administration, about 30 minutes; in subjects with advanced renal failure the plasma half-life is about 10 hours and in patients with renal failure and liver disease the half-life may be as long as 20 hours.

DISTRIBUTION. High concentrations are found in the liver and kidneys; volume of distribution, about 11.4% of body-weight which may be increased in patients with advanced renal failure to about 17.8% of body-weight; protein binding, about 95% bound to plasma proteins.

METABOLIC REACTIONS. Metabolised to a small extent by cleavage of the side chain and glucuronic acid conjugation; the main metabolite appears to be 4-chloro-5-sulphamoylanthranilic acid.

EXCRETION. After an oral dose, 20 to 55% is excreted in the urine in 24 hours and about 2% is excreted in the faeces; after intramuscular or intravenous administration, 70 to 90% is excreted in the urine; unchanged drug and 4-chloro-5-sulphamoylanthranilic acid are detectable in urine.

FURTHER INFORMATION. Protein binding—F. Andreasen and P. Jakobsen, Acta pharmac. tox., 1974, **35**, 49; absorption and excretion—B. Calesnick et al., Proc. Soc. exp. Biol. Med., 1966, **123**, 17; pharmacokinetics—R. E. Cutler et al., Clin. Pharmac. Ther., 1974, **15**, 588 and C. M. Huang et al., Clin. Pharmac. Ther., 1974, **16**, 659; binding to human albumin and plasma—J. Prandota and A. W. Pruitt, Clin. Pharmac. Ther., 1975, **17**, 159; distribution and urinary excretion in rats—S. Seno et al., J. pharm. Sci., 1969, **58**, 935.

Actions and uses. Frusemide is a loop diuretic which reduces the resorption of electrolytes by the proximal and distal renal tubules and by the loop of Henle. Excretion of sodium, potassium, and chloride ions is increased and as a consequence water excretion is enhanced. It has no effect on carbonic anhydrase in the renal tubular cells and urinary pH during the phase of diuresis may be

temporarily lowered; it does not appreciably alter the acid-base balance. Serum-uric-acid concentrations may be increased after administration of frusemide.

Frusemide is rapidly absorbed when given by mouth and provokes an intense diuresis lasting for 4 to 6 hours; this initial diuresis is greater than with equivalent dosage of the thiazide derivatives, although the total volume of fluid excreted over a period of 24 hours may not be greatly different.

Frusemide is used for the treatment of the same conditions as chlorothiazide. It may be effective when tolerance to thiazide diuretics has developed; its action is not enhanced by the thiazides.

It is usually given by mouth in a dosage of 40 milligrams once to 3 times a day. As its action is intense and of short duration it is usually possible to ensure that treatment does not disturb the patient's normal sleep. Once diuresis is adequately established, frusemide may be given every other day or on 3 successive days in a week. In refractory cases the doses may, in exceptional circumstances, be increased to 500 milligrams a day, but careful biochemical control is necessary.

Frusemide is also used in doses of up to 2 grams by injection or infusion for the prophylaxis of incipient and the treatment of established acute renal failure.

The usual dose of frusemide for children is 1 to 3 milligrams per kilogram body-weight daily by mouth or 0.5 to 1.5 milligrams per kilogram body-weight daily by injection.

Frusemide enhances the effect of hypotensive drugs and the dose of these may have to be adjusted to suit the needs of the patient when given concurrently for the control of mild or moderate hypertension. In cerebral oedema, it is given by intravenous injection and produces effects comparable with those following intravenous infusion of osmotically active substances.

Undesirable effects. Prolonged and regular administration may produce hypokalaemia. This intensifies the effect of digitalis on cardiac muscle and the dosage of cardiac glycosides may have to be adjusted or administration temporarily suspended. It may precipitate hepatic coma in patients with impaired liver function.

Precautions. As with chlorothiazide treatment, potassium depletion may occur when treatment with frusemide is prolonged; potassium supplements should be given.

Contra-indications. Frusemide is contra-indicated in acute nephritis, acute renal failure, and when the blood-potassium concentration is low; it should be used with caution in cirrhosis of the liver.

Drug interactions. Frusemide may increase the nephrotoxicity of cephaloridine given concurrently.

Veterinary uses. Frusemide is a diuretic which is used in animals in the treatment of pulmonary oedema. The usual dosage by mouth for horses and cattle is 0.5 to 1 milligram per kilogram body-weight daily and for dogs and cats 5 milligrams per kilogram body-weight daily. It is also administered in similar dosage by intramuscular or intravenous injection as the sodium salt. Potassium supplements may be given to reduce the risk of hypokalaemia.

Preparations

FRUSEMIDE INJECTION: a sterile solution of frusemide sodium, prepared by the interaction of frusemide with sodium hydroxide, in water for injections. It is sterilised by heating in an autoclave or by filtration. Available in 2-, 5-, and 25-ml ampoules containing frusemide sodium equivalent to 10 mg of frusemide per ml.

A standard for this injection is given in the British Pharmacopoeia Addendum 1975

Containers: see the entry on Injections for general information on containers.

Labelling: see the entry on Injections for general information on labelling. In addition, the label on the container should state the amount of the medicament as the equivalent amount of frusemide in a suitable dose-volume.

Storage: it should be protected from light.

FRUSEMIDE TABLETS: available as tablets containing 20, 40, and 500 mg of frusemide, and veterinary tablets containing 1 g of frusemide.

A standard for these tablets is given in the British Pharmacopoeia 1973

Containers and Storage: see the entry on Tablets for general information on containers and storage.

Advice for patients: daily doses should preferably be taken in the morning.

OTHER PREPARATIONS available include an ELIXIR containing frusemide 5 mg in 5 ml when reconstituted; an INJECTION containing the diethanolamine salt of frusemide equivalent to 50 mg of frusemide per ml in 10-ml bottles; TABLETS containing frusemide 20 mg with potassium chloride 750 mg (K⁺ 10 mmol) in a slow-release formulation, tablets containing frusemide 40 mg with potassium chloride 600 mg (K⁺ 8 mmol) in a slow-release formulation, tablets containing frusemide 40 mg, with tablets containing potassium chloride 750 mg (K⁺ 10 mmol) in a slow-release formulation, in a combination pack and tablets containing frusemide 40 mg with sachets containing potassium chloride 1.5 g (K⁺ 20 mmol) in effervescent granules, in a combination pack.

Furazolidone

3-(5-Nitrofurfurylideneamino)oxazolidin-2-one

$C_8H_7N_3O_5 = 225.2$

OTHER NAMES: Coryzium®; Furoxone®; Neftin® Furaphen® (with chloramphenicol); Bifuran® (with nitrofurazone)

A standard is given in the British Pharmacopoeia Addendum 1977 and in the British Pharmacopoeia (Veterinary)

Description. A yellow crystalline odourless powder.

Solubility. Very slightly soluble in water, in alcohol, and in chloroform; practically insoluble in ether.

Storage. It should be protected from light.

Identification. TEST. Dissolve about 1 mg in 1 ml of dimethylformamide and add 1 drop of 1N alcoholic potassium hydroxide; a deep blue colour is produced.

MELTING-POINT. About 259°, with decomposition.

INFRA-RED ABSORPTION. Major peaks at 741, 1020, 1099, 1235, 1250, and 1754 cm⁻¹ (see Appendix 2b: Infra-red Spectra).

Actions and uses. Furazolidone is a bactericide which is absorbed only slightly from the intestinal mucosa and has

therefore been used in the treatment of bacterial diarrhoea and gastro-enteritis. It is also active against Giardia lamblia.

It is rarely used in human medicine but the usual dosage is 100 milligrams 4 times a day for 2 to 5 days and for children 5 milligrams per kilogram body-weight daily in divided doses.

Undesirable effects. Mild toxic symptoms, including headache, nausea, and vomiting may occur; vesicular or morbilliform rashes occur with high dosage but usually subside on reduction of the dose. High doses of furazolidone may also cause haemolysis in genetic groups with glucose-6-phosphate-dehydrogenase deficiency, a condition which is prevalent among dark-skinned people. Flushing and dyspnoea may occur if alcohol is consumed.

Precautions and contra-indications. Furazolidone should not be given to infants under one month of age. Since furazolidone is a potential monoamine-oxidase inhibitor it should be used with caution in patients undergoing treatment with sympathomimetics and anti-depressants and foods with a high tyramine content should be avoided as described under Phenelzine Sulphate.

Veterinary uses. Furazolidone is used in animals as an antibacterial agent and for the prevention and treatment of histomoniasis.

The usual dose for the treatment of salmonella infections of large animals is 10 to 12 milligrams per kilogram body-weight for 5 to 7 days. For Escherichia coli and salmonella infections in weaned pigs the usual prophylactic dosage is 100 parts per million in the feed, and the usual therapeutic dosage is 300 parts per million in the feed for 7 days; these doses may be doubled in unweaned pigs.

For histomoniasis in poultry, the usual prophylactic dosage is 100 parts per million in the feed and the usual therapeutic dosage is 400 parts per million in the feed for 10 days.

Preparations

FURAZOLIDONE MIXTURE (Syn. Furazolidone Drench; Furazolidone Suspension): an aqueous suspension of furazolidone mixed with suitable suspending, dispersing, and preservative agents. Available as a mixture containing 5% of furazolidone and as a mixture containing 7.5% of furazolidone. This mixture should not be diluted.

A standard for this mixture is given in the British Pharmacopoeia (Veterinary)

Labelling: a direction should be given on the label to shake the bottle. In addition, the label on the container should state that the prescribed dosage should not be exceeded, that the preparation should not be administered to calves in process of being introduced to a high barley diet, that calves and piglets should not be slaughtered for human consumption within 7 days after cessation of treatment, and that the preparation should not be diluted.

Storage: it should be protected from light.

FURAZOLIDONE PREMIX: consisting of furazolidone mixed with a suitable inert diluent. This preparation is stable to suitable hot pelleting processes. It must be diluted before administration by mixing thoroughly with the feed. Available as a premix containing 4% of furazolidone and as a premix containing 20% of furazolidone.

A standard for this premix is given in the British Pharmacopoeia (Veterinary)

Containers and Storage: see the entry on Premixes for general information on containers and storage.

Labelling: the label on the container should state that pigs should not be slaughtered for human consumption within 7 days after cessation of treatment.

OTHER PREPARATIONS available include CAPSULES containing furazolidone 20 mg; TABLETS containing furazolidone 100 mg, tablets containing furazolidone 16 mg with nitrofurazone 110 mg, and tablets containing furazolidone 250 mg with chloramphenicol 500 mg.

Furunculosis

see BOILS

Fusidic Acid

ent - 16α - Acetoxy - 3β,11β - dihydroxy - 4β,8β,14α - trimethyl-18-nor-5β,10α-cholesta-(17Z)-17(20),24-dien-21-oic acid hemihydrate, an antimicrobial substance produced by the growth of certain strains of Fusidum coccineum (K. Tubaki).

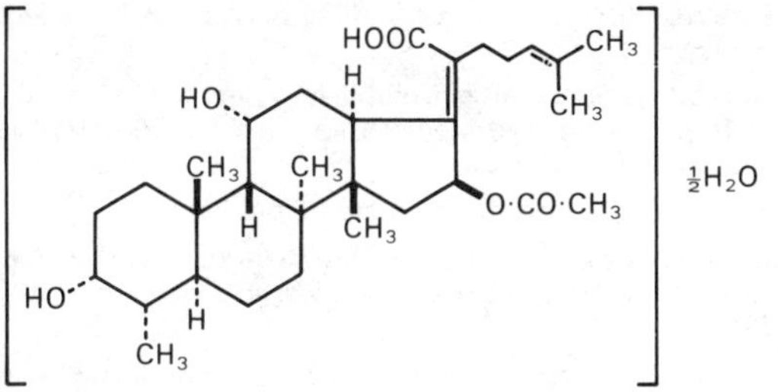

$C_{31}H_{48}O_6, \frac{1}{2}H_2O = 525.7$

OTHER NAME: Fucidin®

A standard is given in the British Pharmaceutical Codex 1973

Description. A white, crystalline, odourless powder.

Solubility. Practically insoluble in water; soluble, at 20°, in 5 parts of alcohol, in 60 parts of ether, and in 4 parts of chloroform.

Moisture content. 1.4 to 2%, determined by Fischer titration.

Specific rotation. −7° to −11°, determined on a 3% solution in chloroform.

Storage. It should be stored in airtight containers, protected from light.

Metabolism. See under Sodium Fusidate.

Actions and uses. Fusidic acid has the actions, uses, and undesirable effects described under Sodium Fusidate. It is used for the preparation of aqueous suspensions for oral administration.

The usual dose for an adult is 1 to 2 grams daily in divided doses; for a child under one year 125 milligrams, from 1 to 5 years 250 milligrams, and from 6 to 12 years 500 milligrams, 3 times daily.

Preparations

FUSIDIC ACID MIXTURE (Syn. Fusidic Acid Suspension): a suspension of fusidic acid in a suitable coloured flavoured aqueous vehicle. This mixture should not be diluted. The general direction given in the entry on Mixtures that the preparation should be diluted so that

the dose is contained in 5 ml does not apply to this mixture; it may be necessary for a dose of 2.5 ml to be measured by the patient in a 5-ml spoon; if a dose smaller than 2.5 ml is required, the dose should be measured by means of a graduated pipette.

Available as a mixture containing 250 mg of fusidic acid in 5 ml.

When Fusidate Mixture is prescribed, Fusidic Acid Mixture is supplied.

A standard for this mixture is given in the British Pharmaceutical Codex 1973

Containers and Labelling: see the entry on Mixtures for general information on containers and labelling.

Storage: it should be protected from light.

Advice for patients: the mixture should be taken at regular intervals, preferably after meals. The prescribed course should be completed.

OTHER PREPARATIONS available include a GEL containing fusidic acid 2% and a gel containing fusidic acid 2% with hydrocortisone acetate 1%.

Galactosaemia

Galactosaemia (inherited galactose intolerance) is an autosomal inborn error of metabolism due to absence of the enzyme galactose-1-phosphate uridyl transferase and consequent inability to metabolise galactose to glucose. Galactose-1-phosphate accumulates in the tissues and results in vomiting, jaundice, and hepatomegaly following milk foods. The weight gain is poor and there may be diarrhoea and increased tendency to bleed. If untreated it may result in cataracts and mental retardation. Galactosaemia may be treated by lactose-free milk substitutes, such as those prepared from soya bean, and the avoidance of lactose. In addition, the administration of progesterone is said to increase the metabolism of galactose, an example of enzyme induction.

Gallamine Triethiodide

2,2′,2″-(Benzene-1,2,3-triyltrioxy)tris(tetraethylammonium) tri-iodide

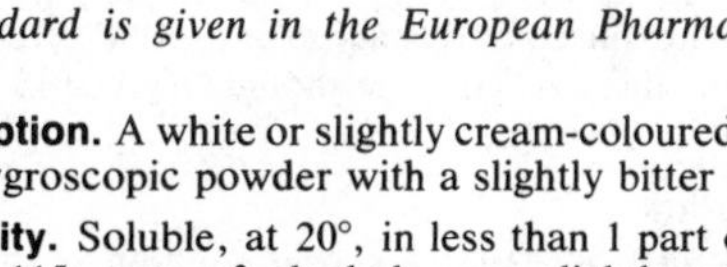

$C_{30}H_{60}I_3N_3O_3 = 891.5$

OTHER NAMES: Flaxedil®; Gallamini Triethiodidum

A standard is given in the European Pharmacopoeia Vol. II

Description. A white or slightly cream-coloured, odourless, hygroscopic powder with a slightly bitter taste.

Solubility. Soluble, at 20°, in less than 1 part of water and in 115 parts of alcohol; very slightly soluble in chloroform; practically insoluble in ether.

Moisture content. Not more than 3%, determined by drying at 105°.

Sterilisation. Solutions for injection are sterilised by heating in an autoclave or by filtration.

Storage. It should be stored in airtight containers, protected from light.

Identification. TESTS. 1. Mix about 500 mg with a few ml of sulphuric acid and heat; violet fumes are produced.

2. Dissolve about 50 mg in 5 ml of water and add 1 ml of *potassium mercuri-iodide solution*; a yellow precipitate is produced.

ULTRAVIOLET ABSORPTION. In 0.01N hydrochloric acid, maximum at 225 nm (E1%, 1cm = 525).

Actions and uses. Gallamine triethiodide has actions and uses similar to those described under Tubocurarine Chloride. It causes paralysis of voluntary muscle by blocking the transmission of impulses at the myoneural junction; this action can be counteracted by neostigmine. Gallamine also causes blockade of the cardiac vagus nerve and associated ganglia. The muscle-relaxant effect of 80 milligrams of gallamine triethiodide is approximately equivalent to that of 15 milligrams of tubocurarine chloride; muscular relaxation occurs in about 4 minutes after intravenous injection and the effect passes off in about 20 minutes.

Gallamine triethiodide is not broken down in the body but is largely eliminated unchanged in the urine within two hours of intravenous injection.

In conjunction with light anaesthesia, gallamine triethiodide is used to produce muscular relaxation during surgical procedures and operations and to reduce the risk of traumatic and other complications of electroconvulsive therapy. It is suitable for use with the usual anaesthetic agents, including nitrous oxide and oxygen, thiopentone sodium, ether, and cyclopropane.

Aqueous solutions of gallamine triethiodide are miscible with those of thiopentone sodium, and the two solutions may be injected simultaneously from the same syringe if desired.

For short operative procedures, 60 to 80 milligrams may be given by intravenous injection to an adult; subsequently, smaller doses, such as 40 milligrams, may be given if required, up to a total dose not exceeding 160 milligrams.

Undesirable effects. The most important undesirable effect is tachycardia, which may develop within one minute of intravenous injection and persist for longer than the relaxant effect of the drug.

Precautions and contra-indications. Gallamine triethiodide is contra-indicated in myasthenia gravis and should be used with care in patients with impaired renal function, hypertension, or cardiac insufficiency.

Poisoning. Assisted respiration with adequate oxygenation should be instituted. Facilities for this should always be available where muscle relaxants are used. Neostigmine methylsulphate should be given intravenously in doses of 2.5 to 5 milligrams; 0.5 to 1 milligram of atropine sulphate should be given at the same time and repeated if necessary. A similar procedure may be used to terminate muscular relaxation at the end of an operation, but in this case atropine should be given 15 minutes before neostigmine.

Preparation

GALLAMINE INJECTION: a sterile solution of gallamine triethiodide, with sodium sulphite equivalent to 0.2% of Na_2SO_3, in water for injections. It is sterilised by heating in an autoclave or by filtration. Available in 2- and 3-ml ampoules and in 10-ml vials containing 40 mg of gallamine triethiodide per ml.
A standard for this injection is given in the British Pharmacopoeia 1973

Containers and *Labelling:* see the entry on Injections for general information on containers and labelling.
Storage: it should be protected from light.

Gamma Benzene Hexachloride

1α,2α,3β,4α,5α,6β-Hexachlorocyclohexane

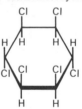

$C_6H_6Cl_6 = 290.8$

OTHER NAMES: Gamma-BHC; Lindane; *Lorexane®*; *Quellada®*
Asuntol® (with coumaphos); *Esoderm®* (with dicophane); *Canolene®* (with rotenone)

A standard is given in the British Pharmacopoeia 1973

Description. A white crystalline powder with a slight odour.

Solubility. Practically insoluble in water; soluble, at 20°, in 19 parts of dehydrated alcohol, in 5.5 parts of ether, and in 2 parts of acetone.

Storage. It should be protected from light.

Determination in body fluids. GAS CHROMATOGRAPHY. In blood—N. C. Jain *et al.*, *J. Pharm. Pharmac.*, 1965, 17, 362.

Actions and uses. Gamma benzene hexachloride is an acaricide, insecticide, and larvicide. It has a more rapid action than dicophane and is effective in lower concentrations, but as it is more volatile it has significantly less residual action.

Used as residual sprays, solutions in kerosene and other suitable solvents containing 0.1 to 0.5% are lethal to dipterous flies, including house flies. Gamma benzene hexachloride may be combined with other insecticides, such as a pyrethrum extract, to obtain a more rapid lethal effect.

A 0.2% alcoholic solution or a 0.1% application is effective against head lice and a 1% emulsion is employed in the treatment of scabies and pediculosis. The method of application is as described under Benzyl Benzoate. The development of resistant strains has been reported in species of insects which are normally susceptible.

Undesirable effects. Gamma benzene hexachloride is not especially toxic when applied externally in the concentrations usually employed, but when ingested it may cause convulsions and liver and kidney damage.

Poisoning. In cases of acute poisoning, after gastric lavage and the administration of a saline cathartic, diazepam should be administered to control convulsions. As there may be subsequent depression of the central nervous system after the convulsions, with respiratory failure and pulmonary oedema, sedation should be stopped should this occur and respiration assisted if necessary.

Veterinary uses. Gamma benzene hexachloride is an ingredient of preparations for the elimination of ticks and other ectoparasites on cattle, horses, sheep, and other animals.

Preparations

DICHLOFENTHION AND GAMMA BENZENE HEXA-
CHLORIDE DIP CONCENTRATE: a solution consisting of
dichlofenthion and gamma benzene hexachloride mixed
with suitable pharmaceutical adjuvants to produce an
emulsifiable concentrate. It may contain a suitable
preservative. Available as a dip concentrate containing
2.5% of dichlofenthion and 2% of gamma benzene
hexachloride. It must be diluted before use.
*A standard for this dip concentrate is given in the British
Pharmacopoeia (Veterinary)*
Replenishment of baths: see the entry on Dip Concentrates for general information on the replenishment of
baths.

GAMMA BENZENE HEXACHLORIDE APPLICATION:

Gamma benzene hexachloride	1 g
Emulsifying wax	40 g
Lavender oil	10 ml
Xylene, of commerce	150 ml
Water for preparations	to 1000 ml

Dissolve the gamma benzene hexachloride and the
lavender oil in the xylene and mix the solution with
the emulsifying wax, previously melted at a low temperature; pour the warm mixture into most of the water,
previously warmed to the same temperature, stir
thoroughly, add sufficient water to produce the required
volume, and mix.
*A standard for this application is given in the British
Pharmaceutical Codex 1973*
Containers and *Labelling:* see the entry on Applications
for general information on containers and labelling.
Advice for patients: a tablespoonful of the application
should be rubbed well into the hair and roots of the hair
and allowed to dry. The hair should not be washed for
the next 24 hours. Immediately after washing the hair it
should be finely combed to remove dead parasites. The
application does not kill parasites immediately; some
may persist for a few days.
It should not be applied to broken or inflamed skin;
contact with the eyes, ears, and lips should be avoided.

GAMMA BENZENE HEXACHLORIDE CREAM: a dispersion
of gamma benzene hexachloride in a suitable basis. It
may contain a suitable bactericide. It may be prepared
according to the following formula:

Gamma benzene hexachloride	a sufficient quantity
Liquid paraffin	80 g
Cetomacrogol emulsifying wax	140 g
Purified water, freshly boiled and cooled	to 1000 g

Dissolve the cetomacrogol emulsifying wax in the liquid
paraffin at a temperature of 60°; dissolve the gamma
benzene hexachloride in the mixture and gradually add
the warm mixture, with rapid stirring, to 750 ml of the
water at the same temperature; cool, add sufficient of the
water to produce the required weight, mix, and stir gently
until cold. Available as a cream containing 1% of gamma
benzene hexachloride.
*A standard for this cream is given in the British
Pharmacopoeia Addendum 1977*
Containers, Labelling, and *Storage:* see the entry on
Creams for general information on containers, labelling,
and storage.
Advice for patients: for the treatment of scabies, a hot
bath should be taken and the body thoroughly dried
before application. The cream should be applied over the

whole body and rubbed in but it should not be applied
to the head and face.
For the treatment of pediculosis, the affected area should
be thoroughly washed and dried prior to application. The
cream should be rubbed lightly on the affected and
adjacent areas and should not be washed off for the next
24 hours. It should not be applied to broken or inflamed
skin; contact with the eyes, ears, and lips should be
avoided.

GAMMA BENZENE HEXACHLORIDE DIP CONCENTRATE: a
solution consisting of gamma benzene hexachloride
mixed with suitable pharmaceutical adjuvants to produce
an emulsifiable concentrate. It may contain a suitable
preservative. Available as a dip concentrate containing
20% of gamma benzene hexachloride. It must be diluted
before use.
*A standard for this dip concentrate is given in the British
Pharmacopoeia (Veterinary)*
Replenishment of baths: see the entry on Dip Concentrates for general information on the replenishment of
baths.

GAMMA BENZENE HEXACHLORIDE DUSTING-POWDER: a
mixture of gamma benzene hexachloride with suitable
inert diluents. It may be perfumed. Available as a
dusting-powder containing 0.5, 0.6, and 0.625% of
gamma benzene hexachloride.
*A standard for this dusting-powder is given in the British
Pharmacopoeia (Veterinary)*
Containers, Labelling, and *Storage:* see the entry on
Dusting-powders for general information on containers,
labelling, and storage.

OTHER PREPARATIONS available include an APPLICATION
containing gamma benzene hexachloride 1% in a shampoo formulation, an application containing gamma
benzene hexachloride 2% in a shampoo formulation, a
veterinary application containing gamma benzene hexachloride 0.1% with rotenone 0.12%, an application containing gamma benzene hexachloride 1% with dicophane
1%; a DIP CONCENTRATE containing gamma benzene
hexachloride 6.4% with carbophenothion 16.8%, a dip
concentrate containing gamma benzene hexachloride
6.4% with chlorpyrifos 5%, a dip concentrate containing
gamma benzene hexachloride 30% with coumaphos
30%; a LOTION containing gamma benzene hexachloride
1%, and a lotion containing gamma benzene hexachloride 1% with dicophane.

Gangrene

Gangrene is the death of tissue, usually in considerable
mass, and usually followed by bacterial invasion and
putrefaction. It is usually associated with loss of blood
supply to the tissue, for example, gangrene of a limb may
be due to arteriosclerosis. It may be due to bacterial
infection, as in gas-gangrene, and also as a complication
of diabetes where it is accompanied by neuropathy and
vascular problems. Drug-induced gangrene is a frequent
complication of Raynaud's disease.

Gas-gangrene is due to the infection of a wound with
anaerobic bacteria of the genus *Clostridium*, usually
Cl. perfringens (*Cl. welchii*). Clostridial infection is
most often seen when wounds are infected with soil.
Gas-gangrene is liable to develop in deep, heavily contaminated wounds involving muscle with retained
foreign bodies or necrotic tissue, especially when
ischaemia is also present. In hospital, gas-gangrene may
follow operation on ischaemic limbs, operation around

the hip joint, or abdominal surgery. When the clostridia start to grow they produce toxins which seep into the surrounding tissues where they produce tissue necrosis. The wound becomes increasingly painful and peripheral circulatory failure is liable to occur.

Prevention of gas-gangrene. The adequate care of wounds likely to be contaminated, the use of penicillin in above-knee amputations, and the avoidance of measures liable to produce ischaemia should prevent the occurrence of gas-gangrene. Before operations on potentially infected sites, for example, ischaemic limbs, or in the hip region, it is desirable to use a sporicidal agent such as povidone-iodine for skin disinfection and to administer benzylpenicillin as a prophylactic.

Treatment of gas-gangrene. Gas-gangrene is treated by antibiotics, incision, and drainage, or amputation of the affected area. Benzylpenicillin is usually employed as the first choice antibiotic. Hyperbaric oxygen may be of value if a suitable chamber is available.

Gas-gangrene antitoxins. For the use of gas-gangrene antitoxins in the prevention and treatment of gas-gangrene see under Gas-gangrene Antitoxins.

Gargles

A gargle is an aqueous solution, usually in concentrated form, intended for use, after dilution, as a prophylactic or in the treatment of an infection of the throat. A quantity of the liquid is taken and suspended in the throat by slowly exhaling through it. The liquid is then rejected, unless the patient has been directed to swallow the liquid after gargling.

The particular method of using a gargle is intended to bring it into intimate contact with the membranous lining of the throat. It is not intended to act as a protective covering to the membrane and therefore oily substances requiring suspending agents and drugs of a mucilaginous nature should not be used.

Containers. Gargles should be dispensed in fluted bottles and labelled in a manner which clearly distinguishes them from preparations intended for internal administration, except when directed to be swallowed after gargling, in which case they should be dispensed in bottles similar to those used for mixtures; if the gargle needs protection from light, the bottle should be coloured.

Labelling. Directions for diluting the gargle should be given on the label.

Gas Chromatography

Gas chromatography is a chromatographic method of separating mixtures of substances in which the mobile phase is a gas and the stationary phase is either a solid or a liquid, the processes being known, respectively, as gas-solid and gas-liquid chromatography. Gas-liquid chromatography has a much wider application than gas-solid chromatography, and the generic term 'gas chromatography' usually refers to the gas-liquid system.

In the conventional gas-liquid system, the liquid phase is held stationary on an inactive solid support packed in a column. A stream of carrier gas is passed through the heated column, and when a sample is injected into the column it is vaporised and, as it moves along the column with the carrier gas, chromatographic separation is achieved. The separated components, as they emerge, are passed through a detector which is connected to a suitable amplifying and recording device.

Commercially available gas chromatographs vary in design, but their essential features are: a control system for the carrier gas, an injection system for the sample, the chromatographic column, an oven for controlling the temperature of the column, a detector, an amplifier and electronic control for the detector, and a potentiometric recorder for making a permanent record of some characteristic of the separated components.

Carrier-gas Control

Control of the flow of the gas through the column is necessary because the rate of flow affects the efficiency of the column (see below under Gas Chromatographic Process). There are two methods of control which are normally used. A pressure regulator may be used, but control of flow by controlling the pressure relies on there being a constant pressure drop across the column. This pressure drop can vary, due to variations in the temperature of the column or variations in the viscosity of the gas at column temperatures. However, if there is a minor leakage of gas between the regulator and the column, which is most likely to occur at the injection port, the flow in the column will not be affected.

Alternatively, a mass-flow control can be used. This maintains a constant flow of gas irrespective of the pressure drop across the column. However, care must be taken to avoid leakage in the system.

Most commercial gas chromatographs are equipped with a mass-flow control, but some have optional pressure control as well. The gas flow should be set according to the manufacturer's instructions, but the optimum flow rate is readily determined by experiment (see below under Gas Chromatographic Process).

Injection System

Injection of the sample is usually made by means of a syringe and needle through a silicone-rubber septum. The sample may be injected either directly into the column or into a heated zone in the gas stream before it enters the column. The latter method is known as flash injection and the temperature of the heated zone is separately controlled.

Some commercial gas chromatographs only allow flash injection, some only allow on-column injection, and some have "straight-through" injection chambers which can be used in either mode by choosing the correct length of needle. Some injectors may also include a removable liner which is used for trapping any non-volatile residue from the sample.

The injection septum is usually of silicone rubber and should be renewed at regular intervals to avoid leakage of carrier gas. For optimum performance the septum should be carefully chosen to produce a tight fit, and thus be held in radial compression, since the axial compression required to seal the injection port induces a radial tension which, if not compensated for, will give rise to gas leakage.

INJECTION TECHNIQUE. This is particularly important because poor technique is by far the greatest single cause of inaccuracy and lack of reproducibility. Practice is required in order to achieve good results and the following points should be noted:

1. The syringe and its needle must not contain any air or vapour bubble.

2. A worn syringe will allow gas pressure to force the sample between the plunger and the barrel before it can be injected. A loose-fitting needle will have the same effect.

3. The needle may become blocked with a "slug" of the

septum material. Special needles for gas chromatography are available.

4. Any material that remains in the needle after injection of the sample will be evaporated by the heat and fractionation of the components will result. This problem occurs even in syringes having a plunger inside the needle. The effect may be reduced by withdrawing the needle immediately after injection and also, where applicable, by using a high boiling-point solvent.

5. There is also the possibility that a droplet of the sample may be retained on the end of the needle after injection and, unless it is removed either by evaporation or mechanically before the needle is withdrawn, it will be coated on the inner surface of the septum and give badly tailing peaks. This effect can be minimised by inserting a loose plug of glass wool, which serves to wipe the needle, inside the injection port.

All these difficulties may be reduced by injecting "on-column", but this may create other problems if the injection site is for some reason cooler than the rest of the column. This may occur in some designs of instrument where the column passes through the insulation of the oven. A suitable length of needle is essential.

6. Repeated injections of solvent "on-column" will wash off the stationary phase and this gives tailing peaks.

7. Injection of samples in a solvent gives a large volume of vapour and, if the expansion of this is greater than the carrier flow, it will diffuse back in the injector and give an excessively wide solvent peak which may mask sample peaks in the early part of the chromatogram. This problem may be reduced by injecting at a controlled rate. If flash injection is used, the temperature of the heated zone should be set about 50° higher than the column temperature, or at the maximum temperature reached during programmed temperature operation (*see* below under Temperature Control of the Column). The temperature of the injection chamber should not be set higher than the upper temperature limit of the stationary phase being used. If thermal degradation in the injection chamber is suspected then the temperature must be lowered or the "on-column" technique adopted.

The Column

The conventional column consists of a tube packed with the solid support upon which is held the stationary phase. The tube is usually either stainless steel or glass and most instruments allow interchangeability of both types. Glass is preferred because of its inert nature but it has the disadvantage of being easily broken. Also, it is difficult to pack a long precoiled length of glass and to seal it to the injection system. However, packing is made easier by the use of large radius coils, and polymers which resist high temperatures can be used to produce a reliable junction between the glass and the injector. Stainless steel columns may cause decomposition of certain compounds.

SOLID SUPPORT. The solid support for the stationary phase is usually a diatomaceous earth which has been calcined, crushed, and graded with reference to the particle size. The support material should have a narrow range of particle size, usually 180 to 150 μm or 150 to 125 μm. The support material should be inert and, in order to reduce active adsorption sites, it should be silanised, a process which involves treatment with a solution of dimethylchlorosilane or hexamethyldisilazane, substances which react with hydroxyl groups on the surface of the particles.

STATIONARY PHASE. The stationary phase should be chosen to be compatible with the sample being analysed.

The choice is usually based on the maxim that "like dissolves like", and polar stationary phases are chosen to separate polar compounds, whilst non-polar stationary phases are usually chosen to separate non-polar or high-boiling compounds. If the qualitative composition of the sample is known, then an appropriate stationary phase may be chosen by reference to published tables of retention indices (see below under Qualitative Determinations).

A very wide range of stationary phases is available. The most commonly used are *Carbowax 20M* and *Apiezon L*, *OV1*, *OV17*, and *SE30*, all of which have very good temperature stability and are obtainable in consistent quality, an important factor when similar analyses may be done with different batches of the stationary phase. *Carbowax 20M* has the wider application since it is of intermediate polarity and is compatible with almost all types of sample. It has a lower temperature limit than the other stationary phases but it is usually considered as the first choice and alternatives are only used if it fails to give a particular resolution or if the analyst requires a higher temperature than its upper limit.

A range of silicone polymers also have a wide use as stationary phases. In particular, the OV range has a very high temperature stability and is consistent in quality and purity. The range includes, in order of increasing polarity, methyl silicones, phenyl silicones, fluoropropyl silicones, and cyano silicones.

A further range of stationary phases is the polyester group, but these must be chosen carefully as they may vary from batch to batch and have a lower temperature stability than the other types. Succinate polyesters are suitable for the separation of methyl esters and, for best results, the "pre-tested, catalyst-free" variety should be used.

In addition to upper temperature limits, stationary phases also have lower temperature limits, since they will not operate if they become solid.

Lists of stationary phases giving their applications and upper temperature limits are provided by most laboratory suppliers.

PREPARATION OF THE COLUMN PACKING. The loading of the stationary phase on the solid support must be high enough to cope with the amount of sample to be separated and low enough to maintain only a thin film on the support. The loading may vary from about 1% to 15% according to requirements. Although there is an optimum loading to give the best resolving power, other factors are often more important. Low loadings give shorter retention times and allow the use of lower temperatures. However, low-loaded columns are more readily overloaded with the sample, and the solid support has to be particularly inactive to avoid tailing of the peaks. Stationary phase tends to be lost from the column during use and packings with high loadings of stationary phase are less likely to show the early effects due to this loss.

Two methods may be used for coating the solid support with the stationary phase. The first is the solution-coating method in which the support is percolated by a solution of the stationary phase in a volatile solvent. The excess solution is allowed to drain off and the wet packing is allowed to dry in air. The method is based on the fact that the solid support will absorb a fixed proportion of the stationary phase solution. For instance, *Chromosorb W* or its equivalent will yield about 3.8% loading from a 2% solution of stationary phase. Other types of support will give different values. In the second method, a calculated amount of stationary phase is dissolved in an excess of volatile solvent and the appropriate amount of the support is added. The slurry is agitated to remove air bubbles and evaporated to dryness with gentle heat under reduced pressure.

In both methods the support must be handled with care to avoid breaking the fragile particles.

PACKING THE COLUMN. The coated support must be packed into the tube in such a way that it is uniformly filled without either leaving "dead spaces" or creating "fines" by crushing the particles. Straight or precoiled columns must be plugged at one end before packing. In the case of precoiled columns a vacuum is applied at the plugged end. In all cases the prepared packing is added a little at a time through a funnel attached to the open end of the column. The column is then tapped lightly working from the top to the bottom to consolidate the packing before the next amount is added. This is continued until the column is filled. The tapping must not be so severe that the particles of material are broken or crushed, and final plugging of the column must not compress the packing or be so tight as to form a resistance to the carrier gas flow.

Temperature Control of the Column

The column is situated inside an oven and this is nearly always of the high velocity air bath type. Temperature control is often better than $\pm 0.5°$, although the resettability may be as low as $\pm 2.5°$. Before beginning an analysis, sufficient time must be allowed for the column temperature to come to equilibrium with the oven temperature.

ISOTHERMAL OPERATION. If a constant temperature is used during an analysis, this is known as isothermal operation and is usually used for quantitative analysis. Increasing the temperature decreases the elution time of a compound; for example, a 30° increase in temperature decreases the elution time by about one half. The elution time should not be reduced to less than 4 times the elution time for an air peak.

The temperature should be adjusted to give an optimum resolution for the compound of interest. A general guide to the appropriate temperature may be obtained by carrying out a temperature-programmed run on the sample.

PROGRAMMED TEMPERATURE OPERATION. Most instruments have the capability of increasing the oven temperature at a predetermined rate during the analysis and this is known as programmed temperature operation. The column temperature is slowly raised, at a controlled rate, until it reaches a predetermined maximum which will be limited by the characteristics of the particular stationary phase being used. In order to determine the best temperature for the analysis of a sample in a particular column under isothermal operation, the sample may be run in a temperature-programmed system and the elution temperature of the compound observed. The best isothermal temperature for its analysis is then given by the relationship:

$$\text{Isothermal temperature} = \frac{t_2° - t_1°}{2} + t_1°$$

where, $t_1° = $ starting temperature and $t_2° = $ elution temperature.

In order to obtain reproducible results from programmed temperature operation, it is important that the column is given plenty of time to restabilise at the lower temperature before starting the next analysis.

See under Qualitative Analysis, below, for further uses of programmed temperature operation.

The Detector

The three main types of detector in common use are the flame ionisation detector (F.I.D.), the thermal conductivity detector (katharometer), and the electron capture detector (E.C.D.).

The flame ionisation detector is very sensitive, has a wide linear range, and is usually specified for use in standard methods. It requires an auxiliary supply of pure hydrogen and of air, and the flows of these gases require careful adjustment to give the optimum response.

The thermal conductivity detector is responsive to all types of compound and is non-destructive, but it is less sensitive than the flame ionisation detector.

The electron capture detector is the most sensitive detector available, but it is only responsive to certain classes of compounds such as those containing two or more electron-capturing groups. This applies particularly to polyhalogenated compounds and this detector is widely used for the determination of pesticide residues at very low levels. Some types of electron capture detector require a special carrier gas mixture, or a separate "purge" gas. All have a β-emitting radioactive source and must be treated with caution.

The performance of these detectors, and the methods used with them, vary widely, and the manufacturer's manual should be studied carefully before use.

DETECTOR TEMPERATURE. Some instruments do not have a separate control of the detector temperature but position the detector so that it is heated by the oven. For those instruments which do have a separate control, the temperature should be adjusted so that the separated components do not condense in the detector and so give rise to tailing peaks. Electron capture detectors have defined upper temperature limits, and they always have their own separate heater control with a built-in thermal trip.

Amplifier and Recorder

The electrical output from the detector is very small and an electronic amplifier must be used. The amplifier can be adjusted to vary the apparent sensitivity. The signal from the detector is amplified and fed to a high-speed potentiometric recorder. The passage of a component into the detector results in the recorder pen rising and falling in a manner corresponding to the concentration of the component arriving at the detector. This part of the recorder trace is known as a peak and, ideally, will be Gaussian in shape. Under ideal conditions the area of this peak will be proportional to the amount of the component.

The Gas Chromatographic Process

All chromatographic processes rely on differential partitions between two phases of the components being separated. The separation procedure may be conveniently considered as a sequential series of equilibria followed by dynamic changes of conditions and the re-establishment of new equilibria.

PARTITION. If a small sample of volatile material is introduced into the static system, partition of the sample will be established between the gas and liquid phases. If the portion of the gas phase containing the equilibrium concentration of sample is then moved into contact with a fresh portion of the liquid phase, a new equilibrium will be established at that point. However, the movement of this portion of the gas phase will allow fresh gas to come into contact with the portion of the liquid phase containing its original equilibrium concentration of the sample. This creates conditions for the establishment of another equilibrium in the rear of the advancing sample. Thus, if the flow of gas is continuous it will create conditions in which the sample is progressively moved through the column. In so doing, it is spread through a continuously increasing length of the liquid/gas phase. This spreading takes the form of a Gaussian distribution and is an inherent feature of the chromatographic process.

Under the dynamic conditions of practical gas chromatography the establishment of ideal partitions never occurs due to the finite time which is available. This results in a spreading of the sample band beyond that of the theoretical Gaussian distribution. Furthermore, the sample will diffuse in the gas phase and contribute further to the band spreading.

EFFICIENCY OF THE COLUMN. The ability of the column to pass a band of sample with the minimum deviation from the theoretical Gaussian distribution is a measure of its efficiency. This may be calculated, in terms of the number of theoretical "plates", from the formula:

$$N = 16 \left[\frac{tR}{W} \right]^2$$

where N = number of plates, tR = retention distance (distance between the point of injection and the maximum intensity of the peak), and W = the width of the base of the peak. Each theoretical plate corresponds to one theoretical stage of the equilibrium process described above.

Because gas chromatography is a compromise between the necessity for moving a sample through a column and at the same time attempting to achieve an ideal partition, it follows that conditions should be such that the time taken to establish partition is reduced to a minimum. This may be achieved by using a thin film of stationary phase with a low viscosity, operating at elevated temperatures, and controlling the gas flow at an optimum value. However, these factors are also subject to conditions of compromise.

Effect of stationary phase. The use of a thin film of stationary phase results in a reduction of the total amount of liquid phase in the system and this reduces the amount of sample which can be accepted without overloading the column.

Effect of temperature. Operation at elevated temperatures increases the rate of diffusion of the sample, particularly in the gas phase, and this increases the rate of band spreading and hence reduces the efficiency.

Effect of gas flow. When the carrier gas flow is high, the comparative rate of diffusion of the sample in the gas is low but partition equilibrium is not achieved. Conversely, when the carrier gas flow is low, partition equilibrium is nearly achieved but the comparative rate of diffusion in the gas is high. There is, therefore, an optimum gas flow rate. This optimum may be determined experimentally by plotting the column efficiencies against a series of gas flow rates. A characteristic curve is obtained which shows the optimum value for the gas flow.

If the gas flow rate is measured as a function of its average linear velocity over the stationary phase, then the optimum value will be independent of the column dimensions. However, as the gas flow rate is usually measured as a bulk property, then it must be related to the column dimensions and the packing density of the stationary phase on its support.

RESOLUTION. So far, consideration has only been given to the behaviour of a single component in the system, but it can be seen that a pair of compounds with different partition coefficients between the chosen phases may be separated under dynamic conditions, provided that their partition coefficients are sufficiently different and that the column has a sufficient number of theoretical plates. The degree of resolution obtained between a pair of compounds may be calculated from measurements taken from the chromatogram. The resolution may be expressed in two ways as illustrated in FIGS. 1 and 2.

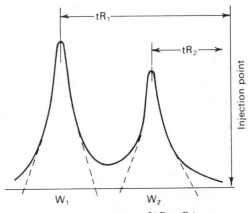

FIG. 1: Resolution $= \dfrac{2(tR_2 - tR_1)}{W_1 + W_2}$

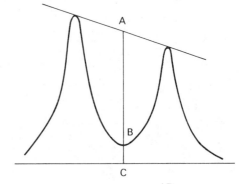

FIG. 2: Resolution $= \dfrac{AB}{AC}$

The method illustrated in Fig. 1 involves measurement of the width of the base of the peak by means of extrapolation of tangents to the baseline. This process becomes more difficult as the resolution decreases. In addition, the assumption is made that all compounds will be passed through a particular column with equal efficiencies, and this does not happen in practice.

The resolution between a pair of compounds may be increased by (a) increasing the length of the column, (b) improving the efficiency of the column, and (c) changing to a stationary phase which shows greater differences in the partition coefficients for the compounds.

OVERLOADING. Most determinations use a dilution of the sample in a suitable solvent. The degree of dilution and the amount of sample injected must be such that the column is not overloaded, which will usually occur before the detector is overloaded. In extreme cases, overloading will be apparent by the non-Gaussian shape of the peak which will rise slowly to the top of the peak and then drop sharply back to the baseline. The top of the peak may be either sharp or curved according to the degree of overloading. However, column overloading with consequent loss of linearity occurs well before it becomes apparent from the peak shape, and it can only be detected by determining the linearity of the response against the amount of sample added.

Qualitative Determinations

Simple mixtures may usually be examined under conditions of *isothermal operation*, and suitable conditions may often be found in the literature, if something is known about the nature of the sample. If the sample is completely unknown or known to be complex, then *programmed temperature operation* will give more useful results.

The best separation of any particular pair of compounds is only achieved by operating under closely controlled, optimised conditions. If a sample contains a range of different compounds then the optimum conditions for separating one pair of compounds may not allow separation of a second pair. However, this second pair may be separated by changing the conditions, and progressive alteration of the column temperature produces progressive alteration in the partition conditions. In this way, a range of compounds with widely differing vapour pressures may be separated.

The initial temperature should be as low as practicable (e.g. 65° for *Carbowax 20M* and 50° for *Apiezon L*), and this temperature should be held for 10 minutes after injection of the sample. The programming of the temperature should then be started at about 3° per minute up to the upper temperature limit for the stationary phase (e.g. 225° for *Carbowax 20M* and 250° for *Apiezon L*). These conditions will give the best practical resolution, but subsequent analyses may be speeded up if the initial chromatogram shows a greater resolution than necessary.

The identity of peaks may be indicated by comparison with retention times of known samples, or by the Kovats retention index system.

RETENTION INDICES. Under the conditions of a linear temperature programme, a homologous series of compounds will be eluted in a regular manner with a constant difference of elution time between each successive pair. The retention time is the difference between injection time and the time at which the intensity reaches a maximum for the peak. When isothermal conditions are used the differences between each successive pair increase logarithmically.

These retention characteristics of a homologous series form the basis of the Kovats system of retention indices. In this system the "retention index" of any particular compound is related to the retention index of the immediately preceding aliphatic hydrocarbon. Thus n-octane has a retention index of 800 and n-nonane 900. Under conditions of linear temperature programming the interval between two hydrocarbons may be divided in a linear fashion and the retention index of any compound in between may be defined.

The determination of retention indices requires the measurement of the retention volume V. This is the volume of carrier gas required, from the injection point to the point of maximum response. It may be calculated by multiplying the retention time by the average flow rate, the latter being corrected for the temperature and pressure of the column.

The Kovats retention index of a compound with a retention volume V, eluting between alkanes containing Z and Z+1 carbon atoms, is given by the formula:

$$\text{Retention index} = 100Z + \frac{\log V - \log V_Z}{\log V_{Z+1} - \log V_Z}$$

where V_Z and V_{Z+1} are the retention volumes of the alkanes Z and Z+1 under isothermal conditions. For temperature programmed operation the formula approximates to:

$$\text{Retention index} = 100[Z + (V - V_Z) \div (V_{Z+1} - V_Z)]$$

The advantage to be gained from programmed temperature operation is that a multicomponent mixture may be separated and the complex chromatogram produced may be used as a "fingerprint" for the mixture. This is particularly valuable in the case of essential oils. However, the method is rarely used for quantitative determination of a particular component of a mixture. For such an analysis it is usual to adopt an optimum isothermal temperature.

Quantitative Determinations

Many published methods do not give rigid specifications for some of the operating conditions such as the stationary phase loading, the method of injection, and the column diameter and associated gas flow, if it has been found that a reasonable variation in the details will still give acceptable results. However, published methods usually recommend the method of peak measurement, and this should be followed if comparable results are to be obtained. The method may be by measurement of peak height or by measurement of peak area, which is defined as the product of the peak height and the width of the peak at half peak height.

The recommended conditions for a quantitative method must fall within the linear range of the apparatus being used. It should also be shown that the component being measured is free from interfering compounds, and all proposed methods must include this evaluation before they can be accepted as reliable. Variation in results can usually be traced to faulty injection technique.

The three main methods of quantitative determination are by the use of an internal standard, by standard additions, and by peak normalisation.

INTERNAL STANDARD. In order to avoid the difficulty caused by non-reproducibility of injected volumes, the response of the substance to be measured is compared with the response of an added suitable compound known as the internal standard. The compound selected as the internal standard must not elute at the same time as any component of the mixture being examined. The method requires the calculation of a response factor for the substance being measured against the internal standard, and this factor is independent of the volume injected. A mixture containing known concentrations of the substance and the internal standard is chromatographed and the response of each component is determined.

$$\frac{\text{Response of substance}}{\text{Response of standard}} \times \frac{\text{Weight of standard}}{\text{Weight of substance}}$$

The unknown sample is then mixed with a known weight of the internal standard, the mixture is chromatographed, and the response of each substance again measured. The percentage of the substance in the sample is then given by the expression:

$$\frac{100}{f} \times \frac{\text{Response of substance}}{\text{Response of standard}} \times \frac{\text{Weight of standard}}{\text{Weight of sample}}$$

The method assumes that a linear relationship exists between the sample content and the response. This may not always be so and in such cases a calibration curve should be prepared and used for the actual determination.

STANDARD ADDITIONS. In this method, the substance to be determined in the sample is measured against another sample containing a known amount of the same added substance.

PEAK NORMALISATION. In this method, the peak height or the peak area due to the substance to be measured is compared to the sum total of the same parameter for all peaks. The method assumes that all the separated compounds have the same response factor and that the entire sample is volatile. The method is only used in certain specified cases.

Gas-gangrene

see under GANGRENE

Gas-gangrene Antitoxins

Preparations from native sera containing the antitoxic globulins that have the specific power of neutralising the alpha toxins formed by the respective clostridial organisms—*Clostridium oedematiens*, *Cl. perfringens* (=*Cl. welchii*, type A), and *Cl. septicum*—and rendering them harmless to susceptible animals. They are as follows.

Gas-gangrene Antitoxin (Oedematiens)

OTHER NAMES: Immunoserum Anticlostridium Oedematiens; Oed/Ser

Gas-gangrene Antitoxin (Perfringens)

OTHER NAMES: Gas-gangrene Antitoxin (Welchii); Immunoserum Anticlostridium Perfringens; Perf/Ser

Gas-gangrene Antitoxin (Septicum)

OTHER NAMES: Immunoserum Anticlostridium Septicum; Sep/Ser

Mixed Gas-gangrene Antitoxin

Prepared by mixing gas-gangrene antitoxin (oedematiens), gas-gangrene antitoxin (perfringens), and gas-gangrene antitoxin (septicum).

OTHER NAMES: Gas/Ser; Immunoserum Anticlostridium Mixtum

Standards for these antitoxins are given in the European Pharmacopoeia Vol. II

Storage. They should be stored as described under Antisera.

Actions and uses. Mixed gas-gangrene antitoxin should be given, as soon as possible after the infliction of a wound, as a prophylactic measure against the development of gas-gangrene. Intravenous injection ensures rapid distribution of the antitoxin but if this route is impracticable the injection may be given intramuscularly into healthy tissue. Mixed gas-gangrene antitoxin has been given with tetanus antitoxin.

The usual prophylactic dose is 25 000 units, but the dose may be doubled or repeated if the clinical condition of the patient deteriorates or if an operation is necessary. The therapeutic dose is not less than 75 000 units and is administered by intravenous injection in order to neutralise the toxaemia with a minimum of delay. Repeated administration may be required every 4 to 6 hours according to the response of the patient.

As soon as the infecting micro-organism has been identified, monovalent antitoxin may be substituted for polyvalent antitoxin, although this course is seldom possible in practice; the suggested initial therapeutic dose of gas-gangrene antitoxin (oedematiens) or (perfringens) is 30 000 units and of gas-gangrene antitoxin (septicum) is 15 000 units.

Serum reactions. See under Antisera.

Gastro-enteritis

Gastro-enteritis is a clinical syndrome characterised by nausea, vomiting, and diarrhoea with abdominal pain and, in severe cases, prostration, collapse, and signs of dehydration.

When the condition is due to the consumption of poisonous or chemically contaminated food the onset is sudden, vomiting occurring within half an hour, but recovery usually occurs within 24 hours.

The symptoms after consumption of bacterial toxins are similar but usually take 1 to 12 hours to develop. When the condition is due to live bacteria such as salmonellae it is slower in onset, taking 12 to 48 hours to develop; the body temperature may be raised and the patient may be ill for several days.

Treatment consists in rest and the administration of antidiarrhoeal agents, when required, and of fluids to prevent dehydration; intravenous administration of electrolyte solutions may be necessary in severe cases. Antibacterial agents are not usually administered even when a bacterial infection is present as their use may prolong the illness and the carrier state in, for example, salmonella infections. However, when bacteraemia accompanies salmonella infections, parenteral antibiotic therapy is indicated.

Gastro-enteritis in infants may result in an intolerance to disaccharides such as the lactose in milk. The lactose is converted in the gut to lactic acid which results in further diarrhoea. When this occurs the infant should be given a disaccharide-free diet and vitamin supplements until recovery is complete.

Enteric fever caused by *Salmonella typhi* and *S. paratyphi* is a systemic infection in which bacteraemia and other manifestations are serious and require prompt treatment usually with chloramphenicol. Carriers are often treated with ampicillin over a long period.

Cholera is manifested by severe diarrhoea, which rapidly causes dehydration, and fluid loss must be corrected early in the illness. Tetracycline may reduce the severity of the disease.

When poisoning is due to chemical agents it should be treated appropriately—see under Poisoning. See also the entries on Cholera, Diarrhoea, and Salmonella Infections.

Gelatin

A protein obtained from collagenous material such as animal skins, tendons, ligaments, and bones. The material is boiled with water and the resulting liquid is skimmed, strained, and evaporated at low temperature after purification. The product is dried by exposure to air.

A standard is given in the British Pharmacopoeia 1973

The viscosity of solutions and the strength and melting-point of jellies prepared from different batches of gelatin may vary. These variations are dependent on the source of the material and on the process used to prepare the gelatins.

Grading is usually by jelly strength, expressed as a "Bloom strength", which is the weight in grams which, when applied under controlled conditions to a plunger 12.7 mm in diameter, will produce a depression exactly 4 mm deep in a matured jelly containing 6.66% w/w of gelatin in water.

The British Pharmacopoeia specifies a jelly strength of not less than 150 g, which is suitable for most pharmaceutical work, but grades are available giving lower and higher figures, up to 230 g. High jelly strength is preferable for gelatin capsules and for bacteriological culture media, in the latter case to allow for the inevitable lowering of the melting-point during sterilisation.

Description. Colourless or pale yellowish translucent sheets, shreds, powder, or granules, with a slight odour.

Solubility. Practically insoluble in cold water, but swells and softens when immersed, gradually absorbing 5 to 10 times its own weight of water; soluble in hot water, forming a viscous liquid which sets to a jelly on cooling; this property is much less marked after prolonged heating of the solution.

Practically insoluble in alcohol, in ether, and in chloroform.

Stability. It is stable in air when dry, but putrefies rapidly when moist or in solution.

FURTHER INFORMATION. Stability in aqueous solution—W. C. Ling, *J. pharm. Sci.*, 1978, **67**, 218.

Sterilisation. It is sterilised by dry heat.

Storage. It should be stored in airtight containers.

Uses. Gelatin is an ingredient of pastilles, pastes, pessaries, bougies, and glycerol suppositories.

Solutions containing 0.5 to 0.7% of gelatin in an isotonic vehicle containing a suitable bactericide may be used as artificial tears.

Gelatin is used as the main constituent of hard and flexible capsule shells. It is also used for the microencapsulation of drugs and flavouring agents.

A solution of hydrolysed gelatin is used as a vehicle in corticotrophin gelatin injection.

In the form of absorbable gelatin sponge, gelatin is used as a haemostatic.

When preparations containing gelatin are to be applied to abraded surfaces, the material should be sterilised, but prolonged heating reduces the strength of the gel.

Gelatin Sponge, Absorbable

A sterile, absorbable, water-insoluble, gelatin-base sponge, prepared by whisking a warm solution of gelatin to a uniform foam and drying.

OTHER NAMES: Gelatin Sponge; Sterispon®

A standard is given in the British Pharmacopoeia 1973

Description. A white or almost white, tough, light, finely porous, sponge-like material which may be wetted by kneading with moistened fingers.

Solubility. Practically insoluble in water. It is completely digested by acid solutions of pepsin.

Sterilisation. It is sterilised by dry heat.

Storage. It should be stored in containers sealed to exclude micro-organisms. It cannot be satisfactorily resterilised and, if a portion only of the contents of a container is used on any one occasion, strict aseptic precautions should be taken to avoid contamination.

Actions and uses. Absorbable gelatin sponge is a haemostatic which depends for its action upon its physical structure. Owing to its porosity it is capable of absorbing many times its weight of blood.

When absorbable gelatin sponge is applied with pressure to a bleeding surface, the blood is absorbed and rapid clotting usually occurs. The mechanically supported coagulum adheres to the tissue surface and permits the formation of fibrin plugs at the underlying capillary ends. As it is not antigenic it may be left in a wound; it is completely absorbed in 4 to 6 weeks.

Although it is an effective haemostatic in capillary oozing or venous bleeding, the sponge should not be relied upon for the control of haemorrhage from the larger vessels.

Absorbable gelatin sponge may be used either in the dry state or moistened with normal saline, a solution of an antibiotic or, to accelerate clotting in the case of a defective clotting mechanism, a solution of thrombin (100 units per ml). If it is to be used in the moistened condition, a piece of sponge is soaked in the chosen medium, squeezed to remove air and excess of solution, moulded with the fingers to the required shape, and then applied with firm pressure to the bleeding point or area until adherent.

The absence of any but very mild cellular reaction permits the use of absorbable gelatin sponge after all types of surgical procedure. In dental and oral surgery it is of value both as a haemostatic agent and in the obliteration of "dead space".

Gels

Gels are semi-solid aqueous preparations, prepared with the aid of a suitable gelling agent such as gelatin, tragacanth, gelatinised starch, or a cellulose derivative. They may also be made with non-aqueous liquids such as mineral or fixed oils. Gels are often used when a non-greasy preparation is required for application to the scalp or skin.

Gentamicin Sulphate

A complex mixture of the sulphates of gentamicin C_1, gentamicin C_{1A}, and gentamicin C_2, antimicrobial substances produced by *Micromonospora purpurea*.

OTHER NAMES: *Cidomycin®*; *Genticin®*
Genticin HC® and *Gentisone HC®* (both with hydrocortisone acetate)

A standard is given in the British Pharmacopoeia 1973

Description. A white to cream-coloured powder.

Solubility. Soluble in water; practically insoluble in alcohol, in ether, and in chloroform.

Acidity. A 4% solution has a pH of 3.5 to 5.5.

Moisture content. Not more than 15%, determined by Fischer titration.

Specific rotation. +107° to +121°, determined on a 10% solution.

Storage. It should be stored in airtight containers.

Determination in body fluids. RADIO-IMMUNOASSAY. In serum—P. Longmore *et al.*, *Med. J. Aust.*, i/1976, 738.

HIGH PRESSURE LIQUID CHROMATOGRAPHY. In serum—S. K. Maitra *et al.*, *Clin. Chem.*, 1977, **23**, 2275.

Metabolism. ABSORPTION. Poorly absorbed after oral administration; rapidly absorbed after intramuscular administration although the absorption may vary according to the injection site used; gentamicin is absorbed systemically following topical application to wounds.

BLOOD CONCENTRATION. After intramuscular doses of 160, 240, and 320 mg, peak serum concentrations at 1 hour reach 5 to 8, 5 to 17, and about 16 μg/ml respectively; after an intravenous dose of 40 mg/m^2 body-surface, serum concentrations of about 4.5 μg/ml are attained which may reach 11 μg/ml in patients with renal function impairment; no gentamicin is detectable in serum following oral administration; serum concentrations appear to be decreased in febrile when compared with non-febrile subjects.

HALF-LIFE. Serum half-life, 1 to 4 hours; in patients with advanced renal failure, the serum half-life is increased to about 35 hours; in children, the half-life appears to be inversely related to age and, in neonates, the half-life is 2.3 to 3.3 hours, in infants over 20 months, 1.5 to 2.5 hours, and in older children about 1 hour.

DISTRIBUTION. Widely distributed throughout the body; it enters the cerebrospinal fluid when the meninges are inflamed; it crosses the placenta but does not appear in the milk in significant amounts; following intramuscular administration, effective bacteriostatic concentrations are achieved in the bronchopulmonary tract; in renal failure gentamicin may accumulate; *protein binding*, 25 to 30% bound to plasma proteins; it is also 10% bound to red blood cells.

METABOLIC REACTIONS. Conjugation.

EXCRETION. Rapidly excreted with 30 to 80% appearing in the urine in 24 hours; most of this is excreted in the first 9 hours; urinary excretion varies slightly according to urinary pH values; in the newborn about 12% of a dose is excreted in the urine in 2 days; nearly all of the urinary excreted material is unchanged; small amounts are excreted in the bile.

FURTHER INFORMATION. Correlation of serum-creatinine concentration and gentamicin half-life—R. E. Cutler *et al.*, *J. Am. med. Ass.*, 1972, **219**, 1037; transport of gentamicin into synovial fluid—D. C. Marsh *et al.*, *J. Am. med. Ass.*, 1974, **228**, 607; pharmacokinetics—T. Dume *et al.*, *Dt. med. Wschr.*, 1971, **96**, 734, J. E. Pennington *et al.*, *J. infect. Dis.*, 1975, **132**, 270, C. Regamey *et al.*, *Clin. Pharmac. Ther.*, 1973, **14**, 396, and H. Regula *et al.*, *Int. J. clin. Pharmac.*, 1973, **7**, 95; distribution in body fluids—V. Rodriguez *et al.*, *Clin. Pharmac. Ther.*, 1970, **11**, 275; bronchial excretion—O. Wieser *et al.*, *Dt. med. Wschr.*, 1971, **96**, 870; elimination—T. W. Wilson, *Clin. Pharmac. Ther.*, 1973, **14**, 815; placental transfer—H. Yoshioka *et al.*, *J. Pediat.*, 1972, **80**, 121.

Actions and uses. Gentamicin sulphate is a broad spectrum aminoglycoside antibiotic which is effective against a wide range of Gram-positive and Gram-negative bacteria, including *Staphylococcus aureus*, species of *Pseudomonas* and *Proteus*, and many coliform bacilli. It is bactericidal and acts by interfering with the synthesis of bacterial proteins.

The principal use of gentamicin is for the treatment of severe, life-threatening infections before bacteriological results are available and of infections caused by organisms resistant to less toxic antibiotics but requiring systemic therapy, for example, *Pseudomonas aeruginosa*.

Resistance may develop, especially among Gram-negative organisms, and cross-resistance with other aminoglycoside antibiotics such as kanamycin, neomycin, streptomycin, and tobramycin may occur. To delay development of resistance, gentamicin may be given in conjunction with carbenicillin, with which it acts synergistically, for the treatment of infections that are sensitive to both these antibiotics. As gentamicin is not absorbed when given by mouth, it is administered by intramuscular and occasionally by intravenous injection. Peak levels are attained about 30 minutes after administration by intramuscular injection and levels remain high for approximately 2 hours and fall towards zero in 8 to 12 hours. As free gentamicin is excreted through the kidney, high antibacterial concentrations are reached in the urine. Excretion is delayed when renal function is impaired.

The usual daily dosage is the equivalent of 3 to 5 milligrams of gentamicin (3000 to 5000 units) per kilogram body-weight and for children up to 6 milligrams (6000 units) per kilogram body-weight in divided doses every 8 hours by intramuscular injection; similar doses may also be given by intravenous injection. These doses should only be given if kidney function is adequate. When gentamicin is given for urinary tract infections the urine should be made alkaline.

Serum concentrations above 10 units per millilitre should be avoided because of the potential toxicity of the drug and it should only be used against organisms sensitive to much lower concentrations. Treatment should not be continued for more than 7 days.

Gentamicin does not readily cross the blood-brain barrier unless the meninges are inflamed and intrathecal therapy is usually required for the treatment of meningitis and intraventricular injection for the treatment of ventriculitis. For this purpose the dose for adults is the equivalent of 1 to 2 milligrams (1000 to 2000 units) of gentamicin daily and for children and neonates the equivalent of 1 milligram of gentamicin daily by intrathecal or intraventricular injection; intramuscular injections may be given at the same time.

Local applications of the equivalent of 0.1 to 0.3% of gentamicin are used for the treatment of infections of the eyes, ears, and skin.

Undesirable effects. Gentamicin may affect the vestibular and auditory branches of the eighth cranial nerve, giving rise to loss of hearing, vertigo, and tinnitus which may be permanent; this rarely occurs in patients with normal renal function and may be related to persistently high trough levels just before the next dose is due, a characteristic of patients with renal failure. Ototoxicity is more likely to occur in patients over 40 years.

Nephrotoxicity may occur but this is unusual. Allergic rashes and fevers may occur but seldom interfere with the treatment of patients who have not received the drug previously. Topical application of gentamicin may give rise to local allergy.

Precautions. Gentamicin is mainly eliminated through the kidneys and therefore patients with impaired renal function must have the dosage adjusted accordingly and monitoring of blood levels attained is mandatory.

Short courses of gentamicin of 5 to 7 days duration may be given in pregnancy or infancy if no safer treatment is available, but prolonged courses should not be given as damage to the eighth cranial nerve in the foetus may occur.

Administration of gentamicin should be discontinued if tinnitus, a sensation of fullness of the ears, or hearing loss occurs.

Drug interactions. Ethacrynic acid, frusemide, and other potent antibiotics may increase the ototoxicity and nephrotoxicity of gentamicin. The cephalosporins, especially cephaloridine, may potentiate nephrotoxicity if used in conjunction with gentamicin. The activity of neuromuscular blocking agents is increased by gentamicin.

Preparations

GENTAMICIN EYE-DROPS: consisting of a sterile solution containing gentamicin sulphate equivalent to 0.3% (3000 units per ml) of gentamicin, with benzalkonium chloride and borax, in purified water.
This preparation is also suitable for use as ear-drops.
Containers and *Labelling:* see the entry on Eye-drops for general information on containers and labelling.
Storage: it should be stored at room temperature; it should not be allowed to freeze.
Advice for patients: see the entry on Eye-drops for general information of the use of eye-drops. The prescribed course should be completed.

GENTAMICIN INJECTION: a sterile solution of gentamicin sulphate, with suitable stabilising agents, in water for injections. It is sterilised by filtration. Available in 2-ml vials containing gentamicin sulphate equivalent to 10 mg (10 000 units) of gentamicin per ml, and in 2-ml vials containing gentamicin sulphate equivalent to 40 mg (40 000 units) of gentamicin per ml.
A standard for this injection is given in the British Pharmacopoeia 1973
Containers: see the entry on Injections for general information on containers.
Labelling: see the entry on Injections for general information on labelling. In addition, the label on the container should state the amount of the medicament as the number of units in a suitable dose-volume.

GENTAMICIN OINTMENT (*Syn.* Gentamicin Sulphate Ointment): a dispersion of finely powdered gentamicin sulphate in a suitable anhydrous greasy basis. Available as an ointment containing gentamicin sulphate equivalent to 0.3% of gentamicin.
A standard for this ointment is given in the British Pharmaceutical Codex 1973
Containers, Labelling, and *Storage:* see the entry on Ointments for general information on containers, labelling, and storage.
Advice for patients: the ointment should be applied sparingly to the affected area.

OTHER PREPARATIONS available include a CREAM containing gentamicin sulphate equivalent to 0.3% of gentamicin and a cream containing gentamicin sulphate equivalent to 0.3% of gentamicin with hydrocortisone acetate 1%; EAR-DROPS containing gentamicin sulphate equivalent to 0.3% of gentamicin with hydrocortisone acetate 1%; an INJECTION containing gentamicin sulphate equivalent to 1 mg (1000 units) of gentamicin with sodium chloride 8.5 mg per ml in 2-ml ampoules (for intrathecal administration); an OINTMENT containing gentamicin sulphate equivalent to 0.3% of gentamicin with hydrocortisone acetate 1%; and a (sterile) POWDER in bottles containing gentamicin sulphate equivalent to 1 g (1 mega unit) and 10 g (10 mega units) of gentamicin.

Gentian

The dried rhizome and root of *Gentiana lutea* L. (Fam. Gentianaceae), a herbaceous perennial indigenous to central Europe, Yugoslavia, France, and Spain. The rhizome and root are collected from the end of May to the beginning of October. The fresh rhizome and root are yellowish-white internally, but become darker during the drying process, when partial fermentation occurs and the characteristic odour of the drug is developed.

OTHER NAMES: Gentian Root; Gentianae Radix

A standard is given in the European Pharmacopoeia Vol. I

Constituents. The fresh drug contains about 2% of the bitter glycoside gentiopicroside (also known as gentiamarin and gentiopicrin), which yields on hydrolysis the lactone gentiogenin and glucose; it is decomposed during the drying of the drug. The trisaccharide gentianose and the disaccharides gentiobiose (about 2%) and sucrose are present, together with pectin and fixed oil. The sugars are partially hydrolysed during slow drying into glucose and fructose.
A number of enzymes, including emulsin, gentiobiase, an oxidase, and a peroxidase have been identified. The alkaloids gentianine and gentialutine [4-(2-hydroxyethyl)-3-vinylpyridine], in total amount about 0.03%, are also present in the root. The dried root contains, in addition, the glycoside gentioside (3-p-primeverosidoisogentisin), the flavonoid gentisin (1,7-dihydroxy-3-methoxyxanthone), other xanthone colouring matters, and gentisic acid (2,5-dihydroxybenzoic acid).
Gentian yields to water 33 to 40% of extractive; overfermented gentian root may yield to cold water as little as 13% of extractive.
Up to 5% of sulphated ash may be present.

Description. UNGROUND DRUG. *Macroscopical characters:* sub-cylindrical pieces either entire or split longitudinally, from 150 to 200 mm or more long and from 3 to 40 mm thick, occasionally up to 80 mm at the crown; outer surface of rhizome and root yellowish-brown to dark brown; root longitudinally wrinkled; rhizome occasionally branched, frequently terminating in a bud and bearing numerous encircling leaf-scars appearing as transverse annulations. When moist, tough and flexible, when dry, brittle, breaking with a short fracture; smoothed, transversely cut surface reddish-yellow, well-marked cambium showing as a dark ring separating a moderately wide bark from a large, mainly parenchymatous xylem lacking a distinctly radiate structure.
It has a characteristic odour and a sweetish taste which afterwards becomes intensely bitter.

Microscopical characters: the diagnostic characters are: *cork cells* yellowish-brown; *parenchyma* abundant, with moderately thickened walls, containing small *oil globules* and in some cells *crystals* of calcium oxalate either as minute needles or slender prisms about 3 to 6 μm long; *vessels* infrequent, with reticulate wall pitting or annular or spiral thickening; *starch* granules small, rounded, very infrequent; *fibres* and *sclereids* absent.

POWDERED DRUG. Powdered Gentian. A light brown or yellowish-brown powder possessing the diagnostic microscopical characters, odour, and taste of the unground drug.

Incompatibility. It is incompatible with iron salts.

Storage. It should be stored in a dry place protected from light.

Actions and uses. Gentian is a bitter and is used to stimulate the appetite. It is usually administered as the compound infusion.

Preparations

ALKALINE GENTIAN MIXTURE (*Syn.* Mistura Gentianae cum Soda):

Concentrated compound gentian infusion	100 ml
Sodium bicarbonate	50 g
Chloroform water, double-strength	500 ml
Water for preparations	to 1000 ml

It should be recently prepared.

A standard for this mixture is given in the British Pharmaceutical Codex 1973
Dose: 10 to 20 millilitres.

COMPOUND GENTIAN INFUSION:

Concentrated compound gentian infusion	100 ml
Purified water, freshly boiled and cooled	to 1000 ml

Mix. For dispensing purposes, it should be used within 12 hours of preparation.
Dose: 15 to 40 ml.

CONCENTRATED COMPOUND GENTIAN INFUSION:

Gentian, cut small and bruised..	125 g
Dried bitter-orange peel, cut small	125 g
Dried lemon-peel, cut small	125 g
Alcohol (25%)	1200 ml

Macerate the gentian, the dried bitter-orange peel, and the dried lemon peel in 1000 ml of the alcohol in a covered vessel for 48 hours and press out the liquid. To the marc add the remainder of the alcohol, macerate for 24 hours, press out the liquid, and add it to the product of the first pressing. Allow the mixed liquids to stand for not less than 14 days and filter.
A standard for this concentrated infusion is given in the British Pharmacopoeia 1973
Dose: 1.5 to 4 ml.

German Measles

see RUBELLA

Giant-cell Arteritis

Polymyalgia Rheumatica; Temporal Arteritis

Polymyalgia rheumatica and temporal arteritis are names given to two clinical syndromes which are probably manifestations of one process, giant-cell arteritis. They often occur together but the clinical picture may be dominated by one or other group of symptoms.

Giant-cell arteritis is a subacute panarteritis usually affecting the larger arteries especially the temporal and occipital vessels. The media of the arteries is damaged most by necrosis and granulomatous inflammation and characteristically giant cells are present.

Polymyalgia rheumatica affects the elderly and rarely occurs before 50 years of age. There is often a sudden onset of muscle and joint pain with malaise, loss of weight, depression, and fever. Symptoms are mainly localised to the shoulder and pelvic girdles and accompanied by severe morning stiffness. There is painful restriction of movement of affected joints particularly those of the shoulder and pelvic girdle.

Temporal arteritis may be preceded by a polymyalgic illness. Headache often occurs later and may sometimes be abrupt in onset with pain of great intensity and tenderness of the scalp usually in the temporal region. The temporal arteries may be thickened, tender, and non-pulsatile with reddening of the overlying skin (temporal arteritis). Diffuse arterial occlusion may lead to actual necrosis of the skin. About half the patients with temporal arteritis have ocular disturbances which may result in loss of vision. Once blindness has occurred there is little chance of improvement.

The erythrocyte sedimentation rate is always raised in giant-cell arteritis.

Early treatment with corticosteroids is of the greatest importance as this will control headache, fever, and myalgia and prevent ocular complications. Treatment must be continued for at least 2 years.

Giant-cell arteritis is a self-limiting disease with a tendency to gradual improvement and complete subsidence within a few years.

Giardiasis

Giardiasis is an infection of the small intestine by the flagellate *Giardia lamblia*. It is commonly reported in visitors returning from eastern Europe. The disease is spread by the faecal-oral route, water being an important souce of infection. Frequently, the infection causes no symptoms, but heavy infection may cause chronic diarrhoea, dyspepsia, malabsorption, and occasionally cholecystitis.

Substances used in the treatment of *Giardia lamblia* infections include chloroquine, furazolidone, mepacrine, and metronidazole.

Ginger

The rhizome of *Zingiber officinale* Roscoe (Fam. Zingiberaceae), scraped to remove the dark outer layer and dried in the sun. It is known in commerce as unbleached Jamaica ginger. The plant is indigenous to Asia, but is cultivated in the West Indies, Africa, Australia, and Taiwan.

OTHER NAME: Zingiber

A standard is given in the British Pharmacopoeia 1973

Constituents. Ginger contains about 1 to 2% of volatile oil, of which the sesquiterpene zingiberene is the principal constituent and in which many other terpenes and terpene alcohols have been reported.

The pungency of ginger is due to gingerol, a yellowish oily substance which is a mixture of homologues of zingerone (4-hydroxy-3-methoxyphenethyl methyl ketone) condensed with saturated aliphatic aldehydes, principally *n*-heptaldehyde, and to shogaol, in which the ketone is condensed with hexaldehyde to give an unsaturated side-chain.

Ginger also contains resin and much starch.

Description. UNGROUND DRUG. *Macroscopical characters:* rhizomes known as "races" or "hands", laterally compressed, sometimes broken, bearing short, flattened, obovate, oblique branches on upper side ("fingers"), about 20 mm in length, each having at its apex a depressed stem scar; pieces about 50 to 120 mm long, 15 to 65 (usually 30 to 40) mm wide, and 10 to 15 mm thick; external surface buff-coloured, longitudinally striated, and with occasional loose fibres; fracture short, with projecting fibres; smoothed, transversely cut surface exhibiting a narrow cortex separated by an endodermis from a much wider stele, numerous scattered vascular bundles and scattered oil cells with yellow contents.

It has an agreeable and aromatic odour and strongly pungent taste.

Microscopical characters: the diagnostic characters are: *starch* abundant in the thin-walled cells of the ground tissue, granules simple, flattened, ovate to subrectangular, with hilum frequently in a terminal projection, mostly up to 50 μm long and up to about 25 μm wide and 7 μm thick; *oil cells* with cutinised walls and yellow contents, numerous in ground tissue; *tannin cells* with dark, reddish-brown contents occurring either singly in the ground tissue or in axial rows accompanying the vascular bundles; *vessels* with spiral or reticulate thickening in the scattered *vascular bundles* showing no reaction for lignin; unlignified *fibres* with delicate transverse septa; *cork*, *sclereids*, and calcium oxalate *crystals* absent.

POWDERED DRUG. Powdered Ginger. A light yellow powder possessing the diagnostic microscopical characters, odour, and taste of the unground drug.

Adulterants and substitutes. Jamaica ginger is sometimes limed to whiten it and is then known as "limed" ginger.

Cochin and Calicut gingers are in smaller "hands" and the branches are usually shorter and thicker; they are often imported only partly scraped ("unscraped" or "coated") and may be bleached (limed) or unbleached. African ginger is more pungent but less aromatic; it is usually small, dark, and coated, but may also be found limed.

Nigerian ginger is obtained from *Z. officinale*; it is rather less aromatic than Jamaica ginger.

Japanese ginger is commonly in small flattened pieces; many of the starch granules are compound and the oil differs in its physical characters (weight per ml at 20° about 0.804 g; optical rotation about +9°), these particulars indicating that it is not produced by *Z. officinale*; it has been referred to *Z. mioga* Roscoe.

Ground ginger is often adulterated with exhausted ("spent") ginger, a sophistication that may be detected by a diminution in the water-soluble ash, as well as by the yields of alcohol-soluble and water-soluble extractives.

Storage. It should be stored in a cool dry place.

Powdered ginger should be stored in airtight containers, in a cool place.

Actions and uses. Ginger is a carminative and a flavouring agent.

Preparations

GINGER SYRUP (*Syn.* Syrupus Zingiberis):

Strong ginger tincture	50 ml
Syrup..	to 1000 ml

Mix.

A standard for this syrup is given in the British Pharmaceutical Codex 1973

Dose: 2.5 to 5 millilitres.

STRONG GINGER TINCTURE (*Syn.* Tinct. Zingib. Fort.; Essence of Ginger):

Ginger, in moderately coarse powder ..	500 g
Alcohol (90%)	to 1000 ml

Prepare by percolation as described in the entry on Tinctures.

A standard for this tincture is given in the British Pharmacopoeia 1973

Dose: 0.25 to 0.5 ml.

WEAK GINGER TINCTURE (*Syn.* Tinct. Zingib. Mit.; Ginger Tincture):

Strong ginger tincture	200 ml
Alcohol (90%)	to 1000 ml

Mix. Filter if necessary.

A standard for this tincture is given in the British Pharmacopoeia 1973

Dose: 1.5 to 3 ml.

OTHER PREPARATIONS: ginger is an ingredient of compound rhubarb powder.

Glandular Fever

Glandular fever (Infective mononucleosis) is an acute infection in which abnormal mononuclear cells are present in the blood. The disease is of low infectivity and may be caused by the herpes-like EB (Epstein–Barr) virus.

Symptoms occur mainly in young persons between the ages of 15 and 25 years. Infections in children are often asymptomatic. The incubation period is uncertain but may be several weeks. Onset is characterised by fever, malaise, headache, generalised muscle pains, enlargement of the lymph nodes and spleen, splenic rupture, and sore throat (especially in adults), sometimes with exudate or pseudomembrane on the tonsils and fauces; swallowing is difficult and painful.

Rubelliform rash, hepatitis, and meningitis may occasionally accompany the disease and haemolytic anaemia, pneumonia, myocarditis, conjunctivitis, and thrombocytopenic purpura are rarely present. During the course of the disease the presence of antibody for sheep red blood cells may be detected by the Paul-Bunnell reaction. Recovery may be prolonged.

There is no specific treatment and symptomatic measures should be adopted. Antibiotics should only be given in the case of secondary bacterial infection and a rash invariably occurs as a result of treatment with ampicillin. Corticosteroid therapy has been used to treat severe complications of the infection.

Glaucoma

Glaucoma is a condition in which the intra-ocular tension is raised and if this is not treated it will result in permanent damage to the eyes or even blindness.

Closed-angle or narrow-angle glaucoma usually occurs after middle age in long-sighted subjects and is characterised by misty vision, rainbow haloes around lights, and localised headaches. In acute attacks there may be violent pain and vomiting. The raised intra-ocular pressure is due to mechanical blockage of the outflow channels of the iridocorneal angle.

This type of glaucoma is a medical emergency as blindness results if untreated. Surgical relief of the blockage by iridectomy is required, but the pressure may be temporarily relieved by reducing the inflow of aqueous humour with acetazolamide and the use of miotics. The intra-ocular pressure may be relieved by osmotic agents such as urea, mannitol, and glycerol.

Simple glaucoma may develop insidiously with advancing age, there being a moderate rise in intra-ocular pressure, the cause of which has not been clearly established. Certain drugs such as corticosteroids administered systemically may also give rise to simple glaucoma. This type of glaucoma is initially symptomless but if untreated leads to cupping and atrophy of the optic disk, resulting in mistiness and restriction of the field of vision. The pressure may be reduced by the use of eye-drops that contract the ciliary muscle, such as parasympathomimetics, or anti-cholinesterases; eye-drops of adrenaline are also used. Carbonic acid anhydrase inhibitors which reduce intra-ocular pressure by reducing the inflow of aqueous humour are used systemically.

Glibenclamide

1-{4-[2-(5-Chloro-2-methoxybenzamido)ethyl]benzene-sulphonyl}-3-cyclohexylurea

$C_{23}H_{28}ClN_3O_5S = 494.0$

OTHER NAMES: *Daonil®*; *Euglucon®*; Glyburide

A standard is given in the British Pharmacopoeia Addendum 1975

Description. A white crystalline odourless powder.

Solubility. Very slightly soluble in water and in ether; soluble, at 20°, in 330 parts of alcohol, in 36 parts of chloroform, and in 250 parts of methyl alcohol.

Moisture content. Not more than 1%, determined by drying at 105°.

Identification. MELTING-POINT. About 173°.

ULTRAVIOLET ABSORPTION. In 0.01N methanolic hydrochloric acid, maxima at 275 nm (weak) and 300 nm (E1%, 1cm = 63).

INFRA-RED ABSORPTION. Major peaks at 1163, 1333, 1471, 1515, 1613, and 1724 cm^{-1} (see Appendix 2b: Infrared Spectra).

Metabolism. ABSORPTION. About 45% of a 5-mg dose is absorbed after oral administration.

BLOOD CONCENTRATION. After an oral dose of 5 mg, peak serum concentrations of about 0.04 μg/ml are attained in 2 to 4 hours.

HALF-LIFE. Plasma half-life, 3 to 7 hours; half-life determined from urinary excretion data, about 10 hours.

DISTRIBUTION. Widely distributed throughout the body and does not appear to accumulate; *protein binding*, about 98% bound to plasma proteins.

METABOLIC REACTIONS. Hydroxylation of the cyclohexyl ring at positions 3 and 4; in the rat, rabbit, and dog the 3-*cis*-hydroxy metabolite is formed and in the rat the 4-*trans*-hydroxy metabolite is additionally produced; hydroxylated metabolites may be conjugated.

EXCRETION. In 5 days, 95% of a dose is excreted in the urine and faeces with about 54% excreted as unchanged drug; of the 95% excreted about 75% is found in the faeces and 20% in the urine; excretion of an intravenous dose is more rapid than that from either oral or intramuscular doses.

FURTHER INFORMATION. Pharmacokinetics—L. Balant *et al.*, *Eur. J. clin. Pharmac.*, 1975, **8**, 63; metabolism and kinetics—L. Fuccella *et al.*, *J. clin. Pharmac.*, 1973, **13**, 68.

Actions and uses. Glibenclamide is an oral hypoglycaemic agent with actions and uses similar to those described under Chlorpropamide.

The usual initial daily dosage in mild maturity-onset diabetes inadequately controlled by diet is 5 milligrams taken with or after food. The daily dose should be adjusted in steps of 2.5 milligrams at intervals of about 1 week until a suitable maintenance level is reached; the total daily dose should not normally exceed 20 milligrams.

Patients who have failed to respond to other oral hypoglycaemic drugs may sometimes respond to glibenclamide alone or in conjunction with biguanides such as metformin.

Undesirable effects; Precautions; Contra-indications. As for Chlorpropamide.

Preparation

GLIBENCLAMIDE TABLETS: available as tablets containing 5 mg of glibenclamide.

A standard for these tablets is given in the British Pharmacopoeia Addendum 1975

Containers and *Storage:* see the entry on Tablets for general information on containers and storage. Containers should be airtight.

Advice for patients: the tablets should be taken at regular intervals, preferably after meals. Treatment should not be discontinued without the advice of the prescriber. Intolerance to alcohol may occur.

Glomerulonephritis

Acute glomerulonephritis is a condition in which there is acute glomerular damage, usually accompanied by haematuria and proteinuria. This condition is commonly preceded by infections such as sore throat or acute tonsillitis due to haemolytic streptococci. In children, there is usually rapid onset with oedema, low urinary output, and associated symptoms such as malaise, fever, anorexia, vomiting, and headache. In adults, onset tends to be slower and accompanied by progressive tiredness, slowly developing oedema of the lower limbs, and sometimes arterial hypertension.

Patients should be treated in bed. The diet should be low in sodium to control oedema and low in protein to prevent rise in blood urea. Fluid intake should be maintained. Streptococcal infections should be treated with suitable antibacterial agents such as the penicillins, and in some cases removal of infected foci such as tonsils or tooth abscesses may be of value. Hypertension should be treated if severe.

Chronic glomerulonephritis is a condition of persistent proteinuria, sometimes accompanied by signs of renal failure and arterial hypertension resulting from an earlier episode of acute glomerulonephritis which may have passed unnoticed. Proteinuria and arterial hypertension are early signs. In later stages, renal function deteriorates and uraemia increases. There may be polyuria, thirst, anaemia, weakness, nausea, vomiting, diarrhoea, and headache. Dietary protein intake should be restricted but fluid intake should be maintained.

Glucagon

A polypeptide, obtained from beef or pork pancreas, which increases the blood-glucose concentration as the result of the rapid breakdown of liver glycogen.

A standard is given in the British Pharmacopoeia Addendum 1975

Description. A white odourless powder.

Solubility. Practically insoluble in water and in most organic solvents; soluble in dilute solutions of alkali hydroxides and mineral acids.

Moisture content. Not more than 10%, determined by drying at 105°.

Storage. It should be stored in airtight glass or metal containers at a temperature of 2° to 8°.

Identification. ULTRAVIOLET ABSORPTION. In 0.01N hydrochloric acid, maximum at 276 nm (E1%, 1cm = 23).

Actions and uses. Glucagon is present in the α-cells of the pancreas. It promotes glycogenolysis in the liver. Very small amounts of glucagon cause an appreciable rise in the blood-sugar concentration and before this rise occurs glucagon stimulates the secretion of insulin. In both normal and diabetic subjects, the level of glucagon rises after a 48 hour fast. The hypoglycaemic sulphonyl-ureas suppress the pancreatic release of glucagon.

Glucagon is also lipolytic, stimulating free fatty acid release from peripheral fat deposits and activating liver lipase.

Other physiological effects of glucagon are an increase in renal blood flow and excretion of electrolytes, an increased release of catecholamines from the adrenal medulla, reduction in gastric and pancreatic secretion, inhibition of gastro-intestinal motility, release of growth hormone, and hypercalciuria with hypocalcaemia, possibly by effect on calcitonin.

Glucagon has also important physiological actions on the heart. It increases myocardial contractility, heart rate, maximum rate of left ventricular pressure development, cardiac output, systolic ejection rate, and arterial blood pressure. It increases cardiac output after myocardial infarction. It is of value in the treatment of patients with low cardiac output due to excessive use of β-adrenergic blocking agents, myocardial infarction, or following cardiac surgery. It is not effective in the routine management of heart failure.

As glucagon is inactive when given by mouth, it is administered by injection. It is inactivated by enzymes present in the liver.

Glucagon is used for the treatment of hypoglycaemia after overdosage with insulin and the oral hypoglycaemic drugs, particularly if the patient is unconscious and cannot take carbohydrate by mouth, or venepuncture is difficult or the administration of dextrose injection has caused local thrombophlebitis. The dose of glucagon for this purpose is 0.5 to 1 unit by subcutaneous, intramuscular, or intravenous injection. This dose is repeated in 20 minutes if necessary. Once consciousness returns carbohydrate is given by mouth.

Glucagon is also used for the treatment of resistant heart failure and cardiogenic shock as an infusion in dextrose injection (5%) at the rate of 1 to 7.5 units per hour; usually about 5 units per hour is required.

Undesirable effects. These include allergic reactions, nausea, vomiting, and hypokalaemia. Since glucagon interferes with vitamin-K synthesis it intensifies the effects of some anticoagulants.

Precautions. It should not be given by intravenous infusion or injection for long periods as there is a possibility that it may give rise to pulmonary emboli. Nausea, which almost invariably accompanies the administration of doses suitable for treatment of heart failure, may be controlled by the injection of a suitable anti-emetic such as trifluoperazine.

Preparation

GLUCAGON INJECTION: a sterile solution of glucagon hydrochloride, with lactose, in a suitable solvent. It is prepared by dissolving the contents of a sealed container in the solvent shortly before use. Available as a powder in ampoules or vials containing glucagon hydrochloride equivalent to 1 mg (1 unit) of glucagon and in vials containing glucagon hydrochloride equivalent to 10 mg (10 units) of glucagon.

A standard for this injection is given in the British Pharmacopoeia Addendum 1975

Containers: see the entry on Injections for general information on containers.

Labelling: see the entry on Injections for general information on labelling. In addition, the label on the sealed container should state the weight of lactose contained in it.

Storage: the injection should be used immediately after preparation, unless a bactericide is present when it may be kept for up to 1 week, provided it is stored at 2° to 8°. It should be discarded if it shows signs of gel formation or deposition of insoluble matter.

Gluten Enteropathy

see under COELIAC DISEASE

Glutethimide

2-Ethyl-2-phenylglutarimide

$C_{13}H_{15}NO_2 = 217.3$

OTHER NAME: *Doriden*®

A standard is given in the British Pharmacopoeia 1973

Description. Odourless colourless crystals or white powder with a bitter taste.

Solubility. Practically insoluble in water; soluble, at 20°, in 5 parts of alcohol, in 12 parts of ether, and in less than 1 part of chloroform; very slightly soluble in light petroleum.

Moisture content. Not more than 1%, determined by drying over phosphorus pentoxide *in vacuo*.

Dissociation constant. pK_a 4.5 (20°).

Storage. It should be stored in airtight containers, protected from light.

Identification. TESTS. 1. Mix about 10 mg with 2 ml of water, 100 mg of hydroxylammonium chloride, and 1 ml of *sodium hydroxide solution*, shake, allow to stand for 10 minutes, and then add 1 ml of *ferric chloride test-solution*; a deep brownish-red colour is produced.

2. To about 10 mg add 0.1 ml of a 1% solution of cobalt acetate in methyl alcohol followed by a freshly prepared 1% solution of lithium hydroxide in methyl alcohol, added dropwise; a blue colour quickly changing to blue-green and then to green is produced. Barbiturates give a blue colour with this test.

3. Mix 1 g with 5 ml of *sodium hydroxide solution* and 15 ml of water, heat on a water-bath for 30 minutes, cool, acidify with *dilute hydrochloric acid*, and filter; the

residue, after washing with water and drying at 100°, melts at about 159°.

MELTING-POINT. About 86°.

ULTRAVIOLET ABSORPTION. In dehydrated alcohol, maxima at 252 nm (E1%, 1cm = 16.6), 258 nm (E1%, 1cm = 18.3), and 264 nm (E1%, 1cm = 14.3).

INFRA-RED ABSORPTION. Major peaks at 1200, 1270, 1336, 1352, 1680, and 1713 cm^{-1} (see Appendix 2a: Infra-red Spectra).

Determination in body fluids. SPECTROPHOTOMETRY. In blood or urine: alkaline hydrolysis of piperidine ring —L. R. Goldbaum et al., Analyt. Chem., 1960, **32**, 81.

GAS CHROMATOGRAPHY. In blood: glutethimide and barbiturates—E. Fierick and N. W. Tietz, Clin. Chem., 1971, **17**, 1024; in plasma and urine: glutethimide and an active metabolite—A. R. Hansen and L. J. Fischer, Clin. Chem., 1974, **20**, 236; in serum: rapid determination of glutethimide and of barbiturates in clinical emergencies—H. E. Sine et al., Clin. Chem., 1970, **16**, 587.

Metabolism. ABSORPTION. Rapidly absorbed after oral administration; alcohol, taken at the same time, will enhance absorption.

BLOOD CONCENTRATION. Blood concentrations show wide variations between individuals and after an oral dose of 500 mg, peak plasma concentrations of 18 to 70 µg/ml are attained within 1 to 6 hours.

HALF-LIFE. Plasma elimination half-life, 5 to 22 hours.

DISTRIBUTION. Distributed throughout the body, rapidly enters the liver and kidneys, and is found in high concentration in body fat; protein binding, about 50% bound to plasma proteins.

METABOLIC REACTIONS. Glutethimide is almost completely metabolised by hydroxylation of the glutarimide ring at the 5-position and of the ethyl side-chain at the 1'-position followed by conjugation of the resultant hydroxyl groups; dealkylation may also take place by removal of the ethyl group, once hydroxylated, to form phenylglutarimide.

EXCRETION. About 2% of a dose is excreted unchanged in the urine in 24 hours and about 0.1% is excreted in the bile in 12 hours; small amounts of the drug are excreted in the milk of lactating mothers.

Actions and uses. Glutethimide has a hypnotic action closely resembling that of an intermediate-acting barbiturate, as described under Barbiturates. Sleep lasting 4 to 6 hours is produced within about 20 minutes by an oral dose of 250 to 500 milligrams.

Undesirable effects. Glutethimide may produce nausea, dizziness, and, occasionally, rashes and mental excitement.

Dependence. It may give rise to dependence of the barbiturate-alcohol type as described under Drug Dependence and it may enhance the effects of alcohol.

Drug interactions. Glutethimide stimulates the activity of the hepatic enzymes responsible for the metabolism of many drugs, including glutethimide itself, barbiturates, and warfarin and other anticoagulants.

Preparation

GLUTETHIMIDE TABLETS: available as tablets containing 250 mg of glutethimide.
A standard for these tablets is given in the British Pharmacopoeia 1973
Containers and Storage: see the entry on Tablets for

general information on containers and storage. Containers should be airtight and light resistant.
Advice for patients: hypnotic doses should be taken 20 minutes before bedtime. The tablets may cause drowsiness on the following day; persons affected should not drive or operate machinery. Alcohol should be avoided.

Glycerins

Glycerins consist of solutions of medicinal substances in glycerol with or without the addition of water, for example, compound thymol glycerin and phenol glycerin.

Glycerol

Propane-1,2,3-triol

$$HOCH_2 \cdot \overset{\displaystyle OH}{\underset{\displaystyle |}{CH}} \cdot CH_2OH$$

$C_3H_8O_3 = 92.09$

OTHER NAMES: Glycerin; Glycerolum

A standard is given in the European Pharmacopoeia Vol. III

Description. A clear, colourless, hygroscopic, syrupy, odourless liquid with a sweet taste.

Solubility. Miscible with water and with alcohol; practically insoluble in ether, in chloroform, and in fixed oils.

Weight per ml. At 20°, 1.255 to 1.260 g.

Refractive index. At 20°, 1.470 to 1.475.

Sterilisation. It is sterilised by dry heat.

Storage. It should be stored in airtight containers.

Identification. TESTS. 1. When heated on a borax bead in a Bunsen flame, it gives a green flame.
2. Mix 1 ml with 10 drops of nitric acid and carefully add 10 drops of potassium dichromate solution; a blue ring is formed at the interface of the two liquids which, after 10 minutes, does not diffuse into the lower layer.

Actions and uses. Given by mouth, glycerol is demulcent. It is an ingredient of some linctuses and pastilles and is used as a sweetening agent in mixtures. It absorbs moisture when applied undiluted to mucous membranes. It promotes peristalsis when administered by rectum, doses of 4 to 16 millilitres being given undiluted as an enema; glycerol suppositories are also used for this purpose. It is used as a water-retaining and emollient ingredient in dermatological preparations, toilet creams, and jellies. Glycerol, with dried magnesium sulphate, in the form of magnesium sulphate paste, is used in the treatment of septic wounds and boils.
Some surgeons prefer sterile glycerol to liquid paraffin for lubricating gastroscopes and similar instruments.
Glycerol is used as a preservative in some pharmaceutical preparations, but a concentration of at least 50% v/v is required to dehydrate contaminating organisms. It is used as a preservative in certain biological preparations and in "non-alcoholic" extracts and tinctures.

Veterinary uses. Glycerol has been used in the treatment of bovine ketosis and pregnancy toxaemia in sheep. The usual dose for cattle is 350 to 500 millilitres and for sheep 100 to 150 millilitres daily for 3 to 4 days.

Preparations

COMPOUND THYMOL GLYCERIN:

Thymol	.. ..	0.50 g
Glycerol	.. ..	.. 100.00 ml
Carmine	.. ..	0.30 g
Menthol	.. ..	0.30 g
Sodium metabisulphite	.. ..	0.35 g
Sodium salicylate ..	.. ..	5.20 g
Sodium benzoate ..	.. ..	8.00 g
Sodium bicarbonate	.. ..	10.00 g
Borax..	.. ..	20.00 g
Methyl salicylate ..	.. ..	0.30 ml
Pumilio pine oil	.. ..	0.50 ml
Dilute ammonia solution..	.. .. ..	0.75 ml
Cineole	.. ..	1.30 ml
Alcohol (90%)	.. ..	.. 25.00 ml
Water for preparations	.. .. ..	to 1000.00 ml

Dissolve the salts in 800 ml of the water and add the glycerol; dissolve the menthol, the thymol, the cineole, the methyl salicylate, and the pumilio pine oil in the alcohol, triturate with 25 g of sterilised purified talc or kaolin, add the mixture gradually to the solution of the salts, and filter. Dissolve the carmine by stirring it into the dilute ammonia solution, warm gently to dissipate most of the ammonia, mix the two solutions, add sufficient water to produce the required volume, and mix.

In making this preparation the alcohol (90%) may be replaced by industrial methylated spirit diluted so as to be of equivalent alcoholic strength, provided that the law and the statutory regulations governing the use of industrial methylated spirit are observed.

A standard for this glycerin is given in the British Pharmaceutical Codex 1973

Containers and *Labelling:* see the entries on Gargles and Mouth-washes for general information on containers and labelling.

Storage: it should be protected from light.

Advice for patients: when used as a gargle or mouth-wash, it should be diluted with about 3 times its volume of warm water and the diluted solution should be used 3 or 4 times daily as required. It should preferably not be swallowed. Diluted solutions should be used immediately and any unused portion discarded.

GLYCEROL SUPPOSITORIES (*Syn.* Glycerin Suppositories):

Glycerol	.. ..	70 g
Gelatin	.. ..	14 g
Purified water	.. .. ..	a sufficient quantity

Add the gelatin to about 30 ml of the water heated nearly to boiling, add the glycerol, previously heated to 100°, and heat the mixture on a water-bath for 15 minutes or until solution is complete; adjust the weight of the product to 100 g by the addition of hot purified water or by evaporation on the water-bath, as appropriate, and pour into suitable moulds. In tropical and subtropical countries the proportion of gelatin may be increased to 18%.

Available as small (1-g mould), medium (2-g mould), and large (4-g mould) size.

A standard for these suppositories is given in the British Pharmacopoeia 1973

Containers: see the entry on Suppositories for general information on containers.

Advice for patients: see the entry on Suppositories for general information on the use of suppositories. They should be moistened with water before insertion.

ICHTHAMMOL GLYCERIN (*Syn.* Glycerin of Ammonium Ichthosulphonate):

Ichthammol..	.. ..	100 g
Glycerol	.. ..	900 g

MAGNESIUM SULPHATE PASTE (*Syn.* Morison's Paste):

Dried magnesium sulphate	..	a sufficient quantity
Phenol	.. ..	0.5 g
Glycerol, previously heated at 120° for 1 hour and cooled	.. .. ..	55 g

Dry about 70 g of the dried magnesium sulphate for 1½ hours at 150° or for 4 hours at 130° and allow to cool in a desiccator; mix 45 g of this powder in a warm mortar with the phenol dissolved in the glycerol.

In preparing larger quantities of the paste the period of heating the dried magnesium sulphate should be increased, if necessary, to ensure that the dried powder contains at least 85% of magnesium sulphate, calculated as $MgSO_4$.

A standard for this paste is given in the British Pharmaceutical Codex 1973

Containers and *Storage:* it should be stored and supplied in airtight glass jars or other suitable containers.

Labelling: the label on the container should state that the paste should be stirred before use.

Advice for patients: the paste may be applied liberally to the affected area with a suitable applicator. It should not be used repeatedly.

PHENOL EAR-DROPS:

Phenol glycerin	.. ..	40 ml
Glycerol	.. ..	to 100 ml

CAUTION. *Dilution with water renders this preparation caustic; it may be diluted with glycerol, if desired.*

A standard for these ear-drops is given in the British Pharmaceutical Codex 1973

Containers and *Labelling:* see the entry on Ear-drops for general information on containers and labelling.

Advice for patients: the preparation should be protected from water. The ear should be dried and the preparation applied undiluted.

PHENOL GLYCERIN:

Phenol	.. ..	160 g
Glycerol	.. ..	840 g

Dissolve the phenol in the glycerol, with the aid of gentle heat if necessary.

CAUTION. *Dilution with water renders this preparation caustic; it may be diluted with glycerol, if desired.*

A standard for this glycerin is given in the British Pharmaceutical Codex 1973

Storage: it should be stored in airtight containers.

OTHER PREPARATIONS: glycerol is an ingredient of pastille basis (see under Pastilles) and, as an adjuvant, of many other preparations.

Glyceryl Trinitrate

$$
\begin{array}{l}
CH_2 \cdot O \cdot NO_2 \\
| \\
CH \cdot O \cdot NO_2 \\
| \\
CH_2 \cdot O \cdot NO_2
\end{array}
$$

$C_3H_5N_3O_9 = 227.1$

OTHER NAMES: *Nitrocontin®*; Nitroglycerin; *Sustac®*; Trinitrin; Trinitroglycerin

CAUTION. *Because of its dangerous nature, glyceryl*

trinitrate is only used in the form of a solution, usually in alcohol.

Description. A clear colourless oily liquid which explodes on rapid heating or concussion.

Solubility. Soluble in 800 parts of water, in 4 parts of alcohol, and in 6 parts of almond oil; miscible with chloroform, with ether, and with acetone; soluble in glycerol and in light petroleum.

Stability. Rapid loss of glyceryl trinitrate may occur from tablets in the presence of cork, cotton wool, paper, plastics, and rubber, especially at elevated temperatures. Tablets containing glyceryl trinitrate should be protected from light and stored at a temperature not exceeding 25° in a glass container closed by means of a screw closure lined with aluminium or tin foil; the use of additional packing that absorbs glyceryl trinitrate should be avoided.

FURTHER INFORMATION. Stability of tablets in containers—R. F. Shangraw, *Am. J. hosp. Pharm.*, 1972, **29**, 286; V. A. Russell *et al.*, *Pharm. J.*, i/1973, 466; D. P. Page *et al.*, *J. pharm. Sci.*, 1975, **64**, 140.

Determination in body fluids. GAS CHROMATOGRAPHY. In plasma—M. T. Rosseel and M. G. Bogaert, *J. pharm. Sci.*, 1973, **62**, 754.

Metabolism. ABSORPTION. Readily absorbed through mucous membranes; it is rapidly absorbed from the buccal cavity but less rapidly absorbed in the gastrointestinal tract; after a dose of 0.6 to 2.5 mg, about 60% is absorbed buccally when held in the mouth for 3 to 4 minutes; it is well absorbed through the skin.

BLOOD CONCENTRATION. After doses of 800 μg absorbed buccally, plasma concentrations of 4 to 7.5 ng/ml are attained in 6 minutes.

HALF-LIFE. Plasma half-life, about 30 minutes.

DISTRIBUTION. In rabbits, rapidly taken up by all tissues; *protein binding*, in the rat, 60% bound to plasma proteins.

METABOLIC REACTIONS. Rapidly metabolised by hydrolysis to the 1,3- and 1,2-dinitrates, mononitrate, and glycerol; in the rabbit, the 1,2-dinitrate does not appear to be formed.

EXCRETION. In the rat, excreted in the urine mainly as the dinitrates, along with small amounts of unchanged drug and the mononitrate; the major urinary metabolite in man is the mononitrate.

FURTHER INFORMATION. Concentrations in plasma after buccal administration—M. G. Bogaert and M. T. Rosseel, *J. Pharm. Pharmac.*, 1972, **24**, 737; aspects of metabolism—M. H. Litchfield, *J. pharm. Sci.*, 1971, **60**, 1599.

Actions and uses. Glyceryl trinitrate causes the relaxation of involuntary muscle. Its effects are most pronounced on the circulatory system; the arterioles dilate and, with therapeutic doses, the systolic blood pressure falls by 10 to 25 millimetres of mercury. The onset of its effect is delayed for 3 to 5 minutes and its action lasts for 30 to 40 minutes, but preparations with a prolonged action are available.

Tolerance may develop with daily use; withdrawal for a week re-establishes the original sensitivity.

Glyceryl trinitrate is used chiefly in the prophylaxis and treatment of angina of effort. The usual dose is 0.5 to 1 milligram. It is also used for the relief of renal and gall-bladder colic.

Undesirable effects. Flushing and headache due to vasodilatation occur commonly. Dizziness and weakness due to postural hypotension and hypersensitivity may occur.

Precautions and contra-indications. Glyceryl trinitrate should be used with caution in patients with glaucoma as intra-ocular pressure is increased. Tolerance may develop with daily use and cross-resistance to other nitrates and nitrites may occur. It should not be used in patients with coronary thrombosis and in those who are sensitive to nitrates.

Poisoning. The patient should be placed in a recumbent position with the legs elevated and oxygen given. Artificial respiration may be necessary. A sympathomimetic vasoconstrictor may be given to restore the blood pressure.

Preparations

CONCENTRATED GLYCERYL TRINITRATE SOLUTION: containing 10% of glyceryl trinitrate in alcohol (95%).
A standard for this solution is given in the British Pharmacopoeia Addendum 1978
Storage: it should be stored in airtight containers, in a cool place, protected from light.

GLYCERYL TRINITRATE TABLETS (*Syn.* Trinitrin Tablets; Nitroglycerin Tablets): prepared by adding concentrated glyceryl trinitrate solution to dried granules of mannitol, mixing intimately, drying without the aid of heat or at a temperature not exceeding 50° for not more than 4 hours, and compressing.
Available as tablets containing 300, 500, and 600 micrograms of glyceryl trinitrate.
A standard for these tablets is given in the British Pharmacopoeia Addendum 1978
Containers and *Storage:* see the entry on Tablets for general information on containers and storage. Containers should be airtight and light resistant. The tablets should be stored at a temperature not exceeding 25° in a glass container closed by means of a screw closure lined with aluminium or tin foil; additional packing that absorbs glyceryl trinitrate should be avoided.
Glyceryl trinitrate tablets should be issued for patients in containers of not more than 100 tablets.
Labelling: the label on the container should state the date after which the tablets are not intended to be used and that the tablets should be allowed to dissolve slowly in the mouth.
Advice for patients: the tablets should be allowed to dissolve slowly under the tongue, when necessary. They should be stored in the original container which should be kept tightly closed. A fresh tablet should produce a slight tingling sensation when placed under the tongue.

OTHER PREPARATIONS available include TABLETS containing glyceryl trinitrate 2.6 and 6.4 mg in slow-release formulations.

Glycine

Aminoacetic acid

$$NH_2 \cdot CH_2 \cdot COOH$$

$C_2H_5NO_2 = 75.07$

OTHER NAMES: *Paynocil*® (with aspirin); *Titralac*® (with calcium carbonate)

A standard is given in the British Pharmacopoeia Addendum 1978

Description. A white crystalline odourless powder with a sweet taste.

Solubility. Soluble, at 20°, in 4 parts of water; very slightly soluble in alcohol and in ether.

Acidity. A 5% solution has a pH of 5.9 to 6.3.

Sterilisation. Solutions are sterilised by heating in an autoclave.

Identification. TESTS. 1. Prepare a 10% solution and to 5 ml add 5 drops of *dilute hydrochloric acid* and 1 ml of *sodium nitrite solution*; gas is evolved vigorously.
2. To 2 ml of a 10% solution add 1 ml of *ferric chloride test-solution*; a red colour is produced. Add excess hydrochloric acid; the solution becomes colourless. Add excess ammonia; the solution becomes red again.
3. To 2 ml of a 10% solution add 1 drop of *liquefied phenol*, shake, and add carefully without shaking 5 ml of *dilute sodium hypochlorite solution*; a blue colour is produced.

Actions and uses. Glycine is the simplest amino acid and is a constituent of many proteins. It is used for its buffering properties in antacid preparations and in some aspirin preparations to reduce gastric irritation. A 15% solution has been used as a bladder irrigation during operations for transurethral section of the prostate.

Preparations

Preparations available include TABLETS containing glycine 180 mg with calcium carbonate 420 mg and tablets containing glycine 300 mg with aspirin 600 mg.

Glymidine

The sodium salt of 5-(methoxyethoxy)-2-phenylsulphonylaminopyrimidine *or* N-[5-(2-methoxyethoxy)pyrimidin-2-yl]benzenesulphonamide sodium

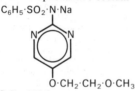

$C_{13}H_{14}N_3NaO_4S = 331.3$

OTHER NAMES: Glycodiazine; Glymidine Sodium; *Gondafon*®

Description. A white crystalline powder.

Solubility. Soluble in water; very slightly soluble in alcohol.

Identification. MELTING-POINT. About 223°.

Metabolism. HALF-LIFE. About 4 hours.

METABOLIC REACTIONS. Demethylation and oxidation to form 2-benzenesulphonamido-5-(2-hydroxyethoxy)pyrimidine and 2-benzenesulphonamido-5-carboxymethoxypyrimidine.

EXCRETION. After an oral dose, glymidine is excreted almost entirely in the urine as the above metabolites.

FURTHER INFORMATION. Estimations in plasma and urine—H. Held *et al.*, *Arzneimittel-Forsch.*, 1970, **20**, 1927 and J. C. Soyfer *et al.*, *Chim. Ther.*, 1969, **4**, 131.

Actions and uses. Glymidine is an oral hypoglycaemic agent with actions and uses similar to Chlorpropamide. It is used for the control of mild to moderate diabetes where dietary treatment alone has failed.
The usual initial daily dose taken at breakfast is 500 milligrams which may be increased to a maximum of 1.5 grams as necessary.

Undesirable effects. Skin sensitisation and gastro-intestinal disturbances may occur and, rarely, leucopenia and purpura.

Precautions and contra-indications. It should be used with caution in elderly patients. It is contra-indicated in severe hepatic and renal disease.

Preparations

Preparations available include TABLETS containing glymidine 500 mg.

Gold (^{198}Au) Injection

A sterile colloidal solution of gold-198 stabilised with gelatin. It may be prepared by reducing a salt of gold-198 with a suitable reducing agent, such as dextrose in alkaline solution, in the presence of gelatin.

OTHER NAMES: Auri Colloidalis (^{198}Au) Solutio Iniectabilis; Colloidal Gold (^{198}Au) Injection

A standard is given in the European Pharmacopoeia Vol. III

CAUTION. *This material is radioactive and any regulations in force must be complied with.*

Gold-198 is a radioactive isotope of gold which decays by emission of β^--radiation mainly of maximum energy 0.961 MeV and γ-radiation mainly of energy 0.412 MeV. It has a half-life of 2.70 days. It may be prepared by neutron irradiation of gold. It contains not more than 10% of gold-199.

Description. A deep red colloidal solution. About 80 per cent of the radioactivity is present in particles between 5 and 50 nm in diameter unless a narrower range within these limits is prescribed or ordered.

Acidity or alkalinity. pH 4.0 to 8.0.

Sterilisation. It is sterilised by heating in an autoclave.

Storage. It should be stored in an area assigned for the purpose. The storage conditions should be such that the maximum radiation-dose-rate to which persons may be exposed is reduced to an acceptable level. Glass containers may darken under the effects of radiation.

Labelling. The label on the container should state (1) the content of gold-198 expressed in microcuries or millicuries at a given date and hour, (2) that the injection is radioactive, and (3) that it does not contain a bactericide, or the name and proportion of any added bactericide.
The label on the package states (1) the total volume in the container and (2) the content of total gold.

Actions and uses. Gold (^{198}Au) injection is used mainly to control malignant effusions in the peritoneal, pleural, or pericardial cavities.
The usual dose is 75 millicuries for a pleural cavity or 130 millicuries for a peritoneal cavity, administered after most of the effusion has been aspirated; it is usual to attempt redistribution of the dense colloidal metal particles within the body cavity by subsequently tilting the patient.
The treatment, when successful, slows down or prevents fluid accumulation, and it may be repeated after an interval of about 8 weeks.
Gold (^{198}Au) injection is also used by intralymphatic infiltration in the treatment of malignant melanoma involving the limbs or of lymph nodes involved by tumours of lymphoid tissue. It is occasionally administered by intra-articular injection for the treatment of persistent joint effusions, usually in rheumatoid arthritis.

Gold (^{198}Au) injection has also been used for diagnostic purposes such as determination of liver blood flow and scanning of the reticulo-endothelial system. The usual dose is 10 to 250 microcuries by intravenous injection. It has also been used in the estimation of reticulo-endothelial activity, the usual dose being 10 to 100 microcuries by intravenous injection. For both these purposes it has been superseded by colloidal preparations of technetium-99m.

Gold (^{198}Au) has also been used in a dosage of 100 to 250 microcuries by intravenous injection for scanning the liver to delineate anatomical abnormalities but ^{99m}Tc colloids are now used for this purpose.

Gonadorelin

see under HYPOTHALAMIC RELEASING FACTORS

Gonadotrophin, Chorionic

A dry sterile preparation of the gonad-stimulating substance obtained from the urine of pregnant women.

OTHER NAMES: *Chorulon®*; *Gonadotraphon LH®*; *Pregnyl®*
Apocrine-S® and *Ovocept®* (both with oestradiol benzoate); *Nymfalon®* (with progesterone); *PG600®* (with serum gonadotrophin); *Apocrine-E®* (with alpha tocopheryl acetate)

A standard is given in the British Pharmacopoeia 1973

Description. A white powder.

Solubility. Soluble in water.

Storage. It should be stored in containers sealed to exclude micro-organisms, at a temperature not exceeding 20°, and protected from light. Under these conditions it may be expected to retain its potency for 3 years.

Actions and uses. The action of chorionic gonadotrophin differs from that of the gonadotrophic hormone of the anterior pituitary gland. In the female, the action of the former is predominantly luteinising and that of the latter mainly follicle-stimulating. In the male, chorionic gonadotrophin stimulates the interstitial cells of the testes and consequently the secretion of androgens and the development of the secondary sexual characteristics. It is of value in cryptorchidism.

In the female, its most important use is in inducing ovulation after pretreatment with follicle-stimulating hormone. The results of treatment of other conditions with chorionic gonadotrophin have been disappointing. It has been used in the preventive treatment of habitual abortion, in metropathia haemorrhagica, and in secondary amenorrhoea.

For the treatment of cryptorchidism, the usual dose is 1500 units intramuscularly 3 times a week; in male secondary hypogonadism, 4000 units intramuscularly 3 times a week initially, reducing thereafter according to the clinical response.

For the induction of ovulation, a single injection of 5000 to 10000 units is given after pretreatment with follicle stimulating hormone as described under Menotrophin.

Veterinary uses. Chorionic gonadotrophin is used to stimulate ovulation of ripe follicles and for the treatment of follicular cysts. The usual dose by intramuscular or intravenous injection for horses, cattle, and pigs is 3 to 10 units per kilogram body-weight as a single dose.

Preparations

CHORIONIC GONADOTROPHIN INJECTION: a sterile solution of chorionic gonadotrophin in water for injections. It is prepared by dissolving the contents of a sealed container in water for injections immediately before use. The sealed container may also contain added inert substances.

Available as a powder in ampoules containing 100, 500, 1000, 1500, and 5000 units of chorionic gonadotrophin.
A standard for this injection is given in the British Pharmacopoeia 1973
Containers and *Labelling:* see the entry on Injections for general information on containers and labelling.
Storage: the sealed container should be stored at a temperature not exceeding 20°, protected from light. Under these conditions it may be expected to retain its potency for at least 3 years. The injection decomposes on storage and should be used immediately after preparation.

OTHER PREPARATIONS available include a veterinary INJECTION containing chorionic gonadotrophin 200 units with oestradiol benzoate 1 mg per ml in 25-ml vials, a veterinary injection containing chorionic gonadotrophin 250 units with oestradiol benzoate 1 mg per ml in 20-ml vials, a veterinary injection reconstituted from vials of powder containing chorionic gonadotrophin 200 units with serum gonadotrophin 400 units, a veterinary injection containing chorionic gonadotrophin 200 units with alpha tocopheryl acetate 30 mg per ml in 25-ml vials, and a veterinary injection reconstituted from vials of powder containing chorionic gonadotrophin 3000 units with progesterone 125 mg.

Gonadotrophin, Human Menopausal

see MENOTROPHIN

Gonadotrophin, Serum

A dry sterile preparation of the follicle-stimulating glycoprotein fraction obtained from the plasma of mares in the 60th to 75th days of pregnancy.

OTHER NAMES: *Apocrine-A®*; *Folligon®*; *Gestyl®*; *Gonadotraphon FSH®*; Gonadotrophinum Sericum; Pregnant Mares' Serum
PG600® (with chorionic gonadotrophin)

A standard is given in the British Pharmacopoeia Addendum 1977 and in the British Pharmacopoeia (Veterinary)

Description. A white or pale grey amorphous powder.

Solubility. Soluble in water.

Uses. Serum gonadotrophin has been used in conditions associated with a deficiency of gonadotrophins. Doses of 500 to 3000 units daily by intramuscular injection have been used.

Veterinary uses. Serum gonadotrophin is used to promote follicular growth and for the control of oestrus. The usual dose by subcutaneous or intramuscular injection for cattle is 1000 to 3000 units and for sheep 750 units.

Preparations

SERUM GONADOTROPHIN INJECTION: a sterile solution of serum gonadotrophin in water for injections. It is prepared by dissolving the contents of a sealed container in water for injections immediately before use. The sealed container may also contain added inert substances and buffering agents.

Available as a powder in vials containing 400, 1000, 3000, and 18 750 units of serum gonadotrophin.
A standard for this injection is given in the British Pharmacopoeia Addendum 1977 and in the British Pharmacopoeia (Veterinary)
Containers and *Labelling:* see the entry on Injections for general information on containers and labelling.
Storage: the sealed container should be stored at a temperature not exceeding 15°, protected from light. Under these conditions it may be expected to retain its potency for at least 2 years.

OTHER PREPARATIONS available include a veterinary injection containing serum gonadotrophin 200 units per ml in 25-ml vials, and a veterinary injection reconstituted from vials of powder containing serum gonadotrophin 400 units with chorionic gonadotrophin 200 units.

Gonorrhoea

Gonorrhoea is due to infection with the Gram-negative coccus *Neisseria gonorrhoeae*. It has an incubation period of 3 to 10 days.
In the male, there is usually inflammation of the urinary meatus, dysuria, and a purulent white discharge.
In the female, the disease is often symptomless but there may be inflammation of the cervix uteri, the vaginal fornices, and the urethra. Inflammation may extend to the fallopian tubes (salpingitis) and may resemble appendicitis.
Proctitis may occur in either sex and is marked by anal discharge, burning rectal pain, and blood and pus in the stools.
Diagnosis of gonorrhoea is made by examination of smears and cultures from the affected areas.
The condition is treated with benzylpenicillin or other substances to which the organism is sensitive.

Gout

Gout is a disorder of purine metabolism which results in the deposition of urate crystals in and around joints. It is characterised by recurrent attacks of pain and swelling in joints, the big toe being most often affected. Later, deposits of urate (tophi) may appear adjacent to the joints, in other soft tissues, and in the kidney. The disorder occurs more commonly in men than in women and is often familial. It may also be secondary to renal tubular disease, neoplasia, or the effects of drugs, particularly the thiazide diuretics and frusemide.
Anti-inflammatory agents (such as indomethacin and phenylbutazone) or colchicine relieve the pain of gout and can be used to cut short or prevent the acute attack. In refractory cases, corticosteroids or corticotrophin may be effective.
For long-term treatment, uricosuric agents such as probenecid and sulphinpyrazone increase the urinary excretion rate of uric acid and will cause a gradual resorption of tophi and disappearance of the symptoms of gout. The xanthine-oxidase inhibitor allopurinol likewise causes the gradual disappearance of tophi and the symptoms of gout by blocking the conversion of xanthine to uric acid. These drugs should not be given in acute gout.

Grand Mal

see under EPILEPSY

Granules

Granules are preparations of medicinal substances usually in the form of small irregular particles ranging from 2 to 4 millimetres in diameter.
Effervescent granules evolve carbon dioxide when added to water.
Some granules are intended to be dissolved or dispersed in water before taking; others are placed on the tongue and swallowed with a draught of water.

Graves' Disease

see HYPERTHYROIDISM

Green Monkey Disease

see under MARBURG VIRUS (GREEN MONKEY) DISEASE

Green S and Tartrazine Solution

Consists of a solution containing 0.5% of green S, food grade of commerce, and 0.5% of tartrazine, food grade of commerce, in chloroform water.

A standard is given in the British Pharmaceutical Codex 1973

Uses. Green S and tartrazine solution is used as a green colouring agent for pharmaceutical preparations. It is an ingredient of piperazine citrate elixir.

Griseofulvin

(2S,6'R)-7-Chloro-2',4,6-trimethoxy-6'-methylbenzo-furan-2-spiro-1'-cyclohex-2'-ene-3,4'-dione

$C_{17}H_{17}ClO_6 = 352.8$

OTHER NAMES: *Fulcin*®; Griseofulvinum; *Grisovin*®

A standard is given in the European Pharmacopoeia Vol. II

Description. A white to pale cream, odourless, tasteless powder the particles of which are generally up to 5 μm in maximum dimension, although larger particles, which may occasionally exceed 30 μm, may be present.

Solubility. Very slightly soluble in water; soluble, at 20°, in 300 parts of dehydrated alcohol, in 25 parts of chloroform, in 20 parts of acetone, in 250 parts of methyl alcohol, and in 3 parts of tetrachloroethane.

Moisture content. Not more than 1%, determined by drying at 105°.

Specific rotation. +354° to +364°, determined on a 1% solution in dimethylformamide.

Identification. TEST. Dissolve about 5 mg in 1 ml of sulphuric acid and add 5 mg of powdered potassium dichromate; a wine-red colour is produced.

MELTING-POINT. About 221°.

ULTRAVIOLET ABSORPTION. In alcohol (95%), maximum at 291 nm (E1%, 1cm = 686).

INFRA-RED ABSORPTION. Major peaks at 1135, 1210, 1220, 1350, 1583, and 1611 cm⁻¹ (see Appendix 2a: Infra-red Spectra).

Determination in body fluids. ULTRAVIOLET SPECTRO-PHOTOMETRY. In urine: metabolite of griseofulvin—M. Rowland and S. Riegelman, *J. pharm. Sci.*, 1973, **62**, 2030.

SPECTROFLUORIMETRY. In blood—M. Kraml *et al.*, *J. pharm. Sci.*, 1965, **54**, 655.

GAS CHROMATOGRAPHY. In plasma—H. J. Schwarz *et al.*, *J. pharm. Sci.*, 1976, **65**, 370.

HIGH PRESSURE LIQUID CHROMATOGRAPHY. In urine: determination of 6-demethylgriseofulvin—E. Papp *et al.*, *J. pharm. Sci.*, 1976, **65**, 441.

Metabolism. ABSORPTION. Irregularly and incompletely absorbed after oral administration; absorption of griseofulvin is particle-size dependent; its absorption is increased when administered with fatty meals or milk and decreased when administered concomitantly with phenobarbitone.

BLOOD CONCENTRATION. After an oral daily dose of 0.5 to 1.0 g, peak plasma concentrations of 1 to 3 μg/ml are attained; after single oral doses of 0.25 to 3 g, peak plasma concentrations of 0.3 to 1.7 μg/ml are attained in 4 hours.

HALF-LIFE. Plasma half-life for the α-phase, about 1 hour and for the β-phase, 9 to 22 hours.

DISTRIBUTION. Localised in the skin, nails, and hair roots; secreted in the sweat and crosses the placenta.

METABOLIC REACTIONS. O-Demethylation at the 4- and 6-positions and glucuronic acid conjugation of the de-methylated metabolites.

EXCRETION. After an oral dose, about 35% is excreted in the urine as the 6-demethylated metabolite in 8 days; after an intravenous dose about 65% is excreted in the urine as the same metabolite in 72 hours; large amounts of an oral dose are eliminated unchanged in the faeces but less than 1% is excreted unchanged in the urine; the urinary excretion of 6-demethylgriseofulvin appears to be pH-dependent; small amounts of the 4-demethylated metabolite are excreted in the urine.

FURTHER INFORMATION. Absorption characteristics—W. L. Chiou and S. Riegelman, *J. pharm. Sci.*, 1971, **60**, 1376; absorption, metabolism, and excretion—C.-C. Lin *et al.*, *J. Pharmac. exp. Ther.*, 1973, **187**, 415; urinary excretion—M. Rowland and S. Riegelman, *J. pharm. Sci.*, 1973, **62**, 2030; in skin, plasma and sweat—V. P. Shah *et al.*, *J. pharm. Sci.*, 1972, **61**, 634.

Bioavailability. The absorption of griseofulvin is dependent upon particle size, dissolution rate, and on inter- and intra-subject variations. The use of a small particle size (about 5 μm) has improved bioavailability but it is still poorly absorbed with only about 50% reaching the circulation in 30 to 40 hours. Various methods have been attempted to improve absorption, of which the use of dispersions in polyethylene glycol and in a mixture with microcrystalline cellulose have been successful.

FURTHER INFORMATION. Use of urinary excretion data to assess bioavailability—T. R. Bates and J. A. L. Sequeira, *J. pharm. Sci.*, 1975, **64**, 709; dissolution rate and bioavailability—K. Yamamoto *et al.*, *J. Pharmacokin. Biopharm.*, 1974, **2**, 487.

Actions and uses. Griseofulvin is an antibiotic which when administered by mouth has an antifungal action against a wide range of dermatophytoses. After absorption from the gastro-intestinal tract, it is deposited in the keratin of the nails, hair, and skin, thus preventing fungal invasion of newly formed cells.

Griseofulvin is effective against infections caused b various species of *Trichophyton*, *Epidermophyton*, and *Microsporum*, including ringworm and onychomycosis. It is ineffective against infections caused by yeasts or *Candida albicans* and against most systemic fungal infections.

The usual daily dosage is 0.5 to 1 gram for adults and the usual dose for children is 10 milligrams per kilogram body-weight daily in single or divided doses. For superficial forms of ringworm, treatment should be continued for 3 to 6 weeks and, for infections of the nails, up to 12 months.

Undesirable effects. Headache, skin rashes, and gastro-intestinal disturbances may occur but these are usually mild and transient and do not necessitate interruption of treatment.

Drug interactions. Griseofulvin may decrease the response to warfarin and other oral anticoagulants, and barbiturates may reduce the effectiveness of griseofulvin.

Veterinary uses. Griseofulvin is an antifungal agent used in the treatment of ringworm in horses, cattle, pigs, dogs, and cats. The usual dose for horses, cattle and pigs is 7.5 to 10 milligrams daily for 7 days, and for dogs and cats 15 to 20 milligrams per kilogram body-weight daily for 10 to 14 days but in small animals, especially long-haired breeds, treatment may be needed for 6 to 12 weeks.

Preparations

GRISEOFULVIN TABLETS: available as tablets containing 125 and 500 mg; they may be film coated.

A standard for these tablets is given in the British Pharmacopoeia 1973

Containers and *Storage:* see the entry on Tablets for general information on containers and storage. Containers should be airtight.

Labelling: the label on the container should state the date after which the tablets are not intended to be used and the conditions under which they should be stored.

Advice for patients: the tablets should preferably be taken after meals and daily doses after the main meal. Treatment should not be discontinued without the advice of the prescriber.

OTHER PREPARATIONS available include a MIXTURE containing griseofulvin 125 mg in 5 ml, diluent syrup, life of diluted mixture 14 days; and a PREMIX containing griseofulvin 7.5%.

Guaiphenesin

3-(2-Methoxyphenoxy)propane-1,2-diol

$C_{10}H_{14}O_4 = 198.2$

OTHER NAMES: Glyceryl Guaiacolate; Guaifenesin; *Robitussin*®

A standard is given in the British Pharmaceutical Codex 1973

Description. Odourless white crystals or crystalline aggregates.

Solubility. Soluble, at 20°, in 33 parts of water, in 11 parts of alcohol, in 200 parts of ether, in 11 parts of chloroform, and in 15 parts of propylene glycol; soluble, with warming, in 15 parts of glycerol.

Acidity. A 1% solution has a pH of 5 to 7.

Identification. ULTRAVIOLET ABSORPTION. In water, maximum at 272 nm (E1%, 1cm = 120).

INFRA-RED ABSORPTION. Major peaks at 746, 1000, 1020, 1042, 1235, and 1250 cm^{-1} (see Appendix 2b: Infra-red Spectra).

Determination in body fluids. GAS CHROMATOGRAPHY. In blood—W. R. Maynard and R. B. Bruce, *J. pharm. Sci.*, 1970, **59**, 1346.

Metabolism. ABSORPTION. Readily absorbed after oral administration.

BLOOD CONCENTRATION. After an oral dose of 600 mg as a solution given to fasting subjects, a peak plasma concentration of about 1.4 μg/ml is attained in 15 minutes.

HALF-LIFE. Plasma half-life, about 1 hour.

METABOLIC REACTIONS. Rapidly metabolised by oxidation to β-(2-methoxyphenoxy)lactic acid and also, in rabbits, to the acetic acid form, and by hydroxylation to β-(4-hydroxy-2-methoxyphenoxy)lactic acid.

EXCRETION. The only detectable urinary metabolite in man is β-(2-methoxyphenoxy)lactic acid.

FURTHER INFORMATION. W. R. Maynard and R. B. Bruce, *J. pharm. Sci.*, 1970, **59**, 1346; W. J. A. Vandenheuvel *et al.*, *J. pharm. Sci.*, 1972, **61**, 1997.

Actions and uses. Guaiphenesin is said to reduce the viscosity of tenacious sputum and is used as an expectorant in cough mixtures and tablets. In large doses, it has a muscle-relaxant effect similar to that of mephenesin, but it is not used for this purpose.
The usual dose is 100 to 200 milligrams every 2 to 4 hours.

Preparations

Preparations available include an ELIXIR containing guaiphenesin 100 mg in 5 ml, diluent syrup, life of diluted elixir 14 days, and a number of compound preparations in which guaiphenesin is an ingredient.

Guanethidine Monosulphate

1-[2-(Perhydroazocin-1-yl)ethyl]guanidine monosulphate

$C_{10}H_{24}N_4O_4S = 296.4$

OTHER NAMES: Guanethidine Sulphate; *Ismelin*®
Ganda® (with adrenaline)

A standard is given in the British Pharmacopoeia 1973

Description. A colourless, crystalline, almost odourless powder.

Solubility. Soluble, at 20°, in 1.5 parts of water; very slightly soluble in alcohol; practically insoluble in ether and in chloroform.

Acidity. A 2% solution has a pH of 5 to 6.

Dissociation constants. pK$_a$ 8.3, 11.4 (20°).

Sterilisation. Solutions are sterilised by heating in an autoclave or by filtration.

Storage. It should be stored in airtight containers, protected from light.

Identification. TESTS. 1. Dissolve about 25 mg in 5 ml of water and add 1.5 ml of *sodium hydroxide solution*, 1 ml of *1-naphthol solution*, and, dropwise with shaking, 0.5 ml of *dilute sodium hypochlorite solution*; a vivid pink precipitate is produced which becomes red on standing.
2. Dissolve about 25 mg in 25 ml of water and add 20 ml of *trinitrophenol solution*; a precipitate is produced which, after washing with water, melts at about 153°.

MELTING-POINT. About 253°.

Determination in body fluids. GAS CHROMATOGRAPHY. In plasma or urine—P. Erdtmansky and T. J. Goehl, *Analyt. Chem.*, 1975, **47**, 750 and J. H. Hengstmann *et al.*, *Analyt. Chem.*, 1974, **46**, 34.

Metabolism. ABSORPTION. Poor and variable after oral administration.

BLOOD CONCENTRATION. After an oral dose equivalent to 41 mg of the base, peak plasma concentrations for total drug (drug plus metabolites) of about 20 ng/ml are attained within 2 hours; after an intravenous dose of about 12 mg, initial plasma concentrations of about 315 ng/ml are obtained which decline to 2 ng/ml after 72 hours; after an intramuscular dose, peak concentrations are attained within about 5 minutes.

HALF-LIFE. The decline in plasma concentration after an intravenous dose shows a triphasic decline and the half-life for each phase is about 12 minutes, 3 hours, and 40 hours respectively; the overall half-life based upon urinary excretion data is about 9 days.

DISTRIBUTION. Highly localised within the tissues and only slowly released; guanethidine does not cross the blood/brain barrier and it is not excreted into the milk.

METABOLIC REACTIONS. Ring fission to form 2-(6-carboxyhexylamino)ethylguanidine which may then cyclise to form 1-(6-carboxyhexyl)-2-iminoimidazolidine; in addition, N-oxidation occurs at the nitrogen atom in the azocine ring.

EXCRETION. After an oral dose, 3 to 27% is excreted in the urine and 20 to 50% in the faeces; after an intravenous dose, 20 to 40% is excreted in the urine in 24 hours and up to 90% in 10 days; of the excreted material, up to 60% is unchanged; after an intramuscular dose, 50% is excreted in the urine and 3% in the faeces in 2 to 3 days; following an intravenous dose to subjects with renal function impairment, about 18% of the dose is excreted in the urine in 24 hours and 80% in 17 days; in these subjects, the ratio of unchanged to metabolised drug in the urine is decreased.

Actions and uses. Guanethidine is a hypotensive agent which lowers the blood pressure by selectively blocking transmission in post-ganglionic adrenergic nerves, thus preventing the release of noradrenaline from the nerve endings.

It does not reduce, but may enhance, the effects of injected adrenaline and noradrenaline, and does not prevent the release of these amines from the suprarenal medulla; it may therefore cause a rise in blood pressure in patients with phaeochromocytoma.

Guanethidine is used to control hypertension. Treatment is started with an oral dosage of 10 to 30 milligrams of guanethidine monosulphate daily, and this is increased by 10 milligrams every 5 to 7 days, to a maximum which rarely exceeds 75 milligrams, until the desired reduction in blood pressure is attained.

Doses of 10 to 20 milligrams may be given by intramuscular injection to control hypertensive crises; the resulting fall in blood pressure usually reaches a maximum in 1 to 2 hours.

The effect of the drug may persist for several days after withdrawal. Tolerance rarely develops. A thiazide diuretic may be given with guanethidine to enhance the hypotensive effect.

Guanethidine eye-drops give rise to an initial mydriasis and increased aqueous outflow followed by miosis and reduced aqueous secretion. The eye-drops are used for the reduction of intra-ocular pressure in open-angle glaucoma and for the treatment of exophthalmos and lid retraction due to endocrine imbalance.

Undesirable effects. Severe postural hypotension, especially with exercise, and diarrhoea may occur.

Precautions. Guanethidine should not be given to patients who are being treated with a monoamine-oxidase inhibitor, such as isocarboxazid, nialamide, phenelzine, or tranylcypromine, or within about 2 weeks of the discontinuation of such treatment.

Drug interactions. The antihypertensive effect of guanethidine is prevented or reversed by simultaneous treatment with antidepressant drugs of the imipramine and amitriptyline ("tricyclic") type which block the neuronal uptake of guanethidine.

Guanethidine potentiates the pressor action of directly-acting sympathomimetic amines such as noradrenaline and phenylephrine.

Preparations

GUANETHIDINE EYE-DROPS: consisting of a sterile solution containing up to 5% of guanethidine monosulphate in a suitable aqueous vehicle.

Containers and *Labelling:* see the entry on Eye-drops for general information on containers and labelling.

Advice for patients: see the entry on Eye-drops for general information on the use of eye-drops. Treatment should not be discontinued without the advice of the prescriber.

GUANETHIDINE TABLETS: available as tablets containing 10 and 25 mg of guanethidine monosulphate; they may be coloured.

A standard for these tablets is given in the British Pharmacopoeia 1973

Containers and *Storage:* see the entry on Tablets for general information on containers and storage. Containers should be airtight and light resistant.

Advice for patients: the tablets should be taken at regular intervals. Treatment should not be discontinued without the advice of the prescriber.

OTHER PREPARATIONS available include EYE-DROPS containing guanethidine monosulphate 3% with adrenaline 0.5%, eye-drops containing guanethidine monosulphate 5% with adrenaline 0.5%, eye-drops containing guanethidine monosulphate 5% with adrenaline 1%, and an INJECTION containing guanethidine monosulphate 10 mg per ml in 1-ml ampoules.

Gumboro Disease Vaccine

see INFECTIOUS BURSAL DISEASE VACCINE, LIVING

Haemodialysis

see under DIALYSIS

Haemophilia

Haemophilia is an inherited haemorrhagic disorder occurring almost exclusively in males and characterised by a tendency to excessive haemorrhage in response to trivial injury.

When an X-chromosome-linked recessive character gives rise to a deficiency of functional antihaemophilic factor (factor VIII) in the blood, the haemorrhagic disorder is known as **haemophilia A.** The extent of this inherited deficiency varies from family to family and some symptoms of haemophilia may be exhibited by an individual in whom the capacity of factor VIII to take part in haemostasis is reduced below about 30 to 40% of normal. In infancy, the bleeding tendency may be manifest by the appearance of cutaneous ecchymoses or haematomata in the soft tissues.

In severely affected patients whose factor VIII level is 2% or less, joint bleeds (haemarthroses) are likely to occur as soon as the child begins to crawl or walk. Unchecked, these bleeds result in increasing deformity, limitation of movement, and destruction of joints.

The knees, elbows, and ankles are most commonly affected. Bleeding into soft tissue also occurs. As it is unrestricted, blood may spread widely through subcutaneous tissues. Excessive bleeding is the rule after dental extractions and other minor surgery, and tonsillectomy and other major operations may give rise to fatal haemorrhage.

When bleeding occurs, the intravenous infusion of human antihaemophilic fraction provides factor VIII so that normal haemostasis can occur. Treatment should be given as soon as possible after the start of a bleed. Intravenous human antihaemophilic fraction, to maintain a level of above 40% of normal, allows even major surgery to be done. In about 10% of haemophiliacs antibodies against factor VIII are produced; such patients should undergo surgery only in extreme circumstances as infusion of factor VIII is likely to be ineffective.

For dental extractions the level of factor VIII in the patient is raised to 50% of normal with dried antihaemophilic fraction, followed by a plasminogen inhibitor such as aminocaproic acid or tranexamic acid. Dried human thrombin for topical use is used to dry the socket and sometimes a dental splint may be applied. Oral tranexamic acid may be given for 7 to 10 days. Further factor VIII is given after a simple extraction only if bleeding occurs. For multiple or difficult extractions further doses of factor VIII may be advisable 24 to 36 hours after operation.

There are many other heritable defects of blood coagulation, each due to hereditary deficiency of one or other factor essential for blood coagulation. They are all characterised by the tendency to bleed more readily than is normal.

Haemophilia B (Christmas Disease) is a congenital deficiency of factor IX and occurs in about 10% of haemophiliacs. Treatment is similar to that for haemophilia A but dried human factor IX fraction is used.

Blood preparations used in haemophilia. The principal preparations used for treating bleeding in haemophilia A are concentrates of human factor VIII—see Antihaemophilic Fraction, Human, Dried.

Freeze-dried concentrates of animal factor VIII (porcine and bovine) have a high potency but are antigenic. They are therefore indicated mainly for the emergency treatment of patients with high titre factor VIII antibodies in whom the human concentrate is ineffective, or when there are insufficient quantities of human factor VIII available. Since thrombocytopenia and severe allergic reactions may occur, corticosteroids and antihistamines are usually given at the same time.

Cryoprecipitate, prepared from fresh-frozen plasma, is rich in factor VIII and fibrinogen. It is widely used for the treatment of haemophilia but has the disadvantage that its potency is not known, preparation for use is tedious, and it must be stored in a deep-freezer. Where possible material of the same ABO and Rh groups as the patients should be used.

Human plasma and dried human plasma were formerly used but their potency is insufficient to cover surgical procedures.

The dose in units of antihaemophilic factor VIII or IX may be calculated by multiplying the patient's weight in kilograms by the percentage rise in factor VIII or IX concentration and dividing by the constant for the material used. The constant for plasma is 2.0; for human antihaemophilic fraction 1.5, for human factor IX fraction 0.7, and for concentrate of animal factor VIII 1.0.

Haemorrhoids

Haemorrhoids (Piles) are varicosities of the superior rectal vein. They cause soreness and pain on defaecation, but the principal symptom is bleeding of bright red blood which at first occurs only on defaecation, and later may occur independently of bowel action. Persistent blood loss may lead to a secondary anaemia. Haemorrhoids which have prolapsed and thrombosed are painful and may become infected or gangrenous.

Treatment may consist in the regulation of the diet to produce soft stools which pass through the anus with a minimum of irritation and the application of soothing ointment or suppositories. Patients should be instructed to take hygienic measures and when necessary to replace protruding piles after defaecation.

Uncomplicated haemorrhoids which bleed may be treated with oily phenol injection as described under Phenol. The aim is to produce fibrosis around the pile, thereby obliterating the lumen of the vessel and drawing up the haemorrhoid. In the presence of complications, for example prolapse, haemorrhoids require surgical treatment.

Halibut-liver Oil

The fixed oil obtained from the fresh or suitably preserved livers of the halibut species belonging to the genus *Hippoglossus* (Fam. Pleuronectidae). It may be obtained by treatment of the livers with weak alkali and separation of the oil. It contains not less than 30000 units of vitamin-A activity per gram.

A standard is given in the British Pharmacopoeia 1973

Constituents. Halibut livers yield oils with vitamin-A activities varying from about 15000 to 250000 units per

g. The antirachitic activity (vitamin D) is less variable, being up to about 3000 units per g. The composition of the fatty acids of halibut-liver oil is similar to that of the fatty acids of cod-liver oil, but the proportion of unsaturated fatty acids is lower.

Description. A pale to golden yellow liquid with a fishy but not rancid odour.

Solubility. Very slightly soluble in alcohol; miscible with ether, with chloroform, and with light petroleum.

Weight per ml. At 20°, 0.915 to 0.925 g.

Storage. It should be stored in well-filled airtight containers, protected from light.

Actions and uses. Halibut-liver oil is used as a means of administering vitamins A and D; the proportion of vitamin A to vitamin D is usually higher in halibut-liver oil than in cod-liver oil. Gross overdosage can lead to vitamin-A and vitamin-D poisoning.

The usual dose for adults and children is 0.15 millilitre (prophylactic) to 0.5 millilitre daily.

Undesirable effects. As for Calciferol and Concentrated Vitamin A Solution.

Preparation

HALIBUT-LIVER OIL CAPSULES: consisting of halibut-liver oil, which may be mixed with a suitable fixed vegetable oil as diluent, if necessary, to give a volume of 0.15 ml per capsule, enclosed in a soft capsule. Each capsule contains about 4000 units of vitamin-A activity; vitamin-D activity is also present.

A standard for these capsules is given in the British Pharmacopoeia 1973

Containers: see the entry on Capsules for general information on containers.

Labelling: the label on the container should state that each capsule contains 4000 units of vitamin-A activity and the label on the container or the label on the package should state the date of preparation.

Storage: see the entry on Capsules for general information on storage. They should be stored at a temperature not exceeding 20°, protected from light. Under these conditions they may be expected to retain their potency for at least 3 years.

Advice for patients: the capsules should not be taken for prolonged periods without medical advice.

Haloperidol

4-[4-(4-Chlorophenyl)-4-hydroxypiperidino]-4'-fluoro-butyrophenone

$C_{21}H_{23}ClFNO_2 = 375.9$

OTHER NAMES: *Haldol®; Serenace®*

A standard is given in the British Pharmacopoeia 1973

Description. An odourless, tasteless, white to faintly yellowish, amorphous or microcrystalline powder.

Solubility. Practically insoluble in water; soluble, at 20°, in 50 parts of alcohol, in 200 parts of ether, and in 20 parts of chloroform.

Identification. MELTING-POINT. About 149°.

ULTRAVIOLET ABSORPTION. In a mixture of 1 volume of 1N hydrochloric acid and 99 volumes of methyl alcohol, maximum at about 245 nm (E1%, 1cm = 340).

INFRA-RED ABSORPTION. Major peaks at 827, 998, 1137, 1158, 1218, and 1598 cm^{-1} (see Appendix 2a: Infra-red Spectra).

Determination in body fluids. GAS CHROMATOGRAPHY. In plasma: avoids interference from chlorpromazine and its metabolites—I. A. Zingales, *J. Chromat.*, 1971, **54**, 15.

Metabolism. ABSORPTION. Readily absorbed after oral administration.

BLOOD CONCENTRATION. On a daily dosage of 50 μg/kg by mouth, steady-state plasma concentrations of about 2 ng/ml are obtained.

HALF-LIFE. The decline in plasma concentration is biphasic, the initial phase having a half-life of about 30 minutes and the second phase, 12 to 22 hours.

DISTRIBUTION. Highly localised in the tissues and rapidly taken up by the brain; volume of distribution, 1200 to 2000 litres.

METABOLIC REACTIONS. Oxidative *N*-dealkylation to β-(4-fluorobenzoyl)propionic acid.

EXCRETION. 24 to 60% of a dose is excreted in the urine and faeces in 7 to 28 days; small amounts may be excreted in the bile.

ENZYME INDUCTION. Haloperidol induces the metabolism of pentobarbitone.

Actions and uses. Haloperidol is a selective central nervous system depressant of the butyrophenone group with properties resembling those of trifluoperazine hydrochloride. As it is almost devoid of peripheral anti-adrenergic effects, it does not cause hypotension and hypothermia is unlikely to occur; it is a powerful anti-emetic. It enhances the action of barbiturates, analgesics, and other depressants of the central nervous system.

Haloperidol is usually of more value in acute psychomotor episodes such as mania, hypomania, and acute schizophrenia than in more chronic psychoses. It is inactive in depression but may help withdrawn apathetic patients to accept treatment. High doses may lead to abnormal wakefulness. Akathisia is a common phenomenon, especially in the elderly, even with moderate dosage.

The usual initial dosage in psychiatric conditions is 6 to 12 milligrams daily, up to 15 milligrams daily in acutely disturbed patients, by mouth or by intramuscular or intravenous injection; the dosage for maintenance is usually in the range 1.5 to 3 milligrams daily. The usual dosage for anxiety neuroses is 500 micrograms daily.

Haloperidol is used in neuroleptanalgesia, usually in combination with potent analgesics, to achieve sedation and analgesia without loss of patient co-operation and with little interference with vital functions, especially in poor-risk cases.

Undesirable effects. Extrapyramidal syndromes are particularly likely to occur. Dystonic reactions and akathisia are common and may not be recognised when they do not resemble classical parkinsonism; dyskinesias may become irreversible. Occasionally, depression may occur during treatment and weight loss may occur during high-dosage treatment.

Precautions and contra-indications. Haloperidol should not be given to patients with disease of the basal ganglia. The effect of oral anticoagulants may be unpredictably reduced by haloperidol.

Poisoning. Heat loss should be prevented and blood pressure maintained by changing posture. Drugs such as benzhexol may be required for the treatment of dystonic effects.

Preparations

HALOPERIDOL INJECTION: a sterile solution of haloperidol as a soluble salt, with suitable pharmaceutical adjuvants, in water for injections. Available in 1- and 2-ml ampoules containing 5 mg of haloperidol per ml and in 2-ml ampoules containing 10 mg of haloperidol per ml. *Containers* and *Labelling:* see the entry on Injections for general information on containers and labelling.

HALOPERIDOL TABLETS: available as tablets containing 0.5, 1.5, 5, 10 and 20 milligrams of haloperidol; they may be coloured.

A standard for these tablets is given in the British Pharmacopoeia 1973

Containers and *Storage:* see the entry on Tablets for general information on containers and storage. Containers should be airtight.

Advice for patients: the tablets may cause drowsiness; persons affected should not drive or operate machinery. Alcohol should be avoided.

OTHER PREPARATIONS available include CAPSULES containing haloperidol 500 micrograms, an ELIXIR containing haloperidol 2 mg per ml, diluent water, life of diluted elixir 14 days—for *Serenace*® with freshly boiled and cooled purified water as the diluent in dilutions containing 50% of the elixir, life of diluted elixir 2 months, and a MIXTURE containing haloperidol 10 mg per ml, to be diluted before administration, preferably with water for preparations containing 0.05% of methyl hydroxybenzoate and 0.005% of propyl hydroxybenzoate.

Halothane

2-Bromo-2-chloro-1,1,1-trifluoroethane, containing 0.01% w/w of thymol as a preservative.

$$CHBrCl \cdot CF_3$$

$C_2HBrClF_3 = 197.4$

OTHER NAMES: *Fluothane*®; Halothanum

A standard is given in the European Pharmacopoeia Vol. III

Description. A colourless mobile heavy liquid with a characteristic odour.

Solubility. Soluble, at 20°, in 400 parts of water; miscible with dehydrated alcohol, with ether, with chloroform, with trichloroethylene, and with fixed and volatile oils.

Weight per ml. At 20°, 1.867 to 1.872 g.

Boiling-point. About 50°.

Stability. On prolonged exposure to ultraviolet radiation, it is decomposed with the formation of halogen acids and free halogens.

Storage. It should be stored in airtight containers, at a temperature not exceeding 25°, protected from light.

Determination in body fluids. GAS CHROMATOGRAPHY. In blood—M. K. Tham et al., Anesthesiology, 1972, **37**, 647.

Metabolism. ABSORPTION. Rapidly absorbed upon inhalation.

BLOOD CONCENTRATION. During the inhalation of 0.5% halothane with continuous ventilation, arterial concentrations are about 16 μg/ml and venous concentrations are 6 to 9 μg/ml, 30 to 60 minutes after beginning anaesthesia.

DISTRIBUTION. Rapidly enters the blood and accumulates in adipose tissue.

METABOLIC REACTIONS. Debromination, dechlorination, and replacement of 1 fluorine atom by a methoxy group followed by glucuronic acid conjugation; about 12% of the absorbed halothane is metabolised to trifluoroacetic acid and bromide; a mercapturic acid is also formed.

EXCRETION. 4 to 23% of a dose is excreted in the urine as trifluoroacetic acid and its salts.

Actions and uses. Halothane is a volatile anaesthetic which is about twice as potent as chloroform and about 4 times as potent as ether. It is not inflammable, is not explosive when mixed with oxygen, and is stable in contact with soda lime. It is not irritant to the skin or mucous membrane, nor does it produce necrosis when spilt on tissues.

Halothane may be administered by any of the usual methods of inducing anaesthesia, although open-mask administration is uneconomical. Because of the high vapour pressure of halothane, vapours saturated with it at 20° contain much too high a concentration, and the use of an apparatus specially calibrated for the administration of halothane is therefore recommended. The patient should be premedicated with an adequate dose of an atropine-like drug.

Anaesthesia can be induced by a concentration of 1.5 to 3% v/v or more of halothane and can be maintained with 0.5 to 1.5% v/v. Induction is rapid, usually without signs of excitement; ventricular tachycardia and other cardiac irregularities rarely occur. Muscular relaxation is obtained at moderately deep levels of anaesthesia with halothane.

As halothane blocks the transmission of nerve impulses through ganglia, ganglion-blocking agents, if used, should be given with caution; however, suxamethonium may be given to increase muscular relaxation if necessary.

Halothane suppresses salivary, mucous, bronchial, and gastric secretions. A substantial fall in blood pressure may occasionally occur during anaesthesia. The pulse rate is usually slow and severe bradycardia is occasionally encountered; this may be controlled by reducing the dosage of the anaesthetic and by the intravenous administration of atropine.

Halothane sensitises the heart to adrenaline and noradrenaline, but to a lesser extent than cyclopropane. Respiratory depression occurs in the deeper planes of anaesthesia and should be regarded as a sign of overdosage. Both blood pressure and respiratory minute volume increase quickly if the concentration administered is decreased.

Recovery from anaesthesia is rapid, but shivering and laryngeal spasm occasionally occur; vomiting is unusual.

Undesirable effects. Liver damage may occur occasionally and caution is necessary in using this anaesthetic for patients who have previously shown this effect after halothane anaesthesia. The incidence of jaundice increases with repeated exposure to halothane.

Poisoning. Signs of overdosage with halothane are bradycardia and profound hypotension, which respond respectively to 500 micrograms of atropine sulphate and up to 10 milligrams of methoxamine hydrochloride, both by intravenous injection. Respiratory depression may also occur, and this should be treated by reducing the concentration of the anaesthetic and giving oxygen.

Haloxon

Bis(2-chloroethyl)   3-chloro-4-methylcoumarin-7-yl phosphate

$C_{14}H_{14}Cl_3O_6P = 415.6$

OTHER NAMES: Equilox®; Loxon®; Whithelmin® Haloxil® (with oxyclozanide)

A standard is given in the British Pharmacopoeia (Veterinary)

Description. A white odourless powder.

Solubility. Practically insoluble in water; soluble, at 20°, in 9 parts of alcohol, in 2 parts of chloroform, and in 4 parts of acetone.

Moisture content. Not more than 1%, determined by drying at 80° in vacuo.

Identification. TEST. Mix 100 mg with 5 ml of sodium hydroxide solution, dissolve with the aid of heat, cool, acidify 1 ml of the solution to litmus paper with dilute nitric acid, and add 1 ml of silver nitrate solution; a white precipitate is produced which is soluble in dilute ammonia solution giving a brown solution which exhibits a green fluorescence when viewed under screened ultraviolet radiation.

MELTING-POINT. About 90°.

ULTRAVIOLET ABSORPTION. In a solution prepared by dissolving in 10 ml of dioxan, adding 0.5 ml of 0.1N hydrochloric acid, and diluting to volume with methyl alcohol, maxima at 290 nm (E1%, 1cm = 262) and at 310 to 315 nm (poorly defined) (E1%, 1cm = 287).

Veterinary Uses. Haloxon is used for the treatment of intestinal nematode infections. The usual dosage given by mouth as a single dose in horses is 75 milligrams per kilogram body-weight, cattle 40 milligrams per kilogram body-weight, sheep 35 to 50 milligrams per kilogram body-weight, pigs 50 milligrams per kilogram body-weight, and poultry 50 to 75 milligrams per kilogram body-weight.

Preparations

COMPOUND HALOXON ORAL PASTE: consisting of haloxon, with cobalt sulphate and copper sulphate, mixed with a suitable edible diluent. Available as an oral paste containing 50% of haloxon and cobalt sulphate and copper sulphate equivalent to 2.1% each of cobalt and copper. In certain parts of the world an oral paste containing 62% of haloxon but without cobalt sulphate or copper sulphate is available.

A standard for this oral paste is given in the British Pharmacopoeia (Veterinary)

Labelling: the label on the container should state the

content of cobalt and copper and that the preparation should not be administered within 7 days of treatment for fluke. This preparation contains an organophosphorus compound and labelling statements (1), (2)(a), (3)(e) and (g), and (4)(j) relating to such preparations given in the entry on Dip Concentrates are applicable. The minimum period that must elapse between cessation of treatment and slaughter of the animals for human consumption is 7 days.

HALOXON DISPERSIBLE POWDER: consisting of haloxon mixed with suitable non-toxic wetting and suspending agents. Available as a dispersible powder containing 75% of haloxon.
A standard for this dispersible powder is given in the British Pharmacopoeia (Veterinary)
Containers and *Storage:* it should be stored in well-filled airtight containers.
Labelling: the label on the container should state the proportion of haloxon in the preparation and the method of use. This preparation contains an organophosphorus compound and labelling statements (1), (2)(a), (3)(d), (e), and (g), and (4)(h), (j), and (k) relating to such preparations given in the entry on Dip Concentrates are applicable.

HALOXON MIXTURE (*Syn.* Haloxon Drench; Haloxon Suspension): an aqueous suspension of haloxon mixed with suitable suspending, dispersing, and preservative agents. It may contain suitable colouring matter. Available as a mixture containing 9.5% of haloxon.
A standard for this mixture is given in the British Pharmacopoeia (Veterinary)
Labelling: the label on the container should state that the container should be shaken before use, that the mixture should be administered undiluted, and that it should not be administered within 7 days of treatment for fluke. This preparation contains an organophosphorus compound and labelling statements (1), (2)(a), (3)(d), (e), and (g), and (4)(h), (j), and (k) relating to such preparations given in the entry on Dip Concentrates are applicable. The minimum period that must elapse between cessation of treatment and slaughter of the animals for human consumption is 7 days.
Storage: contact with metals should be avoided; it should not be allowed to freeze.

HALOXON PELLETS: consisting of haloxon mixed with a suitable cereal diluent and made into pellets for administration by mouth. Available as pellets containing 8% of haloxon.
A standard for these pellets is given in the British Pharmacopoeia (Veterinary)
Containers and *Storage:* they should be stored in airtight containers.
Labelling: this preparation contains an organophosphorus compound and labelling statements (1), (2)(a), (3)(e) and (g), and (4)(h), (j), and (k) relating to such preparations given in the entry on Dip Concentrates are applicable. The minimum period that must elapse between cessation of treatment and slaughter of the animals for human consumption is 7 days.

HALOXON PREMIX: consisting of haloxon mixed with maize flour or other suitable diluent. This preparation is not stable to hot pelleting processes. It must be diluted before administration, by mixing thoroughly with the feed, to give a concentration appropriate to the feeding rate of the animal concerned. Available as a premix containing 8% of haloxon.
A standard for this premix is given in the British Pharmacopoeia (Veterinary)

Containers and *Storage:* see the entry on Premixes for general information on containers and storage.
Labelling: this preparation contains an organophosphorus compound and labelling statements (1), (2)(a), (3)(e) and (g), and (4)(h), (j), and (k) relating to such preparations given in the entry on Dip Concentrates are applicable. The minimum period that must elapse between cessation of treatment and slaughter of the animals for human consumption is 7 days.

OTHER VETERINARY PREPARATIONS include a MIXTURE containing haloxon 10.4% with oxyclozanide 3.05%.

Halquinol

A mixture resulting from the chlorination of quinolin-8-ol. It consists of 5,7-dichloroquinolin-8-ol (57 to 74%), 5-chloroquinolin-8-ol (23 to 40%), and 7-chloroquinolin-8-ol (up to 4%).

OTHER NAMES: *Quixalin®; Quixalud®*
Remiderm®, Remotic®, and *Vetalog®* (all with triamcinolone acetonide)

A standard is given in the British Pharmacopoeia Addendum 1975

Description. A yellowish-white to yellowish-grey voluminous powder with a faint odour characteristic of cresol.

Solubility. Very slightly soluble in water; soluble, at 20°, in 250 parts of alcohol, in 130 parts of ether, and in 50 parts of chloroform.

Storage. It should be stored free from contact with metal and protected from light.

Identification. TEST. Mix 5 mg with 5 ml of water and add, dropwise, a 5% solution of ferric chloride, shaking after each addition; a pale bluish-green colour is produced.

Actions and uses. Halquinol has anti-amoebic, antibacterial, and antifungal activity. It is used in the treatment of intestinal amoebiasis and bacillary dysentery. The usual dose for amoebiasis is 3 to 4 grams daily in divided doses for adults for up to 5 days. Children over 1 year may be given 50 milligrams per kilogram body-weight daily in divided doses. Where there is no improvement within 24 hours alternative treatment should be considered. One month should elapse before a further course of treatment is given.
Halquinol has also been administered in doses of 500 milligrams 3 or 4 times daily up to a maximum total dose of 7.5 grams for the treatment of non-specific diarrhoeas; the corresponding dose for children over 1 year is 30 milligrams per kilogram body-weight daily in divided doses.
Halquinol is also used in topical preparations containing 0.75% in conjunction with corticosteroids for the treatment of skin disorders.

Undesirable effects. Skin rashes and nausea may occur occasionally.

Precautions. It should not be given to children under 1 year of age.

Preparations

Preparations available include an APPLICATION containing halquinol 31.2 mg with triamcinolone acetonide 4.95 mg in 75 g in an aerosol pack, a CREAM and a veterinary cream containing halquinol 0.75% with triamcinolone acetonide 0.025%, EAR-DROPS containing halquinol 0.75% with triamcinolone acetonide 0.025% in 0.3-ml single-dose units, a DISPERSIBLE POWDER containing halquinol 18.5%, an OINTMENT containing halquinol 0.75% with triamcinolone acetonide 0.025%, TABLETS containing halquinol 250 mg and veterinary tablets containing halquinol 1.5 g.

Hamamelis

The dried leaves of *Hamamelis virginiana* L. (Fam. Hamamelidaceae), a shrub indigenous to the United States of America and to Canada; produced mainly in the eastern United States.

OTHER NAMES: Hamamelis Leaves; Witch Hazel Leaves

A standard is given in the British Pharmaceutical Codex 1973

Constituents. Hamamelis contains tannins, principally β-hamamelitannin, the digalloyl ester of hamamelose (2-hydroxymethyl ribose), gallic acid, a bitter principle, and a trace of volatile oil. It yields to alcohol (45%) 20 to 30% of extractive.

Up to 2% of foreign organic matter and up to 3% of stems and fruits may be present.

Description. UNGROUND DRUG. *Macroscopical characters:* Leaves about 70 to 150 mm long, brittle, dark green or brownish-green, broadly oval or rhomboid-ovate; petiole about 10 to 15 mm long, margin coarsely crenate to sinuate, apex acute or rounded, base cordate and unequal and venation pinnate, lateral veins straight, prominent on the under surface, each ending in a marginal crenation; trichomes stellate, scattered on under surface, numerous on young leaves.

Stems and fruits present in small amounts; stems pale reddish-brown or greyish-brown, smooth or slightly warty and up to about 4 mm thick, with alternate leaf scars; fruit a woody capsule, about 15 mm long when mature, splitting at the apex into 2 halves each containing a single seed.

It has an odour which is not marked, and a bitter as-tringent taste.

Microscopical characters: the diagnostic characters are: Leaf: *epidermal cells* with wavy anticlinal walls, *stomata* paracytic, numerous on abaxial surface; *trichomes* stellate, consisting of 4 to 12 slender conical cells, each about 150 to 250 and up to 500 μm long, united at their bases; *spongy mesophyll* appearing as network of cells with intercellular meshes as viewed through abaxial epidermis; *idioblastic sclereids*, large, lignified, linear or sometimes slightly branched, stretching across the thickness of lamina and about 150 to 180 μm long, many with *tannin-like* contents turned black by *ferric chloride solution; midrib* prominent on abaxial surface, with a vascular strand consisting of a cylinder of *phloem* encircling a *xylem* cylinder with a central pith, a shallow adaxial arc of xylem with phloem below and a small group of *fibres* above; near leaf apex this is replaced by a simple shallow arc of phloem and xylem; sclerenchyma cylinder of *fibres* surrounding the vascular strands, this in turn surrounded by an *endodermoid sheath* with many cells containing prismatic *crystals* of calcium oxalate about 10 to 35 μm long.

Stem: rounded or polygonal *sclereids* and small *vessels* and *tracheids* with bordered pits, separated by uniseriate *medullary rays.*

Fruit: large groups of fibrous *sclereids, epidermis* of the persistent calyx bearing numerous stellate *trichomes.*

POWDERED DRUG. Powdered Hamamelis. A green

to greenish-brown powder, possessing the diagnostic microscopical characters, odour, and taste of the unground drug.

Actions and uses. Hamamelis has astringent properties and its preparations are used in the treatment of haemorrhoids. It is used in toilet preparations.

Preparations

HAMAMELIS DRY EXTRACT (*Syn.* Hamamelis Extract): *Small-scale preparation*

Hamamelis, in moderately coarse powder   1000 g
Alcohol (45%)   ..   ..   ..   a sufficient quantity

Exhaust the hamamelis with the alcohol by percolation, remove the alcohol by evaporating to dryness at a low temperature, and reduce the residue to a fine powder.

Manufacture. Prepare the extract by the above method, appropriately scaled up.

In making this preparation the alcohol (45%) may be replaced by industrial methylated spirit diluted so as to be of equivalent alcoholic strength, provided that the law and the statutory regulations governing the use of industrial methylated spirit are observed.

A standard for this extract is given in the British Pharmaceutical Codex 1973

Storage: it should be stored in airtight containers, in a cool place.

HAMAMELIS SUPPOSITORIES: prepared as described in the entry on Suppositories by incorporating hamamelis dry extract in theobroma oil or other suitable basis. Approximately 1.5 g of hamamelis dry extract displaces 1 g of theobroma oil.

Containers and *Storage:* see the entry on Suppositories for general information on containers and storage.

Advice for patients: see the entry on Suppositories for general information on the use of suppositories. They should be used night and morning and after defaecation unless otherwise directed.

HAMAMELIS WATER (*Syn:* Aqua Hamamelidis; Distilled Witch Hazel; Liquor Hamamelidis): prepared by macerating recently cut and partially dried dormant twigs of *Hamamelis virginiana* L. (Fam. Hamamelidaceae) in water, distilling, and adding the requisite quantity of alcohol to the distillate.

A standard for this aromatic water is given in the British Pharmaceutical Codex 1973

Uses: Hamamelis water is used to alleviate minor affections of the skin such as irritation, roughness, or soreness. It has also been employed, well diluted, as a constituent of eye lotions.

Hay Fever

see ALLERGIC RHINITIS AND HAY FEVER

Headache

Headache may appear in the absence of pathological changes or it may appear as a manifestation of serious disease. It may arise from acute systemic infections, meningitis, intracranial tumours, head injuries, severe hypertension, neuralgia, and giant cell arteritis or from disease of the nose, paranasal spaces, eyes, ears, or teeth. Most headaches are due to muscle tension which is related to anxiety, emotional tension, and fatigue. Headache due to migraine may also be associated with emotional factors.

Migraine. Migraine is characterised by paroxysmal headache which is usually but not necessarily unilateral. It may be preceded by an initial aura with visual disturbances, photophobia, nausea, vomiting, facial flushing or pallor, or vertigo. Attacks may last from minutes to days. Migraine is commonly associated with dilatation and distension of cranial arteries. It may be triggered by chocolate, tyramine-containing foods, hunger, smoking, and alcohol.

Mild attacks may be treated by the administration of analgesics and more severe attacks may frequently be controlled by the administration of ergotamine tartrate or dihydroergotamine. The use of anti-emetic drugs at the onset of an attack may be of value and metoclopramide has the advantage of increasing the rate of gastric emptying.

Drugs such as methysergide and clonidine may be effective in preventing attacks of migraine. Medicines may also be required to treat conditions known to precipitate attacks, such as depression, anxiety, stress, and dietary and endocrine disturbances such as those caused by withdrawal of progestogen-oestrogen contraceptive treatment for 7 days of the menstrual cycle.

In prolonged attacks of migraine corticotrophin injection may be of value. Propranolol is effective in some patients.

Tension headache. Tension headache is due to sustained contraction of skeletal muscle of the head. It is characterised by a steady nonpulsatile ache which may be unilateral or bilateral in the temporal, occipital, parietal, or frontal regions. It may last for hours or intermittently for years.

Tension headache may be treated with analgesics such as aspirin or paracetamol or by removal of any underlying anxiety or fatigue.

Heart Block

see under CARDIAC ARRHYTHMIAS

Heart Failure

Heart failure is an acute or chronic condition in which the heart fails to maintain an adequate supply of blood to the tissues. It may occur in the left heart (left ventricular failure) or the right heart (congestive or right ventricular failure) or on both sides. Since coronary atherosclerosis, systemic arterial hypertension, and rheumatic heart disease affect mainly the left heart, left ventricular failure is more common than right.

Failure of one side of the heart leads to congestion and oedema in its venous supply. Thus left heart failure produces breathlessness due to pulmonary congestion and oedema and pulmonary hypertension. Right heart failure produces hepatic enlargement and tenderness, oedema, particularly of the ankles and sacrum, and sometimes ascites. Pulmonary hypertension resulting from left-heart failure frequently causes the right heart to fail. The inadequate cardiac output leads to a disproportionate reduction in renal blood flow, resulting in salt and water retention.

Causes of heart failure include myocardial and valvular disease, arterial hypertension, and dysrhythmias. Right-side failure may be secondary to lung disease such as chronic cor pulmonale or chronic bronchitis. The underlying cause should be treated if possible, patients should have physical and mental rest to reduce the work load

on the heart, and cardiotonic drugs such as digitalis may be administered. Salt and water retention should be reduced by the use of diuretics in conjunction with potassium supplements if required.

Helium

He = 4.003

A standard is given in the British Pharmacopoeia 1973

Description. A colourless odourless tasteless gas with a relative density not greater than 0.16. For convenience in use it is compressed in metal cylinders.

Solubility. One volume, measured at normal temperature and pressure, dissolves, at 20°, in about 70 volumes of water.

Storage, labelling, and colour-markings. It should be stored in metal cylinders designed to hold compressed gases. Cylinders should be stored in a special room free from materials of an inflammable nature. The room should be cool.

The whole of the cylinder should be painted brown and the name of the gas or chemical symbol "He" should be stencilled in paint on the shoulder of the cylinder. The name or chemical symbol of the gas should be clearly and indelibly stamped on the cylinder valve.

Mixtures of helium with oxygen are in cylinders painted in the colours described under Oxygen.

Actions and uses. A mixture of 1 volume of helium and 2 volumes of air diffuses more rapidly than air itself. Breathing such a mixture requires less effort and an air–helium mixture, or a mixture of 21 volumes of oxygen and 79 volumes of helium, has been used in treating prolonged asthmatic attacks resistant to other therapy, for avoiding caisson disease, and in the treatment of oedema and spasm of the larynx.

Henoch–Schönlein Purpura

see PURPURA, HENOCH-SCHÖNLEIN

Heparin Calcium

A preparation containing the calcium salt of a sulphated polysaccharide acid present in mammalian tissues and having the characteristic property of delaying the clotting of blood. It may be obtained from ox lung [Heparin Calcium (Lung)] or from the intestinal mucosa of oxen, pigs, or sheep [Heparin Calcium (Mucous)]

OTHER NAMES: *Calciparine®*; *Pularin Calcium®*

A standard is given in the British Pharmacopoeia Addendum 1978

Description. A white or creamy-white, moderately hygroscopic powder.

Solubility. Soluble, at 20°, in less than 5 parts of water.

Moisture content. Not more than 8%, determined by drying at 60° in vacuo.

Stability; Storage. See under Heparin Sodium.

Metabolism. See under Heparin Sodium.

Actions and uses. Heparin calcium has the actions and

undesirable effects described under Heparin Sodium. It is administered by subcutaneous injection in the prophylaxis or treatment of thrombo-embolic disorders, particularly in the prevention of deep vein thrombosis after surgery; the dosage is as described under Heparin Sodium. It may cause less bruising at the injection site than the sodium salt.

Preparation

HEPARIN INJECTION: see under Heparin Sodium.

Heparin Sodium

A preparation containing the sodium salt of a sulphated polysaccharide acid present in mammalian tissues and having the characteristic property of delaying the clotting of blood. It may be obtained from ox lung [Heparin Sodium (Lung)] or from the intestinal mucosa of oxen, pigs, or sheep [Heparin Sodium (Mucous)].

OTHER NAMES: *Minihep®*; *Pularin®*

A standard is given in the British Pharmacopoeia Addendum 1978

Description. A white or creamy-white, moderately hygroscopic powder.

Solubility. Soluble, at 20°, in 2.5 parts of water.

Moisture content. Not more than 8%, determined by drying at 60° *in vacuo*.

Stability. In aqueous solution at 25° and at pH 7 to 8, heparin is stable for at least 7 years. The stability is markedly reduced if the pH falls below pH 5. Heparin is sometimes added to intravenous infusions containing sodium chloride and such solutions are stable for 24 hours. The stability of heparin in intravenous infusions containing dextrose or lactates is a subject of controversy. Some workers claim that rapid inactivation (40 to 55% in 24 hours) occurs, whereas others assert that there is no detectable loss in potency in 24 hours.

FURTHER INFORMATION. Stability of heparin injection —J. Pritchard, *J. Pharm. Pharmac.*, 1964, **16**, 487; stability in intravenous infusions—J. M. Chessels *et al.*, *Br. med. J.*, ii/1972, 81; J. W. Hadgraft, *Lancet*, ii/1970, 1254; J. Jacobs *et al.*, *J. clin. Path.*, 1973, **26**, 742; S. L. Stock and N. Warner, *Br. med. J.*, ii/1971, 307.

Sterilisation. Solutions for injection are sterilised by filtration.

Storage. It should be stored in containers sealed to exclude micro-organisms and, as far as possible, moisture.

Metabolism. BLOOD CONCENTRATION. Blood concentrations of 5 to 10 units/ml are maintained in patients undergoing haemodialysis after a 50000-unit dose administered as an infusion at the rate of 300 units/minute.

HALF-LIFE. The blood anticoagulant half-life of heparin is 37 minutes after an intravenous dose of 0.6 unit/ml of blood volume and 22 minutes after a dose of 0.3 unit/ml; these times are increased in renal function impairment.

DISTRIBUTION. Localised to some extent in mast cells; it does not appear in the milk nor does it cross the placenta; *protein binding*, extensively bound to plasma proteins.

METABOLIC REACTIONS. Metabolised in the liver to inactive metabolites.

EXCRETION. Excreted in the urine mainly as uroheparin.

FURTHER INFORMATION. H. D. Johnson, *Am. J. Hosp. Pharm.*, 1968, **25**, 60; P. J. Perry *et al.*, *Clin. Pharmac. Ther.*, 1974, **16**, 514.

Actions and uses. Heparin sodium inhibits the clotting of blood *in vivo* and *in vitro* by combining with certain fractions of the plasma proteins. This action can be rapidly prevented by neutralising its electronegative charge with basic substances such as protamine. It has been shown that the heparin–protein complex inhibits the conversion of prothrombin to thrombin, antagonises thromboplastin, and prevents thrombin from reacting with fibrinogen to form fibrin. The prothrombin ratio is increased but this is not a reliable measure of the anticoagulant effect. The inhibition of the conversion of prothrombin to thrombin is probably responsible for the prevention of platelet agglutination.

Heparin is ineffective when taken by mouth and to obtain its full effect it must be given by intravenous injection or infusion.

When injected intravenously, heparin has a rapid but transient action, the extent and duration of its effect on the clotting-time depending on the dose administered. It disappears rapidly from the blood and intravenous or intramuscular injections should be given at intervals not exceeding 4 to 6 hours.

Heparin has no effect on a clot *in vitro*, but there is a more rapid resolution of a clot in a heparinised patient than in an untreated one; heparin also prevents further clotting. It is used as an anticoagulant in vascular surgery and, occasionally, in blood transfusion, but its chief use is in the treatment of arterial and venous thrombosis. In certain selected cases it may be used prophylactically after surgery to prevent thrombo-embolic complications.

The usual practice is to give an initial intravenous injection of 12 500 units of heparin sodium followed by doses of about 10 000 units at four-hourly intervals to keep the clotting-time, tested not less than 3 hours after the last injection of heparin, at about 3 times the pre-treatment figure; the intravenous dose needed to maintain this figure varies from 6000 to 12 000 units. Regular treatment is essential and doses must not be omitted at night; an indwelling needle is therefore frequently used.

In cases of coronary thrombosis, an anticoagulant such as warfarin sodium is commonly given by mouth at the same time as the heparin, which is discontinued after 36 to 48 hours when the action of the oral anticoagulant has developed.

In an emergency, 12 500 units of heparin sodium may be given by intramuscular injection, although haematoma, pain, and severe bruising may occur; if necessary, a second dose should follow after an interval of 6 to 12 hours. Long-acting forms of heparin have been evolved which need only be given at intervals of 12 hours by deep subcutaneous or intramuscular injection.

Doses of 5000 units by subcutaneous injection every 8 to 12 hours, beginning before surgery takes place, have been used to prevent post-operative thrombosis.

If blood transfusions are required during anticoagulant therapy, 3 units of heparin sodium per millilitre may be added to the transfused blood in addition to the dose already being administered.

Bleeding from the site of operation is unlikely if heparin therapy is started after the fourth post-operative or post-partum day.

Menstruation, unless excessive, is no contra-indication to the use of heparin.

Undesirable effects. Complications of therapy are bleeding in various sites (haematuria, haemothorax, retroperitoneal haematoma, subarachnoid haemorrhage) and, rarely, febrile or anaphylactic reactions. Occasionally, there is tachyphylaxis, possibly from an endogenous antagonist. Slight epistaxis, microscopic haematuria, and bruising are signs of overdosage.

More severe bleeding may be reduced by giving intravenously for each 1000 units of heparin to be neutralised 1 millilitre of protamine sulphate injection (1%).

Preparation

HEPARIN INJECTION: a sterile solution of heparin calcium or heparin sodium in water for injections. The pH of the solution may be adjusted by the addition of a suitable alkali. It is sterilised by filtration. Available in 0.2-ml ampoules containing 5000 units of heparin calcium; in 0.2-ml ampoules containing 5000 units of heparin sodium; in 1-ml ampoules containing 1000, 5000, and 12 500 units of heparin sodium per ml; in 5-ml ampoules and 5-ml vials containing 1000 and 5000 units per ml; and in 5-ml vials containing 25 000 units per ml; the vial packs contain preservative.

A standard for this injection is given in the British Pharmacopoeia Addendum 1978

Containers: see the entry on Injections for general information on containers.

Labelling: see the entry on Injections for general information on labelling. In addition, the label on the container should state the amount of the medicament as the number of units in a suitable dose-volume except that for multiple-dose containers, the label on the container should state the amount of the medicament as the number of units per ml, the type of heparin present and whether it is the calcium or sodium salt, and, when no bactericide is present, "Contains no bactericide; any portion of the contents not used at once should be discarded".

Storage: it should be stored at a temperature not exceeding 25°, preferably in containers sealed by fusion of the glass. When stored in a container sealed by a rubber closure, a satisfactory concentration of bactericide may not be maintained for more than 3 years.

Hepatitis

Hepatitis is an inflammation of the liver due to infection, toxic chemicals, or drugs or to autoimmune mechanisms. The infecting agent is usually hepatitis virus A or B or, rarely, yellow fever, glandular fever, or rubella viruses.

Infectious hepatitis. This is usually spread by contaminated human faeces and enters by the oral route; it can also be transmitted by blood transfusion. It occurs sporadically but small epidemics may occur in institutions and larger outbreaks may accompany large movements of population, as in wartime. The incubation period is from 1 to 6 weeks.

The first phase of the condition is the pre-icteric period which is usually rapid in onset and characterised by fever, malaise, anorexia, nausea, vomiting, and abdominal distension. There may also be skin rashes, arthralgia, and symptoms of meningism.

After 3 to 7 days jaundice rapidly develops, the fever subsides, and the patient feels better; the stools are pale, the urine is dark, and the liver is enlarged and tender. In elderly patients there may be disorientation and confusion. The jaundice usually subsides after 2 weeks.

The patient should be confined to bed and a diet low in fat and high in protein and carbohydrate should be instituted. Where the jaundice is prolonged, corticosteroid therapy may be necessary. The prognosis is usually good but complications such as acute hepatic necrosis, hepatic cirrhosis, and aplastic anaemia may occur.

The condition is infectious during the pre-icteric period and contacts may be given human normal immunoglobulin for prophylaxis; protection extends for about 4 months.

Serum hepatitis (post-transfusion hepatitis). This is usually transmitted in transfused blood or plasma, by the use of non-sterile needles and syringes, or by oro-genital contact. The incubation period is from two to twenty-four weeks. Symptoms are insidious in onset and may include urticarial skin lesions and arthritis. The illness tends to be prolonged, mortality is greater than in infective hepatitis, and protection by human normal immunoglobulin poor. Hepatitis B antigen has been detected in the serum of patients with infective serum hepatitis.

Treatment is as described above under Infectious Hepatitis.

A wide variety of substances may cause liver damage as described under Jaundice.

Herpes Simplex

Herpes simplex is a virus infection usually of the skin or adjacent mucous membranes characterised by the formation of groups of vesicles surrounded by erythema. The vesicles later rupture and dry to form a crust which separates several days later.

Primary infection may be asymptomatic or associated with fever and malaise. The virus remains in the tissues at the site of entry and gives rise to recurrent attacks which are associated with the characteristic lesions. Attacks may be precipitated by sunshine, intercurrent infection, menstruation, pregnancy, or emotional strain. The face, mainly around the mouth, is usually affected, but sometimes the genital region is involved. Herpes simplex lesions on the lips are known as *cold sores*.

Infection of the eye with herpes simplex may result in vesiculation of the eyelids and conjunctiva and ulceration of the cornea leading to keratitis.

The application to the skin of a 5% solution of idoxuridine in dimethyl sulphoxide may be successful in aborting attacks of herpes simplex. Corticosteroids should not be used owing to the danger of spreading the infection to other areas and to the increased likelihood of perforation of corneal ulcers. Antibacterial creams may be applied to prevent secondary infection of the lesions.

Hexachlorophane

2,2'-Methylenebis(3,4,6-trichlorophenol)

$C_{13}H_6Cl_6O_2 = 406.9$

OTHER NAMES: *Coopaphene*®; Hexachlorophene; *PhisoMed*®; *Steridermis*®; *Ster-Zac*®; *Zalpon*®

A standard is given in the British Pharmacopoeia 1973

Description. A white or pale buff crystalline powder which is odourless or has a slight phenolic odour.

Solubility. Practically insoluble in water; soluble, at 20°, in 3.5 parts of alcohol, and in less than 1 part of ether and of acetone; soluble in dilute solutions of alkali hydroxides.

Moisture content. Not more than 1%, determined by drying at 105°.

Sterilisation. It is sterilised by dry heat.

Storage. It should be stored in airtight containers, protected from light.

Preparation and storage of solutions. See statement on aqueous solutions of antiseptics in the entry on Solutions.

Identification. TESTS. 1. Heat 0.1 g in a dry tube; a colourless to amber liquid is produced which, after further heating, becomes green, blue, and finally purple. 2. Dissolve about 5 mg in 5 ml of alcohol (95%) and add 1 drop of *ferric chloride solution*; a transient purple colour is immediately produced. 3. Dissolve 0.1 g in 0.5 ml of acetone, add *titanous chloride solution*, and shake; a yellowish-orange oil separates, which is soluble in chloroform and in ether.

MELTING-POINT. About 164°.

ULTRAVIOLET ABSORPTION. In 0.1N sodium hydroxide, maxima at 249 nm (E1%, 1cm = 400) and 320 nm (E1%, 1cm = 300).

Metabolism. ABSORPTION. Absorbed through the skin and after oral administration.

BLOOD CONCENTRATION. Application of a 5% solution topically to the newborn resulted in cord-blood concentrations of 3 to 182 ng/ml and venous blood concentrations of 9 to 646 ng/ml; application of 2 ml of a 3% emulsion to the skin resulted in blood concentrations of 50 to 140 ng/ml.

Actions and uses. Hexachlorophane has antibacterial properties against a wide variety of Gram-positive organisms but is generally less effective against Gram-negative organisms. It has the advantage over many other antiseptics of retaining its activity in the presence of soap. Hexachlorophane is used in soaps and creams in a concentration of 0.25 to 3%. When these preparations are used daily there is a marked diminution of the bacterial flora of the hands due to accumulation of hexachlorophane on the skin. Such preparations are useful in reducing cross-infection in hospital operating theatres and wards and contamination of food during handling.

Dusting-powders containing 0.3% may be used for application to the umbilical stump to reduce the risk of infection with susceptible organisms.

The presence of serum reduces the activity of hexachlorophane but the concentration normally used is sufficient to allow for this.

Undesirable effects. Skin sensitisation has been known to occur after the repeated use of hexachlorophane. Preparations are liable to contamination with Gram-negative organisms such as species of *Pseudomonas* and *Salmonella* which are resistant to its antibacterial action. Absorbed hexachlorophane may damage the central nervous system, especially in infants.

Precautions. As hexachlorophane can be absorbed after application to the skin, preparations should not be used for total body bathing or application to large areas of the skin except in accordance with medical advice. It should not be applied to weeping or broken skin or under occlusive dressings. Particular caution should be exercised in applying preparations containing hexachlorophane to infants.

Veterinary uses. Hexachlorophane is used mainly in sheep for the treatment of chronic liver fluke infection. The usual dosage by mouth is 10 to 15 milligrams per kilogram body-weight as a single dose; this dose may be given monthly to sheep during the period of risk (September to January in the United Kingdom) and to cattle in October and November.

Preparations

CONCENTRATED HEXACHLOROPHANE SOLUTION:

Hexachlorophane ..	..	..	..	..	100 g
Sodium hydroxide..	..	..	..	..	10 g
Alcohol (95%)	..	..	..	..	400 ml
Purified water, freshly boiled and cooled					to 1000 ml

Dissolve the hexachlorophane in the alcohol. Dissolve the sodium hydroxide in 500 ml of the water, mix the two solutions, add sufficient of the water to produce the required volume, and mix.

In making this preparation the alcohol (95%) may be replaced by industrial methylated spirit, provided that the law and the statutory regulations governing the use of industrial methylated spirit are observed.

A standard for this solution is given in the British Pharmaceutical Codex 1973

Containers: it should not be dispensed in types of containers that are normally used for medicinal products taken internally. Containers should be thoroughly cleansed before being filled. Closures should be such that the solution does not come into contact with cork.

Labelling: the container should be labelled ''30 ml (1 fl. oz.) to be added to a bath of about 100 to 150 litres (20 to 30 gallons) of water''. In addition, if the preparation is to be used in a hard water area, the label should state that a suitable water softener should be added to the water before adding the solution. The label also states that this preparation should only be used in accordance with medical advice.

Storage: it should be protected from light.

Advice for patients: it should not be used for prolonged periods.

HEXACHLOROPHANE DUSTING-POWDER:

Hexachlorophane ..	..	..	..	..	..	3 g
Zinc oxide ..	..	..	..	..	..	30 g
Sterilisable maize starch ..	..	..	..			967 g

Prepare as described in the entry on Powders. Distribute, in quantities of not more than 30 g, into suitable glass containers with reclosable perforated lids or into other suitable containers, and heat for a sufficient length of time to ensure that the whole of the powder is maintained at 150° to 155° for 1 hour.

A standard for this dusting-powder is given in the British Pharmaceutical Codex 1973

Labelling: the directions given in the entry on Dusting-powders should be followed. In addition, the label on the container should state that the preparation should not be applied to infants or to large areas of skin except in accordance with medical advice.

Advice for patients: the dusting-powder should be dusted lightly onto the affected area. It should not be applied to open wounds or raw surfaces. It should not be used for prolonged periods.

HEXACHLOROPHANE MIXTURE (*Syn.* Hexachlorophane Drench):

Hexachlorophane ..	..	..	..	..	50 g
Liquid paraffin	..	..	..	..	150 ml
Arachis oil, or other suitable vegetable oil					to 1000 ml

Dissolve the hexachlorophane in 750 ml of the vegetable

oil with the aid of heat and cool; add the liquid paraffin and sufficient of the vegetable oil to produce the required volume, and mix. It contains, in 1 ml, 50 mg of hexachlorophane.

A standard for this mixture is given in the British Pharmacopoeia (Veterinary)

Storage: it should be stored in airtight containers, protected from light.

OTHER PREPARATIONS available include a number of preparations containing hexachlorophane, in concentrations of up to about 3%, usually in saponaceous or detergent bases, for antiseptic washing purposes.

Hexoestrol

4,4'-(1,2-Diethylethylene)diphenol

$C_{18}H_{22}O_2 = 270.4$

OTHER NAME: Hexestrol

A standard is given in the British Pharmacopoeia (Veterinary)

Description. Colourless crystals or a white crystalline powder.

Solubility. Very slightly soluble in water and in chloroform; soluble in alcohol, in ether, in acetone, and in solutions of alkali hydroxides.

Identification. TESTS. 1. To about 250 mg add 1 ml of acetic anhydride and 2 ml of dehydrated pyridine, boil under a reflux condenser for 15 minutes, cool, add 50 ml of water, and shake thoroughly; a precipitate is produced which, after washing with water and drying, melts at about 138°.

2. Dissolve about 10 mg in 5 ml of sulphuric acid; the solution is colourless (distinction from stilboestrol, which gives a golden-yellow colour).

MELTING-POINT. About 186°.

ULTRAVIOLET ABSORPTION. In dehydrated alcohol, maximum at 279 nm (E1%, 1cm = 130).

Veterinary uses. Hexoestrol is an oestrogen used in animals as a growth promoter. It is administered by implantation in a non-edible part of the body, the usual total implantation dose for cattle being up to 45 milligrams and for poultry 15 milligrams.

Preparation

HEXOESTROL IMPLANTS: they may be prepared by fusion or compression.

A standard for these implants is given in the British Pharmacopoeia (Veterinary)

Containers and *Labelling:* see the entry on Implants for general information on containers and labelling.

Hexylresorcinol

4-Hexylresorcinol

$C_{12}H_{18}O_2 = 194.3$

A standard is given in the British Pharmacopoeia 1973

Description. White needles, crystalline powder, plates, or plate aggregates composed of needle masses, with a pungent odour and a taste which is sharp and astringent, accompanied by a sensation of numbness. It becomes brownish-yellow on exposure to light and air.

Solubility. Soluble, at 20°, in 2000 parts of water; soluble in alcohol, in ether, in chloroform, in glycerol, and in fixed oils.

Storage. It should be stored in airtight containers, protected from light.

Identification. TESTS. 1. Dissolve about 100 mg in 10 ml of alcohol (90%) and add 0.2 ml of *ferric chloride test-solution*; a green colour is produced.

2. To 1 ml of a saturated solution add 1 ml of nitric acid; a light red colour is produced.

3. To 1 ml of a saturated solution add 1 ml of *bromine solution*; a yellow flocculent precipitate is produced which dissolves on the addition of 2 ml of *dilute ammonia solution* to give a yellow solution.

MELTING-POINT. About 67°.

Metabolism. ABSORPTION. Incompletely absorbed after oral administration.

EXCRETION. 20 to 30% of an oral dose is excreted unchanged in the urine and 60 to 70% is eliminated in the faeces.

Actions and uses. Hexylresorcinol is an anthelmintic used for the expulsion of hookworms, roundworms, dwarf tapeworms, and fish tapeworms. It is administered by mouth as a single dose, which for an adult is usually 1 gram and for a child 100 milligrams for each year of age up to 10 years. A saline purgative should be given 2 hours after the dose, and no food should be allowed for 5 hours. Because the drug is irritant, tablets and capsules of hexylresorcinol should not be chewed. The treatment may be safely repeated after 3 days, if necessary.

For the expulsion of hookworms, 3 courses of treatment at intervals of 3 days may be necessary.

For the expulsion of dwarf tapeworms, treatment may be given weekly for 3 weeks to ensure that autoinfection does not occur.

Hexylresorcinol has antiseptic properties and it has been used in the form of lozenges for the treatment of mild throat infections.

High Pressure Liquid Chromatography

High pressure liquid chromatography, also known as "high performance liquid chromatography", is a development of classical column chromatography in which the column packing material has a very small particle size (5 to 10 μm). Columns packed with such materials allow very rapid and efficient separations but they have a very low permeability with the result that the mobile phase has to be supplied by means of a high pressure pump. The high speed of analysis requires the use of instrumentation for the detection of components eluted from the column.

A number of features of high pressure liquid chromatography are similar to those of gas chromatography, particularly column efficiency, resolution, column overloading, and quantitative determinations—see under Gas Chromatography.

High pressure liquid chromatography has an advantage

over gas chromatography because it can be used for the analysis of non-volatile, highly polar, or heat-sensitive materials. However, gas chromatography is more sensitive for some compounds and is the method of choice for temperature-volatile compounds.

The equipment for high pressure liquid chromatography consists of a pumping system for the mobile phase, a sample injection device, a column, and a detector coupled to a potentiometric recorder.

Pumping Systems

Constant pressure pumps. These pumps deliver the mobile phase at a predetermined pressure irrespective of the flow rate used, and two types are available. One type is a simple system consisting of a solvent reservoir pressurised by gas from a cylinder. The other type is a more complex pump in which air is fed into a large cylinder the piston of which drives a second piston of smaller cross-sectional area which, in turn, pressurises the mobile phase, thus separating the driving gas from the mobile phase and amplifying the available pressure. Constant pressure pumps are simple to operate and give pulse-free solvent delivery, but they have the disadvantage that any change in resistance to flow through the system changes the rate of flow of the mobile phase, and hence changes the retention time and column efficiency. For the most accurate work with these pumps it is important to control the temperature of the column, because of the change in viscosity of the mobile phase with temperature.

From the point of view of safety, constant pressure pumps do not produce a dangerous build-up of pressure in the event of a blockage, but if a sudden depressurisation of the system occurs, due to accident or failure of a component, the contents will be discharged in a high pressure jet.

Constant flow pumps. There are two types, the reciprocating pump and the syringe pump. Single piston reciprocating pumps give a pulsating solvent flow which has to be smoothed by a pulse-damping system because pressure pulses can disturb the column packing and can also affect the operation of the detector. The use of dual-piston reciprocating pumps reduces the pulsations. Syringe pumps are large volume cylinders with a piston driven by an electric motor at a constant forward speed. These pumps give a pulseless flow but they can be adversely affected by mobile phase compressibility effects at high operating pressures.

Because of the low flow rates involved, constant flow pumps do not give rise to as great a hazard as constant pressure pumps in the event of a sudden system depressurisation, but pressure can build up rapidly following a blockage in the system and pressure cut-out switches are usually incorporated.

Gradient elution. If a sample consists of a mixture of substances of widely differing polarity it may be impossible to find a suitable combination of column and mobile phase which will allow elution of all the components within a reasonable time and which will also give good resolution. This problem may be overcome by changing the proportions of the components in a multi-component mobile phase during the course of the analysis. The change may be in the form of discontinuous "steps" or it may vary continuously with time, and most pumping systems incorporate facilities for this technique.

Injection System

Samples may be introduced into the column by means of a valve or a syringe. There are two types of valve, one of which delivers a fixed volume and the other of which is loaded with a syringe and can deliver variable quantities of sample. Valves are usually positioned in the solvent feed to the column with a minimum of dead volume lying between the valve and the top of the column packing. Syringe injection is carried out either under stopped flow conditions or through a high pressure injection port. For highest column efficiency, the sample must be introduced directly on to the column packing. For stopped-flow injection, the syringe needle is introduced through a valve at the top of the column whilst the flow of mobile phase is stopped.

High pressure injection ports take the form either of a simple septum similar to that used in gas chromatography or of a port which has an air-lock to allow the introduction of a syringe under full system pressure. The elastomers used in septum injectors are prone to be attacked by many of the usual solvents used as mobile phases and they must not be too elastic because they must withstand high pressures. In consequence, the life of the septum is often short.

Syringe injection usually allows higher column efficiency but gives slightly lower quantititative reproducibility than a valve delivering a fixed volume.

The Column and Column Packing

The column is usually constructed from seamless stainless steel tubing and it may vary in length between 10 and 500 mm and in diameter between 2 and 10 mm. The dimensions depend on the particle size of the column packing, the efficiency required to give adequate resolution in the particular analysis being undertaken, and the scale of the chromatography to be carried out. The column is packed under high pressure (about 34 MPa, 5000 pounds force per square inch) with a slurry of the packing material in a suitable solvent. For column packings of particle size in excess of 20 μm, dry-packing techniques similar to those used for gas chromatography may be used.

The necessity for control of the temperature of the column is very much less in liquid chromatography than in gas chromatography because of the much lower enthalpy changes on adsorption or partition, and temperature control is usually devoted to maintaining the column at a steady temperature near to ambient temperature. The exceptions to this are when a constant pressure pump is employed under certain circumstances (see under Pumping Systems) and when the column packing is either polymeric in nature (such as polystyrene-based ion-exchangers or exclusion packings) or is coated with a layer of polymeric bonded material. In these cases, high temperatures ease problems of mass transfer through the polymer matrices. Temperature control is achieved by an air-blown oven or water-jacket, although simple lagging of the column often suffices.

The material used for packing the column is appropriate to the mode of chromatography and at least 6 modes are possible.

Adsorption chromatography. The column packing is usually silica gel although alumina is also occasionally used. The mobile phase dissolves the sample and separation occurs by competition between the solute and the mobile phase for the polar adsorption sites on the packing material. The more polar the sample is the more strongly it is retained and solutes are eluted more rapidly by more polar mobile phases. Thin-layer chromatographic analyses may be adapted for use in this mode of high pressure liquid chromatography with minimal modification.

Liquid–liquid partition chromatography. The column packing is usually silica gel which has been coated with a liquid which is insoluble, or has poor solubility, in the mobile phase. The liquid is referred to as the stationary phase. The coating process is normally carried out in the column in order to avoid difficulties involved in packing coated materials from a slurry; if the particle size of the packing is large enough to allow it to be packed in the dry state, then the coating process may be carried out prior to packing. The solutes partition between the mobile and stationary phases and their chromatographic retention is related to the partition coefficient in the static partition system. The disadvantage of this mode of chromatography is that the stationary phase usually has finite solubility in the mobile phase and therefore bleeds from the column. This effect may be avoided by saturating the mobile phase with the stationary phase, but this is inconvenient because equilibrium between the phases is slow and good temperature control is needed.

Bonded phase partition chromatography. A method of dealing with the problems of liquid–liquid partition chromatography is to bond the stationary phase to the support material by chemical means. The procedure most frequently used is to react silica gel with an organochlorosilane. This produces an organic bonded phase material linked to silica gel through siloxane bridges.

The reaction conditions may be chosen to produce packings with either a monomolecular or a polymeric layer of bonded phase. The former gives the best chromatographic performance whilst the latter may contain higher loadings of stationary phase and has been used with support materials having a low surface area.

The bonded phase functions in the same way as the stationary phase in liquid–liquid partition chromatography described above, but it is not affected by the solvent action of the mobile phase.

Some materials, for instance silica gel to which octadecyl groups have been bonded, are used with more polar mobile phases (such as mixtures of water and methyl alcohol or acetonitrile); this is a reversal of the usual partition mode and the technique is known as reversed-phase chromatography.

Other bonded-phase partition materials are available, such as those bearing amino or cyanopropyl groups, and these can be used for both normal and reversed-phase partition.

Ion-exchange chromatography. The column packing is a material which bears ionic sites of the opposite charge to the ions to be separated. The traditional material is based upon polystyrene resin beads which bear the ionic groups, but this type of packing is prone to changes in volume with ionic strength which may lead to the formation of voids in the column or to a blockage. In addition, large volumes of stagnant mobile phase are trapped within the swollen resin which greatly reduces the efficiency of separation.

Alternatively, packing material based on resin-coated glass beads may be used, but this has the disadvantage of low capacity and a particle diameter greater than 30 μm which results in a column efficiency lower than that attainable with a microparticulate silica column.

Packing materials based upon microparticulate silica gel are also available and these have capacities only slightly lower than resin-based materials and have high separation efficiency.

Elution from ion-exchange columns occurs by competition for the ionic sites between the solute ions and those in the mobile phase. The nature and concentration of the ionic species in the mobile phase affects the separation, as does the pH and, in some cases, the presence of an organic modifier such as alcohol or methyl alcohol, which affects partition or adsorption.

Ion-pair partition chromatography. This is based on the formation of ion pairs between oppositely charged ions and the solubility of certain ion pairs in organic media.

For normal chromatography the stationary phase is an aqueous solution of the relevant counter-ion and the mobile phase is an organic solvent; the ionic species migrate as ion pairs and are retained as the free ion.

Reversed-phase chromatography uses a non-polar organic stationary phase (often a bonded phase packing) and an aqueous mobile phase; in this case the ion pair is retained.

Exclusion chromatography. This is used for the separation of molecules of high molecular weight such as polymers and macromolecules. The separation is on the basis of molecular size and depends only on the physical intrusion of the molecules into pores in the column packing. Column packing materials include swollen gels (which are not very stable to pressure), cross-linked polystyrene beads, rigid porous glasses, and controlled-pore silica gel.

Detectors

The two most widely used detectors are the ultraviolet detector and the differential refractometer. Other systems with limited applications have been used.

Ultraviolet detector. This may be used for any compound which absorbs radiation in the wavelength range available. The detector may either be at a fixed wavelength (usually 254 nm with an optional extra wavelength of 280 nm) or the wavelength may be variable. Many detectors allow wavelengths below 200 nm to be selected and upper limits vary between 380 and 1000 nm.

Both single and dual beam variable wavelength detectors are used and the ultimate sensitivity of either type is similar, being limited mainly by lamp noise. The flow cell volume is usually about 8 μl (10 mm in length and 1 mm in diameter), the small volume being essential for high efficiency operation, and the maximum sensitivity is usually 0.01 absorbance unit although some detectors are capable of higher sensitivities. For a material with a reasonable extinction coefficient, a detection limit of about 1 ng is typical.

Refractive index detector. Differential refractometers monitor the refractive index of the mobile phase and respond to anything that changes this parameter. They are, therefore, of general applicability but their sensitivity is limited by temperature or pressure fluctuations.

Three types of refractometer are commonly used. The first type uses a prismatic cell and measures the deflection of a light beam passing through it, the second type records the amount of light reflected from a glass/mobile phase interface, and the third type measures changes in the speed of light by means of an interferometer. The first two types have a maximum sensitivity (equivalent to noise level) of 10^{-7} refractive index units, whilst the third type is limited by temperature effects to about 10^{-8} refractive index units.

Refractive index detectors are between 100 and 1000 times less sensitive than ultraviolet detectors.

Other detectors. Fluorescence detectors are the most sensitive detectors but they are limited to fluorescent compounds or those compounds which react readily with fluorogenic reagents. Polarographic, conductivity, and electron-capture detectors may be used for special purposes and other systems which have been used include mass spectrometer interfaces, a capacitance detector, and post-column reaction systems.

Histamine Receptors

The actions of histamine are mediated by two types of receptor, designated H_1 and H_2.

H_1-receptor effects. Histamine contracts smooth muscle of the intestine, bronchioles, uterus, and large blood vessels. It causes dilatation of small blood vessels, especially venules, which generally leads to a marked fall in blood pressure and is often accompanied by a throbbing headache. Histamine also causes small vessels to become permeable to blood proteins and the resulting leakage of fluid into the interstitial spaces causes oedema. Histamine may also stimulate nerve endings to produce pain. In this way histamine mediates many of the characteristic phenomena of inflammation and tissue injury.

The effects noted above are generally antagonised by H_1-receptor blockers such as diphenhydramine, mepyramine, and promethazine, which may be used to antagonise the effects of tissue histamine released in allergic conditions such as urticaria and hay fever.

H_2-receptor effects. Histamine stimulates the acid-secreting cells in the gastric mucosa, producing a profuse flow of gastric juice with a high acidity but a relatively low content of pepsin. This action is mediated by H_2 receptors which are sensitive to histamine. H_2 receptors are also found in the heart and uterus but their clinical significance has not been established. The effect of histamine on H_2 receptors is not antagonised by classical antihistamines but by specific antagonists such as cimetidine.

Hodgkin's Disease

see under LYMPHOPROLIFERATIVE DISEASES

Homatropine Hydrobromide

($1R,3r,5S$)-3-(2-Hydroxy-2-phenylacetyloxy)tropanium bromide

$C_{16}H_{22}BrNO_3 = 356.3$

OTHER NAMES: Homatr. Hydrobrom.; Homatropini Hydrobromidum

A standard is given in the European Pharmacopoeia Vol. III

Description. Odourless colourless crystals or a white crystalline powder.

Solubility. Soluble, at 20°, in 6 parts of water and in 60 parts of alcohol, the solubility increasing rapidly with increase of temperature; very slightly soluble in chloroform; practically insoluble in ether.

Acidity. A 2% solution has a pH of 5.5 to 7.

Dissociation constant. pK_a 9.9 (20°).

Stability. In aqueous solution, homatropine hydrolyses to tropine and mandelic acid. Hydrolysis is catalysed by hydrogen ions and hydroxide ions. At 25°, the rate of hydrolysis is a minimum at pH 3.7.

FURTHER INFORMATION. Stability in aqueous solution —M. H. Krasowska *et al.*, *Dansk Tidsskr. Farm.*, 1968, **42**, 170; stability in frozen solution—S. S. Larsen, *Arch. Pharm. Chemi. scient. Edn*, 1973, **1**, 61.

Sterilisation. Solutions are sterilised by heating in an autoclave, by heating with a bactericide, or by filtration.

Identification. TESTS. 1. Dissolve a few mg in 5 ml of water, and add 1 ml of *potassium iodobismuthate solution*; an orange or orange-red precipitate is produced.
2. Dissolve 10 mg in 1 ml of water, add 1 ml of *dilute ammonia solution*, shake with chloroform, and evaporate the chloroform layer to dryness; to the residue add 1.5 ml of a 2% solution of mercuric chloride in alcohol (60%); a yellow colour is produced which becomes red on gently warming (distinction from most other alkaloids except atropine and hyoscyamine).

MELTING-POINT. About 215°, with decomposition.

ULTRAVIOLET ABSORPTION. In 0.1N hydrochloric acid, maxima at 254 nm (E1%, 1cm = 5), 259 nm (E1%, 1cm = 5.2), and 266 nm.

INFRA-RED ABSORPTION. Major peaks at 697, 732, 1026, 1157, 1167, and 1756 cm^{-1} (see Appendix 2a: Infra-red Spectra).

THIN-LAYER CHROMATOGRAPHY. See under Thin-Layer Chromatography, System 8.

Actions and uses. Homatropine has actions similar to those described under Atropine. It is less powerful than atropine and is seldom used internally; its chief use is in ophthalmology to dilate the pupil. It produces mydriasis more rapidly than atropine, but its effect persists for a shorter time, passing off within 24 hours, and may be readily terminated by the action of physostigmine. It has less tendency than atropine to increase the intra-ocular pressure, but produces a less satisfactory mydriasis in children.

Its mydriatic action may be enhanced by the simultaneous local administration of cocaine.

Precautions. It should be used with caution in patients with raised intra-ocular pressure.

Poisoning. As for Atropine.

Veterinary uses. Eye-drops of homatropine are used to dilate the pupil for ophthalmological examinations.

Preparations

COCAINE AND HOMATROPINE EYE-DROPS: consisting of a sterile solution containing 2% of cocaine hydrochloride and 2% of homatropine hydrobromide, with 0.01% of chlorhexidine acetate, in purified water. It is prepared by method B or C described in the entry on Eye-drops.

A standard for these eye-drops is given in the British Pharmaceutical Codex 1973

Containers: see the entry on Eye-drops for general information on containers. This solution is adversely affected by alkali.

Labelling: see the entry on Eye-drops for general information on labelling.

HOMATROPINE EYE-DROPS: consisting of a sterile solution containing up to 2% of homatropine hydrobromide, with 0.02% v/v of benzalkonium chloride solution or 0.01% of chlorhexidine acetate, in purified water. It is prepared by method A, B, or C described in the entry on Eye-drops.

A standard for these eye-drops is given in the British Pharmacopoeia Addendum 1977 and in the British Pharmacopoeia (Veterinary)

Containers: see the entry on Eye-drops for general information on containers. This solution is adversely affected by alkali.

Labelling: see the entry on Eye-drops for general information on labelling.

Advice for patients: see the entry on Eye-drops for general information on the use of eye-drops. Blurring of vision and sensitivity to light may occur for up to 24 hours after instillation of the eye-drops.

Homidium Bromide

3,8-Diamino-5-ethyl-6-phenylphenanthridinium bromide

$C_{21}H_{20}BrN_3 = 394.3$

OTHER NAME: *Ethidium®*

A standard is given in the British Pharmacopoeia (Veterinary)

Description. An almost odourless, dark-purple, crystalline or amorphous powder with a persistently bitter taste.

Solubility. Soluble, at 20°, in 20 parts of water and in 750 parts of chloroform.

Acidity. A 2% solution has a pH of 4 to 7.

Moisture content. Not more than 10%, determined by drying at 130°.

Storage. It should be stored in airtight containers.

Identification. TEST. Dissolve about 50 mg in 20 ml of water, add 1 ml of hydrochloric acid, cool in ice, add 1 ml of *sodium nitrite solution*, and add to a cold solution of 100 mg of 2-naphthol in 20 ml of *dilute sodium hydroxide solution*; an intense dark blue colour is produced.

MELTING-POINT. About 245°, with decomposition.

ULTRAVIOLET ABSORPTION. In 0.1N hydrochloric acid, maxima at 242 nm (E1%, 1cm = 750) and 283 nm (E1%, 1cm = 812).

INFRA-RED ABSORPTION. Major peaks at 1260, 1310, 1400, 1462, 1492, and 1628 cm^{-1} (see Appendix 2c: Infra-red Spectra).

Veterinary uses. Homidium bromide is used in animals as a trypanocide. It is administered by subcutaneous or intramuscular injection to cattle, in a single dose of 1 milligram per kilogram body-weight. In addition to its curative properties, a single dose acts as a prophylactic for about 1 month.

Preparation

HOMIDIUM SOLUTION-TABLETS FOR INJECTION: available as solution-tablets containing 250 mg of homidium bromide.

A standard for these solution-tablets is given in the British Pharmacopoeia (Veterinary)

Labelling: the label on the container should state the amount of homidium bromide in each tablet and that the solution for injection is prepared by dissolving the solution-tablet in boiling water and allowing to cool before administration.

Honey, Purified

Obtained from the honey in the comb of the hive bee, *Apis mellifera* L. and other species of *Apis* (Fam. Apidae). The honey is melted at a temperature not exceeding 80° and allowed to stand, the impurities which rise to the surface are skimmed off, and the liquid diluted with water until the product has a weight per ml at 20° of 1.355 g.

Most of the honey of commerce is extracted from the comb by centrifugation or by pressure.

OTHER NAME: Mel Depuratum

A standard is given in the British Pharmaceutical Codex 1973

Constituents. Purified honey contains 70 to 80% of glucose and fructose, the ratio of fructose to glucose usually being slightly greater than 1 to 1, together with water, sucrose, dextrin, wax, proteins, volatile oil, and formic acid.

Pollen and flocculent matter are usually present in suspension and tend to induce fermentation.

Description. A thick, syrupy, translucent, pale yellow or yellowish-brown liquid. It has a pleasant characteristic odour; when heated on a water-bath the odour becomes more pronounced but is otherwise unchanged. The taste is sweet and characteristic, varying according to the floral origin.

Weight per ml. At 20°, 1.35 to 1.36 g.

Optical rotation. +0.6° to −3°, determined, at 20°, on a 20% solution in water containing 0.2 ml of *strong ammonia solution*, after decolorising with decolorising charcoal if necessary.

Adulterants and substitutes. Invert sugar is sometimes offered as honey, while sucrose and glucose may occur as adulterants. If prepared by acid hydrolysis, both invert sugar and glucose contain traces of furfuraldehyde.

Dissolve 20 g in 20 ml of water and extract with 40 ml of ether; evaporate the ether extract to dryness and dissolve the residue in 10 ml of ether. To 2 ml of the ether solution at room temperature add 2 ml of *resorcinol and hydrochloric acid solution*; the development of a colour deeper than faint pink in the acid layer, changing to cherry-red on standing, indicates the presence of invert sugar. Evaporate the remainder of the ether solution, obtained above, to dryness at room temperature and to the residue add 2 ml of *aniline acetate solution*; the development of a pink to orange colour after allowing the solution to stand for 15 minutes indicates the presence of invert sugar.

Honey derived from some species of *Eucalyptus* or of

Banksia, or of both, has a strong unpleasant aromatic odour and taste; it may be identified by finding the triangular lenticular pollen grains of *Eucalyptus* spp., measuring about 20 μm, or the sausage-shaped pollen grains of *Banksia* spp., measuring about 50 μm in length, or both these pollens.

Honey-dew honey is dark in colour, congeals with difficulty, and contains hardly any pollen, but commonly unicellular algae of the *Pleurococcus* type are present. Honey-dew does not come from flowers, but is secreted by various aphids, and occurs upon the epidermis of the leaves of conifers and other plants.

Actions and uses. Purified honey is used as a demulcent and sweetening agent, especially in linctuses and cough mixtures.

Preparations

OXYMEL:

Acetic acid	150 ml
Purified water, freshly boiled and cooled ..	150 ml
Purified honey	to 1000 ml

Mix thoroughly.
A standard for oxymel is given in the British Pharmaceutical Codex 1973
Dose: 2.5 to 10 millilitres.

OTHER PREPARATIONS: purified honey is an ingredient of squill oxymel.

Hookworm

see ANCYLOSTOMIASIS

Horsesickness Vaccine

see AFRICAN HORSESICKNESS VACCINE

Hyaluronidase

A mucolytic enzyme having a specific action on the mucopolysaccharide, hyaluronic acid.

OTHER NAMES: *Hyalase*®
Xylodase® (with lignocaine)

A standard is given in the British Pharmaceutical Codex 1973

Hyaluronidase may be prepared from the testes and semen of mammals by fractional precipitation of an aqueous extract, followed by dialysis, sterilisation by a process of filtration, and freeze-drying of the resulting solution. Hydrolysed gelatin or a suitable non-protein stabilising agent may be added.

Description. An odourless white or yellowish-white powder.

Solubility. Soluble in water; practically insoluble in alcohol, in ether, and in acetone.

Acidity or alkalinity. A 0.03% solution has a pH of 4.5 to 7.5.

Storage. It should be stored in single-dose containers, sealed to exclude micro-organisms, in a cool dry place.

Actions and uses. Hyaluronidase is an enzyme which breaks down the hyaluronic acid of the mucoprotein ground substance or tissue cement, thereby reducing its viscosity and rendering the tissues more readily permeable to injected fluids.

When the intravenous administration of fluids is difficult, as in infants, the addition of 500 to 1000 units of hyaluronidase to 500 to 1000 millilitres of fluid will enable the injection to be given by the subcutaneous route at the rate of 10 millilitres per minute. Hyaluronidase may be mixed with the fluid to be injected or it may be injected into the site before the fluid is administered.

The diffusion of local anaesthetics is accelerated by the addition of 1000 to 1500 units to each 20 millilitres of the anaesthetic solution. This is of value in the reduction of fractures and in pudendal block in midwifery.

Substances used in radiography are rapidly absorbed from the site of intramuscular injection with the aid of hyaluronidase, thus providing an alternative to the commoner intravenous technique in pyelography.

It is also used, dissolved with sodium chloride injection, to promote resorption of excess fluids and blood in the tissues.

It may be used to accelerate the absorption of drugs given intramuscularly when a rapid action is desired. Thus it is injected in doses of 1500 units with ergometrine maleate for the prevention of post-partum haemorrhage. As an aid to local anaesthesia in ophthalmology, 150 units may be added to each 5 millilitres of local anaesthetic solution.

Aqueous solutions of hyaluronidase prepared by dissolving the freeze-dried material in water for injections are unstable. Stabilised solutions are available.

Precautions. Hyaluronidase should not be administered intravenously.

Preparations

HYALURONIDASE INJECTION: a sterile solution of hyaluronidase in water for injections. It is prepared by dissolving the contents of a sealed container in water for injections immediately before use. Available in ampoules of powder containing 1500 units of hyaluronidase.
A standard for this injection is given in the British Pharmaceutical Codex 1973
Containers: see the entry on Injections for general information on containers.
Labelling: see the entry on Injections for general information on labelling. In addition, the label on the container should state that the contents are not to be used for intravascular injection.
Storage: the sealed container should be stored in a cool place. The injection decomposes on storage and should be used immediately after preparation.

OTHER PREPARATIONS available include a CREAM containing hyaluronidase 50 units and lignocaine 50 mg per g.

Hydrallazine Hydrochloride

1-Hydrazinophthalazine hydrochloride

$C_8H_9ClN_4 = 196.6$

OTHER NAMES: *Apresoline*®; Hydralazine Hydrochloride

Description. An odourless white crystalline powder with a bitter saline taste.

Solubility. Soluble, at 20°, in 25 parts of water and in 500 parts of alcohol; very slightly soluble in ether.

Acidity. A 2% solution has a pH of 3 to 4.

Dissociation constant. pK_a 7.0 (20°).

Storage. It should be stored in airtight containers.

Identification. TEST. Dissolve about 500 mg in a mixture of 100 ml of water and 8 ml of *dilute hydrochloric acid*, add 20 ml of a 1% solution of sodium nitrite, and allow to stand for 10 minutes; a precipitate is produced which, after washing with water, melts at about 210°.

MELTING-POINT. About 275° with decomposition.

ULTRAVIOLET ABSORPTION. In 0.1N hydrochloric acid, maxima at 260 nm (E1%, 1cm = 466) and 304 nm (E1%, 1cm = 243). In water, maxima at 240 nm (E1%, 1cm = 580), 260 nm (E1%, 1cm = 540), 303 nm (E1%, 1cm = 270), and 315 nm (E1%, 1cm = 210).

Determination in body fluids. ULTRAVIOLET SPECTRO-PHOTOMETRY. In plasma or urine—S. B. Zak *et al.*, *J. pharm. Sci.*, 1974, 63, 225.

GAS CHROMATOGRAPHY. In plasma—D. B. Jack *et al.*, *J. Chromat.*, 1975, 115, 87.

Metabolism. ABSORPTION. Rapidly absorbed after oral administration.

BLOOD CONCENTRATION. After a single oral dose of 50 mg, peak serum concentrations of 265 to 580 ng/ml are attained in 30 minutes in fast acetylators and peak serum concentrations of 310 to 670 ng/ml are attained in 1 to 2 hours in slow acetylators; during therapy with an oral dose of 25 mg administered thrice daily, minimum serum concentrations at the steady state are about 57 ng/ml and 33 ng/ml for slow and fast acetylators respectively; maximum serum concentrations at the steady state for the same dose reach 228 ng/ml and 147 ng/ml for slow and fast acetylators respectively.

HALF-LIFE. Serum half-lives do not correspond with the acetylator phenotype and are in the range 2 to 8.5 hours; the serum half-life is increased in patients with renal function impairment.

METABOLIC REACTIONS. Polymorphic *N*-acetylation, hydroxylation, glucuronic acid conjugation, and removal of the hydrazine group to form phthalazine which may be further metabolised; *N*-acetylation is the major reaction and influences systemic availability of the drug since hydrallazine undergoes first-pass metabolism and rapid acetylators metabolise more of the drug during the first-pass phase.

EXCRETION. 3 to 14% of a dose is excreted unchanged in the urine and 10% is excreted in the faeces; the major urinary metabolite has been suggested as 1-(2-acetylhydrazino)phthalazine but this has been disputed and it has been suggested that 3-methyl-1,2,4-triazolo[3,4-*a*]phthalazine may be the major urinary metabolite.

FURTHER INFORMATION. Hydrallazine elimination—M. M. Reidenberg *et al.*, *Clin. Pharmac. Ther.*, 1973, 14, 970; metabolism—T. Talseth, *Eur. J. clin. Pharmac.*, 1976, 10, 183 and 311; concentrations in plasma and urine—S. B. Zak *et al.*, *J. pharm. Sci.*, 1974, 63, 225; identification of a hydrallazine metabolite—H. Zimmer *et al.*, *Arzneimittel-Forsch.*, 1973, 23, 1028.

Actions and uses. Hydrallazine hydrochloride lowers blood pressure. Its exact mechanism of action is unclear but it acts mainly on the cardiovascular system causing relaxation of the vascular smooth muscle and peripheral vasodilatation resulting in a decreased arterial blood pressure and peripheral vascular resistance and an increase in heart rate, stroke volume, and cardiac output. Hydrallazine is usually given in conjunction with other antihypertensive agents.

The usual initial dose given by mouth in conjunction with other antihypertensive agents is 25 milligrams 3 times daily increasing to 50 milligrams 4 times daily if necessary. In the treatment of hypertensive crises associated with pre-eclampsia and of hypertension with renal complications a dose of 20 to 40 milligrams may be administered by slow intravenous injection or infusion and repeated as necessary.

Undesirable effects. Tachycardia, severe headache, anorexia, nausea, vomiting, and postural hypotension may occur. Fever, vertigo, flushing or sweating, dyspnoea, malaise, and urticaria may also occur. Occasionally, angina, localised areas of oedema, urinary retention, paraesthesia, emotional depression, and tremor occur. The prolonged use of large doses may give rise to a condition resembling either early rheumatoid arthritis or acute systemic lupus erythematosus; the condition usually disappears on withdrawal of the drug.

Precautions. Treatment with hydrallazine should be withdrawn if rheumatic symptoms, skin reactions, and fever similar to systemic lupus erythematosus occur. It should be given with caution to patients with coronary disease or to those undergoing anaesthesia or taking tricyclic antidepressants or monoamine-oxidase inhibitors.

Contra-indications. Hydrallazine should not be given to patients with tachycardia.

Preparations

Preparations available include an INJECTION reconstituted from ampoules of powder containing hydrallazine hydrochloride 20 mg and TABLETS containing hydrallazine hydrochloride 25 and 50 mg.

Hydrochloric Acid

HCl = 36.46

OTHER NAMES: Acidum Hydrochloricum Concentratum; Concentrated Hydrochloric Acid

A standard is given in the European Pharmacopoeia Vol. II

Hydrochloric acid contains about 36.5% w/w of HCl. When heated, hydrochloric acid gas is evolved until the strength of the solution falls to approximately 20% w/w; this forms a constant-boiling mixture with a boiling-point of about 110°.

Impure hydrochloric acid of commerce is popularly known as "spirits of salt" and as "muriatic acid".

Description. A clear, colourless, fuming liquid with a pungent odour.

Weight per ml. At 20°, about 1.18 g.

Storage. It should be stored in a stoppered or otherwise suitably closed container of glass or other inert material at a temperature not exceeding 30°.

Actions and uses. Hydrochloric acid is a powerful corrosive although less so than sulphuric acid or nitric acid. The acid is secreted in the body by the oxyntic cells of the stomach; it is essential for the activation of pepsin during the digestion of protein.

Dilute hydrochloric acid, well diluted, is given by mouth in the treatment of achlorhydria, hypochlorhydria, and gastrogenous diarrhoea. Not more than about 20 millilitres, well diluted, should be given during a period of 24 hours.

Poisoning. As for Acetic Acid.

Preparation

DILUTE HYDROCHLORIC ACID (*Syn.* Acidum Hydrochloricum Dilutum):

Hydrochloric acid ..	..	..	..	..	274 g
Purified water, freshly boiled and cooled	..	..	..	..	726 g

Mix.

A standard for this acid is given in the European Pharmacopoeia Vol. II

Storage: it should be stored in a stoppered or otherwise suitably closed container of glass or other inert material at a temperature not exceeding 30°.

Advice for patients: the dose should be taken well diluted with water and sipped slowly through a straw during the course of a meal.

Hydrochlorothiazide

6-Chloro-3,4-dihydro-2*H*-benzo-1,2,4-thiadiazine-7-sulphonamide 1,1-dioxide

$C_7H_8ClN_3O_4S_2 = 297.7$

OTHER NAMES: *Direma®*; *Esidrex®*; *HydroSaluric®*; *Vetidrex®*

Moduretic® (with amiloride hydrochloride); *Hydromet®* (with methyldopa); *Co-Betaloc®* (with metoprolol tartrate); *Esidrex K®* (with potassium chloride); *Dyazide®* (with triamterene)

A standard is given in the British Pharmacopoeia 1973

Description. A white crystalline odourless powder with a slightly bitter taste.

Solubility. Very slightly soluble in water, in ether, and in chloroform; soluble, at 20°, in 200 parts of alcohol and in 20 parts of acetone; soluble in solutions of alkali hydroxides.

Moisture content. Not more than 1%, determined by drying at 105°.

Dissociation constants. pK_a 7.9, 9.2.

Storage. It should be stored in airtight containers.

Identification. TEST. To about 10 mg add 10 mg of chromotropic acid sodium salt and 1 ml of water, and then cautiously add 5 ml of sulphuric acid and mix; a purple colour is produced (distinction from chlorothiazide).

MELTING-POINT. About 267°, with decomposition.

ULTRAVIOLET ABSORPTION. In 0.1N sodium hydroxide, maxima at 273 nm (E1%, 1cm = 500) and 323 nm (E1%, 1cm = 95); in alcohol (95%), maxima at 273 nm (E1%, 1cm = 645) and 320 nm (E1%, 1cm = 101).

INFRA-RED ABSORPTION. Major peaks at 1062, 1128, 1157, 1172, 1324, and 1340 cm^{-1} (see Appendix 2a: Infra-red Spectra).

THIN-LAYER CHROMATOGRAPHY. See under Thin-layer Chromatography, System 6.

Determination in body fluids. COLORIMETRY. In urine —H. Sheppard *et al.*, *J. Am. pharm. Ass., scient. Edn*, 1960, **49**, 722.

GAS CHROMATOGRAPHY. In blood or plasma—W. J. A. Vandenheuvel *et al.*, *J. pharm. Sci.*, 1975, **64**, 1309; in

plasma or urine—B. Lindstroem *et al.*, *J. Chromat.*, 1975, **114**, 459.

Metabolism. ABSORPTION. Well absorbed after oral administration.

BLOOD CONCENTRATION. After an oral dose of 65 mg, peak serum concentrations of about 0.8 μg/ml are attained after 4 hours.

HALF-LIFE. Serum half-life, about 3 hours and, based on urinary excretion, about 6 hours.

METABOLIC REACTIONS. Not significantly metabolised in man.

EXCRETION. After an intravenous dose, 54% is excreted in the urine in 4.5 hours and 100% within 24 hours; after an oral dose in tablet form, up to 80% is excreted in the urine in 24 hours; after an oral dose in capsule form, about 30% is excreted in the urine.

FURTHER INFORMATION. Bioavailability—M. C. Meyer and P. L. Whyatt, *J. Am. pharm. Ass.*, 1976, **16**, 47; influence of formulation and processing on dissolution rates of tablets—P. Seth, *Pharm. Acta Helv.*, 1972, **47**, 457; influence of dosage form on activity—P. J. Tannenbaum *et al.*, *Clin. Pharmac. Ther.*, 1968, **9**, 598.

Actions and uses. Hydrochlorothiazide is a thiazide diuretic which has actions and uses similar to those described under Chlorothiazide, but it is effective in smaller doses.

For the treatment of oedema, the dosage is 50 to 200 milligrams by mouth daily or on alternate days, but as an adjunct to hypotensive drugs in the treatment of hypertension 25 to 50 milligrams may be sufficient.

Undesirable effects; Precautions. As for Chlorothiazide.

Veterinary uses. Hydrochlorothiazide is used in animals as a diuretic. The usual dose by mouth for dogs and cats is 1.25 to 2.5 milligrams per kilogram body-weight daily. It is also administered by intramuscular injection as the sodium salt, the usual dose for horses and cattle being 200 to 500 micrograms per kilogram body-weight daily, for pigs 150 to 500 micrograms per kilogram body-weight daily, and for dogs and cats 250 micrograms per kilogram body-weight daily. The doses for horses and cattle may also be given by intravenous injection.

Preparations

HYDROCHLOROTHIAZIDE TABLETS: available as tablets containing 25 and 50 mg of hydrochlorothiazide.

A standard for these tablets is given in the British Pharmacopoeia 1973

Containers and *Storage:* see the entry on Tablets for general information on containers and storage. Containers should be airtight.

Advice for patients: daily doses should preferably be taken in the morning. Treatment should not be discontinued without the advice of the prescriber.

OTHER PREPARATIONS available include a veterinary INJECTION containing hydrochlorothiazide 50 mg per ml in 10-ml vials; veterinary dispersible TABLETS containing hydrochlorothiazide 250 mg, tablets containing hydrochlorothiazide 12.5 mg with potassium chloride 600 mg (K^+ 8.1 mmol) in a slow-release formulation, tablets containing hydrochlorothiazide 12.5 mg with metoprolol tartrate 100 mg, tablets containing hydrochlorothiazide 15 mg with methyldopa equivalent to 250 mg of anhydrous methyldopa, tablets containing hydrochlorothiazide 25 mg with triamterene 50 mg, and tablets containing hydrochlorothiazide 50 mg with amiloride hydrochloride 5 mg.

Hydrocortisone

11β,17α,21-Trihydroxypregn-4-ene-3,20-dione

$C_{21}H_{30}O_5 = 362.5$

OTHER NAMES: *Cobadex*®; *Cortenema*®; Cortisol; *Cortril*®; *Dioderm*®; *Dome-Cort*®; *Efcortelan*®; Hydrocort.; Hydrocortisonum; *Hydrocortistab*®; *Hydrocortisyl*®; *Hydrocortone*®; *Topisone*® *Otosporin*® (with neomycin sulphate and polymyxin B sulphate); *Terra-Cortril*® (with oxytetracycline hydrochloride); hydrocortisone is an ingredient of a number of other preparations and names for compound preparations with one other ingredient will usually be found in the monograph describing that substance.

A standard is given in the European Pharmacopoeia Vol. II

Description. An odourless white crystalline powder.

Solubility. Practically insoluble in water; soluble, at 20°, in 40 parts of alcohol and in 80 parts of acetone; very slightly soluble in chloroform and in ether.

Moisture content. Not more than 1%, determined by drying at 105°.

Specific rotation. +150° to +156°, determined on a 1% solution in dioxan.

Storage. It should be protected from light.

Identification. TESTS. 1. It complies with Test 1 described under Betamethasone.
2. To 2 ml of a 0.1% solution in alcohol (95%) add 2 ml of sulphuric acid; the solution becomes intensely yellow with a green fluorescence and remains the same after the addition of 16 ml of water.

MELTING-POINT. About 214°, with decomposition.

ULTRAVIOLET ABSORPTION. In alcohol (95%), maximum at 240 nm (E1%, 1cm = 435).

INFRA-RED ABSORPTION. Major peaks at 1114, 1242, 1435, 1612, 1642, and 1710 cm⁻¹ (see Appendix 2a: Infrared Spectra).

THIN-LAYER CHROMATOGRAPHY. See under Thin-layer Chromatography, System 10.

Determination in body fluids. ULTRAVIOLET SPECTROPHOTOMETRY. In plasma—H. E. Hadd, *Biochem. Med.*, 1975, **13**, 353.

SPECTROFLUORIMETRY. In plasma—E. W. Kwarts *et al.*, *Pharm. Weekbl. Ned.*, 1973, **108**, 765.

HIGH PRESSURE LIQUID CHROMATOGRAPHY. In plasma—F. K. Trefz *et al.*, *J. Chromat.*, 1975, **107**, 181.

Metabolism. ABSORPTION. Well absorbed after oral administration of hydrocortisone or acetate; the acetate, however, is more slowly absorbed than hydrocortisone; absorption occurs through the skin after topical application and is increased when hydrocortisone is administered with dimethyl sulphoxide; the acetate is poorly absorbed after intramuscular injection.

BLOOD CONCENTRATION. After an intravenous dose of 100 mg as a soluble compound, plasma concentrations of up to 1 μg/ml are attained in 30 minutes. Endogenous plasma hydrocortisone exhibits a circadian rhythm; in the morning, concentrations are in the range 8 to 20 μg/ml and, in the evening, in the range 4 to 10 μg/ml; it has been suggested that exogenous hydrocortisone in plasma is subject to similar fluctuations possibly as a result of changes in the activities of the drug-metabolising enzymes.

HALF-LIFE. Plasma half-life, 80 to 120 minutes which may be increased in patients with liver disease, hypothyroidism, or in patients undergoing oestrogen therapy.

DISTRIBUTION. Widely distributed throughout the body; *protein binding*, about 90% bound to plasma proteins, mainly to corticosteroid-binding globulin and also to albumin.

METABOLIC REACTIONS. Metabolised in the liver and other tissues by ring-A reduction, 20-ketone reduction, side-chain cleavage, ring-A hydroxylation, and conjugation with glucuronic acid or sulphate.

EXCRETION. About 90% of a dose is excreted in the urine in 24 hours; less than 1% is excreted unchanged, 40% is the 5α- and 5β-forms of tetrahydrocortisol and the 5β-form of tetrahydrocortisone, 17% is a mixture of the 5α- and 5β- and 20α- and 20β-cortols and cortolones, 6% is 11-hydroxy- and 11-keto-etiocholanolone; most of the metabolites are excreted as conjugates; at plasma concentrations of greater than 0.2 μg/ml, the amount of unchanged drug excreted in the urine is increased.

FURTHER INFORMATION. Metabolism—D. K. Fukushima *et al.*, *J. biol. Chem.*, 1960, **235**, 2246 and P. L. Morselli *et al.*, *Biochem. Pharmac.*, 1970, **19**, 1643.

Actions and uses. Hydrocortisone is a normal secretion of the adrenal cortex in man. It has actions, uses, and undesirable effects similar to those described under Cortisone Acetate and it is given in similar dosage; 20 milligrams of hydrocortisone is approximately equivalent in glucocorticoid activity to 5 milligrams of prednisolone.
In emergencies such as Addisonian or postadrenalectomy crises the equivalent of 100 milligrams of hydrocortisone may be given by intravenous infusion followed by similar doses every 6 to 8 hours; a water-soluble derivative of hydrocortisone such as hydrocortisone sodium succinate or hydrocortisone sodium phosphate is used for intravenous administration. When only an anti-inflammatory effect is required prednisolone is to be preferred.
A suspension of 100 milligrams of hydrocortisone in 60 to 120 millilitres of sodium chloride solution may be used as a retention enema in the treatment of ulcerative colitis; hydrocortisone acetate and hydrocortisone sodium succinate are also used for this purpose but prednisolone enema is usually preferred.
Hydrocortisone may be applied externally in ointments, creams, and lotions.

Precautions and contra-indications. As for Cortisone Acetate.

Preparations

HYDROCORTISONE AND CLIOQUINOL OINTMENT:

Hydrocortisone, or hydrocortisone acetate, in ultra-fine powder		10 g
Clioquinol, in very fine powder		30 g
Wool fat		100 g
White soft paraffin		860 g

Melt together the wool fat and white soft paraffin and stir until cold. Incorporate the clioquinol and the hydrocortisone, or hydrocortisone acetate, in the cold basis. The ointment may be prepared with any other suitable basis.

A standard for this ointment is given in the British Pharmaceutical Codex 1973

Containers and *Labelling*: see the entry on Ointments for general information on containers and labelling. The ointment should be protected from light. When collapsible tubes are used they should preferably be made of plastic material. If made of aluminium, the inner surface of the tubes should be lacquered.

Advice for patients: the ointment should be applied sparingly to the affected area. It stains the skin, hair, and fabric; a dressing may be applied.

HYDROCORTISONE AND NEOMYCIN CREAM:

Hydrocortisone, in ultra-fine powder .. .. .. 5 g
Neomycin cream .. .. 995 g

Incorporate the hydrocortisone in the neomycin cream. A phosphate buffer may be included.

A standard for this cream is given in the British Pharmaceutical Codex 1973

Containers, Labelling, and *Storage:* see the entry on Creams for general information on containers, labelling, and storage.

Advice for patients: the cream should be applied sparingly to the affected area.

HYDROCORTISONE AND OXYTETRACYCLINE OINTMENT: a dispersion of hydrocortisone and oxytetracycline hydrochloride in a suitable anhydrous greasy basis. It contains 10 mg of hydrocortisone and oxytetracycline hydrochloride equivalent to 30 mg of oxytetracycline per g.

Containers and *Labelling:* see the entry on Ointments for general information on containers and labelling.

Advice for patients: the ointment should be applied sparingly to the affected area.

HYDROCORTISONE CREAM:

Hydrocortisone or hydrocortisone acetate in ultra-fine powder .. .. 10 g
Chlorocresol .. .. 1 g
Cetomacrogol emulsifying ointment .. .. 300 g
Purified water, freshly boiled and cooled .. 689 g

Dissolve the chlorocresol in the water with the aid of gentle heat; melt the cetomacrogol emulsifying ointment on a water-bath, add the chlorocresol solution at the same temperature, stir until cold, and incorporate the hydrocortisone or hydrocortisone acetate. A phosphate buffer may be included.

A standard for this cream is given in the British Pharmaceutical Codex 1973

Containers and *Storage:* see the entry on Creams for general information on containers and storage.

Labelling: see the entry on Creams for general information on labelling. In addition, the label on the container should state whether the cream contains hydrocortisone or hydrocortisone acetate.

Advice for patients: the cream should be applied sparingly to the affected area.

HYDROCORTISONE LOTION:

Hydrocortisone, in ultra-fine powder .. .. 10.0 g
Chlorocresol .. .. 0.5 g
Self-emulsifying monostearin .. .. .. 40.0 g
Glycerol .. .. 63.0 g
Purified water, freshly boiled and cooled .. .. to 1000 g

Dissolve the chlorocresol in 850 ml of the water with the aid of gentle heat, add the self-emulsifying monostearin, heat to 60°, and stir until completely dispersed. Triturate the hydrocortisone with the glycerol, incorporate, with constant stirring, in the warm basis, allow to cool slowly, stirring until cold, add sufficient of the water to produce the required weight, and mix. Hydrocortisone lotion may be prepared with any other suitable basis. If prepared extemporaneously, the lotion should not be used later than 1 month after preparation.

A standard for this lotion is given in the British Pharmaceutical Codex 1973

Containers and *Labelling:* see the entry on Lotions for general information on containers and labelling.

Advice for patients: the lotion should be applied sparingly to the affected area.

HYDROCORTISONE, NEOMYCIN, AND POLYMYXIN EARDROPS: consisting of hydrocortisone, neomycin sulphate, and polymyxin B sulphate in an aqueous vehicle. It contains 10 mg of hydrocortisone, 3400 units of neomycin sulphate, and 10000 units of polymyxin B sulphate per ml.

Containers and *Labelling:* see the entry on Ear-drops for general information on containers and labelling.

Storage: it should be stored in a cool place, protected from light.

Advice for patients: the ear canal should be cleansed without the use of soap before the drops are instilled. The prescribed course should be completed.

HYDROCORTISONE OINTMENT (*Syn.* Ung. Hydrocort.): prepared by incorporating hydrocortisone, in very fine powder, in either white soft paraffin or a mixture of liquid paraffin and white soft paraffin. Available as an ointment containing 0.5, 1, or 2.5%.

A standard for this ointment is given in the British Pharmacopoeia 1973

Containers: see the entry on Ointments for general information on containers. The ointment should be protected from light.

Advice for patients: the ointment should be applied sparingly to the affected area.

HYDROCORTISONE SUPPOSITORIES: prepared as described in the entry on Suppositories by incorporating hydrocortisone or hydrocortisone acetate, in ultra-fine powder, in theobroma oil or other suitable basis. Approximately 1.5 g of hydrocortisone or hydrocortisone acetate displaces 1 g of theobroma oil.

Available as suppositories containing 25 mg of hydrocortisone or of hydrocortisone acetate.

A standard for these suppositories is given in the British Pharmaceutical Codex 1973

Containers and *Storage:* see the entry on Suppositories for general information on containers and storage.

Advice for patients: see the entry on Suppositories for general information on the use of suppositories. They should be used after defaecation unless otherwise directed.

HYDROCORTISONE TABLETS: available as tablets containing 10 and 20 mg of hydrocortisone.

Containers and *Storage:* see the entry on Tablets for general information on containers and storage. Containers should be airtight and light resistant.

Advice for patients: in long-term use, treatment should not be discontinued without the advice of the prescriber. Patients may carry an identification card giving details of their treatment and the name of the prescriber who should be contacted in the event of accident, feverish illness, diarrhoea, vomiting, or alimentary disturbances.

In short-term treatment the prescribed course should be completed.

OTHER PREPARATIONS available include numerous compound preparations in which hydrocortisone is an ingredient.

Hydrocortisone Acetate

$11\beta,17\alpha,21$-Trihydroxypregn-4-ene-3,20-dione 21-acetate

$C_{23}H_{32}O_6 = 404.5$

OTHER NAMES: *Colifoam* ®; Cortisol Acetate; Hydrocort. Acet.; Hydrocortisoni Acetas; *Hydrocortistab* ®; *Hydrocortone* ®; *Pabracort* ®

Neo-Cortef (with neomycin sulphate); hydrocortisone acetate is an ingredient of a number of other preparations and names for compound preparations with one other ingredient will usually be found in the monograph describing that substance; many names used for preparations of hydrocortisone acetate are also applied to preparations of hydrocortisone.

A standard is given in the European Pharmacopoeia Vol. II

Description. An odourless white crystalline powder.

Solubility. Practically insoluble in water; soluble, at 20°, in 230 parts of alcohol and in 150 parts of chloroform.

Moisture content. Not more than 1%, determined by drying at 105°.

Specific rotation. +157° to +167°, determined on a 1% solution in dioxan.

Preparation of solid dosage forms. In order to achieve a satisfactory rate of dissolution, hydrocortisone acetate in the form of an ultra-fine powder should be used.

Storage. It should be protected from light.

Identification. TESTS. 1. It complies with Test 1 described under Betamethasone.
2. It complies with Test 2 described under Hydrocortisone.
3. It complies with Test 3 under Cortisone Acetate (acetyl groups).

MELTING-POINT. About 220°, with decomposition.

ULTRAVIOLET ABSORPTION. In alcohol (95%), maximum at 240 nm (E1%, 1cm = 390).

INFRA-RED ABSORPTION. Major peaks at 1233, 1272, 1377, 1629, 1723, and 1745 cm^{-1} (see Appendix 2a: Infra-red Spectra).

THIN-LAYER CHROMATOGRAPHY. See under Thin-layer Chromatography, System 10.

Determination in body fluids; Metabolism. See under Hydrocortisone.

Actions and uses. Hydrocortisone acetate has actions, uses, and undesirable effects similar to those described under Cortisone Acetate.

It is given by intra-articular injection into joints affected by rheumatoid and other arthritic conditions; a dose of 5 to 50 milligrams, depending on the size of the joint to be injected, may relieve pain and swelling for several days or weeks. It may also be injected into painful lesions of ligaments and muscle, such as tennis elbow, and into bursae.

Hydrocortisone acetate is applied to the skin for the treatment of inflammatory conditions accompanied by irritation of the skin, such as pruritus ani. It may also be used for the treatment of inflammatory conditions of the eye, but it should be used with the utmost caution, as hydrocortisone may mask the development of infection; an antibacterial substance, such as neomycin, may be used in conjunction with hydrocortisone to minimise this danger.

Hydrocortisone acetate is given in a retention enema in the treatment of ulcerative colitis, the equivalent of 100 milligrams of hydrocortisone suspended in 60 to 120 millilitres of sodium chloride solution being a suitable dose; prednisolone enema is usually preferred for this purpose.

Precautions and contra-indications. As for Cortisone Acetate.

Preparations

HYDROCORTISONE ACETATE INJECTION: a sterile suspension of hydrocortisone acetate, in very fine particles, with suitable dispersing agents, in water for injections. It is prepared by means of an aseptic technique.
Available in 1-ml ampoules and 5-ml vials containing 25 mg of hydrocortisone acetate per ml.
A standard for this injection is given in the British Pharmacopoeia 1973
Containers: see the entry on Injections for general information on containers.
Labelling: see the entry on Injections for general information on labelling. In addition, the label on the container should state the names of the dispersing agents and the words "By injection, for local action".
Storage: it should be protected from light.

HYDROCORTISONE ACETATE OINTMENT (*Syn.* Ung. Hydrocort. Acet.): prepared by incorporating hydrocortisone acetate, in very fine powder, in either white soft paraffin or a mixture of liquid paraffin and white soft paraffin.
Available as an ointment containing 0.5, 1, or 2.5%.
A standard for this ointment is given in the British Pharmacopoeia 1973
Containers: see the entry on Ointments for general information on containers. The ointment should be protected from light.
Advice for patients: the ointment should be applied sparingly to the affected area.

HYDROCORTISONE AND CLIOQUINOL OINTMENT: see above under Hydrocortisone.

HYDROCORTISONE AND NEOMYCIN EAR-DROPS: consisting of a suspension of hydrocortisone acetate, in ultra-fine powder with appropriate pharmaceutical adjuvants, in a solution of neomycin sulphate in freshly boiled and cooled purified water.
Available as ear-drops containing 1.5% of hydrocortisone acetate and 0.5% of neomycin sulphate and as veterinary ear-drops containing 0.5% of hydrocortisone acetate and 0.5% of neomycin sulphate.
A standard for these ear-drops is given in the British Pharmaceutical Codex 1973
Containers: see the entry on Ear-drops for general information on containers.

Labelling: see the entry on Ear-drops for general information on labelling. In addition, the label on the container or package should state the date after which the ear-drops are not intended to be used, and a direction to shake the bottle.

Storage: it should be stored in a cool place; it should not be allowed to freeze.

Advice for patients: the prescribed course should be completed.

HYDROCORTISONE AND NEOMYCIN EYE-DROPS: consisting of a sterile suspension containing up to 1.5% of hydrocortisone acetate, in ultra-fine powder, in a solution containing 0.5% of neomycin sulphate, with 0.002% of phenylmercuric acetate or nitrate or other suitable preservatives, in purified water.

Available as eye-drops containing 1.5% of hydrocortisone acetate and 0.5% of neomycin sulphate and as veterinary eye-drops containing 0.5% of hydrocortisone acetate and 0.5% of neomycin sulphate.

A standard for these eye-drops is given in the British Pharmaceutical Codex 1973

Containers: see the entry on Eye-drops for general information on containers.

Labelling: see the entry on Eye-drops for general information on labelling. In addition, a direction to shake the bottle should be given on the label.

Storage: it should be stored in a cool place; it should not be allowed to freeze.

Advice for patients: see the entry on Eye-drops for general information on the use of eye-drops. The prescribed course should be completed.

HYDROCORTISONE AND NEOMYCIN EYE OINTMENT: prepared by incorporating hydrocortisone acetate and neomycin sulphate, both in ultra-fine powder, in eye ointment basis, or any other suitable basis, by method B described in the entry on Eye Ointments.

Available as an eye ointment containing 1.5% of hydrocortisone acetate and 0.5% of neomycin sulphate.

A standard for this eye ointment is given in the British Pharmaceutical Codex 1973

Labelling: see the entry on Eye Ointments for general information on labelling.

Advice for patients: see the entry on Eye Ointments for general information on the use of eye ointments. The prescribed course should be completed.

HYDROCORTISONE CREAM: see above under Hydrocortisone.

HYDROCORTISONE EYE-DROPS: consisting of a sterile suspension containing up to 1% of hydrocortisone acetate, in ultra-fine powder, with suitable preservatives, in purified water. It may also contain appropriate pharmaceutical adjuvants. The eye-drops are not generally suitable for extemporaneous preparation.

Available as eye-drops containing 1% of hydrocortisone acetate.

Adsorption: it is known that benzalkonium chloride can be adsorbed and partially inactivated by the hydrocortisone acetate in this preparation. The extent of adsorption of other preservatives is not known. These factors should be recognised in the selection of a suitable preservative system for the eye-drops.

A standard for these eye-drops is given in the British Pharmaceutical Codex 1973

Containers: see the entry on Eye-drops for general information on containers.

Labelling: see the entry on Eye-drops for general information on labelling. In addition, a direction to shake the bottle should be given on the label.

Storage: it should be stored in a cool place; it should not be allowed to freeze.

Advice for patients: see the entry on Eye-drops for general information on the use of eye-drops.

HYDROCORTISONE EYE OINTMENT (*Syn.* Hydrocortisone Acetate Eye Ointment): prepared by incorporating hydrocortisone acetate, in ultra-fine powder, in eye ointment basis, or any other suitable basis, by method B described in the entry on Eye Ointments.

Available as an eye ointment containing 2.5% of hydrocortisone acetate.

A standard for this eye ointment is given in the British Pharmaceutical Codex 1973

Labelling: see the entry on Eye Ointments for general information on labelling.

Advice for patients: see the entry on Eye Ointments for general information on the use of eye ointments.

HYDROCORTISONE SUPPOSITORIES: see above under Hydrocortisone.

OTHER PREPARATIONS available include an APPLICATION containing hydrocortisone acetate 10% in an aerosol pack (formulated to produce a foam for rectal application); an INSUFFLATION in cartridges containing hydrocortisone acetate 15 mg; and numerous compound preparations in which hydrocortisone acetate is an ingredient.

Hydrocortisone Hydrogen Succinate

11β,17α,21-Trihydroxypregn-4-ene-3,20-dione 21-(hydrogen succinate)

$C_{25}H_{34}O_8 = 462.5$

OTHER NAME: Hydrocort. Hydrogen Succ.

A standard is given in the British Pharmacopoeia 1973

Description. An odourless white crystalline powder.

Solubility. Very slightly soluble in water; soluble, at 20°, in 40 parts of alcohol, in 7 parts of dehydrated alcohol, and in 25 parts of sodium bicarbonate solution; soluble, with decomposition, in sodium hydroxide solution.

Moisture content. Not more than 5%, determined by drying at 100° *in vacuo.*

Specific rotation. +147° to +153°, determined on a 1% solution in dehydrated alcohol.

Storage. It should be protected from light.

Identification. TESTS. 1. It complies with Test 1 described under Betamethasone.
2. Mix about 25 mg with 10 ml of *dilute hydrochloric acid,* boil for 10 minutes, and evaporate to dryness on a water-bath; add 5 ml of *dilute ammonia solution,* evaporate to dryness in a small dish, and dry at 100° for 30 minutes; mix the residue with 2.5 g of zinc powder, transfer to a test-tube, and heat gently over a flame whilst exposing to the vapours a pine wood shaving which has been moistened with hydrochloric acid; the shaving becomes red to brownish-red.

MELTING-POINT. About 168°; it may also occur in a form which melts at about 200°.

ULTRAVIOLET ABSORPTION. In alcohol (95%), maximum at 240 nm (E1%, 1cm = 338).

INFRA-RED ABSORPTION. Major peaks at 1163, 1178, 1304, 1625, 1719, and 1753 cm⁻¹ (see Appendix 2a: Infra-red Spectra).

THIN-LAYER CHROMATOGRAPHY. See under Thin-layer Chromatography, System 10.

Determination in body fluids; Metabolism. See under Hydrocortisone.

Actions and uses. Hydrocortisone hydrogen succinate has actions, uses, and undesirable effects similar to those described under Cortisone Acetate. It is used in the preparation of hydrocortisone sodium succinate injection.

Precautions and contra-indications. As for Cortisone Acetate.

Hydrocortisone Sodium Phosphate

11β,17α,21-Trihydroxypregn-4-ene-3,20-dione 21-(disodium phosphate)

$C_{21}H_{29}Na_2O_8P = 486.4$

OTHER NAME: *Efcortesol*®

A standard is given in the British Pharmaceutical Codex 1973

Description. An odourless white hygroscopic powder.

Solubility. Soluble, at 20°, in 4 parts of water; very slightly soluble in dehydrated alcohol; practically insoluble in chloroform.

Alkalinity. A 0.5% solution has a pH of 7.5 to 9.

Storage. It should be stored in airtight containers, protected from light.

Identification. TEST. Dissolve about 2 mg in 2 ml of sulphuric acid; a yellowish-green fluorescence is immediately produced (distinction from betamethasone sodium phosphate and prednisolone sodium phosphate).

ULTRAVIOLET ABSORPTION. In alcohol (95%), maximum at 240 nm (E1%, 1cm = 308).

INFRA-RED ABSORPTION. Major peaks at 985, 997, 1115, 1147, 1683, and 1719 cm⁻¹ (see Appendix 2a: Infra-red Spectra).

Determination in body fluids; Metabolism. See under Hydrocortisone.

Actions and uses. Hydrocortisone sodium phosphate has actions, uses, and undesirable effects similar to those described under Cortisone Acetate. As it is soluble in water, it is suitable for the preparation of intravenous or intramuscular injections; 134 mg of the ester is approximately equivalent to 100 mg of hydrocortisone.

Intravenous infusion of hydrocortisone may be life-saving in Addisonian crisis or severe status asthmaticus. The usual dose for this purpose is the equivalent of 100 to 500 milligrams of hydrocortisone.

Precautions and contra-indications. As for Cortisone Acetate.

Preparation

HYDROCORTISONE SODIUM PHOSPHATE INJECTION: a sterile solution of hydrocortisone sodium phosphate, with suitable buffering and stabilising agents, in water for injections. It is sterilised by filtration.

Available in 1- and 5-ml ampoules containing hydrocortisone sodium phosphate equivalent to 100 mg of hydrocortisone per ml.

A standard for this injection is given in the British Pharmaceutical Codex 1973

Containers: see the entry on Injections for general information on containers.

Labelling: see the entry on Injections for general information on labelling. In addition, the label on the container and the label or wrapper on the package should state that the injection should not be administered intrathecally.

Storage: it should be stored in a cool place, protected from light.

Hydrocortisone Sodium Succinate

11β,17α,21-Trihydroxypregn-4-ene-3,20-dione 21-(sodium succinate)

$C_{25}H_{33}NaO_8 = 484.5$

OTHER NAMES: *Corlan*®; *Efcortelan*®; Hydrocort. Sod. Succ.; *Solu-Cortef*®

A standard is given in the British Pharmacopoeia 1973

Description. An odourless, white, hygroscopic, crystalline powder.

Solubility. Soluble, at 20°, in 3 parts of water, in 34 parts of alcohol, and in 200 parts of dehydrated alcohol; practically insoluble in ether and in chloroform.

Moisture content. Not more than 3%, determined by drying at 100° *in vacuo*.

Specific rotation. +136° to +144°, determined on a 1% solution in alcohol (95%).

Storage. It should be stored in airtight containers, protected from light.

Identification. TESTS. 1. It complies with Test 1 described under Betamethasone.
2. It complies with Test 2 described under Hydrocortisone Hydrogen Succinate.

MELTING-POINT. About 170°.

Determination in body fluids; Metabolism. See under Hydrocortisone.

Actions and uses. Hydrocortisone sodium succinate has actions, uses, and undesirable effects similar to those described under Cortisone Acetate. As it is soluble in water, it is suitable for the preparation of intravenous or intramuscular injections; 100 mg of the ester is approximately equivalent to 75 mg of hydrocortisone.

Intravenous administration of hydrocortisone may be life-saving in Addisonian crisis or severe status asthmaticus. The usual dose for this purpose is the equivalent of 100 to 500 milligrams of hydrocortisone.

Hydrocortisone sodium succinate is of value in the withdrawal syndrome of long-term cortisone therapy. As an aerosol spray, it has also been used in asthma and, as lozenges, in the treatment of aphthous ulceration.

Precautions and contra-indications. As for Cortisone Acetate.

Preparations

HYDROCORTISONE SODIUM SUCCINATE INJECTION: a sterile solution of hydrocortisone sodium succinate, with suitable buffering agents, in water for injections. It is prepared by dissolving the contents of a sealed container in water for injections immediately before use. The sealed container contains hydrocortisone sodium succinate, or the contents are made from hydrocortisone hydrogen succinate with the aid of a suitable alkali.

Available as a powder in vials containing hydrocortisone sodium succinate equivalent to 100 mg of hydrocortisone.

A standard for this injection is given in the British Pharmacopoeia 1973

Containers: see the entry on Injections for general information on containers.

Labeling: see the entry on Injections for general information on labelling. In addition, the label on the container should state the amount of the medicament as the equivalent amount of hydrocortisone.

Storage: the sealed container should be protected from light. The injection decomposes on storage and should be used immediately after preparation.

HYDROCORTISONE LOZENGES (*Syn.* Hydrocortisone Sodium Succinate Lozenges): may be prepared by moist granulation and compression, as described in the entry on Lozenges. Each lozenge weighs about 100 mg. Available as lozenges containing hydrocortisone sodium succinate equivalent to 2.5 mg of hydrocortisone.

A standard for these lozenges is given in the British Pharmaceutical Codex 1973

Containers: see the entry on Lozenges for general information on containers. Containers should be airtight.

Storage: they should be stored in a cool place.

Advice for patients: the lozenge should be retained near the ulcer and allowed to dissolve slowly in the mouth. It should not be sucked.

Hydroflumethiazide

3,4-Dihydro-6-trifluoromethyl-2H-benzo-1,2,4-thiadiazine-7-sulphonamide 1,1-dioxide

$C_8H_8F_3N_3O_4S_2 = 331.3$

OTHER NAMES: *Hydrenox®*
Rautrax Sine K® (with rauwolfia serpentina); *Aldactide®* (with spironolactone)

A standard is given in the British Pharmacopoeia 1973

Description. Odourless, tasteless, white, glistening crystals or crystalline powder.

Solubility. Very slightly soluble in water, in ether, and in chloroform; soluble, at 20°, in 50 parts of alcohol.

Acidity or alkalinity. A 1% dispersion has a pH of 4.5 to 7.5.

Dissociation constants. pK_a 8.5, 10.0 (20°).

Identification. TEST. To about 10 mg add 10 mg of chromotropic acid sodium salt and 1 ml of water, add cautiously 5 ml of sulphuric acid, and mix; a purple colour is produced (distinction from bendrofluazide).

MELTING-POINT. About 271°.

ULTRAVIOLET ABSORPTION. In 0.01N sodium hydroxide, maxima at 274 nm (E1%, 1cm = 460) and 333 nm (E1%, 1cm = 95).

INFRA-RED ABSORPTION. Major peaks at 1139, 1151, 1182, 1326, 1341, and 1385 cm^{-1} (see Appendix 2a: Infra-red Spectra).

THIN-LAYER CHROMATOGRAPHY. See under Thin-layer Chromatography, System 6.

Determination in body fluids. SPECTROFLUORIMETRY. In plasma or urine—R. B. Smith *et al., J. pharm. Sci.,* 1976, **65**, 1208.

Metabolism. ABSORPTION. Well absorbed after oral administration.

DISTRIBUTION. *Protein binding,* about 74% bound to plasma proteins.

METABOLIC REACTIONS. Not significantly metabolised in man.

EXCRETION. Up to 85% of a dose may be excreted in the urine in 24 hours.

FURTHER INFORMATION. Pharmacokinetics—G. J. Yakatan *et al., J. clin. Pharmac.,* 1977, **17**, 37.

Actions and uses. Hydroflumethiazide is a thiazide diuretic which has actions and uses similar to those described under Chlorothiazide, but it is effective in smaller doses.

For the treatment of oedema, the dosage is 25 to 100 milligrams by mouth once or twice daily or on alternate days, but as an adjunct to hypotensive drugs in the treatment of hypertension 25 to 50 milligrams may be sufficient.

Undesirable effects; Precautions. As for Chlorothiazide.

Preparations

HYDROFLUMETHIAZIDE TABLETS: available as tablets containing 50 mg of hydroflumethiazide.

A standard for these tablets is given in the British Pharmacopoeia 1973

Containers and *Storage:* see the entry on Tablets for general information on containers and storage. Containers should be airtight.

Advice for patients: daily doses should preferably be taken in the morning. Treatment should not be discontinued without the advice of the prescriber.

OTHER PREPARATIONS available include TABLETS containing 25 mg of hydroflumethiazide with 25 mg of spironolactone, tablets containing hydroflumethiazide 50 mg with rauwolfia serpentina 50 mg, and tablets containing 50 mg of hydroflumethiazide with 50 mg of spironolactone.

Hydrogen Peroxide Solution

An aqueous solution containing about 6% w/v of hydrogen peroxide, H_2O_2.

OTHER NAMES: *Genoxide®*; Hydrogen Peroxide Solution (20-volume)

When Hydrogen Peroxide is prescribed or demanded Hydrogen Peroxide Solution is dispensed or supplied.

A standard is given in the British Pharmacopoeia 1973

Description. An odourless colourless liquid with a slightly acid taste.

Stability. It is comparatively stable in the presence of a slight excess of acid but readily decomposes when alkaline and when in contact with oxidisable substances or certain metals.

When it is prepared by dilution of a strong solution, the acidity should be appropriately adjusted by the addition of dilute phosphoric acid or dilute sulphuric acid. Limited amounts of a suitable stabiliser are sometimes added.

Incompatibility. As for Strong Hydrogen Peroxide Solution.

Storage. It should be stored protected from light, in a cool place, in bottles closed with glass stoppers, paraffined corks, or plastic or protected metal screw caps.

Identification. TESTS. It complies with Test 1 (with the aid of heat) and Test 2 described under Strong Hydrogen Peroxide Solution.

Actions and uses. Hydrogen peroxide solution is an antiseptic and deodorant which owes its efficacy to the readiness with which it evolves oxygen in the presence of living or dead tissue and bacteria; however, because of the rapidity of the evolution of oxygen, its antiseptic action is brief. It does not combine with albumin and is non-poisonous.

It is useful for detaching dead tissue and bacterial nests from dirty wounds and purulent lesions and for removing adherent blood-stained dressings.

It is used, diluted with 3 to 8 parts of water, as a deodorant gargle or mouth-wash and as ear-drops for the removal of wax. For bleaching hair and for removing superficial stains from the teeth, it should be mixed with an equal volume of water.

Undesirable effects. Strong solutions of hydrogen peroxide produce irritating "burns" on the skin but the pain disappears in about an hour.

Preparations

HYDROGEN PEROXIDE EAR-DROPS:

Hydrogen peroxide solution	..	..	..	25 ml
Water for preparations ..	..	..	.. to 100 ml

A standard for these ear-drops is given in the British Pharmaceutical Codex 1973

Containers and *Labelling:* see the entry on Ear-drops for general information on containers and labelling.

HYDROGEN PEROXIDE MOUTH-WASH: consisting of hydrogen peroxide solution.

Containers and *Labelling:* see the entry on Mouth-washes for general information on containers and labelling.

Advice for patients: 15 ml should be used in half a tumblerful of warm water. The diluted solution should be retained in the mouth for 2 to 3 minutes before spitting out.

Hydrogen Peroxide Solution, Dilute

An aqueous solution containing about 3% w/w of hydrogen peroxide, H_2O_2.

OTHER NAMES: Hydrogen Peroxide (10-volume); Hydrogenii Peroxidum Dilutum

A standard is given in the European Pharmacopoeia Vol. I

Description. An odourless colourless liquid.

Stability; Storage. As for Hydrogen Peroxide Solution.

Incompatibility. As for Strong Hydrogen Peroxide Solution.

Identification. TESTS. It complies with Test 1 (with the aid of heat) and Test 2 described under Strong Hydrogen Peroxide Solution.

Actions and uses. Dilute hydrogen peroxide solution is used for the purposes described under Hydrogen Peroxide Solution.

Hydrogen Peroxide Solution, Strong

An aqueous solution containing about 30% w/w of hydrogen peroxide, H_2O_2.

OTHER NAMES: Hydrogen Peroxide Solution (100-volume)

When Hydrogen Peroxide is prescribed or demanded Hydrogen Peroxide Solution is dispensed or supplied.

Standards for two strong solutions of hydrogen peroxide containing 27% and 30% w/w of H_2O_2 are given in the European Pharmacopoeia Vol. III Supplement

Strong hydrogen peroxide solution is a strong oxidising agent which decomposes vigorously in contact with oxidisable organic matter or with certain metals and their compounds. Limited amounts of a suitable stabiliser are usually added.

It is known as "100-volume", the number indicating the volumes of oxygen obtainable from 1 volume of the solution. The strength of diluted solutions may be indicated in a similar manner.

When used to make dilute solutions the products should be adjusted to the appropriate acidity by the addition of dilute phosphoric acid or dilute sulphuric acid.

Description. An odourless colourless liquid.

Weight per ml. About 1.11 g.

Incompatibility. It is incompatible with most organic substances and with alkalis, iodides, permanganates, and oxidisable substances.

Storage. It should be stored protected from light, in a cool place, in bottles closed with glass stoppers or suitable plastic caps and provided with a vent.

Identification. TESTS. 1. Cautiously make the solution alkaline; it decomposes vigorously with effervescence, evolving oxygen.

2. To 1 drop add 2 ml of *dilute sulphuric acid*, 2 ml of ether, and 1 drop of *potassium chromate solution* and shake; the ethereal layer is coloured deep blue.

Actions and uses. Strong hydrogen peroxide solution is used to prepare weaker solutions. It should never be used undiluted; if used without dilution for bleaching hair, it may produce gangrene of the scalp.

Hydroxocobalamin

$Co\alpha$-[α-(5,6-Dimethylbenzimidazolyl)]-$Co\beta$-hydroxo-cobamide

$C_{62}H_{89}CoN_{13}O_{15}P = 1346.4$

OTHER NAMES: *Cobalin-H®*; *Neo-Cytamen®*

A standard is given in the British Pharmacopoeia 1973

In acid solutions, hydroxocobalamin takes up a hydrogen ion which converts the hydroxyl group to a coordinated water molecule, and in this form it is known as aquocobalamin, which is basic and forms salts with acids. In solution, aquocobalamin exists in equilibrium with hydroxocobalamin and, since it is more stable in acid solution, it usually occurs commercially in the form of aquocobalamin, either as aquocobalamin chloride ($C_{62}H_{90}ClCoN_{13}O_{15}P = 1382.8$) or as aquocobalamin sulphate ($C_{124}H_{180}Co_2N_{26}O_{34}P_2S = 2790.8$).

Description. Odourless, tasteless, dark red crystals or crystalline powder.

Solubility. Soluble in water.

Moisture content. 8 to 12% for aquocobalamin chloride or 8 to 16% for aquocobalamin sulphate, determined by drying at 100° *in vacuo*.

Sterilisation. Solutions for injections are sterilised by filtration.

Storage. It should be stored in airtight containers, protected from light.

Identification. TEST. Fuse about 1 mg with 50 mg of potassium hydrogen sulphate, cool, and break up the mass and boil with 3 ml of water until dissolved; make the solution alkaline with *sodium hydroxide solution* using *phenolphthalein solution* as indicator, add 500 mg of sodium acetate, 0.5 ml of *dilute acetic acid*, and 0.5 ml of a 0.2% solution of disodium 1-nitroso-2-naphthol-3,6-disulphonate; a red or red-orange colour is immediately produced; Add 0.5 ml of hydrochloric acid and boil for 1 minute; the red colour persists.

ULTRAVIOLET ABSORPTION. In acetic acid, maxima at 274 nm (E1%, 1cm = 162), 351 nm (E1%, 1cm = 190), and at 525 nm (E1%, 1cm = 57).

Metabolism. ABSORPTION. Irregularly absorbed after oral administration.

BLOOD CONCENTRATION. During therapy with weekly intramuscular doses of 500 μg, serum vitamin-B$_2$ concentrations of over 0.8 ng/ml are attained in 2 weeks and of 5 ng/ml in 8 weeks, rising in some cases to 15 ng/ml; these concentrations are higher than those achieved after an equivalent dose of cyanocobalamin.

DISTRIBUTION. *Protein binding*, more firmly bound to serum proteins than cyanocobalamin.

EXCRETION. 50 to 63% of a dose is excreted after a dose of 1 mg; the excretion of hydroxocobalamin occurs more slowly than that of cyanocobalamin.

FURTHER INFORMATION. Blood levels and urinary excretion—G. B. J. Glass *et al.*, *Blood*, 1961, **18**, 511, 522 and G. B. J. Glass and D. H. Lee, *J. Am. med. Ass.*, 1963, **183**, 425; serum concentrations—M. S. Bourne *et al.*, *Lancet*, ii/1964, 173 and J. N. M. Chalmers and N. K. Shinton, *Lancet*, ii/1965, 1305.

Actions and uses. Hydroxocobalamin is an important member of a group of similar compounds which influence erythropoiesis and which represent the "anti-pernicious anaemia principle" of purified liver extracts. It is bound more firmly to serum proteins than cyanocobalamin and hence has a longer action.

Hydroxocobalamin is effective in the treatment of pernicious anaemia and its neurological complication, subacute combined degeneration of the spinal cord. It is given by intramuscular injection, the dose depending on the clinical state of the patient and the response to treatment; it should not be given by mouth because of its variable absorption.

The dose for children is the same as that for adults.

In uncomplicated pernicious anaemia and for patients in relapse, a weekly dose of not less than 250 micrograms will usually produce a satisfactory response, but a much higher dosage consisting of 5 injections, each of 1 milligram within the first week, has been recommended with the object of restoring the depleted reserve in the liver. A dose of 250 micrograms every 3 or 4 weeks is usually adequate for maintenance, but doses of 1 milligram are often given at longer intervals. In all cases the dosage must be related to the patient's response; in patients with neurological abnormalities, the doses should be doubled.

Hydroxocobalamin is also used in conjunction with folic acid in the treatment of other macrocytic anaemias associated with nutritional deficiencies and sprue. It is used in massive doses in the treatment of neuroblastoma in children, tobacco amblyopia, and Leber's optic atrophy. It may be necessary to give hydroxocobalamin in cases of vitamin-B$_{12}$ deficiency, due, for example, to gastrectomy, disease or resection of the ileum, or conditions resulting in abnormal bacterial flora. Strict vegetarians may be deficient in vitamin B$_{12}$ and may require hydroxocobalamin or other vitamin-B$_{12}$ analogues for the correction of megaloblastic anaemia.

Vitamin-B$_{12}$ analogues are sometimes used in tonics, but this practice has no scientific basis.

Precautions. Hydroxocobalamin should not be given before a diagnosis has been fully established, because of its ability to mask symptoms of subacute combined degeneration of the spinal cord.

Veterinary uses. Hydroxocobalamin is used in animals in the treatment of vitamin-B$_{12}$ deficiency. The usual dose by intramuscular or intravenous injection for all species is 5 to 10 micrograms per kilogram body-weight once or twice weekly according to the severity of the condition.

Preparation

HYDROXOCOBALAMIN INJECTION: a sterile solution of hydroxocobalamin in water for injections. It contains sufficient acetic acid or hydrochloric acid to adjust the pH to about 4. It may also contain a suitable buffering agent. It is sterilised by filtration. Available in 1-ml ampoules containing 250 micrograms and 1 milligram per ml of hydroxocobalamin. Also available for veterinary use in 30-ml vials containing 250 micrograms of hydroxocobalamin per ml and in 10-ml vials containing 1 milligram of hydroxocobalamin per ml.

A standard for this injection is given in the British Pharmacopoeia 1973

Containers: see the entry on Injections for general information on containers.

Labelling: see the entry on Injections for general information on labelling. In addition, the label on the container should state the amount of the medicament as the equivalent amount of anhydrous hydroxocobalamin in a suitable dose-volume.

Storage: it should be protected from light.

Hydroxychloroquine Sulphate

2-{N-[4-(7-Chloroquinol-4-ylamino)pentyl]-N-ethyl-amino}ethanol sulphate

$$C_{18}H_{28}ClN_3O_5S = 433.9$$

OTHER NAME: *Plaquenil®*

A standard is given in the British Pharmacopoeia 1973

Description. An odourless white crystalline powder with a bitter taste.

Solubility. Soluble, at 20°, in 5 parts of water; very slightly soluble in alcohol, in ether, and in chloroform.

Acidity. A 1% solution has a pH of 3.5 to 5.5.

Moisture content. Not more than 2%, determined by drying at 105°.

Storage. It should be protected from light.

Identification. TEST. Dissolve about 200 mg in 10 ml of water, add 30 ml of hot *trinitrophenol solution*, and allow to cool; a precipitate is produced which, after washing with water, melts at about 189°.

MELTING-POINT. It occurs in two forms, one of which melts at about 198° and the other at about 240°.

ULTRAVIOLET ABSORPTION. In 0.01N hydrochloric acid, maxima at 236 nm, 257 nm (E1%, 1cm = 390), 329 nm (E1%, 1cm = 430), and 343 nm (E1%, 1cm = 470).

Determination in body fluids. ULTRAVIOLET SPECTRO-PHOTOMETRY. In blood or urine—R. A. Dalley and D. Hainsworth, *J. forens. Sci. Soc.*, 1965, **5**, 99.

SPECTROFLUORIMETRY. In plasma—E. W. McChesney et al., *Antibiotics Chemother.*, 1962, **12**, 583.

Metabolism. ABSORPTION. Rapidly and almost completely absorbed after oral administration either as the sulphate or diphosphate salt.

BLOOD CONCENTRATION. After an oral dose of 310 mg of the sulphate, peak plasma concentrations of up to 0.2 μg/ml are attained in 3 hours; after an oral dose of 1240 mg of the sulphate administered in 3 divided doses, peak plasma concentrations of up to 0.3 μg/ml are attained in 3 to 6 hours.

HALF-LIFE. Plasma half-life, about 3 days.

DISTRIBUTION. Distribution is similar to that of chloro-quine; largest concentrations are achieved in liver, spleen, kidneys, lungs, skin, and leucocytes.

METABOLIC REACTION. De-ethylation.

EXCRETION. 25% of a dose is excreted in the faeces and 6% is excreted in the urine in 10 days.

FURTHER INFORMATION. Plasma levels, absorption, and excretion—E. W. McChesney and J. P. McAuliff, *Antibiotics Chemother.*, 1961, **11**, 800 and E. W. McChesney et al., *Antibiotics Chemother.*, 1962, **12**, 583.

Actions and uses. Hydroxychloroquine sulphate has antimalarial actions similar to those described under Chloroquine Phosphate, but it is used mainly in the treatment of rheumatoid arthritis and lupus erythema-tosus, both the discoid and the systemic form, when the skin is markedly involved.

The initial dose for the treatment of rheumatoid arthritis is 400 to 600 milligrams daily in divided doses taken with meals. This dosage is taken for 4 to 12 weeks and the result is assessed. Dosage may then be reduced to a maintenance level of 200 to 400 milligrams daily.

The dosage in lupus erythematosus depends on the severity of the condition; the initial dosage range is 400 to 800 milligrams daily in divided doses for several weeks, reducing to a maintenance dose of 200 to 400 milligrams daily.

The usual dose for the suppression of malaria is 400 milligrams weekly. For the treatment of an acute attack 800 milligrams is given initially, 400 milligrams 6 to 8 hours later, and 400 milligrams on each of the two following days. A single dose of 800 milligrams has been used to treat *Plasmodium falciparum* infections and to terminate an acute attack of *Plasmodium vivax* infection. Hydroxychloroquine should not be given to children.

Undesirable effects. Prolonged treatment with large doses sometimes results in nausea, diarrhoea, and intestinal cramps; if the period of administration exceeds 1 year, irreversible retinal damage may be caused. Therefore, an initial ophthalmological examination should be made in all patients on long-term treatment with hy-droxychloroquine and repeated every 2 or 3 months; treatment should be stopped if retinal changes occur.

Other untoward effects that may result from treatment with hydroxychloroquine include skin reactions, bleaching of the hair, alopecia, weakness, vertigo, tinnitus, peripheral neuropathy, and toxic psychosis. Patients receiving hydroxychloroquine therefore require careful supervision. Most reactions are reversible but retinal changes may be permanent.

Precautions. Hydroxychloroquine should be used with caution in patients with liver disease, quinine sensitivity, and glucose-6-phosphate dehydrogenase deficiency, in whom it may cause haemolytic anaemia.

Contra-indications. Hydroxychloroquine should only be used in pregnancy for malaria prophylaxis and only when the need outweighs the possible risk. It should not be given to children or to patients with severe gastro-intestinal, neurological, or blood diseases, or to patients with porphyria or psoriasis.

Poisoning. The stomach should be emptied and convulsions if present should be controlled with diazepam. If the patient becomes anoxic, controlled respiration with oxygen should be applied and a suitable vasopressor administered in the event of shock or hypotension. The excretion of hydroxychloroquine may be hastened by the administration of ammonium chloride to acidify the urine.

Preparation

HYDROXYCHLOROQUINE TABLETS: available as tablets containing 200 mg of hydroxychloroquine sulphate; they are sugar coated; the coat may be coloured. 200 mg of hydroxychloroquine sulphate is approximately equivalent to 156 mg of hydroxychloroquine.

A standard for these tablets is given in the British Pharmacopoeia 1973

Containers and *Storage:* see the entry on Tablets for general information on containers and storage. Containers should be airtight.

Advice for patients: the tablets should be taken at regular intervals, preferably after meals. For the suppression (or prophylaxis) of malaria, doses should be taken during the period at risk and for 4 weeks thereafter. For treatment, the prescribed course should be completed.

For the treatment of chronic diseases, therapy should not be discontinued without the advice of the prescriber.

Hydroxyprogesterone Hexanoate

3,20-Dioxopregn-4-en-17α-yl hexanoate

$C_{27}H_{40}O_4 = 428.6$

OTHER NAMES: Hydroxyprogesterone Caproate; *Primolut-Depot*®

A standard is given in the British Pharmacopoeia 1973

Description. A white, crystalline, almost odourless powder.

Solubility. Practically insoluble in water; soluble, at 20°, in 10 parts of alcohol, in 10 parts of ether, and in less than 1 part of chloroform; soluble in fixed oils and esters.

Specific rotation. +44° to +49°, determined on a 2% solution in dioxan.

Sterilisation. Oily solutions are sterilised by dry heat.

Storage. It should be protected from light.

Identification. TESTS. 1. Dissolve about 1 mg in 1 ml of sulphuric acid and allow to stand for 5 minutes; a faint yellow colour is produced. Add 0.5 ml of water; the colour changes first to green, then to red, and finally to reddish-violet with a blue fluorescence.
2. It complies with Test 3 described under Fluocortolone Hexanoate.

MELTING-POINT. About 122°.

ULTRAVIOLET ABSORPTION. In alcohol (95%), maximum at 239 nm (E1%, 1cm = 388).

INFRA-RED ABSORPTION. Major peaks at 1177, 1188, 1224, 1354, 1670, and 1728 cm^{-1} (see Appendix 2a: Infrared Spectra).

THIN-LAYER CHROMATOGRAPHY. See under Thin-layer Chromatography, System 10.

Metabolism. ABSORPTION. Slowly absorbed after intramuscular injection.

BLOOD CONCENTRATION. Five days after an intramuscular dose, 15% of the dose is present in the total plasma volume; of this, about 12% is conjugated; the blood concentration falls more slowly and remains higher than the corresponding value for progesterone.

HALF-LIFE. During the first 2 hours after administration, the half-life for free drug is about 10 minutes and during the second 2 hours it is about 100 minutes.

DISTRIBUTION. Less than 15% of a dose is taken up by adipose tissue.

METABOLIC REACTIONS. The hexanoic acid moiety ap-

pears to remain attached to the steroid nucleus since no change is observed in blood concentrations of 17α-hydroxyprogesterone or its metabolites (pregnanetriol, 3,17-dihydroxypregnan-20-one, or 17-oxosteroids) following intramuscular injection of the hexanoate ester; much of the drug appears to be conjugated; hydroxyprogesterone hexanoate is metabolised more slowly than progesterone.

EXCRETION. After an intramuscular dose, small amounts appear in the urine; after an intravenous dose, 30% appears in the urine and 50% in the faeces in 2 to 15 days; of the urinary material, 56 to 83% is extracted after hydrolysis, 40 to 50% after enzyme hydrolysis, and 20% by solvolysis.

FURTHER INFORMATION. K. Fotherby and F. James, Metabolism of synthetic steroids, *Advances in Steroid Biochemistry and Pharmacology*, M. H. Briggs and G. H. Christie (Eds), Vol. 3, London, Academic Press, 1972, p. 67.

Actions and uses. Hydroxyprogesterone hexanoate is a synthetic progestational steroid hormone and has actions similar to those of progesterone. It is used in threatened and habitual abortion and in functional uterine disorders and amenorrhoea. It may be used in doses of 250 to 500 milligrams once or twice weekly by intramuscular injection.

Preparation

HYDROXYPROGESTERONE INJECTION: a sterile solution of hydroxyprogesterone hexanoate in a suitable ester or in a suitable fixed oil, or in any mixture of these. It is sterilised by dry heat. Available in 1- and 2-ml ampoules and 1-ml disposable syringes containing 250 mg of hydroxyprogesterone hexanoate per ml.

A standard for this injection is given in the British Pharmacopoeia 1973

Containers: see the entry on Injections for general information on containers.

Labelling: see the entry on Injections for general information on labelling. In addition, the label on the container should state the composition of the solvent and that the injection is for intramuscular injection only.

Storage: it should be protected from light.

Hydroxystilbamidine Isethionate

2-Hydroxystilbene-4,4'-dicarboxamidine 2-hydroxyethanesulphonate

$C_{20}H_{28}N_4O_9S_2 = 532.6$

Description. An odourless, fine, yellow, crystalline powder. It becomes discoloured on exposure to light.

Solubility. Soluble in 8 parts of water and in 300 parts of alcohol; practically insoluble in ether.

Acidity. A 1% solution has a pH of 3.3 to 5.3.

Identification. TESTS. 1. To 10 ml of a 1% solution add

1 ml of *dilute sulphuric acid*; a yellow precipitate is produced.

2. To 10 ml of a 1% solution add 4 drops of *sodium hydroxide solution*; an orange-brown precipitate is produced.

3. To 0.5 ml of a 1% solution add 10 ml of water, 2 ml of a solution containing 0.4% of glyoxal sodium bisulphite and 1.2% of chloral hydrate, and 10 ml of a hot 15% solution of borax, and heat on a water-bath for 10 minutes; a magenta colour is produced.

MELTING-POINT. About 280°, but the melting-point is very indefinite.

ULTRAVIOLET ABSORPTION. In 0.01N hydrochloric acid, maximum at 344 nm (E1%, 1cm = 580).

Actions and uses. Hydroxystilbamidine isethionate has antifungal and antiprotozoal properties. It has a suppressive effect against *Blastomyces dermatitidis* and is used in the treatment of North American blastomycosis. It is also used in other systemic fungal infections such as pulmonary and oesophageal candidiasis and in the treatment of leishmaniasis.

Hydroxystilbamidine isethionate is administered by intravenous infusion over a period of 45 to 120 minutes, the dose being dissolved immediately before use in 200 millilitres of sodium chloride injection or dextrose injection (5%). The usual adult dose is 250 milligrams given daily or on alternate days, but individual dosage may be calculated on the basis of 3 to 5 milligrams per kilogram body-weight for adults or 3 milligrams per kilogram body-weight for children.

Undesirable effects. Hypotension may occur if hydroxystilbamidine isethionate is administered too rapidly by intravenous infusion. Dizziness, headache, nausea, vomiting, breathlessness, tachycardia, fainting, pruritus, and neuropathies may also occur. Concentrated solutions may cause thrombophlebitis.

Precautions. Hydroxystilbamidine isethionate should be given with caution to patients with impaired hepatic and renal function. Before and during treatment with hydroxystilbamidine isethionate, hepatic and renal function should be monitored.

Preparation

HYDROXYSTILBAMIDINE INJECTION: a sterile solution of hydroxystilbamidine isethionate in water for injections, in dextrose injection (5%), or in sodium chloride injection. It is prepared by dissolving the contents of a sealed container in the vehicle immediately before use. Available as a powder in vials containing 250 mg of hydroxystilbamidine isethionate.

Containers: see the entry on Injections for general information on containers.

Labelling: see the entry on Injections for general information on labelling. In addition, the label on the container should state that the solution must not be used if it is cloudy.

Storage: the injection decomposes on storage and should be used immediately after preparation.

Hyoscine Hydrobromide

(−)-(1S,3s,5R,6S,7R)-6,7-Epoxy-3-[(S)-tropoyloxy]tropanium bromide trihydrate, the hydrobromide trihydrate of (−)-hyoscine, an alkaloid obtained from various solanaceous plants, particularly species of *Datura*, *Scopolia*, and *Duboisia*.

$C_{17}H_{22}BrNO_4,3H_2O = 438.3$

OTHER NAMES: Hyoscini Hydrobromidum; *Quick Kwells*®; Scopolamine Hydrobromide; Scopolamini Hydrobromidum

Omnopon-Scopolamine® (with papaveretum)

A standard is given in the European Pharmacopoeia Vol. II

Description. Odourless, slightly efflorescent, colourless crystals or white crystalline powder.

Solubility. Soluble, at 20°, in 3.5 parts of water and in 30 parts of alcohol; very slightly soluble in ether and in chloroform.

Acidity. A 5% solution has a pH of 4 to 5.5.

Moisture content. 10 to 13%, determined by drying for 1 hour *in vacuo* followed by drying at 105°.

Specific rotation. −24° to −27°, determined on a 5% solution and calculated with reference to the dry substance.

Dissociation constant. pK_a 7.6 (23°).

Sterilisation. Solutions are sterilised by heating in an autoclave, by heating with a bactericide, or by filtration.

Storage. It should be stored in airtight containers, in a cool place, protected from light.

Identification. TESTS. 1. Dissolve a few mg in 5 ml of water and add 1 ml of *potassium iodobismuthate solution*; an orange or orange-red precipitate is produced.

2. To about 1 mg add 4 drops of fuming nitric acid, evaporate to dryness, dissolve the residue in 2 ml of acetone and add 4 drops of a 3% solution of potassium hydroxide in methyl alcohol; a violet colour is produced.

3. Carry out Test 1 described under Homatropine Hydrobromide; a white precipitate is produced which dissolves on warming (distinction from atropine and hyoscyamine).

MELTING-POINT. About 197°, with decomposition.

ULTRAVIOLET ABSORPTION. In 0.1N hydrochloric acid, maxima at 254 nm, 258 nm (E1%, 1cm = 4), and 266 nm.

INFRA-RED ABSORPTION. Major peaks at 705, 736, 853, 1047, 1166, and 1730 cm⁻¹ (see Appendix 2a: Infra-red Spectra).

THIN-LAYER CHROMATOGRAPHY. See under Thin-layer Chromatography, System 8.

Determination in body fluids. GAS CHROMATOGRAPHY. In plasma or urine—W. F. Bayne *et al.*, *J. pharm. Sci.*, 1975, **64**, 288.

Metabolism. ABSORPTION. Readily absorbed after oral administration.

BLOOD CONCENTRATION. After an oral dose of 906 µg of hyoscine, peak plasma concentrations of about 1.1 ng/ml are attained in about 1 hour.

METABOLIC REACTIONS. In animal studies, the major metabolite is the glucuronide; minor metabolites are scopine and aposcopolamine.

EXCRETION. 4 to 5% of an oral dose is excreted in the urine as unchanged drug.

FURTHER INFORMATION. Concentrations in plasma and urine—W. F. Bayne *et al.*, *J. pharm. Sci.*, 1975, **64**, 288.

Actions and uses. Hyoscine has peripheral and central actions. Like atropine, it antagonises the muscarinic effects of acetylcholine. It produces mydriasis and relaxes accommodation more quickly but for a shorter time than atropine.

The central action of hyoscine differs from that of atropine; it usually produces immediate depression of the cerebral cortex, especially of the motor areas. Hyoscine is therefore used in mania and in cerebral excitement and delirium such as occur in alcoholism, when, as a rule, it produces a sensation of fatigue and drowsiness which is quickly followed by sleep. For this purpose 1.2 milligrams of hyoscine hydrobromide and 20 milligrams of morphine sulphate may be given by subcutaneous or intramuscular injection.

For pre-operative medication, 600 micrograms of hyoscine hydrobromide and 10 to 15 milligrams of morphine sulphate or an equivalent amount of papaveretum is given by subcutaneous injection about 1 hour before operation. In obstetrics, similar doses have been used for the induction of "twilight sleep"; subsequent injections containing smaller doses of hyoscine and no morphine may be sufficient. Hyoscine is similarly used in conjunction with pethidine.

Hyoscine hydrobromide is given by mouth in doses of 600 micrograms for the prevention and treatment of motion-sickness. It also reduces the tremor of paralysis agitans and chorea and relieves the salivation and, to a lesser extent, the muscular rigidity of postencephalitic parkinsonism; for these purposes it is given by mouth, usually in a dosage of 300 to 600 micrograms 3 times daily; sometimes, however, the dosage may be considerably higher.

In ophthalmology, hyoscine hydrobromide may be used in eye-drops or eye ointment for its peripheral action on the eye.

Undesirable effects. Dryness of the mouth, temporary loss of accommodation, and tachycardia may occur.

Precautions and contra-indications. As for Atropine.

Veterinary uses. Hyoscine hydrobromide is a parasympatholytic and in dogs it is also a central nervous system depressant used in pre-anaesthetic medication. The usual dose in dogs and cats is 30 to 60 micrograms per kilogram body-weight by subcutaneous injection.

Preparations

HYOSCINE EYE-DROPS: consisting of a sterile solution containing up to 0.5% of hyoscine hydrobromide, with 0.02% v/v of benzalkonium chloride solution or 0.01% of chlorhexidine acetate, in purified water. It is prepared by method A, B, or C described in the entry on Eye-drops.
A standard for these eye-drops is given in the British Pharmaceutical Codex 1973
Containers: see the entry on Eye-drops for general information on containers. This solution is adversely affected by alkali.
Labelling: see the entry on Eye-drops for general information on labelling.
Advice for patients: see the entry on Eye-drops for general information on the use of eye-drops. Blurring of vision and sensitivity to light may occur for several days after instillation of the drops.

HYOSCINE EYE OINTMENT (*Syn.* Oculent. Hyoscin.): prepared by incorporating hyoscine hydrobromide in eye ointment basis by method A described in the entry on Eye Ointments.
A standard for this eye ointment is given in the British Pharmacopoeia 1973
Containers and *Labelling:* see the entry on Eye Ointments for general information on containers and labelling.
Advice for patients: see the entry on Eye Ointments for general information on the use of eye ointments. Blurring of vision and sensitivity to light may occur for several days after application of the eye ointment.

HYOSCINE INJECTION: a sterile solution of hyoscine hydrobromide in water for injections. It is sterilised by heating in an autoclave or by filtration. Available in 1-ml ampoules containing 400 micrograms of hyoscine hydrobromide.
A standard for this injection is given in the British Pharmacopoeia 1973
Containers and *Labelling:* see the entry on Injections for general information on containers and labelling.
Storage: it should be protected from light.

HYOSCINE TABLETS: the usual strength is 300 micrograms of hyoscine hydrobromide.
A standard for these tablets is given in the British Pharmacopoeia 1973
Containers and *Storage:* see the entry on Tablets for general information on containers and storage. Containers should be airtight.
Advice for patients: when used in parkinsonism, treatment should not be discontinued without the advice of the prescriber.

OTHER PREPARATIONS available include an INJECTION containing hyoscine hydrobromide 400 micrograms with papaveretum 20 mg per ml in 1-ml ampoules.

Hyoscyamus

The dried leaves, or leaves and flowering tops, of *Hyoscyamus niger* L. (Fam. Solanaceae), an erect herb distributed throughout Europe and cultivated in England and elsewhere.

OTHER NAMES: Henbane Leaf; Hyoscy.; Hyoscyami Folium; Hyoscyamus Leaf

A standard is given in the European Pharmacopoeia Vol. I

Varieties. Hyoscyamus occurs both as an annual and as a biennial and the corresponding leaves are available in commerce. Annual hyoscyamus is smaller than the biennial; the leaves are less hairy and less incised; the corolla is not so deeply purple-veined and the commercial drug frequently contains a large proportion of stem. The leaves of the first year's growth of the biennial plant are large, petiolate, and may be up to 300 mm or more in length; they are free from admixture with the flowers. Second-year biennial hyoscyamus consists of the flowering tops of the biennial variety. These three varieties are approximately equal in alkaloidal content.

Constituents. Hyoscyamus contains the alkaloid (−)-hyoscyamine, together with smaller quantities of atropine [(±)-hyoscyamine] and (−)-hyoscine [(−)-scopolamine]. The proportion of alkaloid in the carefully dried leaf varies from 0.045 to 0.14%. Larger yields of alkaloid (up to 0.27%) have been reported, but these are exceptional. Volatile bases, similar to those in belladonna leaf, are also present.

Up to 2.5% of stem with a diameter exceeding 7 mm may be present. It may yield up to 20% of sulphated ash and up to 12% of acid-insoluble ash.

Description. UNGROUND DRUG. *Macroscopical characters:* laminae pale green, up to about 250 mm long; first year leaves of the biennial plants ovate-lanceolate, petiole flat, about 50 mm long; second-year leaves shorter, sessile and ovate-oblong to triangular-ovate; margin dentately lobed, apex acute, midrib broad, yellowish, and conspicuous; secondary veins leaving midrib at a wide angle and terminating in the apices of the lobes; trichomes abundant on both surfaces, long, soft, many secreting a resinous substance rendering the leaves clammy to the touch.

Flowers crowded together, arising in the axils of large hairy bracts; calyx gamosepalous, having 5 lobes, each with an apical spine, green, hairy; corolla slightly zygomorphic, infundibuliform, yellow with purple veins; stamens 5, epipetalous, anthers purple; ovary superior, 2-celled, containing numerous ovules.

Fruit a pyxis, about 15 mm long, enclosed by the persistent calyx; seeds brownish-grey, flattened reniform-quadrangular, about 1.75 mm long; testa with wavy reticulate surface.

It has a strong characteristic odour and a bitter, slightly acrid taste.

Microscopical characters: the diagnostic characters are: Leaf: *epidermal cells* with wavy anticlinal walls, *cuticle* smooth; *stomata* anisocytic, on both surfaces; *trichomes* uniseriate, up to 500 μm long, of two kinds, some simple, 2- to 4-celled, the majority terminating in an ovoid multicellular gland; *crystals* of calcium oxalate either as single prisms, twin crystals, clusters of few components, or microsphenoidal sand, occurring in cells of mesophyll; *fibres* absent.

Pollen grains, when examined in chloral hydrate solution, subspherical, 35 to **48** to 56 μm diameter, *extine* marked with fine pits in a scattered arrangement, 3 *germinal furrows*, 3 *pores* each about 15 μm in diameter.

Seeds having a *testa* with *epidermal cells* about 100 to 150 μm in diameter, with lignified, wavy anticlinal walls.

POWDERED DRUG: Powdered Hyoscyamus. A green or greyish-green powder possessing the diagnostic microscopical characters, odour, and taste of the unground drug.

Adulterants and substitutes. Egyptian henbane consists of the dried leaves, flowering tops, immature fruits, and smaller stems of *H. muticus* L., a desert perennial collected chiefly in Egypt. The thick, somewhat fleshy leaves are brittle when dry, lanceolate to ovate-lanceolate, the lower and radical ones being petiolate and the upper ones sessile; the fruit is a cylindrical pyxis, about 15 mm long and 6 mm wide, enclosed by a persistent calyx, having 5 broad triangular non-spiny lobes. The drug contains about 0.6 to 1% of total alkaloids, of which about 90% is hyoscyamine.

H. albus L., a perennial plant growing in Mediterranean countries and in the Indian subcontinent, has leaves 50 to 100 mm long, with a slender petiole 20 to 60 mm long and a coarsely toothed margin, yellow flowers, and simple and glandular trichomes, each of the latter having a unicellular spherical head. It contains similar alkaloids to those in *H. niger*.

Some Indian henbane is derived from *H. reticulatus* L. and contains about 0.12 to 0.24% of (−)-hyoscyamine and (−)-hyoscine.

Storage. It should be stored in a cool dry place protected from light.

Identification. TEST. Mix 1 g of powdered drug with 10 ml of 0.1N sulphuric acid, shake, filter, add to the filtrate 1 ml of *strong ammonia solution* and add 5 ml of water, and extract with 15 ml of ether, taking care to avoid formation of an emulsion; dry the ether layer over anhydrous sodium sulphate, filter, evaporate to dryness in a porcelain dish, add 10 drops of fuming nitric acid, evaporate to dryness over a small flame, and add 10 ml of acetone and, dropwise, a 3% solution of potassium hydroxide in alcohol; a violet colour is produced.

Actions and uses. Hyoscyamus has actions similar to those described under Belladonna Herb, but the hyoscine which it contains makes it less likely to give rise to cerebral excitement. Preparations of hyoscyamus are used to counteract the griping action of purgatives and to relieve spasm in the urinary tract.

Precautions and contra-indications; Poisoning. As for Atropine.

Preparations

HYOSCYAMUS DRY EXTRACT:

Small-scale preparation

Hyoscyamus, in moderately
coarse powder .. .. 1000 g

Hyoscyamus, in fine powder, ⎫ of each a
dried at 80° .. .. ⎬ .. .. sufficient
Alcohol (70%) .. .. ⎭ .. .. quantity

Percolate the hyoscyamus in moderately coarse powder with the alcohol until 4000 ml of percolate has been obtained. Determine the proportion of total solids in the percolate by evaporating 20 ml, drying the residue at 80°, and weighing. Determine also the proportion of alkaloids in the percolate, using 100 ml, and the proportion of alkaloids present in the hyoscyamus in fine powder.

From the results of the three determinations, calculate the amount of hyoscyamus in fine powder that must be added to the percolate to produce a dry extract containing 0.3% of alkaloids, calculated as hyoscyamine.

Add to the percolate a somewhat smaller amount of the hyoscyamus in fine powder than calculation has shown to be necessary, remove the alcohol by evaporating to dryness under reduced pressure at a temperature not exceeding 60°, and dry in a current of air at 80°.

Powder the residue, add the final necessary amount of hyoscyamus in fine powder, and triturate in a dry, slightly warmed mortar until thoroughly mixed.

Pass the powdered extract through a No. 710 sieve and mix.

Manufacture. Prepare the extract by the above method, appropriately scaled up.

In making this preparation, the alcohol (70%) may be replaced by industrial methylated spirit diluted so as to be of equivalent alcoholic strength, provided that the law and the statutory regulations governing the use of industrial methylated spirit are observed.

Hyoscyamus dry extract contains, in 60 mg, 180 micrograms of total alkaloids, calculated as hyoscyamine.

A standard for this extract is given in the British Pharmaceutical Codex 1973

Storage: it should be stored in small, wide-mouthed, airtight containers, in a cool place.

Dose: 15 to 60 milligrams.

HYOSCYAMUS LIQUID EXTRACT:

Small-scale preparation

Hyoscyamus, in moderately
coarse powder .. .. 1000 g

Alcohol (70%) .. .. .. a sufficient quantity

Exhaust the hyoscyamus by percolation with the alcohol, reserving the first 850 ml of the percolate. Remove the alcohol from the remainder of the percolate by evaporation under reduced pressure at a temperature not exceeding 60°, evaporate the residue to a soft extract at a temperature not exceeding 60°, and dissolve this in the reserved portion.

Determine the proportion of alkaloids in the liquid thus obtained. To the remainder of the liquid add sufficient alcohol (70%) to produce a hyoscyamus liquid extract of the required strength.

Allow to stand for not less than 24 hours; filter if necessary.

Manufacture. Prepare the extract by the above method, appropriately scaled up, or by the alternative method described in the entry on Extracts.

Hyoscyamus liquid extract contains, in 0.5 ml, 250 micrograms of total alkaloids, calculated as hyoscyamine.

A standard for this extract is given in the British Pharmaceutical Codex 1973

Dose: 0.2 to 0.5 millilitre.

HYOSCYAMUS TINCTURE:

Hyoscyamus, in moderately
coarse powder ..   ..   100 g
Alcohol (70%)   ..   ..   .. a sufficient quantity

Prepare about 900 ml of a tincture by the percolation process and determine the proportion of total alkaloids present in 250 ml of the percolate; dilute the remainder of the percolate, if necessary, with sufficient of the alcohol to produce a tincture of the specified strength. Hyoscyamus tincture contains, in 5 ml, 250 micrograms of total alkaloids, calculated as hyoscyamine.

A standard for this tincture is given in the British Pharmacopoeia 1973

Dose: 2 to 5 millilitres.

POTASSIUM CITRATE AND HYOSCYAMUS MIXTURE:

Potassium citrate	300 g
Hyoscyamus tincture	200 ml
Citric acid monohydrate..	50 g
Lemon spirit	5 ml
Quillaia tincture	10 ml
Syrup..	250 ml
Chloroform water, double-strength	200 ml
Water for preparations	to 1000 ml

It must be freshly prepared.

Containers: see the entry on Mixtures for general information on containers.

Labelling: directions to shake the bottle and to dilute the dose well with water before administration should be given on the label.

Dose: 10 millilitres, well diluted with water.

Hyperaldosteronism

Hyperaldosteronism, or excessive secretion of aldosterone by the adrenal cortex, may be due to a tumour or to hyperplasia of the zona glomerulosa (Conn's syndrome) or it may be a response to abnormal metabolic situations associated with oedema, reduction of the intravascular space and loss of sodium, for example in chronic heart failure or the nephrotic syndrome.

It is characterised by a raised serum sodium, a lowered serum potassium, and alkalosis, resulting in hypertension, muscular weakness, polyuria, polydipsia, and tetany.

Hyperaldosteronism may be treated by removal of the causal adenoma, adrenalectomy in hyperplasia of the zona glomerulosa, or by administration of the specific aldosterone antagonist spironolactone.

Hypermenorrhoea

see under UTERINE BLEEDING, ABNORMAL

Hyperparathyroidism

Hyperparathyroidism is the excessive secretion of hormone by the parathyroid gland and is characterised by hypercalcaemia, hyperphosphaturia, tissue calcification, and bone disease, the most advanced form of which is osteitis fibrosa cystica.

Primary hyperparathyroidism is usually caused by an adenoma of the parathyroid gland but may also be due to hyperplasia and rarely carcinoma of the parathyroid gland.

Secondary hyperparathyroidism arises as a result of an abnormal physiological state that leads to hypocalcaemia, for example, deficiency of vitamin D, vitamin-D-resistant osteomalacia or rickets, malabsorption of calcium, chronic renal disease, or renal tubular acidosis. In this situation the serum calcium may be normal or low.

Occasionally, longstanding hypocalcaemia may give rise to autonomous parathyroid hormone-secreting adenomata (tertiary hyperparathyroidism).

In primary hyperparathyroidism there is a raised serum calcium level and a lowered serum phosphate level. Resorption of calcium from bones is increased and results in skeletal rarefaction, the formation of cysts, and weakness of the bones. Hypercalcaemia results in an increased excretion of calcium in the urine, with the risk of formation of calculi, and the deposition of calcium in the tissues of the body, particularly the kidneys, which may result in renal damage. Hypercalcaemia may also result in weakness, anorexia, nausea, constipation, ileus, abdominal pain, nocturia, polyuria, and thirst.

Hyperparathyroidism is usually of many years standing before it produces clinical manifestations. Acute hypercalcaemia due to hyperparathyroidism may be treated by the parenteral infusion of sodium chloride injection, dilute sodium phosphate solution, calcitonin, or salcatonin. Hyperparathyroidism is treated by surgical removal of parathyroid tissue or treatment of any underlying condition.

Hypertension, Arterial

Hypertension is a condition of abnormally high blood pressure.

The blood pressure of healthy individuals may extend over a wide range of values and tends to increase with age but is considered to be abnormally high in the young or middle aged when the resting systolic pressure exceeds 150 mmHg or the diastolic pressure exceeds 95 or 100 mmHg, although these pressures apparently have no ill effects in some subjects. Periodic examination of heart size and the retina and the testing of the urine for proteins is desirable in such subjects to assess deterioration of the cardiovascular system and kidneys.

When the cause of the elevated blood pressure may be detected the condition is referred to as secondary hypertension. Renal disorders, coarctation of the aorta,

Cushing's syndrome, primary aldosteronism, and phaeochromocytoma are possible causes of secondary hypertension.

In most subjects there is no known cause and the condition is referred to as primary or essential hypertension. The condition may continue unchanged for many years or it may become rapidly worse in which case it is described as malignant hypertension. Obesity may be a predisposing factor. Anxiety may be involved in some instances. Hypertension may also be a complication of pregnancy (as described in the entry on Toxaemias of Pregnancy).

Complications arising from hypertension include heart failure, coronary thrombosis, rupture of blood vessels, particularly where atherosclerosis is present, disturbances in retinal circulation giving rise to blurred vision, and degenerative changes in the kidneys which may lead to renal failure.

Treatment of hypertension. Attempts should be made to reduce stress and anxiety and the administration of sedative drugs may be justified in patients where these characteristics are pronounced. Patients should be taught to organise their lives so as to take sufficient rest. Moderate (but not strenuous) amounts of exertion are to be encouraged. Where obesity is present, weight reduction is desirable.

A wide selection of drugs is available for the treatment of mild hypertension, and thiazide diuretics, alone or in combination with other antihypertensive drugs are commonly used as the side-effects are minimal. In treating more severe cases, more pronounced side-effects may have to be tolerated. Restriction of dietary sodium is sometimes used as an adjunct to drug treatment.

Apart from sedatives and diuretics, the drugs used in antihypertensive treatment act by depleting stores of pressor amines or by antagonising their action, by blocking adrenergic receptors, by ganglion-blocking action, or by peripheral vasodilatation. In many cases, more than one mechanism is involved, for example, the antihypertensive actions of clonidine, methyldopa, and propranolol may be partly due to an effect on the central nervous system.

Substances acting principally by depleting stores of pressor amines or antagonising their action include methyldopa, rauwolfia, and reserpine.

Substances acting principally by blocking adrenergic neurones include bethanidine, debrisoquine, and guanethidine.

Substances acting principally by blocking adrenergic receptors include oxprenolol, pindolol, and propranolol. Substances acting principally by ganglion-blocking action include pentolinium.

Substances acting principally by direct action on the arterioles include diazoxide, hydrallazine, prazosin, and sodium nitroprusside.

Hypertension, Pulmonary

Pulmonary hypertension is a condition of abnormally high blood pressure in the pulmonary circulation. Pulmonary blood pressure is considered to be abnormal when the systolic blood pressure rises above 25 mmHg or the diastolic pressure rises above 12 mmHg. Lung disease and multiple emboli cause chronic hypoxic increase in pulmonary vascular resistance which results in pulmonary hypertension followed by right ventricular hypertrophy and subsequent failure and is known as **cor pulmonale.**

Pulmonary hypertension has been caused by administration of certain drugs such as aminorex but it may also be due to pulmonary fibrosis caused by busulphan. Pulmonary hypertension is characterised by increasing fatigue and breathlessness on effort together with angina or syncope if severe.

Treatment of pulmonary hypertension is directed toward underlying heart or lung disease.

Hyperthyroidism

Hyperthyroidism (Thyrotoxicosis; Graves' disease), or an abnormally high circulating level of thyroid hormone, is characterised by a high metabolic rate with increased appetite and weight loss, tachycardia, retraction of the upper eyelid, and nervous and emotional excitability. There may also be amenorrhoea, diarrhoea, or muscle weakness and wasting.

Thyrotoxicosis is usually due to the presence of thyroid stimulating immunoglobulins (Graves' disease) and less commonly to a single toxic nodule, or to autonomous nodules within a multinodular goitre. Most cases of hyperthyroidism are associated with goitre and exophthalmos. Sometimes thyrotoxicosis occurs as a result of excessive circulating liothyronine (tri-iodothyronine) rather than thyroxine.

Hyperthyroidism is treated by the administration of thyroid antagonists such as carbimazole or, in the event of hypersensitivity, propylthiouracil, by surgical removal of thyroid tissue, or by partial inactivation of the thyroid gland by the administration of radioactive preparations of iodine—see Sodium Iodide (^{131}I) Solution.

Beta-adrenergic blocking agents may also be used for symptomatic treatment. Thyroid antagonists and iodides are used pre-operatively as described under Carbimazole. During thyroid crises, following surgery, potassium iodide and beta-adrenergic blocking agents may be given.

Hypogonadism

Hypogonadism is the deficiency or absence of testicular function in men or of ovarian function in women. It may be due to the hereditary Turner's or Klinefelter's syndromes, to the destruction of the gonads by radiation or infections such as tuberculosis, syphilis, or mumps, or to the removal of the gonads by surgery. It may also be secondary to lesions in the hypothalamus or pituitary gland when lack of gonadotrophins results in gonadal atrophy.

If hypogonadism occurs before puberty, the expected pubertal changes do not take place during adolescence. If it occurs in the adult, there is regression of some of the secondary sexual characteristics. In the prepubertal female, this results in the failure of menstruation to occur, the absence of mammary development or growth of body hair, and failure of the bony epiphyses to close. In the adult female, there is atrophy of the breasts and external genitalia and loss of libido.

In the prepubertal male, hypogonadism results in non-development of the genitalia or musculature, the absence of erection or seminal emission, failure of the voice to break or the bony epiphyses to close, and absence of facial and body hair. In the adult male, there is regression of muscle development, smoothing of the skin, loss of beard and body hair, atrophy of the external genitalia, and also the development of obesity and of mental lethargy. A reversible state of hypogonadism also occurs in patients with anorexia nervosa.

Hypogonadism is treated by substitution therapy with androgens or oestrogens, as appropriate. This will bring about the changes of puberty or return of secondary sexual characteristics but will not confer fertility. If the hypogonadism is due to hypothalamic or pituitary disease, it is sometimes possible to restore fertility by treatment with gonadotrophins.

Hypoparathyroidism

Hypoparathyroidism is a deficiency of secretion of parathyroid hormone characterised by low serum calcium and high serum phosphate levels. It is usually the result of removal of parathyroid tissue during thyroidectomy, but may be due to congenital absence of parathyroid tissue or to autoimmune disease of the parathyroid glands.

Hypoparathyroidism results in a decreased resorption of skeletal calcium and a reduced absorption of calcium from the intestine. The immediate effect of hypoparathyroidism is a low serum calcium which results in tetany or spontaneous tonic contractions of muscles due to neuromuscular instability. This may result in laryngeal spasm. Longer term consequences of hypoparathyroidism include psychotic disorders, epilepsy, cataracts, loss of scalp hair, brittle deformed nails, and dry skin. Papilloedema and other signs of raised intracranial pressure indicate calcification of the basal ganglia.

Hypoparathyroidism is treated initially by injections of calcium gluconate or other calcium salts. Serum calcium is maintained in the long term by the administration of calciferol, cholecalciferol, or dihydrotachysterol.

Hypopituitarism

Hypopituitarism (Simmonds' disease) is a reduced activity of the pituitary gland. There may be a deficiency of only one or of all pituitary hormones (panhypopituitarism).

Deficiency of a single pituitary hormone will result in deficient function of the target organ of that hormone. Panhypopituitarism results in a syndrome characterised by the total lack of pituitary hormones and of hormones from the target glands. Lack of thyrotrophin results in lethargy and cold intolerance (see Hypothyroidism); lack of corticotrophin results in hypotension, water retention, and a tendency to the development of coma from hypoglycaemia (see Addison's disease); lack of gonadotrophin results in atrophy of the genitalia and loss of body hair (see Hypogonadism); lack of antidiuretic hormone results in the passage of large volumes of dilute urine (see Diabetes Insipidus). Patients become weak and easily fatigued and personality changes may occur.

Hypopituitarism in the adult usually occurs as a result of destruction of the pituitary gland. Tumours in the region of the pituitary, such as chromophobe adenoma or craniopharyngioma, cause pressure on the gland resulting in its destruction; associated pressure on the optic chiasma may result in visual impairment. Pituitary damage may occur as a result of tuberculous caseation, granulomatous disease such as sarcoid infiltration, syphilitic gummata, or other destructive processes in the pituitary. In women, pituitary infarction and necrosis may occur in association with post-partum haemorrhage. When this occurs lack of prolactin results in failure of lactation and lack of gonadotrophin results in persistent amenorrhoea. Hypopituitarism may also occur following pituitary ablation for the treatment of hormone-dependent neoplastic disease.

When hypopituitarism occurs before puberty, it is usually partial rather than complete and is dominated by a lack of growth hormone which results in short stature. Also, the onset of puberty is delayed or may not occur. Hypopituitarism is treated by the replacement of hormones together with surgical removal of any tumour or treatment of any infection which is causing destruction of the pituitary gland.

Hypothalamic Releasing Factors

Hypothalamic hormones are peptides or monoamines that stimulate or inhibit the release of hormones from the anterior lobe of the pituitary gland.

The peptides are secreted and stored within the hypothalamus; their release is regulated neurologically and is also affected by the level of circulating anterior pituitary hormones. The principal hypothalamic hormones are listed below.

Corticotrophin-releasing factor (CRF). This hormone stimulates the release of corticotrophin and hence the secretion of corticosteroids from the adrenal cortex.

Gonadorelin (gonadotrophin-releasing factor; GRF). This hormone stimulates the release of the two gonadotrophic hormones, that is, follicle-stimulating hormone (FSH) or interstitial-cell-stimulating hormone (ICSH) and luteinising hormone (LH).

Melanostatin (melanocyte-stimulating hormone release-inhibiting factor). This hormone inhibits the release of melanocyte-stimulating hormone (melanotrophin; intermedine).

Somatostatin (growth hormone release-inhibiting factor; GHRIF). This hormone inhibits the release of growth hormone (somatotrophin). Unlike the other hypothalamic releasing factors its inhibitory effects are not restricted to the pituitary. It also influences the secretion of insulin, glucagon, gastrin, gastric acid, pepsin, and also prolactin and thyrotrophic hormones. Its therapeutic potential in Zollinger-Ellison syndrome, diabetic retinopathy, and somatostatin-dependent tumours such as insulinoma, glucagonoma, and breast tumours, has not yet been fully evaluated.

Protirelin (thyrotrophin-releasing factor; TRF). This hormone stimulates the release of thyrotrophin and hence the secretion of thyroid hormones.

Dopamine. This monoamine is now accepted as an important hypothalamic prolactin-release-inhibiting factor (PRIF).

Bromocriptine, a long-acting dopamine agonist, acts on the pituitary as a functional analogue of endogenous PRIF.

Hypothalamic hormones may be administered in tests of the function of the pituitary and glands affected by the appropriate pituitary secretion.

Hypothyroidism

Hypothyroidism (cretinism; myxoedema) or deficient thyroid function may occur congenitally (cretinism) or may arise later in life.

Cretinism may be due to iodine deficiency, absence of the thyroid gland, a defect in hormone synthesis, or ingestion of antithyroid drugs by the mother. It is characterised by constipation and lethargy. In babies it causes feeding difficulties and the absence of normal growth and mental development.

Hypothyroidism in later life may be due to disease of the thyroid gland, to hypopituitarism, or to prolonged treatment with antithyroid drugs such as carbimazole, sodium aminosalicylate, lithium salts, iodides, or topical resorcinol. It may also be due to too radical a thyroidectomy or irradiation of the thyroid. Onset is insidious and is characterised by a gradual increase in physical and mental lethargy with cold intolerance, gain in weight, and constipation. There may also be swelling of the skin with mucoid infiltration (myxoedema).

Hypothyroidism is treated by replacement therapy with thyroxine sodium or liothyronine sodium (tri-iodothyronine). Caution should be exercised in treating patients with ischaemic heart disease. In congenital hypothyroidism, early diagnosis and treatment are essential if permanent mental deficiency is to be avoided. Treatment of hypothyroidism must always be lifelong, except in those reversible cases due to the ingestion of drugs.

Hypromellose

A mixed ether of cellulose in which the ether groupings are mainly methoxyl groups with a small proportion of hydroxypropoxyl groups.

The name "hypromellose" is followed by a number indicating the approximate viscosity, in centistokes, of a 2% solution.

OTHER NAMES: *Celacol HPM*®; Hydroxypropylmethyl-cellulose; *Isopto (Alkaline/Plain)*®; *Methocel HG*®

A standard is given in the British Pharmaceutical Codex 1973

Description. An odourless white or creamy-white powder.

Solubility. Soluble in cold water, forming a viscous colloidal solution; practically insoluble in alcohol, in ether, and in chloroform.

Moisture content. Not more than 10%, determined by drying at 105°.

Uses. Hypromellose has properties similar to those of methylcellulose but produces aqueous solutions having higher gel-points; for example, a 2% solution of methylcellulose 4500 gels at about 50° and a 2% solution of hypromellose 4500 gels at about 65°.

Because aqueous solutions of hypromellose usually have greater clarity and a lower proportion of undispersed fibres, it is used in preference to methylcellulose to increase the viscosity of ophthalmic solutions; an antimicrobial agent such as benzalkonium chloride should be incorporated.

Hypromellose has also been used in the preparation of anhydrous adhesive ointments for the protection of the skin surrounding ileostomies, fistulas, and exuding ulcers. In the preparation of Plaster of Paris Bandage, hypromellose is used for the same purpose as methylcellulose.

Preparation

HYPROMELLOSE EYE-DROPS (*Syn.* Alkaline Eye-drops; Artificial Tears):

Hypromellose 4000, or 4500, or 5000	0.30 g
Borax..	0.19 g
Boric acid	0.19 g
Potassium chloride	0.37 g
Sodium chloride	0.45 g
Benzalkonium chloride solution	0.02 ml
Purified water	to 100 ml

Add the hypromellose to about 15 ml of the water at 80° to 90° and, when the powder is thoroughly hydrated, add a further 35 ml of the water, preferably in the form of ice, and stir until homogeneous. Dissolve the sodium chloride, the potassium chloride, the borax, and the boric acid in 40 ml of the water and add the benzalkonium chloride solution. Mix the two solutions, add sufficient of the water to produce the required volume, and mix. Allow to stand overnight, and decant and filter the supernatant liquid.

Transfer the filtered solution to the final containers, close the containers so as to exclude micro-organisms, and sterilise by heating in an autoclave or by maintaining at 98° to 100° for 30 minutes. Redisperse the coagulated hypromellose by shaking on cooling.

Alternatively, the filtered solution may be sterilised in bulk, the coagulated hypromellose redispersed by shaking on cooling, and the solution distributed, by an aseptic technique, into the final sterile containers, which are then closed so as to exclude micro-organisms.

When Methylcellulose Eye-drops are ordered or prescribed without qualification, hypromellose eye-drops are supplied.

When the solution is supplied for use in gonioscopy procedures, the amount of hypromellose 4000, 4500, or 5000 may be increased; a concentration between 0.7 and 1.5% may be suitable.

A standard for these eye-drops is given in the British Pharmaceutical Codex 1973

Containers: see the entry on Eye-drops for general information on containers. If the eye-drops are transferred to the final containers before sterilisation, the container should be closed with a screw cap, and a sterile dropper, suitably wrapped, supplied separately.

Labelling: see the entry on Eye-drops for general information on labelling.

Uses: hypromellose eye-drops may be used to replace lachrymal secretion where this is deficient. The solution is not intended as a vehicle for other drugs.

The choice of thickening agent, grade, and concentration is frequently a matter of the personal preference of the ophthalmologist, who may request a formulation other than that specified above.

Some workers stipulate that the viscosity should be about 15 to 20 centistokes (1.5×10^{-5} to 2.0×10^{-5} m² s⁻¹), which would require a content of hypromellose 4000, 4500, or 5000, of 0.45 to 0.5%. Although it is theoretically possible to use various grades of thickening agent at concentrations which result in production of a solution of the required viscosity, difficulty may arise if too high a concentration of viscoliser is used. This is because evaporation of the vehicle after application to the eye may render the preparation sticky and it may be necessary to incorporate a humectant in a formulation to compensate for this.

Advice for patients: see the entry on Eye-drops for general information on the use of eye-drops.

Ibuprofen

2-(4-Isobutylphenyl)propionic acid

$CH_3 \cdot CH \cdot COOH$

$CH_2 \cdot CH(CH_3)_2$

$C_{13}H_{18}O_2 = 206.3$

OTHER NAME: *Brufen®*

A standard is given in the British Pharmacopoeia Addendum 1975

Description. White powder or crystals with a characteristic odour.

Solubility. Very slightly soluble in water; soluble, at 20°, in 1.5 parts of alcohol, in 2 parts of ether, in 1 part of chloroform, and in 1.5 parts of acetone; soluble in aqueous solutions of alkali hydroxides and carbonates.

Identification. MELTING-POINT. About 76°.

ULTRAVIOLET ABSORPTION. In 0.1N hydrochloric acid, maxima at 222 nm (E1%, 1cm = 381), 265 nm (E1%, 1cm = 13), and 274 nm (E1%, 1cm = 9.6).

INFRA-RED ABSORPTION. Major peaks at 779, 1185, 1232, 1384, 1418, and 1721 cm^{-1} (see Appendix 2a: Infra-red Spectra).

THIN-LAYER CHROMATOGRAPHY. See under Thin-layer Chromatography, System 3.

Determination in body fluids. GAS CHROMATOGRAPHY. In plasma or urine: determination of enantiomers of ibuprofen—G. J. VanGiessen and D. G. Kaiser, *J. pharm. Sci.*, 1975, **64**, 798. In serum—D. J. Hoffmann, *J. pharm. Sci.*, 1977, **66**, 749.

Metabolism. ABSORPTION. Readily absorbed after oral administration.

BLOOD CONCENTRATION. After an oral dose of 200 to 800 mg, peak plasma concentrations of 11 to 26 μg/ml are attained in 1 to 2 hours.

HALF-LIFE. Plasma half-life, about 2 hours.

DISTRIBUTION. *Protein binding*, about 99% bound to plasma proteins.

METABOLIC REACTIONS. Oxidation to form 2-p-(2-hydroxy-2-methylpropyl)phenylpropionic acid and 2-p-(carboxypropyl)phenylpropionic acid. The metabolites of ibuprofen are in the (+)-form and are conjugated.

EXCRETION. About 60% is excreted in the urine and 30% in the faeces; of the urinary excreted material 9% is the hydroxy metabolite, 17% is the conjugated hydroxy metabolite, 16% is the carboxy metabolite, and 19% is the conjugated carboxy metabolite.

FURTHER INFORMATION. Pharmacology, metabolism, and toxicology—S. S. Adams *et al.*, *Rheumatol. phys. Med.*, 1970, **10** Suppl., 9; tolerance and pharmacology —C. D. Brooks *et al.*, *Curr. ther. Res.*, 1973, **15**, 180; plasma concentrations—D. G. Kaiser and G. J. VanGiessen, *J. pharm. Sci.*, 1974, **63**, 219; metabolism —R. F. N. Mills *et al.*, *Xenobiotica*, 1973, **3**, 589; plasma concentrations and urinary excretion—G. J. VanGiessen and D. G. Kaiser, *J. pharm. Sci.*, 1975, **64**, 798.

Actions and uses. Ibuprofen is an analgesic with minor anti-inflammatory properties. When compared with aspirin in high dosage ibuprofen has a similar analgesic effect, a somewhat less marked anti-inflammatory effect, and a much lower incidence of gastro-intestinal side-effects. It is used for the relief of pain and inflammation in rheumatic disease.

When given by mouth, it is rapidly absorbed and the excretion of ibuprofen and its major metabolites through the kidneys is complete within 24 hours.

The usual dose is 1.2 grams daily in divided doses. In some cases, higher doses of up to 1.6 grams daily in divided doses may be required but it is sometimes possible, after 2 to 4 weeks' treatment, to reduce the daily dosage to a lower maintenance dose. The usual dose for children is 20 milligrams per kilogram body-weight daily but for children weighing less than 30 kilograms the daily dose should not exceed 500 milligrams.

Undesirable effects. Ibuprofen may give rise to occasional gastro-intestinal upsets or rashes. Gastro-intestinal haemorrhage may rarely occur. Bronchospasm may be precipitated in patients suffering from or with a previous history of bronchial asthma or allergic disease.

Precautions. It may be used with caution in patients with gastro-intestinal disease and is often tolerated by patients with peptic ulcer or intolerance to major anti-inflammatory drugs such as indomethacin, phenylbutazone, or aspirin. If ibuprofen is given to patients receiving anticoagulants, prothrombin times should be monitored at least daily for the first few days of combined treatment.

Preparations

IBUPROFEN TABLETS: available as tablets containing 200 and 400 mg of ibuprofen; they are sugar coated; the coat may be coloured.
A standard for these tablets is given in the British Pharmacopoeia Addendum 1975
Containers and *Storage:* see the entry on Tablets for general information on containers and storage. Containers should be airtight.
Advice for patients: the tablets should preferably be taken after meals.

OTHER PREPARATIONS available include a MIXTURE containing ibuprofen 100 mg in 5 ml, diluent tragacanth mucilage, life of diluted mixture 14 days.

Ichthammol

Consists mainly of the ammonium salts of the sulphonic acids prepared by sulphonating the oily substances resulting from the destructive distillation of a bituminous schist or shale. It contains in addition, 5 to 7% of ammonium sulphate.

OTHER NAME: Ammonium Ichthosulphonate

A standard is given in the British Pharmaceutical Codex 1973

Description. A black viscid liquid with a strong characteristic odour.

Solubility. Soluble in water; partly soluble in alcohol and in ether; completely soluble in a mixture of equal parts of alcohol and ether.

Moisture content. Not more than 50%, determined by drying at 105°.

Incompatibility. It is incompatible with alkaloids.

Actions and uses. Ichthammol has only slight bacteriostatic properties; it is slightly irritant to the skin. It has been used in ointments and creams in the treatment of some chronic skin diseases.

Ichthammol glycerin has been used to reduce the inflammation of lymphadenitis and thrombophlebitis; it has also been used in pessaries and tampons for the treatment of cervicitis.

Preparations

ICHTHAMMOL GLYCERIN (*Syn.* Glycerin of Ammonium Ichthosulphonate):

Ichthammol ..	..	..	..	..	..	100 g
Glycerol	..	..	..	..	..	900 g

ICHTHAMMOL OINTMENT:

Ichthammol ..	..	..	..	..	..	100 g
Wool fat	..	..	..	..	..	450 g
Yellow soft paraffin		..	..	..	..	450 g

Melt together the wool fat and the yellow soft paraffin, incorporate the ichthammol, and stir until cold.

Containers: see the entry on Ointments for general information on containers.

Advice for patients: the ointment should be rubbed lightly on the affected area. It should not be applied to broken skin.

ZINC AND ICHTHAMMOL CREAM (*Syn.* Zinc Oxide and Ichthammol Cream):

Zinc cream ..	..	..	..	..	..	820 g
Ichthammol ..	..	..	..	..	..	50 g
Cetostearyl alcohol		..	..	..	..	30 g
Wool fat	..	..	..	..	..	100 g

Melt together the wool fat and the cetostearyl alcohol with the aid of gentle heat; triturate the warm mixture with the zinc cream until smooth and incorporate the ichthammol.

A standard for this cream is given in the British Pharmaceutical Codex 1973

Containers, Labelling, and *Storage:* see the entry on Creams for general information on containers, labelling, and storage.

Advice for patients: the cream should be rubbed lightly on the affected area. It should not be applied to broken skin.

Icterus

see JAUNDICE

Identification of Drugs

The positive identification of drug substances requires a considerable amount of equipment and expertise and is rarely attempted except for research purposes. In practice, reliance is placed on careful labelling and checking at all stages of production. Confirmatory tests and verification of compliance with an analytical standard may be carried out as required. In the pharmacy, material is normally used only if it has been obtained from a reliable source, is clearly labelled, and appears to comply with the description on the label.

The identification of unknown tablets, capsules etc. is sometimes required in cases of poisoning and as an aid in establishing the nature of a course of treatment when the original prescriber is unknown or cannot be contacted. Some information may be gained by comparing the size and code markings or colour with those given on published charts or by means of a reference collection of such preparations. The appearance, taken in conjunction with simple tests, will indicate the possible or probable identity in many cases. A list of tablet diameters is given in the entry on Tablets.

In the entries on medicinal substances and under the heading "identification", information is given, where available, on chemical tests, melting-point, ultraviolet absorption, infra-red absorption, and thin-layer chromatography. This information is given as an aid to identification but it should be noted that compliance with the given data may not by itself constitute complete evidence of identity.

FURTHER INFORMATION. Tablet identification charts— *The Chemist and Druggist Directory and Tablet and Capsule Identification Guide*, London, Benn Publishing (published annually).

Idoxuridine

5-Iodo-2'-deoxyuridine

$C_9H_{11}IN_2O_5 = 354.1$

OTHER NAMES: *Dendrid®*; *Herpid®*; *Kerecid®*; *Ophthalmidine®*

A standard is given in the British Pharmacopoeia 1973

Description. Odourless tasteless colourless crystals or white powder.

Solubility. Soluble, at 20°, in 500 parts of water, in 400 parts of alcohol, and in 230 parts of methyl alcohol; very slightly soluble in ether, in chloroform, and in acetone.

Moisture content. Not more than 1%, determined by drying at 60° *in vacuo.*

Specific rotation. +28° to +32°, determined on a 1% solution in 1N sodium hydroxide.

Stability of solutions. Aqueous solutions are most stable when the pH is adjusted to between 2 and 6; they should be freshly prepared and kept in a refrigerator. Some decomposition products are more toxic than idoxuridine and may reduce its antiviral activity.

If idoxuridine is required for intravenous infusion, a 0.5% solution may be prepared from the following formula:

Idoxuridine ..	..	..	..	..	..	.. 5 g
Sodium carbonate ..		..	1 g (or a sufficient quantity)			
Dilute sulphuric acid		..	..	a sufficient quantity		
Dextrose injection (5%) ..		..	..			to 1000 ml

Adjust the alkalinity of the dextrose injection to pH 10 by the addition of sodium carbonate and add the idoxuridine, previously ground to a fine powder. Stir mechanically, again measure the pH, and add more sodium carbonate if necessary to re-adjust to pH 10. When solution is complete, adjust the pH to 9.0, using either the dilute sulphuric acid or a further quantity of sodium carbonate, as appropriate.

Sterilise the solution by filtration, distribute, by means of an aseptic technique, into sterile containers, and seal. When stored at a temperature of 0° to 4° it should be used within 6 weeks of preparation. If storage at room temperature is necessary, it should be used within 3 days. Solutions should not be used if there is evidence of deposition.

FURTHER INFORMATION. Stability in aqueous solution— L. J. Ravin *et al., J. pharm. Sci.,* 1964, **53**, 976; L. J. Ravin *et al., J. pharm. Sci.,* 1964, **53**, 1064; E. R. Garrett *et al., Chem. pharm. Bull., Tokyo.,* 1965, **13**, 1113.

Storage. It should be stored in airtight containers, protected from light.

Identification. ULTRAVIOLET ABSORPTION. In 0.01N sodium hydroxide, maximum at 279 nm (E1%, 1cm = 163).

INFRA-RED ABSORPTION. Major peaks at 1050, 1070, 1089, 1262, 1604, and 1665 cm^{-1} (see Appendix 2a: Infrared Spectra).

Metabolism. DISTRIBUTION. Enters the cerebrospinal fluid when the meninges are inflamed; *protein binding*, not significantly bound to serum proteins.

METABOLIC REACTIONS. Deamination and deiodination to form iodouracil, uracil, and iodide.

EXCRETION. Rapidly excreted in the urine; small amounts of active drug are present in the urine.

FURTHER INFORMATION. Concentrations in serum, urine, and cerebrospinal fluid—A. M. Lerner and E. J. Bailey, *J. clin. Invest.*, 1972, **51**, 45.

Actions and uses. Idoxuridine is a thymidine analogue which competes with thymidine both for incorporation into deoxyribonucleic acid and as a substrate for enzymes such as thymidine kinase and thymidylate kinase. It thus acts as an antiviral agent by inhibiting the replication of deoxyribonucleic acid viruses such as herpes simplex, vaccinia, cytomegalovirus, and adenovirus.

Idoxuridine is used in the treatment of herpetic keratitis, particularly the dendritic corneal ulcer type. Cases with deep stromal involvement respond much less satisfactorily than others. Idoxuridine is usually applied as eye-drops containing 0.1%, applications being made every hour during the day and every 2 hours at night; it may also be applied every 4 hours as an eye ointment containing 0.5%.

Herpetic lesions of the skin have been treated by the local application of idoxuridine 5% in dimethyl sulphoxide but the response is variable. Some success has been obtained in disseminated herpes zoster by injecting idoxuridine into the lesions.

In the treatment of systemic viral infections, such as herpes simplex encephalitis and congenital cytomegalovirus infection, the intravenous infusion of idoxuridine has been used when other methods of treatment have proved to be ineffective. Doses of up to a total of 600 milligrams per kilogram body-weight have been given over a period of 5 days.

Undesirable effects. Like any other cytotoxic agent idoxuridine may be teratogenic.

Poisoning. The systemic effects of idoxuridine may be at least partially reversed by the intravenous injection of a solution containing 50 milligrams of thymidine.

Preparations

IDOXURIDINE EYE-DROPS: consisting of a sterile solution of idoxuridine in purified water. Solutions for use on more than one occasion also contain a suitable bactericide. Available as eye-drops containing 0.1% of idoxuridine in containers of up to 15-ml capacity.
A standard for these eye-drops is given in the British Pharmacopoeia Addendum 1977
Containers: see the entry on Eye-drops for general information on containers.
Labelling: see the entry on Eye-drops for general information on labelling. In addition, the label on the container should state that the eye-drops should not be used for continuous periods of treatment exceeding 21 days.

Storage: it should be stored at a temperature not exceeding 8°; it should not be allowed to freeze. Any unused contents should be discarded one month after the container is first opened.
Advice for patients: see the entry on Eye-drops for general information on the use of eye-drops. The eye-drops should be instilled at regular intervals. The prescribed course should be completed. Preparations containing boric acid should be avoided.

IDOXURIDINE PAINT: consisting of the solution used to prepare idoxuridine eye-drops (see above). Available as a paint containing 0.1% of idoxuridine.
CAUTION. *Idoxuridine paint is intended for the treatment of oral lesions. Another preparation of idoxuridine, consisting of a 5% solution in dimethyl sulphoxide is unsuitable for this purpose.*
Containers, Labelling, and Storage: see the entry on Paints for general information on containers, labelling, and storage.
Advice for patients: the paint should be applied sparingly to the affected area at regular intervals. Contact with normal skin should be avoided. The prescribed course should be completed.

OTHER PREPARATIONS available include an EYE OINTMENT containing idoxuridine 0.5%; and a PAINT containing idoxuridine 5% in dimethyl sulphoxide.

Ileitis, Regional

see CROHN'S DISEASE

Imipramine Hydrochloride

10,11-Dihydro-5-(3-dimethylaminopropyl)-5H-dibenz-[b,f]azepine hydrochloride

$C_{19}H_{25}ClN_2 = 316.9$

OTHER NAMES: *Berkomine®*; *Dimipressin®*; Imipramini Hydrochloridum; *Norpramine®*; *Oppanyl®*; *Praminil®*; *Tofranil®*

A standard is given in the European Pharmacopoeia Vol. II

Description. A white or slightly yellow, crystalline, almost odourless powder with a bitter taste followed by a sensation of numbness.

Solubility. Soluble, at 20°, in 2 parts of water and in 1.5 parts of alcohol; very slightly soluble in ether; soluble in chloroform.

Dissociation constant. pK$_a$ 9.4 (24°).

Acidity. A 10% solution has a pH of about 4.7.

Stability. Imipramine hydrochloride is stable for several years when stored at room temperature provided that moisture is absent and that it is protected from light. Solutions of imipramine hydrochloride in water are stable provided that oxygen is absent and the solutions are protected from light.
In the presence of water and oxygen, degradation occurs,

accelerated by light and increase in temperature. Reactions which may occur are loss of the basic alkyl chain with the formation of iminodibenzyl, hydroxylation in position 10 followed by dehydration to the iminostilbene derivative, and ring contraction with the formation of the highly fluorescent acridine and acridone derivatives.

Hygroscopicity. It absorbs insignificant amounts of moisture at 23° at relative humidities up to about 60%, but under damper conditions it absorbs significant amounts.

Sterilisation. Solutions for injection are sterilised by heating in an autoclave or by filtration.

Storage. It should be stored in airtight containers, protected from light.

Identification. TESTS. 1. Dissolve a few mg in 2 ml of nitric acid; an intense blue colour is produced (also given by desipramine).
2. Dissolve about 50 mg in 3 ml of water, and add 1 drop of a 2.5% solution of quinhydrone in methyl alcohol; no red colour is produced within 15 minutes (distinction from desipramine).
3. Dissolve 500 mg in 20 ml of alcohol, boil, add 5 ml of a saturated solution of trinitrophenol in alcohol, and allow to cool; the precipitate, after washing with alcohol and drying, melts at about 140°.

MELTING-POINT. About 172°.

ULTRAVIOLET ABSORPTION. In 0.01N hydrochloric acid, maximum at about 251 nm (E1%, 1cm = 265).

INFRA-RED ABSORPTION. Major peaks at 740, 747, 765, 1445, 1455, and 1483 cm^{-1} (see Appendix 2a: Infra-red Spectra).

Determination in body fluids. COLORIMETRY. In blood or urine—J. E. Wallace and J. D. Biggs, *J. forens. Sci.*, 1969, **14**, 528.

SPECTROPHOTOMETRY. The ultraviolet absorption of imipramine is not suitable for determinations as it may be difficult to distinguish from background absorption and from other drugs, such as phenothiazines, which have similar absorption.

THIN-LAYER CHROMATOGRAPHY. In urine: imipramine (also desipramine and trimipramine)—A. Viala *et al.*, *Annls pharm. fr.*, 1972, **30**, 445.

GAS CHROMATOGRAPHY. In plasma—L. A. Gifford *et al.*, *J. Chromat.*, 1975, **105**, 107. In serum: imipramine and its metabolite desipramine—S. F. Reite, *Meddr. norsk farm. Selsk.*, 1975, **37**, 76. In urine—see Viala *et al.*, above.

Metabolism. ABSORPTION. Readily absorbed after oral administration.

BLOOD CONCENTRATION. 150 mg administered daily in 3 divided doses results in steady-state plasma concentrations of 10 to 100 ng/ml for imipramine and 16 to 570 ng/ml for desipramine (the major metabolite which is also active) 1 week after beginning therapy; minimum effective concentrations for imipramine and desipramine in plasma are about 45 ng/ml and 75 ng/ml respectively.

HALF-LIFE. Plasma half-life, 3 to 4 hours.

DISTRIBUTION. Widely distributed throughout body tissues and may accumulate upon repeated dosage; enters the cerebrospinal fluid in concentrations greater than those in plasma; in rats, imipramine and desipramine cross the placenta; imipramine and many of its metabolites are detectable in brain; *protein binding*, 90 to 95% bound to plasma proteins.

METABOLIC REACTIONS. N-Demethylation, N-oxidation, hydroxylation of the aromatic and alicyclic rings, side-chain removal, and glucuronic acid conjunction; the major reaction is N-demethylation to form desipramine and didesmethylimipramine; hydroxylation occurs at positions 2 and 10 of imipramine and its demethylated metabolites and is a relatively minor reaction as is N-oxidation; imipramine undergoes first pass metabolism mainly by demethylation.

EXCRETION. About 70% of a dose is excreted in the urine in 72 hours and about 20% is excreted in the faeces in a similar period; of the urinary excreted material, about 15% is unconjugated and 35% is composed of conjugates which may be hydrolysed enzymically; when the urine is acidified there is an increase in excretion of 10 to 40% due to a 50 to 100% increase in the excretion of imipramine or its unconjugated metabolites; urinary metabolites include desipramine, 2-hydroxydesipramine, 2-hydroxyimipramine, 2-hydroxyiminodibenzyl, and their conjugates, iminodibenzyl, 10-hydroxydesipramine, and didesmethylimipramine.

FURTHER INFORMATION. Buccal absorption—M. H. Bickel and H. J. Weder, *J. Pharm. Pharmac.*, 1969, **21**, 160; urinary metabolites—J. L. Crammer *et al.*, *Psychopharmacologia*, 1969, **15**, 207; first-pass metabolism—L. F. Gram and J. Christiansen, *Clin. Pharmac. Ther.*, 1975, **17**, 555; distribution and urinary excretion—L. F. Gram *et al.*, *Clin. Pharmac. Ther.*, 1971, **12**, 239; plasma concentrations—L. F. Gram *et al.*, *Clin. Pharmac. Ther.*, 1976, **19**, 318; comparison of observed and predicted first-pass metabolism—S. Niazi, *J. pharm. Sci.*, 1976, **65**, 1063.

Actions and uses. Imipramine hydrochloride is a tricyclic antidepressant with actions and uses similar to those of Amitriptyline Hydrochloride but it has weaker anticholinergic activity and a less tranquillising action. The usual dosage of imipramine hydrochloride necessary to re-establish a normal mood varies between 25 and 75 milligrams by mouth, usually 3 times a day, but only 10 to 30 milligrams daily may be necessary for elderly patients. The relief of symptoms is slow in onset and the patient may show little response until after 2 or 3 weeks of treatment; sometimes, however, there is a good response within a few days.

Imipramine may be used to control nocturnal enuresis. Children from 6 to 10 years may be given 10 milligrams and older children 25 milligrams by mouth twice or thrice daily. When a satisfactory response has been obtained, the drug should be gradually withdrawn but relapse usually occurs.

Undesirable effects; Precautions and contraindications; Drug interactions. As for Amitriptyline Hydrochloride.

Preparations

IMIPRAMINE TABLETS: available as tablets containing 10 and 25 mg of imipramine hydrochloride; they are sugar coated; the coat may be coloured.
A standard for these tablets is given in the British Pharmacopoeia 1973
Containers and *Storage:* see the entry on Tablets for general information on containers and storage. Containers should be airtight.
Advice for patients: when initiating treatment there may be a time-lag of up to 3 weeks before a full therapeutic effect is obtained. The tablets may cause drowsiness; persons affected should not drive or operate machinery. Alcohol should be avoided.

OTHER PREPARATIONS available include CAPSULES containing imipramine hydrochloride 25 mg, capsules containing imipramine hydrochloride 25 mg with promazine hydrochloride 50 mg; an INJECTION containing imipramine hydrochloride 12.5 mg per ml in 2-ml ampoules; and a MIXTURE containing the equivalent of 25 mg of imipramine hydrochloride in 5 ml, diluent water for preparations for dilutions containing 15 to 20 mg in 5 ml, and a diluent of equal parts of syrup and freshly prepared tragacanth mucilage for dilutions containing less than 15 mg in 5 ml, life of diluted mixture 14 days.

Immunoglobulin, Human Rabies

Contains specific antibodies against rabies virus.

OTHER NAMES: Human Antirabies Immunoglobulin; Human Antirabies Immunoglobulin Injection

A standard is given in the British Pharmacopoeia Addendum 1978

Human rabies immunoglobulin is prepared from a pool of plasma from persons who have been vaccinated with rabies vaccine. It contains not less than 80 units of antirabies immunoglobulin per ml.

Storage. It should be protected from light and stored at 2° to 8°.

Actions and uses. Human rabies immunoglobulin is used to protect patients who have been bitten by rabid animals or otherwise exposed to the danger of infection with rabies. The usual dose by intramuscular injection and infiltration around wounds is 20 units per kilogram body-weight.

Immunoglobulin, Human Tetanus

Contains specific antibodies against the toxin of *Clostridium tetani*.

OTHER NAME: Immunoglobulinum Humanum Antitetanicum

A standard is given in the European Pharmacopoeia Vol. II

Human tetanus immunoglobulin is prepared from a pool of plasma from persons immunised against tetanus. It contains not less than 50 units of tetanus antitoxin per ml.

Storage. As for Immunoglobulin Injection, Human Normal.

Actions and uses. Human tetanus immunoglobulin is used to protect unimmunised individuals at risk who are known to be sensitive to the animal preparation (tetanus antitoxin). When available in sufficient amounts it is the preparation of choice for the protection of unimmunised individuals at risk. The usual dose is 250 units by intramuscular injection.

Immunoglobulin, Human Vaccinia

Contains specific antibodies against the vaccinia virus.

OTHER NAME: Immunoglobulinum Humanum Antivaccinicum

A standard is given in the European Pharmacopoeia Vol. II

Human vaccinia immunoglobulin is prepared from a pool of plasma from persons recently vaccinated against smallpox. It contains not less than 500 units of vaccinia antibody per ml.

Storage. As for Immunoglobulin Injection, Human Normal.

Actions and uses. Human vaccinia immunoglobulin is used to treat patients with generalised vaccinia and also those in whom localised vaccinial infection endangers the eye. It is also given simultaneously with smallpox vaccination when this has to be done under circumstances which increase the attendant risks. When the time since exposure is too long for vaccination alone to protect smallpox contacts, this form of immunoglobulin may be given as a prophylactic likely to be of value as a supplement to smallpox vaccine.

The usual dose by intramuscular injection for generalised vaccinia, vaccinial lesions of the eye, and smallpox vaccination in the presence of contra-indications is, in children under 1 year 500 milligrams, 1 to 6 years 1 gram, 7 to 14 years 1.5 grams, and adults and children over 14 years 2 grams. For previously unvaccinated contacts of cases of smallpox, the dose is, in children under 1 year 500 milligrams, 1 to 6 years 1 gram, and adults and children over 6 years 1.5 grams.

Immunoglobulin Injection, Anti-D (Rh$_0$)

A preparation of the incomplete antibody against the rhesus D antigen of human red blood cells.

A standard is given in the British Pharmacopoeia Addendum 1975

Anti-D (Rh$_0$) immunoglobulin injection is prepared from not less than 50 litres of pooled human plasma, from persons who have been artificially or naturally immunised against the rhesus D antigen, by precipitation with organic solvents under controlled conditions of pH, ionic concentration, and temperature.

The separated globulins are dissolved in a 0.8% solution of sodium chloride or other suitable vehicle containing a suitable preservative such as 0.01% w/v of thiomersal. If necessary, human normal immunoglobulin is added to bring the total protein concentration above 3.0%. The solution is sterilised by filtration and distributed aseptically into containers which are then sealed to exclude micro-organisms.

In addition to incomplete anti-D (Rh$_0$) antibody it may contain incomplete antibodies against rhesus C and E antigens, traces of saline haemagglutinating antibodies against rhesus D, C, E, or c antigens and of immunoglobulin G antibodies against the A and B antigens of human red cells, and small amounts of saline haemagglutinating antibodies against the A and B antigens. It is a clear, pale yellow or light brown liquid in which a slight turbidity or occasional particles may appear on keeping. It contains not less than 3% of protein. It has a pH of 6.4 to 7.2.

Storage. It should be protected from light and stored at 2° to 8°.

Actions and uses. Anti-D (Rh$_0$) immunoglobulin injection is used to prevent sensitisation of rhesus (D)-negative women by rhesus (D)-positive foetal red-blood cells which may enter the maternal circulation during delivery of a Rh-positive child and thus to reduce the risk of haemolytic disease of the newborn in Rh-positive children conceived subsequently. A similar risk occurs during termination of an Rh-positive pregnancy in an Rh-negative woman.

It is also used to prevent sensitisation following transfusion of Rh-positive red cells to a Rh-negative recipient.

The usual dose for the prevention of sensitisation of D(Rh₀)-negative women following premature delivery after the twentieth week of pregnancy or following normal delivery of a D(Rh₀)-positive infant is the equivalent of 100 micrograms of antibody, by intramuscular injection, within 60 hours of delivery. This dose should be increased when the transplacental haemorrhage is estimated to exceed 10 ml.

For the prevention of sensitisation of D(Rh₀)-negative women following abortion, the equivalent of 50 micrograms of antibody may be given within 60 hours by intramuscular injection, up to and including the twentieth week of pregnancy and the equivalent of 100 micrograms of antibody after the twentieth week.

For the treatment of incompatible transfusion [D(Rh₀)-positive donor, D(Rh₀)-negative recipient] the equivalent of 10 micrograms of antibody may be given per millilitre of blood transfused or until free anti-D(Rh₀) antibody is detectable in the recipient's plasma.

Immunoglobulin Injection, Human Normal

A sterile preparation containing almost all the gamma-G globulins of human plasma together with smaller amounts of other plasma proteins.

OTHER NAMES: Human Gamma Globulin Injection; Human Gamma-G Immunoglobulin; Human Normal Immunoglobulin; Immunoglobulinum Humanum Normale

A standard is given in the European Pharmacopoeia Vol. II

Human normal immunoglobulin injection is usually prepared from pooled human plasma by precipitation with organic solvents such as alcohol under controlled conditions of pH, ionic concentration, and temperature.

The separated globulins are dissolved in a 0.8% solution of sodium chloride or other suitable vehicle containing a suitable preservative such as 0.01% of thiomersal.

The solution is sterilised by filtration and distributed into single-dose containers; it may also be prepared as a freeze-dried product.

Human normal immunoglobulin injection is also sometimes prepared from saline extracts of intact placentae from healthy women or from retroplacental blood obtained from such placentae.

Human normal immunoglobulin injection is prepared from pools of not less than 1000 donations.

The liquid preparation is a clear pale yellow to light brown liquid, free from turbidity and particulate matter at the time of preparation; during storage, slight turbidity or a small amount of particulate matter may form.

The freeze-dried preparation is a white to slightly yellowish powder or friable solid which is completely soluble in water.

The liquid preparation and the reconstituted freeze-dried material contain 10.0 to 17.0% of protein and specific precipitation tests show that they contain proteins of human origin only.

Storage. The liquid preparation should be protected from light and stored at 2° to 8°; under these conditions it may be expected to retain its potency for 3 years.

The freeze-dried preparations should be stored in an atmosphere of nitrogen, at a temperature below 25°, and protected from light; under these conditions it may be expected to retain its potency for 5 years.

The reconstituted solution should be used immediately after preparation and should be discarded if not used within 3 hours.

Actions and uses. Human normal immunoglobulin injection is used to protect susceptible contacts against hepatitis A and measles and to a lesser extent rubella and poliomyelitis. It is unlikely to be of value in the prevention of chicken pox, mumps, hepatitis B, smallpox, or whooping-cough. It should be administered by intramuscular injection as soon as possible after exposure is thought to have occurred. Protection is achieved in a proportion of subjects and lasts for not more than 4 to 6 weeks.

Human normal immunoglobulin injection is also used for the treatment of congenital or acquired hypogammaglobulinaemia and other immune deficiency states in which immunoglobulin G is diminished or absent.

Infectious hepatitis. Human normal immunoglobulin injection is used to control outbreaks of the disease in institutions or to modify the disease in known contacts for whom an attack would be dangerous. It is also used to protect persons travelling to countries where hepatitis A is endemic.

It is administered by intramuscular injection. The usual dose for prevention in children under 1 year is 250 milligrams; 1 to 2 years, 500 milligrams, 3 years or over 750 milligrams; for attenuation, 250 milligrams.

Measles. Human normal immunoglobulin injection is used for controlling outbreaks of the disease in hospitals and institutions and for preventing or attenuating the disease in children under 3 years of age or in persons suffering from intercurrent illness or living in an unfavourable environment, for whom an attack of measles might be dangerous.

It is administered by intramuscular injection. The usual dose for prevention in children under 1 year is 250 milligrams, 1 to 2 years 500 milligrams, 3 years and over 750 milligrams; for attenuation, 250 milligrams.

Rubella. Human normal immunoglobulin has been used to treat pregnant women who have been exposed to rubella during the early months of pregnancy, for the purpose of protecting the foetus from the effects of infection with rubella virus. Its value has not been unequivocally established. It is not necessary to give immunoglobulin if antibodies to rubella virus are already present, and about 90% of adult women have such antibodies.

The usual dose by intramuscular injection is 0.75 to 1.5 grams.

Hypogammaglobulinaemia and other immune deficiency states. The usual initial dose is 50 milligrams per kilogram body-weight for 5 successive days and the maintenance dose 25 to 50 milligrams per kilogram bodyweight per week, depending upon the severity of the condition.

Impetigo

Impetigo is a bacterial infection of the epidermis characterised by the appearance of weeping red areas with crusts. Usually, the infecting organisms are staphylococci or streptococci and there may be a predisposing condition such as scabies or infection with lice.

Systemic treatment with antibiotics may be required,

especially if the disease is widespread. Crusts and exudate are removed from the skin with the aid of an antiseptic solution such as 0.01% potassium permanganate and an antibiotic cream may be applied to the affected area. Measures to avoid cross-infection should be instituted.

Implants

Sterile disks or cylinders containing one or more medicaments for introduction into body tissues, such that the medicaments are released gradually over an extended period of time. They are prepared by fusion or by compression. Implants prepared by fusion consist of the appropriate quantity of the medicament only but when prepared by compression they may contain suitable absorbable adjuvants.

Containers. Implants are supplied in sterile containers, sealed to exclude micro-organisms.

Labelling. The label on the container should state the name and weight of the medicament(s) in each implant. Any limitation on the use of the preparation should also be specified.

Incompatibility

Incompatibility occurs when the components of a medicine interact in such a way that the properties of that medicine are adversely affected. Incompatibility may be pharmaceutical or therapeutic.

Therapeutic incompatibility arises when, for example, a medicine contains a depressant and a stimulant, the effects of which counteract each other, or when the action of one component in the body affects the action of another component (see under Interaction of Drugs).

Pharmaceutical incompatibility arises when the components of a medicine interact physically or chemically to give an unsuitable product.

Types of pharmaceutical incompatibility. Physical incompatibility may be due to immiscibility or insolubility of phases. Physico-chemical incompatibilities include changes of state such as liquefaction or precipitation arising from chemical interactions. Chemical incompatibilities include interactions of acids and bases, sometimes with the evolution of gas and change in colour or general appearance. Hydrolysis may occur when a substance is dissolved in water or when a strong solution is diluted, as with zinc chloride which forms an insoluble basic salt. Oxidation and reduction may result in changes in the valency of metal ions, liberation of metals, and inactivation of many organic drugs. Dyes may fade or change colour according to the pH of the medicine.

Occurrence of incompatibilities. Incompatibilities may be encountered when compounding medicines according to a prescription or recipe or when a new formula is under investigation. They do not usually occur in well-established formulated products unless they are modified in some way, for example, by addition of other substances or by dilution.

Detection of incompatibilities. When compounding a medicine in accordance with a recipe the pharmacist should consider whether, in view of the physical and chemical properties of the ingredients, an incompatibility is likely to occur.

A quantity of the medicine may be prepared to confirm the presence or absence of incompatibility, but it should be noted that interactions may result in the delayed formation of precipitates, discoloration, etc.

Methods of dealing with incompatibilities. In liquid medicines, an emulsifying or suspending agent may be required. Discoloration or precipitation may sometimes be avoided by adjustment of pH or by issuing the medicine in a diluted form or by dividing the ingredients between two medicines to be mixed immediately before use or taken separately. Powders which liquefy when mixed may be issued separately or diluted with a suitable adsorbent basis and then mixed together.

Incompatibility may occur without visible sign and if it is considered likely that such incompatibility may occur in a medicine it should not be dispensed unless a complete investigation has been carried out to ensure its efficacy.

MANUFACTURED PRODUCTS. Many manufactured products are issued without a full statement of their composition. They should be mixed with other products only in accordance with the recommendations of the manufacturer.

DANGEROUS INCOMPATIBILITIES. Medicines that may give rise to hazards should not be dispensed. Examples include mixtures that may form potent precipitates (e.g. barbiturates) and preparations liable to form gases or explode while in the hands of the patient.

THERAPEUTIC INCOMPATIBILITIES. The prescriber should be informed of any important therapeutic incompatibilities that he may possibly have overlooked.

Interpretation of data on incompatibility. The degree of interaction between the ingredients of a medicine may be dependent on the concentration, pH, temperature, etc. The statement that "x" is incompatible with "y" means that incompatibility has been observed under some conditions but does not necessarily mean that it will always occur.

Indomethacin

1 - (4 - Chlorobenzoyl) - 5 - methoxy - 2 - methylindol - 3 - yl-acetic acid

$C_{19}H_{16}ClNO_4 = 357.8$

OTHER NAMES: *Imbrilon*®; *Indocid*®

A standard is given in the British Pharmacopoeia 1973

Description. A pale yellow to brownish-yellow, crystalline, odourless, almost tasteless powder.

Solubility. Very slightly soluble in water; soluble, at 20°, in 50 parts of alcohol, in 45 parts of ether, and in 30 parts of chloroform.

Storage. It should be protected from light.

Identification. TESTS. 1. Dissolve 300 mg in 15 ml of methyl alcohol and to 5 ml of this solution add 100 mg of sodium hydroxide, shake, and allow to stand for 5 minutes; the colour changes from deep yellow to greenish-yellow to colourless and finally becomes very pale yellow. To another 5 ml of the solution add 2.5 ml of hydrochloric acid; a copious white precipitate is produced and the supernatant liquid becomes very pale yellow.

2. Dissolve 100 mg in 100 ml of water containing 0.5 ml of *dilute sodium hydroxide solution* and to 1 ml of the solution add 1 ml of a 0.1% solution of sodium nitrite, allow to stand for 5 minutes, and add 0.5 ml of sulphuric acid; a deep yellow colour is produced. To another 1 ml of the solution add 1 ml of a 0.1% solution of sodium nitrite, allow to stand for 5 minutes, and add 0.5 ml of hydrochloric acid; a green colour is produced.

MELTING-POINT. About 160°.

ULTRAVIOLET ABSORPTION. In a mixture containing 1 volume of 1N hydrochloric acid and 9 volumes of methyl alcohol, maximum at 318 nm (E1%, 1cm = 180). In 0.1N sodium hydroxide, maxima at 230 nm (E1%, 1cm = 1006) and 284 nm (E1%, 1cm = 225).

INFRA-RED ABSORPTION. Major peaks at 1226, 1236, 1307, 1478, 1690, and 1714 cm^{-1} (see Appendix 2a: Infrared Spectra).

THIN-LAYER CHROMATOGRAPHY. See under Thin-layer Chromatography, System 3.

Determination in body fluids. SPECTROFLUORIMETRY. In serum—L. P. J. Holt and C. F. Hawkins, *Br. med. J.*, i/1965, 1354.

HIGH PRESSURE LIQUID CHROMATOGRAPHY. In plasma: aspirin and frusemide stated not to interfere—G. G. Skellern and E. G. Salole, *J. Chromat.*, 1975, **114**, 483.

SPECTROFLUORIMETRY. In plasma or urine—B. K. Kim and R. T. Koda, *J. pharm. Sci.*, 1977, **66**, 1632.

Metabolism. ABSORPTION. Readily absorbed after oral administration; absorption is delayed but not decreased by antacids.

BLOOD CONCENTRATION. After an oral dose of 50 mg, peak blood concentrations of 2 to 4 μg/ml are attained within 1 to 2 hours.

HALF-LIFE. The decline in blood concentration is biphasic, the initial phase having a half-life of about 20 minutes and the second a half-life of about 70 minutes.

DISTRIBUTION. Indomethacin appears to be distributed according to a 2-compartment model; it is not taken up by red cells and it enters the synovial fluid; *protein binding*, 75 to 90% bound to plasma proteins.

METABOLIC REACTIONS. O-Demethylation and N-deacylation followed by glucuronic acid conjugation; deacylation may occur directly or after demethylation; the metabolites so formed are desmethylindomethacin (DMI), deschlorobenzoylindomethacin (DBI), and desmethyldeschlorobenzoylindomethacin (DMBI).

EXCRETION. About 66% of a dose is excreted in the urine and 33% in the faeces; of the dose excreted in the urine, 11% is unchanged, 22% is indomethacin glucuronide, 15% is either free or conjugated DMI, 12% is free or conjugated DBI, and 2.5% is free or conjugated DMBI; of the dose excreted in the faeces, 1% is unchanged, 14% is DMI, 1% is DBI, and 15% is DMBI; probenecid reduces the renal excretion of indomethacin and in so doing may increase the peak blood concentration by 50%.

Actions and uses. Indomethacin is an anti-inflammatory, antipyretic substance with analgesic properties. It is rapidly absorbed when taken by mouth and is excreted largely by the kidneys. Its action begins within 2 hours of ingestion.

It is effective in relieving pain and swelling in cases of gout and of rheumatoid and allied forms of arthritis and painful symptoms in other disorders of bone and joint, such as osteoarthritis and ankylosing spondylitis. It may also reduce fever and relieve symptoms in febrile inflammatory conditions such as glandular fever.

The usual dosage by mouth is 25 milligrams, 2, 3, or 4 times a day with meals, but the dose may be increased if necessary to 200 milligrams daily if the drug is well tolerated.

A suppository of 100 milligrams may be administered rectally once or twice daily. When 100 milligrams is given by rectum on retiring, symptomatic relief is obtained through the night and ease from pain and stiffness the following morning; 75 to 100 milligrams given by mouth with food at bedtime may prove equally effective.

Undesirable effects. The most common undesirable effects are headache and various unpleasant cerebral sensations such as fullness and dizziness. These are dose-related and usually appear early in the course of treatment and lessen or disappear as dosage is reduced or stopped.

Dyspepsia may occur at any time during treatment and is not always dose-related; peptic ulceration with bleeding may occur and is usually, but not always, accompanied by dyspepsia. Prepyloric ulcers may sometimes be mistaken for malignant lesions on X-ray films but they heal within 3 to 4 weeks of stopping the drug.

Blood dyscrasias, particularly thrombocytopenia may occur.

Bronchospasm may be precipitated in patients suffering from or with a previous history of bronchial asthma or allergic disease.

Rashes, including purpuric eruptions, are uncommon.

Precautions and contra-indications. Indomethacin should be used with caution in the presence of diminished renal function. Peptic ulceration is usually considered to be a contra-indication.

Preparations

INDOMETHACIN CAPSULES: consisting of indomethacin, in powder, which may be mixed with a suitable inert diluent, enclosed in a hard capsule. The capsule shells may be coloured. Available as capsules containing 25 and 50 mg of indomethacin.

A standard for these capsules is given in the British Pharmacopoeia 1973

Containers and *Storage:* see the entry on Capsules for general information on containers and storage.

Advice for patients: the capsules should be taken after meals.

INDOMETHACIN MIXTURE (*Syn.* Indomethacin Suspension): a suspension of indomethacin in a suitable coloured flavoured vehicle. It may contain a suitable preservative. The general direction given in the entry on Mixtures that the preparation should be diluted so that the dose is contained in 5 ml does not apply to this mixture; where necessary, the dose should be measured by means of a graduated pipette.

Available as a mixture containing 25 mg of indomethacin in 5 ml.

A standard for this mixture is given in the British Pharmaceutical Codex 1973

Containers and *Labelling:* see the entry on Mixtures for general information on containers and labelling.

Storage: it should be stored in a cool place; it should not be allowed to freeze.

Advice for patients: the mixture should be taken after

meals. If an antacid is prescribed together with the mixture, they should not be taken mixed together.

INDOMETHACIN SUPPOSITORIES: prepared as described in the entry on Suppositories by incorporating indomethacin in a macrogol or other suitable basis. Available as suppositories containing 100 mg of indomethacin.
A standard for these suppositories is given in the British Pharmacopoeia 1973
Containers and *Storage:* see the entry on Suppositories for general information on containers and storage.
Advice for patients: see the entry on Suppositories for general information on the use of suppositories.

OTHER PREPARATIONS available include CAPSULES containing indomethacin 75 mg in a slow-release formulation.

Infectious Bursal Disease Vaccine, Living

A freeze-dried preparation of attenuated infectious bursal disease virus which has been grown in embryonated eggs. It is reconstituted immediately before use with an appropriate volume of a suitable sterile liquid.

OTHER NAME: Gumboro Disease Vaccine, Living

A standard is given in the British Pharmacopoeia (Veterinary)

Storage. The dried vaccine should be protected from light and stored at 2° to 8°, when it may be expected to retain its potency for 12 months. It should be used immediately after reconstitution.

Veterinary uses. It is administered either by intramuscular injection or in drinking water or by eye-drops to chickens for prophylaxis against infectious bursal disease.

Influenza

Influenza is due to infection by the myxoviruses, influenza virus type A and type B. Infection spreads rapidly and, because the antigenic pattern of the virus constantly changes, epidemics may occur when a large number of susceptible persons are present in the population.
Immunity to individual viruses is of long duration but when major shifts occur in the virus antigens the immune mechanisms are no longer protective. The changes occur in influenza A about every 10 years. Changes in influenza B occur less frequently and generally this virus attacks mainly children. A major change in influenza B occurred in 1973.
The disease is characterised by fever and pains in the head, back, and limbs, and may be followed by complications due to secondary bacterial infection of the respiratory system.
Patients should remain in bed while fever is present. Analgesics and antipyretic drugs may be used to reduce pain and fever and cough suppressants may be required to relieve the unproductive cough which may arise later.

Influenza Vaccine

An aqueous suspension of a suitable strain or strains of influenza virus, inactivated so that they are non-infective but retain their antigenic properties. Suitable strains of influenza virus are those currently recommended by the World Influenza Centre of the World Health Organisation.

OTHER NAMES: Flu/Vac; Influenza Vaccine (Inactivated); Vaccinum Influenzae Inactivatum

A standard is given in the European Pharmacopoeia Vol. II

Storage. It should be stored protected from light at 2° to 10°. It should not be allowed to freeze. Under these conditions it may be expected to retain its potency for 18 months.

Actions and uses. Influenza vaccine is used for active immunisation against epidemic influenza. It is usually given by deep subcutaneous injection as a single dose of 1 millilitre during the autumn, when it may be expected to give substantial protection against infection by the same antigenic variety of virus. Protection develops in 2 to 3 weeks but is, however, short-lived.
As a rule, influenza vaccination is not prescribed annually, except for persons considered to be under special risk, for example, patients with chronic cardiac disease provided they are not suffering from respiratory impairment. It may be given during an influenza epidemic, particularly to such people as medical and nursing staff who are required to remain at work during the epidemic.

Influenza Vaccine, Live (Intranasal)

An aqueous suspension of a suitable live attenuated strain of influenza virus of either type A or type B grown in embryonated eggs. The strains used should possess antigens relevant to protection against currently prevalent influenza viruses. The vaccine is prepared in embryonated eggs and freeze dried. It is reconstituted immediately before use with an appropriate volume of a suitable sterile liquid.

OTHER NAME: *Nasoflu®*

A standard is given in the British Pharmacopoeia Addendum 1978

Storage. The freeze-dried vaccine should be stored between 2° and 8°; under these conditions it may be expected to retain its potency for 1 year.
The reconstituted vaccine should be used immediately after preparation.

Actions and uses. Influenza vaccine, live (intranasal) is used for immunisation against influenza due to strains of influenza virus possessing surface antigens related to those from which the vaccine was prepared.
It may be used annually for persons considered to be under special risk, for example, patients with chronic cardiac or pulmonary insufficiency. A single dose of the quantity indicated on the label is administered by nasal instillation; for maximum protection the dose should be repeated after 1 or 2 weeks.

Infra-red Spectrophotometry

Infra-red spectrophotometry is a technique for examining the absorption by chemical substances of radiation at wavelengths longer than those of visible light. The infra-red region of the spectrum extends from wavelength 0.8 to 1000 μm, but the usual range examined for identification purposes is 5 to 15 μm (2000 to 667 cm^{-1}). In the infra-red region, absorption bands may be found which correspond to vibrations of bonds and groupings

within molecules, but the spectrum is usually complex and difficult to interpret because some bands cannot be assigned to specific groups and some may be due to skeletal vibrations or other effects. However, each compound produces a characteristic absorption spectrum and the method is, therefore, of value as a means of confirming the identity of a given compound.

Infra-red spectrophotometry has the advantage over ultraviolet spectrophotometry for purposes of identification since the ultraviolet absorption spectrum is not usually specific for a particular substance. Infra-red absorption is less suitable than ultraviolet absorption for quantitative determinations.

A number of types of infra-red spectrophotometer are available. Details of construction differ considerably but the most significant points of difference are in the methods of handling the radiation beam and the methods of recording the spectrum. Instruments may be either single or double beam; in the latter case, the radiation beam is switched alternately to pass through the sample and through a reference cell, thus compensating for unwanted absorption in solvents etc. The monochromator may be either a sodium chloride prism or a grating. The recorded spectrum may have either a linear wavelength (λ μm) scale or a linear wavenumber ($10^4/\lambda$ cm^{-1}) scale. Spectra recorded in these two ways have a different appearance and are not easy to compare. Most modern instruments have a linear wavenumber scale.

Identification by infra-red spectrophotometry. Because of the complexity of the spectra and the difficulty of comparing spectra recorded on different instruments it is usual to compare spectra with those obtained on the same or a similar instrument under the same conditions with samples known to be genuine.

It may also be possible to identify a substance by measuring the characteristics and comparing them with tabulated data.

It has been shown (A. S. Curry *et al.*, *J. Pharm. Pharmac.*, 1969, **21**, 224; P. H. B. Ingle and D. W. Mathieson, *Pharm. J.*, 1976, **216**, 73) that an infra-red spectrum of a particular substance can be retrieved from a collection, with some degree of confidence, by reference to its six major absorption bands. This forms the basis for a system of identification, the ultimate confirmation being comparison with a reference spectrum as noted above.

Preparation of infra-red spectra. The resolution of an infra-red spectrum depends partly on the rate at which the spectrum is scanned and this may be limited by the sensitivity of the instrument and the density of the sample.

When it is necessary to distinguish between closely similar compounds, an instrument of high resolving power may be necessary. Solid samples may be examined in solution, in liquid paraffin mulls, or in pressed disks. It is also possible to examine samples in the liquid or gaseous states.

In *solution*, portions of the spectrum may be masked by absorption due to the solvent. The spectrum may be affected by interaction between specimen and solvent, and in some cases, especially when polar solvents are used, association of molecules of the sample may alter the spectrum.

Liquid paraffin mulls are fine suspensions prepared by grinding the substance in liquid paraffin. Portions of the spectrum, mainly in the region 6.8 to 7.3 μm (1460 to 1374 cm^{-1}), are masked by absorption due to the liquid paraffin but the interaction and association effects observed with solutions are absent.

Potassium bromide disks are prepared by mixing the sample with potassium bromide in fine powder and compressing to form a disk for insertion into the spectrophotometer. Disks do not have the disadvantages of solutions and mulls but different polymorphic forms of the sample may give rise to different spectra and suitable techniques must be adopted to ensure that samples and reference substances are in the same polymorphic form.

Infra-red data. Data consisting of six major absorption bands which have been selected from the recorded spectrum are included in a number of the entries on medicinal substances in this volume. The spectra are reproduced, in a reduced size, in Appendix 2. The selected peaks are the six most intense peaks and they are stated in increasing order of wavenumber. Shoulders have been chosen only if they are clearly resolved and the point of maximum absorption can be easily determined. Where there is more than one peak of the same intensity at the sixth intensity level, the choice has been arbitrary. It should be noted that, because of variations in instruments and conditions, other determinations of the spectrum may not give peaks with the same relative intensities.

Where the spectrum has been recorded in a liquid paraffin mull, peaks in the region of 6.8 to 7.3 μm (1460 to 1374 cm^{-1}) have been ignored.

Infusions

Infusions are dilute solutions containing the readily soluble constituents of crude drugs.

Formerly, fresh infusions, prepared by macerating the drug, in a suitable state of comminution, for a short period in cold or boiling water, were used. Now, infusions are usually prepared by diluting 1 volume of a concentrated infusion to 10 volumes with water.

Prior to 1968, concentrated infusions were formulated for dilution to 8 volumes with water and those earlier concentrated infusions that have not been included in the 1968 or subsequent editions of the British Pharmacopoeia or the British Pharmaceutical Codex may still be available at that strength.

Infusions are liable to fungous and bacterial growth and it is necessary to dispense them within 12 hours of their preparation.

Preparation of infusions. *Concentrated infusions* are prepared on a small scale by the methods described in the individual entries for these infusions—see Index. When they are manufactured in larger quantities, the same method, appropriately scaled up, is used; alternatively, for certain concentrated infusions, they may be prepared by the alternative method described for liquid extracts—see under Extracts.

Details of a method for preparing *fresh infusions* were given in the British Pharmaceutical Codex 1949.

Infusions, Intravenous

see under INJECTIONS

Inhalations

Inhalations are liquid preparations composed of or containing volatile ingredients which, when vaporised in a suitable manner, are intended to be brought into contact with the lining of the respiratory tract. The ingredients may be volatile at room temperature, in which case they may be inhaled from an absorbent pad on which they have been placed, or they may require to be added to hot (about 65°) but not boiling water and the vapour inhaled for 5 to 10 minutes—the quantity usually employed is one teaspoonful of the inhalation to one pint of hot water.

Inhalations intended to be added to hot water may consist of alcoholic solutions or of mixtures with water to which a diffusing agent such as light magnesium carbonate has been added.

Containers. Inhalations should be dispensed in white fluted bottles.

Labelling. When an inhalation containing an insoluble diffusing agent is dispensed, a direction to shake the bottle before use should be given on the label.

Injections

Injections are sterile solutions, suspensions, or emulsions which contain one or more medicaments in a suitable aqueous or non-aqueous vehicle; they are intended to be administered parenterally to produce a localised or systemic, rapid or sustained response. The parenteral route of administration is often adopted for medicaments which cannot be given orally because of patient intolerance or because of instability, therapeutic inactivity, or poor absorption. In an emergency, an injection can provide a rapid and effective response.

Preparation of injections. Those which contain thermostable medicaments in solution or suspension are prepared in the appropriate vehicle and, after clarification by filtration (if the injection is a solution) are usually sterilised in the final containers. Injections of medicaments which are unstable in solution are prepared by dissolving or suspending the sterile medicament in the required amount of sterile vehicle by means of an aseptic technique.

All solid and liquid components of the injection should be of high quality and free from micro-organisms, pyrogens, particles, and other foreign matter. High standards of cleanliness are required for all glassware and equipment used in processing and filling; procedures for cleaning and sterilising apparatus, containers, and closures are given in the entry on Sterilisation. All operations should be carried out in an environment which is as free as possible from particulate and microbial contamination arising from dust, droplets, or skin and clothing.

Aqueous injections must be prepared with water for injections. This is sterile water prepared from potable water by distillation under special conditions and immediately sterilised by autoclaving in sealed containers; it is free from pyrogens.

Water for injections may be replaced by unsterilised water prepared freshly by the method for preparing water for injections, provided that the injection is sterilised immediately after preparation. "Immediately" is generally interpreted as within 4 hours of the collection of the water unless special precautions are taken. To minimise the risk of pyrogen formation the freshly distilled water is often maintained at 80° in suitable bulk containers until required for preparing the injection.

When an injection is required to be prepared with water for injections free from dissolved air or carbon dioxide, freshly prepared water for injections is used. It is boiled for 10 minutes, cooled, and used to prepare the injection, precautions being taken to exclude air or carbon dioxide during these procedures.

There are few non-aqueous or water-miscible solvents which are free from toxic effects or of such low potential as irritants or sensitisers as to be considered suitable vehicles for injections. Even fewer can be injected intravenously, so that their main application is in injections administered in small volume subcutaneously or intramuscularly.

Fixed oils of vegetable origin, such as arachis, cottonseed, sesame, and maize are used as vehicles, but only after careful purification; they are also used in some intravenous emulsions. Other immiscible solvents which are sometimes used instead of fixed oils include esters such as ethyl oleate or isopropyl myristate. Water-miscible materials are mainly used as co-solvents to dissolve water-insoluble materials, the most useful being propylene glycol and liquid macrogols. Ethyl alcohol, glycerol, and benzyl alcohol have also been used but have limited application.

Addition of bactericides. Injections supplied in multiple-dose containers should contain a bactericide in a concentration sufficient to prevent the development of micro-organisms, unless the medicament itself is sufficiently bactericidal. A multiple-dose injection sterilised by the process of heating with a bactericide should not require additional bactericide.

Bactericides must not be included in intravenous injections of volumes greater than 15 millilitres, or in intra-arterial, intracardiac, or intraspinal injections (see classification of injections, below).

Provided there is no therapeutic or chemical incompatibility with the medicament or other constituents of the injection, suitable bactericides and their concentrations for aqueous injections include phenol (0.5%), cresol (0.3%), chlorbutol (0.5%), chlorocresol (0.1%), and phenylmercuric acetate or nitrate (0.001%). Any other substance used must have a bactericidal activity at least equivalent to that of an aqueous solution containing phenol (0.5%), or it should be capable of sterilising the injection within 3 hours after inoculation with 10^6 vegetative organisms per ml.

Bactericides included in oily injections in multiple-dose containers include phenol (0.5%), cresol (0.3%), or chlorocresol (0.1%); these bactericides may afford some protection from contamination with vegetative micro-organisms, but are ineffective against sporing organisms.

Because the effectiveness of a bactericide in a preparation may be modified by other components of that preparation, or even by components of the container, it is particularly important that any assessment of antimicrobial effectiveness should be made on the complete preparation taken from the proposed container.

Sterilisation of injections. Methods for the sterilisation of solutions and suspensions are described in the entry on Sterilisation. The methods suitable for a particular injection are given in the entry which includes a description of the preparation.

NOTE. *If an emergency precludes the application of a specific method of sterilisation to a substance or preparation, it is the duty of the pharmacist to obtain the prescriber's approval for any other course taken.*

Pyrogens. Administration of an injection which contains pyrogens, especially if given intravenously and in large volume, may produce a pyrogenic reaction in the patient. Typical reactions are erythema at the injection site, high temperature, pain in the legs and back, and general discomfort.

Pyrogens are lipids associated with polysaccharides and proteins of high molecular weight; they are produced by many micro-organisms but the most potent forms originate from Gram-negative bacteria. The main sources of pyrogens are contaminated tap water, medicaments, containers, and processing equipment. Because pyrogens are water-soluble, thermostable, unaffected by bactericides, and unlikely to be destroyed by autoclaving, it is desirable that their formation should be prevented during the preparation of injections.

The non-volatility of pyrogens aids their elimination by distillation. Other methods for the destruction of pyrogens include exposure to dry heat at 180° for 3 to 4 hours or for shorter periods at higher temperatures. Pyrogens may also be removed by oxidising agents or by adsorbents such as charcoal, aluminium hydroxide gel, and certain ion-exchange resins.

Formulation of injections. Although it is sometimes possible for an injection to be presented as a simple sterile solution of the active compound in water, it is often necessary to formulate a more complex system in order to improve acceptability to the patient, to increase the effectiveness or duration of action of the medicament, or to minimise degradative effects during processing and storage. Some of the more important factors to be taken into account when formulating injections are given below.

Vehicles. Water is the most common solvent or vehicle for injections and is the solvent of choice when rapid absorption of a medicament is required. Alternative non-aqueous solvents may have to be considered for water-insoluble or unstable compounds, or in instances where delayed absorption is desirable.

Isotonicity. Injection of some medicaments in aqueous solution can produce discomfort to patients or damage if the solution is not isotonic, that is, iso-osmotic with blood serum. Adjustment of the tonicity of such solutions may be achieved by the addition of sodium chloride or other suitable substance. However it may not always be feasible, or therapeutically desirable, to make the solution isotonic.

Solutions for subcutaneous injection should preferably be made isotonic to reduce pain on injection.

Solutions for intramuscular injection should preferably be isotonic or slightly hypertonic to increase penetration of the surrounding tissue.

Solutions for intravenous injection should preferably be isotonic, especially when large volumes are to be given, as otherwise if they are administered rapidly they may cause haemolysis of red blood corpuscles and damage to the walls of the veins. If it is not possible to make an intravenous injection isotonic, the solution must be injected slowly.

Solutions for intrathecal injection must be isotonic.

A method for calculating the quantity of adjusting substance to be added to solutions of various medicaments to render them isotonic with blood serum is given in the entry on Isotonic and Isosmotic Solutions.

Hydrogen ion concentration. Controlled conditions of pH may be necessary in aqueous injections for several reasons; to maintain the medicament in solution, to minimise decomposition, to enhance absorption, or to reduce discomfort to the patient. Simple addition of acid or alkali is often used for pH-adjustment or to form the more soluble salts of a less-soluble acidic or basic medicament. Buffers must be non-toxic and carefully selected for compatibility, pH range, and buffer capacity. To minimise pain or irritation on injection, it is desirable that aqueous solutions administered intramuscularly or subcutaneously should be of pH 7.0. Intravenous infusions and all intraspinal injections should, ideally, be of pH 7.4.

Stabilisers for injections. Decomposition of medicaments in aqueous systems is frequently due to hydrolytic, oxidative, or photolytic reactions. The rates at which these reactions occur can be affected by pH conditions, temperature, exposure to atmospheric gases, and the presence of catalysts, so that special consideration may have to be given to these aspects during formulation, preparation, packaging, and subsequent storage.

To retard or prevent decomposition, injections may include buffers, antioxidants, chelating agents, synergists, or special stabilising agents. Such additives must be carefully selected on the grounds of freedom from toxicity and pharmacological effect and of compatibility with the medicament and other components, including the container.

Buffers commonly used in injections include citrates, phosphates, and acetates. Antioxidants for aqueous systems include sodium metabisulphite, sodium sulphite, sodium thiosulphate, ascorbic acid, and dextrose; oily injections may contain propyl gallate, butylated hydroxyanisole, butylated hydroxytoluene, or alpha tocopherol. Injections which are subject to oxidative changes may also be filled and sealed into containers under an inert gas such as nitrogen or less commonly carbon dioxide. Enhancement of the stabilising effect of antioxidants can sometimes be achieved by the inclusion of chelating agents; typical examples are disodium and calcium edetates, and citric and tartaric acids.

Suspensions for injection. Medicaments which are insoluble in the vehicle are administered as suspensions or dispersions, usually in a complex vehicle containing various additives. Because additives must be non-toxic, capable of sterilisation, and suitable for injection, their number is limited. In most suspensions, the particle size of the medicament is small and the size range is closely controlled to ensure that particles pass readily through the bore of a hypodermic needle and do not increase in size or "cake" on storage.

To aid dispersion or subsequent dissolution of the medicament, surface-active agents such as lecithin, polysorbate 80, or sorbitan esters are often included together with hydrophilic colloids (sodium carboxymethylcellulose, gelatin, methylcellulose) to increase viscosity. A vehicle which has thixotropic properties may be ideal if it provides a stable dispersion during storage and is sufficiently fluid to pass through a syringe on injection.

Suspensions in oily vehicles are less frequently used; they provide a "depot" effect when injected intramuscularly. Aluminium monostearate has been included in oily vehicles to produce thixotropic gels.

Emulsions for injection. Occasionally oils or solutions of medicaments in oil are administered intravenously as emulsions. The oil should form the internal phase of the emulsion and, ideally, few of the oil globules should exceed 3 micrometres in diameter.

Nutrient injections which contain up to 15% of emulsified vegetable oil together with dextrose have a limited use in intravenous feeding. Such emulsions require careful formulation and stabilisation to ensure that coalescence of oil globules does not occur during stabilisation and storage.

Emulsifiers and stabilisers for intravenous emulsions must be non-toxic; materials which have been used include lecithin, polysorbate 80, gelatin, methylcellulose, and serum albumin.

Absorption from injections. A medicament in aqueous solution injected by an intravenous or intraspinal route usually produces a rapid therapeutic effect since no absorption mechanism is involved before the medicament is transported by the body fluids. However, in some instances, there may be a short delay until the medicament is present in the blood in its pharmacologically active form and until an equilibrium is established between the concentration of medicament in the blood and that in the tissues. An aqueous solution injected subcutaneously, intradermally, or intramuscularly may still act fairly rapidly but in these instances the medicament must be absorbed from the injection site before a response occurs. The rates at which such absorption occurs follow similar kinetics to those for medicaments administered orally.

From subcutaneous and muscular tissues, absorption is mainly into blood capillaries and the lymphatic system; the absorption mechanism may be by simple diffusion of lipid-soluble forms according to Fick's law, although there is some evidence that small drug particles may be ingested and transported by phagocytes.

Absorption of small molecules is more rapid and mainly through capillary walls; larger molecules and colloids appear to be primarily absorbed and transported via the lymphatic vessels.

Other local factors which affect the rate and extent of absorption include capillary blood flow, hydrostatic and osmotic pressure differences, bodily movement, the extent of dissociation of the medicament, and the nature of the vehicle.

An injection which produces a rapid onset of activity may be inactivated or eliminated at a similar rate and frequent injections may, therefore, be necessary. It is often desirable that a more steady and sustained effect should be achieved.

One approach to producing sustained effects is to reduce the rates of metabolism or excretion of the medicament but the most convenient method is by slowing absorption.

Slow absorption of a medicament from simple aqueous solutions is readily obtained by administration over quite long periods as an intravenous infusion or by a subcutaneous or intramuscular drip; the limitations of this technique are discussed under Intravenous Additives.

Chemical modification, pharmaceutical formulation, and the utilisation of the many physical and physiological factors which influence absorption, have all been employed to retard the rates at which medicaments are absorbed in the circulating body fluids.

Medicaments which are relatively insoluble in water are usually only slowly absorbed and therefore chemical modification of a compound to a less soluble form is likely to retard its absorption. Injection of an active compound as the ester is also a means of slowing absorption; release of the active compound in the region of the injection site is largely controlled by the rate of hydrolysis of the ester. Even further retardation, or a depot effect, can be obtained when the insoluble medicament is suspended in an oily vehicle and injected intramuscularly. Water-soluble medicaments may also be suspended in non-aqueous vehicles.

Absorption of any medicament presented as a suspension or dispersion and injected into the tissues will be affected by the physico-chemical characteristics of both the medicament and the vehicle. Important aspects are the polymorphic form, crystal size and habit, size distribution, surface area, and concentration of the solid component; the volume, pH, tonicity, viscosity, and the presence of adsorbents can also affect release from the vehicle.

Physical actions such as the application of pressure or a reduction in the amount of body movements or local lowering of body temperature can all reduce the rate of drug absorption.

Additives such as histamine or atropine also retard absorption but are infrequently used; adrenaline, however, is still added to injections of local anaesthetics such as lignocaine to prolong their local anaesthetic activity.

Classification of Injections

Injections may be classified according to their route of administration.

General Injections

Intradermal or intracutaneous injections are usually aqueous solutions or suspensions injected between the dermis and the epidermis in small doses (0.1 to 0.2 ml); they are mainly used in diagnostic tests for allergy or immunity.

Subcutaneous or hypodermic injections are usually aqueous isotonic solutions injected under the skin in volumes not greater than 1 millilitre. When intravenous infusion is contra-indicated, larger volumes (3 to 4 litres per day) may be given by the subcutaneous route provided that tissue permeability is enhanced by the enzyme hyaluronidase, administered concomitantly; this infusion technique is termed hypodermoclysis.

Intramuscular injections are solutions or suspensions in aqueous or oily vehicles injected into the large areas of muscle tissue in volumes which should not exceed 4 millilitres at any one site. Unless given slowly, or in small volumes, intramuscular injections can cause considerable pain.

Intravascular injections include both intravenous and intra-arterial injections.

Intravenous injections are usually aqueous solutions injected into a prominent vein, either in volumes from 1 to 10 millilitres or in larger volumes which are termed intravenous infusions. Sterile oil-in-water emulsions may also be administered intravenously if careful control is exercised over globule size. Preparations in which the continuous phase is an oil must not be given by this route. If the single-dose volume exceeds 15 millilitres, the injection should not contain an added bactericide except in special circumstances, and if greater than 10 millilitres, should be free from pyrogens.

Intra-arterial injections are similar to intravenous injections but are administered directly into an artery; their main use is when an immediate effect is required in the control of a peripheral condition. They must not contain an added bactericide.

Intracardiac injections are aqueous solutions used in emergency treatment only and injected directly into the cardiac muscle or ventricle. They must not contain an added bactericide.

Intraspinal injections are aqueous solutions injected into the area of the spinal column in volumes not normally exceeding 20 millilitres; they are further divided into *intrathecal or subarachnoid*, *intracisternal*, and *peridural* injections, depending upon the location of the injection site. They must not contain a bactericide and must be presented in single-dose containers.

To localise the action of the medicament, the weight per ml may be adjusted by the addition of suitable substances.

Intra-articular injections are aqueous solutions or suspensions which are injected into the synovial fluid in a joint cavity.

Intrabursal injections are similar to intra-articular injections but they are injected into a bursa; commonly used sites for injection are the shoulder (subacromial bursa) and the elbow (olecranon bursa).

Other routes for injections used to produce specific effects include intracerebral, intraperitoneal, and intrapleural.

Ophthalmic Injections

These are aqueous solutions or suspensions injected into various regions of the eye for surgical or therapeutic purposes; the volume injected does not usually exceed 1 millilitre.

Ophthalmic injections include *subconjunctival* (beneath Tenon's capsule close to the eye but not into it), *intracameral* (into the anterior chamber), *intravitreous* (into the vitreous chamber), and *retrobulbar* (into the posterior segment of the globe).

Bactericides may be included in subjunctival but not in intracameral or intravitreous injections.

Containers for Injections

Injections, or the sterile ingredients for the preparation of injections, should be supplied in single-dose or multiple-dose containers which are sealed to exclude micro-organisms.

Containers are made of glass or suitable plastic material and, where possible, single-dose containers sealed by fusion should be supplied. Cartridge packs and unit-dose syringes are also available. A multiple-dose container usually consists of a glass bottle or vial sealed by a rubber closure which permits the withdrawal of successive doses, and fitted with a protective overcap; it should not contain an excessive number of doses.

Glass containers should comply with the requirements of the European Pharmacopoeia for Glass Containers for Injectable Preparations.

Plastic containers should be colourless and of sufficient clarity to permit inspection of the contents. The plastic material used should not yield more than a minimum of soluble matter. Additives in plastic materials such as stabilisers, antoxidants, plasticisers, and lubricants must not be toxic.

The rubber closures used with multiple-dose containers should be made from suitably compounded natural or synthetic rubber of good quality; closures which meet British Standard 3263: 1960 and the modified requirements of the British Pharmacopoeia Addendum 1977 are suitable. Closures should be impregnated with any bactericide or preservative included in the injection following the procedure described in the entry on Sterilisation, under Sterilisation of Rubber and Plastics. Containers of oily injections should be fitted with closures made of oil-resistant material.

Large-volume injections should be supplied in bottles which comply with British Standard 2463: 1962, or in other glass or plastic bottles of an appropriate standard. Plastic containers of capacity exceeding 50 ml comply with the tests for metallic additives in plastic containers and the injections contained in them should comply with the tests for toxicity and for ether-soluble extractive referred to in the British Pharmacopoeia 1973 under Injections.

Labelling of Injections

The label on the container should state the strength of the injection as the amount of active ingredient in a suitable dose-volume.

The label on the container or the label on the package states: (1) the name and proportion of any added bactericide; (2) the name of any added buffering or stabilising agent; (3) the date after which the preparation is not intended to be used; and (4) the conditions under which it should be stored.

The label on the sealed container of a powdered medicament intended for the preparation of an injection states: (1) the name of the medicament, followed by the words "for Injection"; (2) the nominal weight or number of units of medicament(s) in the container; (3) the volume and composition of the solvent to be used; (4) the concentration of medicament(s) in the solution when prepared as directed; (5) the date after which the powder is not intended to be used; and (6) the conditions under which the powder should be stored.

The label on the containers of solvent to be used with the powdered medicament states the volume and composition of the solvent.

The label on the sealed container of powdered medicament or the label on the carton states: (1) the name and proportion of any added bactericide; (2) the name of any added buffering or stabilising agent; (3) directions for preparing the injection; (4) the conditions under which the injection should be stored; and (5) the period during which the injection may be expected to be suitable for use when stored under the stated conditions.

Insect Bites and Stings

Midges and *mosquitoes* cause bites of varying severity, usually with immediate irritation, which may be followed by a delayed reaction after several hours. A hard persistent swelling may occur after the bites of *blackflies*. *Horseflies* produce a relatively large incision with oedema, oozing blood, and blister formation; these bites are particularly prone to sepsis. Stiffness and swelling of glands may occur as a result of bites of the insects mentioned above, especially when they are located on the face or limbs.

Ants, bees, hornets and *wasps* produce painful stings. In addition to the local reaction, patients who have been previously sensitised to the stings may develop anaphylactic reactions including generalised urticaria, angioneurotic oedema, nausea, vomiting, and respiratory collapse.

Treatment. Soothing lotions may be applied and antihistamines may be given by mouth to reduce the risk of irritation and swelling. Topical antihistamines, if used, should be restricted to one or two applications for the treatment of acute effects, owing to the risk of hypersensitivity reactions.

Bee stings usually remain in the wound and should be carefully removed without releasing more venom. As bee stings contain formic acid, bathing the affected area in sodium bicarbonate solution or diluted ammonia solution is sometimes recommended.

Anaphylactic shock, occurring in sensitised subjects, may require treatment with adrenaline or corticosteroids. If bites become infected, appropriate treatment should be given, including antibiotics if required.

Prevention. The incidence of bites and stings may be reduced by avoiding heavily infested areas, the use of adequate clothing, and the application of insect repellent preparations such as dimethyl phthalate.

For snake bites and scorpion stings see under Snake Venom Antiserum and Scorpion Venom Antiserum.

Insomnia

Insomnia or sleeplessness may be a difficulty in falling asleep, an early awakening, or an intermittent waking throughout the period of attempted sleep. It may be caused by pain, mental depression, or certain physical illnesses such as acute infections or Sydenham's chorea. Drug treatment is not always necessary for insomnia. Some patients who complain may be found on enquiry to have adequate sleep and others may sleep better if they avoid excitement or stimulant drinks such as coffee or tea or adjust the room temperature. Treatment of troublesome symptoms such as cough or indigestion which disturb the onset of sleep may also be of value. Patients with depression may have sleep disturbances. Treatment of depression with tricyclic antidepressants or monoamine-oxidase inhibitors, as described under Depression, may be effective.

Sedative drugs may be used in patients who have difficulty in getting to sleep or whose sleep is disturbed early in the night. These drugs have the disadvantage that their effect continues into the following day, leading to loss of alertness, and that their use leads to habituation and the need to increase dosage. For these reasons the routine administration of sedative drugs in hospitals and other institutions should be avoided. Enzyme induction during long-term treatment may also lead to a need for increased dosage, especially in the case of barbiturates. A number of drugs have a sedative action similar to the barbiturates although they differ structurally from them. Methaqualone, used in conjunction with an antihistamine drug such as diphenhydramine has the disadvantages of unpredictability and rapidity of onset and the tendency for dependence to develop; moreover, overdosage may give rise to both coma and convulsions for which treatment is difficult. Overdosage with nitrazepam on the other hand does not usually lead to serious effects.

Sedatives and hypnotics should not be used in patients with renal failure or severe hepatic insufficiency.

Analgesics such as morphine are used in the treatment of pain, but are not effective in the treatment of sleeplessness due to any other cause.

Insufflations

Insufflations are powders containing medicinal substances usually diluted with a suitable inert powder such as lactose. They are intended for introduction into the ear, nose, throat, body cavities, or wounds. They are administered by means of an insufflator or, when intended for the nose, they may be used in the same way as snuff.

Insufflations are sometimes supplied in hard capsules (cartridges) intended for use in an inhaler designed so that the flow of powder is controlled by the patient's own inspiratory effort.

Insulin

The properties of insulin are described under Insulin Injection, and other preparations are described in the entries that follow.

Highly purified insulins. Some insulin preparations are available in a highly purified form, variously described as "monocomponent" (MC), "fractionated", "rarely immunogenic" (RI), or "highly purified". These forms are insulins from which most of the pancreatic impurities such as pro-insulin have been removed. Less highly refined bovine or porcine insulins are known as "pro-insulin free". Many of the immunogenic side-effects, such as antibody formation, lipoatrophy, and allergy, associated with ordinary insulins are greatly reduced but it has not been established that the incidence of degenerative changes is decreased when highly purified insulins are used.

Stable diabetics are unlikely to benefit from a change to highly purified insulins but newly diagnosed diabetics, patients with insulin allergy, lipoatrophy, insulin resistance, high daily insulin requirements, or requiring intermittent insulin therapy should preferably be treated with highly purified insulins. The change from ordinary to highly purified insulins must be carefully supervised to avoid possible hypoglycaemic reactions as insulin requirements are often unpredictably reduced either immediately or gradually over a period of months.

Label colours. The following colours are used on labels of insulin preparations used in the United Kingdom: 20 units per millilitre, brown; 40 units per millilitre, blue; 80 units per millilitre, green. It should be noted that insulin preparations containing 100 units per millilitre are available in some countries such as Canada and U.S.A.

An additional colour is used on labels of forms other than soluble insulin: biphasic insulin, turquoise; globin zinc insulin, orange; isophane insulin, white; neutral insulin, brown; protamine zinc insulin, pink; insulin zinc suspension, magenta; insulin zinc suspension (amorphous), red; insulin zinc suspension (crystalline), yellow.

To identify "highly purified" preparations, a white stripe inserted along the diagonal separating the two colours signifying the type of insulin and the strength indicates "monocomponent" insulin, while a white stripe on the diagonal across the two colours indicates "rarely immunogenic" insulin.

Insulin Injection

A sterile solution of the protein insulin, the specific antidiabetic principle of the mammalian pancreas.

OTHER NAMES: Insulin; Insulini Solutio Iniectabilis; Soluble Insulin; Unmodified Insulin.

A standard is given in the European Pharmacopoeia Vol. III

Insulin injection may be prepared by dissolving crystalline insulin having a potency of not less than 23 units per milligram, calculated with reference to the anhydrous material, in water for injections containing 1.6 per cent w/v of glycerol, sufficient hydrochloric acid to adjust the pH to 3 to 3.5, and sufficient bactericide to prevent the growth of micro-organisms.

The solution is sterilised by filtration, assayed, adjusted to the required strength, and distributed aseptically into sterile containers, which are then sealed.

Insulin injection is usually made from ox pancreas.

Description. A colourless liquid, free from turbidity and from matter which deposits on standing, and contains 20, 40, or 80 units per ml, the potency being determined biologically. It has a pH of 3.0 to 3.5.

Containers. The containers are glass vials, sealed so as to allow the withdrawal of successive doses on different occasions.

Storage. It should be stored at 2° to 10°; it should not be allowed to freeze. Under these conditions it may be expected to retain its potency for at least 2 years.

Metabolism. ABSORPTION. Inactive when administered orally; subcutaneous doses are better absorbed from the arms than from the thighs; protamine-zinc forms are slowly but steadily absorbed.

BLOOD CONCENTRATION. During an intravenous infusion of 2 to 12 units/hour, blood concentrations of 20 to 200 microunits/ml are attained; endogenous concentrations under fasting conditions in normal subjects are about 500 pg/ml (12 microunits/ml) in the peripheral circulation and 2 to 4 ng/ml (50 to 100 microunits/ml) in the portal vein; during absorption of food, peripheral blood concentrations increase 10 to 15 times; concentrations in treated diabetics remain at a fairly low but stable level and do not reach the high concentration peaks obtained in normal subjects; blood concentrations of 1 to 2 ng/ml are normally maintained in these subjects.

HALF-LIFE. After intravenous administration, 4 to 9 minutes, after subcutaneous administration, about 4 hours, and after intramuscular administration, about 2 hours; the half-life does not appear to be increased in diabetics.

DISTRIBUTION. Circulates in the blood as a polymer with a molecular weight of 17 000 to 43 000; it is rapidly taken up by the tissues and binds to specific receptors on cell membranes; volume of distribution, approximately equal to extracellular fluid volume but may be increased in diabetes; *protein binding*, bound to a small extent in the blood to globulins; bovine or porcine insulin become bound to circulating antibodies in a few weeks and this binding delays and prolongs the response to injected doses.

METABOLIC REACTIONS. Rapidly metabolised in the liver and other tissues by reduction and hydrolysis; two enzymes have been detected which metabolise insulin, namely insulinase, which is an insulin-specific protease, and glutathione-insulin dehydrogenase; 40 to 50% of endogenous insulin is removed from the portal system by the liver and metabolised.

EXCRETION. Insulin is small enough to be removed from the blood by glomerular filtration but it is reabsorbed and metabolised in the renal tubules; small amounts may appear in the urine; it is also eliminated in the bile.

FURTHER INFORMATION. See J. A. Parsons, Endocrine pharmacology, and G. F. Cahill, Insulin and glucagon, *Peptide Hormones*, J. A. Parsons (Ed.), London, Macmillan, 1976, pp. 67 and 85; measurement of insulin levels in peripheral blood—P. H. Sönksen *et al.*, *Lancet*, ii/1972, 600; insulin metabolism—*Postgrad. med. J.*, 1973, **49**, Suppl. (7).

Actions and uses. Insulin is the hormone, secreted by the beta cells of the islets of Langerhans of the pancreas, that not only regulates carbohydrate metabolism but is also concerned with the synthesis of protein and fat and with the storage of the latter. Secretion of insulin is primarily regulated by the level of the blood sugar, although it is modified by other hormones such as adrenaline, glucagon, hydrocortisone (cortisol), and growth hormone.

In the juvenile diabetic insulin secretion is reduced; in the middle-aged obese diabetic it is present, but largely unavailable, possibly because of the presence of insulin antagonists, or because binding prevents its access to body cells.

Insulin is rapidly inactivated by the enzymes of the gastro-intestinal tract. In a normal person, the fasting blood-sugar level is maintained in the region of 80 to 120 milligrams per 100 millilitres; a store of glucose, as glycogen, is maintained in the liver and muscles. As the blood-sugar level falls, the liver glycogen is mobilised and converted into glucose, which passes into the blood. If insufficient insulin is available to the tissues, as in diabetes mellitus, a rise in the blood-sugar level occurs and, when the renal threshold for sugar is exceeded, glycosuria occurs; in addition, glycogen is not stored in the liver, the respiratory quotient does not rise with increased carbohydrate intake and fat metabolism, and the production of glucose from non-carbohydrate sources (gluconeogenesis) is markedly reduced. Oxidation of some of the fat is incomplete, resulting in the formation of ketones, such as acetone and acetoacetic acid, and β-hydroxybutyric acid, which appear in the urine.

When administered parenterally, insulin causes a fall in the blood-sugar level and increased storage of glycogen in the liver. In the diabetic, it raises the respiratory quotient after a carbohydrate meal and prevents the formation of ketones.

Insulin is used chiefly for the control of diabetes mellitus in diabetics not responding to dietary control. It is ineffective by mouth and is usually administered by deep subcutaneous injection, although the intravenous route may be used when particularly rapid effects are required, as in diabetic coma.

The dose depends upon the patient's diabetic condition. The action of insulin begins within 20 to 30 minutes of subcutaneous injection and reaches its maximum in 4 to 6 hours. Injections are usually given twice a day, 15 to 30 minutes before breakfast and the evening meal; a third dose may be necessary before the midday meal. The number of injections required can be reduced by the simultaneous injection of a slow-acting insulin before breakfast.

Overdosage with insulin causes hypoglycaemia. The early symptoms, such as weakness, giddiness, pallor, sweating, a sinking feeling in the stomach, palpitations, irritability and tremor, resemble those of sympathetic stimulation. Later, the higher centres may be affected, with the onset of either depression or euphoria, inability to concentrate, lack of judgment and self-control, and amnesia. Other symptoms are ataxia, diplopia, and paraesthesia. Convulsions occur if the blood-sugar level falls below 35 milligrams per 100 millilitres and if this is not corrected permanent brain damage may occur and, finally, death.

In the emergency treatment of diabetic coma, insulin injection, but not one of the delayed-acting preparations, is used. In the pre-comatose condition the patient should be given 20 to 50 units of insulin every 2 to 4 hours, depending on the blood-sugar level and intensity of ketosis, although larger doses may often be needed in individual cases. Should the patient be comatose, 100 units of insulin may be given, approximately half of it intramuscularly and half intravenously; if the insulin requirement normally exceeds 80 units daily, or if severe infection, dehydration, or circulatory collapse is present, or if the blood-sugar level is over 600 milligrams per 100 millilitres, the initial dose should be increased up to 200 units.

Frequent determinations of sugar in the blood and urine serve as a guide for further dosage of insulin, which may then be given subcutaneously every 2 to 4 hours. Urine estimations are less reliable as a guide than blood estimations unless specimens are obtained frequently.

Dehydration and acidosis are treated by the rapid intravenous infusion of 1000 millilitres of a solution containing 5.85 grams of sodium chloride and 3.36 grams of sodium lactate or of sodium chloride injection or sodium bicarbonate injection, depending upon the metabolic state; further quantities may be given if required, but at a slower rate. After diuresis has set in and the blood-sugar level has begun to fall, supplements of potassium and magnesium are frequently required. If peripheral circulatory failure has occurred, 1000 millilitres of plasma may be given intravenously.

Low-dose insulin regimens may be used in the treatment of diabetic ketosis or during surgical procedures on insulin-dependent patients. Soluble insulin should preferably be administered by infusion pump. In keto-acidosis it is given at a rate of about 6 units per hour until the blood glucose level has fallen below 280 milligrams per 100 millilitres and then the rate is reduced to 3 units per hour.

During surgery or labour a dose of 2 units is given hourly in dextrose injection (5%); 1000 millilitres of dextrose injection (5%) given over 8 hours will provide 6 grams of carbohydrate per hour.

Insulin injection may be mixed with isophane insulin injection but should preferably not be mixed with protamine zinc insulin injection since a variable amount of the soluble form is converted to protamine zinc insulin. Any mixing should be done in the syringe immediately before injection.

Undesirable effects. In addition to the effects of overdosage described above, insulin may give rise to allergic reactions and atrophy of fat at the site of injection.

Precautions. Thiazide diuretics and corticosteroids may increase insulin requirements.

The hypoglycaemic effect may be enhanced in patients being treated with β-adrenergic blocking drugs, phenylbutazone, or monoamine-oxidase inhibitors, or by excessive alcohol intake.

Poisoning. In the early stages, when the patient can swallow, 3 or 4 lumps of sugar may be given, and again in 10 to 15 minutes if there is no improvement. If consciousness is lost, food cannot be given by mouth and treatment is by the intravenous administration of 10 to 50 millilitres of strong dextrose injection.

Preparations

Available in 10-ml vials containing 20, 40, and 80 units of insulin per ml.

Insulin Injection, Biphasic

A sterile buffered suspension of crystals containing the specific antidiabetic principle of the pancreas of the ox in a solution of the specific antidiabetic principle of the pancreas of the pig.

OTHER NAMES: Biphasic Insulin; *Insulin Novo Rapitard MC®*

A standard is given in the British Pharmacopoeia 1973

Biphasic insulin injection may be prepared from crystalline ox insulin, with a potency of not less than 23 units per milligram, calculated with reference to the anhydrous material and containing about 0.8% of zinc, by dissolving in a dilute hydrochloric acid, sterilising the solution by filtration, and mixing the filtrate aseptically, with constant stirring, with one third of its volume of a sterile solution containing 5.44% of sodium acetate, 28% of sodium chloride, and sufficient sodium hydroxide to produce a pH of 5.4 to 5.5 in the mixture. The stirring is continued for about 20 hours, or until the precipitated insulin is converted into rhombohedral crystals.

The suspension is then added aseptically to eight times its volume of a sterile aqueous solution of a suitable bactericide, and the mixture diluted with sufficient of a solution of sodium hydroxide to produce a preparation containing either 40 or 80 units per ml and having a pH of about 7.

To this preparation is added a sterile solution of insulin, containing either 40 or 80 units per millilitre, until a quarter of the insulin present is in soluble form. This sterile solution of insulin may be prepared from crystalline pig insulin with a potency of not less than 23 units per milligram, calculated with reference to the anhydrous material, and containing about 0.8% of zinc, by dissolving in a dilute hydrochloric acid, sterilising the solution by filtration, diluting the filtrate aseptically with 8 times its volume of a sterile aqueous solution of a suitable bactericide and with one volume of a sterile solution containing 1.36% of sodium acetate, 7% of sodium chloride, and sufficient sodium hydroxide to produce a pH of about 7. The suspension is distributed aseptically into sterile containers which are then sealed.

Description. An almost colourless turbid liquid in which, on examination under a microscope, the majority of the particles are seen as rhombohedral crystals with a maximum dimension greater than 10 μm but rarely exceeding 40 μm.

Containers. The containers are glass vials, sealed so as to allow the withdrawal of successive doses on different occasions.

Storage. It should be stored at 2° to 10°; it should not be allowed to freeze. Under these conditions it may be expected to retain its potency for at least 2 years.

Actions and uses. Biphasic insulin injection produces a rapid hypoglycaemic effect within half an hour of subcutaneous injection due to the soluble insulin fraction, while the insulin crystals, being slowly absorbed, produce a depot effect with an action beginning about 3 hours after subcutaneous injection and reaching a maximum 4 to 12 hours after administration. The total duration of action is from 18 to 22 hours.

Biphasic insulin injection thus combines the properties of a quick-acting soluble insulin and the prolonged action of an insulin of intermediate duration.

Biphasic insulin is administered by subcutaneous injection twice daily, except in mild cases of diabetes when one injection daily may suffice. The first injection is usually given half an hour before breakfast to control the hyperglycaemia occurring shortly afterwards, and the second injection, which should be 30 to 50% of the morning dose, is given half an hour before the evening meal. A more potent initial hypoglycaemic effect may be obtained by mixing neutral insulin with biphasic insulin; other forms of insulin should not be used for this purpose.

The usual dose is from 20 to 80 units daily, but much more than this may be needed. When changing from another insulin to biphasic insulin it is seldom necessary to alter the total dose.

Biphasic insulin should never be given intravenously and is not suitable for the emergency treatment of diabetic coma. It is not always effective in the treatment of juvenile diabetes and brittle diabetes.

Poisoning. The procedure as described under Protamine Zinc Insulin Injection should be adopted.

Preparations

Available in 10-ml vials containing 30 units of insulin crystals (ox) with 10 units of insulin (pig) in solution per ml and in 10-ml vials containing 60 units of insulin crystals (ox) with 20 units of insulin (pig) in solution per ml; these preparations are available in conventional form and in monocomponent form derived from ox and pig.

Insulin Injection, Globin Zinc

A sterile preparation of the protein insulin, the specific antidiabetic principle of the mammalian pancreas, with a suitable globin and zinc chloride.

OTHER NAMES: Globin Insulin; Globin Zinc Insulin

A standard is given in the British Pharmacopoeia 1973

Globin zinc insulin injection may be prepared from crystalline insulin having a potency of not less than 23 units per milligram, calculated with reference to the anhydrous material, by adding aseptically to a sterile solution in hydrochloric acid, the strength of which has been suitably adjusted, the following sterile materials: a solution of globin in the proportion of 3.6 to 4.0 milligrams of globin for each 100 units; zinc chloride equivalent to 0.3 milligram of zinc for each 100 units; 1.6% of glycerol; and sufficient bactericide to prevent the growth of micro-organisms.

The preparation is distributed aseptically into sterile containers, which are then sealed.

Globin zinc insulin injection is usually made from ox pancreas.

Description. An almost colourless liquid substantially free from turbidity and from matter which deposits on standing.

Containers. The containers are glass vials, sealed so as to allow the withdrawal of successive doses on different occasions.

Storage. It should be stored at 2° to 10°; it should not be allowed to freeze. Under these conditions it may be expected to retain its potency for at least 2 years.

Actions and uses. Globin zinc insulin has actions which are essentially the same as those described under Insulin Injection. It has, however, a delayed action which is intermediate in onset between that of unmodified insulin and that of protamine zinc insulin. The onset of activity occurs 2 to 4 hours and the maximum effect 6 to 12 hours after injection; the duration of action is 12 to 18 hours.

Globin zinc insulin is used to reduce the number of injections required for the control of diabetes mellitus, as compared with the use of unmodified insulin alone, especially in patients showing hypersensitivity to protamine zinc insulin. It is usually administered by subcutaneous injection half an hour before breakfast. In some severe cases of diabetes, 2 injections of globin zinc insulin a day may be necessary. The dose is determined by the physician in accordance with the needs of the patient.

Hypoglycaemic reactions, if they occur while a patient is receiving globin zinc insulin, usually take place in the late afternoon or early evening. They can be avoided by reducing the dose or redistributing the carbohydrate intake between the morning, midday, and evening meals in the proportions of one-fifth, two-fifths, and two-fifths respectively. Alternatively, or in addition, a light carbohydrate meal may be taken in the afternoon.

Globin zinc insulin should never be given by intravenous injection, and it is not suitable for the emergency treatment of diabetic coma, for which insulin injection should be used.

Undesirable effects. Globin zinc insulin may occasionally produce cutaneous and allergic reactions.

Poisoning. The procedure as described under Protamine Zinc Insulin Injection should be adopted.

Preparation

Available in 10-ml vials containing 80 units of globin zinc insulin per ml.

Insulin Injection, Isophane

A sterile buffered crystalline suspension of the protein insulin, the specific antidiabetic principle of the mammalian pancreas, with a suitable protamine and zinc.

OTHER NAMES: *Insulin Leo Retard*®; Insulini Isophani Protaminati Suspensio Iniectabilis; Isophane Insulin; Isophane Insulin (NPH); Isophane Protamine Insulin Injection

Mixtard® (with neutral insulin injection)

A standard is given in the European Pharmacopoeia Vol. III

Isophane insulin injection may be prepared from crystalline insulin having a potency of not less than 23 units per milligram, calculated with reference to the anhydrous material. It contains a suitable protamine in the proportion of 0.3 to 0.6 milligram of protamine sulphate for each 100 units and a zinc salt equivalent to not more than 0.04 milligram of zinc for each 100 units, together with 1.6% of glycerol, 0.15 to 0.17% of *m*-cresol, 0.06 to 0.07% of phenol, and sodium phosphate as a buffering agent.

Isophane insulin injection is usually made from ox pancreas.

Description. A white suspension, the particles in which, on examination under a microscope, are seen to be rod-shaped crystals about 20 μm long, free from large aggregates.

Containers. The containers are glass vials, sealed so as to allow the withdrawal of successive doses on different occasions.

Storage. It should be stored at 2° to 10°; it should not be allowed to freeze. Under these conditions it may be expected to retain its potency for at least 2 years.

Actions and uses. Isophane insulin injection has actions which are essentially the same as those described under Insulin Injection. It has a delayed action which begins about 2 hours after subcutaneous injection, becomes maximal after 10 hours, and declines after about 28 hours. Duration of action depends partly on the dosage given.

It is usually administered once a day, before breakfast, in a dosage determined by the physician in accordance with the needs of the patient. When insulin requirements are high it can be given in two doses, two-thirds of the total dose in the morning and one-third in the late afternoon. It should not be given intravenously.

Isophane insulin injection may be given together with unmodified insulin when the combined effect of quick-acting and slow-acting insulin is required; they may be mixed and given in the same syringe. When used in such mixtures, it has the advantage over protamine zinc insulin that it does not affect the rapid action of the unmodified insulin. It may also be mixed with neutral insulin injection, but not with any other forms of insulin.

Poisoning. The procedure as described under Protamine Zinc Insulin Injection should be adopted.

Preparations

Available in 10-ml vials containing 40 and 80 units of isophane insulin per ml; these preparations are available in conventional form derived from the ox and pig and in rarely immunogenic form derived from the pig.

OTHER PREPARATIONS available include an INJECTION containing isophane insulin 28 units with neutral insulin 12 units per ml and an injection containing isophane insulin 56 units with neutral insulin 24 units per ml in 10-ml vials; these preparations are in rarely immunogenic form derived from the pig.

Insulin Injection, Neutral

A sterile buffered solution of the protein insulin, the antidiabetic principle of the mammalian pancreas.

OTHER NAMES: *Actrapid MC®*; *Insulin Leo Neutral®*; Neutral Insulin; *Nuso Neutral Insulin®* *Mixtard®* (with isophane insulin injection)

A standard is given in the British Pharmacopoeia 1973

Neutral insulin injection may be prepared by dissolving crystalline ox or pig insulin with a potency of not less than 23 units per milligram, calculated with reference to the anhydrous material and containing about 0.4% of zinc, in a dilute hydrochloric acid, sterilising the solution by filtration, mixing the filtrate aseptically with a sterile aqueous solution of a suitable bactericide, and adding aseptically sufficient of a sterile solution of sodium acetate, sodium chloride, and sodium hydroxide so that the final preparation contains 0.136% of sodium acetate, 0.7% of sodium chloride, and the requisite number of units, and has a pH of about 7.

The solution is distributed aseptically into sterile containers, which are then sealed.

Description. A colourless liquid free from turbidity; during storage traces of very fine sediment may deposit.

Containers. The containers are glass vials, sealed so as to allow the withdrawal of successive doses on different occasions.

Storage. It should be stored at 2° to 10°; it should not be allowed to freeze. Under these conditions it may be expected to retain its potency for at least 2 years.

Actions and uses. Neutral insulin injection has actions and uses similar to those described under Insulin Injection, but when given subcutaneously it is slightly more rapidly absorbed. The dose of neutral insulin injection is the same as that of insulin injection and is determined by the physician in accordance with the needs of the patient. The first dose of the day is given 20 to 30 minutes before breakfast. After injection, it continues to produce a fall in the blood-sugar level for about 5½ hours and maintains its hypoglycaemic effect for 8 to 9 hours, or slightly longer than insulin injection.

Neutral insulin injection may be given alone or simultaneously with biphasic insulin injection or isophane insulin injection. It is sometimes mixed in the same syringe with globin zinc insulin injection, insulin zinc suspension (amorphous), or insulin zinc suspension (crystalline) but the mixture must be injected immediately after preparation. The effect of these mixtures on the blood-sugar level is very similar to that of mixtures of these preparations with insulin injection. It should preferably not be mixed with protamine zinc insulin injection since a variable amount of the soluble form is converted to protamine zinc insulin. Any mixing should be done in the syringe immediately before injection.

Neutral insulin injection should not be mixed with insulin injection.

Neutral insulin may be used in the emergency treatment of diabetic coma and pre-coma. Patients hypersensitive to bovine insulin may be treated with neutral insulin injection prepared from pig pancreas.

Undesirable effects. These are as described under Insulin Injection.

Poisoning. The procedure as described under Insulin Injection should be followed.

Preparations

Available in 10-ml vials containing 40 and 80 units of neutral insulin per ml; these preparations are available in conventional form and as rarely immunogenic and monocomponent preparations derived from the pig.

OTHER PREPARATIONS available include an INJECTION containing neutral insulin 12 units with isophane insulin 28 units per ml and an injection containing neutral insulin 24 units with isophane insulin 56 units per ml in 10-ml vials ; these preparations are in rarely immunogenic form derived from the pig.

Insulin Injection, Protamine Zinc

A sterile suspension of the protein insulin, the specific antidiabetic principle of the mammalian pancreas, with a suitable protamine and zinc chloride.

OTHER NAMES: Insulini Zinci Protaminati Suspensio Iniectabilis; Protamine Zinc Insulin.

A standard is given in the European Pharmacopoeia Vol. III

Protamine zinc insulin injection may be prepared from crystalline insulin having a potency of not less than 23 units per milligram, calculated with reference to the anhydrous material, by adding aseptically to a sterile aqueous solution, the strength of which has been suitably adjusted, the following sterile materials: a suitable protamine in the proportion of 1.0 to 1.7 milligrams of protamine sulphate for each 100 units; zinc chloride equivalent to 0.2 milligram of zinc for each 100 units; 1.6% of glycerol; and sufficient bactericide to prevent the growth of micro-organisms.

The suspension is distributed aseptically into sterile containers and a sterile solution of sodium phosphate, containing, if necessary, either sodium hydroxide or phosphoric acid, is added so that the final mixture contains 10 to 11 milligrams of sodium phosphate for each 100 units and has a pH of 6.9 to 7.4, within which range most of the active principle is precipitated. The containers are then sealed.

Protamine zinc insulin injection is usually made from ox pancreas.

Description. An almost colourless turbid liquid.

Containers. The containers are glass vials, sealed so as to allow the withdrawal of successive doses on different occasions.

Storage. It should be stored at 2° to 10°; it should not be allowed to freeze. Under these conditions it may be expected to retain its potency for at least 2 years.

Actions and uses. Protamine zinc insulin has actions which are essentially the same as those described under Insulin Injection. It has, however, a delayed action which allows a slow but steady activity of insulin throughout the day.

Protamine zinc insulin is used to reduce the number of

injections needed to control diabetes mellitus as compared with the use of unmodified insulin alone. It is usually administered once a day by subcutaneous injection 30 to 60 minutes before breakfast. A dose of unmodified insulin is often given at the same time to tide over the period until the protamine zinc insulin is absorbed; the two insulins are sometimes mixed in the syringe immediately before injection but this practice should be discouraged as the onset and duration of action of the resulting mixture differ from those of the two insulin preparations injected separately because some of the unmodified insulin is converted by the excess protamine in the protamine zinc insulin into the latter. The onset of action of protamine zinc insulin given alone is from 4 to 7 hours, the maximum effect is obtained in 15 to 20 hours, and the total duration of action is 24 to 36 hours, depending on total dosage.

Intramuscular injection of protamine zinc insulin may cause pain, and it should never be given intravenously. In some patients its action following large doses is sufficiently delayed to render the next morning specimen of urine sugar-free; such patients do not require unmodified insulin.

The dose of protamine zinc insulin is adjusted to suit the needs of the patient; more than 80 units should rarely be given, because of the severe nocturnal hypoglycaemia that may result. If the patient has previously been treated with unmodified insulin, the initial dose of protamine zinc insulin should be from two-thirds to the same number of units. Because protamine zinc insulin lowers the blood-sugar level over a long period, a redistribution of the carbohydrate intake more evenly over the waking hours may be necessary. An increased carbohydrate intake at bedtime may prevent early morning hypoglycaemia.

Because it is slowly absorbed, protamine zinc insulin should never be given in the treatment of diabetic coma. For the same reason, hypoglycaemic attacks resulting from protamine zinc insulin are insidious and tend to occur during the night or early morning. They require immediate and continued treatment for some hours.

Undesirable effects. These are as described under Insulin Injection. Allergic reactions to the protamine may also occur.

Poisoning. The treatment is the same as that for the hypoglycaemic attacks caused by overdosage of unmodified insulin, as described under Insulin Injection, except that when the patient has recovered consciousness and is able to swallow, glucose drinks and a slowly digestible form of carbohydrate, such as bread, must be given until the more prolonged action of the protamine zinc insulin has ceased.

Preparations

Available in 10-ml vials containing 40 and 80 units of protamine zinc insulin per ml.

Insulin Zinc Suspension

A sterile buffered suspension of the protein insulin, the specific antidiabetic principle of the mammalian pancreas, with zinc chloride.

OTHER NAMES: Insulin Lente; Insulin Zinc Suspension (mixed); Insulini Zinci Suspensio Iniectabilis Mixta; I.Z.S.; *Lentard MC®*; *Monotard MC®*

A standard is given in the European Pharmacopoeia Vol. III

Insulin zinc suspension may be prepared by mixing aseptically 3 volumes of insulin zinc suspension (amorphous) and 7 volumes of insulin zinc suspension (crystalline). The suspension is distributed aseptically into sterile containers, which are then sealed. Two forms of insulin zinc suspension, one made from pig pancreas and the other from ox pancreas, are available.

Description. An almost colourless turbid liquid in which, on examination under a microscope, the majority of the particles are seen as rhombohedral crystals with a maximum dimension greater than 10 μm but rarely exceeding 40 μm; a considerable proportion of the particles can be seen under high-power magnification to have no uniform shape and not to exceed 2 μm in maximum dimension.

Containers. The containers are glass vials, sealed so as to allow the withdrawal of successive doses on different occasions.

Storage. It should be stored at 2° to 10°; it should not be allowed to freeze. Under these conditions it may be expected to retain its potency for at least 2 years.

Actions and uses. Insulin zinc suspensions have actions which are essentially the same as those described under Insulin Injection. They have, however, a delayed action which varies in duration from 12 to 30 hours or longer, depending upon the amount of zinc present and the particle size of the insulin.

Insulin zinc suspension (amorphous) has a relatively short duration of action; its effect begins in 30 minutes and is maximal in 2 to 3 hours and persists for 12 to 16 hours. The effect of insulin zinc suspension (crystalline) begins a few hours after injection, is maximal 7 hours after subcutaneous injection, and may persist for 36 hours. These two suspensions are miscible in all proportions without any modification of the one by the other, and in many diabetics good control is maintained by a single daily injection of such a mixture in the form of insulin zinc suspension. Because they are free from foreign protein, these preparations are less likely than protamine zinc insulin injection and globin zinc insulin injection to produce local and allergic reactions.

For the average diabetic, insulin zinc suspension gives suitable control; its onset of action is gradual, with a maximum lowering of blood-sugar level 4 to 5 hours after subcutaneous injection and a total duration of action of 24 hours. The onset of action of the usual morning dose is sufficiently rapid to control the rise of blood-sugar level after breakfast. Most diabetics needing insulin are satisfactorily controlled by one injection a day of this preparation; a small proportion need the addition of insulin zinc suspension (amorphous) or insulin zinc suspension (crystalline) for optimal control.

These insulin zinc suspensions are not suitable for the treatment of diabetic emergencies or diabetic coma, for which insulin injection should be used. They should not be given intravenously or, because they are incompatible with the buffering agents, mixed with other insulin preparations; they are, however, mutually miscible. They are administered by subcutaneous injection, usually 30 to 45 minutes before breakfast.

The dosage varies according to the condition of the patient and usually lies between 20 and 100 units daily. The initial dose is 10 to 16 units daily, increased by 4 units daily until the blood sugar is controlled.

Some diabetics cannot be controlled with insulin zinc suspension alone. In such cases additional insulin zinc suspension (crystalline) or insulin zinc suspension (amorphous) may be added to the mixture. Alternatively, insulin injection may be given in the evening. Before each dose of insulin zinc suspension is withdrawn from the vial it should be shaken gently; vigorous shaking may cause excessive frothing.

Severe diabetes is first brought under control with insulin injection and an insulin zinc suspension is then substituted in the same or slightly larger daily dosage.

Poisoning. The procedure as described under Protamine Zinc Insulin Injection should be adopted.

Preparations

Available in 10-ml vials containing 40 and 80 units of insulin zinc suspension; these preparations are available in conventional form and monocomponent form derived from the ox and pig (crystalline) and pig (amorphous).

Insulin Zinc Suspension (Amorphous)

A sterile buffered suspension of the protein insulin, the specific antidiabetic principle of the mammalian pancreas, with zinc chloride.

OTHER NAMES: Amorph. I.Z.S.; Insulin Semilente; Insulini Zinci Amorphi Suspensio Iniectabilis; *Semitard MC®*

A standard is given in the European Pharmacopoeia Vol. III

Insulin zinc suspension (amorphous) may be prepared from crystalline insulin having a potency of not less than 23 units per milligram, calculated with reference to the anhydrous material, by dissolving it in 0.02N hydrochloric acid containing zinc chloride equivalent to 0.01% of zinc; the solution is sterilised by filtration and diluted aseptically with 8 times its volume of a sterile solution containing, for the 40 units per millilitre preparation, zinc chloride equivalent to 0.00875% of zinc, or, for the 80 units per millilitre preparation, zinc chloride equivalent to 0.01375% of zinc, together with sufficient bactericide to prevent the growth of micro-organisms in the final preparation. A sterile solution of sodium acetate, sodium chloride, and sodium hydroxide is added, with constant stirring, to give a preparation containing 0.136% of sodium acetate and 0.7% of sodium chloride and having a pH of about 7.3.

The preparation is distributed aseptically into sterile containers, which are then sealed.

Two forms of insulin zinc suspension (amorphous), one made from pig pancreas and the other from ox pancreas, are available.

Description. An almost colourless turbid liquid in which, on examination under a microscope, the particles are seen to have no uniform shape and rarely exceed 2 μm in maximum dimension.

Containers. The containers are glass vials, sealed so as to allow the withdrawal of successive doses on different occasions.

Storage. It should be stored at 2° to 10°; it should not be allowed to freeze. Under these conditions it may be expected to retain its potency for at least 2 years.

Actions and uses. Insulin zinc suspension (amorphous) has the actions and uses described under Insulin Zinc Suspension. It may be mixed with insulin zinc suspension or insulin zinc suspension (crystalline) but not with any other form of insulin.

Poisoning. The procedure as described under Protamine Zinc Insulin Injection should be adopted.

Preparations

Available in 10-ml vials containing 40 and 80 units of

insulin zinc suspension (amorphous) per ml; these preparations are available in conventional form and in monocomponent form derived from the pig.

Insulin Zinc Suspension (Crystalline)

A sterile buffered suspension of the protein insulin, the specific antidiabetic principle of the mammalian pancreas, with zinc chloride.

OTHER NAMES: Cryst. I.Z.S.; Insulin Ultralente; Insulini Zinci Crystallisati Suspensio Iniectabilis; *Ultratard MC®*

A standard is given in the European Pharmacopoeia Vol. III

Insulin zinc suspension (crystalline) may be prepared from crystalline insulin having a potency of not less than 23 units per milligram, calculated with reference to the anhydrous material, by dissolving it in 0.02N hydrochloric acid containing, for the 40 units per millilitre preparation, zinc chloride equivalent to 0.0133% of zinc, or, for the 80 units per millilitre preparation, zinc chloride equivalent to 0.0266% of zinc; the solution is sterilised by filtration and is mixed aseptically, with constant stirring, with one-third of its volume of a sterile solution containing 5.44% of sodium acetate, 28% of sodium chloride, and sufficient sodium hydroxide to produce a pH of 5.4 to 5.5. The stirring is continued for about 24 hours or until the insulin is converted into regular crystals.

The suspension is then added aseptically, with constant stirring, to 9 times its volume of a sterile solution containing sufficient bactericide to prevent the growth of micro-organisms, and, for the 40 units per millilitre preparation, 0.014% of sodium hydroxide and zinc chloride equivalent to 0.0077% of zinc, or, for the 80 units per millilitre preparation, 0.017% of sodium hydroxide and zinc chloride equivalent to 0.0111% of zinc. The final preparation has a pH of about 7.3.

The preparation is distributed aseptically into sterile containers, which are then sealed.

Insulin zinc suspension (crystalline) is usually made from ox pancreas.

Description. An almost colourless turbid liquid, the particles in which, on examination under a microscope, are seen to be rhombohedral crystals, the majority having a maximum dimension greater than 10 μm but rarely exceeding 40 μm.

Containers. The containers are glass vials, sealed so as to allow the withdrawal of successive doses on different occasions.

Storage. It should be stored at 2° to 10°; it should not be allowed to freeze. Under these conditions it may be expected to retain its potency for at least 2 years.

Actions and uses. Insulin zinc suspension (crystalline) has the actions and uses described under Insulin Zinc Suspension. It may be mixed with insulin zinc suspension or with insulin zinc suspension (amorphous) but not with any other forms of insulin.

Poisoning. The procedure as described under Protamine Zinc Insulin Injection should be adopted.

Preparations

Available in 10-ml vials containing 40 and 80 units of insulin zinc suspension (crystalline) per ml; these preparations are available in conventional form and monocomponent form derived from the ox.

Interactions of Drugs

It is common for patients to be treated with more than one drug at the same time and there are several different ways in which they may interact for the patient's good or harm.

Important interactions are described in this volume in the entries on individual drugs but for more detailed information reference should be made to the original literature cited therein and to the reference works such as *Evaluations of Drug Interactions*, 2nd Edn, Washington DC, American Pharmaceutical Association, 1976; P. D. Hansten, *Drug Interactions*, 3rd Edn, Philadelphia, Lea and Febiger, 1975; and I. Stockley, *Drug Interactions*, London, Pharmaceutical Press, 1974.

The following is a general summary of the principal mechanisms involved.

Bioavailability and incompatibility. The formulation of medicinal products may affect the rate and extent of their absorption in the body (as described in the entry on Bioavailability). Drugs which are admixed with each other, as for example when solutions are mixed in the same syringe, may interact with each other and with a vehicle in which they are infused (as described in the entry on Incompatibility).

Absorption. For mechanisms of drug absorption and transport across membranes see Absorption in the entry on Metabolism of Drugs; for drug formulations and their effects on absorption see the entry on Bioavailability.

Drugs which influence the rate of gastric emptying may modify the rate of absorption of other drugs. For example, metoclopramide which increases and propantheline which reduces gastric emptying rate have been shown to increase and decrease respectively the rate of absorption of paracetamol. Chelation or the binding of drugs within the gastro-intestinal tract may reduce their absorption, as in the case of tetracyclines which are less readily absorbed from the gut in the presence of salts of aluminium, calcium, iron, and magnesium.

Vasoconstrictor drugs are combined with local anaesthetic agents in some parenteral formulations to restrict their area of action at the injection site. On the other hand, a drug, such as the enzyme hyaluronidase may be given with another drug such as diodone to increase its rate of intramuscular absorption.

Protein binding. For descriptions of mechanisms involved in tissue and plasma protein binding see Plasma Protein Binding and Tissue Binding in the entry on Metabolism of Drugs.

Drugs may compete for tissue or plasma protein binding sites. Protein binding is likely to be of clinical significance with drugs such as warfarin which are more than 97% plasma-protein bound. A small change in binding produced, for example, by phenylbutazone may increase the unbound fraction of warfarin and so markedly lengthen the prothrombin time. Similarly, long-acting sulphonamides such as sulphadimethoxine are also highly protein bound, and may induce hypoglycaemia in diabetics receiving chlorpropamide, glibenclamide, or tolbutamide.

Enzyme induction. For mechanisms of metabolism of drugs see Metabolic Reactions in the entry on Metabolism of Drugs.

The magnitude and duration of action of many drugs as well as endogenously produced substances are dependent on their rate of biotransformation by metabolising enzymes in the liver. The activity of these enzymes may be increased by treatment with some commonly used drugs, including barbiturates and phenytoin, as well as by some common pesticides. An important interaction depending on this mechanism is the increased rate of metabolism of warfarin in patients treated with barbiturates, leading to a reduced anticoagulant effect and difficulty in control of prothrombin time. A list of drugs which will induce metabolising enzymes in the liver is given under Other Factors Affecting Drug Metabolism in the entry on Metabolism of Drugs.

Enzyme inhibition. See also other factors affecting drug metabolism in the entry on Metabolism of Drugs.

Some drugs, such as sulthiame, may inhibit hepatic drug metabolising enzymes and so prolong the plasma half-lives of some other drugs. Treatment with monoamine-oxidase inhibitors leads to accumulation of monoamines such as adrenaline, noradrenaline, dopamine, and 5-hydroxytryptamine within the central and autonomic nervous systems, but also prevents the metabolism of other exogenous monoamines such as tyramine. This is the basis of the important interactions between monoamine-oxidase inhibitors and certain drugs and foodstuffs.

Enzyme inhibition is also the basis of action of many chemotherapeutic agents used in treatment of infection and neoplastic conditions.

Synergism between drugs may occur if they act on different enzyme systems within the cells of an infecting organism or in a neoplastic cell. For example, in the combination product co-trimoxazole, sulphamethoxazole inhibits the conversion of 4-aminobenzoic acid to folic acid and trimethoprim inhibits the conversion of folic acid to folinic acid, sequential steps in the same metabolic pathway. Sulphamethoxazole and trimethoprim are bacteriostatic when used alone but in combination are bactericidal.

Excretion. For principal routes of drug excretion see under Excretion in the entry on Metabolism of Drugs. Also see Assessment of Bioavailability under Bioavailability.

Many drugs are actively excreted by the renal tubules. The excretion of weakly acidic substances such as penicillin can be inhibited by probenecid.

Changes in urinary pH induced by drugs such as ammonium chloride, sodium bicarbonate, or acetazolamide can markedly influence the rate of excretion of weakly basic and acidic drugs. Normally, the urine is slightly acid and favours the excretion of weakly basic drugs such as amphetamine and pethidine. Further acidification of the urine by administration of ammonium chloride demonstrably shortens their action while urinary alkalisation with sodium bicarbonate prolongs their effects. The reverse applies for weakly acidic drugs such as aspirin. These interactions are used in the treatment of poisoning by certain weakly basic or acidic drugs.

Electrolyte changes. Drug-induced changes in electrolyte concentrations may influence the action of some other drugs. The best known example of such an interaction is the enhancement of action of digitalis glycosides by diuretic-induced hypokalaemia which may lead to digitalis intoxication.

Blockade of neuronal uptake. An important mechanism in the termination of action of noradrenaline is its active reuptake into noradrenergic neurones. Blockade of the reuptake process increases the pressor action of noradrenaline and adrenaline and of other substances that also depend on the same uptake process, such as phenylephrine. Among the groups of drugs which may block neuronal uptake are the tricyclic antidepressants such as imipramine and some adrenergic neurone blocking drugs such as guanethidine and bethanidine.

Some indirectly acting sympathomimetic amines such as tyramine and some adrenergic neurone blocking drugs such as guanethidine and bethanidine which are used in the treatment of hypertension depend for their pharmacological effects on being taken up into the neurone through the same uptake process as noradrenaline. Their action may, therefore, be prevented or reversed by treatment with tricyclic antidepressant drugs, with loss of blood pressure control.

Transmitter depletion. The effects of drugs which depend for their action on release of neurotransmitter substances may be reduced by the administration of other drugs which cause neurotransmitter depletion. For example, pressor responses to indirectly acting sympathomimetics such as tyramine are reduced in reserpinised subjects.

Receptor blockade. The development of drugs that block selectively receptors, particularly those of the autonomic nervous system and its effector organs, has led to several important clinical interactions. For example, α-adrenergic-receptor blockade with phenoxybenzamine prevents the pressor effects of sympathomimetic amines such as noradrenaline. β-Receptor blockade with, for example, propranolol reduces or abolishes the cardiac-stimulating activity of sympathomimetic amines such as adrenaline and isoprenaline.

Similarly the anticholinergic action of several different classes of drugs (for example, tricyclic antidepressants and antihistamines) reduces the effects of cholinomimetic agents.

Functional summation of effects. Drugs which produce a pharmacological effect by different biochemical mechanisms may have a synergistic interaction, for example, the mutual enhancement in the central nervous system depressant activity of anaesthetics, hypnotics, sedatives, tranquillisers, and narcotic analgesics.

Other examples include the potentiation of the action of oral anticoagulant drugs by broad spectrum antibiotics which reduce vitamin-K absorption and by aspirin which inhibits prothrombin synthesis as well as competing for plasma-protein binding sites.

Intramammary Injections

Sterile aqueous or oily solutions or suspensions of medicaments intended for injection into the mammary glands of cows through the teat canal.

There are two types of preparation. For administration to lactating animals they are formulated so that the vehicle and the medicament disperse rapidly in the mammary tissue and are rapidly excreted in the milk; the medicament should not be detectable in the milk after the withholding period stated on the label. For administration to animals that are not lactating they are formulated to release the active ingredients over a longer period.

Preparation of intramammary injections. They are usually prepared, by means of an aseptic technique, by dissolving or suspending the sterile medicaments in the sterilised basis. The injections are transferred to clean sterilised final containers (see the entry on Sterilisation).

Containers. Intramammary injections should be dispensed in sterile containers of metal or other suitable material which do not react with the ingredients of the preparation and which are closed to exclude micro-organisms. The containers are fitted with a smooth tapered nozzle to facilitate insertion into the teat canal. Intramammary injections should preferably be dispensed in single-dose containers to minimise the risk of cross-infection.

Labelling. The label on the container should state:
(1) the names of the active ingredients and the total weight or total number of units of activity of the active ingredients in the container; and
(2) for intramammary injections (slow release), that the preparation is not intended for use in lactating animals. The label on the container or the label on the package should state:
(1) for preparations to be used in lactating animals, the minimum period between cessation of treatment and the resumption of the supply of milk for human consumption from treated animals;
(2) for intramammary injections (slow release), the minimum period between cessation of treatment and the expected date of parturition, and the period after parturition, during which the milk must be withheld from human consumption should birth occur earlier than expected;
(3) the conditions under which the preparation should be stored; and
(4) the date after which the preparation is not intended to be used.

Intravenous Additives

Medicinal substances intended for administration by the intravenous route are sometimes added to an intravenous infusion fluid or injected into the giving set or cannula which is being used to administer an intravenous infusion. The advantages and limitations of these methods of administration should be recognised and the appropriate procedure chosen in each case.

Addition of Drugs to Intravenous Infusion Fluids

In some instances it is essential to administer a drug substance in one of these ways but in other cases it has been used simply as a matter of convenience and without regard to the limitations and possible hazards.

Hazards arise because of changes in stability and solubility resulting from interaction between the drug and the infusion fluid or between two or more added drugs. In addition, strict asepsis cannot be observed when drugs are added to infusion fluids in hospital wards and infection may result in bacterial growth in the solutions during administration.

In view of the hazards, additions should be made to intravenous infusion containers only when necessary, as in the following circumstances: (1) when direct intravenous injection is dangerous because the concentrated solution is corrosive or has some other deleterious effect on the blood vessels; (2) when a drug is toxic unless administered in dilute solution at a controlled rate, as for example with potassium chloride; and (3) when it is desirable to maintain a constant blood concentration, as in electrolyte replacement therapy, resuscitation, maintenance of blood pressure, etc.

FURTHER INFORMATION. *Addition of Drugs to Intravenous Infusion Fluids*, Health Circular HC(76)9, Department of Health and Social Security, 1976; J. M. Neil, *The Prescribing and Administration of IV Additives to Infusion Fluids*, Thetford, Travenol Laboratories Ltd., 1976.

TABLE 1. Compatible Intravenous Infusion Solutions

Substance	*Usual Vial Size*	*Compatible Intravenous Solutions*
Amphotericin (for intravenous use)	50 mg	Dextrose injection (5%) of pH above 4.2 (the solid should be dissolved in water for injections before adding to the dextrose injection)
Co-trimoxazole (for infusion)	trimethoprim 80 mg and sulphamethoxazole 400 mg	Dextrose injection (5 or 10%) Sodium chloride injection Sodium chloride and dextrose injection Dextran 40 injection Dextran 70 injection Laevulose injection (5%) Ringer's solution for injection
Frusemide (injection)	250 mg in 25 ml	Sodium chloride injection Ringer's solution for injection
Isoprenaline hydrochloride (injection)	2 mg in 2 ml	Dextrose injection (5%)
Lignocaine hydrochloride (injection)	5 ml (20%)	*Dextrose injection (5%)
Lincomycin hydrochloride (injection)	600 mg in 2 ml	Dextrose injection (5%) Sodium chloride injection
Methyldopate hydro-chloride (injection)	250 mg in 5 ml	Dextrose injection (5%)
Oxytetracycline (injection)	250 and 500 mg	Dextrose injection (5%) Sodium chloride injection (the solid should be dissolved in water for injections before adding to the infusion solution)
Oxytocin (injection)	2 units in 2 ml, 5 units in 1 ml, 10 units in 1 ml, and 50 units in 5 ml	Dextrose injection (5%)
Phenoxybenzamine hydrochloride (injection)	100 mg in 2 ml	Sodium chloride injection
Potassium chloride (injection)	1.5 g (20 mmol) in 10 ml	*Dextrose injection (5%) *Sodium chloride injection
Sodium fusidate (as diethanolamine fusidate for intravenous infusion)	500 mg	Sodium chloride injection (the solid should be dissolved in the buffer provided by the manufacturer before adding to the infusion solution)
Streptokinase	100000, 250000, 600000, and 750000 units	Dextrose injection (5%) Sodium chloride injection (the solid should be dissolved in water for injections before adding to the infusion solution)
Tetracycline hydrochloride (for intravenous use)	250 and 500 mg	Dextrose injection (5%) Sodium chloride injection Sodium chloride and dextrose injection Sodium lactate compound injection

* These solutions are sufficiently stable to be prepared and stored as sterile solutions ready for use.

PRECAUTIONS. Certain precautions should be taken when making additions to intravenous fluids. The procedure should be performed under the control of a pharmacist who should have ascertained that the components are compatible and stable and that continuous infusion is the most appropriate method of administration. The addition should be made by an aseptic technique in an appropriately controlled environment, the components should be mixed thoroughly, and the final container should be labelled with the names and quantities of drugs added, the time of addition, and the time after which the container should not be used.

Drugs should not normally be added to blood, plasma, lipid emulsions, saturated solutions of mannitol or sodium bicarbonate, or solutions of amino acids or dextrans, as these infusion liquids are particularly likely to be degraded by additives.

Preferably, not more than one drug should be added to an infusion solution because multiple additions greatly increase the chances of interaction and degradation.

Compatible intravenous infusion solutions. When the substances in the accompanying TABLE 1 are to be given intravenously they must be diluted in large volume by addition to the container of an intravenous solution, mixed thoroughly, and administered at the prescribed rate.

Intravenous Administration by Giving Set or Cannula

Substances may be administered intravenously by introducing an injection solution into an infusion apparatus by (1) puncturing the injection site of the infusion set, (2) using a set incorporating a burette, (3) injecting into a fixed needle or cannula, (4) injecting via a diaphragm in the side arm of a three-way tap, or (5) using a second infusion container and set, linked to the main infusion line by a Y-piece.

These methods of administration are suitable for many substances. For many antibiotics and similar drugs they have the advantage that higher blood concentrations are attained than by addition to the infusion fluid. The dose may usually be administered over a period of 3 to 5 minutes. The safest method is to give about one-tenth of the dose and then wait 1 or 2 minutes; if there is no adverse reaction the remainder of the dose should be administered over the recommended period.

Method of preparation. The accompanying TABLE 2 describes the method of preparation of some drugs that may be administered via a giving set or cannula.

Inulin

Consists of polysaccharide granules obtained from the tubers of *Dahlia variabilis* Desf., *Helianthus tuberosus* L., and other genera of the family Compositae.

A standard is given in the British Pharmacopoeia 1973

Description. It is a white, amorphous, granular, hygroscopic, odourless powder.

Microscopical characters: small particles, mostly spherules about 2 to 6 μm in diameter, many of them clumped into irregularly shaped granular flakes or masses about 30 to 160 μm in size; when viewed between crossed polars, it shines brightly and the rarely found larger spherules, about 20 μm in diameter, exhibit a black cross.

Solubility. Very slightly soluble in water; more soluble in hot water; very slightly soluble in organic solvents.

Specific rotation. $-36.5°$ to $-40.5°$, determined on a 2% solution, prepared with the aid of heat.

Moisture content. Not more than 5%, determined by drying at 105°.

Sterilisation. Solutions for injection are sterilised by filtration.

Storage. It should be stored in airtight containers.

Identification. TESTS. 1. Dissolve 10 mg in 2 ml of hot water, add 3 ml of a 0.15% solution of resorcinol in alcohol (95%) followed by 3 ml of hydrochloric acid, mix, and heat; a red colour is produced.
2. Boil 5 ml of a 10% solution for 2 minutes with 0.5 ml of hydrochloric acid, cool, neutralise to litmus paper with *sodium hydroxide solution*, add 0.5 ml of *potassium cupritartrate solution*, and heat; a red precipitate is produced.

Actions and uses. Inulin is a saccharide polymer which is not degraded by any mammalian enzyme. It has a half-life in the body of about 1 hour and is excreted almost entirely in the urine and neither secreted nor resorbed by the nephron. The only pharmacological effect of inulin is an osmotic diuresis when it is given in large amounts. Inulin is used to measure the glomerular filtration rate. A primary dose of 30 millilitres of warm inulin injection is injected into a forearm vein and a mixture of 70 millilitres of inulin injection and 500 millilitres of sodium chloride injection is given by intravenous drip into the other forearm, the infusion being made at a steady rate so that the plasma concentration is kept as nearly constant as possible. A depot injection may be made into the subcutaneous tissue for the same purpose but is much less satisfactory than the intravenous infusion method. The inulin content of the plasma and urine is determined after the removal of glucose and proteins. The test measures the clearance of inulin from the plasma and allows the other inferences to be made. For example, substances with a clearance greater than inulin are secreted and those with a smaller clearance resorbed by the nephron.

Preparation

INULIN INJECTION:

Inulin	10.0 g
Sodium chloride	0.8 g
Water for injections	to 100 ml

Dissolve the inulin and the sodium chloride in the water with the aid of heat. Sterilise the solution by filtration; distribute, by means of an aseptic technique, into sterile ampoules, and seal.

A standard for this injection is given in the British Pharmacopoeia 1973

Containers: see the entry on Injections for general information on containers.

Labelling: see the entry on Injections for general information on labelling. In addition, the label on the container should state the amount of the medicament as the percentage w/v of inulin.

Storage: it deposits on storage. Before use solid matter should be completely redissolved by heating for not more than 15 minutes; the solution should be cooled to a suitable temperature before administration and should not be reheated.

TABLE 2. Methods of Preparation for Intravenous Administration by Giving Set or Cannula

Substance	Usual Vial Size	Method of Preparation
Ampicillin sodium	100, 250, and 500 mg ampicillin	dissolve in 10 ml of water for injections
Ampicillin-cloxacillin	250 mg ampicillin with 250 mg cloxacillin	dissolve in 10 ml of water for injections
Azathioprine sodium	50 mg azathioprine	dissolve in not less than 5 ml of water for injections[1]
Benzylpenicillin (without buffer)	500000 units	dissolve in not less than 5 ml of dextrose injection (5%), sodium chloride injection, or water for injections[2]
	1 mega unit	dissolve in 10 to 20 ml of dextrose injection (5%), sodium chloride injection, or water for injections[2]
Carbenicillin sodium	1 g carbenicillin	dissolve in 5 ml of water for injections and then dilute to 10 ml
	5 g	dissolve in at least 20 ml of water for injections
Cephaloridine	250 mg, 500 mg, and 1 g	dissolve in 10 to 20 ml of dextrose injection (5%) or sodium chloride injection
Cephalothin sodium	1 g cephalothin	dissolve in 5 ml of water for injections
Cephradine	250 and 500 mg	dissolve in 5 ml of water for injections
	1 g	dissolve in 10 ml of water for injections
Cloxacillin sodium	250 and 500 mg	dissolve in 10 ml of water for injections
Dexamethasone sodium phosphate (injection)	5 mg dexamethasone sodium phosphate in 1 ml	use undiluted
	8 mg dexamethasone in 2 ml	use undiluted
	8 mg dexamethasone phosphate in 2ml	use undiluted
	100 mg dexamethasone in in 5 ml	use undiluted
Dextrose injection (50%)	50 ml	use undiluted at a rate not exceeding 50 ml in 6 minutes
Flucloxacillin sodium	250 and 500 mg	dissolve in 10 ml of water for injections
Frusemide (injection)[3]	20 mg in 2 ml	use undiluted
	50 mg in 5 ml	use undiluted
Gentamicin sulphate	20 mg gentamicin in 2 ml	use undiluted
	80 mg gentamicin in 2 ml	use undiluted
Heparin sodium	1000 and 5000 units in 1 ml	use undiluted
Hydrocortisone sodium succinate	100 mg hydrocortisone	dissolve in 2 ml of water for injections
Prednisolone sodium phosphate	32 mg prednisolone in 2 ml	use undiluted and administer over a period of at least 5 minutes
Strong vitamins B and C injection for intravenous use	pair of ampoules	mix the two solutions in the syringe before injection

1. The solution is alkaline and very irritant and must therefore be given slowly, preferably by injecting it into the tubing of an intravenous drip of sodium chloride injection or sodium chloride and dextrose injection while the fluid is being infused. It is essential that the infusion solution is injected correctly into the vein.

2. The rate of infusion should not exceed 500000 units per minute.
3. Frusemide injection 250 mg in 25 ml is not suitable for administration by this method; it should be administered by addition to an intravenous infusion.

Invert Syrup

Invert syrup contains a mixture of glucose and fructose. It may be prepared by hydrolysing sucrose with a mineral acid, such as hydrochloric acid, and neutralising the solution with, for example, calcium carbonate or sodium carbonate.

A standard is given in the British Pharmaceutical Codex 1973

The standard refers to a syrup corresponding to at least 95% inversion of a 66.7% w/w solution of sucrose. Syrups are available commercially at strengths corresponding to up to 84% w/w of sugars and to various degrees of inversion.

Description. A clear, colourless to pale straw-coloured, odourless, syrupy liquid with a sweet taste.

Solubility. Miscible with water, forming a clear solution; partly soluble in alcohol.

Weight per ml. At 20°, 1.338 to 1.344 g.

Acidity. pH 5 to 6.

Refractive index. 1.4608 to 1.4630.

Storage. It should be stored at a temperature between 35° and 45°.

Uses. Invert syrup, when mixed in suitable proportions with syrup, prevents the deposition of crystals of sucrose under most conditions of storage. It is an ingredient of ephedrine elixir, paediatric tolu linctus, and paediatric paracetamol elixir.

Iodinated (^{125}I) Human Albumin Injection

A sterile solution in a saline solution isotonic with blood and containing a suitable bactericide, such as benzyl alcohol in a concentration of 0.9% v/v, of human albumin which has been iodinated with iodine-125 and subsequently freed from ^{125}I iodide.

OTHER NAME: IHA (^{125}I) Inj.

A standard is given in the British Pharmacopoeia 1973

CAUTION. *This material is radioactive and any regulations in force must be complied with.*

Iodine-125 is a radioactive isotope of iodine which decays by electron capture with emission of photons mainly of energy 0.028 MeV (X-radiation). It has a half-life of 60 days. It may be prepared by neutron irradiation of xenon-124.

Description. A clear colourless or faintly yellow solution.

Acidity or alkalinity. pH 6.5 to 8.5.

Sterilisation. It is sterilised by filtration.

Storage. It should be stored in an area assigned for the purpose at a temperature between 2° and 10°. The storage conditions should be such that the maximum radiation-dose-rate to which persons may be exposed is reduced to an acceptable level.

Labelling. The label on the container should state (1) the content of iodine-125 expressed in microcuries or millicuries at a given date, (2) the weight of human albumin in the container, (3) that the injection is radioactive, and (4) the date after which the injection should not be used. The label on the package should state (1) the total volume in the container, (2) the nature and proportion of salts and bactericide present, (3) that the injection is not necessarily suitable for metabolic studies, and (4) that it should be stored at a temperature between 2° and 10°.

Actions and uses. Iodinated (^{125}I) human albumin injection has actions and uses similar to those described under Iodinated (^{131}I) Human Albumin Injection.

As the radiation from iodine-125 is less penetrating than that from iodine-131 its use reduces the risk to workers carrying out diagnostic procedures and, in the estimation of blood and plasma volumes, it reduces the radiation dose to the patient, but it is of little value for techniques which depend on radiation measurements at the body surface.

The usual dose for the determination of blood and plasma volumes is 5 microcuries. In other investigations up to 100 microcuries may be required.

Precautions and contra-indications. As for Iodinated (^{131}I) Human Albumin Injection.

Iodinated (^{131}I) Human Albumin Injection

A sterile solution in a saline solution isotonic with blood and containing a suitable bactericide, such as benzyl alcohol in a concentration of 0.9% v/v, of human albumin which has been iodinated with iodine-131 and subsequently freed from ^{131}I iodide.

OTHER NAME: IHA (^{131}I) Inj.

A standard is given in the British Pharmacopoeia 1973

CAUTION. *This material is radioactive and any regulations in force must be complied with.*

Iodine-131 is a radioactive isotope of iodine which decays by emission of β^--radiation mainly having a maximum energy of 0.606 MeV with emission of γ-radiation mainly of energy 0.364 MeV. It has a half-life of 8.06 days. It may be prepared by neutron irradiation of tellurium-130.

Description. A clear colourless or faintly yellow solution.

Acidity or alkalinity. pH 6.5 to 8.5.

Sterilisation. It is sterilised by filtration.

Storage. It should be stored in an area assigned for the purpose at a temperature betwen 2° and 10°. The storage conditions should be such that the maximum radiation-dose-rate to which persons may be exposed is reduced to an acceptable level.

Labelling. The label on the container should state (1) the content of iodine-131 expressed in microcuries or millicuries at a given date and hour, (2) the weight of human albumin in the container, (3) that the injection is radioactive, and (4) the date after which the injection should not be used.
The label on the package should state (1) the total volume in the container, (2) the nature and proportion of salts and bactericide present, (3) that the injection is not necessarily suitable for metabolic studies, and (4) that it should be stored at a temperature between 2° and 10°.

Actions and uses. ^{131}I-labelled human albumin is used to estimate the blood volume and plasma volume by measuring the dilution of an injected sample, and in many respects this procedure is simpler than dye-dilution methods. A dose of 5 microcuries may be used for this purpose. The volume of fluid accumulations, such as ascites or gastric residues, can also be measured.

Circulation times, which provide an approximate measure of the velocity of blood flow between various parts of the body, have also been estimated using injected ^{131}I-labelled human albumin in doses up to 50 microcuries and a suitable detection and recording device at a distal site. Elaboration of such techniques with recording of dilution curves of radioactivity provides one method of estimating cardiac output when the other data provided by cardiac catheterisation are not required.

[131]I-labelled human albumin has also been used in isotope ventriculography, cisternography, and myeloscintigraphy, and for the investigation of hydrocephalus and other disorders. It may be injected intrathecally or directly into the brain cavities for this purpose. The β-energy of iodine-131 and the protein content of the injection make it less than ideal for this purpose and an injection of indium-111 diethylenetriaminepenta-acetic acid is preferable for these investigations of the cerebrospinal system.

Iodine

A solid non-metallic element, the chief source of which is the Chilean nitrate ore, caliche, which contains from 0.15% in the form of iodates. It is also obtained from inorganic iodides present in some natural brine wells and in the ashes of seaweed (kelp). It is purified by sublimation.

I = 126.9

OTHER NAMES: *Iodex* ®; Iodum

A standard is given in the European Pharmacopoeia Vol. I

Description. Greyish-violet brittle plates or small crystals with a metallic sheen and an irritant odour. It is slowly volatile at room temperature and when heated is completely volatilised, giving off violet-coloured vapours which may be condensed as a bluish-black crystalline sublimate.

Solubility. Soluble in alcohol, in ether, and in aqueous solutions of iodides, producing a reddish-brown solution; soluble in chloroform and in carbon disulphide producing a violet-coloured solution.

Incompatibility. It is incompatible with alkalis and alkali carbonates.

Storage. It should be stored in glass stoppered bottles, or in glass or earthenware containers with well waxed bungs.

Metabolism. ABSORPTION. Iodine is slightly absorbed when applied topically to the skin; iodide is readily absorbed after oral administration.

DISTRIBUTION. Iodide is taken up by the thyroid gland and appears in saliva, sweat, and milk; iodide crosses the placenta.

EXCRETION. Excreted mainly in the urine.

Actions and uses. When taken by mouth, iodine is absorbed as iodide and is stored in the thyroid gland as thyroglobulin.

In the treatment of thyrotoxicosis, iodine is given as aqueous iodine solution for 10 to 14 days prior to thyroidectomy in order to produce a firm texture suitable for operation and its administration is continued post-operatively for a few days to avert thyrotoxic crises. For these purposes, 0.1 to 0.3 millilitre of the aqueous solution is administered by mouth 3 times a day in milk or water; larger dosages, such as 2 to 3 millilitres daily,

are given in thyrotoxic crises. The use of iodine in this way has no advantage over the use of iodides.

Iodine is an effective bactericide and is used in solution as a sterilising agent for unbroken skin.

For the pre-operative sterilisation of skin, weak iodine solution or a 2% solution of iodine in isopropyl alcohol or 75% industrial methylated spirit is suitable. When industrial methylated spirit is used as the solvent it should be free from acetone, with which iodine forms an irritant and lachrymatory compound which inconveniences the surgeon.

Weak iodine solution has been used as an antiseptic application to small wounds, but it is rapidly inactivated by combining with tissue substances and it delays healing.

Iodine ointments have been applied as counter-irritants and a compound paint (Mandl's paint) has been used as a throat paint in the treatment of pharyngitis and follicular tonsillitis.

Precautions. Iodine and iodides should not be administered during pregnancy and lactation. They interfere with tests for thyroid function. Some patients show skin sensitivity to iodine.

Poisoning. Large draughts of milk and starch mucilage are given to stop absorption after emptying the stomach by gastric lavage with starch mucilage and 1% sodium thiosulphate. Intravenous solutions of sodium chloride and dextrose should be given to replenish fluids and electrolyte lost.

Veterinary uses. Iodine is used as an antiseptic. A weak aqueous solution of iodine (0.1%) is used in cattle for uterine irrigation.

Preparations

AQUEOUS IODINE SOLUTION (*syn.* Liq. Iod. Aquos.; Lugol's Solution):

Iodine	50 g
Potassium iodide	100 g
Purified water, freshly boiled and cooled	to 1000 ml

Dissolve the potassium iodide and the iodine in 100 ml of the water and add sufficient of the water to produce the required volume. It contains, in 1 ml, 50 mg of iodine and about 130 mg of total iodine, free and combined.

A standard for this solution is given in the British Pharmacopoeia 1973

Storage: it should be stored in airtight containers the materials of which are resistant to iodine.

Advice for patients: the solution should be taken mixed with water or milk. When used prior to thyroidectomy, the prescribed course should be completed.

WEAK IODINE SOLUTION (*Syn.* Iodine Tincture; Liq. Iod. Mit.):

Iodine	25 g
Potassium iodide	25 g
Purified water, freshly boiled and cooled	25 ml
Alcohol (90%)	to 1000 ml

Dissolve the potassium iodide and the iodine in the water and add sufficient of the alcohol to produce the required volume.

A standard for this solution is given in the British Pharmacopoeia 1973

Storage: it should be stored in airtight containers, the materials of which are resistant to iodine.

Advice for patients: when used in the treatment of cuts and grazes it should be applied to the skin undiluted.

A dressing should not be applied. The solution stains the skin, hair, and fabric. Stains may be removed with dilute alkali or sodium thiosulphate solution.

OTHER PREPARATIONS available include an OINTMENT containing iodine 4% and an ointment containing iodine 4% with methyl salicylate 5%.

Iodipamide Meglumine Injection

A sterile solution of the bis(1-methylamino-1-deoxy-D-glucitol) salt of 3,3'-adipoyldiaminobis(2,4,6-tri-iodobenzoic acid).

$C_{34}H_{48}I_6N_4O_{16} = 1530.2$.

OTHER NAME: Iodipamide Methylglucamine Injection

A standard is given in the British Pharmacopoeia 1973

Description. A clear colourless to pale yellow solution.

Sterilisation. It is sterilised by heating in an autoclave.

Actions and uses. Iodipamide meglumine injection is a radio-opaque contrast medium which is used in solutions containing 30, 50, and 70% w/v. The 70% solution has been used for hysterosalpingography and sinography. The 30 and 50% solutions have been used by intravenous injection for radiography of the biliary tract, a suitable dose being 20 millilitres.

The injection should be given slowly over a period of 10 minutes to minimise undesirable effects. After injection, the compound is rapidly excreted in the bile and the hepatic and common bile ducts may frequently be visualised within 20 minutes. With normal liver function, about 90% of the dose is excreted in the bile and the remainder in the urine.

For infusion cholangiography, the contrast medium is diluted and administered as a slow intravenous drip over a period of 30 minutes. This results in improved visualisation of the duct system and a decreased incidence of side-effects. A dose of 20 to 40 millilitres of the 50 per cent solution is commonly used in the infusion techniques; larger doses have been advocated but they are probably undesirable except in special circumstances. With the infusion technique, the common bile duct may often be satisfactorily visualised with only 10 millilitres of the 50% solution.

Intravenous cholangiography is sometimes performed immediately after an oral cholangiogram. However, hepatic excretion appears to be less efficient under these circumstances and the incidence of side-effects is probably increased.

In the presence of jaundice, intravenous cholangiography is frequently disappointing, particularly if the serum bilirubin is above 3 mg per 100 ml, and the risk of the examination is also likely to be increased.

Undesirable effects. Transient restlessness, sensations of warmth, abdominal pain, nausea, and vomiting may occur, particularly if the injection has been given too rapidly. Major side-effects are as described under Sodium Diatrizoate but the toxicity of iodipamide is approximately 6 times that of sodium diatrizoate. Iodipamide has a uricosuric action similar to that of probenecid and adequate hydration is therefore advisable. Rare cases of renal failure have been reported. Predisposing factors have been liver damage, hypotensive collapse, excessive dosage, and previous oral cholangiography.

Precautions. Caution is required in debilitated patients and in the presence of coronary artery disease. Iodipamide should not be mixed in the same syringe with antihistamines since precipitation may occur.

Iodised Oil Fluid Injection

A sterile iodine-addition product of the ethyl esters of the fatty acids obtained from poppy-seed oil, the oil expressed from the ripe seeds of *Papaver somniferum* L. (Fam. Papaveraceae). It is distributed into sterile single-dose containers which are then hermetically sealed.

OTHER NAME: *Lipiodol Ultra-Fluid*®

When Iodised Oil Injection or Iodised Oil is prescribed or demanded, Iodised Oil Fluid Injection is dispensed or supplied.

A standard is given in the British Pharmacopoeia 1973

Description. A straw-coloured or yellow, clear, oily liquid which is odourless or has a slightly alliaceous odour.

Solubility. Immiscible with water; miscible with ether, with chloroform, and with light petroleum.

Weight per ml. At 20°, 1.28 to 1.30 g.

Stability. It decomposes on exposure to air and sunlight, becoming dark brown in colour.

Storage. It should be stored, protected from light, in an atmosphere of carbon dioxide or nitrogen.

Actions and uses. Iodised oil fluid injection is a contrast medium which is now used almost solely for lymphography and sialography.

Iopanoic Acid

2-(3-Amino-2,4,6-tri-iodobenzyl)butyric acid

$C_{11}H_{12}I_3NO_2 = 570.9$

OTHER NAME: *Telepaque*®

A standard is given in the British Pharmacopoeia 1973

Description. A white to cream-coloured, odourless, almost tasteless powder.

Solubility. Practically insoluble in water; soluble, at 20°, in 25 parts of alcohol; soluble in acetone and in solutions of alkali hydroxides.

Storage. It should be protected from light.

Identification. TESTS. 1. Heat strongly; violet vapours of iodine are produced.
2. Carry out Test 2 described under Butyl Aminobenzoate for primary aromatic amines; a deep orange-red precipitate is produced.

MELTING-POINT. About 155°.

ULTRAVIOLET ABSORPTION. In 0.01N sodium hydroxide, maximum at 230 nm (E1%, 1cm = 680).

Metabolism. ABSORPTION. Well absorbed after oral administration.

DISTRIBUTION. Taken up by the liver and peak concentrations in the gall bladder appear 14 to 19 hours after ingestion; *protein binding*, about 97% bound to plasma proteins.

METABOLIC REACTIONS. Conjugation with glucuronic acid.

EXCRETION. 35% of a dose is excreted in the urine mostly in conjugated form, and about 65% is excreted in the faeces via the bile.

FURTHER INFORMATION. Absorption, transport, distribution, and excretion—R. N. Berk et al., New Engl. J. Med., 1974, 290, 204.

Actions and uses. Iopanoic acid is a radio-opaque substance which is absorbed from the gastro-intestinal tract and excreted in the bile, being eliminated in the faeces and, to some extent, in the urine. It is used as a contrast medium in radiography of the gall bladder. Iopanoic acid is given by mouth with a light fat-free meal about 10 to 15 hours before X-ray examination, the usual dose being 3 grams. After two or three exposures have been made, an emulsion or a meal rich in fat is given to test gallbladder reflex contraction and further exposures are made after 10 minutes and, if necessary, after 30 minutes or 1 hour.

Undesirable effects. Diarrhoea is not uncommon and occasionally this may be severe enough to cause collapse. Other side-effects include nausea, vomiting, headache, dysuria, and skin rashes.

Iopanoic acid and other cholecystographic media have a uricosuric action similar to that of probenecid and adequate hydration is therefore advisable.

Rare cases of renal failure have been reported, usually associated with excess dosage in patients suffering from jaundice or liver damage.

Precautions and contra-indications. Pre-existing renal disease may be a contra-indication to cholecystography, particularly if liver damage is suspected. It should not be administered to patients who are hypersensitive to iodine-containing contrast media. In acute gastro-intestinal disorders, the substance may not be absorbed.

Caution should be exercised in patients with severe coronary artery disease or thyrotoxicosis and in pregnancy.

Preparation

IOPANOIC ACID TABLETS: available as tablets containing 500 mg of iopanoic acid.

A standard for these tablets is given in the British Pharmacopoeia 1973

Containers and Storage: see the entry on Tablets for general information on containers and storage. Containers should be airtight and light resistant.

Iophendylate Injection

A sterile mixture of isomers of ethyl 10-(4-iodophenyl)-undecanoate, 4-I.C₆H₄.CH(CH₃).[CH₂]₈.CO.O.C₂H₅ ($C_{19}H_{29}IO_2 = 416.3$). It is distributed in sterile single-dose containers which are then hermetically sealed.

OTHER NAMES: Ethyl Iodophenylundecanoate Injection; Myodil®

A standard is given in the British Pharmacopoeia 1973

Description. A clear, almost colourless to pale yellow, viscous liquid.

Solubility. Very slightly soluble in water; soluble in 2 parts of alcohol; miscible with ether and with chloroform.

Weight per ml. At 20°, 1.245 to 1.260 g.

Refractive index. 1.525 to 1.527.

Storage. It should be protected from light.

Actions and uses. Iophendylate injection is used as a contrast medium for myelography. It is almost completely resorbed from the spinal canal, its rate of disappearance being about 1 millilitre a year.

Iophendylate is used in the radiological diagnosis and localisation of tumours of the spinal cord, displaced intervertebral disks, and any condition in which obstructions in the cerebrospinal canal or compression of the cord are suspected.

The dose depends upon the diagnostic procedure and up to 9 millilitres may be required. The injection is usually made in the mid-lumbar region; to determine the upper level of the lesion an intracisternal injection may be necessary. Plastic syringes should not be used.

Undesirable effects. Although its toxicity is low, cases of allergic reaction and arachnoiditis have occasionally been reported.

Iothalamic Acid

5-Acetamido-2,4,6-tri-iodo-N-methylisophthalamic acid

$C_{11}H_9I_3N_2O_4 = 613.9$

OTHER NAME: Conray®

A standard is given in the British Pharmacopoeia 1973

Description. A white odourless powder.

Solubility. Soluble, at 20°, in 400 parts of water and in 330 parts of alcohol; very slightly soluble in chloroform; very soluble in solutions of sodium hydroxide.

Sterilisation. Solutions for injection are sterilised by heating in an autoclave.

Storage. It should be protected from light.

Identification. TESTS. 1. Heat a small quantity; violet vapours of iodine are evolved.

2. Mix 500 mg with 2 ml of alcohol (95%) and 1 ml of sulphuric acid; the odour of ethyl acetate is produced.

ULTRAVIOLET ABSORPTION. In methyl alcohol, maximum at 243 nm (E1%, 1cm = 530).

Actions and uses. Iothalamic acid is a contrast medium for diagnostic radiology. It is used in the form of its meglumine and its sodium salts. Sodium iothalamate has properties similar to those of Sodium Diatrizoate and is used in similar dosage.

Sodium iothalamate is more soluble in water than sodium diatrizoate and very concentrated solutions may be prepared without the inclusion of organic bases, thus enabling solutions of high iodine content and low viscosity to be obtained.

A 70% solution is used for abdominal and intravenous aortography and an 80% solution is used for angiography. When left-heart studies are carried out, a combined solution of sodium iothalamate 26% and meglumine iothalamate 52% is used.

Undesirable effects; Precautions and contra-indications. As for Sodium Diatrizoate. In addition sodium iothalamate is unsuitable for cerebral angiography.

Preparations

MEGLUMINE IOTHALAMATE INJECTION: a sterile solution of the N-methylglucamine salt of iothalamic acid, containing suitable stabilising agents. It is sterilised by heating in an autoclave.

Available in 10-ml ampoules containing 35% of meglumine iothalamate and in 20-ml ampoules and 50-ml bottles containing 60% of meglumine iothalamate.

A standard for this injection is given in the British Pharmacopoeia 1973

Containers: see the entry on Injections for general information on containers.

Labelling: see the entry on Injections for general information on labelling. In addition, the label on the container should state the amount of the medicament as the percentage w/v of meglumine iothalamate.

Storage: it should be protected from light.

SODIUM IOTHALAMATE INJECTION: a sterile solution of the sodium salt of iothalamic acid, containing suitable stabilising agents. It is sterilised by heating in an autoclave.

Available in 20-ml ampoules and 50-ml bottles containing 54 and 70% of sodium iothalamate and in 20-ml ampoules containing 80% of sodium iothalamate.

A standard for this injection is given in the British Pharmacopoeia 1973

Containers: see the entry on Injections for general information on containers.

Labelling: see the entry on Injections for general information on labelling. In addition, the label on the container should state the amount of the medicament as the percentage w/v of sodium iothalamate.

Storage: it should be protected from light.

OTHER PREPARATIONS available include an INJECTION containing meglumine iothalamate 52% with sodium iothalamate 26%; and a SOLUTION containing sodium iothalamate 60%.

Ipecacuanha

The dried root, or the rhizome and root, of *Cephaëlis ipecacuanha* (Brot.) A. Rich. (Fam. Rubiaceae), known in commerce as Matto Grosso (Rio) and Minas ipecacuanha, or of *C. acuminata* Karsten, known in commerce as Colombia, Nicaragua, or Costa Rica ipecacuanha, or of a mixture of both species. The former is indigenous to and cultivated in Brazil; the latter is imported from Colombia and Central America.

OTHER NAMES: Ipecac.; Ipecacuanha Root; Ipecacuanhae Radix

When Ipecacuanha Powder, Ipecacuanha, or Ipecacuanhae Pulvis is prescribed, Prepared Ipecacuanha is dispensed.

A standard is given in the European Pharmacopoeia Vol. I

Constituents. Ipecacuanha contains the isoquinoline alkaloids emetine and cephaëline (demethylemetine) and small proportions of psychotrine (dehydrocephaëline), methylpsychotrine, and emetamine. The root contains, in addition, ipecacuanhic acid, and the glycoside ipecacuanhin, a saponin, and about 30 to 40% of starch.

The total alkaloidal content of the root varies considerably, Matto Grosso ipecacuanha yielding from 2 to 2.4%, of which about 60 to 75% is emetine and about 26% is cephaëline, while psychotrine, methylpsychotrine, and emetamine form only about 2%. Colombia ipecacuanha contains 2.1 to 2.45% of total alkaloids, Nicaraguan 2.65 to 3.0%, and Costa Rican 2.9 to 3.5%; emetine constitutes between 30 and 50% of the total alkaloids in these three varieties.

Ipecacuanha may contain up to 1% of foreign matter, and may yield up to 6% of sulphated ash, and up to 3% of acid-insoluble ash.

Description. UNGROUND DRUG. *Macroscopical characters:* root of *C. ipecacuanha* occurring in slender somewhat tortuous pieces, rarely exceeding 150 mm in length or 6 mm in thickness and varying from dark brick-red, partly due to adhering earth, to dark brown, showing characteristic annulations resembling wedge-shaped disks, from 1 to 2 mm thick, closely applied to one another, with rounded projecting ridges; fracture short and even in the bark but splintery in the wood; smooth, transversely cut surface showing a thick starchy grey bark and a small dense radiate wood, but no pith.

Rhizome cylindrical, up to 2 mm in diameter, with fine longitudinal wrinkles; the transverse surface showing a narrow bark, a dense xylem cylinder, and a central pith about one-sixth of the diameter of the rhizome.

Root of *C. acuminata* closely resembling that of *C. ipecacuanha*, but distinguished by its larger size, up to 9 mm in thickness, by the absence of annulations and the presence of transverse ridges only partially encircling the root and by its grey or reddish-brown colour, externally. It has a faint odour and a bitter taste.

Microscopical characters: the diagnostic characters are: *C. ipecacuanha* root: cork cells narrow, elongated; *phelloderm* composed of thin-walled parenchyma mostly filled with starch granules, but including scattered cells containing bundles of acicular *crystals* of calcium oxalate, 30 to 80 μm long; *starch* granules simple or more usually compound with 2 to 5 or up to 8 components, individual granules oval, rounded or muller-shaped, rarely more than 15 μm in diameter; *xylem* with *tracheids*, narrow *vessel elements* with lateral perforations and bordered pits, and occasional *fibres; medullary rays* of the xylem with lignified parenchyma, this and many cells of xylem parenchyma containing starch granules. Rhizome: thick-walled rectangular *sclereids* in the outer part of the phloem.

C. acuminata resembles in general characters *C. ipecacuanha* but the *starch* granules are larger, measuring up to 22 μm.

POWDERED DRUG: Powdered Ipecacuanha. A light grey to yellowish-brown powder possessing the diagnostic microscopical characters, odour, and taste of the unground drug.

Adulterants and substitutes. Ipecacuanha is now rarely adulterated, but a number of different roots have been reported from time to time as adulterants; the majority of these do not contain emetine and can be distinguished from ipecacuanha by one or more of the following characters; the presence of a violet colour in the bark, the presence of large vessels in the xylem, and the absence of starch.

Storage. It should be stored in airtight containers, protected from light.

Actions and uses. The actions of ipecacuanha are those of its principal alkaloids, emetine and cephaëline. In small doses it is a reflex expectorant; its action lasts several hours. Large doses are irritant to the whole gastro-intestinal tract, and produce vomiting and diarrhoea. The powdered drug is irritating to the nasal and laryngeal mucous membrane, causing violent sneezing and coughing.

Ipecacuanha is used in small doses as an expectorant in acute and chronic bronchitis, and in cough when secretion is scanty. For an emetic action, larger doses are required.

To produce diaphoresis in the treatment of incipient colds, ipecacuanha and opium powder (consisting of prepared ipecacuanha 10% and powdered opium 10% in lactose) has been given, often in conjunction with aspirin.

Preparations

AMMONIA AND IPECACUANHA MIXTURE (*Syn*. Mistura Expectorans):

Ammonium bicarbonate	20 g
Ipecacuanha tincture	30 ml
Concentrated anise water	5 ml
Concentrated camphor water	10 ml
Liquorice liquid extract	50 ml
Chloroform water, double-strength	500 ml
Water for preparations	to 1000 ml

It should be recently prepared.
A standard for this mixture is given in the British Pharmaceutical Codex 1973
Containers and *Labelling*: see the entry on Mixtures for general information on containers and labelling.
Dose: 10 to 20 millilitres.
Advice for patients: the mixture should not be used for longer than a few days without medical advice.

IPECACUANHA AND MORPHINE MIXTURE (*Syn*. Mistura Tussi Nigra):

Ipecacuanha tincture	20 ml
Chloroform and morphine tincture	40 ml
Liquorice liquid extract	100 ml
Water for preparations	to 1000 ml

It should be recently prepared.
A standard for this mixture is given in the British Pharmaceutical Codex 1973
Containers and *Labelling*: see the entry on Mixtures for general information on containers and labelling.
Dose: 10 millilitres.
Advice for patients: the mixture should not be used for longer than a few days without medical advice.

IPECACUANHA LIQUID EXTRACT:

Small-scale preparation

Ipecacuanha, in fine powder	1000 g
Alcohol (80%)	a sufficient quantity

Exhaust the ipecacuanha by percolation with the alcohol, reserving the first 750 ml of the percolate. Remove the alcohol from the remainder of the percolate by evaporation under reduced pressure at a temperature not exceeding 60° and dissolve the residue in the reserved portion.
Determine the proportion of alkaloids in the liquid thus obtained and to the remainder of the liquid add sufficient alcohol (80%) to produce an ipecacuanha liquid extract of the required strength.
Allow to stand for not less than 24 hours, and filter.

Manufacture. Prepare the extract by the above method, appropriately scaled up, or by the alternative method described in the entry on Extracts.
It contains, in 0.1 ml, 2 mg of total alkaloids, calculated as emetine.
A standard for this extract is given in the British Pharmacopoeia 1973
Dose: as an expectorant, 0.025 to 0.1 ml.

IPECACUANHA TINCTURE:

Ipecacuanha liquid extract	100 ml
Dilute acetic acid	16.5 ml
Glycerol	200 ml
Alcohol (90%)	210 ml
Purified water	to 1000 ml

Mix the alcohol and the dilute acetic acid with the glycerol and 450 ml of the water; add the ipecacuanha liquid extract and sufficient water to produce the required volume.
Allow to stand for not less than 24 hours, and filter.
It contains, in 1 ml, 2 mg of total alkaloids, calculated as emetine.
When Ipecacuanha Wine or Vinum Ipecacuanhae is prescribed or demanded, Ipecacuanha Tincture is supplied.
A standard for this tincture is given in the British Pharmacopoeia 1973
Dose: as an expectorant, 0.25 to 1 ml.

PAEDIATRIC BELLADONNA AND IPECACUANHA MIXTURE:

Belladonna tincture	30 ml
Ipecacuanha tincture	20 ml
Sodium bicarbonate	20 g
Tolu syrup	200 ml
Chloroform water, double-strength	500 ml
Water for preparations	to 1000 ml

It must be freshly prepared.
Containers and *Labelling*: see the entry on Mixtures for general information on containers and labelling.
Dose: CHILD: Up to 1 year, 5 millilitres; 1 to 5 years, 10 millilitres.
Advice for patients: the mixture should not be used for longer than a few days without medical advice.

PAEDIATRIC IPECACUANHA AND AMMONIA MIXTURE:

Ipecacuanha tincture	20 ml
Ammonium bicarbonate	6 g
Sodium bicarbonate	20 g
Tolu syrup	100 ml
Chloroform water, double-strength	500 ml
Water for preparations	to 1000 ml

It should be recently prepared.
A standard for this mixture is given in the British Pharmaceutical Codex 1973
Containers and *Labelling*: see the entry on Mixtures for general information on containers and labelling.
Dose: CHILD: Up to 1 year, 5 millilitres; 1 to 5 years, 10 millilitres.
Advice for patients: the mixture should not be used for longer than a few days without medical advice.

PAEDIATRIC IPECACUANHA AND SQUILL LINCTUS:

Ipecacuanha tincture	20 ml
Squill tincture	30 ml
Compound orange spirit	1.5 ml
Black currant syrup	500 ml
Syrup..	to 1000 ml

When a dose less than or not a multiple of 5 ml is prescribed, the linctus may be diluted, as described in the entry on Linctuses, with syrup.
A standard for this linctus is given in the British Pharmaceutical Codex 1973
Containers: see the entry on Linctuses for general information on containers.
Storage: it should be stored in a cool place.

Dose: CHILD: 5 millilitres.
Advice for patients: the linctus should be sipped and swallowed slowly. It should not be used for longer than a few days without medical advice.

PAEDIATRIC IPECACUANHA EMETIC DRAUGHT (*Syn.* Ipecacuanha Emetic):

Ipecacuanha liquid extract	70 ml
Hydrochloric acid..	2.5 ml
Glycerol	100 ml
Syrup..	to 1000 ml

It has a weight per ml at 20° of about 1.29 g.
This preparation should only be given in the emergency treatment of poisoning under medical supervision. It should not be supplied for use in first-aid kits.
A standard for this draught is given in the British Pharmaceutical Codex 1973
Dose: CHILD: 6 months to 18 months, 10 millilitres; 18 months to 5 years, 15 millilitres.
The dose should be followed by a tumblerful of water and, if there is no response after 20 minutes, a further dose and a tumblerful of water should be given.

PREPARED IPECACUANHA (*Syn.* Ipecacuanhae Pulvis Normatus): obtained by reducing ipecacuanha to a fine powder and adjusting, if necessary, to the required alkaloidal content. When adjustment is necessary, powdered lactose or powdered ipecacuanha of lower alkaloidal content is added.
It contains, in 100 mg, 2 mg of total alkaloids, calculated as emetine.
A standard for this powder is given in the European Pharmacopoeia Vol. I
Storage: it should be stored in airtight containers, in a cool place, protected from light.
Actions and uses: prepared ipecacuanha has the actions and uses described under Ipecacuanha.
Dose: as an expectorant, 25 to 100 milligrams.

Iritis

Iritis is a condition in which the eyes are red and painful and vision is impaired. The pupil is constricted and inflammatory exudates in the eye result in photophobia and sometimes adhesions between the iris and lens. Causative organisms include staphylococci, streptococci, and rarely *Pseudomonas aeruginosa*.
The condition is treated by the local application of atropine and corticosteroids and the use of suitable antibiotics, given by injection or by mouth and also subconjunctivally.

Iron Dextran Injection

A sterile colloidal solution containing a complex of ferric hydroxide with dextrans of weight average molecular weight between 5000 and 7500. It contains approximately 5% of iron.

OTHER NAMES: *Imferon®; Ironorm®*

When Iron Dextran Injection is ordered for veterinary use Iron Dextran Injection (10 per cent) is supplied.
A standard is given in the British Pharmacopoeia 1973

Description. A dark brown solution.

Acidity. It has a pH of 5.2 to 6.5.

Sterilisation. It is sterilised by heating in an autoclave or by filtration.

Actions and uses. Iron dextran injection is used for the treatment of iron-deficiency anaemia when oral administration of iron fails to correct it, when oral medication is impracticable or undesirable, in some cases of rheumatoid arthritis, and when a rapid rise of serum-iron is essential as in emergency surgery on iron-deficient patients, when iron deficiency is diagnosed in late pregnancy, and in premature iron-deficient infants. In gastro-intestinal bleeding, oral iron therapy may mask melaena, and the administration of iron parenterally may be desirable.

Absorption from the injection site is virtually complete and maximum serum levels are reached within 24 to 48 hours of administration. The iron complex is transported from the muscle to the blood and then to the liver, where the dextran fraction is removed and metabolised or excreted. The iron is then stored in the form of ferritin and haemosiderin and metabolised as required.

The usual method of administration is by deep intramuscular injection into the ventrolateral aspect of the upper and outer quadrant of the buttock, care being taken to avoid leakage of fluid through the needle track. The initial dose is usually 1 millilitre (equivalent to 50 milligrams of iron) on the first day and then 2 millilitres is given daily or at longer intervals, according to the haemoglobin response. Up to 5 millilitres may be given as a single dose.

The total number of millilitres of iron dextran injection required may be calculated from the formula $\dfrac{0.66\,WD}{50}$ in which W is the body-weight in kilograms and D the percentage haemoglobin deficiency on the Haldane scale. This formula makes allowance for the replenishment of body iron stores. Alternatively, periodic intramuscular injections are given until the haemoglobin level has returned to normal. For an adult weighing 70 kilograms, approximately 45 milligrams of iron is needed (approximately 1 millilitre is needed for each 1% deficiency in the haemoglobin scale). The dose for a child over 10 kilograms body-weight is up to 2 millilitres, up to 1 millilitre for a child between 4 and 10 kilograms, and up to 0.5 millilitre for a child under 4 kilograms.

Iron dextran injection may also be administered as a single large dose, calculated as above, given by slow intravenous infusion over a period of 6 to 8 hours. For this treatment, it is diluted with sodium chloride injection or dextrose injection.

Undesirable effects. Iron dextran injection may cause staining of the skin by leakage through the needle track into subcutaneous fat.

Anaphylactoid reactions have occurred after the intravenous infusion of a large dose; if these occur, administration should be stopped and treatment given for shock.

Allergic reactions and transient local thrombophlebitis at the site of venepuncture, nausea, vomiting, flushing, sweating, pyrexia, leucocytosis, lymphadenopathy, dyspnoea, and circulatory collapse may occur.

In cases of severe dyspnoea with collapse, an antihistamine or 0.25 to 0.5 millilitre of adrenaline injection may be given subcutaneously.

Precautions. When iron dextran injection is administered in large doses by intravenous infusion, measures for the treatment of anaphylactoid and allergic reactions should be at hand. If it is given by slow infusion, the patient should be kept under observation while the infusion is being given and for at least an hour afterwards.

Iron dextran injection should not be given to patients with severe liver disease or acute kidney infection. Patients with a known history of allergy should be given a graded series of injections, starting with a small dose. Large single doses should not be given to patients with rheumatoid arthritis, but repeated small doses may be given.

Preparations

Available in 2-, 5-, and 20-ml ampoules and in 2- and 5-ml disposable syringes.

Iron Dextran Injection (10 per cent)

A sterile colloidal solution containing a complex of ferric hydroxide with dextrans of weight average molecular weight between 5000 and 7500. It contains approximately 10% of iron.

OTHER NAMES: *Imposil®*; *Injex®*; *Iroflex®*; *Tendex®*

When Iron Dextran Injection is ordered for veterinary use Iron Dextran Injection (10 per cent) is supplied.

A standard is given in the British Pharmacopoeia (Veterinary)

Description. A dark brown, slightly viscous solution.

Acidity. It has a pH of 5.2 to 6.5.

Sterilisation. It is sterilised by heating in an autoclave or by filtration.

Veterinary uses. Iron dextran injection (10 per cent) is used in the prophylaxis and treatment of iron-deficiency anaemia in piglets. Usually a single dose of 1 to 2 millilitres is given by intramuscular injection to piglets aged 3 to 7 days.

Preparations

Available in 20- and 100-ml vials.

Iron Sorbitol Injection

A sterile colloidal solution of a complex of ferric iron, sorbitol, and citric acid, stabilised with dextrin and sorbitol.

OTHER NAMES: Iron Sorbitex Injection; *Jectofer®*

A standard is given in the British Pharmacopoeia 1973

Description. A clear brown solution.

Weight per ml. At 20°, 1.17 to 1.19 g.

Alkalinity. It has a pH of 7.2 to 7.9.

Sterilisation. It is sterilised by heating in an autoclave.

Storage. It should be stored at a temperature between 15° and 30°; it should not be stored at a low temperature or allowed to freeze.

Actions and uses. Iron sorbitol injection is used for the correction of iron deficiency when the oral administration of iron is not possible or not desirable for the reasons stated under Iron Dextran Injection. It contains in 2 millilitres the equivalent of 100 milligrams of iron. After intramuscular injection into the iron-deficient subject, half the dose of iron enters the blood stream within three-quarters of an hour, and after 10 hours no significant amount remains. Some of the iron is made available almost immediately for haemoglobin synthesis in the bone marrow, the rest being stored in the liver. About 30% of an injected dose appears in the urine, the actual amount depending upon the iron stores of the individual.

It turns the urine a dark colour but this is of no pathological significance and is due to chemical changes in the excreted iron. Iron sorbitol injection is rarely antigenic and does not cause blood haemolysis.

Iron sorbitol injection should be given by deep intramuscular injection into the ventrolateral aspect of the upper and outer quadrant of the buttock, taking care to prevent leakage of the solution along the needle track. It is not suitable for intravenous injection.

The initial dose is a quantity corresponding to 1.5 milligrams of iron per kilogram body-weight for both children and adults; this corresponds to 2 millilitres of the injection for an adult of average weight. The total dose depends upon the haemoglobin level of the patient and is calculated on the basis that in women about 200 milligrams of iron and in men about 250 milligrams of iron is required to increase the haemoglobin by 1 gram per 100 millilitres of blood. Repeated haemoglobin estimations should be made to determine whether the response to treatment is satisfactory. Injections of 1 to 2 millilitres are given daily, according to body-weight. An additional amount of iron sorbitol injection, corresponding to 0.5 to 1 gram of iron, is given to replenish iron stores. In the case of children, injections of the equivalent of 1.5 milligrams of iron per kilogram body-weight may be given daily or on alternate days. The very small volumes needed by young children may be diluted with sodium chloride injection. In pregnancy, five additional injections of 2 millilitres are given after the haemoglobin has been restored to the normal level.

Undesirable effects. Nausea, vomiting and a metallic taste or loss of taste may occur about half an hour after the injection if too high a dose is given or if iron is being erroneously given by mouth concurrently. Localised or generalised urticaria may occur but this is rare.

Precautions and contra-indications. At least 24 hours should elapse between taking iron orally and receiving an injection of iron sorbitol. Oral iron therapy should never be given concurrently. If another injectable iron preparation has been administered previously, a week should elapse between the last injection of this and the first injection of iron sorbitol.

Iron sorbitol injection is contra-indicated in liver disease and kidney disease, particularly pyelonephritis, and in untreated urinary tract infections.

Preparations

Available in 2-ml ampoules and disposable syringes.

Isocarboxazid

2'-Benzyl-5-methylisoxazole-3-carbohydrazide

$C_{12}H_{13}N_3O_2 = 231.3$

OTHER NAME: *Marplan®*

A standard is given in the British Pharmacopoeia 1973

Description. A tasteless, white or creamy-white, crystalline powder with a faint characteristic odour.

Solubility. Very slightly soluble in water; soluble, at 20°, in 150 parts of alcohol, in 50 parts of ether, and in 3 parts of chloroform.

Identification. TESTS. 1. Dissolve 10 mg in 10 ml of acetone and add 0.2 ml of water and 0.2 ml of a 1% solution of ammonium molybdate in *dilute hydrochloric acid*; an orange colour is produced.

2. Dissolve 10 mg in 5 ml of alcohol (95%) and add 1 ml of a 1% solution of dimethylaminobenzaldehyde in alcohol containing 1% of hydrochloric acid; a yellow colour is produced.

MELTING-POINT. About 106°.

INFRA-RED ABSORPTION. Major peaks at 702, 747, 868, 1448, 1480, and 1670 cm^{-1} (see Appendix 2a: Infra-red Spectra).

Metabolism. ABSORPTION. Rapidly absorbed after oral administration.

BLOOD CONCENTRATION. Peak plasma concentrations are attained about 4 hours after oral administration.

HALF-LIFE. The plasma concentration decreases biphasically with a half-life of 2 to 3 hours for the α-phase and 36 hours for the β-phase.

DISTRIBUTION. In the rat, high concentrations are detectable in the blood, the liver, and the kidneys; significant amounts are taken up by red blood cells.

METABOLIC REACTIONS. Oxidation to benzoic acid followed by glycine conjugation to form hippuric acid and also hydrolysis to an active metabolite, benzhydrazine; evidence for benzhydrazine formation however comes from studies in the guinea-pig and rat and, although it is suspected that it is formed in man, this has not been confirmed.

EXCRETION. About 60% of a dose is excreted in the urine in 24 hours and about 70% after 8 days; 95% of the excreted material is hippuric acid.

FURTHER INFORMATION. Metabolism—B. A. Koechlin *et al.*, *J. Pharmac. exp. Ther.*, 1962, **138**, 11 and T. Satoh and K. Moroi, *Archs int. Pharmacodyn. Ther.*, 1971, **192**, 128; monoamine oxidase inhibition by isocarboxazid —M. A. Schwartz, *J. Pharmac. exp. Ther.*, 1962, **135**, 1.

Actions and uses. Isocarboxazid is an antidepressant drug which inhibits monoamine oxidase. It has actions and uses similar to those described under Phenelzine Sulphate.

The usual initial dose is 30 milligrams daily in divided doses and the usual maintenance dose is 10 to 20 milligrams daily in single or divided doses.

Undesirable effects; Precautions and drug interactions. As for Phenelzine Sulphate.

Preparation

ISOCARBOXAZID TABLETS: available as tablets containing 10 mg of isocarboxazid; they may be coloured.

A standard for these tablets is given in the British Pharmacopoeia 1973

Containers and *Storage:* see the entry on Tablets for general information on containers and storage. Containers should be airtight.

Advice for patients: treatment should not be discontinued without the advice of the prescriber. The tablets may affect mental concentration; persons affected should not drive or operate machinery.

Patients should be advised, during treatment and for 2 weeks thereafter, to avoid certain foodstuffs containing pressor agents such as cheese, pickled herrings, broad bean pods, and certain protein extracts prepared from meat or yeast, and medicines containing sympathomimetic drugs such as ephedrine, methoxamine, phenylephrine, phenylpropanolamine, and pseudoephedrine as found in cough and cold remedies, analgesics, and tonics. Warning cards, containing this advice may be carried by the patient during treatment and shown when further medical or dental treatment is required or when other medicines are needed.

Isoniazid

Isonicotinohydrazide *or* pyridine-4-carbohydrazide

$C_6H_7N_3O = 137.1$

OTHER NAMES: Isoniazidum; Isonicotinic Acid Hydrazide; *Rimifon*®
Mynah® (with ethambutol); *Trescazide*® (with ethionamide); *Rifinah*® and *Rimactazid*® (both with rifampicin); *Inapasade*® (with sodium amino salicylate)

A standard is given in the European Pharmacopoeia Vol. I

Description. Odourless, colourless crystals or white crystalline powder with a taste which is sweet at first then bitter.

Solubility. Soluble, at 20°, in 8 parts of water, in 45 parts of alcohol, and in 1000 parts of chloroform; very slightly soluble in ether.

Dissociation constants. pK_a 1.8, 3.5, 10.8 (20°).

Sterilisation. Solutions for injection are sterilised by heating in an autoclave or by filtration.

Storage. It should be stored in airtight containers, protected from light.

Identification. TESTS. 1. Heat with anhydrous sodium carbonate; the odour of pyridine is produced.

2. Dissolve about 50 mg in 1 ml of water with the aid of heat, cool, and add 4 ml of *cupro-citric solution*; a greenish precipitate is produced. Warm the mixture; gas is evolved and the precipitate becomes reddish-brown.

3. Dissolve 100 mg in 2 ml of water, add a warm solution of 100 mg of vanillin in 10 ml of water, allow to stand, and induce crystallisation; a yellow precipitate is produced which, after recrystallisation from alcohol (70%), melts at about 227°.

MELTING-POINT. About 172°.

ULTRAVIOLET ABSORPTION. In 0.01N hydrochloric acid, maximum at 265 nm (E1%, 1cm = 420); in 0.5N sodium hydroxide, maximum at 296 nm (E1%, 1cm = 292).

INFRA-RED ABSORPTION. Major peaks at 676, 1316, 1408, 1538, 1613, and 1639 cm^{-1} (see Appendix 2b: Infra-red Spectra).

Determination in body fluids. COLORIMETRY. In urine; certain metabolites—H. G. Boxenbaum and S. Riegelman, *J. pharm. Sci.*, 1974, **63**, 1191.

SPECTROFLUORIMETRY. In whole blood—H. G. Boxenbaum and S. Riegelman, *J. pharm. Sci.*, 1974, **63**, 1191; in serum—J. N. Miceli *et al.*, *Biochem. Med.*, 1975, **12**, 348.

GAS CHROMATOGRAPHY. In urine; isoniazid and its acetylated metabolite—M. Frater-Schroeder and G. Zbinden, *Biochem. Med.*, 1975, **14**, 274.

HIGH PRESSURE LIQUID CHROMATOGRAPHY. In plasma or urine—S. J. Saxena *et al.*, *J. pharm. Sci.*, 1977, **66**, 813.

Metabolism. ABSORPTION. Readily and completely absorbed after oral administration.

BLOOD CONCENTRATION. After an oral dose of 300 mg, peak plasma concentrations of about 4 and 6 μg/ml are attained within 1 hour for rapid and slow acetylators respectively; after an oral dose of 300 mg in a sustained release preparation, peak plasma concentrations of 0.5 to 0.7 μg/ml at 2 to 6 hours and 3.0 to 6.5 μg/ml at 2 to 4 hours are attained for the rapid and slow acetylators respectively; concentrations after intramuscular doses are very similar to those after oral administration.

HALF-LIFE. Plasma elimination half-life, in rapid acetylators about 1.2 hours and in slow acetylators about 3.5 hours.

DISTRIBUTION. Readily diffuses into all tissues and fluids including the cerebrospinal fluid; isoniazid is retained in the skin and in infected tissue; it crosses the placenta and is secreted in the milk of lactating mothers; *protein binding*, isoniazid does not appear to be bound in the blood.

METABOLIC REACTIONS. Acetylation, hydrolysis and glycine conjugation, hydrazone formation, and N-methylation; acetylation is polymorphic and two groups of acetylators have been identified, rapid and slow acetylators; approximately 40% of the population are rapid acetylators; the rate of hydrolysis appears to be more rapid in rapid acetylators than in the slow ones; the metabolites formed include acetylisoniazid, isonicotinic acid, isonicotinuric acid, and isonicotinoylhydrazones of pyruvic and glutaric acids, and N-methylisoniazid.

EXCRETION. Over 90% of a dose is excreted in the urine in 24 hours, most being excreted in the first 12 hours; of the excreted material 5 to 76% is acetylisoniazid and 4 to 32% is unchanged; no more than 10% of the dose is excreted in the faeces.

ENZYME INHIBITION. Isoniazid inhibits the acetylation of phenytoin and p-aminosalicylic acid inhibits the acetylation of isoniazid.

DISEASE STATES. In liver disease the half-life of isoniazid is increased and in Down's syndrome high serum concentrations are attained as a consequence of reduced acetylation.

FURTHER INFORMATION. Pharmacokinetics of isoniazid and some metabolites—H. G. Boxenbaum and S. Riegelman, *J. Pharmacokin. Biopharm.*, 1976, **4**, 287. Serum concentrations and bioavailability of isoniazid and rifampicin—J. C. Garnham et al., *Br. J. clin. Pharmac.*, 1976, **3**, 897.

Actions and uses. Isoniazid has no significant antibacterial action against any micro-organisms except the mycobacteria; against *Mycobacterium tuberculosis* it is bacteriostatic in extremely low concentrations.

Isoniazid is used mainly in the treatment of pulmonary tuberculosis but it appears to be effective also in the treatment of extrapulmonary lesions, including meningitis and genito-urinary disease.

Bacterial resistance may develop within a few weeks of starting treatment with isoniazid alone, but when it is administered concurrently with ethambutol or rifampicin, or with intramuscular injections of streptomycin, the proportion of patients in whom the infecting organisms develop resistance during 6 months of treatment is greatly reduced. Isoniazid therapy should, therefore, always be supplemented by the administration of other antituberculous drugs.

Isoniazid is administered by mouth, the initial dosage being usually about 4 milligrams per kilogram body-weight daily, in two or more divided doses; up to 10 milligrams per kilogram body-weight has been given daily, particularly during the first 1 or 2 weeks, in the treatment of tuberculous meningitis. The corresponding daily doses for children are 5 to 20 milligrams per kilogram body-weight (150 to 600 milligrams per square metre body-surface). An effective level of isoniazid in the cerebrospinal fluid usually follows oral administration.

When isoniazid cannot be given by mouth, similar doses may be administered by intramuscular injection.

Isoniazid has been used with success in the treatment of lupus vulgaris, for which the dosage may be up to 300 milligrams or more daily in divided doses. Treatment must be continued for several months.

Undesirable effects. Peripheral neuropathy, constipation, difficulty in starting urination, dryness of the mouth, and sometimes vertigo and hyperreflexia may be troublesome with doses of 10 milligrams per kilogram body-weight. The onset of peripheral neuritis should be expected with doses of 10 milligrams per kilogram body-weight and prophylactic doses of 100 milligrams of pyridoxine hydrochloride should be given daily.

Although isoniazid usually has a mood-elevating effect, mental disturbances, ranging from minor personality changes to major mental derangements have been reported; these are usually reversed on withdrawal of the drug.

Withdrawal symptoms, which may occur on the cessation of treatment, include headache, insomnia, excessive dreaming, irritability, and nervousness.

Precautions. When isoniazid is administered to nursing mothers, breast-fed infants should be monitored for possible signs of isoniazid toxicity.

Preparations

ISONIAZID ELIXIR (*Syn.* Isoniazid Syrup):

Isoniazid	10.0 g
Citric acid monohydrate	2.5 g
Sodium citrate	12.0 g
Concentrated anise water	10 ml
Compound tartrazine solution	10 ml
Glycerol	200 ml
Chloroform water, double-strength	400 ml
Water for preparations	to 1000 ml

Dissolve the sodium citrate, the citric acid, and the isoniazid in 300 ml of the water, add the double-strength chloroform water, the glycerol, the compound tartrazine solution, and the concentrated anise water, mix, and add sufficient water to produce the required volume.

Alternatively, the double-strength chloroform water may be omitted and the preparation preserved with methyl hydroxybenzoate, 0.1%, together with propyl hydroxybenzoate, 0.02%. Dissolve these substances in 600 ml of the water with the aid of heat, cool, and dissolve the sodium citrate, the citric acid, and the isoniazid in solution; add the glycerol, the compound tartrazine solution, and the concentrated anise water, mix, and add sufficient water to produce the required volume.

It has a weight per ml at 20° of about 1.07 g.

When a dose less than or not a multiple of 5 ml is prescribed, the elixir may be diluted, as described in the entry on Elixirs, with chloroform water. The diluted elixir must be freshly prepared.

Syrup must not be used as diluent as isoniazid is unstable in the presence of sugars.

A standard for this elixir is given in the British Pharmaceutical Codex 1973

Containers and *Labelling:* see the entry on Elixirs for general information on containers and labelling.

Storage: it should be protected from light. When stored in filled unopened containers at a temperature not exceeding 25°, it may be expected to retain its potency for 1 year. When dispensed, each container should be filled and the contents should represent not more than 1 month's supply.

Advice for patients: the elixir should be taken at regular intervals, preferably after meals. Treatment should not be discontinued without the advice of the prescriber.

ISONIAZID INJECTION: a sterile solution of isoniazid in water for injections. The acidity of the solution is adjusted to pH 5.6 to 6.0 by the addition of 0.1N hydrochloric acid. The solution is sterilised by heating in an autoclave or by filtration. Available in 2-ml ampoules containing 25 mg of isoniazid per ml.

A standard for this injection is given in the British Pharmaceutical Codex 1973

Containers and *Labelling:* see the entry on Injections for general information on containers and labelling.

ISONIAZID TABLETS: available as tablets containing 50 and 100 mg of isoniazid.

A standard for these tablets is given in the British Pharmacopoeia 1973

Containers and *Storage:* see the entry on Tablets for general information on containers and storage. Containers should be airtight and light resistant.

Advice for patients: the tablets should be taken at regular intervals, preferably after meals. Treatment should not be discontinued without the advice of the prescriber.

SODIUM AMINOSALICYLATE AND ISONIAZID GRANULES: prepared by incorporating sodium aminosalicylate and isoniazid in a suitable basis and granulating the product. The granules may be coated and the coat may be coloured. Available as granules in sachets containing 50 mg of isoniazid with 2 g of sodium aminosalicylate and 150 mg of isoniazid with 6 g of sodium aminosalicylate.

A standard for these granules is given in the British Pharmaceutical Codex 1973

Storage: they should be stored in airtight containers, in a cool place, protected from light.

Advice for patients: the granules should be placed on the tongue and swallowed with water, preferably after meals, or alternatively may be sprinkled on cool food. Doses should be taken at regular intervals and treatment should not be discontinued without the advice of the prescriber.

SODIUM AMINOSALICYLATE AND ISONIAZID POWDER: consisting of sodium aminosalicylate and isoniazid mixed with a suitable coloured flavoured basis. The ingredients are usually in the proportion of 1 g of sodium aminosalicylate to each 25 mg of isoniazid.

Storage: it should be stored in airtight containers, in a cool place, protected from light.

Advice for patients: the powder should be taken dissolved in water or other fluid, preferably after meals. Doses should be taken at regular intervals and treatment should not be discontinued without the advice of the prescriber.

OTHER PREPARATIONS available include TABLETS containing isoniazid 100 mg with ethambutol 200, 250, 300 and 365 mg, tablets containing isoniazid 75 mg with ethionamide 125 mg, tablets containing isoniazid 100 mg with rifampicin 150 mg, and tablets containing isoniazid 150 mg with rifampicin 300 mg.

Isoprenaline Hydrochloride

N-[2-(3,4-Dihydroxyphenyl)-2-hydroxyethyl]-N-isopropylammonium chloride
$C_{11}H_{18}ClNO_3 = 247.7$

OTHER NAMES: Isoprenalini Hydrochloridum; Isoproterenol Hydrochloride; *Saventrine®*; *Suscardia® Brontisol®* (with deptropine citrate); *Duo-Autohaler®* and *Medihaler-Duo®* (with phenylephrine acid tartrate); *PIB®* (with atropine methonitrate)

A standard is given in the British Pharmacopoeia Addendum 1975

Description. An odourless white crystalline powder.

Solubility. Soluble, at 20°, in less than 1 part of water and in 55 parts of alcohol; practically insoluble in ether and in chloroform.

Moisture content. Not more than 1%, determined by drying *in vacuo*.

Dissociation constants. pK_a 8.6, 10.1, 12.0 (20°).

Stability. It gradually darkens on exposure to air and light. Aqueous solutions become pink to brownish-pink, on exposure to air, and almost immediately when made alkaline. Solutions should contain an antoxidant such as sodium metabisulphite and contact with metals should be avoided as it causes discoloration and loss of activity.

Sterilisation. Solutions for injection are sterilised by filtration.

Storage. It should be stored in airtight containers, protected from light.

Identification. TESTS. 1. Dissolve about 10 mg in 1 ml of water and add 1 drop of *ferric chloride test-solution*; an intense green colour is produced. Add, dropwise, *sodium bicarbonate solution*; the colour changes first to blue and then to red.

2. Dissolve about 10 mg in 1 ml of water and add 1 drop of *phosphotungstic acid solution*; a white precipitate is produced which becomes brown on standing (distinction from adrenaline).

3. Dissolve about 10 mg in 10 ml of water, dilute 1 ml of this solution to 10 ml with water, add 2 drops of 0.1N hydrochloric acid, followed by 1 ml of 0.1N iodine, allow to stand for 5 minutes, and add 2 ml of 0.1N sodium thiosulphate; a red-brown colour is produced (distinction from noradrenaline which gives no more than a faint pink colour under these conditions).

MELTING-POINT. About 168°.

ULTRAVIOLET ABSORPTION. In 0.1N hydrochloric acid, maxima at 222 nm (E1%, 1cm = 257) and 281 nm (E1%, 1cm = 113); in water, maximum at 280 nm (E1%, 1cm = 100).

Metabolism. ABSORPTION. Readily absorbed after inhalation and after oral or parenteral administration; most of an inhaled dose is swallowed, only about 10% reaching the lungs.

BLOOD CONCENTRATION. After a dose of 500 μg, administered by an aerosol inhalation, a plasma concentration of about 0.03 ng/ml is attained in 5 minutes.

HALF-LIFE. Plasma half-life, after rapid intravenous injection, 3 to 5 minutes, and after an intravenous infusion, about 2 hours; more detailed studies in children show the decline in plasma concentration to be biphasic, the α-phase having a half-life of 2 to 5 minutes and the β-phase, a half-life of 3 to 7 hours.

METABOLIC REACTIONS. *O*-Methylation and sulphate conjugation; after oral administration or inhalation most of the drug is conjugated but after intravenous or intrabronchial administration it is mostly in the *O*-methylated form; after oral administration isoprenaline is extensively metabolised by conjugation by the gut wall prior to absorption but the extent of conjugation may be reduced by pretreatment with salicylamide; the sulphate conjugate is inactive but the methylated metabolite exhibits weak activity.

EXCRETION. After intravenous administration, about 90% of a dose is excreted in the urine in 24 hours, mostly as the 3-*O*-methylated metabolite with about 15% being excreted unchanged; after inhalation or oral administration, 80 to 95% of a dose is excreted in the urine mainly as the sulphate conjugate, with about 10% as the 3-*O*-methylated conjugate, 1 to 2% as unchanged drug, and 1 to 2% as the free methylated metabolite; small amounts of a dose are excreted in the bile, mainly as metabolites.

FURTHER INFORMATION. Metabolism—M. E. Conolly *et al.*, *Br. J. Pharmac.*, 1972, **46**, 458, C. F. George *et al.*, *J. Pharm. Pharmac.*, 1974, **26**, 265, and D. Kadar *et al.*, *Clin. Pharmac. Ther.*, 1974, **16**, 789.

Actions and uses. Isoprenaline hydrochloride has the actions and undesirable effects of isoprenaline, as described under Isoprenaline Sulphate. It is usually administered in the form of slow-release tablets.

The usual initial dosage is 30 milligrams 3 times a day and this may be increased until the heart rate is sufficiently accelerated. The maximum daily dosage is 750 milligrams.

Isoprenaline hydrochloride is also used as an aerosol inhalation, as described under Isoprenaline Sulphate.

Isoprenaline hydrochloride is occasionally administered by intravenous infusion in the emergency treatment of cardiogenic or endotoxic shock states, heart block, or severe bradycardia, and in the evaluation of cardiac function. It is given by slow intravenous infusion, usually in dextrose injection (5%), under electrocardiographic surveillance. The usual dose is 0.5 to 10 micrograms of isoprenaline hydrochloride per minute, adjusted according to the response of the patient. Higher doses, up to 40 micrograms per minute, may be necessary in the treatment of heart block.

Precautions and contra-indications. As for Isoprenaline Sulphate.

Preparations

ISOPRENALINE HYDROCHLORIDE INJECTION: a sterile solution of isoprenaline hydrochloride, with suitable stabilisers, in water for injections. It is sterilised by filtration and, by means of an aseptic technique, distributed into sterile ampoules, the air in the ampoules being replaced with sterile nitrogen or other suitable gas, and sealed.

Available in 2-ml ampoules containing 1 mg of isoprenaline hydrochloride per ml.

A standard for this injection is given in the British Pharmacopoeia Addendum 1975

Containers and *Labelling:* see the entry on Injections for general information on containers and labelling.

Storage: it should be stored in a cool place, protected from light.

SLOW ISOPRENALINE TABLETS: available as tablets containing 30 mg of isoprenaline hydrochloride, in a slow-release formulation.

Containers and *Storage:* see the entry on Tablets for general information on containers and storage. Containers should be airtight.

Advice for patients: the tablets should be swallowed whole. Doses should be taken at regular intervals. Treatment should not be discontinued without the advice of the prescriber.

OTHER PREPARATIONS available include an AEROSOL INHALATION containing isoprenaline hydrochloride 0.3% with deptropine citrate 0.2% providing isoprenaline hydrochloride 150 micrograms with deptropine citrate 100 micrograms per metered dose, an aerosol inhalation containing isoprenaline hydrochloride 0.8% with phenylephrine acid tartrate 1.2% providing isoprenaline hydrochloride 160 micrograms with phenylephrine acid tartrate 240 micrograms per metered dose, an aerosol inhalation containing isoprenaline hydrochloride 0.35% with atropine methonitrate 0.1% providing isoprenaline hydrochloride 180 micrograms with atropine methonitrate 50 micrograms per metered dose, and an aerosol inhalation containing isoprenaline hydrochloride 1% with atropine methonitrate 0.1% providing isoprenaline hydrochloride 500 micrograms with atropine methonitrate 50 micrograms per metered dose.

Isoprenaline Sulphate

N-[2-(3,4-Dihydroxyphenyl)-2-hydroxyethyl]-*N*-isopropylammonium sulphate dihydrate

$$\left[HO \cdot CH \cdot CH_2 \cdot \overset{+}{N}H_2 \cdot CH(CH_3)_2 \right]_2 \quad SO_4^{2-}, 2H_2O$$

$C_{22}H_{36}N_2O_{10}S,2H_2O = 556.6$

OTHER NAMES: *Aleudrin*®; *Iso-Autohaler*®; Isoprenalini Sulfas; Isoproterenol Sulphate; *Lomupren*®; *Medihaler Iso*®; *Prenomiser*®

A standard is given in the European Pharmacopoeia Vol. III Supplement

Description. An odourless white crystalline powder with a taste somewhat bitter and astringent.

Solubility. Soluble, at 20°, in 4 parts of water; very slightly soluble in alcohol, in ether, and in chloroform.

Acidity. A 1% solution has a pH of 4 to 5.5.

Moisture content. 5 to 7.5%, determined by Fischer titration.

Stability; Sterilisation; Storage. As for Isoprenaline Hydrochloride.

Identification. TESTS. It complies with the tests described under Isoprenaline Hydrochloride.

MELTING-POINT. About 128°, with decomposition.

ULTRAVIOLET ABSORPTION. In 0.1N hydrochloric acid, maxima at 224 nm (E1%, 1cm = 239) and 281 nm (E1%, 1cm = 96); in water, maximum at 280 nm (E1%, 1cm = 100).

Metabolism. See under Isoprenaline Hydrochloride.

Actions and uses. Isoprenaline, like adrenaline, is a directly-acting sympathomimetic amine but it acts almost exclusively on beta receptors, as described under Adrenergic Receptors, producing bronchial relaxation, peripheral vasodilatation, tachycardia, and myocardial stimulation. It is used in the treatment of bronchial asthma, but other drugs such as salbutamol and terbutaline, which do not markedly stimulate the heart, are usually preferred for this purpose. Isoprenaline is also used to counteract the effects of excessive dosage with beta-adrenergic receptor blocking agents.

Isoprenaline is such a potent cardiac stimulant that it is not usually given by injection except in cardiac surgery to combat heart block and also in the treatment of shock.

Isoprenaline sulphate is usually administered by inhalation but it may also be given sublingually. When swallowed, its activity in markedly impaired; the tablets should therefore be allowed to dissolve under the tongue without being sucked and as little saliva as possible should be swallowed.

The usual initial dosage is 10 to 20 milligrams three times a day. Very mild asthmatic spasm may require only 5 milligrams and very severe spasm up to 40 milligrams or even more; relief is felt after 2 to 4 minutes.

A more rapid and selective effect is produced when the drug is given by inhalation of a spray containing from 0.5 to 3% of isoprenaline hydrochloride or sulphate, about 1 millilitre being inhaled.

Doses of up to 1.2 milligrams may be given in the form of an aerosol inhalation and repeated if necessary after 30 minutes up to a maximum of 8 doses in 24 hours. Doses of 15 milligrams may be administered by mouth in the treatment of heart block.

Undesirable effects. Reactions such as tachycardia, headache, dizziness, and vigorous myocardial stimulation, together with a fall in arterial pressure may occur; these effects quickly subside on withdrawal of the drug.

Precautions and contra-indications. Isoprenaline should not be given in hyperthyroidism and cardiac disease. It should be given with caution to patients with diabetes as it can cause a rise in blood sugar.

The excessive use of sprays containing isoprenaline should be avoided as it may lead to fatal results. Isoprenaline should not be given simultaneously with adrenaline but it may be used simultaneously with phenylephrine. It should be used with caution in patients taking monoamine-oxidase inhibitors.

Preparations

ISOPRENALINE AEROSOL INHALATION: a suspension of isoprenaline sulphate, in sufficiently fine powder to meet the requirements of the standard, in a suitable mixture of aerosol propellents, which may contain a surface-active agent, stabilising agents, and other adjuvants. It is packed in a pressurised container fitted with a special metering valve, delivering 80 micrograms of isoprenaline sulphate to the patient each time it is actuated, and an oral adapter.

A standard for this aerosol inhalation is given in the British Pharmaceutical Codex 1973

Containers, Labelling, and *Storage:* see the entry on Aerosol Inhalations for general information on containers, labelling, and storage.

Advice for patients: see the entry on Aerosol Inhalations for general information on the use of aerosol inhalations.

The patient should be advised verbally to read the instructions on the leaflet enclosed with the product. If more than 1 inhalation is taken at a time, at least 1 minute should elapse between any 2 inhalations. An interval of at least 30 minutes should elapse between any 2 doses unless otherwise directed.

When used in conjunction with beclomethasone or other corticosteroid aerosol inhalation, isoprenaline should be given first and the corticosteroid administered 5 minutes later.

Excessive use of the preparation should be avoided.

ISOPRENALINE TABLETS: available as tablets containing 20 mg of isoprenaline sulphate with 1% each of citric acid and sodium metabisulphite.

A standard for these tablets is given in the British Pharmacopoeia 1973

Containers and *Storage:* see the entry on Tablets for general information on containers and storage. Containers should be airtight and light resistant.

Advice for patients: the tablets should be allowed to dissolve under the tongue when required.

STRONG ISOPRENALINE AEROSOL INHALATION: a suspension of isoprenaline sulphate, in sufficiently fine powder to meet the requirements of the standard, in a suitable mixture of aerosol propellents, which may contain a surface-active agent, stabilising agents, and other adjuvants.

It is packed in a pressurised container fitted with a special metering valve, delivering 400 micrograms of isoprenaline sulphate to the patient each time it is actuated, and an oral adapter.

This preparation is 5 times the strength of isoprenaline aerosol inhalation.

A standard for this aerosol inhalation is given in the British Pharmaceutical Codex 1973

Containers, Labelling, and *Storage:* see the entry on Aerosol Inhalations for general information on containers, labelling, and storage.

Advice for patients: see above under Isoprenaline Aerosol Inhalation.

OTHER PREPARATIONS available include an AEROSOL INHALATION containing isoprenaline sulphate 1% providing 100 micrograms of isoprenaline sulphate per metered dose; CARTRIDGES (for use with a suitable inhaler) containing isoprenaline sulphate 100 micrograms, cartridges containing isoprenaline sulphate 100 micrograms with sodium cromoglycate 20 mg; and a SPRAY containing isoprenaline sulphate 1%.

Isopropyl Alcohol

$(CH_3)_2CHOH = 60.10$

OTHER NAMES: *Avantine®; IPS/C®; IPS.1®;* Isopropanol; 2-Propanol

A standard is given in the British Pharmacopoeia 1973

Description. A clear, colourless, highly inflammable liquid with a characteristic alcoholic odour.

Solubility. Miscible with water, with ether, and with chloroform. The alcohol may be salted out from aqueous mixtures by the addition of salts or sodium hydroxide.

Weight per ml. At 20°, 0.784 to 0.786 g.

Boiling point. About 82°.

Refractive index. 1.377 to 1.378.

Storage. It should be stored in airtight containers.

Metabolism. ABSORPTION. Readily absorbed after oral administration and slowly absorbed through the skin.

METABOLIC REACTIONS. Oxidation to form acetone, formic acid, and acetic acid together with conjugation with glucuronic acid.

EXCRETION. Unchanged drug and metabolites are excreted in the urine.

Actions and uses. Isopropyl alcohol taken by mouth has an action similar to that of ethyl alcohol. Its toxicity is about twice that of ethyl alcohol and because of this and its unpleasant taste, its oral administration is inadvisable. Isopropyl alcohol is used extensively as a solvent, especially in perfumery and cosmetics, and externally it may be used as a substitute for industrial methylated spirit and surgical spirit.

Isopropyl alcohol is more effective as an antibacterial preservative than ethyl alcohol at concentrations greater than 70% v/v. It may be used in place of ethyl alcohol for preserving pathological specimens and for dehydrating tissues. Stock solutions of chlorhexidine and cetrimide may contain 4% v/v of isopropyl alcohol as a precaution against bacterial contamination. When mixed with a small proportion of water, it is a suitable storage fluid for surgical sutures.

It is a useful non-aqueous moistening agent for tablet granulation, especially as its water content is low. It is also used in hair preparations, lotions and liniments.

Isopropyl Myristate

$$CH_3 \cdot [CH_2]_{12} \cdot CO \cdot O \cdot CH(CH_3)_2$$
$$C_{17}H_{34}O_2 = 270.5$$

OTHER NAME: *Crodamol IPM®*

A standard is given in the British Pharmaceutical Codex 1973

Description. An odourless colourless mobile liquid.

Solubility. Soluble, at 20°, in 3 parts of alcohol; practically insoluble in water and in glycerol; miscible with liquid hydrocarbons and with fixed oils.

Weight per ml. At 20°, 0.850 to 0.855 g.

Refractive index. At 20°, 1.434 to 1.437.

Incompatibility. Isopropyl myristate is incompatible with hard paraffin, producing a granular mixture.

Uses. Isopropyl myristate may be used in external preparations in place of vegetable oils. It is resistant to oxidation and hydrolysis, does not become rancid, is free from irritant and sensitising properties, and is absorbed fairly readily by the skin.

Isopropyl myristate is used in emollient ointments and creams, giving preparations which are relatively free from greasiness. It is a solvent for many substances applied externally and is of value as a vehicle when direct contact and penetration of the medicament are required.

Isotonic and Isosmotic Solutions

The following table lists the freezing-point depression values for 1% aqueous solutions of various substances described in this volume for use in calculating the quantity of an adjusting substance to be added to an aqueous solution to render it isosmotic with a 0.9% solution of sodium chloride and thus, in most cases, isotonic with blood serum and lachrymal secretion.

The amount of adjusting substance required may be calculated from the equation:

$$W = \frac{0.52 - a}{b}$$

where W = the weight, in g, of the added substance in 100 millilitres of the final solution, a = the depression of the freezing-point of water produced by the medicament already in solution, calculated by multiplying the value for b for the medicament by the strength of the solution expressed as a percentage w/v, and b = the depression of the freezing-point of water produced by 1% of the adjusting substance (for example sodium chloride).

Substance	b
Adrenaline acid tartrate	0.098
Amethocaine hydrochloride	0.109
Aminocaproic acid	0.148
Aminophylline	0.098
Amitriptyline hydrochloride	0.100
Amphetamine sulphate	0.129
Ampicillin sodium	0.090
Amylobarbitone sodium	0.143
Antazoline hydrochloride	0.132
Antimony potassium tartrate	0.106
Antimony sodium tartrate	0.075
Apomorphine hydrochloride	0.080
Ascorbic acid	0.105
Atropine methonitrate	0.100
Atropine sulphate	0.074
Benzalkonium chloride solution (50%)	0.046
Benztropine mesylate	0.115
Benzyl alcohol	0.094
Benzylpenicillin (potassium salt)	0.102
Benzylpenicillin (sodium salt)	0.100
Borax	0.241
Boric acid	0.288
Bupivacaine hydrochloride	0.096
Calcium chloride	0.298
Calcium gluconate	0.091
Calcium lactate	0.135
Capreomycin sulphate	0.020
Carbachol	0.205
Carbenicillin sodium	0.118
Cephaloridine	0.041
Cephalothin sodium	0.095
Cetrimide	0.051
Chloramphenicol sodium succinate	0.080
Chlordiazepoxide hydrochloride	0.125
Chloroquine phosphate	0.082
Chloroquine sulphate	0.050
Chlorpheniramine maleate	0.085
Chlorpromazine hydrochloride	0.058
Chlortetracycline hydrochloride	0.061
Cinchocaine hydrochloride	0.074
Cocaine hydrochloride	0.090
Codeine phosphate	0.080
Colistin sulphomethate sodium	0.085
Copper sulphate	0.100
Cyclopentolate hydrochloride	0.115
Cyclophosphamide	0.061
Cytarabine	0.066
Desferrioxamine mesylate	0.047
Dexamethasone sodium phosphate	0.095
Dexamphetamine sulphate	0.134
Dextrose (anhydrous)	0.101
Dextrose (monohydrate)	0.091
Diethylcarbamazine citrate	0.083
Diphenhydramine hydrochloride	0.161

Substance	b	Substance	b
Disodium edetate	0.132	Paraldehyde	0.142
Doxapram hydrochloride	0.070	Pentobarbitone sodium	0.145
Ecothiopate iodide	0.090	Pentolinium tartrate	0.098
Edrophonium chloride	0.179	Pethidine hydrochloride	0.125
Emetine hydrochloride	0.058	Phenazone	0.093
Ephedrine hydrochloride	0.165	Phenobarbitone sodium	0.135
Ergometrine maleate	0.089	Phentolamine mesylate	0.096
Ethanolamine	0.306	Phenylephrine hydrochloride	0.184
Ethylenediamine hydrate	0.253	Phenylpropanolamine hydrochloride	0.219
Ethylmorphine hydrochloride	0.088	Physostigmine salicylate	0.090
Fluorescein sodium	0.181	Physostigmine sulphate	0.074
Fluphenazine hydrochloride	0.082	Pilocarpine hydrochloride	0.138
Gallamine triethiodide	0.046	Pilocarpine nitrate	0.132
Gentamicin sulphate	0.030	Polymyxin B sulphate	0.052
Glycerol	0.203	Potassium chloride	0.439
Glycine	0.235	Potassium iodide	0.196
Heparin sodium	0.042	Potassium nitrate	0.324
Histamine acid phosphate	0.149	Potassium permanganate	0.223
Homatropine hydrobromide	0.097	Prilocaine hydrochloride	0.125
Hydroxyamphetamine hydrobromide	0.156	Procainamide hydrochloride	0.127
Hydroxystilbamidine isethionate	0.090	Procaine hydrochloride	0.122
Hyoscine hydrobromide	0.068	Promazine hydrochloride	0.077
Imipramine hydrochloride	0.110	Promethazine hydrochloride	0.104
Isoniazid	0.144	Propylene glycol	0.262
Isoprenaline sulphate	0.078	Pyridostigmine bromide	0.125
Kanamycin sulphate	0.041	Pyridoxine hydrochloride	0.213
Lactic acid	0.239	Quinine dihydrochloride	0.130
Lactose	0.040	Quinine hydrochloride	0.077
Laevulose	0.099	Resorcinol	0.161
Levallorphan tartrate	0.073	Silver nitrate	0.190
Levorphanol tartrate	0.067	Sodium acetate	0.265
Lignocaine hydrochloride	0.130	Sodium acid phosphate	0.207
Lincomycin hydrochloride	0.090	Sodium aminosalicylate	0.170
Magnesium chloride	0.259	Sodium benzoate	0.230
Magnesium sulphate	0.094	Sodium bicarbonate	0.380
Mannitol	0.098	Sodium carboxymethylcellulose	0.017
Mephenesin	0.109	Sodium chloride	0.576
Mepyramine maleate	0.108	Sodium citrate	0.178
Mersalyl acid	0.069	Sodium diatrizoate	0.049
Methacholine chloride	0.184	Sodium iodide	0.222
Methadone hydrochloride	0.101	Sodium metabisulphite	0.386
Methicillin sodium	0.099	Sodium nitrite	0.480
Methoxamine hydrochloride	0.150	Sodium salicylate	0.210
Methyldopate hydrochloride	0.122	Sodium sulphate	0.148
Minocycline hydrochloride	0.058	Sodium thiosulphate	0.181
Morphine hydrochloride	0.086	Streptomycin sulphate	0.036
Morphine sulphate	0.079	Strychnine hydrochloride	0.104
Naloxone hydrochloride	0.083	Sucrose	0.047
Neomycin sulphate	0.063	Sulphacetamide sodium	0.132
Neostigmine bromide	0.127	Sulphadiazine sodium	0.137
Neostigmine methylsulphate	0.115	Sulphobromophthalein sodium	0.034
Nicotinamide	0.148	Suramin	0.058
Nicotinic acid	0.144	Suxamethonium chloride	0.115
Nikethamide	0.100	Tartaric acid	0.143
Noscapine hydrochloride	0.058	Tetracycline hydrochloride	0.081
Novobiocin sodium	0.046	Thiamine hydrochloride	0.139
Orphenadrine citrate	0.074	Thiopentone sodium	0.155
Oxytetracycline hydrochloride	0.075	Thiotepa	0.090
Papaverine hydrochloride	0.061	Tolazoline hydrochloride	0.196

Substance	b
Trifluoperazine hydrochloride	0.100
Trimeprazine tartrate	0.035
Tropicamide	0.050
Tubocurarine chloride	0.076
Urea	0.341
Vancomycin hydrochloride	0.028
Viomycin sulphate	0.047
Xylometazoline hydrochloride	0.121
Zinc chloride	0.351
Zinc sulphate	0.086

Ispaghula Husk

The epidermis and the collapsed adjacent layers removed from the dried ripe seeds of *Plantago ovata* Forssk. (Fam. Plantaginaceae). The plant is a herbaceous annual indigenous to the Indian subcontinent and Iran.

OTHER NAMES: *Fybogel*®; Isapgol Husk; *Isogel*®; *Vi-Siblin*®

A standard is given in the British Pharmaceutical Codex 1973

Constituents. Ispaghula husk contains mucilage and hemicelluloses. Cold water extraction yields a polysaccharide which on hydrolysis yields D-xylose (46%), L-arabinose (7%), and the aldobiouronic acid, 2-O-α-D-galactopyranosyluronic acid L-rhamnose (40%). Subsequent extraction with hot water removes a xylan composed of D-xylose (80%) and L-arabinose (14%).

Description. *Macroscopical characters:* pale buff brittle flakes, more or less lanceolate, up to 2 mm long and 1 mm wide at the centre, much broken into smaller fragments; many of the flakes have a small brownish oval spot, about 0.8 to 1.0 mm long, in the centre; the drug swells rapidly in water, forming a stiff mucilage.

Microscopical characters: mounted in cresol, the particles are transparent and angular, the edges straight or curved and sometimes rolled. They are composed of polygonal prismatic cells with 4 to 6 straight or slightly curved walls; the cells vary in size in different parts of the seed-coat, being about 25 to 60 μm at the summit of the seed, that is, near and over the brown spot, to 25 to 100 μm for the remainder of the epidermis except at the edges of the seed, where the cells are again smaller, about 45 to 70 μm.

Mounted in alcohol (95%) and irrigated with water, the mucilage in the outer part of the epidermal cells swells rapidly and goes into solution, while the two inner layers of mucilage are more resistant and swell to form rounded papillae.

Mounted in *iodine water*, occasional single and 2- to 4-compound starch granules, about 2 to 10 μm, can be seen in some of the cells.

Endosperm, if present, is dark and dense.

Moisture content. Not more than 12%, determined by drying at 105°.

Adulterants and substitutes. Fragments of the endosperm of ispaghula seed are usually dark and dense, the cells being chiefly polyhedral with thick cellulosic walls, about 2.5 to 7.0 μm thick and perforated by simple pits; the cells are about 30 to 60 μm in diameter, a few from the radicle pocket being subcylindrical and about 18 μm in diameter. All the cells contain fixed oil and aleurone grains.

Actions and uses. Ispaghula husk has the laxative actions and uses described under Psyllium. The usual dose is 3 to 5 grams.

Preparations

Preparations available include GRANULES containing ispaghula husk 66% and 90%.

Jaundice

Jaundice (also called icterus) is a yellow discoloration of the skin, conjunctivae, and mucous membranes caused by accumulation of bile pigment. All tissues and fluids of the body are affected except the mucous secretions.

Haemolytic jaundice. In this condition excessive destruction of red corpuscles results in the release of more bilirubin than the liver can metabolise. It may be due to excessive fragility of the red cells as in certain congenital diseases such as spherocytosis, sickle-cell anaemia, or thalassaemia, to infections with organisms that produce haemolytic toxins, to haemolytic poisons, or to circulating red-cell antibodies. It occasionally occurs in patients treated with methyldopa. The urine and stools may be darker than normal and there may be enlargement of the spleen.

Treatment depends on the cause of the disease but surgery and administration of corticosteroids may be required.

Hepatocellular jaundice. In this condition the parenchymal cells of the liver have been damaged, usually by virus infections or by toxic substances such as carbon tetrachloride, halothane, paracetamol, or hydrazines such as hydrallazine, isoniazid, and phenelzine, so that they fail to take up bilirubin, conjugate it, and pass the product to the bile ducts. The condition may also be due to congenital abnormalities or deficient enzyme systems. Onset is usually rapid and the disease varies from mild to severe.

Treatment depends on the underlying cause but generally surgery is of no value and should be avoided.

Obstructive jaundice. This type of jaundice is caused by obstruction, either in the bile ducts or between the liver cells and the bile ducts.

It is usually insidious in onset, of variable intensity, and characterised by pruritus, anorexia, and a metallic taste in the mouth. Bradycardia is sometimes present, the stools are pale or clay coloured and contain excessive amounts of fat, and the urine is dark.

Numerous drugs and chemicals affect bilirubin metabolism and may cause obstructive jaundice particularly phenothiazine derivatives and more rarely oral contraceptives, indanedione-type anticoagulants, phenylbutazone, chlorpropamide, ibufenac, norethandrolone, methyltestosterone, norethynodrel, methandienone, and amitriptyline.

Treatment is related to the cause and in the case of extrahepatic obstruction surgery may be necessary.

Johnin Purified Protein Derivative

A preparation of the heat-treated products of growth and lysis of *Mycobacterium paratuberculosis.*

OTHER NAME: Johnin P.P.D.

A standard is given in the British Pharmacopoeia (Veterinary)

Storage. It should be protected from light and stored at

2° to 8° when it may be expected to retain its potency for 5 years.

Veterinary uses. It is administered as an aid in the diagnosis of Johne's disease in cattle by intradermal injection in a dose of 0.1 ml.

Kala-azar

see under LEISHMANIASIS

Kanamycin Acid Sulphate

A form of kanamycin sulphate prepared by adding sulphuric acid to a solution of kanamycin sulphate and drying by a suitable method.

OTHER NAME: *Kannasyn®*

A standard is given in the British Pharmacopoeia Addendum 1975

Description. An odourless white hygroscopic powder.

Solubility. Soluble at 20°, in 1 part of water; very slightly soluble in alcohol, in ether, and in chloroform.

Acidity or alkalinity. A 1% solution has a pH of 6 to 8.5.

Moisture content. Not more than 5%, determined by drying *in vacuo*.

Specific rotation. +103° to +115°, determined on a 5% solution.

Labelling. If the material is not intended for parenteral administration, the label on the container states that the contents are not to be injected.

Storage. It should be stored in airtight containers, protected from light.

Identification. It complies with the tests described under Kanamycin Sulphate.

Determination in body fluids; Metabolism. As for Kanamycin Sulphate.

Actions and uses. Kanamycin acid sulphate has the actions, uses, and undesirable effects described under Kanamycin Sulphate, and is used in similar dosage.

Precautions; Drug interactions. As for Kanamycin Sulphate.

Preparation

KANAMYCIN INJECTION: a sterile solution of either kanamycin sulphate with sulphuric acid and suitable buffering and stabilising agents, or of kanamycin acid sulphate, in water for injections. If the injection is made from kanamycin acid sulphate, it is prepared by dissolving the contents of a sealed container in water for injections shortly before use. Available as a powder in vials containing kanamycin acid sulphate equivalent to 1 g (1 mega unit) of kanamycin; and as a solution in 3-ml vials containing kanamycin sulphate equivalent to 1 g (1 mega unit) of kanamycin (334 mg of kanamycin per ml) and in 4-ml vials containing kanamycin sulphate equivalent to 250 mg (250 000 units) of kanamycin per ml.
A standard for this injection is given in the British Pharmacopoeia Addendum 1975
Containers and *Labelling*: see the entry on Injections for general information on containers and labelling.
Storage: it should be protected from light. The injection prepared from kanamycin acid sulphate by dissolving the contents of a sealed container in water for injections

contains no bactericide and should be used as soon as possible after preparation, but solutions of kanamycin acid sulphate may be expected to retain their potency for up to 14 days after preparation, provided they are stored at 2° to 10°. The injection prepared from kanamycin sulphate may be stored at room temperature.

Kanamycin Sulphate

The sulphate of 6-O-(3-amino-3-deoxy-α-D-gluco-pyranosyl)-4-O-(6-amino-6-deoxy-α-D-glucopyranosyl)-2-deoxystreptamine, an antimicrobial substance produced by *Streptomyces kanamyceticus*.

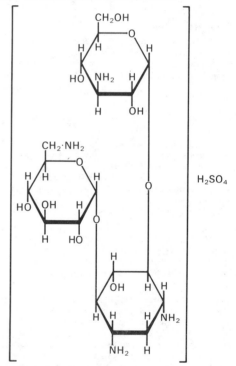

$C_{18}H_{38}N_4O_{15}S = 582.6$

OTHER NAMES: *Kannasyn®*; *Kantrex®*

A standard is given in the British Pharmacopoeia 1973

Description. An odourless, white, crystalline powder.

Solubility. Soluble, at 20°, in 8 parts of water; very slightly soluble in alcohol, in ether, and in chloroform.

Acidity or alkalinity. A 1% solution has a pH of 6 to 8.5.

Moisture content. Not more than 3%, determined by drying *in vacuo*.

Specific rotation. +112° to +123°, determined on a 5% solution.

Labelling. If the material is not intended for parenteral administration the label on the container states that the contents are not to be injected.

Storage. It should be stored in airtight containers, protected from light, at a temperature not exceeding 20°.

Identification. TESTS. 1. Dissolve about 10 mg in 1 ml of water, add 1 ml of a 0.2% solution of ninhydrin in

2-butyl alcohol, then add 0.5 ml of pyridine, heat for 5 minutes on a water-bath, and add 10 ml of water; a deep purple colour is produced.

2. Dissolve 500 mg in 5 ml of water, add 5 ml of *trinitrophenol solution*, stir to induce crystallisation, and filter; a precipitate is produced which, after washing with water and drying at 105°, melts at about 235° with decomposition.

Determination in body fluids. THIN-LAYER CHROMATOGRAPHY. In serum or urine—D. M. Benjamin *et al.*, *Analyt. Chem.*, 1973, **45**, 1531.

Metabolism. ABSORPTION. Poorly absorbed after oral administration and well absorbed after intramuscular or subcutaneous injection.

BLOOD CONCENTRATIONS. Following an intramuscular dose of 0.6 g, a peak concentration of about 20 μg/ml is obtained within 1 to 2 hours; following an intravenous infusion of 3.33 mg/kg per hour, serum levels of about 15 μg/ml are attained.

HALF-LIFE. Serum half-life, about 3 hours in normal subjects and 3 to 4 days in oliguria; in premature infants and infants from 5 to 21 days old, the half-life is increased to 18 and 6 hours respectively and in the elderly it is increased to about 6 hours. There appears to be a linear relationship between serum creatinine concentration and the half-life of kanamycin and therefore creatinine concentrations may be used to calculate dose adjustments in subjects with renal dysfunction.

DISTRIBUTION. Kanamycin appears in the peritoneal, synovial, and pleural fluids, and also in small amounts in prostatic and amniotic fluids; negligible amounts are found in the cerebrospinal fluid of adults but in children these levels may be 10 to 20% of that of the corresponding blood level; apparent volume of distribution, 20 to 25% body-weight; *protein binding*, about 1% bound to plasma proteins. It may accumulate when renal function is impaired.

EXCRETION. Excreted mainly in the urine but small amounts may be found in the bile; 40 to 100% of a dose is excreted in the urine in 24 hours.

FURTHER INFORMATION. Pharmacokinetics—J. T. Clarke *et al.*, *Clin. Pharmac. Ther.*, 1974, **15**, 610; J. T. Doluisio *et al.*, *J Pharmacokinet. Biopharm.*, 1973, **1**, 253.

Actions and uses. Kanamycin sulphate is an aminoglycoside antibiotic and has a spectrum of antibacterial activity similar to that of gentamicin sulphate but it is more toxic and resistance develops more rapidly. It is bactericidal in action. It is used primarily in the treatment of systemic and urinary infections caused by organisms insensitive to less toxic antibiotics. It is also occasionally used as a second line drug against tuberculosis.

Absorption from the gut is poor and in systemic infections kanamycin is given by injection. It may however be administered by mouth for the treatment of diarrhoea of bacterial origin and in the preparation of the gut for large bowel surgery. Resistance is fairly readily induced and cross-resistance with other aminoglycosides, particularly streptomycin and neomycin, is common.

For intestinal infections kanamycin sulphate is given by mouth in doses of the equivalent of 30 milligrams of kanamycin per kilogram body-weight daily in divided doses and for pre-operative bowel preparation the equivalent of 90 milligrams of kanamycin may be given daily in divided doses for a few days.

The dose for systemic and urinary infections is the equivalent of 0.5 to 1 gram of kanamycin daily in 2 to 4 divided doses by intramuscular injection for an adult, or the equivalent of 15 milligrams of kanamycin per kilogram body-weight daily in divided doses for children. Kanamycin sulphate may also be given by slow intravenous infusion of 3 to 4 millilitres per minute of a 0.25% solution up to a total dose equivalent to 15 to 30 milligrams of kanamycin per kilogram body-weight daily in 2 or 3 divided doses; the total dose should not exceed a maximum of 1 gram of kanamycin daily.

The dose by intrathecal injection is the equivalent of 25 to 50 milligrams of kanamycin daily for an adult or 2.5 to 12.5 milligrams daily for a child.

1.2 grams of kanamycin sulphate is equivalent to 1 gram of kanamycin.

Undesirable effects. As for Gentamicin Sulphate. The margin between therapeutic and toxic levels is narrower. The principal toxic effect is on the eighth cranial nerve resulting in vertigo and deafness. Pain at the site of intramuscular injection sometimes occurs. Skin eruptions, nausea, and vomiting usually disappear quickly on withdrawing treatment.

Precautions. As for Gentamicin Sulphate.

Caution should be exercised during prolonged usage of kanamycin (as in tuberculosis) and in patients with impaired renal function the dosage should be reduced in accordance with published nomograms (G. E. Mawer *et al.*, *Lancet*, i/1972, 12).

Kanamycin impairs neuromuscular transmission and while this action is too weak to cause symptoms in normal subjects caution should be exercised in patients with myasthenia gravis.

Drug interactions. As for Gentamicin Sulphate. In addition, kanamycin may potentiate the neuromuscular blocking action of procainamide.

Preparations

KANAMYCIN INJECTION: see above under Kanamycin Acid Sulphate.

OTHER PREPARATIONS available include CAPSULES containing kanamycin sulphate equivalent to 250 mg (250 000 units) of kanamycin.

Kaolin, Heavy

A purified native hydrated aluminium silicate, powdered, and freed from gritty particles by elutriation.

OTHER NAME: Kaolinum Ponderosum

When Kaolin or Light Kaolin is prescribed or demanded, Light Kaolin is supplied, unless it has been ascertained that Light Kaolin (Natural) is required.

A standard is given in the European Pharmacopoeia Vol. III

The native clay is derived from the decomposition of the felspar of granite rocks and contains about 47% of silica, 40% of alumina, and 13% of water. It is mined in large quantities in Cornwall.

Description. *Macroscopical characters:* a fine, white or greyish-white, odourless, almost tasteless powder, unctuous to the touch.

Microscopical characters: irregularly angular particles, up to about 60 μm in width, intermixed with innumerable minute fragments, about 1 or 2 μm in width. With *alcoholic methylene blue solution*, kaolin stains deep blue but, with *safranine solution*, only a very faint pink or not at all; mounted in cresol, it is clearly visible and shines brightly on a dark field under crossed polars.

Solubility. Practically insoluble in water and in mineral acids.

Sterilisation. It is sterilised by heating at a temperature not lower than 160° for sufficient time to ensure that the whole of the powder is maintained at that temperature for 1 hour.

Uses. Heavy kaolin is used in the preparation of kaolin poultice.

Preparation

KAOLIN POULTICE (*Syn.* Cataplasma Kaolini):

Heavy kaolin, finely sifted,

dried at 100°	527.0 g
Thymol	0.5 g
Boric acid, finely sifted	45.0 g
Peppermint oil	0.5 ml
Methyl salicylate	2.0 ml
Glycerol	425.0 g

Mix the heavy kaolin and the boric acid with the glycerol, heat at 120° for 1 hour, stirring occasionally, and allow to cool. Add the thymol, previously dissolved in the methyl salicylate, and the peppermint oil, and mix thoroughly.

A standard for this poultice is given in the British Pharmaceutical Codex 1973

Containers and *Storage:* it should be stored and supplied in well-closed containers which prevent evaporation.

Advice for patients: for use in reducing pain and inflammation. It should be warmed and applied liberally to the affected area, either directly or between layers of muslin.

Kaolin, Light

A purified native hydrated aluminium silicate, free from gritty particles, obtained by elutriating powdered native kaolin and collecting the fraction having the required particle size. It contains a suitable dispersing agent.

OTHER NAMES: Kaolinum Leve; *Kaopectate®*; *Kaylene® Kaylene-Ol®* (with liquid paraffin)

When Kaolin or Light Kaolin is prescribed or demanded, Light Kaolin is supplied, unless it has been ascertained that Light Kaolin (Natural) is required.

A standard is given in the British Pharmacopoeia 1973

Description. *Macroscopical characters:* a light white, odourless, tasteless powder free from gritty particles and unctuous to the touch.

Microscopical characters: irregularly angular particles, up to about 10 μm in width, intermixed with innumerable minute fragments, about 1 to 2 μm in width. With *alcoholic methylene blue solution*, kaolin stains deep blue but, with *safranine solution*, only a very faint pink or not at all; mounted in cresol it is clearly visible and shines brightly on a dark field under crossed polars.

Solubility. Practically insoluble in water and in mineral acids.

Moisture content. Not more than 1.5%, determined by drying at 105°.

Hygroscopicity. At relative humidities between about 15 and 65% the equilibrium moisture content at 25° is about 1%, but at relative humidities above about 75%, it absorbs small amounts of moisture.

Sterilisation. As for Kaolin, Heavy.

Actions and uses. Light kaolin is an adsorbent. It is administered by mouth in the symptomatic treatment of enteritis, colitis, and dysentery associated with food poisoning and alkaloidal poisoning. It may be administered suspended in water.

The usual daily dose for adults is 15 to 75 grams of kaolin. Infants under one year may be given 1 gram and children aged 1 to 5 years, 2 grams one to three times daily, as necessary.

Light kaolin is applied externally as a dusting-powder, either undiluted or mixed with other protectives. It is an ingredient of toilet powders and a basis of disinfectant powders. It is also used for clarification purposes.

Veterinary uses. Light kaolin is used in animals as an adsorbent in the treatment of diarrhoea, the usual single dose for all species being 0.5 to 1 gram per kilogram body-weight.

Preparations

KAOLIN AND MORPHINE MIXTURE (*Syn.* Mistura Kaolini Sedativa):

Light kaolin or light kaolin (natural) ..		..	200 g
Chloroform and morphine tincture		..	40 ml
Sodium bicarbonate	..	.. ..	50 g
Water for preparations ..	..	..	to 1000 ml

It should be recently prepared, unless the kaolin has been sterilised.

A standard for this mixture is given in the British Pharmaceutical Codex 1973

Containers: see the entry on Mixtures for general information on containers.

Labelling: see the entry on Mixtures for general information on labelling. A direction to shake the bottle should be given on the label.

Dose: 10 millilitres.

Advice for patients: the mixture should not be used for longer than a few days without medical advice.

KAOLIN AND MORPHINE POWDER FOR MIXTURE:

Light kaolin or light kaolin (natural) ..		..	800 g
Sodium bicarbonate	..	.. ..	200 g

Mix, as described in the entry on Powders.

Labelling: the directions given under Powders for Mixtures should be followed.

Preparation of 1000 ml of kaolin and morphine mixture: add 250 g of the powder for mixture to about 500 ml of water for preparations and shake. Add 40 ml of chloroform and morphine tincture, shake, add sufficient water for preparations to produce 1000 ml and again shake.

KAOLIN MIXTURE (*Syn.* Mistura Kaolini Alkalina):

Light kaolin or light kaolin (natural) ..		..	200 g
Light magnesium carbonate	..	..	50 g
Sodium bicarbonate	..	.. ..	50 g
Peppermint emulsion, concentrated ..		..	25 ml
Chloroform water, double-strength ..		..	500 ml
Water for preparations ..	..	..	to 1000 ml

It should be recently prepared, unless the kaolin has been sterilised.

A standard for this mixture is given in the British Pharmaceutical Codex 1973

Containers: see the entry on Mixtures for general information on containers.

Labelling: see the entry on Mixtures for general information on labelling. A direction to shake the bottle should be given on the label.

Dose: 10 to 20 millilitres.

Advice for patients: the mixture should not be used for longer than a few days without medical advice.

KAOLIN POWDER FOR MIXTURE:

Light kaolin or light kaolin (natural) ..	..	666.6 g
Light magnesium carbonate ..	.. ..	166.7 g
Sodium bicarbonate ..	.. .. ..	166.7 g

Mix, as described in the entry on Powders.
Labelling: the directions given under Powders for Mixtures should be followed.
Preparation of 1000 ml of kaolin mixture: add 300 g of the powder for mixture to 500 ml of double-strength chloroform water and shake. Add 25 ml of concentrated peppermint emulsion, shake, add sufficient water for preparations to produce 1000 ml and again shake.

KAOLIN VETERINARY MIXTURE:

Light kaolin or light kaolin (natural)	200 g
Light magnesium carbonate	50 g
Sodium bicarbonate	50 g
Water for preparations	to 1000 ml

It should be freshly prepared, unless the kaolin has been sterilised, in which case it may be recently prepared.
A standard for this mixture is given in the British Pharmacopoeia (Veterinary)
Containers: see the entry on Mixtures for general information on containers.
Labelling: see the entry on Mixtures for general information on labelling. A direction to shake the bottle should be given on the label.

PAEDIATRIC KAOLIN MIXTURE:

Light kaolin or light kaolin (natural)	200 g
Amaranth solution	10 ml
Benzoic acid solution	20 ml
Raspberry syrup	200 ml
Chloroform water, double-strength	500 ml
Water for preparations	to 1000 ml

It should be recently prepared, unless the kaolin has been sterilised.
A standard for this mixture is given in the British Pharmaceutical Codex 1973
Containers: see the entry on Mixtures for general information on containers.
Labelling: see the entry on Mixtures for general information on labelling. A direction to shake the bottle should be given on the label.
Dose: CHILD: up to 1 year, 5 millilitres; 1 to 5 years, 10 millilitres.
Advice for patients: the mixture should not be used for longer than a few days without medical advice.

OTHER PREPARATIONS available include an EMULSION containing light kaolin 7.5% with liquid paraffin 22.5% and a MIXTURE containing light kaolin 1.03 g in 5 ml, diluent water, life of diluted mixture 14 days.
Light kaolin is an ingredient of compound calcium carbonate powder and of compound magnesium carbonate powder. It is also an ingredient of numerous compound preparations for the treatment of diarrhoea.

Kaolin, Light (Natural)

A purified native hydrated aluminium silicate, free from gritty particles; it differs from light kaolin in that it does not contain a dispersing agent.
When Kaolin or Light Kaolin is prescribed or demanded, Light Kaolin is supplied unless it has been ascertained that Light Kaolin (Natural) is required.
A standard is given in the British Pharmacopoeia 1973
Description; Solubility; Moisture content. As for Kaolin, Light.
Sterilisation. As for Kaolin, Heavy.
Actions and uses. Light kaolin (natural) may be used for the same purposes as light kaolin. Kaolin mixtures may be prepared with light kaolin or with light kaolin (natural).

Preparations
See above under Light Kaolin.

Ketoprofen
2-(3-Benzoylphenyl)propionic acid

$C_{16}H_{14}O_3 = 254.3$
OTHER NAMES: *Alrheumat®; Orudis®*
Description. A white to off-white powder.
Identification. MELTING-POINT. About 93°.
ULTRAVIOLET ABSORPTION. In 0.1N hydrochloric acid, maximum at 260 nm (E1%, 1cm = 665).
INFRA-RED ABSORPTION. Major peaks at 690, 714, 1226, 1284, 1656, and 1693 cm^{-1} (see Appendix 2a: Infra-red Spectra).
THIN-LAYER CHROMATOGRAPHY. See under Thin-layer Chromatography, System 3.
Metabolism. ABSORPTION. Well absorbed after parenteral, rectal, or oral administration.
BLOOD CONCENTRATION. After intramuscular administration of 50 mg, peak serum concentrations of 5 to 12 µg/ml are attained in 10 to 30 minutes; after rectal administration of 150 mg, peak serum concentrations of 2 to 8 µg/ml are attained in 2 to 3 hours; after oral administration of 100 mg, as capsules, peak serum concentrations of 3 to 12 µg/ml are attained in about 2 hours; and after the same dose in enteric-coated capsules, peak serum concentrations of 2 to 8 µg/ml are attained in 2 to 3 hours.
HALF-LIFE. Serum half-life, 1.5 to 2 hours.
DISTRIBUTION. *Protein binding,* 60 to 95% bound to plasma proteins.
METABOLIC REACTIONS. Mainly glucuronic acid conjugation and also some hydroxylation.
EXCRETION. After oral, rectal, or intramuscular doses, 30 to 90% is excreted in the urine in 24 hours.
FURTHER INFORMATION. Pharmacological activity—R. N. Brogden *et al., Drugs,* 1974, **8**, 168; metabolism—P. Populaire *et al., Annls pharm. Fr.,* 1973, **31**, 679, 735.
Actions and uses. Ketoprofen is an analgesic with anti-inflammatory properties and has the actions and uses described under Ibuprofen but it has a greater incidence of gastro-intestinal side-effects.
The usual dosage is 50 milligrams 3 times daily which may be increased to 50 milligrams 4 times daily or decreased

to 50 milligrams twice daily depending on the size and condition of the patient and the severity of the disease.

Undesirable effects; Precautions. As for Ibuprofen.

Preparations

Preparations available include CAPSULES containing ketoprofen 50 mg.

Klinefelter's Syndrome

A hereditary form of male hypogonadism (see under Hypogonadism).

Lachesine Chloride

(2-Benziloyloxyethyl)ethyldimethylammonium chloride

$$
\left[\begin{array}{cc} C_6H_5 & CH_3 \\ | & |+ \\ HO\cdot C\cdot CO\cdot O\cdot [CH_2]_2\cdot N\cdot C_2H_5 \\ | & | \\ C_6H_5 & CH_3 \end{array} \right] \; Cl^-
$$

$C_{20}H_{26}ClNO_3 = 363.9$

OTHER NAMES: Laches. Chlor.; Lachesine

A standard is given in the British Pharmaceutical Codex 1973

Description. An odourless white amorphous powder.

Solubility. Soluble, at 20°, in 3 parts of water and in 10 parts of alcohol (90%); very slightly soluble in ether, in chloroform, and in acetone.

Incompatibility. Lachesine chloride is incompatible in aqueous solution at concentrations of 1% or above with 0.01% of benzalkonium chloride; at concentrations of 2% and above, it is incompatible with 0.002% of phenylmercuric salts and with 0.01% of chlorhexidine acetate if the solution is boiled or autoclaved.

Sterilisation. Solutions are sterilised by heating in an autoclave, by heating with a bactericide, or by filtration.

Identification. TESTS. 1. Mix about 10 mg with 4 drops of sulphuric acid; an orange-red colour is produced, which quickly changes to rose-pink.
2. To a solution in water add *gold chloride solution*; a precipitate is produced which, after washing with water and drying, melts at about 148°.

MELTING-POINT. After drying at 105°, it melts at about 214°, darkening and shrinking at 2° or 3° below the melting-point.

ULTRAVIOLET ABSORPTION. In 0.1N hydrochloric acid, maxima at 254 nm, 259 nm (E1%, 1cm = 12), and 265 nm.

INFRA-RED ABSORPTION. Major peaks at 699, 743, 1176, 1241, 1449, and 1739 cm^{-1} (see Appendix 2a: Infra-red Spectra).

Actions and uses. Lachesine has mydriatic and cycloplegic actions similar to those described under Atropine. The degree and duration of the cycloplegic effect are about midway between those produced by homatropine and atropine; in old people, however, the response to miotics is slower and less complete after lachesine than when homatropine has been used. The mydriatic action of lachesine is neither so rapid nor so prolonged as that of atropine; it reaches a maximum in about an hour and begins to subside after 5 or 6 hours.
Lachesine is particularly useful in patients with hypersensitivity to atropine and hyoscine, as it does not give

rise to irritation of the conjunctiva or to eczema of the eyelids. It is usually administered as a 1% aqueous solution, 2 drops delivered into the conjunctival sac being the usual dose.

Precautions. As for Cyclopentolate Hydrochloride.

Preparation

LACHESINE EYE-DROPS: consisting of a sterile solution containing up to 1% of lachesine chloride, with 0.002% of phenylmercuric acetate or nitrate, in purified water. It is prepared by method A, B, or C described in the entry on Eye-drops.
A standard for these eye-drops is given in the British Pharmaceutical Codex 1973
Containers: see the entry on Eye-drops for general information on containers. This solution is adversely affected by alkali.
Labelling: see the entry on Eye-drops for general information on labelling.
Advice for patients: see the entry on Eye-drops for general information on the use of eye-drops. Blurring and sensitivity to light may occur for up to 24 hours after instillation of the eye-drops.

Lactic Acid

2-Hydroxypropionic acid
$CH_3 \cdot CH(OH) \cdot CO_2H = 90.08$

OTHER NAMES: Acidum Lacticum
Duofilm® (with salicylic acid)

A standard is given in the European Pharmacopoeia Vol. III

Lactic acid consists of a mixture of 2-hydroxypropionic acid, its condensation products, such as lactoyl-lactic acid and polylactic acids, and water. The equilibrium between lactic acid and polylactic acids depends on the concentration and the temperature.
Lactic acid is usually in the form of the racemate (*RS*-lactic acid), but sometimes the (+)-*S*-isomer is predominant.

Description. A colourless or slightly yellow, syrupy, hygroscopic liquid which is odourless or has a slight but not unpleasant odour and a taste which, in dilute aqueous solution, is mildly acid.

Solubility. Miscible with water, with alcohol, and with ether.

Weight per ml. At 20°, about 1.20 g.

Dissociation constant. pK_a 3.9 (25°).

Storage. It should be stored in airtight containers.

Actions and uses. Lactic acid is used in the preparation of compound sodium lactate injection and other solutions containing sodium lactate which are given by intravenous injection in the treatment of diabetic coma as described under Insulin Injection. Compound sodium lactate injection is given also by mouth for infantile gastro-enteritis. Lactate is converted slowly into bicarbonate in the blood and restores diminished alkali reserve without the danger of producing alkalosis.
Lactic acid milk may be given in infantile gastro-enteritis; it may check the vomiting but not the diarrhoea. It has also been used for infant feeding when breast milk is not available. It is prepared by adding lactic acid to whole milk in the proportion of 5 to 7 millilitres to the litre; the acid should be added drop by drop to the cold milk, stirring vigorously to prevent the formation of clots. A

fine flocculent curd results, which will flow through an ordinary rubber teat. Sugar or honey is then added. After the addition of the acid the milk must not be unduly heated or thick clots will form.

Lactic acid, which is normally present in the vaginal secretion, is used in the treatment of leucorrhoea as a 0.5 to 2% vaginal douche or in pessaries prepared with glycerol suppositories mass.

Preparations

COMPOUND SODIUM LACTATE INJECTION (*Syn.* Hartmann's Solution for Injection; Ringer-Lactate Solution for Injection):

Lactic acid	2.4 ml
Sodium hydroxide..	1.15 g
Dilute hydrochloric acid	a sufficient quantity
Calcium chloride	0.27 g
Potassium chloride	0.4 g
Sodium chloride	6.0 g
Water for injections	to 1000.0 ml

Dissolve the sodium hydroxide in 200 ml of the water, add the lactic acid, and heat in an autoclave at 115° to 116° for 1 hour. Cool, and cautiously add sufficient of the dilute hydrochloric acid (about 1 ml is normally required) until a few drops of the solution give a full orange colour with 1 drop of *phenol red solution*. Dissolve the other ingredients in 700 ml of the water, mix the two solutions, and add sufficient of the water to produce the required volume. Clarify by filtration and immediately sterilise by heating in an autoclave.

A standard for this injection is given in the British Pharmacopoeia 1973

Containers: see the entry on Injections for general information on containers.

Labelling: see the entry on Injections for general information on labelling. In addition, when the injection is intended for intravenous infusion, the label on the container should state that the injection contains, in millimoles per litre, the following approximate amounts of ions: Na^+ 131, K^+ 5, Ca^{2+} 2, HCO_3^- (as lactate) 29, and Cl^- 111.

Storage: it may, on storage, cause the separation of small solid particles from a glass container. A solution containing such particles must not be used.

SODIUM LACTATE INJECTION:

Lactic acid	14 ml
Sodium hydroxide..	6.7 g
Dilute hydrochloric acid	a sufficient quantity
Water for injections	to 1000 ml

Dissolve the sodium hydroxide in 400 ml of the water, add the lactic acid, and heat in an autoclave at 115° to 116° for 1 hour. Cool, and cautiously add sufficient of the dilute hydrochloric acid (about 2 ml is normally required) until a few drops of the solution give a full orange colour with 1 drop of *phenol red solution*. Add sufficient of the water to produce the required volume, clarify by filtration, and immediately sterilise by heating in an autoclave.

A standard for this injection is given in the British Pharmacopoeia 1973

Containers: see the entry on Injections for general information on containers.

Labelling: see the entry on Injections for general information on labelling. In addition, when the injection is intended for intravenous infusion, the label on the container should state that the injection is one-sixth molar and contains, in 1 litre, approximately 167 millimoles each of Na^+ and HCO_3^- (as lactate) ions.

Storage: it may, on storage, cause the separation of small solid particles from a glass container. A solution containing such particles must not be used.

OTHER PREPARATIONS available include a COLLODION containing lactic acid 16.7% with salicylic acid 16.7%.

Lactose

4-*O*-β-D-Galactopyranosyl-α-D-glucopyranose monohydrate

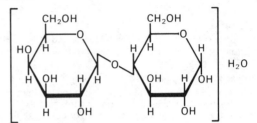

$C_{12}H_{22}O_{11},H_2O = 360.3$

OTHER NAMES: Lactosum; Milk Sugar

A standard is given in the European Pharmacopoeia Vol. II

Description. An odourless white crystalline powder with a slightly sweet taste.

Solubility. Soluble, at 20°, in 6 parts of water; soluble in 1 part of boiling water; very sightly soluble in alcohol, in ether, and in chloroform.

Specific rotation. +52.2° to +52.8°, determined on a solution prepared by dissolving 10 g in 80 ml of water, adding 1 drop of *dilute ammonia solution*, allowing to stand for 15 to 30 minutes and diluting to 100 ml with water.

Hygroscopicity. It absorbs insignificant amounts of moisture at 25° at relative humidities up to about 90%.

Sterilisation. It is first dried at 105° and then sterilised by dry heat.

Identification. TESTS. 1. To 5 ml of a 1% solution add 2 ml of *dilute sodium hydroxide solution* and 3 drops of *copper sulphate solution*; the solution is blue and clear. Heat to boiling; an abundant red precipitate is produced. 2. Mix 5 ml of a 5% solution with 5 ml of *dilute ammonia solution* and heat on a water-bath at 80° for 10 minutes; a red colour is produced.

Actions and uses. Lactose is less sweet than sucrose and less liable to cause intestinal fermentation in infants. It is added to diluted cows' milk for infant feeding to adjust the carbohydrate content to that of human milk.

Lactose is used as a diluent for standardised vegetable products and to give bulk to powders, particularly those which are to be compressed into tablets intended to dissolve completely.

Precautions. Lactose intolerance may occur in persons deficient in intestinal lactase. They should avoid lactose and preparations containing it which may cause abdominal distension, cramps, diarrhoea, and flatulence.

Lactulose

4-O-β-D-Galactopyranosyl-D-fructose, a synthetic sugar.

$C_{12}H_{22}O_{11} = 342.3$

OTHER NAMES: *Duphalac*® (with lactose and galactose); *Gatinar*® (with lactose, galactose, tagatose, and other ketonic sugars)

Solubility. Soluble in water.

Actions and uses. Lactulose is used in the treatment of constipation. It is degraded to organic acids such as lactic acid by the action of saccharolytic enzymes in the flora of the colon. It stimulates peristalsis and softens the faeces by osmotic action. Lactulose is not absorbed and may be given to diabetics and during late pregnancy.

Lactulose is available as an elixir containing about 67% w/v of lactulose in conjunction with other sugars such as lactose and galactose. The initial dose of lactulose elixir for an adult is 15 millilitres, twice daily. For children under one year 2.5 millilitres is administered twice daily, 1 to 5 years 5 millilitres twice daily, and 6 to 10 years 10 millilitres twice daily.

In the treatment of portal systemic encephalopathy 30 to 50 millilitres of the elixir may be given 3 times a day; the dose is adjusted so that soft stools are produced 2 or 3 times a day.

Contra-indications. Lactulose should not be given to patients with galactosaemia.

Preparations

Preparations available include an ELIXIR containing lactulose 3.325 g with lactose 33.25 mg and galactose 532 mg in 5 ml, diluent water, life of diluted elixir 14 days; and an elixir containing lactulose 3.35 g with lactose, galactose, tagatose, and other ketonic sugars 1.34 g in 5 ml, which should not be diluted.

Laevulose

D-(−)-Fructopyranose

$C_6H_{12}O_6 = 180.2$

OTHER NAMES: Fructose; *Laevuflex*®; Laevulosum; *Levugen*®
Ethulose® (with alcohol)

A standard is given in the European Pharmacopoeia Vol. II

Description. An odourless white crystalline powder with a very sweet taste.

Solubility. Soluble, at 20°, in less than 1 part of water and in 15 parts of alcohol; very slightly soluble in ether.

Specific rotation. −91.0° to −93.5°, determined by dissolving 10 g in 80 ml of water, adding 1 drop of *dilute ammonia solution*, allowing to stand for 2 hours, and diluting to 100 ml.

Sterilisation. Solutions for injection are sterilised immediately after preparation by heating in an autoclave.

Storage. It should be stored in airtight containers, in a cool place.

Identification. TESTS. 1. Mix 1 ml of a 10% solution with 5 ml of *cupro-citric solution* and heat at 40° for 30 minutes; an orange-yellow precipitate is produced.
2. To 1 ml of a 10% solution add 10 ml of water and 5 ml of hydrochloric acid and heat at 70°; the solution turns brown.
3. To 1 drop of a 50% solution add 200 mg of resorcinol and 9 ml of hydrochloric acid and heat on a water-bath for 2 minutes; a red colour is produced.

Actions and uses. Laevulose is sweeter than sucrose. In contrast to dextrose, it does not require insulin for its utilisation and conversion into glycogen. When administered intravenously it is metabolised nearly twice as rapidly as dextrose, but the rate of absorption after oral administration is less than half that of dextrose. Laevulose is mainly metabolised in the liver, where it is first phosphorylated and then partially converted into dextrose; it is probable that some laevulose is also metabolised in adipose tissue. Owing to its rapid metabolism by the liver, laevulose has little effect on the blood-sugar level, except in diabetics who convert it largely into dextrose. When administered intravenously in conjunction with amino-acids, laevulose has a protein-sparing action.

Laevulose accelerates the metabolism of ethyl alcohol and is used in the treatment of alcohol poisoning; for this purpose 500 millilitres of a 40% solution may be given by intravenous infusion. It should not be used for the treatment of methyl alcohol poisoning as it accelerates the oxidation of methyl alcohol to formaldehyde.

Laevulose is given intravenously, in preference to dextrose, as a source of carbohydrate in the treatment of renal failure, in which condition dextrose tolerance is impaired, whereas laevulose tolerance is not.

It is also useful in the management of neonatal hypoglycaemia, which may occur in newborn infants of diabetic mothers receiving large doses of insulin; laevulose given by the umbilical vein in these infants produces a more prolonged rise in blood-sugar level than an equivalent quantity of dextrose.

Laevulose offers no advantage over dextrose as a source of carbohydrate for the diabetic or in diabetic emergencies because it is largely converted into dextrose in the diabetic liver, the degree of conversion increasing with the severity of the diabetes.

Laevulose has been used as a source of carbohydrate in debilitated patients suffering from a variety of conditions, including muscular dystrophy, vomiting of pregnancy, senility, and chronic alcoholism, but there is no evidence that it has any advantage over other carbohydrates or carbohydrate-containing foods for such patients.

Laevulose has been used as a diagnostic agent for assessing liver function.

The dosage of laevulose depends upon the condition being treated. Up to 150 grams of laevulose or even more may be given by mouth daily in divided doses of 2 to 25 grams. It may also be given by slow intravenous infusion of a 20 or 40% solution in doses up to 200 grams.

Undesirable effects. Large doses given by mouth may cause abdominal distress and diarrhoea, probably as a result of an osmotic effect. Large infusions may cause sweating, flushing, and epigastric discomfort or pain. Thrombophlebitis may occur from too rapid intravenous injection of strong solutions.

Contra-indications. Laevulose should not be given to patients with familial laevulose intolerance, which is due to a congenital absence of the enzyme breaking down phosphorylated laevulose; in such subjects, laevulose causes hypoglycaemia and accumulation of laevulose in the liver, which may suffer damage. Sucrose produces a similar effect in such subjects.

Preparations

LAEVULOSE INJECTION: a sterile solution of laevulose in water for injections. It is sterilised, immediately after preparation, by heating in an autoclave. Available in 500-ml glass bottles containing 20% of laevulose and in 500-ml plastic packs containing 5, 10, and 20% of laevulose.
A standard for this injection is given in the British Pharmacopoeia 1973
Containers: see the entry on Injections for general information on containers.
Labelling: see the entry on Injections for general information on labelling. In addition, the label on the container should state the amount of the medicament as the number of grams of laevulose per litre.
Storage: it should be stored at a temperature not exceeding 25°.

OTHER PREPARATIONS available include an INJECTION containing laevulose 15% with alcohol 5% w/w.

Lamb Dysentery Antiserum

see CLOSTRIDIUM PERFRINGENS TYPE B ANTITOXIN

Lanatoside C

3-[(O-β-D-Glucopyranosyl-(1 → 4)-O-3-acetyl-2,6-dideoxy-β-D-*ribo*-hexopyranosyl-(1 → 4)-O-2,6-dideoxy-β-D-*ribo*-hexopyranosyl-(1 → 4)-O-2,6-dideoxy-β-D-*ribo*-hexopyranosyl)oxy]-12,14-dihydroxy-3β,5β,12β,14β-card-20(22)enolide

$C_{49}H_{76}O_{20} = 985.1$

OTHER NAME: *Cedilanid®* (this name is also applied to a preparation of deslanoside)

A standard is given in the British Pharmacopoeia 1973

Description. An odourless, white, crystalline, hygroscopic powder or colourless crystals.

Solubility. Very slightly soluble in water and in ether; soluble, at 20°, in 20 parts of methyl alcohol.

Moisture content. Not more than 7.5%, determined by drying over phosphorus pentoxide *in vacuo*.

Specific rotation. +31.5° to +34.5°, determined on a 2% solution in methyl alcohol.

Storage. It should be stored in airtight containers, protected from light.

Identification. TESTS. It complies with the tests described under Deslanoside.

MELTING-POINT. Above 240°, with decomposition.

Metabolism. ABSORPTION. Poorly absorbed after oral administration; it is converted to digoxin in the gastrointestinal tract by acid hydrolysis and by the action of gut flora which results in a second absorption phase—that of digoxin. The administration of antacids reduces the acid hydrolysis and hence reduces the amount of digoxin formed.

BLOOD CONCENTRATION. Two peaks of plasma concentration occur for drug plus metabolites, one at 90 minutes due to the absorption of digoxin, and the other at 5 hours due to the absorption of lanatoside C.

DISTRIBUTION. Crosses the placenta; *protein binding*, weakly bound to plasma proteins.

METABOLIC REACTIONS. Hydrolysis to derivatives of digoxigenin and also deacetylation to deslanoside.

EXCRETION. After an oral dose, about 18% is excreted in the urine, and of the excreted material, about 80% is digoxin and a small amount includes other derivatives of digoxigenin; after an intravenous dose, about 25% is excreted in the urine in 24 hours, and of the excreted material, 70% is unchanged and the remainder is digoxin and desacetyl lanatoside C (deslanoside).

Actions and uses. Lanatoside C has the actions and uses described under Digitalis Leaf. Its rate of onset and duration of action are similar to those of oral digoxin. The usual digitalising dose is 1 to 1.5 milligrams daily in divided doses with a maintenance dose of 250 to 750 micrograms daily when the desired therapeutic effect has been obtained.

Undesirable effects. The undesirable effects described under Digitalis Leaf may occur, but as lanatoside C is excreted more rapidly than most other cardiac glycosides it is less likely to give rise to cumulative effects.

Precautions; Poisoning. As for Digitalis Leaf.

Preparations

Preparations available include TABLETS containing lanatoside C 250 micrograms

Laryngitis

Acute laryngitis is characterised by hoarseness or loss of voice accompanied by local discomfort. It may be due to virus infection which is also producing infection of the nose and nasopharynx. Sometimes *Haemophilus influenzae* is the infecting organism. Excessive use of the voice, particularly shouting, may be a precipitating factor. Laryngitis may also occur in a chronic form with similar characteristics to the acute form and with throat irritation and spasmodic coughing.

Chronic laryngitis has similar causes to the acute disease and frequently occurs after repeated attacks of acute laryngitis; heavy smoking and nasal congestion are additional precipitating factors.

Warmth, rest, and steam inhalations may relieve the symptoms, and a cough suppressant may be given if required. Antibacterial treatment may be required if laryngitis is due to bacterial infection.

Laryngotracheitis Vaccine, Living

A freeze-dried preparation of naturally occurring or modified virus strains of low pathogenicity. The dried preparation is reconstituted immediately before use with an appropriate quantity of a suitable sterile liquid.

OTHER NAME: Infectious Laryngotracheitis Vaccine, Living

A standard is given in the British Pharmacopoeia (Veterinary)

Storage. The dried vaccine should be protected from light and stored at $-20°$ to $-30°$ when it may be expected to retain its potency for 2 years. If stored at $2°$ to $8°$ the vaccine will retain its potency for not longer than 6 months. It should be used immediately after reconstitution.

Veterinary uses. It is administered by eye-drops to chickens for prophylaxis of laryngotracheitis.

Lassa Fever

Lassa fever is an infectious disease now recognised to be caused by a virus of the *Arenavirus* group. It was first described in north-east Nigeria and is thought to be widely distributed throughout western Africa. Lassa fever has never occurred naturally outside this area; the only cases reported are laboratory infections and patients who contracted the disease in Africa and travelled elsewhere.

The reservoir of infection is thought to be a rodent, and man may become infected by direct contact or by inhalation of excretions or secretions of infected animals. When man is infected, the virus is found in the blood, urine, and secretions. The disease is spread by personal contact but in primary cases seems to be more frequently fatal than in secondary contacts.

The incubation period for lassa fever is 3 to 17 days and the onset is gradual; the severity of the symptoms increases after 3 to 5 days. Fever, myalgia, sore throat, and pharyngitis are prominent. There is relative bradycardia and there may be respiratory symptoms, a macular or papular rash, conjunctivitis, and bleeding from the skin or mucous membranes.

By the second week, if recovery does not occur, the patient may progress to shock, serous effusions, and severe haemorrhage and may succumb from renal or cardiac failure. Hepatomegaly with or without hepatitis occurs but never jaundice. The mortality is 30 to 50% but subclinical infection undoubtedly occurs.

Diagnosis is carried out in specially equipped laboratories. There are no known prophylactic measures and the only form of treatment involves the use of immune plasma or immunoglobulin prepared from the blood of a patient recovered from lassa fever. Such treatment is probably ineffective if begun after 6 days and this poses problems as the onset of disease is insidious and laboratory diagnosis of the virus takes at least 4 to 5 days. Wherever possible, suspected cases in an endemic area should be admitted to specially equipped isolation centres. Outside these areas the risk of spreading the disease and of infecting medical staff is far greater. Rodent control may be of value in specific areas.

Lavender Oil

Obtained by distillation from the fresh flowering tops of *Lavandula intermedia* Loisel. (English oil) or of *L. angustifolia* P. Miller (foreign oil) (Fam. Labiatae).

OTHER NAME: Oleum Lavandulae

A standard is given in the British Pharmaceutical Codex 1973

English lavender oil, which is usually considered to have the finer odour, contains little linalyl acetate. On the other hand, the fresh floral note of the French oil is enhanced in those oils having higher contents of linalyl acetate. The English oil is sometimes described as being easily distinguished from the French oil by its odour, which has a camphoraceous note.

Constituents. French lavender oil contains chiefly linalol and linalyl acetate, with small amounts of ethyl pentyl ketone, geraniol, and terpenes. English oil contains chiefly free linalol and little linalyl acetate, the total amount of linalol being similar to that in French oil. Cineole occurs in some quantity in English oil, but only in traces in French oil.

Description. A colourless, pale yellow, or yellowish-green liquid. The odour is reminiscent of the flowers.

Solubility. Soluble at $20°$, English oil, in 3 parts of alcohol (80%); foreign oil, in 4 parts of alcohol (70%). The solutions may be slightly opalescent and the oils become less soluble with age.

Weight per ml. At $20°$, English oil, 0.875 to 0.895 g; foreign oil, 0.878 to 0.892 g.

Refractive index. English oil, 1.460 to 1.474; foreign oil, 1.457 to 1.464.

Optical rotation. English oil, $-5°$ to $-13°$; foreign oil, $-5°$ to $-12°$.

Adulterants and substitutes. Adulterants of lavender oil include spike lavender oil, lavandin oil, linalol, and synthetic esters. Spike lavender oil decreases the ester content and increases the cineole content.

Storage. It should be stored in well-filled airtight containers, in a cool place, protected from light.

Uses. Lavender oil is used largely in perfumery and occasionally to cover disagreeable odours in ointments and other preparations. Its value as a preservative is equivocal.

Preparation

Lavender oil is an ingredient of gamma benzene hexachloride application.

Laxatives

see under CONSTIPATION

Leishmaniasis

Leishmaniasis is a chronic disease caused by protozoa of the genus *Leishmania* and transmitted by the sandfly (*Phlebotomus* spp.). *L. donovani* gives rise to a generalised disease known as visceral leishmaniasis (kala-azar). *L. tropica* and *L. brasiliensis* give rise to localised infections of the skin, or skin and mucous membranes respectively, known as cutaneous leishmaniasis.

Visceral leishmaniasis (kala-azar) is found around the Mediterranean and in the Sudan, East Africa, and India. The parasites invade and cause proliferation of the cells of the reticuloendothelial system within which they may be found as Leishman-Donovan bodies. Rapid enlargement of the liver, spleen, and lymph nodes results. Erythrophagocytosis, caused by immunologically mediated haemolytic anaemia may also contribute to these effects. Leucopenia and bone-marrow hyperplasia occasionally occur.
Onset of the disease is marked by tiredness and a fever which subsides spontaneously but reappears irregularly. The skin may become pigmented and there is lack of resistance to other infections.
Drugs used in the treatment of visceral leishmaniasis include amphotericin, pentamidine, sodium stibogluconate, and other compounds of antimony.

Cutaneous leishmaniasis (oriental sore) due to infection with *L. tropica* is characterised by the formation of an irritable papule which gradually enlarges, becomes indurated, and later ulcerates. The ulcer takes months to heal and leaves a scar resembling a vaccination mark. Infection with *L. tropica major* results in immunity to both major and minor varieties and deliberate infection of the leg with local live strains of *L. tropica major* has been practised as a means of preventing the unsightly lesions on the face.
L. brasiliensis produces a cutaneous lesion similar to that from *L. tropica* but after a quiescent period of up to 2 years there follows a destructive ulcerating lesion of the nasopharynx.
Cutaneous leishmaniasis may be treated with pentamidine or sodium stibogluconate.

Lemon Oil

Expressed from the outer part of the fresh pericarp of the ripe or nearly ripe fruit of *Citrus limon* (L.) Burm. f. (Fam. Rutaceae).

OTHER NAME: Oleum Limonis

A standard is given in the British Pharmaceutical Codex 1973

Constituents. Lemon oil consists chiefly of (+)-limonene which, together with small quantities of other terpenes, constitutes about 90% of the oil. The remaining 10% consists of oxygenated compounds, of which citral is present in the largest amount. The quality of the oil is not determined solely by the citral content.

Description. A pale yellow or greenish-yellow liquid. The odour is reminiscent of lemon.

Solubility. Soluble, at 20°, in 12 parts of alcohol (90%), the solution showing a slight opalescence; miscible with dehydrated alcohol.

Weight per ml. At 20°, 0.850 to 0.856 g.

Refractive index. 1.474 to 1.476.

Optical rotation. +57° to +65°.

Adulterants and substitutes. Lemon oil is sometimes adulterated with distilled lemon oil, with terpenes

obtained as residues in the preparation of terpeneless oils, with low-grade orange oil, and with citral obtained from lemon grass oil.

Storage. It should be stored in well-filled airtight containers, in a cool place, protected from light.

Uses. The principal use of lemon oil is as a flavouring and perfumery agent. It is used to make terpeneless lemon oil.

Preparations
Lemon oil is an ingredient of aromatic ammonia solution, aromatic ammonia spirit, benzalkonium lozenges, formaldehyde lozenges, mouth-wash solution-tablets, and pastille basis.

Lemon Oil, Terpeneless

Prepared by concentrating lemon oil *in vacuo* until most of the terpenes have been removed, or by solvent partition.

OTHER NAME: Oleum Limonis Deterpenatum

A standard is given in the British Pharmaceutical Codex 1973

Constituents. Terpeneless lemon oil consists chiefly of citral, with considerable quantities of esters, chiefly geranyl and linalyl acetates.

Description. A colourless or pale yellow liquid. It has the odour and taste of lemon.

Solubility. Soluble, at 20°, in 1 part of alcohol (80%).

Weight per ml. At 20°, 0.880 to 0.890 g.

Refractive index. 1.478 to 1.485.

Optical rotation. −4° to +1°.

Storage. It should be stored in well-filled airtight containers, in a cool place, protected from light.

Uses. Terpeneless lemon oil is used almost exclusively as a flavouring agent; it has the advantages of being stronger in flavour and odour and more readily soluble in dilute alcoholic solution than the natural oil.
The terpeneless oil is equivalent in flavour to 10 to 15 times its volume of lemon oil; a 1% solution in alcohol (70%) is generally used for culinary purposes.

Preparations

COMPOUND ORANGE SPIRIT (*Syn.* Spiritus Aurantii Compositus):

Terpeneless orange oil	..	..	..	2.50 ml
Terpeneless lemon oil	..	..	..	1.30 ml
Anise oil	..	..	..	..	4.25 ml
Coriander oil	..	..	..	..	6.25 ml
Alcohol (90%)	..	..	..	to 1000.00 ml

A standard for this spirit is given in the British Pharmaceutical Codex 1973

LEMON SPIRIT:

Terpeneless lemon oil	..	..	..	100 ml
Alcohol (95%)	..	..	..	to 1000 ml

A standard for this spirit is given in the British Pharmaceutical Codex 1973

LEMON SYRUP:

Lemon spirit	..	..	..	..	5 ml
Citric acid monohydrate	..	..	..	..	25 g
Invert syrup	..	..	..	..	100 ml
Syrup..	..	..	..	..	to 1000 ml

Dissolve the citric acid in a portion of the syrup, add the

invert syrup, the lemon spirit, and sufficient syrup to produce the required volume, and mix. It has a weight per ml at 20° of about 1.33 g.

A standard for this syrup is given in the British Pharmaceutical Codex 1973

Storage: it should be stored in a cool place.

Dose: 2.5 to 5 millilitres.

Lemon Peel, Dried

The dried outer part of the pericarp of the ripe, or nearly ripe, fruit of *Citrus limon* (L.) Burm. f. (Fam. Rutaceae), obtained principally from Spain, Italy, and Sicily.

OTHER NAME: Limonis Cortex Siccatus

A standard is given in the British Pharmacopoeia 1973

Constituents. Dried lemon peel contains volatile oil, vitamin C, hesperidin and other flavonoid glycosides, a bitter principle, mucilage, pectin, and calcium oxalate.

Description. *Macroscopical characters:* strips or pieces, outer surface yellow and somewhat rough from the presence of numerous minute pits, each corresponding to an oil gland; inner surface with only a small amount of white spongy pericarp; fracture short; some pieces with nipple-shaped apex attached.

It has an aromatic odour and an aromatic and bitter taste.

Microscopical characters: the diagnostic characters are: *epidermis* of small, polyhedral cells; tissue subjacent to the epidermis parenchymatous, many cells containing prismatic *crystals* of calcium oxalate, 15 to 25 μm long; numerous large lysigenous *oil glands* about 0.3 to 0.6 mm in diameter and small *vascular strands* embedded in the parenchyma.

Adulterants and substitutes. Peel which has been scarified by machines is dried and offered as dried lemon peel; it contains very little oil and can be distinguished by the fine lines of scarification or cuts on the outer surface.

Storage. It should be stored in airtight containers.

Actions and uses. Dried lemon peel is used as a flavouring agent.

Leprosy

Leprosy is a chronic disease due to infection with *Mycobacterium leprae*. The incubation period may be long and the disease is characterised by lesions of the skin and peripheral nerves. The disease occurs in two forms, lepromatous and tuberculoid leprosy, but many cases are intermediate in type and exhibit some of the characteristics of both forms.

Tuberculoid leprosy develops in patients with pronounced tissue reaction to the infection. The skin lesions are clearly demarcated and the peripheral nerves are involved early resulting in motor and sensory changes in the affected areas.

Lepromatous leprosy develops in patients with little resistance to the organisms, which are able to multiply and disseminate freely in the tissues resulting in a generalised disease. The skin lesions which may become extensive are at first flushed and shiny but indefinitely demarcated. Later the skin becomes thickened and oedematous and painless nodular lesions occur in the skin, which may become necrotic and ulcerate, releasing large numbers of mycobacteria. The mycobacteria surround the peripheral nerves, but there is little tissue reaction and con-

sequently little neurological damage until late in the disease.

Lepromatous and tuberculoid leprosy may also affect the eyes, testes, regional lymph nodes, bones, and sometimes other structures.

Leprosy is treated with suitable antibacterials but the disease is slow to respond and treatment has to be given for many years and sometimes for life. Care must be taken to prevent too rapid a destruction of *Mycobacterium leprae* since the breakdown products are toxic and may cause extensive tissue reaction.

Substances used in the treatment of leprosy include clofazimine, dapsone, thiacetazone, and thiambutosine.

Leptospira Antiserum

Native serum, or a preparation from native serum, containing the antibodies that give specific protection against strains of *Leptospira icterohaemorrhagiae.*

OTHER NAMES: Lep/Ser; Leptospira Icterohaemorrhagiae Antiserum

A standard is given in the British Pharmaceutical Codex 1973

Storage. It should be stored as described under Antisera.

Actions and uses. Leptospira antiserum is occasionally used in the treatment of spirochaetal jaundice (Weil's disease), mainly as an adjuvant to various forms of chemotherapy. Administration by the intravenous route is preferable in severe cases and by the intramuscular route in patients less severely affected. The usual dose is 20 to 40 millilitres.

Leptospira antiserum is not used routinely in prophylaxis. It is not effective against infections due to *L. canicola*, for which no specific antiserum is available for therapeutic use.

Leukaemia, Acute

Acute leukaemia is an acute proliferative disease of the bone marrow characterised by infiltration with the most primitive form of white-cell precursor. Four different forms may be recognised depending upon the morphology of the blast cell—lymphoblastic, myeloblastic, monoblastic, and those in which the cells are insufficiently differentiated to type.

In acute leukaemia, the bone marrow fails to make the normal elements of blood; this results in anaemia, a haemorrhagic state due to thrombocytopenia, and infections due to neutrophil leucopenia.

During the course of the disease, infiltration of any organ may occur. Infiltration of the central nervous system may result in leukaemic meningitis; there may also be splenomegaly and lymphadenopathy.

Acute lymphoblastic leukaemia responds to treatment much better than the other forms but the principle of the treatment of all forms is the same. *Remission* of acute leukaemia may be induced by corticosteroids together with vincristine or other antimitotic drugs. Prophylactic irradiation of the skull and spinal canal may be carried out to prevent or delay the onset of meningeal leukaemia.

Intermittent *maintenance* treatment with methotrexate or specific or non-specific immunotherapy may be used to delay relapse. When relapse occurs it may be treated with corticosteroids and vincristine or other antimitotic drugs.

Leukaemia, Chronic, Myeloid

see under MYELOPROLIFERATIVE DISEASES

Levallorphan Tartrate

(−)-*N*-Allyl-3-hydroxymorphinanium hydrogen tartrate

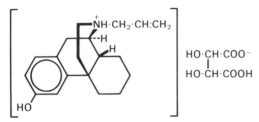

$C_{23}H_{31}NO_7 = 433.5$

OTHER NAMES: *Lorfan®*
Pethilorfan® (with pethidine hydrochloride)

A standard is given in the British Pharmacopoeia 1973

Description. An odourless white crystalline powder with an intensely bitter taste.

Solubility. Soluble, at 20°, in 20 parts of water and in 100 parts of alcohol; very slightly soluble in ether.

Acidity. A 0.2% solution has a pH of 3.2 to 4.

Specific rotation. −37.5° to −39°, determined on a 2% solution.

Dissociation constants. pK_a 4.5, 6.9.

Sterilisation. Solutions for injection are sterilised by heating in an autoclave or by filtration.

Storage. It should be stored in airtight containers, protected from light.

Identification. TESTS. 1. Dissolve about 5 mg in 1 ml of water containing 1 drop of hydrochloric acid and add a mixture of 1 ml of *potassium ferricyanide solution*, 1 drop of *ferric chloride test-solution*, and 4 ml of water; a green or bluish-green colour is produced (distinction from dextromethorphan).
2. Mix a few mg of the sample with an equal quantity of resorcinol, add 1 drop of sulphuric acid, and warm gently; an intense red colour is produced.

MELTING-POINT. About 176°.

ULTRAVIOLET ABSORPTION. In water, màximum at 279 nm (E1%, 1cm = 47); in 0.1N sodium hydroxide, maxima at 240 nm (E1%, 1cm = 204) and 299 nm (E1%, 1cm = 70).

THIN-LAYER CHROMATOGRAPHY. See under Thin-layer Chromatography, System 7.

Metabolism. DISTRIBUTION. Crosses the placenta.

METABOLIC REACTIONS. *N*-Dealkylation and conjugation with glucuronic acid; the major metabolite in most animals is 3-hydroxymorphinan in free and conjugated forms.

EXCRETION. In the rat, 5% is excreted in the urine unchanged in 24 hours, 2% is excreted as 3-hydroxymorphinan mostly in conjugated form, and 7% is excreted as an unidentified metabolite; traces of a dose are detectable in the faeces in the rat.

FURTHER INFORMATION. Metabolism and excretion in animals—G. T. Mannering and L. S. Schanker, *J. Pharmac. exp. Ther.*, 1958, **124**, 296.

Actions and uses. Levallorphan is an antagonist of morphine and similar drugs. Its action resembles that of nalorphine, but it is more potent. It is usually administered in a dosage of 0.2 to 2 milligrams by intravenous injection as a 0.1% solution.
Levallorphan is sometimes used in obstetrics in conjunction with a morphine-like agent such as pethidine with the object of reducing the respiratory depression for a given level of analgesia but there is no convincing evidence that this objective is achieved.

Preparation

LEVALLORPHAN INJECTION: a sterile solution of levallorphan tartrate in water for injections. The acidity of the solution is adjusted to pH 4.5. It is sterilised by heating in an autoclave or by filtration. Available in 1-ml ampoules containing 1 mg of levallorphan tartrate.
A standard for this injection is given in the British Pharmacopoeia 1973
Containers and *Labelling:* see the entry on Injections for general information on containers and labelling.
Storage: it should be protected from light.

OTHER PREPARATIONS include an INJECTION containing levallorphan tartrate 625 micrograms with pethidine hydrochloride 50 mg per ml in 1- and 2-ml ampoules.

Levamisole Hydrochloride

(−)-(*S*)-2,3,5,6-Tetrahydro-6-phenylimidazo[2,1-*b*]thiazole hydrochloride, the laevo-isomer of tetramisole hydrochloride.

$C_{11}H_{13}ClN_2S = 240.8$

OTHER NAMES: *Ketrax®* (available only in certain overseas countries); *Nemicide®*; *Nilverm®*
Nilzan® (with oxyclozanide)

A standard is given in the British Pharmacopoeia Addendum 1977 and the British Pharmacopoeia (Veterinary)

Description. An odourless, white to pale cream-coloured, crystalline powder.

Solubility. Soluble, at 20°, in 2 parts of water, and in 5 parts of methyl alcohol; practically insoluble in ether.

Specific rotation. Not less than −121.5°, determined on a 5% solution, freshly prepared and filtered.

Sterilisation. Solutions for injection are sterilised by filtration.

Storage. It should be stored in a cool place, protected from light.

Identification. TEST. Dissolve 500 mg in 20 ml of water, add 6 ml of 1N sodium hydroxide, extract with 20 ml of dichloromethane, wash the solvent layer with 10 ml of water, dry over anhydrous sodium sulphate, evaporate to dryness at room temperature and dry *in vacuo*; the residue melts at about 59°.

MELTING-POINT. About 228°.

Actions and uses. Levamisole hydrochloride is an anthelmintic that is used in the treatment of gastrointestinal ascariasis, ancylostomiasis, and strongyloidiasis. The usual dose for an adult is the equivalent of 120 to 150 milligrams of levamisole by mouth as a single dose, but patients with ancylostomiasis may be given the equivalent of 2.5 to 5 milligrams per kilogram body-weight of levamisole daily for 3 days or weekly for 3 weeks. 1.2 grams of levamisole hydrochloride is approximately equivalent to 1 gram of levamisole.

Levamisole enhances cell-mediated immunity in certain diseases associated with immunodeficiency states. It is therefore of value in the treatment of recurrent severe infections and, in conjunction with other treatment, in reducing the duration, severity, and frequency of attacks in a variety of chronic recurrent diseases such as rheumatoid arthritis, systemic lupus erythematosus, and aphthous stomatitis. Levamisole may also be of value as an aid in the treatment of some types of malignant disease. It is usually administered in an intermittent regimen; a possible dosage scheme is the equivalent of 150 milligrams of levamisole for 3 days of each week.

Precautions and contra-indications. Neutropenia and granulocytopenia, which may necessitate discontinuation of treatment may occur, especially in the treatment of rheumatoid arthritis. They may occur after only short periods as well as after prolonged treatment and regular blood counts are therefore required. Levamisole is contra-indicated in patients with severe hepatic or renal disease.

Veterinary uses. Levamisole hydrochloride is used in the treatment of parasitic gastro-enteritis and parasitic bronchitis. The usual dose by mouth or by subcutaneous injection for cattle, sheep, and pigs is 7.5 milligrams per kilogram body-weight as a single dose. The usual dose for poultry is 20 milligrams per kilogram body-weight as a single dose incorporated in the drinking water.

Preparations

LEVAMISOLE GRANULES: consisting of levamisole hydrochloride mixed with suitable edible diluents and made into hard, cylindrical granules by a suitable process; they are free-flowing and free from aggregates. Available as granules containing 2.5% of levamisole hydrochloride.
A standard for these granules is given in the British Pharmacopoeia (Veterinary)
Labelling: the label on the container should state the amount of the medicament as the proportion of levamisole hydrochloride in the granules, and the directions for using the preparation.

LEVAMISOLE INJECTION: a sterile solution of levamisole hydrochloride, with suitable stabilising and preservative agents, in water for injections. It may contain suitable colouring matter. It is sterilised by filtration. Available in 500-ml plastic packs containing 75 mg of levamisole hydrochloride per ml.
A standard for this injection is given in the British Pharmacopoeia (Veterinary)
Containers and *Labelling:* see the entry on Injections for general information on containers and labelling.
Storage: it should be stored at a temperature not exceeding 25°, protected from light.

LEVAMISOLE MIXTURE: consisting of an aqueous solution of levamisole hydrochloride containing suitable stabilising agents. It may contain suitable preservatives. Available as a mixture containing 1.5% of levamisole hydrochloride.
A standard for this mixture is given in the British Pharmacopoeia (Veterinary)
Containers and *Labelling:* see the entry on Mixtures for general information on containers and labelling.

OTHER PREPARATIONS available include an ELIXIR containing levamisole hydrochloride 40 mg in 5 ml; veterinary GRANULES containing levamisole hydrochloride 2.5% with oxyclozanide 5%; a veterinary MIXTURE containing levamisole hydrochloride 1.5% with oxyclozanide 3%; and TABLETS containing levamisole hydrochloride 40 mg.

Levodopa

(−)-3-(3,4-Dihydroxyphenyl)-L-alanine

$C_9H_{11}NO_4 = 197.2$

OTHER NAMES: *Berkdopa®*; *Brocadopa®*; *Larodopa®*; L-Dopa; *Levopa®*
Madopar® (with benserazide hydrochloride); *Sinemet®* (with carbidopa)

A standard is given in the British Pharmacopoeia 1973

Description. An odourless, almost tasteless, white, crystalline powder.

Solubility. Soluble, at 20°, in 300 parts of water; very slightly soluble in alcohol, in ether, and in chloroform; soluble in aqueous solutions of mineral acids and alkali carbonates.

Dissociation constants. pK_a 2.3, 8.7, 9.7, 13.4 (25°).

Storage. It should be stored in airtight containers, protected from light.

Identification. TEST. To 5 ml of a 0.1% solution in 0.1N hydrochloric acid add 2 drops of *ferric chloride test-solution*; a green colour is produced. To one half of this solution add excess *dilute ammonia solution*; a purple colour is produced. To the remainder of the solution add excess *dilute sodium hydroxide solution*; a red colour is produced.

MELTING-POINT. Above 270°, with decomposition.

ULTRAVIOLET ABSORPTION. In 0.1N hydrochloric acid, maximum at 280 nm (E1%, 1cm = 140).

INFRA-RED ABSORPTION. Major peaks at 1124, 1250, 1351, 1389, 1562, and 1639 cm⁻¹ (see Appendix 2b: Infra-red Spectra).

Determination in body fluids. GAS CHROMATOGRAPHY. In urine—K. Imai *et al.*, *Chem. pharm. Bull.*, Tokyo, 1972, **20**, 2436.

HIGH PRESSURE LIQUID CHROMATOGRAPHY. In serum: stated to be no interference from carbidopa—R. M. Riggin *et al.*, *Clin. Chem.*, 1976, **22**, 782.

Metabolism. ABSORPTION. Rapidly absorbed after oral administration; the rate of absorption is influenced by the rate of gastric emptying and by diet. Levodopa is decarboxylated in the gastric mucosa and increased contact caused by a slow gastric-emptying time may therefore increase the amount metabolised; anticholinergics administered concomitantly may also decrease absorption of levodopa for the same reason and antacids, which may increase gastric emptying in subjects with low basal gastric pH values, may increase absorption.

Levodopa is absorbed by an active transport process and other amino acids from the diet may compete for the transport process and thus reduce the amount of levodopa absorbed; sustained release preparations are particularly susceptible to decarboxylation in the gastric mucosa.

BLOOD CONCENTRATION. After an oral dose of 1.5 g, peak plasma concentrations of levodopa of about 1 μg/ml are attained at 1 hour; differences between peak concentrations in subjects given levodopa with or without anticholinergics have not been significant in the studies so far undertaken; after an oral dose of 1.5 g, extremes in peak plasma concentrations of up to 10 μg/ml in 1.5 hours to 1 μg/ml in 4 hours have been observed; as yet there has been no successful attempt to correlate blood concentrations of either levodopa or its metabolites with clinical effectiveness; the relationship between these two parameters appears to be extremely variable.

HALF-LIFE. Plasma half-life, about 1 hour which may be increased by concomitant administration of peripheral decarboxylase inhibitors; the half-life of 3-O-methyldopa is about 13 hours.

DISTRIBUTION. Levodopa and its metabolites are widely distributed throughout the body; less than 1% of a dose reaches the brain; levodopa is secreted in the milk; 3-O-methyldopa accumulates in the central nervous system.

METABOLIC REACTIONS. Extensively metabolised mainly by decarboxylation to dopamine, which is further metabolised, and also by methylation to 3-O-methyldopa; most of a dose is decarboxylated by the gastric mucosa before entering the systemic circulation; once in the circulation the remaining levodopa is rapidly decarboxylated by other peripheral decarboxylases. Levodopa decarboxylase activity is enhanced by pyridoxine and inhibited by carbidopa and benserazide.

Dopamine is further metabolised to noradrenaline by hydroxylation, to 3-methoxytyramine by methylation, and to 3,4-dihydroxyphenylacetic acid (DOPAC) and 3-methoxy-4-hydroxyphenylacetic acid (HVA), which are the major metabolites, by oxidative deamination and methylation.

Monoamine-oxidase inhibitors inhibit the metabolism of dopamine resulting in higher circulating levels of dopamine and levodopa; during prolonged therapy the rate of levodopa metabolism appears to increase and this may be due to enzyme induction. In addition, the ratio of the amount of DOPAC produced to that of HVA is increased in prolonged therapy.

EXCRETION. About 80% of a dose is excreted in the urine in 24 hours and very little is found in the faeces. Over 50% of the material in the urine is excreted as DOPAC and HVA, 30% is excreted as 3-O-methyldopa, about 4% is excreted as dopamine, and less than 1% is excreted unchanged.

FURTHER INFORMATION. Absorption and metabolism— S. Bergmann et al., Br. J. clin. Pharmac., 1974, 1, 417; pharmacokinetics—J. R. Bianchine and G. M. Shaw, Clin. Pharmacokinet., 1976, 1, 313; metabolism of dopamine in man and rats—W. J. Louis et al., Clin. exp. Pharmac. Physiol., 1974, 1, 341; metabolism in small intestine in rats—P. T. Mearrick et al., J. Pharmacokinet. Biopharm., 1975, 3, 13.

Actions and uses. Levodopa is a precursor of dopamine, which is depleted from the brain in Parkinson's disease. In the treatment of Parkinson's disease, levodopa is most effective in relieving hypokinesia, and may also decrease rigidity, oculogyric crises, and tremor, but it is ineffective in drug-induced parkinsonism.

Treatment may be commenced with a dosage of 125 milligrams or 250 milligrams 4 or 5 times daily, according to the weight of the patient, and in the absence of adverse effects the dosage may be increased by 250 milligrams per day every second or third day up to a maximum of 8 grams daily. Elderly patients may require a lower initial dosage such as 125 milligrams daily.

Levodopa is commonly administered in conjunction with a dopa decarboxylase inhibitor such as benserazide or carbidopa; the dosage and side-effects of levodopa may then be reduced.

Undesirable effects. Anorexia and nausea are not uncommon. Giddiness due to postural hypotension may occur and palpitations and cardiac arrhythmias have been recorded. The commonest dose-limiting reaction, apart from nausea, is the appearance of involuntary movements, particularly affecting the tongue, jaw, and neck.

A wide variety of psychotic responses to levodopa has been described including confusion, depression, and hypomania.

Precautions. It should not be given to patients who are being treated with pyridoxine or a monoamine-oxidase inhibitor, such as isocarboxazid, nialamide, phenelzine, or tranylcypromine, or within about 2 weeks of the discontinuation of such treatment.

It should be administered with caution to patients being treated with antihypertensive drugs as it may augment their hypotensive effect. It should also be administered with caution in patients with bronchial asthma or renal, hepatic, or cardiac insufficiency. Its use should be avoided in pregnancy, in nursing mothers, and in severe psychosis.

Preparations

LEVODOPA AND BENSERAZIDE CAPSULES: consisting of levodopa and benserazide hydrochloride, which may be mixed with a suitable inert diluent, enclosed in a hard capsule. The capsule shells may be coloured. Available as capsules containing 100 mg of levodopa and benserazide hydrochloride equivalent to 25 mg of benserazide and as capsules containing 200 mg of levodopa and benserazide hydrochloride equivalent to 50 mg of benserazide.

Containers and Storage: see the entry on Capsules for general information on containers and storage. Containers should be light resistant.

Advice for patients: the capsules should be taken after meals. Treatment should not be discontinued without the advice of the prescriber. The capsules may affect mental concentration in the first few days of treatment and the urine may darken.

LEVODOPA AND CARBIDOPA TABLETS: available as tablets containing 100 mg of levodopa and carbidopa (monohydrate) equivalent to 10 mg of anhydrous carbidopa and as tablets containing 250 mg of levodopa and carbidopa (monohydrate) equivalent to 25 mg of anhydrous carbidopa; they may be coloured.

Containers and Storage: see the entry on Tablets for general information on containers and storage. Containers should be airtight and light resistant.

Advice for patients: see above under Levodopa and Benserazide Capsules.

LEVODOPA CAPSULES (Syn. L-Dopa Capsules): consisting of levodopa, in powder, which may be mixed with a suitable inert diluent, enclosed in a hard capsule. Available as capsules containing 125, 250, and 500 mg of levodopa.

A standard for these capsules is given in the British Pharmacopoeia 1973

Containers and *Storage:* see the entry on Capsules for general information on containers and storage.

Advice for patients: see above under Levodopa and Benserazide Capsules.

LEVODOPA TABLETS (*Syn.* L-Dopa Tablets): available as tablets containing 500 mg of levodopa.

A standard for these tablets is given in the British Pharmacopoeia 1973

Containers and *Storage:* see the entry on Tablets for general information on containers and storage. Containers should be airtight.

Advice for patients: see above under Levodopa and Benserazide Capsules.

OTHER PREPARATIONS available include TABLETS containing levodopa 500 mg in a slow-release formulation.

Levorphanol Tartrate

(−)-3-Hydroxy-*N*-methylmorphinanium hydrogen tartrate dihydrate

$C_{21}H_{29}NO_7,2H_2O = 443.5$

OTHER NAME: *Dromoran®*

A standard is given in the British Pharmacopoeia 1973

Description. An odourless white crystalline powder with a bitter taste.

Solubility. Soluble, at 20°, in 45 parts of water, in 110 parts of alcohol, and in 50 parts of ether.

Acidity. A 0.2% solution has a pH of 3.4 to 4.

Moisture content. 7 to 9%, determined by drying at 105°.

Dissociation constant. pK_a 8.2 (20°).

Sterilisation. Solutions for injection are sterilised by heating in an autoclave or by filtration.

Storage. It should be stored in airtight containers.

Identification. TESTS. 1. It complies with Test 1 described under Levallorphan Tartrate.
2. Dissolve about 50 mg in 2 ml of *dilute sulphuric acid*, add 1 ml of a freshly prepared solution containing 700 mg of mercuric nitrate in 4 ml of water and then add 100 mg of sodium nitrite, filter, and heat the filtrate; a red colour is produced immediately.

MELTING-POINT. About 116°.

ULTRAVIOLET ABSORPTION. In water, maximum at 279 nm (E1%, 1cm = 46); in 0.1N sodium hydroxide, maxima at 240 nm (E1%, 1cm = 198) and 299 nm (E1%, 1cm = 70).

Metabolism. ABSORPTION. Well absorbed after oral administration and after injection.

HALF-LIFE. Biological half-life, 75 to 90 minutes in dogs and monkeys.

DISTRIBUTION. Concentrated in liver and kidneys.

METABOLIC REACTIONS. *N*-Demethylation and conjugation with glucuronic acid.

EXCRETION. In the monkey, 2.5% is excreted unchanged and 35% is excreted as conjugates; in the dog, 4.4% is excreted unchanged and 42% as conjugates; very little is excreted in the faeces of either species.

FURTHER INFORMATION. *N*-Demethylation depressed by levorphanol in rats—G. J. Mannering and A. E. Takemori, *J. Pharmac. exp. Ther.*, 1959, **127**, 187; estimation in plasma and urine of dogs and monkeys—L. A. Woods *et al.*, *J. Pharmac. exp. Ther.*, 1958, **124**, 1.

Actions and uses. Levorphanol is an analgesic which has actions, uses, and undesirable effects similar to those described under Morphine Hydrochloride, but it differs from morphine in being almost as effective when given by mouth as by injection. Levorphanol tartrate is given by mouth in doses of 1.5 to 4.5 milligrams, by subcutaneous or intramuscular injection in doses of 2 to 4 milligrams, and by intravenous injection in doses of 1 to 1.5 milligrams; these doses may be repeated in accordance with the needs of the patient. In an emergency, 2 to 4 milligrams may be administered by slow intravenous injection.

Dependence. Prolonged administration of therapeutic doses may lead to the development of dependence of the morphine type, as described under Drug Dependence.

Poisoning. The procedure described under Morphine Hydrochloride should be adopted.

Preparations

LEVORPHANOL INJECTION: a sterile solution of levorphanol tartrate in water for injections. The acidity of the solution is adjusted to pH 5.5. It is sterilised by heating in an autoclave or by filtration. Available in 1-ml ampoules containing 2 mg of levorphanol tartrate.

A standard for this injection is given in the British Pharmacopoeia 1973

Containers and *Labelling:* see the entry on Injections for general information on containers and labelling.

Storage: it should be protected from light.

LEVORPHANOL TABLETS: available as tablets containing 1.5 mg of levorphanol tartrate.

A standard for these tablets is given in the British Pharmacopoeia 1973

Containers and *Storage:* see the entry on Tablets for general information on containers and storage. Containers should be airtight.

Lice

Lice are ectoparasitic arthropods, the species parasitic upon man being *Pediculus capitis* (the head louse), *Pediculus corporis* (the body louse), and *Phthirus pubis* (the crab louse). These species are 1 to 4 millimetres in length and mainly infect the head, the body and clothes, and the pubic hair respectively. They lay several eggs (nits) each day at the bases of hairs. Lice spread by close body contact with an infected person. They may be eliminated by the use of a suitable insecticidal preparation, and contacts such as other members of a patient's family should be treated to stop the spread of infection.

Suitable insecticidal preparations contain carbaryl, gamma benzene hexachloride, or malathion; dicophane has also been used. Carbaryl (0.5%) has a rapid action but malathion (0.5%) should be left in contact with the infected area for 12 hours and gamma benzene hexachloride (0.1 to 0.2%) for at least 24 hours.

Since resistance may develop to some of these insecticides, the preparations effective in the locality should be used.

Lignocaine Hydrochloride

NN-Diethyl[(2,6-dimethylphenyl)carbamoyl]methylammonium chloride monohydrate

$C_{14}H_{23}ClN_2O,H_2O = 288.8$

OTHER NAMES: Lidocaine Hydrochloride; Lidocaini Hydrochloridum; Lignoc. Hydrochlor.; *Xylocard® Lidocaton®; Lidothesin®; Lignol®; Lignostab®; Versicaine®; Xylocaine®; Xylotox®* (these names are also applied to compound preparations of lignocaine hydrochloride with various other medicaments)
Xylodase® (with hyaluronidase)

A standard is given in the European Pharmacopoeia Vol. II

Description. An odourless, white, crystalline powder with a slightly bitter taste followed by numbing.

Solubility. Soluble, at 20°, in less than 1 part of water and in 1.5 parts of alcohol; soluble in chloroform; practically insoluble in ether.

Acidity. A 0.5% solution has a pH of 4 to 5.5.

Moisture content. 5 to 7.5%, determined by Fischer titration.

Dissociation constant. pK_a 7.9 (25°).

Stability. It is extremely stable in the solid state and in solution. Even at extreme pH values and high temperatures hydrolysis to 2,6-xylidine and *NN*-diethylglycine is very slow. It does not degrade by oxidation.

Incompatibility. Lignocaine base may be precipitated from alkaline solutions of lignocaine hydrochloride at concentrations greater than 4 mg per ml.

Hygroscopicity. It absorbs insignificant amounts of water at 25° at relative humidities up to about 80%.

Sterilisation. Solutions for injection are sterilised by heating in an autoclave or by filtration.

Identification. TESTS. 1. To 5 ml of a 5% solution add 5 ml of water, make alkaline with *dilute sodium hydroxide solution*, filter, and wash the precipitate with water; dissolve 100 mg of the precipitate in 1 ml of alcohol, and add 0.5 ml of a 10% solution of cobalt nitrate; a bluish-green precipitate is produced.
2. Dissolve 200 mg in 10 ml of water and add 10 ml of *trinitrophenol solution*; a precipitate is produced which, after washing with water and drying, melts at about 230°.

MELTING-POINT. About 77°.

ULTRAVIOLET ABSORPTION. In 0.1N hydrochloric acid, maxima at 235 nm (E1%, 1cm = 40) and 266 nm (E1%, 1cm = 14.5).

INFRA-RED ABSORPTION. Major peaks at 787, 952, 1031, 1149, 1538, and 1639 cm^{-1} (see Appendix 2b: Infra-red Spectra).

THIN-LAYER CHROMATOGRAPHY. See under Thin-layer Chromatography, System 2.

Determination in body fluids. GAS CHROMATOGRAPHY. In plasma or urine: lignocaine and metabolites—K. K. Adjepon-Yamoah and L. F. Prescott, *J. Pharm. Pharmac.*, 1974, **26**, 889; in plasma—G. Caille *et al.*, *J. pharm. Sci.*, 1977, **66**, 1383; H. B. Hucker and S. C. Stauffer, *J. pharm. Sci.*, 1976, **65**, 926; in blood—T. R. Irgens *et al.*, *J. pharm. Sci.*, 1976, **65**, 608; in plasma: lignocaine and a metabolite—R. L. Nation *et al.*, *J. Chromat.*, 1976, **116**, 188.

Metabolism. ABSORPTION. Rapidly absorbed after intramuscular injection; injection into the deltoid muscle results in better absorption than that from either the vastus lateralis or the gluteus maximus muscles.

BLOOD CONCENTRATION. After an oral dose of 500 mg, peak plasma concentrations of over 10 μg/ml are obtained and concentrations of over 5 μg/ml are maintained for about 2½ hours; after an intravenous injection of 5 to 10 mg/kg body-weight concentrations of 5 to 15 μg/ml are obtained within 15 minutes in the blood and 3 to 11 μg/ml within the same period in the cerebrospinal fluid; after the intramuscular injection of 4.5 mg/kg into the deltoid muscle or the vastus lateralis, peak blood concentrations of 2 to 6 μg/ml at 10 minutes and 1 to 4 μg/ml at 30 minutes are obtained respectively; therapeutic concentrations are usually above 1.4 μg/ml and toxic concentrations above 6 μg/ml.

HALF-LIFE. Plasma elimination half-life after intravenous injection, about 13 minutes; after intramuscular injection, about 90 minutes; the half-life is increased in liver disease.

DISTRIBUTION. Lignocaine enters the cerebrospinal fluid and crosses the placenta.

METABOLIC REACTIONS. *N*-De-ethylation, hydrolysis, and/or ring hydroxylation, possibly followed by conjugation.

EXCRETION. In 24 hours, 3 to 12% of a dose is excreted in the urine as unchanged drug, 70% as 4-hydroxy-2,6-dimethylaniline, 4% as monoethylglycinexylidide, 2% as glycinexylidide, 1% as 2-hydroxylignocaine, 1% as 2,6-xylidine, and 0.3% as 3-hydroxymonoethylglycinexylidide. Glycinexylidide and the hydroxy-metabolites appear to be excreted as acid-hydrolysable conjugates. The renal clearance of lignocaine is affected by urinary pH but not by urinary flow.

Actions and uses. Lignocaine is a local anaesthetic, widely used by injection and for local application to mucous membranes. In equal concentration, it is more effective than procaine and gives a greater area of anaesthesia, but may be more toxic.
Solutions containing 0.5 to 2% of lignocaine hydrochloride, with adrenaline 1 in 100 000 to 1 in 50 000, may be used for infiltration; except under special circumstances the concentration of lignocaine used should not exceed 1% and the total quantity of lignocaine administered should not exceed 200 milligrams unless adrenaline is present, when up to 500 milligrams may be given. Solutions containing adrenaline should not be used for inducing anaesthesia in digits because the profound ischaemia produced may lead to gangrene.
Preparations containing 1 to 4% of lignocaine hydrochloride may be used to anaesthetise the pharynx, larynx, and trachea before endoscopic examination.

A 1 or 4% solution is used for epidural anaesthesia.

In the treatment of cardiac arrhythmias, lignocaine hydrochloride has been given by intravenous injection in doses of 50 to 100 milligrams, administered as 5 to 10 millilitres of a 1% solution over a period of two minutes, followed by intravenous infusion at a rate of 1 to 4 milligrams per minute in accordance with the needs of the patient.

If lignocaine hydrochloride is required for intravenous infusion a suitable solution may be prepared according to the following formula:

Lignocaine hydrochloride .. .. 1 g
(or a sufficient quantity)
Anhydrous dextrose .. .. 50 g
Water for injections .. .. .. to 1000 ml

Dissolve. Adjust the acidity of the solution to pH 4 to 4.5 by the addition of hydrochloric acid or a 20% solution of sodium hydroxide, as appropriate, and clarify by filtration. Distribute the solution into suitable glass or plastic containers, seal, and immediately sterilise by heating in an autoclave.

The solution is colourless and, within the pH range specified, is not subject to discoloration or caramelisation during autoclaving.

Precautions. The use of large doses should be avoided during pregnancy since when plasma levels exceed 3 micrograms per millilitre depression of the foetus may occur.

Poisoning. The procedure as described under Procaine Hydrochloride should be adopted.

Preparations

LIGNOCAINE AND ADRENALINE INJECTION: a sterile solution of lignocaine hydrochloride and adrenaline acid tartrate, with 0.1% of sodium metabisulphite, in water for injections. It is sterilised by heating in an autoclave or by filtration.

Available in 2-, 5-, and 10-ml ampoules and in 20- and 50-ml vials containing 0.5% (5 mg per ml) of lignocaine hydrochloride and 1 in 200 000 of adrenaline; in 10-ml ampoules and 20- and 50-ml vials containing 1% (10 mg per ml) of lignocaine hydrochloride and 1 in 200 000 of adrenaline; in 2-, 5-, and 10-ml ampoules and 20- and 50-ml vials containing 1% of lignocaine hydrochloride and 1 in 100 000 of adrenaline; in 2-ml cartridges containing 2% (20 mg per ml) of lignocaine hydrochloride and 1 in 250 000 of adrenaline; in 2-ml cartridges, 2-, 5-, and 10-ml ampoules, and 20- and 50-ml vials containing 2% of lignocaine hydrochloride and 1 in 100 000 of adrenaline; in 1.8-, 2-, and 2.2-ml cartridges and 20- and 50-ml vials containing 2% of lignocaine hydrochloride and adrenaline 1 in 80 000; in 1.8- and 2.2-ml cartridges containing 2% of lignocaine hydrochloride with adrenaline 1 in 50 000; and in 1.8- and 2-ml cartridges containing 2% of lignocaine hydrochloride and 1 in 80 000 of noradrenaline. Available for veterinary use in 50- and 250-ml vials containing 2% of lignocaine hydrochloride with adrenaline 1 in 100 000, and in 1.8- and 2-ml cartridges and in 50- and 250-ml vials containing 2% of lignocaine hydrochloride with adrenaline 1 in 80 000.

A standard for this injection is given in the British Pharmacopoeia 1973

Containers: see the entry on Injections for general information on containers.

Labelling: see the entry on Injections for general information on labelling. In addition, the label on the container should state the amount of the medicament as the percentage w/v of lignocaine hydrochloride and the proportion of adrenaline base.

Storage: it should be protected from light.

LIGNOCAINE GEL (*Syn.* Lignocaine Hydrochloride Gel): a sterile solution of lignocaine hydrochloride in a suitable water-miscible basis containing chlorhexidine gluconate, or a mixture of the sodium salts of methyl hydroxybenzoate and propyl hydroxybenzoate, as the preservative. It is sterilised by heating in an autoclave.

Available as gels containing 1 and 2% of lignocaine hydrochloride.

A standard for this gel is given in the British Pharmaceutical Codex 1973

Containers: it should be packed in collapsible tubes of suitable metal or plastic material. If metal tubes of capacity 7.5 g or less are used they should comply with British Standard 4230: 1967.

All containers should be as free as possible, consistent with good manufacturing practice, from dirt and particles of the material used in their construction.

Tubes and screw caps, complete with wads if used, should be sterilised before use; the wads should not be of cork. The screw caps should be covered with a readily breakable seal or, alternatively, the tube should be enclosed in a sealed package from which the tube cannot be removed without breaking the seal; suitable outer packages include paperboard cartons with sealed flaps and sealed pouches of paper, plastic, or cellulose film.

LIGNOCAINE HYDROCHLORIDE INJECTION: a sterile solution of lignocaine hydrochloride in water for injections. It is sterilised by heating in an autoclave or by filtration.

Available in 2-, 5-, 10-, and 20-ml ampoules and 20- and 50-ml vials containing 0.5% (5 mg per ml) of lignocaine hydrochloride; in 2-, 5-, 10-, and 20-ml ampoules and 20- and 50-ml vials containing 1% (10 mg per ml) of lignocaine hydrochloride; in 25-ml ampoules containing 1.5% (15 mg per ml) of lignocaine hydrochloride; in 1.8-, 2-, and 2.2-ml cartridges, 2-, 5-, 10-, 20-, and 30-ml ampoules, and 20-, 50-, and 100-ml vials containing 2% (20 mg per ml) of lignocaine hydrochloride; 10-ml ampoules containing 5% (50 mg per ml) of lignocaine hydrochloride; 3-ml disposable syringes containing 10% (100 mg per ml) of lignocaine hydrochloride; and 5-ml disposable syringes containing 20% (200 mg per ml) of lignocaine hydrochloride. Available for veterinary use in 100-ml vials containing 2% of lignocaine hydrochloride.

A standard for this injection is given in the British Pharmacopoeia 1973

Containers and *Labelling:* see the entry on Injections for general information on containers and labelling.

OTHER PREPARATIONS available include EYE-DROPS containing lignocaine hydrochloride 4% with methylcellulose 0.65%; an INJECTION containing lignocaine hydrochloride 20 mg per ml with sodium chloride 0.6% in 5-ml disposable syringes; a viscous SOLUTION containing lignocaine hydrochloride 2%, and a solution containing lignocaine hydrochloride 4%.

Preparations of lignocaine base include an OINTMENT containing 5% in a water-miscible basis.

Lincomycin Hydrochloride

Methyl 6,8-dideoxy-6-[(2S,4R)-(1-methyl-4-propylpyrrolidine-2-carboxamido)]-1-thio-α-D-*erythro*-D-*galacto*-octopyranoside hydrochloride monohydrate, an antimicrobial substance produced by *Streptomyces lincolnensis* var. *lincolnensis*.

$C_{18}H_{35}ClN_2O_6S,H_2O = 461.0$

OTHER NAMES: *Lincocin®*; *Mycivin®*
Linco-Spectin® (with spectinomycin sulphate)

A standard is given in the British Pharmacopoeia 1973

Description. A white crystalline powder with a slight characteristic odour and a bitter taste.

Solubility. Soluble, at 20°, in 1 part of water, in 40 parts of alcohol, and in 20 parts of dimethylformamide; practically insoluble in ether and in chloroform; very slightly soluble in acetone.

Acidity. A 10% solution has a pH of 3 to 5.5.

Moisture content. 3 to 6%, determined by Fischer titration.

Specific rotation. +135° to +150°, determined on a 4% solution.

Dissociation constant. pK_a 7.5.

Labelling. If the material is not intended for parenteral administration, the label on the container states that the contents are not to be injected.

Storage. It should be stored in airtight containers at a temperature not exceeding 30°. If it is intended for parenteral administration, the containers should be sterile and sealed to exclude micro-organisms.

Identification. ULTRAVIOLET ABSORPTION. A solution in 0.1N sulphuric acid exhibits no significant absorption in the range 230 to 360 nm.

INFRA-RED ABSORPTION. Major peaks at 1040, 1075, 1104, 1262, 1564, and 1655 cm⁻¹ (see Appendix 2a: Infra-red Spectra).

Metabolism. ABSORPTION. Lincomycin is incompletely absorbed after oral administration and its rate of absorption is reduced after meals.

BLOOD CONCENTRATION. After an oral dose of 500 mg to fasting subjects, peak serum concentrations of 3 to 10 μg/ml are attained in about 2 hours; after an intramuscular dose of 500 to 600 mg, peak serum concentrations of 1 to 12 μg/ml are attained in 1 to 2 hours; during therapy with intravenous infusions of 5 to 8 g daily, peak concentrations of 25 to 35 μg/ml and minimum concentrations of 10 to 12 μg/ml are attained.

DISTRIBUTION. Widely and rapidly distributed throughout the body tissues and fluids; it appears in peritoneal and pleural fluids, crosses the placenta, and is secreted in milk; it is taken up by bone and enters the cerebrospinal fluid when the meninges are inflamed; *protein binding*, about 70 to 90% bound to plasma proteins.

EXCRETION. Excreted in both urine and bile; 2 to 9% of an oral dose may be excreted in the urine in 24 hours with 30 to 40% appearing in the faeces; up to about 60% of an injected dose is excreted in the urine.

FURTHER INFORMATION. Protein binding in serum—R. C. Gordon et al., *J. pharm. Sci.*, 1973, **62**, 1074; blood

concentrations from intravenous infusion—E. Novak et al., *Clin. Pharmac. Ther.*, 1971, **12**, 793; R. L. Parsons et al., Lincomycin bone concentrations during total hip replacement, *Clinical Aspects of Infection, Chemotherapy*, J. D. Williams and A. M. Geddes (Eds), London, Plenum Press, 1976, p. 195.

Actions and uses. Lincomycin is an antibiotic with a range of antibacterial activity similar to that of erythromycin. It is active against *Streptococcus pyogenes, Str. pneumoniae, Staphylococcus aureus,* and *Bacteroides* spp., but much less active than erythromycin against *Neisseria* spp. and *Haemophilus influenzae*. It is bacteriostatic in low concentrations and bactericidal in high concentrations, and acts by interfering with the synthesis of deoxyribonucleic acid.

Lincomycin is used chiefly for the treatment of susceptible infections in patients allergic to penicillins and for the treatment of infections that are not susceptible to penicillins. As it penetrates bone, it is also used for the treatment of osteomyelitis. Resistance is induced relatively easily; there is partial cross-resistance with erythromycin.

The usual dosage for adults is the equivalent of 1.5 grams of lincomycin daily in divided doses 30 minutes before food, 0.6 to 1.2 grams of lincomycin by intramuscular injection daily in two doses, or 600 milligrams in dextrose injection (5%) or sodium chloride injection every 8 to 12 hours by intravenous infusion.

Children may be given the equivalent of 25 to 50 milligrams of lincomycin per kilogram body-weight daily in 3 or 4 divided doses by mouth or the equivalent of 10 to 20 milligrams per kilogram daily by injection in 2 divided doses or by intravenous infusion in 2 or 3 divided doses. 1.1 grams of lincomycin hydrochloride is approximately equivalent to 1 gram of lincomycin.

Undesirable effects. Diarrhoea, allergic reactions, and supra-infection with yeasts may occur, and, rarely, liver damage. Pseudomembranous colitis may be a very serious complication of treatment with lincomycin.

Precautions. Lincomycin should be administered with caution to patients with renal failure as accumulation may occur and the substance cannot be removed by dialysis.

Veterinary uses. Lincomycin hydrochloride is an antibacterial agent. The usual dose by mouth for dogs and cats is the equivalent of 50 milligrams of lincomycin per kilogram body-weight daily in divided doses. The usual dose for all species by intramuscular injection is the equivalent of 20 milligrams of lincomycin per kilogram body-weight daily and by intravenous injection the equivalent of 10 to 20 milligrams per kilogram daily.

Preparations

LINCOMYCIN CAPSULES: consisting of lincomycin hydrochloride, in powder, which may be mixed with a suitable inert diluent, enclosed in a hard capsule. The capsule shells may be coloured. Available as capsules containing lincomycin hydrochloride equivalent to 500 mg of lincomycin.

A standard for these capsules is given in the British Pharmacopoeia 1973

Containers and *Storage*: see the entry on Capsules for general information on containers and storage.

Labelling: the label on the container should state the amount of the medicament as the equivalent amount of lincomycin, the date after which the capsules are not intended to be used, and the conditions under which they should be stored.

Advice for patients: the capsules should be taken at regular intervals, preferably half to 1 hour before meals. The prescribed course should be completed.

LINCOMYCIN INJECTION: a sterile solution of lincomycin hydrochloride in water for injections. It is sterilised by filtration. Available in 20-ml vials containing lincomycin hydrochloride equivalent to 100 mg of lincomycin per ml, in 2-ml ampoules containing lincomycin hydrochloride equivalent to 300 mg of lincomycin per ml, and in 6.67-ml vials containing lincomycin hydrochloride equivalent to 2 g of lincomycin (300 mg per ml).

A standard for this injection is given in the British Pharmacopoeia 1973

Containers: see the entry on Injections for general information on containers.

Labelling: see the entry on Injections for general information on labelling. In addition, the label should state the amount of the medicament as the equivalent amount of lincomycin in a suitable dose-volume.

Storage: it should be stored at a temperature not exceeding 20°, protected from light. Under these conditions, it may be expected to retain its potency for at least 3 years.

LINCOMYCIN TABLETS: available as tablets containing lincomycin hydrochloride equivalent to 100 and 500 mg of lincomycin.

A standard for these tablets is given in the British Pharmacopoeia (Veterinary)

Containers and *Storage:* see the entry on Tablets for general information on containers and storage. Containers should be airtight.

Labelling: the label on the container should state the amount of the medicament as the equivalent amount of lincomycin, and the date after which the tablets are not intended to be used.

OTHER PREPARATIONS available include an ELIXIR containing lincomycin hydrochloride equivalent to 250 mg of lincomycin in 5 ml, diluent syrup, life of diluted elixir 14 days; a veterinary MIXTURE containing lincomycin hydrochloride equivalent to 50 mg of lincomycin per ml and a veterinary soluble POWDER containing lincomycin hydrochloride equivalent to 33.3 g of lincomycin with spectinomycin sulphate equivalent to 66.7 g of spectinomycin per pack.

Linctuses

Viscous liquid preparations, usually containing sucrose and medicinal substances and possessing demulcent, expectorant, or sedative properties; they are usually used for the relief of cough. They are administered in doses of small volume and should be sipped and swallowed slowly without the addition of water.

Dilution of linctuses. When a dose ordered or prescribed is less than or not a multiple of 5 millilitres, the linctus should be diluted with the vehicle recommended in the entry describing the preparation concerned, so that the dose to be measured for the patient is one 5-millilitre spoonful or multiple thereof.

Diluted linctuses must always be freshly prepared and not more than 2 weeks' supply should be issued at a time unless otherwise specified in the entry describing the preparation.

Containers. Linctuses should be dispensed in plain bottles of colourless or amber glass.

Liniments

Liniments are usually liquid or semi-liquid preparations which are intended for external application and may contain substances possessing analgesic, rubefacient, soothing, or stimulating properties. Analgesic and soothing liniments may be applied to the skin on warmed flannel or other suitable material, or by means of a camel-hair brush; stimulating liniments should be applied to the skin with considerable friction by massaging with the hand. Liniments should not be applied to broken skin.

Containers. Liniments should be dispensed in coloured fluted bottles.

Labelling. The containers should be labelled "For external use only".

Linseed Oil

The fixed oil obtained by expression from the ripe seeds of *Linum usitatissimum* L. (Fam. Linaceae), and subsequently clarified.

OTHER NAMES: Flaxseed Oil; Oleum Lini

A standard is given in the British Pharmacopoeia (Veterinary)

Constituents. Linseed oil consists of glycerides, the fatty acid constituents of which are chiefly linolenic, linoleic and oleic acids, with smaller amounts of stearic and palmitic acids.

Description. It is a clear yellowish-brown oil with a characteristic odour and a bland taste. Much commercial oil has a marked odour and an acrid taste. Linseed oil gradually thickens when exposed to the air and a thin film of the oil dries to a hard transparent varnish. It does not congeal until cooled to about −15°.

Solubility. Slightly soluble in alcohol (95%); miscible with ether, with chloroform, with carbon disulphide, with light petroleum (boiling range 40° to 60°), and with turpentine.

Weight per ml. At 20°, 0.925 to 0.930 g.

Refractive index. 1.479 to 1.484.

Storage. It should be stored in well-filled airtight containers.

Veterinary uses. Linseed oil is a laxative which is also used in conjunction with turpentine oil in the treatment of cattle bloat (ruminal tympany). The usual dose for horses, cattle, sheep, and pigs is 1.5 to 2 millilitres per kilogram body-weight.

Liothyronine Sodium

The sodium derivative of O^4-(4-hydroxy-3-iodophenyl)-3,5-di-iodotyrosine.

$C_{15}H_{11}I_3NNaO_4 = 673.0$

OTHER NAMES: *Tertroxin®*; L-Tri-iodothyronine Sodium

A standard is given in the British Pharmacopoeia 1973

Description. An odourless white or buff-coloured solid.

Solubility. Very slightly soluble in water, in ether, and in chloroform; soluble, at 20°, in 500 parts of alcohol; soluble in solutions of alkali hydroxides.

Moisture content. Not more than 4%, determined by drying at 105°.

Specific rotation. +18° to +22°, determined on a 2% solution in a mixture containing 1 volume of 1N hydrochloric acid and 4 volumes of alcohol (95%).

Storage. It should be stored in airtight containers, protected from light.

Identification. TEST. Dissolve about 5 mg in 2 ml of alcohol (50%) containing 1 drop of hydrochloric acid, add 1 drop of a 10% solution of sodium nitrite and boil; a yellow colour is produced. Cool the solution and make alkaline with *dilute ammonia solution*; the colour changes to red.

ULTRAVIOLET ABSORPTION. In 0.1N sodium hydroxide, maximum at 319 nm (E1%, 1cm = 65).

Determination in body fluids. RADIO-IMMUNOASSAY. In serum—M. L. Brown and J. Metheany, *J. pharm. Sci.*, 1974, **63**, 1214.

Metabolism. ABSORPTION. Absorbed after oral or intramuscular administration.

BLOOD CONCENTRATION. About 5% of endogenous organic iodine in the blood is in the form of liothyronine and normal plasma concentrations are about 70 ng/ml.

HALF-LIFE. Liothyronine has a half-life in the blood circulation of about 2 days.

DISTRIBUTION. Widely distributed throughout the body tissues and fluids; tissue concentrations of liothyronine may be derived from deiodination of thyroxine; liothyronine is subject to enterohepatic circulation; it does not appear to cross the placenta or to be secreted into the milk; *protein binding*, highly bound in plasma but to a lesser extent than thyroxine.

METABOLIC REACTIONS. Conjugation with glucuronic acid or sulphate, deiodination, oxidative deamination, decarboxylation, and possibly cleavage of the ether linkage; it is metabolised more rapidly than thyroxine.

EXCRETION. Excreted mainly in the bile and faeces although iodide may be excreted in the urine.

FURTHER INFORMATION. V. A. Galton, The physiological role of thyroid hormone metabolism, *Recent Advances in Endocrinology*, V. H. T. James (Ed.), London, Churchill, 1968, p. 181; J. Robbins and J. E. Rall, The iodine containing compounds, *Hormones in Blood*, R. H. Gray and H. L. Bacharach (Eds), Vol. 1, London, Academic Press, 1967, p. 383.

Actions and uses. Liothyronine has the actions and uses described under Thyroxine Sodium. It is an active principle of the thyroid gland and is believed to be the activated form of the thyroid hormone which has a stimulant effect on cellular metabolism. It is effective in smaller doses than thyroid or thyroxine and its action is quicker in onset but of shorter duration. It has the advantage over thyroid that it is of constant composition and biological assay is not necessary. 20 micrograms of liothyronine is approximately equivalent in activity to 100 micrograms of thyroxine.

Liothyronine sodium is used in the treatment of severe hypothyroidism when a rapid therapeutic action is required, but it is less suitable than thyroxine for maintenance therapy, because of its shorter duration of action. It is given by mouth in an initial dosage of 10 to 20 micrograms daily, which is gradually increased by

10-microgram increments every 3 to 7 days up to a total of 80 to 100 micrograms daily. A child may be given 5 micrograms increasing if necessary to up to 40 micrograms daily according to age and similar dosage may be required for elderly patients.

In hypothyroid coma a dose of 100 micrograms may be given by intravenous injection followed by 25 micrograms every 6 hours until improvement is noted.

Liothyronine is used in a tri-iodothyronine suppression test for the diagnosis of thyrotoxicosis; for this purpose it is given in a daily dosage of 80 micrograms for 7 days.

Undesirable effects. Effects similar to those described under Thyroxine Sodium may occur, but rapidly disappear if treatment is stopped or the dosage reduced.

Veterinary uses. Liothyronine sodium is used in the treatment of thyroid hormone deficiency. The usual dose by mouth for dogs is 1 to 2 micrograms per kilogram body-weight twice daily.

Preparations

LIOTHYRONINE INJECTION: a sterile solution of liothyronine sodium in water for injections. It is prepared by dissolving the contents of a sealed container in water for injections immediately before use. Available as a powder in ampoules containing 20 micrograms of liothyronine sodium.

Containers and *Labelling:* see the entry on Injections for general information on containers and labelling.

Storage: the sealed container should be protected from light. The injection decomposes on storage and should be used immediately after preparation.

LIOTHYRONINE TABLETS (*Syn.* L-Tri-iodothyronine Sodium Tablets): available as tablets containing 20 micrograms of liothyronine sodium.

A standard for these tablets is given in the British Pharmacopoeia 1973

Containers and *Storage:* see the entry on Tablets for general information on containers and storage. Containers should be airtight and light resistant.

Advice for patients: the tablets should be taken at regular intervals. For the treatment of hypothyroidism the tablets should not be discontinued without the advice of the prescriber. For the diagnosis of thyrotoxicosis the prescribed course should be completed.

Liquorice

The dried peeled or unpeeled root and stolon of various species of *Glycyrrhiza* (Fam. Leguminosae), yielding a drug having a sweet taste and almost free from bitterness.

OTHER NAMES: Glycyrrhiza; Liquiritiae Radix; Liquorice Root; *Ulcedal®*

A standard is given in the European Pharmacopoeia Vol. II

The more important species of *Glycyrrhiza* are *G. glabra* L. and *G. glabra* var. *glandulifera* (Waldst. et Kit.) Regel and Herd. *G. glabra* is a tall erect herbaceous perennial, widely distributed over southern Europe. It is imported chiefly from Russia, Turkey, Syria, and Iran.

Varieties. Russian liquorice is obtained from *G. glabra* var. *glandulifera*, which grows abundantly in southern Russia; it consists mainly of root and is usually imported in the unpeeled condition. The pieces are often much larger than those of *G. glabra* and are usually split longitudinally. The cork, when present, is somewhat purplish in colour and frequently scaly. The taste is sweet but has a slight bitterness; unpeeled Russian liquorice yields about 25 to 30% of water-soluble extractive.

Persian liquorice, from Iran, is obtained from *G. glabra* var. *glandulifera* and is usually imported unpeeled; it resembles unpeeled Russian root in appearance.

Anatolian liquorice, from Turkey, and Syrian liquorice are derived from *G. glabra*; the pieces, which may be peeled or unpeeled, are sometimes of a very large size, up to 80 mm in diameter.

Constituents. Liquorice contains about 7% of glycyrrhizin, a sweet white crystalline powder consisting of the calcium and potassium salts of glycyrrhizinic acid. The acid, which forms colourless crystals melting at 222°, is the diglucopyranosiduronic acid of the triterpenoid glycyrrhetic acid (glycyrrhetinic acid) (3β-hydroxy-11-oxo-18β-olean-12-en-30-oic acid).

Liquorice also contains glucose, sucrose, starch (about 30%), other triterpenoid acids, and numerous flavonoid glycosides including isoliquiritin, which imparts a yellow colour to the peeled drug.

A bitter principle, glycyramarin is particularly abundant in the outer tissues and therefore largely absent from the peeled drug. Liquorice may yield up to 10% of sulphated ash and up to 2% of acid insoluble ash.

Description. UNGROUND DRUG. *Macroscopical characters:* pieces nearly cylindrical, about 5 to 30 mm in diameter and up to about 1 m in length, sometimes cut into lengths of about 100 to 150 mm. Unpeeled external surface longitudinally wrinkled, covered with a reddish-brown or purplish-brown corky layer, bearing small circular roots scars and, on pieces of stolon, occasional small dark buds. Peeled drug: external surface smooth, yellow, and fibrous. Fracture fibrous in the bark and splintery in the wood. Smoothed, transversely cut surface showing a distinct cambium line at a depth of about one-third of the radius, separating the yellowish-grey bark from the finely radiate yellow wood; central pith only in the stolon. Xylem wedges narrow, finely porous, each with a phloem strand opposite, with groups of included fibres visible as a radial row of dark points. It has a faint characteristic odour and a sweet taste which is almost free from bitterness.

Microscopical characters: the diagnostic characters are: *fibres* with thick, lignified or partially lignified walls present in groups of 10 to 50 in both phloem and xylem, often accompanied by rows of small rectangular cells each containing a prismatic *crystal* of calcium oxalate about 10 to 15 to 25 to 35 μm long; *vessels* large, walls with closely arranged bordered pits, frequently associated with lignified parenchyma; *starch* granules simple, oval, and rounded, 2 to 4 to 10 to 20 μm in diameter. In the unpeeled drug, *cork cells* brownish, polyhedral, tabular.

POWDERED DRUG: Powdered Liquorice. A brownish-yellow powder possessing the diagnostic characters, odour, and taste of the unground drug. It is prepared from the unpeeled drug unless the peeled drug is specified.

Adulterants and substitutes. Manchurian liquorice, possibly from *G. uralensis* Fisch. ex DC., has a pale chocolate-brown, readily exfoliated cork, a lacunar xylem, and conspicuously wavy medullary rays. It contains glycyrrhizin but is practically free from sugars.

Liquorice derived from *G. glabra* has been imported from India: it varies considerably in thickness and is usually cut into short lengths.

Storage. It should be stored in airtight containers, protected from light.

Identification. TEST. Mix the powdered drug with 1 drop of sulphuric acid (80% v/v); an orange-yellow colour is produced and many particles slowly develop a pink-red colour.

Actions and uses. Liquorice is a demulcent and mild expectorant. Extracts of liquorice with sedatives and other expectorants are used in cough lozenges and cough pastilles; the liquid extract is used in cough mixtures.

Liquorice is used as a flavouring agent in the compound powder, and the liquid extract will disguise the taste of nauseous medicines, especially the alkali iodides, ammonium chloride, quinine, creosote, and cascara liquid extract.

Liquorice extract from which most of the glycyrrhizinic acid has been removed is used in the treatment of peptic ulceration.

Preparations

LIQUORICE EXTRACT (*Syn.* Extractum Glycyrrhizae): *Small-scale preparation*

Liquorice, unpeeled,
  in coarse powder   ..   ..   1000 g
Chloroform water ..   ..   .. a sufficient quantity

Exhaust the liquorice with the chloroform water by percolation, boil the percolate for 5 minutes, and allow to stand for not less than 12 hours; decant the clear liquid and filter the remainder; mix the two liquids and evaporate to the consistency of a soft extract.

Manufacture. Prepare the extract by the above method, appropriately scaled up.

Storage: it should be stored in a cool place.

Dose: 0.6 to 2 grams.

LIQUORICE LIQUID EXTRACT (*Syn.* Ext. Glycyrrh. Liq.): *Small-scale preparation*

Liquorice, unpeeled, in
  coarse powder ..   ..   1000 g
Chloroform water }
Alcohol (90%)   } .. of each a sufficient quantity

Exhaust the liquorice with the chloroform water by percolation, boil the percolate for 5 minutes, and allow to stand for not less than 12 hours; decant the clear liquid and filter the remainder; mix the two liquids and evaporate until the weight per ml of the liquid is 1.198 g; allow to cool, and add to the liquid one-fourth of its volume of the alcohol; allow to stand for not less than 4 weeks, and filter.

Manufacture. Prepare the extract by the above method, appropriately scaled up.

A standard for this extract is given in the British Pharmacopoeia 1973

Dose: 2 to 5 ml.

OTHER PREPARATIONS available include CAPSULES containing an extract of liquorice (containing not more than 3% of glycyrrhizinic acid) 450 mg.

Lithium Carbonate

$Li_2CO_3 = 73.89$

OTHER NAMES: *Camcolit*®; Lithii Carbonas; *Phasal*®; *Priadel*®

A standard is given in the European Pharmacopoeia Vol. III Supplement

Description. An odourless white crystalline powder.

Solubility. Soluble, at 20°, in 100 parts of water; less soluble in boiling water; practically insoluble in alcohol.

Metabolism. ABSORPTION. Readily absorbed after oral administration.

BLOOD CONCENTRATION. After an oral dose of 3 g (40.6 mmol), peak plasma concentrations of about 1.7 mmol/litre are attained in 1 to 3 hours; effective concentrations are in the range 0.6 to 1.6 mmol/litre above which side effects may occur; plasma concentrations of up to 0.9 mmol/litre appear to be adequate to treat acute mania and there is no advantage if the concentration is increased to 1.4 mmol/litre.

HALF-LIFE. The decline in plasma concentration is biphasic with a half-life for the α-phase of 4 to 6 hours and a half-life for the β-phase of 14 to 25 hours.

DISTRIBUTION. Widely distributed throughout the body and concentrations in the cerebrospinal fluid may reach 50% of those in the plasma; lithium is taken up by red blood cells and this uptake appears, to some extent, to be genetically determined; it crosses the placenta and is secreted in the milk and saliva; saliva concentrations are higher than and parallel those in the plasma; volume of distribution, 650 to 850 ml/kg body-weight; *protein binding*, lithium is not bound to plasma proteins.

EXCRETION. Excreted mainly in the urine and about 50% or more of a dose may be excreted by this route in 24 hours; the urinary excretion of lithium appears to be slower in the elderly than the young and also appears to occur more slowly at night, resulting in a diurnal rhythm in excretion rate; its excretion is also markedly influenced by sodium and, possibly, potassium status; in subjects where the sodium intake is reduced lithium is reabsorbed by the renal tubules and in subjects who have a high sodium intake the excretion of lithium is increased.

FURTHER INFORMATION. Distribution: study in twins —E. Dorus *et al.*, *Archs gen. Psychiat.*, 1974, **31**, 463; excretion in saliva and urine—U. Groth *et al.*, *Clin. Pharmac. Ther.*, 1974, **16**, 490; influence of age on lithium dosage—D. S. Hewick and P. A. Newbury, *Br. J. clin. Pharmac.*, 1976, **3**, 354P.

Bioavailability. The absorption of standard tablets results in peak plasma concentrations which, being high, may result in the development of side effects; by reducing the dose, a reduction in the time at which effective concentrations are present in the blood occurs. Thus sustained release preparations have been used to provide a steadier release of the drug. However, the slower the release of the drug from the formulation, the greater appears the incidence of diarrhoea and the faster the release, the greater appears the incidence of nausea.

FURTHER INFORMATION. Dissolution rate and side effects—K. O. Borg *et al.*, *Acta pharm. suec.*, 1974, **11**, 133; absorption from sustained-release tablets—U. Otto *et al.*, *Acta pharm. suec.*, 1972, **9**, 595.

Actions and uses. Lithium carbonate is used as a source of lithium ions, which may act by competing with sodium at various sites. It causes changes in the composition of electrolytes in body fluids and increases the intracellular and total body water content.

Lithium carbonate is used in the treatment of acute mania and in the prevention of both mania and depression. It is more effective against manic than depressive swings.

The initial dose in affective disorders is 250 milligrams daily and this may be gradually increased to 750 milligrams daily in divided doses; in the treatment of mania these doses may be doubled. It is advisable to control treatment by measurement of the plasma lithium level, which should be maintained between 0.6 and 1.5 millimoles per litre, above which side-effects commonly occur.

Undesirable effects. Side-effects depend upon the dose and the degree of accumulation and usually develop slowly over a period of several days; they include sluggishness, drowsiness, loss of memory, coarse tremor, loss of appetite, diarrhoea, vomiting, polyuria, and polydipsia. The electrocardiogram may show flattening of the T-wave.

Administration of lithium carbonate may cause goitre and less frequently hypothyroidism requiring treatment with thyroxine.

Sodium depletion or the use of diuretics increases the toxicity of lithium compounds.

Contra-indications. Lithium carbonate should not be administered to patients with renal or cardiac disease. It should preferably be avoided during pregnancy, especially in the first trimester, and in nursing mothers.

Preparations

LITHIUM CARBONATE TABLETS: available as tablets containing 250 and 400 mg of lithium carbonate.

A standard for these tablets is given in the British Pharmacopoeia 1973

Containers and *Storage:* see the entry on Tablets for general information on containers and storage. Containers should be airtight.

Advice for patients: the tablets should be taken at regular intervals. Treatment should not be discontinued without the advice of the prescriber. The tablets may affect mental concentration; persons affected should not drive or operate machinery. Adequate salt and fluid intake should be maintained.

SLOW LITHIUM CARBONATE TABLETS: available as tablets containing 300 and 400 mg of lithium carbonate in slow release formulations.

A standard for these tablets is given in the British Pharmacopoeia 1973

Containers and *Storage:* see the entry on Tablets for general information on containers and storage. Containers should be airtight.

Advice for patients: the tablets should be taken at regular intervals and swallowed whole. Treatment should not be discontinued without the advice of the prescriber. The tablets may affect mental concentration; persons affected should not drive or operate machinery. Adequate salt and fluid intake should be maintained.

Loaiasis

see under FILARIASIS

Lonchocarpus

The dried roots of *Lonchocarpus utilis* A. C. Smith, *L. urucu* Killip and Smith, and possibly other species of *Lonchocarpus* (Fam. Leguminosae).

OTHER NAMES: Barbasco; Cube Root; Timbo

A standard is given in the British Pharmacopoeia (Veterinary)

Lonchocarpus utilis, formerly regarded as *L. nicou* (Aubl.) DC., is grown in Peru, and *L. urucu* in Brazil. Over 70 species of *Lonchocarpus* have been identified, some of which are known to contain rotenone. Among those that possess insecticidal properties but do not contain significant amounts of rotenone are *L. flori-bundus* Benth., *L. rariflorus* Mart., and *L. sylvestris* A. C. Smith.

Constituents. The active constituents are similar to those described under Derris. It contains from 3 to 10% of rotenone.

Description. *Macroscopical characters:* whole root, up to about 3 m long but usually in pieces from 40 to 300 mm in length and 15 to 25 mm in diameter; externally, brownish-grey with fine longitudinal reticulated wrinkles and occasional round or oval scars left by side roots, older pieces having transverse lenticels at intervals of 10 to 20 mm; lenticels about 2 to 5 mm long, 2 mm wide and rounded-oblong in outline; fracture short and irregular in the wood and fibrous in the bark; xylem porous and traversed by fairly numerous medullary rays which continue across the phloem where they widen towards the periphery; rays of phloem laminated by the alternation of strips of starch-containing parenchyma with strips of keratenchyma and fibres; blackened parts of certain roots result from the presence of very dark-coloured fungous hyphae penetrating the tissues of the root. When viewed in screened ultraviolet radiation, the transversely cut surface and the powder vary in appearance from yellow through greenish-yellow to orange-yellow; a filtered ether extract (1 in 20) appears blue to bluish-green. It has a slight odour and a taste which is slight at first becoming acrid and producing an unpleasant, numbing sensation in the mouth and throat.

Microscopical characters: the diagnostic characters are: numerous *starch* grains in all the parenchymatous tissues, most abundant in the medullary rays but absent from those cells containing a yellow-brown *resinous secretion*; starch mostly in simple circular to ovoid grains and to a less extent in compound grains of 2, frequently unequal, or rarely 3, components, individual grains being 6 to **15** to **25** to 35 μm in diameter; *xylem vessels* chiefly large, scattered and isolated, about 300 to 500 μm in diameter, their walls being covered with numerous bordered pits, with occasional small vessels adjacent to the larger ones; smaller *vessels* about 30 to 100 μm in diameter, in small groups associated with the groups of *xylem fibres*, which number about 25 to 35 in each group; *vessels* and bundles of *fibres* embedded in parenchyma having strongly pitted walls where the cells surround the vessels, similar bundles of fibres occurring in the phloem, associated with yellowish bands of *keratenchyma*; adjacent to the bundles of fibres, both of xylem and of the phloem, a few files of subcubical *parenchyma*, each cell containing a *crystal* of calcium oxalate in the form of a prism, about 20 to 30 μm in diameter; vessels lignified; *fibres* of the *phloem* largely unlignified except for the middle lamellae, those of the xylem being slightly more lignified; a few rectangular *sclereids* present in the phelloderm and pericyclic parenchyma; *cork cells*, thin walled and slightly lignified.

Incompatibility. Rotenone is readily oxidised in the presence of alkali, and materials of this nature should be avoided in preparing sprays, dip concentrates, and dusts containing lonchocarpus.

Storage. It should be stored in a dry place at a temperature not exceeding 25°.

Actions and uses. Lonchocarpus owes its action to the presence of constituents similar to those of derris and is used for the purposes described under Derris.

Lonchocarpus may be supplied when derris is demanded; derris may be supplied when lonchocarpus is demanded.

Preparations

LONCHOCARPUS DUSTING-POWDER: consisting of powdered lonchocarpus root, powdered derris root, or a mixture of the two, mixed with suitable inert diluents. Available as a dusting-powder containing 1% of rotenone. When Derris Dusting-powder is demanded, lonchocarpus dusting-powder may be supplied.

A standard for this dusting-powder is given in the British Pharmacopoeia (Veterinary)

PREPARED LONCHOCARPUS (*Syn.* Prepared Lonchocarpus Powder; Lonchocarpus Praeparata): consisting of lonchocarpus or derris, or a mixture of the two, which has been reduced to a fine powder and adjusted, if necessary, by the addition of fine powder prepared from lonchocarpus or derris of lower or higher rotenone content, to produce a powder of the required strength. It contains 5% of rotenone. When Prepared Derris, Prepared Derris Powder, or Derris Praeparata is demanded, Prepared Lonchocarpus may be supplied.

A standard for this powder is given in the British Pharmacopoeia (Veterinary)

Description: a cream to buff powder with a slight odour and a bitter or acrid taste causing a persistent sensation of numbness in the mouth and throat. The diagnostic characters are: *sclereids, fibres, parenchymatous cells* and *cork cells*, described under Derris and Lonchocarpus; if prepared from lonchocarpus only, or from a mixture of lonchocarpus and derris, it contains in addition bordered pitted *vessels* up to 500 μm in diameter, *crystals* of calcium oxalate in the form of prisms up to 30 μm long and *starch* granules up to 25 μm in diameter; if prepared from derris only it contains in addition bordered pitted *vessels* up to 220 μm in diameter, *crystals* of calcium oxalate in the form of prisms up to 20 μm long and *starch* granules up to 20 μm in diameter.

Incompatibility: rotenone is readily oxidised in the presence of alkali and materials of this nature should be avoided in preparing sprays, dip concentrates, and dusting-powders containing lonchocarpus or derris.

Storage: it should be stored in airtight containers, at a temperature not exceeding 25°, protected from light.

Actions and uses: prepared lonchocarpus depends for its action on the presence of rotenone and other constituents of the drugs and is used as described under Derris.

Lotions

Lotions are liquid preparations intended for application to the skin. The inclusion of alcohol in a lotion hastens its drying and accentuates its cooling effect, whilst the inclusion of glycerol keeps the skin moist for a considerable time.

Lotions are applied, without friction, on lint or other soft absorbent fabric and covered with waterproof material, or dabbed on the skin.

Avoidance of microbial contamination. Microorganisms may grow in certain lotions if no preservative is included; even if a preservative is present, care should be taken to avoid contaminating the lotions during their preparation. If a lotion is likely to be applied to broken or inflamed skin, the directions for preparation and dilution given under Creams should be followed.

Containers. Lotions should be dispensed in coloured fluted bottles or in suitable plastic containers.

Labelling. The container should be labelled "For external use only". The label on a diluted lotion should also state that the lotion should not be used later than one month after issue for use.

Louping-ill Vaccine

An emulsion in liquid paraffin or other suitable vehicle of cell-culture liquids containing louping-ill virus which has been inactivated in such a manner that immunogenic activity is retained.

A standard is given in the British Pharmacopoeia (Veterinary)

Storage. The vaccine should be protected from light and stored at 2° to 8° when it may be expected to retain its potency for 12 months.

Veterinary uses. It is administered by subcutaneous injection to cattle and sheep for prophylaxis of louping-ill.

Lozenges

Lozenges consist of medicaments incorporated in a flavoured basis and are intended to dissolve or disintegrate slowly in the mouth. They are prepared either by moulding and cutting or by compression.

Moulded Lozenges
These are usually prepared by mixing the medicaments, in powder or solution, with the basis, usually sucrose and acacia or tragacanth, making the mixture into a uniform paste with water, acacia mucilage, and the other ingredients, cutting the mass into uniform shapes, and drying the lozenges in a hot-air chamber at a moderate temperature.

Lozenges with Simple Basis
For 100 lozenges take:

Acacia, in fine powder .. .. 7 g
Sucrose, in fine powder .. .. 100 g
Water for preparations .. .. a sufficient quantity

Mix the medicaments intimately with the sucrose and the acacia, make the mixture into a paste with water, divide into 100 equal lozenges, and dry.

Compressed Lozenges
These are prepared by the method for compressed tablets described under Tablets. Heavy compression is necessary in order to ensure slow disintegration in the mouth. Each lozenge is made up to the weight specified in the individual monograph with an inert excipient which usually contains not less than 50% of sucrose.

Containers. Lozenges should be stored in well-closed containers which provide adequate protection against moisture and crushing. They should be supplied in wide-mouthed glass jars or plastic containers, or aluminium containers, suitably protected; lined screw-cap closures or plastic caps should be used.

Lungworm (Dictyocaulus viviparus) Oral Vaccine, Living

An aqueous preparation containing larvae of *Dictyocaulus viviparus* modified by exposure to X-rays.

OTHER NAME: Oral Husk Vaccine, Living

A standard is given in the British Pharmacopoeia (Veterinary)

Storage. The vaccine deteriorates rapidly and should be used as soon as possible after preparation. When stored at as low a temperature as possible above 0° the parasites may be expected to survive for 10 days.

Veterinary uses. It is administered by mouth to cattle for prophylaxis of parasitic bronchitis attributable to the helminth *Dictyocaulus viviparus*.

Lymecycline

A soluble tetracycline incorporating lysine, formaldehyde, and tetracycline, and having a molecular weight of approximately 603.

OTHER NAME: *Tetralysal*®

A standard is given in the British Pharmacopoeia 1973

Description. A yellow, very hygroscopic powder.

Solubility. Soluble, at 20°, in less than 1 part of water; very slightly soluble in alcohol; practically insoluble in ether, in chloroform, and in acetone.

Alkalinity. A 1% solution has a pH of 7.8 to 8.1.

Moisture content. Not more than 5%, determined by Fischer titration.

Specific rotation. −180° to −210°, determined on a 0.5% solution.

Stability. It is inactivated in solutions with a pH less than 2 and is slowly destroyed at pH 7 or above.

Labelling. If the material is not intended for parenteral administration the label on the container indicates that the contents are not to be injected.

Storage. It should be stored in airtight containers, protected from light, at a temperature not exceeding 25°.

Identification. TESTS. 1. To about 500 μg add 2 ml of sulphuric acid; a purple-red colour is produced.
2. Dissolve about 50 mg in 5 ml of water, add 50 mg of ninhydrin, boil, and add 15 ml of water; a blue-violet colour is produced.
3. Dissolve about 200 mg in 5 ml of water, add 300 mg of phosphoric acid and distil the mixture, collecting about 1 ml of distillate in a receiver containing 10 ml of *chromotropic acid solution*; a violet colour is produced.

MELTING-POINT. Above 200°, with slow decomposition.

ULTRAVIOLET ABSORPTION. In 0.1N hydrochloric acid, maxima at 220 nm (E1%, 1cm = 272), 272 nm (E1%, 1cm = 304), and 360 nm (E1%, 1cm = 181). In 0.1N sodium hydroxide, maxima at 240 nm (E1%, 1cm = 318) and 390 nm (E1%, 1cm = 224).

Metabolism. ABSORPTION. Well absorbed after oral administration; it is better absorbed than tetracycline and its absorption is only slightly affected by the presence of food; absorption of lymecycline may be reduced by the presence of metal ions such as aluminium, calcium, iron, and magnesium.

BLOOD CONCENTRATION. After an oral dose of approximately 200 mg, peak serum concentrations of about 0.6 to 2.0 μg/ml tetracycline are attained in about 4 hours; during therapy with 300 mg twice daily for 3 days serum concentrations of about 1.5 μg/ml are attained on the first day, rising to about 3.7 μg/ml by the third day.

HALF-LIFE. Serum half-life about 7 hours in children, 10 hours in infants, and 16 hours in the newborn.

DISTRIBUTION. Appears to be widely distributed throughout the body and has been detected in prostate, kidneys, liver, and lungs in concentrations higher than those in serum; it is secreted in the saliva in concentrations much lower than those in serum and it crosses the placenta; therapeutic concentrations are attained in the cerebrospinal fluid.

EXCRETION. 20 to 40% of a dose is excreted in the urine in 24 hours rising to about 65% in 48 hours; it is also excreted in high concentration in the bile.

FURTHER INFORMATION. Blood and urine concentrations—I. de Carneri and N. Manfredi, *Arzneimittel-Forsch.*, 1962, **12**, 1174, M. Parravicini, *Rif. med.*, 1964, **78**, 712 and J. L. Whitby and H. J. Black, *Br. med. J.*, ii/1964, 1491; transplacental diffusion—A. Prakash *et al.*, *J. Obstet. Gynaec. Br. Commonw.*, 1970, **77**, 247; twice-daily administration—L. Vitartali and A. Pisani-Ceretti, *Lancet*, i/1968, 923.

Actions and uses. Lymecycline is an antibiotic with the actions and uses described under Tetracycline Hydrochloride but when taken by mouth it is more rapidly absorbed and with doses containing the same amount of tetracycline a substantially higher concentration is produced in the blood.

Salts of aluminium, calcium, iron, and magnesium, antacids and milk which may decrease the absorption of tetracyclines from the gut should not be given with lymecycline.

The usual oral dose for an adult is 200 to 400 milligrams of lymecycline 4 times a day; in general, tetracyclines should not be given to children but when considered essential the usual oral dose for a child is 12 to 36 milligrams of lymecycline per kilogram body-weight (approximately equivalent to 9 to 27 milligrams of tetracycline) daily in divided doses. 200 milligrams of lymecycline is approximately equivalent to 150 milligrams of tetracycline or 160 milligrams of tetracycline hydrochloride. For intramuscular injection lymecycline is preferred to tetracycline hydrochloride because it is readily soluble at the pH of body fluids and so does not precipitate at the injection site to the same degree as tetracycline. The dose for adults is 135 milligrams of lymecycline (equivalent to 100 milligrams of tetracycline) 2 or 3 times daily. The usual dose for children is 6.5 milligrams of lymecycline per kilogram body-weight (approximately equivalent to 5 milligrams of tetracycline) daily in 2 divided doses.

Undesirable effects; Precautions and contra-indications; Drug interactions. As for Tetracycline Hydrochloride.

Preparations

LYMECYCLINE AND PROCAINE INJECTION: a sterile solution of lymecycline and procaine hydrochloride, with tartaric acid and magnesium ascorbate, in water for injections. It is prepared by dissolving the contents of a sealed container (containing the lymecycline, tartaric acid, and magnesium ascorbate) in the solvent (consisting of a solution of the procaine hydrochloride with tartaric acid in water for injections), immediately before use.

A standard for this injection is given in the British Pharmacopoeia 1973

Containers: see the entry on Injections for general information on containers.

Labelling: see the entry on Injections for general information on labelling. In addition, the label on the sealed container should state that the injection is for intramuscular use only, the date after which the contents are not intended to be used, and the conditions under which it should be stored. The label on the container of the solvent should state the composition of the solution.

Storage: the sealed container should be stored at a temperature not exceeding 25°, protected from light. The injection decomposes on storage and should be used immediately after preparation.

LYMECYCLINE CAPSULES: consisting of lymecycline, in powder, which may be mixed with a suitable inert diluent, enclosed in a hard capsule. The capsule shells may be coloured. Available as capsules containing 204 mg of lymecycline (equivalent to 150 mg of tetracycline).

A standard for these capsules is given in the British Pharmacopoeia 1973

Containers and *Storage:* see the entry on Capsules for general information on containers and storage.

Labelling: the label on the container should state the date after which the capsules are not intended to be used, and the conditions under which they should be stored.

Advice for patients: the capsules should be taken at regular intervals and salts of aluminium, calcium, iron, and magnesium, and antacids and milk should not be taken within 1 hour of administration. The prescribed course should be completed.

Lymphadenoma

see under LYMPHOPROLIFERATIVE DISEASES

Lymphocytic Leukaemia, Chronic

see under LYMPHOPROLIFERATIVE DISEASES

Lymphoproliferative Diseases

The lymphoproliferative diseases are malignant neoplastic diseases of the lymphoid tissue. They are classified according to the cell type which has undergone neoplastic change. They include the acute and chronic lymphatic (lymphocytic) leukaemias, multiple myeloma, macroglobulinaemia of Waldenström, Hodgkin's disease, lymphosarcoma, reticulum cell sarcoma, giant follicular lymphoma, and Burkitt's lymphoma.

Acute lymphatic leukaemia (acute lymphoblastic leukaemia) is described under Leukaemia, Acute.

Chronic lymphocytic leukaemia is a malignant proliferation of lymphocytes with infiltration of the bone marrow and, frequently, the blood. It is characterised by malaise and lassitude, localised or generalised lymphadenopathy, and anaemia. Patients with chronic lymphocytic leukaemia fail to form antibodies to foreign antigens; this renders them unusually prone to infections, particularly in the respiratory tract and skin. Infiltration of any organ or haemolytic anaemia may also occur.

Chronic lymphocytic leukaemia may be treated by radiotherapy, cytotoxic drugs, and corticosteroids. The aim is to control the disease rather than bring about radical cure. When infections occur, appropriate antibiotics must be given as soon as possible.

Multiple myeloma (myelomatosis) is a malignant proliferation of plasma cells within the bone marrow resulting in the excessive production of immunoglobulins. Multiple myeloma is characterised by erosion of cortical bone giving rise to pain and pathological fractures, bone-marrow infiltration causing anaemia and sometimes leucopenia or thrombocytopenia, renal failure, hypercalcaemia, and a haemorrhagic state as in macroglobulinaemia. Patients with multiple myeloma are particularly prone to infection because of their inability to form antibodies against foreign antigens. Multiple myeloma has been treated by corticosteroids to lower serum calcium, local radiotherapy for the relief of bone pain, and cytotoxic drugs.

Macroglobulinaemia of Waldenström is a group of diseases characterised by the presence of a high concentration of macroglobulins in the serum proteins. It is usually associated with a lymphoproliferative disorder such as lymphosarcoma or lymphocytic leukaemia. Macroglobulinaemia is commonly associated with lymphadenopathy or splenomegaly.

The symptoms present will be those of the underlying condition and those of macroglobulinaemia. Macroglobulinaemia causes an increased viscosity of blood which may result in heart failure, retinopathy, a haemorrhagic state, or haemolytic anaemia.

Treatment is aimed at the underlying condition, but in addition plasmapheresis and replacement with normal plasma proteins may be lifesaving.

Hodgkin's disease (lymphadenoma) is a neoplastic proliferation of lymphoreticular tissue characterised by painless enlargement of lymph nodes and spleen and the presence of Reed-Sternberg cells. There may be malaise, weakness, weight loss, anaemia, pruritus, fever, splenomegaly, and hepatomegaly. Infiltration of any organ of the body may also occur and there is an increased risk of infection.

Localised disease may be treated by radiotherapy of the area involved and local lymph nodes. For generalised disease, chemotherapy and corticosteroids are usually tried.

Lymphosarcoma and **Reticulum cell sarcoma** (reticulosarcoma) are characterised by a malignant proliferation of lymphocytes and reticular cells respectively in lymph nodes, spleen, and other organs.

Giant follicular lymphoma is a malignant disease arising in the lymph nodes or spleen characterised by the presence of giant pseudofollicles. Lymphadenopathy and splenomegaly may occur. It is treated by irradiation or surgical removal of lymph nodes or spleen or by cytotoxic drugs.

Burkitt's lymphoma is a particular form of lymphosarcoma occurring chiefly in Africa. The Epstein Barr virus has been isolated from the tumour cells grown in tissue culture. Burkitt's lymphoma responds well to cytotoxic drugs.

Lymphosarcoma

see under LYMPHOPROLIFERATIVE DISEASES

Lynoestrenol

19-Nor-17α-pregn-4-en-20-yn-17β-ol

$C_{20}H_{28}O = 284.4$

OTHER NAME: *Minilyn*® (with ethinyloestradiol)

A standard is given in the British Pharmacopoeia 1973

Description. An odourless white crystalline powder.

Solubility. Very slightly soluble in water; soluble, at 20°, in 15 parts of alcohol and of dehydrated alcohol, in 12 parts of ether and of acetone, and in 8 parts of chloroform.

Specific rotation. $-8°$ to $-12°$, determined on a 5% solution in dioxan.

Storage. It should be stored in airtight containers, protected from light.

Identification. MELTING-POINT. About 162°.

ULTRAVIOLET ABSORPTION. In methyl alcohol, it exhibits no significant absorption in the range 230 to 350 nm.

INFRA-RED ABSORPTION. Major peaks at 650, 683, 1014, 1040, 1053, and 1450 cm⁻¹ (see Appendix 2a: Infra-red Spectra).

THIN-LAYER CHROMATOGRAPHY. See under Thin-layer Chromatography, System 10.

Actions and uses. Lynoestrenol is a synthetic progestational steroid which has actions similar to those described under Norethisterone. It is used, chiefly in conjunction with oestrogens, as an oral contraceptive to inhibit ovulation. For this purpose doses of 2.5 milligrams are given daily, with ethinyloestradiol, from the fifth to the twenty-fourth day of each menstrual cycle. The course is repeated after an interval of one week. Regular administration is essential.

Lynoestrenol may also be used in doses of 5 milligrams daily for the treatment of dysfunctional uterine bleeding and in endometriosis; therapy in the latter condition must be continuous for 9 to 12 months.

Undesirable effects. Lynoestrenol may give rise to headaches and tension, mental depression, nausea and vomiting, breast engorgement, fluid retention, and weight gain; a state of pseudopregnancy and premenstrual tension may be aggravated. It may give rise to breakthrough bleeding, and may cause hirsutism, acneiform skin rashes, and deepening of the voice. Prolonged use may lead to impairment of liver function. When taken without oestrogens it may not prevent conception.

Regular use of progestational oral contraceptives combined with oestrogens increases the risk of intravascular thrombosis and thromboembolic accidents.

Precautions. These are as described under Norethisterone.

Contra-indications. It is contra-indicated in patients with hepatic disturbances.

Preparations

Preparations available include TABLETS containing lynoestrenol 2.5 mg with ethinyloestradiol 50 micrograms.

Lypressin

[8-Lysine]vasopressin, a cyclic octapeptide having the structure C̲ys-Tyr-Phe-Gln-Asn-C̲ys-Pro-Lys-Gly-NH₂.

It may be extracted from the posterior pituitary of pigs or prepared synthetically.

$C_{46}H_{65}N_{13}O_{12}S_2 = 1056.2$

OTHER NAME: *Syntopressin*®

Solubility. Soluble in water.

Actions and uses. Lypressin has the actions and uses described under Vasopressin Injection and is used in the treatment of polyuria and diabetes insipidus. It is administered as a nasal spray in a dosage of 5 to 20 units to one or both nostrils 3 to 7 times daily according to the patient's response.

Undesirable effects. Nasal congestion and ulceration of the nasal mucosa may occur.

Precautions. It should be administered with caution during pregnancy and to patients with coronary ischaemia, peripheral vascular disease, and hypertension.

Preparation

LYPRESSIN SPRAY: a solution of lypressin in a suitable vehicle. Available in 5-ml bottles containing 50 units of lypressin per ml. Approximately 5 units of lypressin is available to the patient each time the bottle is squeezed. *Storage:* when stored at temperatures between 4° and 25°, it may be expected to retain its potency for 2 years. *Advice for patients:* the bottle should be held vertically, and the inside of one or both nostrils sprayed by squeezing the bottle firmly one or more times at intervals in accordance with the dose required.

Macroglobulinaemia of Waldenström

see under LYMPHOPROLIFERATIVE DISEASES

Macrogol 300

A mixture of the polycondensation products of ethylene oxide and water obtained under controlled conditions. It is represented by the formula $CH_2(OH).(CH_2.O.CH_2)_m.CH_2OH$, where m may be 5 or 6. It has an average molecular weight of 285 to 325.

OTHER NAMES: *Carbowax*®; Liquid Macrogol; Polyethylene Glycol 300

A standard is given in the British Pharmacopoeia 1973

Description. A clear colourless viscous liquid with a faint characteristic odour.

Solubility. Miscible with water, with alcohol, and with glycols; practically insoluble in ether.

Weight per ml. At 20°, 1.120 to 1.130 g.

Acidity. A 5% solution has a pH of 4 to 7.

Moisture content. Not more than 1% w/w, determined by Fischer titration.

Viscosity. At 25°, 59 to 73 centistokes (5.9 to 7.3×10^{-5} m^2 sec^{-1}).

Refractive index. 1.462 to 1.466.

Sterilisation. Aqueous solutions are sterilised by heating in an autoclave or by filtration.

Storage. It should be stored in airtight containers.

Uses. The macrogols are strongly hydrophilic substances that are stable and non-irritant to the skin. They do not readily penetrate the skin, but as they are water-soluble and easily removed by washing, they are useful as ointment bases. An example is macrogol ointment which is a suitable mixture of macrogols 300 and 4000. Macrogols 1540 and 4000 are used as water-soluble bases for pessaries and suppositories. The hardness, melting-point, and dissolution rate of the product can be modified by varying the proportions of the macrogols used. Since suppositories made with macrogols dissolve in water drawn from the rectal mucosa by osmosis, irritation may occur where the tissues are sensitive; to minimise irritant effects, about 20% of water is often included in the basis.
Macrogol 4000 is employed as a binding agent and lubricant for tablets and, in alcoholic solution, for the film-coating of tablets.

Mixtures of the various liquid and solid grades of macrogol are used in the preparation of water-soluble bases for gauze dressings.
Macrogol 300 is used in preparations for external application as a solvent for drugs such as hydrocortisone and undecenoic acid which are relatively insoluble in water. It has also been used as a vehicle for injections.

Preparation

MACROGOL OINTMENT:

Macrogol 4000	..	..	..	..	.. 350 g
Macrogol 300	..	..	..	..	.. 650 g

Melt the macrogol 4000, add the macrogol 300, and stir continuously until cold.
Containers and *Storage:* see the entry on Ointments for general information on containers and storage.

Macrogol 1540

A mixture of the polycondensation products of ethylene oxide and water obtained under controlled conditions. It is represented by the formula $CH_2(OH).(CH_2.O.CH_2)_m.CH_2OH$, where m may be 28 to 36. It has an average molecular weight of 1300 to 1600.

OTHER NAMES: *Carbowax*®; Polyethylene Glycol 1540

A standard is given in the British Pharmacopoeia 1973

Description. A creamy-white soft wax-like solid with a faint characteristic odour.

Solubility. Soluble in 1 part of water, in 3 parts of chloroform, and in 100 parts of dehydrated alcohol; practically insoluble in ether.

Acidity. A 5% solution has a pH of 4 to 7.

Freezing-point. 42° to 46°.

Uses. These are described under Macrogol 300.

Macrogol 4000

A mixture of the polycondensation products of ethylene oxide and water obtained under controlled conditions. It is represented by the formula $CH_2(OH).(CH_2.O.CH_2)_m.CH_2OH$, where m may be 69 to 84. It has an average molecular weight of 3100 to 3700.

OTHER NAMES: *Carbowax*®; Hard Macrogol; Polyethylene Glycol 4000

A standard is given in the British Pharmacopoeia 1973

Description. A creamy-white, hard, wax-like solid or flakes with a faint characteristic odour.

Solubility. Soluble in 3 parts of water, in 2 parts of alcohol, and in 2 parts of chloroform; practically insoluble in ether.

Acidity or alkalinity. A 5% solution has a pH of 4.5 to 7.5.

Freezing-point. 53° to 56°.

Incompatibility. Macrogol 4000 has been reported to form a complex of low solubility with phenobarbitone and is therefore unsuitable for use in the preparation of tablets of phenobarbitone.

Sterilisation. It is sterilised by dry heat.

Uses. These are described under Macrogol 300.

Preparation

MACROGOL OINTMENT: see above under Macrogol 300.

Macrosalb (^{131}I) Injection

Macrosalb (^{131}I) Injection is a sterile suspension of human albumin which has been iodinated with iodine-131 and which has been denatured in such a way as to form insoluble aggregates. The aggregates are suspended in a saline solution isotonic with blood. The injection contains a suitable bactericide such as benzyl alcohol 0.9% v/v.

OTHER NAMES: MAA (^{131}I) Injection; Macroaggregated Iodinated (^{131}I) Human Albumin Injection; Macrisalb (^{131}I) Injection

A standard is given in the British Pharmacopoeia 1973

CAUTION. *This material is radioactive and any regulations in force must be complied with.*

Iodine-131 is a radioactive isotope of iodine which decays by emission of β^{-}-radiation mainly having a maximum energy of 0.606 MeV with emission of γ-radiation mainly of energy 0.364 MeV. It has a half-life of 8.06 days. It may be prepared by neutron irradiation of tellurium-130.

Description. A dilute suspension of white or faintly yellow particles which may settle on standing. The radioactivity is virtually all present in irregular particles with mean linear dimensions in the range 10 to 100 μm.

Acidity or alkalinity. pH 5.0 to 8.5.

Labelling. The label on the container should state (1) the content of iodine-131 expressed in microcuries or millicuries at a given date and hour, (2) the weight of human albumin in the container, (3) that the injection is radioactive, and (4) the date after which the injection is not intended to be used. The label on the package states (1) the total volume in the container, (2) the conditions under which it should be stored, and (3) the name of the bactericide.

Storage. It should be stored in an area assigned for the purpose at a temperature between 2° and 10°. The storage conditions should be such that the maximum radiation-dose-rate to which persons may be exposed is reduced to an acceptable level. Glass containers may darken under the effects of radiation.

Actions and uses. Macrosalb (^{131}I) Injection is used mainly in the investigation of lung perfusion by external visualisation of the organ by scintiscanner or gamma-ray camera.

It is administered by intravenous injection, the usual dose being 300 microcuries. After injection, almost all the particles are trapped in the capillaries of the lung, the number in any region being dependent on the blood supply of that region. Only a very small percentage of the capillaries are occluded and within 24 hours all particles have been cleared.

Pulmonary embolism is suggested by a silent area on the scan, indicating a reduced blood supply to the region. The emphysematous lung may show a patchy uptake. Tumours may produce large silent areas by pressure on the blood vessels.

Magnesium Acetate

$(CH_3 . CO_2)_2Mg, 4H_2O = 214.5$

A standard is given in the British Pharmaceutical Codex 1973

Description. Odourless colourless crystals or a white crystalline powder.

Solubility. Soluble, at 20°, in 1.5 parts of water and in 4 parts of alcohol.

Alkalinity. A 5% solution has a pH of 7.5 to 8.5.

Storage. It should be stored in airtight containers.

Uses. Magnesium acetate is a source of magnesium ions and may be used to adjust the magnesium content of solutions for haemodialysis.

Magnesium Carbonate, Heavy

A hydrated basic magnesium carbonate of varying composition. It corresponds approximately to the formula $3MgCO_3, Mg(OH)_2, 4H_2O$.

OTHER NAMES: Heavy Mag. Carb.; Magnesii Subcarbonas Ponderosus

A standard is given in the European Pharmacopoeia Vol. I

It may be prepared by mixing boiling concentrated aqueous solutions of magnesium sulphate and sodium carbonate, evaporating to dryness, and washing the product.

Description. *Macroscopical characters:* an odourless white powder.

Microscopical characters: mounted in *dilute glycerol* it is seen to consist mainly of subspherical particles, about 10 to 20 μm in diameter, many being arranged in clumps of 4 to 20; small numbers of particles resembling light magnesium carbonate occur amongst the spherites. Between crossed polars each particle shows a well-marked black cross.

Solubility. Very slightly soluble in water; practically insoluble in alcohol; soluble with effervescence in dilute acids.

Apparent volume. 15 g occupies a volume of about 30 ml.

Hygroscopicity. At relative humidities between about 15 and 65%, the equilibrium moisture content at 25° is about 1%, but at relative humidities above about 75%, the powder absorbs small amounts of moisture.

Actions and uses. Heavy magnesium carbonate has the actions and uses described under Light Magnesium Carbonate, but its smaller bulk renders it more suitable as an ingredient of antacid powders.

It is usually given as an antacid, in a dosage of 250 to 500 milligrams repeated in accordance with the needs of the patient. As a laxative the usual dose is 2 to 5 grams.

Preparations

COMPOUND MAGNESIUM CARBONATE POWDER:

Heavy magnesium carbonate	400 g
Light kaolin or light kaolin (natural)	100 g
Sodium bicarbonate	300 g
Calcium carbonate	400 g

Mix, as described in the entry on Powders.

A standard for this powder is given in the British Pharmaceutical Codex 1973

Containers and *Storage:* see the entry on Powders for general information on containers and storage.

Dose: 1 to 5 grams.

Advice for patients: the powder should be taken mixed with a little water or other fluid between meals. Treatment should not be continued for longer than a few days without medical advice.

OTHER PREPARATIONS: heavy magnesium carbonate is an ingredient of compound calcium carbonate powder, compound magnesium trisilicate powder, and compound rhubarb powder.

Magnesium Carbonate, Light

A hydrated basic magnesium carbonate of varying composition. It corresponds approximately to the formula $3MgCO_3,Mg(OH)_2,3H_2O$.

OTHER NAMES: Light Mag. Carb.; Magnesii Subcarbonas Levis

A standard is given in the European Pharmacopoeia Vol. I

It may be prepared by boiling a mixture of dilute aqueous solutions of magnesium sulphate and sodium carbonate.

Description. *Macroscopical characters:* a very light, white, odourless powder.

Microscopical characters: mounted in *dilute glycerol* it is seen to consist of small acicular crystals, about 7 μm long and 1 to 2 μm thick, partly in clumps of about 10 to 200 crystals.

Solubility. Very slightly soluble in water; practically insoluble in alcohol; soluble with effervescence in dilute acids.

Apparent volume. 15 g occupies a volume of about 200 ml.

Actions and uses. Light magnesium carbonate has antacid and laxative actions. It is less effective for neutralising gastric acidity than magnesium hydroxide and has the disadvantage of liberating carbon dioxide. As an antacid, the usual dose is 250 to 500 milligrams, repeated in accordance with the needs of the patient. The usual laxative dose is 2 to 5 grams.

Light magnesium carbonate is more suitable for use in mixtures and the heavy variety for powders. It is used for dispersing volatile oils in inhalations having an aqueous vehicle.

Veterinary uses. Light magnesium carbonate is used as an antacid. The usual dose by mouth for all species is 15 to 30 milligrams per kilogram body-weight.

Preparations

AROMATIC MAGNESIUM CARBONATE MIXTURE (*Syn.* Mistura Carminativa):

Light magnesium carbonate	30 g
Aromatic cardamom tincture	30 ml
Sodium bicarbonate	50 g
Chloroform water, double-strength	500 ml
Water for preparations	to 1000 ml

It should be recently prepared.
A standard for this mixture is given in the British Pharmaceutical Codex 1973
Containers: see the entry on Mixtures for general information on containers.
Labelling: see the entry on Mixtures for general information on labelling. A direction to shake the bottle should be given on the label.
Dose: 10 to 20 millilitres.
Advice for patients: the mixture may be taken alone or with water or other fluid between meals. It should not be used for longer than a few days without medical advice.

AROMATIC MAGNESIUM CARBONATE POWDER FOR MIXTURE:

Light magnesium carbonate	375 g
Sodium bicarbonate	625 g

Mix, as described in the entry on Powders.
Labelling: the directions given under Powders for Mixtures should be followed.
Preparation of 1000 ml of aromatic magnesium carbonate mixture: add 80 g of the powder for mixture to 500 ml of double-strength chloroform water and shake. Add 30 ml of aromatic cardamom tincture, shake, add sufficient water for preparations to produce 1000 ml and again shake.

MAGNESIUM CARBONATE MIXTURE:

Light magnesium carbonate	50 g
Sodium bicarbonate	80 g
Peppermint emulsion, concentrated	25 ml
Chloroform water, double-strength	500 ml
Water for preparations	to 1000 ml

It should be recently prepared.
A standard for this mixture is given in the British Pharmaceutical Codex 1973
Containers: see the entry on Mixtures for general information on containers.
Labelling: see the entry on Mixtures for general information on labelling. A direction to shake the bottle should be given on the label.
Dose: 10 to 20 millilitres.
Advice for patients: the mixture may be taken alone or with water or other fluid between meals. It should not be used for longer than a few days without medical advice.

MAGNESIUM CARBONATE POWDER FOR MIXTURE:

Light magnesium carbonate	384.6 g
Sodium bicarbonate	615.4 g

Mix, as described in the entry on Powders.
Labelling: the directions given under Powders for Mixtures should be followed
Preparation of 1000 ml of magnesium carbonate mixture: add 130 g of the powder for mixture to 500 ml of double-strength chloroform water and shake. Add 25 ml of concentrated peppermint emulsion, shake, add sufficient water for preparations to produce 1000 ml and again shake.

OTHER PREPARATIONS: light magnesium carbonate is an ingredient of paediatric compound calcium carbonate mixture, kaolin mixture, kaolin veterinary mixture, magnesium sulphate mixture, magnesium trisilicate mixture, magnesium trisilicate and belladonna mixture, and compound rhubarb powder.

Magnesium Chloride

$MgCl_2,6H_2O = 203.3$

OTHER NAMES: Mag. Chlor.; Magnesii Chloridum

A standard is given in the European Pharmacopoeia Vol. III

Description. Odourless colourless hygroscopic crystals with a bitter taste.

Solubility. Soluble, at 20°, in 1 part of water and in 2 parts of alcohol.

Stability. When heated at 100°, it loses two molecules of water of crystallisation; at 110° it begins to lose hydrogen chloride, forming basic salts.

Storage. It should be stored in airtight containers.

Veterinary uses. Magnesium chloride is used in conjunction with calcium salts in the treatment of hypomagnesaemia associated with hypocalcaemia. The usual dose by subcutaneous injection for cattle and sheep is 150 milligrams per kilogram body-weight.

Magnesium Chloride for Dialysis

$MgCl_2,6H_2O = 203.3$

OTHER NAME: Mag. Chlor. for Dialysis

A standard is given in the British Pharmacopoeia 1973

Description; Solubility; Stability; Storage. As for Magnesium Chloride (above).

Uses. Magnesium chloride for dialysis is used to adjust the concentration of magnesium ions in preparing solutions for haemodialysis and peritoneal dialysis.

Magnesium Hydroxide

$Mg(OH)_2 = 58.32$

OTHER NAMES: *Aquamag*®; Mag. Hydrox.

A standard is given in the British Pharmaceutical Codex 1973

Description. An odourless white amorphous powder.

Solubility. Very slightly soluble in water; readily soluble in dilute acids.

Storage. It should be stored in airtight containers.

Actions and uses. Magnesium hydroxide is an antacid, and owing to the formation of magnesium chloride in the stomach, it also acts as a mild saline laxative. It does not produce alkalosis.
The usual dose as an antacid is 500 to 750 milligrams, repeated in accordance with the needs of the patient. The usual laxative dose is 2 to 4 grams.

Preparations

LIQUID PARAFFIN AND MAGNESIUM HYDROXIDE MIXTURE (*Syn.* Liquid Paraffin and Magnesium Hydroxide Emulsion):

Liquid paraffin	250 ml
Magnesium hydroxide mixture..	735 ml
Chloroform spirit	15 ml

Mix the chloroform spirit with the magnesium hydroxide mixture, add to the liquid paraffin, and pass through a homogeniser.
A standard for this mixture is given in the British Pharmaceutical Codex 1973
Containers: see the entry on Mixtures for general information on containers. It should be supplied in wide-mouthed bottles.
Labelling: see the entry on Mixtures for general information on labelling. A direction to shake the bottle should be given on the label.
Dose: 5 to 20 millilitres.
Advice for patients: the mixture should preferably not be taken within 30 minutes of mealtimes and should preferably be taken on an empty stomach. It should not be used for longer than a few days without medical advice.

MAGNESIUM HYDROXIDE MIXTURE (*Syn.* Cream of Magnesia): consisting of an aqueous suspension of hydrated magnesium oxide containing the equivalent of 7.9% w/w

of $Mg(OH)_2$. It may be prepared from a suitable grade of light magnesium oxide, or according to the following formula:

Light magnesium oxide	52.5 g
Sodium hydroxide..	15.0 g
Magnesium sulphate	47.5 g
Chloroform water, double-strength	500 ml
Purified water, freshly boiled and cooled	to 1000 ml

Dissolve the sodium hydroxide in 150 ml of purified water, add the light magnesium oxide, mix to form a smooth cream, and add sufficient purified water to produce 2500 ml. Pour this suspension, in a thin stream, into a solution prepared by dissolving the magnesium sulphate in 2500 ml of purified water, stirring continuously. Allow the precipitate to subside, remove the clear liquid, and transfer the residue to a calico strainer. Allow to drain and wash the precipitate with purified water until the washings give only a slight reaction when tested for the presence of sulphates. Mix the washed precipitate with purified water, add the double-strength chloroform water, and sufficient purified water to produce the required volume. It contains, in 10 ml, the equivalent of 550 mg of magnesium oxide.
A standard for this mixture is given in the British Pharmacopoeia 1973
Containers: see the entry on Mixtures for general information on containers. It should be supplied in wide-mouthed bottles.
Labelling: see the entry on Mixtures for general information on labelling. A direction to shake the bottle should be given on the label.
Storage: it should *not* be stored in a cold place.
Dose: as an antacid: 5 to 10 ml, repeated in accordance with the needs of the patient.
As a laxative: 25 to 50 ml.
Advice for patients: when used as an antacid the mixture may be taken alone or with water or other fluid between meals. When used as a laxative the mixture should be taken well diluted with water on an empty stomach. It should not be used for longer than a few days without medical advice.

OTHER PREPARATIONS available include a PASTE containing magnesium hydroxide 28% (approximately) suitable for dilution to prepare magnesium hydroxide mixture.

Magnesium Oxide, Light

$MgO = 40.30$

OTHER NAMES: Light Mag. Ox.; Light Magnesia; Magnesii Oxidum Leve

A standard is given in the European Pharmacopoeia Vol. I

It may be prepared by heating light magnesium carbonate to dull redness.

Description. An odourless, very light, white, fine amorphous powder. It forms a gelatinous mass on standing for about 30 minutes with 15 times its weight of water.

Solubility. Very slightly soluble in water; practically insoluble in alcohol; soluble in dilute acids.

Apparent volume. 20 g occupies a volume of about 150 ml.

Hygroscopicity. On exposure to air it rapidly absorbs moisture and carbon dioxide.

Storage. It should be stored in airtight containers.

Actions and uses. Light magnesium oxide has the actions and uses described under Magnesium Hydroxide. Because of its lightness, light magnesium oxide is suitable for inclusion in mixtures.

The usual dose as an antacid is 250 to 500 milligrams, repeated in accordance with the needs of the patient. The usual laxative dose is 2 to 5 grams.

Preparation

MAGNESIUM HYDROXIDE MIXTURE: see above under Magnesium Hydroxide.

Magnesium Stearate

A mixture of varying proportions of magnesium stearate $[(C_{17}H_{35}COO)_2Mg = 591.3]$ and magnesium palmitate $[(C_{15}H_{31}COO)_2Mg = 535.1]$.

OTHER NAME: Magnesii Stearas

A standard is given in the European Pharmacopoeia Vol. III

Description. A fine, white, impalpable, tasteless powder, which is unctuous and readily adherent to the skin, and has a faint characteristic odour.

Solubility. Practically insoluble in water, in alcohol, and in ether.

Moisture content. Not more than 6%, determined by drying at 105°.

Storage. It should be stored in airtight containers.

Actions and uses. Magnesium stearate is used as dusting-powder in the treatment of skin diseases, and in creams as a barrier to chemical irritants. It is also used as a lubricant for granules in the manufacture of tablets.

Magnesium Sulphate

$MgSO_4,7H_2O = 246.5$

OTHER NAMES: Epsom Salts; Mag. Sulph.; Magnesii Sulfas

A standard is given in the European Pharmacopoeia Vol. I

Description. Odourless brilliant colourless crystals or white crystalline powder with a bitter taste.

Solubility. Soluble, at 20°, in 1.5 parts of water; soluble in less than 0.2 part of boiling water; very slightly soluble in alcohol.

Moisture content. 48 to 52%, determined by drying first at 110° to 120° for 1 hour and then at 400°.

It effloresces in warm dry air and when heated at 150° to 160° is converted into the monohydrate; the last molecule of water of crystallisation is expelled at about 280°.

Incompatibility. It is incompatible with alkali carbonates and bicarbonates; strong solutions are incompatible with potassium and ammonium bromides, the double sulphates crystallising out.

Sterilisation. Solutions for injection are sterilised by heating in an autoclave or by filtration.

Storage. It should be stored in airtight containers, in a cool place.

Actions and uses. Magnesium sulphate is a saline purgative. Such purgatives are not readily absorbed from

the intestine. When taken by mouth in dilute solution they reduce the normal absorption of water from the intestine, with the result that the bulky fluid contents distend the bowel, active reflex peristalsis is excited, and evacuation of the contents of the intestine occurs in 1 to 2 hours. If hypertonic solutions are given by mouth the osmotic pressure in the bowel is raised and water is withdrawn from the tissues to restore the balance; the purgative action is then delayed.

Saline purgatives are often given in habitual constipation due to deficient peristalsis, the best results being obtained by taking the dose in a half to one tumblerful of water, preferably before breakfast.

The usual dose of magnesium sulphate is 5 to 15 grams. The purgative dose for children is from one-quarter to three-quarters the dose for adults.

A 50% solution in water, in a dose of 60 to 180 millilitres, may be given as an enema.

In the treatment of cholecystitis, 50 millilitres of a 25% solution of magnesium sulphate, administered directly into the duodenum by means of a duodenal tube, or given by mouth on an empty stomach, has been used to promote evacuation of the gall-bladder. The intravenous injection of 10 to 25 millilitres of a 10% solution has been used to lower intracranial pressure and to control the convulsions in acute uraemia and eclampsia.

In cases of magnesium deficiency 5 to 10 millilitres of a 50% solution of magnesium sulphate is given daily, by intramuscular injection or by intravenous infusion well diluted with dextrose injection.

Wet dressings of a 25% solution of magnesium sulphate are sometimes used in the treatment of carbuncles and boils.

Magnesium sulphate is a common ingredient of aperient mineral waters.

Veterinary uses. Magnesium sulphate is used as a purgative. The usual dose by mouth for all species except cats is 0.5 to 1 gram per kilogram body-weight. It is also used in the treatment of hypomagnesaemia in cattle and sheep by subcutaneous, intraperitoneal, or slow intravenous injection in doses up to 200 milligrams per kilogram body-weight.

Preparations

MAGNESIUM SULPHATE INJECTION: a sterile solution of magnesium sulphate in water for injections. It is sterilised by heating in an autoclave or by filtration. Available in 400-ml bottles containing 25% of magnesium sulphate.

A standard for this injection is given in the British Pharmacopoeia (Veterinary)

Containers: see the entry on Injections for general information on containers.

Labelling: see the entry on Injections for general information on labelling. In addition, the label on the container should state the amount of the medicament as the percentage w/v of magnesium sulphate.

MAGNESIUM SULPHATE MIXTURE (*Syn.* Mistura Alba):

Magnesium sulphate	400 g
Light magnesium carbonate	50 g
Peppermint emulsion, concentrated	25 ml
Chloroform water, double-strength	300 ml
Water for preparations .. ., ..	to 1000 ml

It should be recently prepared.

A standard for this mixture is given in the British Pharmaceutical Codex 1973

Containers: see the entry on Mixtures for general information on containers.

Labelling: see the entry on Mixtures for general information on labelling. A direction to shake the bottle should be given on the label.

Dose: 10 to 20 millilitres.

Advice for patients: the mixture should be taken well diluted with water or other fluid, preferably on an empty stomach. It should not be used for longer than a few days without medical advice.

Magnesium Sulphate, Dried

Magnesium sulphate which has been dried at 100° until it has lost approximately 25% of its weight.

OTHER NAMES: Dried Epsom Salts; Dried Mag. Sulph.; Exsiccated Magnesium Sulphate

A standard is given in the British Pharmacopoeia 1973

Description. An odourless white powder with a saline and bitter taste.

Solubility. Soluble, at 20°, in 2 parts of water; more rapidly soluble in hot water.

Storage. It should be stored in airtight containers.

Actions and uses. Dried magnesium sulphate has the actions and uses described under Magnesium Sulphate, but it is employed only when the use of the hydrated salt would be disadvantageous. It is one of the chief ingredients of effervescent and non-effervescent aperient powders or granules. The usual dose is 2 to 12 grams, as a single dose.

As magnesium sulphate paste it is used as an application to carbuncles and boils but prolonged or repeated use may damage the surrounding skin and predispose to further boils.

Preparation

MAGNESIUM SULPHATE PASTE (*Syn.* Morison's Paste):

Dried magnesium sulphate ..	a sufficient quantity
Phenol	0.5 g
Glycerol, previously heated at 120° for 1 hour and cooled	55 g

Dry about 70 g of the dried magnesium sulphate for 1½ hours at 150° or for 4 hours at 130° and allow to cool in a desiccator; mix 45 g of this powder in a warm mortar with the phenol dissolved in the glycerol. In preparing larger quantities of the paste the period of heating the dried magnesium sulphate should be increased, if necessary, to ensure that the dried powder contains at least 85% of magnesium sulphate, calculated as $MgSO_4$.

A standard for this paste is given in the British Pharmaceutical Codex 1973

Containers and *Storage:* it should be stored and supplied in airtight glass jars or other suitable containers.

Labelling: the label on the container should state that the paste should be stirred before use.

Advice for patients: the paste may be applied liberally to the affected area. It should not be used repeatedly.

Magnesium Trisilicate

A hydrated magnesium silicate corresponding approximately to the formula $2MgO,3SiO_2$, with water of crystallisation.

OTHER NAMES: Mag. Trisil.; Magnesii Trisilicas; *Magsorbent®; Trisillac®*

A standard is given in the European Pharmacopoeia Vol. III Supplement

Description. *Macroscopical characters:* an odourless, white, slightly hygroscopic powder.

Microscopical characters: consists of irregular rounded particles, from about 10 by 15 μm to 40 by 60 μm, and thin flat lamellae, 10 by 10 μm up to 25 by 80 μm, together with numerous particles about 5 to 10 μm across. With *safranine solution,* it stains deep red, and with *alcoholic methylene blue solution,* deep blue.

Solubility. Practically insoluble in water.

Hygroscopicity. At relative humidities between about 15 and 65%, the equilibrium moisture content at 25° is between about 17 and 23%; at relative humidities between about 75 and 95%, the equilibrium moisture content is between about 24 and 30%.

Storage. It should be stored in airtight containers.

Actions and uses. Magnesium trisilicate has adsorbent and antacid properties and is non-toxic even in very large doses. Its action is exerted slowly, so that it does not give such rapid symptomatic relief as the alkali carbonates, bicarbonates, and oxides. However, the action continues for some time, and the substance is therefore of value in the treatment of dyspepsia. It does not give rise to alkalosis.

During neutralisation, magnesium chloride and a hydrated silica gel are formed; the latter also possesses adsorbent properties, although inferior in this respect to the original substance. The formation of magnesium chloride sometimes causes diarrhoea, but this is seldom severe.

Magnesium trisilicate is usually given in a dosage of 0.5 to 2 grams, repeated in accordance with the needs of the patient.

Preparations

COMPOUND MAGNESIUM TRISILICATE POWDER:

Magnesium trisilicate ..	..	..	..	250 g
Chalk, in powder ..	..	..	..	250 g
Heavy magnesium carbonate ..	..	..	250 g
Sodium bicarbonate ..	..	..	..	250 g

Mix, as described in the entry on Powders.

A standard for this powder is given in the British Pharmaceutical Codex 1973

Containers and *Storage:* see the entry on Powders for general information on containers and storage.

Dose: 1 to 5 grams.

Advice for patients: the powder should be taken mixed with a little water or other fluid between meals. Treatment should not be continued for longer than a few days without medical advice.

COMPOUND MAGNESIUM TRISILICATE TABLETS (*Syn.* Aluminium Hydroxide and Magnesium Trisilicate Tablets):

For each tablet take:

Magnesium trisilicate ..	..	..	250 mg
Dried aluminium hydroxide gel	..	..	120 mg
Peppermint oil ..	..	..	0.003 ml

Mix the solid ingredients and granulate by moist granulation as described in the entry on Tablets; dry the granules at a suitable temperature, which should not exceed 30° if a drying oven is used, mix with the peppermint oil previously dissolved in a small quantity of alcohol (95%), and prepare by compression.

A standard for these tablets is given in the British Pharmaceutical Codex 1973

Containers and *Storage:* see the entry on Tablets for general information on containers and storage. Containers should be airtight. The tablets should be stored at a temperature not exceeding 25°.

Labelling: a direction to chew the tablets before they are swallowed should be given on the label.

Dose: 1 to 2 tablets.

Advice for patients: the tablets should be chewed half an hour after meals. They should not be used for longer than a few days without medical advice.

MAGNESIUM TRISILICATE AND BELLADONNA MIXTURE:

Belladonna tincture	..	..	..	50 ml
Magnesium trisilicate mixture	..	..		to 1000 ml

It must be freshly prepared.

Containers and *Labelling:* see the entry on Mixtures for general information on containers and labelling.

Dose: 10 to 20 millilitres.

Advice for patients: the mixture may be taken alone or with water or other fluid between meals. It should not be used for longer than a few days without medical advice.

MAGNESIUM TRISILICATE MIXTURE (*Syn.* Compound Magnesium Trisilicate Mixture):

Magnesium trisilicate	..	..	..	50 g
Light magnesium carbonate	..	..	..	50 g
Sodium bicarbonate	..	..	..	50 g
Peppermint emulsion, concentrated	..	..	25 ml
Chloroform water, double-strength	..	..	500 ml
Water for preparations	..	..	..	to 1000 ml

It should be recently prepared.

A standard for this mixture is given in the British Pharmaceutical Codex 1973

Containers: see the entry on Mixtures for general information on containers.

Labelling: see the entry on Mixtures for general information on labelling. A direction to shake the bottle should be given on the label.

Dose: 10 to 20 millilitres.

Advice for patients: the mixture may be taken alone or with water or other fluid between meals. It should not be used for longer than a few days without medical advice.

MAGNESIUM TRISILICATE POWDER FOR MIXTURE:

Magnesium trisilicate	..	..	..	333.3 g
Light magnesium carbonate	..	..	..	333.3 g
Sodium bicarbonate	..	..	..	333.4 g

Mix, as described in the entry on Powders.

Storage: it should be stored in airtight containers.

Labelling: the directions given under Powders for Mixtures should be followed.

Preparation of 1000 ml of magnesium trisilicate mixture: add 150 g of the powder for mixture to 500 ml of double-strength chloroform water and shake. Add 25 ml of concentrated peppermint emulsion, shake, add sufficient water for preparations to produce 1000 ml and again shake.

OTHER PREPARATIONS available include a MIXTURE containing magnesium trisilicate 600 mg in 5 ml.

Maize Oil

The fixed oil obtained from the embryos of maize, *Zea mays* L. (Fam. Gramineae), which are separated during the preparation of maize starch.

OTHER NAME: Corn Oil

A standard is given in the British Pharmacopoeia 1973

Constituents. Maize oil consists of glycerides, the fatty acid constituents of which are mainly oleic and linoleic acids, with smaller proportions of palmitic and stearic acids.

Description. A pale yellow to golden yellow oil with a faint characteristic odour.

Solubility. Very slightly soluble in alcohol; miscible with ether, with chloroform, and with light petroleum.

Weight per ml. At 20°, 0.915 to 0.923 g.

Refractive index. 1.472 to 1.475.

Adulterants and substitutes. Arachis oil, cottonseed oil, and sesame oil may be present. The tests for arachis oil, cottonseed oil, and sesame oil are described under Almond Oil.

Sterilisation. Maize oil is sterilised by dry heat.

Storage. It should be stored in well-filled containers, protected from light, in a cool place.

Actions and uses. Maize oil has properties similar to those of olive oil. It is used, because of its high content of glycerides of unsaturated acids, as a constituent of diets intended to reduce high blood-cholesterol levels.

Maize Starch, Pregelatinised

Maize starch which has been treated by heating as an aqueous slurry and subsequently removing the water from the resulting paste.

OTHER NAME: *National 1551*®

A standard is given in the British Pharmacopoeia Addendum 1975

Description. *Macroscopical characters:* a white to pale cream-coloured, almost odourless powder which disperses in cold water.

Microscopical characters: irregular, translucent, cream-coloured flakes with a reticulated surface and numerous fragmented flakes; very occasional starch grains with a well-marked cross when viewed between crossed polars.

Acidity or alkalinity. A 20% dispersion in water has a pH of 5.5 to 8.

Moisture content. Not more than 15%, determined by drying at 105°.

Storage. It should be stored in airtight containers.

Uses. Pregelatinised maize starch is incorporated in tablet formulations as a binding agent and disintegrating agent. It has an advantage over other agents in that it may be intimately mixed, in the dry state, with other ingredients and granulation is effected by addition of water only.

Maize Starch, Sterilisable

Maize starch which has been treated by chemical and physical means so that it does not gelatinise on exposure to moisture or steam sterilisation. It contains up to 2.2% of magnesium oxide.

OTHER NAMES: Absorbable Dusting-powder; *Bio-Sorb*®; Modified Starch Dusting-powder

A standard is given in the British Pharmacopoeia 1973

Description. *Macroscopical characters:* an odourless white free-flowing powder.

Microscopical characters: it exhibits polyhedral or

rounded granules, about 5 to 10 to 20 to 30 μm in diameter, having in the centre a distinct cavity or a 2- to 5-rayed cleft.

Alkalinity. A 10% suspension has a pH of 9.5 to 10.8.

Moisture content. Not more than 12%, determined by drying at 105°.

Sterilisation. It may be sterilised by heating at 150° to 160° for sufficient time to ensure that the whole of the powder is maintained at this temperature for one hour or by autoclaving, in thin layers, at 115° to 116° for thirty minutes.

Labelling. The label on the container states that care should be taken to avoid the use of excessive amounts of the powder on surgeons' gloves.

Uses. Sterilisable maize starch is used as a lubricant for surgeons' gloves; the lubricant properties are not affected by autoclaving. Unlike talc and similar substances it is completely absorbed by body tissues. It should, however, be used sparingly to minimise the possibility of inflammatory tissue reactions.

Malaria

Malaria is a disease caused by infection with protozoa of the genus *Plasmodium*, transmitted by the bite of mosquitoes of the genus *Anopheles*. Causal organisms include *P. falciparum* (malignant tertian malaria; falciparum malaria), *P. malariae* (quartan malaria; malariae malaria), *P. ovale* (ovale tertian malaria; ovale malaria), and *P. vivax* (benign tertian malaria; vivax malaria). The commonest and most important of these infections are those caused by *P. falciparum* and *P. vivax*.

Malaria is characterised by intermittent fever, anaemia, and spleen enlargement. There is an incubation period of from 12 days (*P. falciparum*) to up to a month (*P. malariae*). The malarial attack starts with headache, nausea, and vomiting followed by febrile paroxysms which are characterised by shivering at first followed by profuse sweating. The attacks may recur every second day (vivax malaria), every third day (malariae malaria), or daily or irregularly (falciparum malaria).

Complications of malaria may occur in the brain, gastro-intestinal system, kidneys, or lungs. Falciparum malaria may be fatal if not treated promptly and returning travellers should therefore seek medical assistance if they feel unwell.

Prophylaxis for travellers (suppressive treatment)

When visiting areas where malaria is endemic precautions against infection should be taken. Persons staying in the open after sunset should be suitably protected from mosquitoes and openings in living quarters should be screened or alternatively mosquito nets should be used. Prophylactic dosage of antimalarial drugs should begin before entering a malarious area and should continue until 4 weeks after leaving. Drugs commonly used in the prophylaxis of malaria include amodiaquine, chloroquine, proguanil, and pyrimethamine. To maintain protection, doses should be taken regularly at the same hour for drugs taken daily or on the same day for drugs taken weekly. The dose should be taken with liquid after meals to minimise gastro-intestinal disturbances, particularly when chloroquine or amodiaquine is given. Pregnancy is not a contra-indication.

Chloroquine and amodiaquine will generally eliminate *P. falciparum* infections, but acute attacks due to *P. vivax* and *P. malariae* may occur later. Chloroquine-resistant falciparum infections may occur in some Central and South American and far-eastern countries, and these are publicised every 6 months in *Weekly Epidemiological Record*.

Treatment of attacks of malaria

Acute attacks occur when the schizont form of the parasite is released in the body, and the attacks can therefore be terminated by schizontocidal drugs such as the 4-aminoquinolines amodiaquine and chloroquine. Quinine is usually reserved for the treatment of *P. falciparum* infections that are resistant to other drugs.

Radical cure. To prevent the recurrence of attacks it is necessary to eliminate exo-erythrocytic forms of the parasite. For *P. falciparum* infections this may be accomplished using the 4-aminoquinolines but for *P. vivax* infections primaquine is required.

Interruption of transmission. Transmission of malaria may be prevented by elimination of the mosquito vector or by treating all malaria cases. To eliminate re-infection of mosquitoes the destruction of the gametocytes is necessary. The 4-aminoquinolines (amodiaquine and chloroquine) destroy *P. vivax* gametocytes, and primaquine destroys those of all species.

Countries where there may be a risk of malaria

Details of the areas of risk may be found from tables in *Weekly Epidemiological Record*, 1978, **53**, pp. 181–196. The tables also show any altitudes and times of year that are free from risk and indicate where malaria has been eliminated from urban areas. The main countries at risk are shown below:

Africa	The *whole of Africa* except as follows: Chagos Archipelago; French Southern and Antarctic Territory; Lesotho; Mauritius; Reunion; St Helena; Seychelles; Western Sahara
Asia	The *whole of Asia* except as follows: Brunei; Cyprus; Hong Kong; Israel; Japan; Democratic people's republic of Korea; Kuwait; Lebanon; Macao; Mongolia
North America	Belize; Costa Rica; Dominican Republic; El Salvador; Guatemala; Haiti; Honduras; Mexico; Nicaragua; Panama (excluding canal zone)
South America	Argentina; Bolivia; Brazil; Colombia; Ecuador; French Guiana; Guyana; Paraguay; Peru; Surinam; Venezuela
Others	British Solomon Is.; New Hebrides; Papua New Guinea.

Malathion

Diethyl 2-(dimethoxyphosphinothioylthio)succinate

$C_{10}H_{19}O_6PS_2 = 330.4$

OTHER NAMES: *Derbac*®; *Prioderm*®; *Taskil*®

Description. A colourless to light amber liquid with a characteristic odour.

Solubility. Very slightly soluble in water; miscible with alcohol, with ether, and with chloroform.

Storage. Contact with certain metals, including copper, iron, lead, and tin, should be avoided as malathion corrodes them.

Actions and uses. Malathion is a pesticide which is used in the treatment of head and pubic louse infections; it kills both lice and eggs very rapidly.

Malathion is applied to the scalp or pubic hair as a shampoo containing 1% or as an application containing 0.5% in volatile alcoholic solution. It is also used as an application containing 0.5% in a non-inflammable basis for the treatment of head louse infections. Malathion scalp application is probably more effective than malathion shampoo, because it gives better penetration of the waxy cuticle of the insect and prolongs contact time; the active ingredient is rapidly concentrated by evaporation of the solvent but the preparation has the disadvantage of being inflammable.

Malathion treatment may be repeated if necessary after 7 to 9 days.

Undesirable effects. Mild stinging may occur when malathion solutions are applied to the pubic area.

Precautions. Caution should be exercised in treating children under 6 months of age.

Preparations

MALATHION SCALP APPLICATION: a solution of malathion in an alcoholic vehicle. Available as an application containing 0.5% of malathion.

Containers: see the entry on Applications for general information on containers.

Labelling: see the entry on Applications for general information on labelling. In addition, the container should be labelled "CAUTION. This preparation is inflammable. Keep away from a naked flame".

Storage: it should be stored in a cool place.

Advice for patients: the application should be rubbed gently into the hair and the roots of the hair and allowed to dry without the aid of heat. The hair should not be washed for the next 12 hours. Immediately after washing the hair it should be finely combed to remove dead parasites. The preparation should not be applied to broken or inflamed skin; contact with the eyes should be avoided.

OTHER PREPARATIONS available include an APPLICATION, in a shampoo basis, containing malathion 1%, an application containing malathion 0.5% in a non-inflammable basis; and a veterinary DUSTING-POWDER containing malathion 3.5%.

Male Fern

The rhizome, frond-bases, and apical bud of *Dryopteris filix-mas* agg., which includes *D. filix-mas* (L.) Schott. s. str., *D. borreri* Newm., and *D. abbreviata* (DC.) Newm. (Fam. Polypodiaceae).

OTHER NAME: Filix Mas

A standard is given in the British Pharmacopoeia 1973

Male fern is indigenous to Great Britain, other temperate regions, and the Indian subcontinent. It is usually collected late in the autumn, divested of its roots and dead portions, and then carefully dried. Internally, the freshly collected rhizome is green in colour, but during storage the green colour of the interior gradually disappears, often after a lapse of 6 months, and such drug is unfit for medicinal use.

Varieties. European male fern yields about 6 to 10% of ethereal extractive of which about 25% is filicin. Indian male fern yields about 8 to 9.5% of ethereal extractive, of which about 30% is filicin.

Constituents. The drug contains a number of ether-soluble derivatives of phloroglucinol, some of which contribute to the anthelmintic action.

The phloroglucides are substituted partly with methyl or methoxyl groups and always with an acyl side-chain, mainly butyryl but also acetyl or propionyl, and occur as polymers linked by methylene bridges.

The active polymers are readily broken down in alkaline conditions to inactive monomers; aspidinol (2,6-dihydroxy-4-methoxy-3-methylbutyrophenone), a monomer with a butyryl side-chain, may be found in large amounts in *D. filix-mas*, but is not always present in *D. borreri* or *D. abbreviata*.

The proportions of different compounds vary but filicic acid (a trimer) and flavaspidic acid (a dimer) are invariably present as the major components, the latter being mainly responsible for the pharmacological activity of the drug.

Filicic acid is a mixture of 6 homologues which vary in the length of the acyl side chains of the two filicinic acid units which are linked by methylene bridges to a butyrylphoroglucinol residue.

Flavaspidic acid is the methylene-bridge-linked dimer of butyrylfilicinic acid and methyl butyrylphloroglucinol.

Albaspidin is usually present and there may be small proportions of desaspidin, which, if present, contributes to the anthelmintic activity.

In addition to the phoroglucinol derivatives, tannin (filicitannic acid) and volatile and fixed oils are present.

Filicin is the name given to the mixture of ether-soluble substances obtained in the assay of the drug and the extract.

It may yield up to 2% of acid-insoluble ash.

Description. UNGROUND DRUG. *Macroscopical characters:* pieces 70 to 150 mm or more in length and about 50 mm wide, oblique in direction and ending in a large bud, the fronds showing circinate vernation; rhizome proper, about 20 mm in diameter, entirely covered with hard, persistent, ascending, hemicylindrical, dark brown bases of the fronds, about 30 to 60 mm long and 6 to 8 mm thick; phyllotaxis 5:8; rhizome and frond bases densely covered with ramenta; frond bases green internally; rhizome yellowish-green; transversely cut surface of both rhizome and each frond base showing a circle of about 7 to 9 pale yellowish vascular strands of various sizes.

It has a slight odour and a taste which is at first sweetish and astringent, later becoming bitter and nauseous.

Microscopical characters: the diagnostic characters are: *ramenta*, with marginal teeth of 2 or occasionally more cells, *glands* present at base only, usually 2, small, unicellular; *hypodermis* composed of yellowish-brown, longitudinally elongated cells with thickened walls; *ground tissue* composed of cellulosic parenchyma, cells filled with small *starch* granules up to 25 µm in diameter; *trichomes* glandular, short-stalked, pear-shaped, projecting into some intercellular spaces in ground tissue; *vascular system* dictyostelic, xylem with large lignified prismatic scalariform *tracheids* with pointed ends; cells of *endodermis* with thin, sinuous walls, surrounding each vascular strand.

POWDERED DRUG: Powdered Male Fern. A brown powder possessing the diagnostic microscopical characters, odour, and taste of the unground drug.

Adulterants and substitutes. The rhizomes and frond bases of several other ferns may occur as substitutes. Lady-fern, *Athyrium filix-femina* (L.) Roth. is distinguished by the presence of only two dumb-bell shaped vascular strands in each frond base and by the absence of internal glandular trichomes and active phloroglucides.

Several European buckler ferns, including *D. villarii* (Bell.) Woynar, *D. aemula* (Ait.) O. Kuntze and members of the "*Dryopteris spinulosa*" complex [*D. carthusiana* (Vill.) H. P. Fuchs, *D. dilatata* (Hoffm.) A. Gray, *D. assimilis* S. Walker, and *D. cristata* (L.) A. Gray], as well as various hybrids belonging to the genus *Dryopteris*, all yield rhizomes and frond bases resembling those of male fern although some are more slender and elongated, with narrower rhizomes. The shape of the ramenta and the microscopical appearance of the ramental margins may distinguish some of these taxa. All contain characteristic mixtures of phloroglucides which vary both qualitatively and quantitatively. Flavaspidic acid is present, usually with smaller amounts of desaspidin, tridesaspidin, para-aspidin, albaspidin, aspidinol, and, sometimes, phloropyrone; aspidin (not present in male fern) is a major active component in most of these taxa except *D. villarii* and *D. cristata*.

Actions and uses. Male fern has been used, as the extract or draught, for the expulsion of tapeworms, but as safer drugs are available for the purpose there seems little justification for its continued use.

The patient should be given a low-residue diet on the day before the extract is administered and a saline purgative during the evening. Next morning the extract should be given to the fasting patient in one dose or in several equal portions at half-hourly intervals, followed 2 hours after the last portion by a saline purgative. Male fern extract may be administered in capsules but is more effective as a draught.

Undesirable effects. Toxic effects, which are rare, include headache, nausea, vomiting, severe abdominal cramp, diarrhoea, albuminuria, and dyspnoea. In severe cases, convulsions, loss of reflexes, and optic neuritis, leading to temporary or permanent blindness, may occur. Death sometimes ensues from respiratory or cardiac failure. Since absorption of male fern extract may be increased by the presence of fat in the intestine, fatty meals and purgatives such as castor oil should not be given.

Contra-indications. It is contra-indicated in anaemia and pregnancy and in old people and infants.

Preparations

MALE FERN EXTRACT (*Syn*. Ext. Filic.): a suitable extract may be prepared according to the following method:

Small-scale preparation

Exhaust male fern, in moderately coarse powder, by percolation with ether; remove the ether and evaporate the remainder of the percolate on a water-bath until an oily extract remains. Determine the proportion of filicin in a portion of the extract and to the remainder add, if necessary, sufficient arachis oil, or other suitable fixed oil, to produce an extract of the required strength.

Manufacture. Prepare the extract by the above method, appropriately scaled up.

It contains 22% w/w of filicin.

A standard for this extract is given in the British Pharmacopoeia 1973

Storage: it should be stored in airtight containers, protected from light; it should be thoroughly stirred before use.

Dose: 3 to 6 ml.

Advice for patients: see above under Actions and uses.

MALE FERN EXTRACT DRAUGHT (*Syn*. Haustus Filicis; Male Fern Draught):

Male fern extract	4 g
Acacia, in powder..	4 g
Water for preparations	to 50 ml

Triturate the male fern extract with the acacia, add in one quantity 10 ml of water, and stir briskly until emulsified. Add sufficient water to produce the required volume and mix. It should be recently prepared.

Dose: 50 millilitres.

Advice for patients: see above under Actions and uses.

Maleic Acid

(*Z*)-But-2-ene-1,4-dioic acid

$C_4H_4O_4 = 116.1$

A standard is given in the British Pharmacopoeia 1973

Description. An odourless white crystalline powder with a strongly acid taste.

Solubility. Soluble, at 20°, in 1.5 parts of water, in 2 parts of alcohol, and in 12 parts of ether.

Moisture content. Not more than 1.5%, determined by drying over phosphorus pentoxide *in vacuo*.

Identification. TEST. Dissolve 500 mg in 1 ml of water, neutralise with *sodium hydroxide solution*, using *phenolphthalein solution* as indicator, add 1 g of 4-nitrobenzyl bromide dissolved in 10 ml of alcohol (95%), and heat under a reflux condenser for 2 hours, cool, and filter; the residue, after recrystallisation from diluted alcohol melts at about 90°.

MELTING-POINT. About 136°.

Uses. Maleic acid is used in the preparation of ergometrine injection and methylergometrine injection.

Mallein Purified Protein Derivative

A preparation of the heat-treated products of growth and lysis of *Actinobacillus mallei* (*Pseudomonas mallei*).

OTHER NAME: Mallein P.P.D.

A standard is given in the British Pharmacopoeia (Veterinary)

Storage. It should be protected from light and stored at 2° to 8°, when it may be expected to retain its potency for 6 months.

Veterinary uses. It is administered by intradermal injection into the lower eyelid in a dose of 0.1 ml as an aid to the diagnosis of glanders in horses, donkeys, and mules.

Malt Extract

Obtained from sound malted grain of barley, *Hordeum distichon* L. or from *H. vulgare* L. (Fam. Gramineae), or a mixture of this with not more than 33.0% of sound malted grain of wheat, *Triticum aestivum* L. or *T.*

turgidum L. (Fam. Gramineae). It contains 50% or more of maltose, together with dextrin, glucose, and small amounts of other carbohydrates, and protein.

A standard is given in the British Pharmaceutical Codex 1973

It may be prepared by digesting at a suitable temperature, for an hour or more, a mixture of crushed malt with 2 to 3 times its weight of hot water, allowing to settle, drawing off the strained liquid, and extracting the mass with more hot water.

In order to obtain a product devoid of enzymic activity, the mixed liquids are heated at a convenient stage and kept at about 90° for an hour before finally evaporating under reduced pressure until a viscous product is obtained. Care must be taken not to overheat and darken the product.

Description. An amber or yellowish-brown viscous liquid with an agreeable and characteristic odour.

Solubility. Miscible with water, giving a translucent solution.

Weight per ml. At 20°, 1.39 to 1.42 g.

Refractive index. 1.489 to 1.498.

Actions and uses. Malt extract is used chiefly as a vehicle for cod-liver oil and halibut-liver oil. It also has nutritive properties. It is a useful flavouring agent for masking bitter tastes. A diastatic malt extract, which is usually administered undiluted to children, is easily digested.

Preparation

MALT EXTRACT WITH COD-LIVER OIL (*Syn.* Extractum Malti cum Oleo Morrhuae):

Malt extract..	900 g
Cod-liver oil	100 g

Mix thoroughly, with the aid of gentle heat. The extract may be flavoured. It contains, in 30 ml, about 4.5 ml of cod-liver oil.

A standard for this extract is given in the British Pharmaceutical Codex 1973

Storage: it should be stored in well-filled airtight containers, in a cool place, protected from light.

Dose: 10 to 30 millilitres daily.

Advice for patients: it should not be taken for prolonged periods without medical advice.

Malta Fever

see BRUCELLOSIS

Manganese Sulphate

$MnSO_4,4H_2O = 223.1$

OTHER NAME: Mang. Sulph.

A standard is given in the British Pharmaceutical Codex 1973

Description. Odourless, pale pink crystals or crystalline powder.

Solubility. Soluble, at 20°, in 1 part of water; practically insoluble in alcohol.

Sterilisation. Solutions are sterilised by heating in an autoclave or by filtration.

Actions and uses. Manganese sulphate is given for its supposed effect in increasing the haematinic action of iron in the treatment of microcytic anaemia. The usual dose is 2.5 milligrams daily.

Veterinary uses. Manganese sulphate is used for the prevention and treatment of manganese deficiency. The usual dose by mouth for cattle is 8 milligrams per kilogram body-weight. Poultry may be given 120 parts per million in the feed.

Preparation

Manganese sulphate is an ingredient of compound ferrous sulphate tablets.

Mannitol

A hexahydric alcohol related to mannose; it is isomeric with sorbitol.

$$
\begin{array}{c}
CH_2OH \\
|\\
HO-C-H \\
|\\
HO-C-H \\
|\\
H-C-OH \\
|\\
H-C-OH \\
|\\
CH_2OH
\end{array}
$$

$C_6H_{14}O_6 = 182.2$

OTHER NAME: *Osmitrol*®

A standard is given in the British Pharmacopoeia 1973

Description. An odourless white crystalline powder with a sweetish taste.

Solubility. Soluble, at 20°, in 6 parts of water; very slightly soluble in alcohol; practically insoluble in ether.

Specific rotation. +23° to +24°, determined on a solution prepared by dissolving 5 g of the sample and 6.4 g of borax in sufficient water to give 45 ml, allowing to stand for 1 hour, and diluting to 50 ml.

Sterilisation. Solutions for injection are sterilised by heating in an autoclave or by filtration.

Identification. TESTS. 1. To 1 ml of a saturated solution add 0.5 ml of *ferric chloride test-solution* followed by 0.25 ml of *sodium hydroxide solution* and shake well; a clear solution is obtained which remains clear after the further addition of *sodium hydroxide solution.*

2. Mix 500 mg with 2.5 ml of acetyl chloride, cautiously add 0.5 ml of pyridine, keep the mixture warm until it becomes turbid and cool in ice; a precipitate is produced which, after filtering on a sintered glass filter and recrystallising several times from ether, melts at about 123°.

MELTING-POINT. About 167°.

Actions and uses. Mannitol, when given by intravenous injection, acts as an osmotic diuretic. It is administered as a 20% solution in a dosage of 50 to 100 grams daily to supplement the action of more potent diuretics; it is of little value when given alone.

A 2.5% solution is used for irrigation of the bladder during transurethral resection of the prostate.

A 20 or 25% solution is given by slow intravenous injection, in volumes up to 500 millilitres, to produce decompression in concussion and cerebral injury.

The 20 and 25% solutions are supersaturated and may require warming before use to redissolve any crystals that have formed.

Mannitol is used as a basis for glyceryl trinitrate tablets.

Preparation

MANNITOL INJECTION: a sterile solution of mannitol in water for injections. It is sterilised by heating in an autoclave.

Available in 50-ml ampoules containing 25% (250 mg per ml) of mannitol and in 500-ml plastic packs containing 10 and 20% (100 and 200 mg per ml respectively) of mannitol. Also available as an injection containing 15% (150 mg per ml) of mannitol.

A standard for this injection is given in the British Pharmacopoeia 1973

Containers: see the entry on Injections for general information on containers.

Labelling: see the entry on Injections for general information on labelling. In addition, the label on the container should state the amount of the medicament as the percentage w/v of mannitol.

Storage: it should be stored at a temperature between 20° and 30°. Exposure to lower temperatures may result in the deposition of crystals. If this occurs, the crystals should be redissolved by warming before using the injection.

Mannomustine Hydrochloride

1,6-Bis(2-chloroethylamino)-1,6-dideoxy-D-mannitol dihydrochloride

$$
\left[
\begin{array}{c}
CH_2 \cdot NH \cdot CH_2 \cdot CH_2Cl \\
| \\
HO-C-H \\
| \\
HO-C-H \\
| \\
H-C-OH \\
| \\
H-C-OH \\
| \\
CH_2 \cdot NH \cdot CH_2 \cdot CH_2Cl
\end{array}
\right] \quad 2HCl
$$

$C_{10}H_{24}Cl_4N_2O_4 = 378.1$

A standard is given in the British Pharmaceutical Codex 1973

Description. An odourless white crystalline powder.

Solubility. Soluble, at 20°, in 2 parts of water; very slightly soluble in alcohol; practically insoluble in dehydrated alcohol, in ether, and in chloroform.

Acidity. A 2.5% solution has a pH of 2 to 3.5.

Moisture content. Not more than 1%, determined by drying at 105°.

Specific rotation. +17° to +22°, determined on a 2% solution.

Identification. TEST. Dissolve about 20 mg in 2 ml of a 2% solution of periodic acid, allow to stand for 30 seconds and add 0.5 ml of *barium chloride solution*; a white precipitate is produced.

MELTING-POINT. About 241°, with decomposition.

INFRA-RED ABSORPTION. Major peaks at 1010, 1064, 1299, 1389, 1429, and 1449 cm^{-1} (see Appendix 2b: Infra-red Spectra).

Actions and uses. Mannomustine is a cytotoxic agent with the actions, uses, and undesirable effects described under Mustine Hydrochloride.

It is used for the treatment of neoplastic disease, particularly of the lymphoid and haemopoietic systems. It is used for the palliative symptomatic treatment of chronic lymphatic leukaemia, Hodgkin's disease, reticulosarcoma, multiple myeloma, polycythaemia, and Brill-Symmers disease. When given in generalised carcinomatosis, pain may be relieved and metastases in lymph nodes may regress, but these effects may be accompanied by severe bone-marrow depression.

Mannomustine may be useful in the treatment of acute leukaemia, particularly of the monocytic type, if the white-cell count is considerably increased.

Mannomustine hydrochloride is given by intravenous injection or infusion, or orally in enteric-coated tablets. It may also be given directly into body cavities, such as the pleural space. The parenteral dose is 0.5 to 1.5 milligrams per kilogram body-weight dissolved in sodium chloride injection. It may be given daily or on alternate days until a total dose of 8.5 to 11.5 milligrams per kilogram body-weight has been administered; total doses of twice this quantity have been given.

Mannomustine hydrochloride may be given orally in enteric-coated tablets in doses of 50 to 100 milligrams.

Precautions. Dosage should be controlled by response to the treatment, by periodic white-cell and red-cell counts, and also by observations on the bone marrow during the treatment of leukaemia and polycythaemia. Bone-marrow depression, when it occurs, may be prolonged.

Preparations

MANNOMUSTINE INJECTION (*Syn.* Mannomustine Hydrochloride Injection): a sterile solution of mannomustine hydrochloride in sodium chloride injection. It is prepared by dissolving the contents of a sealed container in sodium chloride injection shortly before use. Available as a powder in ampoules containing 50 mg of mannomustine hydrochloride.

A standard for this injection is given in the British Pharmaceutical Codex 1973

Containers and *Labelling:* see the entry on Injections for general information on containers and labelling.

Storage: the injection contains no bactericide and should be used as soon as possible after preparation, but solutions of mannomustine hydrochloride retain their potency for up to 24 hours provided they are stored at 2° to 10°.

Marburg Virus (Green Monkey) Disease

Marburg virus was first described in 1967. It is larger than known viruses and of a different shape. Antigenically it is unrelated to other known viruses but is closest to the *Rhabdovirus* group. Since the initial outbreak, all cases have originated in the central equatorial region of Africa.

No reservoir, host, or vector has as yet been described. Current thought points to it not being a true monkey disease but that of a rare animal or plant host. Primary cases, as with lassa fever, seem more likely to be fatal than secondary contacts.

Infection occurs by direct contact with blood, organs, or semen, through the skin, conjunctiva, respiratory tract mucosa, and possibly the gastro-intestinal tract. When man is infected, an intense viraemia occurs; the virus is also present in the urine, semen, and throat.

The incubation period for Marburg virus disease is 3 to 9 days and is characterised by an acute onset of fever (often biphasic), malaise, nausea, vomiting, and a watery diarrhoea. There is a distinctive maculopapular rash and scrotal and labial erythema accompanied by deep erythema of the face, limbs, and trunk. Generalised lymphadenopathy, hepatomegaly with relapses of acute hepatitis, orchitis, pancreatitis, myocarditis, encephalitis, and haemorrhagic manifestations are some of the presenting features. In addition, renal failure occurs more often than in lassa fever. Diagnosis is carried out in specially equipped laboratories.

As with lassa fever there are no known prophylactic measures and the treatment is carried out in suitable isolation units. Supportive measures, such as electrolyte and fluid balance control, together with intensive care are particularly important. Specific antiviral chemotherapy is not available but treatment using interferon is currently being investigated; the use of immune serum prepared from the blood of a recovered case of Marburg virus disease may be of value.

Marek's Disease Vaccine, Living (Turkey Herpesvirus)

A freeze-dried or deep-frozen preparation of a suitable live strain of turkey herpesvirus grown in suitable cell cultures. The vaccine is prepared immediately before use by reconstitution with an appropriate volume of a suitable liquid, either from the dried vaccine or, for cell-bound vaccine from a thawed deep-frozen suspension of live cultured cells infected with turkey herpesvirus.

OTHER NAME: Marek's Disease Vaccine, Living (HVT)

A standard is given in the British Pharmacopoeia (Veterinary)

Storage. The dried vaccine should be protected from light and stored at 2° to 8° when it may be expected to retain its potency for 6 months. Cell-bound vaccine is stored in liquid nitrogen and may be expected to retain its potency for 2 years. The vaccine should be used immediately after reconstitution.

Veterinary uses. It is administered by intramuscular or subcutaneous injection to chickens for prophylaxis against Marek's disease.

Mastic

A resinous exudation from certain forms of varieties of *Pistacia lentiscus* L. (Fam. Anacardiaceae), a small tree indigenous to the Mediterranean countries.

OTHER NAME: Mastiche

A standard is given in the British Pharmaceutical Codex 1973

Mastic is exported mainly from the island of Chios (Scio) in the Aegean Sea, where it is obtained by puncturing the bark of the trees and allowing the oleoresin to exude and harden. It melts between 105° and 120°.

Constituents. Mastic consists mainly of triterpenoid acids, including mastic-adienonic acid, triterpene alcohols such as tirucallol, and about 2% of volatile oil.

Description. Small hard globular or pyriform pieces, about 4 to 8 mm in diameter, or more rarely in ovoid or nearly cylindrical pieces, up to 20 mm long and 10 mm wide; when fresh, pale yellow, clear, and glassy, the surface becoming dull and dusty on keeping; brittle, and breaking with a conchoidal fracture; when chewed, breaking up into sandy fragments which agglomerate into a plastic mass.

It has a somewhat aromatic odour and agreeable taste.

Solubility. Practically insoluble in water; partly soluble in alcohol and in turpentine oil; soluble, at 20°, in less than 1 part of chloroform and of ether.

Adulterants and substitutes. East Indian or Bombay mastic is obtained from *P. khinjuk* Stocks and possibly other *Pistacia* species; it somewhat resembles genuine mastic, but the tears are darker, less vitreous, and not so clean. It is also more soluble in alcohol, less soluble in turpentine oil, and less disposed to agglomerate when chewed; the acid value varies from 103 to 109.

Uses. A solution of mastic in alcohol, ether, or chloroform is applied on cotton wool as a temporary filling for carious teeth. The compound paint is used as a protective covering for wounds and to hold gauze and radium needles in position. As it contains acetone it should not be used in conjunction with iodine.

Preparation

COMPOUND MASTIC PAINT:

Mastic	..	..	..	..	..	400 g
Castor oil	..	..	..	..	..	12.5 ml

Acetone ⎫ equal
Industrial methylated ⎬ quantities .. to 1000 ml
spirit ⎭ of each

Dissolve and filter or, alternatively, allow to stand in a closed vessel and decant the clear liquid. This preparation was formerly prepared with a vehicle consisting of benzene, nitration grade of commerce, and carried the synonym "Benzo-mastic".

A standard for this paint is given in the British Pharmaceutical Codex 1973

Containers and *Storage*: see the entry on Paints for general information on containers and storage.

Labelling: see the entry on Paints for general information on labelling. In addition, the label on the container should state "This preparation is inflammable. Keep away from a naked flame".

Measles

Measles (morbilli) is a highly contagious viral disease spread by droplet infection and occurring in epidemics; infection may occur at any age but is most prevalent in children under 5 years. The incubation period is between 7 and 14 days and the two days preceding the appearance of the rash are the most infectious period. Initial symptoms include coryza, conjunctivitis, hoarseness, harsh cough, and photophobia with rising fever. This stage is called the catarrhal stage and the disease is most infectious during this period. Small white spots (Koplik's spots) may be detected on the mucous membranes of the mouth.

After 3 to 5 days a red rash appears behind the ears and on the face and spreads rapidly down the trunk and on to the arms and legs. The fever is accentuated. The spots proliferate and fuse into blotches which after 2 to 3 days deepen in colour, then gradually fade into a faint brown stain and slowly desquamate on about the sixth day. The body temperature thereafter returns to normal.

Complications may include convulsions in young children as the rash appears and secondary infection by haemolytic streptococci or pneumococci which may cause otitis media or acute lobular pneumonia. These conditions are most dangerous during the first 18 months of life. Other complications include persistent conjunctivitis followed by corneal ulceration, gastro-enteritis, appendicitis, and encephalitis.

Patients should be confined to bed in a well-ventilated room to reduce the incidence of secondary respiratory infection. Antibiotics should be used only where bacterial complications occur.

Immunoglubulin may be given for the prevention or attenuation of measles (passive inmunisation) as described under Immunoglubulin Injection, Human Normal. For active immunisation see under Vaccines.

Measles, German

see RUBELLA

Measles Vaccine (Live Attenuated)

A freeze-dried preparation of an aqueous suspension of an approved strain of live attenuated measles virus grown in cultures of chick-embryo cells.

OTHER NAMES: Measles Vaccine (Live); Meas/Vac (Live); Vaccinum Morbillorum

A standard is given in the European Pharmacopoeia Vol. II

Storage. It should be stored between 2° and 10°; under these conditions it may be expected to retain its potency for one year.

The reconstituted vaccine should be used immediately after preparation.

Actions and uses. Measles vaccine (live attenuated) is used for active immunisation against measles. Susceptible subjects develop protective antibodies towards the end of the second week after vaccination.

Mild clinical effects, lasting a day or two and consisting mainly of pyrexia, general irritability, and a transient rash, may develop in a minority of patients from 6 to 12 days after vaccination. The clinical effects are not transmissible to other individuals.

The virus present in the vaccine is rendered ineffective by the presence of measles antibodies in the circulation, whether derived transplacentally from the mother or as a result of injection of measles immunoglobulin in prophylactic doses during the previous 6 weeks, or actively stimulated by previous infection with epidemic measles or vaccination previously with measles vaccine (live attenuated). The vaccine is therefore unlikely to be effective in the majority of children under 6 months of age and a substantial proportion of those aged 6 to 12 months. Measles vaccination is therefore usually carried out during the second year of life.

The vaccine is administered by subcutaneous or intramuscular injection in a dose of 0.5 millilitre.

A suitable schedule for the immunisation of children is given under Vaccines.

Precautions and contra-indications. The vaccine should be used with care in individuals having a history of febrile convulsions and in the presence of brain damage; the concurrent administration of human normal immunoglobulin injection with a specific measles content should be considered in these cases. Care should also be exercised in treating individuals with egg-protein sensitivity.

It is contra-indicated in leukaemia, lymphoma, and other generalised malignant diseases, hypogammaglobulinaemia, acute febrile illness, and pregnancy.

It should not be given at the same time as therapy that depresses the immune response.

Caution. The vaccine is readily inactivated by traces of virucidal agents, including chemical disinfectants, antiseptics, spirits, bactericidal soaps, and heavy metals.

Disposable syringes sterilised by gamma-irradiation should preferably be used for reconstituting and administering the vaccine.

Glass syringes and steel needles, if they are used, should be thoroughly cleansed in recently distilled water and sterilised by autoclaving or by dry heat.

Chlorinated or other chemically treated water must be avoided.

Mebeverine Hydrochloride

N- Ethyl -*N*- (4-methoxy-α- methylphenethyl) -*N*-(4-veratroyloxybutyl)ammonium chloride

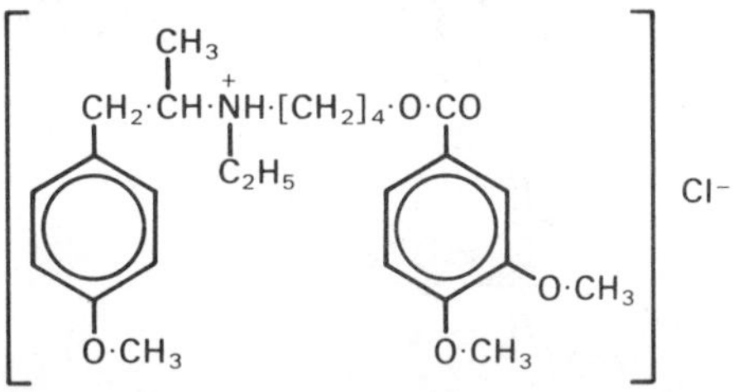

$C_{25}H_{36}ClNO_5 = 466.0$

OTHER NAME: *Colofac®*

Description. A white crystalline powder.

Solubility. Soluble in water and in alcohol.

Identification. MELTING-POINT. About 133°.

ULTRAVIOLET ABSORPTION. In alcoholic 0.01N hydrochloric acid, maximum at 262 nm (E1%, 1cm = 283).

Actions and uses. Mebeverine hydrochloride has an antispasmodic action on smooth muscle and is used in the treatment of abdominal pain and spasm associated with gastro-intestinal disorders such as mucous colitis. The usual dose by mouth for adults and children over 7 years is 135 milligrams 3 times daily, taken 20 minutes before meals; this dose may be progressively reduced according to the response of the patient.

Preparation

MEBEVERINE TABLETS: available as tablets containing 135 mg of mebeverine hydrochloride; they may be sugar coated.

Containers and *Storage:* see the entry on Tablets for general information on containers and storage. Containers should be airtight.

Advice for patients: the tablets should preferably be taken 20 minutes before meals.

Meclozine Hydrochloride

1-(4-Chlorobenzhydryl)-4-(3-methylbenzyl)piperazine dihydrochloride

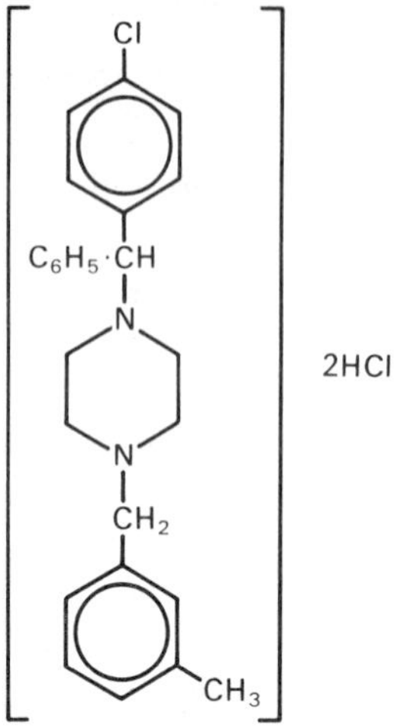

$C_{25}H_{29}Cl_3N_2 = 463.9$

OTHER NAMES: Meclizine Hydrochloride; *Sea-Legs*® *Ancoloxin*® (with pyridoxine hydrochloride)

A standard is given in the British Pharmacopoeia 1973

Description. An almost odourless, tasteless, white, crystalline powder.

Solubility. Soluble, at 20°, in 1000 parts of water, in 25 parts of alcohol, and in 5 parts of chloroform.

Moisture content. Not more than 5%, determined by Fischer titration.

Dissociation constants. pK_a 3.1, 6.2 (25°).

Storage. It should be stored in airtight containers.

Identification. TEST. Dissolve about 100 mg in 100 ml of water, add 10 ml of *trinitrophenol solution* and cool in ice; a precipitate is produced which, after washing with water, melts at about 219° with decomposition.

MELTING-POINT. About 224°, with decomposition.

ULTRAVIOLET ABSORPTION. In alcohol (95%), maximum at 230 nm (E1%, 1cm = 330), and small maxima at 261 nm, 266 nm, and 273 nm.

INFRA-RED ABSORPTION. Major peaks at 700, 720, 760, 805, 940, and 1435 cm^{-1} (see Appendix 2a: Infra-red Spectra).

Metabolism. DISTRIBUTION. Norchlorcyclizine, a metabolite of meclozine, crosses the placenta in rats.

METABOLIC REACTIONS. In rats, meclozine is metabolised to norchlorcyclizine and N-(4-chlorobenzhydryl)ethylenediamine.

FURTHER INFORMATION. Metabolism to an ethylenediamine derivative in the rat—H. J. Gaertner *et al.*, *J. Pharmac. exp. Ther.*, 1973, **185**, 195; metabolism and pharmacokinetics in the rat—S. A. Narrod *et al.*, *J. Pharmac. exp. Ther.*, 1965, **147**, 380.

Actions and uses. Meclozine hydrochloride has the actions and undesirable effects of the antihistamine drugs, as described under Promethazine Hydrochloride. It is used in the treatment of motion-sickness, nausea, and vomiting, particularly that of pregnancy, and for the relief of allergic states. For these purposes 25 to 50 milligrams of meclozine hydrochloride is given by mouth daily in single or divided doses. The usual dose for children under 1 year is 6.25 milligrams daily; 1 to 5 years 12.5 milligrams daily; and 6 to 12 years 12.5 to 25 milligrams daily in divided doses.

The effect of a single dose lasts for 24 hours. For motion sickness the dose is taken one hour before a journey.

Poisoning. As for Promethazine Hydrochloride.

Preparations

MECLOZINE TABLETS: available as tablets containing 12.5 mg of meclozine hydrochloride.

A standard for these tablets is given in the British Pharmacopoeia 1973

Containers and *Storage:* see the entry on Tablets for general information on containers and storage. Containers should be airtight.

Advice for patients: the tablets may cause drowsiness; persons affected should not drive or operate machinery. Alcohol should be avoided.

OTHER PREPARATIONS available include TABLETS containing meclozine hydrochloride 25 mg with pyridoxine hydrochloride 50 mg.

Medroxyprogesterone Acetate

6α-Methyl-3,20-dioxopregn-4-en-17α-yl acetate

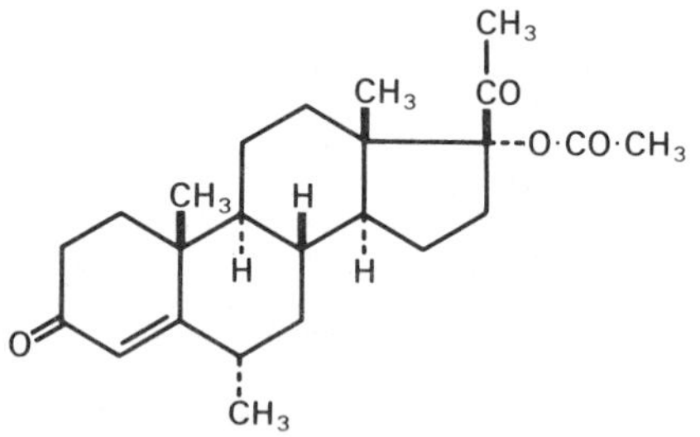

$C_{24}H_{34}O_4 = 386.5$

OTHER NAMES: *Anoestrulin*®; *Depo-Provera*®; *Perlutex*®; *Promone E*®; *Provera*®; *Veramix Sheep Sponge*®

A standard is given in the British Pharmacopoeia Addendum 1977

Description. An odourless white crystalline powder.

Solubility. Practically insoluble in water; soluble, at 20°, in 800 parts of alcohol, in 10 parts of chloroform, in 50 parts of acetone, and in 60 parts of dioxan; very slightly soluble in ether and in methyl alcohol.

Specific rotation. +45° to +51°, determined on a 1% solution in dioxan.

Storage. It should be protected from light.

Identification. MELTING-POINT. About 204°.

THIN-LAYER CHROMATOGRAPHY. See under Thin-layer Chromatography, System 10.

Metabolism. ABSORPTION. Slowly absorbed following subcutaneous or intramuscular injection; it is absorbed after oral administration, the extent being significantly increased if the particle size is reduced.

BLOOD CONCENTRATION. 1 to 3% of a dose is present in the total plasma volume 4 hours after administration, mostly in conjugated form.

HALF-LIFE. Plasma half-life, about 4 hours; half-life determined from urinary excretion data, about 14 hours.

DISTRIBUTION. Small amounts are detectable in the reproductive tract of women and either the drug or its metabolites appear to cross the placenta; neither drug nor metabolites are detectable in milk; bound to some extent to red blood cells.

METABOLIC REACTIONS. Hydroxylation and conjugation with glucuronic acid and sulphate; hydroxylation occurs at the 6- and 21- positions; the 4-en-3-one structure is not reduced; the major metabolite is the glucuronide of $6\beta,17\alpha,21$- trihydroxy-6α-methylpregn-4-ene-3,20-dione 17-acetate; the 21-acetate of the above metabolite has been isolated but is probably formed during the hydrolysis or extraction process and does not appear to be a true metabolite.

EXCRETION. 4 to 8% of an oral dose is excreted in the urine in 24 hours and about 80% is excreted in the faeces; medroxyprogesterone acetate is excreted in conjugated form in the bile; of the urinary excreted material, 50 to 60% is glucuronide conjugates and about 3% is free drug; after an intravenous dose 20 to 40% is excreted in the urine in 4 days and 5 to 13% is excreted in faeces; the excretion rate appears to be higher in non-pregnant than in pregnant women.

FURTHER INFORMATION. Improved absorption from micronised drug—D. L. Smith *et al.*, *J. pharm. Sci.*, 1966, **55**, 398; K. Fotherby and F. James, Metabolism of synthetic steroids, *Advances in Steroid Biochemistry and Pharmacology*, M. H. Briggs and G. A. Christie (Eds), Vol. 3, London, Academic Press, 1972, p. 67; J. H. H. Thijssen, The metabolism of orally active synthetic progestational compounds, *International Encyclopedia of Pharmacology and Therapeutics*, Section 48, M. Tausk (Ed.), Vol. 2, Oxford, Pergamon Press, 1972, p. 217; plasma concentrations in dogs by gas-liquid chromatography—D. G. Kaiser *et al.*, *J. pharm. Sci.*, 1974, **63**, 420.

Actions and uses. Medroxyprogesterone acetate has actions and uses similar to those described under Progesterone. It is used in the treatment of endometriosis, secondary amenorrhoea, functional uterine bleeding, and neoplasms of the kidney and endometrium and for contraception. It may also have a limited use in the treatment of habitual and threatened abortion. In the treatment of habitual abortion, 10 milligrams may be given by mouth daily in the first trimester of pregnancy, increasing to 20 milligrams in the second and 40 milligrams in the third trimester. Alternatively, 50 milligrams of a long-acting preparation may be given weekly by intramuscular injection in the first trimester and 100 milligrams every 2 weeks in the second and third trimesters. Treatment is continued until the end of the thirty-second week or until foetal viability is evident.

Medroxyprogesterone acetate is given, in conjunction with oestrogen, in the treatment of secondary amenorrhoea and functional uterine bleeding; 2.5 to 10 milligrams is given daily for 5 to 10 days, beginning on the sixteenth to the twenty-first day of the menstrual cycle and continuing for three consecutive cycles in secondary amenorrhoea.

In the treatment of endometriosis, 50 milligrams of medroxyprogesterone once a week or 100 milligrams of a long-acting preparation every 2 weeks is given by intramuscular injection for 6 months.

For contraception, 150 milligrams is given as a single intramuscular injection at the beginning of the menstrual cycle. In the treatment of neoplasms of the kidney and endometrium 200 to 400 milligrams is given by mouth daily for 3 months, after which the patient's response is assessed.

Undesirable effects. Clitoral hypertrophy may occur; disturbances of the menstrual cycle and infertility may also occur in patients receiving continuous and prolonged treatment by intramuscular injection.

Precautions. It should not be administered to patients with abnormal uterine bleeding until the absence of genital malignancy has been established.

Contra-indications. Medroxyprogesterone acetate should not be administered by intramuscular injection to patients with thrombophlebitis, pulmonary embolism, liver disease, or neoplasms of the breast or genital organs. It should not be used for contraception over long periods. Its use during pregnancy should be avoided, unless progesterone deficiency is demonstrable, because of the virilising effect on a female foetus.

Veterinary uses. Medroxyprogesterone acetate is a progestational agent used mainly in bitches and cats for the prevention of oestrus. The usual dose is 500 micrograms per kilogram body-weight daily by mouth commencing before full oestrus has developed. It may also be administered by subcutaneous injection in a single dose of 5 to 8 milligrams per kilogram body-weight. It has also been used in sheep and goats for the synchronisation of oestrus in a flock; when 60 milligrams is given as a single dose over 14 days as a vaginal tampon, oestrus occurs after withdrawal of the tampon.

Preparations

Preparations available include a veterinary INJECTION containing medroxyprogesterone acetate 28 mg per ml in 10-ml vials, a veterinary injection containing medroxyprogesterone acetate 50 mg per ml in 5- and 10-ml vials, an injection containing medroxyprogesterone acetate 50 mg per ml in 1-, 3-, and 5-ml vials; veterinary TABLETS containing medroxyprogesterone acetate 5 mg, tablets containing medroxyprogesterone acetate 5 and 100 mg, and veterinary TAMPONS containing medroxyprogesterone acetate 60 mg.

Mefenamic Acid

N-2,3-Xylylanthranilic acid

$C_{15}H_{15}NO_2 = 241.3$

OTHER NAME: *Ponstan*®

A standard is given in the British Pharmacopoeia 1973

Description. An odourless, tasteless, white to greyish-white, microcrystalline powder.

Solubility. Very slightly soluble in water; soluble, at 20°, in 185 parts of alcohol, in 80 parts of ether, and in 150 parts of chloroform.

Identification. TESTS. 1. Dissolve about 25 mg in chloroform and examine under ultraviolet radiation; a strong greenish-yellow fluorescence is exhibited.

2. Dissolve about 5 mg in 2 ml of sulphuric acid and add 1 drop of 0.1N potassium dichromate; an intense blue colour is produced which rapidly fades to brownish-green.

ULTRAVIOLET ABSORPTION. In a mixture containing 1 volume of 1N hydrochloric acid and 99 volumes of methyl alcohol, maxima at 279 nm (E1%, 1cm = 357) and 350 nm (E1%, 1cm = 290); in 0.1N sodium hydroxide, maximum at 288 nm (E1%, 1cm = 432).

INFRA-RED ABSORPTION. Major peaks at 758, 1250, 1449, 1515, 1562, and 1639 cm^{-1} (see Appendix 2b: Infra-red Spectra).

THIN-LAYER CHROMATOGRAPHY. See under Thin-layer Chromatography, System 3.

Determination in body fluids. THIN-LAYER CHROMATOGRAPHY. In urine: detection and identification of mefenamic acid and two metabolites—B. Demetriou and B. G. Osborne, *J. Chromat.*, 1974, **90**, 405.

Metabolism. ABSORPTION. Well absorbed after oral administration.

BLOOD CONCENTRATION. During therapy with 250 mg thrice daily after a loading dose of 500 mg, plasma concentrations of 0.3 to 3.6 μg/ml are attained 2 hours after the morning dose; after a single dose peak plasma concentrations are attained in 2 to 4 hours.

DISTRIBUTION. Does not appear to accumulate in the body; small amounts are secreted in the milk; *protein binding*, extensively bound to plasma proteins.

METABOLIC REACTIONS. Hydroxylation of the 3-methyl group followed by oxidation to produce the 3-carboxymetabolite, and conjugation.

EXCRETION. About 50% of a dose is excreted in the urine in 48 hours mainly as conjugates.

FURTHER INFORMATION. Excretion in breast milk— R. A. Buchanan *et al.*, *Curr. ther. Res.*, 1968, **10**, 592.

Actions and uses. Mefenamic acid is an analgesic with minor anti-inflammatory properties and has the actions and uses described under Ibuprofen. It has a weaker anti-inflammatory effect and is often used as a simple analgesic.

The usual dose for adults is 0.5 to 1.5 grams daily in divided doses and for children over 6 months of age the usual dose is 6.5 milligrams per kilogram body-weight 3 to 4 times daily.

Undesirable effects. As for Ibuprofen. Mefenamic acid may give rise to diarrhoea or rashes which may necessitate discontinuation of treatment. Rarely, leucopenia or haemolytic anaemia may occur.

Precautions. As for Ibuprofen. In addition it should be given with caution to patients with renal impairment. Treatment should not be continued for longer than 7 days in children, except in the treatment of Still's disease.

Contra-indications. It is contra-indicated in pregnancy and lactation and it should be avoided in patients with inflammatory bowel disease.

Preparations

MEFENAMIC ACID CAPSULES: consisting of mefenamic acid, in powder, which may be mixed with a suitable inert diluent, enclosed in a hard capsule. The capsule shells may be coloured. Available as capsules containing 250 mg of mefenamic acid.

A standard for these capsules is given in the British Pharmacopoeia 1973

Containers and *Storage:* see the entry on Capsules for general information on containers and storage.

Advice for patients: the capsules should preferably be taken after meals.

OTHER PREPARATIONS available include a MIXTURE containing mefenamic acid 50 mg in 5 ml, diluent syrup, life of diluted mixture 14 days, and TABLETS containing mefenamic acid 500 mg.

Megestrol Acetate

6-Methyl-3,20-dioxopregna-4,6-dien-17α-yl acetate

$C_{24}H_{32}O_4 = 384.5$

OTHER NAME: *Ovarid*®

A standard is given in the British Pharmacopoeia 1973

Description. An odourless, white to creamy-white, crystalline powder.

Solubility. Very slightly soluble in water; soluble, at 20°, in 55 parts of alcohol, in 130 parts of ether, and in less than 1 part of chloroform; very slightly soluble in fixed oils.

Specific rotation. +9° to +12°, determined on a 5% solution in chloroform.

Storage. It should be protected from light.

Identification. TEST. It complies with Test 3 described under Cortisone Acetate (acetyl groups).

MELTING-POINT. About 217°.

ULTRAVIOLET ABSORPTION. In dehydrated alcohol, maximum at 287 nm (E1%, 1cm = 630).

INFRA-RED ABSORPTION. Major peaks at 1249, 1263, 1272, 1662, 1712, and 1733 cm^{-1} (see Appendix 2a: Infra-red Spectra).

THIN-LAYER CHROMATOGRAPHY. See under Thin-layer Chromatography, System 10.

Metabolism. ABSORPTION. Absorption following administration in a gelatin capsule is slow; as a solution in alcohol it is well absorbed.

BLOOD CONCENTRATION. Peak plasma concentrations are attained in 1 to 3 hours after a single oral dose and reach about 30% of the peak value after 24 hours.

METABOLIC REACTIONS. Hydroxylation at the 6- and 2α-positions, and glucuronic acid conjugation; metabolism of megestrol acetate occurs to a lesser extent than that of medroxyprogesterone and this reduction appears to be a consequence of a protective effect by the double bond at position 6.

EXCRETION. After oral administration as a solution in 10% alcohol, 56 to 78% of a dose is excreted in the urine and 8 to 30% in the faeces in 7 days; the percentage of a dose excreted in the urine appears to increase as the dose is decreased.

FURTHER INFORMATION. Metabolism—J. M. Cooper and A. E. Kellie, *Steroids*, 1968, **11**, 133 and J. H. H. Thijssen, The metabolism of orally active synthetic progestational compounds, *International Encyclopedia of Pharmacology and Therapeutics*, Section 48, M.

Tausk (Ed.), Vol. 2, Oxford, Pergamon Press, 1972, p. 217; plasma concentrations—J. S. Elce *et al.*, *Biochem. J.*, 1967, **104**, 58P.

Actions and uses. Megestrol acetate has been withdrawn from use in human medicine because of the possibility that its use stimulates tumour formation.

Veterinary uses. Megestrol acetate is a progestational agent used mainly for the prevention or postponement of oestrus in bitches; treatment must begin before oestrus has developed. The usual dose by mouth for dogs and cats is 0.5 to 2 milligrams per kilogram body-weight daily, the lower dose being used when treatment continues for several weeks, and the higher for up to 8 days. Megestrol acetate is also used in cats to relieve allergic dermatitis. The initial dose for this purpose is 2.5 milligrams every 2 or 3 days; weekly or fortnightly doses of 2.5 milligrams may be required for maintenance.

Preparation

MEGESTROL TABLETS: available as tablets containing 5 and 20 mg of megestrol acetate; they may contain suitable flavouring.
A standard for these tablets is given in the British Pharmacopoeia (Veterinary)
Containers and *Storage:* see the entry on Tablets for general information on containers and storage. Containers should be airtight and light resistant.

Meglumine

1-Methylamino-1-deoxy-D-glucitol

$$
\begin{array}{c}
CH_2 \cdot NH \cdot CH_3 \\
| \\
H - C - OH \\
| \\
HO - C - H \\
| \\
H - C - OH \\
| \\
H - C - OH \\
| \\
CH_2OH
\end{array}
$$

$C_7H_{17}NO_5 = 195.2$

OTHER NAME: *N*-Methylglucamine

A standard is given in the British Pharmacopoeia 1973

Description. A white microcrystalline powder with a slight odour and a slightly bitter taste.

Solubility. Soluble, at 20°, in 1 part of water and in 100 parts of alcohol; practically insoluble in ether and in chloroform.

Moisture content. Not more than 1%, determined by drying at 105°.

Specific rotation. $-16°$ to $-17°$, determined on a 10% solution.

Dissociation constant. pK$_a$ 9.5 (20°).

Identification. TEST. Dissolve 200 mg in 2 ml of water, add 1 drop of *methyl red solution* and neutralise the solution by the addition of 1N sulphuric acid. To 1 ml of the solution add 2 ml of a freshly prepared mixture of 1 ml of acetaldehyde and 10 ml of *sodium nitroprusside solution* and then add 2 ml of *sodium carbonate solution*; a blue colour is gradually produced. To the remainder of the solution add 0.5 ml of 0.1N sodium hydroxide and 500 mg of boric acid; the solution becomes distinctly acid.

MELTING-POINT. About 129°.

Actions and uses. Meglumine is an organic base which is used for the preparation of soluble salts of iodinated organic acids used as contrast media.
When the limited solubility of the sodium salt does not permit the preparation of the highly concentrated solutions that may be required for diagnostic procedures, the meglumine salts may be suitable for this purpose.
In the case of those contrast media which are available as highly soluble sodium salts, the meglumine salts may nevertheless be preferred for certain purposes on account of their lower toxicity to the heart, kidneys, and nerve tissues.

Meglumine Diatrizoate Injection

A sterile solution of the meglumine salt of 3,5-diacetamido-2,4,6-tri-iodobenzoic acid containing a suitable stabilising agent.

OTHER NAMES: Meglumine Diatriz. Inj.
Gastrografin®; *Hypaque®*; *Urografin®* (all with sodium diatrizoate)

A standard is given in the British Pharmacopoeia 1973

Description. A clear, colourless to pale yellow, slightly viscous liquid.

Sterilisation. It is sterilised by heating in an autoclave.

Storage. It should be protected from light.

Actions and uses. Meglumine diatrizoate injection is used as a contrast medium for angiography. The solution generally used for this purpose contains 65% w/v of meglumine diatrizoate. The strength of the solution and the dose are determined by the physician in accordance with the diagnostic procedure.

Undesirable effects. The effects described under Sodium Diatrizoate may occur but are usually less marked.

Precautions. As for Sodium Diatrizoate.

Preparations

Preparations available include an INJECTION containing meglumine diatrizoate 65% (equivalent to 30.6% of iodine) in 10- and 20-ml ampoules and 50-ml vials, an injection containing meglumine diatrizoate 18% with sodium diatrizoate 40% (equivalent to 32.5% of iodine) in 20-ml ampoules and 50-ml vials, an injection containing meglumine diatrizoate 26.1% with sodium diatrizoate 3.9% (equivalent to 14.6% of iodine) in 10-ml ampoules and 250-ml bottles, an injection containing meglumine diatrizoate 50.46% with sodium diatrizoate 25.23% (equivalent to 39% of iodine) in 20-ml ampoules, an injection containing meglumine diatrizoate 52.1% with sodium diatrizoate 7.9% (equivalent to 29.2% of iodine) in 20-ml ampoules and 50-ml vials, an injection containing meglumine diatrizoate 56.67% with sodium diatrizoate 28.33% (equivalent to 44% of iodine) in 20-ml ampoules, an injection containing meglumine diatrizoate 66% with sodium diatrizoate 10% (equivalent to 37% of iodine) in 20-ml ampoules and 50-, 100-, and 200-ml vials; and a SOLUTION containing meglumine diatrizoate 66% with sodium diatrizoate 10%.

Melanostatin

see under HYPOTHALAMIC RELEASING FACTORS

Melarsoprol Injection

A sterile solution of melarsoprol, 2-[4-(4,6-diamino-1,3,5-triazin-2-ylamino)phenyl]-1,3,2-dithiarsolan-4-ylmethanol ($C_{12}H_{15}AsN_6OS_2 = 398.3$), in propylene glycol containing 5% of water. It contains 3.6% of melarsoprol.

OTHER NAMES: *Arsobal*® (available only in certain overseas countries); Mel B; Melarsoprol Inj.

A standard is given in the British Pharmacopoeia 1973

Description. A clear solution with not more than a slight alliaceous odour.

Sterilisation. It is sterilised by heating in an autoclave.

Actions and uses. Melarsoprol is a trypanocide that has superseded tryparsamide. It is usually reserved for the treatment of advanced sleeping sickness caused by *Trypanosoma rhodesiense* and *T. gambiense* in which the parasites have invaded the central nervous system.

The dosage is 3.6 milligrams per kilogram body-weight for an adult or 1.8 milligrams per kilogram body-weight for a child, given by intravenous injection daily for 3 or 4 days; this course of treatment should be repeated after an interval of 7 to 10 days.

Care should be taken during injection to avoid leakage of the drug into the surrounding tissues.

During the administration of melarsoprol the patient should be kept in hospital.

If recrudescence occurs after adequate treatment with melarsoprol, the infection is usually resistant to all other organic arsenic derivatives. It is necessary to use suramin sodium or pentamidine isethionate in conjunction with melarsoprol to remove trypanosomes from the blood and lymph nodes. Melarsoprol is not used for prophylaxis because of its toxicity.

Undesirable effects. Two kinds of undesirable effect may occur: Herxheimer reactions produced by the effect of the drug on the infection and toxic effects of arsenic such as encephalopathy. The toxic effects of arsenic may be alleviated by injection of dimercaprol and the administration of sedatives.

Melphalan

4-Bis(2-chloroethyl)amino-L-phenylalanine

```
        COOH
         |
NH2—C—H
         |
        CH2
```

(benzene ring structure)

N(CH₂·CH₂·Cl)₂

$C_{13}H_{18}Cl_2N_2O_2 = 305.2$

OTHER NAME: *Alkeran*®

A standard is given in the British Pharmacopoeia 1973

Description. An odourless white powder.

Solubility. Very slightly soluble in water; soluble, at 20°, in 150 parts of methyl alcohol; practically insoluble in ether and in chloroform; soluble in dilute mineral acids.

Moisture content. Not more than 7%, determined by drying at 100° *in vacuo*.

Optical rotation. A 0.5% solution in methyl alcohol is laevorotatory.

Storage. It should be stored in airtight containers, protected from light, at a temperature not exceeding 25°.

Identification. TEST. Dissolve about 20 mg in 50 ml of methyl alcohol with the aid of gentle heat, add 1 ml of a 5% solution of 4-(4-nitrobenzyl)pyridine in acetone, evaporate to dryness, dissolve the residue in 1 ml of hot methyl alcohol, and add 2 drops of *strong ammonia solution*; a red colour is produced.

MELTING-POINT. About 177° with decomposition.

ULTRAVIOLET ABSORPTION. In methyl alcohol, maximum at 260 nm and a less well-defined maximum at 310 nm.

Actions and uses. Melphalan, a cytotoxic drug, has the actions of mustine, from which it is derived. It acts mainly on dividing cells by causing cross linkage of deoxyribonucleic acid during the resting phase of mitosis. Like other cytotoxic drugs melphalan inhibits the growth of neoplastic cells but at the same time depresses bone-marrow activity, producing leucopenia and thrombocytopenia.

It is well absorbed orally and remains for about 6 hours in the bloodstream, from which it is rapidly taken up by the tissues and organs, notably the kidneys.

About half to one-third of cases of myelomatosis treated with melphalan show improvement for 6 months to 2 years and subjective remissions occur in 70 to 80% of cases. In this disease melphalan produces a decrease in abnormal serum globulin, an increase in serum albumin, a reduction in proteinuria, and a rise in haemoglobin.

Melphalan has also been used with variable results in the palliative treatment of Hodgkin's disease, Burkitt's lymphoma, reticulum cell sarcoma, and some other sarcomata (fibro-sarcoma, neurofibrosarcoma, and Kaposi's sarcoma), seminoma, and carcinoma of the ovary and breast.

For the treatment of myelomatosis the initial dose of melphalan is 100 to 150 micrograms per kilogram body-weight daily for the first week. Dosage is then adjusted so that the white cell and platelet counts do not fall below 2000 and 75000 per cubic millimetre respectively. A course of treatment lasts from 4 to 8 weeks. An alternative method is to give 30 to 60 micrograms per kilogram body-weight daily for 3 or 4 months, keeping a careful check on the white-cell and platelet counts. Provided these do not fall below the levels stated above, maintenance doses may be continued for 9 months.

For the treatment of other conditions the dose of melphalan varies from 30 to 60 micrograms per kilogram body-weight, continued until a total dose of 1.5 to 3 milligrams per kilogram body-weight has been given. Melphalan has also been given intravenously in doses of 0.5 to 1 milligram per kilogram body-weight and by intra-arterial perfusion into an isolated limb in doses of 1 to 2 milligrams per kilogram body-weight.

Undesirable effects. Nausea, vomiting, diarrhoea, haemorrhage into the gastro-intestinal tract, temporary alopecia, and ulceration of the mouth and mucous membranes may occur, and may precede depression of the bone marrow, leucopenia, and thrombocytopenia. The bone-marrow depression persists for longer than with other alkylating agents.

Regional perfusion of melphalan may cause oedema, neurotoxic effects, and blistering of the skin.

Precautions. A haematological investigation, including white-cell and platelet counts, should be made before and during treatment with melphalan. It should precede any change of dosage. The dosage for uraemic patients should be reduced.

Contra-indications. Melphalan is contra-indicated in severe anaemia, leucopenia, or thrombocytopenia. It is also contra-indicated in the first trimester of pregnancy.

Preparations

MELPHALAN INJECTION: a sterile solution of melphalan hydrochloride, with alcohol (95%), hydrochloric acid, dipotassium hydrogen phosphate, and propylene glycol, in water for injections. It is prepared by dissolving the contents of a sealed container, which consist of melphalan, first in a mixture of alcohol (95%) and hydrochloric acid, containing 92% v/v of C_2H_5OH and 2% w/v of HCl, and then diluting with a suitable volume of a solution containing 1.2% of dipotassium hydrogen phosphate and 60% v/v of propylene glycol in water for injections, immediately before use.

Available as a powder in ampoules containing 100 mg of melphalan with 1-ml ampoules of a solvent solution containing the alcohol and hydrochloric acid and 9-ml ampoules containing the diluent (dipotassium hydrogen phosphate, propylene glycol, and water for injections).

A standard for this injection is given in the British Pharmacopoeia 1973

Containers: see the entry on Injections for general information on containers.

Labelling: see the entry on Injections for general information on labelling. In addition, the label on the sealed container should state the amount of the medicament as the equivalent amount of anhydrous melphalan contained in it.

Storage: the sealed container should be stored at a temperature not exceeding 25°, protected from light. The injection decomposes on storage and should be used immediately after preparation.

MELPHALAN TABLETS: available as tablets containing 2 and 5 mg of melphalan; they are compression coated or film coated; the coat may be coloured. The method of preparation should be such that water does not come into contact with the medicament at any stage.

A standard for these tablets is given in the British Pharmacopoeia 1973

Containers and *Storage:* see the entry on Tablets for general information on containers and storage. Containers should be airtight. The tablets should be stored at a temperature not exceeding 25°.

Ménière's Disease

Ménière's disease is characterised by tinnitus and progressive nerve deafness accompanied by severe attacks of vertigo usually associated with nausea and vomiting; other possible causes of vertigo are investigated during diagnosis. During attacks of vertigo an anti-emetic drug is usually required and in addition a sedative may be used. Patients who have frequent attacks may benefit from continuous sedation.

Since the disease appears to be associated with an increased amount of endolymph, a low-salt diet and diuretic treatment may be given. Surgical destruction of the inner ear may be required in resistant cases.

Meningitis

Meningitis is an inflammation of the meninges or membranes of the brain and spinal cord. It may be classified according to the aetiology of the inflammatory process —pyogenic, tuberculous, viral, and others, including fungal and syphilitic meningitis.

Pyogenic meningitis. Infecting bacteria include meningococci, pneumococci, staphylococci, streptococci, and *Haemophilus* spp. Bacterial inflammation of the meninges usually results from a similar infection in the upper respiratory tract, lungs, middle ear, or nasopharynx. Onset is usually rapid and characterised by pyrexia, headache, neck stiffness, rigors, and delirium; in meningococcal infections there is usually an associated rash. Cerebrospinal fluid should be obtained immediately for examination by Gram staining and the appropriate cultures must be set up.

Parenteral antibiotic therapy should commence as soon as possible. Fluid and electrolyte balance should be maintained. Symptomatic treatment may be given if required for headaches, restlessness, or fits.

Tuberculous meningitis (see also Tuberculosis). This is usually insidious in onset with a prodromal period of fever, weight loss, vomiting, and mental confusion. Treatment with standard drugs such as streptomycin or isoniazid and ethambutol or rifampicin is required. Where drug resistance is apparent a second-line drug such as ethambutol may be necessary. Treatment is generally continued for a minimum of 2 years.

Viral meningitis. This form may be characterised by myalgia, retro-orbital pain, pain on lateral movement of the eyes, excruciating headache, and photophobia. Most patients recover fully.

There is no specific treatment.

Syphilitic meningitis. Meningitis due to infection with *Treponema pallidum* may occur any time after infection but most cases occur during the first 4 years.

The condition is treated with antibacterial agents (principally benzylpenicillin), as described under Syphilis.

Fungal meningitis. The most common form is due to infection with *Cryptococcus neoformans*; meningitis is usually gradual in onset and may even be asymptomatic. Treatment consists of parenteral and intrathecal administration of antifungal agents such as amphotericin or flucytosine.

Menopause

The menopause is the cessation of menstruation. The time around the menopause when the characteristic endocrinological changes are occurring is called the climacteric. It usually occurs in the late forties. During the climacteric the ovaries progressively secrete less oestrogen and progesterone and in consequence the circulating plasma level of gonadotrophins rises to a high level, and menstrual irregularities arise, culminating in the cessation of menstruation. Changes in the ovary result in the synthesis of small amounts of androgenic hormones which together with the lack of oestrogen result in a loss of femininity in the post-menopausal woman.

During the climacteric, many women complain of symptoms of vasomotor instability such as hot flushes, sweating, headache, fainting, and palpitations. Psychological disturbance at the menopause may manifest itself as insomnia, irritability, anxiety, or depression. Long-term effects of the endocrinological changes, which may become manifest in post-menopausal women combined with the effects of ageing, include obesity, pruritus, osteoporosis, and atrophy of the breasts, endometrium, myometrium, vagina, and vulva. Atrophy of pelvic muscles and ligaments may lead to cystocele, rectocele, or uterine prolapse.

Treatment of menopausal symptoms is symptomatic. Oestrogen therapy may be beneficial in the treatment of hot flushes, and minor tranquillisers and antidepressants may be used in the treatment of anxiety and depression. Dietary control is necessary in the treatment of obesity. All bleeding from the genital tract in postmenopausal women is abnormal and should be investigated to eliminate the possibility of malignancy.

Menorrhagia

see under UTERINE BLEEDING, ABNORMAL

Menotrophin

A dry sterile preparation of a glycoprotein fraction obtained from human post-menopausal urine.

OTHER NAME: *Pergonal*®; Human Menopausal Gonadotrophin; HMG

A standard is given in the British Pharmacopoeia Addendum 1978

Menotrophin contains urinary derivatives of follicle-stimulating hormone and luteinising hormone which stimulate, respectively, the growth and maturation of germinal follicles in the ovary, and ovulation and formation of a corpus luteum.

Description. An off-white or slightly yellow powder.

Solubility. Soluble in water.

Moisture content. Not more than 5%, determined by a gas chromatographic procedure.

Storage. It should be stored in containers sealed to exclude micro-organisms, at a temperature not exceeding 15°, and protected from light. Under these conditions it may be expected to retain its potency for 3 years.

Actions and uses. Menotrophin has the actions of human follicle-stimulating hormone. It promotes follicular growth and maturation and by its effect on oestrogen production it stimulates endometrial proliferation.

Menotrophin is used, in conjunction with human chorionic gonadotrophin, to promote ovulation in patients where infertility is attributed to gonadotrophin deficiency or an insufficient ovarian response to the anterior pituitary gonadotrophins. Patients are usually amenorrhoeic but in menstruating patients treatment is commenced on the third to the fifth day of menstruation and repeated at monthly intervals until pregnancy results. Urinary oestrogen levels should be frequently monitored throughout treatment to evaluate the clinical response. Patient response to treatment varies widely and during the first course the dosage of menotrophin is adjusted according to the pretreatment hormonal status of the patient. In the amenorrhoeic patient the dose during the first course is steadily increased until an adequate oestrogen response is obtained, and in subsequent courses doses are re-evaluated according to the hormonal response to menotrophin in the previous course. The initial course usually consists of 225 units of human follicle-stimulating hormone with 225 units of human luteinising hormone by intramuscular injection given on alternate days, but larger doses of up to 600 units of human follicle-stimulating hormone and 600 units of human luteinising hormone may be given. If excessive oestrogenic stimulation has not occurred an intramuscular dose of 10 000 units of chorionic gonadotrophin is given on the third day after the final injection of menotrophin to stimulate ovulation and corpus luteum formation.

An alternative schedule may be used in which menotrophin is administered by intramuscular injection in a dosage equivalent to approximately 75 to 150 units of human follicle-stimulating hormone with 75 to 150 units of human luteinising hormone daily for up to 14 days or until adequate urinary oestrogen levels have been attained for one week. Chorionic gonadotrophin is then given by intramuscular injection in a dosage of 10 000 units 2 days after cessation of treatment with menotrophin.

Undesirable effects. These are usually associated with excessive oestrogenic responses and include ovarian enlargement, ovarian cyst development, multiple pregnancy, abdominal distension, gastro-intestinal disturbances, ascites, hydrothorax, and haemodynamic disturbances. Death may occasionally occur. Pyrexia, joint pain, and reactions at the site of injection may also occur.

Precautions. Menotrophin treatment should be given under the supervision of physicians who are experienced in the treatment of infertility. It should be used with caution in patients with polycystic ovary syndrome. Urinary oestrogen levels should be frequently monitored and examination of the vagina and cervical mucus should be carried out to avoid the risk of excessive oestrogenic response which may lead to the undesirable effects described above. In the event of ovarian hyperstimulation the dose of chorionic gonadotrophin should be omitted. Pelvic examination should be carried out before and after each course to detect ovarian enlargement.

Preparation

MENOTROPHIN INJECTION (*Syn.* Human Menopausal Gonadotrophin Injection (HMG)): a sterile solution of menotrophin in an aqueous vehicle. It is prepared by dissolving the contents of a sealed container, which may also contain added inert substances, in water for injections or sodium chloride injection immediately before use.

Available as a powder in ampoules containing 75 units of human follicle-stimulating hormone (FSH), 75 units of human luteinising hormone (LH), and 10 mg of lactose, together with a 1-ml ampoule of sodium chloride injection.

A standard for this injection is given in the British Pharmacopoeia Addendum 1978

Containers: see the entry on Injections for general information on containers.

Labelling: see the entry on Injections for general information on labelling. In addition, the label on the sealed container should state the amount of the medicament as the number of units of follicle-stimulating-hormone activity and the number of units of luteinising-hormone activity contained in it.

Storage: the sealed container should be stored at a temperature not exceeding 15°, protected from light. Under these conditions it may be expected to retain its potency for at least 3 years. The injection decomposes on storage and should be used immediately after preparation.

Menthol

p-Menthan-3-ol, either natural or synthetic (−)-menthol, or synthetic (±)-menthol

$C_{10}H_{20}O = 156.3$

A standard is given in the British Pharmacopoeia 1973

Natural (−)-menthol may be obtained from the volatile oils of various species of *Mentha* (Fam. Labiatae), chiefly from *M. arvensis* L. var. *piperascens* Holmes in Japan, var. *glabrata* Holmes in China, and *M. piperita* L. in America; it is separated from the oils by freezing. Synthetic menthol may be obtained by the catalytic hydrogenation of thymol.

Description. Colourless acicular or prismatic crystals with a penetrating odour similar to that of peppermint oil and a taste which is warm and aromatic followed by a sensation of cold.

Solubility. Very slightly soluble in water and in glycerol; soluble in alcohol and in essential oils; soluble, at 20°, in less than 1 part of ether, of chloroform, and of light petroleum, in 6 parts of liquid paraffin, and in 4 parts of olive oil.

Specific rotation. For natural or synthetic (−)-menthol, −49° to −50°, determined on a 10% solution in alcohol (95%).

Storage. It should be stored in airtight containers, protected from light.

Actions and uses. Menthol is used to relieve the symptoms of bronchitis and sinusitis. For this purpose it is used, frequently mixed with camphor and eucalyptus oil, in pastilles, inhalations, and ointments. It is also used as a flavouring agent.

Preparations

MENTHOL AND BENZOIN INHALATION:

Menthol	20 g
Benzoin inhalation	to 1000 ml

A standard for this inhalation is given in the British Pharmaceutical Codex 1973
Containers: see the entry on Inhalations for general information on containers.
Advice for patients: see the entry on Inhalations for general information on the use of inhalations.

MENTHOL AND EUCALYPTUS INHALATION:

Menthol	20 g
Eucalyptus oil	100 ml
Light magnesium carbonate	70 g
Water for preparations	to 1000 ml

Dissolve the menthol in the eucalyptus oil and add the light magnesium carbonate and sufficient of the water to produce the required volume.
A standard for this inhalation is given in the British Pharmaceutical Codex 1973
Containers and *Labelling:* see the entry on Inhalations for general information on containers and labelling.
Advice for patients: see the entry on Inhalations for general information on the use of inhalations.

Menthol is an ingredient of benzalkonium lozenges, compound benzocaine lozenges, compound methyl salicylate ointment, compound thymol glycerin, formaldehyde lozenges, and mouth-wash solution-tablets.

Mepacrine Hydrochloride

4-(3-Chloro-7-methoxyacridin-9-ylamino)-NN-diethylpentylamine dihydrochloride dihydrate

$C_{23}H_{32}Cl_3N_3O,2H_2O = 508.9$

OTHER NAMES: Mepacrini Hydrochloridum; *Quinacrine*®

A standard is given in the European Pharmacopoeia Vol. III

Description. An odourless yellow crystalline powder with a bitter taste.

Solubility. Soluble, at 20°, in 40 parts of water; very slightly soluble in alcohol and in chloroform; practically insoluble in ether.

Acidity. A 2% solution has a pH of 3 to 5.

Moisture content. 5 to 8%, determined by Fischer titration.

Dissociation constants. pK_a 7.7, 10.3 (25°).

Storage. It should be protected from light.

Identification. TESTS. 1. To 2.5 ml of a 2.5% solution add a slight excess of *dilute ammonia solution*; a yellow to orange-coloured pasty precipitate is produced which adheres to the side of the tube and is soluble in ether.
2. To 2.5 ml of a 2.5% solution add 0.5 ml of *dilute nitric acid*; a yellow crystalline precipitate is produced.
3. To 2.5 ml of a 2.5% solution add 0.5 ml of *mercuric chloride test-solution*; a yellow precipitate is produced.

ULTRAVIOLET ABSORPTION. In 0.01N hydrochloric acid, maxima at 220 nm, 279 nm, and 343 nm.

INFRA-RED ABSORPTION. Major peaks at 1245, 1467, 1500, 1560, 1587, and 1627 cm^{-1} (see Appendix 2a: Infra-red Spectra).

Actions and uses. Mepacrine has actions similar to those described under Chloroquine Phosphate but it has been largely replaced by chloroquine for the suppression and treatment of malaria and is now used mainly as a taenicide. It is well absorbed after oral administration. A daily dose of 100 milligrams of mepacrine hydrochloride by mouth in divided doses will suppress the symptoms of malaria and may be safely continued for long periods. Treatment should be continued for 4 weeks after leaving the endemic area. For the treatment of malaria the dosage is 300 milligrams, 3 times on the first day and twice on the second day, followed by 100 milligrams 3 times a day for the next 3 to 5 days. Mepacrine is ineffective for the cure of benign tertian malaria and is not a true causal prophylactic.
In the treatment of giardiasis, 100 milligrams of mepacrine hydrochloride, 3 times a day for 7 days is usually effective, although relapses may occur.
For the expulsion of tapeworms, doses of 100 milligrams

are given at intervals of 5 minutes until a total of 1 gram has been administered. The dose for children, corresponding to an adult dose of 100 milligrams of mepacrine hydrochloride, is: under one year 2.5 to 3 milligrams per kilogram body-weight, 1 to 5 years 25 to 40 milligrams, and 6 to 12 years 45 to 75 milligrams.

Intra-pleural and intra-cavitary instillations of mepacrine hydrochloride are occasionally used to decrease malignant effusions in intra-cavity cancer and other severe conditions, such as pneumothorax in cystic fibrosis, but the incidence of toxic side-effects is high. It may act by causing tissue fibrosis with subsequent diminution of serous fluid production.

Undesirable effects. Mepacrine may occasionally cause gastric pain and headache; large doses may cause nausea, vomiting, diarrhoea and, rarely, transient mental disturbance. Yellow pigmentation of the skin usually accompanies its use and prolonged administration occasionally causes a condition of the skin resembling lichen planus. Exfoliative dermatitis, vertigo, pruritus, and anaemia may also occur.

Contra-indications. Mepacrine is contra-indicated in patients with neurosyphilis.

Preparation

MEPACRINE TABLETS: available as tablets containing 100 mg of mepacrine hydrochloride.

A standard for these tablets is given in the British Pharmacopoeia 1973

Containers and *Storage:* see the entry on Tablets for general information on containers and storage. Containers should be airtight and light resistant.

Advice for patients: the tablets should be taken at regular intervals preferably after meals. For suppression of malaria (prophylaxis), doses should be taken during the period at risk and for 4 weeks thereafter. For therapy the prescribed course should be completed. A yellow colour may be imparted to the urine and, after prolonged use, to the skin, hair, and nails.

Mephenesin

3-*o*-Tolyloxypropane-1,2-diol

$$OH$$
$$CH_2 \cdot CH \cdot CH_2OH$$
$$O$$

$$CH_3$$

$C_{10}H_{14}O_3 = 182.2$

OTHER NAME: *Myanesin*®

A standard is given in the British Pharmaceutical Codex 1973

Description. Odourless white crystals or crystalline aggregates.

Solubility. Soluble, at 20°, in 100 parts of water, in 8 parts of alcohol, in 12 parts of chloroform, and in 7 parts of propylene glycol.

Sterilisation. Solutions for injection are sterilised by heating in an autoclave or by filtration.

Identification. TEST. To about 1 g add 2 ml of methyl carbonate and 0.2 ml of a solution of 500 mg of sodium in 10 ml of dehydrated alcohol, heat on a water-bath until a gelatinous precipitate remains, and remove the last traces of solvent by warming under reduced pressure; extract the residue by warming with 10 ml of dehydrated alcohol, filter, and evaporate the filtrate to dryness; the residue, after drying in a current of air, melts at about 95°.

MELTING-POINT. About 71°.

ULTRAVIOLET ABSORPTION. In water, maximum at 270 nm (E1%, 1cm = 80).

INFRA-RED ABSORPTION. Major peaks at 746, 758, 1053, 1124, 1250, and 1515 cm^{-1} (see Appendix 2b: Infra-red Spectra).

Metabolism. ABSORPTION. Readily absorbed after oral administration.

BLOOD CONCENTRATION. After an intravenous dose, mephenesin disappears from the plasma within 60 to 90 minutes.

DISTRIBUTION. Widely distributed throughout the body.

EXCRETION. Less than 2% is excreted unchanged in the urine.

Actions and uses. Mephenesin is a muscle relaxant which exerts a selective action on the spinal cord, probably through the anterior horn cells. Although it antagonises the action of strychnine on the spinal cord, it is ineffective in preventing leptazol convulsions. In small doses it relaxes hypertonic muscles without appreciably reducing motor power or producing respiratory depression. It lowers response to sensory stimuli and depresses superficial reflexes.

Mephenesin also has a central action, possibly on the basal ganglia and subcortical efferent pathways. Its effects are more prolonged when it is administered by mouth than when given by injection.

Mephenesin has been given by mouth for the treatment of spastic, hypertonic, and hyperkinetic conditions, such as parkinsonism, cerebral palsy, choreoathetosis, and lesions of extrapyramidal origin. The usual dose by mouth is 0.5 to 1 gram once to 6 times daily. For the relief of spasms of tetanus a 10% solution is administered by intramuscular injection. It may also be given by intravenous injection, a 1 or 2% solution being administered slowly or in a drip infusion. The usual dose by intramuscular or intravenous injection is 0.1 to 1 gram.

Undesirable effects. When given by mouth mephenesin may cause drowsiness and, in some cases, nausea.

If a 10% solution is given by intravenous injection, it may give rise to intravascular haemolysis, haemoglobinuria, and local thrombosis at the site of injection; solutions containing more than 2% may give rise to anuria if injected intravenously.

Overdosage with mephenesin may produce coarse nystagmus, blurred vision, and circumoral numbness.

Drug interactions. It may enhance the effect of narcotics and barbiturates.

Preparations

Preparations available include TABLETS containing mephenesin 500 mg.

Meprobamate

2-Methyl-2-propyltrimethylene dicarbamate

$$CH_2 \cdot O \cdot CO \cdot NH_2$$
$$CH_3 \cdot C \cdot [CH_2]_2 \cdot CH_3$$
$$CH_2 \cdot O \cdot CO \cdot NH_2$$

$C_9H_{18}N_2O_4 = 218.3$

OTHER NAMES: *Equanil®*; *Meprate®*; Meprobamatum; *Milonorm®*; *Miltown®*; *Tised®* *Tenavoid®* (with bendrofluazide)

A standard is given in the European Pharmacopoeia Vol. III

Description. An odourless white crystalline powder or granular crystalline aggregates with a bitter characteristic taste.

Solubility. Soluble, at 20°, in 240 parts of water, in 7 parts of alcohol, and in 70 parts of ether.

Identification. TESTS. 1. Dissolve about 20 mg in 2 ml of a 1% solution of dimethylaminobenzaldehyde in sulphuric acid; a yellow colour is produced which changes to orange on standing. Heat the solution on a water-bath for 2 minutes; the colour changes to an intense red. Allow the solution to cool and add, drop-wise, 5 ml of water; the colour changes first to dark red and then to a fairly stable blue-violet.
2. Dissolve about 200 mg in 15 ml of 0.5N alcoholic potassium hydroxide, heat under reflux for 15 minutes, and add 0.5 ml of glacial acetic acid followed by 1 ml of a 5% solution of cobalt nitrate in alcohol (95%); an intense blue colour is produced.

MELTING-POINT. About 105°.

ULTRAVIOLET ABSORPTION. It exhibits no significant absorption in the range 230 to 360 nm.

INFRA-RED ABSORPTION. Major peaks at 1072, 1339, 1380, 1404, 1593, and 1690 cm^{-1} (see Appendix 2a: Infra-red Spectra).

Determination in body fluids. GAS CHROMATOGRAPHY. In plasma—A. Arbin and M.-L. Ejderfjall, *Acta pharm. suec.*, 1974, **11**, 439; in plasma or urine—L. Martis and R. H. Levy, *J. pharm. Sci.*, 1974, **63**, 834.

Metabolism. ABSORPTION. Readily absorbed after oral administration.

BLOOD CONCENTRATION. Peak plasma concentrations of 10 to 20 μg/ml are attained within 1 to 2 hours after the oral administration of 800 mg of meprobamate in solution.

HALF-LIFE. Plasma half-life, 6 to 16 hours, which is decreased by continual ingestion of alcohol; the half-life may be dose-dependent.

DISTRIBUTION. Distributed throughout the body and secreted in the milk.

METABOLIC REACTIONS. Hydroxylation and N-glucuronic acid conjugation; the metabolism of meprobamate is inhibited by glutethimide, imipramine, chlorcyclizine, and barbitone; in rats, the metabolism of meprobamate appears to be age-dependent.

EXCRETION. About 90% of a dose is excreted in the urine in 24 hours and the remaining 10% is excreted in the faeces; 10 to 20% of a dose is excreted in the urine as unchanged drug and the remainder is excreted as metabolites, mainly as 2-(2-hydroxypropyl)-2-methyl-1,3-propanediol.

ENZYME INDUCTION. Meprobamate may induce the drug metabolising enzymes in the rat and in man and may induce its own metabolism.

FURTHER INFORMATION. Absorption, metabolism, and excretion—J. F. Douglas *et al.*, *Proc. Soc. exp. Biol. Med.*, 1963, **112**, 436 and S. S. Walkenstein *et al.*, *J. Pharmac. exp. Ther.*, 1958, **123**, 254; pharmacokinetics —L. E. Hollister and G. Levy, *Chemotherapia*, 1964, **9**, 20 and E. van der Kleijn, *Archs int. Pharmacodyn. Thér.*, 1969, **178**, 457; plasma concentrations and half-life—L. Martis and R. H. Levy, *J. pharm. Sci.*, 1974, **63**, 834.

Actions and uses. Meprobamate has tranquillising, anticonvulsant, and muscle relaxant properties. It is used in the treatment of psychoneurotic disorders when anxiety and nervous tension are present. The usual dosage is 400 milligrams 3 times a day.

Undesirable effects. Meprobamate sometimes provokes excitement instead of sedation. Idiosyncratic reactions may occur after a single dose and the drug should then be discontinued. It may cause hypotension, drowsiness, and blood dyscrasias and may enhance the effects of alcohol.
Meprobamate may give rise to dependence of the barbiturate-alcohol type as described under Drug Dependence.

Precautions. It should be used with caution in nursing mothers.

Poisoning. Overdosage may give rise to coma, respiratory depression, hypotension, and hypothermia. The usual supportive measures should be taken and, as meprobamate is rapidly metabolised, recovery is rapid and is usually complete within 24 hours.

Preparations

MEPROBAMATE TABLETS: available as tablets containing 200 and 400 mg of meprobamate.
A standard for these tablets is given in the British Pharmacopoeia 1973
Containers and *Storage*: see the entry on Tablets for general information on containers and storage. Containers should be airtight.
Advice for patients: the tablets may cause drowsiness; persons affected should not drive or operate machinery. Alcohol should be avoided.

OTHER PREPARATIONS available include CAPSULES containing meprobamate 400 mg in a slow-release formulation; and TABLETS containing meprobamate 200 mg with bendrofluazide 3 mg.

Mepyramine Maleate

2-(N-p-Anisyl-N-2-pyridylamino)ethyldimethylamine hydrogen maleate

$C_{21}H_{27}N_3O_5 = 401.5$

OTHER NAMES: *Anthisan®*; Pyrilamine Maleate
Anthical® (with zinc oxide)

A standard is given in the British Pharmacopoeia 1973

Description. An odourless white or creamy-white powder with a bitter taste.

Solubility. Soluble, at 20°, in less than 1 part of water, in 2.5 parts of alcohol, and in 1.5 parts of chloroform.

Acidity. A 1% solution has a pH of 4.7 to 5.2.

Dissociation constants. pK_a 4.0, 8.9 (25°).

Sterilisation. Solutions for injection are sterilised by heating in an autoclave or by filtration.

Identification. TESTS. 1. Dissolve about 200 mg in 3 ml of water, add 2 ml of *sodium hydroxide solution*, and extract with three 3-ml portions of ether; to the aqueous layer add 2 ml of *bromine solution AsT*, warm in a water-bath for 10 minutes, heat to boiling, cool, add a few drops of this solution to a solution of 10 mg of resorcinol in 3 ml of sulphuric acid and heat in a water-bath for 15 minutes; a blue-black colour is produced.
2. To 2 ml of a 1% solution add 1 ml of *cyanogen bromide solution* and 5 ml of a 2% solution of potassium hydrogen phthalate, mix, allow to stand for 15 minutes, and then add 1 ml of a 4% solution of aniline in alcohol (95%); a yellow colour is produced.

MELTING-POINT. About 100°.

ULTRAVIOLET ABSORPTION. In 0.1N hydrochloric acid, maxima at 240 nm (E1%, 1cm = 415) and 316 nm (E1%, 1cm = 203); in alcohol (95%), maxima at 252 nm (E1%, 1cm = 479) and 312 nm (E1%, 1cm = 116).

INFRA-RED ABSORPTION. Major peaks at 1360, 1443, 1464, 1494, 1510, and 1598 cm^{-1} (see Appendix 2a: Infra-red Spectra).

THIN-LAYER CHROMATOGRAPHY. See under Thin-layer Chromatography, System 4.

Actions and uses. Mepyramine has the actions, uses, and undesirable effects of the antihistamine drugs, as described under Promethazine Hydrochloride, but it is less potent than promethazine and has a shorter duration of action. It is used mainly in the treatment of allergic and anaphylactic conditions, including hayfever, urticaria, and drug reactions.

Mepyramine maleate is usually given by mouth in a dosage of 50 milligrams every 4 to 6 hours; this may be increased gradually, according to the response and tolerance of the patient, but the daily dose should not exceed 1 gram. The usual dose for children up to 5 years is 12.5 to 25 milligrams 3 times daily and for children 6 to 12 years, 25 to 75 milligrams 3 times daily. Mepyramine maleate may also be given by intramuscular or slow intravenous injection in a dose of 25 to 50 milligrams.

Poisoning. As for Promethazine Hydrochloride.

Veterinary uses. Mepyramine maleate is used for the prevention and treatment of allergic reactions. The usual dose by intramuscular injection is for horses and cattle 1 to 3 milligrams per kilogram body-weight, pigs 1.5 to 3 milligrams per kilogram body-weight, sheep 5 to 10 milligrams per kilogram body-weight, and dogs 2.5 to 25 milligrams per kilogram body-weight. The usual dose by mouth for dogs is 5 to 10 milligrams per kilogram body-weight. These doses may be repeated every 6 to 8 hours.

Preparations

MEPYRAMINE ELIXIR: a solution of mepyramine maleate in a suitable coloured flavoured vehicle. When a dose less than or not a multiple of 5 ml is prescribed, the elixir may be diluted, as described in the entry on Elixirs, with syrup. The diluted elixir must be freshly prepared.
Available as an elixir containing 25 mg of mepyramine maleate in 5 ml.
A standard for this elixir is given in the British Pharmaceutical Codex 1973
Containers and *Labelling:* see the entry on Elixirs for general information on containers and labelling.
Storage: it should be protected from light.
Advice for patients: the elixir should preferably be taken after meals. It may cause drowsiness; persons affected should not drive or operate machinery. Alcohol should be avoided.

MEPYRAMINE INJECTION: a sterile solution of mepyramine maleate in water for injections. It is sterilised by heating in an autoclave or by filtration. Available in 2-ml ampoules containing 25 mg of mepyramine maleate per ml. Also available as a veterinary injection containing 50 mg of mepyramine maleate per ml.
A standard for this injection is given in the British Pharmacopoeia 1973
Containers and *Labelling:* see the entry on Injections for general information on containers and labelling.

MEPYRAMINE TABLETS: available as tablets containing 50 and 100 mg of mepyramine maleate; they are sugar coated; the coat may be coloured.
A standard for these tablets is given in the British Pharmacopoeia 1973
Containers and *Storage:* see the entry on Tablets for general information on containers and storage. Containers should be airtight.
Advice for patients: the tablets should preferably be taken after meals. They may cause drowsiness; persons affected should not drive or operate machinery. Alcohol should be avoided.

OTHER PREPARATIONS available include a CREAM containing mepyramine maleate 2%, and a cream containing mepyramine maleate 1.5% with zinc oxide 15%.

Mercaptopurine

Purine-6-thiol monohydrate

$C_5H_4N_4S,H_2O = 170.2$

OTHER NAME: *Puri-Nethol®*

A standard is given in the British Pharmacopoeia 1973

Description. An odourless yellow crystalline powder.

Solubility. Very slightly soluble in water, in ether, and in acetone; soluble, at 20°, in 950 parts of alcohol; soluble in solutions of alkali hydroxides.

Moisture content. 10 to 12%, determined by Fischer titration.

Dissociation constants. pK_a 7.7, 11 (20°).

Storage. It should be stored in airtight containers, protected from light.

Identification. TESTS. 1. Dissolve about 20 mg in 20 ml

of warm alcohol (95%) and add 1 ml of a saturated solution of mercuric acetate in alcohol (95%); a white precipitate is produced.

2. Dissolve about 20 mg in 20 ml of warm alcohol (95%) and add 1 ml of a 1% solution of lead acetate in alcohol (95%); a yellow precipitate is produced.

MELTING-POINT. About 300°, with decomposition.

ULTRAVIOLET ABSORPTION. In a solution prepared by dissolving 50 mg in 5 ml of dimethyl sulphoxide and diluting suitably with 0.1N hydrochloric acid to give a 0.00125% solution, maximum at 325 nm.

INFRA-RED ABSORPTION. Major peaks at 1010, 1220, 1346, 1406, 1570, and 1610 cm^{-1} (see Appendix 2a: Infra-red Spectra).

Determination in body fluids. COLORIMETRY. In plasma or urine—T. L. Loo et al., Clin. Pharmac. Ther., 1968, **9**, 180.

ULTRAVIOLET SPECTROPHOTOMETRY. In urine—A. H. Chalmers, Biochem. Med., 1975, **12**, 234.

GAS CHROMATOGRAPHY. In serum—D. G. Bailey et al., J. Chromat., 1975, **111**, 305.

Metabolism. ABSORPTION. Well, though somewhat variably, absorbed after oral administration.

BLOOD CONCENTRATION. After an intravenous dose of 5 to 77 mg/kg plasma concentrations at 1 hour are in the range 1 to 20 μg/ml.

HALF-LIFE. Plasma half-life, 20 to 90 minutes.

DISTRIBUTION. Widely distributed throughout the body water and enters the cerebrospinal fluid in small amounts; protein binding, about 20% bound to plasma proteins.

METABOLIC REACTIONS. Rapidly and extensively metabolised by oxidation and conjugation to form 6-thiouric acid, its sulphate conjugate, and other metabolites.

EXCRETION. Up to about 40% is excreted in the urine in 12 hours; about 8% of a dose is excreted unchanged.

FURTHER INFORMATION. Absorption and excretion—T. L. Loo et al., Clin. Pharmac. Ther., 1968, **9**, 180; short review of pharmacokinetics—A. H. Chalmers et al., Drugs, 1973, **3**, 227.

Actions and uses. Mercaptopurine is a cytotoxic agent. It is an analogue of adenine, a component of nucleic acid, and is believed to exert its effect in malignant disease by interfering with nucleic acid biosynthesis.

Although various natural purines protect microorganisms from the inhibitory action of mercaptopurine, they do not interfere with its toxic or antitumour activity in animals and in man.

Mercaptopurine is used for the palliative treatment of acute leukaemia or chronic myeloid leukaemia; its value in other forms of cancer has not been fully assessed.

In the treatment of acute leukaemia it produces remissions lasting from a few weeks to several months in a considerable proportion of children. Favourable results cannot be predicted and may be delayed.

Patients with chronic myeloid leukaemia may also react favourably, but the administration of mercaptopurine is advisable only after other forms of treatment, such as irradiation or busulphan, have been fully utilised. However favourable the initial response may be, repeated courses of treatment invariably result in the development of a refractory state. Treatment with mercaptopurine is usually combined with other antineoplastic agents.

Mercaptopurine is also used as an immunosuppressant, for example in the treatment of the nephrotic syndrome and autoimmune haemolytic anaemia, and also with folic acid antagonists for the treatment of choriocarcinoma.

Mercaptopurine is administered by mouth, the usual dosage for a child or for an adult being 2.5 milligrams per kilogram body-weight daily in divided doses; this may have to be reduced or cautiously increased according to the response. Opinion varies about the advisability of maintenance therapy during remission periods.

Undesirable effects. The most serious toxic action of mercaptopurine is the production of hypoplasia of the bone marrow, and careful haematological control should be maintained. Other undesirable effects include oral ulceration and gastro-intestinal symptoms.

As with other cytotoxic agents the toxic effects may be delayed. They are usually quickly relieved by discontinuing treatment with the drug.

The toxicity of mercaptopurine may be increased if given concurrently with allopurinol.

Preparation

MERCAPTOPURINE TABLETS: available as tablets containing 50 mg of mercaptopurine.

A standard for these tablets is given in the British Pharmacopoeia 1973

Containers and Storage: see the entry on Tablets for general information on containers and storage. Containers should be airtight and light resistant.

Mercuric Chloride

$HgCl_2 = 271.5$

OTHER NAMES: Corrosive Sublimate; Hydrargyri Perchloridum

A standard is given in the European Pharmacopoeia Vol. II

Description. Heavy colourless or white crystals or crystalline masses, or a white crystalline powder.

Solubility. Soluble, at 20°, in 15 parts of water and in 3 parts of alcohol; soluble in ether and in glycerol.

Moisture content. Not more than 1%, determined by drying over anhydrous silica gel in vacuo.

Incompatibility. It is incompatible with alkalis, lead acetate, silver nitrate, alkaloids (especially when iodides are present), and vegetable astringents.

Storage. It should be protected from light.

Actions and uses. The mercuric ion forms insoluble complexes with proteins and, by reason of this action on the proteins of bacterial cells, mercuric chloride is an antibacterial substance. To some extent its effect can be reversed by sulphydryl compounds.

Its use is limited by its toxicity, its precipitating action on proteins, its irritant action on raw surfaces, its corrosive action on metals, and by the fact that its activity is greatly reduced in the presence of excreta or body fluids.

Salicylic acid and mercuric chloride lotion is used for the treatment of follicular infections.

Solutions of mercuric chloride for external use should be coloured with indigo carmine as a warning of their toxic nature.

Poisoning. In acute poisoning, death may ensue within a few hours from profound shock and circulatory collapse. Nephritis may sometimes develop if the patient survives and may lead to death several weeks after the original poisoning occurred.

Acute mercurial poisoning should be treated as soon as possible by intramuscular injections of dimercaprol, 5 milligrams per kilogram body-weight being given, but this is an effective antidote only if given in the first hour or two after poisoning. It should be followed by 2 or 3 further injections of half this dose during the next 12 hours. Suitable fluids should be given by intravenous infusion for shock and the infusion should be continued, unless oedema occurs, to minimise kidney damage. If poisoning is mild, it usually responds readily to treatment with demulcents.

Preparation

SALICYLIC ACID AND MERCURIC CHLORIDE LOTION (Syn. Lotio Acidi Salicylici et Hydrargyri Perchloridi):

Salicylic acid	20 g
Mercuric chloride	.. 1 g
Castor oil	10 ml
Acetone	125 ml
Alcohol (95%)	to 1000 ml

Dissolve the mercuric chloride and the salicylic acid in 500 ml of the alcohol, add the castor oil, the acetone, and sufficient of the alcohol to produce the required volume, and mix. In making this preparation the alcohol (95%) may be replaced by industrial methylated spirit, provided that the law and the statutory regulations governing the use of industrial methylated spirit are observed.

A standard for this lotion is given in the British Pharmaceutical Codex 1973

Containers: see the entry on Lotions for general information on containers.

Labelling: see the entry on Lotions for general information on labelling. In addition, the label on the container should state "Caution. This preparation is inflammable Do not use it or dry the hair near a fire or naked flame."

Storage: it should be stored in airtight containers, in a cool place.

Advice for patients: a small amount of the lotion should be rubbed gently into the roots of the hair and allowed to dry without the aid of heat. It should not be applied to broken or inflamed skin; contact with the eyes should be avoided. The lotion should be kept in the original container and contact with metals should be avoided.

Mercury, Ammoniated

$NH_2 . HgCl = 252.1$

OTHER NAMES: Hydrargyrum Ammoniatum; White Precipitate

A standard is given in the British Pharmacopoeia 1973

It may be prepared by pouring a solution of mercuric chloride, with constant stirring, into a dilute solution of ammonia; the resulting precipitate is washed with cold water until the washings are nearly free from chloride, and dried at a low temperature.

Description. An odourless white powder.

Solubility. Practically insoluble in water, in alcohol, and in ether; soluble in warm hydrochloric, nitric, and acetic acids.

Stability. It is decomposed slowly by warm water and rapidly by boiling water, a yellow basic salt of the composition $NH_2 . HgCl,HgO$ being formed.

Storage. It should be protected from light.

Actions and uses. Ammoniated mercury is a mild antiseptic and is sometimes applied to the skin surrounding the perineum to destroy threadworms and to reduce reinfection. It was formerly used in the treatment of low-grade staphylococcal infections of the skin, and in psoriasis.

Precautions. It should not be applied to raw surfaces because of the risk of absorption of mercury.

Preparations

AMMONIATED MERCURY AND COAL TAR OINTMENT (Syn. Unguentum Hydrargyri Ammoniati et Picis Carbonis; Unguentum Picis Carbonis Compositum):

Ammoniated mercury, finely powdered ..	25 g
Strong coal tar solution	25 g
Yellow soft paraffin	950 g

Triturate the ammoniated mercury with a portion of the yellow soft paraffin until smooth, mix with the remainder of the yellow soft paraffin, and incorporate the strong coal tar solution.

A standard for this ointment is given in the British Pharmaceutical Codex 1973

Containers: see the entry on Ointments for general information on containers. Containers should prevent evaporation.

Advice for patients: it should not be applied to broken or inflamed skin. The ointment stains the skin, hair, and fabric.

AMMONIATED MERCURY, COAL TAR, AND SALICYLIC ACID OINTMENT (Syn. Unguentum Hydrargyri Ammoniati et Picis Carbonis cum Acido Salicylico):

Ammoniated mercury and coal tar ointment	980 g
Salicylic acid, in fine powder	20 g

Triturate the salicylic acid with a portion of the ammoniated mercury and coal tar ointment until smooth and gradually incorporate the remainder of the ointment.

A standard for this ointment is given in the British Pharmaceutical Codex 1973

Containers: see the entry on Ointments for general information on containers. Containers should prevent evaporation.

Advice for patients: the ointment should be applied sparingly to the affected area. It should not be applied to broken or inflamed skin. The ointment stains the skin, hair, and fabric. Prolonged use should be avoided and its use should be discontinued if excessive dryness or irritation of the skin occurs.

AMMONIATED MERCURY OINTMENT (Syn. Ung. Hydrarg. Ammon.):

Ammoniated mercury, finely powdered ..	25 g
Simple ointment	975 g

Triturate the ammoniated mercury with a portion of the simple ointment until smooth and gradually incorporate the remainder of the ointment.

A standard for this ointment is given in the British Pharmacopoeia 1973

Containers: see the entry on Ointments for general information on containers.

Advice for patients: it should not be applied to broken or inflamed skin. In threadworm infections its use should not be discontinued without the advice of the prescriber.

Mersalyl Acid

A mixture of [3-(2-carboxymethoxybenzamido)-2-methoxypropyl]hydroxymercury and its anhydrides.

O·CH$_2$·COOH   O·CH$_3$

CO·NH·CH$_2$·CH·CH$_2$·Hg·OH

$C_{13}H_{17}HgNO_6 = 483.9$

A standard is given in the British Pharmacopoeia 1973

Description. An odourless, white, slightly hygroscopic powder.

Solubility. Very slightly soluble in water and in dilute mineral acids; soluble in solutions of alkali hydroxides.

Moisture content. Not more than 2%, determined by drying at 105°.

Sterilisation. Solutions for injection are sterilised by heating with a bactericide, phenylmercuric nitrate being used, or by filtration. Contact with metal must be avoided.

Storage. It should be stored in airtight containers.

Identification. TESTS. 1. Mix 15 ml of water and 5 ml of hydrochloric acid, add about 100 mg of the sample and distil; to 5 ml of the distillate add 2.0 ml of *potassium permanganate and phosphoric acid solution*, allow to stand for 10 minutes, add 2.0 ml of *oxalic acid and sulphuric acid solution* and to the colourless solution add 5 ml of *decolorised magenta solution* and allow to stand at a temperature between 15° and 30° for 30 minutes; a deep violet colour is produced.
2. To 500 mg add 1 ml of water and 1 ml of formic acid, boil under a reflux condenser for 15 minutes, decant while hot, and allow to cool; crystals are produced which, after washing with water and drying *in vacuo*, melt at about 120°.

Metabolism. ABSORPTION. Slowly and incompletely absorbed after oral or rectal administration and rapidly absorbed after intramuscular injection.

EXCRETION. Most of an injected dose is excreted in the urine as a mersalyl-cysteine conjugate.

Actions and uses. Mersalyl acid, in the form of its salts, is a powerful mercurial diuretic which acts directly on the kidneys, increasing the excretion of water and sodium.

Mersalyl acid has been largely superseded by less toxic diuretics but is occasionally used in the treatment of oedema and ascites in cardiac failure and is of value in relieving pulmonary oedema. It is also of value in ascites due to cirrhosis of the liver, in nephrotic oedema, and in carefully selected cases of subacute and chronic nephritis provided that there is no serious impairment of renal function.

Mersalyl acid is usually given, in the form of mersalyl injection, by deep intramuscular injection. Its diuretic action may be increased by producing a mild acidosis before administering the injection by giving 3 doses, each of 2 grams, of ammonium chloride on the previous day. The patient's tolerance to mersalyl injection may be tested by giving a preliminary intramuscular injection of 0.5 millilitre; in the absence of signs of intolerance, such as haematuria, diarrhoea, irritation of the skin, or prostration, 1 or 2 millilitres may be given on the following day. The intervals between injections are based on the therapeutic response; in the absence of a satisfactory diuretic response, repeated injections should not be given.

Overdosage may give rise to dehydration and consequently to uraemia. Some patients are intolerant of mercurial compounds; great care should be taken in the treatment of patients exhibiting numerous extrasystoles, those who have suffered recent myocardial infarction, and those receiving massive digitalis therapy. Intravenous injection is dangerous and may be followed by sudden death.

Undesirable effects. The most frequently occurring toxic effects following the administration of mersalyl acid are stomatitis, gastric disturbance, vertigo, febrile reactions, and skin irritation. To prevent the accumulation of excreted mercury in the intestine, constipation should be avoided. Some patients may be sensitive to mersalyl acid but tolerant to other mercurial compounds.

Contra-indications. It should not be given in acute nephritis.

Preparation

MERSALYL INJECTION (*Syn.* Mersalyl and Theophylline Injection):

Mersalyl acid	..	..	..	..	9.56 g
Theophylline	..	..	..	..	.. 5 g
Sodium hydroxide..	..	..	..	..	.. 1 g
				or a sufficient quantity
Water for injections	..	..	..	.. to 100 ml

Suspend the mersalyl and the theophylline in about 80 ml of the water, prepare an approximately 10% solution of the sodium hydroxide in water for injections and add to the suspension, stirring continuously, until solution is effected; adjust the alkalinity of the solution to pH 8 by the addition of a further quantity of the sodium hydroxide solution, add sufficient of the water to produce the required volume, mix, and clarify by filtration. Distribute the solution into ampoules, seal, and sterilise by heating with a bactericide, using phenylmercuric nitrate as the bactericide.

Alternatively, sterilise the solution by filtration; distribute, by means of an aseptic technique, into sterile ampoules, and seal.

The solution must not be allowed to come into contact with metal.

It contains 10% of $C_{13}H_{16}HgNNaO_6$. It contains, in 1 ml, 100 mg of mersalyl (the sodium salt of mersalyl acid) and 50 mg of theophylline.

A standard for this injection is given in the British Pharmacopoeia 1973

Containers: see the entry on Injections for general information on containers.

Labelling: see the entry on Injections for general information on labelling. In addition, the label on the container should state the amount of the medicament as 10% w/v of mersalyl.

Storage: it should be protected from light.

Mestranol

3 - Methoxy -19- nor -17α- pregna - 1,3,5(10) - trien - 20 - yn-17β-ol

$C_{21}H_{26}O_2 = 310.4$

OTHER NAMES: *Demulen*® and *Metrulen*® (both with ethynodiol diacetate); *Norinyl*®, *Ortho-Novin*®, and *Menophase*® (all with norethisterone); *Enavid*® and *Enavid E*® (both with norethynodrel).

A standard is given in the British Pharmacopoeia 1973

Description. An odourless white crystalline powder.

Solubility. Very slightly soluble in water; soluble, at 20°, in 44 parts of alcohol, in 23 parts of ether, in 4.5 parts of chloroform, in 23 parts of acetone, and in 12 parts of dioxan.

Specific rotation. +2° to +8°, determined on a 1% solution in dioxan.

Storage. It should be protected from light.

Identification. TESTS. 1. It complies with Tests 1, 2, and 3 described under Ethinyloestradiol.
2. It is insoluble in a 5% solution of potassium hydroxide (distinction from ethinyloestradiol).

MELTING-POINT. About 152°.

ULTRAVIOLET ABSORPTION. In methyl alcohol, maximum at 279 nm (É1%, 1cm = 82) and a weak maximum at 287 nm.

INFRA-RED ABSORPTION. Major peaks at 1035, 1060, 1255, 1291, 1449, and 1612 cm^{-1} (see Appendix 2a: Infra-red Spectra).

THIN-LAYER CHROMATOGRAPHY. See under Thin-layer Chromatography, System 10.

Metabolism. ABSORPTION. Readily absorbed after oral administration.

BLOOD CONCENTRATION. 4% of an oral dose is present in the total plasma volume 4 hours after administration which falls to 2% at 24 hours and to 0.3 to 1.6% at 96 hours.

HALF-LIFE. Plasma half-life, 40 to 70 hours.

DISTRIBUTION. Taken up by many tissues and secreted in small amounts in the milk; volume of distribution, 80 to 180 litres.

METABOLIC REACTIONS. Demethylation to ethinyloestradiol and conjugation with glucuronic acid and sulphate.

EXCRETION. 10 to 50% of a dose is excreted in the urine in 5 to 8 days; the major urinary metabolite is ethinyloestradiol in conjugated form; no unchanged drug is detectable in urine.

FURTHER INFORMATION. Excretion in women—B. D. Kulkarni and J. W. Goldzieher, *Contraception*, 1970, **1**, 131; metabolism in women—K. I. H. Williams, *Steroids*, 1969, **13**, 539; metabolism to ethinyloestradiol—R. J. Warren and K. Fotherby, *J. Endocr.*, 1973, **59**, 369; studies during lactation— H. G. Wijmenga and H. J. Van der Molen, *Acta endocr. Copenh.*, 1969, **61**, 665.

Actions and uses. Mestranol has the actions of the oestrogens, as described under Oestradiol Benzoate. It is often included for these actions in amounts of 50 to 100 micrograms in oral contraceptive tablets.

Undesirable effects. Headache, dizziness, nausea, and vomiting may occur, but usually disappear if cyclic contraception is continued.

Preparations

Preparations available include TABLETS containing mestranol 100 micrograms with ethynodiol diacetate 0.5, 1, and 2 mg; tablets containing mestranol 50 micrograms with norethisterone 1 mg, tablets containing mestranol 80 micrograms with norethisterone 1 mg, tablets containing mestranol 100 micrograms with norethisterone 2 mg; tablets containing mestranol 75 micrograms with norethynodrel 5 mg, tablets containing mestranol 100 micrograms with norethynodrel 2.5 mg; and a combination pack providing graded doses of mestranol and norethisterone.

Metabolism of Drugs

Absorption, Distribution, and Elimination

Absorption, distribution, and excretion all involve, to some extent, the transfer of the drug across biological membranes. Biological membranes are complex lipoprotein structures and may vary from a single membrane, such as a cell membrane, to several layers of cells, such as the skin. They permit the passage of lipophilic compounds but present a barrier to all lipid-insoluble compounds unless a specific transport process is available or unless these lipid-insoluble compounds are of sufficiently low molecular weight to be filtered through the membrane.

There are five recognised mechanisms of membrane transfer, the major ones being illustrated in FIG. 1. The most important mechanism is by *passive diffusion*, the basic requirements for which are that the compound should be lipid-soluble and that there should be a concentration gradient across the membrane. Water-soluble compounds of small molecular weight, such as thiourea and urea, and small ions, such as sodium and potassium, may cross membranes by *filtration*, which occurs through membrane pores and which also requires a concentration gradient.

Certain drugs such as antimetabolites and levodopa may be transported by special biological systems evolved for the transport of natural compounds such as amino acids and sugars. These systems involve a carrier which binds with the compound and transports it across the membrane, either in the same direction as the concentration gradient, when it is referred to as *facilitated transport*, or against the gradient when it is referred to as *active transport*, and which additionally requires energy.

The fifth mechanism is *pinocytosis* whereby extracellular material is enveloped and absorbed by a cell. This mechanism is unimportant for drug transfer but it is very important for the transfer of large molecules such as proteins.

Many drugs are weak acids or weak bases and at physiological pH values are not completely ionised. A pH gradient across a membrane will influence the passive diffusion of these drugs since, in general, only the lipid-soluble, non-ionised form may pass. This is particularly important when considering absorption from the gastro-intestinal tract. FIG. 2 demonstrates the effect

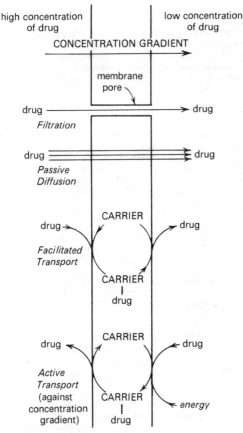

FIG. 1. Main mechanisms of membrane transfer.

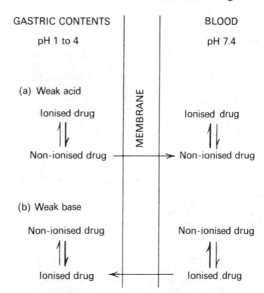

FIG. 2. Passive diffusion across the gastric blood barrier of (a) a weak acid and (b) a weak base. Direction of passive diffusion is dictated by concentration gradient for non-ionised drug.

of pH on the passive diffusion of a weak acid and a weak base across the gastric/blood barrier. In the gastric contents an acid drug is mostly in the non-ionised lipophilic state, and in this form, may cross the membrane. Once it has entered the blood, it is converted to the ionised form. As a result, the concentration gradient for the non-ionised drug is maintained thus enabling more drug to cross the membrane.

A weak base will not diffuse into the blood from the stomach, but if the concentration of the non-ionised form in the blood is greater than that in the stomach contents it would diffuse into the stomach. For example, bases such as quinine, morphine, and nicotine, following parenteral administration, are excreted into the gastric juice.

It is evident therefore that the physicochemical characteristics of the drug, the properties of the membrane, the environmental pH value, and the concentration gradient can influence the degree of transport across biological membranes.

Absorption

The type and number of membranes which a drug must traverse before it is absorbed and distributed is determined by the route of administration. Thus the rates of absorption and distribution will vary according to the route used. The most common route is oral administration, after which absorption may occur at any site in the gastro-intestinal tract. Because the pH values of the regions of the gut vary, different sites will be involved

in the absorption of drugs with different dissociation constants, as shown in FIG. 3.

ORAL ADMINISTRATION. Lipophilic drugs are rapidly absorbed from the mouth (buccal or sublingual absorp-

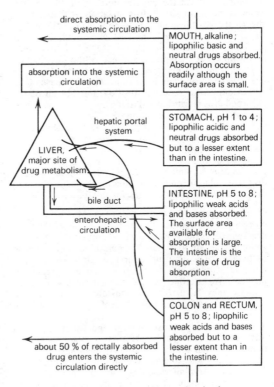

FIG. 3. Sites of drug absorption in the gastro-intestinal tract.

tion) by passive diffusion. Despite the fact that the area for absorption is small this route is used where a rapid effect is required such as that with glyceryl trinitrate, and also for drugs such as the steroids which may be metabolised in the gut or liver before entering the systemic circulation. Many drugs are secreted into the saliva and then swallowed and reabsorbed from other gastro-intestinal sites.

Lipophilic acidic and neutral drugs are absorbed in the stomach, the contents of which have a pH value of 1 to 4, but to a small extent compared with the intestinal sites, because the surface area is very much smaller. Some drugs, such as succinylsulphathiazole, although non-ionised in the stomach, are not absorbed because they are lipid-insoluble. Basic drugs that are ionised at the pH of the stomach are not absorbed.

The small intestine, comprising the duodenum, jejunum, and ileum, is the major site for drug absorption. Most drugs are absorbed in this region of the gut by passive diffusion but some may be absorbed by active transport mechanisms.

The intestine has pH values in the range 5 to 8 and thus permits the passive diffusion of weak acids and weak bases. The surface area available for absorption is very large and only a small amount of non-ionised drug need be present to enable a significant amount of absorption to occur. Some ionised drugs are also absorbed in this region but at an extremely slow rate. Absorption from the colon and rectum is very similar to intestinal absorption. The surface area available is less but absorption may occur readily.

All drugs absorbed from the stomach, intestine, and colon will encounter the enzymes of the gut wall and, in the lower regions of the gastro-intestinal tract, enzymes of the gut microflora, and will, upon absorption, be transported via the hepatic portal vein to the liver which is the major site of drug metabolism. Thus, drugs absorbed from these sites may be substantially metabolised before they reach the systemic circulation. This phenomenon is commonly known as the *first pass effect*. Lignocaine, for example, is subject to first pass metabolism and is 70% metabolised by the gut wall and the liver following oral administration. This first pass effect also occurs after rectal absorption, but not all of the absorbed drug is transported to the liver since about 50% enters the systemic circulation directly.

Other factors which affect gastro-intestinal absorption include gastric emptying time, gastro-intestinal motility, visceral blood flow, gastro-intestinal secretions, the presence of food or other drugs, changes in gut flora, and the drug formulation used. The factors involved in drug formulation and their effects on absorption are described in the entry on Bioavailability.

OTHER ROUTES OF ADMINISTRATION. Many drugs are given by other routes. This may be because they are deactivated in the gut or poorly absorbed (for example capreomycin sulphate and cephaloridine), or because particular rates of drug action or drug release are required (for example the intramuscular injection of medroxyprogesterone acetate for use as a depot), or because they have to be administered at their site of action, as in the case of intrathecal injections or local anaesthetics.

All routes, except those through the gastro-intestinal tract or the lungs avoid first pass metabolism and therefore enable a more reliable correlation to be made between the dose and the blood concentration of the active drug. Administration by some of the routes may result in some metabolism at the site of administration,

for example metabolism of a drug by the skin following percutaneous absorption.

After topical application to the skin the major barrier encountered is the stratum corneum, through which absorption occurs by passive diffusion. The extent of absorption appears to be influenced by the degree of skin hydration. This route is mainly used for local action and has not been used to any great extent for absorption into the blood stream.

Drugs which are inhaled may be absorbed by the nasal mucosa, the trachea, and the lungs. Absorption from the nasal mucosa occurs readily but it is rarely used as a route of administration except for certain polypeptide preparations. Absorption from the trachea and lungs, which is rapid and occurs readily, is important for a number of anaesthetics and for drugs which act locally on the respiratory system. They may be absorbed as solids, liquids, or gases.

Drugs administered as gases and vapours are readily absorbed by the alveoli of the lungs, which are highly permeable, have a large surface area, and have an abundant blood supply. Drugs administered in aerosols are trapped and absorbed at various sites in the respiratory tract depending on their particle size. Inhaled drugs are susceptible to first pass metabolism by the lungs and also by the liver, since 25% of the cardiac output flows through the liver.

Distribution and Pharmacokinetics

The main factors controlling distribution, in addition to those influencing membrane transfer, are plasma protein binding, tissue binding, blood-flow rate, and tissue fat content.

PLASMA PROTEIN BINDING. Many drugs are reversibly bound to plasma proteins, mainly to plasma albumin. The extent of protein binding is dependent upon the concentrations of drug and protein, the number of binding sites, and the affinity of these binding sites for the drug. This affinity may be related to the number of lipophilic groups in the drug molecule. However, both ionised and non-ionised drugs may be protein bound.

Often, more than one drug is bound and one drug may be displaced by another which has a higher binding affinity. For example coumarin anticoagulants will displace sulphonamides, sulphaphenazole will displace tolbutamide, and phenylbutazone, oxyphenbutazone, aspirin, mefenamic acid, and nalidixic acid will displace coumarin anticoagulants. This can lead to toxic reactions; for instance the displacement of coumarin anticoagulants may lead to bleeding since an increased amount of anticoagulant is unbound and therefore able to carry out its pharmacological action. In general, toxic reactions may only be transient because an increase in unbound drug may be compensated by a concomitant increase in tissue uptake and the unbound concentration may remain the same whilst the total blood concentration may be reduced.

Plasma protein binding has two important effects on drug distribution, particularly when the fraction of bound drug is large. Firstly it helps to maintain a concentration gradient for the absorption of drugs from the gastro-intestinal tract. Secondly, it may decrease the amount of drug available for tissue uptake, metabolism, and excretion, although this action depends upon whether or not the process affected is an equilibrium process. In general, the equilibrium between bound and unbound drug is reached very rapidly, in milliseconds; release of drug from the protein is therefore unlikely to be a rate-limiting step unless the process affected is also extremely rapid.

The extent of tissue uptake, which is an equilibrium process, is determined by the relative affinities of the plasma protein and tissue. The extent of a metabolic reaction, which is a non-equilibrium process, is unaffected since the protein-binding equilibrium is continually pulled in one direction.

TISSUE BINDING. Drugs are highly bound to tissues, and to produce their pharmacological action are bound to specific macromolecules, called receptors, which may be enzymes, genetic material, or membrane structures. The amount of drug at a receptor is very small compared to the amount bound to non-pharmacologically-active sites and therefore does not significantly change the overall distribution pattern.

Some drugs bind specifically to tissues in which there are no receptors and this binding may be non-reversible. For example, many drugs are localised in melanin-containing tissues, tetracycline is localised in bone and teeth where it binds with calcium, and phenothiazines and arsenicals are deposited in hair shafts.

BLOOD-FLOW RATE. Tissue uptake is dependent on blood-flow rate in relation to tissue mass. Tissues with high blood-flow rates will equilibrate more rapidly with plasma concentrations of the drug than tissues with low flow rates. However, tissues with low blood-flow rates but high membrane permeabilities will still absorb large quantities of drug. The liver, for example, has a relatively slow blood flow but instead of the blood flowing through blood capillaries, it is transported along the hepatic sinusoids, the walls of which are highly permeable. TABLE 1 shows the variations in blood flow between various tissues.

TABLE 1. Blood Flow to Human Tissues

Tissue	% Body Weight	% Cardiac Output	Blood Flow ml/100 g tissue per minute
Adrenals	0.02	1	550
Kidneys	0.4	24	450
Thyroid	0.04	2	400
Liver Hepatic	2	5	20
Portal	0	20	75
Portal-drained Viscera	2	20	75
Heart (basal)	0.4	4	70
Brain	2	15	55
Skin	7	5	5
Muscle (basal)	40	15	3
Connective Tissue	7	1	1
Fat	15	2	1

After T. C. Butler, in *Proceedings of the First International Pharmacological Meeting*, B. B. Brodie and E. G. Erdos (Eds), Vol. 4, London, Pergamon Press, 1962, p. 197.

FAT CONTENT. Tissues with a high fat content will accumulate lipophilic drugs by simple partitioning, as exemplified by the deposition of thiopentone in adipose tissue.

PHARMACOKINETICS. Pharmacokinetics is the study of the kinetics of drug distribution. It has several important applications and may be used to determine rational dosage schedules in therapeutics, to evaluate absorption and other processes in order to develop more effective drug formulations, to determine the concentration of a drug at its site of action, and to provide information on the variations in drug metabolism and response between individuals and between patients with different disease states.

It is difficult to assess the distribution of a drug because tissue levels cannot usually be measured directly and also because the fate of a drug in the body is determined by a series of dynamic interactions.

To overcome these problems it is possible to use a series of mathematical models, based on a knowledge of the changes in blood concentration and urinary excretion with time, to ascertain the kinetics of drug distribution. In these models a drug is considered to be distributed within a series of interconnected body compartments, which do not necessarily relate precisely to actual anatomical compartments, but which do relate to discrete pools of drug availability. For instance a two-compartment model, as shown in FIG. 4, consists of a central compartment (1) and a peripheral compartment (2).

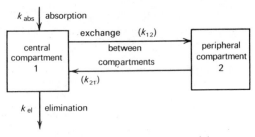

FIG. 4. A two-compartment model.

Drug enters central compartment (1) either by absorption or by direct injection, then equilibrates with peripheral compartment (2) and is eliminated. Generally, transfer from one pool to another is assumed to be governed by first order kinetic equations. Under certain conditions, zero order kinetics may apply. The relationship between drug concentrations in the compartments is expressed in the following equation.

[Rate of change of plasma concentration]
$$= [\text{Rate of absorption } (k_{abs})]$$
$$- [\text{Rate of transfer from 1 to 2 } (k_{12})]$$
$$+ [\text{Rate of transfer from 2 to 1 } (k_{21})]$$
$$- [\text{Rate of elimination } (k_{el})]$$

From this relationship it is possible to derive the various rate constants mathematically.

Differences in the rates of movement of the drug between compartments 1 and 2 in the two-compartment model produce the variations in drug concentrations shown in FIG. 5.

Another mathematical concept is the *volume of distribution* (V_d). This is the volume in which the total amount of drug in the body would be uniformly distributed to give an observed plasma concentration. Since it is an imaginary quantity it is often called the *apparent volume of distribution*. For drugs that are uniformly distributed throughout body water, V_d reflects the actual volume of distribution. For drugs that are localised in tissue, however, V_d is very much greater than the volume of body water. For drugs that are bound to plasma proteins,

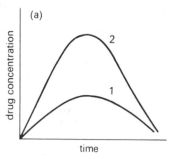

(a) $k_{abs} = k_{el} = k_{21}$, and k_{12} is more than k_{21}

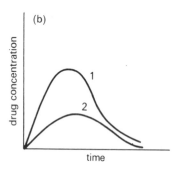

(b) $k_{abs} = k_{el} = k_{12}$, and k_{21} is more than k_{12}

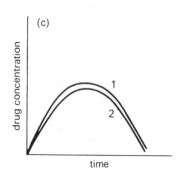

(c) $k_{abs} = k_{el}$, $k_{12} = k_{21}$, and k_{12} and k_{21} are greater than k_{abs} and k_{el}

FIG. 5. Effect of different rate constants on drug distribution between compartments in a two-compartment model. Curves 1 and 2 represent drug concentration/time curves for compartments 1 and 2 respectively; where k_{abs} = rate of absorption, k_{el} = rate of elimination, k_{12} = rate of transfer from 1 to 2, and k_{21} = rate of transfer from 2 to 1.

V_d is less than the actual volume of distribution. The V_d values for some drugs, for example phenazone, may correspond to the volumes of the body water compartments (see TABLE 2) but this does not necessarily mean that the distribution of these drugs is restricted to those particular body compartments.

The volume of distribution is usually quoted in litres. However, it may also be quoted in litres per kilogram of body-weight or as a percentage of body-weight.

TABLE 2. Approximate Volume of the Body Water Compartments for a Person of Average Weight

Compartment	Volume in litres
Interstitial water	12.8
Plasma water	3.2
Transcellular water	1.0
Extracellular water, total	17.0
Intracellular water	25.0
Total body water	42.0

A further important concept is the *plasma half-life*. This is the time required for the plasma concentration to fall by 50%. A short plasma half-life may be a consequence of tissue uptake, rapid metabolism, or excretion, and a long half-life may be a consequence of protein binding, slow metabolism, or poor excretion.

After the intravenous injection of a drug, the rates of the various processes involved in its removal from the blood may be determined from a plasma concentration/time curve. When two or more processes are involved, the curve will show more curvature than when only one process is involved. If the curve is plotted on a semilogarithmic scale the separate processes become evident, provided that the rate constant for each process is different. These rates can be expressed in terms of the *half-life* ($t_\frac{1}{2}$) for each process.

For example, FIG. 6 shows a semilogarithmic plot of the

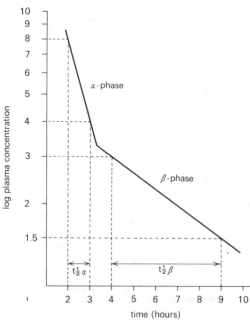

FIG. 6. Semilogarithmic plot of plasma concentration versus time for a drug distributed within 2 compartments.

concentration of a drug which is distributed within a two-compartment model. The biphasic nature of this curve is attributable to two processes—an initial distribution process (α-phase) followed by an elimination process (β-phase) which involves both metabolic reactions and the excretion of the drug. In general, the α-phase is much more rapid than the β-phase. The half-life of the β-phase is often referred to as the *elimination half-life* or *biological half-life*.

Metabolic Reactions

Many drugs are lipophilic and mainly non-ionised at physiological pH values and therefore they are reabsorbed from the renal tubules by passive diffusion. As a result they are not readily excreted. Most metabolic reactions, for example the oxidation of amylobarbitone and of trimethylamine, the glucuronidation of morphine, and the O-dealkylation of phenacetin, convert drugs to more polar metabolites which are readily excreted. However, there are some exceptions. The sulphonamides, for example, are acetylated to form metabolites which are less soluble in water than their parent compounds. Hydrophilic compounds are, in general, poorly metabolised and are excreted unchanged.

There are two groups of reactions by which drugs are metabolised—*preconjugation* reactions, such as oxidation, reduction, or hydrolysis, and *conjugation* reactions in which chemical moieties are added to the drug or metabolite. The former reactions either expose or add functional groups to render the drug more polar and produce sites for conjugation reactions. Many of these reactions are reversible and the products derived from them may undergo re-arrangements or further metabolism. The enzymes responsible for these reactions are found in many tissues, but especially at sites of absorption or excretion such as the liver, gastro-intestinal tract, skin, lungs, and kidneys. In addition the gut flora may metabolise certain drugs.

The liver is the most important organ for the metabolism of drugs and the enzymes concerned are located mainly in the endoplasmic reticuli (microsomes) of the parenchymal cells. These microsomal enzymes include oxidases, reductases, esterases, and a number of enzymes involved in the conjugation reactions. Other enzymes are located in mitochondria or in the soluble fraction of cells.

PRECONJUGATION (PHASE 1) REACTIONS. 1. *Oxidation.* This is one of the most important general metabolic reactions of drugs. The principal enzymes involved are the mixed function oxidases, of which there are several, each capable of catalysing the metabolism of a number of drugs. The enzymes are located in the endoplasmic reticuli (microsomal fraction) of the liver and other tissues and they require oxygen and reduced nicotinamide-adenine dinucleotide phosphate (NADPH). They participate in an electron transport chain in which cytochrome P450 is an important terminal oxygen-transferring enzyme system to which the drug binds. Non-microsomal oxidations are catalysed by enzymes in mitochondria (for example, amine oxidases), cell sap (for example, xanthine oxidase and alcohol dehydrogenase), and in the plasma (for example, amidases, esterases, hydrolases, and amine oxidases).

The wide variety of oxidative reactions is illustrated in the following examples.

At carbon atoms,
  Aliphatic oxidation (for example, glutethimide, tolbutamide, meprobamate, chloral hydrate, and amylobarbitone)

amylobarbitone   hydroxyamylobarbitone

Aromatic oxidation (for example, phenobarbitone and phenylbutazone)

phenobarbitone   p-hydroxyphenobarbitone

Alicyclic oxidation (for example, cyclobarbitone and hexobarbitone)

cyclobarbitone   ketocyclobarbitone

Epoxidation (for example, cyproheptadine, in rats)

cyproheptadine   cyproheptadine epoxide

At nitrogen atoms,
  Primary N-oxidation (for example, amphetamine)

amphetamine   N-(1-phenylprop-2-yl)hydroxylamine

Tertiary N-oxidation (for example, chlorpromazine)

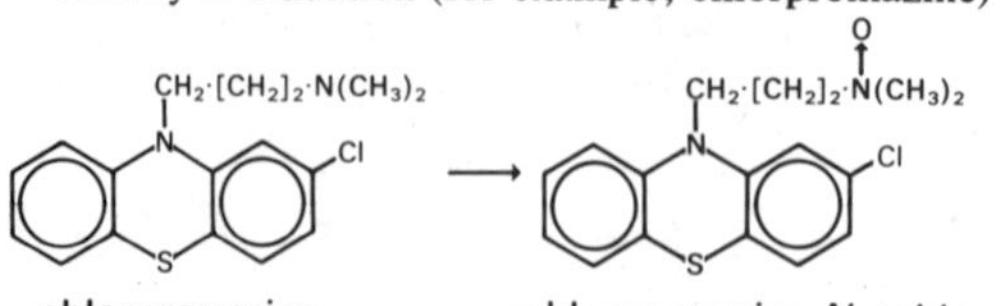

chlorpromazine → chlorpromazine N-oxide

N-Dealkylation (for example, ephedrine, imipramine, and iproniazid)

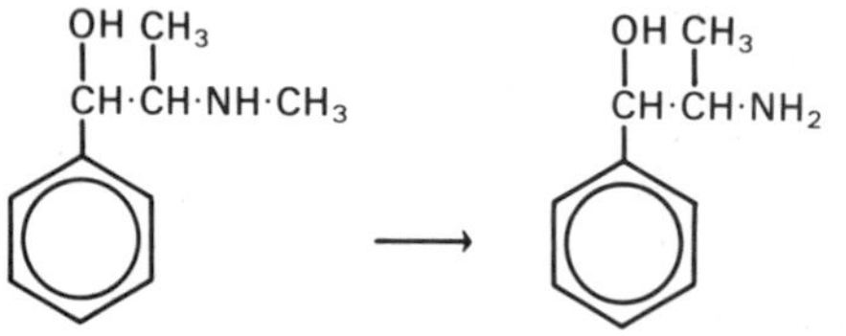

ephedrine → phenylpropanolamine

Deamination (for example, amphetamine and noradrenaline)

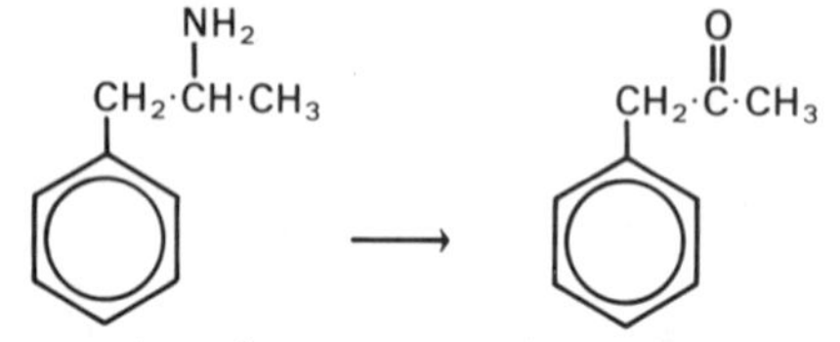

amphetamine → 1-phenylpropan-2-one

At sulphur atoms,
S-Oxidation (for example, chlorpromazine and thioridazine)

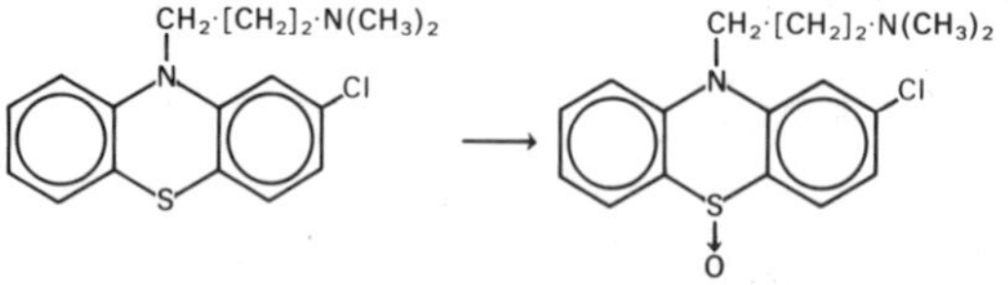

chlorpromazine → chlorpromazine sulphoxide

S-Dealkylation (for example, 6-methylthiopurine)

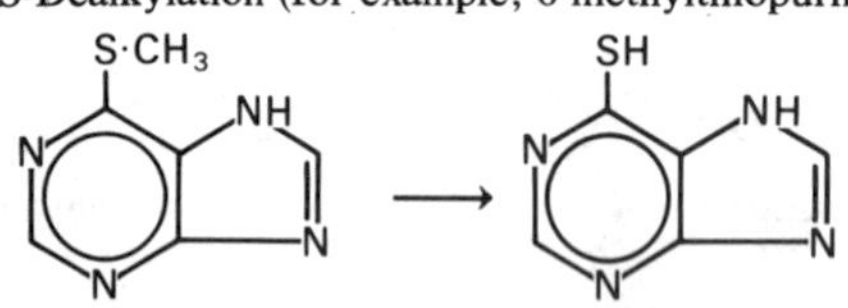

6-methylthiopurine → 6-thiopurine

Desulphuration (for example, thiopentone)

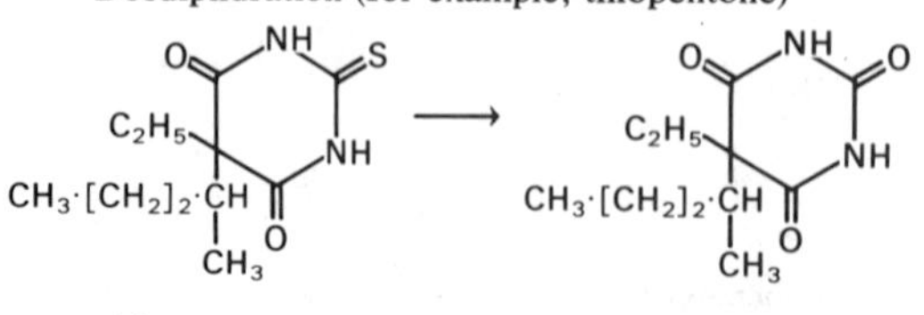

thiopentone → pentobarbitone

At oxygen atoms,
O-Dealkylation (for example, diamorphine and phenacetin)

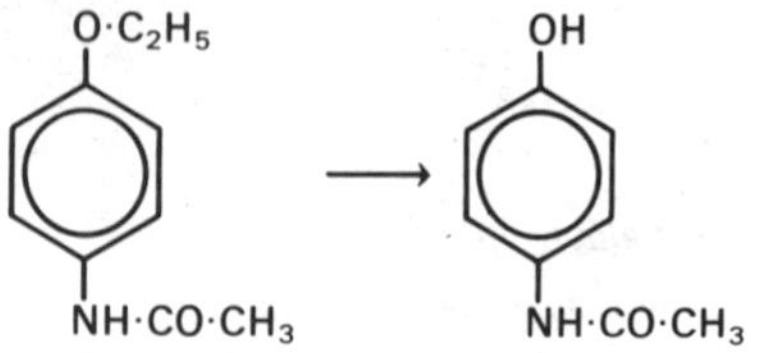

phenacetin → paracetamol

Other oxidation reactions,
Ring fission (for example, catechol)

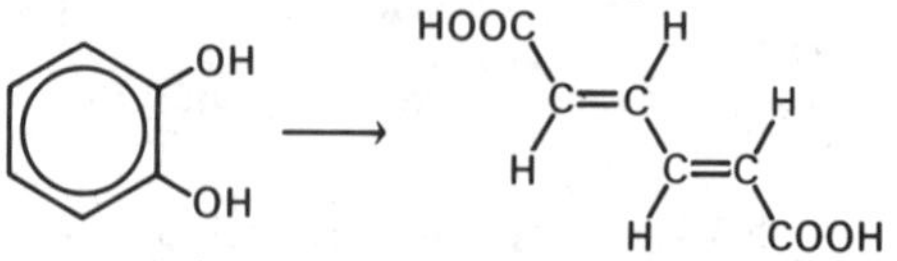

catechol → trans-trans-muconic acid

Ring formation (for example, proguanil)

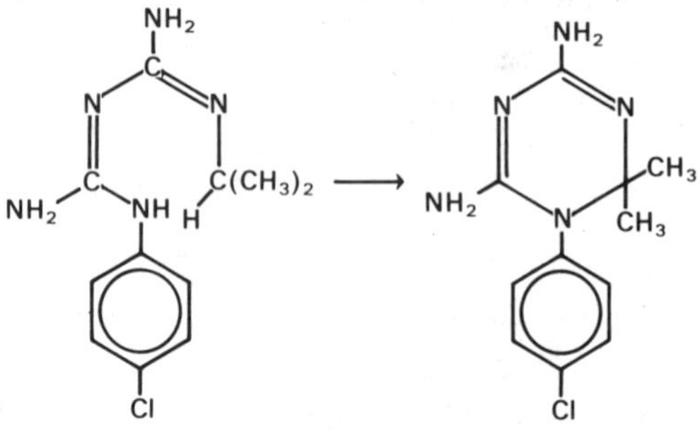

proguanil → cycloguanil

2. *Reduction.* These reactions are less commonly observed than oxidation reactions and sometimes result in the formation of metabolites which are more lipid soluble than their parent compounds. In addition the toxicity of such metabolites may be greater than the toxicity of metabolites derived from oxidation. Toxic amines, for example, are formed by the reduction of azo compounds.
Both microsomal and non-microsomal enzymes will carry out reductions and some reductions are known to be catalysed by enzymes of the gut flora. The microsomal reductases are flavoproteins with flavine-adenine dinucleotide (FAD) as their prosthetic group and they require reduced nicotinamide-adenine dinucleotide phosphate (NADPH). It is possible that the reaction mechanism involves the reduction of FAD by the enzyme, using NADPH or reduced nicotinamide-adenine dinucleotide (NADH) as a cofactor, and then the reduction of the drug non-enzymatically by a reaction with the reduced FAD.
Examples of reduction reactions are illustrated in the following examples.
At carbon atoms,
  Aldehyde reduction (for example, chloral)

$$CCl_3 \cdot CHO \longrightarrow CCl_3 \cdot CH_2OH$$

chloral → trichloroethanol

Ketoreduction (for example, metyrapone)

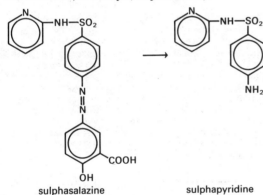

metyrapone → 2-methyl-1,2-di(pyrid-3-yl)propan-1-ol

Dehalogenation (for example, halothane)

$CF_3 \cdot CHBrCl \longrightarrow CF_3 \cdot CH_3$

halothane → 1,1,1-trifluoroethane

At nitrogen atoms,
Nitroreduction (for example, nitrofurantoin)

nitrofurantoin → 1-(5-aminofurfurylidene-amino)hydantoin

Azoreduction (for example, sulphasalazine)

sulphasalazine → sulphapyridine

Hydroxamic acid reduction (for example, salicyl hydroxamic acid)

salicylhydroxamic acid → salicylamide

At sulphur atoms,
sulphoxide reduction (for example, dimethyl sulphoxide)

$(CH_3)_2SO \longrightarrow (CH_3)_2S$

dimethyl sulphoxide → dimethyl sulphide

Disulphide reduction (for example, disulfiram)

disulfiram → diethyldithiocarbamic acid

3. Hydrolysis.
This is a major metabolic reaction of esters and amides. The enzymes involved are present in the microsomes of the liver, gut wall, and other tissues, and in the blood plasma.

Ester hydrolysis (for example, pethidine, procaine, and suxamethonium)

$$CH_2 \cdot CO \cdot O \cdot [CH_2]_2 \cdot \overset{+}{N}(CH_3)_3$$
$$CH_2 \cdot CO \cdot O \cdot [CH_2]_2 \cdot \overset{+}{N}(CH_3)_3 \longrightarrow CH_2 \cdot CO \cdot O \cdot [CH_2]_2 \cdot \overset{+}{N}(CH_3)_3$$
$$CH_2 \cdot COOH$$

suxamethonium → choline hydrogen succinate

$$CH_2 \cdot COOH$$
$$CH_2 \cdot COOH \quad + \quad (CH_3)_3 \cdot \overset{+}{N} \cdot CH_2 \cdot CH_2OH$$

succinic acid + choline

Amide hydrolysis (for example, salicylamide)

salicylamide → salicylic acid

Hydrazide hydrolysis (for example, isoniazid and phenelzine)

isoniazid → isonicotinic acid + hydrazine $+ \ NH_2 \cdot NH_2$

Carbamate hydrolysis (for example, meprobamate)

$$CH_2 \cdot O \cdot CO \cdot NH_2$$
$$CH_3 \cdot C \cdot [CH_2]_2 \cdot CH_3 \longrightarrow CH_3 \cdot C \cdot [CH_2]_2 \cdot CH_3 + 2NH_2 \cdot COOH$$
$$CH_2 \cdot O \cdot CO \cdot NH_2 \qquad CH_2OH$$

meprobamate → 2-hydroxymethyl-2-methylpentan-1-ol + carbamic acid

Deacetylation (for example, phenacetin)

phenacetin → p-ethoxyaniline

Hydrolytic ring fission (for example, hexobarbitone and phenytoin)

phenytoin   α-aminodiphenylacetic acid

CONJUGATION (PHASE 2) REACTIONS. In these reactions a chemical moiety is combined with the drug which generally results in increased polarity and decreased lipid solubility, thereby facilitating elimination. In many conjugation reactions the conjugating group is transferred to the drug or metabolite from an activated coenzyme by the influence of an appropriate transferase enzyme. Glucuronides, sulphates, and methyl and acetyl conjugates are formed in this way, but amino-acid conjugates are formed by the initial production of a coenzyme-drug complex before the conjugating group is added. A few conjugation reactions do not require coenzymes, for example glutathione conjugation and thiocyanate formation.

1. *Glucuronide formation.* This is the most important conjugation reaction since the enzyme systems involved are present in a large number of tissues, especially the liver, kidneys, skin, and gastro-intestinal tract, and will react with a diverse range of compounds. Glucuronides are formed at the N-, O-, or S-positions of many functional groups such as phenols, carboxylic acids, alcohols, aromatic amines, sulphonamides, heterocyclic nitrogen compounds, aliphatic amino groups, carbamyl groups, and thiols. Examples of compounds which form glucuronides are shown in Table 3.
Glucuronides are polar and water soluble and hence readily excreted in the urine or bile. Under conditions of acid hydrolysis, ether glucuronides are more stable than ester glucuronides but the N-glucuronides vary considerably in their stability. The O-glucuronides are hydrolysed by β-glucuronidase but the N-glucuronides are relatively stable to this enzyme.

TABLE 3. Examples of Compounds which Conjugate with Glucuronic Acid

O-*conjugation*	N-*conjugation*	S-*conjugation*
hydrocortisone	meprobamate	NN-diethyldithio-
4-hydroxycoumarin	sulphadimethoxine	carbamic acid
indomethacin	sulphafurazole	2-mercaptobenzo-
morphine	sulphathiazole	thiazole
nicotinic acid		
salicylic acid		

The conjugating enzymes are located in the endoplasmic reticulum of the liver, kidney, and skin but the formation of the coenzyme complex is catalysed by enzymes in the soluble fraction.
The reaction sequence, where ROH represents the drug, is:
Uridine triphosphate (UTP)
    +glucose-1-phosphate → UDP-glucose + 2phosphate
UDP-glucose
    +2NAD → UDP-glucosiduronic acid (UDPGA)
                                        +2NADH$_2$
UDPGA + ROH → RO-glucuronide
                    +uridine diphosphate (UDP)

2. *Sulphate conjugation.* This is an important reaction for phenols, amines, and alcohols. Sulphate conjugation occurs, for example, with chloramphenicol, 3-hydroxy-coumarin, oestrone and other steroids, and catecholamines. The resulting conjugates are relatively strong acids and readily excreted. They are hydrolysed by sulphatases. Sulphate conjugation is catalysed by one of several enzymes, all of which exhibit substrate specificity. Steroids, for example, are converted to sulphates only in the liver, whilst studies *in vitro* show that phenols may be converted by enzymes in the soluble fraction of the liver, kidney, and intestine. The reaction is:

SO_4^{2-} + adenosine triphosphate (ATP)
    → adenosine-5'-phosphosulphate (APS)
                                        +pyrophosphate
APS + ATP
    → phosphoadenosine-5'-phosphosulphate (PAPS)
                        +adenosine diphosphate (ADP)
PAPS + ROH → ROSO$_3$H + ADP

3. *Methylation.* This reaction is important but its effects are not always fully evident because of subsequent demethylation reactions. Methylation is catalysed by many enzymes which are widely distributed throughout the body. These enzymes exhibit substrate specificity and vary in cofactor requirements. Some amines, phenols, and thiols, such as isoniazid, noradrenaline, isoprenaline, dihydroxybenzoic acid, and thiouracil, are conjugated by this reaction.

Methionine + ATP → S-adenosylmethionine
                        +pyrophosphate + phosphate
S-adenosylmethionine + ROH → ROCH$_3$
                        +S-adenosylhomocysteine

In contrast to most other types of metabolite, methylated substances are usually more liposoluble than the compounds from which they are derived.
4. *Acetylation.* This reaction takes place mainly in the liver but also in the spleen, lungs, and many other tissues. It occurs with primary aromatic and primary aliphatic amines, hydrazines, hydrazides, and sulphonamides. Isoniazid and sulphanilamide are two examples of compounds which are acetylated. Sulphonamides form acetyl derivatives at the N^4-position and, in some cases, at both the N^1- and N^4-positions. The acetyl group is attached to coenzyme A (CoA-SH) before transference to the drug.

CH_3CO-S-CoA + RSO$_2$NH$_2$
                    → RSO$_2$NHCOCH$_3$ + CoA-SH

5. *Amino-acid conjugation.* Aromatic and heterocyclic carboxylic acids and certain aliphatic acids with aromatic substituents are conjugated with glycine or, in some cases, taurine or glutamine. Most aliphatic acids, however, are readily oxidised so that conjugation cannot occur. The amino-acid conjugates are strongly acidic, having pK$_a$ values of about 3. They are split by alkali hydrolysis as opposed to the acid hydrolysis of the glucuronides.
Unlike most other reactions, amino-acid conjugation occurs in the mitochondria. The acid is converted to an active form and is attached to coenzyme A before it is converted to the amide.

RCO$_2$H + ATP → RCO-AMP + pyrophosphate
RCO-AMP + CoA-SH → RCO-S-CoA + AMP
RCO-S-CoA + NH$_2$.CH$_2$.CO$_2$H
                → RCONH.CH$_2$.CO$_2$H + CoA-SH

6. *Glutathione conjugation and mercapturic acid formation.* Compounds containing electrophilic centres, such as ethacrynic acid and certain unsaturated hydrocarbons and their halides and nitro-compounds, may be conju-

gated with glutathione. The conjugate so formed may be excreted in the bile together with its catabolites formed by stepwise removal of glutamate and glycine followed by acetylation of the resultant free amino group. The mercapturic acid metabolite (*N*-acetylcysteine derivative) so produced is excreted in the urine and in the bile. The aromatic hydrocarbons are first converted to an epoxide before conjugation with glutathione. The enzymes responsible for both conjugation and the removal of the amino acids are located mainly in the liver and kidneys.

7. *Thiocyanate formation.* Cyanide ions are conjugated by endogenous thiosulphate, which is a sulphur donating compound, to form thiocyanates. This reaction is important as a detoxication mechanism and leads to a 100-fold reduction in toxicity.

$$CN^- + S_2O_3^{2-} \rightarrow SCN^- + SO_3^{2-}$$

Excretion

The principal routes of excretion are via the kidney into the urine and via the liver into the bile, but some drugs may also be excreted in the sweat, milk, saliva, exhalations, or into the gastro-intestinal tract.

RENAL EXCRETION. This depends upon three processes, namely glomerular filtration, passive tubular diffusion, and active transport into the renal tubules.
Glomerular filtration is the simple ultrafiltration of the blood plasma. Lipid-soluble compounds may be excreted into the distal portion of the renal tubule by *passive diffusion*, providing that there is a concentration gradient and a suitable urinary pH value. In addition, lipid-soluble compounds already in the glomerular filtrate may be reabsorbed by the same process. Highly lipid-soluble compounds therefore are slowly excreted.
Since the reabsorption of weak electrolytes is pH dependent—only the non-ionised form may cross the renal tubular wall—the rates of urinary excretion of weak electrolytes will be dependent upon the urinary pH value, which varies over a wide range (pH 5 to 8). Weak acids having pK_a values in the range 3 to 7.5, such as the salicylates and phenobarbitone, will be more readily excreted in alkaline urine, whilst weak bases having pK_a values in the range 7.5 to 10.5, such as amphetamines, will be more readily excreted in acid urine. The effect of pH on overall drug excretion, however, is only significant if the drug is excreted mostly in the unchanged form since most drug metabolites are polar and therefore not readily reabsorbed.
Active transport is associated with the proximal tubule of the kidney and is involved in the secretion of some acids and bases. These compounds are highly ionised and are readily excreted with little or no tubular reabsorption. Although the active transport mechanism exists for the excretion of endogenous substances, such acidic drugs as probenecid, the penicillins, thiazides, and glucuronic acid conjugates and such basic drugs as quinine, mecamylamine, and quaternary ammonium compounds are also excreted by this process.

BILIARY-FAECAL EXCRETION. This route of excretion is governed by both active transport and passive diffusion processes. The major mechanism is active transport which only occurs with drugs or their metabolites that have a molecular weight above about 500. The membranes of the parenchymal cells of the liver are highly permeable and thus drugs and their metabolites may appear in the bile in concentrations equal to those in blood.

In general, biliary excretion is more important for the excretion of metabolites, especially water-soluble conjugates such as the glucuronides and glutathione conjugates; only small amounts of unchanged drug are excreted by this route.
Drugs which are excreted in bile include carbenoxolone, cromoglycate, digitoxin, norethynodrel, pancuronium, rifampicin, and sulphobromophthalein.
Conjugates excreted in the bile may be hydrolysed by biliary enzymes or by the gut flora. The resultant free drugs may then be reabsorbed. This cycle of excretion and reabsorption, the *enterohepatic circulation*, therefore increases the time that a drug will remain in the body. In this situation, however, concentrations in the body still decline since some of the drug will not be reabsorbed and some will be excreted in the urine.
Digitoxin is enterohepatically recycled in man, several antibiotics such as nafcillin and erythromycin are recycled in the dog, and a wide variety of drugs are recycled in the rat. Several drugs are excreted in the faeces and are not involved in enterohepatic cycling. These drugs are usually strongly polar and include cromoglycate and oxyphenonium.

OTHER ROUTES. 1. *Sweat.* Sulphonamides, some amines, and urea are excreted in the sweat by passive diffusion.

2. *Milk.* Excretion into milk occurs primarily by passive diffusion, the extent being dependent upon the concentration gradient between the blood and milk, the pK_a and lipid solubility of the drug, and the pH value of the milk. Milk, being more acid than blood (pH value about 6.8), accumulates weak bases.
Almost any drug administered to a nursing mother will be excreted in milk to some extent, either unchanged or as a metabolite. The size and frequency of the dose and the potency of the drug will determine whether or not the concentration in the milk will be harmful to the infant. Whilst the amount of drug excreted in milk is generally small, the cumulative amount excreted in 24 hours could produce therapeutic or toxic concentrations in the infant.
Chloramphenicol, sulphafurazole, and metronidazole, for example, are excreted in milk in high concentration but whilst sulphafurazole may cause kernicterus and chloramphenicol may cause toxic reactions upon accumulation, metronidazole does not appear to affect the infant adversely. Owing to its high concentration in milk however, it would be appropriate to exercise caution when metronidazole is administered to nursing mothers.
Examples of other drugs which may be excreted in milk in significant amounts include anticoagulants, aspirin, barbiturates, benzodiazepines, caffeine, erythromycin, morphine, nicotine, penicillins, quinine, steroidal hormones, sulphonamides, and tetracyclines.

3. *Exhalations.* The extent of excretion through the lungs is small and occurs with gases, for example the gaseous anaesthetics, by passive diffusion.

4. *Gastro-intestinal tract.* There are three sites of excretion into the gastro-intestinal tract, namely into the saliva, into the stomach, and into the intestine.
Excretion into the saliva is dependent upon passive diffusion. A number of compounds may be excreted by this route such as the sulphonamides, phenobarbitone, clonidine, and many amines. There may be an active transport process because although penicillin and probenecid are each excreted into the saliva when they are given together the amount of penicillin in the saliva is reduced.
Concentrations of drugs in the saliva relate directly to

those in the plasma and, for the monitoring of drug concentrations in the body, saliva may be used as an alternative to plasma.

The drug excreted in saliva is swallowed and may be reabsorbed by other regions of the gut thus setting up an excretion/reabsorption cycle.

A number of basic drugs such as morphine, quinine, and nicotine are excreted into the stomach by pH-dependent passive diffusion processes. Some basic drugs may be excreted in large quantities by this route.

Other Factors Affecting Drug Metabolism

In addition to the factors already described, there are many other variables which may influence drug metabolism. These variables not only result in differences in metabolism between individuals but also result in differences in metabolism by the same individual depending on his or her particular physiological or pathological state.

PHARMACOGENETICS. Discontinuous and continuous variations in drug metabolism arise as a result of genetic factors. Discontinuous variations give rise to recognisable phenotypes and therefore to *polymorphism*. The acetylation of isoniazid is a typical example where there are 2 populations—one which rapidly acetylates the drug and the other which slowly acetylates it. Similar polymorphism has been shown for dapsone, phenelzine, sulphadimidine, and sulphamethoxypyridazine.

Other bimodal distributions in metabolic activity have been shown with the action of plasma cholinesterase on suxamethonium, the hydroxylation of phenytoin, the hydroxylation of debrisoquine, and the metabolism of phenacetin. In the latter case, a single family was shown to have a deficiency of the enzymes which de-ethylate phenacetin to form paracetamol and they produced a toxic metabolite, hydroxyphenetidine, instead.

Evidence of continuous variations has come from studies on identical and non-identical twins with dicoumarol, nortriptyline, phenazone, and phenylbutazone.

SPECIES. There are considerable variations in drug metabolism between species resulting from the presence, absence, or relative deficiency, of a particular enzyme in one species as compared with another. Aromatic hydroxylations, conjugate formation, and biliary excretion, for example, are all subject to wide species variation. As a result of these differences, extrapolation from studies in animals to man may be difficult to accomplish.

AGE. In the newborn, the drug metabolising enzymes are not so well developed as in the adult, and in the elderly the activities of these enzymes tend to be reduced. Thus there will be differences in the metabolism of a particular drug depending on age. The hydroxylation of amylobarbitone is less in neonates than adults, for example, and is decreased in the elderly.

Differences in renal excretion patterns may also be expected between different age groups because renal function deteriorates with age and is not fully developed in neonates.

SEX. Studies in rats have demonstrated that male rats will metabolise drugs more quickly than female rats.

There have not been many studies of sex-linked differences in drug metabolism in man, but studies on methadone, nicotine, and pentazocine have shown that sex-linked differences in drug metabolism do occur.

NUTRITIONAL STATES. Diets low in protein have been shown to reduce amino-acid conjugation and the activity of other microsomal enzymes. The type of food eaten influences the pH of the urine and may therefore influence pH-dependent excretion.

PHYSIOLOGICAL FACTORS. Factors such as stress, pregnancy, and hormonal state may influence drug metabolism. In rats, for example, pretreatment with adrenal steroids has resulted in increased activity of the drug metabolising enzymes. In mice, exposure to cold has increased the microsomal oxidation of naphthylamine and in rats subjected to similar treatment the oxidation of acetanilide has been increased.

In pregnancy, the placenta forms an extra membrane barrier through which a drug may pass. *Placental transfer* is controlled mostly by passive diffusion but there is evidence of an active transport system for certain drugs, for example ampicillin.

Most drugs cross the placenta and those which readily cross the placenta include alcohol, chlorpromazine, anaesthetics, sulphonamides, barbiturates, morphine, and certain antibiotics. Quaternary ammonium compounds do not cross the placenta readily. For information on the possible hazards of drug therapy during pregnancy, see the entry on Pregnancy.

Drug metabolism may also be affected by pregnancy; the conjugation of drugs with glucuronic acid is reduced and the metabolism of pethidine is decreased.

Differences in weight and in the distribution of body fat may lead to quite important differences in drug distribution.

DISEASE STATES. In patients with impaired renal function, drugs which are normally excreted by the kidney will accumulate in the body. This could lead to overdosage and possibly to toxic reactions in the case of chloramphenicol, nitrofurantoin, the tetracyclines, and the cardiac glycosides, for example.

In patients with liver disease, studies of the effects of impaired liver function have been inconclusive and blood concentrations of drugs and metabolites have been similar in both normal individuals and patients. In the case of these patients a correlation does appear to exist between the extent of protein binding and the extent of amylobarbitone metabolism by the liver. In studies where no differences have been shown, the effect of drug therapy must be considered and it is possible that rates of drug metabolism are similar in patients and in normal individuals as a result of enzyme induction.

Many studies on drug metabolism are carried out on normal individuals and it must be borne in mind that the results obtained may be very different from those obtained in studies on patients.

DRUG INTERACTIONS. Drug interactions are discussed in the entry on Interaction of Drugs but their effect on drug metabolism requires some explanation.

There are three basic mechanisms involved in drug metabolism and distribution which may be affected by drug interactions. These are transport across membranes, protein binding, and the activities of the drug metabolising enzymes.

1. *Transport across membranes.* Complex formation between drugs or chelation may increase polarity and decrease lipid solubility and thereby reduce the ability of a drug to cross membranes. Antacids containing aluminium, calcium, and magnesium, for example, will complex with tetracycline and thus reduce its absorption while the absorption of warfarin is reduced by cholestyramine which binds to the ionised form of the anticoagulant. Chymotrypsin appears to increase the

absorption of phenethicillin possibly by reducing the extent of binding to gut proteins.

Another form of interaction which may reduce membrane transfer is competition between drugs for the same active transport process. Probenecid for example competitively inhibits the excretion of penicillin.

2. *Plasma protein and tissue binding.* Competition between drugs for the same sites on plasma albumin may lead to a drug (A) being displaced by another drug (B) which has a higher binding affinity. This may lead to an increased amount of drug A in the blood (see Plasma Protein Binding, above). Similar displacement may occur with tissue-bound drugs.

3. *Activities of the drug metabolising enzymes.* The action of the drug metabolising enzymes may be increased or decreased by a wide variety of drugs and foreign compounds. The liver enzymes are predominantly affected but in animals certain enzymes of the kidney and small intestine may also be affected.

The changes in enzyme activity may be the result of changes in the amount of enzyme present or the activity of the individual enzyme molecules. The former may be affected by drugs which increase or reduce the synthesis of the enzyme involved or may increase or reduce the catabolism of that enzyme. The latter may be affected by the concentration of the substrate or product of the reaction, by isosteric inhibition where the catalytic site of the enzyme is blocked, or by allosteric inhibition where the catalytic site is free but where the activity of the enzyme is influenced by binding to another site on the enzyme molecule. A resultant decrease in enzyme activity is known as *enzyme inhibition* whilst a stimulation of enzyme activity is known as *enzyme induction*. Induction occurs in many species and is generally produced by compounds which are slowly excreted and lipid soluble. TABLE 4 lists some of the drugs whose metabolism is increased in man with its corresponding enzyme inducer. It should be noted that in some instances a drug acts as its own enzyme inducer.

TABLE 4. Examples of Enzyme Induction in Man

Drug affected	*Enzyme inducer*
amidopyrine	phenylbutazone
coumarin anticoagulants	phenobarbitone and other barbiturates
digitoxin	phenobarbitone and other barbiturates
glutethimide	glutethimide
hydrocortisone	phenobarbitone and other barbiturates, phenylbutazone, phenytoin, dicophane
meprobamate	meprobamate
oral contraceptives	rifampicin
phenytoin	phenobarbitone and other barbiturates
testosterone	phenobarbitone and other barbiturates
tolbutamide	alcohol
warfarin	glutethimide

Inhibition of both microsomal and non-microsomal enzymes has been shown in man. Examples of non-microsomal inhibition occur with the monoamine-oxidase inhibitors which increase patient sensitivity to some sympathomimetic amines. An example of microsomal inhibition is the inhibition of tolbutamide metabolism by

dicoumarol, phenylbutazone, phenyramidol, or sulphaphenazole. As a result of this inhibition the plasma elimination half-life of tolbutamide may be increased as much as 5 times.

Metabolism Statements in Drug Monographs

Statements relating to the absorption, distribution, and excretion of individual drugs are given, wherever possible, in the drug monographs under the heading **Metabolism**. The information has been abstracted from published material, and where figures are given for drug concentrations in blood or other body fluids it should be noted that the figures are ranges or approximations deduced from reports of clinical trials or other research projects. The numerous factors which may affect the absorption, distribution, and excretion of drugs, as well as unavoidable analytical inaccuracies, may cause considerable variations in drug concentrations found in individual cases.

In some monographs the information is incomplete, the amount of detail being dependent upon that available in the literature searched, and it should not be assumed that the statements presented reflect the only significant factors in the metabolism of the drug concerned.

Metaraminol Tartrate

$(-)$-1-Hydroxy-1-(3-hydroxyphenyl)prop-2-ylammonium hydrogen tartrate

$C_{13}H_9NO_8 = 317.3$

OTHER NAME: *Aramine®*

A standard is given in the British Pharmacopoeia 1973

Description. An almost odourless, white, crystalline powder.

Solubility. Soluble, at 20°, in 3 parts of water and in 100 parts of alcohol; very slightly soluble in ether and in chloroform.

Acidity. A 5% solution has a pH of 3.2 to 3.5.

Sterilisation. Solutions are sterilised by filtration.

Storage. It should be stored in airtight containers.

Identification. TESTS. 1. To 0.5 ml of a 0.05% solution add 0.5 ml of *lithium and sodium molybdophosphotungstate solution* and 5 ml of *sodium carbonate solution* and allow to stand for 5 minutes; an intense blue colour is produced.

2. Dissolve about 50 mg in 2 ml of water and add 1 ml of acetic acid, 1 drop of *ferrous sulphate solution*, 3 drops of *hydrogen peroxide solution*, and an excess of *sodium hydroxide solution*; a deep red colour is produced.

3. To 4 ml of a 0.05% solution add 5 ml of *solution of standard pH 9.6* and 1 ml of a freshly prepared 0.5% solution of sodium 1,2-naphthaquinone-4-sulphonate, allow to stand for 1 minute, add 4 drops of a 2% solution of *benzalkonium chloride solution* and 5 ml of toluene and shake; the toluene layer becomes mauve (distinction from phenylephrine).

MELTING-POINT. About 176°.

ULTRAVIOLET ABSORPTION. In water, maximum at 272 nm (E1%, 1cm = 60).

Actions and uses. Metaraminol is a sympathomimetic amine with actions similar to those of noradrenaline but it is resistant to the action of monoamine oxidases. It is used as a long-acting vasopressor agent which is given by injection to raise the blood pressure in hypotensive emergencies. Its duration of action varies from 20 to 90 minutes according to the route of administration. When given by subcutaneous or intramuscular injection in a dosage equivalent to 2 to 10 milligrams of metaraminol, a pressor effect is exerted in 5 to 12 minutes, and the peak effect is observed in about 30 minutes. When metaraminol tartrate is given by intravenous injection in a dosage equivalent to 0.5 to 5 milligrams of metaraminol, a pressor effect begins after 1 to 2 minutes, and the peak occurs in about 5 minutes.

Metaraminol may be given by intravenous infusion for the continuous maintenance of blood pressure. For this purpose the equivalent of up to 100 milligrams of metaraminol is dissolved in not less than 500 millilitres of sodium chloride injection or dextrose injection (5%). 1.9 milligrams of metaraminol tartrate is approximately equivalent to 1 milligram of metaraminol.

Precautions. As for Noradrenaline Acid Tartrate.

Preparation

METARAMINOL INJECTION: a sterile solution of metaraminol tartrate, with a suitable stabilising agent, in water for injections. It is sterilised by filtration. Available in 1-ml ampoules and 10-ml vials containing metaraminol tartrate equivalent to 10 mg of metaraminol per ml.

A standard for this injection is given in the British Pharmacopoeia 1973

Containers: see the entry on Injections for general information on containers.

Labelling: see the entry on Injections for general information on labelling. In addition, the label on the container should state the amount of the medicament as the equivalent amount of metaraminol.

Storage: it should be protected from light.

Metformin Hydrochloride

1,1-Dimethylbiguanide hydrochloride

$$\left[\begin{array}{c} \overset{NH}{\underset{\|}{}} \quad \overset{NH}{\underset{\|}{}} \\ (CH_3)_2N \cdot C \cdot NH \cdot C \cdot NH_2 \end{array} \right] HCl$$

$C_4H_{12}ClN_5 = 165.6$

OTHER NAME: *Glucophage*®

A standard is given in the British Pharmacopoeia 1973

Description. An odourless, hygroscopic, white, crystalline powder with a bitter taste.

Solubility. Soluble, at 20°, in 2 parts of water and in 100 parts of alcohol; practically insoluble in ether and in chloroform.

Dissociation constants. pK_a 2.8, 11.5 (32°).

Storage. It should be stored in airtight containers.

Identification. TESTS. 1. Dissolve about 25 mg in 5 ml of water, add 1.5 ml of *sodium hydroxide solution*, 1 ml of *1-naphthol solution* and, dropwise with shaking, 0.5 ml of *dilute sodium hypochlorite solution*; an orange-red colour is produced which darkens on standing.

2. Dissolve about 10 mg in 10 ml of water and add 10 ml of a solution prepared by mixing equal volumes of a 10% solution of sodium nitroprusside, a 10% solution of potassium ferricyanide, and a 10% solution of sodium hydroxide, and allow to stand; a wine-red colour develops in about 3 minutes.

MELTING-POINT. About 225°.

Determination in body fluids. HIGH PRESSURE LIQUID CHROMATOGRAPHY. In urine—M. S. F. Ross, *J. Chromat.*, 1977, **133**, 408.

Metabolism. ABSORPTION. Well absorbed after oral administration.

BLOOD CONCENTRATION. After an oral dose of up to 1 g, plasma concentrations of up to about 8 μg/ml may be attained.

HALF-LIFE. Half-life determined from urinary excretion data, about 3 hours.

DISTRIBUTION. *Protein binding*, about 10% bound to plasma proteins.

EXCRETION. Up to about 70% of an oral dose is excreted in the urine in 24 to 36 hours; very little appears in the faeces.

FURTHER INFORMATION. Excretion in urine—G. Debry and F.-P. Cherrier, *Thérapie*, 1965, **20**, 351; J. Sterne, Pharmacology and mode of action of the hypoglycaemic guanidine derivatives, *Medicinal Chemistry*, Vol. 9, Oral Hypoglycaemic Agents, G. D. Campbell (Ed.), London, Academic Press, 1969, p. 193.

Actions and uses. Metformin is an oral hypoglycaemic agent with actions and uses similar to those of phenformin.

The initial dose is 500 milligrams 2 or 3 times a day with meals, gradually increased if necessary to 3 grams daily over a period of 10 to 14 days. Once control of the blood glucose has been achieved, it may be possible to reduce the dose without loss of control. The usual maintenance dosage is 1.0 to 1.5 grams daily, although more may be required.

Metformin may be given in conjunction with a sulphonylurea.

If the patient is already receiving insulin, the dosage of insulin should be given in full for 2 days and then gradually reduced while the dosage of metformin is increased.

Metformin alone is unsuitable for the treatment of young diabetics.

Undesirable effects. Anorexia, nausea, and vomiting may occur and are usually dose-related. Urticarial reactions, weakness, and loss of weight occur rarely. Lactic acidosis is less common than with phenformin.

Precautions and contra-indications. Metformin should not be given to patients in diabetic coma or with severe acidosis or infection or after operations or trauma. It should be given with caution to patients with hepatic and renal disease and it should not be used during pregnancy.

Poisoning. The procedure for the treatment of hypoglycaemia as described under Phenformin Hydrochloride should be followed.

Preparation

METFORMIN TABLETS: available as tablets containing 500 and 850 mg of metformin hydrochloride; they may be film coated.

A standard for these tablets is given in the British Pharmacopoeia 1973

Containers and *Storage:* see the entry on Tablets for general information on containers and storage. Containers should be airtight.

Advice for patients: the tablets should be taken at regular intervals preferably after meals. Treatment should not be discontinued without the advice of the prescriber. Intolerance to alcohol may occur.

Methacholine Chloride

2-Acetoxypropyltrimethylammonium chloride

$$\left[CH_3 \cdot CO \cdot O \cdot \overset{CH_3}{\underset{}{CH}} \cdot CH_2 \cdot \overset{+}{N}(CH_3)_3 \right] Cl^-$$

$C_8H_{18}ClNO_2 = 195.7$

A standard is given in the British Pharmaceutical Codex 1973

Description. Odourless, deliquescent, colourless or white crystals or white crystalline powder.

Solubility. Soluble, at 20°, in less than 1 part of water and in 1.2 parts of alcohol; soluble in chloroform.

Acidity. A 2% solution has a pH of 4.5 to 5.5.

Moisture content. Not more than 1.5%, determined by drying at 105°.

Sterilisation. Solutions for injection are sterilised by filtration.

Storage. It should be stored in airtight containers.

Identification. TESTS. 1. To 1 ml of a 10% solution add 1 ml of alcohol (95%) and 1 ml of sulphuric acid; the odour of ethyl acetate is produced.
2. To 5 ml of a 10% solution add 2 g of potassium hydroxide and heat gently; the odour of trimethylamine is produced.
3. To 1 ml of a 10% solution add a slight excess of a 10% solution of gold chloride; a precipitate is produced which, after recrystallising from hot water and drying at 105°, melts at about 127°.

MELTING-POINT. About 171°.

Actions and uses. Methacholine chloride has the muscarinic actions of acetylcholine, but is more stable and so provides a more sustained stimulus to cholinergic nerves. It slows the heart, increases peristalsis, dilates peripheral blood vessels, and increases salivary, sweat, and bronchial secretions.

Methacholine chloride has been used to terminate attacks of atrial paroxysmal tachycardia when simpler methods have failed. It has also been used in the treatment of post-operative abdominal distension and retention of urine. The usual dose is 20 milligrams given by subcutaneous injection; this may be repeated in half an hour.

Eye-drops containing 2.5% of methacholine chloride are used for the diagnosis of Adie's pupil; the affected pupil contracts within 15 to 30 minutes of the instillation of the drops whereas the normal pupil does not respond. The eye-drops should be freshly prepared.

Undesirable effects. When given by injection, methacholine chloride may cause a terrifying sensation of choking; this may be stopped immediately by giving 600 micrograms of atropine sulphate by intravenous injection.

Contra-indications. Methacholine chloride is contra-indicated in patients suffering from allergic conditions, especially asthma, as it may cause bronchial spasm and excessive bronchial secretion.

Methadone Hydrochloride

(±)-*NN*-Dimethyl-*N*-(5-oxo-4,4-diphenylheptan-2-yl)-ammonium chloride

$$\left[(CH_3)_2\overset{+}{N}H \cdot \overset{CH_3}{\underset{}{CH}} \cdot CH_2 \cdot \overset{C_6H_5}{\underset{C_6H_5}{C}} \cdot CO \cdot C_2H_5 \right] Cl^-$$

$C_{21}H_{28}ClNO = 345.9$

OTHER NAMES: Amidone Hydrochloride; Methadoni Hydrochloridum; *Physeptone®*

A standard is given in the European Pharmacopoeia Vol. III

Description. Odourless colourless crystals or white crystalline powder with a bitter taste.

Solubility. Soluble, at 20°, in 12 parts of water and in 7 parts of alcohol; soluble in chloroform; practically insoluble in ether.

Acidity. A 1% solution has a pH of 4.5 to 6.5.

Dissociation constant. pK_a 8.3 (20°).

Incompatibility. It is incompatible with some dyes.

Sterilisation. Solutions for injection are sterilised by heating in an autoclave or by filtration. Chlorocresol should not be included as a bactericide.

Identification. TESTS. 1. To 4 drops of a 5% solution add 2 drops of formaldehyde and 2 ml of sulphuric acid; a red colour is produced. Examine the solution under ultraviolet radiation at 365 nm; the solution exhibits a red fluorescence.
2. Add *sodium hydroxide solution* to a 5% solution of the sample, stir, and filter; the residue, after washing with water and drying, melts at about 76°.

MELTING-POINT. About 234°.

ULTRAVIOLET ABSORPTION. In 0.1N sulphuric acid, weak maxima at 253 nm, 259 nm, 265 nm, and 292 nm.

INFRA-RED ABSORPTION. Major peaks at 709, 769, 943, 1111, 1136, and 1695 cm^{-1} (see Appendix 2b: Infra-red Spectra).

THIN-LAYER CHROMATOGRAPHY. See under Thin-layer Chromatography, System 7.

Determination in body fluids. ULTRAVIOLET SPECTRO-PHOTOMETRY. In urine—H. E. Hamilton *et al., J. pharm. Sci.,* 1974, **63**, 741.

THIN-LAYER CHROMATOGRAPHY. In urine: separation of methadone and its primary metabolite in the presence of other drugs—N. C. Jain *et al., J. Chromat.,* 1975, **103**, 85.

GAS CHROMATOGRAPHY. In plasma or urine: methadone and metabolites—C. E. Inturrisi and K. Verebely, *J. Chromat.,* 1972, **65**, 361. In blood, saliva, or urine—R. K. Lynn *et al., J. Chromat.,* 1977, **131**, 329.

Metabolism. ABSORPTION. Rapidly absorbed after oral administration.

BLOOD CONCENTRATION. During therapy with oral maintenance doses of 100 to 120 mg daily, peak plasma concentrations of unchanged drug of about 900 ng/ml are attained 4 hours after dosing and fall to a pre-dose level of about 500 ng/ml; after an intramuscular dose of 10 mg, peak plasma concentrations of about 75 ng/ml are attained in about 1 hour.

HALF-LIFE. Plasma half-life, 15 to 25 hours, which may be increased in methadone-tolerant subjects and decreased in subjects whose urine is acid; after an intramuscular dose, the plasma half-life is about 7 hours.

DISTRIBUTION. Widely distributed and rapidly taken up by the tissues; post-mortem studies show that more drug is concentrated in the liver, lungs, and kidneys than in the blood; methadone is secreted in sweat; in rats, methadone and its metabolites persist in the brain; *protein binding,* 60 to 85% bound to plasma proteins —mostly to albumin but about 15% to immunoglobulin.

METABOLIC REACTIONS. Mainly oxidative *N*-demethylation to form a metabolite which spontaneously cyclises to 2-ethylidene-1,5-dimethyl-3,3-diphenylpyrrolidine; this metabolite may be hydroxylated or demethylated to form 2-ethylidene-1,5-dimethyl-3-*p*-hydroxyphenyl-3-phenylpyrrolidine and 2-ethyl-5-methyl-3-*p*-hydroxyphenyl-3-phenyl-1-pyrroline; other reactions include ketone oxidation and oxidative removal of the ethyl group to form 4-dimethylamino-2,2-diphenylvaleric acid, and side-chain reduction, in which the ketone is reduced to a hydroxyl group, to form methadol which may be demethylated; in rats, methadol may be dealkylated to form the primary amine which may then be acetylated; the reduction process appears to be stereospecific and only the (−) form is produced; glucuronic acid conjugation of methadone metabolites and the formation of *p*-hydroxymethadone occur in rats and the *N*-oxide has been detected in the urine of man; *N*-oxide formation appears to be a spontaneous process which occurs in the urine; the *N*-oxide is not therefore a true metabolite; the *S*-(+)-form of methadone appears to be more extensively metabolised than the *R*-(−)-form; in rats, phenobarbitone appears to induce methadone metabolism.

EXCRETION. Small doses appear to be excreted mainly in the faeces but urinary excretion appears to be the main route for doses over 55 mg; in 96 hours, 17 to 60% of a dose is excreted in the urine as methadone and its metabolites; the percentage of unchanged drug excreted increases with increasing dosage and with decreasing urinary pH values; up to a three-fold increase in excretion may result from acidification of the urine; about 70% of the total dose excreted in urine and faeces is unconjugated; methadone appears to be excreted in high concentrations into the gastric juice.

FURTHER INFORMATION. Excretion in gastric juice—R. K. Lynn *et al., Drug Met. Disp.*, 1976, **4**, 504; excretion in urine—R. C. Baselt and L. J. Casarett, *Clin. Pharmac. Ther.*, 1972, **13**, 64; excretion and metabolism—E. Änggård *et al., Clin. Pharmac. Ther.*, 1975, **17**, 258 and A. H. Beckett *et al., J. Pharm. Pharmac.*, 1968, **20**, 754; *N*-oxide formation in urine—A. H. Beckett *et al., J. Pharm. Pharmac.*, 1972, **24**, 244 and H. R. Sullivan *et al., J. Pharm. Pharmac.*, 1973, **25**, 1009; plasma concentrations in methadone maintenance therapy—W. H. Horns *et al., Clin. Pharmac. Ther.*, 1975, **17**, 636 and C. E. Inturrisi and K. Verebely, *Clin. Pharmac. Ther.*, 1972, **13**, 633.

Actions and uses. Methadone has actions and uses similar to those described under Morphine Hydrochloride.

It is a potent analgesic; the effect begins about 15 minutes after subcutaneous injection and about 45 minutes after oral administration and lasts from 2 to 4 hours.

Its sedative action is much less marked than that of morphine and it is therefore not used as a pre-anaesthetic agent.

Methadone depresses the cough centre. It also depresses the respiratory centre and is therefore undesirable as an obstetric analgesic. Its action on the gastro-intestinal tract is weaker than that of morphine and constipation seldom occurs.

Methadone is used extensively for the relief of pain where sedation is not necessary. For moderately severe pain, 5 to 10 milligrams of methadone hydrochloride by mouth every 4 hours is usually adequate; for a rapid effect it may be given by subcutaneous or intramuscular injection.

To suppress useless coughing, 1 to 2 milligrams of methadone hydrochloride is usually given by mouth in the form of a linctus. The corresponding dose for children is 250 to 500 micrograms, repeated if necessary at intervals of 4 hours.

Morphine addicts may be given methadone orally as substitution therapy; a suitable mixture contains 1 milligram of methadone hydrochloride per millilitre in a vehicle consisting of syrup 250, green S and tartrazine solution 1, tartrazine compound solution 4, and chloroform water double-strength to 500 parts by volume. Methadone effectively controls the symptoms of morphine withdrawal and dependence on methadone is easier to treat than dependence on morphine.

Undesirable effects. Nausea, vomiting, dizziness, faintness, and constriction of the pupil may occur. As with morphine, many of these effects occur more often in ambulant than in recumbent patients.

Dependence. When administered in therapeutic doses for prolonged periods, methadone may lead to the development of dependence of the morphine type, as described under Drug Dependence.

Poisoning. The procedure described under Morphine Hydrochloride should be adopted.

Preparations

METHADONE INJECTION: a sterile solution of methadone hydrochloride in water for injections. It is distributed into ampoules, the ampoules are sealed and it is sterilised by heating in an autoclave. Alternatively, the solution is sterilised by filtration; it is distributed, by means of an aseptic technique, into sterile ampoules, and the ampoules are sealed. Available in 1-ml ampoules containing 10 mg of methadone hydrochloride.

A standard for this injection is given in the British Pharmacopoeia 1973

Containers and *Labelling:* see the entry on Injections for general information on containers and labelling.

METHADONE LINCTUS (*Syn.* Amidone Linctus):

Methadone hydrochloride	..	..	..	0.4 g
Compound tartrazine solution	..	..	..	8 ml
Water for preparations	..	..	..	120 ml
Glycerol	..	..	..	..	250 ml
Tolu syrup	..	..	..	..	to 1000 ml

Dissolve the methadone hydrochloride in the water, add the compound tartrazine solution, the glycerol, and sufficient tolu syrup to produce the required volume, and mix.

When a dose less than or not a multiple of 5 ml is prescribed, the linctus may be diluted, as described in the entry on Linctuses, with syrup.

It contains, in 5 ml, 2 mg of methadone hydrochloride.

A standard for this linctus is given in the British Pharmaceutical Codex 1973

METHADONE TABLETS: available as tablets containing 5 mg of methadone hydrochloride.

A standard for these tablets is given in the British Pharmacopoeia 1973

Containers and *Storage:* see the entry on Tablets for general information on containers and storage. Containers should be airtight.

Methallenoestril

3-(6-Methoxynaphth-2-yl)-2,2-dimethylpentanoic acid

$C_{18}H_{22}O_3 = 286.4$

OTHER NAME: *Vallestril®*

A standard is given in the British Pharmaceutical Codex 1973

Description. An odourless white crystalline powder.

Solubility. Very slightly soluble in water; soluble, at 20°, in 10 parts of alcohol, in 8 parts of ether, and in 2 parts of chloroform; soluble in solutions of alkali hydroxides.

Identification. MELTING-POINT. About 138°.

ULTRAVIOLET ABSORPTION. In methyl alcohol, maxima at 232 nm (E1%, 1cm = 3050), 253 nm (E1%, 1cm = 148), 264 nm (E1%, 1cm = 180), 273 nm (E1%, 1cm = 180), 317 nm (E1%, 1cm = 52), and 332 nm (E1%, 1cm = 68).

INFRA-RED ABSORPTION. Major peaks at 857, 1149, 1232, 1270, 1606, and 1689 cm^{-1} (see Appendix 2a: Infra-red Spectra).

THIN-LAYER CHROMATOGRAPHY. See under Thin-layer Chromatography, System 10.

Actions and uses. Methallenoestril is a synthetic oestrogenic hormone which has actions and uses similar to those described under Oestradiol Benzoate.

For replacement therapy, it is generally given by mouth in a dosage of 3 milligrams 2 or 3 times a day for 2 to 3 weeks. In post-menopausal osteoporosis, this may be followed by a maintenance dosage of 3 milligrams daily. For the suppression of lactation, 12 milligrams may be given 3 times a day for 5 days.

It may also be useful, when stilboestrol therapy is badly tolerated, for the symptomatic treatment of prostatic carcinoma, for which it may be given in a dosage of 3 to 6 milligrams 3 times a day.

Undesirable effects. These are as described under Oestradiol Benzoate. Methallenoestril seldom causes nausea, except when given in large doses, and gives rise to less withdrawal bleeding and gynaecomastia than oestradiol.

Preparation

METHALLENOESTRIL TABLETS: may be prepared by moist granulation and compression as described in the entry on Tablets. Available as tablets containing 3 mg of methallenoestril.

A standard for these tablets is given in the British Pharmaceutical Codex 1973

Containers and *Storage:* see the entry on Tablets for general information on containers and storage. Containers should be airtight.

Advice for patients: the prescribed course should be completed or, where applicable, treatment should not be discontinued without the advice of the prescriber.

Methandienone

17β-Hydroxy-17α-methylandrosta-1,4-dien-3-one

$C_{20}H_{28}O_2 = 300.4$

OTHER NAMES: *Dianabol®*; Methandrostenolone; *Vetanabol®*

A standard is given in the British Pharmacopoeia 1973

Description. An odourless, white or faintly yellowish-white, crystalline powder.

Solubility. Practically insoluble in water; soluble in alcohol, in chloroform, and in glacial acetic acid; very slightly soluble in ether.

Specific rotation. +7° to +11°, determined on a 1% solution in alcohol (95%).

Storage. It should be protected from light.

Identification. TESTS. 1. Dissolve about 10 mg in nitrobenzene, add 500 mg of anhydrous aluminium chloride, and shake for several minutes; a red colour is produced.
2. Dissolve about 50 mg in 9 ml of methyl alcohol, add 1 ml of *dinitrophenylhydrazine solution*, and induce crystallisation; a precipitate is produced which, after washing with water, melts at about 213°.

MELTING-POINT. About 165°.

ULTRAVIOLET ABSORPTION. In dehydrated alcohol, maximum at 245 nm (E1%, 1cm = 516).

INFRA-RED ABSORPTION. Major peaks at 886, 1160, 1374, 1601, 1620, and 1660 cm^{-1} (see Appendix 2a: Infra-red Spectra).

THIN-LAYER CHROMATOGRAPHY. See under Thin-layer Chromatography, System 10.

Actions and uses. Methandienone has actions and uses similar to those described under Testosterone; its anabolic properties are more pronounced than its androgenic effects. It causes nitrogen and calcium retention and promotes protein synthesis, leading to an increase in skeletal weight and growth in bone. It has little progestational action.

Methandienone is used as an anabolic agent in the treatment of osteoporosis, though there is little evidence of its effectiveness. It is also given during post-operative recovery and during convalescence after chronic debilitating disease. It may be used in the palliative treatment of inoperable mammary carcinoma, especially where bone metastases have developed.

When combined with a high-calorie low-protein diet and with or without peritoneal dialysis or haemodialysis, methandienone may be of value in the treatment of acute renal failure by reducing the speed at which the blood urea rises. In patients on chronic dialysis, methandienone may be helpful in preventing anaemia, although testosterone is more often used for this purpose in men.

Methandienone is also used to prevent extensive nitrogen loss after severe burns.

The initial dosage is 15 to 20 milligrams daily by mouth and this is reduced to 2.5 to 10 milligrams daily for maintenance. For long-term treatment, intermittent therapy is usually adequate, courses of 4 to 6 weeks' duration being given with intervals of 2 to 4 weeks. A child usually requires 40 micrograms per kilogram body-weight daily; courses should be limited to 4 weeks and followed by an interval of 1 to 2 months before further treatment is given.

Undesirable effects. When given for prolonged periods, méthandienone may give rise to androgenic effects and there may be some water retention and hypercalcaemia. Jaundice may develop occasionally.

Benign and malignant liver tumours have been reported following the use of methandienone.

Contra-indications. Methandienone is contra-indicated in patients with prostatic carcinoma or hepatic dysfunction or during pregnancy.

Drug interactions. Methandienone may enhance the anticoagulant effect of warfarin and similar anti-coagulants.

Veterinary uses. Methandienone is an anabolic steroid used in the treatment of convalescent or debilitated animals. The usual dose by mouth for dogs is 500 micrograms per kilogram body-weight at intervals of 2 to 14 days according to the response of the animal.

Preparation

METHANDIENONE TABLETS: available as tablets containing 5 mg of methandienone.

A standard for these tablets is given in the British Pharmacopoeia 1973

Containers and *Storage:* see the entry on Tablets for general information on containers and storage. Containers should be airtight and light resistant.

Methaqualone

2-Methyl-3-*o*-tolylquinazolin-4(3*H*)-one

$C_{16}H_{14}N_2O = 250.3$

OTHER NAMES: *Revonal®*
Mandrax® (with diphenhydramine hydrochloride)

A standard is given in the British Pharmacopoeia 1973

Description. An odourless white crystalline powder with a bitter taste.

Solubility. Practically insoluble in water; soluble, at 20°, in 12 parts of alcohol, in 50 parts of ether, and in 1 part of chloroform.

Storage. It should be stored in airtight containers, protected from light.

Identification. TEST. Dissolve about 10 mg in 2 ml of alcohol (95%), add 1 ml of *alcoholic dimethylamino-benzaldehyde solution*, and heat on a water-bath for 5 minutes; a reddish-orange colour is produced.

MELTING-POINT. About 115°.

ULTRAVIOLET ABSORPTION. In 0.1N hydrochloric acid, maxima at 234 nm (E1%, 1cm = 1300) and 269 nm (E1%, 1cm = 320).

INFRA-RED ABSORPTION. Major peaks at 770, 1335, 1465, 1565, 1600, and 1680 cm^{-1} (see Appendix 2c: Infra-red Spectra).

Determination in body fluids. COLORIMETRY. In blood —J. N. Pirl *et al.*, *Analyt. Chem.*, 1972, **44**, 1675.

ULTRAVIOLET SPECTROPHOTOMETRY. In serum—D. N. Bailey and P. I. Jatlow, *Clin. Chem.*, 1973, **19**, 615.

SPECTROFLUORIMETRY. In plasma: barbiturates, mepro-bamate, methyprylone, paracetamol, and salicylates are stated not to interfere—S. S. Brown and G. A. Smart, *J. Pharm. Pharmac.*, 1969, **21**, 466.

GAS CHROMATOGRAPHY. In plasma—A. Noirfalaise, *J. Chromat.*, 1974, **90**, 394. In urine: methaqualone and various hydroxylated metabolites—R. C. Permisohn *et al.*, *J. forens. Sci.*, 1976, **21**, 98.

Metabolism. ABSORPTION. Readily absorbed following oral administration; the hydrochloride salt is more rapidly absorbed than the base and the extent of absorption may vary according to the formulation used.

BLOOD CONCENTRATION. Peak plasma concentrations of 2 to 5 μg/ml are attained within 2 to 3 hours after an oral dose of 300 to 500 mg.

HALF-LIFE. Plasma elimination half-life is 2 to 3 hours.

DISTRIBUTION. Methaqualone is widely distributed and is taken up by the liver, body fat, and brain; about 20% is absorbed by the red cells and it has a large volume of distribution; *protein binding*, about 70% bound to plasma albumin.

METABOLIC REACTIONS. Non-specific hydroxylation, mainly of the tolyl substituent, followed by sulphation, methylation, or glucuronic acid conjugation; *N*-oxidation and ring fission may also occur.

EXCRETION. Slowly excreted in the urine and bile; about 2% of a dose is excreted in the urine unchanged.

ENZYME INDUCTION. Methaqualone stimulates the drug metabolising enzymes of the liver in the rat.

FURTHER INFORMATION. Pharmacokinetics—R. K. Nayak *et al.*, *J. Pharmacokinet. Biopharm.*, 1974, **2**, 107.

Actions and uses. Methaqualone has a hypnotic action resembling that of an intermediate-acting barbiturate, the actions and uses of which are described under Barbiturates.

Sleep lasting 6 to 8 hours is produced within about 15 minutes by an oral dose of 150 to 300 milligrams. The onset of sleep is rapid and may occur abruptly, particularly when methaqualone is given in conjunction with an antihistamine such as diphenhydramine.

Methaqualone has been used as a sedative in doses of 75 milligrams 2 or 3 times a day.

Undesirable effects. When sleep is delayed, a transient paraesthesia of the limbs and face may occur, but this does not appear to be associated with peripheral neuropathy. Headache, drowsiness, dizziness, and skin rashes may occur.

Methaqualone may reduce the ability of patients to drive or work with moving machinery.

Precautions and contra-indications. Methaqualone should not be given to patients with hepatic dysfunction, eclampsia, or epilepsy. It may potentiate the action of neuroleptics, tranquillisers, barbiturates, and alcohol.

Particular care is necessary when methaqualone is prescribed in conjunction with an antihistamine as both stupor and convulsions may occur within the dose-range of both drugs.

Dependence. Methaqualone may give rise to dependence of the barbiturate-alcohol type, as described under Drug Dependence, particularly when it is given in conjunction with an antihistamine.

Poisoning. Methaqualone overdosage, unlike that with barbiturates, may be associated with hypertonia and convulsions. Severe renal damage is uncommon but acute pulmonary oedema may occur. Treatment consists of the usual supportive measures. Haemodialysis and forced diuresis are ineffective.

Preparations

Preparations available include CAPSULES containing methaqualone 250 mg with diphenhydramine hydrochloride 25 mg; TABLETS containing methaqualone 200 mg, and tablets containing methaqualone 250 mg with diphenhydramine hydrochloride 25 mg.

Methicillin Sodium

Sodium (6R)-6-(2,6-dimethoxybenzamido)penicillanate monohydrate

$C_{17}H_{19}N_2NaO_6S,H_2O = 420.4$

OTHER NAME: *Celbenin®*

A standard is given in the British Pharmacopoeia 1973

Description. A white microcrystalline powder.

Solubility. Soluble, at 20°, in 0.6 part of water and in 35 parts of alcohol; practically insoluble in fixed oils and in liquid paraffin.

Acidity or alkalinity. A 10% solution has a pH of 5.5 to 7.5.

Moisture content. Not more than 4.8%, determined by Fischer titration.

Specific rotation. +235° to +245°, determined on a 5% solution in water.

Dissociation constant. pK_a 2.8 (20°).

Stability. In aqueous solution methicillin sodium degrades by hydrolysis. Degradation is catalysed by hydrogen ions and by hydroxide ions. Solutions are most stable at about pH 6.8. Degradation is also catalysed by monohydrogen phosphate ions but not by citrate ions or dihydrogen phosphate ions. At 5°, unbuffered solutions (50%) may be expected to lose 20% of their potency after 7 days; at 23°, 20% of their potency is lost after 2 days. Intravenous infusions in sodium chloride injection or dextrose injection (5%) should be infused within 4 hours of preparation.

FURTHER INFORMATION. Stability in aqueous solution —M. A. Schwartz *et al.*, *J. pharm. Sci.*, 1965, **54**, 149. Stability in intravenous infusions—J. Jacobs *et al.*, *J. clin Path.*, 1973, **26**, 742; B. Lynn, *J. hosp. Pharm.*, 1970, **28**, 71 and 1972, **30**, 81.

Hygroscopicity. It absorbs insignificant amounts of moisture at 25° at relative humidities up to about 65%, but under damper conditions it absorbs significant amounts.

Labelling. If the material is not intended for parenteral administration, the label on the container states that the contents are not to be injected.

Storage. It should be stored in airtight containers at a temperature not exceeding 25°. If it is intended for parenteral administration, the containers should be sterile and sealed to exclude micro-organisms.

Identification. TEST. Mix 2 mg with 2 mg of chromotropic acid sodium salt and 2 ml of sulphuric acid, and immerse in a suitable liquid at 150° for 4 minutes; the colour of the solution changes through greenish-yellow to yellowish-brown and finally chars (distinction from certain other penicillins).

ULTRAVIOLET ABSORPTION. In water, maximum at 280 nm (E1%, 1cm = 55); in 0.1N sodium hydroxide, maximum at 280 nm (E1%, 1cm = 53).

INFRA-RED ABSORPTION. Major peaks at 1093, 1327, 1500, 1607, 1673, and 1766 cm^{-1} (see Appendix 2a: Infra-red Spectra).

Metabolism. ABSORPTION. Inactivated by acid hydrolysis in the stomach after oral administration and therefore administered parenterally.

BLOOD CONCENTRATIONS. After an intramuscular dose of 1 g, serum concentrations of about 20 μg/ml are attained in 30 minutes falling to about 2 μg/ml after 4 hours; after an intravenous dose of 1 g, serum concentrations of about 40 μg/ml are attained within 15 minutes falling to 10 μg/ml after 30 minutes, and to 3 to 4 μg/ml after 2 hours.

HALF-LIFE. Serum half-life, 0.5 to 1 hour in adults, 1 to 3 hours in infants, and about 4 hours in subjects with renal function impairment.

DISTRIBUTION. Widely distributed throughout the body and enters the pericardial and synovial fluids and, when the meninges are inflamed, the cerebrospinal fluid; crosses the placenta; volume of distribution, about 40 litres.

EXCRETION. 60 to 70% is excreted in the urine and about 20% in the bile in about 6 hours after a single oral dose of 1 g; the excretion of methicillin is delayed by probenecid.

FURTHER INFORMATION. Pharmacokinetics in animals —P. Acred *et al.*, *Br. J. Pharmac. Chemother.*, 1961, **17**, 70; pharmacokinetics in renal failure—R. J. Bulger *et al.*, *J. Am. med. Ass.*, 1964, **187**, 319 and M. Gibaldi and D. Perrier, *J. clin. Pharmac.*, 1972, **12**, 201.

Actions and uses. Methicillin is a semi-synthetic penicillin which is not decomposed by staphylococcal penicillinase but which has a reduced antibiotic potency compared with benzylpenicillin. It is not well absorbed when taken by mouth and should be given by injection. Its only use is in the treatment of severe penicillinase-producing staphylococcal infections, when it should be given in a dose of 1 gram every 4 to 6 hours by intramuscular injection. In serious infections the dose can be increased to 2 grams every 4 hours.

The dose for children up to one year is 250 milligrams, 1 to 5 years 500 milligrams, and 6 to 12 years 1 gram; these doses should be repeated every 6 hours. Resistance of staphylococci to methicillin is increasing.

Precautions. The same precautions against allergy

should be taken as for benzylpenicillin. It should not be used topically or in the treatment of non-penicillinase-producing staphylococcal infections. Methicillin should not be mixed with other antibiotics.

Preparation

METHICILLIN INJECTION: a sterile solution of methicillin sodium in water for injections. It is prepared by dissolving the contents of a sealed container in water for injections shortly before use. Available as a powder in vials containing 1 g of methicillin sodium.
A standard for this injection is given in the British Pharmacopoeia 1973
Containers and *Labelling:* see the entry on Injections for general information on containers and labelling.
Storage: the sealed container should be stored at a temperature not exceeding 25°. The injection contains no bactericide and should be used as soon as possible after preparation, but solutions of methicillin sodium may be expected to retain their potency for up to 48 hours after preparation, provided they are stored at 2° to 10°.

Methisazone

1-Methylindoline-2,3-dione 3-thiosemicarbazone

$C_{10}H_{10}N_4OS = 234.3$

OTHER NAME: *Marboran®*

A standard is given in the British Pharmacopoeia Addendum 1975

Description. An orange-yellow powder.

Solubility. Practically insoluble in water; soluble, at 20°, in 2000 parts of methyl alcohol, and in 800 parts of chloroform; soluble in warm dilute solutions of alkali hydroxides and in hot glacial acetic acid.

Moisture content. Not more than 1%, determined by drying at 105° *in vacuo*.

Storage. It should be protected from light.

Identification. MELTING-POINT. About 250°, with decomposition.

INFRA-RED ABSORPTION. Major peaks at 1097, 1340, 1468, 1492, 1605, and 1673 cm^{-1} (see Appendix 2c: Infra-red Spectra).

ULTRAVIOLET ABSORPTION. In alcohol (95%), maxima at 241 nm (E1%, 1cm = 571), 274 nm (E1%, 1cm = 588), and 358 nm (E1%, 1cm = 929).

Determination in body fluids. ULTRAVIOLET SPECTRO-PHOTOMETRY. In serum—C. H. Kempe *et al.*, *Lancet*, i/1965, 824.

Metabolism. ABSORPTION. Absorbed after oral administration.

BLOOD CONCENTRATION. After an oral dose of 40 mg/kg body-weight, administered as a suspension, plasma concentrations of 300 to 800 ng/ml are attained during the period 2 to 8 hours after administration.

FURTHER INFORMATION. Serum concentrations—C. P. Gomez and T. F. Sandeman, *Lancet*, ii/1966, 233.

Actions and uses. Methisazone is an antiviral agent which is effective against viruses of the pox group. It is used mainly for the short-term prophylaxis of smallpox contacts and of persons suspected of being in the early stages of the disease. It may be given at the same time as vaccination or at any time thereafter and rarely interferes with the success of vaccination. Methisazone may also be used for the treatment of eczema vaccinatum and vaccinia gangrenosa.

The usual dose for smallpox prophylaxis in adults is 3 grams followed after 12 hours by a further 3 grams. Children under 3 years may be given 750 milligrams and at 3 to 10 years 1.5 grams; in each case the dose is repeated after 12 hours.

For the treatment of eczema vaccinatum and vaccinia gangrenosa the usual initial dosage is 200 milligrams per kilogram body-weight followed by 8 doses of 50 milligrams per kilogram body-weight at intervals of 6 hours; if necessary the course of treatment may be repeated after 7 days.

Undesirable effects. Nausea and vomiting may occur but can be minimised by administering the dose after meals. Fluid retention may also occur.

Precautions and contra-indications. Its use in patients with liver dysfunction should preferably be avoided. The concurrent use of alcohol should be avoided as it increases the severity of the undesirable effects.

Preparation

METHISAZONE MIXTURE (*Syn.* Methisazone Suspension): a suspension of methisazone in a suitable syrupy vehicle. It contains 6 g of methisazone in 30 ml. Available in 15-ml sachets.
A standard for this mixture is given in the British Pharmacopoeia Addendum 1975
Labelling: see the entry on Mixtures for general information on labelling.
Storage: it should be protected from light.
Advice for patients: the mixture should preferably be taken after meals and the prescribed course completed. Alcohol should be avoided.

Methohexitone Sodium for Injection

A mixture of 100 parts of sodium α-(±)-5-allyl-1-methyl-5-(1-methylpent-2-ynyl)barbiturate with 6 parts of dried sodium carbonate ($C_{14}H_{17}N_2NaO_3 = 284.3$).

OTHER NAMES: *Brietal Sodium®*; Sodium Methohexital

A standard is given in the British Pharmacopoeia 1973 under Methohexitone Injection

Description. An odourless hygroscopic white powder.

Solubility. Soluble in water.

Alkalinity. A 5% solution has a pH of 11 to 11.6.

Stability. Aqueous solutions decompose on keeping and solutions should not be used if they have become cloudy or discoloured. They may usually be stored without undue decomposition for up to 24 hours at temperatures not exceeding 25° when the solvent is water but stability is reduced in the presence of sodium chloride or dextrose and such solutions should be made immediately before use. The use of preservatives should be avoided as they cause precipitation. See also under Barbiturates.

Incompatibility. As with other sodium derivatives of barbiturates, precipitation is liable to occur when solutions of methohexitone sodium are mixed with solutions of acid pH. It has been reported that the mixing of solutions of methohexitone sodium 1% in water for injections with solutions containing the drugs listed below produces the physical changes shown at the times indicated:

	Immedi-ate	15 mins	30 mins	60 mins
Atropine sulphate 0.04%	None	Haze	—	—
Atropine sulphate 0.06%	None	Ppt	—	—
Gallamine triethiodide 1.3%	None	None	None	None
Hyoscine hydrobromide 0.05%	None	None	None	Haze
Suxamethonium chloride 0.05% or 0.1%	None	None	Haze	—
Tubocurarine chloride 0.075%	None	Haze	—	—

Methohexitone sodium is incompatible with compound sodium lactate injection.

Sterilisation. Sterile solutions of methohexitone sodium are prepared from sterile powder, by means of an aseptic technique, using water for injections free from carbon dioxide.

Storage. It should be stored in airtight containers.

Identification. TESTS. 1. Dissolve about 500 mg in 10 ml of water, add 10 ml of *dilute hydrochloric acid*, extract the solution with successive portions of chloroform, and evaporate the chloroform extracts to dryness; the residue, after recrystallisation from alcohol (70%) and drying at 70° *in vacuo*, melts at about 94°.
2. The residue obtained in Test 1, above, complies with general test 1, described under Barbiturates.

ULTRAVIOLET ABSORPTION. See under Barbiturates.

INFRA-RED ABSORPTION. Major peaks at 943, 1042, 1205, 1250, 1316, and 1695 cm^{-1} (see Appendix 2b: Infra-red Spectra).

Determination in body fluids. See under Barbiturates.

Metabolism (see also under Barbiturates).

BLOOD CONCENTRATION. After an intravenous dose of 2 mg/kg body-weight of methohexitone, peak venous blood concentrations of 4 to 8.5 μg/ml are attained within 1 to 3 minutes.

DISTRIBUTION. Methohexitone rapidly enters the brain and upon redistribution is localised in body fat, but to a lesser extent than thiopentone; *protein binding*, 73% bound to plasma albumin.

METABOLIC REACTIONS. In animals, hydroxylation and N-demethylation.

EXCRETION. After a dose of 1 g, less than 1% is excreted unchanged in the urine in 24 hours; in animals, the major urinary metabolite is 5-allyl-5-(4-hydroxy-1-methylpent-2-ynyl)-1-methylbarbituric acid together with a small amount of the demethylated metabolite.

Actions and uses. Methohexitone is a very short-acting barbiturate, the actions and uses of which are described under Barbiturates. It is used as an anaesthetic for intravenous administration, with actions and uses similar to those described under Thiopentone Sodium, but it is more potent, acts for a shorter time, and is more rapidly eliminated from the tissues.

The usual dose for induction is 70 to 120 milligrams, administered in the form of a 1% solution over a period of about 30 seconds. A 0.1% solution may be used for continuous drip anaesthesia.

Precautions and contra-indications. See under Barbiturates. The only contra-indications are those common to all present-day general anaesthetics.

Veterinary uses. Methohexitone sodium is used as a general anaesthetic. The usual dose by intravenous injection for dogs and cats is 10 milligrams per kilogram body-weight.

Preparation

METHOHEXITONE INJECTION: a sterile solution of methohexitone sodium and sodium carbonate in water for injections free from carbon dioxide. It is prepared shortly before use by dissolving the contents of a sealed container in water for injections free from carbon dioxide.
Available as a powder in 10-ml vials containing 100 mg of methohexitone sodium and 6 mg of dried sodium carbonate, in 50-ml vials containing 500 mg of methohexitone sodium and 30 mg of dried sodium carbonate, in 17.5- and 250-ml vials containing 2.5 g of methohexitone sodium and 150 mg of dried sodium carbonate, and in 35-ml vials containing 5 g of methohexitone sodium and 300 mg of dried sodium carbonate.
A standard for this injection is given in the British Pharmacopoeia 1973
Containers and *Labelling:* see the entry on Injections for general information on containers and labelling.
Storage: the injection contains no bactericide and should be used as soon as possible after preparation, but solutions of methohexitone may be expected to retain their potency for up to 24 hours provided they are stored at 2° to 10°.

Methoin

5-Ethyl-3-methyl-5-phenylimidazolidine-2,4-dione

$C_{12}H_{14}N_2O_2 = 218.3$

OTHER NAMES: Mephenytoin; *Mesontoin*®

A standard is given in the British Pharmacopoeia 1973

Description. Odourless, tasteless, colourless, lustrous plates.

Solubility. Very slightly soluble in water; soluble, at 20°, in 13 parts of alcohol, in 85 parts of ether, and 2.3 parts of chloroform; soluble in solutions of alkali hydroxides.

Identification. MELTING-POINT. About 137°.

INFRA-RED ABSORPTION. Major peaks at 735, 1053, 1389, 1449, 1695, and 1754 cm^{-1} (see Appendix 2b: Infra-red Spectra).

Actions and uses. Methoin is an anticonvulsant which has actions similar to those described under Phenytoin Sodium. It is used in the treatment of grand mal. It has also produced satisfactory results in some patients with psychomotor seizures, Jacksonian epilepsy, and behaviour disorders. In some cases the simultaneous administration of methoin and phenobarbitone has given the best results. Methoin is ineffective in controlling petit mal attacks.

The initial daily dosage is 50 to 100 milligrams by mouth, given in divided doses; this may be increased by 50 milligrams at weekly intervals until a daily dosage of 600 milligrams is reached. The maximum daily dosage for a child is 400 milligrams.

Undesirable effects. Methoin gives rise to undesirable effects more frequently than phenytoin sodium, the commonest reactions being drowsiness, dizziness, muscular incoordination, and ataxia. The appearance of a rash indicates the need to reduce the dose or to discontinue the drug, but in some cases treatment can be maintained by reducing the dose of methoin and giving phenobarbitone in addition.

The most serious toxic effect of methoin is on the haemopoietic system, and cases of pancytopenia and aplastic anaemia have been reported. If sore throat or fever occurs the drug should be witheld while investigations are made.

Preparation

METHOIN TABLETS: available as tablets containing 100 mg of methoin; they may be coloured.

A standard for these tablets is given in the British Pharmacopoeia 1973

Containers and *Storage:* see the entry on Tablets for general information on containers and storage. Containers should be airtight.

Advice for patients: when initiating treatment there may be a time-lag of up to 2 weeks before a full therapeutic response is obtained. Treatment should not be discontinued without the advice of the prescriber. The tablets may cause drowsiness; persons affected should not drive or operate machinery. Alcohol should be avoided.

Methoserpidine

Methyl 11-demethoxy-10-methoxy-*O*-(3,4,5-trimethoxybenzoyl)reserpate

$C_{33}H_{40}N_2O_9 = 608.7$

OTHER NAMES: *Decaserpyl®*; Methoserp. *Decaserpyl Plus®* (with benzthiazide)

A standard is given in the British Pharmacopoeia 1973

Description. An odourless, tasteless, hygroscopic, cream-coloured, microcrystalline powder. It darkens on exposure to light.

Solubility. Very slightly soluble in water; soluble, at 20°, in 60 parts of alcohol, in 5 parts of chloroform, and in 8 parts of dioxan.

Moisture content. Not more than 2%, determined by drying at 60° *in vacuo*.

Specific rotation. −144° to −154°, determined on a 1% solution in dioxan.

Storage. It should be stored in airtight containers, protected from light.

Identification. TESTS. 1. Mix about 500 μg with 5 mg of dimethylaminobenzaldehyde and 0.2 ml of glacial acetic acid, and add 0.2 ml of sulphuric acid; a green colour is produced. Add 1 ml of glacial acetic acid; the colour changes to red (this test is also given by reserpine).
2. To about 1 mg add 0.2 ml of a freshly prepared 1% solution of vanillin in hydrochloric acid; a blue colour is produced in about 1 minute (distinction from reserpine which gives a rose-pink colour in about 2 minutes).

MELTING-POINT. About 171°, with decomposition.

ULTRAVIOLET ABSORPTION. In dehydrated alcohol, maxima at 273 nm (E1%, 1cm = 320) and 295 nm (E1%, 1cm = 200).

INFRA-RED ABSORPTION. Major peaks at 1090, 1120, 1220, 1328, 1414, and 1710 cm⁻¹ (see Appendix 2a: Infra-red Spectra).

Actions and uses. Methoserpidine has actions and uses similar to those described under Reserpine.

When methoserpidine is used as a hypotensive agent for the treatment of mild to moderate hypertension, response to treatment is slow in onset, the full effect being observed about the second or third week after treatment is begun.

The initial dosage is up to 30 milligrams daily in divided doses for one week. The daily dosage is then adjusted by 5 or 10 milligrams at intervals of a week until a suitable maintenance dose is established; this should be between 15 and 60 milligrams daily in divided doses.

Undesirable effects. Nasal congestion, mild sedation, and gastro-intestinal disturbances may occur.

Contra-indications. Methoserpidine should not be administered to patients with endogenous depression.

Preparations

METHOSERPIDINE TABLETS: available as tablets containing 5 and 10 mg of methoserpidine; they may be coloured.

A standard for these tablets is given in the British Pharmacopoeia 1973

Containers and *Storage:* see the entry on Tablets for general information on containers and storage. Containers should be airtight and light resistant.

Advice for patients: the tablets should be taken at regular intervals. Treatment should not be discontinued without the advice of the prescriber.

OTHER PREPARATIONS available include TABLETS containing methoserpidine 10 mg with benzthiazide 20 mg.

Methotrexate

A mixture of N-{4-[(2,4-diaminopteridin-6-ylmethyl)methylamino]benzoyl}-L-glutamic acid ($C_{20}H_{22}N_8O_5 = 454.4$) and related substances.

OTHER NAME: Methotrexatum

A standard is given in the European Pharmacopoeia Vol. III

Description. A yellow to orange crystalline powder.

Solubility. Very slightly soluble in water, in alcohol, in ether, and in chloroform; soluble in dilute solutions of alkali hydroxides and carbonates.

Moisture content. Not more than 8%, determined by Fischer titration.

Storage. It should be stored in airtight containers, protected from light.

Identification. ULTRAVIOLET ABSORPTION. In 0.1N sodium hydroxide, maxima at 258 nm (E1%, 1cm = 500), 303 nm (E1%, 1cm = 500), and 365 nm (E1%, 1cm = 200).

Determination in body fluids. SPECTROFLUORIMETRY. In whole blood, plasma, or urine—J. M. Kinkade *et al.*, *Biochem. Med.*, 1974, **10**, 337.

RADIOIMMUNOASSAY. In biological fluids—J. Hendel *et al.*, *Clin. Chem.*, 1976, **22**, 813.

ENZYME INHIBITION. In serum—L. C. Falk *et al.*, *Clin. Chem.*, 1976, **22**, 785.

Metabolism. ABSORPTION. Rapidly absorbed after oral administration; absorption appears to be dose dependent and high doses appear to be less well absorbed; in addition, some subjects appear to absorb methotrexate more slowly than others and this may be due to a deterioration of the gut epithelium.

BLOOD CONCENTRATION. The minimum therapeutic concentration is approximately 0.4 μg/ml; after an intravenous dose of 1 mg/kg body-weight, plasma concentrations of 1 to 4 μg/ml are attained immediately after injection; after an intravenous infusion of 500 mg/m² body-surface over 24 hours, an average serum concentration of 9 μg/ml, and a ventricular fluid concentration of about 0.24 μg/ml are attained; after an intraventricular dose of 6.25 mg/m², therapeutically active concentrations in ventricular fluid are maintained for 48 hours and are attained in lumbar fluid by 4 hours and maintained for a similar period.

HALF-LIFE. Serum half-life, about 27 hours.

DISTRIBUTION. Distributed mainly in the extracellular spaces but does penetrate cell membranes; it is strongly bound to dihydrofolate reductase and this bound methotrexate may be retained in the body for many months; small amounts enter the cerebrospinal fluid from blood and it is taken up to some extent by red blood cells, secreted in milk, and secreted in saliva; volume of distribution at steady state, about 70 litres; *protein binding*, about 50% bound to plasma proteins and this binding is affected by other organic acids.

METABOLIC REACTIONS. About 6% of an intravenous dose is metabolised and about 35% of an oral dose is metabolised; it appears therefore that methotrexate is subject to first pass metabolism; in rats and mice, methotrexate has been shown to be metabolised by intestinal bacteria to form metabolites such as 2,4-diamino-6-carboxypteridine and 2,4-diamino-6-methyl-pteridine; hydroxylation occurs in the guinea-pig and rabbit.

EXCRETION. After an intravenous dose, 50 to 100% is excreted in the urine and up to 9% in the faeces in 96 hours; up to about 15% of a dose may be excreted in the bile although some may be reabsorbed in the intestines.

FURTHER INFORMATION. Analysis of labelled methotrexate in rat plasma—R. E. Kates and T. N. Tozer, *J. pharm. Sci.*, 1973, **62**, 2056; distribution and pharmacokinetics in cerebrospinal fluid—*Lancet*, i/1975, 465 and W. R. Shapiro *et al.*, *New Engl. J. Med.*, 1975, **293**, 161; neoplastic tissue uptake in dogs—R. J. Lutz *et al.*, *J. Pharmacokinet. Biopharm.*, 1975, **3**, 77; pharmacokinetics—D. L. Azarnoff *et al.*, *Clin. Pharmac. Ther.*, 1974, **16**, 884, K. B. Bischoff, *J. Pharmacokinet. Biopharm.*, 1973, **1**, 465, K. B. Bischoff *et al.*, *J. pharm.*

Sci., 1971, **60**, 1128, R. L. Dedrick, *J. Pharmacokinet. Biopharm.*, 1973, **1**, 435, and D. H. Huffman *et al.*, *Clin. Pharmac. Ther.*, 1973, **14**, 572.

Actions and uses. Methotrexate is a cytotoxic antimetabolite. It acts as a folic acid antagonist by combining irreversibly with the enzyme dihydrofolate reductase and inhibiting the formation of tetrahydrofolic acid from dihydrofolic acid. The resultant folic acid deficiency inhibits nucleic acid synthesis and in this way cell division is stopped. Malignant tissue with a high cell turnover may be eliminated but other rapidly dividing normal tissue such as bone marrow, the epithelial lining of the gastro-intestinal tract and the bronchioles, and the cells in the hair follicles may be damaged. In addition, methotrexate induces immunosuppression; if given in early pregnancy it may be teratogenic.

Methotrexate is well absorbed when given by mouth and rapidly excreted through the kidneys. It is usually given by mouth but can be given by intramuscular or intravenous injection as the sodium salt.

Methotrexate is now rarely used to induce remission in acute lymphoblastic leukaemia but is commonly used to maintain remission. Intermittent oral administration, usually once a week, in a dose of 20 milligrams per square metre body-surface, may be given as a maintenance dose and modified if signs of toxicity occur.

Methotrexate either alone or in conjunction with cranial irradiation is of value in the prophylaxis of meningeal leukaemia. It does not cross the blood–brain barrier and therefore needs to be given intrathecally. The prophylactic dose, when used in conjugation with cranial irradiation, is 12 milligrams per square metre body-surface once a week for 4 to 5 weeks. When used without irradiation the dose of methotrexate is 12 milligrams per square metre body-surface every 1 to 3 months. In no instance should a dose of more than 12 milligrams per square metre body-surface be given at one time.

Methotrexate is valuable in the treatment of established leukaemic meningitis when it is used in conjunction with cranio-spinal irradiation. The usual dose is 12 milligrams per square metre body-surface by intrathecal injection, twice a week for 10 doses. To prevent relapse the cerebrospinal fluid must be cleared of blast cells.

Combinations of chemotherapeutic drugs used in the treatment of choriocarcinoma, testicular cancer, and disseminated breast cancer frequently include methotrexate.

An important recent development is the use of intensive high doses, such as 200 to 1000 milligrams of methotrexate per square metre body-surface by intravenous infusion followed by folinic acid (citrovorum factor) infusions for 72 hours or longer as a means of preventing damage to normal tissue. This procedure should only be carried out in special centres and careful monitoring of the liver and renal function is required. Using these methods dramatic improvements are now being obtained for highly lethal tumours such as osteogenic sarcoma, when treated early.

In severe acute pustular psoriasis methotrexate therapy is of value and may be lifesaving. Prolonged treatment is necessary and to lessen the incidence of hepatic toxicity methotrexate should be given every 7 to 14 days in a dosage of 5 to 15 milligrams per square metre body-surface.

The immunosuppressive action of methotrexate has been used in the palliative treatment of dermatomyositis.

Undesirable effects. Anorexia, nausea, vomiting, abdominal cramps, diarrhoea, alopecia, ulceration of the mucous membranes of the mouth, rectum, or vagina, or the onset of bone-marrow depression with anaemia, leucopenia, and thrombocytopenia may occur. Hepatitis, pneumonitis, and renal tubular damage occur more rarely. An increased tendency to fractures of the long bones may occur in patients on long-term treatment with methotrexate. Intrathecal administration may produce symptoms of neurotoxicity such as meningeal irritation and, less commonly, paraplegia, seizures, and encephalopathy.

Precautions. Regular haemoglobin estimations and white-cell and platelet counts are required during methotrexate therapy. Signs of toxicity such as mouth ulceration, gastro-intestinal disturbances, or onset of bone-marrow depression will necessitate modification of the dose. The undesirable effects of methotrexate on the bone marrow and the gut may be minimised by administering the drug in large intermittent doses rather than daily.

As methotrexate is excreted through the kidney the presence of impaired renal function will aggravate the toxic action of the drug. Methotrexate therapy should be withdrawn immediately if there is severe infection.

Contra-indications. Methotrexate should not be given to patients with bone-marrow depression or in early pregnancy.

Poisoning. In the case of inadvertent overdosage calcium folinate should be given by intravenous infusion within 4 hours; a suggested regimen is 12 milligrams per square metre body-surface every 4 hours for 24 hours and every 6 hours for the next 48 hours. Unless renal function is very poor it is unlikely that there will be circulating methotrexate thereafter.

Preparations

METHOTREXATE INJECTION: a sterile solution of methotrexate, with sodium hydroxide, in water for injections. It is sterilised by filtration. Available in 1- and 2-ml ampoules containing 2.5 mg of methotrexate per ml, and in 1-, 2-, and 10-ml ampoules containing 25 mg of methotrexate per ml. These packs contain no bactericides.
A standard for this injection is given in the British Pharmacopoeia Addendum 1975
Containers: see the entry on Injections for general information on containers.
Labelling: see the entry on Injections for general information on labelling. In addition, when a bactericide is present, the label on the container should state that it is not intended for intrathecal injection.
Storage: it should be protected from light.

METHOTREXATE TABLETS: available as tablets containing 2.5 mg of methotrexate.
A standard for these tablets is given in the British Pharmacopoeia 1973
Containers and *Storage:* see the entry on Tablets for general information on containers and storage. Containers should be airtight and light resistant.

OTHER PREPARATIONS available include an INJECTION reconstituted from vials of powder containing methotrexate 50 mg with preservatives (unsuitable for intrathecal injection).

Methotrimeprazine

$(-)$-10-(3-Dimethylamino-2-methylpropyl)-2-methoxy-phenothiazine

$C_{19}H_{24}N_2OS = 328.5$

OTHER NAMES: Levomepromazine
Immobilon® (with etorphine hydrochloride—for small animals)
A standard is given in the British Pharmacopoeia (Veterinary)

Description. An odourless, white or slightly cream-coloured, crystalline powder.

Solubility. Practically insoluble in water; soluble, at 20°, in 140 parts of alcohol; soluble in chloroform and in ether.

Specific rotation. $-15°$ to $-18°$, determined on a 5% solution in chloroform.

Storage. It should be protected from light.

Identification. TEST. Dissolve about 5 mg in 2 ml of sulphuric acid and allow to stand for 5 minutes; a deep purple colour is produced.

MELTING-POINT. About 125°.

ULTRAVIOLET ABSORPTION. In 0.1N hydrochloric acid, maximum at 250 nm (E1%, 1cm = 750), and a less well-defined maximum at 300 nm.

INFRA-RED ABSORPTION. Major peaks at 1170, 1205, 1270, 1445, 1460, and 1590 cm^{-1} (see Appendix 2c: Infra-red Spectra).

Veterinary uses. Methotrimeprazine is a tranquilliser used in conjunction with etorphine to induce neuroleptanalgesia in dogs. The usual dose in conjunction with etorphine is 1 to 2 milligrams per kilogram body-weight.

Preparation

ETORPHINE AND METHOTRIMEPRAZINE INJECTION: a sterile solution of etorphine hydrochloride and methotrimeprazine, with suitable stabilising agents, in water for injections. The acidity of the solution is adjusted to pH 4. The solution is sterilised by heating in an autoclave or by filtration. It contains 74 micrograms of etorphine hydrochloride and 18 mg of methotrimeprazine per ml. Available in 20-ml vials.
A standard for this injection is given in the British Pharmacopoeia (Veterinary)
Containers and *Labelling:* see the entry on Injections for general information on containers and labelling.
Storage: it should be protected from light.
Dose: dogs, 0.1 millilitre per kilogram body-weight by intramuscular injection or 0.05 millilitre per kilogram body-weight by intravenous injection.

Methoxamine Hydrochloride

1-(2,5-Dimethoxyphenyl)-1-hydroxyprop-2-ylammonium chloride

$C_{11}H_{18}ClNO_3 = 247.7$

OTHER NAME: *Vasoxine®*

A standard is given in the British Pharmaceutical Codex 1973

Description. Colourless or white plate-like crystals or white crystalline powder; odourless or with a faint odour.

Solubility. Soluble in 2.5 parts of water and in 12 parts of alcohol; very slightly soluble in ether and in chloroform.

Acidity. A 2% solution has a pH of 4 to 6.

Dissociation constant. pK_a 9.2 (25°).

Sterilisation. Solutions for injection are sterilised by heating in an autoclave or by filtration.

Identification. TEST. Dissolve about 20 mg in 2 ml of water, add 5 ml of *diazotised nitroaniline solution* and 1 ml of *sodium carbonate solution*, allow to stand for 2 minutes, and add 1 ml of 1N sodium hydroxide; a deep red colour is produced which is extractable with butyl alcohol.

MELTING-POINT. About 214°.

ULTRAVIOLET ABSORPTION. In 0.1N hydrochloric acid, maxima at 228 nm (E1%, 1cm = 291) and 294 nm (E1%, 1cm = 134).

INFRA-RED ABSORPTION. Major peaks at 1022, 1179, 1219, 1276, 1461, and 1496 cm⁻¹ (see Appendix 2a: Infra-red Spectra).

Actions and uses. Methoxamine is a synthetic sympathomimetic amine with peripheral actions similar to those described under Noradrenaline Acid Tartrate. It causes prolonged peripheral vasoconstriction and consequently a rise in arterial blood pressure. It has little effect on the heart, although reflex bradycardia may occur. It has a marked pilomotor effect, but does not stimulate the central nervous system or cause bronchodilatation.

Methoxamine hydrochloride is administered by intramuscular injection in doses of 5 to 20 milligrams to maintain or restore the blood pressure during surgical operations and in hypotensive states such as postoperative shock or after ganglion blockade.

In emergencies, or when the systolic blood pressure has fallen to less than 60 mm of mercury, 5 to 10 milligrams may be given by intravenous injection at a rate of about 1 milligram per minute.

Its effect begins almost immediately after intravenous injection and lasts for about one hour; after intramuscular injection it begins within about 15 minutes and lasts for about one and a half hours. A second intramuscular injection should not be given within 15 minutes of the first dose, and the total daily dosage should not normally exceed 60 milligrams; a single intravenous dose should not exceed 10 milligrams. There is no diminution of effect with repeated doses. To prolong the effect of an intravenous dose, it may be supplemented by an intramuscular injection of 10 to 15 milligrams.

Methoxamine is especially suitable for maintaining blood pressure during spinal anaesthesia; a dose of 10 milligrams by intramuscular injection is usually sufficient for operations below the umbilical level and 15 to 20 milligrams for operations above this.

Methoxamine is applied locally for the relief of nasal congestion. It is suitable for infants and children. Applied intranasally as drops or spray it does not produce systemic side-effects, but occasionally may cause rebound congestion.

Undesirable effects. Methoxamine may produce an undesirably high blood pressure with headache and vomiting. Bradycardia may occur, but this may be prevented or abolished by atropine. Methoxamine frequently induces the desire to urinate. After intravenous injection there may be a feeling of coldness.

Precautions and contra-indications. It is contra-indicated in coronary disease, severe hypertension or cardiovascular disease, and should be used with caution in patients with hyperthyroidism. It should not be given to patients who are being treated with a monoamine-oxidase inhibitor, such as isocarboxazid, nialamide, phenelzine, or tranylcypromine, or within about 2 weeks of the discontinuation of such treatment.

Preparation

METHOXAMINE INJECTION (*Syn.* Methoxamine Hydrochloride Injection):

Methoxamine hydrochloride	..	..	2.00 g
Sodium chloride	.. .. ..	..	0.43 g
Water for injections	.. ..	..	to 100 ml

Dissolve and filter. Distribute the solution into ampoules, replace the air in the ampoules with nitrogen or other suitable gas, seal, and sterilise by heating in an autoclave. Available in 1-ml ampoules containing 20 mg of methoxamine hydrochloride.

A standard for this injection is given in the British Pharmaceutical Codex 1973

Containers: see the entry on Injections for general information on containers. The injection should be supplied in single-dose ampoules.

Labelling: see the entry on Injections for general information on labelling.

Methoxyflurane

2,2-Dichloro-1,1-difluoroethyl methyl ether, to which 0.01% of butylated hydroxytoluene has been added.

$$CHCl_2 \cdot CF_2 \cdot O \cdot CH_3$$

$C_3H_4Cl_2F_2O = 165.0$

OTHER NAME: *Penthrane®*

A standard is given in the British Pharmacopoeia 1973

Description. A clear, almost colourless, mobile liquid with a characteristic odour and a sweet and burning taste.

Solubility. Practically insoluble in water; miscible with alcohol, with ether, and with chloroform.

Weight per ml. At 20°, 1.423 to 1.427 g.

Boiling-point. About 105°.

Storage. It should be stored in airtight containers, protected from light, in a cool place.

Determination in body fluids. GAS CHROMATOGRAPHY.

In blood—P. L. Jones *et al.*, *Br. J. Anaesth.*, 1972, **44**, 124.

Actions and uses. Methoxyflurane is a volatile anaesthetic with actions similar to those described under Halothane, but induction is relatively slow. At operating theatre temperatures it is not inflammable or explosive and it may be used in conjunction with a cautery. Methoxyflurane may be administered by any of the usual methods, alone or in combination with thiopentone, muscle relaxants, and other drugs used as aids to anaesthesia. For induction, a concentration of 2 to 2.8% v/v may be given and the anaesthesia maintained with 0.5% v/v in oxygen.

Good muscular relaxation can be obtained. There is some depression of respiration and blood pressure, but vomiting is unusual. The hypnotic effect of methoxyflurane is such that administration may be discontinued half an hour before the completion of operation.

For obstetrical use a concentration of 0.5% v/v in a mixture of nitrous oxide and oxygen may be used for anaesthesia and a concentration of 0.35% v/v in air may be administered intermittently for analgesia; no depression of uterine contractions occurs. Methoxyflurane may cause the skin to look pale although the circulation remains stable.

Precautions and contra-indications. Methoxyflurane is contra-indicated in the presence of liver damage. It enhances the effects of muscle relaxants of the tubocurarine type and of narcotics, which should therefore be used with caution, as also should adrenaline. Methoxyflurane should not be given to patients taking tetracyclines as the risk of renal toxicity is potentiated.

Methyl Benzoquate

Methyl 7-benzyloxy-6-butyl-1,4-dihydro-4-oxoquinoline-3-carboxylate

$C_{22}H_{23}NO_4 = 365.4$

OTHER NAMES: Nequinate; *Statyl®*

A standard is given in the British Pharmacopoeia (Veterinary)

Description. An odourless, white or creamy-white, amorphous powder.

Solubility. Practically insoluble in water; very slightly soluble in alcohol, in chloroform, and in methyl alcohol.

Identification. MELTING-POINT. About 208°.

ULTRAVIOLET ABSORPTION. In 0.1N methanolic hydrochloric acid, maximum at 261 nm (E1%, 1cm = 1960).

INFRA-RED ABSORPTION. Major peaks at 1087, 1220, 1250, 1562, 1639, and 1695 cm⁻¹ (see Appendix 2b: Infra-red Spectra).

Veterinary uses. Methyl benzoquate is used for the prevention of coccidiosis in broiler chickens, the usual dosage being 20 parts per million in the feed from day-old to slaughter.

Preparation

METHYL BENZOQUATE PREMIX: consisting of methyl benzoquate mixed with suitable inorganic diluents. This preparation is stable to hot pelleting processes. It must be diluted before administration by mixing thoroughly with the feed. Available as a premix containing 4% of methyl benzoquate.

A standard for this premix is given in the British Pharmacopoeia (Veterinary)

Containers and *Storage:* see the entry on Premixes for general information on containers and storage.

Labelling: the label on the container should state that the preparation should not be given to birds producing eggs for human consumption.

Methyl Hydroxybenzoate

Methyl 4-hydroxybenzoate

$C_8H_8O_3 = 152.1$

OTHER NAMES: Methyl Parahydroxybenzoate; Methylis Parahydroxybenzoas; Methylparaben; *Nipagin M®*; *Phytodermine®* (with salicylic acid)

A standard is given in the European Pharmacopoeia Vol. III

Description. An odourless, fine, white, crystalline powder with a faintly burning taste.

Solubility. Soluble, at 20°, in 500 parts of water, in 3.5 parts of alcohol, and in 3 parts of acetone; soluble in 20 parts of boiling water; soluble in ether and in solutions of alkali hydroxides; soluble in 60 parts of warm glycerol and in 40 parts of warm vegetable oils, the solutions remaining clear on cooling.

Dissociation constant. pK_a 8.4 (22°).

Identification. TEST. Dissolve about 100 mg in 2 ml of alcohol (95%), boil, and add 0.5 ml of *mercury nitrate solution*; a precipitate is produced and the supernatant liquid becomes red.

MELTING-POINT. About 126°.

ULTRAVIOLET ABSORPTION. In alcohol (95%), maximum at 258 nm.

Uses. Methyl hydroxybenzoate is a preservative which is used mainly for its activity in solutions of pH up to 9 against moulds, fungi, and yeasts; it is less active against bacteria. Methyl hydroxybenzoate is more soluble than the higher esters such as ethyl, propyl, butyl, and benzyl hydroxybenzoates, but they are more active in a given concentration than the methyl compound. A concentration of 0.1 to 0.2% of methyl hydroxybenzoate is often employed to preserve aqueous preparations. It may be incorporated in preparations as a solution in alcohol or dissolved with the aid of heat.

Preparations

Preparations available include a DUSTING-POWDER containing methyl hydroxybenzoate 5% with salicylic acid 5%.

Methyl Nicotinate

Methyl pyridine-3-carboxylate

$C_7H_7NO_2 = 137.1$

A standard is given in the British Pharmacopoeia Addendum 1978

Description. White crystals or crystalline powder with a characteristic odour.

Solubility. Soluble, at 20°, in 0.7 part of water and of alcohol, in 0.4 part of chloroform, and in 1 part of ether.

Storage. It should be stored in airtight containers.

Identification. TEST. To 2 ml of a 0.1% solution add 6 ml of *cyanogen bromide solution* and 1 ml of a 2.5% solution of aniline; a golden-yellow colour is produced.

MELTING-POINT. About 41°.

ULTRAVIOLET ABSORPTION. In water, maximum at 264 nm (E1%, 1cm = 230).

INFRA-RED ABSORPTION. Major peaks at 741, 1020, 1111, 1282, 1429, and 1724 cm^{-1} (see Appendix 2b: Infra-red Spectra).

Actions and uses. Methyl nicotinate has vasodilator properties. It is used in a concentration of 1% as an ingredient of topical rubefacient preparations intended to relieve the pain of muscular and rheumatic conditions and minor circulatory disorders.

Methyl Salicylate

Methyl 2-hydroxybenzoate

$C_8H_8O_3 = 152.1$

OTHER NAMES: Methyl Sal.; Methylis Salicylas
Bengué's Balsam® (with menthol)

When Oil of Wintergreen, Wintergreen, or Wintergreen Oil is prescribed or demanded, Methyl Salicylate is dispensed or supplied.

A standard is given in the European Pharmacopoeia Vol. II

Description. A colourless or slightly yellow liquid with a strong, persistent, characteristic aromatic odour.

Solubility. Very slightly soluble in water; soluble, at 20°, in 10 parts of alcohol (70%); miscible with alcohol (90%), with ether, with chloroform, with carbon disulphide, with glacial acetic acid, and with fixed and volatile oils.

Weight per ml. At 20°, 1.179 to 1.184 g.

Refractive index. 1.535 to 1.538.

Boiling-point. About 221°, with decomposition.

Storage. It should be protected from light.

Identification. TESTS. 1. To a saturated solution add 1 drop of *ferric chloride solution*; a violet colour is produced.

2. Mix 12 drops with 2 ml of a 10% solution of potassium hydroxide, warm on a water-bath for 5 minutes, and add 3 ml of *dilute sulphuric acid*; a precipitate is produced which, after washing with water and then with two 1-ml portions of toluene and drying at 80°, melts at about 160°.

Actions and uses. Methyl salicylate has the actions of salicylates, as described under Sodium Salicylate, but it is seldom given by mouth. It is readily absorbed through the skin and is applied in liniments and ointments for the relief of pain in lumbago, sciatica, and rheumatic conditions.

Poisoning. The procedure as described under Aspirin should be adopted.

Preparations

COMPOUND METHYL SALICYLATE OINTMENT (*Syn.* Analgesic Balm; Unguentum Methylis Salicylatis Compositum Forte):

Methyl salicylate	500 g
Cajuput oil	25 g
Cineole	25 g
Water for preparations	45 g
Menthol	100 g
Wool fat	105 g
White beeswax	200 g

Melt together the white beeswax and the wool fat and add the menthol previously dissolved in the methyl salicylate, the cineole, and the cajuput oil. Incorporate the water at the same temperature, and stir until cold.

A standard for this ointment is given in the British Pharmaceutical Codex 1973

Containers: see the entry on Ointments for general information on containers. Containers should prevent evaporation. Certain plastic containers, such as those made from polystyrene, are unsuitable for use with this ointment.

Advice for patients: the ointment should be massaged well into the skin. It should not be applied to broken or inflamed skin or near to the eyes or mucous membranes. The container should be kept tightly closed.

METHYL SALICYLATE LINIMENT:

Methyl salicylate	250 ml
Arachis oil	to 1000 ml

A standard for this liniment is given in the British Pharmacopoeia Addendum 1977 and in the British Pharmacopoeia (Veterinary)

Containers and *Labelling:* see the entry on Liniments for general information on containers and labelling. Certain plastic containers, such as those made from polystyrene, are unsuitable for use with this liniment.

Storage: it should be stored in airtight containers, in a cool place.

Advice for patients: the liniment should be applied to the skin with considerable friction. It should not be applied to broken or inflamed skin or near to the eyes or mucous membranes. The container should be kept tightly closed.

METHYL SALICYLATE OINTMENT (*Syn.* Unguentum Methylis Salicylatis Forte; Strong Methyl Salicylate Ointment):

Methyl salicylate	500 g
White beeswax	250 g
Hydrous wool fat	250 g

Melt together the beeswax and the hydrous wool fat, add the methyl salicylate, and stir until cold.

A standard for this ointment is given in the British

Pharmacopoeia Addendum 1977 and in the British Pharmacopoeia (Veterinary)

Containers: see the entry on Ointments for general information on containers. Containers should prevent evaporation. Certain plastic containers, such as those made from polystyrene, are unsuitable for use with this ointment.

Advice for patients: see above under Compound Methyl Salicylate Ointment.

OTHER PREPARATIONS available include a CREAM containing methyl salicylate 15% with menthol 10%; and an OINTMENT containing methyl salicylate 20% with menthol 20%.

Methylated Spirit, Industrial

A mixture, made by a legally authorised methylator, of 19 volumes of alcohol (95%) with 1 volume of approved wood naphtha.

OTHER NAMES: I.M.S.; Industrial Methylated Spirits; *Methasept®*

A standard is given in the British Pharmacopoeia 1973

Industrial methylated spirit is of the quality known as "66 O.P. Industrial Methylated Spirits". Other strengths are available such as "Absolute Industrial Methylated Spirits", which is 74 O.P. and contains less than 1% of water, and "64 O.P. Industrial Methylated Spirits".

Industrial Methylated Spirit (Acetone-free), for which a standard is given in the *British Pharmaceutical Codex 1973*, is similar in all respects to Industrial Methylated Spirit, but is required to contain less than 500 parts per million of acetone. Most industrial methylated spirit is now produced free of acetone.

Description. A clear, colourless, mobile, volatile liquid with an odour of alcohol and wood naphtha, and a burning taste. It is highly inflammable, burning with a blue smokeless flame.

Identification. TEST. Dilute 0.5 ml to 5 ml with water, add 2.0 ml of *potassium permanganate and phosphoric acid solution*, allow to stand for 10 minutes, and add 2.0 ml of *oxalic acid and sulphuric acid solution*; to the colourless solution add 5 ml of *decolorised magenta solution*; a deep violet colour is produced.

Actions and uses. Industrial methylated spirit is applied externally for its astringent action, but mucous membranes and excoriated skin surfaces must be protected from such application. It is usually applied externally as surgical spirit.

The United Kingdom Board of Customs and Excise permit, subject to the observance of the conditions laid down in their regulations, the use of industrial duty-free spirit in the preparation of a range of specified preparations intended for external use only. These scheduled preparations include certain inhalations, liniments, lotions, sprays, spirits, and solutions of the British Pharmacopoeia and the British Pharmaceutical Codex, in addition to a formulary of medicinal, surgical, toilet, and other preparations.

Industrial methylated spirit may also be used in the preparation of certain extracts, resins, and surgical dressings, provided that in each case no alcohol remains in the finished product.

Provisions governing the dispensing, on the prescriptions of medical practitioners, dentists, and veterinary surgeons and practitioners, of industrial methylated spirit or of preparations of which it is an ingredient, and its use in ways other than those mentioned, are also contained in the regulations issued by the United Kingdom Board of Customs and Excise.

Industrial methylated spirit from some sources may contain small amounts of acetone and should not be used for the preparation of iodine solutions, as an irritating compound is formed by reaction between the iodine and acetone; for such preparations industrial methylated spirit (acetone-free) is used.

Undesirable effects. Industrial methylated spirit must not be taken by mouth, as its methyl alcohol content renders it poisonous. Symptoms include visual disturbances which often proceed to blindness, severe acidosis, and prolonged coma which may terminate in death from respiratory failure.

Poisoning. Gastric lavage should be employed and the usual means adopted for the treatment of shock and respiratory failure. Acidosis should be treated by the administration of compound sodium lactate injection or sodium bicarbonate injection, and delirium, if it occurs, by diazepam. In severe cases haemodialysis may be effective.

Preparations

SURGICAL SPIRIT (*Syn.* Spiritus Chirurgicalis; Surgical Spirit No. 1):

Methyl salicylate	..	..	..	..	5 ml
Diethyl phthalate	..	..	..	..	20 ml
Castor oil	..	..	..	..	25 ml
Industrial methylated spirit		..	..	to 1000 ml

A standard for this spirit is given in the British Pharmaceutical Codex 1973

Labelling: the label on the container should state "Caution. This preparation is inflammable. Keep away from a naked flame".

Advice for patients: it should not be applied to broken or inflamed skin.

OTHER PREPARATIONS available include an APPLICATION containing absolute industrial methylated spirit with a lubricant in an aerosol pack.

Methylcellulose

A methyl ether of cellulose. The name "methylcellulose" is followed by a number indicating the approximate viscosity in centistokes of a 2.0% solution.

OTHER NAMES: *Celacol M®*; *Celevac®*; *Cellucon®*; *Cologel®*; *Methocel A®*
Nilstim® (with microcrystalline cellulose)

Standards for Methylcellulose 20, Methylcellulose 2500, and Methylcellulose 4500 are given in the British Pharmaceutical Codex 1973. A standard for Methylcellulose 450 is given in the British Pharmacopoeia 1973.

Description. An odourless white or creamy-white powder.

Solubility. Soluble in cold water, forming a viscous colloidal solution; practically insoluble in hot water, in alcohol, in ether, and in chloroform.

Storage. It should be stored in airtight containers, in a cool place.

Identification. TESTS. 1. Add 1 g to 100 ml of water; the powder swells and disperses, forming a viscous colloidal solution. Boil; a white precipitate is produced which redissolves on cooling.

2. To 10 ml of the cold solution prepared in Test 1 add 0.5 ml of a 0.05% solution of brilliant yellow, 1 drop of 0.1N sodium hydroxide and 10 ml of a saturated solution of sodium sulphate; a voluminous, flocculent, red precipitate is produced. Filter; the filtrate is colourless.

3. Soak in *iodine water* for a few minutes and remove the excess of reagent with the aid of a filter paper; the powder is stained yellow. Add 2 drops of sulphuric acid (66% v/v); it is stained dark brown (distinction from microcrystalline cellulose).

Actions and uses. Methylcellulose disperses slowly in cold water to form a viscous colloidal solution. A mucilage may be prepared by adding the methylcellulose to about one-third the required amount of boiling water and, when the powder is thoroughly hydrated, adding the remainder of the water, preferably in the form of ice, and stirring until homogeneous.

Various viscosity grades of methylcellulose are available. High-viscosity grades, such as methylcellulose 2500 and 4500, are used as thickening agents for medicated jellies and creams, as dispersing agents in suspensions, and as binding and disintegrating agents in tablets. A 0.5 to 1% solution of a high-viscosity grade of methylcellulose is sometimes used to increase the viscosity of ophthalmic solutions, but for this purpose hypromellose is usually preferred; an antimicrobial agent such as benzalkonium chloride should be incorporated. Special grades with a high content of methoxyl, or having hydroxypropyl groups in place of some of the methyl groups (hypromellose) are used as adhesives in plaster of Paris bandage.

A low-viscosity grade, such as methylcellulose 20, is used as an emulsifying agent for liquid paraffin and other mineral oils and also for arachis and olive oils; it is less efficient for emulsifying cod-liver oil. Emulsions are prepared by mixing the oil with a methylcellulose mucilage, preferably using a mechanical stirrer.

Medium- and high-viscosity grades, such as methylcellulose 450, 2500, and 4500, are used as bulk laxatives, usually in the form of granules or tablets. The usual dose for this purpose is 1 to 4 grams daily in divided doses well diluted with water. Methylcellulose is also used as a bulk-forming agent to relieve hunger in dieting patients.

Methylcellulose is also used in doses of 2 grams taken with the minimum of liquid to relieve simple diarrhoea or to prevent diarrhoea in patients on a liquid diet.

Preparations

METHYLCELLULOSE GRANULES:

Methylcellulose 2500 *or* 4500, in powder	..	64.00 g
Amaranth, food grade of commerce ..	..	0.02 g
Saccharin sodium ..	.. ..	0.10 g
Vanillin	.. ..	0.20 g
Acacia, powdered ..	.. ..	4.00 g
Lactose	.. ..	31.68 g

Mix the powdered ingredients, add sufficient water for preparations to form a coherent mass suitable for granulation, and pass through a No. 2.80 sieve; place the granules upon a No. 710 sieve and discard the powder which passes through. Dry the granules at a temperature not exceeding 60°.

A standard for these granules is given in the British Pharmaceutical Codex 1973

Containers and *Storage:* they should be stored in airtight containers. They should preferably be stored and supplied in wide-mouthed glass or plastic containers or in lined aluminium containers closed with lined screw caps or plastic caps.

Advice for patients: the granules should be placed on the tongue and swallowed with water. When used as an antidiarrhoeal agent they should be taken with the minimum of fluid and fluid should not be taken within 30 minutes. For the treatment of constipation, the granules should be taken well diluted with water. When used as an appetite suppressant the dose should be taken well diluted with water about half an hour before meals and between meals when necessary.

OTHER PREPARATIONS available include an ELIXIR containing methylcellulose 9%, diluent water, life of diluted elixir 14 days; TABLETS containing methylcellulose (450) 500 mg, tablets containing methylcellulose (2500) 500 mg, and tablets containing methylcellulose (2500) 400 mg with microcrystalline cellulose 220 mg.

Methyldopa

(−)-3-(3,4-Dihydroxyphenyl)-2-methyl-L-alanine sesquihydrate

$C_{10}H_{13}NO_4, 1\frac{1}{2}H_2O = 238.2$

OTHER NAMES: *Aldomet®; Dopamet®; Medomet® Hydromet®* (with hydrochlorothiazide)

A standard is given in the British Pharmacopoeia 1973

Description. An odourless, almost tasteless, white to yellowish-white fine powder which may contain friable lumps.

Solubility. Soluble, at 20°, in 100 parts of water, in 400 parts of alcohol, and in less than 1 part of dilute hydrochloric acid; very slightly soluble in ether.

Moisture content. 10 to 13%, determined by Fischer titration.

Dissociation constants. pK_a 2.2, 9.2, 10.6, 12 (25°).

Storage. It should be stored in airtight containers, protected from light.

Identification. TESTS. 1. It complies with Test 1 described under Levodopa.

2. To about 10 mg add 3 drops of a 0.4% solution of ninhydrin in sulphuric acid; a dark purple colour develops in 5 to 10 minutes. Add 3 drops of water; the colour changes to pale brownish-yellow.

MELTING-POINT. About 290°.

ULTRAVIOLET ABSORPTION. In 0.1N hydrochloric acid, maximum at 280 nm (E1%, 1cm = 115).

INFRA-RED ABSORPTION. Major peaks at 1250, 1282, 1370, 1389, 1493, and 1613 cm⁻¹ (see Appendix 2b: Infra-red Spectra).

Determination in body fluids. SPECTROFLUORIMETRY. In blood—J. W. Meilink, *Pharm. Weekbl. Ned.*, 1971, **106**, 385. In plasma or urine—B. K. Kim and R. T. Koda, *J. pharm. Sci.*, 1977, **66**, 1632.

Metabolism. ABSORPTION. Poorly absorbed after oral administration.

BLOOD CONCENTRATION. After an oral dose of 1 g, a peak plasma concentration of unchanged methyldopa of 3 to 13 μg/ml is attained in 1 to 6 hours; after an intravenous dose of 250 mg as the hydrochloride, plasma concentrations of about 7 μg/ml are obtained after 40 minutes for unchanged and conjugated methyldopa.

HALF-LIFE. Biological half-life after intravenous administration, 3 to 12 hours; during the period 1 to 4 hours following intravenous administration the plasma half-life is about 2 hours.

DISTRIBUTION. Volume of distribution, 30 to 35 litres.

METABOLIC REACTIONS. Mainly sulphate conjugation with O-methylation and decarboxylation; the (+)-form does not appear to be decarboxylated however; metabolites include 3-O-methylmethyldopa, methyldopamine, 3-O-methyldopamine, sulphate conjugates, and ketones consisting mainly of 3,4-dihydroxybenzyl methyl ketone; sulphate conjugation varies considerably, appears to occur in the gastro-intestinal tract, and is stimulated by barbiturates; following intravenous administration very little sulphate conjugation occurs.

EXCRETION. 20 to 60% of a dose is excreted in the urine and the remainder is eliminated in the faeces; the major urinary metabolite is conjugated or unconjugated methyldopa and this accounts for 20 to 35% of the dose; urinary 3-O-methylmethyldopa accounts for about 4%, amine metabolites account for about 6%, and ketones account for about 3%; only unchanged drug is found in the faeces.

FURTHER INFORMATION. Enhancement of metabolism by phenobarbitone—A. Káldor *et al.*, *Br. med. J.*, iii/1971, 518; metabolism in normal and hypertensive subjects —W. Y. W. Au *et al.*, *Biochem. J.*, 1972, **129**, 1; plasma concentrations after oral and intravenous administration —J. A. Saavedra *et al.*, *Eur. J. clin. Pharmac.*, 1975, **8**, 381.

Actions and uses. Methyldopa is an antihypertensive agent which has a depressant action on the central nervous system. It inhibits the conversion of dopa to dopamine by competing for the enzyme dopa decarboxylase. In consequence, after the administration of methyldopa there is a reduction in the amount of noradrenaline formed from dopamine, but it has not been proved that this is entirely responsible for its hypotensive effect. Postural hypotension, although it occurs after administration of methyldopa, is never severe, nor does the blood pressure fall much on exercise.

Methyldopa is used in the treatment of moderate to severe hypertension. A thiazide diuretic may be given concurrently to potentiate the hypotensive effect.

The daily dosage of methyldopa is usually the equivalent of 0.5 to 2 grams of anhydrous methyldopa in divided doses; 1.13 grams of methyldopa is approximately equivalent to 1 gram of anhydrous methyldopa. Occasionally, the daily dosage may be increased to the equivalent of 4 grams.

Undesirable effects. Tolerance to methyldopa is rarely progressive and can usually be overcome by increasing the dose.

Undesirable effects include drowsiness, depression, dryness of the mouth, diarrhoea, and hyperpyrexia; liver damage, thrombocytopenia, and granulocytopenia have been reported.

Cases of acquired haemolytic anaemia have rarely occurred, but some patients have developed a positive direct Coombs test without evidence of haemolysis, anaemia, or related clinical effects.

Drowsiness is particularly liable to occur following a rapid increase in dosage.

Oedema resulting from sodium retention may occur; this requires the administration of a diuretic.

Contra-indications. Methyldopa is contra-indicated in patients with liver damage or dysfunction or with phaeochromocytoma.

Preparations

METHYLDOPA TABLETS: available as tablets containing methyldopa equivalent to 125, 250, and 500 mg of anhydrous methyldopa; they are film coated. The method of preparation should be such that water does not come into contact with materials used to make the tablets at any stage.

A standard for these tablets is given in the British Pharmacopoeia 1973

Containers and *Storage:* see the entry on Tablets for general information on containers and storage. Containers should be airtight and light resistant.

Labelling: the label on the container should state the amount of the medicament as the equivalent amount of anhydrous methyldopa.

Advice for patients: the tablets should be swallowed whole and should preferably be taken after meals. Treatment should not be discontinued without the advice of the prescriber. They may cause drowsiness; persons affected should not drive or operate machinery; Alcohol should be avoided. Methyldopa may cause the urine to darken.

OTHER PREPARATIONS available include TABLETS containing methyldopa equivalent to 250 mg of anhydrous methyldopa with hydrochlorothiazide 15 mg.

Methyldopate Hydrochloride

(2S)-1-(3,4-Dihydroxyphenyl)-2-ethoxycarbonylprop-2-ylammonium chloride

$C_{12}H_{18}ClNO_4 = 275.7$

OTHER NAME: *Aldomet*®

A standard is given in the British Pharmacopoeia Addendum 1975

Description. An odourless white crystalline powder.

Solubility. Soluble, at 20°, in 1 part of water, in 3 parts of alcohol, and in 2 parts of methyl alcohol; very slightly soluble in chloroform and in ether.

Acidity. A 1% solution has a pH of 3 to 5.

Specific rotation. $-7°$ to $-8.8°$, determined on a 2% solution in 0.1N hydrochloric acid.

Sterilisation. Solutions for injection are sterilised by filtration.

Storage. It should be protected from light.

Identification. ULTRAVIOLET ABSORPTION. In 0.1N hydrochloric acid, maximum at 280 nm (E1%, 1cm = 100).

INFRA-RED ABSORPTION. Major peaks at 1192, 1241, 1286, 1342, 1511, and 1720 cm^{-1} (see Appendix 2a: Infra-red Spectra).

Metabolism. BLOOD CONCENTRATION. After an intravenous dose of 250 mg, plasma concentrations of about 1.7 μg/ml for the total of conjugated, unconjugated, and esterified forms of methyldopa are attained in about 1 hour.

HALF-LIFE. During the period 1 to 4 hours after intravenous administration, the plasma half-life is about 4 hours.

DISTRIBUTION. Volume of distribution, about 145 litres.

METABOLIC REACTIONS. De-esterification to methyldopa, a small amount of sulphate conjugation, and other reactions similar to those for methyldopa; de-esterification appears to occur in both plasma and tissues.

FURTHER INFORMATION. Plasma concentrations of methyldopate and methyldopa from intravenous doses— J. A. Saavedra, *Eur. J. clin. Pharmac.*, 1975, **8**, 381.

Actions and uses. Methyldopate hydrochloride is a soluble compound which has actions and uses similar to those described under Methyldopa, and is suitable for intravenous administration in hypertensive crises; 1.16 milligrams of methyldopate hydrochloride is equivalent to 1 milligram of methyldopa.
The usual dosage for an adult is 250 to 500 milligrams administered by intravenous infusion in 100 millilitres of dextrose injection (5%) over a period of half to one hour and repeated every 6 hours if required, but doses of up to 1 gram every 6 hours may be necessary in severe cases.

Undesirable effects; Contra-indications. As for Methyldopa.

Preparation

METHYLDOPATE INJECTION: a sterile solution prepared by dissolving methyldopate hydrochloride, with suitable stabilising agents, in water for injections. Hydrolysis of the methyldopate hydrochloride may occur resulting in the presence of a variable amount of methyldopa. It is sterilised by filtration. It is distributed, by means of an aseptic technique, into sterile ampoules, and the ampoules are then sealed.
Available in 5-ml ampoules containing 50 mg of methyldopate hydrochloride per ml.
A standard for this injection is given in the British Pharmacopoeia Addendum 1975
Containers and *Labelling:* see the entry on Injections for general information on containers and labelling.
Storage: it should be protected from light.

Methylene Blue

3,7-Bisdimethylaminophenazathionium chloride dihydrate (Colour Index No. 52015)

$C_{16}H_{18}ClN_3S,2H_2O = 355.9$

OTHER NAME: Methylthionine Chloride

A standard is given in the British Pharmacopoeia 1973

Description. An almost odourless, hygroscopic, dark greenish, crystalline powder with a metallic lustre or dull, dark green or brown powder.

Solubility. Soluble, at 20°, in 40 parts of water, in 110 parts of alcohol, and in 450 parts of chloroform.

Moisture content. 8 to 15%, determined by drying at 105°.

Sterilisation. Solutions for injection are sterilised by heating in an autoclave or by filtration.

Storage. It should be stored in airtight containers.

Identification. TESTS. 1. Mix 10 ml of a 0.01% solution with 1 ml of acetic acid and 100 mg of zinc powder and warm; the solution is decolorised. Filter and expose the filtrate to air; the blue colour returns.
2. To 10 ml of a 0.01% solution add a few drops of *potassium iodide solution*; a deep blue flocculent precipitate is produced which separates slowly leaving a pale blue supernatant liquid.
3. To 10 ml of a 0.01% solution add 1 ml of *dilute sulphuric acid* and a few drops of 0.1N potassium dichromate; a reddish-violet colour and a bluish-violet precipitate are produced. Add sulphurous acid; the blue colour is restored.

Metabolism. ABSORPTION. Well absorbed in man but poorly absorbed in dogs.

DISTRIBUTION. Distributed evenly between red cells and plasma.

METABOLIC REACTIONS. Converted to leucomethylene blue.

EXCRETION. 50 to 97% of a dose is excreted in the urine; of the excreted material about 80% is leucomethylene blue and the remainder appears to be unchanged.

FURTHER INFORMATION. Pharmacokinetics in man and dogs—A. R. DiSanto and J. G. Wagner, *J. pharm. Sci.*, 1972, **61**, 1086.

Actions and uses. Methylene blue is used in the treatment of drug-induced methaemoglobinaemia, for which purpose it is administered by intravenous injection as a 1% solution in doses of 1 to 4 milligrams per kilogram body-weight. It has also been used in the treatment of idiopathic methaemoglobinaemia, in a daily dose of 300 milligrams, by mouth, with large doses of ascorbic acid.
Methylene blue is used in a renal function test, especially to compare the function of the two kidneys, but is inferior to indigo carmine for this purpose. For the test, 2 millilitres of a 2.5% solution of methylene blue is injected intramuscularly and the ureteric orifices are examined by cystoscopy. Urine excreted by the normal kidney assumes a greenish colour in about half an hour; a delay in excretion is an indication of impairment of renal function.
Methylene blue has been administered by mouth in doses of 50 to 300 milligrams daily as a urinary antibacterial agent but it is of no value for this purpose.

Stains on the skin caused by methylene blue can be removed with a hypochlorite solution.

NOTE. Commercial methylene blue is the double chloride of tetramethylthionine and zinc and is not suitable for medicinal use.

Methylergometrine Maleate

(+)-N-[(2S)-1-Hydroxybut-2-yl]-D-lysergamide hydrogen maleate

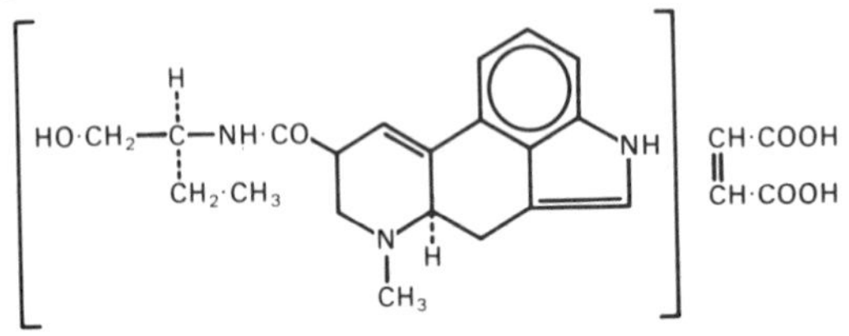

$C_{24}H_{29}N_3O_6 = 455.5$

A standard is given in the British Pharmacopoeia 1973

Description. A white or faintly yellow crystalline powder.

Solubility. Soluble, at 20°, in 200 parts of water and in 140 parts of alcohol.

Moisture content. Not more than 2%, determined by drying at 100° in vacuo.

Specific rotation. +44° to +50°, determined on a 0.5% solution.

Sterilisation. Solutions for injection are sterilised by filtration or by heating in an autoclave in an atmosphere of nitrogen or other suitable gas.

Storage. It should be stored in hermetically sealed containers, protected from light, in an atmosphere of nitrogen.

Identification. TESTS. 1. A solution has a blue fluorescence.
2. Dissolve 250 μg in 1 ml of glacial acetic acid containing a trace of ferric chloride, carefully add 1 ml of sulphuric acid and shake well; a deep blue colour is produced.

MELTING-POINT. About 190°, with decomposition.

ULTRAVIOLET ABSORPTION. In 0.1N sulphuric acid, maxima at 226 nm and 313 nm.

Actions and uses. Methylergometrine has actions and uses similar to those described under Ergometrine Maleate, but it is effective in smaller doses. It must not be given in the first and second stages of labour and, because of its powerful oxytocic action, it is not usually administered before the expulsion of the placenta.
Methylergometrine maleate may be administered by mouth in a dose of 250 to 500 micrograms, or by intramuscular or subcutaneous injection in a dose of 100 to 200 micrograms. It may also be given intravenously in a dose of 50 to 100 micrograms. If the patient is anaesthetised, 200 micrograms may be given intravenously, or 200 to 400 micrograms intramuscularly. If uterine inertia or haemorrhage persists, the dose may be repeated at intervals of 2 to 4 hours.
For the treatment of subinvolution or during post-partum convalescence, 250 micrograms may be given by mouth 3 or 4 times a day.

Preparations

METHYLERGOMETRINE INJECTION: a sterile solution of methylergometrine maleate in water for injections, free from dissolved air. The acidity of the solution is adjusted to pH 3.2 by the addition of maleic acid. The solution is distributed into ampoules, the air in the ampoules being replaced with nitrogen or other suitable gas, and the ampoules are sealed and sterilised by heating in an autoclave. Alternatively, the solution is sterilised by filtration, distributed, by means of an aseptic technique, into sterile ampoules, the air in the ampoules being replaced with sterile nitrogen or other suitable gas, and the ampoules are sealed.
A standard for this injection is given in the British Pharmacopoeia 1973
Containers and Labelling: see the entry on Injections for general information on containers and labelling.
Storage: it should be protected from light.

METHYLERGOMETRINE TABLETS: containing methylergometrine maleate; they are sugar coated. The usual strength is 125 micrograms of methylergometrine maleate.
A standard for these tablets is given in the British Pharmacopoeia 1973
Containers and Storage: see the entry on Tablets for general information on containers and storage. Containers should be airtight.

Methylprednisolone

11β,17α,21 - Trihydroxy - 6α - methylpregna - 1,4 - diene - 3,20-dione

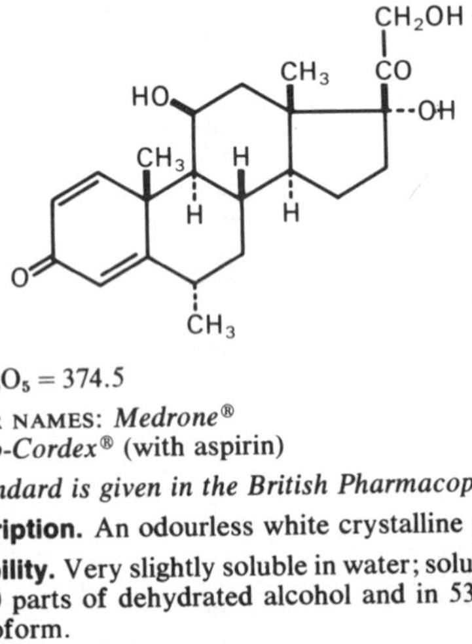

$C_{22}H_{30}O_5 = 374.5$

OTHER NAMES: Medrone®
Medro-Cordex® (with aspirin)

A standard is given in the British Pharmacopoeia 1973

Description. An odourless white crystalline powder.

Solubility. Very slightly soluble in water; soluble, at 20°, in 100 parts of dehydrated alcohol and in 530 parts of chloroform.

Specific rotation. +79° to +86°, determined on a 1% solution in dioxan.

Storage. It should be protected from light.

Identification. TEST. It complies with Test 1 described under Betamethasone.

MELTING-POINT. About 243°, with decomposition.

ULTRAVIOLET ABSORPTION. In dehydrated alcohol, maximum at 240 nm (E1%, 1cm = 400).

INFRA-RED ABSORPTION. Major peaks at 914, 1114, 1313, 1396, 1595, and 1650 cm^{-1} (see Appendix 2a: Infra-red Spectra).

THIN-LAYER CHROMATOGRAPHY. See under Thin-layer Chromatography, System 10.

Actions and uses. Methylprednisolone has the actions,

uses, and undesirable effects described under Prednisolone; it is effective in a slightly lower dosage, 4 milligrams being approximately equivalent in glucocorticoid effect to 5 milligrams of prednisolone. It is used in a dosage of 8 to 80 milligrams daily in divided doses.

Precautions and contra-indications. As for Cortisone Acetate.

Preparations

METHYLPREDNISOLONE TABLETS: available as tablets containing 2, 4, and 16 mg of methylprednisolone; they may be coloured.

A standard for these tablets is given in the British Pharmacopoeia 1973

Containers and *Storage:* see the entry on Tablets for general information on containers and storage. Containers should be airtight and light resistant.

Advice for patients: in long-term use, treatment should not be discontinued without the advice of the prescriber. Patients may carry an identification card giving details of their treatment and the name of the prescriber who should be contacted in the event of an accident, feverish illness, diarrhoea, vomiting, or alimentary disturbances. In short-term treatment, the prescribed course should be completed.

OTHER PREPARATIONS available include TABLETS containing methylprednisolone 1 mg with aspirin 300 mg.

Methylprednisolone Acetate

$11\beta,17\alpha,21$-Trihydroxy-6α-methylpregna-1,4-diene-3,20-dione 21-acetate

$C_{24}H_{32}O_6 = 416.5$

OTHER NAMES: *Depo-Medrone®*; *Medrone®*
Neo-Medrone® (with neomycin sulphate)

A standard is given in the British Pharmacopoeia Addendum 1977 and the British Pharmacopoeia (Veterinary)

Description. An odourless white, crystalline powder.

Solubility. Practically insoluble in water; soluble, at 20°, in 100 parts of dehydrated alcohol and in 1000 parts of ether.

Moisture content. Not more than 1%, determined by drying at 105°.

Specific rotation. +97° to +105°, determined on a 1% solution in dioxan.

Storage. It should be stored in airtight containers, protected from light.

Identification. ULTRAVIOLET ABSORPTION. In dehydrated alcohol, maximum at 240 nm (E1%, 1cm = 355).

Actions and uses. Methylprednisolone acetate has the actions described under Methylprednisolone but it is less soluble and less readily metabolised and has a more sustained effect.

For the treatment of localised allergic and inflammatory conditions, an aqueous suspension of methylprednisolone acetate is injected at the site of inflammation. It is injected in a dosage of 4 to 80 milligrams to alleviate pain, inflammation, and swelling, by intracutaneous injection in severe inflammatory skin disorders, into soft tissues in conditions such as bursitis, and intra-articularly into swollen joints in rheumatoid arthritis.

Methylprednisolone acetate is also administered by intramuscular injection to produce a sustained systemic effect in allergic and inflammatory conditions in a dosage of 40 to 120 milligrams approximately every 2 weeks.

Methylprednisolone acetate may be administered rectally, in a retention enema or by continuous rectal drip, in the treatment of ulcerative colitis. The usual dose is 40 to 120 milligrams, 3 to 7 times weekly for 2 weeks. Ointments containing 0.25% of methylprednisolone acetate are used in inflammatory skin disorders and it is used in conjunction with other ingredients as a 0.25% lotion in the treatment of acne vulgaris.

Undesirable effects; Precautions and contra-indications. As for Cortisone Acetate.

Veterinary uses. Methylprednisolone acetate is a glucocorticoid used to reduce inflammatory reactions especially in the skin and locomotor systems. The usual dose by intramuscular injection for horses, dogs, and cats is 0.4 to 1 milligram per kilogram body-weight weekly.

Preparations

METHYLPREDNISOLONE ACETATE INJECTION: a sterile suspension of methylprednisolone acetate, in very fine particles, with suitable dispersing agents, in water for injections. It is prepared by means of an aseptic technique. Available in 1-, 2-, and 5-ml vials, and in 2-ml disposable syringes containing 40 mg of methylprednisolone acetate per ml.

A standard for this injection is given in the British Pharmacopoeia Addendum 1977 and the British Pharmacopoeia (Veterinary)

Containers: see the entry on Injections for general information on containers.

Labelling: see the entry on Injections for general information on labelling. In addition, the label on the container should state "Not to be given by intravenous injection".

Storage: it should be stored at a temperature not exceeding 30°, protected from light. It should not be allowed to freeze.

OTHER PREPARATIONS available include a CREAM containing methylprednisolone acetate 0.25%, and a cream containing methylprednisolone acetate 0.25% with neomycin sulphate 0.5%.

Methyltestosterone

17β-Hydroxy-17α-methylandrost-4-en-3-one

$C_{20}H_{30}O_2 = 302.5$

OTHER NAMES: Methyltestosteronum; *Orandrone®*; *Perandren®*; *Virormone-Oral®*
Climatone®; *Declimone®*; *Menolet®*; *Mixogen®* (all with ethinyloestradiol)

A standard is given in the European Pharmacopoeia Vol. II

Description. An odourless, white or slightly yellowish-white, crystalline powder.

Solubility. Very slightly soluble in water; soluble, at 20°, in 5 parts of alcohol, in 10 parts of acetone, and in 160 parts of arachis oil; very slightly soluble in ether.

Moisture content. Not more than 1%, determined by drying at 105°.

Specific rotation. +79° to +85°, determined on a 1% solution in alcohol (95%).

Storage. It should be stored in airtight containers, protected from light.

Identification. TESTS. 1. Dissolve about 1 mg in 1 ml of sulphuric acid; a yellowish colour with a slight green fluorescence develops. Add 1 ml of water; the solution becomes dark yellow and shows a faint green fluorescence.
2. Mix about 50 mg with 0.5 ml of acetic anhydride and 1 drop of dehydrated pyridine, boil gently for 1 hour under a reflux condenser, cool in ice-water, add 10 ml of ice-cold water and allow to stand for 30 minutes; a precipitate is produced which, after washing with water and recrystallising from dilute alcohol, melts at about 176°.

MELTING-POINT. About 165°.

ULTRAVIOLET ABSORPTION. In alcohol (95%), maximum at 239 nm (E1%, 1cm = 525).

INFRA-RED ABSORPTION. Major peaks at 1160, 1239, 1377, 1454, 1612, and 1664 cm^{-1} (see Appendix 2a: Infra-red Spectra).

THIN-LAYER CHROMATOGRAPHY. See under Thin-layer Chromatography, System 10.

Metabolism. ABSORPTION. Absorbed from the gastro-intestinal tract and from the oral mucosa; sublingual absorption is faster than absorption from the gastro-intestinal tract.

BLOOD CONCENTRATION. After an oral dose of 10 mg, peak serum concentrations of 25 to 40 ng/ml are attained in 1 to 2 hours; after an oral dose of 10 mg absorbed sublingually, peak serum concentrations of about 45 ng/ml are attained in about 1 hour.

HALF-LIFE. Serum half-life, about 3.5 hours; methyltestosterone displays dose-independent kinetics.

METABOLIC REACTIONS. Slowly metabolised mainly by hydroxylation of ring A and conjugation.

EXCRETION. About 3% of a dose is excreted unchanged and the remainder as polar metabolites in the urine.

FURTHER INFORMATION. Bioavailability from oral and sublingual tablets—D. Alkalay *et al.*, *J. clin. Pharmac.*, 1973, **13**, 142; spectrophotofluorimetric estimation in plasma after oral administration—D. Alkalay *et al.*, *J. pharm. Sci.*, 1972, **61**, 1746.

Actions and uses. Methyltestosterone has the actions and uses described under Testosterone. It has the advantage of being absorbed when given orally or sublingually. When given by mouth it has one-third to one-quarter of the androgenic activity of the same weight of testosterone propionate administered intra-muscularly.

In the male, methyltestosterone has been used for maintenance therapy after the full androgenic effect has been produced by parenteral administration of testosterone propionate. The dosage required varies considerably; it is usual to begin with 30 to 50 milligrams of methyltestosterone daily, in divided doses.
The usual dosage for a woman is 5 to 20 milligrams daily. For mammary carcinoma, 50 to 100 milligrams may be given daily.

Undesirable effects. Jaundice may occur when the drug is given for long periods. Prolonged administration to women may give rise to excessive libido and, with large dosage, virilism may be produced. Benign and malignant liver tumours have been reported following the use of methyltestosterone.

Precautions and contra-indications. The precautions described under Testosterone should be observed.
Methyltestosterone is contra-indicated in patients with impaired liver function and in pregnancy.

Veterinary uses. Methyltestosterone is an androgen that is effective when given by mouth. It is used for the treatment of male hypogonadism, to suppress certain hormone-dependent tumours, and to promote healing or growth. The usual dose for dogs and cats is 250 micrograms per kilogram body-weight daily.

Preparations

METHYLTESTOSTERONE TABLETS: available as tablets containing 5, 10, 25, and 50 mg of methyltestosterone.
A standard for these tablets is given in the British Pharmacopoeia 1973
Containers and *Storage:* see the entry on Tablets for general information on containers and storage. Containers should be airtight and light resistant.
Advice for patients: sublingual tablets should be allowed to dissolve slowly under the tongue; oral tablets should be swallowed whole. The prescribed course should be completed or, where applicable, treatment should not be discontinued without the advice of the prescriber.

OTHER PREPARATIONS available include TABLETS containing methyltestosterone 2.5 mg with ethinyloestradiol 5 micrograms, tablets containing methyltestosterone 3.6 mg with ethinyloestradiol 4.4 micrograms, tablets containing methyltestosterone 5 mg with ethinyloestradiol 5 micrograms, and tablets containing methyltestosterone 5 mg with ethinyloestradiol 15 micrograms.

Methyprylone

3,3-Diethyl-5-methylpiperidine-2,4-dione

$C_{10}H_{17}NO_2 = 183.2$

OTHER NAME: *Noludar®*

A standard is given in the British Pharmacopoeia 1973

Description. A white crystalline powder with a slight characteristic odour and a burning taste with a bitter after-taste.

Solubility. Soluble, at 20°, in 14 parts of water, in less than 1 part of alcohol and of chloroform, and in 3.5 parts of ether.

Storage. It should be stored in airtight containers, protected from light.

Identification. TEST. Mix 2 ml of 1N sodium hydroxide and 5 ml of water and add about 50 mg of the sample followed by 0.5 ml of *potassium ferricyanide solution*; the solution shows a green fluorescence under ultraviolet radiation.

MELTING-POINT. About 75°.

ULTRAVIOLET ABSORPTION. In alcohol (95%), a weak maximum at 290 nm (E1%, 1cm = 2).

Determination in body fluids. COLORIMETRY. In serum or urine—G. Xanthaky *et al.*, *J. Am. med. Ass.*, 1966, **198**, 1212.

Actions and uses. Methyprylone is used as a hypnotic and, less often, as a sedative. The usual hypnotic dose is 200 to 400 milligrams; the effect develops in half to one hour and persists for about 6 hours. The usual dose as a sedative is 50 to 100 milligrams, repeated as required.

Undesirable effects. It may give rise to dependence of the barbiturate-alcohol type, as described under Drug Dependence, enhance the effects of alcohol, and reduce the ability to drive motor cars and operate moving machinery.

The higher hypnotic doses, when given at night, may result in giddiness or drowsiness the next morning.

Poisoning. In severe poisoning, treatment should follow that recommended for barbiturate poisoning as described under Barbiturates and may need to be supplemented by vasopressor drugs. There is little evidence to support the use of forced diuresis or dialysis.

Preparation

METHYPRYLONE TABLETS: available as tablets containing 200 mg of methyprylone; they may be sugar coated.

A standard for these tablets is given in the British Pharmacopoeia 1973

Containers and *Storage:* see the entry on Tablets for general information on containers and storage. Containers should be airtight and, if the tablets are not sugar coated, light resistant.

Advice for patients: hypnotic doses should be taken 30 minutes before bedtime. The tablets may cause drowsiness on the following day; persons affected should not drive or operate machinery. Alcohol should be avoided.

Methysergide Maleate

(−)-N-[(2S)-1-Hydroxybut-2-yl]-1-methyl-D-lysergamide hydrogen maleate

$C_{25}H_{31}N_3O_6 = 469.5$

OTHER NAME: *Deseril*®

A standard is given in the British Pharmacopoeia Addendum 1977

Description. An odourless, white to creamy-white, crystalline powder which may have a yellow or pink tinge.

Solubility. Soluble, at 20°, in 500 parts of water, in 10000 parts of chloroform, and in 125 parts of methyl alcohol; practically insoluble in ether.

Acidity. A 0.2% solution has a pH of 3.7 to 4.7.

Moisture content. Not more than 7%, determined by drying at 120° *in vacuo*.

Specific rotation. +35° to +45°, determined on a 0.25% solution.

Storage. It should be stored in airtight containers, protected from light, at 2° to 6°.

Identification. TEST. Dissolve about 1 mg in 1 ml of alcohol (95%) and add 1 ml of *dimethylaminobenzaldehyde solution*; a brownish-red to violet colour is produced.

Actions and uses. Methysergide selectively antagonises the effects of 5-hydroxytryptamine (serotonin). Its main use is in the prophylactic treatment of severe or recurrent migraine, where the patient's social or economic life is seriously disrupted. As the role of 5-hydroxytryptamine in this condition is not yet known, the mechanism of action is obscure. Methysergide may also control the profuse diarrhoea associated with some cases of the carcinoid syndrome. Methysergide is ineffective in the treatment of acute attacks of migraine.

Treatment is started with the equivalent of 1 milligram of methysergide daily, increasing to a maximum of 6 milligrams daily in divided doses. Daily doses should not exceed 4 milligrams for continuous periods, which should not exceed 3 months, and it is advisable to reduce dosage gradually before discontinuing treatment. 1.3 milligrams of methysergide maleate is approximately equivalent to 1 milligram of methysergide.

Undesirable effects. Undesirable effects occur in about 25% of patients, and appear most commonly when doses of more than 8 milligrams daily are given. The most frequent effects are vertigo, nausea, vomiting, drowsiness, abdominal discomfort, unsteadiness, water retention and weight gain, loss of scalp hair, skin eruptions, and psychic reactions.

Cardiovascular reactions including coronary artery spasms may occur. The most serious side-effect is an abnormal fibrotic reaction, most commonly retroperitoneal, but pleuropulmonary and endocardial fibrosis may also occur. The fibrosis may be reversible if methysergide is discontinued at an early stage, and therefore patients taking the drug should be carefully examined at frequent intervals.

Precautions. Because of its potential toxicity, methysergide should only be used in severe recurrent cases of migraine where other drugs are ineffective. It should not be given to patients with known or suspected cardiovascular disease, impaired hepatic or renal function, pulmonary or collagen disorders, or states of sepsis, or to pregnant or nursing mothers. It should not be given during an established attack.

Preparation

METHYSERGIDE TABLETS: available as tablets containing methysergide maleate equivalent to 1 mg of methysergide; they are sugar coated; the coat may be coloured.

A standard for these tablets is given in the British Pharmacopoeia Addendum 1977

Containers and *Storage:* see the entry on Tablets for general information on containers and storage. Containers should be airtight and light resistant.

Advice for patients: the tablets should preferably be taken after meals. When initiating treatment, the first dose should preferably be taken at night. Treatment should not be discontinued without the advice of the prescriber.

Metoclopramide Hydrochloride

4-Amino-5-chloro-*N*-(2-diethylaminoethyl) - 2 - methoxy-benzamide hydrochloride monohydrate

$C_{14}H_{23}Cl_2N_3O_2,H_2O = 354.3$

OTHER NAMES: *Maxolon®*; *Primperan®*

A standard is given in the British Pharmacopoeia Addendum 1977

Description. An odourless white crystalline powder.

Solubility. Soluble, at 20°, in 0.7 part of water, in 3 parts of alcohol, and in 55 parts of chloroform; practically insoluble in ether.

Acidity. A 10% solution has a pH of 4.5 to 6.5.

Moisture content. 4.5 to 5.5%, determined by Fischer titration.

Sterilisation. Solutions for injection are sterilised by heating in an autoclave or by filtration.

Storage. It should be protected from light.

Identification. TEST. Dissolve about 50 mg in 5 ml of water and add 5 ml of a 1% solution of dimethylamino-benzaldehyde in 1N hydrochloric acid; a yellow-orange colour is produced.

ULTRAVIOLET ABSORPTION. In 0.01N hydrochloric acid, maxima at 273 nm (E1%, 1cm = 395) and 309 nm (E1%, 1cm = 345).

INFRA-RED ABSORPTION. Major peaks at 1254, 1311, 1496, 1530, 1590, and 1614 cm^{-1} (see Appendix 2a: Infra-red Spectra).

Determination in body fluids. THIN-LAYER CHROMA-TOGRAPHY. In plasma: metoclopramide and its principal metabolite—O. M. Bakke and J. Segura, *J. Pharm. Pharmac.*, 1976, **28**, 32.

HIGH PRESSURE LIQUID CHROMATOGRAPHY. In plasma —L. Teng *et al.*, *J. pharm. Sci.*, 1977, **66**, 1615.

Metabolism. ABSORPTION. In animals, well absorbed after oral or intramuscular administration.

BLOOD CONCENTRATION. After an intramuscular dose of 40 mg, no drug is detectable at 1 hour but concentrations of 0.02 to 0.2 μg/ml are detectable at 2 to 3 hours; in rabbits, plasma concentrations of about 90 μg/ml are attained after 30 to 120 minutes after an oral dose of 200 mg/kg.

HALF-LIFE. In rats and dogs, plasma half-life, 60 to 90 minutes; in rabbits about 2 hours.

DISTRIBUTION. In mice, widely distributed throughout the body with highest concentrations appearing in the liver, intestinal mucosa, and biliary tract, and lesser concentrations appearing in the heart, adrenal glands, thymus, fat, bone marrow, and central nervous system;

in animals, metoclopramide appears to be subject to enterohepatic circulation; volume of distribution in rats, rabbits, and dogs, greater than 1.1 litres/kg body-weight; *protein binding*, moderately bound to plasma proteins in man.

METABOLIC REACTIONS. In rats and dogs, metabolised by *O*-demethylation, *N*-de-ethylation, and amide hy-drolysis then conjugated with glucuronic acid and sulphate; in rabbits, possibly the formation of N^4-acetyl derivatives; in animals there appears to be significant first pass metabolism in the liver.

EXCRETION. After an oral dose of 10 mg, 50% is excreted unchanged in 8 hours; after an intramuscular dose of 40 mg, about 24% is excreted in the urine unchanged in 24 hours; in rats and dogs about 50% is excreted as unchanged drug and the remainder is excreted mainly as *N*-dealkylated or *O*-demethylated metabolites.

FURTHER INFORMATION. Review of effects and phar-macokinetics—R. M. Pinder *et al.*, *Drugs*, 1976, **12**, 81.

Actions and uses. Metoclopramide increases gastric motility and accelerates gastric emptying. This action is antagonised by atropine. It also has an anti-emetic action that is due partly to its local action on the gastro-intestinal tract and partly to a direct action on the central nervous system.

Metoclopramide is used in the radiographic examination of the stomach and duodenum, to promote rapid emp-tying of the stomach, and as an aid to duodenal intuba-tion. It is used to prevent nausea and vomiting induced by drugs, radiation, anaesthesia, or disease. It is also used to restore gastric motility in vagotomised patients and in post-operative conditions.

Doses are expressed in terms of the equivalent of anhydrous metoclopramide hydrochloride; 1.05 milli-grams of metoclopramide hydrochloride is approxi-mately equivalent to 1 milligram of anhydrous meto-clopramide hydrochloride. The usual dose for an adult is 10 milligrams 3 times a day by mouth or by intramuscular or intravenous injection.

The usual daily dosage given by mouth in divided doses for children under 1 year is 2 milligrams, 1 to 5 years 2 to 6 milligrams, and 6 to 12 years 8 to 15 milligrams. The total daily dosage, especially in children and young adults, should not exceed 500 micrograms per kilogram body-weight.

Undesirable effects. Drowsiness and constipation may occur. Metoclopramide may rarely give rise to extra-pyramidal effects such as dystonias which disappear soon after the drug is withdrawn.

Precautions and contra-indications. To minimise the possibility of extrapyramidal effects the recommended dosage should not be exceeded and treatment should begin with reduced dosage. Metoclopramide should preferably not be given in conjunction with phenothia-zine derivatives.

Preparations

METOCLOPRAMIDE INJECTION: a sterile solution of meto-clopramide hydrochloride in water for injections free from dissolved air. It is sterilised by heating in an autoclave or by filtration.

Available in 2-ml ampoules containing metoclopramide hydrochloride equivalent to 5 mg of anhydrous meto-clopramide hydrochloride per ml.

A standard for this injection is given in the British Pharmacopoeia Addendum 1977

Containers and *Labelling*: see the entry on Injections for general information on containers and labelling.

Storage: it should be protected from light. Solutions showing a yellow discoloration should be discarded.

METOCLOPRAMIDE TABLETS: available as tablets containing metoclopramide hydrochloride equivalent to 10 mg of anhydrous metoclopramide hydrochloride.
A standard for these tablets is given in the British Pharmacopoeia Addendum 1977
Containers and *Storage:* see the entry on Tablets for general information on containers and storage. Containers should be airtight and light resistant.

OTHER PREPARATIONS available include a paediatric ELIXIR containing metoclopramide hydrochloride equivalent to 1 mg of anhydrous metoclopramide hydrochloride per ml, diluent water for preparations, life of diluted elixir 7 days; and an elixir containing metoclopramide hydrochloride equivalent to 5 mg of anhydrous metoclopramide hydrochloride in 5 ml, diluent for *Maxolon*® water for preparations, life of diluted elixir 7 days, and diluent for *Primperan*® syrup, life of diluted elixir 14 days.

Metronidazole

2-(2-Methyl-5-nitroimidazol-1-yl)ethanol

$C_6H_9N_3O_3 = 171.2$

OTHER NAMES: *Flagyl*®
Flagyl Compak® (with nystatin)
A standard is given in the British Pharmacopoeia 1973

Description. A white or creamy-white crystalline powder with a slight odour and a bitter and saline taste.

Solubility. Soluble, at 20°, in 100 parts of water, in 200 parts of alcohol, and in 250 parts of chloroform; very slightly soluble in ether.

Identification. TESTS. 1. Mix about 10 mg with 10 mg of zinc powder, 1 ml of water, and 0.25 ml of hydrochloric acid, heat in a water-bath for 5 minutes, cool in ice, add 0.5 ml of *sodium nitrite solution*, and remove the excess of nitrite with sulphamic acid; add 0.5 ml of the product to a mixture of 0.5 ml of *2-naphthol solution* and 2 ml of *sodium hydroxide solution*; an orange-red colour is produced.
2. Dissolve about 100 mg in 4 ml of 1N sulphuric acid, add 10 ml of *trinitrophenol solution* and allow to stand; a precipitate is produced which, after washing with water and drying at 105°, melts at about 150°.

MELTING-POINT. About 160°.

ULTRAVIOLET ABSORPTION. In 0.1N hydrochloric acid, maximum at 277 nm (E1%, 1cm = 380).

Determination in body fluids. COLORIMETRY. In urine —P. Durel *et al.*, *Br. J. vener. Dis.*, 1967, **43**, 111.

GAS CHROMATOGRAPHY. In plasma—K. K. Midha *et al.*, *J. Chromat.*, 1973, **87**, 491; N. F. Wood, *J. pharm. Sci.*, 1975, **64**, 1048.

Metabolism. ABSORPTION. Readily absorbed after oral administration.

BLOOD CONCENTRATION. After an oral dose of 200 mg, peak serum concentrations of about 5 to 7 µg/ml are

attained in 1 to 2 hours; during therapy with 400 mg daily, steady state serum concentrations are in the range 2 to 6 µg/ml; effective serum concentrations are in the range 2 to 20 µg/ml.

HALF-LIFE. Serum half-life, about 6 hours.

DISTRIBUTION. Widely distributed throughout the body; in blood it is evenly distributed between serum and red blood cells; metronidazole enters the cerebrospinal fluid and crosses the placenta; it is secreted in the milk in concentrations similar to those in serum and small amounts are secreted in the saliva; *protein binding*, in concentrations of 2 to 70 µg/ml, metronidazole is 1 to 4% bound to plasma proteins.

METABOLIC REACTIONS. Oxidation of the hydroxyethyl group to form 2-methyl-5-nitroimidazole-1-acetic acid, oxidation of the methyl group to form the hydroxymethyl and carboxylic acid metabolites, and glucuronic acid conjugation. Reduction of metronidazole may occur under anaerobic conditions, giving rise to reactive toxic metabolites.

EXCRETION. 50 to 80% of a dose is excreted in the urine as metronidazole and its metabolites; most of the dose is excreted unchanged; about 14% is eliminated in the faeces.

FURTHER INFORMATION. Absorption and excretion—J. A. McFadzean, *Medicine Today*, 1969, **3**, 10; metabolism and excretion in urine—J. E. Stambaugh *et al.*, *J. Pharmac. exp. Ther.*, 1968, **161**, 373; pharmacokinetics —D. E. Schwartz and F. Jaunet, *Chemotherapy*, *Basle*, 1976, **22**, 19 and P. G. Welling and A. M. Monro, *Arzneimittel-Forsch.*, 1972, **22**, 2128; plasma concentrations—N. F. Wood, *J. pharm. Sci.*, 1975, **64**, 1049; protein binding—D. R. Sanvordeker *et al.*, *J. pharm. Sci.*, 1975, **64**, 1797.

Actions and uses. Metronidazole is used in the treatment of trichomoniasis and amoebiasis and in the prophylaxis and treatment of anaerobic infections. It has activity against *Trichomonas vaginalis, Entamoeba histolytica, Giardia lamblia,* and the causative organisms of acute ulcerative gingivitis. Metronidazole is inactive against aerobic and facultatively anaerobic bacteria but it is used in the treatment of infections caused by anaerobic organisms, particularly species of *Bacteroides.*
It is well absorbed when given by mouth and about half the dose is excreted by the kidneys, so an effective concentration of the drug appears in the urine. Its presence in the vagina does not interfere with the normal acidophilic flora and it has no effect on *Candida* species.
In the treatment of infections due to *Trichomonas vaginalis,* metronidazole is given by mouth in a dosage of 200 milligrams 3 times a day for 7 days or alternatively 800 milligrams in the morning and 1.2 grams in the evening for 2 successive days; children may be given 10 to 15 milligrams per kilogram body-weight daily in divided doses for 7 days.
Microscopical examinations of the vaginal secretion should be made to confirm the diagnosis and cure and to eliminate the possibility of a gonorrhoeal infection. Many relapses may be due to reinfection by the male partner, who may show no clinical signs of infection but may also need treatment. In elderly patients hormone therapy may be necessary in order to clear up any concomitant vaginitis. In mixed trichomonal-candidial infections, a course of nystatin pessaries may be given concurrently.
Vincent's disease may also be treated with a 7-day course of metronidazole as described above.

For the treatment of intestinal and hepatic infections with *Entamoeba histolytica*, metronidazole is given in a dosage of 400 to 800 milligrams 3 times a day for 5 to 10 days. Children may be given 50 milligrams per kilogram body-weight daily in divided doses.

In the treatment of giardiasis, metronidazole is given as a single oral dose of 2 grams. The usual dose for children is 40 milligrams per kilogram body-weight.

Metronidazole is used, alone or in conjunction with other antimicrobials, in the treatment of infections involving susceptible anaerobic organisms, including septicaemia, brain abscesses, necrotising pneumonia, puerperal sepsis, pelvic abscesses, cellulitis, and post-operative wound infections. It is also used to prevent post-operative anaerobic infections after surgery.

The usual adult dose by mouth for the treatment of infections is 400 milligrams, 3 times a day for at least 7 days; the corresponding dose for children is 7 milligrams per kilogram body-weight 3 times a day.

For prophylaxis, an oral dose of 2 grams of metronidazole is given to adults 24 to 48 hours before surgery followed by 200 milligrams 3 times daily before and up to 7 days after surgery. The corresponding dose for children is 3.7 to 7.5 milligrams per kilogram body-weight every 8 hours.

If oral administration is not convenient metronidazole may be administered rectally as suppositories in a dosage of 1 gram 3 times a day for adults, and for children aged 6 to 12 years 500 milligrams 3 times a day for 3 days or until oral administration can be substituted.

Metronidazole may be administered by intravenous infusion for the prevention and treatment of anaerobic infections. A buffered intravenous infusion containing 0.5% of metronidazole may be administered in a dosage equivalent to 500 milligrams of metronidazole, infused over 20 minutes, every 8 hours and oral treatment substituted as soon as possible. The corresponding dose for children is 7.5 milligrams of metronidazole per kilogram body-weight every 8 hours.

Undesirable effects. Metronidazole may cause headache, malaise, transient rashes, anorexia, nausea, and gastro-intestinal disturbances. Consumption of alcohol increases nausea. The urine of patients taking large doses of the drug is stained brown. Metronidazole may cause peripheral neuropathy, especially at high doses; this slowly disappears after discontinuing treatment.

Precautions. Prolonged courses of treatment should be avoided as animal experiments have indicated that metronidazole is mutagenic. Alcohol should be avoided. It should be used with caution in nursing mothers.

Drug interactions. Metronidazole may enhance the activity of warfarin and other anticoagulants.

Veterinary uses. Metronidazole is used for the treatment of certain infections of the mouth in dogs and cats. The usual dose by mouth is 20 milligrams per kilogram body-weight daily for 10 to 20 days.

Preparations

METRONIDAZOLE TABLETS: available as tablets containing 200 and 400 mg of metronidazole; they may be coloured.

A standard for these tablets is given in the British Pharmacopoeia 1973

Containers and *Storage:* see the entry on Tablets for general information on containers and storage. Containers should be airtight.

Advice for patients: the tablets should be swallowed whole followed by a tumblerful of water and taken preferably after meals. They should be taken at regular intervals and the prescribed course completed. Intoler-

ance to alcohol may occur. Metronidazole may cause the urine to darken.

OTHER PREPARATIONS available include an INJECTION containing metronidazole 5 mg per ml in 100-ml bottles; SUPPOSITORIES containing metronidazole 500 mg and 1 g; and a special pack of TABLETS containing 21 tablets of metronidazole 200 mg with 14 pessaries containing nystatin 100 000 units.

Metropathia Haemorrhagica

see under UTERINE BLEEDING, ABNORMAL

Metrorrhagia

see under UTERINE BLEEDING, ABNORMAL

Metyrapone

2-Methyl-1,2-di(pyrid-3-yl)propan-1-one

$C_{14}H_{14}N_2O = 226.3$

OTHER NAME: *Metopirone®*

A standard is given in the British Pharmacopoeia 1973

Description. A white to light amber crystalline powder with a characteristic odour.

Solubility. Soluble, at 20°, in 100 parts of water, in 3 parts of alcohol, and in 3 parts of chloroform; soluble in dilute mineral acids.

Storage. It should be protected from light.

Identification. TEST. To 5 ml of a 1% solution in 1N sulphuric acid add a few drops of *potassium mercuri-iodide solution*; a cream-coloured precipitate is produced.

MELTING-POINT. About 51°.

ULTRAVIOLET ABSORPTION. In 0.1N hydrochloric acid, maximum at 260 nm (E1%, 1cm = 500).

Determination in body fluids. COLORIMETRY. In plasma: separation by thin-layer or paper chromatography—S. Szeberenyi *et al.*, *J. Chromat.*, 1969, **40**, 417.

GAS CHROMATOGRAPHY. In urine—D. M. Hannah and J. G. Sprunt, *J. Pharm. Pharmac.*, 1969, **21**, 877.

SPECTROFLUORIMETRY. In plasma—A. Meikle, *et al.*, *J. Lab. clin. Med.*, 1969, **74**, 515.

Metabolism. DISTRIBUTION. Metyrapone crosses the placenta in rabbits.

METABOLIC REACTIONS. Reduction to an active metabolite, 2-methyl-1,2-di(pyrid-3-yl)propan-1-ol followed by conjugation of both the metabolite and unchanged drug with glucuronic acid; metyrapone also appears to be oxidatively metabolised, the oxidation, in rats, being stimulated by phenobarbitone; the oxidised metabolites are unknown.

EXCRETION. After 6 doses of 750 mg given every 4 hours, about 40% is recovered in the urine in 48 hours; of the excreted material about 80% is the conjugated metabolite, 12% is the non-conjugated metabolite, 7% is metyrapone glucuronide, and 1% is unchanged.

Actions and uses. Metyrapone is a diagnostic agent used to investigate the function of the anterior lobe of the pituitary gland and in the investigation and treatment of Cushing's Syndrome. It inhibits 11β-hydroxylase, an enzyme necessary for the formation of cortisone and hydrocortisone from their precursors, and the resultant fall in the glucocorticoid blood level stimulates the anterior pituitary gland to secrete corticotrophin. This in turn stimulates production of further glucocorticoid precursors by the adrenal cortex and since metyrapone blocks conversion of these to cortisone and hydrocortisone they are excreted in the urine.

Estimation of urinary 17-hydroxycorticosteroids over the period of the test indicates whether or not the anterior pituitary is functioning effectively with regard to corticotrophin secretion.

Metyrapone also interferes with the formation of aldosterone but to a much lesser extent.

In the assessment of anterior pituitary lobe function and the diagnosis of hypopituitarism, it is usually administered by mouth in doses of 250 to 750 milligrams every 4 hours for 6 doses; children may be given up to 15 milligrams per kilogram body-weight every 4 hours for 6 doses.

In the treatment of resistant oedema the usual dosage is 2.5 to 4.5 grams daily in divided doses.

Undesirable effects. Nausea and vomiting may occur, with or without epigastric pain. Giddiness and hypotension may be experienced if adrenal function is impaired.

Precautions. Metyrapone may precipitate acute adrenal failure and should be used with great caution in patients with gross hypopituitarism. Metyrapone may impair the biosynthesis of foetal-placental steroids and should preferably be avoided during pregnancy.

Preparation

METYRAPONE CAPSULES: consisting of metyrapone, in powder, which may be mixed with a suitable inert diluent, enclosed in a soft capsule. The capsule shells may be coloured. Available as capsules containing 250 mg of metyrapone.
A standard for these capsules is given in the British Pharmacopoeia 1973
Containers and Storage: see the entry on Capsules for general information on containers and storage. Containers should be light resistant.

Mexenone

2-Hydroxy-4-methoxy-4'-methylbenzophenone

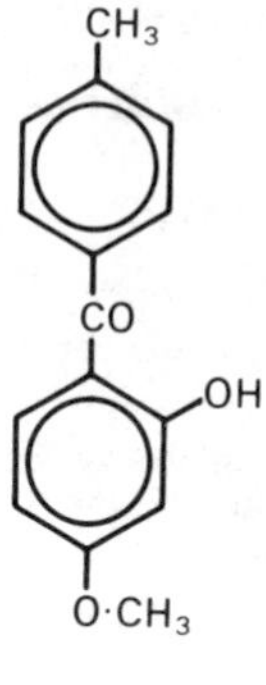

$C_{15}H_{14}O_3 = 242.3$

OTHER NAME: Uvistat®

A standard is given in the British Pharmaceutical Codex 1973

Description. An odourless, pale yellow, crystalline powder.

Solubility. Practically insoluble in water; soluble, at 20°, in 70 parts of alcohol and in 7 parts of acetone.

Identification. ULTRAVIOLET ABSORPTION. In methyl alcohol, maximum at 287 nm (E1%, 1cm = 600).

Actions and uses. Mexenone is characterised by its ability to absorb ultraviolet radiation over a wide range of wavelengths and even in low concentrations shows a sharp cut-off at about 350 nanometres, as the wavelength approaches that of visible light.

It is used as a sun-screening compound in preparations designed to reduce the risk of sunburn and other light-induced dermatoses.

It is applied in a concentration of 4% in an aqueous cream basis. Owing to its low solubility it is not easily washed off the skin or removed by perspiration.

Preparations

MEXENONE CREAM: a dispersion of mexenone in a suitable water-miscible basis. Available as a cream containing 4% of mexenone.
A standard for this cream is given in the British Pharmaceutical Codex 1973
Containers, Labelling, and Storage: see the entry on Creams for general information on containers, labelling, and storage.
Advice for patients: the cream should be applied liberally and rubbed well into the skin when necessary and immediately after bathing.

OTHER PREPARATIONS available include a lipstick APPLICATION containing mexenone 4%.

Miconazole Nitrate

1-[2,4 - Dichloro - β - (2,4 - dichlorobenzyloxy) phenethyl]-imidazole nitrate

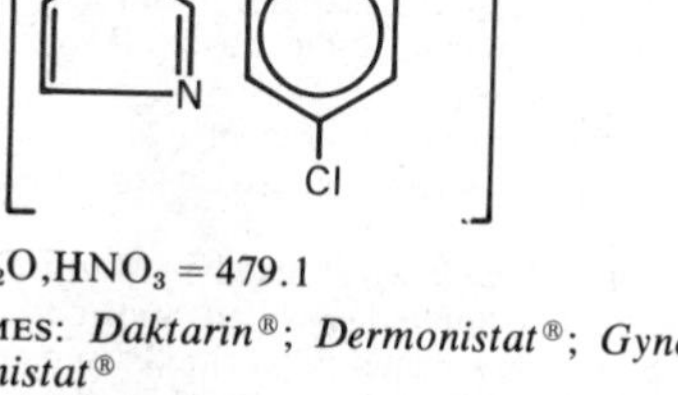

$C_{18}H_{14}Cl_4N_2O,HNO_3 = 479.1$

OTHER NAMES: Daktarin®; Dermonistat®; Gyno-Daktarin®; Monistat®
Daktacort® (with hydrocortisone)

A standard is given in the British Pharmacopoeia Addendum 1978

Description. An odourless white microcrystalline powder.

Solubility. Very slightly soluble in water; soluble in 140 parts of alcohol; very slightly soluble in ether and in chloroform.

Storage. It should be stored in airtight containers, protected from light.

Identification. TEST. To about 3 mg add 2 drops of sulphuric acid and 1 drop of a solution containing 500 mg of diphenylamine in a cooled mixture of 50 ml of sulphuric acid and 10 ml of water; an intense blue colour is produced.

MELTING-POINT. About 182°.

ULTRAVIOLET ABSORPTION. In a mixture of 1 volume of 0.1N hydrochloric acid and 9 volumes of methyl alcohol, maxima at 264 nm (E1%, 1cm = 10), 272 nm (E1%, 1cm = 14.5), and 280 nm (E1%, 1cm = 12).

INFRA-RED ABSORPTION. Major peaks at 826, 1087, 1299, 1316, 1370, and 1408 cm^{-1} (see Appendix 2b: Infra-red Spectra).

Metabolism. ABSORPTION. Very little is absorbed systemically following topical application.

BLOOD CONCENTRATION. After an intravenous infusion of about 500 mg of miconazole administered as the nitrate, serum concentrations of about 2 to 9 μg/ml are obtained after 15 minutes, falling to about 1 μg/ml at 4 hours; in subjects with renal function impairment, serum concentrations are increased.

HALF-LIFE. Biological half-life, about 25 hours.

DISTRIBUTION. Volume of distribution, about 1500 litres which is reduced to about 800 litres in renal function impairment.

METABOLIC REACTIONS. The principal urinary metabolites are 2,4-dichloromandelic acid and 2-(2,4-dichlorobenzyloxy)-2-(2,4-dichlorophenyl)acetic acid.

EXCRETION. In 6 days, about 14% to 20% of an oral dose is excreted in the urine and about 50% is eliminated in the faeces as unchanged drug and metabolites.

FURTHER INFORMATION. Absorption and excretion—J. Brugmans *et al.*, *Eur. J. clin. Pharmac.*, 1972, **5**, 93; pharmacokinetics—P. J. Lewi *et al.*, *Eur. J. clin. Pharmac.*, 1976, **10**, 49.

Actions and uses. Miconazole is an antifungal agent which also has antibacterial activity against some Gram-positive bacteria.
It is applied topically as a cream containing 2% in the treatment of superficial fungal infections of the skin, hair, and nails. A vaginal cream containing 2% is used in the treatment of vulvo-vaginal candidiasis.

Undesirable effects. Local irritation and occasionally sensitisation may occur at the site of application.

Preparations

MICONAZOLE CREAM: a dispersion of miconazole nitrate in a suitable water-miscible basis. It contains 2% of miconazole nitrate.
Containers, Labelling, and *Storage:* see the entry on Creams for general information on containers, labelling, and storage.
Advice for patients: when used in skin infections, the cream should be applied sparingly and gently rubbed into the affected area. The prescribed course should be completed. When used in nail infections, the cream should be applied sparingly to the affected nail and a non-porous dressing applied. Treatment should not be discontinued without the advice of the prescriber. For the treatment of vaginal infections, the cream should be applied high into the vagina with a suitable applicator, preferably at night. The prescribed course should be completed.

OTHER PREPARATIONS available include a CREAM containing miconazole nitrate 2% with hydrocortisone 1%; PESSARIES containing miconazole nitrate 100 mg; a combination pack consisting of a cream and a POWDER each containing miconazole nitrate 2%; and a combination pack consisting of a cream containing miconazole nitrate 2% with pessaries containing miconazole nitrate 100 mg.

Migraine

see under HEADACHE

Millimoles and Milliequivalents

The strengths of intravenous infusion fluids are sometimes expressed in terms of the number of millimoles or milliequivalents.
A *mole* (mol) is the basic unit of amount of substance of a specified chemical formula, containing the same number of formula units (atoms, molecules, ions, electrons, quanta, or other entities) as there are in 12 g of the pure nuclide ^{12}C. A *millimole* (mmol) is one thousandth of this amount and for ions it is the ionic weight, that is, the sum of the atomic weights of the elements of an ion, expressed in milligrams. A *milliequivalent* (mEq) is this quantity divided by the valency of the ion, that is, the number of milliequivalents in a given amount of ion is equal to the number of millimoles multiplied by the valency of that ion.
An *osmol* is the molecular weight of a substance divided by the number of chemical species (ions or non-ionised substances) formed from a molecule of the substance on dissolution. In ideal solutions of electrolytes the milliosmol (mosmol) has the same value as the milliequivalent.
The *osmolarity* of a solution is expressed as the number of osmols (or of milliosmols) per litre. Solutions containing approximately 300 milliosmols per litre are isotonic with blood serum and tears.

Use of Table of Millimoles and Milliequivalents

EXAMPLE. To prepare a solution containing 67 mmol sodium, 6 mmol potassium, 2 mmol calcium, and 77 mmol chloride.

Millimoles required				Salts and quantities used
Ca^{2+}	K$^+$	Na$^+$	Cl$^-$	
2			4	CaCl$_2$,2H$_2$O 2×147 mg = 0.294 g
	6		6	KCl 6×74.5 mg = 0.447 g
		67	67	NaCl 67×58.5 mg = 3.920 g

Conversion Equations

To convert percentage strength w/v of a solution of a salt to millimoles or milliequivalents per litre of the specified ion the following equations may be used:

$$\text{Millimoles per litre} = \frac{C \times 10\,000}{W_1}$$

$$\text{Milliequivalents per litre} = \frac{C \times 10\,000}{W_2}$$

and to convert millimoles or milliequivalents per litre to percentage strength w/v, the following equations:

$$\text{Percentage strength w/v} = \frac{W_1 \times M}{10\,000} \text{ or} \frac{W_2 \times E}{10\,000}$$

Ion	Weight of Millimole (mmol) in mg	Weight of Milliequivalent (mEq) in mg	Salt	Milligrams of salt containing	
				1 mmol = W_1*	1 mEq = W_2*
				of specified ion	
Ca^{2+}	40.0	20.0	Calcium Acetate, $C_4H_6CaO_4$	158	79
			Calcium Chloride, $CaCl_2,2H_2O$	147	73.5
			Calcium Gluconate, $C_{12}H_{22}CaO_{14},H_2O$	448	224
			Calcium Lactate, $C_6H_{10}CaO_6,5H_2O$	308	154
K^+	39.1	39.1	Potassium Acetate, $C_2H_3KO_2$	98	98
			Potassium Bicarbonate, $KHCO_3$	100	100
			Potassium Bromide, KBr	119	119
			Potassium Chloride, KCl	74.5	74.5
			Potassium Citrate, $C_6H_5K_3O_7,H_2O$	108	108
			Potassium Gluconate, $C_6H_{11}KO_7$	234	234
Mg^{2+}	24.3	12.15	Magnesium Acetate, $C_4H_6MgO_4,4H_2O$	214	107
			Magnesium Chloride, $MgCl_2,6H_2O$	203	101.5
			Magnesium Sulphate, $MgSO_4,7H_2O$	246	123
Na^+	23.0	23.0	Sodium Acetate, $C_2H_3NaO_2,3H_2O$	136	136
			Sodium Acid Citrate, $C_6H_6Na_2O_7,1½H_2O$	131	131
			Sodium Acid Phosphate, $NaH_2PO_4,2H_2O$	156	156
			Sodium Bicarbonate, $NaHCO_3$	84	84
			Sodium Chloride, $NaCl$	58.5	58.5
			Sodium Citrate, $C_6H_5Na_3O_7,2H_2O$	98	98
			Sodium Hydroxide, $NaOH$	40	40
			Sodium Lactate†	112	112
			Sodium Phosphate, $Na_2HPO_4,12H_2O$	179	179
			Sodium Salicylate, $C_7H_5NaO_3$	160	160
			Sodium Sulphate, $Na_2SO_4,10H_2O$	161	161
NH_4^+	18.0	18.0	Ammonium Chloride, NH_4Cl	53.5	53.5
Cl^-	35.5	35.5	Ammonium Chloride, NH_4Cl	53.5	53.5
			Calcium Chloride, $CaCl_2,2H_2O$	73.5	73.5
			Magnesium Chloride, $MgCl_2,6H_2O$	101.5	101.5
			Potassium Chloride, KCl	74.5	74.5
			Sodium Chloride, $NaCl$	58.5	58.5
$C_2H_3O_2^-$ (Acetate)	59.0	59.0	Calcium Acetate, $C_4H_6CaO_4$	79	79
			Magnesium Acetate, $C_4H_6MgO_4,4H_2O$	107	107
			Potassium Acetate, $C_2H_3KO_2$	98	98
			Sodium Acetate, $C_2H_3NaO_2,3H_2O$	136	136
$C_6H_5O_7^{3-}$ (Citrate)	189.1	63.0	Potassium Citrate, $C_6H_5K_3O_7,H_2O$	324	108
			Sodium Citrate, $C_6H_5Na_3O_7,2H_2O$	294	98
$C_6H_6O_7^{2-}$ (Acid citrate)	190.1	95.0	Sodium Acid Citrate, $C_6H_6Na_2O_7,1½H_2O$	263	131.5
$C_3H_5O_3^-$ (Lactate)	89.0	89.0	Calcium Lactate, $C_6H_{10}CaO_6,5H_2O$	154	154
			Sodium Lactate†	112	112
HCO_3^-	61.0	61.0	Potassium Bicarbonate, $KHCO_3$	100	100
			Sodium Bicarbonate, $NaHCO_3$	84	84
HPO_4^{2-}	96.0	48.0	Sodium Phosphate, $Na_2HPO_4,12H_2O$	358	179
$H_2PO_4^-$	97.0	97.0	Sodium Acid Phosphate, $NaH_2PO_4,2H_2O$	156	156

* W_1 may be calculated by dividing the molecular weight of the salt used by the number of the specified ions in a molecule of the salt. W_2 may be obtained by dividing W_1 by the valency of the specified ion.

† Prepared in solution by neutralising lactic acid with sodium hydroxide; 1.0 ml of 1M sodium lactate contains the equivalent of 112 mg.

where C = percentage strength w/v,
W_1 = milligrams of salt containing 1 mmol of the specified ion,
W_2 = milligrams of salt containing 1 mEq of specified ion,
E = milliequivalents per litre, and
M = millimoles per litre.

Concentration of Ions in Intravenous Fluids

Intravenous fluid	Approximate number of millimoles per litre					
	Ca^{2+}	K^+	Na^+	H^+†	Cl^-	HCO_3^-*
Sodium Bicarbonate Injection (1.4%)			167			167
Sodium Chloride Injection (0.9%)			154		154	
Sodium Chloride (0.18%) and Dextrose (4.3%) Injection			31		31	
Compound Sodium Lactate Injection	2	5	131		112	29
M/6 Ammonium Chloride				167	167	
M/6 Sodium Lactate			167			167

† H^+ equivalent   * HCO_3^- (or equivalent as lactate)

Mineral Deficiencies

Calcium. The treatment of calcium deficiency is described under Calcium Gluconate.
Other salts used as calcium supplements include calcium chloride, calcium lactate, and calcium sodium lactate.

Iron. See Anaemia.

Potassium. Deficiency of potassium ions gives rise to muscular weakness, paraesthesia, and cardiac arrhythmias. It is therefore desirable to give potassium supplements to replace loss as a result of diarrhoea, vomiting, or the use of diuretics that cause potassium loss. The treatment of potassium deficiency is described under Potassium Chloride.

Sodium. Sodium ions play an important part in maintaining the osmotic effect of the blood and hence the distribution of fluid in the cellular tissues. It is thus essential to replace any excessive loss of sodium salts due to severe sweating or to deficiency of corticosteroids, as in Addison's disease. The treatment of sodium deficiency is described under Sodium Chloride.

Fluorine. The use of fluoride for the prophylaxis of dental caries is described under Sodium Fluoride.

Iodine. Deficiency of iodide gives rise to simple goitre (enlargement of the thyroid gland which is not associated with clinical hypothyroidism or hyperthyroidism). It may be treated by the use of salt iodised with sodium iodide or iodate, or alternatively by small doses of potassium iodide.

Minocycline Hydrochloride

6 - Demethyl - 6 - deoxy - 7 - dimethylaminotetracycline hydrochloride

$C_{23}H_{28}ClN_3O_7 = 493.9$

OTHER NAME: *Minocin*®

Description. A yellow crystalline powder.

Solubility. Soluble in water; very slightly soluble in alcohol; practically insoluble in chloroform and in ether; soluble in solutions of alkali hydroxides and carbonates.

Storage. It should be stored in airtight containers, protected from light.

Identification. INFRA-RED ABSORPTION. Major peaks at 1220, 1400, 1466, 1520, 1590, and 1647 cm^{-1} (see Appendix 2a: Infra-red Spectra).

Metabolism. ABSORPTION. Readily and almost completely absorbed after oral administration; it is more rapidly absorbed than tetracycline and its absorption is less influenced by milk and foods than other tetracycline analogues; absorption is reduced by the presence of iron, aluminium, calcium, or magnesium salts.

BLOOD CONCENTRATION. After a single dose of 200 mg peak serum concentrations of 2 to 3 µg/ml are attained in about 2 hours; during therapy with 200 mg followed by 100 mg every 12 hours, plasma concentrations of 1 to 3 µg/ml are maintained; concentrations in resting subjects appear to be higher than those in ambulatory subjects; serum concentrations after oral or intravenous administration appear to be similar; therapeutic serum concentrations are in the range 0.5 to 3 µg/ml.

HALF-LIFE. Plasma half-life, 10 to 17 hours which may increase during continuous therapy or in subjects with renal function impairment.

DISTRIBUTION. Widely distributed throughout the body tissues and fluids; concentrations in cerebrospinal fluid are 25 to 30% of those in the serum; minocycline crosses the placenta and is secreted in milk, sebum, and sweat; it is taken up by skin and is stored in fat and adipose tissue; *protein binding*, 60 to 76% bound to plasma proteins.

METABOLIC REACTIONS. Partly metabolised to inactive metabolites; in dogs and rats, 20% of a dose is converted to 4-epiminocycline.

EXCRETION. Up to about 11% of a dose is excreted in the urine in 96 hours and about 35% is excreted in the faeces; excretion is increased by the administration of diuretics; minocycline is excreted to some extent in the bile.

FURTHER INFORMATION. Review of actions, uses, and pharmacokinetics—R. N. Brogden *et al.*, *Drugs*, 1975, **9**, 251.

Actions and uses. Minocycline has the actions and uses described under Tetracycline Hydrochloride but it is active against some strains that are resistant to tetracycline, including some pneumococci, *Haemophilus influenzae*, and methicillin-resistant staphylococci.
In the treatment of susceptible infections an initial dose of the equivalent of 200 milligrams of minocycline is given by mouth followed by 100 milligrams every 12 hours. A single dose of the equivalent of 200 to

400 milligrams of minocycline is effective in gonorrhoeal urethritis in the male. Minocycline should not be administered to children or in pregnancy.

Minocycline is rapidly absorbed after oral administration, peak blood concentrations being attained within 2 or 3 hours. The drug is partially metabolised within the body and readily diffuses into the tissues and fluids including the cerebrospinal fluid.

Salts of aluminium, calcium, iron, and magnesium and antacids which may decrease the absorption of tetracyclines from the gut, should not be given at the same time as minocycline.

Undesirable effects. As for Tetracycline Hydrochloride. In addition it may give rise to nausea, ataxia, dizziness, and vertigo. It may therefore reduce ability to drive motor cars or operate moving machinery.

Precautions and contra-indications. As for Tetracycline Hydrochloride.

Drug interactions. As for Tetracycline Hydrochloride.

Preparations

Preparations available include TABLETS containing minocycline hydrochloride equivalent to 100 mg of minocycline.

Mixtures

Mixtures are liquid preparations intended for administration by mouth. They consist of one or more medicaments dissolved or suspended in an aqueous vehicle or occasionally in a suitable non-aqueous vehicle.

Suspending agents. Insoluble substances which do not diffuse evenly throughout the aqueous vehicle when shaken should be finely powdered and mixed with compound tragacanth powder, sodium carboxymethylcellulose, or other suitable suspending agent; sodium starch glycollate and certain pregelatinised starches may be suitable in some cases.

FURTHER INFORMATION. Suspending agents as alternatives to tragacanth—C. A. Farley and W. Lund, *Pharm. J.*, i/1976, 562.

Preservation of mixtures. Mixtures, in common with other aqueous preparations, are liable to growth of bacteria and moulds unless adequately preserved. Mixtures that are prepared extemporaneously (including those for which complete recipes are given in this book) are not usually formulated to keep for long periods, but they are prepared with water of low bacterial content and most formulae include a preservative such as chloroform. When so indicated they should be recently prepared. Some mixtures are also subject to chemical decomposition and an expiry date may be specified; in some cases they must be freshly prepared.

FURTHER INFORMATION. Chloroform as a preservative in aqueous systems—M. Lynch *et al.*, *Pharm. J.*, ii/1977, 507.

FRESHLY PREPARED. The direction that a preparation must be freshly prepared indicates that it must be made not more than 24 hours before it is issued for use.

RECENTLY PREPARED. The direction that a preparation should be recently prepared indicates that deterioration is likely if the preparation is stored for longer than a few weeks under temperate room conditions.

Unless the keeping properties of a mixture under the appropriate conditions have been specially investigated it is suggested that the mixtures should be prepared

freshly or that (i) stock mixtures made up and stored in full airtight unopened bottles should be stored for not more than 3 months; (ii) stock mixtures in opened containers being used up progressively in the pharmacy should be used for not more than 2 weeks; and (iii) mixtures prepared freshly or dispensed from stock mixtures should not be used by patients for more than about 2 weeks from the date of issue.

WATER. Unless otherwise specified water for preparations is used. In some districts, the water supply may be unsuitable for preparing certain mixtures because of chemical incompatibility. A note is included in the formula where known that the preparation in question is likely to be affected in this manner.

Manufacture of mixtures. A number of entries provide a complete formula and directions for preparing a mixture that is required to be recently prepared. Manufacturers may add suitable preservatives and stabilising agents to these mixtures to extend the shelf life, but the preparations should not otherwise differ significantly in appearance and composition from mixtures prepared as directed in the relevant entries. Such additions should not interfere with any procedure which may be specified for checking the quality of a preparation.

Dilution of mixtures. Unless otherwise indicated in the entry describing a preparation, when a dose prescribed or ordered is less than or not a multiple of 5 millilitres, the mixture should be diluted with the vehicle used in the preparation of the mixture or that specified in the relevant entry as a diluent, so that the dose to be measured for the patient is one 5-ml spoonful or multiple thereof.

Advice on the stability of diluted mixtures is given, if known, in the relevant entries. In the absence of such advice, it should be assumed that the diluted mixture is less stable than the undiluted preparation.

Dilution should therefore be carried out immediately before the mixture is issued for use and not more than 2 weeks' supply should be issued at a time, unless otherwise indicated in the entry describing the preparation concerned.

Containers. Mixtures should be dispensed in plain bottles of colourless or amber glass.

Labelling of mixtures

A. The label on the container of a mixture, other than one which is directed to be freshly or recently prepared, should state: (1) the name and concentration of the active ingredient for mixtures other than those for which a full recipe is given in the entry describing the preparation; and (2) directions for storage.

If the mixture is one which is to be prepared freshly before issue to the patient from dry powder or granules, the label on the container of powder or granules should state: (1) the name of the preparation in the form of "Granules (or Powder) for the Mixture", as specified in the entry concerned; (2) the name and concentration of the active ingredient in the mixture when prepared according to the manufacturer's instructions; (3) directions for storage; and (4) the date after which the granules or powder should not be used.

The label on the container or on the package leaflet or the label on the carton should state: (1) the directions for preparing the mixture; (2) the directions for storage of the mixture; and (3) the period during which the mixture may be expected to retain its potency when stored under the stated conditions.

The label on the container of a mixture directed to be

recently prepared, but to which suitable preservatives and stabilising agents have been added should state: (1) the name and concentration of the added adjuvants; and (2) the date after which the preparation is not intended to be used.

B. The label on the container of a mixture issued to the patient on a prescription should state, in addition to the prescriber's directions: (1) any special storage directions as directed in the entry describing the preparation; (2) for suspensions, a direction to shake the bottle; (3) if such a recommendation is made by the manufacturer, the date after which the mixture should not be used; and (4) if the mixture has been diluted before issue "The contents to be discarded if not taken before ...... [a date 2 weeks, or other period specified by the manufacturer or in the entry describing the preparation, after the date of issue]".

Moniliasis

see CANDIDIASIS

Mononucleosis, Infective

see GLANDULAR FEVER

Monostearin, Self-emulsifying

A mixture consisting principally of mono-, di-, and tri-glyceryl esters of stearic and palmitic acids, with small quantities of the corresponding esters of oleic and other fatty acids; it also contains free fatty acids, free glycerol, and a small percentage of potassium, sodium, or triethanolamine oleate or stearate.

OTHER NAMES: *Abracol GMS®*; *Empilan SE 32®*; *Empilan SE 40®*; Glyceryl Monostearate Self-emulsifying; *Imwitor (Emulsifier) 960®*

A standard is given in the British Pharmaceutical Codex 1973

Description. A white to cream-coloured hard fat of waxy appearance with a faint fatty odour.

Solubility. Dispersible in hot water; soluble in hot dehydrated alcohol, in hot liquid paraffin, and, subject to turbidity at concentrations below 20%, in hot vegetable oils.

Incompatibility. Owing to the presence of soap, it is incompatible with acids, high concentrations of ionisable salts, with zinc oxide, and oxides of heavy metals.

Uses. Self-emulsifying monostearin is used as an emulsifying agent for oils, fats, solvents, and waxes in the preparation of bases of the non-emulsified, emulsified, and vanishing-cream types.

It produces stable, fine-grained creams, which are reasonably resistant to extremes of temperature. For ointments and more viscous creams, 5 to 20% of self-emulsifying monostearin may be used. It is not intended for inclusion in preparations for internal use. Aqueous preparations containing self-emulsifying monostearin should contain a preservative to prevent fungous or bacterial growth.

Preparation

Self-emulsifying monostearin is an ingredient of hydrocortisone lotion.

Monosulfiram

Tetraethylthiuram monosulphide

$$(C_2H_5)_2N \cdot \overset{\overset{S}{\|}}{C} \cdot S \cdot \overset{\overset{S}{\|}}{C} \cdot N(C_2H_5)_2$$

$C_{10}H_{20}N_2S_3 = 264.5$

OTHER NAME: *Tetmosol®*

A standard is given in the British Pharmacopoeia Addendum 1977 and the British Pharmacopoeia (Veterinary)

Description. A yellow or yellowish-brown solid with a sulphurous odour.

Solubility. Practically insoluble in water, in acids, and in alkali hydroxides; soluble in organic solvents.

Moisture content. Not more than 1%, determined by Fischer titration.

Storage. It should be stored in a cool place, protected from light.

Identification. TESTS. 1. Mix a small quantity with *dilute hydrochloric acid* and boil; hydrogen sulphide is evolved.
2. Dissolve about 100 mg in 5 ml of alcohol (95%) containing 3 drops of a 1% solution of copper sulphate, evaporate on a water-bath and dissolve the residue in chloroform; a deep yellowish-brown colour is produced.

ULTRAVIOLET ABSORPTION. In methyl alcohol, maximum at 281 nm (E1%, 1cm = 650).

Actions and uses. Monosulfiram is a parasiticide which is active against *Sarcoptes scabiei* and is used in the prophylaxis and treatment of scabies in adults and children. It is applied as a 25% solution in industrial methylated spirit; the solution is diluted with 2 to 3 parts of water before use. The patient's body is washed and dried and then the entire body except the face and scalp is painted with the dilute solution which is rubbed in well and left to dry.

This treatment may be repeated on 2 or 3 successive days.

Undesirable effects. Erythematous rashes may rarely occur.

Precautions. Alcohol should not be taken before and for at least 48 hours after the application of monosulfiram as there is a possibility that reactions similar to those caused by disulfiram may occur.

Contra-indications. It should not be used on patients who are hypersensitive to it or to disulfiram.

Poisoning. Solutions containing alcohol and monosulfiram may produce a disulfiram-like reaction when taken by mouth. The reaction includes vomiting, drowsiness, and sleep. Tachycardia, hypotension, and myocardial ischaemia may also occur. Symptomatic treatment may be required.

Veterinary uses. Monosulfiram is an insecticide. It is used as the soap and as an application prepared by diluting the 25% solution with 9 times its volume of water, for the treatment of mange in dogs and cats.

Preparations

MONOSULFIRAM SOAP: consisting of monosulfiram in a suitable toilet-soap basis. It may be perfumed. Available as a soap containing 5% of monosulfiram.
A standard for this soap is given in the British Pharmacopoeia (Veterinary)

Labelling: the label on the container, or the label on the immediate wrapper, should state the amount of the medicament as the proportion of monosulfiram in the preparation, and the directions for use.

MONOSULFIRAM SOLUTION: consisting of a solution of monosulfiram, with a suitable dispersing agent, in alcohol (95%). In making this preparation the alcohol (95%) may be replaced by industrial methylated spirit, provided that the law and the statutory regulations governing the use of industrial methylated spirit are observed. Available as a solution containing 25% w/w of monosulfiram.
A standard for this solution is given in the British Pharmacopoeia Addendum 1977 and the British Pharmacopoeia (Veterinary)
Labelling: the label on the container should state the amount of the medicament as the percentage w/w of monosulfiram, and the directions for use.
Advice for patients: the solution should be diluted with 2 to 3 parts of water before use. A hot bath should be taken and the body thoroughly dried prior to application. The diluted preparation should be applied to the entire body with the aid of a suitable brush. It should not be applied to the head and face or to broken or inflamed skin. It should not be applied near a naked flame. Alcohol should be avoided before and for 48 hours after application of monosulfiram.

Morbilli

see MEASLES

Morning Sickness

see under NAUSEA AND VOMITING

Morphine Hydrochloride

(4aR, 5S, 7aR, 8R, 9cS)-4a, 5, 7a, 8, 9, 9c-Hexahydro-12-methyl-8, 9c-iminoethanophenanthro[4, 5-*bcd*]furan-3, 5-diol hydrochloride trihydrate, a salt of the principal alkaloid of opium.

HCl, 3H$_2$O

$C_{17}H_{20}ClNO_3,3H_2O = 375.8$

OTHER NAMES: Morph. Hydrochlor.; Morphinii Chloridum

A standard is given in the European Pharmacopoeia Vol. I

Description. Odourless, colourless, silky crystals, crystalline powder, or cubical white masses, with a bitter taste.

Solubility. Soluble, at 20°, in 24 parts of water, in 100 parts of alcohol, and in 10 parts of glycerol; practically insoluble in ether and in chloroform.

Moisture content. 12 to 15%, determined by drying at 130°.

Dissociation constants. pK$_a$ 8.0, 9.9 (20°).

Incompatibility. It is incompatible with solutions of ammonia.

Sterilisation. Solutions for injection are sterilised by heating with a bactericide or by filtration.

Storage. It should be stored in airtight containers, protected from light.

Identification. TESTS. 1. Add a small amount of powdered sample to 0.5 ml of sulphuric acid containing 1 drop of *formaldehyde solution* in a porcelain dish; a purple colour is produced which changes to violet.
2. Dissolve a small amount in 5 ml of water and add 3 drops of a freshly prepared 1% solution of potassium ferricyanide and 1 drop of *ferric chloride solution*; a bluish-green colour is produced.
3. Dissolve about 20 mg in 5 ml of 0.1N sulphuric acid and add 0.5 ml of a saturated solution of potassium iodate; an amber colour is produced which reaches a maximum in about 5 minutes. Add 0.5 ml of *strong ammonia solution*; the colour darkens almost to black (distinction from codeine and diamorphine).

ULTRAVIOLET ABSORPTION. In water, maximum at 285 nm (E1%, 1cm = 41); in 0.1N sodium hydroxide, maximum at 298 nm (E1%, 1cm = 70).

THIN-LAYER CHROMATOGRAPHY. See under Thin-layer Chromatography, System 7.

Determination in body fluids. COLORIMETRY. In plasma or urine—L. A. Woods *et al.*, *J. Pharmac. exp. Ther.*, 1954, **111**, 64.

GAS CHROMATOGRAPHY. In urine—D. E. Fry *et al.*, *Clinica chim. Acta*, 1974, **51**, 183.

THIN-LAYER CHROMATOGRAPHY. In urine: detection and isolation of metabolites—U. Boerner *et al.*, *J. Pharm. Pharmac.*, 1974, **26**, 393.

HIGH PRESSURE LIQUID CHROMATOGRAPHY. In urine—I. Jane and J. F. Taylor, *J. Chromat.*, 1975, **109**, 37.

RADIOIMMUNOASSAY. In serum—S. Spector, *J. Pharmac. exp. Ther.*, 1971, **178**, 253.

Metabolism. ABSORPTION. Variably absorbed after oral administration; rapidly absorbed after subcutaneous or intramuscular administration.

BLOOD CONCENTRATION. After an oral dose of 10 mg as the sulphate, peak serum concentrations of free morphine of about 10 ng/ml are attained in 15 to 60 minutes; after an intramuscular dose of 10 mg, peak serum concentrations of 70 to 80 ng/ml are attained in 10 to 20 minutes; after an intravenous dose of 10 mg, serum concentrations of about 60 ng/ml are obtained in 15 minutes falling to 30 ng/ml after 30 minutes and to 10 ng/ml after 3 hours; subcutaneous doses give similar concentrations to intramuscular doses at 15 minutes but remain slightly higher during the following 3 hours; serum concentrations measured soon after administration correlate closely with the ages of the subjects studied and are increased in the aged.

HALF-LIFE. Serum half-life in the period 10 minutes to 6 hours following intravenous administration, 2 to 3 hours; serum half-life in the period 6 hours onwards, 10 to 44 hours.

DISTRIBUTION. Widely distributed throughout the body, mainly in the kidneys, liver, lungs, and spleen; lower concentrations appear in the brain and muscles; morphine crosses the placenta and traces are secreted in sweat and milk; *protein binding*, about 35% bound to albumin and to immunoglobulins at concentrations within the therapeutic range.

METABOLIC REACTIONS. Mainly glucuronic acid conjugation to form morphine-3- and 6-glucuronides, with sulphate conjugation, N-demethylation, O-methylation and N-oxide formation; glucuronide formation occurs in the intestinal mucosa and liver; N-demethylation occurs to a greater extent after oral than parenteral administration; the O-methylation pathway to form codeine has been challenged and codeine and norcodeine metabolites in urine may be formed from codeine impurities in the morphine sample studied.

EXCRETION. After an oral dose, about 60% is excreted in the urine in 24 hours, with about 3% excreted as free morphine in 48 hours; after a parenteral dose, about 90% is excreted in 24 hours, with about 10% as free morphine, 65 to 70% as conjugated morphine, 1% as normorphine and 3% as normorphine glucuronide; after the administration of large doses to addicts about 0.1% of a dose is excreted as norcodeine; urinary excretion of morphine appears to be pH dependent to some extent: as the urine becomes more acid more free morphine is excreted and as the urine becomes more alkaline more of the glucuronide conjugate is excreted; up to about 10% of a dose may be excreted in the bile.

FURTHER INFORMATION. Absorption and excretion—R. G. Twycross et al., Br. J. clin. Pharmac., 1974, **1**, 491; effects of amiphenazole and tacrine on metabolism—J. T. C. Woo et al., J. Pharm. Pharmac., 1968, **20**, 763; no interaction with propranolol—S. F. Brunk et al., Clin. Pharmac. Ther., 1974, **16**, 1039; no interaction with guanethidine—S. F. Brunk et al., J. clin. Pharmac., 1974, **14**, 581; metabolism to codeine and norcodeine—U. Boerner and R. L. Roe, J. Pharm. Pharmac., 1975, **27**, 215 and S. Y. Yeh, J. Pharm. Pharmac., 1975, **27**, 214; pharmacokinetics—B. A. Berkowitz et al., Clin. Pharmac. Ther., 1975, **17**, 629; protein binding—G. B. Olsen, Clin. Pharmac. Ther., 1974, **17**, 31.

Actions and uses. Morphine is a powerful analgesic and narcotic, but it also has central stimulant actions. It especially depresses the thalamus, sensory cortex, and respiratory and cough centres. It stimulates the spinal cord, the vagus and vomiting centres, and the third-nerve nucleus. Occasionally the stimulant actions are seen before or without the usual narcotic effects.

Morphine increases tone in involuntary muscle, especially the sphincters of the gastro-intestinal tract. It reduces secretions, except those of the skin glands. It dilates skin vessels, but, in therapeutic doses, it has little effect on the circulation as a whole.

Morphine is used to relieve pain, anxiety, and sleeplessness due to pain. It reduces all disagreeable sensations apart from skin irritation. Where sleeplessness is not due to pain, dyspnoea, or cough, morphine usually fails to induce sleep when used in ordinary doses. Its analgesic action reaches a maximum in about an hour and persists for 3 or 4 hours. It is more effective when injected than when taken by mouth.

Morphine is invaluable in such emergencies as cardiac asthma and acute abdominal conditions such as perforation, and in the treatment of severe trauma, for which it should be given in doses of 15 to 20 milligrams by mouth or by subcutaneous or intramuscular injection. Children up to one year may be given 200 micrograms per kilogram body-weight, 1 to 5 years 2.5 to 5 milligrams, and 6 to 12 years 5 to 7.5 milligrams.

These doses may be repeated every 4 to 6 hours. Since it masks warning symptoms and physical signs, it is not given until a diagnosis has been made.

As a sedative and for pre-operative medication morphine is usually administered with atropine or hyoscine.

A dose of 5 to 10 milligrams of morphine hydrochloride often checks coughing, but for this action codeine is more commonly used. When the constipating effect of morphine is desired, it is often prescribed in a mixture containing kaolin.

Morphine has no local analgesic action and its use in local applications has no sound basis.

Undesirable effects. Tolerance is rapidly acquired and morphine produces marked euphoria and dependence (see below). Very young children are particularly susceptible to opiates; atypical and alarming effects sometimes occur in the elderly.

Morphine crosses the placenta and is secreted in the milk; it may cause respiratory depression and dependence in the newborn.

Precautions. Morphine should not be given to patients who are being treated with a monoamine-oxidase inhibitor, such as isocarboxazid, nialamide, phenelzine, or tranylcypromine, or within about 2 weeks of the discontinuation of such treatment.

Dependence. It may give rise to dependence of the morphine type, as described under Drug Dependence.

Poisoning. If the drug has been taken by mouth, the stomach should be washed out; a 0.2% solution of potassium permanganate is commonly used for this purpose. A saline purgative may then be administered to reduce absorption from the gastro-intestinal tract.

The most important aspect of treatment is to guard the patient from respiratory failure; for this reason naloxone or levallorphan should be used only when respiration is dangerously depressed. Artificial respiration may be required.

Preparations

AMMONIUM CHLORIDE AND MORPHINE MIXTURE (Syn. Mistura Tussi Sedativa):

Ammonium chloride	30 g
Chloroform and morphine tincture	30 ml
Ammonium bicarbonate	20 g
Liquorice liquid extract	50 ml
Water for preparations	to 1000 ml

It should be recently prepared.

A standard for this mixture is given in the British Pharmaceutical Codex 1973

Containers and Labelling: see the entry on Mixtures for general information on containers and labelling.

Dose: 10 to 20 millilitres.

Advice for patients: the mixture should not be used for longer than a few days without medical advice.

CHLOROFORM AND MORPHINE TINCTURE (Syn. Chlorodyne; Tinct. Chlorof. et Morph., B.P. '85):

Chloroform	125.0 ml
Morphine hydrochloride	2.29 g
Peppermint oil	1.0 ml
Anaesthetic ether	30.0 ml
Water for preparations	50.0 ml
Alcohol (90%)	125.0 ml
Liquorice liquid extract	125.0 ml
Treacle, of commerce	125.0 ml
Syrup	to 1000.0 ml

Dissolve the peppermint oil in the alcohol, add the water,

dissolve the morphine hydrochloride in the mixture, and add the chloroform and the anaesthetic ether. Mix the liquorice extract and the treacle with 400 ml of the syrup, add to the previously formed solution, mix thoroughly, add sufficient syrup to produce the required volume, and mix.

A standard for this tincture is given in the British Pharmacopoeia Addendum 1977 and in the British Pharmacopoeia (Veterinary)

Labelling: a direction to shake the bottle well before use should be given on the label.

Storage: it should be stored in airtight containers.

Dose: 0.3 to 0.6 millilitre.

Veterinary dose: horses and cattle 30 to 60 millilitres; foals and calves 15 to 30 millilitres; dogs 0.3 to 1.5 millilitres.

IPECACUANHA AND MORPHINE MIXTURE (*Syn.* Mistura Tussi Nigra):

Ipecacuanha tincture	20 ml
Chloroform and morphine tincture	40 ml
Liquorice liquid extract	100 ml
Water for preparations	to 1000 ml

It should be recently prepared.

A standard for this mixture is given in the British Pharmaceutical Codex 1973

Containers and *Labelling:* see the entry on Mixtures for general information on containers and labelling.

Dose: 10 millilitres.

Advice for patients: the mixture should not be used for longer than a few days without medical advice.

KAOLIN AND MORPHINE MIXTURE (*Syn.* Mistura Kaolini Sedativa):

Light kaolin or light kaolin (natural)	200 g
Chloroform and morphine tincture	40 ml
Sodium bicarbonate	50 g
Water for preparations	to 1000 ml

It should be recently prepared, unless the kaolin has been sterilised.

A standard for this mixture is given in the British Pharmaceutical Codex 1973

Containers: see the entry on Mixtures for general information on containers.

Labelling: see the entry on Mixtures for general information on labelling. A direction to shake the bottle should be given on the label.

Dose: 10 millilitres.

Advice for patients: the mixture should not be used for longer than a few days without medical advice.

KAOLIN AND MORPHINE POWDER FOR MIXTURE: see under Kaolin, Light

MORPHINE HYDROCHLORIDE SOLUTION:

Morphine hydrochloride	10 g
Dilute hydrochloric acid	20 ml
Alcohol (90%)	250 ml
Purified water, freshly boiled and cooled	to 1000 ml

Mix the alcohol with an equal volume of the water, add the dilute hydrochloric acid, dissolve the morphine hydrochloride in the mixture, add sufficient of the water to produce the required volume, and mix. It contains, in 2 ml, 20 mg of morphine hydrochloride.

A standard for this solution is given in the British Pharmaceutical Codex 1973

Storage: it should be protected from light.

MORPHINE SUPPOSITORIES: prepared as described in the entry on Suppositories by incorporating morphine hydrochloride or morphine sulphate in theobroma oil or

other suitable basis. Approximately 1.5 g of morphine hydrochloride or of morphine sulphate displaces 1 g of theobroma oil. The strength of the suppositories and the morphine salt contained in them must be specified by the prescriber.

Available as suppositories containing 15 and 30 mg of morphine sulphate.

A standard for these suppositories is given in the British Pharmaceutical Codex 1973

Containers and *Storage:* see the entry on Suppositories for general information on containers and storage.

OTHER PREPARATIONS: morphine hydrochloride is an ingredient of two of the four variants of diamorphine and cocaine elixir (see under Diamorphine Hydrochloride).

Morphine Sulphate

(4a*R*,5*S*,7a*R*,8*R*,9c*S*) - 4a,5,7a,8,9,9c - Hexahydro - 12-methyl-8,9c-iminoethanophenanthro[4,5-*bcd*]furan-3,5-diol sulphate pentahydrate, a salt of the principal alkaloid of opium.

$(C_{17}H_{19}NO_3)_2,H_2SO_4,5H_2O = 758.8$

OTHER NAME: Morph. Sulph.

A standard is given in the British Pharmacopoeia 1973

Description. Odourless, white, acicular crystals, cubical masses, or crystalline powder, with a bitter taste.

Solubility. Soluble, at 20°, in 21 parts of water and in 1000 parts of alcohol; practically insoluble in ether and in chloroform.

Moisture content. 9 to 12%, determined by drying at 145°.

Incompatibility. It is incompatible with solutions of ammonia.

Sterilisation. Solutions for injection are sterilised by heating with a bactericide or by filtration.

Storage. It should be stored in airtight containers, protected from light.

Identification. TESTS. It complies with the tests described under Morphine Hydrochloride.

ULTRAVIOLET ABSORPTION. As for Morphine Hydrochloride.

INFRA-RED ABSORPTION. Major peaks at 786, 1070, 1108, 1175, 1313, and 1500 cm^{-1} (see Appendix 2a: Infra-red Spectra).

THIN-LAYER CHROMATOGRAPHY. See under Thin-layer Chromatography, System 7.

Determination in body fluids; Metabolism. As for Morphine Hydrochloride.

Actions and uses. Morphine sulphate has the actions and uses described under Morphine Hydrochloride and is used in similar dosage.

Undesirable effects; Precautions; Dependence; Poisoning. As for Morphine Hydrochloride.

Preparations

MORPHINE AND ATROPINE INJECTION:

Morphine sulphate	1.00 g
Atropine sulphate	0.06 g
Sodium metabisulphite	0.10 g
Sodium chloride	0.69 g
Water for injections	to 100.0 ml

Dissolve, and clarify by filtration. Sterilise by heating with a bactericide or by filtration.
A standard for this injection is given in the British Pharmaceutical Codex 1973
Containers and *Labelling:* see the entry on Injections for general information on containers and labelling.
Storage: it should be protected from light.
Dose: 0.5 to 1 millilitre by subcutaneous injection.

MORPHINE SULPHATE INJECTION (*Syn.* Morphine Injection): a sterile solution of morphine sulphate, with 0.1% of sodium metabisulphite, in water for injections. It is sterilised by heating with a bactericide or by filtration. Available in 1-ml ampoules containing 10, 15, 20, and 30 mg of morphine sulphate and in 2-ml ampoules containing 30 mg of morphine sulphate per ml.
A standard for this injection is given in the British Pharmacopoeia 1973
Containers and *Labelling:* see the entry on Injections for general information on containers and labelling.
Storage: it should be protected from light.

MORPHINE SUPPOSITORIES: see above under Morphine Hydrochloride.

Motion Sickness

see under NAUSEA AND VOMITING

Mouth-washes

Mouth-washes are usually aqueous solutions, in concentrated form, of substances with deodorant, antiseptic, local analgesic, or astringent properties.

Containers. Mouth-washes should be dispensed in white fluted bottles.

Labelling. When mouth-washes are dispensed, a direction should be given on the label, where appropriate, for diluting the mouth-wash before use. They should be labelled in a manner which clearly distinguishes them from preparations intended for internal administration.

Mumps

Mumps (Epidemic Parotitis) is an infectious disease occurring mainly in children and young adults. The causative organism is a myxovirus and is spread in infected droplets. The condition is infective from 2 to 3 days before the appearance of swollen parotids until 7 days after they return to normal size. The incubation period is between 12 and 28 days.
Swelling of the salivary glands, especially the parotid glands, is usually the first sign of the disease, and moderate fever may arise at onset and continue for a few days. In children the condition is often mild but in adults complications are more common. No specific treatment is required in uncomplicated cases.
Complications include viral infection of the pancreas accompanied by pain, vomiting, and anorexia. Infection of the central nervous system may give rise to meningo-encephalitis with intense headache and, in severe cases, delirium and hallucinatory disturbances. In men, orchiditis may occur with swelling of the testicles accompanied by pain, high fever, mild delirium, and, frequently, mental depression; in women, oophoritis may occur. Corticosteroids in large dosage and appropriate analgesics are usually required in such cases.

Mustine Hydrochloride

Bis(2-chloroethyl)methylammonium chloride

$$\left[CH_3 \cdot \overset{+}{N}H(CH_2 \cdot CH_2Cl)_2 \right] Cl^-$$

$C_5H_{12}Cl_3N = 192.5$

OTHER NAMES: Chlormethine; Mechlorethamine Hydrochloride; Nitrogen Mustard

A standard is given in the British Pharmacopoeia 1973

CAUTION. *Mustine hydrochloride is highly toxic; it is a powerful vesicant and a strong nasal irritant.*

Description. A white, crystalline, vesicant, hygroscopic powder or mass.

Solubility. Soluble in water.

Dissociation constant. pK_a 6.4 (25°).

Storage. It should be stored in airtight containers, in a cool place.

Identification. TESTS. 1. Dissolve about 50 mg in 5 ml of water and add 1 ml of *sodium hydroxide solution*; oily globules are formed, which dissolve on warming.
2. Dissolve about 50 mg in 5 ml of water and add 0.02 ml of *potassium mercuri-iodide solution*; a cream-coloured precipitate is produced.

MELTING-POINT. About 108°.

Metabolism. ABSORPTION. Absorbed to some extent from serous surfaces.

METABOLIC REACTIONS. After intravenous administration, mustine is rapidly metabolised to an ethylene-immonium ion which is very reactive and alkylates deoxyribonucleic acid.

Actions and uses. Mustine is a cytotoxic agent which acts mainly on proliferating cells by alkylating the nucleic acids of the chromosomes. When administered by intravenous injection it causes a fall in the number of circulating lymphocytes and depresses the activity of the bone marrow, resulting in granulocytopenia, thrombocytopenia, and anaemia.
Mustine is used in conjunction with other drugs such as prednisolone, procarbazine, vinblastine, and vincristine, in the treatment of Hodgkin's disease; it brings about a temporary remission of symptoms, but relapse may occur after a period of several months or years. Subsequent courses of treatment are usually less effective than the first. In the treatment of leukaemias and polycythaemia vera, mustine has been used as an alternative to irradiation.
The recommended dosage is 100 micrograms of mustine hydrochloride per kilogram body-weight by intravenous injection daily on 4 consecutive days, after which there should be a rest period of at least 6 weeks. Regardless of body-weight, a single dose should not exceed 10 milligrams. The response should be assessed by examination of bone-marrow smears and blood counts. Necrosis may occur if the solution is not sufficiently diluted and not carefully administered directly into the vein.
A solution containing 1 milligram per millilitre in sodium chloride injection is suitable for intravenous injection and a solution containing 1 milligram in 50 millilitres of sodium chloride injection may be given by slow intravenous infusion.

Undesirable effects. Mustine commonly causes nausea and vomiting; 0.5 to 1 milligram of hyoscine hydrobromide by subcutaneous injection or 4 to 8 milligrams of perphenazine by mouth may relieve these symptoms.

Other possible undesirable effects of mustine include liver damage, skin reactions, transient anorexia, light-headedness, drowsiness, and temporary amenorrhoea in women. Diarrhoea and gastric erosions may occur in some patients. Thrombophlebitis is a potential hazard if mustine is insufficiently diluted.

Mustine has a vesicant action on skin and mucous membrane, and care must be taken to avoid extravasation during injection. Should this occur, isotonic sodium thiosulphate solution (3%) should be infiltrated into the affected area, and ice compresses then applied.

Overdosage with mustine causes severe haemopoietic depression, leading to severe anaemia, lymphocytopenia, granulocytopenia, and thrombocytopenic purpura. The last mentioned may cause bleeding from mucous membranes, and the granulocytopenia may be severe enough to be fatal.

Precautions and contra-indications. Mustine hydrochloride should not be given to patients with acute leukaemia, or with severe bone-marrow depression. Dosage should be controlled by blood counts. It should not be used in pregnancy.

Preparation

MUSTINE INJECTION: a sterile solution of mustine hydrochloride in water for injections. It is prepared by dissolving the contents of a sealed container in water for injections immediately before use. Available as a powder in vials containing 10 mg of mustine hydrochloride.

A standard for this injection is given in the British Pharmacopoeia 1973
Containers: see the entry on Injections for general information on containers.
Labelling: see the entry on Injections for general information on labelling. In addition, the label on the sealed container should state that the contents are strongly vesicant.
Storage: the sealed container should be stored in a cool place. The injection decomposes on storage and should be used immediately after preparation.

Myasthenia Gravis

Myasthenia gravis is a condition in which muscles become fatigued too readily as a result of a defect in neuromuscular transmission. Transmission through the neuromotor end-plate is interrupted either because the quantity of acetylcholine released on stimulation is insufficient to ensure adequate contraction or because the presence of an excessive amount of cholinesterase renders it ineffective. All muscles including the respiratory muscles may be involved but the first to be affected are usually those controlled by the cranial nerves, resulting in ptosis, diplopia, and weakness of mastication, phonation, articulation, and deglutition.

The cause of the disorder has not been established, but there is some evidence of a breakdown in immune tolerance which may be related to a disorder of the thymus gland since a thymoma is often present. It has been suggested that antibodies to constituents of skeletal muscle, which have been found in the serum of many patients, may cause damage to acetylcholine receptors. Remissions commonly occur, and relapses may be precipitated by emotional disturbances, infection, pregnancy, or severe muscular effort.

Neuromuscular transmission may be restored by the administration of an anticholinesterase. Short-acting anticholinesterases such as edrophonium are used for the diagnosis of myasthenia gravis and longer-acting agents, including ambenonium, neostigmine, and pyridostigmine, are used for treatment.

An atropine-like drug will reverse the muscarinic effects of the anticholinesterases; 500 micrograms of atropine sulphate will reverse the effects of one milligram of neostigmine. Thymectomy will sometimes alleviate the disease but corticosteroids or plasmapheresis with immunosuppressants are sometimes used in subsequent treatment.

Myelofibrosis

see under MYELOPROLIFERATIVE DISEASES

Myeloid Leukaemia, Chronic

see under MYELOPROLIFERATIVE DISEASES

Myeloma, Multiple

see under LYMPHOPROLIFERATIVE DISEASES

Myelomatosis

see under LYMPHOPROLIFERATIVE DISEASES

Myeloproliferative Diseases

The myeloproliferative diseases are malignant neoplastic diseases of the cells of the bone marrow. They are classified according to the cell type which has undergone neoplastic change. They include acute and chronic myeloid leukaemia, myelofibrosis, polycythaemia vera, and primary thrombocythaemia.

Acute myeloid leukaemia (acute myeloblastic leukaemia) is described under Leukaemia, Acute.

Chronic myeloid leukaemia is a malignant proliferation of the bone marrow involving all the developing cells of the granulocyte series. It is characterised by general malaise, lassitude and weakness, splenomegaly, weight loss, anaemia, and a greatly raised white-cell count.
Chronic myeloid leukaemia is treated with antineoplastic drugs and radiotherapy. Busulphan is the drug of choice in inducing remission; it may later be used in lower dosage for maintenance therapy.
Chronic myeloid leukaemia may enter an acute blastic phase and should then be treated as described under Leukaemia, Acute.

Myelofibrosis (myelosclerosis) is a chronic myeloproliferative disease due to hyperplasia of the fibrous tissue in the bone marrow. It is associated with failure of erythropoiesis, splenomegaly, hepatomegaly, and extramedullary erythropoiesis. There is a resultant anaemia which is due to both bone-marrow failure and haemolysis. There may also be weakness, fatigue, anorexia, weight loss, and pallor.
The anaemia of myelofibrosis may be treated by blood transfusion, stimulation of the bone marrow with androgens, or splenectomy. If the white-cell count becomes high, busulphan may be given or the spleen may be irradiated.

Polycythaemia vera (polycythaemia rubra vera) is due to abnormal hyperplasia of the bone marrow and is characterised by an increase in concentration of all cells in the circulation particularly the reticulocytes (red cells). The patient develops a brick red or purplish complexion, prominent engorged veins, and splenomegaly. The viscosity of the blood is increased and lassitude, headache, dysphagia, breathlessness, or anginal pain may occur. There is also a tendency to arterial and venous thrombosis and haemorrhage.

The acute effects of polycythaemia rubra may be controlled by venesection, but this may result in a rise in the platelet count and in iron deficiency. The excessive bone-marrow proliferation may be depressed by the beta radiation of phosphorus-32 administered in the form of sodium phosphate (^{32}P) or by antineoplastic agents such as busulphan. Polycythaemia vera may develop into acute myeloblastic leukaemia or myelofibrosis.

Primary thrombocythaemia is a myeloproliferative disease characterised by a marked rise in the number of circulating platelets. This frequently produces a haemorrhagic state, commonly in the gastro-intestinal tract. There may also be splenomegaly. Primary thrombocythaemia is usually treated with sodium phosphate (^{32}P) as in polycythaemia vera. It follows a similar clinical course and may end in myelofibrosis.

Myelosclerosis

see under MYELOPROLIFERATIVE DISEASES

Myocardial Infarction

Myocardial infarction is a condition in which occlusion of a coronary vessel leads to destruction of heart muscle. The occlusion is usually due to thrombosis in atheromatous vessels (coronary thrombosis). If the affected area is not too large the remainder of the myocardium continues to function, but there is a decrease in cardiac output which may cause hypotension and shock. This may be accompanied by severe prolonged chest pain resembling anginal pain but differing in that it cannot be relieved by rest and the administration of coronary vasodilators. Nausea and vomiting may also occur.

Analgesics of the morphine type are required for relief of pain, and anti-emetics such as cyclizine are required for relief of vomiting. Shock, when present, should be treated as described under Circulatory Failure, Acute, and failure of the functional portion of the myocardium may be treated with cardiotonic drugs such as digitalis. Anti-arrhythmic drugs such as lignocaine may be required if serious arrhythmias occur.

Pressor drugs may be given to correct hypotension and atropine to reverse serious bradycardia. In serious cases, treatment with heparin followed by an oral anticoagulant may be of value in preventing mural thrombus, venous thrombosis, and embolisation.

Myoclonic Jerks

see under EPILEPSY

Myrrh

An oleo-gum-resin obtained from the stem of *Commiphora molmol* (Engl.) Engl. and possibly other species of *Commiphora* (Fam. Burseraceae), shrubs or small trees growing in north-eastern Africa and southern Arabia.

A standard is given in the British Pharmaceutical Codex 1973

Constituents. Myrrh contains 25 to 40% of resin, 57 to 61% of gum, 7 to 17% of volatile oil, a bitter principle, and 3 to 4% of impurities. The resin contains several complex acids including α-, β-, and γ-commiphoric, commiphorinic, α- and β-heerabomyrrholic acids and also resin phenols α- and β-heerabomyrrhol and heeraboresene. The gum has been likened to acacia and yields pentosans, galactan, xylan, and araban, an oxidising enzyme system, and protein.

The volatile oil contains eugenol, *m*-cresol, cuminaldehyde, cinnamaldehyde, pinene, dipentene, and esters of formic, acetic, and myrrholic acids.

Both volatile oil and resin yield the same characteristic violet reaction with bromine vapour. It may yield up to 9% of ash. Up to 4% of foreign organic matter may be present.

Description. Rounded or irregular tears, about 15 to 25 mm in diameter, or masses of agglutinated tears, up to about 100 mm across. Externally it is reddish-brown or reddish-yellow in colour, dry, and often covered with a fine dust. It breaks with a brittle fracture, exhibiting a granular, somewhat translucent surface, which is oily and of a rich brown colour and frequently exhibits whitish spots or veins.

Myrrh has an agreeably aromatic odour and an aromatic bitter acrid taste. When triturated with water, a yellowish emulsion is produced.

Adulterants and substitutes. Fahdli or Arabian myrrh occurs in small masses of agglutinated tears with a less dusty surface and free from whitish markings on the fractured surface. It is less bitter in taste and also less fragrant than genuine Somali myrrh.

Yemen myrrh occurs in large dusty pieces. It does not exhibit whitish streaks, does not exude oil when pressed with the finger-nail, and is less aromatic than myrrh.

Perfumed bdellium or bissabol closely resembles myrrh. It breaks with a waxy fracture and gives an oily exudate when pressed with the finger-nail. The whitish markings on the fractured surface are traversed by brown resin patches. It differs from myrrh both in odour and taste and does not respond to the colour test; it is probably obtained from *C. erythraea* (Ehrenb.) Engl. var. *glabrescens* Engl.

Opaque bdellium is a very hard, yellowish-brown, opaque gum-resin with a slight odour and a bitter taste. African bdellium occurs in hard pieces, translucent in thin layers and breaking with a dull slaty fracture; it has a bitter taste and an odour recalling that of pepper.

Indian bdellium occurs in irregular, reddish-brown masses. The fractured surface is hard and, like the outer surface, covered with minute, shiny points of resin. It has a slight cedar-like odour, which develops on keeping, and an acrid but not bitter taste.

Gum hotai occurs in liver-coloured opaque masses. It contains an acid resin and a saponin.

Finely powdered myrrh is deficient in volatile oil and may yield as much as 13% of ash.

Storage. It should be stored in a cool dry place.

Identification. TEST. Triturate 100 mg with 500 mg of sand, shake with 3 ml of ether, filter, allow the filtrate to evaporate to a thin film, and pass the vapour of bromine over the film; a violet colour is produced.

Actions and uses. Myrrh is astringent to the mucous membranes; the tincture is used in mouth-washes and gargles for application to ulcers in the mouth and pharynx.

Preparation

MYRRH TINCTURE:

Myrrh, crushed	..	..	..	..	200 g
Alcohol (90%)	..	..	..	..	to 1000 ml

Macerate the myrrh with 800 ml of the alcohol in a closed vessel for 7 days, with frequent shaking; filter, and pass sufficient of the alcohol through the filter to produce the required volume.
A standard for this tincture is given in the British Pharmaceutical Codex 1973
Dose: 2.5 to 5 millilitres.

Myxoedema

see HYPOTHYROIDISM

Nalidixic Acid

1-Ethyl-7-methyl-4-oxo -1,8-naphthyridine- 3 -carboxylic acid

$C_{12}H_{12}N_2O_3 = 232.2$

OTHER NAME: *Negram*®

A standard is given in the British Pharmaceutical Codex 1973

Description. An odourless, almost white or very pale yellow, crystalline powder.

Solubility. Practically insoluble in water; very slightly soluble in alcohol; soluble, at 20°, in 25 parts of chloroform and in 350 parts of acetone; very slightly soluble in solutions of alkali hydroxides.

Dissociation constant. pK_a 6.0.

Storage. It should be stored in airtight containers, protected from light.

Identification. MELTING-POINT. About 228°.

ULTRAVIOLET ABSORPTION. In 0.1N sodium hydroxide, maxima at 258 nm (E1%, 1cm = 1125) and 334 nm (E1%, 1cm = 492).

INFRA-RED ABSORPTION. Major peaks at 806, 1250, 1429, 1471, 1613, and 1695 cm^{-1} (see Appendix 2b: Infra-red Spectra).

Determination in body fluids. HIGH PRESSURE LIQUID CHROMATOGRAPHY. In plasma or urine: nalidixic acid and hydroxynalidixic acid—L. Shargel *et al.*, *J. pharm. Sci.*, 1973, **62**, 1452.

Metabolism. ABSORPTION. Readily absorbed after oral administration but absorption appears to be delayed in subjects with shigellosis; administration of bicarbonate appears to increase absorption.

BLOOD CONCENTRATION. After an oral dose of 1 g, peak plasma concentrations of unchanged drug plus hydroxy-

lated nalidixic acid in conjugated or unconjugated form reach about 20 to 35 µg/ml in 1 to 2 hours; about 85% of this is unchanged drug; after 2 days' therapy with 1 g 4 times daily, plasma concentrations are about twice those obtained after a single 1-g dose; therapeutic concentrations are in the range 4 to 30 µg/ml.

HALF-LIFE. Plasma half-life of free nalidixic acid plus hydroxynalidixic acid, about 90 minutes.

DISTRIBUTION. Negligible amounts enter the cerebrospinal fluid and very little is secreted in milk; *protein binding*, nalidixic acid together with its hydroxylated metabolite are 75 to 95% bound to plasma proteins and may displace warfarin.

METABOLIC REACTIONS. Hydroxylation and glucuronic acid conjugation; hydroxynalidixic acid is an active metabolite.

EXCRETION. 80% of a dose is excreted in the urine in 24 hours mostly as glucuronide conjugate; 11 to 33% is excreted in active form; active urinary concentrations are still attained in renal function impairment.

FURTHER INFORMATION. Absorption by infants in acute shigellosis—J. D. Nelson *et al.*, *Clin. Pharmac. Ther.*, 1972, **13**, 879; plasma concentrations and excretion—P. T. Männistö *et al.*, *Clin. Pharmac. Ther.*, 1976, **19**, 37.

Actions and uses. Nalidixic acid is an antibacterial agent which is effective against infections by Gram-negative organisms, including *Escherichia coli, Enterobacter aerogenes, Klebsiella pneumoniae, Salmonella typhimurium, Shigella flexneri,* and species of *Proteus.* After oral administration it is rapidly absorbed and excreted by the kidneys, so that antibacterial concentrations are not reached in the tissues.
Nalidixic acid is used for the treatment of infections of the urinary tract and gastro-intestinal tract when these are due to susceptible organisms. The usual dose for adults is 1 gram 4 times a day; children may be given 60 milligrams per kilogram body-weight daily in divided doses. When treatment is prolonged in chronic conditions these doses should be halved.
Nalidixic acid has also been used in the treatment of brucellosis.

Undesirable effects. Nausea, vomiting, dizziness, drowsiness, weakness, pruritus, and rashes may occur.
Disturbances of the central nervous system, including visual disturbances, excitement, depression, confusion, and hallucinations, may occur but these reactions are transient and reversible.
Photosensitivity reactions may occur.

Precautions and contra-indications. It should not be given to neonates and should be used with caution in young children.

Preparations

NALIDIXIC ACID MIXTURE: a suspension of nalidixic acid in a suitable coloured flavoured vehicle. It may contain a suitable preservative.
When a dose less than or not a multiple of 5 ml is prescribed, the mixture may be diluted, as described in the entry on Mixtures, with syrup. The diluted mixture must be freshly prepared. Available as a mixture containing 300 mg of nalidixic acid in 5 ml.
A standard for this mixture is given in the British Pharmaceutical Codex 1973
Containers and *Labelling:* see the entry on Mixtures for general information on containers and labelling.
Advice for patients: the mixture should be taken at regular intervals, preferably after meals. For the treat-

ment of acute infections the prescribed course should be completed. In chronic conditions treatment should not be discontinued without the advice of the prescriber. The mixture may affect mental concentration; persons affected should not drive or operate machinery. Direct exposure to sunlight should be avoided during treatment.

NALIDIXIC ACID TABLETS: may be prepared by moist granulation and compression as described in the entry on Tablets. Available as tablets containing 500 mg of nalidixic acid; they may be coloured.

A standard for these tablets is given in the British Pharmaceutical Codex 1973

Containers and *Storage:* see the entry on Tablets for general information on containers and storage. Containers should be airtight and light resistant.

Advice for patients: the advice given under Nalidixic Acid Mixture (above) should be followed.

Nalorphine Hydrobromide

N-Allylnormorphine hydrobromide

$C_{19}H_{22}BrNO_3 = 392.3$

OTHER NAME: *Lethidrone®*

A standard is given in the British Pharmacopoeia 1973

Description. An odourless, white to creamy-white, crystalline powder.

Solubility. Soluble, at 20°, in 24 parts of water and in 35 parts of alcohol. Crystals of the dihydrate may be deposited from aqueous solutions; the anhydrous salt separates from solutions of the dihydrate in dehydrated alcohol.

Moisture content. Not more than 1%, determined by drying at 100° *in vacuo.*

Specific rotation. −100° to −105°, determined on a 1% solution in methyl alcohol.

Dissociation constant. pK_a 7.8 (20°).

Sterilisation. Solutions for injection are sterilised by heating in an autoclave or by filtration.

Storage. It should be stored in airtight containers, protected from light.

Identification. TESTS. 1. To 5 ml of a 3% solution add 1 drop of *dilute ammonia solution;* a bulky white precipitate is produced. Add *sodium hydroxide solution;* the precipitate dissolves.

2. To 5 ml of a 3% solution add 1 drop of *ferric chloride test-solution;* a blue colour is produced.

MELTING-POINT. About 260°, with decomposition.

ULTRAVIOLET ABSORPTION. In water, maximum at 285 nm (E1%, 1cm = 39); in 0.1N sodium hydroxide, maximum at 298 nm (E1%, 1cm = 60).

THIN-LAYER CHROMATOGRAPHY. See under Thin-layer Chromatography, System 7.

Metabolism. ABSORPTION. Poorly absorbed after oral administration but rapidly absorbed after subcutaneous injection.

BLOOD CONCENTRATION. Peak concentrations are attained in 15 to 30 minutes.

DISTRIBUTION. Rapidly taken up by the brain and at a faster rate than morphine; crosses the placenta.

METABOLIC REACTIONS. In rats and cats, *N*-dealkylation; in rats, dogs, and cats glucuronic acid conjugation; and in rabbits and cats glucuronic acid and sulphate conjugation.

EXCRETION. 2 to 6% of a dose is excreted unchanged in the urine.

FURTHER INFORMATION. Urinary metabolites in cats and dogs—S. Y. Yeh and L. A. Woods, *J. pharm. Sci.,* 1971, **60**, 148.

Actions and uses. Nalorphine reduces or abolishes most of the characteristic actions of morphine, other opiates, and many related synthetic substances, such as pethidine and methadone, and thus substantially lessens the toxicity of such drugs. It has no comparable action against the toxic effects of ether, cyclopropane, and barbiturates.

Nalorphine has analgesic properties similar to those described under Morphine Hydrochloride, but it is unsuitable for use as an analgesic because of its unpleasant side-effects. Because of the side-effects it has been largely replaced as a narcotic antagonist by naloxone which is now the drug of choice for this purpose.

Nalorphine hydrobromide is given by intravenous injection in doses of 5 to 10 milligrams in the treatment of poisoning by morphine or its substitutes. It acts within 20 seconds, and the dose may have to be repeated, depending on the severity of the intoxication, up to a total of 40 milligrams.

It is also used in the treatment of respiratory depression due to opiates and in opiate-induced respiratory depression in the newborn. Ten minutes or so before the expected time of delivery, nalorphine hydrobromide may be given to the mother in a dose of 10 milligrams, intravenously, or it may be injected into the umbilical vein of the newborn infant in a dose of 0.25 to 1 milligram. The dose for children from 1 to 12 years is 200 micrograms per kilogram body-weight by intravenous injection, up to a maximum of 10 milligrams.

Nalorphine is used in the diagnosis of drug dependence, as it provokes prompt and possibly severe withdrawal symptoms in the addict.

Undesirable effects. These include sweating, restlessness, pallor, nausea, bradycardia, hypotension, and disturbing psychotic effects. Although it antagonises respiratory depression due to morphine and similar drugs, nalorphine is itself a potent respiratory depressant.

Veterinary uses. Nalorphine hydrobromide is used as an antagonist to morphine and other drugs with a similar action. The usual dose by subcutaneous, intramuscular, or intravenous injection for dogs is 2 to 3 milligrams per kilogram body-weight.

Preparation

NALORPHINE INJECTION: a sterile solution of nalorphine hydrobromide in water for injections. The acidity of the solution is adjusted to pH 3 by the addition of hydrobromic acid. The solution is sterilised by heating in an autoclave or by filtration.

Available in 1-ml ampoules containing 10 mg of nalorphine hydrobromide, in 5-ml vials containing 1 mg of nalorphine hydrobromide per ml, and in 5-ml packs for veterinary use containing 20 mg of nalorphine hydrobromide per ml.

A standard for this injection is given in the British Pharmacopoeia 1973

Containers and *Labelling:* see the entry on Injections for general information on containers and labelling.

Storage: it should be protected from light.

Naloxone Hydrochloride

(−)-*N*-Allyl-7,8-dihydro-14-hydroxynormorphinone hydrochloride

$C_{19}H_{22}ClNO_4 = 363.8$

OTHER NAME: *Narcan*®

Description. A white or slightly off-white powder.

Solubility. Soluble in water, in alcohol, and in dilute acids and strong alkalis; practically insoluble in chloroform and in ether.

Storage. It should be stored in airtight containers, protected from light.

Identification. TEST. To 1 ml of a 1% solution add 1 drop of *ferric chloride solution*; a purplish-blue colour is produced.

MELTING-POINT. About 202°.

INFRA-RED ABSORPTION. As naloxone, major peaks at 922, 940, 1050, 1244, 1460, and 1728 cm⁻¹ (see Appendix 2a: Infra-red Spectra).

Determination in body fluids. GAS CHROMATOGRAPHY. In urine—G. J. DiGregorio and C. O'Brien, *J. Chromat.*, 1974, **101**, 424.

Metabolism. ABSORPTION. Rapidly absorbed after oral administration.

HALF-LIFE. Plasma half-life, 70 to 100 minutes.

DISTRIBUTION. Volume of distribution, about 200 litres.

METABOLIC REACTIONS. *N*-Dealkylation, keto-reduction at the 6 position, and glucuronic acid conjugation; naloxone appears to be subject to extensive first-pass metabolism.

EXCRETION. Up to about 70% of a dose is excreted in the urine in 72 hours, mainly as conjugates; metabolites in urine include the glucuronides of naloxone and of 7,8-dihydro-14-hydroxynormorphinone and *N*-allyl-7,8-dihydro-14-hydroxynormorphine.

FURTHER INFORMATION. Pharmacokinetics—J. Fishman *et al.*, *J. Pharmac. exp. Ther.*, 1973, **187**, 575 and S. H. Weinstein *et al.*, *J. pharm. Sci.*, 1973, **62**, 1416.

Actions and uses. Naloxone is an antagonist of morphine and other narcotic analgesics. Its action resembles that of nalorphine and levallorphan but it is more potent and it does not give rise to respiratory depression. It is used to reduce or abolish the actions of natural and synthetic narcotics, pentazocine, and dextropropoxyphene and so reduce their toxicity.

In the treatment of narcotic overdosage, the usual initial dose administered to adults by subcutaneous, intramuscular, or intravenous injection is 400 micrograms, repeated at intervals of 2 to 3 minutes if the respiratory function does not improve. If improvement does not occur after 2 to 3 doses, causes other than narcotic overdosage may be responsible for the patient's condition. The initial dose of naloxone for children is 5 to 10 micrograms per kilogram body-weight; doses may be repeated at intervals of 2 to 3 minutes if necessary. As naloxone is more rapidly eliminated than long-acting narcotics such as methadone, further doses may be required at intervals to maintain reversal of the effects of the narcotic.

When naloxone hydrochloride is administered postoperatively the dose should be calculated for each patient to obtain or retain optimum respiratory function whilst maintaining analgesia. The usual initial intravenous dose is 1.5 to 3 micrograms per kilogram body-weight, and further doses of 1.5 micrograms per kilogram body-weight may be given at intervals of not less than 2 minutes. Doses may be given by intramuscular injection after 1 to 2 hours if required.

Naloxone should be given to mothers during the second stage of labour to correct respiratory depression in the newborn caused by narcotics used to produce obstetric analgesia.

Precautions. It should be administered with caution to patients who are pregnant or who have received large doses of narcotics. In patients physically dependent on narcotics an acute withdrawal syndrome may be induced by too rapid a reversal of narcotic effects.

Contra-indications. Naloxone hydrochloride should not be administered to patients who are known to be hypersensitive to it.

Preparation

NALOXONE INJECTION: a sterile solution of naloxone hydrochloride in water for injections. Available in 1-ml ampoules containing 400 micrograms of naloxone hydrochloride, and in 2-ml ampoules containing 20 micrograms of naloxone hydrochloride per ml.

Containers and *Labelling:* see the entry on Injections for general information on containers and labelling.

Storage: it should be protected from light.

Nandrolone Decanoate

3-Oxoestr-4-en-17β-yl decanoate

$C_{28}H_{44}O_3 = 428.7$

OTHER NAME: *Deca-Durabolin*®

A standard is given in the British Pharmacopoeia 1973

Description. A white to creamy-white crystalline powder with a faint characteristic odour.

Solubility. Very slightly soluble in water; soluble, at 20°, in 1 part of alcohol; soluble in ether, in chloroform, in fixed oils, and in esters.

Specific rotation. +32° to +36°, determined on a 2% solution in dioxan.

Sterilisation. Oily solutions for injection are sterilised by dry heat.

Storage. It should be stored under nitrogen at a temperature between 2° and 10° and protected from light.

Identification. TEST. Dissolve about 25 mg in 1 ml of methyl alcohol, add 2 ml of *semicarbazide acetate solution*, heat under a reflux condenser for 30 minutes, and cool; a precipitate is produced which, after recrystallisation from acetone, melts at about 175°.

MELTING-POINT. About 35°

ULTRAVIOLET ABSORPTION. In dehydrated alcohol, maximum at 240 nm (E1%, 1cm = 407).

THIN-LAYER CHROMATOGRAPHY. See under Thin-layer Chromatography, System 10.

Actions and uses. Nandrolone decanoate has the actions, uses, undesirable effects, and contra-indications described under Methandienone, but it is not active when given by mouth. It is usually given by intramuscular injection in doses of 50 to 100 milligrams and its action lasts for 3 or 4 weeks. For infants the dose is 400 micrograms per kilogram body-weight every 3 weeks. Jaundice has not been reported after its use.

Drug interactions. Nandrolone decanoate may enhance the anticoagulant effect of warfarin and similar anticoagulants.

Preparation

NANDROLONE DECANOATE INJECTION: a sterile solution of nandrolone decanoate in ethyl oleate or other suitable ester, in a suitable fixed oil, or in any mixture of these. It is sterilised by dry heat. Available in 1-ml ampoules and 1-ml disposable syringes containing 25 and 50 mg of nandrolone decanoate.
A standard for this injection is given in the British Pharmacopoeia 1973
Containers: see the entry on Injections for general information on containers.
Labelling: see the entry on Injections for general information on labelling. In addition, the label on the package should state the composition of the solvent, and that the injection is for intramuscular use only.
Storage: it should be protected from light.

Nandrolone Laurate

3-Oxoestr-4-en-17β-yl dodecanoate

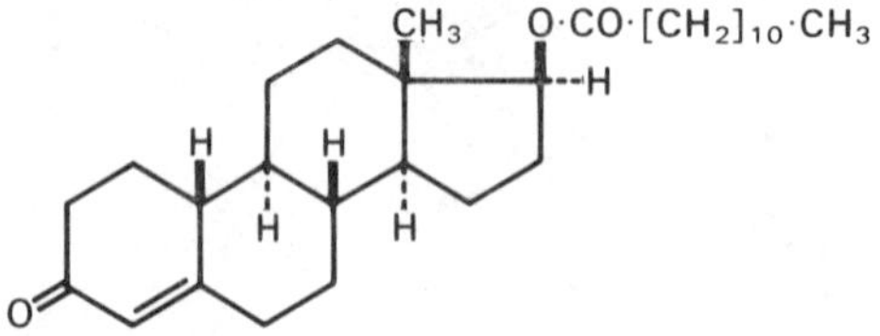

$C_{30}H_{48}O_3 = 456.7$

OTHER NAME: *Laurabolin®*

A standard is given in the British Pharmacopoeia (Veterinary)

Description. A white to creamy-white crystalline powder with a faint characteristic odour.

Solubility. Practically insoluble in water; soluble, at 20°, in 1 part of alcohol; soluble in chloroform, in ether, in fixed oils, and in esters of fatty acids.

Specific rotation. +31° to +35°, determined on a 2% solution in dioxan.

Sterilisation. Oily solutions for injection are sterilised by dry heat.

Storage. It should be protected from light.

Veterinary uses. Nandrolone laurate is an anabolic steroid used in the treatment of convalescent or debilitated animals. The usual dose by subcutaneous or intramuscular injection for all species is 0.2 to 1 milligram per kilogram body-weight, repeated every 2 or 3 weeks according to the response of the animal.

Preparation

NANDROLONE LAURATE INJECTION: a sterile solution of nandrolone laurate in ethyl oleate or other suitable ester, in a suitable fixed oil, or in any mixture of these. It is sterilised by dry heat. Available in 10-ml vials containing 25 and 50 mg of nandrolone laurate per ml.
A standard for this injection is given in the British Pharmacopoeia (Veterinary)
Containers and *Labelling:* see the entry on Injections for general information on containers and labelling.
Storage: it should be stored at a temperature of 2° to 8°, protected from light.

Nandrolone Phenylpropionate

3-Oxoestr-4-en-17β-yl phenylpropionate

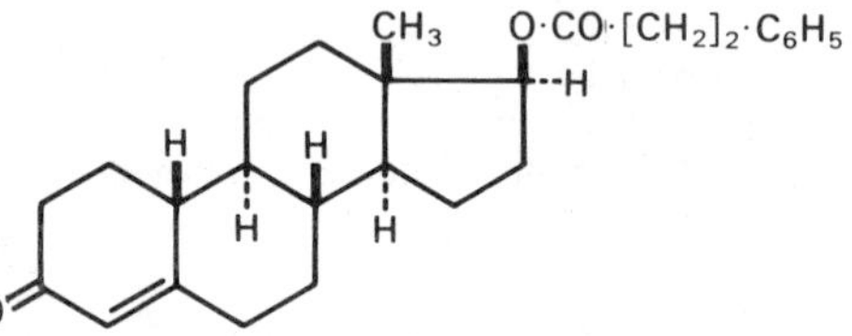

$C_{27}H_{34}O_3 = 406.6$

OTHER NAMES: *Durabolin®*; *Nandrolin®*; Nandrolone Phenpropionate

A standard is given in the British Pharmacopoeia 1973

Description. A white to creamy-white crystalline powder with a characteristic odour.

Solubility. Very slightly soluble in water; soluble, at 20°, in 20 parts of alcohol.

Specific rotation. +48° to +51°, determined on a 1% solution in dioxan.

Sterilisation. Oily solutions for injection are sterilised by dry heat.

Storage. It should be protected from light.

Identification. TEST. Carry out the test described under Nandrolone Decanoate; the precipitate melts at about 182°.

MELTING-POINT. About 97°.

ULTRAVIOLET ABSORPTION. In dehydrated alcohol, maximum at 240 nm (E1%, 1cm = 430).

INFRA-RED ABSORPTION. Major peaks at 999, 1052, 1254, 1282, 1495, and 1614 cm⁻¹ (see Appendix 2a: Infra-red Spectra).

THIN-LAYER CHROMATOGRAPHY. See under Thin-layer Chromatography, System 10.

Actions and uses. Nandrolone phenylpropionate has the actions, uses, undesirable effects, and contra-indications described under Methandienone, but it is not active when given by mouth. It is usually given by intramuscular injection in a dosage of 25 to 50 milligrams weekly. Jaundice has not been reported after its use.

Drug interactions. Nandrolone phenylpropionate may enhance the anticoagulant effect of warfarin and similar anticoagulants.

Veterinary uses. As for Nandrolone Laurate. Doses are repeated every 1 to 2 weeks according to the response of the animal.

Preparation

NANDROLONE PHENYLPROPIONATE INJECTION: a sterile solution of nandrolone phenylpropionate in ethyl oleate or other suitable ester, in a suitable fixed oil or in any mixture of these. It is sterilised by dry heat. Available in 1-ml ampoules and 1-ml disposable syringes containing 25 mg of nandrolone phenylpropionate, in 1-ml disposable syringes containing 50 mg of nandrolone phenylpropionate, and, for veterinary use, in 10-ml vials containing 25 mg of nandrolone phenylpropionate per ml and in 25-ml vials containing 50 mg of nandrolone phenylpropionate per ml.
A standard for this injection is given in the British Pharmacopoeia 1973
Containers: see the entry on Injections for general information on containers.
Labelling: see the entry on Injections for general information on labelling. In addition, the label on the package should state the composition of the solvent and that the injection is for intramuscular use only.
Storage: it should be protected from light.

Naphazoline Nitrate

2-(Naphth-1-ylmethyl)-2-imidazoline nitrate

$C_{14}H_{15}N_3O_3 = 273.3$

OTHER NAME: *Antistin-Privine*® (with antazoline sulphate)

A standard is given in the British Pharmacopoeia 1973

Description. An odourless white crystalline powder with a bitter taste.

Solubility. Soluble, at 20°, in 36 parts of water and in 16 parts of alcohol; very slightly soluble in ether and in chloroform.

Acidity. A 1% solution has a pH of 5 to 6.5.

Dissociation constant. pK_a 10.9 (20°).

Sterilisation. Solutions are sterilised by heating with a bactericide or by filtration.

Storage. It should be stored in airtight containers, protected from light.

Identification. TEST. Dissolve about 300 mg in 25 ml of water, add 3 ml of *sodium hydroxide solution*, extract

with two 25-ml portions of chloroform, and evaporate the chloroform extracts to dryness; the residue, after drying for 1 hour at 80°, melts at about 120°.

MELTING-POINT. About 168°.

ULTRAVIOLET ABSORPTION. In 0.01N hydrochloric acid, maxima at 271 nm (E1%, 1cm = 215), 281 nm (E1%, 1cm = 250), 288 nm (E1%, 1cm = 175), and 291 nm (E1%, 1cm = 170).

Actions and uses. Naphazoline has a potent vasoconstrictor action comparable with that of adrenaline, but it does not produce prolonged vasoconstriction at the site of subcutaneous or intramuscular injection.
Naphazoline nitrate is applied in the form of nasal drops containing 0.05 or 0.1% to reduce local swelling and congestion in cases of acute or chronic rhinitis of allergic or inflammatory origin, vasomotor rhinitis, and rhinosinusitis.
It is also used as eye-drops containing 0.05% to relieve inflammation of the cornea.

Undesirable effects. Naphazoline differs from the sympathomimetic amines in producing some central nervous depression after overdosage or accidental oral ingestion; drowsiness or even coma may result.

Precautions. Frequent or prolonged use of naphazoline is undesirable as it usually gives rise to congestion of the mucosa and a return of symptoms; for this reason the smallest effective concentration should be used at intervals of not less than 4 to 6 hours.

Preparations

Preparations available include a SOLUTION containing naphazoline nitrate 0.025% with antazoline sulphate 0.5%.

Naproxen

(+)-2-(6-Methoxynaphth-2-yl)propionic acid

$C_{14}H_{14}O_3 = 230.3$

OTHER NAME: *Naprosyn*®

A standard is given in the British Pharmacopoeia Addendum 1978

Description. An odourless, white, crystalline powder.

Solubility. Practically insoluble in water; soluble, at 20°, in 25 parts of alcohol, in 15 parts of chloroform, in 40 parts of ether, and in 20 parts of methyl alcohol.

Specific rotation. +63° to +68.5°, determined on a 4-dm layer of a 1% solution in chloroform.

Storage. It should be protected from light.

Identification. MELTING-POINT. About 156°.

ULTRAVIOLET ABSORPTION. In methyl alcohol, maxima at 262 nm (E1%, 1cm = 227), 271 nm (E1%, 1cm = 230), 316 nm (E1%, 1cm = 65), and 331 nm (E1%, 1cm = 75).

INFRA-RED ABSORPTION. Major peaks at 820, 1160, 1178, 1196, 1386, and 1729 cm⁻¹ (see Appendix 2a: Infra-red Spectra).

THIN-LAYER CHROMATOGRAPHY. See under Thin-layer Chromatography, System 3.

Metabolism. ABSORPTION. Readily absorbed after oral administration or as suppositories; administration of bicarbonate appears to increase the rate of absorption whilst the administration of magnesium or aluminium hydroxides appears to delay absorption; the absorption of naproxen appears to be only slightly delayed in non-fasting subjects.

BLOOD CONCENTRATION. After an oral dose of 500 mg, peak plasma concentrations of 60 to 80 μg/ml are attained in about 2 hours; after administration of 500 mg rectally, peak concentrations of about 65 μg/ml are attained in 2 hours; the plasma concentration is dose-dependent at concentrations up to about 90 μg/ml.

HALF-LIFE. Plasma half-life, 10 to 15 hours.

DISTRIBUTION. Naproxen has a small volume of distribution, it is secreted in milk in concentrations of about 1% of those in plasma, and it crosses the placenta; naproxen appears to be subject to enterohepatic circulation; *protein binding*, about 99% bound to plasma proteins at concentrations within the therapeutic range but at high doses the percentage bound is decreased.

METABOLIC REACTIONS. *O*-Demethylation and conjugation mainly with glucuronic acid.

EXCRETION. After an intravenous dose, about 95% is excreted in the urine in 5 days with about 1 to 2% in the faeces; about 10% is excreted unchanged, 60% is conjugated naproxen, 5% is desmethylnaproxen, and about 20% is conjugated desmethylnaproxen.

FURTHER INFORMATION. Absorption in children—B. M. Ansell *et al.*, *Curr. med. Res. Opinion*, 1975, **3**, 46; absorption in man—J. P. Desager *et al.*, *J. clin. Pharmac.*, 1976, **16**, 189; metabolism—E. J. Segre, *J. clin. Pharmac.*, 1975, **15**, 316; review—R. N. Brogden *et al.*, *Drugs*, 1975, **9**, 326.

Actions and uses. Naproxen is an analgesic with anti-inflammatory properties and has the actions and uses described under Ibuprofen but is more effective.

When given by mouth, naproxen is well absorbed and as it has a relatively long half-life it is effective when doses are given twice daily.

The usual dose for adults is 250 milligrams twice daily, the first dose being taken with the morning meal and the second dose 12 hours later. The dose may be increased to 375 to 750 milligrams daily according to the response. The usual dose for children between the ages of 5 and 16 years is 5 milligrams per kilogram body-weight twice daily.

Undesirable effects; Precautions. As for Ibuprofen. Gastro-intestinal haemorrhage is a rare complication and it is often tolerated by patients with peptic ulcer or intolerance to major anti-inflammatory drugs. Naproxen may prolong bleeding time owing to a decrease in platelet aggregation.

Preparations

NAPROXEN TABLETS: available as tablets containing 250 mg of naproxen; they may be coloured.
A standard for these tablets is given in the British Pharmacopoeia Addendum 1978
Containers and *Storage:* see the entry on Tablets for general information on containers and storage. Containers should be airtight and light resistant.
Advice for patients: the tablets should preferably be taken after meals.

OTHER PREPARATIONS available include a MIXTURE containing naproxen 125 mg in 5 ml, diluents water for preparations or a mixture of equal volumes of this and syrup, life of diluted mixture 14 days; and SUPPOSITORIES containing naproxen 500 mg..

Nasal Drops

Nasal drops are liquid preparations for instillation into the nostrils by means of a dropper. They may be aqueous or oily solutions and usually contain substances with antiseptic, local analgesic, or vasoconstrictor properties.

Oily nasal drops should not be used over long periods, as the oil retards the ciliary action of the nasal mucosa; drops of oil may enter the trachea and cause lipoid pneumonia.

Containers. Nasal drops should be supplied in coloured fluted glass bottles fitted with a plastic screw cap incorporating a glass dropper tube fitted with a rubber teat or in a plastic squeeze bottle fitted with a plastic cap incorporating a dropper device.

Nausea and Vomiting

Nausea and vomiting are common symptoms occurring as a result of various disturbances such as gastric irritation, irradiation ("radiation sickness"), or travel ("motion sickness") or in conditions such as pregnancy ("morning sickness").

Nausea and vomiting may also occur post-operatively or following the administration of certain drugs. They may be prevented or treated by the administration of anticholinergic drugs such as hyoscine, of antihistamines with an anti-emetic effect, or of metoclopramide. Metoclopramide may, however, produce, dystonic reactions in children. The most powerful of these drugs may also be effective in the treatment of post-operative vomiting and of radiation sickness.

Persistant nausea and vomiting may be an indication of a serious condition such as appendicitis, and if this is suspected it may be desirable to withhold treatment with·anti-emetic drugs until a diagnosis has been made.

Most anti-emetic drugs have a sedative action and are liable to affect the patient's ability to drive motor cars or operate moving machinery.

Neomycin Sulphate

A mixture of the sulphates of the antimicrobial substances produced by the growth of certain selected strains of *Streptomyces fradiae*. 500 milligrams of neomycin sulphate is approximately equivalent to 350 000 units of neomycin.

OTHER NAMES: *Mycifradin®*; *Myciguent®*; *Neobiotic®*; *Neojectin®*; *Neomin®*; Neomycini Sulfas; *Nivemycin®*; *Oranecin®*; *Tampovagan N®*; *Vonamycin®*
Antidiar with Neomycin® (with aluminium hydroxide gel); *Betnesol-N®* and *Betsolan®* (both with betamethasone sodium phosphate); *Dermamed®* (with bacitracin); *Gargon®* (with thiostrepton); *Graneodin®* (with gramicidin); *Hydromycin-D®* (with prednisolone acetate); *Ivax®*, *Kaomycin®*; and *Neovax®* (all with kaolin); *Mastikort 500/300®* (with procaine penicillin); *Nebacetin®* and *Neobacrin®* (both with zinc bacitracin); *Synalar-N®* (with fluocinolone acetonide); *Vetsovate®* (with betamethasone valerate). Names for some other preparations containing neomycin sulphate and one other medicament

are stated in the entries describing the relevant substances.

A standard is given in the European Pharmacopoeia Vol. II

Description. An almost odourless, hygroscopic, white or yellowish-white powder.

Solubility. Soluble in 3 parts of water; slowly soluble in 1 part of water; very slightly soluble in alcohol; practically insoluble in ether, in chloroform, and in acetone.

Acidity or alkalinity. A 10% solution has a pH of 5 to 7.5.

Moisture content. Not more than 6%, determined by drying at 60° over phosphorus pentoxide *in vacuo*.

Storage. It should be stored in airtight containers, protected from light, at a temperature not exceeding 30°.

Identification. TEST. Dissolve about 10 mg in 5 ml of water, add 2 drops of pyridine and 2 ml of a 0.1% solution of ninhydrin and heat on a water-bath at a temperature between 65° and 70° for 10 minutes; a deep violet colour is produced.

Metabolism. ABSORPTION. Only about 1 to 6% of an oral dose is absorbed; the remainder is eliminated unchanged in the faeces. Absorption does not appear to be affected by intestinal ulceration, by enteritis, or by antacids; absorption from enemas is similar to that following an oral dose; neomycin is not absorbed percutaneously.

BLOOD CONCENTRATION. After an oral dose of 2 g, plasma concentrations of about 1 μg/ml are attained in about 2 hours; after an intramuscular dose of 2 g, plasma concentrations of about 1 μg/ml are attained in about 2 hours; after an intramuscular dose of 0.5 to 1 g, plasma concentrations of about 20 μg/ml are attained which are maintained for about 8 hours.

HALF-LIFE. Biological half-life, about 2 hours.

DISTRIBUTION. May enter the cerebrospinal fluid; may accumulate in renal function impairment.

EXCRETION. Absorbed neomycin appears to be completely excreted in the urine in active form.

FURTHER INFORMATION. Absorption—K. J. Breen *et al.*, *Ann. intern. Med.*, 1972, **76**, 211; release from chewing gum—F. Wertalik and R. Bonorden, *J. pharm. Sci.*, 1968, **57**, 530.

Actions and uses. Neomycin is an aminoglycoside antibiotic belonging to the same group as gentamicin and having a wide antibacterial spectrum similar to that described under Gentamicin Sulphate. Other aminoglycoside antibiotics such as gentamicin, kanamycin, streptomycin, and tobramycin are preferred for systemic therapy as they have a greater margin of safety.

Neomycin is used typically for the control of staphylococcal infections and staphylococcal carriage. It is not absorbed after oral administration but may be administered by mouth for the suppression of bacterial growth in the large bowel prior to colonic surgery. However, because of the increasing prevalence of resistance in staphylococci and large bowel flora these uses are being abandoned.

As an intestinal antiseptic in gastro-intestinal infections the usual dose for an adult is 1 to 3 grams by mouth daily in divided doses. The usual dose for children aged 6 to 12 years is 500 milligrams 3 or 4 times daily (50 to 80 milligrams per kilogram body-weight daily).

For pre-operative bowel preparation the usual dose is 1 gram of neomycin sulphate every 4 hours; at least 6 doses are given. In the treatment of hepatic coma 1 gram may be given by mouth every 4 hours to reduce the absorption of protein breakdown products and up to 12 grams daily has been given, but continued use may cause serious malabsorption.

Neomycin is used locally in a concentration of 0.25% to 0.5%, often with other antibiotics such as bacitracin or polymyxin, which may reduce the chance of resistant strains developing.

Undesirable effects. Continued oral use of neomycin may result in supra-infection with *Candida albicans*.

Precautions. Neomycin should not be used in the systemic treatment of infections because of its toxic effect on the kidneys and eighth cranial nerve and its liability to give rise to hypersensitivity. Application to extensive raw areas, wounds, and cavities and oral administration for long periods should be avoided, especially in the presence of ulceration, in the elderly, and in patients with renal disease, as it may give rise to symptoms of ototoxicity.

Local application should be limited to the treatment of neomycin-sensitive staphylococcal infections and prolonged topical use should be avoided as it leads to skin sensitisation which may be obscured but not prevented by the concomitant use of corticosteroids.

Veterinary uses. Neomycin sulphate is an antibacterial used mainly in the control of enteritis due to *Escherichia coli*. The usual dose by mouth for all species is 10 milligrams per kilogram body-weight daily but it should not be administered by mouth to adult ruminants. The usual dosage by intramuscular injection for all species is 10 milligrams per kilogram body-weight daily.

Preparations

CHLORHEXIDINE AND NEOMYCIN CREAM: containing 0.1% of chlorhexidine hydrochloride with 0.5% of neomycin sulphate in a suitable water-miscible basis. This cream should not be diluted.

Containers and Labelling: see the entry on Creams for general information on containers and labelling.

Storage: it should be stored at a temperature not exceeding 25°.

Advice for patients: a small quantity of cream should be placed on the tip of the finger and applied to the inside of each nostril; the cream may be spread further inward by squeezing the nares. For prophylaxis, application should not be discontinued without the advice of the prescriber. For therapy the prescribed course should be completed. Contact with the eyes and ears should be avoided. Fabric which has been in contact with chlorhexidine may subsequently stain if washed in solutions containing hypochlorite but solutions containing perborate may be used in laundering.

HYDROCORTISONE AND NEOMYCIN CREAM:

Hydrocortisone, in ultra-fine powder ..	..	.. 5 g
Neomycin cream	..	995 g

Incorporate the hydrocortisone in the neomycin cream. A phosphate buffer may be included.

A standard for this cream is given in the British Pharmaceutical Codex 1973

Containers, Labelling, and Storage: see the entry on Creams for general information on containers, labelling, and storage.

Advice for patients: the cream should be applied sparingly to the affected area.

HYDROCORTISONE AND NEOMYCIN EAR-DROPS: consisting of a suspension of hydrocortisone acetate, in ultra-fine powder, with appropriate pharmaceutical adjuvants, in a solution of neomycin sulphate in freshly boiled and cooled purified water. Available as ear-drops containing 1.5% of hydrocortisone acetate and 0.5% of neomycin sulphate.

A standard for these ear-drops is given in the British Pharmaceutical Codex 1973

Containers: see the entry on Ear-drops for general information on containers.

Labelling: see the entry on Ear-drops for general information on labelling. In addition, the label on the container or package should state the date after which the ear-drops are not intended to be used, and a direction to shake the bottle.

Storage: it should be stored in a cool place; it should not be allowed to freeze.

Advice for patients: the prescribed course should be completed.

HYDROCORTISONE AND NEOMYCIN EYE-DROPS: consisting of a sterile suspension containing up to 1.5% of hydrocortisone acetate, in ultra-fine powder, in a solution containing 0.5% of neomycin sulphate, with 0.002% of phenylmercuric acetate or nitrate or other suitable preservatives, in purified water. Available as eye-drops containing 1.5% of hydrocortisone acetate and 0.5% of neomycin sulphate.

A standard for these eye-drops is given in the British Pharmaceutical Codex 1973

Containers: see the entry on Eye-drops for general information on containers.

Labelling: see the entry on Eye-drops for general information on labelling. In addition, a direction to shake the bottle should be given on the label.

Storage: it should be stored in a cool place; it should not be allowed to freeze.

Advice for patients: see the entry on Eye-drops for general information on the use of eye-drops. The prescribed course should be completed.

HYDROCORTISONE AND NEOMYCIN EYE OINTMENT: prepared by incorporating hydrocortisone acetate and neomycin sulphate, both in ultra-fine powder, in eye ointment basis, or any other suitable basis, by method B described in the entry on Eye Ointments. Available as an eye ointment containing 1.5% of hydrocortisone acetate and 0.5% of neomycin sulphate.

A standard for this eye ointment is given in the British Pharmaceutical Codex 1973

Labelling: see the entry on Eye Ointments for general information on labelling.

Advice for patients: see the entry on Eye Ointments for general information on the use of eye ointments. The prescribed course should be completed.

HYDROCORTISONE, NEOMYCIN, AND POLYMYXIN EAR-DROPS: consisting of hydrocortisone, neomycin sulphate, and polymyxin B sulphate in an aqueous vehicle. It contains 10 mg of hydrocortisone, 3400 units of neomycin sulphate, and 10 000 units of polymyxin B sulphate per ml.

Containers: see the entry on Ear-drops for general information on containers.

Storage: it should be stored in a cool place, protected from light.

Advice for patients: the ear canal should be cleansed without the use of soap before the drops are instilled. The prescribed course should be completed.

NEOMYCIN AND BACITRACIN OINTMENT:

Neomycin sulphate	5 g
Bacitracin zinc	500 000 units
Liquid paraffin	100 g
White soft paraffin	to 1000 g

Melt the white soft paraffin, incorporate the liquid paraffin, and stir until cold. Triturate the neomycin sulphate and the bacitracin zinc with a portion of the basis and gradually incorporate the remainder of the basis. The ointment may be expected to retain its potency for 2 years provided that the moisture content of the ointment does not exceed 0.2%. When materials complying with B.P.C. 1973 requirements are used, the moisture content may be expected to be below this figure.

A standard for this ointment is given in the British Pharmaceutical Codex 1973

Containers: see the entry on Ointments for general information on containers. Containers should be airtight.

Advice for patients: the ointment should be applied sparingly to the affected area.

NEOMYCIN CREAM:

Neomycin sulphate	5.0 g
Disodium edetate	0.1 g
Chlorocresol	1.0 g
Cetomacrogol emulsifying ointment	300.0 g
Purified water, freshly boiled and cooled	693.9 g

Dissolve the disodium edetate and the chlorocresol in about 650 ml of the water with the aid of gentle heat; melt the cetomacrogol emulsifying ointment on a water-bath, add the aqueous solution at the same temperature, and stir until cold. Incorporate the neomycin sulphate dissolved in the remainder of the water. A phosphate buffer may be included.

A standard for this cream is given in the British Pharmaceutical Codex 1973

Containers, Labelling, and *Storage:* see the entry on Creams for general information on containers, labelling, and storage.

Advice for patients: the cream should be applied sparingly to the affected area.

NEOMYCIN ELIXIR (*Syn.* Neomycin Mixture):

Neomycin sulphate	20.0 g
Disodium edetate	0.5 g
Saccharin sodium	0.9 g
Benzoic acid	2.0 g
Citric acid	a sufficient quantity
Compound tartrazine solution	6.0 ml
Sorbitol solution	385.0 ml
Purified water, freshly boiled and cooled	to 1000.0 ml

The mixture may be lime-flavoured. The compound tartrazine solution may be replaced by another suitable dye or mixture of dyes, provided that any dye used is of food grade of commerce and that its use for colouring food is permitted in the country concerned. If the mixture is recently prepared, the disodium edetate may be omitted.

Dissolve the benzoic acid, the saccharin sodium, and the disodium edetate in 500 ml of water with the aid of gentle heat, cool, and dissolve the neomycin sulphate in the solution. Add the sorbitol solution and mix; add the colouring, the flavouring, and sufficient of the water to produce the required volume, and mix. If necessary, add sufficient citric acid to adjust to pH 4 to 5.

When a dose less than or not a multiple of 5 ml is prescribed, the elixir may be diluted, as described in the entry on Elixirs, with syrup. The diluted elixir must be freshly prepared. It contains 400 mg (approximately 250 000 units) of neomycin sulphate in 20 ml.

A standard for this elixir is given in the British Pharmaceutical Codex 1973

Containers and *Labelling:* see the entry on Elixirs for general information on containers and labelling.

Storage: it should be stored in a cool place, protected from light.

Advice for patients: the elixir should be taken at regular intervals. The prescribed course should be completed.

NEOMYCIN EYE-DROPS: consisting of a sterile solution containing up to 0.5% of neomycin sulphate, with 0.7% of sodium acid phosphate, 0.7% of sodium phosphate, and 0.002% of phenylmercuric acetate or nitrate, in purified water. It may also contain 0.01% of disodium edetate. It is prepared by method B or C described in the entry on Eye-drops. Available as eye-drops containing 0.5% of neomycin sulphate.

A standard for these eye-drops is given in the British Pharmaceutical Codex 1973

Containers and *Labelling:* see the entry on Eye-drops for general information on containers and labelling.

Storage: it should be protected from light.

Advice for patients: see the entry on Eye-drops for general information on the use of eye-drops. The prescribed course should be completed.

NEOMYCIN EYE OINTMENT: prepared by incorporating neomycin sulphate in eye ointment basis by method B described in the entry on Eye Ointments. Available as an eye ointment containing 0.5% of neomycin sulphate.

A standard for this eye ointment is given in the British Pharmaceutical Codex 1973

Labelling: see the entry on Eye Ointments for general information on labelling.

Advice for patients: see the entry on Eye Ointments for general information on the use of eye ointments. The prescribed course should be completed.

NEOMYCIN TABLETS: available as tablets containing 500 mg (approximately 350 000 units) of neomycin sulphate, and, for veterinary use, containing 100 mg (approximately 70 000 units) of neomycin sulphate.

A standard for these tablets is given in the British Pharmacopoeia 1973

Labelling: the label on the container should state the date after which the tablets are not intended to be used and the conditions under which they should be stored.

Containers and *Storage:* see the entry on Tablets for general information on containers and storage. Containers should be airtight and light resistant. The tablets should be stored at a temperature not exceeding 30°.

Advice for patients: the tablets should be taken at regular intervals. The prescribed course should be completed.

OTHER PREPARATIONS available include numerous compound preparations in which neomycin sulphate is an ingredient.

Neoplastic Disease

A *neoplasm* or *tumour* is an abnormal growth which may be benign or malignant. Benign tumours are usually surrounded by a fibrous capsule. They lack the property of invasion and metastasis. They have a lesser degree of anaplasia or loss of cell differentiation than malignant tumours. Malignant tumours (cancers) are not surrounded by a capsule and they may invade and destroy the tissue in which they arise. They have an unlimited power of disorderly reproduction, showing loss of differentiation and a tendency to become primitive in nature. They are capable of producing metastases or secondary growths at a distance from the primary site. Malignant growth is often classified according to the site of primary growth, as in osteoma, hepatoma, etc.

Carcinoma is a malignant growth derived from epithelial cells (or cells similar to the skin or the mucous membrane lining the stomach, bowels, or glands) and it tends to infiltrate the surrounding tissues and to give rise to metastases.

Sarcoma is a malignant tumour developing in the connective tissues of the bone, muscle, and tendon.

Factors affecting the Incidence of Neoplastic Disease

The incidence of neoplastic disease increases with age, and is related to factors such as diet and smoking, and genetic factors. Some types of neoplasm are associated with viruses (as in Burkitt's lymphoma) and with occupational exposure to carcinogens such as X-rays, radioactive substances, and certain chemicals, such as asbestos, benzpyrene, and vinyl chloride.

Immunosuppression gives rise to an increased incidence of tumours.

Early signs of neoplastic disease. Early diagnosis of cancer is advantageous and patients should therefore be encouraged to seek advice at an early stage.

Medical advice should be sought by any person who experiences any of the following signs: unusual bleeding or discharge from any body orifice; a sore that does not heal; a change in bladder or bowel habits; a lump or thickening in the breast or elsewhere; persistent hoarseness, cough, or spitting of blood; persistent indigestion or difficulty in swallowing; a change in a wart or mole.

Treatment. The aim of treatment of neoplastic disease is to destroy tumour cells selectively without producing irreversible changes in other tissues. Surgical removal of neoplasms is possible in many cases especially in the early stages. Irradiation with suitable X-rays or with radiation from radioactive preparations such as gold-198, sodium iodide (^{131}I), and sodium phosphate (^{32}P) may be administered to the patient. Some radioactive preparations are preferentially absorbed by certain organs or tissues. In selected cases hormone therapy is of value, for example administration of oestrogens in prostatic carcinoma. Cytotoxic agents, including alkylating agents such as busulphan, chlorambucil, cyclophosphamide, mannomustine, melphalan, mustine, and thiotepa and antimetabolites such as azathioprine, cytarabine, mercaptopurine, and methotrexate may also be used, alone or in combination with irradiation. Such treatment affects all rapidly dividing cells in the body including neoplastic cells. Therefore careful control is required to avoid undue effects on other rapidly dividing cells such as the bone-marrow.

See also Leukaemia, Acute, Lymphoproliferative Diseases, and Myeloproliferative Diseases.

Neostigmine Bromide

3 - (Dimethylcarbamoyloxy) - *NNN* - trimethylanilinium bromide

$C_{12}H_{19}BrN_2O_2 = 303.2$

OTHER NAMES: Neostig. Brom.; Neostigminii Bromidum; *Prostigmin*®

A standard is given in the European Pharmacopoeia Vol. II

Description. Odourless colourless crystals or white crystalline powder.

Solubility. Soluble, at 20°, in less than 1 part of water and in 8 parts of alcohol; soluble in chloroform; practically insoluble in ether.

Moisture content. Not more than 1%, determined by drying at 105°.

Storage. It should be stored in airtight containers, protected from light.

Identification. TEST. To 2 drops of a 1% solution add 0.5 ml of *sodium hydroxide solution* and evaporate to dryness on a water-bath; heat quickly on an oil-bath to about 250°, maintain at this temperature for 30 seconds, cool, dissolve the residue in 1 ml of water, cool in ice water, and add 1 ml of *diazoaminobenzenesulphonic acid*; a cherry-red colour is produced.

MELTING-POINT. About 167°, with decomposition.

ULTRAVIOLET ABSORPTION. In 1N sulphuric acid, maxima at 226 nm and 260 nm.

Metabolism. ABSORPTION. Poorly absorbed after oral administration.

METABOLIC REACTIONS. Ester hydrolysis to form active 3-hydroxytrimethylanilinium bromide.

EXCRETION. 20% of an oral dose is excreted in the urine and 50% in the faeces; less than 5% of the oral dose is excreted in the urine unchanged; following intramuscular administration about 65% of a dose is excreted in the urine unchanged.

FURTHER INFORMATION. Metabolism and excretion in man—P. T. Nowell *et al.*, *Br. J. Pharmac.*, 1962, **18**, 617; metabolism and excretion in rats—M. A. Husain *et al.*, *Br. J. Pharmac.*, 1969, **35**, 344 and S. M. Somani *et al.*, *Eur. J. Pharmac.*, 1970, **12**, 114.

Actions and uses. Neostigmine bromide has the actions described under Neostigmine Methylsulphate. It is given by mouth in the treatment of myasthenia gravis. The usual dose is 15 to 30 milligrams by mouth, the frequency of the dose being determined in accordance with the needs of the patient.

Undesirable Effects. As for Physostigmine Salicylate. In addition, neostigmine bromide, by increasing intestinal motility, may cause disruption of intestinal suture lines.

Poisoning. As for Neostigmine Methylsulphate.

Preparation

NEOSTIGMINE TABLETS: available as tablets containing 15 mg of neostigmine bromide.
A standard for these tablets is given in the British Pharmacopoeia 1973
Containers and *Storage:* see the entry on Tablets for general information on containers and storage. Containers should be airtight and light resistant.

Neostigmine Methylsulphate

3 - (Dimethylcarbamoyloxy) - *NNN* - trimethylanilinium methylsulphate
$C_{13}H_{22}N_2O_6S = 334.4$

OTHER NAMES: Neostig. Methylsulph.; *Prostigmin*®

A standard is given in the British Pharmacopoeia 1973

Description. Odourless colourless crystals or white crystalline powder.

Solubility. Soluble, at 20°, in less than 1 part of water and in 6 parts of alcohol.

Moisture content. Not more than 1%, determined by drying at 105°.

Sterilisation. Solutions are sterilised by heating in an autoclave or by filtration.

Storage. It should be stored in airtight containers, protected from light.

Identification. TEST. It complies with the test described under Neostigmine Bromide.

MELTING-POINT. About 143°.

Actions and uses. Neostigmine inhibits cholinesterase activity and has actions similar to those described under Physostigmine Salicylate but it does not act on the central nervous system. Its nicotinic action is more pronounced and its muscarinic action less pronounced than that of physostigmine. It is used mainly for its action on voluntary muscle and less frequently to increase the activity of involuntary muscle.

Neostigmine methylsulphate is used in the diagnosis and treatment of myasthenia gravis. For diagnosis, 1 to 1.5 milligrams is given by intramuscular or intravenous injection; relief of signs and symptoms usually occurs within 15 minutes in true cases of myasthenia. In the treatment of myasthenia gravis, doses of 1 to 2.5 milligrams are given by subcutaneous, intramuscular, or intravenous injection several times a day, according to the severity of the condition. Oral administration of neostigmine bromide or of pyridostigmine bromide are other methods of treatment. If the muscarinic effect of neostigmine is troublesome, it can be controlled by prior administration of atropine by mouth or by injection.

Neostigmine methylsulphate is also used to curtail the muscular relaxation produced by non-depolarising neuromuscular-blocking drugs such as tubocurarine and gallamine triethiodide; 2.5 to 5 milligrams is given intravenously after an injection of 0.5 to 1 milligram of atropine sulphate.

In the treatment of paralytic ileus and post-operative urinary retention, neostigmine methylsulphate is given by subcutaneous or intramuscular injection in doses of 0.5 to 1 milligram.

A dose of 500 micrograms is sometimes used to promote the expulsion of intestinal flatus before radiography of the gall-bladder, kidneys, or ureters.

Eye-drops containing 3% are used in the treatment of glaucoma.

Undesirable effects. As for Physostigmine Salicylate. In addition, neostigmine methylsulphate, by increasing intestinal motility, may cause disruption of intestinal suture lines.

Poisoning. Atropine sulphate should be given subcutaneously in doses of 1 to 2 milligrams and further doses may be given by intramuscular injection when required. It may be necessary to give artificial respiration until atropine can be administered.

Preparations

NEOSTIGMINE INJECTION: a sterile solution of neostigmine methylsulphate in water for injections. It is sterilised by heating in an autoclave or by filtration. Available in 1-ml ampoules containing 500 micrograms and 2.5 milligrams of neostigmine methylsulphate.

A standard for this injection is given in the British Pharmacopoeia 1973
Containers and *Labelling:* see the entry on Injections for general information on containers and labelling.
Storage: it should be protected from light.

OTHER PREPARATIONS available include EYE-DROPS containing neostigmine methylsulphate 3%.

Nephrotic Syndrome

The nephrotic syndrome consists of excessive protein-uria and the resultant hypoproteinaemia and oedema. It may be due to nephritis but the cause is often unknown and may be part of an autoimmune phenomenon. Drugs such as penicillamine, phenylbutazone, sodium auro-thiomalate, and probenecid may produce a similar clinical picture. A high-protein low-sodium diet should be given and oedema controlled by the use of appropriate diuretics. Corticosteroids and immunosuppressants may also be required.

Neuralgia

Neuralgia is a paroxysmal pain which extends along the course of one or more nerves in the absence of evidence of organic change in the nerve. It should be noted that the term neuralgia is often used in a wider sense to refer to any chronic pain.
Trigeminal neuralgia (Tic douloureux) is a syndrome characterised by brief attacks of severe pain over an area of the face supplied by one or more branches of the trigeminal nerve. The pain may be triggered by touching a hypersensitive area on the skin. Analgesics do not give prolonged relief of trigeminal neuralgia but drugs such as carbamazepine decrease the frequency of attacks. Glossopharyngeal neuralgia may also be treated with drugs such as carbamazepine.

Newcastle Disease and Avian Infectious Bronchitis Vaccine, Living

A mixture of a strain of Newcastle disease virus and a strain of avian infectious bronchitis virus.

A standard is given in the British Pharmacopoeia (Veterinary)

Storage. The dried vaccine should be protected from light and stored at 2° to 8° when it may be expected to retain its potency for 12 months. The vaccine should be used immediately after reconstitution.

Veterinary uses. It is administered in drinking water to chickens for prophylaxis of Newcastle disease and avian infectious bronchitis attributable to the Massachusetts type of virus.

Newcastle Disease Vaccine, Inactivated

A suspension or an emulsion of Newcastle disease virus which has been inactivated in such a manner that immunogenic activity is retained.

A standard is given in the British Pharmacopoeia (Veterinary)

Storage. The vaccine should be protected from light and stored at 2° to 8° when it may be expected to retain its potency for 12 months. It should not be allowed to freeze.

Veterinary uses. It is administered by subcutaneous or intramuscular injection to turkeys, chickens, and game birds for prophylaxis of Newcastle disease.

Nialamide

N'-(2-Benzylcarbamoylethyl)isonicotinohydrazide

$CO\cdot NH\cdot NH\cdot CH_2\cdot CH_2\cdot CO\cdot NH\cdot CH_2\cdot C_6H_5$

$C_{16}H_{18}N_4O_2 = 298.3$

A standard is given in the British Pharmacopoeia 1973

Description. An almost odourless, white, crystalline powder with a bitter taste.

Solubility. Soluble, at 20°, in 400 parts of water, in 40 parts of alcohol, in 10 parts of methyl alcohol, and in 150 parts of chloroform.

Identification. TEST. Dissolve about 10 mg in 10 ml of a 1% solution of sodium carbonate and add 1 ml of *sodium nitroprusside solution*; the solution is yellow, then deepens to orange and finally becomes red within 10 minutes.

MELTING-POINT. About 152°.

ULTRAVIOLET ABSORPTION. In 0.1N sulphuric acid, maximum at 266 nm (E1%, 1cm = 185).

INFRA-RED ABSORPTION. Major peaks at 670, 698, 1408, 1520, 1547, and 1625 cm⁻¹ (see Appendix 2a: Infra-red Spectra).

Actions and uses. Nialamide is an antidepressant drug which inhibits monoamine oxidase. It has actions and uses similar to those described under Phenelzine Sulphate. It is used for the treatment of depression, especially when associated with phobic anxiety.
As an antidepressant, the usual initial dose is 150 milligrams daily by mouth in divided doses, and this may need to be increased to 300 milligrams daily in some cases. When a satisfactory response has been obtained the dose should be gradually reduced to the minimum which provides relief from symptoms; this may be as little as 75 milligrams daily.

Undesirable effects. The most frequently occurring reactions are headache, nausea, vertigo, dryness of the mouth, and excessive perspiration.

Precautions and drug interactions. As for Phenelzine Sulphate. Although nialamide appears to be free from hepatotoxicity, the fact that analogous compounds have given rise to hepatic reactions should be borne in mind when giving nialamide to patients with a history of liver damage or impaired liver function.

Preparation

NIALAMIDE TABLETS: they may be coloured. The usual strength is 25 mg of nialamide.
A standard for these tablets is given in the British Pharmacopoeia 1973
Containers and *Storage:* see the entry on Tablets for

general information on containers and storage. Containers should be airtight.

Advice for patients: treatment should not be discontinued without the advice of the prescriber. The tablets may affect mental concentration; persons affected should not drive or operate machinery.

Patients should be advised, during treatment and for 2 weeks thereafter, to avoid certain foodstuffs containing pressor agents such as cheese, pickled herrings, broad bean pods, and certain protein extracts prepared from meat or yeast and medicines containing sympathomimetics such as ephedrine, methoxamine, phenylephrine, phenylpropanolamine, and pseudoephedrine as found in cough and cold remedies, analgesics, and tonics. Warning cards, containing this advice, may be carried by the patient during treatment and shown when further medical or dental treatment is required or when other medicines are needed.

Niclosamide

2′,5-Dichloro-4′-nitrosalicylanilide

$C_{13}H_8Cl_2N_2O_4 = 327.1$

OTHER NAMES: *Mansonil*®; *Yomesan*®

A standard is given in the British Pharmacopoeia 1973

Description. An odourless tasteless cream-coloured powder.

Solubility. Very slightly soluble in water; soluble, at 20°, in 150 parts of alcohol, in 350 parts of ether, and in 400 parts of chloroform.

Identification. TEST. Mix about 50 mg with 5 ml of 1N hydrochloric acid and 100 mg of zinc powder, heat in a water-bath for 10 minutes, cool, filter, and to the filtrate add 0.5 ml of a 1% solution of sodium nitrite, allow to stand for 10 minutes, add 2 ml of a 2% solution of ammonium sulphamate, shake, allow to stand for 10 minutes, and add 2 ml of a 0.5% solution of N-(1-naphthyl)ethylenediamine hydrochloride; a deep red colour is produced.

MELTING-POINT. About 228°.

ULTRAVIOLET ABSORPTION. In alcohol (95%), maximum at 335 nm (E1%, 1cm = 470).

INFRA-RED ABSORPTION. Major peaks at 1282, 1333, 1351, 1515, 1562, and 1613 cm⁻¹ (see Appendix 2b: Infra-red Spectra).

Actions and uses. Niclosamide is a taenicide; it is effective against all the species of tapeworm that infect man. As with dichlorophen, the worms are partially digested before they are expelled, and the scolices cannot be found in the stools. A stool examination should be made after 8 weeks to ensure that the worm has been killed.

The use of niclosamide against *Taenia solium* may predispose to cysticercosis, as there is a possibility of ova from a partially digested worm migrating into the stomach. A purge should therefore be given 1 or 2 hours

after the drug. In *T. saginata* infection there is no risk of cysticercosis.

The usual dose for adults and children over 6 years is 2 grams on an empty stomach or after a light breakfast. Children from 2 to 5 years are given 1 gram and children under 2 years 500 milligrams. Niclosamide is administered as a single dose.

The tablets must be crushed or thoroughly chewed and washed down with water. A saline purge should be given 2 hours after treatment; if the patient is constipated it is advisable to purge on the day before treatment.

Niclosamide is not appreciably absorbed from the intestine and therefore has no effect in cysticercosis. *Hymenolepis nana* completes its life-cycle in man without passing through an intermediate host, and cysticerci of this tapeworm embedded in the intestinal mucosa escape the action of the drug and later develop into adults.

For the treatment of *H. nana* infection adults and children over 6 years are given 2 grams on the first day, children 2 to 5, 1 gram, and children under 2 years, 500 milligrams. Half these doses are given daily for a further 6 days.

Veterinary uses. Niclosamide is an anthelmintic used mainly for the control of tapeworms. The usual dose for cattle is 50 milligrams per kilogram body-weight, for sheep and goats 75 milligrams per kilogram body-weight, and for dogs and cats 100 milligrams per kilogram body-weight. Niclosamide is administered by mouth as a single dose.

Preparations

NICLOSAMIDE DISPERSIBLE POWDER: consisting of niclosamide mixed with suitable non-toxic wetting, dispersing, and suspending agents. Available as a dispersible powder containing 75% of niclosamide.

A standard for this dispersible powder is given in the British Pharmacopoeia (Veterinary)

Containers and *Storage:* it should be stored in well-filled airtight containers, in a cool place.

Labelling: the label on the container should state the amount of the medicament as the proportion of niclosamide in the preparation, the method of use, that it should not be administered to lactating cattle and goats, and that any unused suspension should be discarded.

NICLOSAMIDE TABLETS: available as tablets containing 500 mg of niclosamide; they contain suitable sweetening and flavouring agents.

A standard for these tablets is given in the British Pharmacopoeia 1973

Containers and *Storage:* see the entry on Tablets for general information on containers and storage. Containers should be airtight.

Advice for patients: the tablets should be chewed thoroughly and swallowed with water. The dose should be taken on an empty stomach, preferably in the morning. When applicable the prescribed course should be completed.

Nicotinamide

Pyridine-3-carboxamide

$C_6H_6N_2O = 122.1$

OTHER NAMES: Niacinamide; Nicotinamidum
Amisyn® (with acetomenaphthone)

A standard is given in the European Pharmacopoeia Vol. II

Description. Colourless crystals or white crystalline powder with a faint characteristic odour and a bitter taste.

Solubility. Soluble; at 20°, in 1 part of water, in 1.5 parts of alcohol, and in 10 parts of glycerol; very slightly soluble in ether.

Dissociation constant. pK_a 3.3 (20°).

Hygroscopicity. It absorbs insignificant amounts of moisture at 25° at relative humidities up to about 90%.

Sterilisation. Solutions for injection are sterilised by heating in an autoclave or by filtration.

Storage. It should be stored in airtight containers.

Identification. TESTS. 1. Mix about 100 mg with 1 ml of *dilute sodium hydroxide solution* and boil; ammonia is evolved (distinction from nicotinic acid).
2. To 2 ml of a 0.1% solution add 6 ml of *cyanogen bromide solution* and 1 ml of a 2.5% solution of aniline; a golden yellow colour is produced (also given by nicotinic acid).

MELTING-POINT. About 129°.

ULTRAVIOLET ABSORPTION. In 0.1N sulphuric acid, maxima at 261 nm (E1%, 1cm = 478) and 317 nm (E1%, 1cm = 46).

Actions and uses. Nicotinamide has the actions described under Nicotinic Acid but it has no vasodilator action. It is used as an alternative to nicotinic acid for the treatment of pellagra.
The usual prophylactic dose for children and adults is 15 to 30 milligrams daily by mouth. The usual therapeutic dose for children and adults is 50 to 250 milligrams daily by mouth or by intravenous injection.

Preparations

NICOTINAMIDE TABLETS (*Syn.* Niacinamide Tablets): may be prepared by moist granulation and compression as described in the entry on Tablets. Available as tablets containing 50 mg of nicotinamide.
A standard for these tablets is given in the British Pharmaceutical Codex 1973
Containers and *Storage:* see the entry on Tablets for general information on containers and storage. Containers should be airtight and light resistant.

OTHER PREPARATIONS available include TABLETS containing nicotinamide 50 mg with acetomenaphthone 10 mg.
Nicotinamide is an ingredient of compound vitamin B tablets, strong compound vitamin B tablets, vitamins B and C injection, and vitamins capsules.

Nicotinic Acid

Pyridine-3-carboxylic acid

$C_6H_5NO_2 = 123.1$

OTHER NAMES: Acidum Nicotinicum; Niacin
Chilblain Treatment Dellipsoids D27® and *Pernivit®* (both with acetomenaphthone)

A standard is given in the European Pharmacopoeia Vol. III

Description. An odourless white crystalline powder with a feebly acid taste.

Solubility. Soluble, at 20°, in 55 parts of water; soluble in boiling water and in boiling alcohol; very slightly soluble in ether; soluble in solutions of alkalis.

Acidity. A 1.3% solution has a pH of 3 to 3.5.

Moisture content. Not more than 1%, determined by drying at 105°.

Dissociation constants. pK_a 2.0, 4.8 (25°).

Sterilisation. Solutions of the sodium salt for injection are sterilised by heating in an autoclave or by filtration.

Identification. TESTS. 1. Mix about 100 mg with 1 ml of *dilute sodium hydroxide solution* and boil; no ammonia is evolved (distinction from nicotinamide).
2. Mix about 100 mg with 10 mg of citric acid and 3 drops of acetic anhydride and heat on a water-bath; a red-violet colour is produced.

MELTING-POINT. About 235°.

Metabolism. ABSORPTION. Readily absorbed after oral administration.

BLOOD CONCENTRATION. After an intravenous infusion of 10 to 100 μg/kg per minute for 20 to 180 minutes, an increase of 0.1 to 0.4 μg/ml is attained in the plasma concentration of free nicotinic acid; plasma concentrations of nicotinic acid decline rapidly.

DISTRIBUTION. Widely distributed throughout the body and enters the cerebrospinal fluid; trace amounts are taken up by red blood cells.

METABOLIC REACTIONS. N'-Methylation, amino-acid conjugation, and nicotinamide formation.

EXCRETION. After an intravenous dose, about 40% is excreted in the urine in 19 days mainly as metabolites; the major metabolite appears to be nicotinuric acid with smaller amounts of nicotinamide and N'-methyl-nicotinamide.

FURTHER INFORMATION. Absorption of nicotinic acid and pentaerythritol tetranitrate—N. Svedmyr and L. Harthon, *Acta pharmac. tox.*, 1970, **28**, 66.

Actions and uses. Nicotinic acid is essential for human nutrition, the normal daily requirement being probably about 6.6 to 8.8 milligrams per 1000 kilocalories or approximately 17 to 22 milligrams, depending on the protein intake. Its amide (nicotinamide) is a constituent of diphosphopyridine nucleotide (DPN) and triphosphopyridine nucleotide (TPN), two coenzymes associated with hydrogen transport in many biological oxidation-reduction processes.
A deficiency of nicotinic acid is one factor in the aetiology of pellagra, and the acid or its amide is used in the prophylaxis and treatment of this condition. Pellagra is characterised by dermatitis, enteritis, a red swollen tongue, and mental symptoms.
For the treatment of acute exacerbations of pellagra, up to 500 milligrams is given daily in divided doses by mouth. The amide, which is devoid of vasodilator action, may be given instead. The prophylactic or maintenance dose is 50 milligrams daily. If the patient is unable to swallow or absorb the nicotinic acid, it may be injected as a solution of the sodium salt in a dose not exceeding 50 milligrams, which may be repeated hourly; if nicotinamide is used, much larger doses may be given. The dose for children is the same as for adults.

When taken with food absorption is delayed but the undesirable vasodilator action may be reduced.

Nicotinic acid and its amide produce improvement in the mental, cutaneous, and alimentary manifestations of pellagra, but they have little influence on the neuropathy or the lesions of the lips and face that are frequently seen in pellagrins; foods or concentrates rich in the vitamin-B group should therefore be administered as well as nicotinic acid or its amide in the treatment of pellagra.

It has a transient fibrinolytic action and in large doses lowers blood cholesterol, although it impairs liver function at the same time. Nicotinamide has no such action. In addition to its action as a vitamin, nicotinic acid has a vasodilator action. When given by mouth or by injection in therapeutic doses, it may cause flushing of the face, a sensation of heat, and a pounding in the head; these symptoms are transient and harmless and may be avoided by substituting nicotinamide. Tolerance to the vasodilator effect develops rapidly when large doses are taken. Nicotinic acid has been employed for its vasodilator action in the treatment of peripheral vascular disease.

Undesirable effects. Nicotinic acid may cause dryness of the skin, anorexia, nausea, vomiting, diarrhoea, activation of peptic ulcer, hepatic disease, hyperuricaemia, and circulatory collapse after rapid intravenous injection.

Preparations

NICOTINIC ACID TABLETS: available as tablets containing 50 and 100 mg of nicotinic acid.

A standard for these tablets is given in the British Pharmacopoeia 1973

Containers and *Storage:* see the entry on Tablets for general information on containers and storage. Containers should be airtight.

Advice for patients: the tablets should preferably be taken after meals.

OTHER PREPARATIONS available include TABLETS containing nicotinic acid 25 mg with acetomenaphthone 7 mg.

Nicoumalone

4-Hydroxy-3-(1-*p*-nitrophenyl-3-oxobutyl)coumarin

$C_{19}H_{15}NO_6 = 353.3$

OTHER NAMES: Acenocoumarol; *Sinthrome*®

A standard is given in the British Pharmacopoeia 1973

Description. An odourless almost white to buff powder with a slightly sweet taste becoming bitter.

Solubility. Very slightly soluble in water and in ether; soluble, at 20°, in 400 parts of alcohol and in 200 parts of chloroform; soluble in solutions of alkali hydroxides.

Identification. Mix about 50 mg with 2.5 ml of glacial acetic acid, 0.5 ml of hydrochloric acid and 200 mg of zinc powder, heat on a water-bath for 5 minutes, cool, filter, and to the filtrate add 0.5 ml of 0.1M sodium nitrite followed by 10 ml of a 1% solution of 2-naphthol containing 3 ml of *sodium hydroxide solution;* a bright red precipitate is produced.

MELTING-POINT. About 198°.

ULTRAVIOLET ABSORPTION. In a mixture containing 1 volume of 1N hydrochloric acid and 9 volumes of methyl alcohol, maxima at 283 nm (E1%, 1cm = 650) and 306 nm (E1%, 1cm = 500).

INFRA-RED ABSORPTION. Major peaks at 1068, 1344, 1387, 1507, 1612, and 1680 cm^{-1} (see Appendix 2a: Infra-red Spectra).

Metabolism. ABSORPTION. Readily absorbed after oral administration.

HALF-LIFE. Plasma half-life, about 24 hours.

DISTRIBUTION. Crosses the placenta and is secreted in milk.

EXCRETION. Excreted in the urine mainly as unchanged drug.

Actions and uses. Nicoumalone has the actions and uses described under Warfarin Sodium. A therapeutic effect is obtained 24 to 48 hours after the initial dose has been given and continues until about 36 to 48 hours after the last dose. The initial dose is 8 to 16 milligrams by mouth on the first day, followed on the second day by 4 to 12 milligrams; thereafter the dose is carefully controlled by daily determinations of the prothrombin time.

Nicoumalone is sometimes tolerated by patients intolerant of other oral anticoagulants.

Undesirable effects. As for Warfarin Sodium. Nausea, loss of appetite, headache, and giddiness rarely occur.

Precautions and contra-indications; Drug interactions. As for Warfarin Sodium.

Preparation

NICOUMALONE TABLETS: available as tablets containing 1 and 4 mg of nicoumalone; they may be coloured.

A standard for these tablets is given in the British Pharmacopoeia 1973

Containers and *Storage:* see the entry on Tablets for general information on containers and storage. Containers should be airtight.

Advice for patients: the tablets should be taken at regular intervals. Treatment should not be discontinued without the advice of the prescriber. Patients may carry an identification card giving details of their treatment and the name of the prescriber who should be contacted in the event of accident or illness. Patients should not take other medicine (including aspirin) without medical or pharmaceutical advice. Preparations containing liquid paraffin should preferably be avoided.

Nikethamide

NN-Diethylpyridine-3-carboxamide

$C_{10}H_{14}N_2O = 178.2$

OTHER NAME: Nicethamidum

A standard is given in the European Pharmacopoeia Vol. II

Description. A colourless or slightly yellow oily liquid or crystalline mass with a slight characteristic odour and a taste which is slightly bitter, then burning, and leaves a faint warm sensation on the tongue.

Solubility. Miscible with water, with alcohol, with ether, and with chloroform.

Acidity or alkalinity. A 25% solution has a pH of 6.5 to 7.8.

Refractive index. 1.524 to 1.526.

Dissociation constant. pK_a 3.5 (20°).

Sterilisation. Solutions for injection are sterilised by heating in an autoclave or by filtration.

Identification. TESTS. 1. Mix about 100 mg with 1 ml of *dilute sodium hydroxide solution* and heat; diethylamine, recognisable by its odour, is produced; the vapour turns red litmus paper blue.
2. Mix about 100 mg with 500 mg of sodium carbonate and heat until charring begins; pyridine, recognisable by its odour, is produced.
3. Mix about 100 mg with 0.5 ml of *copper sulphate solution*; an intense blue colour is produced. Add *potassium thiocyanate solution*; a voluminous green precipitate is produced.

INFRA-RED ABSORPTION. Major peaks at 1290, 1414, 1436, 1460, 1590, and 1635 cm^{-1} (see Appendix 2c: Infra-red Spectra).

Metabolism. ABSORPTION. Rapidly absorbed after oral administration.

METABOLIC REACTION. Converted to nicotinamide by N-dealkylation.

EXCRETION. Rapidly excreted in the urine.

Actions and uses. Nikethamide is a respiratory stimulant, its site of action being the medullary centres of the brain. It increases the rate and depth of respiration and produces slight peripheral vasoconstriction, although in man it has very little effect on blood pressure. Any beneficial effect it has on the circulation is probably due to an improvement in the respiration. An increasing coronary flow has been demonstrated in animals, but there is no clinical evidence of the value of nikethamide in coronary and myocardial diseases, and there appears to be little justification for its use in cardiac conditions unless these are due to respiratory distress.

In emergencies, nikethamide is given by slow intravenous injection; the usual dose is 0.5 to 2 grams repeated as necessary but doses as high as 2.5 grams may be necessary.

Convulsive movements occur before the toxic dose is reached.

Preparation

NIKETHAMIDE INJECTION:

Nikethamide	..	..	..	..	.. 25 g
Water for injections	..	..	..		.. to 100 ml

Dissolve, and clarify by filtration. Distribute the solution into ampoules, seal the ampoules, and sterilise by heating in an autoclave. Alternatively, sterilise the solution by filtration; distribute, by means of an aseptic technique, into sterile ampoules, and seal the ampoules. It contains, in 8 ml, 2 g of nikethamide. Available in 2-ml ampoules.

A standard for this injection is given in the British Pharmacopoeia 1973

Containers and *Labelling:* see the entry on Injections for general information on containers and labelling.

Niridazole

1-(5-Nitrothiazol-2-yl)imidazolidin-2-one

$C_6H_6N_4O_3S = 214.2$

OTHER NAME: *Ambilhar*®

Description. An odourless, tasteless, yellow, crystalline powder.

Solubility. Practically insoluble in water, in alcohol, in ether, in chloroform, and in acetone; soluble in dimethyl sulphoxide, in dimethylformamide, and in pyridine.

Identification. ULTRAVIOLET ABSORPTION. In alcohol (95%), maximum at 359 nm (E1%, 1cm = 670).

Determination in body fluids. HIGH PRESSURE LIQUID CHROMATOGRAPHY. In serum or urine—J. J. Miller *et al.*, *J. Chromat.*, 1978, **147**, 507.

Metabolism. ABSORPTION. Slowly absorbed after oral administration.

BLOOD CONCENTRATION. After an oral dose of 25 mg/kg, peak blood concentrations of unchanged drug of about 3 µg/ml are attained in 6 hours; the concentration may be higher in advanced bilharziasis.

HALF-LIFE. Plasma half-life, 12 to 15 hours.

DISTRIBUTION. Widely distributed throughout the body; *protein binding*, highly bound to plasma proteins.

METABOLIC REACTIONS. Rapidly metabolised in the liver; in advanced bilharziasis the metabolism of niridazole is reduced; this is caused by the development of a portal systemic shunt arising from the infection, through which the drug may pass and so bypass liver metabolism.

EXCRETION. 50% of a dose is excreted in the urine as metabolites in 48 hours; niridazole is also excreted as metabolites in bile.

FURTHER INFORMATION. Blood concentration and liver function—J. W. Faigle, *Acta pharmac. tox.*, 1971, **29**, *Suppl.* 3, 233.

Actions and uses. Niridazole is active against all forms of schistosomal worms in man. When given by mouth it is slowly absorbed from the gastro-intestinal tract and is rapidly metabolised in the liver; it exerts a toxic effect on the parasites in the mesenteric veins (*S. mansoni* and *S. japonicum*) or in the bladder veins (*S. haematobium*). It damages the vitellogenous cells of the female schistosome and in successfully treated patients all schistosomal oviproduction ceases. The worms then lose their hold on the venous wall to which they had been attached and are carried to the liver where they die; at the site of their death areas of granulomatous reaction form.

The cure rate is higher in patients infected with *Schistosoma haematobium* than in those with *S. mansoni*; the drug is also active against *S. japonicum* but experience with niridazole in this infection is limited.

The usual dose is 25 milligrams per kilogram body-weight daily in 2 divided doses given morning and evening for 7 days; this may be increased to 10 days when treating an infection due to *S. mansoni* and reduced to 5 days when treating an infection due to *S. japonicum*. The total daily dose should not exceed 1.5 grams. Treatment may be repeated if required after an interval of 4 to 6 months. Niridazole is also used in infections caused by the guinea worm (*Dracunculus medinensis*) in a dosage of 25 milligrams per kilogram body-weight for 7 to 10 days.

The urine of patients taking niridazole becomes a deep brown colour.

Undesirable effects. Headache, dizziness, asthma, muscle pains, anorexia, nausea, vomiting, and abdominal discomfort or cramps may occur. The electrocardiogram may show flattening or even inversion of the T-wave but serious cardiac complications are very rare. A transient depression of spermatogenesis may occur. Central nervous system changes include psychological upset, anxiety, and occasionally mania; epileptiform attacks have been reported and electroencephalographic tracings may exhibit hypersynchronous bursts. Allergic reactions may follow destruction of the parasites.

Precautions and contra-indications. Niridazole is conjugated in the liver and children tolerate the drug relatively well because they usually have good liver function, but particular care should be taken when treating adults, and it should not be given to patients with evidence of liver damage, epilepsy, or psychological instability. Niridazole should not be given in conjunction with isoniazid. Treatment of schistosomiasis in pregnant women should be postponed until pregnancy is over.

Preparation

NIRIDAZOLE TABLETS: available, in certain countries only, as tablets containing 100 and 500 mg of niridazole. *Containers* and *Storage:* see the entry on Tablets for general information on containers and storage. Containers should be airtight.

Advice for patients: the tablets should be taken at regular intervals after meals. The prescribed course should be completed. Niridazole may darken the urine.

Nitrazepam

1,3-Dihydro-7-nitro-5-phenyl-2*H*-1,4-benzodiazepin-2-one

$C_{15}H_{11}N_3O_3 = 281.3$

OTHER NAMES: *Mogadon®*; Nitrazepamum; *Nitrados®*; *Remnos®*; *Somnased®*; *Somnite®*

A standard is given in the European Pharmacopoeia Vol. III Supplement

Description. An odourless yellow crystalline powder.

Solubility. Very slightly soluble in water; soluble, at 20°, in 120 parts of alcohol, in 900 parts of ether, and in 45 parts of chloroform.

Dissociation constants. pK_a 3.2, 10.8 (20°).

Stability. Nitrazepam degrades by hydrolysis through an intermediate compound to 2-amino-5-nitrobenzophenone and 3-amino-6-nitro-4-phenyl-2(1*H*)-quinoline. In the dry state there is preferential formation of the quinoline derivative but in the presence of water the benzophenone is the main product.

FURTHER INFORMATION. Effect of temperature and relative humidity—D. Genton and U. W. Kesselring. *J. pharm. Sci.*, 1977, **66**, 676.

Storage. It should be stored in airtight containers, protected from light.

Identification. TEST. To about 10 mg add 5 ml of hydrochloric acid and 10 ml of water, heat on a water-bath for 15 minutes, filter, and to the filtrate add 1 ml of a 0.1% solution of sodium nitrite, allow to stand for 3 minutes, add 1 ml of a 0.5% solution of sulphamic acid, allow to stand for 3 minutes, and add 1 ml of a 0.1% solution of N-(1-naphthyl)ethylenediamine hydrochloride; a red colour is produced.

MELTING-POINT. About 227°.

ULTRAVIOLET ABSORPTION. In a mixture containing 1 volume of 1N hydrochloric acid and 9 volumes of methyl alcohol, maximum at 280 nm (E1%, 1cm = 910).

INFRA-RED ABSORPTION. Major peaks at 698, 1340, 1482, 1536, 1610, and 1690 cm⁻¹ (see Appendix 2a: Infra-red Spectra).

Determination in body fluids. SPECTROFLUORIMETRY. In plasma or urine: nitrazepam and main metabolites—J. Rieder, *Arzneimittel-Forsch.*, 1973, **23**, 207.

GAS CHROMATOGRAPHY. In serum—K. M. Jensen, *J. Chromat.*, 1975, **111**, 389.

REVIEWS OF METHODS FOR BENZODIAZEPINES. See under Chlordiazepoxide Hydrochloride.

Metabolism. ABSORPTION. Readily absorbed after oral administration.

BLOOD CONCENTRATION. After an oral dose of 10 mg, peak plasma concentrations of 70 to 110 ng/ml are attained in 2 hours; during therapy with 5 mg daily, steady state plasma concentrations of about 40 ng/ml are attained within 4 days.

HALF-LIFE. Plasma half-life, 17 to 28 hours.

DISTRIBUTION. Secreted in milk; *protein binding*, about 85% bound to plasma proteins.

METABOLIC REACTIONS. Nitroreduction and acetylation of the resultant amino group, hydroxylation, ring fission and hydroxylation, and glucuronic acid conjugation; the major metabolite is the 7-acetamido derivative and the fission products are 2-amino-5-nitrobenzophenone and 2-amino-3-hydroxy-5-nitrobenzophenone; nitroreduction appears to be the main pathway.

EXCRETION. After oral administration, 65 to 71% of a dose is excreted in the urine and 14 to 20% is excreted in the faeces; after intravenous administration, about 90% is excreted in the urine and 2 to 10% is excreted in the faeces; about 5% of a dose is excreted unchanged.

FURTHER INFORMATION. Pharmacokinetics—J. Rieder, *Arzneimittel-Forsch.*, 1973, **23**, 212.

Actions and uses. Nitrazepam has properties similar to those described under Chlordiazepoxide Hydrochloride. It possesses marked sedative properties and is used principally as a hypnotic agent.

Sleep lasting 6 to 8 hours is produced within 30 to 60 minutes of an oral dose of 5 to 10 milligrams. The dose should be reduced in elderly patients to 2.5 to 5 milligrams.

Undesirable effects. Nitrazepam may cause hangover and light-headedness. In elderly patients it may cause confusion. It may reduce the patient's ability to drive motor cars or operate moving machinery. Long-term administration of nitrazepam in late pregnancy may cause sedation in the offspring.

Precautions. Caution should be exercised in using nitrazepam in conjunction with alcohol and other drugs that act on the central nervous system. It should be used with caution in chronic airways obstruction.

Dependence. Nitrazepam may give rise to dependence of the barbiturate-alcohol type, as described under Barbiturates.

Preparations

NITRAZEPAM TABLETS: available as tablets containing 5 and 10 mg of nitrazepam.
A standard for these tablets is given in the British Pharmacopoeia 1973
Containers and *Storage:* see the entry on Tablets for general information on containers and storage. Containers should be airtight and light resistant.
Advice for patients: hypnotic doses should be taken half to 1 hour before bedtime. They may cause drowsiness on the following day; persons affected should not drive or operate machinery. Alcohol should be avoided.

OTHER PREPARATIONS available include CAPSULES containing nitrazepam 5 mg.

Nitrofurantoin

1-(5-Nitrofurfurylideneamino)imidazolidine-2,4-dione

$C_8H_6N_4O_5 = 238.2$

OTHER NAMES: *Berkfurin®*; *Furadantin®*; *Furan®*; *Macrodantin®*; *Urantoin®*
Ceduran® (with block liquorice)

A standard is given in the British Pharmacopoeia 1973

Description. Odourless yellow crystals or fine powder with a bitter taste.

Solubility. Very slightly soluble in water, in alcohol, and in glycerol; soluble, at 20°, in 200 parts of acetone, in 16 parts of dimethylformamide, and in 70 parts of macrogol 300.

Moisture content. Not more than 1%, determined by drying at 105°.

Dissociation constant. pK_a 7.2.

Storage. It should be stored in airtight containers, protected from light, at a temperature not exceeding 25°.

Identification. TEST. Dissolve about 5 mg in 5 ml of 0.1N sodium hydroxide; a deep yellow solution is produced which becomes deep orange-red.

MELTING-POINT. About 271°.

ULTRAVIOLET ABSORPTION. Dissolve 30 mg in 50 ml of dimethylformamide, dilute to 500 ml with water, and then dilute 10 ml of this solution to 100 ml with a solution containing 1.8% of sodium acetate and 0.14% of acetic acid; maxima at 266 nm and 367 nm (E1%, 1cm = 767).

INFRA-RED ABSORPTION. Major peaks at 1205, 1235, 1333, 1370, 1429, and 1724 cm⁻¹ (see Appendix 2b: Infra-red Spectra).

Determination in body fluids. ULTRAVIOLET SPECTROPHOTOMETRY. In blood or urine—G. L. Mattok *et al.*, *Clin. Chem.*, 1970, **16**, 820.

HIGH PRESSURE LIQUID CHROMATOGRAPHY. In plasma or urine—M. B. Aufrere *et al.*, *Clin. Chem.*, 1977, **23**, 2207.

Metabolism. ABSORPTION. Nitrofurantoin is readily absorbed after oral administration; the rate of absorption is delayed by food but peak body concentrations of the macrocrystalline form are increased by the presence of food in the gastro-intestinal tract; in addition, the presence of food in the gut increases the time that therapeutic concentrations are present in the urine; after intramuscular injection, nitrofurantoin is well absorbed but it is not absorbed after rectal administration.

BLOOD CONCENTRATION. After 100 mg orally 3 times daily, mean plasma concentrations of about 2 μg/ml are obtained; after a single oral dose, peak plasma concentrations are attained within 1 to 2 hours and do not exceed 2.5 μg/ml.

HALF-LIFE. Plasma half-life, about 20 minutes.

DISTRIBUTION. Small amounts cross the placenta and are also detectable in the milk of lactating mothers; *protein binding*, 25 to 60% bound to plasma proteins.

METABOLIC REACTIONS. Metabolised rapidly to inactive metabolites by most tissues.

EXCRETION. Nitrofurantoin is excreted in the urine by glomerular filtration and by active tubular secretion; after an oral dose of 100 mg of macro- and microcrystalline forms given to fasting subjects, about 20% and 35% of the doses are excreted in the urine respectively; after a similar dose of the two forms to non-fasting subjects about 40 and 50% of the doses are excreted in the urine respectively; about 50% of an intravenous dose is excreted in the urine and a higher proportion of an intravenous dose of the sodium salt is excreted in the same manner; the rate of urinary excretion of nitrofurantoin is increased by an increase in urinary pH or urinary flow but the activity is higher in acid urine since in this situation it is reabsorbed; small amounts of nitrofurantoin are excreted in the bile of dogs; supersaturation of the urine with nitrofurantoin does not result in crystalluria.

DISEASE STATES. In uraemics and azotaemics very little or no drug is excreted in the urine.

Bioavailability. The absorption of nitrofurantoin is influenced by particle size. Large (macro) crystals are more slowly absorbed than small (micro) crystals. In fasting patients, the bioavailabilities of the macro and micro forms are increased by 80 and 30% respectively.

Actions and uses. Nitrofurantoin is a broad-spectrum antibacterial agent whose mode of action on bacteria is unknown. It is well absorbed after oral administration but it is not possible to achieve effective concentrations in the tissues without intolerable side-effects. It is excreted in high concentration in the urine and its sole use is in the treatment of urinary infections.
Nitrofurantoin may not be as effective in the eradication of urinary infections as agents that can be used to produce high tissue concentrations but it is useful as a long-term suppressive agent in chronic infections that cannot be treated by other means. Bacterial resistance does not develop readily but many strains of coliform organisms encountered in hospitals are now resistant. *Pseudomonas* strains are naturally resistant and infections with *Proteus* strains respond poorly to treatment because of their alkalising action on the urine.

The usual dose for adults is 100 milligrams 4 times daily. The dose for children is 5 to 8 milligrams per kilogram body-weight daily in divided doses, but for the treatment of severe infections 10 milligrams per kilogram body-weight may be given. Treatment is usually continued for 7 to 14 days.

Undesirable effects. Nausea, abdominal discomfort, dizziness, and drowsiness may occur on full dosage but the symptoms usually subside when the dose is reduced. Serious complications are uncommon but include rashes and an alarming acute pulmonary syndrome that resembles pulmonary oedema. Polyneuritis may occur after prolonged administration, especially in patients with impaired renal function.

Undesirable effects may be minimised by adjusting the dose according to body-weight and administering the dose after meals.

Precautions and contra-indications. Nitrofurantoin should not be used in patients with a history of allergy to it or of the pulmonary syndrome or in those with glucose-6-phosphate-dehydrogenase deficiency in whom it may cause haemolytic anaemia. It should be used with caution in patients with renal impairment.

Preparations

NITROFURANTOIN MIXTURE (*Syn.* Nitrofurantoin Suspension): a homogeneous suspension of nitrofurantoin in a suitable flavoured vehicle. It has a pH at 20° of about 5.4.

This mixture should not be diluted. The general direction given in the entry on Mixtures that the preparation should be diluted so that the dose is contained in 5 ml does not apply to this mixture; it may be necessary for a dose of 2.5 ml to be measured by the patient in a 5-ml spoon; if a dose smaller than 2.5 ml is required, the dose should be measured by means of a graduated pipette.

Available as a mixture containing 25 mg of nitrofurantoin in 5 ml.

A standard for this mixture is given in the British Pharmaceutical Codex 1973

Containers and *Labelling:* see the entry on Mixtures for general information on containers and labelling.

Storage: it should be stored in a cool place, protected from light.

Advice for patients: the mixture should be taken at regular intervals after meals. The prescribed course should be completed. Nitrofurantoin may darken the urine.

NITROFURANTOIN TABLETS: available as tablets containing 50 and 100 mg of nitrofurantoin.

A standard for these tablets is given in the British Pharmacopoeia 1973

Containers and *Storage:* see the entry on Tablets for general information on containers and storage. Containers should be airtight and light resistant. The tablets should be stored at a temperature not exceeding 25°.

Advice for patients: the advice given under Nitrofurantoin Mixture (above) should be followed.

OTHER PREPARATIONS available include CAPSULES containing nitrofurantoin 50 and 100 mg; a veterinary POWDER containing nitrofurantoin 50% (in packs containing nitrofurantoin 1 g); and TABLETS containing nitrofurantoin 100 mg with block liquorice 250 mg (containing not more than 3% of glycyrrhizinic acid).

Nitrofurazone

5-Nitro-2-furaldehyde semicarbazone

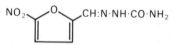

$$C_6H_6N_4O_4 = 198.1$$

OTHER NAMES: *Furacin*®
Bifuran® (with furazolidone); *Neovagon*® (with neomycin sulphate)

A standard is given in the British Pharmacopoeia Addendum 1977 and the British Pharmacopoeia (Veterinary)

Description. An odourless, yellow or brownish-yellow, crystalline powder with a bitter taste. It darkens in colour on exposure to light.

Solubility. Very slightly soluble in water; soluble, at 20°, in 600 parts of alcohol.

Storage. It should be stored in airtight containers, protected from light.

Identification. TEST. Dissolve about 1 mg in 1 ml of dimethylformamide and add 1 drop of 1N alcoholic potassium hydroxide; a ruby-red colour is produced.

MELTING-POINT. It turns yellow-black on heating and decomposes at about 238°.

INFRA-RED ABSORPTION. Major peaks at 971, 1020, 1205, 1250, 1587, and 1724 cm^{-1} (see Appendix 2b: Infra-red Spectra).

Determination in body fluids. ULTRAVIOLET SPECTROPHOTOMETRY. In urine—F. Fontani *et al.*, *J. pharm. Sci.*, 1972, **61**, 1502.

Actions and uses. Nitrofurazone has an antibacterial action against a number of Gram-negative and Gram-positive bacteria. It may be effective against strains which have become resistant to sulphonamides or penicillin. It is used as a local application for superficial wounds, burns, ulcers, and skin and mucous membrane infections and for the preparation of surfaces before skin grafting. It is usually applied in a concentration of 0.2% in a non-greasy ointment basis. A solution of this strength has been used in the treatment of otitis of the middle and external ear. Nitrofurazone has also been employed in infections of the eye.

Veterinary uses. Nitrofurazone is used as a coccidiostat and as an antibacterial agent. The usual dose for the treatment of coccidiosis in chickens is 100 parts per million in the drinking water or 200 parts per million in the feed for 7 days; for prophylaxis nitrofurazone is given continuously in the feed in a dosage of 67 to 100 parts per million. The usual dose for the treatment of necrotic enteritis in pigs is 500 parts per million in the feed for 7 days.

Preparations

Preparations available include an OINTMENT containing nitrofurazone 0.2%; a SOLUTION containing nitrofurazone 0.2%, diluent water for preparations; veterinary PESSARIES containing nitrofurazone 120 mg with neomycin sulphate 100 mg; and veterinary TABLETS containing nitrofurazone 110 mg with furazolidone 16 mg.

Nitrous Oxide

$$N_2O = 44.01$$

OTHER NAMES: Nitrogenii Oxidum

A standard is given in the European Pharmacopoeia Vol. II

Description. An odourless colourless tasteless gas which is heavier than air.

Solubility. One volume, measured at normal temperature and pressure, dissolves, at 20°, in about 1.5 volumes of water.

Storage, labelling, and colour-markings. It should be stored in metal cylinders designed to hold compressed gases. Cylinders should be stored in a special room free from materials of an inflammable nature. The room should ideally be cool but in any case the temperature should not exceed 36°.
The whole of the cylinder should be painted blue and the name of the gas or chemical symbol "N₂O" should be stencilled in paint on the shoulder of the cylinder. The name or chemical symbol of the gas should be clearly and indelibly stamped on the cylinder valve.

Identification. TEST. When mixed with nitric oxide, no red fumes are produced (distinction from oxygen).

Metabolism. ABSORPTION. Rapidly absorbed after inhalation; diffuses into skin at a higher rate than halothane or cyclopropane.

BLOOD CONCENTRATION. During intermittent therapy with 50% nitrous oxide to pregnant subjects during the first stage of labour, arterial blood concentrations of 80 to 280 µg/ml are attained at the end of each inhalation; once administration ceases, arterial concentrations rapidly fall to less than 5 µg/ml by 1 hour.

DISTRIBUTION. Rapidly crosses the placenta.

EXCRETION. Rapidly eliminated.

FURTHER INFORMATION. Arterial concentrations during labour—I. P. Latto *et al.*, *Br. J. Anaesth.*, 1973, **45**, 1029.

Actions and uses. Nitrous oxide is the oldest of the anaesthetics and is still the safest anaesthetic known. When given alone, it produces anaesthesia lasting only for about 45 seconds, recovery occurring within 1 to 2 minutes. When administered without air or oxygen, it produces complete anaesthesia in about one minute, with cyanosis, slow snoring respiration, dilated pupils, and raised blood pressure. These symptoms of anoxia disappear when air is breathed; they do not occur if mixtures containing 10% of oxygen are used. Almost the only complications following the use of nitrous oxide are those due to varying degrees of oxygen lack.
Nitrous oxide is used extensively in dental and obstetric practice for producing both analgesia and light anaesthesia. In the production of full surgical anaesthesia nitrous oxide is usually used only for induction and as a vehicle for, or an adjuvant to, other anaesthetics. It is often used in conjunction with local anaesthetics and muscle relaxants.

Poisoning. In the event of poisoning by nitrous oxide resulting in collapse and asphyxia, the procedure described under Chloroform should be adopted.

Nitroxynil

4-Hydroxy-3-iodo-5-nitrobenzonitrile

$C_7H_3IN_2O_3 = 290.0$

OTHER NAME: *Trodax*®

A standard is given in the British Pharmacopoeia (Veterinary)

Description. An odourless yellow powder.

Solubility. Practically insoluble in water; soluble, at 20°, in 120 parts of alcohol and in 60 parts of ether; soluble in solutions of alkali hydroxides.

Moisture content. Not more than 1%, determined by drying at 105°.

Storage. It should be protected from light.

Identification. TEST. Heat with sulphuric acid; iodine vapour is evolved.

MELTING-POINT. About 137°.

ULTRA-VIOLET ABSORPTION. In 0.01N sodium hydroxide, maxima at 225 nm and 271 nm (E1%, 1cm = 650).

INFRA-RED ABSORPTION. Major peaks at 730, 1124, 1250, 1316, 1333, and 1538 cm⁻¹ (see Appendix 2b: Infra-red Spectra).

Veterinary uses. Nitroxynil is used in the treatment of liver fluke infection in cattle and sheep. The usual dose is 10 milligrams per kilogram body-weight administered as the eglumine salt by subcutaneous injection and repeated if necessary at intervals of not less than 4 weeks.

Preparation

NITROXYNIL INJECTION: a sterile solution of the N-ethylglucamine salt of nitroxynil in water for injections. It is sterilised by heating in an autoclave or by filtration. Available in 50- and 250-ml packs containing the equivalent of 200 mg of nitroxynil per ml, and in 100- and 250-ml packs containing the equivalent of 340 mg of nitroxynil per ml.
A standard for this injection is given in the British Pharmacopoeia (Veterinary)
Containers: see the entry on Injections for general information on containers.
Labelling: see the entry on Injections for general information on labelling. In addition, the label on the container should state that animals should not be slaughtered for human consumption within 30 days after cessation of treatment, that the preparation should not be administered to lactating cows, and that the preparation should be washed from the eyes or exposed skin immediately if splashed.
Storage: it should be protected from light.

Noradrenaline Acid Tartrate

(R)-β,3,4-Trihydroxyphenethylammonium hydrogen tartrate monohydrate

$C_{12}H_{17}NO_9,H_2O = 337.3$

OTHER NAMES: Levarterenol Bitartrate; *Levophed*®; Noradren. Tart.; Noradrenaline Tartrate; Noradrenalini Tartras

A standard is given in the European Pharmacopoeia Vol. II

Description. An odourless white crystalline powder with a bitter taste. It slowly darkens on exposure to air and light.

Solubility. Soluble, at 20°, in 2.5 parts of water and in 300 parts of alcohol; very slightly soluble in ether and in chloroform.

Acidity. A 1% solution has a pH of 3 to 5.

Moisture content. 4.5 to 5.8%, determined by Fischer titration.

Specific rotation. $-10°$ to $-13°$, determined on a 5% solution.

Dissociation constants. pK_a 8.6, 9.8, 12 (20°).

Sterilisation. The strong solution containing 0.1% of sodium metabisulphite and 0.8% of sodium chloride is sterilised by heating in an autoclave or by filtration.

Storage. It should be stored in airtight containers, protected from light. It darkens on exposure to air and light.

Identification. TESTS. 1. To 1 ml of a 0.1% solution add 10 ml of *solution of standard pH 3.6* and 1 ml of 0.1N iodine, allow to stand for 5 minutes and add 2 ml of 0.1N sodium thiosulphate; not more than a very faint red colour is produced. Repeat the test using *solution of standard pH 6.6*; a strong reddish-violet colour is produced (distinction from adrenaline and isoprenaline).
2. Dissolve a few mg in 2 ml of water, add 5 ml of a 20% solution of sodium acetate and 2 drops of a 1% solution of mercuric chloride; a reddish-violet colour is produced.
3. Dissolve about 10 mg in 1 ml of water and add 1 drop of *ferric chloride test-solution*; an intense green colour is produced. Add *sodium bicarbonate solution*; the colour changes first to blue and then to red (also given by adrenaline and isoprenaline).

MELTING-POINT. About 102°.

ULTRAVIOLET ABSORPTION. In 0.01N hydrochloric acid, maximum at 279 nm (E1%, 1cm = 80).

INFRA-RED ABSORPTION. Major peaks at 1066, 1200, 1216, 1265, 1293, and 1395 cm^{-1} (see Appendix 2a: Infra-red Spectra).

Determination in body fluids. See under Adrenaline.

Metabolism. ABSORPTION. Rapidly metabolised before reaching the systemic circulation and therefore ineffective after oral administration; subcutaneous injections are poorly absorbed.

BLOOD CONCENTRATIONS. Endogenous plasma concentrations are approximately in the range 0.12 to 0.3 ng/ml.

HALF-LIFE. Plasma half-life for the distribution phase (α-phase) 1 to 6 minutes.

DISTRIBUTION. Widely distributed throughout the body.

METABOLIC REACTIONS. *O*-Methylation catalysed by catechol-*O*-methyltransferase to form normetanephrine, followed by oxidative deamination catalysed by monoamine oxidase, to form 4-hydroxy-3-methoxymandelic aldehyde which is converted to 4-hydroxy-3-methoxymandelic acid (vanillylmandelic acid) and to 4-hydroxy-3-methoxyphenyl glycol; the reaction sequence also occurs in reverse with the action of monoamine oxidase producing 3,4-dihydroxymandelic acid which is methylated to 4-hydroxy-3-methoxymandelic acid; the metabolites are conjugated with glucuronic acid or sulphate or further metabolised.

EXCRETION. Up to about 16% of an intravenous dose is excreted unchanged in the urine with methylated and deaminated metabolites in free and conjugated forms; negligible amounts of endogenous noradrenaline are excreted in the urine in normal subjects but may reach about 15 mg per day in subjects with phaeochromocytoma.

FURTHER INFORMATION. Metabolic reactions—J. Axelrod, *Science*, 1971, **173**, 598; uptake and metabolism in animals—L. L. Iversen *et al.*, *Br. J. Pharmac.*, 1971, **43**, 845; metabolism in man—J. W. Maas and D. H. Landis, *J. Pharmac. exp. Ther.*, 1971, **177**, 600; pharmacokinetics—G. Bufano *et al.*, *Eur. J. clin. Pharmac.*, 1973, **6**, 88.

Actions and uses. Noradrenaline is the neurohormone released at the terminations of post-ganglionic adrenergic nerve fibres when they are stimulated; it is also present in the adrenal medulla, from which it is liberated with adrenaline.

In its effect it differs from adrenaline in having little or no bronchodilator or vasodilator action (beta-effect). Its alpha-receptor actions are vasoconstriction, dilatation of the pupil, inhibition of the movements of the stomach, intestine, and bladder, and liberation of glucose from the liver.

The vasoconstrictor action of noradrenaline may be used to diminish the absorption and localise the effects of local anaesthetics, and to reduce haemorrhage during the subsequent operation; it should not, however, be used with cocaine. For these purposes it is given in solutions containing concentrations of noradrenaline of 1 in 100 000 to 1 in 50 000.

When applied to mucous membranes it produces ischaemia by constricting the vessels. For the control of capillary bleeding, local application of a 1 in 5000 solution is usually effective.

Noradrenaline is preferred to adrenaline in the treatment of peripheral vasomotor collapse in which the blood volume is adequate, such as after the removal of phaeochromocytomata, sometimes following the use of ganglion-blocking drugs, in surgical shock, and in acute myocardial infarction.

In man, noradrenaline produces the desired pressor response mainly by peripheral vasoconstriction and with little myocardial stimulation; coronary flow is usually increased, and the diastolic interval is lengthened because of the compensatory vagal slowing which follows the increased arterial pressure.

Noradrenaline acid tartrate is usually administered by intravenous infusion as a solution containing 8 micrograms, equivalent to 4 micrograms of the base, per millilitre in dextrose injection (5% w/v) or sodium chloride and dextrose injection; the solution is usually given initially at a rate of 1 millilitre per minute and subsequently at a rate sufficient to maintain the desired blood pressure, up to a maximum of 2.5 millilitres per minute. The infusion may be continued for days, if necessary, although there is a risk of gangrenous changes, especially at the site of infusion, and for this reason metaraminol is often preferred. Administration must not be stopped suddenly, but should be withdrawn gradually to guard against a disastrous fall in blood pressure.

Undesirable effects. As for Adrenaline.

Precautions. Noradrenaline should not be used in the presence of ventricular hyperexcitability produced by chloroform, trichloroethylene, cyclopropane, mercurial diuretics, quinidine, or large dosage of digitalis.

Drug interactions. As for Adrenaline.

Veterinary uses. Noradrenaline acid tartrate is a sympathomimetic. It is given by injection to control hypotension in acute circulatory collapse. However intravenous injections may give rise to cardiac arrhythmias especially when noradrenaline is given in conjunction with certain anaesthetics. The usual dosage by intravenous injection for all species is 0.5 microgram per kilogram body-weight per minute, adjusted in accordance with the response of the animal.

Preparations

NORADRENALINE INJECTION (*Syn.* Noradrenaline Acid Tartrate Injection): a sterile solution of noradrenaline acid tartrate in dextrose injection (5%) or in sodium chloride and dextrose injection. It is prepared immediately before use by diluting sterile strong noradrenaline solution (see below) to 250 times its volume with dextrose injection (5%) or sodium chloride and dextrose injection. Noradrenaline injection contains, in 1 ml, 8 micrograms of noradrenaline acid tartrate, equivalent to approximately 4 micrograms of noradrenaline; it contains, in 0.06 ml, 0.5 microgram of noradrenaline acid tartrate, equivalent to 0.25 microgram of noradrenaline.

STERILE STRONG NORADRENALINE SOLUTION:

Noradrenaline acid tartrate	..	..	..	0.2 g
Sodium metabisulphite	..	..	..	0.1 g
Sodium chloride	..	..	..	..	0.8 g
Water for injections	..	..	..	to 100.0 ml

It is prepared as described in the entry on Solutions. Sterilise by heating in an autoclave or by filtration. Available in 2- and 4-ml ampoules.
A standard for this solution is given in the British Pharmacopoeia Addendum 1977 and the British Pharmacopoeia (Veterinary)
Containers: see the entry on Injections for general information on containers. The solution is supplied in single-dose ampoules.
Labelling: the label on the container should state "Sterile Strong Noradrenaline Solution" and "This solution must be diluted before use"; the label on the container or the label or wrapper on the package should state "Sterile Strong Noradrenaline Solution for the preparation of Noradrenaline Injection", and "One volume of this solution diluted to 250 volumes with Dextrose Injection (5 per cent w/v) or with Sodium Chloride and Dextrose Injection produces Noradrenaline Injection, which must be used immediately after preparation".
Storage: it should be protected from light; it should not be used if it is brown in colour.

OTHER PREPARATIONS available include a sterile SOLUTION containing noradrenaline acid tartrate 200 micrograms per ml, equivalent to approximately 100 micrograms of noradrenaline per ml, in 2-ml ampoules.

Norethandrolone

17β-Hydroxy-19-nor-17α-pregn-4-en-3-one

$C_{20}H_{30}O_2 = 302.5$

OTHER NAME: *Nilevar®*

A standard is given in the British Pharmacopoeia 1973

Description. A white crystalline powder.

Solubility. Practically insoluble in water; soluble, at 20°, in 8 parts of alcohol, in 5 parts of chloroform, and in 3 parts of methyl alcohol.

Specific rotation. +20° to +22.6°, determined on a 2% solution in methyl alcohol.

Storage. It should be protected from light.

Identification. MELTING-POINT. About 135°.

ULTRAVIOLET ABSORPTION. In methyl alcohol, maximum at 240 nm (E1%, 1cm = 565).

INFRA-RED ABSORPTION. Major peaks at 894, 1210, 1263, 1583, 1612, and 1650 cm^{-1} (see Appendix 2a: Infra-red Spectra).

THIN-LAYER CHROMATOGRAPHY. See under Thin-layer Chromatography, System 10.

Metabolism. METABOLIC REACTIONS. Glucuronic acid conjugation and reduction.

EXCRETION. Small amounts are excreted in the urine as the glucuronide and about 10% is excreted as the glucuronides of 2 metabolites.

FURTHER INFORMATION. Metabolism—P. M. Adhikary and R. A. Harkness, *Acta endocr. Copenh.*, 1971, **67**, 721.

Actions and uses. Norethandrolone has actions and uses similar to those described under Methandienone. It is given by mouth in a dosage of 25 to 50 milligrams daily. A child usually requires a daily dosage of 500 micrograms per kilogram body-weight.

Undesirable effects. Because of its progestational activity, amenorrhoea and uterine bleeding may result from its withdrawal. It may also give rise to water retention and to jaundice.

Contra-indications; Drug interactions. As for Methandienone.

Preparation

NORETHANDROLONE TABLETS: available as tablets containing 10 mg of norethandrolone.
A standard for these tablets is given in the British Pharmacopoeia 1973
Containers and *Storage:* see the entry on Tablets for general information on containers and storage. Containers should be airtight and light resistant.

Norethisterone

17β-Hydroxy-19-nor-17α-pregn-4-en-20-yn-3-one

$C_{20}H_{26}O_2 = 298.4$

OTHER NAMES: *Micronor®*; Norethindrone; *Noriday®*; *Primolut N®*
Brevinor® and *Ovysmen®* (both with ethinyloestradiol); *Norinyl®*, *Ortho-Novin®*, and *Syntex Menophase®* (all with mestranol)

A standard is given in the British Pharmacopoeia 1973

Description. An odourless, white or creamy-white, crystalline powder.

Solubility. Practically insoluble in water; soluble, at 20°, in 150 parts of alcohol, in 30 parts of chloroform, in 80 parts of acetone, and in 5 parts of pyridine; very slightly soluble in vegetable oils.

Specific rotation. $-23°$ to $-27°$, determined on a 1% solution in chloroform.

Storage. It should be protected from light.

Identification. MELTING-POINT. About 203°.

ULTRAVIOLET ABSORPTION. In dehydrated alcohol, maximum at 240 nm (E1%, 1cm = 570).

INFRA-RED ABSORPTION. Major peaks at 660, 689, 1068, 1272, 1617, and 1649 cm^{-1} (see Appendix 2a: Infra-red Spectra).

THIN-LAYER CHROMATOGRAPHY. See under Thin-layer Chromatography, System 10.

Metabolism. DISTRIBUTION. In rats, there does not appear to be any selective tissue uptake; appears to cross the placenta.

METABOLIC REACTIONS. Norethisterone esters are hydrolysed to norethisterone; norethisterone is metabolised by ring A reduction to form 3-hydroxytetrahydro metabolites which are conjugated with glucuronic acid or sulphate; ethinyloestradiol has been detected in urine as a metabolite but aromatisation probably occurs as an artefact; 10β-hydroxylation may also occur.

EXCRETION. After an oral dose 35 to 50% is excreted in the urine in 5 to 10 days and 35 to 40% is eliminated in the faeces in 10 days; after an intravenous dose 37 to 80% is excreted in the urine in 5 days; a small amount is excreted unchanged and the major metabolites are glucuronic acid conjugates; urinary metabolites include the glucuronides of 17α-ethinyl-5β-estrane-3α,17β-diol, 17α-ethinyl-5β-estrane-3β,17β-diol, and 17α-ethinyl-5α-estrane-3α,17β-diol and the sulphate of 17α-ethinyl-5β-estrane-3β,17β-diol.

FURTHER INFORMATION. K. Fotherby, Metabolism of synthetic steroids by animals and man, *Pharmacological Models in Contraceptive Development*, M. H. Briggs and E. Diczfalusy (Eds), Geneva, World Health Organisation, 1974, p. 119; metabolism in man—E. Gerhards *et al.*, *Acta endocr. Copenh.*, 1971, **68**, 219; J. H. H. Thijssen, The metabolism of orally active synthetic progestational compounds, *International Encyclopedia of Pharmacology and Therapeutics*, Sect. 48, M. Tausk, (Ed.), Vol. 2, Oxford, Pergamon Press, 1972, p. 217.

Actions and uses. Norethisterone is a synthetic progestational steroid which converts the proliferative uterine endometrium to the secretory phase. It has slight oestrogenic and androgenic activities. Norethisterone is active when taken by mouth and is generally used in conjunction with oestrogens.

In the treatment of primary and secondary amenorrhoea 10 to 20 milligrams is given daily, in divided doses, from the fifth day to the twenty-fourth day of each menstrual cycle; withdrawal bleeding usually occurs one to three days after discontinuing treatment.

Norethisterone is also used for the treatment of menorrhagia, metrorrhagia, and endometriosis; in endometriosis, therapy must be continuous for 9 to 12 months. It has also been used to reduce premenstrual tension and relieve dysmenorrhoea. To delay or prevent menstruation, it is given in a dosage of up to 20 milligrams daily in divided doses, beginning 3 days before the expected onset of menstruation.

Norethisterone is used in conjunction with oestrogens as an oral contraceptive to inhibit ovulation. For this purpose doses of 1 to 2 milligrams are given daily, usually with ethinyloestradiol or mestranol, from the fifth to the twenty-fourth day of each menstrual cycle. The course is repeated after an interval of 1 week. Regular administration is essential. Norethisterone is also administered continuously in daily doses of 350 micrograms without oestrogen as an oral contraceptive.

Undesirable effects. Norethisterone may give rise to headache and tension, mental depression, nausea and vomiting, breast engorgement, fluid retention, and weight gain; a state of pseudopregnancy and premenstrual tension may be aggravated.

It may give rise to break-through bleeding and may cause hirsutism, acneiform skin rashes, and deepening of the voice. Virilisation of the female foetus may occur when doses of more than 15 milligrams daily of norethisterone are given. Prolonged use may lead to impairment of liver function. When taken without oestrogens it may not prevent conception.

Regular use of progestational oral contraceptives combined with oestrogens increases the risk of intravascular thrombosis and thromboembolic accidents. Progestogen-only contraceptives have little or no effect on clotting mechanisms.

Precautions and contra-indications. Care is necessary when liver function is impaired. Like other oral contraceptives, it is not reliable as a suppressant of ovulation in the first 10 to 12 days of the first regular course. It should not be used in pregnancy and should be used with caution in nursing mothers. Ectopic pregnancies have been reported with progestogen-only contraceptives.

Preparations

NORETHISTERONE TABLETS: available as tablets containing 350 micrograms and 5 mg of norethisterone; they may be coloured.

A standard for these tablets is given in the British Pharmacopoeia 1973

Containers and *Storage:* see the entry on Tablets for general information on containers and storage. Containers should be airtight and light resistant.

Advice for patients: the prescribed course should be completed or, where applicable, treatment should not be discontinued without the advice of the prescriber.

OTHER PREPARATIONS available include TABLETS containing norethisterone 500 micrograms with ethinyloestradiol 35 micrograms; tablets containing norethisterone 1 mg with mestranol 50 micrograms; tablets containing norethisterone 1 mg with mestranol 80 micrograms; tablets containing norethisterone 2 mg with mestranol 100 micrograms; and a combination pack providing graded doses of mestranol and norethisterone.

Norethisterone Acetate

3-Oxo-19-nor-17α-pregn-4-en-20-yn-17β-yl acetate

$C_{22}H_{28}O_3 = 340.5$

OTHER NAMES: Norethindrone Acetate; *SH420*®
Anovlar®; *Controvlar*®; *Gynovlar*®; *Loestrin*®; *Minovlar*®; *Norlestrin*®; *Orlest*® (all with ethinyloestradiol)

A standard is given in the British Pharmacopoeia 1973

Description. An odourless white or creamy-white crystalline powder.

Solubility. Very slightly soluble in water; soluble, at 20°, in 12.5 parts of alcohol, and in 4 parts of acetone; very slightly soluble in ether; soluble in chloroform.

Specific rotation. $-32°$ to $-38°$, determined on a 2% solution in dioxan.

Storage. It should be protected from light.

Identification. TEST. It complies with Test 3 described under Cortisone Acetate (presence of acetyl groups).

MELTING-POINT. About 163°.

ULTRAVIOLET ABSORPTION. In alcohol (95%), maximum at 240 nm (E1%, 1cm = 505).

INFRA-RED ABSORPTION. Major peaks at 1016, 1035, 1227, 1256, 1661, and 1752 cm^{-1} (see Appendix 2a: Infra-red Spectra).

THIN-LAYER CHROMATOGRAPHY. See under Thin-layer Chromotography, System 10.

Metabolism. See under Norethisterone.

Actions and uses. Norethisterone acetate has the actions, uses, and undesirable effects described under Norethisterone.
The usual dosage of norethisterone acetate is 2.5 to 20 milligrams daily in divided doses. As an oral contraceptive, 1 to 4 milligrams may be given daily.

Precautions and contra-indications. As for Norethisterone.

Preparations

Preparations available include TABLETS containing norethisterone acetate 10 mg, tablets containing norethisterone acetate 1 mg with ethinyloestradiol 20 micrograms, tablets containing norethisterone acetate 1 mg with ethinyloestradiol 50 micrograms, tablets containing norethisterone acetate 2.5 mg with ethinyloestradiol 50 micrograms, tablets containing norethisterone acetate 3 mg with ethinyloestradiol 50 micrograms, and tablets containing norethisterone acetate 4 mg with ethinyloestradiol 50 micrograms.

Norethynodrel

17β-Hydroxy-19-nor-17α-pregn-5(10)-en-20-yn-3-one. It contains not more than 1% of mestranol.

$C_{20}H_{26}O_2 = 298.4$

OTHER NAME: *Enavid*® and *Enavid-E*® (both with mestranol)

A standard is given in the British Pharmacopoeia 1973

Description. An odourless white crystalline powder.

Solubility. Practically insoluble in water; soluble, at 20°,

in 30 parts of alcohol, in 60 parts of ether, and in 7 parts of chloroform.

Specific rotation. $+120°$ to $+125°$, determined on a 1% solution in dioxan.

Labelling. The label on the container states the percentage of mestranol present.

Storage. It should be protected from light.

Identification. TEST. Dissolve about 2 mg in 0.3 ml of a 0.5% solution of dinitrobenzene in alcohol (95%), add 2 drops of *benzalkonium chloride solution*, mix, and add 2 ml of *dilute ammonia solution*; an intense magenta colour is produced immediately, changing to reddish-brown after about 5 minutes.

MELTING-POINT. About 175°.

ULTRAVIOLET ABSORPTION. In alcohol (95%), maximum at 240 nm (E1%, 1cm = 560).

INFRA-RED ABSORPTION. Major peaks at 644, 1066, 1140, 1390, 1690, and 1729 cm^{-1} (see Appendix 2a: Infra-red Spectra).

THIN-LAYER CHROMATOGRAPHY. See under Thin-layer Chromatography, System 10.

Metabolism. HALF-LIFE. Plasma half-life for free norethynodrel and free metabolites, about 9 hours.

DISTRIBUTION. In the rat, rapidly taken up by neural, genital, and other tissues; about 1% of a dose is secreted in milk.

METABOLIC REACTIONS. After oral administration, rapidly metabolised by reduction of ring A, hydroxylation, glucuronic acid conjugation, and conversion to norethisterone; metabolites include estrenes or 5α- or 5β-estranes possessing combinations of 3α,17β- or 3β,17β-dihydroxy substituents or combinations of 3α or 3β,10β,17β-trihydroxy substituents; all metabolites appear to retain the 17α-ethinyl group.

EXCRETION. After an oral dose, 28 to 40% is excreted in the urine in 5 days and 27 to 37% is eliminated in the faeces; 20% of the dose is excreted in the urine in conjugated form and about 10% is excreted as hydroxylated metabolites.

FURTHER INFORMATION. C. E. Cook *et al.*, *J. Pharmac. exp. Ther.*, 1972, **183**, 197; K. H. Palmer *et al.*, *J. Pharmac. exp. Ther.*, 1969, **167**, 207; J. H. H. Thijssen, The metabolism of orally active synthetic progestational compounds, *International Encyclopedia of Pharmacology and Therapeutics*, Sect. 48, M. Tausk (Ed.), Vol. 2, Oxford, Pergamon Press, 1972, p. 217.

Actions and uses. Norethynodrel is a synthetic progestational steroid which has actions similar to those described under Norethisterone. It is active when taken by mouth and is generally used in conjunction with oestrogens.
In the treatment of primary and secondary amenorrhoea it is given daily in a dosage of 5 to 10 milligrams from the fifth day to the twenty-fourth day of each menstrual cycle; withdrawal bleeding usually occurs 1 to 3 days after discontinuing treatment.
Norethynodrel is also used for the treatment of other dysfunctional uterine bleeding. For the treatment of endometriosis, doses of 20 to 30 milligrams daily are usually given continuously for 9 to 12 months.
Norethynodrel is used in conjunction with oestrogens as an oral contraceptive to inhibit ovulation. For this purpose doses of 2.5 or 5 milligrams are given daily, usually with mestranol, from the fifth to the twenty-fourth day of each menstrual cycle. The course is repeated

after an interval of one week. Regular administration is essential.

Undesirable effects. Norethynodrel may give rise to headache and tension, mental depression, nausea and vomiting, breast engorgement, fluid retention, and weight gain; a state of pseudopregnancy and pre-menstrual tension may be aggravated.

It may give rise to break-through bleeding, and may cause hirsutism, acneiform skin rashes, and deepening of the voice. Prolonged use may lead to impairment of liver function. When taken without oestrogens it may not prevent conception.

Regular use of progestational oral contraceptives combined with oestrogens increases the risk of intravascular thrombosis and thromboembolic accidents.

Precautions and contra-indications. As for Norethisterone.

Preparations

Preparations available include TABLETS containing norethynodrel 2.5 mg with mestranol 100 micrograms, and tablets containing norethynodrel 5 mg with mestranol 75 micrograms.

Nortriptyline Hydrochloride

N-10,11-Dihydro-5H-dibenzo[a,d]cyclohepten-5-ylidenepropyl-N-methylammonium chloride

$C_{19}H_{22}ClN = 299.8$

OTHER NAMES: *Allegron®*; *Aventyl®*
Motipress®; *Motival®* (both with fluphenazine hydrochloride)

A standard is given in the British Pharmacopoeia 1973

Description. A white powder with a slight characteristic odour and a taste which is burning and bitter followed by a sensation of numbness.

Solubility. Soluble, at 20°, in 50 parts of water, in 10 parts of alcohol, and in 5 parts of chloroform; practically insoluble in ether.

Dissociation constant. pK_a 10 (20°).

Storage. It should be protected from light.

Identification. TEST. Dissolve about 50 mg in 3 ml of warm water, cool, and add 1 drop of a 2.5% solution of quinhydrone in methyl alcohol; a red colour is slowly produced (distinction from amitriptyline).

MELTING-POINT. About 218°.

ULTRAVIOLET ABSORPTION. In methyl alcohol, maximum at 239 nm (E1%, 1cm = 480).

INFRA-RED ABSORPTION. Major peaks at 742, 758, 769, 1442, 1476, and 1488 cm^{-1} (see Appendix 2a: Infra-red Spectra).

Determination in body fluids. See under Amitriptyline Hydrochloride.

Metabolism. ABSORPTION. Readily and completely absorbed after oral administration.

BLOOD CONCENTRATION. Plasma concentrations vary considerably between individuals, are influenced by exposure to other drugs, and show no relationship with therapeutic effect; during therapy with 50 mg thrice daily, plasma concentrations of 30 to 280 ng/ml are attained; these concentrations are reduced when patients are also treated with anticonvulsants.

HALF-LIFE. Plasma half-life after intravenous administration, 18 to 60 hours.

DISTRIBUTION. Volume of distribution, 1400 to 2000 litres; nortriptyline enters the cerebrospinal fluid and crosses the placenta; *protein binding*, about 95% bound to plasma proteins which may be slightly decreased in the presence of phenytoin.

METABOLIC REACTIONS. 40 to 50% of an oral dose is subject to first pass metabolism; reactions are hydroxylation and N-demethylation to form 10-hydroxynortriptyline, desmethylnortriptyline, and 10-hydroxydesmethylnortriptyline; nortriptyline and its metabolites are conjugated with glucuronic acid; hydroxylamines of nortriptyline and desmethylnortriptyline are formed *in vitro*.

EXCRETION. 50 to 98% of a dose is excreted in the urine in 24 hours; less than 5% of a dose is excreted unchanged and 5 to 50% is excreted as 10-hydroxynortriptyline in free or conjugated form.

FURTHER INFORMATION. Metabolism—A. H. Beckett and S. Al-Sarraj, *J. Pharm. Pharmac.*, 1973, **25**, 335, L. F. Gram and K. F. Overø, *Clin. Pharmac. Ther.*, 1975, **18**, 305, D. R. Knapp *et al.*, *J. Pharmac. exp. Ther.*, 1972, **180**, 784, and S. Niazi, *J. pharm. Sci.*, 1976, **65**, 1535; plasma concentrations in twins—B. Alexanderson *et al.*, *Br. med. J.*, iv/1969, 764; plasma concentrations reduced by anticonvulsants—R. A. Braithwaite *et al.*, *Br. J. clin. Pharmac.*, 1975, **2**, 469; plasma concentrations in depression—P. Kragh-Sørensen *et al.*, *Lancet* i/1973, 113; renal excretion—F. Sjöqvist *et al.*, *Clin. Pharmac. Ther.*, 1969, **10**, 826.

Actions and uses. Nortriptyline is a tricyclic antidepressant with actions and uses as described under Amitriptyline Hydrochloride but it is less sedative. It is effective in similar dosage to amitriptyline, the usual dose by mouth being the equivalent of 30 to 100 milligrams of nortriptyline base daily in divided doses. 1.15 grams of nortriptyline hydrochloride is approximately equivalent to 1 gram of nortriptyline.

Undesirable effects; Precautions and contra-indications; Drug interactions. As for Amitriptyline Hydrochloride.

Preparations

NORTRIPTYLINE CAPSULES: consisting of nortriptyline hydrochloride, which may be mixed with a suitable inert diluent, enclosed in a hard capsule. The capsule shells may be coloured. Available as capsules containing nortriptyline hydrochloride equivalent to 10 and 25 mg of nortriptyline.

A standard for these capsules is given in the British Pharmacopoeia 1973

Containers and *Storage*: see the entry on Capsules for general information on containers and storage.

Labelling: the label on the container should state the amount of the medicament as the equivalent amount of nortriptyline.

Advice for patients: when initiating treatment there may be a time-lag of up to 2 weeks before a full therapeutic response is obtained. The capsules may cause drowsiness; persons affected should not drive or operate machinery. Alcohol should be avoided.

NORTRIPTYLINE TABLETS: available as tablets containing nortriptyline hydrochloride equivalent to 10 and 25 mg of nortriptyline; they are film coated; the coat may be coloured.

A standard for these tablets is given in the British Pharmacopoeia 1973

Containers and *Storage:* see the entry on Tablets for general information on containers and storage. Containers should be airtight.

Labelling: the label on the container should state the amount of the medicament as the equivalent amount of nortriptyline.

Advice for patients: see above under Nortriptyline Capsules.

OTHER PREPARATIONS available include a SOLUTION containing nortriptyline hydrochloride equivalent to 10 mg of nortriptyline in 5 ml, diluent syrup, life of diluted solution in both cases 14 days; TABLETS containing nortriptyline hydrochloride equivalent to 10 mg of nortriptyline with fluphenazine hydrochloride 500 micrograms, and tablets containing nortriptyline hydrochloride equivalent to 30 mg of nortriptyline with fluphenazine hydrochloride 1.5 mg.

Noscapine

(3*S*)-6,7-Dimethoxy-3-[(5*R*)-5,6,7,8-tetrahydro-4-methoxy-6-methyl-1,3-dioxolo[4,5-g]isoquinolin-5-yl]-phthalide

$C_{22}H_{23}NO_7 = 413.4$

OTHER NAMES: Narcotine; Noscapinum

A standard is given in the European Pharmacopoeia Vol. III

Description. An odourless, tasteless, almost white, fine, crystalline powder.

Solubility. Practically insoluble in water; very slightly soluble in alcohol and in ether; soluble in chloroform.

Moisture content. Not more than 1%, determined by drying at 105°.

Specific rotation. −196° to −201°, determined on a 4% solution in chloroform; +42° to +48°, determined on a 2% solution in 0.1N hydrochloric acid.

Dissociation constant. pK_a 6.2 (20°).

Storage. It should be stored in airtight containers.

Identification. TESTS. 1. Mix about 100 mg with a few drops of sulphuric acid in a porcelain dish and stir; a greenish-yellow solution is produced. Warm; the solution becomes red and finally violet.

2. Dissolve about 50 mg in 5 ml of 0.5N hydrochloric acid, add 10 ml of a mixture of equal volumes of alcohol (95%) and a saturated solution of sodium acetate, mix, and allow to stand; after about 3 minutes shining crystals separate.

MELTING-POINT. About 175°, with decomposition.

ULTRAVIOLET ABSORPTION. In alcohol (95%), maxima at 291 nm (E1%, 1cm = 92), and 310 nm (E1%, 1cm = 117).

INFRA-RED ABSORPTION. Major peaks at 1010, 1042, 1087, 1282, 1493, and 1754 cm⁻¹ (see Appendix 2b: Infra-red Spectra).

THIN-LAYER CHROMATOGRAPHY. See under Thin-layer Chromatography, System 7.

Determination in body fluids. SPECTROFLUORIMETRY. In plasma or urine—S. Vedsø, *Acta pharmac. tox.*, 1961, **18**, 119.

Metabolism. BLOOD CONCENTRATION. After oral doses of 250 to 300 mg of the chloride, peak plasma concentrations of 0.8 to 1.5 μg/ml are attained within 1 hour.

EXCRETION. About 1% of a dose is excreted in the urine partly in free and partly in conjugated forms.

FURTHER INFORMATION. Absorption and excretion— S. Vedsø, *Acta pharmac. tox.*, 1961, **18**, 157.

Actions and uses. Noscapine has an antitussive action similar to that described under Codeine Phosphate. It has no analgesic or narcotic action, it does not produce euphoria or drowsiness, and its use is unlikely to lead to dependence.

Noscapine is given by mouth to suppress irritant dry cough. It may also be used to suppress the cough of bronchitis and for the relief of whooping-cough in children.

The usual dose for adults is 15 to 30 milligrams and for children up to one year 1 milligram; 2 to 5 years 2 to 5 milligrams, and 6 to 12 years 6 to 12 milligrams. These doses may be given up to 4 times a day.

Preparation

NOSCAPINE LINCTUS:

Noscapine	.. 3 g
Citric acid monohydrate	10 g
Compound tartrazine solution	3 ml
Chloroform spirit	75 ml
Water for preparations	100 ml
Syrup..	to 1000 ml

Add the noscapine and the citric acid monohydrate to the water, previously heated to about 50°, and stir until dissolved; cool, add 800 ml of the syrup, followed by the compound tartrazine solution, the chloroform spirit, and sufficient syrup to produce the required volume, and mix. When a dose less than or not a multiple of 5 ml is prescribed, the linctus may be diluted, as described in the entry on Linctuses, with syrup.

It contains, in 5 ml, 15 mg of noscapine.

A standard for this linctus is given in the British Pharmaceutical Codex 1973

Containers: see the entry on Linctuses for general information on containers.

Storage: it should be stored in a cool place.

Advice for patients: the linctus should not be used for longer than a few days without medical advice.

Novobiocin Calcium

The calcium salt of 4-hydroxy-3-[4-hydroxy-3-(3-methyl-but-2-enyl)benzamido]-8-methylcoumarin-7-yl 3-*O*-carbamoyl-5,5-di-*C*-methyl-α-L-lyxofuranoside, an antimicrobial substance from *Streptomyces niveus* or related organisms.

$(C_{31}H_{35}N_2O_{11})_2Ca = 1263.3$

OTHER NAME: *Albamycin T Paediatric*® (with tetracycline)

A standard is given in the British Pharmacopoeia 1973

Description. An odourless, white or yellowish-white, crystalline powder with a taste which is sweet at first becoming bitter.

Solubility. Soluble, at 20°, in 300 parts of water, in 8 parts of alcohol, in 60 parts of acetone, in 100 parts of butyl acetate, and in 8 parts of methyl alcohol.

Alkalinity; Moisture content. As for Novobiocin Sodium.

Storage. It should be stored in airtight containers, protected from light.

Metabolism. See under Novobiocin Sodium.

Actions and uses. Novobiocin calcium has the antibacterial actions, uses, and undesirable effects of novobiocin, as described under Novobiocin Sodium. It is more stable in the presence of water than the sodium compound and can be used in the form of liquid suspensions for administration by mouth; 265 milligrams of novobiocin calcium is approximately equivalent to 250 milligrams of novobiocin.
Dosage is as for novobiocin sodium.

Precautions and contra-indications. As for Novobiocin Sodium.

Preparations

NOVOBIOCIN MIXTURE (*Syn.* Novobiocin Syrup): a suspension of novobiocin calcium, in a powder of suitable particle size, in a suitable flavoured vehicle, which may be coloured. When a dose less than or not a multiple of 5 ml is prescribed, the mixture may be diluted, as described in the entry on Mixtures, with syrup. The diluted mixture must be freshly prepared.
Available as a mixture containing novobiocin calcium equivalent to 125 mg of novobiocin in 5 ml.
A standard for this mixture is given in the British Pharmaceutical Codex 1973
Containers and *Labelling:* see the entry on Mixtures for general information on containers and labelling.
Storage: it should be stored in a cool place, protected from light.
Advice for patients: the mixture should be taken at regular intervals preferably after meals. The prescribed course should be completed.

NOVOBIOCIN TABLETS: containing novobiocin calcium or novobiocin sodium; they may be sugar coated or compression coated.
A standard for these tablets is given in the British Pharmacopoeia 1973
Containers and *Storage:* see the entry on Tablets for general information on containers and storage. Containers should be airtight.
Labelling: the label on the container should state the amount of the medicament as the equivalent amount of novobiocin, the date after which the tablets are not intended to be used, and the conditions under which they should be stored.
Advice for patients: see above under Novobiocin Mixture.

OTHER PREPARATIONS available include granules to prepare a MIXTURE containing novobiocin calcium equivalent to 62.5 mg of novobiocin with tetracycline 62.5 mg in 5 ml, when reconstituted, diluent water for preparations, life of mixture and diluted mixture 7 days.

Novobiocin Sodium

The monosodium salt of 4-hydroxy-3-[4-hydroxy-3-(3-methylbut-2-enyl)benzamido]-8-methylcoumarin-7-yl 3-O-carbamoyl-5,5-di-C-methyl-α-L-lyxofuranoside, an antimicrobial substance from *Streptomyces niveus* or related organisms.

$C_{31}H_{35}N_2NaO_{11} = 634.6$

OTHER NAME: *Albamycin T*® (with tetracycline hydrochloride)

A standard is given in the British Pharmacopoeia 1973

Description. An odourless, white or yellowish-white, crystalline powder with a taste which is sweet at first becoming bitter.

Solubility. Soluble, at 20°, in 5 parts of water, in 7 parts of alcohol, and in 3 parts of methyl alcohol; very slightly soluble in butyl acetate.

Alkalinity. A 2.5% suspension has a pH of 7 to 8.5.

Moisture content. Not more than 5%, determined by Fischer titration.

Dissociation constants. pK_a 4.2, 9.1 (25°).

Labelling. If the material is not intended for parenteral administration, the label on the container states that the contents are not to be injected.

Storage. It should be stored in airtight containers, protected from light. If it is intended for parenteral administration, the containers should be sterile and sealed to exclude micro-organisms.

Metabolism. ABSORPTION. Well absorbed after oral administration.

BLOOD CONCENTRATION. After oral doses of 150 to 700 mg, peak serum concentrations of up to 40 µg/ml are attained in 1 to 4 hours; therapeutic concentrations may be maintained for a further 24 hours; on repeated dosage, for example 500 mg every 6 hours, novobiocin may accumulate and serum concentrations of about 100 µg/ml may be attained.

HALF-LIFE. Serum half-life, 2 to 3 hours; in children the half-life appears to be dose dependent with a half-life of about 1.5 hours at low doses and a half-life of about 4 hours at high doses.

DISTRIBUTION. Slowly diffuses throughout most body tissues and enters pleural and ascitic fluids, and when the meninges are inflamed, enters the cerebrospinal fluid in small amounts; secreted in milk; subject to enterohepatic cycling; *protein binding*, about 96% bound to plasma proteins.

EXCRETION. Excreted mainly in the bile with about 30% of a dose appearing in the faeces and about 3% in the urine in active form.

FURTHER INFORMATION. Blood concentrations—S. Furesz, *Antibiotics Chemother.*, 1958, **8**, 446; review —A. Kucers and N. M. Bennett, *The Use of Antibiotics. A Comprehensive Review with Clinical Emphasis*, 2nd edn, London, Heinemann Medical Books Ltd, 1975, p. 325; pharmacokinetics—J. G. Wagner and R. E. Damiano, *J. clin. Pharmac.*, 1968, **8**, 102.

Actions and uses. Novobiocin is an antibiotic which is

active against a number of Gram-positive organisms, especially *Staphylococcus aureus*; in general, it has no significant action against Gram-negative bacteria, except some strains of *Proteus* species. The antibacterial range of activity of novobiocin is similar to that of penicillin. Its action is primarily bacteriostatic, but it is bactericidal in high concentrations against highly sensitive strains. Novobiocin is used in the treatment of staphylococcal infections, but its value is limited by the frequent occurrence of undesirable effects and the readiness with which bacterial resistance is acquired. Its use should be restricted to the treatment of staphylococcal infections in which the organisms are resistant to other antibiotics but have been proved to be sensitive to novobiocin, to the treatment of biliary tract infections by sensitive bacteria, and to the treatment of *Proteus* infections not suitable for treatment with other drugs. It is advisable to administer novobiocin with another antibiotic, such as erythromycin, to diminish the chance of acquired resistance.

Novobiocin is usually given by mouth as the sodium or calcium salt, the dosage for an adult being 250 milligrams every 6 hours or 500 milligrams every 12 hours; if tolerated, these doses may be doubled in severe or resistant infections; 260 milligrams of novobiocin sodium is approximately equivalent to 250 milligrams of novobiocin. The usual dose of novobiocin for children up to 1 year is 62.5 to 125 milligrams, 1 to 5 years 125 to 250 milligrams, and 6 to 12 years 250 to 500 milligrams; these doses are given twice daily.

Novobiocin, in the form of the sodium salt, has been given by the slow intravenous injection of a solution containing the equivalent of 500 milligrams of novobiocin in 30 millilitres of sodium chloride injection over a period of 5 to 10 minutes, or a more dilute solution may be given by intravenous infusion; solutions containing dextrose are incompatible with novobiocin sodium and should not be used as diluents. For a child the intravenous dosage is 15 milligrams per kilogram body-weight every 12 hours. Intramuscular injection is painful.

A yellow pigment which may appear in the serum of patients treated with novobiocin is a metabolite of the drug and does not indicate liver damage.

Undesirable effects. Nausea and vomiting may occur during treatment and skin rashes and fever are relatively common. Leucopenia sometimes occurs when treatment is prolonged. It may cause skin sensitisation, eosinophilia, and a temporary yellow discoloration of the skin and sclerae.

Precautions and contra-indications. The administration of novobiocin should be discontinued if jaundice develops. Novobiocin should not be given to children under 6 months, as it may interefere with the conjugation of bilirubin. It should not be given in pregnancy, particularly just before parturition.

Preparations

NOVOBIOCIN TABLETS: see above under Novobiocin Calcium.

OTHER PREPARATIONS available include CAPSULES containing novobiocin sodium equivalent to 125 mg of novobiocin with tetracycline hydrochloride equivalent to 125 mg of tetracycline.

Nutmeg

The dried kernels of the seeds of *Myristica fragrans* Houtt. (Fam. Myristicaceae), a tree indigenous to the Moluccas and cultivated in Indonesia and the West Indies (Grenada).

OTHER NAME: Myristica

A standard is given in the British Pharmaceutical Codex 1973

The seed is divested of the arillus (mace) and slowly dried, an operation which takes from 8 to 10 weeks; the testa is then broken and the kernel removed.

Constituents. Nutmeg contains about 5 to 15% of volatile oil and about 35% of solid fat, the chief fatty acid constituents of which are myristic acid (about 60%) and smaller amounts of palmitic, oleic, linoleic, and lauric acids. It also contains small amounts of myristicin, elemicin, safrole, phytosterin, starch, amylodextrin, colouring matter, and a saponin. It yields up to 3% of ash.

Description. UNGROUND DRUG. *Macroscopical characters:* kernels ovoid, about 20 to 30 mm long and 15 to 20 mm broad; surface light brown, showing network of shallow reticulate grooves and marked with numerous small, dark brown points and lines; slight circular elevation about 5 mm in diameter, somewhat eccentrically placed at wider end, indicating tip of radicle, connected by a broad shallow groove to the chalaza showing as a slight circular depression at the opposite end; kernel consisting of a pale brown endosperm covered by a thin darker brown perisperm penetrating the endosperm by numerous infoldings, producing the characteristic ruminate appearance of the cut surface; embryo small, embedded in the endosperm near the micropyle; when pressed by the finger-nail the cut surface exudes oil. It has an aromatic characteristic odour and an aromatic somewhat bitter taste.

Microscopical characters: the diagnostic characters are: peripheral *perisperm* composed of strongly flattened polyhedral cells with brown contents and occasional prismatic *crystals;* inner ruminate portion of perisperm consisting of parenchyma containing isolated groups of yellow *oil cells; endosperm* of polyhedral cells each containing a single *aleurone grain* with a large crystalloid, about 12 by 20 μm, and *starch* granules, 2- to 10-compound or simple, the latter up to about 20 μm in width, all frequently embedded in a dark brown, *fatty mass;* the fat forms radiating groups of feathery crystals when a preparation in hot *chloral hydrate solution* is allowed to cool.

POWDERED DRUG. Powdered Nutmeg. A reddish-brown powder possessing the diagnostic microscopical characters, odour, and taste of the unground drug.

Adulterants and substitutes. Bombay nutmegs, from *M. malabarica* Lam., are longer, narrower, and almost devoid of odour.

Macassar or Papua nutmegs, from *M. argentea* Warb., are also longer and narrower and have a uniform scurfy surface, a safrole-like odour, and an acrid taste.

Limed nutmegs are nutmegs which have been dipped in milk of lime and subsequently dried, a process which is intended to protect them from the attacks of insects.

Storage. It should be stored in airtight containers, in a cool place.

Actions and uses. Nutmeg is a carminative and a

Undesirable effects. In large doses, it excites the motor cortex and produces epileptiform convulsions.

Preparation

Powdered nutmeg is an ingredient of aromatic chalk powder.

Nutmeg Oil

Obtained by distillation from nutmeg.

OTHER NAMES: Myristica Oil; Oleum Myristicae

A standard is given in the British Pharmaceutical Codex 1973

Constituents. Nutmeg oil consists chiefly of terpenes, including α- and β-pinene. It also contains myristicin (4-allyl-6-methoxy-1,2-methylenedioxybenzene) and safrole. East Indian nutmeg oil contains 1.9 to 2.9% of safrole and 14.0 to 15.8% of myristicin. West Indian nutmeg oil contains 0.28 to 0.38% of safrole and 1.8 to 2.6% of myristicin. Nutmeg oil may contain up to 3% of non-volatile matter.

Description. A colourless, pale yellow, or pale green liquid. The odour is that of nutmeg.

Solubility. Soluble at 20°, East Indian oil, in 3 volumes of alcohol (90%); West Indian oil, in 4 volumes of alcohol (90%).

Weight per ml. At 20°, East Indian oil, 0.885 to 0.915 g; West Indian oil, 0.860 to 0.880 g.

Refractive index. East Indian oil, 1.475 to 1.488; West Indian oil, 1.472 to 1.477.

Optical rotation. East Indian oil, +10° to +25°; West Indian oil, +25° to +45°.

Storage. It should be stored in well-filled airtight containers, in a cool place, protected from light.

Actions and uses. Nutmeg oil has been used in a dose of 0.05 to 0.2 millilitre for its carminative properties; it is also used as a flavouring agent. When absorbed, large doses stimulate the cerebral cortex and may induce epileptiform convulsions.

Preparations

Nutmeg oil is an ingredient of aromatic ammonia solution and aromatic ammonia spirit.

Nux Vomica

Consists of the dried ripe seeds of *Strychnos nux-vomica* L. (Fam. Loganiaceae), a small tree widely distributed over the Indian subcontinent and south-east Asia.

A standard is given in the British Pharmacopoeia 1973

The ripe fruit, which externally resembles an orange, contains a whitish bitter pulp, in which are embedded 3 to 5 seeds; the seeds are removed when ripe, washed free from pulp, and dried in the sun.

Constituents. Nux vomica contains strychnine and brucine as major alkaloids together with lesser amounts of the closely related alkaloids α- and β-colubrine, 4-hydroxystrychnine, pseudostrychnine, pseudobrucine, pseudo-α-colubrine, pseudo-β-colubrine, icajine, novacine, vomicine, and N-methyl-sec-pseudo-β-colubrine. The total alkaloid ranges from 1.8 to 5.3%, about half of which is strychnine, although the proportion is subject to variation. The iridoid glycoside loganin together with very small amounts of loganic acid, deoxyloganin, seco-

loganin, and ketologanin are also present, as are fatty material (3%) and chlorogenic acid.

Nux vomica may also contain up to 1% of foreign organic matter and yield up to 3% of ash.

Description. UNGROUND DRUG. *Macroscopical characters*: seeds grey to greenish-grey, disk-shaped, nearly flat, umbonate, sometimes irregularly curved, 10 to 30 mm in diameter and 4 to 6 mm thick, edge rounded or subacute; umbo connected to micropyle by a radial ridge; trichomes crowded, radiating from centre of both flat faces, and appressed, giving seed a silky surface; endosperm abundant, translucent, horny, with a central disk-shaped cavity; embryo situated in central cavity next to micropyle, having 2 small, thin, cordate cotyledons and a cylindrical radicle.

It has no odour; it has an extremely bitter taste.

Microscopical characters: the diagnostic characters are: *trichomes* with strongly thickened, pitted, lignified bases and cylindrical limbs, up to about 1 mm long; limbs with several lignified *ribs* and breaking up in powder to form rod-like fragments; *endosperm* consisting of thick-walled unlignified polyhedral cells with well-marked plasmodesmata and containing *oil-plasma* and *aleurone grains*, the grains up to 30 μm in diameter; *starch* and *crystals* of calcium oxalate absent; length of lignified rib per mg of seed 1.67 to **1.84** to 2.06 m.

POWDERED DRUG. Powdered Nux Vomica. A yellowish-grey powder possessing the diagnostic microscopical characters and taste of the unground drug; odourless.

Adulterants and substitutes. The following have been imported as nux vomica.

Seeds of *S. nux-blanda* A. W. Hill. The seeds may be distinguished by their regular shape, paler colour, and the presence of a distinct ridge on the edge of the seeds; the alkaloid content of the seeds is about 0.1% and the alkaloid composition resembles that of *S. nux-vomica* seeds; strychnine and brucine are the major alkaloids.

Seeds of *S. potatorum* L.f., are Indian seeds known as clearing nuts. They are smaller and thicker in appearance and contain about 0.3% of total alkaloids of which diaboline and acetyldiaboline are the major alkaloids. Small amounts of strychnine and brucine may occur in some seeds.

Seeds of *S. wallichiana* Steud ex DC. (*S. cinnamomifolia* Thwaites) var. *wightii* (A. W. Hill) are similar to nux vomica but are fawn rather than grey in colour; the alkaloidal content and composition is very similar to that of *S. nux-vomica*. Seeds of a south Indian sample have been shown to contain 4-hydroxy-3-methoxystrychnine as the major alkaloid with smaller amounts of strychnine, 4-hydroxystrychnine, brucine, vomicine, 4-hydroxy-3-methoxy-N-methyl-sec-pseudostrychnine and novacine.

Actions and uses. Nux vomica has the actions, uses, and undesirable effects described under Strychnine Hydrochloride.

Poisoning. The procedure described under Strychnine Hydrochloride should be adopted.

Preparations

NUX VOMICA LIQUID EXTRACT:

Small-scale preparation

Nux vomica, in moderately

coarse power   ..   ..   1000 g

Alcohol (45%) }

Alcohol (70%) }   ..   ..   ..   of each sufficient quantity

Exhaust the nux vomica with alcohol (70%) by percolation. Remove the alcohol from the percolate and concentrate the liquid until it measures 250 ml. To this liquid, while still hot, add 15 g of hard paraffin, heat to 60°, and shake vigorously. Allow to cool, perforate the solidified waxy layer, and pour off the liquid. Determine the proportion of strychnine in the liquid, and to the remainder of the liquid add sufficient alcohol (45%) to produce an extract of the required strength; allow to stand for not less than 24 hours and filter.

Manufacture. Prepare the extract by the above method, appropriately scaled up, or by the alternative method described in the entry on Extracts.

It contains, in 0.2 ml, 3 mg of strychnine.

A standard for this extract is given in the British Pharmacopoeia 1973

Dose: 0.05 to 0.2 ml.

NUX VOMICA TINCTURE:

Nux vomica liquid extract	..	..	..	83.4 ml
Alcohol (45%)	..	..	..	to 1000.0 ml

Mix; filter, if necessary.

It contains, in 2 ml, 2.5 mg of strychnine.

A standard for this tincture is given in the British Pharmacopoeia 1973

Dose: 0.5 to 2 ml.

Nystatin

An antifungal substance produced by the growth of *Streptomyces noursei.* It has a potency of not less than 4400 units per milligram.

OTHER NAMES: *Nystan®*; *Nystavescent®*
Mysteclin® (with tetracycline hydrochloride); *Nysta-dermal®* (with triamcinolone acetonide); *Nystaform®* (with clioquinol); *Flagyl Compak®* (with metronidazole); *Tinaderm-M®* (with tolnaftate)

A standard is given in the British Pharmacopoeia 1973

Description. A yellow to light brown hygroscopic powder with a characteristic odour.

Solubility. Very slightly soluble in water, in alcohol, and in methyl alcohol; practically insoluble in ether and in chloroform.

Moisture content. Not more than 5%, determined by drying at 60° *in vacuo.*

Storage. It should be stored in airtight containers, protected from light, at a temperature not exceeding 5°. Under these conditions the potency may fall at the rate of about 1% per month.

Actions and uses. Nystatin is an antibiotic which is active against a wide range of fungi and yeasts. It is poorly absorbed after oral administration and is not absorbed through skin or mucous membranes.

The chief use of nystatin is in the local treatment of candidal infections of the mucous membrane and of the skin and nails. In the treatment of candidal infections of the mouth, nystatin is used in the form of tablets which are allowed to dissolve slowly in the mouth or it is applied topically as a suspension. For intestinal candidiasis it is given by mouth in the form of tablets in a dosage of 500000 to 1000000 units 3 times a day. Vaginal candidiasis may be treated by means of soluble tablets or pessaries containing 100000 units; local treatment may be supplemented by oral administration of nystatin with a view to reducing the risk of reinfection from the intestinal tract. In candidal infections of the skin, nystatin is applied several times daily as an oint-

Undesirable effects. Oral administration of nystatin may give rise to diarrhoea, nausea, and vomiting, but these effects are rare and usually transient.

Veterinary uses. Nystatin is an antifungal agent. It is administered to cattle by intramammary injection, the usual dose being 20 milligrams (100000 units) into each infected quarter daily.

Preparations

NYSTATIN MIXTURE (*Syn.* Nystatin Suspension): a suspension of nystatin in a suitable flavoured vehicle. This mixture should not be diluted. The general direction given in the entry on Mixtures that the preparation should be diluted so that the dose is contained in 5 ml does not apply to this mixture; the dose should be measured by means of a graduated pipette.

Available as a ready-prepared mixture containing 100000 units of nystatin per ml.

A standard for this mixture prepared freshly from granules is given in the British Pharmaceutical Codex 1973. Granules for nystatin mixture are no longer generally available in the United Kingdom but supplies of the granules, which contain no sugar, may be available for the treatment of sugar-intolerant patients.

Containers and *Labelling:* see the entry on Mixtures for general information on containers and labelling.

Advice for patients: the dose should be retained in the mouth for as long as possible before swallowing. The prescribed course should be completed.

NYSTATIN OINTMENT: a dispersion of nystatin, in powder of suitable particle size, in a polyethylene-mineral-oil gel or other suitable anhydrous basis. Available as an ointment containing 100000 units of nystatin per g.

A standard for this ointment is given in the British Pharmaceutical Codex 1973

Containers and *Labelling:* see the entry on Ointments for general information on containers and labelling.

Advice for patients: the ointment should be applied sparingly to the affected area.

NYSTATIN PESSARIES: may be prepared by moist granulation and compression as described in the entry on Tablets. Available as pessaries containing 100000 units of nystatin. The pessaries may also be suitable for use as lozenges.

A standard for these pessaries is given in the British Pharmaceutical Codex 1973

Containers and *Storage:* see the entry on Tablets for general information on containers and storage. Containers should be airtight.

Advice for patients: the pessaries should be moistened with water and inserted high into the vagina with a suitable applicator, preferably at night. When used as lozenges the pessaries should be allowed to dissolve slowly in the mouth. The prescribed course should be completed.

NYSTATIN TABLETS: available as tablets containing 500000 units of nystatin; they are sugar coated; the coat may be coloured.

A standard for these tablets is given in the British Pharmacopoeia 1973

Containers and *Storage:* see the entry on Tablets for general information on containers and storage. Containers should be airtight. The tablets should be stored at a temperature not exceeding 25°. Under these conditions they may be expected to retain their potency for at least 3 years.

Advice for patients: the tablets should be taken at regular intervals. The prescribed course should be completed.

OTHER PREPARATIONS available include CAPSULES containing nystatin 250 000 units with tetracycline hydrochloride 250 mg; a CREAM containing nystatin 25 000 units per g, a cream containing nystatin 100 000 units per g, a cream containing nystatin 100 000 units per g with clioquinol 1%, a cream containing nystatin 100 000 units per g with tolnaftate 1%, a cream containing nystatin 100 000 units per g with triamcinolone acetonide 0.1%; a DUSTING-POWDER containing nystatin 100 000 units per g; a GEL containing nystatin 100 000 units per g; an OINTMENT containing nystatin 100 000 units per g with clioquinol 1%, an ointment containing nystatin 100 000 units per g with triamcinolone acetonide 0.1%; PESSARIES containing nystatin 100 000 units in an effervescent basis; TABLETS containing nystatin 250 000 units with tetracycline hydrochloride 250 mg; a combination pack consisting of pessaries containing nystatin 100 000 units in an effervescent basis, tablets containing nystatin 500 000 units, and a gel containing nystatin 100 000 units per g, and a combination pack consisting of 14 pessaries containing nystatin 100 000 units with 21 tablets containing metronidazole 200 mg.

Nystatin, Dermatological

A grade of nystatin (see above) that is suitable for preparations for use on the skin but not for oral administration. A standard is given in an addition to the British Pharmacopoeia 1973, *Pharm. J.*, i/1978, 354. It is similar to the standard of the British Pharmacopoeia 1973 for Nystatin but Nystatin (Dermatological) is not required to comply with a test for abnormal toxicity.

Description; Solubility; Moisture content; Storage. As for Nystatin (above).

Obesity

Obesity is the condition in which there is an excessive accumulation of fat in storage areas of the body due to dietary intake in excess of requirements for tissue repair, vital functions, and physical activities. The additional burden creates a mechanical disability with an increased liability to skeletal problems such as flat feet and osteoarthrosis of the knees, and to varicose veins, abdominal hernias, and bronchitis.

Overweight subjects are also more likely to develop cardiovascular defects such as hypertension, angina pectoris, and cardiac failure than subjects of average weight. Obesity may lead to diabetes in middle age. Body weight may be reduced by restricting diet to below the individual's energy requirements. A diet providing 1000 kilocalories (4 megajoules) daily should cause a loss of about 1 kg weekly in a sedentary worker with a daily requirement of 2000 to 2500 kilocalories (8 to 10 megajoules) daily. A similar negative balance can be arranged by giving about 1500 kilocalories (6 megajoules) daily to a person doing light work or 3000 kilocalories (13 megajoules) daily to a heavy manual worker.

Endocrine disorders are rarely the cause of obesity except insulin-secreting tumours of the pancreas, Cushing's disease, and, occasionally, myxoedema. There may be genetic factors involved in obesity but evidence for this is inconclusive. Overeating is often a sign of emotional disturbance which may require treatment.

Treatment of obesity by turkish baths, massage, diuretics, or purgation with hypertonic saline solutions is unsatisfactory as the weight reduction achieved is merely due to fluid loss which is quickly replaced. The use of drugs should be avoided except in the most resistant cases where dietary measures alone have proved unsuccessful.

Amphetamine has anorectic activity but is also a central nervous stimulant and drug of abuse and should not be used for this purpose. This is also true of some related compounds such as phenmetrazine.

Diethylpropion has only slight central stimulant properties and is useful in some patients when given in courses of up to three months' duration, after which its effectiveness appears to diminish.

Fenfluramine tends to have a central depressant rather than stimulant action and should not be used in patients with a past history of depression. Studies *in vitro* and *in vivo* have suggested that at least part of its anti-obesity action is due to peripheral metabolic effects.

Thyroxine has been used as a "slimming drug" but in small doses it is ineffective and in large doses it is dangerous.

Methylcellulose is a substance which is not absorbed from the alimentary tract and which swells in water. When administered with water before a meal it increases the bulk of the gastric contents and so gives rise to a feeling of satiety leading to decreased food intake. Its value in the treatment of obesity has not, however, been confirmed.

Octaphonium Chloride

Benzyldiethyl-2-[4-(1,1,3,3-tetramethylbutyl)phenoxy]-ethylammonium chloride monohydrate

$C_{27}H_{42}ClNO,H_2O = 450.1$

OTHER NAME: Phenoctide

A standard is given in the British Pharmacopoeia Addendum 1975

Description. An odourless white crystalline powder.

Solubility. Soluble, at 20°, in 5 parts of water; soluble in alcohol and in chloroform.

Acidity. A 1% solution has a pH of 5 to 6.

Moisture content. 3.5 to 4.5%, determined by Fischer titration.

Identification. TESTS. 1. 10 ml of a 1% solution complies with Test 1 described under Benzalkonium Chloride Solution.

2. Dissolve about 250 mg in 1 ml of sulphuric acid; the solution complies with Test 2 described under Benzalkonium Chloride Solution, commencing with the words "add 100 mg of potassium nitrate".

ULTRAVIOLET ABSORPTION. In alcohol (95%), maxima at 263 nm (E1%, 1cm = 25), 269 nm (E1%, 1cm = 30), 274 nm (E1%, 1cm = 29), and 282 nm (E1%, 1cm = 25).

Actions and uses. Octaphonium chloride has the actions

and uses of the quaternary ammonium compounds, as described under Cetrimide. In addition it has antifungal activity.

A solution with methacrylate polymers is used as a waterproof antiseptic covering for fistulas and dry skin lesions. It has been used as a 0.5 or 1% solution for general antiseptic purposes. A 0.5% solution in alcohol (50%) has been used for pre-operative sterilisation of the skin.

Precautions. As for Cetrimide.

Octyl Gallate

Octyl 3,4,5-trihydroxybenzoate

$$CO \cdot O \cdot CH_2 \cdot [CH_2]_6 \cdot CH_3$$

$C_{15}H_{22}O_5 = 282.3$

OTHER NAME: *Progallin O*®

A standard is given in the British Pharmacopoeia 1973

Description. An odourless white or creamy-white powder.

Solubility. Practically insoluble in water; soluble, at 20°, in 2.5 parts of alcohol, in 3 parts of ether, in 30 parts of chloroform, in 1 part of acetone, in 33 parts of arachis oil, in 0.7 part of methyl alcohol, and in 7 parts of propylene glycol.

Storage. It should be stored in airtight containers, protected from light, contact with metals being avoided.

Identification. TESTS. It complies with the tests described under Dodecyl Gallate.

MELTING-POINT. About 101°.

ULTRAVIOLET ABSORPTION. In methyl alcohol, maximum at 275 nm (E1%, 1cm = 375).

Uses. Octyl gallate is used as an antoxidant for preserving oils and fats, as described under Dodecyl Gallate.

Oedema

Oedema is swelling due to the presence of abnormally large amounts of fluid in the intercellular tissue spaces of the body. It is usually detected by the accumulation of fluid in the subcutaneous tissues. Swelling of the ankles is characteristic of oedema in the ambulant patient. When a patient is confined to bed oedema may be detected around the sacrum. Oedema of the lungs (pulmonary oedema) occurs in left-heart failure and is characterised by breathlessness.

Oedema is accompanied by retention of sodium and chloride ions. It may be caused by any process which causes retention of water or sodium and chloride ions in the body, for example glomerulonephritis, the nephrotic syndrome, or heart failure. The excess fluid causing oedema may be removed by treatment of the underlying disorder or by the use of diuretics. A negative sodium balance may be produced by increasing sodium excretion or decreasing dietary intake of sodium.

Oestradiol Benzoate

Estra-1,3,5(10)-trien-3,17β-diol 3-benzoate

$C_{25}H_{28}O_3 = 376.5$

OTHER NAMES: *Benztrone*®; Oestradiol Monobenzoate; Oestradioli Benzoas

Apocrine® and *Ovocept*® (both with chorionic gonadotrophin); *Declimone*® (with testosterone propionate)

A standard is given in the European Pharmacopoeia Vol. II

Description. Odourless colourless crystals or white crystalline powder.

Solubility. Practically insoluble in water and in solutions of alkali hydroxides; soluble, at 20°, in 150 parts of alcohol, in 50 parts of acetone, in 500 parts of arachis oil, and in 200 parts of ethyl oleate.

Specific rotation. +57° to +63°, determined on a 1% solution in dioxan.

Sterilisation. Oily solutions for injection are sterilised by dry heat.

Storage. It should be protected from light.

Identification. TEST. Mix about 1 mg with 3 drops of *sulphomolybdic reagent*; a yellowish-green colour with an intense green fluorescence is produced. Add 1 ml of sulphuric acid followed by 9 ml of water; the solution becomes pink with a yellowish fluorescence.

MELTING-POINT. About 194°.

ULTRAVIOLET ABSORPTION. In alcohol (95%), maximum at 231 nm (E1%, 1cm = 490).

INFRA-RED ABSORPTION. Major peaks at 704, 709, 1075, 1220, 1250, and 1724 cm⁻¹ (see Appendix 2b: Infra-red Spectra).

THIN-LAYER CHROMATOGRAPHY. See under Thin-layer Chromatography, System 10.

Metabolism. ABSORPTION. Oestradiol is readily absorbed after oral administration but to varying extents; esters of oestradiol are absorbed to varying extents depending upon the polarity of the ester; well absorbed through mucous membranes and skin; oestradiol benzoate is slowly absorbed after intramuscular injection.

BLOOD CONCENTRATION. Endogenous oestradiol plasma concentrations are variable and under hormonal control; during the menstrual cycle plasma concentrations are about 10 to 100 ng/ml in the early follicular phase, 47 to 70 ng/ml in the late follicular phase, 130 to 720 ng/ml at the pre-ovulatory peak, 30 to 390 ng/ml in the early luteal phase, and 25 to 260 ng/ml at the mid-luteal phase; in men, endogenous oestradiol concentrations are about 20 pg/ml; during pregnancy oestrogens are synthesised in large amounts by the placenta resulting in high circulating concentrations especially of oestriol.

DISTRIBUTION. Widely distributed throughout the body and secreted in milk; *protein binding*, bound to both albumin and globulins.

METABOLIC REACTIONS. Oxidation of oestradiol (E_2) to oestrone (E_1), hydroxylation at positions 16, 2, 6, 15, and 18 to produce a large number of metabolites, dehydrogenation at position 11, methylation of the 2-hydroxylated metabolite, and conjugation with glucuronic acid or sulphate; the major reaction is the formation of oestrone (E_1) which is hydrated to form oestriol (E_3); the other important metabolite is 2-hydroxy-E_1; other metabolites include 6α- and 6β-hydroxy forms of E_1 and of E_2, 16β-hydroxy E_2 (epioestriol), 2-methoxyoestrogens, 15α- and 15β-hydroxy forms of E_1 and of E_2, and the 18-hydroxy form and the 11-dehydro form of E_2; most of the urinary metabolites are conjugated, mainly with glucuronic acid; rifampicin and phenobarbitone stimulate oestradiol hydroxylation; after oral administration oestradiol is subject to first pass metabolism.

EXCRETION. About 50 to 80% of a dose is excreted in the urine in 5 to 6 days, and about 18% is excreted in the faeces; of the urinary excreted material, 55 to 80% is conjugated with glucuronic acid; about 20% of the excreted material is oestrone, 20% oestradiol, 20% 2-hydroxyoestrone, and about 5% 2-methoxyoestrone; less than 4% is unconjugated; oestradiol and its metabolites are excreted as conjugates in the bile, hydrolysed, and reabsorbed. Urinary concentrations of endogenously derived oestrogens during the menstrual cycle are as follows: onset of cycle 4.7(E_1), 0.3(E_2), and 0.15(E_3) μg/24 hours; follicular phase, 6(E_1), 3(E_2), and 8(E_3) μg/24 hours; ovulation, 11–31(E_1), 4–14(E_2), and 13–54(E_3) μg/24 hours; luteal phase, 10–23(E_1), 4–10(E_2), and 8–72(E_3) μg/24 hours.

FURTHER INFORMATION. Effect of rifampicin on oestradiol metabolism—H. M. Bolt *et al.*, *Eur. J. clin. Pharmac.*, 1975, **8**, 301; metabolism of oral oestradiol—J. Fishman *et al.*, *J. clin. Endocr. Metab.*, 1969, **29**, 41; K. Fotherby and F. James, Metabolism of synthetic steroids, *Advances in Steroid Biochemistry and Pharmacology*, M. H. Briggs and G. A. Christie (Eds), Vol. 3, London, Academic Press, 1972, p. 67.

Actions and uses. Oestradiol is the most active of the naturally occurring oestrogens. These substances are concerned in producing the oestrous changes in animals and in controlling certain functions of the human uterus and accessory organs, particularly the proliferation of the endometrium, the development of the decidua, and the cyclic changes in the cervix and vagina. They also influence the development of the secondary sex characters and mammary glands and affect the contractility of the uterus and its response to oxytocic drugs.

Large doses of oestrogens depress the activities of the anterior lobe of the pituitary gland.

The oestrogens are mainly used in therapeutics for replacement therapy in conditions in which there is a deficiency of them; for the treatment of conditions associated with hypoplasia of the genital tract, such as primary amenorrhoea and delayed onset of puberty; for the treatment of the menopausal syndrome, particularly the vasomotor disturbances and psychological upsets; for the treatment of conditions such as senile vaginitis, vulvitis, and kraurosis vulvae; and for the treatment, in conjunction with progesterone, of some disturbances of menstruation, including secondary amenorrhoea due to ovarian deficiency, some types of dysmenorrhoea, and functional uterine bleeding.

Oestrogens are also used to inhibit lactation; for this purpose large doses are required, which act by inhibiting release of prolactin by the anterior pituitary. They are also used in the palliative treatment of carcinoma of the prostate and breast to diminish pain and to produce temporary subjective improvement, particularly in bone metastases.

Oestrogens are administered orally, intramuscularly, and topically by inunction and in pessaries, tampons, and suppositories. The oral dose of the naturally occurring oestrogens is 5 to 10 times that required by intramuscular injection.

Oestradiol benzoate is given by intramuscular injection to provide a depot from which the drug is slowly liberated during 2 to 5 days. The dosage is 1 to 5 milligrams at intervals of 1 to 14 days; smaller doses may be used for maintenance therapy.

Undesirable effects. Oestrogens may sometimes cause undesirable uterine growth and proliferation and withdrawal bleeding in the menopause. If bleeding occurs following the use of oestrogens in the menopause, action should be taken to exclude cancer as a cause. The effects of the oestrogens on the uterus are enhanced by alternating courses of treatment with oestrogens and progesterone.

Veterinary uses. Oestradiol benzoate is used in the control of breeding in all species and as an anti-androgen in dogs. The dose as an oily injection by subcutaneous or intramuscular injection varies from 1 microgram to 1.5 milligrams per kilogram body-weight depending on the response required. Oestradiol benzoate is also administered to cattle as a single uterine infusion of 50 milligrams.

Preparations

OESTRADIOL BENZOATE INJECTION: a sterile solution of oestradiol benzoate in ethyl oleate or other suitable ester, in a suitable fixed oil, or in any mixture of these. It is sterilised by dry heat. Available in 1-ml ampoules containing 1 and 2 mg of oestradiol benzoate, and in 1- and 2-ml ampoules containing 5 mg of oestradiol benzoate per ml. Also available for veterinary use in 10-ml vials containing 5 mg of oestradiol benzoate per ml.

A standard for this injection is given in the British Pharmacopoeia 1973

Containers: see the entry on Injections for general information on containers.

Labelling: see the entry on Injections for general information on labelling. In addition, the label on the package should state the composition of the solvent, and that the injection is for intramuscular use only.

Storage: it should be protected from light. On standing, solid matter may separate; it should be redissolved by heating before use.

OTHER PREPARATIONS available include an INJECTION containing oestradiol benzoate 500 micrograms with testosterone propionate 25 mg per ml in 1-ml ampoules, a veterinary injection containing oestradiol benzoate 1 mg with chorionic gonadotrophin 200 units per ml in 25-ml vials, and a veterinary injection containing oestradiol benzoate 1 mg with chorionic gonadotrophin 250 units per ml in 20-ml vials.

Ointments

Ointments are semisolid preparations intended for application to the skin; they usually contain a medicament or mixture of medicaments dissolved, dispersed, or emulsified in a suitable basis. The consistency of the basis is such that it spreads and softens when stress is applied. Bases are often anhydrous and comprise fats, oils, and waxes of animal, vegetable, or mineral origin; non-oleaginous and synthetic substances are also used as bases.

Ointments are used as vehicles for medicaments intended to produce a pharmacological effect at or near the application site; they are also applied as emollients and skin protectives.

Ideally, an ointment basis should not produce irritation or sensitisation of the skin, nor should it retard wound healing; it should be smooth, inert, odourless, physically and chemically stable, and compatible with the skin and with dermatological medicaments.

Classification of Ointment Bases

Ointment bases can be classified in terms of their physico-chemical properties into four main types—fatty or oleaginous, "absorption", emulsion, and water-soluble.

Fatty bases are usually anhydrous and may contain water-insoluble vegetable oils, animal fats and waxes, hydrocarbons, silicones, or certain synthetic esters. Such bases exert an occlusive effect by limiting the evaporation of moisture from the skin; they have a low capacity to absorb water and are usually used as emollients or as inert vehicles. Because of their greasiness they tend to be cosmetically unattractive.

Absorption basis is the name given to a basis which absorbs water; the name does not describe the mode of action of the basis. Absorption bases are often anhydrous and, typically, consist of a hydrophobic fatty basis in which a water-in-oil emulsifier has been incorporated to render it hydrophilic. Additional water can be incorporated into the basis to form the internal phase of an emulsion, with a consequent increase in the viscosity of the system. Bases of this type are used as vehicles for aqueous liquids or solutions of medicaments; they are not always easily removed from the skin.

Emulsion bases are semisolid emulsified systems which can be either water-in-oil or oil-in-water emulsions; in each case additional water can be incorporated until the consistency is that of a soft cream. Water-in-oil bases have occlusive properties and because of their oily external phase are less readily removed by water than the oil-in-water bases. Oil-in-water bases are easily spread on the skin and readily form vanishing-type creams on admixture with water.

Most *water-soluble* ointment bases are made by blending macrogols of high and low molecular weight; water is not usually included as it dissolves the base and promotes softening. Consistency is varied by adjusting the proportion of the liquid and solid macrogols. Water-soluble medicaments can usually be dissolved in macrogol bases but because these bases are less occlusive than absorption or fatty bases, rates of drug release from them may differ and require evaluation.

Rheology

The term ointment is applied to semisolid systems which usually behave as viscoelastic materials when shear stress is applied. The rheological behaviour of ointments is closely related to their structure; for example, at microscopic level soft paraffins consist of solid and liquid fractions in the form of a fibrous crystal matrix of the waxy components to which the liquid components are held by sorption. A gel-like matrix can also form in the continuous phase of emulsified bases and in absorption bases, especially those which contain emulsifiers based on surface-active agents and long-chain alcohols. The flow properties of ointments are controlled mainly by the rigidity of the matrix and the concentration of the waxy constituents.

Percutaneous Absorption

Percutaneous absorption is the term used to describe the penetration of a substance through the skin and its subsequent passage into the blood-stream. Medicaments applied in ointments are usually intended to exert a local effect; where the desired effect is simply protective or emollient, penetration of the medicament may not be necessary.

Some medicaments do not appear to be absorbed percutaneously, but in instances where absorption does occur, it is usually desirable that the rate of absorption should be slow in order that the medicament is retained at the site of action for as long as possible. Appreciable absorption of medicaments such as corticosteroids can give rise to side effects.

The properties of the medicament are an important factor in determining the extent of percutaneous absorption. Absorption is also affected by the nature of the ointment basis but to a lesser extent than was formerly considered to be the case.

Percutaneous absorption and the properties of the skin, medicament, and basis which affect it, are discussed in the entry on Creams.

Constituents of Ointment Bases

Hydrocarbons (hard, soft, and liquid paraffins)

Paraffins are the most widely used constituents of ointment bases. They are relatively inert and show few incompatibilities with dermatological medicaments. Soft paraffin is easily spread at normal temperature but its rheological properties can change after heating and cooling, or after mechanical treatment; modification to more liquid or solid consistency is made by the addition of liquid or hard paraffin.

Soft paraffin is commercially available which exhibits a "fibrous" internal appearance. The "long fibre" type is considered to enhance stability in emulsified systems and to produce better occlusion than the "short fibre" type. Liquid paraffin can be mixed with hard paraffin to form semisolid bases, some of which tend to become crystalline on storage; it has also been formed into an ointment-like gel (*Plastibase®*) by heating with polyethylene and cooling under special conditions.

Vegetable oils (almond, arachis, castor, coconut, cottonseed, maize, olive)

Except for coconut oil, these are all liquids and are used to modify the consistency of ointments and for their emollient properties. Vegetable oils tend to vary in composition and they are readily oxidised, especially if contaminated with trace metals. Butylated hydroxyanisole, butylated hydroxytoluene or alkyl gallates are often incorporated to retard oxidation, sometimes in conjunction with organic acids (citric, phosphoric, and tartaric) to chelate metal ions; these are usually added by the suppliers of vegetable oils.

Wool fat

Wool fat has both emollient properties and the ability to absorb about 30% of water. Thus, wool fat and its derivatives are widely used in absorption bases. Limitations of wool fat are its tendency to oxidise, its sticky texture, its odour, and its capacity to induce skin sensitivity in occasional patients.

Fatty acids and alcohols (stearic and oleic acids; ceto-stearyl, stearyl, and cetyl alcohols)

Because fatty acids are of natural origin, their composition varies; their main use is to form soap emulsifiers with alkalis, but an excess of acid can also increase the stiffness and change the appearance of emulsified systems. Fatty alcohols act as secondary emulsifiers and also as bodying agents; stearyl alcohol tends to form harder bases than cetyl alcohol.

Other substances

Other raw materials used in ointments include macrogols, beeswax, propylene glycol, cholesterol, isopropyl myristate, carbomer, silicones, and some colloidal clays. Emulsifying agents such as esters of macrogols and sorbitan are included in emulsion bases.

Preparation of Ointments

The method selected for the preparation of ointments usually depends on the properties of the medicament, the type of basis, and the quantity of ointment required. For small quantities of a relatively soft ointment, trituration on a slab with a spatula of flexible metal, plastic, or bone is one of the easiest methods for the mixing and incorporation of liquids or solids. Before incorporation, insoluble powders must be finely powdered and levigated either with some of the melted basis or a suitable liquid. Water-soluble salts are dissolved in a small amount of water and incorporated with the aid of a small amount of lanolin. A mortar and pestle is more convenient when liquids are to be incorporated or for the preparation of larger amounts of ointment.

Fusion is the method usually adopted for large-scale manufacture or for ointments in which waxes or solids of high melting-point are to be mixed with semisolids or oils; it is also used when large volumes of water are to be incorporated.

Constituents are melted successively in decreasing order of melting-point and the fluid mixture stirred until cooled, avoiding aeration. If not stirred effectively, fatty alcohols and acids may crystallise from systems which contain paraffins. Volatile medicaments are usually added when the ointment has cooled to below 40°. Insoluble powders in the form of a levigated dispersion are often incorporated when the ointment begins to thicken. Soluble solids which are heat-stable can be dissolved in the melted basis before it congeals.

For quantities of less than 500 g, further treatment of the ointment to improve homogeneity may not be feasible, but for larger amounts, roller mills or colloid mills aid the uniform distribution of insoluble solids and the elimination of particles larger than about 50 μm.

In making ointments which are intended to be used in tropical or sub-tropical climates, a more satisfactory consistency may be obtained by altering the proportions of paraffins, oils, fats, and waxes given in published formulae; in all cases, the amounts of active ingredients must be maintained.

Preservation and Sterilisation of Ointments

Preservatives are not commonly included in anhydrous ointments because, although micro-organisms may survive in such systems, they rarely proliferate. In polyphasic ointments which contain water, effective antimicrobial systems should be included to prevent both spoilage and the growth of pathogenic organisms.

Important factors which can reduce antimicrobial action in polyphasic systems are the partitioning of the anti-microbial agent between the oil and water phases, and the inactivation of the antimicrobial in the presence of surface-active agents, especially nonionic surfactants.

In investigations of formulae it is usual to assess the effectiveness of systems by submitting the preserved ointment to challenge tests with appropriate pathogenic and spoilage organisms.

Preservatives most widely used commercially in water-containing ointments are mixtures of hydroxybenzoate esters, sorbic acid, phenethyl alcohol, organic mercurials, and quaternary ammonium compounds.

Bacterial filtration or sterilisation by exposure to dry heat for one hour at a temperature not lower than 150° can be applied to some anhydrous ointments or their constituents, but these procedures are not usually practicable for polyphasic ointments or for those which contain water. For the latter, an aseptic technique is necessary.

Dilution of Ointments

For certain specific ointments, when a strength of ointment not available from a manufacturer is prescribed, a stronger ointment should be diluted to the required strength with the diluent suggested in the relevant entry. When the specified diluent is soft paraffin, a portion of it may be replaced by hard paraffin or liquid paraffin to obtain an ointment of suitable consistency.

Containers

Ointments should be stored and supplied in containers which prevent evaporation and contamination of the contents. The materials of construction should be resistant to sorption or diffusion of the contents. Collapsible tubes of metal (to British Standard 4230:1967) or flexible plastic tubes may be used. The internal surface of metal tubes may be coated with a lacquer of a heat-cured epoxy resin. Collapsible tubes may also be lined near the base with a suitable pressure-sensitive sealing coat.

Ointments may also be supplied in wide-mouth jars of glass or plastic fitted with plastic screw caps with impermeable liners or with close-fitting slip-on lids. Plastic containers may be unsuitable for ointments which contain methyl salicylate, phthalate esters, or similar substances.

Labelling

The container should be labelled "for external use only". If a preservative is included, the name and concentration should appear on the label.

FURTHER INFORMATION. B. W. Barry, Rheology of pharmaceutical semisolids, *Advances in Pharmaceutical Sciences*, H. S. Bean *et al.*, (Eds), Vol. 4, London, Academic Press, 1974; review of the literature on lanolin hypersensitivity—E. W. Clark, *J. Soc. cosmet. Chem.*, 1975, **26**, 323.

Oleic Acid

(*Z*)-Octadec-9-enoic acid

$$CH_3 \cdot [CH_2]_7 - \overset{\overset{\displaystyle H}{|}}{C} = \overset{\overset{\displaystyle H}{|}}{C} - [CH_2]_7 \cdot COOH$$

$C_{18}H_{34}O_2 = 282.5$

OTHER NAME: *Priolene 6986*®

A standard is given in the British Pharmacopoeia 1973

Oleic acid also contains some stearic and palmitic acids and usually traces of iron, probably derived from the vessels in which it is stored.

Description. A yellowish to pale brown oily liquid with a characteristic tallow-like odour.

Solubility. Practically insoluble in water; soluble in alcohol, in ether, in chloroform, and in light petroleum.

Weight per ml. At 20°, 0.889 to 0.895 g.

Stability. On exposure to air it darkens in colour and the odour becomes more pronounced.

Storage. It should be stored in well-filled airtight containers, protected from light, contact with iron being avoided.

Uses. Oleic acid forms soaps with alkaline substances and is used in the preparation of injections, liniments, and lotions.

Preparations

Oleic acid is an ingredient of chloroxylenol solution, ethanolamine oleate injection, soap liniment, and white liniment.

Olive Oil

The fixed oil obtained by expression from the ripe fruits of *Olea europea* L. (Fam. Oleaceae), a small tree cultivated in Spain, Portugal, Italy, and other countries bordering on the Mediterranean Sea, California, and South Australia; the oil may be refined.

OTHER NAME: Oleum Olivae

A standard is given in the British Pharmacopoeia 1973

Constituents. Olive oil consists of glycerides, the chief fatty acid of which is oleic acid, with smaller amounts of palmitic, linoleic, stearic, and myristic acids.

Description. A pale yellow or greenish-yellow oil with a slight but not rancid odour; at low temperatures it may be solid or partly solid.

Solubility. Very slightly soluble in alcohol; miscible with ether, with chloroform, and with light petroleum.

Weight per ml. At 20°, 0.910 to 0.916 g.

Refractive index. 1.468 to 1.471.

Adulterants and substitutes. Possible adulterants of olive oil include cottonseed oil, arachis oil, tea-seed oil, obtained from *Camellia sasanqua* Thunb. and sometimes other species of *Camellia* (Fam. Theaceae), and sesame oil. Tests for the presence of arachis, cottonseed, and sesame oils are given under Almond Oil.
Olive oil is sometimes prepared by refining oil obtained by solvent-extraction processes and such oil is often sold for edible or technical purposes.

Sterilisation. It is sterilised by dry heat.

Storage. It should be stored in well-filled airtight containers. If it has solidified, it should be completely melted and mixed before use.

Actions and uses. Olive oil is nutritious, demulcent, and mildly laxative. In the form of an emulsion, it may be given as a nitrogen-free diet during the treatment of renal failure.
Olive oil (100 to 500 millilitres) warmed to body temperature is injected per rectum to facilitate removal of impacted faeces.
Externally, olive oil is emollient and soothing to inflamed surfaces. It is applied to the skin to remove incrustations in eczema and psoriasis and is used as a lubricant in massage. Olive oil is employed in the preparation of liniments, ointments, plasters, and soaps and as a vehicle in oily suspensions for injection.

Onchocerciasis

see under FILARIASIS

Ophthalmia neonatorum

This is an infection of the eyes of the newborn baby and is usually acquired during its passage through the birth canal. The eyelids are swollen and there is a profuse purulent discharge. Sight may be lost if the condition is left untreated. The infecting organism may be the gonococcus or Chlamydia, or in later or less severe cases, other organisms such as staphylococci.
Gonococcal ophthalmia is treated by the very frequent instillation of penicillin drops into the eye, every 5 minutes at first, then half-hourly and finally 2 hourly; penicillin is also given intramuscularly. Silver nitrate solution has also been used for instillation. The strength should not be more than 1%, and even this concentration may produce a chemical conjunctivitis, so that penicillin is preferred. Penicillin may be used prophylactically as well as in treatment.
Chlamydia infection is best treated with tetracycline locally and by mouth. Infections due to bacteria other than the gonococcus may be treated locally with chloramphenicol.

Opium

The dried or partly dried latex obtained from the unripe capsules of *Papaver somniferum* L. (Fam. Papaveraceae).

OTHER NAME: Raw Opium
When Opium is prescribed, Powdered Opium is dispensed.

A standard is given in the British Pharmacopoeia 1973

Opium is collected principally in the Indian subcontinent. It has also been collected in Bulgaria, Iran, Japan, Turkey, U.S.S.R., and Yugoslavia. The exuded latex is partially dried by spontaneous evaporation together with artificial heat, and is manipulated to form cakes of uniform composition, variously shaped according to the country of origin. Usually only Indian opium is now available in commerce.

Varieties. Indian opium: cubical or rectangular blocks or masses, weighing from 1 to 10 kg, wrapped in greaseproof paper or plastic material, varying in consistence from brittle to plastic; internally dark brown to almost black, smooth and homogeneous.
Manipulated Turkish opium: brick-shaped masses, about 130 to 150 mm long, 100 to 120 mm wide, and 100 to 120 mm thick, usually bearing on one surface an indented monogram consisting of the letters T and M inside an O, covered with roughly powdered poppy leaves, weighing usually about 2 kg; outer surface firm, plastic, or very rarely brittle; internally softer, chocolate-brown or dark brown, and somewhat granular.

Constituents. Opium contains about 25 alkaloids; morphine, which occurs in commercial varieties in proportions varying from about 9 to 17%, exists in combination with meconic and sulphuric acids in the form of salts readily soluble in water. Turkish opium contains about 10 to 16% of morphine and Indian about 9 to 12%.

The proportion of noscapine [(−)-narcotine], which exists partly in the free state and partly as a salt, is usually about 2 to 9%.

Codeine is present to the extent of about 0.3 to 4% in combination with acids, Indian opium containing the highest proportion and Turkish opium the lowest.

The remaining alkaloids constitute about 2.5 to 6% of the drug; they include thebaine (0.5 to 2%), papaverine (0.5 to 2.5%) and other alkaloids of the 1-benzyltetra-hydroisoquinoline, morphinane, protropine, phthalide-isoquinoline, and papaverrubine types.

Starch, tannin, calcium oxalate, and fat do not normally occur and their presence therefore indicates sophistication.

When exhausted with water, undried opium gives an infusion which is acid and yields from 40 to 55% of dry aqueous extract which contains most of the morphine present in the drug (constituting about 25% of the extract).

Description. UNGROUND DRUG. *Macroscopical characters:* see under Varieties (above).
Opium has a strong characteristic odour and a bitter taste.

Microscopical characters: the diagnostic characters are: *latex* in abundant brown, granular, amorphous masses amongst which occur small quantities of structures insoluble in water: *Outer epidermis of capsule* of poppy plant in fragments composed of polyhedral tabular cells in surface view, about 20 to 50 μm in either direction with strongly thickened unlignified walls sometimes strongly pitted, giving the lumen a stellate form; outer wall thick as seen in transverse section; *stomata* anomocytic, oval, about 17 μm wide and 25 μm long or sometimes circular and about 20 μm in diameter; *epidermis of leaf* of poppy plant present as rare fragments composed of thin-walled polyhedral cells; *stomata* anomocytic, confined to abaxial surface; *starch* almost absent, but a few small granules present measuring about 4 to 8 μm in diameter; *pollen grains* occasional, subspherical, with 3 pores, 16 to 20 to 30 to 40 μm in diameter.

Adulterants and substitutes. Powdered poppy capsule sometimes occurs as an adulterant and can be identified by the characters of the inner epidermis of the pericarp, which is composed of subrectangular and often slightly sinuous cells, as seen in surface view, about 85 to 245 μm long and 18 to 50 μm wide, with lignified and pitted anticlinal walls, about 7 μm thick; fairly numerous stomata, usually 5- or 6-sided and about 25 to 35 μm in diameter.

Actions and uses. The actions, uses, and undesirable effects of opium are substantially those of the morphine it contains and are described under Morphine Hydrochloride. The other alkaloids have little, if any, of the effects of morphine on pain and anxiety, and claims that they enhance the actions of morphine, other than its constipating actions, are not convincing.

The action of opium is exerted less rapidly than that of morphine, as absorption appears to take place less readily. Noscapine and papaverine relax intestinal muscle, in contrast to morphine and codeine which increases its tone; this action contributes to the greater constipating effect of opium as compared with that of morphine. Preparations of opium are therefore preferred

in the treatment of diarrhoea and intestinal disorders, but their use in these conditions is diminishing.

For the action of opium on the intestine, aromatic chalk powder with opium is employed. Camphorated opium tincture is used to relieve coughing.

Opium has been given as a diaphoretic in the form of ipecacuanha and opium powder or tablets in the early stages of colds.

Although preparations containing opium have been used in a variety of local applications, the opium alkaloids have no action on motor or sensory nerve endings and there is no evidence that they are absorbed after local application in sufficient amount to produce any characteristic effect.

Precautions. As for Morphine Hydrochloride.

Dependence. Opium may give rise to dependence of the morphine type, as described under Drug Dependence.

Poisoning. The procedure described under Morphine Hydrochloride should be adopted.

Preparations

AROMATIC CHALK WITH OPIUM MIXTURE (*Syn.* Chalk and Opium Mixture; Mistura Cretae Aromatica cum Opio):

Aromatic chalk powder	130 g
Opium tincture	50 ml
Tragacanth, in powder	.. 2 g
Aromatic ammonia solution	50 ml
Compound cardamom tincture..	50 ml
Catechu tincture	50 ml
Chloroform water, double-strength	500 ml
Water for preparations	to 1000 ml

It should be recently prepared.
A standard for this mixture is given in the British Pharmaceutical Codex 1973
Containers and *Labelling:* see the entry on Mixtures for general information on containers and labelling.
Dose: ADULT: 10 to 20 millilitres.
CHILD: Up to 1 year, 1 millilitre; 1 to 5 years, 2 to 5 millilitres.
Advice for patients: the mixture should not be used for longer than a few days without medical advice.

AROMATIC CHALK WITH OPIUM POWDER (*Syn.* Pulvis Cretae Aromaticus cum Opio):

Aromatic chalk powder	975 g
Powdered opium	25 g

Mix, as described in the entry on Powders.
A standard for this powder is given in the British Pharmaceutical Codex 1973
Containers and *Storage:* see the entry on Powders for general information on containers and storage. Containers should be airtight.
Dose: 0.5 to 5 grams.
Advice for patients: the powder should be taken mixed with a little water or other fluid. It should not be used for longer than a few days without medical advice.

CAMPHORATED OPIUM TINCTURE (*Syn.* Paregoric):

Opium tincture	50 ml
Camphor	.. 3 g
Benzoic acid	.. 5 g
Anise oil	3 ml
Alcohol (60%)	to 1000 ml

Dissolve the benzoic acid, the camphor, and the anise oil in 900 ml of the alcohol, add the opium tincture and sufficient alcohol to produce the required volume, mix, and filter if necessary.

It contains, in 10 ml, 5 mg of morphine, calculated as anhydrous morphine.

A standard for this tincture is given in the British Pharmacopoeia 1973

Dose: 2 to 10 ml.

CONCENTRATED CAMPHORATED OPIUM TINCTURE (*Syn.* Liquor Opii Camphoratus Concentratus):

Opium tincture	400 ml
Camphor	24 g
Benzoic acid	40 g
Anise oil	24 ml
Alcohol (95%)	400 ml
Water for preparations	to 1000 ml

Dissolve the benzoic acid, the camphor, and the anise oil in the alcohol, add the opium tincture and sufficient water to produce the required volume, mix, and filter if necessary. It is approximately 8 times as strong as camphorated opium tincture.

A standard for this tincture is given in the British Pharmaceutical Codex 1973

Dose: 0.25 to 1.25 millilitres.

OPIUM TINCTURE:

Opium, sliced	200 g
Alcohol (90%) ⎫ .. .. .. of each a sufficient	
Purified water ⎭	quantity

Pour 500 ml of boiling purified water on to the opium and allow to stand for 6 hours; add 500 ml of alcohol (90%), mix thoroughly, and allow to stand in a covered vessel for 24 hours; strain, press the marc, mix the liquids, and allow to stand for not less than 24 hours; filter. Determine the proportion of morphine, calculated as anhydrous morphine, in the tincture so prepared, using 40 ml. To the remainder of the liquid add sufficient of a mixture of equal volumes of the alcohol and water to produce a tincture of the required strength.

It contains, in 2 ml, 20 mg of morphine, calculated as anhydrous morphine.

A standard for this tincture is given in the British Pharmacopoeia 1973

Dose: 0.25 to 2 ml.

POWDERED OPIUM (*Syn.* Opium Pulveratum): obtained by reducing opium, dried at a moderate temperature, to a fine or moderately fine powder and adjusting, if necessary, to the required strength. When adjustment is necessary, powdered lactose, coloured with burnt sugar, or powdered cocoa husk is added.

It contains 10% of morphine, calculated as anhydrous morphine.

A standard for this powder is given in the British Pharmacopoeia 1973

Description: a light brown powder consisting of yellowish-brown or brownish-red particles. It possesses the diagnostic microscopical characters, odour, and taste described above under Opium. If powdered cocoa husk is present, the following characters are also exhibited: spiral, thickened *vessels* about 10 to 20 μm wide, in groups of 1 to 6, embedded in spongy *parenchyma* composed of thin-walled cells about 40 to 60 μm long and wide, with arm-like *projections;* projections from adjacent cells united to one another to enclose almost circular intercellular spaces; *stone-cells* derived from a single sclerenchymatous layer, individual cells thick-walled, about 5 to 10 μm wide and 10 to 30 μm long, rectangular to polyhedral in shape; *mucilage* as fragments staining in *ruthenium red solution.*

Storage: it should be stored in airtight containers.

Actions and uses: powdered opium has the actions, uses, and undesirable effects described above under Opium. The usual dose is 25 to 200 milligrams.

Precautions: as for Morphine Hydrochloride.

Dependence: powdered opium may give rise to dependence of the morphine type, as described under Drug Dependence.

Poisoning: the procedure as described under Morphine Hydrochloride should be adopted.

OTHER PREPARATIONS: opium, in the form of camphorated opium tincture, is an ingredient of opiate squill linctus and of paediatric opiate squill linctus and, in the form of concentrated camphorated opium tincture, of opiate squill pastilles.

Oral Medicines

A medicine should be administered in such a way that it produces the maximum therapeutic effect with a minimum of side-effects. In some cases this depends upon the intervals between doses and their relationship to mealtimes.

Factors that Influence the Effectiveness of Medicines Administered by Mouth

Medicines taken before food. Absorption is most rapid and complete when medicines are taken at least half an hour before food except in a few instances where food may increase the rate of absorption through the stomach (see below). Medicines that are relatively poorly absorbed or which are intended to produce high peak blood concentrations are best taken before meals.

Medicines taken with or after food. Although the presence of food may make absorption slower and less complete, it minimises gastric irritation, nausea, and vomiting. It is therefore preferable to take irritant or nauseant substances after food.

Interactions between medicines and food. Foods containing salts of calcium, magnesium, iron, etc. form insoluble compounds with medicines containing, for example, fluorides and tetracyclines, thus reducing absorption. Some foods may increase the absorption of drugs; for example griseofulvin absorption is increased in the presence of fat. As antacids affect the absorption of many medicines they should preferably be taken alone and no other medicines taken within two hours. Cholestyramine chelates with many drugs and also interferes with the absorption of fat.

Regular administration with consistent intervals between doses is necessary when it is desired to maintain a concentration of medicament in the tissues.

Dilution. Irritant substances should be well diluted before administration.

Enteric-coated and sustained-release preparations. These dosage forms should be swallowed whole as otherwise the protective structure will be destroyed. Antacids that can destroy the enteric coating should not be taken at the same time.

Sublingual administration. Some preparations are intended to be dissolved under the tongue, and have a greater effect than when swallowed. This may be because of improved absorption or because the drug appears in the circulation without first passing through the liver where some of it may be metabolised.

Examples of Oral Administration

Antibiotics and other antibacterial agents should generally be given before meals to produce high peak blood concentrations. Doses should be given at regular intervals chosen to maintain an inhibitory concentration in the blood and tissues, and in many cases a prescribed course should be completed to minimise recurrence or emergence of resistant strains. Milk, antacids, iron salts, and other preparations containing aluminium, calcium, iron, and magnesium should not be administered with tetracyclines.

Anthelmintics are generally given on an empty stomach to improve contact with the parasites.

Mucosal protectants such as silicones are given before meals.

Salicylates, and other anti-inflammatory drugs should preferably be administered after food to reduce nausea, vomiting, and erosion of the gastric mucosa.

Progestogen–oestrogen contraceptives, malaria prophylactics, anticoagulants, and anticonvulsants should be administered regularly and care should be taken to avoid the accidental omission of any doses.

Chloral, paraldehyde, and potassium chloride solutions should be well diluted to minimise gastric irritation.

Oral Pastes

OTHER NAME: Electuaries

Oral pastes are semi-solid veterinary preparations intended for internal use. They consist of the medicament, in powder, mixed with a suitable edible diluent. They are usually supplied in a container specially designed to provide the paste in measured quantities for direct delivery to the back of the mouth. They may also be administered by smearing on the tongue or wall of the buccal cavity by means of a wooden or plastic spatula.

Containers. Oral pastes are supplied in suitable containers which prevent the loss of volatile ingredients.

Labelling. The label on the container should state the names and amounts of the active ingredients in the container. The label on the container or the label on the package should state the recommended method of use.

Orange Oil

Obtained by mechanical means from the fresh peel of the sweet orange, *Citrus sinensis* (L.) Osbeck (Fam. Rutaceae).

OTHER NAMES: Sweet Orange Oil; Oleum Aurantii

A standard is given in the British Pharmaceutical Codex 1973

It is produced in many tropical and subtropical countries.

Constituents. Orange oil contains at least 90% of (+)-limonene. It also contains up to 3% of aldehydes, calculated as decanal.

Description. It is a yellow to yellowish-brown liquid with a characteristic odour.

Solubility. Soluble, at 20°, in 7 parts of alcohol (90%), but rarely with formation of bright solutions on account of the presence of waxy non-volatile substances.

Weight per ml. At 20°, 0.842 to 0.848 g.

Refractive index. 1.472 to 1.476.

Optical rotation. +94° to +99°. When distilled, the first 10% of the distillate has an optical rotation the same as, or only slightly lower than, the original oil.

Adulterants and substitutes. Distilled orange oil is an inferior article, the effect of heat and steaming being detrimental to the oxygenated compounds.

Bitter orange oil, from *C. aurantium* L., is chemically almost identical with sweet orange oil, but can be distinguished by its odour and bitter taste. The optical rotation varies from +92° to +97°, the weight per ml at 20° from 0.845 to 0.851 g, and the aldehyde content from 0.3 to 1%, calculated as decanal.

Stability. Orange oil deteriorates on keeping, acquiring a disagreeable terebinthinate taste.

Storage. It should be stored in well-filled airtight containers, in a cool place, protected from light.

Uses. Orange oil is employed as a flavouring agent, in perfumery, and for the preparation of the terpeneless oil.

Orange Oil, Terpeneless

Prepared by concentrating orange oil *in vacuo* until most of the terpenes have been removed, or by solvent partition.

OTHER NAME: Oleum Aurantii Deterpenatum

A standard is given in the British Pharmaceutical Codex 1973

Constituents. Terpeneless orange oil consists chiefly of the free alcohols, (+)-linalol and (+)-terpineol, with considerable quantities of aldehydes, chiefly decanal, and smaller amounts of esters.

Description. A yellow or orange-yellow liquid with a characteristic odour.

Solubility. Soluble, at 20°, in 1 part of alcohol (90%).

Weight per ml. At 20°, 0.860 to 0.880 g.

Refractive index. 1.461 to 1.473.

Optical rotation. Up to +55°.

Storage. It should be stored in well-filled airtight containers, in a cool place, protected from light.

Uses. Terpeneless orange oil is used as a flavouring agent. It has a stronger flavour and odour and is more readily soluble than orange oil; 1 millilitre of terpeneless oil is equivalent in flavour to about 15 millilitres of the natural oil.

Preparation

COMPOUND ORANGE SPIRIT (*Syn.* Spiritus Aurantii Compositus):

Terpeneless orange oil	2.50 ml
Terpeneless lemon oil	1.30 ml
Anise oil	4.25 ml
Coriander oil	6.25 ml
Alcohol (90%)	to 1000.00 ml

A standard for this spirit is given in the British Pharmaceutical Codex 1973

Bitter-Orange Peel, Dried

The dried outer part of the pericarp of the ripe or nearly ripe fruit of *Citrus aurantium* L. (Fam. Rutaceae).

OTHER NAME: Aurantii Cortex Siccatus

A standard is given in the British Pharmacopoeia 1973

It is imported chiefly from Spain and other Mediterranean countries and from the West Indies.

Constituents. Dried bitter-orange peel contains volatile oil, the bitter glycoside aurantiamarin, the glycosides hesperidin and isohesperidin, hesperic acid, aurantiamaric acid, and an eriodictyol glycoside.

The peel also contains the carotenoid pigments kryptoxanthin, zeaxanthin, xanthophyll, citraurin, and violaxanthin. Pectin and a little fixed oil are also present, as well as small quantities of vitamins A, B_1, and C. The bitter constituents occur chiefly in the white "zest" of the peel.

It yields to alcohol (60%) about 30 to 40% of extractive.

Description. *Macroscopical characters:* strips, ribbons, or quarters; outer surface red to dark orange-red and somewhat rough from the presence of numerous minute pits each corresponding to an oil gland; inner surface with only a small amount of white spongy pericarp; fracture short.

It has an aromatic odour and aromatic and bitter taste.

Microscopical characters: the diagnostic characters are: epidermis, small polyhedral cells about 5 to 13 μm wide with numerous circular *stomata* about 25 to 28 μm in diameter; tissues subjacent to epidermis parenchymatous, many cells containing prismatic *crystals* of calcium oxalate; numerous large *oil glands* and some small *vascular strands* embedded in the parenchyma.

Adulterants and substitutes. Owing to excessive rupturing of the oil glands, peel in narrow machine-cut strips (gelatin-cut) is not equal in aroma to hand-cut dried peel and the volatile oil content is usually only about 1%. Dried sweet-orange peel may be distinguished by its paler, more yellowish colour and by being much less bitter in taste.

Indian orange peel is the fresh or the dried outer part of the pericarp of varieties of *C. aurantium* L. grown in the Indian sub-continent and Ceylon.

Storage. It should be stored in airtight containers.

Actions and uses. Dried bitter-orange peel is used as a flavouring agent.

Preparations

CONCENTRATED ORANGE PEEL INFUSION (*Syn.* Infusum Aurantii Concentratum):

Dried bitter-orange peel, cut
small .. .. 500 g
Alcohol (25%) .. .. 1350 ml

Macerate the dried bitter-orange peel in 1000 ml of the alcohol in a covered vessel for 48 hours and press out the liquid. To the marc, add the remainder of the alcohol, macerate for 24 hours, press out the liquid, and add it to the product of the first pressing. Allow the mixed liquids to stand for not less than 14 days and filter.

Orange peel infusion is prepared by diluting concentrated orange peel infusion with 9 times its volume of water for preparations.

A standard for this infusion is given in the British Pharmaceutical Codex 1973

Dose: 2.5 to 5 millilitres.

ORANGE SYRUP (*Syn.* Syrupus Aurantii):

Orange tincture .. .. 60 ml
Syrup.. .. .. to 1000 ml
Mix.

A standard for this syrup is given in the British Pharmaceutical Codex 1973

Dose: 2.5 to 5 millilitres.

ORANGE TINCTURE (*Syn.* Tinctura Aurantii):

Dried bitter-orange peel, in moderately
fine powder .. .. 110 g
Alcohol (70%) .. .. .. a sufficient quantity

Prepare 1000 ml of tincture by the percolation process.

A standard for this tincture is given in the British Pharmaceutical Codex 1973

Dose: 1 to 2 millilitres.

Orciprenaline Sulphate

N-Isopropyl-N-3,5,β-trihydroxyphenethylammonium sulphate

$(C_{11}H_{17}NO_3)_2,H_2SO_4 = 520.6$

OTHER NAME: *Alupent*® (this name is also applied to preparations containing orciprenaline sulphate with bromhexine hydrochloride); Metaproterenol Sulfate

A standard is given in the British Pharmacopoeia 1973

Description. An odourless white crystalline powder with a bitter taste.

Solubility. Soluble, at 20°, in 2 parts of water and in 1 part of alcohol; very slightly soluble in chloroform and in ether.

Acidity. A 10% solution has a pH of 4 to 5.5.

Moisture content. Not more than 2%, determined by Fischer titration.

Dissociation constants. pK_a 9.0, 10.1, 11.4 (25°).

Stability. It is more stable than adrenaline and other 3,4-substituted phenylalkanolamines but it is oxidised by atmospheric oxygen, especially in neutral or alkaline solution, in the presence of light and of heavy metal ions.

Sterilisation. Solutions are sterilised by heating in an autoclave or by filtration.

Storage. It should be protected from light.

Identification. TEST. To 1 ml of a 1% solution add a few drops of a saturated solution of mercuric acetate; a yellow colour is produced.

MELTING-POINT. About 205°.

ULTRAVIOLET ABSORPTION. In 0.1N hydrochloric acid, maximum at 280 nm (E1%, 1cm = 69); in 0.1N sodium hydroxide, maxima at 222 nm (E1%, 1cm = 655) and 297 nm (E1%, 1cm = 124).

Actions and uses. Orciprenaline is a directly acting sympathomimetic amine with actions similar to those described under Isoprenaline Sulphate. It differs in having a longer duration of action and in being effective when taken by mouth and swallowed.

In the treatment of bronchial asthma a rapid effect is obtained by the use of an aerosol inhalation in a dosage of 670 to 1340 micrograms up to 6 times daily. The usual dose for children is 670 micrograms 4 times daily. Orciprenaline sulphate is also administered by subcutaneous or deep intramuscular injection in doses of 500 micrograms. It may also be administered by mouth in a dosage of 20 milligrams 4 times a day; children up to 1 year may be given 5 to 10 milligrams 3 times daily, 1 to 3 years 5 to 10 milligrams 4 times daily, and 4 to 12 years 40 to 60 milligrams daily in divided doses.

Undesirable effects. Tachycardia, headache, and dizziness are usually associated with overdosage, but are transient and seldom so severe as to necessitate withdrawal of the drug. Nausea may occur and, occasionally, difficulty in micturition.

Precautions and contra-indications. As for Isoprenaline Sulphate.

Preparations

ORCIPRENALINE AEROSOL INHALATION: a suspension of orciprenaline sulphate, in powder of a suitable particle size, in a suitable mixture of aerosol propellents, which may contain a surface-active agent, stabilising agents, and other adjuvants. Available as a preparation delivering 670 micrograms of orciprenaline sulphate to the patient each time the valve is actuated.
A standard for this aerosol inhalation is given in the British Pharmaceutical Codex 1973
Containers, Labelling, and Storage: see the entry on Aerosol Inhalations for general information on containers, labelling, and storage.
Advice for patients: see the entry on Aerosol Inhalations for general information on the use of aerosol inhalations. The patient should be advised verbally to read the instructions on the leaflet enclosed with the product. If more than one inhalation is taken at a time at least 1 minute should elapse between any 2 inhalations, and not less than 30 minutes between any 2 doses. When used in conjunction with beclomethasone or other corticosteroid inhalation, orciprenaline should be given first and the corticosteroid preparation used 5 minutes later. Excessive use of the inhalation should be avoided.

ORCIPRENALINE ELIXIR (*Syn.* Orciprenaline Sulphate Elixir; Orciprenaline Syrup): a solution of orciprenaline sulphate in a suitable flavoured vehicle. Available as an elixir containing 10 mg of orciprenaline sulphate in 5 ml. When a dose less than or not a multiple of 5 ml is prescribed, the elixir may be diluted, as described in the entry on Elixirs, with syrup. The diluted elixir must be freshly prepared.
A standard for this elixir is given in the British Pharmaceutical Codex 1973
Containers and *Labelling:* see the entry on Elixirs for general information on containers and labelling.
Storage: it should be stored in a cool place, protected from light.

ORCIPRENALINE INJECTION: a sterile solution of orciprenaline sulphate, with suitable stabilising agents, in water for injections. It is distributed into ampoules and the ampoules are sealed and sterilised by heating in an autoclave; alternatively it is sterilised by filtration and distributed by means of an aseptic technique into sterile ampoules which are then sealed. Available in 1-ml ampoules containing 500 micrograms of orciprenaline sulphate.
A standard for this injection is given in the British Pharmacopoeia 1973
Containers and *Labelling:* see the entry on Injections for general information on containers and labelling.
Storage: it should be protected from light.

ORCIPRENALINE TABLETS: available as tablets containing 20 mg of orciprenaline sulphate.

A standard for these tablets is given in the British Pharmacopoeia 1973
Containers and *Storage:* see the entry on Tablets for general information on containers and storage. Containers should be airtight and light resistant.

OTHER PREPARATIONS available include a MIXTURE containing orciprenaline sulphate 10 mg with bromhexine hydrochloride 4 mg in 5 ml, diluent sorbitol solution or syrup, life of diluted mixture 14 days; a SPRAY containing orciprenaline sulphate 5%; and TABLETS containing orciprenaline sulphate 20 mg with bromhexine hydrochloride 8 mg.

Orf Vaccine

see CONTAGIOUS PUSTULAR DERMATITIS VACCINE, LIVING

Oriental Sore

see under LEISHMANIASIS

Orphenadrine Citrate

NN-Dimethyl-*N*-2-(2-methylbenzhydryloxyethyl)ammonium dihydrogen citrate

$$\left[\begin{array}{c} C_6H_5\cdot CH\cdot O\cdot[CH_2]_2\cdot \overset{+}{N}H(CH_3)_2 \\ CH_3 \end{array} \right] \quad \begin{array}{c} CH_2\cdot COO^- \\ HO\cdot C\cdot COOH \\ CH_2\cdot COOH \end{array}$$

$C_{24}H_{31}NO_8 = 461.5$

OTHER NAMES: *Norflex®*
Norgesic® (with paracetamol)

A standard is given in the British Pharmacopoeia 1973

Description. An almost odourless white crystalline powder with a taste which is bitter followed by a sensation of numbness.

Solubility. Soluble, at 20°, in 70 parts of water; very slightly soluble in alcohol; practically insoluble in ether and in chloroform.

Storage. It should be protected from light.

Identification. TESTS. 1. Dissolve about 50 mg in 10 ml of *alcohol (50%)*, add 10 ml of *trinitrophenol solution* and allow to stand; a precipitate is produced which, after recrystallisation from alcohol (95%), melts at about 89° or at about 107°.
2. Dissolve a few mg in 2 ml of sulphuric acid; an orange-red colour is produced.

MELTING-POINT. About 136°.

ULTRAVIOLET ABSORPTION. In alcohol (95%), maxima at 258 nm (E1%, 1cm = 11.3), 264 nm (E1%, 1cm = 12), and 271 nm (E1%, 1cm = 7.8).

THIN-LAYER CHROMATOGRAPHY. See under Thin-layer Chromatography, System 8.

Determination in body fluids. GAS CHROMATOGRAPHY. In plasma or urine—J. J. M. Labout *et al.*, *J. Chromat.*, 1977, **144**, 201.

Metabolism. ABSORPTION. Readily absorbed after oral administration.

HALF-LIFE. Half-life of drug plus metabolite, 14 to 25 hours.

DISTRIBUTION. Rapidly distributed.

METABOLIC REACTIONS. N-Demethylation, deamination and oxidation, O-dealkylation, and conjugation with glucuronic acid or sulphate.

EXCRETION. Up to about 60% of an oral dose is excreted in the urine in 3 days; of the urinary excreted dose, about 8% is unchanged, 8% is N-demethylorphenadrine, 4% is NN-didemethylorphenadrine, 13% is a conjugate of α-o-tolylbenzyloxyacetic acid, 8% is a conjugate of α-o-tolylbenzyl alcohol, and less than 1% is composed of α-o-tolylbenzyl alcohol and α-o-tolylbenzyloxyacetic acid; the excretion of orphenadrine is both urinary-pH and urinary-volume dependent and at a urinary pH of 5, about 30% is excreted unchanged, 5% is excreted as N-demethylorphenadrine, and 4% is excreted as orphenadrine N-oxide.

FURTHER INFORMATION. Metabolism—A. H. Beckett and F. Khan, *J. Pharm. Pharmac.*, 1971, **23**, *Suppl.*, 222S and T. Ellison *et al.*, *J. Pharmac. exp. Ther.*, 1971, **176**, 284.

Actions and uses. By its action on the central nervous system orphenadrine reduces spasm of voluntary muscle, and it is used, usually in conjunction with other drugs, in the treatment of parkinsonism; it relieves mental depression and reduces excessive salivation and perspiration. It is also used to reduce spasm and associated pain resulting from injury to voluntary muscle.

The daily dosage is 200 milligrams of orphenadrine citrate by mouth, gradually increased to up to 400 milligrams according to the response of the patient. The usual dosage by intramuscular or intravenous injection is 60 milligrams once or twice daily.

There is some evidence that, with continued use, treatment with orphenadrine may become less effective.

Orphenadrine has anticholinergic activity. It has a chemical structure closely related to that of diphenhydramine, but has only a weak antihistamine action and produces euphoria without sedation.

Undesirable effects. Insomnia, mental excitement, increased tremor, and nausea may occur, but these usually disappear if the dosage is reduced.

Precautions and contra-indications. As for Atropine.

Preparations

SLOW ORPHENADRINE CITRATE TABLETS: available as tablets containing 100 mg of orphenadrine citrate in a slow-release formulation.

A standard for these tablets is given in the British Pharmacopoeia 1973

Containers and *Storage:* see the entry on Tablets for general information on containers and storage. Containers should be airtight and light resistant.

Advice for patients: the tablets should be swallowed whole. Doses should be taken before meals if the patient is inconvenienced by dryness of the mouth or after meals if there are gastro-intestinal disturbances. Treatment should not be discontinued without the advice of the prescriber.

OTHER PREPARATIONS available include an INJECTION containing orphenadrine citrate 30 mg per ml in 2-ml ampoules; and TABLETS containing orphenadrine citrate 35 mg with paracetamol 450 mg.

Orphenadrine Hydrochloride

NN-Dimethyl-*N*-2-(2-methylbenzhydryloxyethyl)ammonium chloride
$C_{18}H_{24}ClNO = 305.8$

OTHER NAME: *Disipal*®

A standard is given in the British Pharmacopoeia 1973

Description. An odourless white crystalline powder with a taste which is bitter followed by a sensation of numbness.

Solubility. Soluble, at 20°, in 1 part of water, in 1 part of alcohol, and in 2 parts of chloroform; practically insoluble in ether.

Storage. It should be stored in airtight containers, protected from light.

Identification. TESTS. It complies with the tests described under Orphenadrine Citrate.

MELTING-POINT. About 160°.

ULTRAVIOLET ABSORPTION. In alcohol (95%), maxima at 258 nm (E1%, 1cm = 17.8), 264 nm (E1%, 1cm = 18.8), and 271 nm (E1%, 1cm = 12.2).

Metabolism. See under Orphenadrine Citrate.

Actions and uses. Orphenadrine hydrochloride has the actions, uses, and undesirable effects described under Orphenadrine Citrate.

The usual dose is 200 to 400 milligrams daily in divided doses by mouth or up to 40 milligrams 3 times a day by intramuscular injection.

Precautions and contra-indications. As for Atropine.

Preparations

ORPHENADRINE HYDROCHLORIDE TABLETS: available as tablets containing 50 mg of orphenadrine hydrochloride; they are sugar coated; the coat may be coloured.

A standard for these tablets is given in the British Pharmacopoeia 1973

Containers and *Storage:* see the entry on Tablets for general information on containers and storage. Containers should be airtight.

Advice for patients: the tablets should be taken before meals if the patient is inconvenienced by dryness of the mouth or after meals if there are gastro-intestinal disturbances. Treatment should not be discontinued without the advice of the prescriber.

OTHER PREPARATIONS available include an INJECTION containing orphenadrine hydrochloride 20 mg per ml in 2-ml ampoules.

Osteitis Deformans

see PAGET'S DISEASE OF BONE

Osteoarthritis

Osteoarthritis is a disease occurring mainly in the elderly. There is degeneration of the articular cartilage and the formation of bony outgrowths (osteophytes) at the edges of the affected joints which are most frequently in the spine (spondylosis), hips, knees, and hands. Usually only one or two of the large joints are involved. Disease or injury to joints, obesity, postural defects, and certain manual occupations are predisposing factors. It results in pain and loss of joint mobility which may finally result in deformities.

Treatment may include rest, gentle exercises, heat treatment, and hydrotherapy. Analgesics and anti-inflammatory drugs may be required for the relief of pain. Surgery may be beneficial in severe cases.

Osteomalacia

Osteomalacia is a disease in which bones become soft and easily deformed owing to loss of calcium and phosphorus. The causative factors include deficiency of vitamin D or resistance to its effects (as, for example, in certain forms of renal disease), low dietary calcium intake, poor calcium absorption (as, for example, after partial gastrectomy), and drugs including phenytoin and phenobarbitone. The softening of bone in osteomalacia results in bony deformities and aches and pains beginning in the spine and then extending symmetrically to other bones. Decreased muscle tone and weakness may also occur.

Treatment is described under Calciferol and Dihydrotachysterol.

Osteoporosis

Osteoporosis is a condition in which the bones are abnormally porous and brittle. The bone mass is reduced but its chemical composition is unchanged.

Osteoporosis may be due to changes in the metabolism of bone or of calcium resulting from nutritional deficiency, endocrine disturbance, immobility, or confinement to bed, but it occurs most commonly in women who have passed the menopause and in old age. In osteoporosis the bones are readily fractured, and multiple fractures in the vertebrae lead to vertebral compression which, together with dorsal kyphosis, results in a shortening of the trunk height.

The changes of osteoporosis are generally irreversible, except in childhood or after temporary immobilisation, and the aim of treatment is to arrest the progress of the disease. A dietary intake of calcium in excess of 500 milligrams (12.5 millimoles of Ca^{2+}) daily may be expected to produce a suitable positive calcium balance and small doses of vitamin D are often given to facilitate the absorption of calcium. Supplements of gonadal hormones, oestrogens in the female and androgens in the male, may sometimes improve calcium balance.

Intensive physiotherapy is of value since osteoporosis is a common feature of disuse.

Ovine Enzootic Abortion Vaccine

An emulsion in liquid paraffin or other suitable vehicle of the yolk-sac membranes of eggs infected with a laboratory strain of *Chlamydia* organisms which has subsequently been inactivated in such a manner that immunogenic activity is retained.

OTHER NAME: Kebbing Vaccine

A standard is given in the British Pharmacopoeia (Veterinary)

Storage. The vaccine should be protected from light and stored at 2° to 8° when it may be expected to retain its potency for 1 year.

Veterinary uses. It is administered by subcutaneous injection to sheep for prophylaxis of enzootic abortion.

Oxidised Cellulose

A sterilised polyanhydroglucuronic acid, prepared by oxidation of cotton, usually in the form of surgical gauze or lint, with nitrogen dioxide.

OTHER NAMES: Oxycel®; Surgicel®

A standard is given in the British Pharmacopoeia 1973

Description. A white or creamy-white gauze, lint, or knitted material with a faint odour.

Solubility. Practically insoluble in water and in mineral acids; soluble in solutions of alkali hydroxides.

Moisture content. Not more than 15%, determined by drying over phosphorus pentoxide *in vacuo*.

Storage. It should be stored in containers sealed to exclude micro-organisms, protected from light, in a cool place. It cannot be satisfactorily resterilised and if a portion only of the contents of a container is used on any one occasion, strict aseptic precautions should be taken to avoid contamination.

Actions and uses. Oxidised cellulose is an absorbable haemostatic, the action of which depends on the formation of a coagulum consisting of salts of polyanhydroglucuronic acid and haemoglobin.

When oxidised cellulose is applied to a bleeding surface it swells and forms a brown gelatinous mass which is gradually absorbed, usually within 2 to 7 days of application. The rate of absorption depends on the size of the piece used and the vascularity of the area. Complete absorption of large amounts of blood-soaked material may take 6 weeks or longer.

The haemostatic effect of oxidised cellulose is greater when dry material is used, hence moistening with water or saline is undesirable. If used with thrombin solution, however, it should first be neutralised by moistening with a solution of sodium bicarbonate in order to prevent inactivation of the thrombin.

Oxidised cellulose is used as a haemostatic in many types of surgery, including brain surgery. It is useful for packing cavities after surgical excisions and as a haemostatic uterine packing. Since it is non-irritant and completely absorbable, oxidised cellulose may be enclosed without drainage in a clean wound but not in the presence of gross contamination or infection. In dental surgery it is used to pack bleeding tooth sockets.

Except when used as a haemostatic, oxidised cellulose should not be used as a surface dressing for open wounds because it inhibits epithelialisation and, since it delays the formation of callus, it is contra-indicated in clean bone surgery. It inactivates penicillin.

Oxprenolol Hydrochloride

N-(3-o-Allyloxyphenoxy-2-hydroxypropyl)-N-isopropyl ammonium chloride

$C_{15}H_{24}ClNO_3 = 301.8$

OTHER NAME: *Trasicor*®

A standard is given in the British Pharmacopoeia Addendum 1975

Description. An almost odourless, white to slightly cream-coloured crystalline powder.

Solubility. Soluble, at 20°, in less than 1 part of water and in 1.5 parts of alcohol; very slightly soluble in ether.

Acidity. A 5% solution has a pH of 4 to 6.

Identification. TEST. Dissolve about 200 mg in 10 ml of water, make alkaline with *dilute sodium hydroxide solution*, extract with two 5-ml portions of ether, wash the combined extracts with water until free from alkali, dry over anhydrous sodium sulphate, filter, and evaporate to dryness; the residue melts at about 76°.

MELTING-POINT. About 107°.

ULTRAVIOLET ABSORPTION. In 0.01N hydrochloric acid, maximum at 273 nm (E1%, 1cm = 75).

INFRA-RED ABSORPTION. Major peaks at 750, 1037, 1092, 1120, 1258, and 1500 cm^{-1} (see Appendix 2a: Infra-red Spectra).

Determination in body fluids. GAS CHROMATOGRAPHY. In blood or plasma—P. H. Degen and W. Riess, *J. Chromat.*, 1976, **121**, 72.

Metabolism. ABSORPTION. Readily absorbed after oral administration.

BLOOD CONCENTRATION. After 40, 80, and 160 mg doses given orally, peak plasma concentrations of about 260, 560, and 700 ng/ml respectively, are attained; up to a 5-fold variation in plasma concentration may occur.

HALF-LIFE. Plasma half-life, 80 to 120 minutes after oral administration.

METABOLIC REACTIONS. Oxidative N-dealkylation and N-methylation followed by glucuronic acid conjugation; in the dog the major metabolites are 1-(*o*-allyloxyphenoxy)-3-aminopropan-2-ol, 1-(*o*-allyloxyphenoxy)-3-methylaminopropan-2-ol, and oxprenolol glucuronide; oxprenolol appears to be subject to extensive first pass metabolism.

EXCRETION. About 90% of a dose is excreted in the urine, partly as conjugates.

FURTHER INFORMATION. Cardiac effects and plasma concentration—L. Brunner *et al.*, *Eur. J. clin. Pharmac.*, 1975, **8**, 3; N-methylation in the dog—G. A. Leeson *et al.*, *Drug Met. Disp.*, 1973, **1**, 565; metabolism —W. Riess *et al.*, *Postgrad. med. J.*, 1970, **46** (Nov.), Suppl., 32.

Actions and uses. Oxprenolol is a beta-adrenergic blocking agent with actions similar to those described under Propranolol Hydrochloride.

In the treatment of cardiac arrhythmias 20 to 40 milligrams of oxprenolol hydrochloride may be given by mouth 2 or 3 times a day and the dosage increased if necessary. In urgent cases 1 to 2 milligrams may be given slowly by intravenous or intramuscular injection and repeated if necessary every 10 to 20 minutes until 12 milligrams has been given.

In the treatment of angina pectoris the usual dosage is 40 to 80 milligrams of oxprenolol hydrochloride by mouth 3 times a day, increased if necessary according to the needs of the patient up to a maximum of 2 grams daily. Oxprenolol is also used in the treatment of arterial hypertension. Treatment is started with a dosage of 160 milligrams of oxprenolol hydrochloride by mouth daily in divided doses and the dosage gradually increased until the condition is controlled; a dosage of 1 gram daily should not normally be exceeded.

Undesirable effects. As for Propranolol Hydrochloride.

Precautions and contra-indications. Oxprenolol should be given with caution in patients with a history of bronchial asthma and cardiac failure. It is not suitable for the treatment of hyperthyroidism because of its intrinsic sympathomimetic activity. It is contra-indicated in atrioventricular block or marked bradycardia.

Preparations

OXPRENOLOL TABLETS: available as tablets containing 20, 40, 80, and 160 mg of oxprenolol hydrochloride; they are film coated; the coat may be coloured.
A standard for these tablets is given in the British Pharmacopoeia Addendum 1975
Containers and *Storage:* see the entry on Tablets for general information on containers and storage. Containers should be airtight.
Advice for patients: treatment should not be discontinued without the advice of the prescriber. The tablets may affect mental concentration; persons affected should not drive or operate machinery.

OTHER PREPARATIONS available include an INJECTION reconstituted from a powder in ampoules containing oxprenolol hydrochloride 2 mg; and as TABLETS containing oxprenolol hydrochloride 160 mg in a slow-release formulation.

Oxyclozanide

3,3′,5,5′,6-Pentachloro-2′-hydroxysalicylanilide

$C_{13}H_6Cl_5NO_3 = 401.5$

OTHER NAMES: *Zanil*®
Haloxil® (with haloxon); *Nilzan*® (with levamisole hydrochloride)

A standard is given in the British Pharmacopoeia (Veterinary)

Description. An odourless cream powder.

Solubility. Very slightly soluble in water; soluble, at 20°, in 20 parts of alcohol, in 600 parts of chloroform, and in 5 parts of acetone.

Moisture content. Not more than 1%, determined by drying at 60° *in vacuo*.

Identification. MELTING-POINT. About 208°.

ULTRAVIOLET ABSORPTION. In alcohol (95%), maximum at 302 nm (E1%, 1cm = 188).

INFRA-RED ABSORPTION. Major peaks at 1163, 1205, 1408, 1471, 1538, and 1587 cm^{-1} (see Appendix 2b: Infra-red Spectra).

Veterinary uses. Oxyclozanide is used in the treatment of liver fluke infections. The usual dosage by mouth is 10 milligrams per kilogram body-weight for cattle and 15 milligrams per kilogram body-weight for sheep as a single dose. In the treatment of acute fascioliasis, sheep may be given 45 milligrams per kilogram body-weight as a single dose.

Preparations

OXYCLOZANIDE GRANULES: consisting of oxyclozanide mixed with suitable edible diluents. Available as granules containing 5% of oxyclozanide.

A standard for these granules is given in the British Pharmacopoeia (Veterinary)

Labelling: the label on the container should state the amount of the medicament as the proportion of oxyclozanide in the granules, the method of use, and that cattle and sheep should not be slaughtered for human consumption within 14 days after cessation of treatment.

OXYCLOZANIDE MIXTURE (*Syn.* Oxyclozanide Drench; Oxyclozanide Suspension): an aqueous suspension of oxyclozanide mixed with suitable suspending and dispersing agents. Available as a mixture containing 3.4% of oxyclozanide.

A standard for this mixture is given in the British Pharmacopoeia (Veterinary)

Containers: see the entry on Mixtures for general information on containers.

Labelling: see the entry on Mixtures for general information on labelling. In addition, the label on the container should state that cattle and sheep should not be slaughtered for human consumption within 14 days after cessation of treatment. A direction to shake the bottle should be given on the label.

OTHER PREPARATIONS available include veterinary GRANULES containing oxyclozanide 5% with levamisole 2.5%; a veterinary MIXTURE containing oxyclozanide 3.05% with haloxon 10.4% and a veterinary mixture containing oxyclozanide 3% with levamisole 1.5%.

Oxygen

$O_2 = 32.00$

OTHER NAME: Oxygenium

A standard is given in the European Pharmacopoeia Vol. II

Oxygen may be obtained by the fractional distillation of liquid air, when it will contain a small proportion of argon and a trace of nitrogen, or by the electrolysis of water, when it will contain a small proportion of hydrogen.

Description. An odourless colourless gas.

Solubility. One volume, measured at normal temperature and pressure, dissolves, at 20°, in 32 volumes of water.

Storage, labelling, and colour-markings. It should be stored in metal cylinders designed to hold compressed gases. Cylinders should be stored in a special storage room which should be cool and free from materials of an inflammable nature. The valve end of the cylinder should be painted white down to the shoulder, and the remainder of the cylinder black; the name of the gas or chemical symbol "O_2" should be stencilled in paint on the shoulder of the cylinder. The name or chemical symbol of the gas should be clearly and indelibly stamped on the cylinder valve.

Oxygen and carbon dioxide mixtures should be stored in a similar manner. The valve end of the cylinder should be painted white and grey in four segments, two of each colour, down to the shoulder, and the remainder of the cylinder black; the names or chemical symbols of the gases should be stencilled in paint on the shoulder of the cylinder. The names or chemical symbols of the gases should be clearly and indelibly stamped on the cylinder valve.

Oxygen and helium mixtures should be stored in a similar manner. The valve end of the cylinder should be painted white and brown in four segments, two of each colour, down to the shoulder, and the remainder of the cylinder black; the names or chemical symbols of the gases should be stencilled in paint on the shoulder of the cylinder. The names or chemical symbols of the gases should be clearly and indelibly stamped on the cylinder valve.

Identification. TEST. When mixed with nitric oxide, red fumes are produced (distinction from nitrous oxide).

Actions and uses. Oxygen inhalation is indicated in anoxia in such conditions as pneumonia, post-operative pulmonary complications, pulmonary oedema, shock, asphyxia neonatorum, congestive heart failure, and in poisoning due to carbon monoxide or to barbiturates and other depressants.

The concentration of oxygen for inhalation over long periods should be about 50% at sea level; it should not as a rule exceed 60%, except at high altitudes when as much as 80% may be necessary or when the administration is for short periods only. The continued inhalation of oxygen at concentrations above 70% may cause blindness. The administration of concentrations above 50% to premature infants may interfere with the development of a normal retinal blood supply and cause blindness.

The withdrawal of oxygen treatment should be gradual, especially in cases of chronic cyanosis.

Oxygen is administered by means of an oxygen tent, face mask, or nasal catheter. If a catheter is used the oxygen should be passed through a humidifier before inhalation. A flow rate of 5 to 8 litres per minute through a nasal catheter gives an oxygen concentration of 40 to 60%; increasing the rate of flow beyond this does not result in an increased oxygen concentration in the lungs. To obtain concentrations above 60% a mask must be used. A mask is not suitable for prolonged administration, as the percentage of oxygen in the inspired air depends on the depth of respiration and at low flow rates resistance to breathing increases. An oxygen tent is used for children and those unable to tolerate catheters or masks; a flow rate up to 7 litres per minute will maintain an oxygen concentration of 60%; it is impracticable to maintain concentrations higher than this.

In the treatment of patients with chronic bronchitis it is desirable to maintain constant concentrations of inspired oxygen of 24 to 32%; special masks for controlled oxygen therapy are used for this purpose.

Oxygen under pressure is used in the treatment of carbon monoxide poisoning, in some types of vascular injury, and to increase the effectiveness of irradiation in the treatment of malignant disease. For such purposes the patient is enclosed in a special high-pressure (hyperbaric) chamber.

Metal cylinders containing oxygen should be fitted with a reducing valve by which the rate of flow can be controlled. It is important that the reducing valve should be free from all traces of oil, as otherwise a violent explosion may occur. Also, if the reducing valve is of the rubber-bellows type, the tap of the reducer should always be opened before opening the main oxygen tap on the cylinder; opening the main tap with the reducing valve tap closed has been known to cause spontaneous fire.

Oxymel

see under ACETIC ACID, GLACIAL

Oxymetholone

17β - Hydroxy - 2 - hydroxymethylene - 17α - methyl - 5α-androstan-3-one

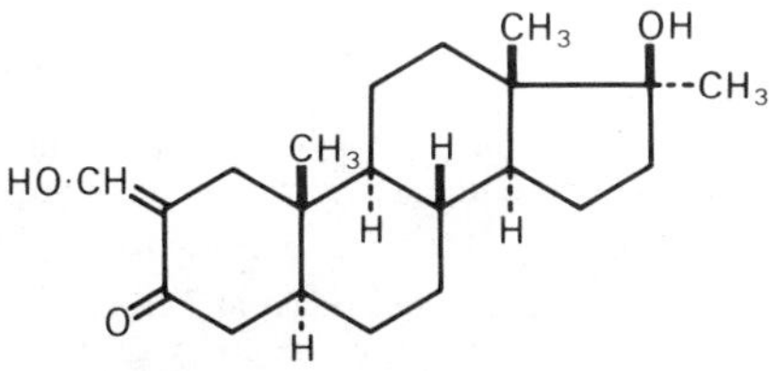

$C_{21}H_{32}O_3 = 332.5$

OTHER NAME: *Anapolon*®

A standard is given in the British Pharmacopoeia Addendum 1978

Description. An odourless, white to creamy-white crystalline powder.

Solubility. Practically insoluble in water; soluble, at 20°, in 50 parts of alcohol, in 9 parts of chloroform, and in 200 parts of ether.

Specific rotation. +34° to +38°, determined on a 2% solution in dioxan.

Storage. It should be protected from light. Contact with ferrous metals should be avoided.

Identification. MELTING-POINT. About 177°.

ULTRAVIOLET ABSORPTION. In 0.01N alcoholic hydrochloric acid, maximum at 277 nm (E1%, 1cm = 300); in 0.01N sodium hydroxide, maximum at 315 nm (E1%, 1cm = 550).

INFRA-RED ABSORPTION. Major peaks at 1149, 1190, 1220, 1235, 1316, and 1613 cm^{-1} (see Appendix 2b: Infra-red Spectra).

THIN-LAYER CHROMATOGRAPHY. See under Thin-layer Chromatography, System 10.

Actions and uses. Oxymetholone has the actions and uses described under Methandienone. The usual dosage by mouth is 5 to 10 milligrams daily. For long-term treatment intermittent therapy is usually adequate, courses of 4 to 6 weeks duration being given with intervals of 1 to 2 weeks.

Children may be given 2.5 to 5 milligrams daily with an interval of 3 weeks after each month of treatment. Higher doses such as 2 to 5 milligrams per kilogram body-weight for adults and 2 to 4 milligrams per kilogram body-weight for children daily in divided doses may be given for prolonged periods in aplastic anaemia and similar conditions.

Undesirable effects. As for Methandienone.

Precautions and contra-indications. It should be used with caution in cardiac disease, hepatic dysfunction, and nephritis. It is contra-indicated in prostatic carcinoma and in pregnancy.

Drug interactions. The prothrombin time is prolonged in patients using warfarin and other anticoagulants.

Preparation

OXYMETHOLONE TABLETS: available as tablets containing 5 and 50 mg of oxymetholone.

A standard for these tablets is given in the British Pharmacopoeia Addendum 1978

Containers and *Storage:* see the entry on Tablets for general information on containers and storage. Containers should be airtight and light resistant and the tablets should not be in contact with ferrous metals.

Oxyphenbutazone

4-Butyl-2-(4-hydroxyphenyl)-1-phenylpyrazolidine-3,5-dione monohydrate

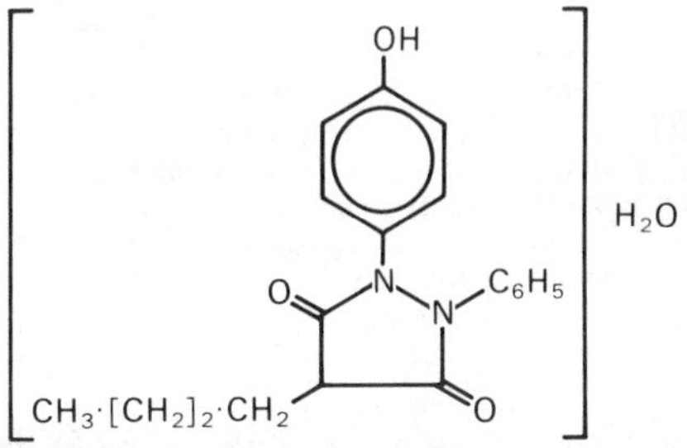

$C_{19}H_{20}N_2O_3, H_2O = 342.4$

OTHER NAMES: *Tandacote*®; *Tanderil*®
Tandalgesic® (with paracetamol); *Tanderil-Chloramphenicol*®

A standard is given in the British Pharmacopoeia 1973

Description. An odourless white crystalline powder with a bitter taste.

Solubility. Very slightly soluble in water; soluble, at 20°, in 3 parts of alcohol, in 20 parts of chloroform, in 20 parts of ether, and in 6 parts of acetone; soluble in solutions of alkali hydroxides.

Moisture content. 5 to 6%, determined by Fischer titration.

Identification. TEST. To about 100 mg add 1 ml of glacial acetic acid and 2 ml of hydrochloric acid, heat on a water-bath for 30 minutes, cool, add 10 ml of water, filter, and to the filtrate add 3 ml of 0.1M sodium nitrite; a yellow colour is produced. Add 1 ml of this solution to 5 ml of *2-naphthol solution*; a bright orange precipitate is produced. Add alcohol (95%); the precipitate dissolves giving an orange solution.

MELTING-POINT. About 96°.

ULTRAVIOLET ABSORPTION. In 0.01N sodium hydroxide, maximum at 254 nm (E1%, 1cm = 750).

INFRA-RED ABSORPTION. Major peaks at 1277, 1350, 1383, 1513, 1685, and 1736 cm^{-1} (see Appendix 2a: Infra-red Spectra).

THIN-LAYER CHROMATOGRAPHY. See under Thin-layer Chromatography, System 3.

Determination in body fluids. See under Phenylbutazone.

Metabolism. ABSORPTION. In rats, absorption is delayed by tricyclic antidepressants.

HALF-LIFE. Plasma half-life, 27 to 64 hours.

DISTRIBUTION. *Protein binding*, extensively bound to plasma proteins.

METABOLIC REACTIONS. Mainly hydroxylation.

EXCRETION. Very little unchanged drug is excreted in the urine.

FURTHER INFORMATION. Absorption inhibited by tricyclic antidepressants in rats—S. Consolo and H. Ladinsky, *Archs int. Pharmacodyn. Thér.*, 1971, **192**, 265; half-life and metabolism—W. Hammer *et al.*, *Clin. Pharmac. Ther.*, 1969, **10**, 44; plasma and urinary concentrations in animals—R. B. Bruce *et al.*, *J. pharm. Sci.*, 1974, **63**, 446.

Actions and uses. Oxyphenbutazone has the actions, uses, and undesirable effects described under Phenylbutazone, of which it is a metabolite. It may be used in acute gout, active rheumatoid arthritis, and related diseases, when they do not respond to safer medication. Oxyphenbutazone is even more slowly excreted than phenylbutazone and does not appear to have any advantage over it.

The usual initial dosage is 300 to 400 milligrams daily in divided doses after meals, usually for 2 days, after which it may be reduced to a maintenance dose of 200 to 300 milligrams daily. The usual dose for children is 5 to 10 milligrams per kilogram body-weight daily. Oxyphenbutazone may also be administered rectally in a dosage of 250 to 500 milligrams daily.

The eye ointment is used in inflammatory conditions of the eye.

Precautions and contra-indications. As for Phenylbutazone.

Preparations

OXYPHENBUTAZONE EYE OINTMENT: prepared by incorporating oxyphenbutazone in eye ointment basis, or any other suitable basis, by Method B described in the entry on Eye Ointments. It contains 10% of oxyphenbutazone.

Labelling: see the entry on Eye Ointments for general information on labelling.

Advice for patients: see the entry on Eye Ointments for general information on the use of eye ointments.

OXYPHENBUTAZONE TABLETS: available as tablets containing 100 mg of oxyphenbutazone; they are sugar coated; the coat may be coloured.

A standard for these tablets is given in the British Pharmacopoeia 1973

Containers and *Storage:* see the entry on Tablets for general information on containers and storage. Containers should be airtight.

Advice for patients: the tablets should be taken after meals.

OTHER PREPARATIONS available include an EYE OINTMENT containing oxyphenbutazone 10% with chloramphenicol 1%; SUPPOSITORIES containing oxyphenbutazone 250 mg; TABLETS (enteric coated) containing oxyphenbutazone 100 mg, and tablets containing oxyphenbutazone 50 mg with paracetamol 500 mg.

Oxyphencyclimine Hydrochloride

1,4,5,6-Tetrahydro-1-methylpyrimidin-2-ylmethyl α-cyclohexylmandelate hydrochloride

$C_{20}H_{29}ClN_2O_3 = 380.9$

A standard is given in the British Pharmacopoeia 1973

Description. An odourless white crystalline powder with a bitter taste.

Solubility. Soluble, at 20°, in 100 parts of water, in 60 parts of alcohol, in 20 parts of methyl alcohol, and in 200 parts of chloroform; very slightly soluble in ether.

Identification. TEST. Mix about 200 mg with 5 ml of hydrochloric acid and 100 mg of zinc powder, heat on a water-bath for 5 minutes, cool, add 1 ml of *copper sulphate solution* and sufficient *strong ammonia solution* to give a blue colour, and then add 10 ml of a mixture of 1 volume of carbon disulphide and 3 volumes of toluene and shake; the upper layer is coloured yellow.

MELTING-POINT. About 230° with decomposition.

INFRA-RED ABSORPTION. Major peaks at 705, 1201, 1227, 1322, 1656, and 1737 cm^{-1} (see Appendix 2a: Infra-red Spectra).

THIN-LAYER CHROMATOGRAPHY. See under Thin-layer Chromatography, System 8.

Actions and uses. Oxyphencyclimine is an anticholinergic drug with actions, uses, and undesirable effects similar to those described under Propantheline Bromide, but it has a prolonged action so that its effects may be obtained throughout the day with only 2 doses. Treatment should commence with 10 to 20 milligrams of oxyphencyclimine hydrochloride daily in divided doses; this should be reduced to a maintenance dose of 10 milligrams daily.

Precautions and contra-indications. As for Atropine.

Preparation

OXYPHENCYCLIMINE TABLETS: they may be coloured. The usual strength is 5 milligrams of oxyphencyclimine hydrochloride.

A standard for these tablets is given in the British Pharmacopoeia 1973

Containers and *Storage:* see the entry on Tablets for general information on containers and storage. Containers should be airtight.

Oxytetracycline Dihydrate

5β-Hydroxytetracycline dihydrate

$C_{22}H_{24}N_2O_9,2H_2O = 496.5$

OTHER NAMES: *Abbocin®*; *Berkmycen®*; *Clinimycin®*; *Galenomycin®*; *Imperacin®*; *Oppamycin®*; *Oxydon®*; *Oxymycin®*; *Oxytetracyclini Dihydras*; *Salamycin®*; *Stecsolin®*; *Terramycin®*

A standard is given in the European Pharmacopoeia Vol. II

Description. An odourless yellow crystalline powder with a slightly bitter taste.

Solubility. Very slightly soluble in water; soluble in dilute acids and alkalis.

Acidity or alkalinity. A 1% suspension has a pH of 5 to 7.5.

Moisture content. 4 to 7.5%, determined by Fischer titration.

Specific rotation. − 203° to − 216°, determined on a 1% solution in 0.1N hydrochloric acid, after standing for 1 hour.

Dissociation constants. pK$_a$ 3.3, 7.3, 9.1 (25°).

Storage. It should be stored in airtight containers, protected from light.

Identification. TESTS. 1. To about 500 μg add 2 ml of sulphuric acid; a deep crimson colour is produced. Add 1 ml of water; the colour changes to yellow.
2. Dissolve about 2 mg in 5 ml of a 1% solution of sodium carbonate and add 2 ml of *diazoaminobenzenesulphonic acid*; a light brown colour is produced.

ULTRAVIOLET ABSORPTION. In *solution of standard pH 2.0*, maximum at 353 nm (E1%, 1cm = 280).

INFRA-RED ABSORPTION. Major peaks at 1243, 1312, 1386, 1462, 1590, and 1622 cm^{-1} (see Appendix 2a: Infra-red Spectra).

Determination in body fluids. SPECTROFLUORIMETRY. In blood or plasma—B. Scales and D. A. Assinder, *J. pharm. Sci.*, 1973, **62**, 913.

Metabolism. ABSORPTION. Not completely absorbed after oral administration; absorbed to about the same extent as tetracycline; absorption is delayed by milk, iron compounds, and antacids.

BLOOD CONCENTRATION. After an intravenous dose of 250 mg, serum concentrations of 5 to 10 μg/ml are obtained in about 1 hour; after a single oral dose of 250 mg, peak serum concentrations of about 1.5μg/ml are attained in 2 to 3 hours; during therapy with 250 mg administered 4 times daily, peak serum concentrations of about 3 μg/ml are attained.

HALF-LIFE. Serum half-life, 9 to 10 hours, which may be increased in renal function impairment.

DISTRIBUTION. Widely distributed throughout the body, secreted in milk and saliva, and crosses the placenta; oxytetracyline binds to calcium to a lesser extent than other tetracyclines and does not accumulate in bone and teeth to the same extent; *protein binding*, 20 to 35% bound to plasma proteins.

EXCRETION. About 70% of a dose is excreted in the urine; it is also excreted, in active form, in the bile and eliminated in the faeces.

FURTHER INFORMATION. Review—M. M. Musselman, *Terramycin (Oxytetracycline)*, Antibiotics Monograph, No. 26, New York, Medical Encyclopedia Inc., 1956.

Bioavailability. Several studies have demonstrated differences in bioavailability in commercial preparations. The variations have been associated with differences in particle size and hence dissolution rate, with differences in conditions of storage, and with differences in tablet age.

FURTHER INFORMATION. Bioavailability and bioequivalence—H. E. Barber *et al.*, *Br. J. clin. Pharmac.*, 1974, **1**, 405, T. Bergan *et al.*, *Acta pharmac. tox.*, 1973, **33**, 138, W. G. Crouthamel, *The Bioavailability of Drug Products*, Washington, American Pharmaceutical Association, 1975, p. 27, and T. M. Jones *et al.*, *J. Pharm. Pharmac.*, 1974, **26**, 116P.

Actions and uses. Oxytetracycline dihydrate has the actions and uses described under Tetracycline Hydrochloride and is given in similar dosage. The usual oral dose for an adult is 250 to 500 milligrams every 6 hours,

but up to 3 grams daily may be given in more severe infections. In general, tetracyclines should not be given to children, but when considered essential the usual dose is 2.5 to 7.5 milligrams per kilogram body-weight every 6 hours.

Salts of aluminium, calcium, iron, and magnesium, and antacids and milk which may decrease the absorption of tetracyclines from the gut should not be given with oxytetracycline.

Undesirable effects; Precautions and contra-indications; Drug interactions. As for Tetracycline Hydrochloride.

Veterinary uses. Oxytetracycline dihydrate is an antibacterial. The usual dose by mouth for all species is 15 to 50 milligrams per kilogram body-weight daily in divided doses but it should not be administered by mouth to adult ruminants. The usual dose by intra-uterine administration for mares and cows is 0.5 to 1 gram daily.

Preparation

OXYTETRACYCLINE TABLETS: available as tablets containing 100, 250, and 500 mg of oxytetracycline dihydrate; they are film coated or sugar coated; the coat may be coloured. Also available as veterinary tablets in the same strengths; they may be film coated or sugar coated and the coat may be coloured; veterinary tablets containing 500 mg of oxytetracycline dihydrate need not be circular in shape.
A standard for these tablets is given in the British Pharmacopoeia 1973 and in the British Pharmacopoeia (Veterinary)
Containers and *Storage:* see the entry on Tablets for general information on containers and storage. Containers should be airtight.
Labelling: the label on the container should state the date after which the tablets are not intended to be used, and the conditions under which they should be stored.
Advice for patients: the tablets should be taken at regular intervals and salts of aluminium, calcium, iron, and magnesium, and antacids and milk should not be taken within 1 hour. The prescribed course should be completed.

Oxytetracycline Hydrochloride

5β-Hydroxytetracycline hydrochloride
$C_{22}H_{25}ClN_2O_9 = 496.9$

OTHER NAMES: *Berkmycen®*; *Duphacycline®*; *Engemycin®*; *Occrycetin®*; Oxytetracyclini Hydrochloridum; *Oxytracyl®*; *Salamycin®*; *Terramycin®*; *Unimycin® Bisolvomycin®* (with bromhexine hydrochloride); *Dispray Oxytetracycline and Hydrocortisone Spray®* and *Terra-Cortril®* (with hydrocortisone); *Neo-Occrycetin®* (with neomycin sulphate); *Terramycin with Polymyxin B Sulphate®*

A standard is given in the European Pharmacopoeia Vol. II

Description. An odourless, yellow, crystalline, hygroscopic powder with a bitter taste.

Solubility. Soluble, at 20°, in 2 parts of water, giving a clear solution which becomes turbid on standing, and in 45 parts of alcohol; soluble in propylene glycol.

Acidity. A 1% solution has a pH of 2.3 to 2.9.

Moisture content. Not more than 2%, determined by Fischer titration.

Specific rotation. − 188° to − 200°, determined on a 1%

solution in 0.1N hydrochloric acid, after standing for 1 hour.

Storage. It should be stored in airtight containers, protected from light.

Labelling. If the material is not intended for parenteral administration, the label on the container states that the contents are not to be injected.

Identification. TESTS. It complies with the tests described under Oxytetracycline Dihydrate.

ULTRAVIOLET ABSORPTION. In *solution of standard pH 2.0*, maximum at 353 nm (E1%, 1cm = 280).

INFRA-RED ABSORPTION. Major peaks at 1235, 1359, 1454, 1584, 1616, and 1665 cm^{-1} (see Appendix 2a: Infra-red Spectra).

Determination in body fluids; Metabolism. As for Oxytetracycline Dihydrate.

Actions and uses. Oxytetracycline hydrochloride has the actions and uses described under Tetracycline Hydrochloride and is given in similar dosage.

The usual dose by mouth for an adult is 250 to 500 milligrams every 6 hours, but up to 3 grams daily in divided doses may be given in severe infections. In general, tetracyclines should not be given to children, but when considered essential the usual dose is 2.5 to 7.5 milligrams per kilogram body-weight every 6 hours. Salts of aluminium, calcium, iron, and magnesium, and antacids and milk which may decrease the absorption of the tetracyclines from the gut should not be given with oxytetracycline.

Oxytetracycline hydrochloride may also be given by intravenous infusion in severe acute infections. For adults, up to 1 gram may be given every 12 hours by slow intravenous infusion of a solution containing not more than 0.1%. The usual dose for children is 10 to 20 milligrams per kilogram body-weight daily in divided doses. Oral treatment should be substituted as soon as possible.

Undesirable effects; Precautions and contra-indications; Drug interactions. As for Tetracycline Hydrochloride.

Veterinary uses. Oxytetracycline hydrochloride is an antibacterial. The usual dose by mouth for all species is 15 to 50 milligrams per kilogram body-weight daily in divided doses but it should not be administered by mouth to adult ruminants. The usual dose by intramuscular injection as a solution of the magnesium complex is for horses and cattle 2 to 5 milligrams per kilogram body-weight daily, for sheep 2 to 7 milligrams per kilogram body-weight daily, and for dogs and cats 7 to 11 milligrams per kilogram body-weight daily; these doses may also be given by intravenous injection except to dogs and cats.

Oxytetracycline hydrochloride may be administered in the feed for pigs at a rate of 200 to 700 parts per million and for poultry at a rate of 100 to 600 parts per million. Alternatively it may be given in the drinking water at a rate of 110 to 280 parts per million for pigs or 60 to 260 parts per million for poultry, according to age and weight. The usual dose by intra-uterine administration for mares, cows, ewes, sows, and goats is 0.5 to 1 gram daily.

Preparations

HYDROCORTISONE AND OXYTETRACYCLINE OINTMENT: a dispersion of hydrocortisone and oxytetracycline hydrochloride in a suitable anhydrous greasy basis. It contains 10 mg of hydrocortisone and oxytetracycline hydrochloride equivalent to 30 mg of oxytetracycline per g.

Containers, *Labelling*, and *Storage:* see the entry on Ointments for general information on containers, labelling, and storage.

Advice for patients: the ointment should be applied sparingly to the affected area.

OXYTETRACYCLINE CAPSULES: consisting of oxytetracycline hydrochloride, in powder, which may be mixed with suitable inert diluents, enclosed in a hard capsule. The capsule shells may be coloured. Available as capsules containing 250 mg of oxytetracycline hydrochloride.

A standard for these capsules is given in the British Pharmacopoeia 1973

Containers and *Storage:* see the entry on Capsules for general information on containers and storage.

Labelling: the label on the container should state the date after which the capsules are not intended to be used and the conditions under which they should be stored.

Advice for patients: the capsules should be taken at regular intervals and salts of aluminium, calcium, iron, and magnesium, and antacids and milk should not be taken within 1 hour. The prescribed course should be completed.

OXYTETRACYCLINE INJECTION: a sterile solution of oxytetracycline hydrochloride, with a suitable buffering agent, in water for injections. It is prepared by dissolving the contents of a sealed container (containing the oxytetracycline hydrochloride and the buffering agent) in water for injections shortly before use.

Available as a powder in vials containing oxytetracycline hydrochloride equivalent to 250 and 500 mg of anhydrous oxytetracycline.

A standard for this injection is given in the British Pharmacopoeia 1973

Containers: see the entry on Injections for general information on containers.

Labelling: see the entry on Injections for general information on labelling. In addition, the label on the sealed container should state that the contents are to be used for intravenous injection only, in a well-diluted solution.

Storage: the sealed container should be protected from light. The injection contains no bactericide and should be used as soon as possible after preparation but solutions of oxytetracycline hydrochloride may be expected to retain their potency for up to 72 hours after preparation, provided that a buffering agent is present and that it is stored at a temperature not exceeding 4°.

OXYTETRACYCLINE SOLUBLE POWDER: consisting of oxytetracycline hydrochloride, with a suitable yellow dye, in a water-soluble diluent consisting of lactose or other suitable diluent. Available as soluble powders containing 5, 5.5, 11, and 13.2% of oxytetracycline hydrochloride.

A standard for this powder is given in the British Pharmacopoeia (Veterinary)

Containers and *Storage:* see the entry on Powders for general information on containers and storage. Containers should be airtight. The powder should be stored in a cool place.

Labelling: the label on the container should state the amount of the medicament in terms of the concentration of oxytetracycline hydrochloride, the date after which the powder is not intended to be used, and the conditions under which it should be stored.

OTHER PREPARATIONS available include an APPLICATION containing oxytetracycline hydrochloride 150 mg with hydrocortisone 50 mg in 30 ml, in an aerosol pack; an application containing oxytetracycline hydrochloride equivalent to 200 mg of anhydrous oxytetracycline with hydrocortisone 100 mg in 60 ml, in an aerosol pack; CAPSULES containing oxytetracycline hydrochloride 250 mg with bromhexine hydrochloride 8 mg; an EYE OINTMENT containing oxytetracycline hydrochloride equivalent to 5 mg of anhydrous oxytetracycline with polymyxin B sulphate 10000 units per g; an INJECTION containing, when reconstituted from vials of powder to prepare 2 ml of solution, oxytetracycline hydrochloride equivalent to 50 mg of anhydrous oxytetracycline with procaine hydrochloride 20 mg (2%) per ml; an OINTMENT containing oxytetracycline hydrochloride equivalent to 30 mg of anhydrous oxytetracycline per g; and an ointment containing oxytetracycline hydrochloride equivalent to 30 mg of anhydrous oxytetracycline with hydrocortisone 10 mg per g.

OTHER VETERINARY PREPARATIONS available include an APPLICATION containing oxytetracycline hydrochloride 2% (with crystal violet as marker) in an aerosol pack; an application containing oxytetracycline hydrochloride 2.5% (with crystal violet as marker), in an aerosol pack; an application containing oxytetracycline hydrochloride equivalent to 150 mg of anhydrous oxytetracycline with hydrocortisone 50 mg in 30 ml, in an aerosol pack; an application containing oxytetracycline hydrochloride equivalent to 300 mg of oxytetracycline with hydrocortisone 100 mg in 60 ml, in an aerosol pack; an INJECTION containing oxytetracycline hydrochloride 50 mg per ml in 100-ml vials; and injection containing oxytetracycline hydrochloride equivalent to 50 mg of anhydrous oxytetracycline per ml (in an aqueous solution containing povidone) in 50- and 100-ml packs; an injection containing oxytetracycline hydrochloride equivalent to 100 mg of oxytetracycline per ml (in an aqueous solution containing povidone) in 100-ml packs; an injection containing the equivalent of 50 mg of oxytetracycline hydrochloride per ml in 40- and 100-ml vials; an injection containing the equivalent of 100 mg of oxytetracycline hydrochloride per ml in 50- and 100-ml vials; an injection containing the equivalent of 125 mg of oxytetracycline hydrochloride with lignocaine hydrochloride 10 mg per ml in 30-ml vials; an INTRAMAMMARY INJECTION containing the equivalent of 30 mg of oxytetracycline hydrochloride per g in 14.2-g tubes; a PREMIX containing the equivalent of 5, 10, and 20% of oxytetracycline hydrochloride; a soluble POWDER containing oxytetracycline hydrochloride 5.5% with neomycin sulphate 5.5%; TABLETS containing oxytetracycline hydrochloride 100 mg, and bolus tablets containing oxytetracycline hydrochloride 250 mg with neomycin sulphate 250 mg.

Oxytocin Injection

A sterile aqueous solution containing the oxytocic principle of the posterior lobe of the pituitary body prepared by a process of fractionation from mammalian pituitary glands or by synthesis. Oxytocin is a cyclic peptide having the structure Cys-Tyr-Ile-Gln-Asn-Cys-Pro-Leu-Gly-NH$_2$.

OTHER NAMES: Oxytocini Solutio Iniectabilis; *Pitocin*®; *Syntocinon*®
Syntometrine® (with ergometrine maleate)

A standard is given in the European Pharmacopoeia Vol. III

Description. A clear colourless liquid.

Acidity. It has a pH of 3.5 to 4.5.

Sterilisation. It is sterilised by filtration.

Storage. It should be stored between 2° and 10°. Under these conditions it may be expected to retain its potency for 3 years from the date of manufacture. When stored at a temperature not exceeding 25° it may be expected to retain its potency for 2 years from the date of manufacture.

Actions and uses. Oxytocin injection has the oxytocic action of the posterior lobe of the pituitary gland, but has little pressor or antidiuretic action. It causes contraction of the uterus by direct stimulation of the uterine muscle, the effect varying with the phase in the menstrual cycle when it is given and depending on whether or not the uterus is pregnant and on the stage of pregnancy. Small doses increase the tone and amplitude of the uterine contractions; large or repeated doses result in tetany lasting for 5 to 10 minutes; oestrogens intensify and progestogens diminish the effect. Oxytocin is used for the induction of labour and to overcome uterine inertia.

For the induction of labour, 2 to 5 units in 1000 millilitres of dextrose injection (5%) may be given by slow intravenous infusion, and to overcome uterine inertia in labour, 1 to 5 units similarly diluted may be given by intravenous infusion at a rate of 30 drops per minute until the inertia is overcome.

Oxytocin injection is used to control post-partum haemorrhage, a dose of 2 to 5 units being given by subcutaneous or intramuscular injection or slow intravenous infusion; it may also be used in conjunction with ergometrine.

Oxytocin is also administered in buccal tablets and as a nasal spray, but it is then less effective and its action is more difficult to control.

Precautions. The dosage, regardless of the route of administration, should be adjusted to the requirements of the patient. Excessive doses give rise to violent contractions, with danger of uterine rupture or foetal asphyxiation and to water retention.

Veterinary uses. Oxytocin is used as a uterine stimulant at parturition and in the treatment of retained membranes in cattle. It is also used to stimulate milk release. The usual dose by intramuscular injection for horses, cattle, sheep, goats, pigs, and dogs is up to 0.05 unit per kilogram body-weight repeated if necessary at intervals of not less than 1 hour.

Preparations

Available in 2-ml ampoules containing 1 unit of oxytocin per ml, in 1-ml ampoules containing 5 units of oxytocin, and in 0.5-, 1-, and 5-ml ampoules containing 10 units of oxytocin per ml.

OTHER PREPARATIONS available include ERGOMETRINE AND OXYTOCIN INJECTION, see under Ergometrine Maleate; and a SPRAY containing oxytocin 40 units per ml.

Oxytocin Tablets

Oxytocin tablets contain synthetic oxytocin.

OTHER NAME: *Pitocin*®

A standard is given in the British Pharmacopoeia 1973

Actions and uses. The actions and uses of oxytocin are described under Oxytocin Injection. The tablets are intended to be dissolved slowly in the mouth and the oxytocin absorbed through the buccal mucosa. Absorption is incomplete and the effect is less reliable than when oxytocin is injected.

The usual dose by buccal administration for the induction of labour is 100 units every 30 minutes.

Precautions. As for Oxytocin Injection.

Preparation

Available as tablets containing synthetic oxytocin citrate equivalent to 200 units of oxytocin.

Oxyuriasis

see ENTEROBIASIS

Packaging, Stability, and Storage

Packaging

The function of a container for a medicinal preparation is to maintain the quality, safety, and stability of its contents.

A container should withstand the mechanical hazards of handling and transport, prevent leakage, and provide an appropriate level of protection from environmental conditions. Ideally, the materials of construction should have no chemical or physical effect on the preparation, and, for liquid preparations, should be sufficiently transparent to permit inspection of the contents whilst providing protection from incident radiation when necessary.

Not all these criteria can be met by the packaging materials currently available and the pharmacist should therefore select a container which most closely conforms to these requirements.

Packaging Materials

Glass. For medicinal preparations, particularly liquids, glass containers offer certain advantages over containers made from other materials. Glass can be moulded and sealed either hermetically or by a removable closure; it is transparent but can be coloured to resist ultraviolet radiation. Containers of glass are rigid, impermeable to atmospheric gases and moisture, and can be sterilised by heat; they are easily labelled.

Disadvantages of glass are its brittleness, its weight, and its ability to release alkali to aqueous contents. Solutions of soluble citrates, phosphates, and bicarbonates kept or heated in glass containers may degrade the inner surface of the container to produce a deposit of glass flakes or spicules.

Plastics. Several polymeric materials used for containers are collectively described as plastics; they may comprise single polymers with few additives or complex mixtures of polymers with resins, fillers, plasticisers, stabilisers, and antistatic agents. Although the properties of plastic materials vary with their composition, they are generally more flexible, lighter in weight, and less brittle than glass, and not all plastics are transparent. Like glass, plastics can be moulded and some can be sealed hermetically but only a few will withstand the temperatures required for heat sterilisation without softening or distortion.

Permeability to water vapour and atmospheric gases varies considerably between materials, for example, polyethylene is an effective barrier to water vapour while polyvinyl chloride is sufficiently permeable to preclude its use in containers for moisture-sensitive products. Although plastics are resistant to most chemicals, certain organic materials such as phthalates, esters of salicylic acid, paraldehyde, and essential oils rapidly interact with plastics to cause softening or distortion. Sorption effects whereby materials, notably preservatives, are removed from preparations by the container have also been observed. Leaching of additives such as plasticisers and stabilisers from plastic containers into their liquid contents can occur; this problem has been most evident in compound plastic materials such as flexible polyvinyl chloride.

Metals. Metal containers used for medicinal products include rigid cans or tubes of aluminium or tinplate, collapsible tubes made of aluminium, tin, lead, or tin-coated lead, and metal cylinders for medicinal gases. Rigid cans are used for solid dosage forms and collapsible tubes for ointments and creams.

Metal containers are usually robust, light in weight, and impermeable to gases and water vapour; their disadvantages include chemical and electrochemical activity, their opacity, and a tendency to contain metallic particles, especially near the screw threads of collapsible tubes. The inner surfaces of aluminium containers are often coated with lacquer or epoxy-resins to reduce electrolytic and chemical reactions. Further sealing at the crimped ends of collapsible tubes may be provided by an internal coating of latex.

Paper and paperboard. Because of their low strength, lack of rigidity, and high permeability to water vapour, containers of paper or paperboard are unsuitable as primary packaging for pharmaceutical preparations with the exception of certain powders dispensed in individual doses. Cartons or wallets of paperboard may, however, be suitable as outer containers to provide additional mechanical protection, for example, to solid dosage forms enclosed in strip or blister packs.

Films and laminates. By forming laminates from combinations of paper, aluminium foil, plastics, and cellulose films, and additional coating it is possible to produce flexible packaging materials with barrier properties to suit the needs of particular preparations. Laminates and foil-film combinations can be readily sealed into units to contain single doses of solids, liquids, and semi-solids; examples include strip and blister packs for solid dose forms and sachets for powders or liquids.

Simple cellulose films may offer little protection from moisture whereas the laminates which include aluminium foil, polyethylene film, or a coating of polyvinylidene usually provide an effective moisture barrier. Because only a few plastic materials can be formed into trays for blister packs and these materials are all highly permeable to water vapour, the provision of a moisture barrier in such packs usually entails additional coatings or enclosure within a moisture-resistant overwrap.

Rubber. Rubber is a compounded product based on natural or synthetic polymers. To improve the mechanical properties of rubber, other materials are incorporated which include vulcanisers, accelerators, activators, and fillers. Pigments, antioxidants, and lubricants may also be added.

The main pharmaceutical use of rubber is in the construction of closures for containers, including plugs, disks, and liners to fit containers for sterile fluids, and teats for eye-drop bottles. Rubber is strong and resilient and has the property of re-sealing itself after penetration by a needle; furthermore, many rubbers can be sterilised by heat. The limitations of rubber are similar to those of plastics in that when in contact with solutions it has an ability to absorb materials from such solutions.

Preservatives and antoxidants included in injections and in eye-drops present a particular problem. To some extent this problem of sorption can be met by pretreatment of the rubber closures before use.

Like plastics, rubber also is subject to leaching, and constituents of the rubber compound may migrate into the contents of the container. Different types of rubber exhibit different degrees of permeability to gases and water vapour. Synthetic silicone rubber is permeable to water vapour and eye-drops kept in containers fitted with silicone rubber teats therefore have a limited shelf-life.

Selection of Containers

Containers should be sufficiently rigid to protect their contents from damage due to ordinary conditions of handling, storage, and transport; they should be effectively sealed to prevent leakage and the ingress of contaminants, and when necessary should be capable of being opened and reclosed repeatedly.

FURTHER INFORMATION. Recommendations of the Council of the Pharmaceutical Society on containers for dispensing, *Pharm. J.*, i/1972, 80.

Containers which provide additional protection are described below.

Airtight container. This container protects the contents from contamination with extraneous solids, liquids, and vapours, from loss of volatile constituents, and from changes due to efflorescence, deliquescence, and evaporation under ordinary conditions of handling, storage, and transport.

Securely closed container. This is an airtight container fitted with some means of preventing the unintentional displacement of the closure.

Hermetically sealed container. This container is impervious to air and other gases under ordinary conditions of handling, storage, and transport. It is usually a glass ampoule sealed by fusion of the glass.

Light-resistant container. Preparations which are subject to oxidation, and in some cases hydrolysis, may require protection from light. To reduce the passage of ultraviolet radiation containers are made from coloured glasses or from plastic materials which contain ultraviolet absorbing substances. A light-resistant container is defined as one which does not transmit more than 10% of incident radiation at any wavelength between 290 and 450 nm.

Single-dose containers. Special sealing techniques are necessary to prevent the ingress of micro-organisms, particularly into containers for parenteral solutions. Ideally, all injections should be supplied in single-dose containers, that is, containers which are hermetically sealed and contain only a single dose of an injection solution; when once opened such containers cannot be resealed. For single-dose injections of larger volume glass containers with composite closures of rubber, metal, and sometimes plastic are still widely used.

Multiple-dose containers. A multiple-dose container prevents as far as possible the access of moisture and is fitted with a closure, usually of rubber, that prevents the access of micro-organisms and allows the withdrawal of successive doses of an injection solution. Because of the risk of microbial contamination during use and the limitations of the closure system the continuing use of multiple-dose containers should be discouraged.

Child-resistant container. A container designed to prevent children gaining access to its contents. Such containers may be used when supplying medicines for domiciliary use especially for substances known to be dangerous to children.

Containers for Preparations for External Use

Medicinal preparations for external use should not be supplied in the same types of containers as are normally used for medicinal preparations taken internally. For example, liquid products for external use should preferably be dispensed in fluted bottles, although in special instances, other suitable containers may be used, provided that such containers are clearly distinguishable from types normally used for medicinal preparations taken internally.

Stability

The stability of a medicine is its ability to resist deterioration. For a packaged medicinal preparation, stability is usually considered in terms of shelf-life, that is, the period under specified storage conditions during which the properties and characteristics of the original preparation can be expected to remain within acceptable limits.

Deterioration may take several forms arising from changes in the chemical, physical, and microbiological properties of a medicament or preparation. These changes may affect the therapeutic value of a preparation or increase its toxicity.

Chemical deterioration. Provided that degradation products are not toxic a preparation is generally considered to be of acceptable quality until its potency or content of active medicament has fallen to not less than 90% of the labelled value. A closer tolerance is required when degradation products are more toxic than the active medicament and conversely a wider tolerance may be acceptable if the degradation products have an action closely similar to that of the active ingredient.

Physical changes. A limit may be placed on the extent of changes in colour, flavour, or particle size range, or the development of undesirable rheological properties.

Microbiological stability. Microbiological stability is often assessed on the effectiveness of the preparation in maintaining its sterility or in the retention of its antimicrobial properties.

Causes of Instability

In many instances, rates of chemical breakdown of medicaments are affected by environmental conditions such as temperature, atmospheric gases, humidity, light, and the presence of micro-organisms. Non-active adjuvants may also degrade or be involved in the reaction and pH and the nature of the solvent can be important factors in liquid systems. As a general rule, it may be assumed that because chemical reactions tend to take place more rapidly in liquid systems than in the dry state, solutions are less stable than suspensions which in turn are less stable than solid dosage forms.

The most common degradation reactions found in medicinal products are hydrolysis, oxidation, and photolysis; less frequent occurrences are racemisation, complexation, reduction, and biochemical reactions.

An increase in the temperature of a medicinal preparation may provide the activation necessary to promote an oxidation reaction; it may also increase the rates of existing oxidation or hydrolytic reactions. In liquid systems, pH is important since both hydrolysis and oxidation reactions can be catalysed by hydrogen or hydroxyl ions; there is often an optimum pH range within which a medicament in solution exhibits maximum stability.

Atmospheric oxygen, even in low concentration, can initiate oxidation of a medicament; such reactions are often catalysed by traces of heavy metals and ultraviolet radiation from light sources. In general, hydrolytic reactions are less sensitive than oxidation reactions to light and atmospheric gases. Medicaments which are rapidly hydrolysed are usually supplied in the dry state and require protection from conditions of high humidity. Physical changes and their rates of development in preparations are often less predictable than chemical changes although in some instances the two types may be interdependent. However, independent physical changes can occur as a direct result of conditions such as temperature, humidity, or exposure to radiation.

Microbial proliferation may develop in water-containing preparations which do not include a suitable antimicrobial substance or in which the antimicrobial substance has become inactivated by physico-chemical interaction with other constituents or with components of the container.

Indications of Deterioration

Chemical degradation may not necessarily be accompanied by obvious physical changes so undue reliance should not be placed on the absence of organoleptic changes as a positive indication of chemical stability.

Assay methods for the determination of chemical stability or potency must be capable of measuring the content of the active constituent in the presence of its breakdown products. Although such methods are used by manufacturers during stability testing of their products, they are not readily applied by pharmacists in general practice to detect chemical breakdown. However, when untoward physical changes have occurred in a preparation, it is reasonable to assume, in most instances, that other forms of deterioration have developed and to reject the preparation as unsuitable.

Many untoward physical effects which appear in solid dosage forms and powders are due to the presence of excessive moisture; typical examples are loss of effervescent properties, swelling, cracking, and adhesion of coated tablets, and the discoloration, caking, and fusion of powders and granules. Instability in water-containing semi-solids may be evident as "drying-out" due to water loss by evaporation under low humidity conditions. Rheological changes, discoloration, and microbial spoilage also occur in ointments, lotions, and creams.

In simple liquid preparations, instability is usually indicated by the formation of a haze, turbidity, or a precipitate; discoloration may also be present and if microbial proliferation has occurred there may be gas formation and organoleptic changes. The more complex systems such as emulsions may show evidence of cracking or thickening, while suspensions become caked.

Maintenance of Stability

During the development of a new medicinal preparation the manufacturer should establish the formulation, package, and processing conditions which together yield a safe, acceptable product of the required therapeutic efficiency and stability. The appropriate storage conditions for the preparation should also be defined by the manufacturer and related to the shelf-life or expiry date. In order to maintain stability, the preparation, in its original package, should be stored under the specified conditions and issued or dispensed, in rotation, in accordance with the expiry date. At intervals, stock should be examined for evidence of deterioration.

In dispensing it may be necessary to transfer a manufactured medicinal preparation from its original package to another container; in these circumstances the protection offered by the container should be that recommended by the manufacturer or should be at least equivalent to that of the original package. In selecting the container any recommendations of the manufacturer should be taken into consideration.

If dilution or admixture of a liquid or semi-solid preparation has to be undertaken consideration should be given not only to the possibility of incompatibilities and modification of absorption characteristics in the case of an admixture, but also to the possible effect on the stability of the original preparation. Changes of solvent and pH may induce instability while the dilution of adjuvants such as preservatives, antoxidants, and chelating agents is likely to reduce their effectiveness. In the case of a manufactured product the shelf-life period originally specified by the manufacturer would no longer be relevant and, ideally, a new, shorter, shelf-life should be assigned to the new preparation.

Unless the necessary information on the stability characteristics and composition of a proprietary medicinal product is available, extemporaneous admixture is not recommended; dilutions should be prepared in accordance with the entry on Dilution.

As a further safeguard, it is desirable that when any medicinal product is supplied, the patient should be informed of suitable storage conditions for the preparation and when relevant given an indication of the time after which the preparation should be discarded.

Storage

Rates at which most hydrolytic and oxidation reactions occur are reduced as the temperature is lowered, and the growth of micro-organisms is likewise generally slower at low temperatures. As a general rule, therefore, high temperatures should be avoided when storing raw materials and medicinal products.

Medicinal products should not be exposed to conditions of high temperature or humidity, and extreme fluctuations of temperature should be avoided. Suspensions in particular should be stored at an even temperature as otherwise crystal growth may occur. Containers should not be exposed to direct sunlight even when they are light resistant.

Any specific storage directions should be followed. *Cool place* is usually defined as a space in which the temperature does not exceed 15°. When a cool place is not available in ordinary storage areas a refrigerator may be used, but care should be taken to avoid freezing aqueous preparations which deteriorate when frozen and thawed.

FURTHER INFORMATION. Stability of pharmaceutical products—J. A. Mollica *et al.*, *J. pharm. Sci.*, 1978, **67**, 443.

Padimate

A mixture of pentyl, isopentyl, and 2-methylbutyl 4-dimethylaminobenzoates.
$C_{14}H_{21}NO_2 = 235.3$

OTHER NAMES: *Escalol 506*®; Padimate A; *Spectraban*®

Description. A yellow liquid with a faint aromatic odour.

Solubility. Soluble in alcohol, in chloroform, and in liquid paraffin.

Actions and uses. Padimate is used as a sunscreen agent. It helps to prevent sunburn by absorbing ultraviolet radiation of wavelength 290 to 320 nm which is mainly responsible for the production of sunburn. It is applied to exposed skin as a 2.5% alcoholic lotion, avoiding contact with the eyes.

Preparations

Preparations available include a LOTION containing padimate 2.5%.

Paget's Disease of Bone

Paget's disease (osteitis deformans) is a chronic progressive disease of bone characterised by deformity and weakness of bones and deep bone pain. Initially, decalcification and softening of bones result in deformations such as kyphosis, flattening of the vertebrae, broadening of the pelvis, and bowing of the legs. This is followed by uncontrolled recalcification which results in loss of bone structure with thickening and enlargement of the deformed bones.

Onset is insidious and is rarely noted before the age of 50. Localised lesions may be noted during X-ray examination for other reasons. The changes of Paget's disease are asymmetrical and most commonly affect weight-bearing bones, especially the pelvis and sacrum. The serum calcium is normal and serum phosphate is normal or slightly raised. However, alkaline phosphatase and urinary hydroxyproline are elevated. The lesions of Paget's disease are highly vascular and act as arterio-venous shunts which eventually lead to strain on the left ventricle and high-output heart failure.

There is no specific treatment for Paget's disease, but calcitonin and salcatonin may be used to reduce severe pain unresponsive to analgesics. In selected cases mithramycin is used.

Pain

Pain may be due to organic or psychological disturbances or a combination of both. It may be characteristic of a disease and is sometimes the only factor that reveals the presence of a disease.

Diagnostic value of pain. Pain varies in many ways and the characteristics of a particular pain may help in the diagnosis of the underlying condition.

Site. The location of a pain may indicate the part of the body affected. However, pain felt in one position may sometimes be referred from pathology in another part of the body. This occurs when pain cannot be felt in the affected area (for example, the viscera) or when it causes pressure on a nerve. Some pains do not remain localised in one area but move from one place to another.

Radiation. The pain may be felt most in one particular place but there may be a characteristic region where discomfort is felt. For example, cardiac pain is felt most as central chest pain but often radiates to the shoulders and left arm.

Severity. A pain may be anything from a mild discomfort to a severe pain which fills consciousness.

Timing. Pain may be continuous or it may only appear at certain times of the day or night. It may last only briefly or for many hours.

Character. A pain may have a particular characteristic which is described by the patient as stabbing, crushing, gnawing, burning, throbbing, etc. It may be localised to a particular place or it may be a generalised discomfort.

Aggravating and relieving factors. Certain factors may be found to aggravate a pain, and these may be avoided by the patient. Other factors may be found to bring relief from pain. Consideration of these factors may be helpful in the treatment of pain.

Relief of pain

Pain may resolve itself with reassurance or appropriate treatment of an underlying condition, or rest, warming, cooling, or changing position may provide relief. In other cases drug treatment may be required. Local anaesthetics may be used to control local pain. Pain from musculoskeletal disorders may be treated as described under Rheumatoid Arthritis and related conditions.

Minor pains, including some headaches, may be treated with mild peripherally acting analgesics such as aspirin or paracetamol. More intense pain may require the use of centrally acting analgesics. The mildest effective substance should be used but the dose should be regulated to provide adequate relief and the interval between doses should be adjusted so as to prevent the re-emergence of pain.

Major tranquillisers and corticosteroids may increase the effects of analgesics; benzodiazepines may relieve anxiety, and antidepressives may relieve the depression associated with pain. Strong analgesics may cause nausea and vomiting, and tolerance and dependence may occur. In certain cases of intractable pain, relief may be obtained only by surgical division of the posterior root of the posterolateral column of the spinal cord.

Narcotic analgesics used in the relief of pain include codeine, dextromoramide, dextropropoxyphene, diamorphine, dihydrocodeine, dipipanone, fentanyl, levorphanol, methadone, morphine, opium, papaveretum, pentazocine, pethidine, and phenazocine.

Non-narcotic analgesics used in the relief of pain include alclofenac, aloxiprin, aspirin, benorylate, fenoprofen, flufenamic acid, ibuprofen, indomethacin, ketoprofen, mefenamic acid, naproxen, oxyphenbutazone, paracetamol, phenacetin, phenazone, and phenylbutazone.

See also Gout, Headache, Neuralgia, and Rheumatoid Arthritis.

Paints

Paints are liquid preparations for application to the skin or mucous surfaces. They are usually medicated with substances possessing antiseptic, astringent, caustic, or analgesic properties. Resinous substances such as benzoin, prepared storax, or tolu balsam in ethereal solution are employed as bases of medicated varnishes.

Containers. They should be dispensed in coloured fluted bottles in order that they may be distinguished from preparations intended for internal administration.

Labelling. The containers of paints (with the exception of throat paints) should be labelled "For external use only".

Storage. They should be stored in airtight containers.

Palm Kernel Oil, Fractionated

Obtained by expression of the natural oil from the kernels of *Elaeis guineensis* Jacquin (Fam. Palmae) followed by selective solvent fractionation and hydrogenation.

OTHER NAMES: *Extracoa®*; *Supercoa®*

A standard is given in the British Pharmacopoeia 1973

Description. A white, solid, brittle, odourless fat.

Solubility. Insoluble in water; very slightly soluble in alcohol; miscible with ether, with chloroform, and with light petroleum.

Melting-point. 31° to 36°.

Refractive index. At 50°, 1.445 to 1.447.

Storage. It should be stored in a cool place.

Uses. Fractionated palm kernel oil is used instead of theobroma oil as a fatty basis for the preparation of suppositories.

Pancreatin

A preparation of mammalian pancreas containing enzymes having protease, lipase, and amylase activity. It may contain sodium chloride as a diluent. It contains in 1 milligram not less than 1.4 B.P. units of free protease, 20 B.P. units of lipase, and 24 B.P. units of amylase activity. It corresponds to the preparation described as "strong pancreatin powder" in the British National Formulary 1976–78.

OTHER NAMES: *Panar®*; *Pancrex®*; *Zypanar®*
Phazyme® (with silica in dimethicone); *Panteric Compound®* (with sodium tauroglycocholate)

A standard is given in the British Pharmacopoeia Addendum 1978

Description. A white or buff-coloured amorphous powder.

Solubility. Soluble or partly soluble in water, forming a slightly turbid solution; practically insoluble in alcohol and in ether.

Moisture content. Not more than 5%, determined by drying at 105°.

Stability. Its proteolytic activity is destroyed by treatment with more than traces of mineral acids and it is thereby distinguished from pepsin, which is active only in acid solution; all enzymic activity of pancreatin is destroyed by strong alkalis and by heat. When dissolved in water, it is precipitated by heat, acids, metallic salts, strong alcohol, and tannic acid, but not by a saturated solution of sodium chloride, differing in this last respect from pepsin.

Storage. It should be stored in airtight containers, in a cool place.

Actions and uses. Pancreatin may be administered by mouth in the form of a powder, tablets, or enteric-coated tablets or granules to assist the digestion of starch, fat, and protein in patients with pancreatic deficiency.

The enzymatic activity of pancreatin is now expressed in units and the minimum specified in the British Pharmacopoeia Addendum 1978 for each component is approximately 1½ times the minimum of the British Pharmacopoeia 1973 and about 5 times the minimum potency required by the British Pharmacopoeia 1968.

The usual dose for an adult is 2 to 8 grams daily in divided doses with meals. The dose for infants up to one year is 500 to 750 milligrams with each feed, and for children 1 to 12 years 0.75 to 1 gram 4 times daily before each meal.

Pancreatin is also used for the preparation of predigested protein foods. For peptonising milk, pancreatin is added to tepid water, and milk, previously heated to 38°, is then added; the mixture is stirred and maintained at 38° for

15 minutes longer if complete peptonisation is desired, and then raised to boiling-point, after which it should be transferred to a cool place. The peptonised milk should be used within 24 hours of preparation. Gruel, arrowroot, and other farinaceous foods may be similarly predigested.

Precautions. If pancreatin is mixed with liquids or feeds the resulting mixture should not be allowed to stand for more than one hour prior to use.

Veterinary uses. Pancreatin is administered by mouth in replacement therapy for dogs and cats that are deficient in pancreatic enzymes, the usual dose being 0.3 to 0.6% in the feed, adjusted in accordance with the response of the animal.

Preparations

PANCREATIN GRANULES: consisting of pancreatin. They may contain suitable entero-protective substances. Available as granules containing at least 41 000 U.S.N.F. units (equivalent to 650 B.P. units) of free protease activity, 10 000 B.P. units of amylase, and 7150 B.P. units of lipase per g, and as granules containing at least 75 000 U.S.N.F. units (equivalent to 1200 B.P. units) of free protease activity, 18 000 B.P. units of amylase, and 11 100 B.P. units of lipase per g.

A standard for these granules is given in the British Pharmacopoeia Addendum 1978

Containers and *Storage:* they should be stored in airtight containers in a cool place.

Labelling: the label on the container should state the minimum number of units of free protease activity, of lipase activity, and of amylase activity per g.

Advice for patients: the granules should be swallowed dry or taken mixed with a little fluid before meals or mixed with the food; excessive heat will destroy its effect. See also under Strong Pancreatin Capsules (below).

PANCREATIN TABLETS: available as tablets containing 110 B.P. units of free protease activity and 1900 B.P. units of lipase activity, and as tablets containing 330 B.P. units of free protease activity and 5600 B.P. units of lipase activity; they are enteric coated and sugar coated. The Strong Pancreatin Tablets described in the British National Formulary 1976–78 correspond to the tablets containing 330 B.P. units of free protease activity and 5600 B.P. units of lipase activity.

A standard for these tablets is given in the British Pharmacopoeia Addendum 1978

Containers and *Storage:* see the entry on Tablets for general information on containers and storage. Containers should be airtight. The tablets should be stored in a cool place.

Labelling: the label on the container should state the minimum number of units of free protease activity, of lipase activity, and of amylase activity per g.

Advice for patients: the tablets should be swallowed whole and taken before meals. See also under Strong Pancreatin Capsules.

STRONG PANCREATIN CAPSULES: consisting of pancreatin, in powder, which may be mixed with a suitable inert diluent, enclosed in a suitable capsule. They are intended to be opened before administration of the contents (see advice below). Available as capsules containing not less than 430 B.P. units of free protease activity and not less than 8000 B.P. units of lipase activity.

Containers and *Storage:* see the entry on Capsules for general information on containers and storage. The capsules should be stored in a cool place.

Advice for patients: the capsules should be opened and

the contents sprinkled on the food or taken mixed with fluid before meals; excessive heat will destroy its effect. Treatment should not be discontinued without the advice of the prescriber. Pancreatin may irritate the skin surrounding the mouth and anus; a barrier cream may be applied.

STRONG PANCREATIN POWDER: see opening statement on Pancreatin above; the advice for patients is similar to that given under Pancreatin Granules.

OTHER PREPARATIONS available include TABLETS containing pancreatin 240 mg with silica in dimethicone 60 mg, and veterinary tablets containing pancreatin 300 mg with sodium tauroglycocholate 100 mg.

Pancreatitis

Pancreatitis is inflammation of the pancreas and may be either acute or chronic.

Acute pancreatitis is an acute inflammatory and sometimes haemorrhagic process in the pancreas; there is ischaemia and activation of proteolytic enzymes, resulting in damage to the pancreas and surrounding tissues. It is characterised by severe upper abdominal pain radiating to the back and by peripheral circulatory collapse. The abdominal wall is rigid and there are signs of peritoneal irritation.

The cause of acute pancreatitis is unknown but it may be associated with biliary-tract disease or a bout of excessive alcoholic drinking. Recurrent pancreatic disease is almost always associated with biliary-tract disease.

Treatment should be conservative and laparotomy should be performed only if there is diagnostic difficulty or if there is underlying biliary-tract disease. No fluids or solids are given by mouth and any shock should be treated. The stomach should be aspirated and anticholinergic drugs given to minimise the production of secretin which stimulates pancreatic activity. A protease inhibitor (aprotinin) may also be given to reduce the effects of released pancreatic enzymes. Glucagon has also been used.

Chronic pancreatitis is characterised by the progressive destruction and fibrosis of pancreatic glandular tissue, resulting in the failure of endocrine and exocrine pancreatic function. Episodes of severe epigastric pain lasting for 24 to 48 hours occur and these may be aggravated by a heavy meal or by alcohol. They may be accompanied by vomiting and diarrhoea and are not relieved by antacids. Chronic pancreatitis results in a reduction in pancreatic size and a dilatation of the pancreatic ducts. Lack of pancreatic enzyme gives rise to malabsorption from the intestine. Initially the endocrine function of the pancreas may continue but eventually a mild diabetes occurs.

Chronic pancreatitis may be due to chronic alcoholism, chronic protein malnutrition, or hyperparathyroidism. It may also result from treatment with drugs such as corticosteroids and diuretics, including thiazides and frusemide.

Chronic pancreatitis is treated symptomatically. Acute attacks are treated with analgesics, intravenous fluids, and gastric aspiration. A low-fat, high-protein diet should be given, alcohol forbidden, and replacement therapy with pancreatic enzymes such as pancreatin provided when required. Insulin may be needed for the treatment of diabetes as oral hypoglycaemic agents are unlikely to be effective.

Pancuronium Bromide

1,1'-(3α,17β-Diacetoxy-5α-androstan-2β,16β-ylene)-bis(1-methylpiperidinium) dibromide

$C_{35}H_{60}Br_2N_2O_4 = 732.7$

OTHER NAME: *Pavulon®*

A standard is given in the British Pharmacopoeia Addendum 1978

Description. Odourless hygroscopic white crystals or crystalline powder.

Solubility. Soluble, at 20°, in 1 part of water, in 5 parts of alcohol, in 5 parts of chloroform, in 4 parts of dichloromethane, and in 1 part of methyl alcohol; practically insoluble in ether.

Moisture content. 5 to 8%, determined by Fischer titration.

Specific rotation. +38° to +42°, determined on a 3% solution.

Storage. It should be stored in airtight containers at a temperature between 2° and 8°.

Identification. TEST. Dissolve about 5 mg in 10 ml of water, add 10 ml of ethylene chloride and 1 ml of *methyl orange solution*, shake, centrifuge, allow to separate, and acidify the solvent layer with *dilute sulphuric acid*; a red colour is produced.

MELTING-POINT. About 215°.

INFRA-RED ABSORPTION. Major peaks at 1031, 1053, 1235, 1370, 1449, and 1754 cm⁻¹ (see Appendix 2b: Infra-red Spectra).

Metabolism. BLOOD CONCENTRATION. After an intravenous dose of 4 mg, plasma concentrations of about 600 ng/ml are obtained in 5 minutes, falling to about 65 ng/ml in 4 hours; in subjects with renal function impairment the decrease in concentration is much less, falling from 460 ng/ml at 5 minutes to 180 ng/ml at 4 hours.

HALF-LIFE. Plasma half-life, α-phase, 7 to 19 minutes; β-phase, 90 to 160 minutes.

DISTRIBUTION. Volume of distribution 0.15 to 0.4 litre/kg which may be increased in renal function impairment; in rats, high concentrations appear in the liver and kidneys with smaller amounts appearing in the spleen, lungs, muscles, and bile; pancuronium crosses the placenta.

METABOLIC REACTIONS. Hydrolysis; in cats the 3-hydroxy-, 17-hydroxy-, and 3,17-dihydroxy-metabolites are produced.

EXCRETION. About 10% of an intravenous dose is excreted unchanged in the urine in about 90 minutes.

FURTHER INFORMATION. Metabolism—S. Agoston *et al.*, *Acta anaesth. scand.*, 1973, **17**, 129 and 267; pharmacokinetics—K. McLeod *et al.*, *Br. J. Anaesth.*,

1976, **48**, 341 and A. A. Somogyi *et al.*, *Eur. J. clin. Pharmac.*, 1976, **10**, 367; review—T. M. Speight and G. S. Avery, *Drugs*, 1972, **4**, 163.

Actions and uses. Pancuronium bromide is a muscle relaxant of the non-depolarising type which is used to secure muscular relaxation during surgery and in the intensive treatment of conditions characterised by muscular spasm. It has actions and uses similar to those described under Tubocurarine Chloride.

For intubation procedures the usual dose administered to adults is 60 to 80 micrograms per kilogram body-weight by intravenous injection over 120 to 150 seconds or 80 to 100 micrograms per kilogram body-weight over 60 to 90 seconds; subsequent doses of 30 to 40 micrograms per kilogram body-weight may be given when necessary. The usual dose for children is 60 to 80 micrograms per kilogram body-weight by intravenous injection; subsequently doses of 30 to 40 micrograms per kilogram body-weight may be given. Neonates may be given 30 to 40 micrograms per kilogram body-weight by intravenous injection with subsequent doses of 15 to 20 micrograms per kilogram body-weight.

In the intensive treatment of conditions such as intractable status asthmaticus and tetanus, 30 to 60 micrograms per kilogram body-weight may be given by intramuscular or intravenous injection every 1 to 2 hours. When given by intramuscular injection the onset of action occurs in about 10 minutes.

Drug interactions. The neuromuscular blocking action of pancuronium bromide may be increased by the concurrent administration of anaesthetics, such as cyclopropane, ether, halothane, methohexitone, methoxyflurane, and thiopentone, and decreased by propanidid. Diazepam, kanamycin, monoamine-oxidase inhibitors, neomycin, propranolol, protamine, quinidine, streptomycin, and high doses of thiamine may also increase the neuromuscular blocking action. High doses of corticosteroids, adrenaline, calcium chloride, potassium chloride, and sodium chloride may decrease the neuromuscular blocking action.

Poisoning. Neostigmine methylsulphate should be given by intravenous injection in a dose of 1 to 5 milligrams together with 0.5 to 1 milligram of atropine sulphate and the dose of atropine may be repeated as required. Controlled respiration is essential until spontaneous breathing is resumed.

Preparation

PANCURONIUM INJECTION: a sterile solution of pancuronium bromide, with a suitable stabilising agent, in sodium chloride injection. It may contain a suitable bactericide. It is sterilised by filtration. Available in 2-ml ampoules containing 2 mg of pancuronium bromide per ml; this preparation contains 1% of benzyl alcohol.
A standard for this injection is given in the British Pharmacopoeia Addendum 1978
Containers and *Labelling:* see the entry on Injections for general information on containers and labelling.
Storage: it should be stored at a temperature of 2° to 8°. Under these conditions it may be expected to retain its potency for 2 years.

Panhypopituitarism

see under HYPOPITUITARISM

Papaveretum

A mixture of the hydrochlorides of alkaloids of opium, prepared either from opium or by mixing suitable proportions of the hydrochlorides of morphine, codeine, noscapine (narcotine), and papaverine. It contains approximately 50% of morphine, 3% of codeine, 20% of noscapine, and 5% of papaverine.

OTHER NAMES: *Omnopon®*; Opium Concentratum *Omnopon-Scopolamine®* (with hyoscine hydrobromide); *Nepenthe®* injection (with morphine hydrochloride)

A standard is given in the British Pharmaceutical Codex 1973

Description. A white, light brown, or brownish-grey powder.

Solubility. Soluble, at 20°, in 15 parts of water; less soluble in alcohol.

Identification. TESTS. 1. To about 10 mg add 4 drops of *sulphomolybdic acid solution;* a purple colour is produced.
2. Dissolve about 10 mg in 1 ml of water and add 1 drop of *ferric chloride test-solution;* a blue or greenish-blue colour is produced.
3. Mix about 10 mg with sulphuric acid containing a trace of ferric chloride and heat; a violet to purple colour is produced.

Actions and uses. Papaveretum has the sedative and soporific actions described under Morphine Hydrochloride but it produces milder secondary effects.
It is used as a means of administering the total alkaloids of opium by parenteral injection; it is given with hyoscine as a sedative before the administration of a general anaesthetic. It has also been given with hyoscine and atropine to produce light anaesthesia. Papaveretum is also given by mouth.
The usual dose by mouth or by injection is 10 to 20 milligrams. Children may be given the following doses by intramuscular injection: up to one year 150 to 200 micrograms per kilogram body-weight; 1 to 5 years 2.5 to 5 milligrams; and 6 to 12 years 5 to 10 milligrams.

Undesirable effects; Poisoning. As for Morphine Hydrochloride.

Dependence. It may give rise to dependence of the morphine type as described under Drug Dependence.

Preparations

PAPAVERETUM INJECTION:

Papaveretum	..	..	..	..	2.0 g
Glycerol	..	..	..	..	1.4 g
Water for injections	..	..	..	to 100.0 ml

Dissolve the papaveretum in the bulk of the water, add the glycerol and sufficient of the water to produce the required volume, mix, and clarify the solution by filtration. Distribute the solution into the final containers, seal, and sterilise by heating with a bactericide; phenylmercuric nitrate is a suitable bactericide.
Alternatively, sterilise the solution by filtration; distribute, by means of an aseptic technique, into sterile final containers, and seal.
It contains, in 1 ml, approximately 10 mg of anhydrous morphine.

A standard for this injection is given in the British *Pharmaceutical Codex 1973*
Containers: see the entry on Injections for general information on containers. The injection should be supplied in single-dose containers.
Labelling: see the entry on Injections for general information on labelling.
Storage: it should be protected from light.

PAPAVERETUM TABLETS: may be prepared by moist granulation and compression as described in the entry on Tablets. Available as tablets containing 10 mg of papaveretum.
A standard for these tablets is given in the British *Pharmaceutical Codex 1973*
Containers and *Storage:* see the entry on Tablets for general information on containers and storage. Containers should be airtight.

OTHER PREPARATIONS available include an INJECTION containing papaveretum 30 mg in 1-ml ampoules, an injection containing papaveretum 20 mg with hyoscine hydrobromide 400 micrograms in 1-ml ampoules, and an injection containing papaveretum and morphine hydrochloride equivalent to 0.84% (8.4 mg per ml) of anhydrous morphine, of which 0.05% is derived from the papaveretum and 0.79% from the morphine hydrochloride, in 0.5-ml ampoules.

Papaverine Hydrochloride

6,7-Dimethoxy-1-(3,4-dimethoxybenzyl)isoquinolinium chloride

$C_{20}H_{22}ClNO_4 = 375.9$

OTHER NAMES: Papaver. Hydrochlor.; Papaverinii Chloridum

A standard is given in the European Pharmacopoeia Vol. I

Description. Odourless white crystals or powder with a taste which is bitter at first then pungent.

Solubility. Soluble, at 20°, in 40 parts of water and in 120 parts of alcohol; soluble in chloroform; practically insoluble in ether.

Acidity. A 2% solution has a pH of 3 to 4.5.

Moisture content. Not more than 1%, determined by drying at 105°.

Dissociation constant. pK_a 6.4 (25°).

Sterilisation. Solutions for injection are sterilised by heating in an autoclave or by filtration.

Storage. It should be stored in airtight containers, protected from light.

Identification. TESTS. 1. Dissolve a few mg in 5 ml of water and add 1 ml of *potassium iodobismuthate solution;* an orange or orange-red precipitate is produced.
2. Mix about 10 mg with 3 ml of acetic anhydride, cautiously add 3 drops of sulphuric acid, and heat on a water-bath for 3 to 4 minutes; a yellow colour with a green fluorescence is produced.

ULTRAVIOLET ABSORPTION. In 0.1N sulphuric acid, maxima at 251 nm (E1%, 1cm = 1518), 284 nm (E1%, 1cm = 157), and 309 nm (E1%, 1cm = 202).

INFRA-RED ABSORPTION. Major peaks at 1020, 1266, 1282, 1408, 1429, and 1515 cm^{-1} (see Appendix 2b: Infra-red Spectra).

THIN-LAYER CHROMATOGRAPHY. See under Thin-layer Chromatography, System 7.

Determination in body fluids. GAS CHROMATOGRAPHY. In plasma or urine—D. E. Guttman et al., J. pharm. Sci., 1974, **63**, 1625.

Metabolism. ABSORPTION. Readily and completely absorbed after oral administration.

BLOOD CONCENTRATION. After an intravenous dose of 3 mg/kg of the hydrochloride, plasma concentrations of about 1.9 µg/ml are attained in 30 minutes and 0.6 µg/ml in 2 hours; after an oral dose of 3 mg/kg of the hydrochloride a peak plasma concentration of 0.6 µg/ml is attained in 1 to 2 hours.

HALF-LIFE. Plasma half-life, about 100 minutes.

DISTRIBUTION. In the dog, papaverine is localised in the fat and liver and uniformly distributed in other tissues; *protein binding,* in the dog 66 to 87% bound to plasma proteins.

METABOLIC REACTIONS. Demethylation and glucuronic acid and sulphate conjugation of the phenolic groups so formed; the major metabolite is 4'-hydroxypapaverine, mostly in conjugated form.

EXCRETION. Less than 1% is excreted in the urine unchanged, and about 60% is excreted as conjugated phenolic metabolites.

FURTHER INFORMATION. Metabolism—J. Axelrod et al., J. Pharmac. exp. Ther., 1958, **124**, 9.

Actions and uses. Papaverine has little, if any, hypnotic or analgesic action. It is used occasionally to produce relaxation of involuntary muscle in the treatment of peripheral vascular disease and in the treatment of coronary spasm, of intestinal, ureteric, and biliary colic, and of dysmenorrhoea.
It may be administered by mouth in a dosage of 150 to 300 milligrams 2 or 3 times daily or by subcutaneous or intravenous injection in a dosage of 30 to 100 milligrams. It may be applied to arteries during operations.
It is also used in bronchodilator sprays and as an ingredient of cough mixtures.

Undesirable effects. The intravenous administration of papaverine may give rise to cardiac arrhythmias.

Preparation
Papaverine hydrochloride is an ingredient of compound adrenaline and atropine spray.

Paper Chromatography

Paper chromatography is a method of flat-bed chromatography, analogous to thin-layer chromatography, in which the stationary phase is a strip of filter paper (chromatographic grade). The paper is suspended in the tank, either with its lower end dipping into the mobile phase, in which case the mobile phase migrates up the paper (ascending paper chromatography), or with its upper end dipping into a trough containing the mobile phase, in which case the mobile phase migrates down the paper (descending paper chromatography). In ascending paper chromatography there is limited solvent front movement whereas in descending paper chromatography there is the possibility of unlimited solvent front movement.

The practical details concerning the application of samples, choice of mobile phase, equilibration, chromatographic process, visualisation, and evaluation are similar to those described for thin-layer chromatography.

The predominant mechanism is partition between the water bound to the cellulose fibres and the immiscible mobile phase. This may be accentuated in partition or reverse-phase chromatography by pretreating the paper with a second, immiscible phase.

Paper chromatography has certain advantages and disadvantages when compared with thin-layer chromatography.

Advantages are that (1) Rf values are more reproducible, (2) aqueous mobile phases, which would inactivate many thin-layer systems, can be used, (3) in the descending mode unlimited solvent front movement is possible, and (4) ionic species may be examined, although this advantage is being reduced with the introduction of ion-exchange thin-layer systems.

The disadvantages of paper chromatography are that (1) the spots tend to become more diffuse, (2) many of the spray reagents used in thin-layer chromatography are precluded, especially those dissolved in concentrated acids, and (3) the process takes a longer time; this is dependent on the length of run, for in order to achieve the same degree of separation on paper, the solvent front often has to be run several times as far as would be necessary in thin-layer chromatography.

Paracetamol

4'-Hydroxyacetanilide

$C_8H_9NO_2 = 151.2$

OTHER NAMES: Acetaminophen; *Calpol®*; *Pamol®*; *Panadol®*; *Panasorb®*; Paracetamolum; *Salzone®*; *Ticelgesic®*

Safapryn® (with aspirin); *Veganin®* (with aspirin and codeine phosphate); *Paraseltzer®* (with caffeine); *Cafadol®* (with caffeine citrate); *Lobak®* (with chlormezanone); *Neurodyne®*, *Panadeine Co.®*, *Paracodol®*, and *Parake®* (all with codeine phosphate); *Distalgesic®* (with dextropropoxyphene hydrochloride and napsylate); *Paedosed®* (with dichloralphenazone); *Paramol-118®* (with dihydrocodeine tartrate); *Norgesic®* (with orphenadrine citrate); *Tandalgesic®* (with oxyphenbutazone); *Fortagesic®* (with pentazocine hydrochloride); *Pamol®* Supps for babies (with phenobarbitone); *Parazolidin®* (with phenylbutazone); *Triogesic®* (with phenylpropanolamine hydrochloride)

A standard is given in the European Pharmacopoeia Vol. III

Description. An odourless white crystalline powder with a bitter taste.

Solubility. Soluble, at 20°, in 70 parts of water, in 7 parts of alcohol, in 13 parts of acetone, in 40 parts of glycerol, and in 9 parts of propylene glycol; soluble in solutions of alkali hydroxides.

Dissociation constant. pK_a 9.5 (25°).

Hygroscopicity. It absorbs insignificant amounts of moisture at 25° at relative humidities up to about 90%.

Storage. It should be stored in airtight containers, protected from light.

Identification. TESTS. 1. Dissolve about 100 mg in 10 ml of water and add 1 drop of *ferric chloride test-solution*; a violet-blue colour is produced.
2. Mix about 100 mg with 1 ml of hydrochloric acid, boil for 3 minutes, add 10 ml of water and cool; no precipitate is produced. Add 1 drop of 0.1N potassium dichromate; a violet colour is slowly produced, which does not become red (distinction from phenacetin).

MELTING-POINT. About 170°.

ULTRAVIOLET ABSORPTION. In 0.1N hydrochloric acid, maximum at 245 nm (E1%, 1cm = 661); in 0.1N sodium hydroxide, maximum at 257 nm (E1%, 1cm = 715).

INFRA-RED ABSORPTION. Major peaks at 1263, 1387, 1441, 1506, 1565, and 1657 cm^{-1} (see Appendix 2a: Infra-red Spectra).

THIN-LAYER CHROMATOGRAPHY. See under Thin-layer Chromatography, System 3.

Determination in body fluids. COLORIMETRY. In plasma—K. Weiner, *Ann. Clin. Biochem.*, 1977, **14**, 55.

ULTRAVIOLET SPECTROPHOTOMETRY. In blood—J. Knepil, *Clin. chim. Acta*, 1974, **52**, 369.

GAS CHROMATOGRAPHY. In serum or saliva—W. A. Dechtiaruk *et al.*, *Clin. Chem.*, 1976, **22**, 879. In plasma: in the presence of barbiturates—H. V. Street, *J. Chromat.*, 1975, **109**, 29.

HIGH PRESSURE LIQUID CHROMATOGRAPHY. In urine: paracetamol and metabolites—D. Howie *et al.*, *J. Pharm. Pharmac.*, 1977, **29**, 235. In plasma or urine—L. T. Wong *et al.*, *J. pharm. Sci.*, 1976, **65**, 1064.

Metabolism. ABSORPTION. Small doses are rapidly and completely absorbed but the absorption of larger doses varies considerably. Paracetamol absorption appears to be mainly influenced by gastric emptying rate, the presence of food, especially carbohydrate, and the time of day at which the drug is taken. Administration of propantheline and metoclopramide reduce and increase the absorption of paracetamol respectively by their actions on gastric emptying rate.

BLOOD CONCENTRATION. Plasma paracetamol concentrations vary considerably between subjects. After an oral dose of 1 g to fasting subjects, peak plasma concentrations of 20 to 30 µg/ml are attained in about 20 minutes. After giving the same dose to non-fasting subjects, peak plasma concentrations of 10 to 20 µg/ml are attained in 40 to 120 minutes. After an oral dose of 2 g to fasting subjects, peak plasma concentrations of about 30 to 40 µg/ml are attained in 1 to 3 hours.

HALF-LIFE. The plasma half-life after therapeutic doses is approximately 1 to 4 hours and plasma half-lives greater than 4 hours are indicative of possible liver damage. In neonates, the half-life is increased to about

5 hours; in subjects with functional or surgical anephria, the half-life does not appear to be influenced.

DISTRIBUTION. Widely distributed throughout most body fluids; secreted in the saliva in concentrations paralleling those in the plasma; not taken up by red cells; volume of distribution, about 1 litre/kg body-weight; *protein binding*, 8 to 40% bound to plasma proteins.

METABOLIC REACTIONS. Mainly conjugation to form glucuronides and ethereal sulphates; hydroxylation at position 3 occurs followed by conjugation or O-methylation of the hydroxyl group produced. Oxidation occurs to a small extent after therapeutic doses and becomes more significant after large doses. The metabolite formed by oxidation is conjugated by the glutathione pathway to form mercapturic acid and cysteine conjugates. The nature of the oxidised metabolite is uncertain but may be an epoxide, an N-hydroxylated metabolite, a benzoquinoneimine derived from N-hydroxylation, or a radical. This metabolite appears to be the agent responsible for hepatic necrosis in paracetamol overdosage. Nearly all the metabolic reactions of paracetamol occur at the 3-position.

Neonates produce more of the sulphate conjugate than the glucuronide whilst in the adult the proportions of the two conjugates are either approximately equal or the glucuronide fraction is the larger. The administration of salicylamide appears to block paracetamol conjugation by competitive inhibition.

Enzyme induction stimulates the oxidative metabolism of paracetamol and thereby increases the amount of toxic metabolite without, however, increasing the extent of glutathione conjugation. First pass metabolism is not extensive for paracetamol.

In overdosage, sulphate and glucuronide formation becomes exhausted and more of the drug is oxidised. Mercapturic acid and cysteine conjugation are, as a result, much increased. Depending upon the extent of overdosage, glutathione may become depleted leaving no mechanism for detoxifying the metabolite.

EXCRETION. About 85% of a therapeutic dose is excreted in the urine in 24 hours; of the excreted material in the adult, 1 to 4% is unchanged, 20 to 30% is conjugated with sulphate, 40 to 60% is conjugated with glucuronic acid, 5 to 10% is composed of 3-hydroxy-3-sulphate, 3-methoxyglucuronide, and 3-methoxy-3-sulphate metabolites, and 5 to 10% is composed of mercapturic acid and cysteine conjugates. Larger amounts of the mercapturic acid and cysteine conjugates are excreted in overdosage.

OVERDOSAGE. Plasma concentrations have been used to indicate possible hepatic necrosis, and at 4 hours, hepatic necrosis is possible at concentrations of paracetamol of 120 to 300 μg/ml, probable at concentrations of over 300 μg/ml, and unlikely at concentrations below 120 μg/ml. Similarly, at 12 hours, concentrations above 120 μg/ml indicate probable necrosis, concentrations of 50 to 120 μg/ml indicate that it is possible, and concentrations below 50 μg/ml indicate that it is unlikely. The hepatic necrosis appears to be caused by increased oxidation of paracetamol resulting in the formation of a toxic metabolite. This metabolite is normally detoxified by glutathione conjugation but once sources of glutathione are depleted the free metabolite is available to bind covalently with liver cell protein. This binding occurs some 10 hours after dosing. Thus any treatment must be initiated within about 10 hours after the overdose.

FURTHER INFORMATION. Effects of food—I. J.

McGilveray and G. L. Mattok, *J. Pharm. Pharmac.*, 1972, **24**, 615 and J. M. Jaffe *et al.*, *J. pharm. Sci.*, 1971, **60**, 1646; effects of other drugs on metabolism—G. Levy and C.-G. Regårdh, *J. pharm. Sci.*, 1971, **60**, 608, J. Nimmo *et al.*, *Br. med. J.*, i/1973, 587, B. H. Thomas, *Clin. Pharmac. Ther.*, 1972, **13**, 906, and L. T. Wong *et al.*, *Xenobiotica*, 1976, **6**, 575; excretion in saliva—J. P. Glynn and W. Bastain, *J. Pharm. Pharmac.*, 1973, **25**, 420; first pass effects—W. L. Chiou, *J. pharm. Sci.*, 1975, **64**, 1734; overdosage—*Symposium on Paracetamol in the Liver, J. int. med. Res.*, 1976, **4**, Suppl. 4, and R. B. Payne and P. Sheridan, *Lancet*, ii/1976, 964; pharmacokinetics—K. S. Albert *et al.*, *Pharmacokinet. Biopharm.*, 1974, **2**, 381, J. A. Clements and L. F. Prescott, *J. Pharm. Pharmac.*, 1976, **28**, 707, and D. T. Lowenthal *et al.*, *J. Pharmac. exp. Ther.*, 1976, **196**, 570; protein binding—B. G. Gazzard *et al.*, *J. Pharm. Pharmac.*, 1973, **25**, 964.

BIOAVAILABILITY. Absorption from effervescent tablet formulations is greater than that from non-effervescent tablets and absorption from suppositories varies according to the dielectric properties of the vehicle used.

FURTHER INFORMATION. Bioavailability—K. S. Albert *et al.*, *J. clin. Pharmac.*, 1974, **14**, 264, and A. Richter and S. E. Smith, *Br. J. clin. Pharmac.*, 1974, **1**, 495; bioavailability from suppositories—S. N. Pagay *et al.*, *J. pharm. Sci.*, 1974, **63**, 44.

Actions and uses. Paracetamol has analgesic and antipyretic actions similar to, but weaker than, those described under Aspirin; it has no anti-inflammatory properties.

In the treatment of pain, such as headache, toothache, rheumatism, and neuralgia, paracetamol is given by mouth in a dosage of 0.5 to 1 gram every 3 or 4 hours with a maximum of 4 grams in 24 hours. The usual dose for a child under 1 year is 120 milligrams, and for a child of 1 to 5 years 250 milligrams.

Undesirable effects. Purpura may occur. Rarely, renal damage may occur after long-term usage.

Poisoning. Hepatic damage has been reported after doses of 7 grams but is usually caused by doses exceeding 15 grams. Paracetamol is therefore more hazardous, weight for weight, in suicide attempts than aspirin. Symptoms of hepatic damage will not occur in less than 12 hours but may not appear until 4 to 6 days later. The more rapid the onset of hepatic symptoms, the more severe is likely to be the hepatic damage.

Less frequent complications of paracetamol overdosage include cardiac damage, generalised bleeding, renal damage, and hypoglycaemia.

Gastric lavage should be carried out whenever the patient is seen within 4 hours of ingestion of paracetamol. Charcoal or cholestyramine may be given but should be withheld until any necessary treatment with methionine or cysteamine has been initiated. The measurement of blood-paracetamol concentrations is the best index of risk of paracetamol toxicity and the decision to use antidotes is based on such measurements.

In severe cases treatment with cysteamine (mercaptamine) or methionine should be initiated as soon as possible within the first 10 hours to minimise damage to the liver by toxic metabolites. They should not be given at later stages since they are not effective and may also precipitate hepatic coma.

The advantage of methionine is that it may be given orally and that it appears to have fewer side-effects than cysteamine, which must be given intravenously, but cysteamine appears to be more effective in preventing hepatic damage when more than 8 hours has elapsed before treatment is begun.

Cysteamine hydrochloride may be administered in an initial dose equivalent to 2 grams of cysteamine by intravenous injection over 10 minutes, followed by intravenous infusion of 800 milligrams in dextrose injection (5%) in 4 hours, 400 milligrams in the next 8 hours, and a further 400 milligrams in the next 8 hours. 1.5 grams of cysteamine hydrochloride is approximately equivalent to 1 gram of cysteamine base.

Methionine may be given orally in a dosage of 2.5 grams every 4 hours up to a total dose of 10 grams. To permit absorption in the patient who is vomiting, metoclopramide may be used as an anti-emetic, at least during the first 15 hours after ingestion. Serious paracetamol overdosage in children is rare. A suggested regimen is 4 doses of methionine each of 1 gram by mouth, at intervals of 4 hours.

Only limited information is available on the stability of cysteamine in aqueous solution; there are indications that breakdown to cystamine is accelerated by exposure to oxidation conditions or to strong alkali. Various procedures have been followed in the preparation and sterilisation of solutions for injection. J. B. J. Brouwers and P. Vermeij (*Pharm. Weekbl. Ned.*, 1976, **111**, 204) have indicated that a stable injection can be prepared as follows:

dissolve 2 grams of cysteamine hydrochloride in 100 millilitres of a 0.2% solution of ascorbic acid in water, filter, distribute into vials under nitrogen, and sterilise by heating in an autoclave at 115° for 30 minutes. Samples of the injections showed negligible loss of cysteamine after 8 months at room temperature.

A similar formulation, but without ascorbic acid, has been suggested by F. G. R. Prior, *Lancet*, i/1977, 315. Samples from a batch sterilised by filtration showed no increase in the cystamine content after 30 days at 18°. L. F. Prescott *et al.* (*Lancet*, ii/1976, 109) used injections prepared by reconstitution from freeze-dried cysteamine (without additives). Cysteamine solutions have been freshly prepared in water for injections and sterilised directly from a syringe by filtration through two membranes as described by L. F. Prescott and H. Matthew (*Lancet*, i/1974, 998). The solution is first passed through a coarse filter to remove large particles and then through a bacterial filter.

Veterinary uses. Paracetamol is used as an analgesic in dogs. It is administered by mouth, the usual dose being 20 milligrams per kilogram body-weight.

Preparations

ASPIRIN, PARACETAMOL, AND CODEINE TABLETS: for each tablet take:

Aspirin	250 mg
Paracetamol..	250 mg
Codeine phosphate	9.58 mg

Containers and *Storage:* see the entry on Tablets for general information on containers and storage. Containers should be airtight and light resistant.

Dose: ADULT: 1 or 2 tablets every 4 hours as necessary. CHILD: 6 to 12 years, half a tablet up to 4 times daily as necessary.

Advice for patients: the tablets should preferably be taken after meals. Treatment should not be continued for longer than 2 days without medical advice.

CODEINE AND PARACETAMOL TABLETS: for each tablet take:

Codeine phosphate	8 mg
Paracetamol..	500 mg

Containers and *Storage:* see the entry on Tablets for general information on containers and storage. Containers should be airtight and light resistant.

Dose: 2 tablets up to 4 times daily as necessary.

Advice for patients: the tablets should not be used for longer than 2 days without medical advice.

DIHYDROCODEINE AND PARACETAMOL TABLETS: for each tablet take:

Dihydrocodeine tartrate	10 mg
Paracetamol..	500 mg

Containers and *Storage:* see the entry on Tablets for general information on containers and storage. Containers should be airtight.

Dose: 2 tablets up to 4 times daily as necessary.

Advice for patients: the tablets should preferably be taken after meals.

PAEDIATRIC PARACETAMOL ELIXIR:

Paracetamol..	24 g
Amaranth solution	2 ml
Chloroform spirit	20 ml
Concentrated raspberry juice	25 ml
Alcohol (95%)	100 ml
Propylene glycol	100 ml
Invert syrup	275 ml
Glycerol	to 1000 ml

Dissolve the paracetamol in a mixture of the alcohol, the propylene glycol, and the chloroform spirit, and add the concentrated raspberry juice diluted with the invert syrup, the amaranth solution, and sufficient glycerol to produce the required volume, and mix.

This elixir should not be diluted. The general direction given in the entry on Elixirs that the preparation should be diluted so that the dose is contained in 5 ml does not apply to this elixir; if necessary, the prescribed dose should be measured by means of a graduated pipette.

A standard for this elixir is given in the British Pharmaceutical Codex 1973

Containers: see the entry on Elixirs for general information on containers.

Storage: it should be protected from light.

Advice for patients: the elixir should not be used for longer than 2 days or given to children under 1 year without medical advice.

PARACETAMOL TABLETS: available as tablets containing 500 mg of paracetamol; they may be coloured.

A standard for these tablets is given in the British Pharmacopoeia 1973

Containers and *Storage:* see the entry on Tablets for general information on containers and storage. Containers should be airtight and light resistant.

Advice for patients: the tablets should not be used for longer than 2 days without medical advice.

OTHER PREPARATIONS available include CAPSULES containing paracetamol 500 mg with codeine phosphate 8 mg; an ELIXIR containing paracetamol 120 mg in 5 ml, diluent syrup, life of diluted elixir 14 days, an elixir containing paracetamol 100 mg with dichloralphenazone 200 mg in 5 ml, diluent syrup, life of diluted elixir 14 days, an elixir containing paracetamol 125 mg with phenylpropanolamine hydrochloride 3 mg in 5 ml, diluent water or syrup, life of diluted elixir 14 days; a MIXTURE containing paracetamol 120 mg in 5 ml, diluent syrup, life of diluted mixture 14 days; paediatric SUPPOSITORIES containing paracetamol 200 mg with phenobarbitone 15 mg; TABLETS containing paracetamol 250 mg with aspirin 300 mg, tablets containing paracetamol 500 mg with caffeine 20 mg, tablets containing paracetamol

500 mg with caffeine citrate 30 mg, tablets containing paracetamol 450 mg with chlormezanone 100 mg, tablets containing paracetamol 325 mg with dextropropoxyphene hydrochloride 32.5 mg, tablets containing paracetamol 325 mg with dextropropoxyphene napsylate 50 mg, tablets containing paracetamol 450 mg with orphenadrine citrate 35 mg, tablets containing paracetamol 500 mg with oxyphenbutazone 50 mg, tablets containing paracetamol 500 mg with pentazocine hydrochloride equivalent to 15 mg of pentazocine, tablets containing paracetamol 500 mg with phenylbutazone 50 mg, and tablets containing paracetamol 500 mg with phenylpropanolamine hydrochloride 12.5 mg.

Paraffin, Hard

A mixture of solid hydrocarbons consisting mainly of n-paraffins and, to a lesser extent, of their isomers.

OTHER NAME: Paraffinum Durum

A standard is given in the British Pharmacopoeia 1973

Description. A colourless or white, somewhat translucent, wax-like, odourless solid, frequently showing a crystalline structure; it is slightly unctuous to the touch and burns with a luminous flame.

Solubility. Practically insoluble in water and in alcohol; soluble in ether and in chloroform.

Solidifying-point. Between 50° and 57°.

Sterilisation. It is sterilised by dry heat.

Uses. Hard paraffin is used to stiffen ointment bases. A similar wax, melting at 43° to 46°, is used in the preparation of wax baths in physiotherapy. The wax should be melted in a covered container, over a water-bath. It must be heated gradually to a temperature of about 48°. Several layers are applied to the affected part and left in position for approximately 20 minutes, after which the wax may be readily peeled off. The heat retained by the wax dilates the peripheral blood vessels and improves the blood supply to the area. It is most commonly used for the small joints of the hands and feet, relieving pain, increasing mobility, and softening scar tissue.

Preparations

PARAFFIN OINTMENT: ⎱ see below under Paraffin,
SIMPLE OINTMENT: ⎰ White Soft.

Paraffin, Liquid

A mixture of liquid hydrocarbons obtained from petroleum. The composition varies according to the source of the petroleum. It may contain up to 10 parts per million of tocopherol or of butylated hydroxytoluene as antoxidant.

OTHER NAMES: Mineral Oil
Petrolagar® (with light liquid paraffin); *Agarol*® (with phenolphthalein)

A standard is given in the British Pharmacopoeia 1973

Description. A transparent, colourless, oily, almost odourless liquid.

Solubility. Practically insoluble in water; soluble in ether and in chloroform.

Weight per ml. At 20°, 0.830 to 0.890 g.

Sterilisation. It is sterilised by dry heat.

Storage. It should be protected from light.

Actions and uses. Liquid paraffin, when taken by mouth, keeps the stools soft and is therefore particularly useful in the treatment of chronic constipation and in painful conditions of the anus and rectum, such as haemorrhoids and anal fissure, although excessive doses may result in seepage and anal irritation. Intestinal absorption of small amounts of liquid paraffin may occur, especially if it is emulsified, and if this absorption is long continued paraffinomata may develop; continued use of liquid paraffin may interfere with the absorption of the fat-soluble vitamins especially if it is taken with meals. Liquid paraffin is not irritant when applied to mucous surfaces; it is used as an emollient in irritant skin conditions and for the removal of desquamative crusts. Sterile liquid paraffin is used as an aseptic surgical dressing and as a lubricant for surgical instruments. Liquid paraffin is administered as a laxative in doses of 10 to 30 millilitres as an emulsion, preferably between meals.

Veterinary uses. Liquid paraffin is used as a laxative. The usual dose by mouth for all species is 1 to 2 millilitres per kilogram body-weight.

Preparations

LIQUID PARAFFIN AND MAGNESIUM HYDROXIDE MIXTURE (*Syn.* Liquid Paraffin and Magnesium Hydroxide Emulsion):

Liquid paraffin	250 ml
Magnesium hydroxide mixture	735 ml
Chloroform spirit	15 ml

Mix the chloroform spirit with the magnesium hydroxide mixture, add to the liquid paraffin, and pass through a homogeniser.

A standard for this mixture is given in the British Pharmaceutical Codex 1973

Containers: see the entry on Mixtures for general information on containers. It should be supplied in wide-mouthed bottles.

Labelling: see the entry on Mixtures for general information on labelling. A direction to shake the bottle should be given on the label.

Dose: 5 to 20 millilitres.

Advice for patients: the mixture should not be taken within 30 minutes of mealtimes and preferably on an empty stomach. It should not be used for longer than a few days without medical advice.

LIQUID PARAFFIN AND PHENOLPHTHALEIN MIXTURE (*Syn.* Liquid Paraffin and Phenolphthalein Emulsion; Compound Liquid Paraffin Emulsion):

Phenolphthalein, microcrystalline	3 g
Liquid paraffin mixture	to 1000 ml

Triturate the phenolphthalein with the liquid paraffin mixture.

It is essential to use phenolphthalein in which not more than an occasional particle has a diameter greater than 15 μm; larger particles tend to sediment in this mixture on storage and may prove difficult to redisperse uniformly by shaking the product. If a suitable microcrystalline grade is not obtainable, it may be prepared in small batches from ordinary grades by the following method: Dissolve the phenolphthalein, with the aid of gentle heat if necessary, in sufficient alcohol (95%) to give a 5% solution. Stir, by means of a high-speed stirrer, 25 times this volume of water in a suitable container, add slowly down the vortex the alcoholic phenolphthalein solution, and continue to stir for 5 minutes.

It is essential that an efficient stirrer is used in order to obtain particles of sufficiently small size.

Set the suspension aside for 1½ to 2 hours, collect the precipitated phenolphthalein on a suitable filter, such as a Whatman No. 42, and dry the phenolphthalein to constant weight at 80°. As phenolphthalein is slightly soluble in the diluted alcohol, a sufficient excess of phenolphthalein should be used and the quantity required for preparing the mixture should be weighed from the final dry powder.

A standard for this mixture is given in the British Pharmaceutical Codex 1973

Containers: see the entry on Mixtures for general information on containers. It should be supplied in wide-mouthed bottles.

Labelling: see the entry on Mixtures for general information on labelling. A direction to shake the bottle should be given on the label.

Dose: 5 to 20 millilitres.

Advice for patients: see above under Liquid Paraffin and Magnesium Hydroxide Mixture. The mixture may colour the urine red.

LIQUID PARAFFIN MIXTURE (Syn. Liquid Paraffin Emulsion):

Liquid paraffin	500.0 ml
Saccharin sodium	0.05 g
Vanillin	0.50 g
Methylcellulose 20	20.00 g
Chloroform	2.5 ml
Benzoic acid solution	20.0 ml
Water for preparations	to 1000.0 ml

Mix the methylcellulose with 200 ml of boiling water, allow to stand for 2 hours with constant stirring, add sufficient water to produce 350 ml, and allow to stand for 16 hours.

Alternatively, mix the methylcellulose with 120 ml of boiling water and, when the powder is thoroughly hydrated, add sufficient water in the form of ice to produce 350 ml, and stir until homogeneous.

Dissolve the vanillin in a mixture of the chloroform and the benzoic acid solution, and add, with vigorous stirring for 5 minutes, to the methylcellulose dispersion.

Add the saccharin sodium dissolved in water and sufficient water to produce 500 ml, and mix; add the liquid paraffin, with constant stirring, and pass through a homogeniser.

A standard for this mixture is given in the British Pharmaceutical Codex 1973

Containers: see the entry on Mixtures for general information on containers. It should be supplied in wide-mouthed bottles.

Labelling: see the entry on Mixtures for general information on labelling. A direction to shake the bottle should be given on the label.

Dose: 10 to 30 millilitres.

Advice for patients: see above under Liquid Paraffin and Magnesium Hydroxide Mixture.

OTHER PREPARATIONS available include a MIXTURE (emulsion) containing liquid paraffin 31.9% with phenolphthalein 1.32% and agar, diluent water for preparations, life of diluted mixture 28 days; and a mixture (emulsion) containing liquid paraffin 7% with light liquid paraffin 18% (also available with phenolphthalein 0.35% in addition).

Liquid paraffin is an ingredient of cetomacrogol emulsifying ointment (see under Cetomacrogol 1000), of emulsifying ointment (see note below under Paraffin, White Soft), of eye ointment basis (see entry on Eye Ointments), and of wool alcohols ointment (see note below under Paraffin, White Soft).

Paraffin, White Soft

Bleached yellow soft paraffin.

OTHER NAMES: Paraffinum Molle Album; Vaseline®; White Petroleum Jelly

A standard is given in the British Pharmacopoeia 1973

Description. A white, translucent, soft, unctuous, odourless mass.

Solubility. Practically insoluble in water and in alcohol; soluble in ether, in chloroform, in light petroleum, the solutions sometimes showing a slight opalescence, and in fixed and volatile oils.

Melting-point. Between 38° and 56°.

Sterilisation. It is sterilised by dry heat.

Uses. White soft paraffin has the uses described under Yellow Soft Paraffin.

Preparations

PARAFFIN OINTMENT:

Hard paraffin	..	..	..	..	30 g
White soft paraffin	..	..	..	..	900 g
White beeswax	..	..	..	..	20 g
Cetostearyl alcohol	..	..	..	..	50 g

Melt together and stir until cold.

Containers and Storage: see the entry on Ointments for general information on containers and storage.

SIMPLE OINTMENT (Syn. Ung. Simp.):

Cetostearyl alcohol	..	..	..	50 g
Hard paraffin	..	..	..	50 g
Wool fat	..	..	..	..	50 g
White soft paraffin or yellow soft paraffin	..			850 g

Melt together and stir until cold. Simple ointment is made with white soft paraffin to prepare white ointments and with yellow soft paraffin to prepare coloured ointments, except where otherwise stated.

OTHER PREPARATIONS: white soft paraffin is an ingredient of cetomacrogol emulsifying ointment (see under Cetomacrogol 1000), of emulsifying ointment and hence of aqueous cream and buffered cream (see under Cetostearyl Alcohol), and of wool alcohols ointment and hence of oily cream (see under Wool Alcohols).

Paraffin, Yellow Soft

A purified mixture of semi-solid hydrocarbons obtained from petroleum.

OTHER NAMES: Paraffinum Molle Flavum; Vaseline®; Yellow Petroleum Jelly

A standard is given in the British Pharmacopoeia 1973

Description. A pale yellow to yellow, translucent, soft, unctuous, odourless mass.

Solubility. Practically insoluble in water and in alcohol; soluble in ether, in chloroform, in light petroleum, the solutions sometimes showing a slight opalescence, and in fixed and volatile oils.

Melting-point. Between 36° and 56°.

Sterilisation. It is sterilised by dry heat.

Uses. Yellow soft paraffin is bland, neutral, and non-irritant to the skin, but is poorly absorbed. It is used as a basis for ointments which are not intended to be absorbed. Sterile dressings containing yellow soft paraffin or its preparations are often used as wound dressings because they are easily removed.

Samples of yellow soft paraffin vary in rheological and other physical properties; in some samples hard waxy lumps are produced and there may be an excessive separation of liquid components. Differences in physical properties depend upon the chemical composition which varies according to the source, the type and degree of refining, and the blending processes.

Preparations

SIMPLE OINTMENT: see above under Paraffin, White Soft.

OTHER PREPARATIONS: yellow soft paraffin is an ingredient of eye ointment basis (see entry on Eye Ointments), of hydrous wool fat ointment (see under Wool Fat), and of wool alcohols ointment (see note above under Paraffin, White Soft and under Wool Alcohols).

Paraformaldehyde

A solid polymer of formaldehyde.

A standard is given in the British Pharmaceutical Codex 1973

Paraformaldehyde volatilises at 100° and is readily converted into formaldehyde when heated to this temperature or in the presence of water. A solution of paraformaldehyde in hot water exhibits the chemical properties of formaldehyde.

Description. A white amorphous powder or friable amorphous mass with a pungent odour.

Solubility. Practically insoluble in water; soluble in solutions of alkali hydroxides.

Storage. It should be stored in airtight containers.

Uses. Paraformaldehyde is used as a source of formaldehyde. For disinfecting rooms it is vaporised by heating on an electric hot-plate or by interaction with potassium permanganate, as described under Formaldehyde Solution, but as it produces a dry gas it is less satisfactory for this purpose than formaldehyde solution. Tablets prepared for disinfecting rooms by vaporisation should be coloured by the addition of a suitable blue dye.

In dentistry, it has been used as an obtundent for sensitive dentine and as an antiseptic in mummifying pastes and for root canals.

Paraformaldehyde is also used in lozenges.

Preparations

FORMALDEHYDE LOZENGES (*Syn.* Formalin Throat Lozenges; Formamint Tablets):
The general use of the names "Formalin" and "Formamint" for formaldehyde lozenges is limited, and in any country in which the words "Formalin" and "Formamint" are trade marks they may be used only when applied to the products made by the owners of the trade marks.

For each lozenge take:

Paraformaldehyde	10.0 mg
Menthol	2.5 mg
Citric acid monohydrate	20.0 mg
Lemon oil	0.0006 ml

Prepare by moist granulation and compression, as described in the entry on Lozenges, adding the paraformaldehyde, followed by the menthol and the lemon oil dissolved in a little alcohol (95%), to the dried granules. Each lozenge weighs about 1 gram.

A standard for these lozenges is given in the British Pharmaceutical Codex 1973
Containers: see the entry on Lozenges for general information on containers. The containers should be airtight.
Storage: they should be stored in a cool place. They are liable to deteriorate on storage.
Advice for patients: the lozenges should be allowed to dissolve slowly in the mouth.

Paraldehyde

The trimer of acetaldehyde. It contains a suitable amount of an antioxidant.
$(CH_3.CHO)_3 = 132.2$

OTHER NAME: Paraldehydum

A standard is given in the European Pharmacopoeia Vol. I

CAUTION. *Paraldehyde decomposes with increase in toxicity on storage, particularly when the container has been opened. It must not be used if it has a brownish colour or if an odour of acetic acid has developed.*

Description. A clear colourless or slightly yellow liquid with a strong characteristic odour.

Solubility. Soluble, at 20°, in 9 parts of water; miscible with alcohol, with ether, with chloroform, and with volatile oils.

Weight per ml. At 20°, about 0.991 g.

Refractive index. 1.404 to 1.406.

Sterilisation. It is sterilised by filtration; contact with rubber and plastics should be avoided.

Storage. It should be stored in small, well-filled, airtight bottles, in complete darkness, in a cool place, avoiding contact with cork and plastics. If it has solidified, the whole contents of the bottle should be liquefied by warming and well mixed before use.

Determination in body fluids. GAS CHROMATOGRAPHY. In blood, plasma, serum, urine, or stomach contents— R. Maes *et al., J. forens. Sci.,* 1969, **14**, 235. In blood or gastric fluid—J. P. Hancock *et al., J. analyt. Toxicol.,* 1977, **1**, 161.

Metabolism. ABSORPTION. Readily absorbed after oral, intramuscular, and rectal administration.

BLOOD CONCENTRATION. After an intramuscular dose of 0.25 ml/kg to children, serum concentrations of 0.2 to 0.3 ng/ml are attained in 1 hour, falling to 0.1 to 0.2 ng/ml at 6 hours.

HALF-LIFE. Serum half-life, 3 to 10 hours.

DISTRIBUTION. Widely distributed throughout the body, crosses the placenta, and cerebrospinal fluid concentrations are about 60 to 75% those of plasma; volume of distribution, 80 to 120% of body-weight at 6 hours after an intramuscular dose.

METABOLIC REACTIONS. Depolymerisation to acetaldehyde which is oxidised to acetic acid and ultimately to carbon dioxide.

EXCRETION. About 7% of an oral dose is exhaled unchanged in 4 hours and about 80% is excreted in urine as metabolites; in hepatic function impairment, elimination is slowed and the amount of unchanged drug exhaled may be increased.

FURTHER INFORMATION. Blood and cerebrospinal fluid concentrations—R. Maes *et al., J. forens. Sci.,* 1969, **14**,

235 and J. H. Thurston *et al.*, *J. Lab. clin. Med.*, 1968, **72**, 699; pulmonary excretion—D. W. Lang and H. H. Borgstedt, *Toxic. appl. Pharmac.*, 1969, **15**, 269.

Actions and uses. Paraldehyde is a powerful and quick-acting hypnotic and anticonvulsant. Because of its objectionable odour and taste and slow part-excretion by the lungs, it is now rarely used as a hypnotic. The usual dose by mouth for this purpose is 5 to 10 millilitres, suitably diluted. It is irritant to mucous membranes unless it has been well diluted.

In the treatment of convulsions, paraldehyde is usually given by intramuscular injection in doses of 2 to 10 millilitres; not more than 5 millilitres should be injected into any one site. The injection is painful, and care should be taken to avoid the neighbourhood of nerve trunks. It has also been given by intravenous injection as a 10% solution in water, but this is not recommended. Plastic syringes should not be used.

Paraldehyde is sometimes used as a basal anaesthetic, especially in children. The dose is 0.5 millilitre per kilogram body-weight, with an upper limit of 30 millilitres, as an enema containing up to 10% v/v in isotonic sodium chloride solution; 1 millilitre of benzyl alcohol may be added to the enema to reduce local irritation. Children under 1 year may be given 0.5 to 1.5 millilitres and children from 1 to 5 years 2 to 4 millilitres of paraldehyde.

Dependence. In spite of the unpleasantness of paraldehyde, dependence of the barbiturate-alcohol type, as described under Drug Dependence, has occurred, especially among alcoholics.

Poisoning. In cases of poisoning by paraldehyde, which may cause death by respiratory failure, oxygen should be administered and respiration assisted if necessary.

Preparation

PARALDEHYDE INJECTION: consisting of sterile paraldehyde. It is sterilised by filtration. No bactericide should be added. Available in 5- and 10-ml ampoules.
A standard for this injection is given in the British Pharmaceutical Codex 1973
Containers: see the entry on Injections for general information on containers. The injection should be supplied in single-dose ampoules; contact with rubber and plastics should be avoided.
Labelling: see the entry on Injections for general information on labelling. In addition, the label on the container and the label or wrapper on the package should state that plastic syringes should not be used for the administration of the injection.
Storage: it should be stored at 15° to 20° in complete darkness.

Paralysis Agitans

see PARKINSONISM

Paramethadione

5-Ethyl-3,5-dimethyloxazolidine-2,4-dione

$C_7H_{11}NO_3 = 157.2$

OTHER NAME: *Paradione*®

A standard is given in the British Pharmacopoeia 1973

Description. A clear colourless liquid with a characteristic odour.

Solubility. Soluble in water, in alcohol, in ether, and in chloroform.

Acidity or alkalinity. A 2.5% solution has a pH of 4 to 7.5.

Refractive index. 1.448 to 1.450.

Metabolism. ABSORPTION. Readily absorbed after oral administration.

BLOOD CONCENTRATION. After an oral dose of 300 mg, peak serum concentrations of about $6 \mu g/ml$ are attained in 1 hour, falling to about 0.3 $\mu g/ml$ in 48 hours; after the same dose, serum concentrations of the metabolite 5-ethyl-5-methyloxazolidine-2,4-dione steadily rise to about 8.5 $\mu g/ml$ after 32 hours.

HALF-LIFE. Serum half-life, about 16 hours.

DISTRIBUTION. Concentrations in cerebrospinal fluid are lower than those in serum; accumulation may occur during continuous therapy.

METABOLIC REACTIONS. Rapid N-demethylation to form 5-ethyl-5-methyloxazolidine-2,4-dione which is an active metabolite.

EXCRETION. Slowly excreted in urine as the N-demethylated metabolite.

FURTHER INFORMATION. Metabolism—T. C. Butler, *J. Pharmac. exp. Ther.*, 1955, **113**, 178; serum concentrations—D. J. Hoffman and A. H. Chun, *J. pharm. Sci.*, 1975, **64**, 1702.

Actions and uses. Paramethadione has an anticonvulsant action similar to that described under Troxidone. It is used to control attacks of petit mal epilepsy, but is less effective than troxidone and less liable to produce severe toxic effects.

The usual initial dose for an adult is 900 milligrams daily in divided doses, with subsequent doses increasing to 1.8 grams daily in accordance with the needs of the patient. The initial dose for a child is 300 milligrams daily in divided doses with subsequent doses increasing to 900 milligrams daily in accordance with the needs of the patient.

Undesirable effects. As for Troxidone.

Precautions and contra-indications. As for Troxidone. Paramethadione may produce renal damage and thrombocytopenic purpura and should not be administered to patients with renal or hepatic disease. It should be used with caution during pregnancy.

Preparation

PARAMETHADIONE CAPSULES: consisting of paramethadione enclosed in a soft capsule. The capsule shells may be coloured. Available as capsules containing 300 mg of paramethadione.
A standard for these capsules is given in the British Pharmacopoeia 1973
Containers and *Storage:* see the entry on Capsules for general information on containers and storage.
Advice for patients: when initiating treatment there may be a time-lag of up to 2 weeks before a full therapeutic response is obtained. Treatment should not be discontinued without the advice of the prescriber. The capsules may cause drowsiness; persons affected should not drive or operate machinery. Alcohol should be avoided.

Paratyphoid Fever

see under SALMONELLA INFECTIONS

Parbendazole

Methyl 5-butylbenzimidazol-2-ylcarbamate

$C_{13}H_{17}N_3O_2 = 247.3$

OTHER NAMES: *Helmatac®*; *Ridhelmin®*

A standard is given in the British Pharmacopoeia (Veterinary)

Description. An odourless white crystalline powder.

Solubility. Practically insoluble in water; soluble, at 20°, in 900 parts of alcohol and in 300 parts of chloroform; very slightly soluble in ether; soluble in dilute mineral acids.

Identification. TEST. Dissolve about 5 mg in 5 ml of 0.1N hydrochloric acid, add 3 mg of *p*-phenylenediamine hydrochloride, shake to dissolve, add 100 mg of zinc powder, mix, allow to stand for 2 minutes, and add 10 ml of *ferric ammonium sulphate solution*; a deep blue or violet-blue colour is produced.

MELTING-POINT. About 225°, with decomposition.

ULTRAVIOLET ABSORPTION. In 0.01N alcoholic hydrochloric acid, maxima at 281 nm (E1%, 1cm = 610) and 288 nm (E1%, 1cm = 760).

Veterinary uses. Parbendazole is used in the treatment of gastro-intestinal nematode infections in cattle, sheep, and pigs. The usual dose by mouth for cattle is 25 to 35 milligrams per kilogram body-weight up to a maximum of 10 grams, for sheep 20 milligrams per kilogram body-weight, and for pigs 35 milligrams per kilogram body-weight as a single dose.

Preparations

PARBENDAZOLE MIXTURE (*Syn.* Parbendazole Drench; Parbendazole Suspension): consisting of an aqueous suspension of parbendazole mixed with suitable suspending and dispersing agents. Available as a mixture containing 4% of parbendazole.
A standard for this mixture is given in the British Pharmacopoeia (Veterinary)
Containers: see the entry on Mixtures for general information on containers.
Labelling: see the entry on Mixtures for general information on labelling. A direction to shake the bottle should be given on the label. In addition, the label on the container should state that pregnant cattle and those producing milk for human consumption should not be treated with parbendazole, that ewes should not be treated with parbendazole during tupping and for 30 days after removal of the ram, that cattle should not be slaughtered for human consumption within 5 days after cessation of treatment with parbendazole, and that sheep should not be slaughtered for human consumption within 6 days after cessation of treatment with parbendazole.

PARBENDAZOLE PREMIX: consisting of parbendazole mixed with a suitable inert diluent. It must be diluted before administration by thoroughly mixing with the feed. Available as a premix containing 30% of parbendazole.
A standard for this premix is given in the British Pharmacopoeia (Veterinary)
Containers and *Storage:* see the entry on Premixes for general information on containers and storage.
Labelling: the label on the container should state that pregnant cattle and those producing milk for human consumption should not be treated with parbendazole, that ewes should not be treated with parbendazole during tupping and for 30 days after removal of the ram, that cattle should not be slaughtered for human consumption within 5 days, sheep within 6 days, and pigs within 16 days after cessation of treatment with parbendazole.

OTHER PREPARATIONS available include veterinary PELLETS containing parbendazole 3.2%.

Parkinsonism

Parkinsonism (Paralysis Agitans) is a disease of the extrapyramidal system of the brain characterised by tremor, muscular rigidity, loss of postural reflexes, and hypokinesia (loss of coordination of movements). It usually begins between the ages of 50 and 65 years and is progressive. In the majority of cases there is no definable cause, although it may be due to poisoning with carbon monoxide, manganese or other metals, brain tumours in the basal ganglia, cerebral trauma, degenerative diseases, or following encephalitis. A parkinsonian-like syndrome may also occur as a result of drug treatment with, for example, phenothiazine derivatives. In parkinsonism there are degenerative changes with loss of cells in the substantia nigra and basal ganglia. There may also be degenerative changes in the brain stem or cranial nerve nuclei or atrophy of the cerebral cortex. Depletion of the neural transmitter dopamine results in an imbalance between the cholinergic and dopaminergic neurones in the extrapyramidal system and symptoms may be relieved by drugs which increase the production of dopamine or reduce cholinergic activity.

Levodopa is a precursor of dopamine and is usually effective in controlling symptoms such as defects in initiation of movement and hypokinesia. It may also control rigidity and tremor and is the drug of choice unless precluded by its many side-effects. Only a small fraction of the dose of levodopa reaches the basal ganglia and is converted into dopamine. The remainder is decarboxylated in the peripheral tissues. Benserazide and carbidopa are decarboxylase inhibitors which do not penetrate the brain, and when either is given with levodopa block its peripheral utilisation without affecting central metabolism. Therefore their use leads to a reduction in the daily dose of levodopa with a reduction in incidence of some of its adverse effects.

Amantadine is less potent but has fewer side-effects than levodopa. Anticholinergic drugs such as atropine and other solanaceous alkaloids have been used to reduce rigidity and to a lesser extent tremor. These drugs have been largely replaced by benztropine, which is structurally similar to atropine, and by benzhexol, biperiden, and procyclidine, which resemble each other in structure and effect. Orphenadrine is also used.

Parotitis, Epidemic

see MUMPS

Partition Coefficients

A partition coefficient is a solubility ratio which is a measure of the distribution of a solute between two immiscible phases. For most purposes these phases are an organic solvent and water.

Partition coefficients are most frequently determined in attempts to correlate the relative lipophilic character of a drug substance with biological properties. A drug substance can exert its influence only if it can reach the active site by a transfer process that involves passage through both hydrophilic and lipophilic barriers in the biological system. As a consequence, an important aspect of drug design is the modification of the hydrophobic character of drugs so as to facilitate their transport to, and binding at, the site of action. In the investigation of this problem, partition in a solvent-water system can act as a useful model of the real situation.

The *partition coefficient* (P) of a solute is defined as the ratio of the concentrations in the two phases at equilibrium, and it is usual to present the ratio as that in favour of the organic phase:

$$P = \frac{Co}{Cw} \tag{1}$$

where Co = the concentration of the solute in the organic phase, and Cw = the concentration of the solute in the aqueous phase.

Owing to the widespread use of partition coefficients in structure-activity studies (see below), it is often convenient to use log P, the logarithm of the partition coefficient, instead of the partition coefficient itself.

Equation (1) assumes that the compound, if it is an ionisable molecule such as an acid or a base, is fully non-ionised under the conditions of the measurement. This usually requires the use of an acidic aqueous phase for an acidic compound, or of an alkaline phase for a base. However, it may be desirable to measure a partition coefficient under conditions where the compound is partially ionised, for example by using a pH 7.4 buffer. In this case, the ratio is termed the *apparent partition coefficient* to distinguish it from the real partition coefficient for the totally non-ionised compound. The term *distribution coefficient* (D) is also used for this quantity. The apparent partition coefficient (P_{app}) is related to the proportion of drug present in solution as the non-ionised species, which in turn depends upon the pH of the aqueous phase used.

$$P_{app} = P \cdot f_u \tag{2}$$

where f_u = the fraction of molecules present in the non-ionised form.

For a monobasic acid,

$$f_u = \frac{1}{(1 + 10^{pH - pK_a})} \tag{3}$$

For a monoacidic base,

$$f_u = \frac{1}{(1 + 10^{pK_a - pH})} \tag{4}$$

Hence, for an acid,

$$P_{app} = \frac{P}{(1 + 10^{pH - pK_a})} \tag{5}$$

and for a base,

$$P_{app} = \frac{P}{(1 + 10^{pK_a - pH})} \tag{6}$$

Thus knowledge of the pK_a and true partition coefficient of a molecule allows calculation of the apparent partition coefficient at any pH. For example, the basic drug amphetamine has a pK_a of 9.70 and an n-heptane/water partition coefficient of 3.4. Using equation (6), its apparent partition coefficient at pH 7.4 is 0.017.

It is assumed here that ions are not extracted into the organic layer. This can occur under some circumstances and precautions have to be taken to prevent it occurring during the determination of apparent partition coefficients (see under Buffer Ratio Method, below).

Determination of Partition Coefficients

The shake-flask method. Partition coefficients are usually determined by the traditional shake-flask method. In this method the compound is dissolved in one phase, the other phase added, the mixture is shaken, allowed to stand, and the phases separated; the concentration of solute in each phase is then determined by a suitable analytical method.

It is useful to pre-equilibrate both phases, which will then separate much faster during the determination. Each phase is saturated with the other by adding 5% v/v, shaking, and allowing to stand overnight. This does not affect the value of the partition coefficient, although equilibrium will probably be attained more rapidly than would otherwise be the case.

Various techniques have been used for mixing the two phases, but hand shaking is efficient and often the most convenient. Lengthy periods of shaking are not required to obtain an equilibrium distribution of solute between the two phases, and partitioning is usually complete after vigorous shaking by hand for 1 to 2 minutes followed by standing for 10 minutes. Alternatively, mixing can be carried out by inverting the container about 100 times during 5 minutes, a method which is useful in cases where vigorous shaking may cause the formation of an emulsion.

After the mixture has been allowed to stand, it is often worthwhile to ensure separation of the two phases by centrifugation, as the apparent clarity of the liquids is not a dependable criterion for the absence of an emulsion. Another useful technique is to filter each phase, after separation, through a filter paper previously saturated with the phase concerned; this prevents entrainment of one phase in the other.

EFFECT OF TEMPERATURE. Partition coefficients are usually measured at room temperature. Although the values will vary with temperature, the effect is usually of the order of 0.01 log unit per degree (either positively or negatively) and, in general, is not large enough for normal fluctuations in room temperature to be significant.

DETERMINATION OF CONCENTRATION OF SOLUTE. A prerequisite for the determination of partition coefficients is the availability of a suitable sensitive method of assaying the compound in one (or preferably both) phases. Measurement of the ultraviolet absorption is usually the most convenient method because it is quick, simple, and applicable to a very large number of organic solutes. When using this method, it cannot be assumed that either the frequency or the intensity are independent of the solvent and so extinction values must be measured in both phases. With compounds which have no suitable ultraviolet spectrum, other analytical techniques will have to be employed.

ADJUSTMENT OF CONCENTRATION. In an ideal determination the following conditions are met: the two phases are transparent to ultraviolet radiation, the solute is a neutral molecule with a strong ultraviolet absorption spectrum, and the ratio of concentration at equilibrium lies within the ratio of 5 to 1 either way. In this situation, absorbances can be measured directly in both phases, the concentrations calculated, and the partition coefficient obtained using equation (1).

However, partition coefficients well outside this range often occur and, with compounds with very high or very low partition coefficients, the equilibrium concentration in the less favoured phase may be below or close to the limits of detection. Modifications to the ideal situation are therefore required.

The concentration ratio method. If, for instance, a partition ratio of 100 is encountered, the amount of compound used is increased by the same ratio, allowing concentrations to be measured directly in the less favoured phase, and in the other phase after dilution. With this technique, the presence of impurities can cause large errors, and it is necessary to investigate this possibility. For instance, with ultraviolet measurements, the spectrum should be inspected for any signs of qualitative discrepancy with the calibration spectrum.

The volume ratio method. As an alternative, the volume ratio of the two phases can be adjusted to enable high partition coefficients to be determined without increasing the amount of material used. For example, if a lipophilic solute has a partition coefficient of 200, and 20 mg was partitioned between 100-ml volumes of the two phases, the less favoured (aqueous) phase would contain only 0.1 mg at equilibrium. This may be close to the limits of the analytical procedure and errors could result. If, however, 200 ml and 5 ml, respectively, of the aqueous and non-aqueous phases were used, the aqueous phase would contain 3.3 mg of solute at equilibrium. This is likely to be within the working range of the analytical procedure.

The buffer ratio method. If the pH of the aqueous phase is selected so that the compound is partially ionised, a double equilibrium exists between the ionised and non-ionised species in water, and between the non-ionised species in both phases (see FIG. 1).

Normal case

Buffer ratio case

FIG. 1. Partitioning situation with non-ionised and ionised species present in the aqueous phase.

With a highly lipophilic compound that is basic or acidic, it is possible, therefore, to reduce the apparent partition coefficient so that it can be determined readily. This method may also be useful because the partition coefficient for some chosen physiological pH, for example that of blood, can be measured directly.

The method depends on the assumption that ions are not extracted into the organic layer. This can happen under some circumstances and precautions have to be taken to prevent it. It requires the careful choice of anion (for basic solutes) or cation (for acidic solutes). For instance, sulphate, phosphate, perchlorate, and other highly oxygenated anions are generally suitable; halides and most organic anions are to be avoided.

Apparent partition coefficients measured in this way are dependent on pH, and a knowledge of the pK_a of the compound is therefore required.

CHOICE OF SOLVENT. A large number of different solvent-water systems have been used for the determination of partition coefficients in connection with drug design and structure-activity studies. In this context the solvent is intended as a model for the lipophilic phase of biological systems, and the water as a model for the hydrophilic phase.

The relative merits of the most widely used solvents are still a matter for dispute. The difficulty arises because biological systems, or parts thereof, are too complicated for a simple two-phase system to be an ideal model. Furthermore, in biological systems, the membranes are associated with significant amounts of water held by the polar and/or ionic areas of the macromolecules of which they are composed. The polar areas and their associated water molecules have a significant effect on the lipophilic nature of these membranes. The physical characteristics of various solvent-water systems used in the measurement of partition coefficients, and their theoretical suitability as models of biological membrane systems, have been reviewed by R. N. Smith *et al.* (*J. pharm. Sci.*, 1975, **64**, 599). These authors stress the importance of regarding partitioning systems as being composed of two binary phases, a water-saturated solvent phase, and a solvent-saturated aqueous phase.

1-Octanol is the solvent for which most partition coefficient values have been published, and with which partition coefficient-activity correlations have most often been obtained. It is claimed that the 1-octanol/water system is a satisfactory model for the biological system because the organic phase is not completely non-polar and contains a significant amount of water in a stable, hydrogen-bonded complex. At the same time, non-polar solvents such as n-heptane and cyclohexane are criticised for not being good theoretical models for biological membranes, and also on the basis that the small amounts of dissolved water which they contain can be greatly altered by the presence of partitioned solute. A further complication is that association of polar solute molecules can occur in non-polar solvents, although correction of measured partition coefficients can be applied to overcome this, as described by A. H. Beckett and A. C. Moffat (*J. Pharm. Pharmac.*, 1969, **21**, Suppl., 144S). Despite these objections, there has been considerable success in correlating biological parameters with partition coefficients which have been determined using non-polar solvents, particularly n-heptane, and there is a firm body of opinion which believes that such solvents give a more realistic indication of the relative lipid solubility of molecules than do the more polar solvents. Choice of the best solvent system for a particular purpose is, therefore, often difficult, although the suitability of a system lies in the correlation obtained between the partition coefficients measured and the biological data concerned. Often, the choice of solvent will be dictated simply by what has been used previously for a similar purpose, as partition coefficients can only be compared when they are measured in the same solvent system.

An organic solvent must also satisfy certain physical criteria in order to be suitable for the measurement of partition coefficients. Firstly, it must be nearly immiscible with water. If this criterion is not satisfied (as for example by diethyl ether) the resultant phases may be undefinable. For similar reasons, the use of mixed solvents is unsuitable. Secondly, the purity of the organic phase must be high and its behaviour reproducible, a factor that has sometimes been in doubt for 1-octanol; chloroform must be washed to remove ethanol, and olive oil, one of the original organic phases used, is unsuitable because of its varying composition and purity.

Chromatographic methods. Most chromatographic techniques depend on partition processes, and new methods for determining partition coefficients have been developed, including the use of thin-layer chromatography, as described by C. B. C. Boyce and B. V. Milborrow (*Nature*, 1965, **208**, 537), and high pressure liquid chromatography, as described by J. M. McCall (*J. Mednl Chem.*, 1975, **18**, 549). The advantages of such methods over the shake-flask method are that they are quicker, less wasteful of compound and solvents, and less demanding in the standard of purity required.

The Significance and Use of Partition Coefficients

Body membranes are mainly lipoid in nature and consequently are more easily penetrated by lipophilic molecules than by hydrophilic molecules. As the partition coefficient between organic solvent and water is an index of the lipid solubility of a compound, there is often a relationship between this and the rate of transfer of a molecule across a biological membrane; this may be evident particularly within a series of structurally related compounds.

It has been concluded that most drugs are absorbed from the gastro-intestinal tract by a process of passive diffusion (see under Metabolism of Drugs) of the non-ionised moiety across the lipoid mucosal membrane, a principle which has become known as the "pH-partition hypothesis". This conclusion was reached primarily on the basis of the demonstration of a relationship between partition coefficient, dissociation constant, and degree of absorption for a series of different compounds.

The principles of the pH-partition hypothesis also apply to absorption in the mouth, and relationships between partition coefficient and buccal absorption rates have been demonstrated for various series of compounds. Similarly, the principle has been shown to apply to the transfer of drugs from, or into, various other tissues or organs including transfer from the blood stream into the saliva, the excretion of drugs via sweat, the secretion of drugs into milk, and the transport of drugs across the cornea, across the placenta, and into and out of cerebrospinal fluid and the brain.

Such a correlation between partition coefficients and transfer across a membrane can apply to relatively simple situations where only one membrane or membrane system is involved, or in much more complex situations such as the metabolism of drugs, or even in drug action where a very large number of membrane systems may be sequentially involved.

The most far-reaching studies in quantifying the biological significance of the lipid solubility of drugs and in the broader area of structure-activity relationships have been made by Hansch and his co-workers. Hansch supposes that biological potency is a function of a number of variables, and may be represented by a general equation of the following type:

$$\log \frac{1}{C} = x \log X + y \log Y + z \log Z \qquad (7)$$

where C = biologically active concentrations defined in suitable terms (e.g. ED_{50}), X, Y, and Z are the relevant variables, and x, y, and z are coefficients which dictate their relative importance. A large number of variables might each have some effect on biological activity, but for simplicity three parameters of the drug molecule are usually taken as being the prime factors controlling action in the biological system; these are hydrophobic, electronic, and steric parameters. The hydrophobic parameter is usually the most significant and is represented by $\log P$, the logarithm of the partition coefficient. An important part of this approach is the recognition that an "additivity principle" applies to partition coefficients. This means that the total partition coefficient of a molecule can be derived by adding together the contributions from separate fragments of the molecule. In a series of compounds consisting of different substituent groups on a common nucleus, the contribution of a particular substituent (the substituent constant, π) is defined as:

$$\pi_x = \log P_x - \log P_H \qquad (8)$$

where P_H refers to the parent molecule, and P_x to its derivative.

For example, in a simple case such as chlorobenzene, π_{Cl} is the logarithm of the partition coefficient of the substituent Cl obtained from the difference in the two $\log P$ values. The use of π values simplifies the use of partition coefficients in structure-activity studies, and, in addition, allows partition coefficients to be calculated by utilising values from a suitable model series of compounds.

The concept represented in equation (7) is used in practice for a series of compounds by comparing biological and physicochemical parameters by means of regression analysis on a computer. An equation which quantifies the correlation between the two sets of data can then be obtained. For example, the equation obtained for the narcosis of goldfish by a series of alcohols was:

$$\log \frac{1}{C} = 1.15(\pm 0.20) \log P + 0.34(\pm 0.11) \qquad (9)$$

in which the number of molecules studied was 8, the correlation coefficient was 0.985, and the standard deviation was 0.106.

The relationship between $\log \frac{1}{C}$ and $\log P$ is often not linear but parabolic. The partition coefficient value corresponding to the maximum of this parabola is denoted P_o, and is the ideal or optimum value for a given series of compounds acting on a given system. P_o (or $\log P_o$) values have been identified for a variety of different biological systems. For example, in testing the hypnotic activity of a series of carbamates in the mouse, $\log P_o$ was found to be 1.6, and in the inhibition of *Glomerella cingulata* by imidazolines, $\log P_o$ was found to be 7.0.

Further information

METHODS. *Shake-flask:* A. Leo et al., *Chemical Reviews*, 1971, **71**, 525.

Thin-layer chromatography: C. B. C. Boyce and B. V. Milborrow, *Nature*, 1965, **208**, 537.

High pressure liquid chromatography: J. M. McCall, *J. mednl Chem.*, 1975, **18**, 549.

RELATIONSHIP BETWEEN PARTITION COEFFICIENT AND TRANSFER ACROSS MEMBRANES. A. H. Beckett and E. J. Triggs, *J. Pharm. Pharmac.*, 1967, **19**, *Suppl.*, 31S;

S. A. Killman and J. H. Thaysen, *Scand. J. clin. Lab. Invest.*, 1955, **7**, 86; Y. C. Martin and C. Hansch, *J. mednl Chem.*, 1971, **14**, 777; L. S. Schanker *et al.*, *J. Pharmac. exp. Ther.*, 1958, **123**, 81; L. S. Schanker, *J. mednl pharm. Chem.*, 1960, **2**, 343; J. G. Wagner, *Biopharmaceutics and Relevant Pharmacokinetics*, Illinois, Drug Intelligence Publications, 1971.

STRUCTURE-ACTIVITY   RELATIONSHIPS.   C. Hansch, Quantitive approaches to pharmacological structure-activity relationships, *Structure-Activity Relationships*, *International Encyclopedia of Pharmacology and Therapeutics*, Sect. 5, C. J. Cavallito (Ed.), Oxford, Pergamon Press, 1973; C. Hansch *et al.*, *J. mednl Chem.*, 1968, **11**, 1; C. Hansch and E. J. Lien, *J. mednl Chem.*, 1971, **14**, 653; C. Hansch *et al.*, *Archs Biochem. Biophys.*, 1968, **128**, 319.

COLLECTION OF DATA. *Hansch Database*, available on subscription from Pomona College, California, U.S.A.

Pastes

Pastes are semisolid preparations for external application. They usually consist of a high proportion of finely powdered medicaments mixed with soft or liquid paraffin or with a non-greasy basis made with glycerol, mucilage, or soap. They are used principally as antiseptic, protective, or soothing dressings which are often spread on lint before being applied.

Containers and storage. Pastes should be stored and supplied in glass or plastic jars fitted with screw caps with impermeable liners or with close-fitting slip-on lids so that absorption or diffusion of the contents is prevented. Alternatively, collapsible tubes of metal or suitable plastic material may be used.

Pastes containing water or other volatile ingredients should be stored and supplied in well-closed containers which prevent evaporation.

Pastilles

Pastilles consist of medicaments incorporated in an inert basis and are intended to dissolve slowly in the mouth. The basis is composed of a preparation containing gelatin and glycerol or a mixture of acacia and sucrose. For extemporaneous preparation, a suitable basis may be prepared from the following formula:

Gelatin	200 g
Sodium benzoate	2 g
Citric acid monohydrate	20 g
Sucrose	50 g
Lemon oil	1 ml
Amaranth solution	20 ml
Glycerol	400 g
Purified water, freshly boiled and cooled	to 1000 g

Soak the gelatin until softened in 300 g of the water at a temperature above 90°, add the glycerol, and heat on a water-bath until the gelatin is dissolved and the mass weighs 850 g; add the sucrose, the citric acid, and the sodium benzoate previously dissolved in 60 ml of the water, and add the lemon oil and the amaranth solution and sufficient water to produce the required weight. Strain and allow to cool.

Care should be taken to minimise microbial contamination by observing the highest standards of cleanliness during preparation. If a pastille which dissolves less rapidly is required, some of the gelatin in the above formula may be replaced by agar, but it should be noted that this will render the pastille basis opaque.

Containers and storage. Pastilles should be stored and supplied in containers that provide adequate protection against moisture and crushing. They should preferably be supplied in wide-mouthed glass or suitable plastic containers, or cylindrical aluminium containers internally coated with a suitable lacquer or lined with paper; lacquered or lined screw-cap closures or plastic caps should be used.

Patients, Advice for

see ADVICE FOR PATIENTS

Pediculosis

see under LICE

Pellagra

Pellagra is due to a deficiency of nicotinic acid and also other B-complex vitamins. It is characterised by a symmetrical erythematous rash with thickening and pigmentation of the skin. There may also be gastrointestinal disturbances and involvement of the central nervous system, with a progressive encephalopathy. Symptoms are rapidly relieved by nicotinic acid or nicotinamide but treatment of deficiencies of other members of the vitamin-B group may be necessary for complete relief. Treatment is described under Nicotinic Acid.

Penicillamine

D-3,3-Dimethylcysteine

$C_5H_{11}NO_2S = 149.2$

OTHER NAMES: *Cuprimine®*; *Depamine®*; *Distamine®*; D-Penicillamine

A standard is given in the British Pharmacopoeia 1973

Description. A white finely crystalline powder with a characteristic odour and a slightly bitter taste.

Solubility. Soluble, at 20°, in 9 parts of water and in 530 parts of alcohol; practically insoluble in ether and in chloroform.

Acidity. A 1% solution has a pH of 4.5 to 5.5.

Specific rotation. −58° to −68°, determined on a 5% solution in 1N sodium hydroxide.

Stability. In aqueous solution penicillamine degrades slowly by first-order or pseudo-first-order kinetics. A 3% solution of penicillamine hydrochloride stored at 20° in a sealed container, the air in which has been replaced by nitrogen, decomposes to the extent of about 10% per year.

FURTHER INFORMATION. J. R. J. B. Brouwers *et al.*, *Pharm. Weekbl. Ned.*, 1977, **112**, 121.

Storage. It should be stored in airtight containers.

Identification. TESTS. 1. Dissolve about 20 mg in 4 ml of water and add 2 ml of *phosphotungstic acid reagent*; a deep blue colour is formed on standing for a few minutes.
2. Dissolve about 10 mg in 5 ml of water and add 1 drop of *sodium hydroxide solution* and 20 mg of ninhydrin; an intense blue or violet-blue colour is produced.

MELTING-POINT. About 210°, with decomposition.

Metabolism. ABSORPTION. Readily absorbed after oral administration.

BLOOD CONCENTRATION. Peak plasma concentrations are attained in about 1 hour.

DISTRIBUTION. *Protein binding*, a small percentage is bound to plasma proteins.

METABOLIC REACTIONS. Penicillamine is relatively stable but is metabolised to some extent by *S*-methylation, by disulphide formation, and by the formation of a cysteine-penicillamine conjugate.

EXCRETION. About 80% of an intravenous dose is excreted in the urine; penicillamine is excreted mainly as the disulphide or cysteine conjugate and 4 to 8% is excreted as the *S*-methylated metabolite.

FURTHER INFORMATION. Metabolism in Wilson's disease—K. Gibbs and J. M. Walshe, *Q. J. Med.*, 1971, **40**, 275; *S*-methylation—D. Perrett *et al.*, *Biochem. Pharmac.*, 1976, **25**, 254; reviews—*Postgrad. Med. J.*, 1974, **50**, *Suppl.* 2.

Actions and uses. Penicillamine is a chelating agent which aids elimination of certain toxic metal ions. It is used mainly in the treatment of hepatolenticular degeneration (Wilson's disease); when it is given by mouth in a dosage of 0.5 to 1.5 grams daily, it increases the urinary output of copper 5- to 20-fold. The corresponding dose for children up to 5 years is 150 milligrams twice daily, from 6 to 12 years 300 milligrams twice daily, and older children 450 milligrams twice daily.

The condition of some patients treated with penicillamine improves dramatically, but other patients, although their copper output increases considerably, show no improvement; improvement probably depends on the amount of permanent and irreversible structural damage. Penicillamine is also of value in the treatment of copper and lead poisoning. It will chelate *in vitro* with antimony, bismuth, chromium, cobalt, silver, and zinc ions, but evidence of its value in poisoning with these ions is limited.

Penicillamine is also used empirically in the treatment of scleroderma and rheumatoid arthritis. Its effect in rheumatoid arthritis is similar to that of gold compounds. Its action is not only anti-inflammatory but it is accompanied by improvement in extra-articular as well as articular features of the disease and by reduction in the titre of rheumatoid factor. The initial dose is 250 milligrams daily taken with food. Dosage is increased every fortnight by 250 milligrams up to a total daily dose of about 1 gram, adjusted according to the response of the patient. Improvement may not begin for up to 8 weeks after the start of treatment; the greatest mean improvement usually occurs in the second month of treatment but improvement may continue to the sixth month. About 80% of patients obtain substantial benefit. Because of its side-effects this treatment should be reserved for patients who are not satisfactorily treated with analgesic and anti-inflammatory drugs or who deteriorate despite such treatment.

Undesirable effects. Penicillamine may give rise to proteinuria. Allergic reactions, nausea, anorexia, loss of taste, leucopenia, thrombocytopenia, mouth ulceration, proteinuria, and the nephrotic syndrome may occur. These side-effects are usually reversible and may not require cessation of therapy.

Precautions. The blood and urine of patients being treated with penicillamine should be examined every 2 to 4 weeks. Penicillamine should be used with caution in pregnancy and in nursing mothers.

Preparations

PENICILLAMINE CAPSULES: consisting of penicillamine or penicillamine hydrochloride, which may be mixed with a suitable inert diluent, enclosed in a hard capsule. The capsule shells may be coloured. Available as capsules containing 125 and 250 mg of penicillamine.
A standard for these capsules is given in the British Pharmacopoeia 1973
Containers and *Storage:* see the entry on Capsules for general information on containers and storage.
Labelling: when the active ingredient is penicillamine hydrochloride, the label on the container should state the amount of the medicament as the equivalent amount of penicillamine.
Advice for patients: the capsules should be taken half to 1 hour before meals. When used in the treatment of rheumatoid arthritis and related diseases the capsules may be taken after meals if there are gastro-intestinal disturbances. Treatment should not be discontinued without the advice of the prescriber.

PENICILLAMINE TABLETS: available as tablets containing 50, 125, and 250 mg of penicillamine; they are film coated.
A standard for these tablets is given in the British Pharmacopoeia 1973
Containers and *Storage:* see the entry on Tablets for general information on containers and storage. The tablets should be stored at a temperature not exceeding 25°.
Advice for patients: see above under Penicillamine Capsules.

Penicillamine Hydrochloride

D-3,3-Dimethylcysteine hydrochloride
$C_5H_{12}ClNO_2S = 185.7$

OTHER NAME: D-Penicillamine Hydrochloride

A standard is given in the British Pharmacopoeia 1973

Description. A white, finely crystalline, hygroscopic powder with a characteristic odour and an acidic taste.

Solubility. Soluble, at 20°, in 1 part of water, in 1.5 parts of alcohol, and in 230 parts of chloroform; practically insoluble in ether.

Acidity. A 1% solution has a pH of 1.6 to 2.2.

Moisture content. Not more than 3%, determined by drying *in vacuo*.

Specific rotation. $-46°$ to $-53°$, determined on a 5% solution in 1N sodium hydroxide.

Stability. See above under Penicillamine.

Storage. It should be stored in airtight containers at a temperature not exceeding 25°.

Identification. TESTS. It complies with the tests described under Penicillamine.

MELTING-POINT. About 162°.

Metabolism. As for Penicillamine.

Actions and uses. Penicillamine hydrochloride has the actions, uses, and undesirable effects described under Penicillamine; 1.25 grams of penicillamine hydrochloride is approximately equivalent to 1 gram of penicillamine.

Precautions. As for Penicillamine.

Preparation

PENICILLAMINE CAPSULES: see above under Penicillamine.

Pentaerythritol Tetranitrate, Diluted

A mixture of pentaerythritol tetranitrate with lactose, or with a mixture of 3 parts of lactose and 1 part of starch. Pentaerythritol tetranitrate is 2,2-bis(hydroxymethyl)-propane-1,3-diol tetranitrate.

OTHER NAMES: *Cardiacap®*; Dil. Pentaerythr. Tetranit.; *Mycardol®*; Pentaerythritol Tetranitrate (20%); *Pentral®*; *Peritrate®*
Cardiacap-A® (with amylobarbitone); *Peritrate with Phenobarbitone®*; *Pentoxylon®* (with *Rauwolfia serpentina* alkaloids)

A standard is given in the British Pharmaceutical Codex 1973

Description. An odourless white crystalline powder.

Storage. It should be stored in airtight containers, protected from light, in a cool place.

Metabolism. ABSORPTION. Incompletely absorbed after oral administration; the trinitrate is more rapidly absorbed than the tetranitrate.

BLOOD CONCENTRATION. After an oral dose of 40 mg, peak plasma concentrations of drug plus metabolites of 0.2 to 0.25 μg/ml are attained in 4 to 8 hours.

DISTRIBUTION. Accumulation of pentaerythritol mononitrate may occur; *protein binding*, about 85% bound to plasma proteins.

METABOLIC REACTIONS. Rapid de-esterification to form the mononitrate and a limited capacity to de-esterify the mononitrate to pentaerythritol; liberated nitrite is oxidised to nitrate.

EXCRETION. About 90% of a dose is excreted in urine and faeces in 48 hours; 50 to 60% is excreted in the urine and 20 to 40% is eliminated in the faeces; small amounts are excreted in the bile.

FURTHER INFORMATION. Absorption, excretion, and metabolism—I. W. F. Davidson *et al.*, *J. Pharmac. exp. Ther.*, 1970, **175**, 42; nitrate ester metabolism—M. H. Litchfield, *J. pharm. Sci.*, 1971, **60**, 1599; pharmacokinetics and metabolism of tetranitrate—I. W. F. Davidson *et al.*, *J. pharm. Sci.*, 1971, **60**, 274; pharmacokinetics and metabolism of trinitrate—I. W. F. Davidson *et al.*, *Clin. Pharmac. Ther.*, 1971, **12**, 972.

Actions and uses. Pentaerythritol tetranitrate has the actions and uses described under Glyceryl Trinitrate. When given by mouth, it is slowly absorbed from the gastro-intestinal tract; its effect commences about 1 hour after administration and lasts for about 5 hours. The usual dose is 10 to 30 milligrams of pentaerythritol tetranitrate 3 or 4 times daily. It is also administered in sustained release tablets in doses of 80 milligrams twice daily.

Contra-indications. It is contra-indicated in coronary thrombosis.

Poisoning. As for Glyceryl Trinitrate.

Preparations

PENTAERYTHRITOL TABLETS: available as tablets containing 10 and 30 mg of pentaerythritol tetranitrate; they may be coloured.
A standard for these tablets is given in the British Pharmacopoeia 1973
Containers and *Storage:* see the entry on Tablets for general information on containers and storage. Containers should be airtight and light resistant. The tablets should be stored in a cool place.
Advice for patients: the tablets should preferably be taken half to 1 hour before meals.

OTHER PREPARATIONS available include CAPSULES containing pentaerythritol tetranitrate 30 mg in a slow-release formulation, capsules containing pentaerythritol tetranitrate 30 mg with amylobarbitone 50 mg in a slow-release formulation, capsules containing pentaerythritol tetranitrate 80 mg in a slow-release formulation; TABLETS containing pentaerythritol tetranitrate 10 mg with phenobarbitone 15 mg, tablets containing pentaerythritol tetranitrate 80 mg in a slow-release formulation, and tablets containing pentaerythritol tetranitrate 10 mg with *Rauwolfia serpentina* alkaloid hydrochlorides 1 mg.

Pentagastrin

N-t-Butoxycarbonyl- β-alanyl - L-tryptophyl - L-methionyl-L-aspartyl-L-phenylalanine amide

$C_{37}H_{49}N_7O_9S = 767.9$

OTHER NAME: *Peptavlon®*

A standard is given in the British Pharmacopoeia 1973

Description. An odourless white powder.

Solubility. Practically insoluble in water; very slightly soluble in alcohol; soluble in dilute ammonia solution and in dimethylformamide.

Specific rotation. $-25°$ to $-29°$, determined on a 1% solution in dimethylformamide.

Sterilisation. Solutions for injection are sterilised by filtration.

Storage. It should be protected from light.

Actions and uses. Pentagastrin stimulates the secretion of gastric acid, pepsin with intrinsic factor, pancreatic juice, and bile, and the segmenting activity of the bowel and sodium diuresis. It is not absorbed from the gut. When it is administered by intramuscular injection the peak effect occurs in 10 to 30 minutes.
Pentagastrin is used as a diagnostic agent to test the acid-secreting function of the stomach and as a means of differentiating between the absolute achylia of pernicious anaemia and the relative achylia of carcinoma of the stomach. For this purpose pentagastrin is administered usually by subcutaneous injection but occasionally by intramuscular injection in a dosage of 6 micrograms per kilogram body-weight. It may also be given by intravenous infusion at a rate of 0.6 micrograms per kilogram body-weight per hour. Pentagastrin is used to determine the maximum acid secretion by recovering the

gastric juice while successively higher doses of pentagastrin are given by intravenous infusion.

Undesirable effects. Mild abdominal discomfort commonly occurs. Occasionally cramps, nausea, palpitation, and tachycardia occur about 10 minutes after injection and these effects are more marked when the drug is administered intravenously.

Preparation

PENTAGASTRIN INJECTION: a sterile solution of pentagastrin, with ammonium hydroxide, in water for injections. It is sterilised by filtration. Available in 2-ml ampoules containing 250 micrograms of pentagastrin per ml.
A standard for this injection is given in the British Pharmacopoeia 1973
Containers and *Labelling:* see the entry on Injections for general information on containers and labelling.
Storage: it should be stored at a temperature below 20°, protected from light.

Pentamidine Isethionate

4,4′-(Pentamethylenedioxy)dibenzamidine di(2-hydroxy-ethanesulphonate)

$C_{23}H_{36}N_4O_{10}S_2 = 592.7$

A standard is given in the British Pharmacopoeia 1973

Description. Odourless white hygroscopic crystals or powder with a very bitter taste.

Solubility. Soluble, at 20°, in 10 parts of water; soluble in glycerol; very slightly soluble in alcohol; practically insoluble in ether, in chloroform, and in liquid paraffin.

Acidity. A 5% solution has a pH of 4.5 to 6.5.

Moisture content. Not more than 4%, determined by drying at 105°.

Storage. It should be stored in airtight containers.

Identification. TESTS. 1. To 10 ml of a 1% solution add 1 ml of *dilute sulphuric acid*; a white precipitate is produced.
2. To 10 ml of a 1% solution add 4 drops of *sodium hydroxide solution*; a white precipitate is produced.
3. Dilute 0.5 ml of a 1% solution to 10 ml with water, add 1 ml of a 0.1% solution of glyoxal sodium bisulphite and 1 ml of a solution prepared by dissolving 4 g of boric acid in a mixture of 27 ml of 1N sodium hydroxide and sufficient water to produce 100 ml, and heat on a water-bath for 10 minutes; a magenta colour is produced.

MELTING-POINT. About 190°.

ULTRAVIOLET ABSORPTION. In 0.01N hydrochloric acid, maximum at 262 nm (E1%, 1cm = 460).

Metabolism. ABSORPTION. Well absorbed after parenteral administration.

BLOOD CONCENTRATION. After an intramuscular dose of 4 mg/kg, plasma concentrations of about 300 to 500 ng/ml are attained in 30 minutes and about 300 to 1400 ng/ml in 1 hour falling to about 300 ng/ml at 3 to 24 hours.

DISTRIBUTION. In animals, stored for long periods in kidneys and liver.

EXCRETION. 10 to 30% of a daily dose is excreted in the urine in 24 hours, 50 to 70% of which is excreted in the first 6 hours.

FURTHER INFORMATION. Plasma and urine concentrations—T. P. Waalkes and V. T. DeVita, *J. Lab. clin. Med.*, 1970, **75**, 871 and T. P. Waalkes *et al.*, *Clin. Pharmac. Ther.*, 1970, **11**, 505.

Actions and uses. Pentamidine is used in the prophylaxis and treatment of African trypanosomiasis. It does not attain a trypanocidal concentration in the cerebrospinal fluid after intramuscular injection and is therefore of little value in the treatment of advanced cases in which the central nervous system is involved.

For the treatment of early trypanosomiasis, 300 milligrams of pentamidine isethionate is given daily as a 10% solution by intramuscular or intravenous injection on 7 to 15 successive days; this treatment is frequently supplemented with melarsoprol.

For prophylaxis, a dose of 300 milligrams is given every 3 to 6 months. Before pentamidine is used for prophylaxis in a community, a careful examination should be made to detect patients in whom the disease has advanced beyond the early stages and these must be given a full course of treatment with a drug such as melarsoprol.

Pentamidine is also used in the treatment of visceral leishmaniasis (kala-azar); it is especially valuable in patients who do not respond to treatment with antimony. A dosage of 300 milligrams is given daily or on alternate days until 12 to 15 doses have been given; a second course of treatment may be given 1 or 2 weeks later.

Pentamidine is also used for the treatment of pneumonia caused by *Pneumocystis carinii*. The dose is 300 milligrams daily for 10 to 14 days administered by intramuscular injection. The corresponding dose for children under 1 year is 7.5 milligrams per kilogram body-weight, 1 to 5 years 75 to 120 milligrams, and 6 to 12 years 135 to 225 milligrams.

When pentamidine isethionate is injected the patient should be recumbent and the injection should be given slowly over a period of about 3 minutes.

Undesirable effects. Intravenous injection, if made too rapidly, may produce a profound fall in blood pressure; this hypotensive effect may be prevented by giving the injection very slowly, or it may be relieved by the injection of a vasopressor drug such as adrenaline, noradrenaline, or metaraminol. Pentamidine is better tolerated by intramuscular injection, although it is more painful and there may be swelling at the site of injection. Pentamidine sometimes causes hypoglycaemia, dizziness, tachycardia, flushing, itching, and an increase in blood urea. Abnormal liver-function tests may develop in patients under treatment with pentamidine.

Preparation

PENTAMIDINE INJECTION: a sterile solution of pentamidine isethionate in water for injections. It is prepared by dissolving the contents of a sealed container in water for injections immediately before use. Available as a powder in ampoules containing 200 mg of pentamidine isethionate.
A standard for this injection is given in the British Pharmacopoeia 1973
Containers and *Labelling:* see the entry on Injections for general information on containers and labelling.
Storage: the injection decomposes on storage and should be used immediately after preparation.

Pentazocine

1,2,3,4,5,6-Hexahydro-6,11-dimethyl-3-(3-methylbut-2-enyl)-2,6-methano-3-benzazocin-8-ol

$C_{19}H_{27}NO = 285.4$

OTHER NAME: *Fortral*®

A standard is given in the British Pharmacopoeia Addendum 1975

Description. An odourless white or creamy-white powder.

Solubility. Very slightly soluble in water; soluble, at 20°, in 15 parts of alcohol, in 33 parts of ether, and in 2 parts of chloroform.

Moisture content. Not more than 1%, determined by drying at 60° *in vacuo*.

Dissociation constants. pK_a 8.5, 10 (20°).

Storage. It should be protected from light.

Identification. TESTS. It complies with the tests described under Pentazocine Hydrochloride.

MELTING-POINT. About 152°.

ULTRAVIOLET ABSORPTION. See under Pentazocine Hydrochloride.

INFRA-RED ABSORPTION. Major peaks at 1238, 1264, 1384, 1435, 1454, and 1609 cm^{-1} (see Appendix 2a: Infra-red Spectra).

THIN-LAYER CHROMATOGRAPHY. As for Pentazocine Hydrochloride under Thin-layer Chromatography, System 3.

Determination in body fluids; Metabolism. See under Pentazocine Hydrochloride.

Actions and uses. Pentazocine has the actions described under Pentazocine Hydrochloride. It is administered as the lactate by injection or rectally in suppositories.

The usual dose by intramuscular injection is 30 to 60 milligrams repeated if necessary every 3 or 4 hours. Children may be given 500 micrograms per kilogram body-weight by intravenous injection or 1 milligram per kilogram body-weight by subcutaneous or intramuscular injection. The dose by rectal administration for an adult is 50 milligrams repeated, if necessary, every 6 hours.

Undesirable effects; Precautions; Poisoning. As for Pentazocine Hydrochloride.

Preparations

PENTAZOCINE LACTATE INJECTION (*Syn.* Pentazocine Injection): a sterile solution of pentazocine lactate in water for injections. It is prepared by the interaction of pentazocine and lactic acid. It is sterilised by heating in an autoclave or by filtration.

Available in 1- and 2-ml ampoules containing pentazocine lactate equivalent to 30 mg of pentazocine per ml. *A standard for this injection is given in the British Pharmacopoeia Addendum 1975*

Containers and *Labelling:* see the entry on Injections for general information on containers and labelling.

Storage: it should be protected from light.

PENTAZOCINE SUPPOSITORIES: prepared as described in the entry on Suppositories by incorporating pentazocine lactate in a suitable basis. Available as suppositories containing pentazocine lactate equivalent to 50 mg of pentazocine.

Containers and *Storage:* see the entry on Suppositories for general information on containers and storage.

Advice for patients: see the entry on Suppositories for general information on the use of suppositories. They may cause drowsiness; persons affected should not drive or operate machinery. Alcohol should be avoided.

Pentazocine Hydrochloride

1,2,3,4,5,6 - Hexahydro - 8 - hydroxy - 6,11 - dimethyl - 3 - (3-methylbut - 2 - enyl) - 2,6 - methano - 3 - benzazocinium chloride

$C_{19}H_{28}ClNO = 321.9$

OTHER NAMES: *Fortral*®
Fortagesic® (with paracetamol)

A standard is given in the British Pharmacopoeia Addendum 1975

Description. An odourless, white or pale cream-coloured powder.

Solubility. Soluble, at 20°, in 30 parts of water, in 16 parts of alcohol, and in 4 parts of chloroform; very slightly soluble in ether.

Acidity. A 1% solution has a pH of 4 to 6.

Moisture content. Not more than 1%, determined by drying at 100° *in vacuo*.

Storage. It should be protected from light.

Identification. TESTS. 1. To about 1 mg in a porcelain crucible add 0.5 ml of a 1% solution of ammonium molybdate in sulphuric acid; an intense blue colour is produced which changes to green and, after standing, to yellow.

2. Dissolve about 5 mg in 5 ml of sulphuric acid, add 1 drop of a 9% solution of ferric chloride and mix; a yellow colour is produced. Warm the solution; the colour deepens in intensity. Add 1 drop of nitric acid; the colour is unchanged.

ULTRAVIOLET ABSORPTION. In 0.01N hydrochloric acid, maximum at 278 nm (E1%, 1cm = 61); in 0.1N sodium hydroxide, maxima at 240 nm (E1%, 1cm = 238) and 300 nm (E1%, 1cm = 94).

THIN-LAYER CHROMATOGRAPHY. See under Thin-layer Chromatography, System 3.

Determination in body fluids. GAS CHROMATOGRAPHY. In plasma or urine: pentazocine and metabolites—K. A. Pittman and C. Davidson, *J. pharm. Sci.*, 1973, **62**, 765. In urine—D. P. Vaughan and A. H. Beckett, *J. Pharm. Pharmac.*, 1974, **26**, 789.

SPECTROFLUORIMETRY. In urine—B. Berkowitz and E. L. Way, *Clin. Pharmac. Ther.*, 1969, **10**, 681.

Metabolism. ABSORPTION. Well absorbed after oral, intramuscular, and rectal administration.

BLOOD CONCENTRATION. Subject to considerable variation; after oral administration of 90 mg as the hydrochloride, peak plasma concentrations of 70 to 300 ng/ml are attained in about 2 hours; after rectal administration, plasma concentrations are approximately within the same range; after an intramuscular dose of 45 mg, a peak plasma concentration of about 140 ng/ml is attained in 15 to 20 minutes; blood concentrations may be erratic and after intramuscular or oral administration more than one plasma peak may occur.

HALF-LIFE. Plasma half-life, 2 to 3 hours after intravenous or intramuscular administration; half-life from urinary excretion data, 1.5 to 6.5 hours.

DISTRIBUTION. Volume of distribution, about 200 litres; pentazocine crosses the placenta, appears in cerebrospinal fluid in concentrations reaching 30 to 50% of those in plasma, and is taken up to some extent by red blood cells; *protein binding*, 50 to 75% bound to plasma proteins.

METABOLIC REACTIONS. Extensive oxidation of the methyl groups of the dimethylallyl side-chain to produce hydroxylated and carboxylated metabolites; in man, the cis-hydroxy and the trans-carboxylic acid metabolites are formed; it appears that the trans-hydroxy metabolite is rapidly oxidised to the acid and is not therefore detectable; glucuronic acid conjugation of metabolites and pentazocine also occurs; there appears to be a wide variation in the rate of metabolism of pentazocine and smokers appear to metabolise 40% more pentazocine than non-smokers; this difference is a consequence of enzyme induction; pentazocine may be subject to first pass metabolism.

EXCRETION. Pentazocine excretion in urine is pH-dependent; after an intramuscular dose, 65 to 76% is excreted in the urine in 48 hours; in acid urine in 32 hours, 8 to 25% is excreted unchanged after intravenous administration and 3 to 15% is excreted unchanged after oral administration; 12 to 30% of a dose is excreted as the glucuronide conjugates of pentazocine and its metabolites; the major metabolite appears to be the trans-carboxylic acid; less than 2% of a dose is eliminated in the faeces unchanged in 48 hours.

FURTHER INFORMATION. Absorption and excretion—R. A. P. Burt and A. H. Beckett, *Br. J. Anaesth.*, 1971, **43**, 427; clinical pharmacology—J. P. Payne, *Drugs*, 1973, **5**, 1; influence of smoking on elimination—D. P. Vaughan and A. H. Beckett, *J. Pharm. Pharmac.*, 1974, **26**, 789 and D. P. Vaughan *et al.*, *Br. J. clin. Pharmac.*, 1976, **3**, 279; pharmacokinetics in cerebrospinal fluid—S. Agurell *et al.*, *J. Pharm. Pharmac.*, 1974, **26**, 1; pharmacokinetics in monkeys—K. A. Pittman and G. A. Portmann, *J. pharm. Sci.*, 1974, **63**, 84; protein binding—M. Ehrnebo *et al.*, *Clin. Pharmac. Ther.*, 1974, **16**, 424; review—R. N. Brogden *et al.*, *Drugs*, 1973, **5**, 6.

Actions and uses. Pentazocine hydrochloride is a narcotic antagonist which has analgesic and sedative actions similar to those described under Morphine Hydrochloride. It depresses the respiratory centre and on parenteral administration may cause a transient fall in blood pressure which may be followed by a significant rise. It does not usually produce the sustained hypotension associated with morphine and it is also less liable to give rise to dependence. When given by mouth it is well absorbed, an oral dose having about one-third of the potency of the same dose given by intramuscular injection. There are individual variations in the rate of metabolism of pentazocine administered by mouth.
The usual adult dose is 25 to 100 milligrams by mouth, and for a child aged 6 to 12 years, 25 milligrams by mouth. These doses may be repeated every 3 to 4 hours as required; 1.1 milligrams of pentazocine hydrochloride is approximately equivalent to 1 milligram of pentazocine. Pentazocine may antagonise the effects of opiates and may provoke withdrawal symptoms when given to narcotic addicts. Tolerance to its action may develop.

Undesirable effects. Drowsiness, sweating, dizziness, nausea, vomiting, nightmares, anxiety, and hallucinations may occur. Drug dependence may rarely occur after prolonged administration.

Precautions. It should be given with caution to patients with depressed respiration, raised intracranial pressure, or severe renal or hepatic insufficiency. The effects of pentazocine may be enhanced by alcohol, depressants of the central nervous system, and monoamine-oxidase inhibitors. Since pentazocine may cause respiratory depression in an infant at birth it should not be used during labour.

Poisoning. Naloxone is a specific antagonist for pentazocine, but nalorphine is ineffective for this purpose.

Preparations

PENTAZOCINE TABLETS: available as tablets containing 25 mg of pentazocine hydrochloride; they may be film coated and the coat may be coloured.
A standard for these tablets is given in the British Pharmacopoeia Addendum 1975
Containers and *Storage*: see the entry on Tablets for general information on containers and storage. Containers should be airtight.
Advice for patients: the tablets should preferably be taken after meals. They may cause drowsiness; persons affected should not drive or operate machinery. Alcohol should be avoided.

OTHER PREPARATIONS available include CAPSULES containing pentazocine hydrochloride 50 mg; and TABLETS containing pentazocine hydrochloride equivalent to 15 mg of pentazocine with paracetamol 500 mg.

Pentobarbitone Sodium

Sodium 5-ethyl-5-(1-methylbutyl)barbiturate

$C_{11}H_{17}N_2NaO_3 = 248.3$

OTHER NAMES: *Anaesleep Forte®*; *Euthatal®*; *Euthesate®*; *Expiral®*; *Lethobarb®*; *Nembutal®*; Pentobarbitalum Natricum; Pentobarbital Sodium; *Sagatal®*; Soluble Pentobarbitone
Carbrital® (with carbromal)

A standard is given in the European Pharmacopoeia Vol. III Supplement

Description. Odourless hygroscopic white granules or crystalline powder.

Solubility. Soluble in water and in alcohol; practically insoluble in ether.

Alkalinity. A 10% solution has a pH of 9.6 to 11.

Moisture content. Not more than 3%, determined by drying at 105°.

Dissociation constant. pK_a 8.2 (25°).

Stability; Incompatibility. See under Barbiturates.

Storage. It should be stored in airtight containers.

Identification. TEST. Acidify an aqueous solution with *dilute hydrochloric acid* and extract with ether. The residue obtained after evaporation of the extract complies with general test 1 described under Barbiturates.

MELTING-POINT. The residue obtained in the test, above, after recrystallisation from alcohol (25%), melts at about 128°.

ULTRAVIOLET ABSORPTION. See under Barbiturates.

INFRA-RED ABSORPTION. As pentobarbitone, major peaks at 855, 1220, 1299, 1695, 1724, and 1754 cm^{-1} (see Appendix 2b: Infra-red Spectra).

THIN-LAYER CHROMATOGRAPHY. See under Thin-layer Chromatography, System 5.

Determination in body fluids. See under Barbiturates.

Metabolism. (See also under Barbiturates.) ABSORPTION. Over 90% of the sodium salt is absorbed after oral administration; absorption is delayed but not reduced by the presence of food.

BLOOD CONCENTRATION. After an oral dose of 50 mg of pentobarbitone sodium, given to fasting patients, peak plasma concentrations of about 0.7 μg/ml are attained within 1 hour and a similar dose, given to non-fasting patients, produces peak plasma concentrations of about 1.0 μg/ml in 2.5 hours; after the intravenous administration of 50 mg of the sodium salt, plasma concentrations of 1.2 μg/ml are obtained within 5 minutes which fall to 0.5 μg/ml within 1 hour and to 0.2 μg/ml within 48 hours.

HALF-LIFE. The plasma half-life of the α-phase is 4 hours and for the β-phase 50 hours.

DISTRIBUTION. Pentobarbitone is not taken up by the brain as rapidly, nor does it accumulate to such an extent, as thiopentone; *protein binding*, 50% to plasma albumin.

METABOLIC REACTIONS. Pentobarbitone is metabolised more slowly than thiopentone, mainly by side-chain hydroxylation at the 3'-position followed by possible further oxidation; some ring fission may also occur.

EXCRETION. Of an oral dose, 80% is excreted in the urine within 5 days, 50% as the two stereoisomers of 5-ethyl-5-(3-hydroxy-1-methylbutyl)barbituric acid; more than 5 times as much of the (+)-isomer is excreted as of the (−)-isomer; both the unchanged drug and 5-(3-carboxy-1-methylpropyl)-5-ethylbarbituric acid are also excreted in the urine.

FURTHER INFORMATION. Pharmacokinetics—R. B. Smith *et al.*, *J. Pharmacokinet. Biopharm.*, 1973, **1**, 5.

Actions and uses. Pentobarbitone sodium is an intermediate-acting barbiturate, the actions and uses of which are described under Barbiturates. The usual hypnotic dose is 100 to 200 milligrams.

Pentobarbitone sodium has been used as a basal anaesthetic before surgical operations, its sedative effect on the patient reducing the amount of general anaesthetic required. For this purpose 100 to 200 milligrams may be given by mouth in the evening preceding the operation, and the dose repeated 2 hours before the operation; this may be repeated again 1 hour before the operation if the sedative effect is inadequate.

Pentobarbitone sodium may be given slowly by intravenous injection as an anticonvulsant in the treatment of tetanus or of strychnine poisoning, the dose being 500 milligrams dissolved in 10 millilitres of water for injections. It is also given by mouth or by rectum. Solutions for injection are prepared by an aseptic technique.

Undesirable effects; Precautions; Contra-indications; Dependence. See under Barbiturates.

Poisoning. As for Barbiturates, but haemodialysis is not effective.

Veterinary uses. Pentobarbitone sodium is used as a general anaesthetic in dogs and cats. The usual dose by intravenous injection is 20 to 35 milligrams per kilogram body-weight. Larger doses are used for euthanasia.

Preparations

PENTOBARBITONE CAPSULES (*Syn.* Soluble Pentobarbitone Capsules; Pentobarbital Sodium Capsules): consisting of pentobarbitone sodium, in powder, which may be mixed with a suitable inert diluent, enclosed in a hard capsule. The capsule shells may be coloured. Available as capsules containing 50 and 100 mg of pentobarbitone sodium.
A standard for these capsules is given in the British Pharmacopoeia 1973
Containers and *Storage:* see the entry on Capsules for general information on containers and storage.
Advice for patients: hypnotic doses should be taken half to 1 hour before bedtime. The capsules may cause drowsiness on the following day; persons affected should not drive or operate machinery. Alcohol should be avoided.

PENTOBARBITONE INJECTION (*Syn.* Pentobarbitone Sodium Injection): a sterile solution of pentobarbitone sodium in a suitable vehicle. It is sterilised by filtration. Available in 100-ml packs containing 60 mg of pentobarbitone sodium per ml. Also available in 100-ml vials containing 200 mg of pentobarbitone sodium per ml for animal euthanasia; such solutions need not be sterile and may be coloured.
A standard for this injection is given in the British Pharmacopoeia (Veterinary)
Containers and *Labelling:* see the entry on Injections for general information on containers and labelling.

PENTOBARBITONE TABLETS (*Syn.* Soluble Pentobarbitone Tablets; Pentobarbital Sodium Tablets).
A standard for these tablets is given in the British Pharmacopoeia 1973
Containers and *Storage:* see the entry on Tablets for general information on containers and storage. Containers should be airtight.
Advice for patients: see above under Pentobarbitone Capsules.

OTHER PREPARATIONS available include CAPSULES containing pentobarbitone sodium 100 mg with carbromal 250 mg.

Pentolinium Tartrate

Pentamethylenebis(1-methylpyrrolidinium hydrogen tartrate)

$C_{23}H_{42}N_2O_{12} = 538.6$

OTHER NAME: *Ansolysen®*

A standard is given in the British Pharmacopoeia 1973

Description. An odourless white powder with an acidic taste.

Solubility. Soluble, at 20°, in less than 1 part of water and in 800 parts of alcohol; practically insoluble in ether and in chloroform.

Acidity. A 1% solution is acid to *litmus solution*.

Moisture content. Not more than 2%, determined by drying at 105°.

Sterilisation. Solutions for injection are sterilised by heating in an autoclave or by filtration.

Storage. It should be stored in airtight containers, in a cool place.

Identification. TEST. Dissolve about 50 mg in 10 ml of water and add 10 ml of *trinitrophenol solution*; a precipitate is produced which, after washing with water, melts at about 270°.

MELTING-POINT. About 206°, with decomposition.

Actions and uses. Pentolinium tartrate is a ganglion-blocking agent which inhibits the transmission of nerve impulses in both sympathetic and parasympathetic ganglia by raising the threshold of the ganglion cell to the acetylcholine released at preganglionic nerve endings. The sympathetic block produces peripheral dilatation, which causes increased blood flow, raised skin temperature, and reduced blood pressure. The parasympathetic block diminishes movement of the gastro-intestinal tract and bladder, reduces gastric and salivary secretion, and produces disturbances of visual accommodation.

Pentolinium has been used in severe or malignant hypertension but it has been largely replaced by drugs that selectively block sympathetic nerve transmission and do not produce the effects of parasympathetic blockade. As it is poorly and erratically absorbed from the gastro-intestinal tract it should not be given by mouth. It may be administered by subcutaneous injection; the usual initial dose is 2.5 milligrams, and this may be increased by amounts of 0.5 to 1 milligram until the dose is effective.

To reduce side-effects, a smaller dose may be given in conjunction with reserpine (100 micrograms) or chlorothiazide (500 milligrams).

Pentolinium tartrate is given in the emergency treatment of hypertensive encephalopathy and eclampsia in a dose of 2 milligrams by subcutaneous injection; this dose may be repeated after 15 minutes if the response is not satisfactory.

Undesirable effects. Constipation, dryness of the mouth, blurring of vision, and retention of urine may occur, but disappear when the drug is withdrawn.

Contra-indications. Pentolinium is contra-indicated in patients with pyloric stenosis. As with all potent hypotensives it may enhance severe renal or cerebral vascular insufficiency.

Poisoning. Patients with severe hypotension should be placed in the supine position with the feet raised, and if necessary the blood pressure should be increased by an infusion of noradrenaline injection or by intramuscular injection of metaraminol.

Preparations

PENTOLINIUM INJECTION: a sterile solution of pentolinium tartrate in water for injections. The acidity of the solution is adjusted to pH 6.5 by the addition of sodium hydroxide. It is sterilised by heating in an autoclave or by filtration. Available in 10-ml bottles containing 5 mg of pentolinium tartrate per ml.

A standard for this injection is given in the British Pharmacopoeia 1973

Containers and *Labelling:* see the entry on Injections for general information on containers and labelling.

Peppermint Oil

Obtained by distillation from the fresh flowering tops of *Mentha* × *piperita* L. (Fam. Labiatae), a herb growing wild throughout Europe and cultivated in England, France, Italy, Bulgaria, Morocco, and America.

OTHER NAMES: Oleum Menthae Piperitae; Menthae Piperitae Aetheroleum

A standard is given in the European Pharmacopoeia Vol. III

Varieties. There are two varieties of peppermint, black peppermint and white peppermint, the former yielding more oil than the latter, but of a less delicate aroma. The oil is rectified if necessary. The odour and taste afford the best indication of the quality of the oil and by this means it is possible to distinguish between English, American, and other types of oils.

Constituents. Peppermint oil contains chiefly menthol, menthone, menthyl acetate, and terpenes. Menthofuran and other minor constituents contribute to the quality of the odour and flavour. Dimethyl sulphide is present in unrectified oil.

Description. A colourless, pale yellow, or greenish-yellow liquid having the odour of peppermint. It has a pungent and aromatic taste, followed by a sensation of cold.

Solubility. Soluble, at 20°, in 4 parts of alcohol (70%) with a slight opalescence, and in 0.5 part of alcohol (90%), the solution sometimes becoming turbid on adding more of the solvent; miscible with dehydrated alcohol.

Weight per ml. At 20°, 0.897 to 0.910 g.

Refractive index. 1.460 to 1.467.

Optical rotation. −16° to −30°.

Adulterants and substitutes. Japanese, Chinese, Formosan (Taiwan), and Brazilian mint oils obtained from varietal forms of *M. arvensis* L. are the richest of all in menthol, sometimes containing 85%. Oils of these varieties are commonly partially dementholised; they still contain about 50% of menthol and may occur as adulterants.

Stability. It darkens in colour and becomes viscous on keeping. On cooling to a low temperature, separation of menthol occurs, especially when a few crystals of this substance are added to start crystallisation.

Storage. It should be stored in well-filled airtight containers, in a cool place, protected from light.

Identification. TEST. Mix in a dry test-tube 3 drops of the oil with 5 ml of a mixture containing 1 volume of nitric acid and 300 volumes of glacial acetic acid, and place the tube in a beaker of boiling water; a blue colour develops within 5 minutes. Continue heating; the colour deepens and shows a copper-coloured fluorescence, and finally fades, leaving a golden-yellow solution (distinction from other mint oils).

Actions and uses. Peppermint oil is a carminative and is used in a dosage of 0.05 to 0.2 millilitre. It may be administered on sugar or in tablets or lozenges. Peppermint oil has mildly antiseptic properties; it is used to flavour dental preparations.

Preparations

CONCENTRATED PEPPERMINT EMULSION:

Peppermint oil	..	..	..	..	20 ml
Polysorbate 20	..	..	..	..	1 ml
Chloroform water, double-strength		..	..	500 ml
Purified water, freshly boiled and cooled	..	..	..	..	to 1000 ml

Shake the peppermint oil with the polysorbate 20.

Add gradually the double-strength chloroform water, and sufficient of the purified water to produce the required volume, shaking well after each addition.

When diluted with 39 times its volume of freshly boiled and cooled purified water, a preparation equivalent in strength to *peppermint water* is produced.

Containers: the general direction to supply emulsions in wide-mouthed bottles does not apply to this preparation.

Labelling: see the entry on Emulsions for general information on labelling.

Dose: 0.25 to 1 millilitre.

CONCENTRATED PEPPERMINT WATER (*Syn.* Aq. Menth. Pip. Conc.):

Peppermint oil	20 ml
Alcohol (90%)	600 ml
Purified water, freshly boiled and cooled	to 1000 ml

Dissolve the peppermint oil in the alcohol and sufficient of the water in successive small quantities to produce the required volume, shaking vigorously after each addition. Add 50 g of sterilised purified talc or other suitable filtering aid, shake, allow to stand for a few hours, shaking occasionally, and filter.

When diluted with 39 times its volume of freshly boiled and cooled purified water, *peppermint water* is produced (*Syn.* Aq. Menth. Pip.).

Dose: 0.25 to 1 millilitre.

PEPPERMINT SPIRIT (*Syn.* Essence of Peppermint; Spiritus Menthae Piperitae):

Peppermint oil	100 ml
Alcohol (90%)	to 1000 ml

Dissolve; if the solution is not clear, shake with sterilised purified talc, and filter.

A standard for this spirit is given in the British Pharmaceutical Codex 1973

Dose: 0.3 to 2 millilitres.

OTHER PREPARATIONS: peppermint oil is an ingredient of compound magnesium trisilicate tablets and compound sodium bicarbonate tablets. It is also an ingredient of many other preparations.

Peptic Ulceration

A peptic ulcer is loss of tissue of the mucosa, submucosa, and muscularis mucosae occurring in regions of the digestive tract exposed to gastric juice.

Peptic ulcers may occur in the lower oesophagus, the stomach, and the duodenum. Stress and trauma may be precipitating factors, as also may aspirin and many other anti-inflammatory drugs that have an irritant effect on the gastric mucosa.

Chronic peptic ulceration is characterised by dyspepsia, pain at varying times in relation to meals or when hungry, and sometimes vomiting and haematemesis. Ulceration is caused by the action of pepsin and hydrochloric acid on the gastric mucosa which may also have a reduced resistance to this condition.

Treatment consists of rest, removal of gastric irritants, restriction of smoking, and the taking of frequent meals which buffer the acid. Treatment with antacids relieves pain and by reducing the activity of pepsin may allow ulcers to heal. Anticholinergic drugs may be used to reduce gastric secretion and spasm especially at night. The minimum effective dose should be administered to reduce troublesome side-effects. There is little evidence that they have a sustained action in reducing stomach acid or that they increase ulcer healing. They should never be used when there is a risk of pyloric obstruction.

Carbenoxolone is used to promote healing of gastric ulcers in the ambulant patient, but because of its adverse effects special care and precautions are needed in the elderly and those with cardiovascular and renal disease. H_2-receptor antagonists such as cimetidine are potent inhibitors of gastric acid secretion and may be used in the treatment of peptic ulceration.

Surgery may be necessary when there is severe haemorrhage, malignancy, stenosis, or failure of ulcers to heal.

Antacids used in the treatment of peptic ulceration include aluminium hydroxide, aluminium phosphate, bismuth carbonate, calcium carbonate, chalk, magnesium carbonate, magnesium hydroxide, magnesium trisilicate, and sodium bicarbonate.

Anticholinergics used in the treatment of peptic ulceration include atropine, belladonna, dicyclomine, hyoscine, mebeverine, hyoscyamus, orphenadrine, oxyphencyclimine, poldine, procyclidine, and propantheline.

Drugs with a healing effect on gastric ulcers include carbenoxolone and liquorice derivatives.

Peritoneal Dialysis

see under DIALYSIS

Perphenazine

2-{4-[3-(2-Chlorophenothiazin-10-yl)propyl]piperazin-1-yl}ethanol

$C_{21}H_{26}ClN_3OS = 404.0$

OTHER NAMES: *Fentazin*®
Triptafen® (with amitriptyline hydrochloride)

A standard is given in the British Pharmacopoeia 1973

Description. An almost odourless white or creamy-white powder with a bitter taste.

Solubility. Very slightly soluble in water; soluble, at 20°, in 20 parts of alcohol, in 80 parts of ether, and in 1 part of chloroform; soluble in dilute hydrochloric acid.

Dissociation constant. pK_a 7.8 (24°).

Sterilisation. Solutions for injection are sterilised by heating in an autoclave or by filtration.

Storage. It should be protected from light.

Identification. TESTS. 1. Dissolve about 5 mg in 2 ml of sulphuric acid and allow to stand for 5 minutes; a red colour is produced.

2. Dissolve about 10 mg in 5 ml of methyl alcohol and add 10 ml of a mixture containing 4 volumes of sulphuric acid and 1 volume of methyl alcohol; a pink colour is

produced. Add 2 drops of *ferric ammonium sulphate solution;* a reddish-purple colour is produced.

MELTING-POINT. About 98°.

ULTRAVIOLET ABSORPTION. In 0.1N hydrochloric acid, maxima at 256 nm (E1%, 1cm = 788) and 307 nm (E1%, 1cm = 106).

INFRA-RED ABSORPTION. Major peaks at 757, 917, 1145, 1294, 1404, and 1456 cm^{-1} (see Appendix 2a: Infra-red Spectra).

THIN-LAYER CHROMATOGRAPHY. See under Thin-layer Chromatography, System 9.

Determination in body fluids. ULTRAVIOLET SPECTRO-PHOTOMETRY. In blood, serum, or urine: general method for phenothiazines—J. E. Wallace and J. D. Biggs, *J. pharm. Sci.,* 1971, **60**, 1346.

GAS CHROMATOGRAPHY. In plasma: perphenazine and its sulphoxide metabolite—N.-E. Larsen and J. Naestoft, *J. Chromat.,* 1975, **109**, 259.

Actions and uses. Perphenazine has the actions and uses described under Chlorpromazine Hydrochloride but it is effective in much smaller doses, produces less sedation, and has a greater tendency to produce parkinsonism.

In psychotic patients the usual effective daily dosage by mouth is 12 to 24 milligrams and 5 to 15 milligrams daily by intramuscular injection. In the treatment of psychoneurosis, nausea, and vomiting, the daily dosage by mouth is usually 2 to 12 milligrams and should not exceed 24 milligrams. For the immediate relief of acute symptoms doses of 5 to 10 milligrams may be given by intramuscular injection at six-hourly intervals, the route being changed as soon as possible to oral administration.

For the prevention of post-operative vomiting 8 milligrams is given by mouth as a single dose prior to induction of anaesthesia. Vomiting arising from radiation therapy or occurring during pregnancy may be controlled by a dosage of 4 milligrams by mouth 3 times a day.

To control acute alcoholic psychosis 5 to 10 milligrams is given by intramuscular injection and to allay withdrawal symptoms during the treatment of addiction to drugs or alcohol 5 milligrams is given by intramuscular injection at six-hourly intervals for 24 hours, followed by 8 milligrams by mouth 3 times a day.

Undesirable effects. At therapeutic dosage levels, perphenazine rarely produces undesirable effects. However, extrapyramidal dysfunction, exhibited as pseudo-parkinsonism, may occur. At higher dosage levels, it may provoke extrapyramidal symptoms, such as dystonia and parkinsonism; these symptoms can be relieved or controlled by reducing the dosage or by using an anti-parkinsonism drug.

Poisoning. The procedure described under Chlorpromazine Hydrochloride should be adopted.

Veterinary uses. Perphenazine is used as a tranquilliser, motion sickness remedy, and pre-anaesthetic medication. The usual dose for dogs and cats is 800 micrograms per kilogram body-weight by mouth twice daily and 300 micrograms per kilogram body-weight by intramuscular injection.

Preparations

PERPHENAZINE INJECTION: a sterile solution of perphenazine, with suitable buffering and stabilising agents, in water for injections free from dissolved air. The solution is distributed into the final containers, the air in the containers is replaced with nitrogen or other suitable gas, and the containers are sealed and sterilised by heating in an autoclave. Alternatively, the solution is sterilised by filtration, distributed by means of an aseptic technique into sterile final containers, the air in the containers is replaced with sterile nitrogen or other suitable gas, and the containers are sealed. Available in 1-ml ampoules containing 5 mg of perphenazine.

A standard for this injection is given in the British Pharmacopoeia (Veterinary)

Containers and *Labelling:* see the entry on Injections for general information on containers and labelling.

Storage: it should be protected from light.

PERPHENAZINE TABLETS: available as tablets containing 2, 4, and 8 mg of perphenazine; they are sugar coated.

A standard for these tablets is given in the British Pharmacopoeia 1973

Containers and *Storage:* see the entry on Tablets for general information on containers and storage. Containers should be airtight.

Advice for patients: the tablets may cause drowsiness; persons affected should not drive or operate machinery. Alcohol should be avoided.

OTHER PREPARATIONS available include a SOLUTION containing perphenazine 10 mg in 5 ml, supplied only to hospitals, for preparing dilutions with unpreserved syrup; TABLETS containing perphenazine 2 mg with amitriptyline hydrochloride 10 mg, tablets containing perphenazine 2 mg with amitriptyline hydrochloride 25 mg, and tablets containing perphenazine 4 mg with amitriptyline hydrochloride 25 mg.

Pertussis Vaccine

A sterile suspension of killed *Bordetella pertussis.* It contains not less than 4 units per ml.

OTHER NAMES: Per/Vac; Vaccinum Pertussis; Whooping-cough Vaccine

A standard is given in the European Pharmacopoeia Vol. II

Storage. It should be stored as described under Vaccines. Under these conditions it may be expected to retain its potency for 2 years.

Actions and uses. Pertussis vaccine is used for active immunisation against whooping-cough, but it is best used in the form of the combined diphtheria, tetanus, and pertussis vaccine. Whooping-cough is most dangerous in early life, and the first dose of the vaccine should be injected when the infant is 3 months old. Pertussis vaccine should not normally be administered after the age of 3 years.

The vaccine is administered by intramuscular or deep subcutaneous injection of 0.5 or 1 millilitre as stated on the label as the dose. A suitable schedule for the immunisation of children is given under Vaccines. Reactions to the vaccine in children are usually mild, but a very few severe reactions such as encephalopathy may occur. The vaccine should therefore not be administered to children with a history or family history of convulsions, epilepsy, disorders of the central nervous system, or severe allergy.

Pessaries

Pessaries are solid bodies suitably shaped for vaginal administration and containing medicaments which are usually intended to act locally. They may be prepared by moulding, as described in the entry on Suppositories, or by compression, as described in the entry on Tablets. Moulded pessaries are usually bluntly conical in shape. Theobroma oil, glycerol suppositories mass of the British Pharmacopoeia, or other suitable basis, such as fractionated palm kernel oil or a hydrogenated vegetable oil, may be used. Bases containing gelatin should be maintained at 100° for 1 hour, replacing any water lost by evaporation, before incorporating the other ingredients. Bases should be formulated so that the pessaries melt at or slightly below 37°.

For pessaries intended to be used in tropical or subtropical climates, the amount of gelatin in the glycerol suppositories mass may be increased to an amount not exceeding 18% w/w to meet conditions of temperature, but the amounts of active ingredients must in all cases be maintained.

Compressed pessaries are usually prepared in the form of a diamond, almond, wedge, disk, or other suitably shaped tablet. They may be manufactured by the moist-granulation or direct-compression techniques using diluents, disintegrating agents, moistening agents, and lubricants as described in the entry on Tablets.

Containers. Moulded pessaries should be dispensed in partitioned boxes, in shallow boxes lined with waxed paper, or in suitable plastic containers. When intended for use in tropical or subtropical climates or when containing volatile ingredients, pessaries should be wrapped separately in metal foil or enclosed in a suitable form of strip packing.

For compressed pessaries the directions given in the entry on Tablets should be followed.

Storage. They should be stored in a cool place.

Administration. The pessary should be inserted high into the vagina with a suitable applicator. It is usually preferable to insert the pessary shortly before retiring to help retain it in the desired position.

Pesticides

Pesticides are substances used to destroy organisms that are a nuisance or cause injury or damage to crops, stored products, livestock, or man. Most pesticides are used to protect plant crops grown for food; such pesticides include insecticides, fungicides, herbicides, and rodenticides. These groups may then be further subdivided according to mode of action or chemical type. In the following pages pesticides are classified in this way and examples of each type are given with brief information on their properties and uses. Usually the LD_{50} by oral administration to rats is given as a guide to toxicity, but undue reliance should not be placed on this information because the toxicity in other species and by other routes may be different.

In this entry the information relates mainly to the use of pesticides in agriculture. Pesticides are, however, widely used in animal treatment. They are also used for the elimination of ectoparasites from human patients. Information on such uses is included in separate entries on selected pesticides.

Storage of pesticides. Pesticides should be stored in a dry place, preferably above floor level, and protected from extremes of temperature, especially frost, which may adversely affect liquid formulations. Most pesticides are formulated to retain efficiency for at least 2 years under normal storage conditions.

They should be stored in containers which do not interact with the pesticide and the label should clearly indicate the toxic nature of the contents. No container should be used which might lead to the pesticide being mistaken for food or drink. Pesticides should be stored in a locked place to prevent access by unauthorised persons, especially children, and by animals and birds.

Disposal of residues. Pesticide containers should be thoroughly washed out and the washings included with the spray solution. Some paper packs and plastic containers, depending on the chemical concerned, may be burned. Those which may not be burned should be buried in an isolated place and the area fenced off if necessary. Containers that have been used for pesticides should never be used for any other purpose.

Unwanted pesticides must be disposed of safely in accordance with any legal restrictions so that they do not cause danger to man or animals or pollute any water supply. The Code of Practice for the Disposal of Unwanted Pesticides and Containers on Farms and Holdings, published by the Ministry of Agriculture, Fisheries, and Food, should be followed.

In certain situations the local authority must be notified, especially with regard to possible contamination of water supplies.

Application of pesticides. The way in which a pesticide is applied depends on the pest itself, the nature of the organism being protected, and the physical properties of the pesticide.

The commonest way in which pesticides are applied is in the form of a spray. The scale ranges in size from a hand aerosol to use of aerial spraying from aircraft. The technique basically consists of forcing a liquid solution, emulsion, or suspension of the pesticide out of orifices designed so that droplets are formed which become a mist and fall onto the crop. Pesticides which are suitable for application by spraying are usually supplied in solid or liquid concentrated forms which are then diluted or suspended in the appropriate liquid. Water is often the most suitable liquid but sometimes others such as kerosene are used. Surface-active agents are usually included in formulations.

Several different spraying techniques are used:

High-volume spraying. It is desirable that the area treated should be covered with a complete film of pesticidal liquid. It is used for pesticides having a direct contact action and where the maximum possible coverage is required.

Low-volume spraying. It is not essential that the area treated should be completely covered with a film of pesticidal liquid. Low-volume spraying at low pressure gives fewer, larger droplets over a given area and can be used for translocated and residual poisons. The advantages of low-volume over high-volume spraying are that it is quicker, less wasteful of water, and easier to handle. There are, however, greater difficulties due to drift onto areas other than the one being sprayed. The problems of ensuring adequate coverage and possible incompatibilities arising from the greater concentration of pesticides present must always be considered.

Pesticides may also be applied in the form of dusts or powders. These are dilutions of the pesticide mixed with or adsorbed upon an inert solid powder, such as kieselguhr, which is then spread over the area to be covered. They are not as useful as sprays when applied to plant foliage but may be used in situations where water is scarce and if the plants are damp with dew or rain.

When applied in dusts, pesticides are usually less phytotoxic than in sprays. There are, however, disadvantages in the use of dusts such as loss of accuracy in dosage, danger of drift, waste, possible caking on storage, and difficulties in dilution.

Granules of inert materials with pesticides absorbed on their surfaces are used for application to soil or foliage. They overcome the problem of drift associated with dusts and sprays but accurate dosage is not possible. Granules are often used for the application of systemic poisons in broadleaf crops and in woodlands.

There are several minor ways in which pesticides may be applied. *Fumigants* are pesticides which are vaporised by burning. They are used in soil or enclosed spaces such as greenhouses. Pesticides are also used as dips and drenches for protecting individual plant seedlings, seed dressings to protect the seed and young seedlings from pest attack, and baits in which pesticides are mixed with appropriate food material attractive to the pest.

For use against parasites such as lice on animals, pesticides are usually incorporated in creams, dips, dusting-powders, liniments, lotions, ointments, and shampoos.

Most pesticides are supplied in a form ready to use or with clear instructions for preparing a usable form. Thorough mixing is necessary if the pesticide has to be diluted.

Metabolism and degradation of pesticides. Most pesticides are converted after application to their degradation products by the effects of the environment. Oxidation is a common reaction and several different types of compounds may be formed such as epoxides and *N*-oxides. Hydrolysis, which often occurs, is also a reaction leading to breakdown of the pesticide, for example the pyrethrum esters, the carbamates, and some organophosphorus compounds readily undergo hydrolysis. Other reactions which occur more slowly are reduction and dehydrochlorination. Applied pesticides may be metabolised in the plant or animal. The products of metabolism are of similar chemical nature to those produced by environmental breakdown. The products formed are usually less toxic than the initial pesticide and eventually are degraded further.

Some pesticides, however, especially the organochlorine compounds, are very resistant to any form of breakdown and may persist in detectable amounts for months or even years.

Hazards in the use of pesticides. *Injury to man and animals.* A degree of risk of direct or indirect injury from a pesticide exists for all those involved at each stage of its use in research, manufacture, formulation, handling, mixing, and application, and for those who consume the crop. Hazards may also arise from thoughtless disposal of residues.

Direct injury can be caused by ingestion, inhalation, or skin contamination and can be acute or chronic. Permanent disability or even death may result from effects like suppression of respiration or excessive stimulation of the central nervous system. Lachrymation, irritation, dermatitis, and allergies are fairly common unpleasant effects following contact with pesticides.

One of the unforeseen effects of the use of pesticides has been the production of infertile eggs by birds of prey due to their ingestion of the organochlorines from the fat of animals which have been fed plants treated with these pesticides. Chronic effects take several years to become apparent and the trend has been in recent years to use less persistent pesticides.

Indirect injury comes through the general contamination of the environment by persistent pesticides and the breakdown products of other pesticides. Some pesticides, particularly the organochlorine compounds, accumulate in fatty tissue whilst others are very resistant to removal from the crops to which they are applied. Pesticide residues may, therefore, become part of the food chain.

Residues can also affect man and animals by contamination of the water supply by run-off from land which has been treated with pesticides. Pesticides have often been the cause of interference and upset of the balance of nature which has led to many ecological problems. Fish are very susceptible to many pesticides and care must be taken to prevent any run-off from the land into water containing them.

Birds which eat insects or seeds which may have been treated with pesticides, and beneficial insects which either eat insect pests or pollinate crops are two other types of wildlife which must be given special consideration when reviewing the possible effects of using a pesticide.

Injury to plants. One of the main hazards involved in the use of pesticides is that of drift. This occurs when a crop is sprayed or dusted with a pesticide and air currents carry the fine droplets or particles to another crop which might be susceptible to the pesticide.

Some pesticides can also have a phytotoxic action on the crop to which they are applied; phytotoxic action is usually seen as a scorched appearance of the foliage. Pesticide residues in the soil may harm the microorganisms present and thus alter many of their activities such as nitrogen fixation. Residues on crops may also cause tainting both directly when the crops are eaten or indirectly in the taste of animal meat or milk obtained from animals which have been fed on the crop.

Some poisonous plants are rendered more palatable to livestock by the action of certain herbicides thus indirectly having an injurious effect upon the animals. Examples are given in individual statements on pesticides.

Injury to property. Property is susceptible to damage by pesticides, especially those which are inflammable or are oxidising agents. Some pesticides may also stain or corrode the machinery used to apply them or the places where they are stored.

Pest resistance. Many pests have become resistant through natural selection to the highly persistent pesticides. Such resistance is more likely to occur with insects having a short life-cycle. Because of the widespread resistance to some of the organochlorine insecticides, their use has been largely discontinued.

Precautions and safety measures. Preparations should be diluted and applied in accordance with official requirements or the manufacturer's recommendations. Between application of the pesticide and permitting access to the area, harvesting of the crop, or other appropriate procedure, sufficient time must elapse for the substance to have been eliminated or for its concentration to have been reduced to a level considered to be safe. Minimum periods may also be necessary for some pesticides which, although much less dangerous, may taint the crop.

Many of the hazards involved in the use of pesticides can be avoided by care and adherence to instructions. Constant vigilance needs to be maintained in order to detect chronic toxic effects due to the pesticide. In the United Kingdom, advisory leaflets on the use of pesticides are issued by the Ministry of Agriculture, Fisheries, and Food. General advice can be summarised as follows:

(i) Carefully read the label and comply with its instructions.

(ii) Use the least persistent effective pesticide for the purpose required and where possible the least toxic to bees.

(iii) Avoid risk of drift by consideration of the weather conditions and prevent contamination of water supplies.

(iv) Dispose of residues and containers safely.

(v) Store pesticides away from general access by public and animals.

(vi) Wash the body and clean the clothes after use of pesticides.

(vii) Carefully maintain the machinery used and keep equipment clean.

The possibility of phytotoxicity, crop tainting, pest resistance and toxicity to wildlife should be checked by reference to a list of approved products and by consultation with an expert adviser.

Legal requirements. In most countries pesticides are subject to legal control, and any statutory regulations covering such matters as manufacture, distribution, storage, labelling, and use must be duly complied with. In addition to legal safeguards the following two schemes are in operation in the United Kingdom.

Pesticides Safety Precautions Scheme. Under this scheme, which was introduced in 1957, manufacturers have undertaken to provide extensive data and information concerning the properties and hazards of any new pesticide or new formulation or new use of an existing pesticide. Clearance for marketing is given when the appropriate authority, advised by the Advisory Committee on Pesticides, is satisfied that the product can be used without risk to people or livestock and with a minimum of risk to wildlife provided that suitable precautions are taken. Appropriate recommendations are then issued by the Ministry of Agriculture, Fisheries, and Food. The scheme provides for the review and possible withdrawal of a permitted substance if necessary.

Agricultural Chemicals Approval Scheme. This deals with the efficiency of pesticides. Proprietary brands are listed as a guide to users and the list is reviewed and published annually as a list of *Approved Products for Farmers and Growers.* Pesticides included in the list must first have been cleared under the pesticides safety precautions scheme. The list emphasises cases where special caution is required such as toxicity to bees and defines the interval between application and harvesting of the crop or between application and access to grazing animals.

Further information on pesticides. British Crop Protection Council, *Insecticide and Fungicide Handbook,* 4th Edn, H. Martin (Ed.), London, Blackwell Scientific Publications, 1972; British Crop Protection Council, *Pesticide Manual,* 5th Edn, H. Martin and C. R. Worthing (Eds), Droitwich, British Crop Protection Council, 1977; British Crop Protection Council, *Weed Control Handbook,* 5th Edn, J. D. Fryers and S. A. Evans (Eds), Oxford, Blackwell Scientific Publications, 1968; Ministry of Agriculture, Fisheries, and Food, *Approved Products for Farmers and Growers,* London, HM Stationery Office, 1978.

Insecticides

These include substances which kill insects or related forms of animal life such as mites. Substances that kill mites are sometimes called acaricides. Insecticides may be classified on the basis of mode of action or chemical type.

Classification According to Mode of Action

(i) *Stomach poisons.* After these are applied to the insect's food plant they are eaten together with the plant material if the insect has biting, chewing, or rasping mouth parts. They enter the blood stream through the thin peritrophic membrane in the mid gut and are thus distributed throughout the insect. Stomach poisons are not very effective against insects that feed by piercing or by sucking plant juice.

(ii) *Contact poisons.* These enter the body of the insect through its skin while it walks or crawls over a surface to which the insecticide has been applied. Although most of the insect is covered by a hard impermeable exoskeleton, it has vulnerable parts, which are the spiracles through which the gaseous exchange takes place and the cracks in the skeleton where the body and limbs are segmented. Soft-bodied insects and especially insect larvae are the most susceptible to this type of insecticide. Some preparations of contact poisons contain an additive which scratches or dissolves the protective surface of the exoskeleton and allows easier penetration of the insecticide.

Residual contact poisons are very resistant to breakdown by environmental factors after they are applied and therefore toxic residues remain for a considerable time. This has been the cause of environmental problems.

(iii) *Fumigants.* Fumigants are released into the atmosphere as a gas, fine-particle suspension, or aerosol so that they enter the insect's respiratory system via the spiracles. They are generally used only in confined spaces in order to achieve a sufficient concentration in the atmosphere.

(iv) *Systemic insecticides.* In this context the term "systemic" refers to the host plant or animal. Systemic insecticides are absorbed by the host plant and consequently, when the insect eats the plant, it also ingests the poison. Limited translocation facilities mean that this method is less suitable for plants than animals, but where it can be applied it is especially useful against sucking insects such as aphids. Other advantages are that only the insect species that feed on the host plants are affected, and further that it is not necessary to spray the entire plant when only a specific part of it may be damaged by the insects.

(v) *Ovicides.* These are especially toxic to the eggs of insects.

Chemical Classification

Several different types of chemical compound are used. The three most widely used groups are the organochlorine, the organophosphorus, and the naturally occurring organic compounds.

Organochlorine compounds. These were one of the first types of synthetic insecticide developed and, especially in the form of dicophane (DDT), have been extensively used. They have a high lipid solubility and owing to their low volatility are very persistent. They act as contact poisons causing stimulation of the central nervous system and lack of co-ordination in the insect. Some organochlorine compounds also act as stomach poisons.

Because of their high persistence and accumulation in lipid tissue, which causes chronic poisoning, the use of organochlorine compounds has been severely restricted in many parts of the world. Use has also been curtailed because of the development of resistance to them in many species of insect pest. This is especially true of dicophane. A more volatile and, therefore, less persistent organochlorine compound which is widely used is gamma benzene hexachloride. As well as being used for agricultural purposes, it is used in human medicine to destroy insect parasites.

The symptoms of acute poisoning by organochlorine compounds are vomiting, giddiness, fatigue, and paraesthesia, followed by tremors, convulsions, and coma. Chronic poisoning is also a hazard and early symptoms are loss of appetite, muscular weakness, and an apprehensive mental state. Continued exposure may lead to liver and kidney damage.

All the organochlorine pesticides consist of chlorinated cyclic compounds which may be saturated or unsaturated. The following examples show the range of chemical structures encountered.

ALDRIN (*Alderstan®*; *Aldrex®*). 1,2,3,4,10,10-Hexachloro-1,4,4a,5,8,8a-hexahydro-*exo*-1,4-*endo*-5,8-dimethanonaphthalene. Practically insoluble in water; soluble in ether. Used as a stomach poison only against insects which attack roots. LD_{50} (rats) 67 mg/kg. Available as a dust containing 2% and as a concentrate containing 30%.

DICOFOL (*Kelthane®*). 2,2,2-Trichloro-1,1-di(4-chlorophenyl)ethanol. Practically insoluble in water. Used as an acaricide against strawberry and red spider mites. LD_{50} (rats) 809 mg/kg. Minimum period between application and harvesting of the crop 7 days. Available as liquid concentrate containing 20%.

DICOPHANE (DDT; *Deestan®*; *Didi-Col®*; *Didimac®*; *Vitanol®*) (see also separate entry). Has been used as a stomach and contact poison against many insects. Very persistent; usage now limited to situations in which no other pesticide is effective. LD_{50} (rats) 113 mg/kg. Harmful to bees, fish, and livestock. May damage certain crops. Minimum period between application and harvesting of the crop or allowing livestock access to treated areas 2 weeks. Available as dusts containing from 1 to 10% and wettable powders containing from 20 to 50%.

DIELDRIN (*Dilstan®*). 1,2,3,4,10,10-Hexachloro-6,7-epoxy-1,4,4a,5,6,7,8,8a-octahydro-*exo*-1,4-*endo*-5,8-dimethanonaphthalene. Practically insoluble in water; soluble, at 25°, in 4 parts of alcohol, in 1 part of methyl alcohol, in 40 parts of carbon tetrachloride, and in most aromatic hydrocarbons. Used against cabbage root fly. LD_{50} (rats) 46 mg/kg. Harmful to fish. Available as a liquid concentrate containing 15%.

ENDOSULFAN (*Thiodan®*). 6,7,8,9,10,10-Hexachloro-1,5,5a,6,9,9a-hexahydro-6,9-methano-2,4,3-benzodioxathiepin 3-oxide. Used as an acaricide especially on black currants and strawberries. LD_{50} (rats) 110 mg/kg. Dangerous to fish, bees, and livestock. Minimum period between application and harvesting of the crop 6 weeks, and between application and allowing livestock access to treated areas 3 weeks. Available as an emulsifiable concentrate containing 35%.

GAMMA BENZENE HEXACHLORIDE (*Gamma-Col®*; *Gammalex®*; *Gammalin®*; *Gammexane®*; *Kotol®*; *Leytosan®*; Lindane; *Mergamma®*; *Strykol®*) (see also separate entry). Used as a systemic and contact poison against many insects and as a seed dressing. Persistent. LD_{50} (rats) 88 mg/kg. Dangerous to bees, fish, and livestock. Minimum period between application and harvesting of the crop or allowing livestock access to treated areas 2 weeks. Available as a dust containing 0.65%, liquid concentrates containing up to 20%, and as smokes.

TETRADIFON (*Tedion®*). 2,4,4',5-Tetrachlorodiphenyl sulphone. Soluble in 5000 parts of water; slightly soluble

in alcohol and acetone; soluble in aromatic hydrocarbons. Used as an acaricide against red spider mites. LD_{50} (rats) more than 14700 mg/kg. Available as liquid concentrate containing 8%.

Organophosphorus compounds. Many types are in current use as insecticides. Although they all have the basic property of inhibiting the action of cholinesterase at the ganglia they enter the insect's body by different routes depending on the properties of the particular compound. Thus the group contains contact, stomach, and systemic insecticides.

Those most suitable for systemic action have a high water solubility and resistance to breakdown and are particularly useful against sucking insects.

Some of the organophosphorus compounds are fairly persistent but less so than organochlorine compounds. Some of the organophosphorus compounds have a high acute toxicity in mammals because of their pharmacological action and considerable care is needed if they are to be used safely. However, malathion, which is one of the most widely used of these compounds, has a very low toxicity and persistence and is, therefore, safe for general use.

Many of the organophosphorus pesticides used are readily absorbed through the skin, respiratory system, and gastro-intestinal tract.

Toxic effects of small doses include nausea, vomiting, anorexia, sweating, salivation, giddiness, restlessness, and tightness of the chest. Larger doses cause, in addition, diarrhoea, lachrymation, blurred vision, respiratory failure, and convulsions.

Chemically, the organophosphorus compounds usually contain a phosphorus atom linked to an atom of sulphur or oxygen which in turn is linked to a further sulphur or oxygen atom. They may be divided into four main groups as shown below. Other groups are attached to the phosphorus (group R) and second oxygen or sulphur atom (group R') to give a very diverse range of compounds.

Phosphorothiolothionates. General formula $R_2PS \cdot SCH_2R'$, where $R = -OCH_3$ or $-OC_2H_5$

Phosphorothiolates. General formula $R_2PO \cdot SR'$, where $R = -OCH_3$

Phosphorothionates. General formula $R_2PS \cdot OR'$, where $R = -OCH_3$, $-OC_2H_5$, or $-CH_3$

Phosphates. General formula $R_2PO \cdot OR'$, where $R = -OCH_3$ or $-OC_2H_5$

The following is a representative selection of organophosphorus pesticides.

AZINPHOS-METHYL (*Gusathion®*). S-(3,4-Dihydro-4-oxobenzo[*d*]-[1,2,3]-triazin-3-ylmethyl) dimethyl phosphorothiolothionate. Used against a wide range of organisms especially on fruit crops. Moderately persistent. LD_{50} (rats) 16.4 mg/kg. Dangerous to bees, fish, livestock, and wildlife. Minimum period between application and harvesting of the crop 3 weeks, and between application and allowing livestock access to treated areas 2 weeks. Available as an emulsifiable concentrate containing 22% and as a wettable powder containing 25%.

CARBOPHENOTHION (*Trithion®*). S-(4-Chlorophenylthiomethyl) diethyl phosphorothiolothionate. Used in seed dressings against wheat bulb fly. LD_{50} (rats) 32.2 mg/kg. Harmful to fish and wildlife. Treated seed is unfit for consumption. Available as a liquid concentrate containing 25%.

CHLORFENVINPHOS (*Birlane®*; *Sapecron®*). 2-Chloro-1-(2,4-dichlorophenyl)vinyl diethyl phosphate. Soluble in 7000 parts of water. Used in seed dressings against various root flies and other soil insects. LD_{50} (rats) 10 to 39 mg/kg. Dangerous to fish. Minimum period between application and harvesting of the crop 3 weeks. Treated seed is unfit for consumption. Available as granules containing 10% and as a liquid concentrate containing 25%.

DEMEPHION (*Atlasetox®*; *Pyracide®*). A mixture of dimethyl 2-(methylthio)ethyl phosphorothionate and dimethyl S-[(2-methylthio)ethyl] phosphorothiolate, known respectively as demephion O and S. Soluble in 1000 parts of water. Used as a systemic insecticide on many crops for the control of aphids. LD_{50} (rats) 138 mg/kg. Harmful to bees, fish, livestock, and wildlife. Minimum period between application and harvesting of the crop 3 weeks, and between application and allowing livestock access to treated areas 2 weeks. Available as a liquid concentrate containing 30%.

DEMETON-S-METHYL (*Azotox®*; *Demetox®*; *DSM®*; *Duratox®*; *Metasystox®*). S-[2-(Ethylthio)ethyl] dimethyl phosphorothiolate. Soluble in 300 parts of water. Used as a systemic insecticide and acaricide on many crops. LD_{50} (rats) 40 mg/kg. Harmful to bees, fish, livestock, and wildlife. Minimum period between application and harvesting of the crop 3 weeks, and between application and allowing livestock access to treated areas 2 weeks. Available as a liquid concentrate containing 50%.

DICHLORVOS (*Nogos®*). 2,2-Dichlorovinyl dimethyl phosphate. Soluble in 100 parts of water. Used as an insecticide and acaricide for the control of aphids, small flies, and some moths where rapid extermination is required close to harvest. Low persistence. LD_{50} (rats) 56 to 80 mg/kg. Dangerous to bees. Minimum period between application and harvesting of the crop 24 hours, and between application and allowing unprotected personnel access to treated areas 12 hours. Should not be used at temperatures below 15°. Available as a liquid concentrate containing 50%.

DIMEFOX (*Terra Sytam®*). NNN'N'-Tetramethylphosphorodiamidic fluoride. Used as a systemic insecticide and acaricide to control aphids and red spider mites on hops. LD_{50} (rats) 1 to 2 mg/kg. Dangerous to fish, livestock, and wildlife. Minimum period between application and harvesting of the crop 24 hours, and between application and allowing unprotected persons and livestock access to treated areas 24 hours and 4 weeks respectively. Available as a liquid concentrate containing 50%.

DIMETHOATE (*Rogor®*). Dimethyl S-(N-methylcarbamoylmethyl) phosphorothiolothionate. Soluble in 40 parts of water. Used as a systemic insecticide and acaricide against aphids and red spider mites. LD_{50} (rats) 500 to 600 mg/kg. Dangerous to bees. Harmful to fish, livestock, and wildlife. Minimum period between application and harvesting of the crop or allowing livestock access to treated areas 1 week. Available as a liquid concentrate containing 40% and as a wettable powder containing 20%.

DIMPYLATE (*Basudin®*; Diazinon; *Diazitol®*). Diethyl (2-isopropyl-6-methylpyrimidin-4-yl) phosphorothionate. Used as an insecticide and acaricide against soil insects and sucking insects. LD_{50} (rats) 600 mg/kg. Dangerous to bees. Harmful to fish, livestock, and wildlife. Minimum period between application and harvesting of the crop when applied by atomising spray 2 days, and for other forms of preparation, 2 weeks. Available as atomising solutions containing 5 and 10% and other liquid preparations containing from 25 to 60%.

DISULFOTON (*Disyston®*; *Granulox®*; *Parsolin®*; *Solvi-*

gran®). Diethyl S-2-(ethylthio)ethyl phosphorothiolothionate. Used as a systemic insecticide for the control of aphids and carrot fly. LD_{50} (rats) 12.5 mg/kg. Dangerous to fish. Minimum period between application and harvesting of the crop 6 weeks. Available as granules containing 7.5 or 10%.

FENITROTHION (*Accothion®*; *Agrothion®*; *Dicofen®*; *Fenstan®*; *Folithion®*; *Verthion®*). Dimethyl 3-methyl-4-nitrophenyl phosphorothionate. Used for the control of many pests especially against sawfly and against beetles and weevils in stored grain. LD_{50} (rats) 250 to 500 mg/kg. Harmful to bees, fish, livestock, and wildlife. Minimum period between application and harvesting of the crop 2 weeks, and between application and allowing livestock access to treated areas 1 week. Available as liquid concentrates containing 20 and 50%.

FONOFOS (*Dyfonate®*). Ethyl S-phenyl ethylphosphonothiolothionate. Miscible with xylene. Used for the control of cabbage root fly. LD_{50} (rats) 8 to 17.5 mg/kg. Dangerous to fish. Minimum period between application and harvesting of the crop 6 weeks. Available as granules containing 5 and 10%.

FORMOTHION (*Anthio®*). S-(N-Formyl-N-methylcarbamoylmethyl) dimethyl phosphorothiolothionate. Soluble in 400 parts of water. Used as a systemic insecticide and acaricide mainly against aphids. LD_{50} (rats) 330 mg/kg. Dangerous to bees. Harmful to fish and livestock. Minimum period between application and harvesting of the crop, or allowing livestock access to treated areas, 1 week. Available as a liquid concentrate containing 25%.

MALATHION (*Malastan®*; *Malathexo®*) (see also separate entry). Used as an insecticide and acaricide against a very wide range of pests. LD_{50} (rats) 2800 mg/kg. Harmful to bees and fish. May taint crops. Minimum period between application and harvesting of the crop 4 days, and between application and processing 7 days. Available as dusts containing 4% and liquid concentrates containing 60%.

MENAZON (*Saphicol®*). S-(4,6-Diamino-1,3,5-triazin-2-ylmethyl) dimethyl phosphorothiolothionate. Soluble in 4000 parts of water. Used as a systemic insecticide against aphids. LD_{50} (rats) 1950 mg/kg. Harmful to bees and livestock. Minimum period between application and harvesting of the crop or allowing livestock access to treated areas 3 weeks. Available as a colloidal product containing 40%.

METHIDATHION (*Supracide®*). S-(2,3-Dihydro-5-methoxy-2-oxo-1,3,4-thiadiazol-3-ylmethyl) dimethyl phosphorothiolothionate. Soluble in 4000 parts of water. Used for the control of aphids on hops. LD_{50} (rats) 25 to 48 mg/kg. Dangerous to fish. Harmful to bees and livestock. Minimum period between application and harvesting of the crop 3 weeks, and between application and allowing livestock access to treated areas 2 weeks. Available as a liquid concentrate containing 40%.

MEVINPHOS (*Phosdrin®*). 2-Methoxycarbonyl-1-methylvinyl dimethyl phosphate. Miscible with water. Used as a systemic insecticide for the control of aphids, caterpillars, and other pests where rapid kill is required close to harvest time. Short persistence. LD_{50} (rats) 6.8 mg/kg. Dangerous to bees, fish, livestock, and wildlife. Minimum period between application and harvesting of the crop 3 days, and between application and allowing unprotected persons and livestock access to treated areas 1 day. Available as liquid concentrates containing from 5 to 50%.

OXYDEMETON-METHYL (*Metasystox®*). S-[2-(Ethylsulphinyl)ethyl] dimethyl phosphorothiolate. Miscible with water. Used as a systemic insecticide and acaricide against a wide variety of pests. LD_{50} (rats) 67 to 75 mg/kg. Harmful to bees, fish, livestock, and wildlife. Minimum period between application and harvesting of the crop 3 weeks, between application and clamping 10 days, and between application and allowing livestock access to treated areas 2 weeks. Available as a liquid concentrate containing 57%.

PARATHION (*Fosfex®*). Diethyl 4-nitrophenyl phosphorothionate. Used as an insecticide, acaricide, and nematocide against a wide variety of pests on crops grown under glass. LD_{50} (rats) 6.4 mg/kg. Dangerous to bees, fish, livestock, and wildlife. Minimum period between application and harvesting of the crop 4 weeks, and between application and allowing livestock and unprotected persons access to treated areas 1 day and 10 days respectively. Available as a liquid concentrate containing 20%.

PHORATE (*Thimet®*). Diethyl S-(ethylthiomethyl) phosphorothiolothionate. Used as a systemic insecticide against a wide range of aphids, capsids, and weevils. Moderately persistent. LD_{50} (rats) 3.7 mg/kg. Dangerous to fish and livestock. Minimum period between application and harvesting of the crop or allowing livestock access to treated areas 6 weeks. Available as granules containing 10%.

PHOSALONE (*Zolone®*). S-(6-Chloro-2-oxobenzoxazolin-3-yl)methyl diethyl phosphorothiolothionate. Soluble in 10000 parts of water; soluble in acetone, in chloroform, and in methanol; insoluble in light petroleum. Used against aphids, caterpillars, and red spider mites on apples and pears. LD_{50} (rats) 120 mg/kg. Harmful to bees, fish, and livestock. Minimum period between application and harvesting of the crop 3 weeks, and between application and allowing livestock access to treated areas 4 weeks. Available as a liquid concentrate containing 33%.

PHOSPHAMIDON (*Dicron 54 SC®*; *Dimecron®*). 2-Chloro-2-diethylcarbamoyl-1-methylvinyl dimethyl phosphate. Miscible with water. Used as a systemic insecticide and acaricide particularly against aphids and red spider mites. LD_{50} (rats) 28.3 mg/kg. Dangerous to bees. Harmful to livestock. Minimum interval between application and harvesting of the crop 3 weeks, and between application and allowing livestock access to treated areas 2 weeks. Available as liquid concentrates containing 20 and 54%.

Carbamates. As with organophosphorus compounds, carbamates have an anticholinesterase action but it is more readily reversible. They have a low mammalian toxicity. Most carbamates are contact poisons. Toxic effects resemble those of organophosphorus compounds but because the anticholinesterase action is more readily reversible the symptoms disappear much more quickly. The general formula for carbamates is $RCO.NHCH_3$, where R may be a wide variety of chemical structures. The following is a representative selection of carbamate pesticides.

CARBARYL (*Murvin®*; *Sevin®*). 1-Naphthyl methylcarbamate. Used to control earthworms and certain caterpillars which later become pests of apples. LD_{50} (rats) 850 mg/kg. Dangerous to bees. Harmful to fish. Minimum period between application and harvesting of the crop 1 week. Available as wettable powder containing 50%.

PIRIMICARB (*Aphox®*; *Pirimor®*). 2-Dimethylamino-5,6-dimethylpyrimidin-4-yl dimethylcarbamate. Soluble in 300 parts of water. Used as a systemic insecticide for the control of aphids. Does not persist for long. LD_{50} (rats) 147 mg/kg. Harmful to livestock. Minimum period between application and harvesting of the crop 2 weeks, and between application and allowing livestock access to treated areas 1 week. Available as dispersible granules containing 5%, wettable powder containing 50%, and as smokes.

PROPOXUR (*Undene®*). 2-Isopropoxyphenyl methylcarbamate. Soluble in 300 parts of water. Used for the control of aphids and adult whitefly under glass and on hops. LD_{50} (rats) 100 mg/kg. Harmful to bees, fish, livestock, and wildlife. Minimum period between application and harvesting of the crop for hops 1 week or for crops under glass 2 days, and between application and allowing livestock access to treated areas 1 week. Available as smokes and as a wettable powder.

Naturally-occurring organic compounds. The chief materials used are derris, lonchocarpus, nicotine, and pyrethrum.

Derris, lonchocarpus, and the roots of some other species of the family Leguminosae contain the insecticide rotenone. This is a stomach and contact poison and causes a slow death by cardiac and respiratory depression. It has a wide range of kill and is non-toxic to mammals. There is little residual action because the rotenone is quickly destroyed by heat and light.

Nicotine is a liquid alkaloid obtained from *Nicotiana* species and is used mainly as a fumigant. In the form of one of its salts it is adsorbed onto a suitable material such as gypsum to produce a dust which is then used as a contact poison. Nicotine has a paralytic action on the insect's nervous system and is non-toxic to plants. Its main disadvantage is its high mammalian toxicity and it is generally used only on a small scale.

Pyrethrum flowers contain esters known as pyrethrins which act very quickly on the nervous system of the insect to give a rapid "knockdown" effect which is, however, reversible. Pyrethrins are contact poisons and are often mixed with other insecticides with which they have a synergistic action. They are used against a wide range of flying insects. Pyrethrum is non-toxic to mammals but quickly loses its insecticidal action. The solvent used for extraction and application is important, petrol (gasoline) giving the best effect.

DERRIS (see also separate entry). Produces unpleasant effects on inhalation. Toxic to fish. Minimum period between application and harvesting of the crop is 24 hours. Available as a powder mixed with a non-alkaline carrier as a dispersible powder.

LONCHOCARPUS (see also separate entry). As for Derris (above).

NICOTINE (*XL All®*). 3-(1-Methyl-2-pyrrolidinyl)pyridine. Soluble in water and in alcohol. Used as a fumigant and contact poison especially against aphids. LD_{50} (rats) 50 to 60 mg/kg. Dangerous to bees, fish, livestock, game, and wildlife. Rapidly absorbed through the skin. Minimum period between application and harvesting of the crop 2 weeks, and between application and allowing livestock access to treated areas 12 hours. Available as a dust containing 3%, a liquid concentrate containing 95%, and a liquid concentrate containing 40% of nicotine sulphate.

PYRETHRUM (see also separate entry). Used as a contact insecticide with a rapid paralysing effect. Low level of persistence. LD_{50} (rats) 200 mg/kg. Pyrethrins may cause dermatitis. Available as a dust consisting of the powdered flowers in a non-alkaline carrier, and as a liquid extract of the flowers. Pyrethrum is often mixed with other insecticides such as derris.

Dinitro compounds. These are used as "winter washes" on dormant fruit trees to kill eggs of insect pests. They have a high acute toxicity to mammals and early detection of symptoms is difficult. The substances may be absorbed through the lungs, skin, or gastro-intestinal tract. Absorption of toxic amounts may give rise to yellow discoloration of the sclera. The metabolic rate is increased and in mild poisoning the feeling of well-being thus produced disguises the other symptoms of sweating and thirst. In more severe poisoning, sweating is profuse, there is fatigue, nausea, restlessness, and loss of weight. If no action is taken, death results from cerebral oedema and failure of heart and respiration.

Dinitro compounds are all derivatives of 1,3-dinitrobenzene of general formula

R and R′ are diverse in character and the following is a representative selection of dinitro compounds.

BINAPACRYL (*Morocide®*). 2-*sec*-Butyl-4,6-dinitrophenyl 3-methylcrotonate. Practically insoluble in water; soluble in 10 parts of alcohol. Used to control powdery mildew on apples. LD$_{50}$ (rats) 150 to 350 mg/kg. Harmful to fish and livestock. Precautions should be taken to prevent drift onto soft fruit. Minimum period between application and harvesting of the crop 1 week, and between application and allowing livestock access to treated areas 4 weeks. Available as colloidal solution containing 40%.

DINOBUTON (*Sytasol®*). 2-*sec*-Butyl-4,6-dinitrophenyl isopropyl carbonate. Used as an acaricide against red spider mites on apples. LD$_{50}$ (rats) 140 mg/kg. Dangerous to fish. Harmful to bees and livestock. Minimum period between application and harvesting of the crop or allowing livestock access to treated areas 3 weeks. Available as liquid concentrates containing 30 and 50%.

DINOCAP (*AM 62®*; *Crotothane®*; *Karathane®*). An isomeric mixture of 2,6-dinitro-4-octylphenyl crotonates and 2,4-dinitro-6-octylphenyl crotonates. Used against powdery mildew on many crops. LD$_{50}$ (rats) 980 mg/kg. Irritating to skin, eyes, and nose. Dangerous to fish. Minimum period between application and harvesting of outdoor crops 1 week, and, for indoor crops, 2 days. Available as liquid concentrate containing 50% and wettable powder containing 25%.

DNOC (*Cresofin®*; Dinitrocresol; DNC; *Ovamort®*). 2-Methyl-4,6-dinitrophenol. Soluble in 7500 parts of water. Used to control overwintering stages of many insects of fruit trees. LD$_{50}$ (rats) 40 mg/kg. Dangerous to fish. Minimum period between application and allowing unprotected persons access to treated areas 1 day, and, for animals and poultry 10 days. Available as 1.35 to 3.5% solutions in petroleum oil.

Oils. Petroleum oils and tar oils are used as insecticides. The action of petroleum oils is thought to be due to a physical rather than chemical effect on the insect's metabolism. Tar oils, however, contain more actively toxic compounds. Both types are used as washes on fruit trees and the high phytotoxicity involved limits their use to winter when the trees are dormant. Neither type is

a hazard as far as toxicity is concerned except that tar oils may cause contact dermatitis in some individuals. Large doses may cause headache, nausea, and vomiting.

Petroleum oils consist of mixtures of hydrocarbons similar in composition to those in liquid paraffin. Tar oils consist mainly of anthracene derivatives.

Inorganic compounds. Salts of arsenic, lead, and mercury have been used as insecticides for a long time. They are stomach poisons and as they are highly toxic to mammals, their use is declining. The heavy metal salts are accumulated in the body and, in consequence, persons using them regularly are liable to chronic poisoning.

Acute poisoning is shown by intense thirst, abdominal pain, vomiting, diarrhoea, and a metallic taste in the mouth. Chronic poisoning gives rise to anorexia, constipation, headache, and weakness. Large doses may produce many irregularities in normal body function.

LEAD ARSENATE. Used for the control of winter and ermine moths, sawfly, and leatherjackets. 10 to 50 mg/kg is fatal. Dangerous to bees. Harmful to fish and livestock. Minimum period between application and harvesting of the crop 6 weeks, and between application and allowing livestock access to treated areas 6 weeks, or in wet weather, 3 weeks. Available as wettable powder containing 40%.

LIME SULPHUR. Consists of calcium polysulphides. Miscible with water. Used as an acaricide against leaf curl, powdery mildew, and apple scab. No evidence of toxicity. May taint fruit. Should not be used on "sulphur-shy" varieties of fruit trees. Available as a liquid, usually as a dilution containing 1% of lime sulphur.

MERCUROUS CHLORIDE (Calomel). Soluble in alcohol. Used as a fungicide and herbicide on turf. LD$_{50}$ (rats) 210 mg/kg. Harmful to fish. Available as a spray for use as a herbicide, a dust containing 4%, and a powder containing 0.65% mixed with ferrous sulphate ("Lawn Sand").

Fungicides

Most plant diseases are caused by fungi or viruses. The latter are difficult to control chemically although some compounds have been used for this purpose. Virus attack is usually controlled by breeding resistant varieties of plants or by controlling the insect vectors of viruses. Attacks by fungi have also been controlled by breeding resistant varieties of plants but many chemicals have been developed as fungicides. However, progress with chemicals has been slow owing to the difficulty of acquiring information about fungal pests, the production of many strains by some species of fungus, and the problem that the metabolism of the host plant may resemble that of the fungus. Fungicides used must therefore be more selective than the insecticides, where the metabolic differences between plants and insects can be exploited more easily.

Classification According to Mode of Action

(i) *Contact fungicides.* These chemicals act by killing fungi exposed on the surface of the plant. However, only a relatively small number can be treated by this type of fungicide because most fungi penetrate deep into the tissues of the host plant.

(ii) *Protective fungicides.* Most commercial products contain this type of fungicide. They are applied to the plant prior to possible attack of fungal spores which are thus killed when they alight on the surface of the plant or are prevented from growing.

(iii) *Systemic fungicides*. These are absorbed by the plant via the roots or aerial parts and are then translocated throughout the plant. Fungal hyphae are then killed when they penetrate the plant tissues.

Chemical Classification

Inorganic compounds. Three elements are used as the basis of fungicidal preparations, namely sulphur, copper, and mercury. Sulphur is used as such or in compounds, and copper and mercury are used in the form of their salts.

Sulphur is the oldest fungicide in use and is still widely used, being cheap and effective. Its mode of action is uncertain but possibly it acts as a hydrogen acceptor to give the toxic compound hydrogen sulphide. Sulphur is used in dust form, as a colloid, or as a wettable powder, and in chemical combination with lime or as a polysulphide. Sulphur has a wide spectrum of activity but some important crop plants are sulphur shy, that is, susceptible to sulphur poisoning. Sulphur exhibits very little toxicity to mammals.

Copper compounds are widely used as fungicides, especially in the form of Bordeaux mixture, a complex of lime and copper sulphate which provides a system slowly releasing cupric ions. Some plants are poisoned by copper compounds.

Mercury compounds have a high toxicity in respect of both plants and animals, mercuric salts being more toxic than mercurous compounds. Both copper and mercury act by interfering with the enzyme systems necessary to the fungus for respiration. Some inorganic fungicides are also used as insecticides, for example, mercurous chloride and lime sulphur. Copper and mercury compounds are used only for the control of soil organisms and as seed dressings.

BORDEAUX MIXTURE. Consists of copper sulphate together with varying proportions of calcium hydroxide, mixed with water to form a suspension immediately before use as it deteriorates on storage. Too high a proportion of lime renders the preparation phytotoxic. The dry powder should be stored in airtight containers. Used as a protective fungicide against potato blight and mildews. Toxicity is low. Available as various combinations of the two ingredients, the usual ones containing, when reconstituted, 1% of copper sulphate with 1.25, 1.5, or 1.6% of calcium hydroxide.

BURGUNDY MIXTURE. A variant of Bordeaux mixture containing copper sulphate and sodium carbonate. As with Bordeaux mixture, it is prepared by mixing the dry ingredients with water immediately before use as it deteriorates on storage. The dry powder should be stored in airtight containers. It is more likely to cause damage to plants than Bordeaux mixture. Available as a mixture containing, when reconstituted, 1% of copper sulphate with 1.25% of sodium carbonate.

PHENYLMERCURIC ACETATE (*Ceresol®*; *Hanresar®*; *Leytosan®*; *Parogen M®*; *Phelam®*) (see also separate entry). Used against apple and pear scab and for control of various seed-borne diseases on root and cereal crops. LD_{50} (rats) 60 mg/kg. May cause rashes and blisters on the skin. Harmful to bees, fish, and livestock. Minimum period between application and harvesting of the crop 6 weeks, and between application and allowing livestock access to treated areas 2 weeks. Treated seed unfit for consumption. Available as dry and liquid seed treatments, and as a spray containing 2.5%. Often mixed with other pesticides such as gamma benzene hexachloride and carboxin.

SULPHUR (see also separate entry). Used as a contact fungicide in a wide variety of situations but especially against powdery mildews. Non-toxic to mammals. Unsuitable for sulphur-shy plants. Available as dust, wettable powder, and colloidal suspension. Formulations should contain not less than 70% of active ingredient.

Dithiocarbamates. These are organic compounds of sulphur, some of which also contain a metal. They were developed to reduce the cost and phytotoxicity associated with some of the simpler sulphur-containing compounds. Their toxic action, which is exerted by their interfering with the fungal respiratory process, is thought to be due to decomposition products which may be isothiocyanates or ethylenethiuram disulphide.

The dithiocarbamates are compatible physico-chemically and biologically with many other pesticides and are often used in conjunction with them. They are generally not very toxic to mammals but may cause tainting of foodstuffs. Consequently a minimum period between application and harvesting of the crop is usually specified. Most of the dithiocarbamates also cause irritation to the skin, eyes, nose, and mouth.

Dithiocarbamates have the general formula

$$\begin{array}{c} R' \quad\; S \\ \backslash \quad \parallel \\ N{\cdot}C{\cdot}S{\cdot}R'' \\ / \\ R \end{array}$$

Most compounds contain a pair of these units in each molecule, where R'' represents the duplicate unit or is a divalent metal linking the two units together. In other cases R' and R may form the link with the second unit but these may also be other groups or hydrogen atoms. Some ring compounds also occur, usually derived by linkage between R'' and either R or R'.

SUBSTANCES CONTAINING NO METAL. DAZOMET (*Basamid®*). Tetrahydro-3,5-dimethyl-2*H*-1,3,5-thiadiazine-2-thione. Soluble in 400 parts of water and in 5 parts of acetone. Used as a soil sterilant. LD_{50} (rats) 500 mg/kg. Irritant to the eyes, skin, nose, and mouth. Minimum period between application and use of the soil for planting 6 weeks. Available as granules containing 98%.

THIRAM (*Ferna-Col®*; *Fernasan®*; *Tripomol®*). Bis(dimethylthiocarbamoyl) disulphide. Practically insoluble in water; slightly soluble in alcohol; soluble in acetone. Used against *Botrytis*, rusts, and downy mildews. Also used as a seed dressing against "damping off" and *Verticillium* wilt. LD_{50} (rats) very high. Irritant to the eyes, skin, nose, and throat. Minimum period between application and harvesting of the crop 1 week. Taints food derived from crops unless they are thoroughly washed. Dressed seed unfit for consumption. Available as colloidal suspension containing 50%, powder containing 50%, and wettable powder containing 80%.

SUBSTANCES CONTAINING A METAL. These can be divided into two groups, the first comprising various compounds of general formula:

$$\begin{array}{c} S \qquad\quad S \\ \parallel \qquad\quad \parallel \\ NH_2{\cdot}C{\cdot}S{\cdot}X{\cdot}S{\cdot}C{\cdot}NH_2 \end{array}$$

where X = Zn, Mn, Cu, or Fe. Examples of preparations of this type of compound are Cufraneb (*Cufram Z®*), *Carmazine®*, *Farmanz®*, *Moromate®*, and *Trimanzone®*; the following notes apply to all the substances in this group.

Practically insoluble in water. Used against potato blight, hop downy mildew, and tulip fire. Irritant to the eyes, skin, and nose. Minimum period between application and harvesting of the crop 1 week. Available as wettable powder.

The second group consists of compounds of more varied structure, mostly containing divalent metals and some of which are polymers. The following are examples.

MANCOZEB (*Dicamate®*; *Dithrane 945®*; *Karamate®*). A zinc complex of manganese ethylene-1,2-bisdithiocarbamate. Practically insoluble in water and most organic solvents. Used against potato blight, various rusts, and spots. Applied as a spray to aerial parts. LD_{50} (rats) 5000 mg/kg. Minimum period between application and harvesting of crops intended for consumption 1 week. Available as wettable powder containing 80%.

MANEB (*Croptex®*; *Manzate®*; *Plantineb®*; *Trimangol®*; *Tubothane®*; *Mazin®*). Manganese ethylene-1,2-bisdithiocarbamate. Practically insoluble in water and most organic solvents. Used against downy mildews, spots, and blights. Applied as a spray. LD_{50} (rats) 4000 mg/kg. Irritant to the eyes, skin, and nose. Minimum period between application and harvesting of outdoor crops 1 week and, for greenhouse crops, 48 hours. Available as wettable powder containing 80%.

METHAM SODIUM (*Maposyl®*; *Sistan®*; *Trimaton®*; *Unifume®*; *Vapam®*; *Vitafume®*). Sodium N-methyldithiocarbamate. Soluble in 1.3 parts of water; practically insoluble in organic solvents. Used as a soil sterilant. LD_{50} (rats) 820 mg/kg. Irritant to the eyes, skin, nose, and mouth. Soil should not be used for sowing until a cress germination test has confirmed that decomposition is complete. Available as a solution containing 35%.

NABAM (*X-Spor®*). Disodium ethylene-1,2-bisdithiocarbamate. Soluble in 5 parts of water. Used on the soil against root rots, and in combination with maneb and zineb. LD_{50} (rats) 395 mg/kg. Irritant to the eyes, skin, and nose. Minimum period between application and harvesting of outdoor crops, 1 week and, for greenhouse crops, 48 hours. Available as solution containing 22% and powder containing 93%.

POLYRAM. A complex of zineb (see below) and polyethylene, thiuram disulphide. Practically insoluble in water. Used against potato blight. Irritant to the eyes, skin, and nose. Available as wettable powder.

PROPINEB (*Antracol®*). Zinc propylenebisdithiocarbamate polymer. Practically insoluble in water and most organic solvents. Used against downy mildew and potato blight. Applied as a spray. LD_{50} (rats) 8500 mg/kg. Available as wettable powder containing 70%.

ZINEB (*Anglian Blue®*; *Dithane wettable®*; *Dyblite®*; *Tiezene®*; *Tritoftorol®*). Zinc ethylene-1,2-bisdithiocarbamate polymer. Practically insoluble in water; soluble in pyridine. Used against downy mildews. LD_{50} (rats) greater than 5200 mg/kg. Minimum period between application and harvesting of the crop 1 month for black currants, 1 week for other outdoor crops, and 48 hours for greenhouse crops. May taint black currants. Available as dusting-powder containing 8 and 15% and as wettable powder containing 65%.

Nitro compounds. These compounds are used for treating sulphur-shy plants such as lettuce. Some are contact fungicides, acting directly on the fungus, and others are protective fungicides. As with dithiocarbamates, nitro compounds interfere with the respiratory process of the fungus but at a different stage. Chlorinated nitrocompounds are more persistent. Some are insecti-

cidal as well as fungicidal, for example binapacryl and dinocap (see above under Insecticides).

The following compounds represent chlorinated nitro compounds.

DICLORAN (*Allisan®*). 2,6-Dichloro-4-nitroaniline. Practically insoluble in water. Used in the control of *Botrytis*. LD_{50} (rats) 1500 to 4000 mg/kg. Minimum period between application and harvesting of the crop (lettuce) 3 weeks. Available as dusting-powder containing 4%.

QUINTOZENE (*Botrilex®*; *Bras-sicol®*; Tri-P.C.N.B.). Pentachloronitrobenzene. Practically insoluble in water; soluble in 50 parts of alcohol; soluble in chloroform. Used to control damping off and other fungal infections. LD_{50} (rats) more than 12000 mg/kg. May damage cucurbit crops or tomatoes if they are planted in treated soil. Available as dusting-powder containing 20% and as wettable powder containing 75%.

Miscellaneous. Other types of organic compound with various properties are in use. These include some systemic fungicides developed only in the last few years which are particularly useful against vascular infection by fungi. Some are used as seed dressings, while others are applied to, and absorbed from, the foliage of the plant. The mode of action of many of the compounds is obscure but some act by interfering with synthesis of deoxyribonucleic acid. There are several chemical types of systemic fungicide, and other fungicidal compounds are also in use.

The two principal types of systemic fungicide are (a) the morpholines of general formula

where R is a long hydrocarbon chain; and (b) the benzimidazoles of general formula

where R and R' are aliphatic groups.

Other substances used as fungicides include compounds containing organically combined sulphur, chlorinated compounds, and organic tin salts.

BENOMYL (*Benlate®*). Methyl N-1-(butylcarbamoyl)-2-benzimidazol-2-ylcarbamate. Practically insoluble in water. Used as a systemic fungicide against many diseases of fruit trees and greenhouse crops. LD_{50} (rats) more than 9590 mg/kg. Available as wettable powder containing 50%.

CAPTAFOL (*Sanspor®*). N-(1,1,2,2-Tetrachloroethylthio)-3a,4,7,7a-tetrahydrophthalimide. Practically insoluble in water. Used in the control of potato blight. LD_{50} (rats) 5000 to 6200 mg/kg. Irritating to the eyes, skin, nose, and throat. Dangerous to fish. Available as wettable powder containing 80%.

CAPTAN. N-(Trichloromethylthio)-3a,4,7,7a-tetrahydrophthalimide. Practically insoluble in water; soluble in 20 parts of acetone; soluble in chloroform. Used in the control of black spot, *Botrytis*, scab, and stem rot. LD_{50}

(rats) 9000 mg/kg. Harmful to fish. Available as wettable powder containing 50%.

CARBOXIN (*Murganic*®). 5,6-Dihydro-2-methyl-1,4-oxathiin-3-carboxanilide. Very slightly soluble in water; soluble in 1 part of acetone. Used as a systemic fungicide in admixture with organic mercury compounds and with gamma benzene hexachloride to control seed-borne diseases of barley and wheat. LD_{50} (rats) 3200 mg/kg. Harmful to fish. Treated seed unfit for consumption. Available as dusting-powders containing 5 and 10% and a liquid preparation containing 75%, all for seed treatment.

CHLOROPICRIN. Trichloronitromethane. Soluble in 50 parts of water. Used as a soil sterilant and for the control of nematodes, fungi, and other soil pests. Strongly irritant to the eyes, skin, nose, mouth, and lungs. Dangerous to fish. Unprotected persons should not be allowed access to treated areas. Available as liquid concentrate containing chloropicrin with methyl isocyanate and a mixture of dichloropropane and dichloropropenes.

DICHLOFLUANID (*Elvaron*®). N′-Dichlorofluoromethyl-thio-NN-dimethyl-N′-phenylsulphamide. Practically insoluble in water; soluble in methyl alcohol and in acetone. Used to control *Botrytis* on soft fruits and several other diseases on tomatoes. LD_{50} (rats) 1000 mg/kg. Harmful to fish. Minimum period between application and harvesting the crop 3 days for tomatoes under glass, and 3 weeks for soft fruits. Available as wettable powder containing 50%.

DITHIANON (*Delan-Col*®). 2,3-Dicyano-1,4-dithia-anthraquinone. Practically insoluble in water; soluble in chloroform. Incompatible with petroleum oil. Used for the control of scab on apples and pears. LD_{50} (rats) 1015 mg/kg. Available as colloidal solution containing 25%.

DRAZOXOLON (*Mil-Col*®). 4-(2-Chlorophenylhydrazono)-3-methyl-5-isoxazolone. Practically insoluble in water; soluble in 10 parts of chloroform. Used as a seed dressing against damping-off and foot rot in peas. Also used to control powdery mildew and leaf spot. LD_{50} (rats) 126 mg/kg. Dangerous to livestock. Harmful to fish. Treated seed unfit for consumption. Minimum period between application and harvesting of the crop or allowing livestock access to treated areas 4 weeks. Available as colloidal mixture containing 40%. Sometimes used in admixture with pirimiphos-ethyl.

ETHIRIMOL (*Milgo*®; *Milstem*®). 5-Butyl-2-ethylamino-4-hydroxy-6-methylpyrimidine. Very slightly soluble in water; soluble in 50 parts of alcohol, in 7 parts of chloroform, and in 200 parts of acetone. Used as a systemic fungicide to control mildew on spring barley. Also used as a seed dressing. LD_{50} (rats) 4000 mg/kg. Treated seed is unfit for consumption. Available as a liquid concentrate containing 20%.

FENTIN HYDROXIDE (*Du-ter*®; *Erithane*®; *Farmatin*®; *Profarma*®; *Tubotin*®; *Vitospor*®). Triphenyltin hydroxide. Practically insoluble in water. Used for the control of potato blight. LD_{50} (rats) 108 mg/kg. Irritating to the eyes, skin, and nose. Harmful to fish and livestock. Available as wettable powder containing 20%.

QUINOMETHIONATE (*Morestan*®). 6-Methyl-2-oxo-1,3-dithiolo[4,5,b]quinoxaline. Practically insoluble in water. Used as an acaricide and fungicide against red spider mites and powdery mildews. LD_{50} (rats) 2500 to 3000 mg/kg. Minimum interval between application and harvesting of the crop 3 weeks, reduced to 2 weeks for

soft fruits, 1 week for marrows, and 48 hours for greenhouse crops. Available as wettable powder containing 25% and as smokes.

TRIDEMORPH (*Calixin*®). 2,6-Dimethyl-4-tridecylmorpholine. Used as a systemic fungicide for the control of mildew on cereal crops. LD_{50} (rats) 1250 mg/kg. Irritating to the eyes and skin. Harmful to fish. Available as liquid concentrate containing 75%.

Herbicides

These are substances used to kill weeds, that is, any plant which becomes a pest. The development of selective herbicides has meant that weeds growing amongst a crop can be killed and non-selective herbicides have facilitated the complete clearance of vegetation from paths, irrigation canals, etc. The mode of action of many herbicides is not known completely but they may interfere with photosynthetic processes or with metabolism and growth.

The means of application and entry into the plant are used to divide herbicides into three classes.

(i) *Contact herbicides.* This type kills all plant parts through the surfaces with which it comes into contact.

(ii) *Translocated herbicides.* This group, when applied to plant foliage, is absorbed and translocated throughout the whole plant. Translocation herbicides are especially useful against perennials which lie dormant, often underground, between growing seasons.

(iii) *Residual herbicides.* These compounds are applied to the soil from which they are absorbed by the roots of plants and translocated within them. They are especially useful against germinating seeds and seedlings. Their efficiency depends on persistence resulting from resistance to biological, chemical, and meteorological causes of breakdown.

Herbicides are often classed as selective or non-selective but this distinction is rather arbitrary as selective herbicides become non-selective at high doses.

Selectivity of herbicides can be due to one or more of the following factors:

Morphology. The effectiveness of many herbicides depends upon the retention of the applied substance by the plant's outer surface. Plants with a large, horizontal surface area, for example broad-leaved rosette weeds, retain more of a solution sprayed on them than those with narrow vertical leaves such as many grain crops. Other characteristics influencing retention and penetration are the nature of the surface, the thickness of the cuticle, and the pubescence of the leaves. The meristematic tissues, in buds especially, are very susceptible to some herbicides and so the degree of protection, for example by a sheath of leaves, will modify the efficiency of a herbicide.

Chronology. By careful timing of planting and spraying, weed seedlings can be killed before the crop seedlings appear above ground.

Ecology. Weed seeds often lie near the surface of the soil while crop seeds are often planted further down. Thus a herbicide which is not leached down through the soil will kill weed seeds but not those of the crop.

Biochemistry. Auxins are plant hormones which influence many aspects of plant metabolism, especially cell division and cell growth. For each plant species there is an optimum concentration of auxins for growth. Excess of auxin causes over-stimulation of growth and then retardation. Many synthetic auxins have been developed and the basis of their use as selective herbicides depends on the varying sensitivity of different species. A plant that is particularly sensitive to auxins is not likely to have an efficient enzyme system for dealing with them. The optimal concentration of auxin to be used in a particular situation is that which kills the largest number of weeds but does not affect the crop adversely to any great extent.

Chemical Classification

Carbamates. This group includes some of the dithio-carbamates mentioned above under Fungicides. Carbamate herbicides act by interfering with mitosis. Persistence and toxicity to mammals are low but some compounds may cause skin irritation.
The general formula for carbamate herbicides is:

$$\begin{array}{c} R \quad\quad X \\ \diagdown \quad\quad \| \\ N\cdot C\cdot Y\cdot R'' \\ \diagup \\ R' \end{array}$$

where, for carbamates X and Y are both oxygen atoms, for thiocarbamates X is an oxygen atom and Y a sulphur atom, for dithiocarbamates X and Y are both sulphur atoms, and R, R', and R" may be either aliphatic or aromatic groups. Either or both R and R' are hydrogen atoms in some compounds.
The following is a representative selection of carbamate herbicides.

ASULAM (*Asulox®*). Methyl N-(4-aminobenzenesulphonyl)carbamate. Soluble in 200 parts of water, in 4 parts of methyl alcohol, in 3 parts of acetone, and in 50 parts of hydrocarbon liquids. Used as a foliage translocated and residual herbicide to control docks and bracken. LD$_{50}$ (mice) greater than 5000 mg/kg. Renders poisonous weeds palatable to livestock. Available as liquid concentrate containing 40%.

BARBAN (*Carbyne®*; *Oatax®*). 4-Chlorobut-2-ynyl N-(3-chlorophenyl)carbamate. Soluble in 100000 parts of water, in 5 parts of xylene and in 2 parts of e'hylene dichloride. Used as a translocated herbicide, absorbed through the leaves, for post-emergence control of weed grasses in cereal crops. LD$_{50}$ (rats) 600 mg/kg. May be irritating to the skin. Harmful to fish. Minimum interval between application and harvesting of the crop 6 weeks. Available as liquid concentrate containing 25% and as wettable powder containing 50%. Often used in combination with MCPB, dichlorprop and mecoprop.

CYCLOATE (*Ro-neet®*). S-Ethyl N-cyclohexyl-N-ethylthiocarbamate. Soluble in 10000 parts of water. Used as a residual herbicide for control of wild oats and other annual weeds in root crops. Not very persistent. LD$_{50}$ (rats) 3100 mg/kg. Irritating to the eyes, skin, nose, and mouth in some cases. Harmful to fish. Available as liquid concentrate. Often mixed with lenacil.

DI-ALLATE (*Avadex®*; DATC). S-2,3-Dichloroallyl NN-di-isopropylthiocarbamate. Soluble in 25000 parts of water. Used as a residual herbicide for the control of blackgrass and wild oats in brassicas and beet. LD$_{50}$ (rats) 393 mg/kg. May be irritating to the skin. Harmful to fish. Incorporation into the soil essential as it is volatile. Available as granules containing 10% and as liquid concentrate containing 40%.

E.P.T.C. (*Eptam®*). S-Ethyl NN-dipropylthiocarbamate. Soluble in 30000 parts of water. Used as a residual herbicide for the control of seedling stages of broad-leaved annual weeds and perennial grass weeds. LD$_{50}$ (rats) 1630 mg/kg. Harmful to fish. Essential that it is incorporated into the soil immediately. Available as a liquid concentrate containing 60%.

PROPHAM (*Herbon®*; Isopropyl Carbanilate; *Premalox®*; *Quintex®*; *Triherbide®*). Isopropyl N-phenylcarbamate. Soluble in 10000 parts of water. Used as a residual herbicide for the control of many germinating weeds especially in beet crops. LD$_{50}$ (rats) 1000 mg/kg. May be irritating to the eyes, skin, nose, and mouth. Dangerous to fish. Available as wettable powder containing 75% and liquid concentrate containing 24%. Often mixed with other pesticides.

Dipyridyl compounds. Two compounds are in use, diquat and paraquat. They have a very quick killing action by contact and translocation with a very widespread use for many types of weed control. The compounds are inactivated by adsorption as soon as they enter the soil and planting can consequently begin very soon after treatment. Toxic effects include a burning sensation in the mouth and abdomen followed by ulceration. Later effects are alveolitis and terminal bronchiolitis. Renal failure may occur followed by death. Vomiting seldom occurs.
Chemically these compounds are based on two cationic pyridine rings and they are used in the form of their salts.

DIQUAT (*Aquacide®*; Diquat-dibromide; *Reglone®*). 9,10-Dihydro-8a,10a-diazoniaphenanthrene dibromide. Very soluble in water; slightly soluble in polar organic solvents; insoluble in non-polar organic solvents. Solutions of diquat should not be allowed to come into contact with metals because the solutions will corrode them. Used as a contact and foliar translocated herbicide mainly for desiccation of foliage in crops prior to harvesting seed and root crops. Also used for the control of weeds in slow-moving water. LD$_{50}$ (rats) 400 mg/kg. Harmful to livestock which should not be allowed access to treated areas for at least 24 hours after application. Available as liquid concentrate containing 14%.

PARAQUAT (*Dextrone X®*; *Esgram®*; *Gramoxone®*; Paraquat-dichloride; *Weedol®*). 1,1'-Dimethyl-4,4'-bipyridylium dichloride. Very soluble in water; slightly soluble in alcohol. Solutions of paraquat should not be allowed to come into contact with metals because the solutions will corrode them. Used as a contact and foliage translocated herbicide for the control of a wide range of broad-leaved weeds and grasses and for controlling water weeds. LD$_{50}$ (rats) 155 to 203 mg/kg. Harmful to animals. Available as liquid concentrates containing 20% and as granules containing 2.5% mixed with 2.5% of diquat.

Substituted phenoxy acids. These are synthetic auxins which act by stopping cell division at the meristems and producing an abnormal structure in leaves, stems, and roots by interfering with the normal processes of cell elongation. The vascular system is disrupted and the plant slowly dies. The synthetic auxins are quickly broken down in the soil and in the plant and are not very toxic to mammals. The main problem in their use lies in the possibility that during spraying operations there may be some drifting onto other crops which are susceptible to the action of synthetic auxins.
Toxic effects seen only after the ingestion of large doses of these substances include weakness, anorexia, and myotonia. Very high doses (of the order of 6 grams) cause death by ventricular fibrillation.

Substituted phenoxy acids used as herbicides have the general formula:

$$O \cdot [CH_2]_n \cdot COOH$$

where n is 1 or 3 and R and R' are CH_3, Cl, or H. The following is a representative selection of substituted phenoxy acid herbicides.

2,4-D (*Cornox D*®; *Destox*®; *Dicotox*®; *Dioweed*®; *Dormone*®; *Fernimine*®; *For-ester*®; *Iso-planotox*®; *Lornox*®; *Palormone D*®; *Silvapron*®; *Syford*®; *Vergemaster*®; *Vigon-DC*®; *Weedone*®). 2,4-Dichlorophenoxyacetic acid. Soluble in 150 parts of water; the sodium salt is soluble in 20 parts of water. Used as a foliar translocated herbicide with some residual action for the control of many broad-leaved weeds in cereal and grass crops and for the control of weeds on verges and in farm buildings. LD_{50} (rats) 500 mg/kg. Available as solution of the free acid in oil, amine salts and esters as 98% liquid concentrate, and as powder mixed with alkali. Often mixed with other herbicides.

2,4-DB (*Butoxone*®; 4-(2,4-DB); *Embutox*®; *Lomnitox*®; *Perselect*®; *Redlegor*®; *Vigon-4B*®). 4-(2,4-Dichlorophenoxy)butyric acid. Soluble in 25000 parts of water; alkali-metal salts are soluble in water; soluble in 10 parts of acetone. Used as a foliar translocated herbicide with some residual action for post-emergence control of many broad-leaved weeds in clover, cereals, and grass. LD_{50} (rats) 700 mg/kg. Renders poisonous weeds more palatable to livestock. Harmful to fish. Livestock should not be allowed access to treated areas for at least 2 weeks after application. Available as solid salts and emulsifiable concentrate containing 40%. Often mixed with 2,4-D, MCPA, or benazolin.

MCPA (*Agritox*®; *Agroxone*®; *Empal*®; *Herbitox*®; *Phenoxylene Plus*®; *Vigon-P*®). 4-Chloro-2-methylphenoxyacetic acid. Soluble in 125 parts of water; the sodium salt is soluble in 4 parts of water. Used as a foliar translocated herbicide with some residual action for post-emergence control of many broad-leaved weeds in cereals and grassland. LD_{50} (rats) 700 mg/kg. Renders poisonous weeds palatable to livestock. Livestock should not be allowed access to treated areas for at least 2 weeks after application. Available as liquid concentrates containing 20 to 50%. Often used in the form of a salt. Formulations often include other herbicides.

MCPB (4-(MCPB); *New Legumex*®; *Tropotox*®). 4-(4-Chloro-2-methylphenoxy)butyric acid. Soluble in 25000 parts of water, in 6 parts of alcohol and in 4 parts of acetone. Used as a translocated herbicide with some residual action for post-emergence treatment of broad-leaved weeds. LD_{50} (rats) 680 mg/kg. Renders poisonous weeds palatable to livestock. Harmful to fish. Livestock should not be allowed access to treated areas for at least 2 weeks after application. Available as concentrated solution containing 40% of the sodium salt. Often mixed with MCPA or benazolin.

MECOPROP (*Chipko*®; *Clovotox*®; CMPP; *Compitox*®; *Gallitox*®; *Herrifex DS*®; *Iso-Cornox 64*®; *Mecodex*®; *Methoxone*®; *Proponex Plus*®; *Supertox*®; *Sydex*®; *Verdone*®). 2-(4-Chloro-2-methylphenoxy)propionic acid. Soluble in 2000 parts of water; salts of mecoprop are soluble in 2 parts of water. Used as a foliar trans-located herbicide with some residual action for post-emergence control of many broad-leaved weeds in cereals, grass, and fruit tree crops. LD_{50} (rats) 930 mg/kg. Renders poisonous weeds palatable to livestock. Livestock should not be allowed access to treated areas for at least 2 weeks after application. Available as aqueous concentrates containing 40 to 60% of the potassium, sodium, and amine salts. Sometimes mixed with 2,4-D or teroprop.

2,4,5-T (*Brushwood Emulsion*®; *Brushwood Killer*®; *Econal*®; *Phortox*®; *Spontox*®; *Stancide*®; *Trioxone 50*®). 2,4,5-Trichlorophenoxyacetic acid. Soluble in 400 parts of water; soluble in polar solvents. Used as a foliar translocated herbicide with some residual action for the control of woody weeds. LD_{50} (rats) 300 mg/kg. Renders poisonous weeds palatable to livestock. Harmful to fish. It should not be diluted with oils when used in conifers. Available as emulsifiable concentrate containing 40% of the esters. Often mixed with 2,4-D.

Ureas and uracils. These compounds are very persistent but of low solubility so that they have a residual action at the surface of the soil. Otherwise they are not selective. They are widely used for killing young seedling plants which germinate after the soil has been treated. They act mainly by inhibition of photosynthesis. All the compounds in this group have a low mammalian toxicity.

Ureas used as herbicides have the general formula $RNH \cdot CO \cdot NR'R''$, where R is a substituted phenyl group and R' and R'' are small aliphatic groups. The following is a representative selection of urea and uracil herbicides.

BROMACIL. 5-Bromo-3-*sec*-butyl-6-methyluracil. Soluble in 12000 parts of water; soluble in polar solvents and strong aqueous bases. Used as a residual and contact herbicide for total weed control and for selective control in cane fruit. LD_{50} (rats) 5200 mg/kg. May be irritating to the eyes, skin, nose, and mouth. Available as wettable powder containing 80%.

CHLOROXURON (*Tenoran*®). 3-[4-(4-Chlorophenoxy)-phenyl]-1,1-dimethylurea. Soluble in 300000 parts of water; slightly soluble in alcohol and acetone. Used as a residual action herbicide to control seedling weeds among strawberries and chrysanthemums. LD_{50} (rats) greater than 3000 mg/kg. Available as wettable powder containing 50%.

DIURON (*Dexuron*®). 3-(3,4-Dichlorophenyl)-1,1-dimethylurea. Soluble in 25000 parts of water and in 20 parts of acetone. Used as a persistent residual herbicide for total non-selective weed control or selective weed control in woody crops. LD_{50} (rats) 3400 mg/kg. May be irritating to the eyes, skin, nose, and mouth. Harmful to fish. Available as wettable powder containing 80%. Mixed with paraquat as liquid concentrate and sometimes mixed with other herbicides.

LENACIL (*Venzar*®). 3-Cyclohexyl-6,7-dihydro-1*H*-cyclopentapyrimidine-2,4-(3*H*,5*H*)-dione. Soluble in 200000 parts of water. Used as a persistent residual herbicide with some contact action for pre-emergence control of germinating weeds in root crops and in some flower crops. LD_{50} (rats) greater than 11000 mg/kg. Available as wettable powder containing 80%.

LINURON (*Afalon*®; *Lanslide*®). 3-(3,4-Dichlorophenyl)-1-methoxy-1-methylurea. Soluble in 13000 parts of water. Used as a residual and contact herbicide for pre-emergence control of corn marigolds in cereals and a wide range of weeds in potatoes and post-emergence control in carrot and other umbelliferous crops. LD_{50} (rats) 1500 mg/kg. Can be irritating to skin, eyes, nose, and mouth. Harmful to fish. Available as liquid concentrates containing 15% and as wettable powder containing 50%. Often mixed with chlorpropham, ioxynil, or lenacil.

MALEIC HYDRAZIDE. 1,2-Dihydropyridazine-3,6-dione. Soluble in 200 parts of water, in 1000 parts of acetone, in 1000 parts of alcohol, and in 2000 parts of xylene. Used as a foliage translocated herbicide with some residual action to suppress grass and sucker growth and to prevent sprouting of onions in stores. LD_{50} (rats) 4000 mg/kg. Harmful to fish. Available as a liquid concentrate containing 30%. Often mixed with 2,4-D.

Triazines. These are persistent non-selective herbicides absorbed through the roots of the plant and translocated to all parts. They act by interfering with photosynthesis. Toxicity to mammals is low. They have the general formula

where R is a variable structure and R' and R" are substituted amines.
The following is a representative selection of triazines.

AMETRYNE (*Gesapax®*). 2-Ethylamino-4-isopropylamino-6-methylthio-1,3,5-triazine. Soluble in 5000 parts of water. Used as a foliar translocated and residual herbicide to control annual weeds in potatoes. LD_{50} (rats) 1405 mg/kg. Harmful to fish. Available as wettable powder containing 80%.

ATRAZINE (*Gesaprim®*; *Residox®*; *Vectal®*; *Weedex A 50 WP®*). 2-Chloro-4-ethylamino-6-isopropylamino-1,3,-5-triazine. Soluble in 15000 parts of water, in 50 parts of methyl alcohol, and in 20 parts of chloroform. Used as a persistent residual and contact herbicide in non-crop situations. It is also used as a selective herbicide for control of many germinating weeds in maize. LD_{50} (rats) 3080 mg/kg. Available as granules containing 4% and as wettable powders containing 50 and 80%.

SIMAZINE (*Herbazin®*; *Gesatop®*; *Simadex®*; *Simasol®*; *Weedex S50®*). 2-Chloro-4,6-bisethylamino-1,3,5-triazine. Soluble in 200000 parts of water and in 2500 parts of methanol. Used as a persistent residual action herbicide for pre-emergence control of many germinating weeds. It is also used for total weed control. LD_{50} (rats) greater than 5000 mg/kg. Available as granules containing 10% and as wettable powder containing 50%.

TERBUTRYNE (*Opogard®*; *Prebane®*). 2-*tert*-Butylamino-4-ethylamino-6-methylthio-1,3,5-triazine. Soluble in 20000 parts of water. Used as a residual herbicide in pre-emergence control of blackgrass and broad-leaved weeds in winter wheat and barley. LD_{50} (rats) 2400 mg/kg. Harmful to fish. Available as wettable powder containing 50%. Sometimes mixed with terbuthylazine.

Substituted aliphatic acids. These are used especially against perennial grass weeds. They have a low level of persistence and are irritant but only moderately toxic. The mode of action has not been established but may involve combination with proteins. The following is a representative selection of substituted aliphatic acid herbicides.

DALAPON (*Basfapon®*; *Dalacide®*; Dalapon Sodium;

Dowpon®; *Hurstmaster®*). Sodium 2,2-dichloropropionate. Soluble in 2 parts of water and in 5 parts of methyl alcohol. Used as a foliar translocated herbicide with some contact and residual action for control of couch and other perennial grasses. LD_{50} (rats) 6000 to 8000 mg/kg. Irritating to the eyes and skin. Available as powder for solution and also as solution with MCPA.

SODIUM MONOCHLORO-ACETATE (*Herbon®*; *Somon®*; *Monoxane®*). Soluble in 1.5 parts of water. Used as a contact herbicide for control of many post-emergence weeds in *Brassica* crops. LD_{50} (rats) 300 to 400 mg/kg. Harmful to bees and livestock, especially poultry. Livestock should not be allowed access to treated areas for at least 2 weeks after application. Available as powder for solution.

TRICHLOROACETIC ACID (*Actan®*; TCA; *Tecane®*; *Varitox®*) (see also separate entry). Used as a residual herbicide with some contact and foliar translocated action for pre-planting control of couch grass and wild oats. LD_{50} (rats) 3200 mg/kg. Irritating to the eyes, nose, mouth, and skin. Not to be used on soil where bulbs are to be grown. Available as the sodium salt for solution.

Phenols. A number of phenols described above as fungicides or insecticides are used as herbicides with a contact action. They are used mainly for crop desiccation or in pre-emergence treatment.

Benzonitriles. Various substituted compounds of benzonitrile are used as herbicides. They have a residual action in the soil and are of low or moderate toxicity to mammals.
The following is a representative selection of benzonitriles.

BROMOXYNIL (*Oxytril®*; *Tetroxone®*). 3,5-Dibromo-4-hydroxybenzonitrile. Soluble in 7500 parts of water, in 10 parts of methyl alcohol, and in 5 parts of acetone; metallic salt derivatives are much more soluble in water. Used as a contact herbicide with some foliar translocated action for control of broad-leaved weeds in cereals. LD_{50} (rats) 190 mg/kg. Harmful to fish. Used only in admixture with other herbicides. Available as liquid concentrates of salts or esters containing 20% of active ingredients.

DICHLOBENIL (*Casoron®*; 2-6 DBN). 2,6-Dichlorobenzonitrile. Soluble in 55000 parts of water. Used as a residual herbicide with some contact activity for total weed control and for selective control of annual weeds in woody crops. Also used to kill weeds in still or slow-moving water. LD_{50} (rats) 3160 mg/kg. Available as granules containing 7.5%.

IOXYNIL (*Totril®*; *Actrilawn®*). 4-Hydroxy-3,5-di-iodo-benzonitrile. Soluble in 20000 parts of water, in 14 parts of acetone, and in 50 parts of methyl alcohol; alkali metal salt derivatives are soluble in 5 parts of water. Used as a contact herbicide for general weed control in newly sown turf, onions, and leeks. LD_{50} (rats) 110 mg/kg. Harmful to fish. Available as aqueous concentrates of metallic salts and emulsifiable concentrates of amines. Often mixed with other herbicides.

Inorganic compounds. Sodium chlorate is the most widely used inorganic herbicide. Toxicity is low but it is explosive and corrosive. Ammonium sulphamate, which is also corrosive, is used particularly to kill woody plants. Sulphuric acid is used as a contact herbicide but not in cereal crops; because of its extremely corrosive properties its use is very limited.

AMMONIUM SULPHAMATE (*Amcide®*). Soluble in water;

insoluble in non-polar solvents. Used as a foliar translocated and residual herbicide with some contact action to control woody plants on non-cropped land. LD_{50} (rats) 4000 mg/kg.

SODIUM CHLORATE (*Atlacide®*; *Atlavar®*; *Chlorea®*). Soluble in 1.5 parts of water; soluble in alcohol and in glycerol. It should be stored away from heat. Containers should not be made of metals liable to corrosion. Materials impregnated with sodium chlorate may become inflammable when dry. Used as a residual poison with foliar translocated and contact action for total weed control. LD_{50} (rats) 1200 mg/kg. Harmful to fish. Available as powder and formulated as dust and granules. Often mixed with atrazine to give a more persistent effect.

SULPHURIC ACID (see also separate entry). Containers should be airtight and corrosion resistant. Used as a contact herbicide for potato haulms and leguminous seed crops. It has a desiccant action. Also used in pre-emergence weed control in crops. Very corrosive. Used diluted.

Chemicals used to Control Mammalian Pests (Rodenticides)

In Great Britain, the chief mammalian pests which destroy growing and stored foodstuffs are rabbits, mice, rats, and grey squirrels. Squirrels are difficult to control by chemical means but the others can be controlled by chemicals, either by mixing the poison with bait or by fumigation of the places where they live.

Because of the similarity in their physiology, mammalian pests, man, and domestic animals are susceptible to the same poisons and so care must be taken when pesticides are used to ensure that only the pests are exposed to the poison.

Warfarin is used extensively against rats and mice. Very little need be put in the bait as it acts as a cumulative poison in the body. In recent years, colonies of rats have become resistant to warfarin in some parts of the country. Calciferol, alone or with warfarin, is effective in warfarin-resistant rodents.

Sodium monofluoroacetate is extremely toxic to man and is difficult to handle safely. The potassium salt occurs in some plants, such as the South African plant *Dichapetalum agmosum*. Sodium monofluoroacetate causes rats to need water and so they leave their hiding places before dying. It is an effective and fast poison.

Alphachloralose and thallium sulphate are also used.

Hydrogen cyanide gas is widely used against rabbits as a fumigant placed at the entrance to the rabbit burrows. Powdered sodium cyanide is used which releases hydrogen cyanide when moistened. Hydrogen cyanide is highly toxic to man.

The following is a representative selection of chemicals used to control mammalian pests.

SODIUM MONOFLUOROACETATE. Soluble in water. Used as a rodenticide. LD_{50} (rats) 0.22 mg/kg. Very toxic to mammals. Toxic effects include vomiting, apprehension, tremors, cardiac irregularities, and convulsions. Coma and death may eventually follow. Available as an aqueous solution containing also 0.5% of nigrosine.

WARFARIN SODIUM (see also separate entry). Used as a rodenticide by utilising its property of preventing coagulation of blood. LD_{50} (rats) 1 mg/kg. Very toxic to all mammals. Symptoms include bleeding from the gums and presence of erythrocytes in the urinary deposit. Available as a dust containing 1% for use on runs and in holes and in a concentration of 0.1% mixed with a suitable bait.

Nematocides and Molluscicides

Nematocides are used for the control of eelworms which live in the soil and attack the roots of some crops. Molluscicides are used for the control of slugs and snails which cause damage mainly by eating new leaves on seedlings.

Two organophosphorus compounds, oxamyl and thionazin, are used as nematocides. The organochlorine compounds dichlorpropene, chlordane, and tetrachlorothiophene are also used.

All nematocides are somewhat persistent and are ploughed into the soil from which they are absorbed by the nematodes. Two compounds are commonly used as molluscicides: methiocarb, a carbamate with anticholinesterase activity, and metaldehyde, the mode of action of which is unknown. Metaldehyde is the more commonly used and is mixed with food as a bait.

The following is a representative selection of nematocides and molluscicides.

ALDICARB (*Temik®*). 2-Methyl-2-(methylthio)propionaldehyde *O*-(methylcarbamoyl)oxime. Soluble in 150 parts of water. Used as a systemic carbamate nematocide and insecticide against millipedes, eelworms, and many insect pests of root crops. LD_{50} (rats) 0.93 mg/kg. Dangerous to fish, game, and wildlife. Available as granules containing 10%.

CHLORDANE (*Sydane®*). 1,2,4,5,6,7,8,8-Octachloro-3a,4,7,7a-tetrahydro-4,7-methanoindane. Practically insoluble in water. Used as a persistent organochlorine earthworm killer for turf. LD_{50} (rats) 457 mg/kg. Harmful to livestock and fish. Livestock should not be allowed access to treated areas for at least 2 weeks after application. Available as liquid concentrate containing 25%.

METALDEHYDE (Metacetaldehyde; Meta; *Sluggex®*; *Slugoids®*). Soluble in 5000 parts of water; slightly soluble in alcohol and ether; soluble in chloroform. Should be stored in airtight containers. Used as a molluscicide for the control of slugs and snails. LD_{50} (dogs) 600 mg/kg. Dangerous to game, wild birds, and animals. Harmful to fish. Children, livestock, and domestic animals should not be allowed access to storage places or treated areas. Available as baits containing 2.5 to 6% in a protein-rich milling offal such as bran.

METHIOCARB (*Draza®*). 4-Methylthio-3,5-xylyl *N*-methylcarbamate. Practically insoluble in water. Used as a molluscicide. LD_{50} (rats) 100 mg/kg. Harmful to fish. Minimum interval between application and harvesting of the crop 7 days; livestock should not be allowed access to treated areas for at least 7 days after application. Available as bait containing 4%.

THIONAZIN (*Nemafos®*). Diethyl 2-pyrazinyl phosphorothionate. Soluble in 900 parts of water. Used as a systemic nematocide against eelworms in some flower crops and also against mites. LD_{50} (rats) 12 mg/kg. Dangerous to fish and livestock. Livestock should not be allowed access to treated areas for at least 8 weeks after application. Available as liquid concentrates containing 25 to 45%.

Pethidine Hydrochloride

4 - Ethoxycarbonyl - 1 - methyl - 4 - phenylpiperidinium chloride

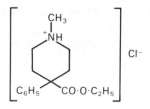

$C_{15}H_{22}ClNO_2 = 283.8$

OTHER NAMES: Meperidine Hydrochloride: Pethidini Hydrochloridum
Pethilorfan® (with levallorphan tartrate); *Pamergan®* (with promethazine hydrochloride)

A standard is given in the European Pharmacopoeia Vol. III

Description. An odourless white crystalline powder with a slightly acid and bitter taste.

Solubility. Soluble in water; soluble, at 20°, in 20 parts of alcohol; soluble in chloroform; very slightly soluble in ether and in acetone.

Acidity. A 2% solution has a pH of 4.5 to 5.5.

Dissociation constant. pK_a 8.7 (20°).

Sterilisation. Solutions for injection are sterilised by heating in an autoclave or by filtration.

Identification. TESTS. 1. Dissolve about 5 mg in 0.5 ml of water and add 2 drops of *formaldehyde solution* and 2 ml of *sulphuric acid*; an orange-red colour is produced.
2. To 5 ml of a 1% solution add 10 ml of *trinitrophenol solution*; a precipitate is produced which, after washing with water, melts at about 190°.

MELTING-POINT. About 188°.

ULTRAVIOLET ABSORPTION. In water or alcohol, weak maxima at 251 nm, 257 nm, and 263 nm.

INFRA-RED ABSORPTION. Major peaks at 735, 1064, 1099, 1176, 1235, and 1724 cm^{-1} (see Appendix 2b: Infra-red Spectra).

THIN-LAYER CHROMATOGRAPHY. See under Thin-layer Chromatography, System 7.

Determination in body fluids. COLORIMETRY. In plasma or urine—J. J. Burns *et al.*, *J. Pharmac. exp. Ther.*, 1955, **114**, 289.

GAS CHROMATOGRAPHY. In plasma—M. A. Evans and R. D. Harbison, *J. pharm. Sci.*, 1977, **66**, 599; H. H. Szeto and C. E. Inturrisi, *J. Chromat.*, 1976, **125**, 503.

Metabolism. ABSORPTION. Readily absorbed after oral administration.

BLOOD CONCENTRATION. After an intravenous dose of 0.8 mg/kg of pethidine hydrochloride to normal subjects, plasma concentrations of about 0.2 μg/ml are obtained in 1 hour falling to 0.1 μg/ml after a further 2 hours; after an intramuscular dose of 100 mg, plasma concentrations of about 0.5 μg/ml are attained in about 1 hour; the administration of anaesthetics appears to cause up to a two-fold increase in plasma concentration of unchanged drug; similarly plasma concentrations appear to vary according to age, concentrations being higher in older subjects.

DISTRIBUTION. Rapidly and extensively distributed throughout the tissues; volume of distribution, 200 to 300 litres; it readily crosses the placenta, is secreted in milk, and taken up to some extent by red blood cells; *protein binding*, 40 to 65% bound to plasma proteins.

METABOLIC REACTIONS. N-Demethylation, hydrolysis, glucuronic acid conjugation, and N-oxidation; the rate of metabolism is decreased in pregnancy and increased in older subjects; pethidine appears to be subject to first pass metabolism after oral administration.

EXCRETION. The excretion of pethidine and its metabolites is influenced by the pH value of the urine; less unchanged drug is excreted in older subjects; in subjects with cirrhosis, excretion of pethidine is delayed; in acid urine, 10 to 30% of a dose is excreted unchanged, 10 to 35% is excreted as norpethidine, and about 1% is excreted as pethidine N-oxide; in alkaline urine less than 5% is excreted as pethidine and norpethidine; in normal subjects, about 70% of a dose is excreted in the urine in 24 hours, up to 10% as unchanged drug, 10% as norpethidine, 20% as pethidinic acid, 16% as conjugated pethidinic acid, 8% as norpethidinic acid, and 10% as conjugated norpethidinic acid; in pregnant women and in women taking oral contraceptives, the urinary excretion of unchanged pethidine appears to be increased.

FURTHER INFORMATION. Bioavailability—K. Chan *et al.*, *J. Pharm. Pharmac.*, 1975, **27**, 235 and J. E. Stambaugh and I. W. Wainer, *J. clin. Pharmac.*, 1975, **15**, 269; effect of ageing on metabolism—K. Chan *et al.*, *Br. J. clin. Pharmac.*, 1975, **2**, 297; metabolites—C. Lindberg *et al.*, *J. Pharm. Pharmac.*, 1975, **27**, 975 and M. Mitchard *et al.*, *J. Pharm. Pharmac.*, 1972, **24**, 915; pharmacokinetics—U. Klotz *et al.*, *Clin. Pharmac. Ther.*, 1974, **16**, 667 and L. E. Mather *et al.*, *Clin. Pharmac. Ther.*, 1975, **17**, 21; secretion into gastric juice—T. Gessner *et al.*, *J. Pharm. Pharmac.*, 1976, **28**, 79.

Actions and uses. Pethidine has analgesic, sedative, spasmolytic, and local anaesthetic actions. Its spasmolytic action is less important than was originally claimed and may be largely dependent on its local effect on nerve fibres and nerve endings.
Pethidine is used to relieve the more severe types of pain which were previously controllable only by opiates; 100 milligrams of pethidine hydrochloride by mouth or by intramuscular or slow intermittent intravenous injection produces relief from pain in most medical or surgical conditions. Intravenous injection often produces undesirable effects. Intramuscular injection is more reliable than oral administration and produces an effect in 10 to 15 minutes which lasts for 2 to 5 hours.
Pethidine has been substituted for morphine in pre- and post-operative medication, but its action is not as powerful or prolonged as that of morphine for the control of severe post-operative pain. It is sometimes used in association with intravenous anaesthetics.
As it reduces the severity of labour pains without seriously diminishing the force of uterine contractions, pethidine is used as an obstetric analgesic; 100 milligrams is given by intramuscular injection as soon as regular contractions begin; the injection may be repeated 1 to 3 hours later if necessary, but more than 4 doses should not be given within 24 hours.
Barbiturates or hyoscine may be given concurrently to enhance sedation and depress memory.
The usual dose of pethidine hydrochloride is 50 to 100 milligrams by mouth, 25 to 100 milligrams by subcutaneous or intramuscular injection, or 25 to 50 milli-

grams by intravenous injection. Children may be given the following doses by intramuscular injection: up to one year 1 to 2 milligrams per kilogram body-weight, 1 to 5 years 12.5 to 25 milligrams, and 6 to 12 years 25 to 50 milligrams.

Undesirable effects. Pethidine rarely produces toxic effects, although dizziness, nausea, and dryness of the mouth may occur. Intravenous injection of pethidine may cause a fall in blood pressure.

The administration of pethidine as an analgesic during labour may give rise to respiratory depression in the infant at birth; levallorphan, 1.25 milligrams for every 100 milligrams of pethidine hydrochloride, has been administered simultaneously with the object of reducing this risk.

Precautions. Pethidine should not be given to patients who are being treated with a monoamine-oxidase inhibitor, such as isocarboxazid, nialamide, phenelzine, or tranylcypromine, or within about 2 weeks of the discontinuation of such treatment. It should not be given in conjunction with meprobamate as the treatment may cause the development of hypotension.

Dependence. Pethidine produces mild euphoria in some patients and may lead to dependence of the morphine type, as described under Drug Dependence.

Poisoning. The procedure described under Morphine Hydrochloride should be adopted.

Veterinary uses. Pethidine hydrochloride is a narcotic analgesic. The usual dose by intramuscular injection for all species is 1 to 5 milligrams per kilogram body-weight.

Preparations

PETHIDINE INJECTION: a sterile solution of pethidine hydrochloride in water for injections. It is sterilised by heating in an autoclave or by filtration. Available in 1- and 2-ml ampoules containing 50 mg of pethidine hydrochloride per ml.
A standard for this injection is given in the British Pharmacopoeia 1973
Containers and *Labelling:* see the entry on Injections for general information on containers and labelling.

PETHIDINE TABLETS: available as tablets containing 50 mg of pethidine hydrochloride.
A standard for these tablets is given in the British Pharmacopoeia 1973
Containers and *Storage:* see the entry on Tablets for general information on containers and storage. Containers should be airtight.

OTHER PREPARATIONS available include an INJECTION containing pethidine hydrochloride 50 mg with levallorphan tartrate 625 micrograms per ml in 1- and 2-ml ampoules, and an injection containing pethidine hydrochloride 50 mg with promethazine hydrochloride 25 mg per ml in 2-ml ampoules.

Petit Mal

see under EPILEPSY

Phaeochromocytoma

A phaeochromocytoma is a catecholamine-producing tumour arising from chromaffin tissue usually in the adrenal medulla but sometimes in other sites. The tumour gives rise to hypertension which may be paroxysmal or, rarely, sustained, according to the pattern of the release of pressor amines, although in some patients hypotension may be the presenting feature. Headaches, palpitations, pain in chest and abdomen, sweating, apprehension, nausea, vomiting, hyperglycaemia, and glycosuria may occur.

In the diagnosis of phaeochromocytoma, an attack may be precipitated by drugs such as histamine, methacholine, or tyramine; however, precipitation of an attack is dangerous and diagnosis should therefore rely on urinary estimation of catecholamines or their metabolites. The effects of released catecholamines may be blocked by α-adrenergic blocking agents such as phenoxybenzamine or phentolamine followed by blockade with β-adrenergic blocking drugs such as propranolol or oxprenolol.

Phaeochromocytoma is treated by the surgical excision of the adenoma. Care should be taken to prevent excessive rises or falls in blood pressure or contraction of plasma volume during induction of anaesthesia, during surgery, or in the immediate post-operative period.

Pharmacy Practice

Good Pharmaceutical Practice in the Preparation of Medicines

The quality of a pharmaceutical product depends primarily on the degree of care taken in its preparation. Final checks carried out on the finished product are useful in confirming that the correct ingredients have been used and that the materials have been correctly processed but it is essential that proper in-process control is exercised and that it is adequately documented to provide reliable evidence that the correct procedures have been followed.

General Principles

Pharmaceutical operations vary from dispensing for individual patients to large-scale manufacture of complex products. Sound practice and some form of quality control are necessary in every case but although widely differing facilities are necessary, the general principles remain the same; however expansion of the scope of operations generally leads to a need for more stringent precautions. Premises have to be clean and suitable (preferably built for the purpose) and there must be adequately trained staff directed by qualified personnel. In all except the smallest operations production and quality control functions are separated, written directions are followed, and records are kept that would enable faulty medicines to be traced and recalled. Stocks of raw materials and medicinal products are kept under optimum storage conditions and used in rotation.

Staff should avoid hazardous methods of working. They should avoid contact with hazardous materials and should not inhale toxic dusts. Suitable arrangements should be made for handling inflammable, explosive, or radioactive materials.

Dispensing Operations

This section covers the preparation of medicines for individual patients.

Quality is dependent on in-process control exercised by the pharmacist who must carry out all operations himself or maintain a close scrutiny and satisfy himself before the medicine is released that the prescription has been correctly interpreted and that procedures have been correctly carried out by selected and trained staff.

Similar considerations apply when medicines are dispensed by or under the supervision of a medical or veterinary practitioner instead of a pharmacist.

Special arrangements should be made to ensure that no mix-up can occur in labelling or in identification of patients. Comprehensive records are not usually justified but it should be possible to trace, for a short period at least, the person who prepared and checked any dispensed medicine, and the origin of the medicine if a manufactured product or the ingredients if it was compounded in the pharmacy. In areas where pharmacies serve a suitable population the keeping of patient records may be a valuable additional safeguard.

Premises and apparatus should be suitable when considered by the criteria of the paragraphs below headed "premises" and "apparatus". In larger dispensaries where many operations are going on simultaneously special vigilance is required and some of the checks described under "manufacturing" are applicable. Dispensaries should be kept as free from disturbance as possible and benches free from all apparatus and materials other than those necessary for the operations being carried out. Where operations have to be interrupted a clear sequence of events should be established to prevent the possibility of duplication or omission.

Finally, the pharmacist should establish that the recipient is aware of the correct method of use of the medicine and should take any other steps to prevent the possibility of misuse and to ensure that there are no inadvertent hazards introduced by the supply of the medicine.

Hospital Pharmacies

It is customary to classify operations as "dispensing" or "manufacturing" and to perform separate quality-control procedures for manufactured products. The procedures to be adopted are those outlined under "dispensing operations" (above) and "manufacturing operations" (below). Some operations are intermediate in scale and an intermediate procedure may sometimes be adopted; such a scheme is given below for small-scale pharmaceutical manufacturing for pharmacists in retail pharmacy business. Pre-packaging from bulk and the preparation of medicines for stock are regarded as manufacturing operations.

Manufacturing Operations

In this category the scale of operations justifies the need for the most complete scheme of recording and checking, and requires that the testing and approval of the final product is carried out by a unit that is separate from the production unit.

The overall arrangements to prepare a satisfactory product may be referred to as quality assurance. This includes product design, development, and good manufacturing practice. Good manufacturing practice itself involves quality control. Tests are carried out on raw materials and at each stage of production, and any batch of material completed is released only if it has the approval of the quality control section; this applies to release of a product for further work or as a finished product. Safeguards such as label counts, area clearance, and yield data are maintained to minimise the possibility of error. Production documentation and quality control results must be reconciled before a batch is released. The release specification should be drawn up bearing in mind the need for the product to comply with pharmacopoeial or other recognised standards at any time during the expected shelf-life.

Precautions should be taken to avoid cross-contamination with other products being manufactured. This may require segregation of manufacture, containment of material in an area by means of airlocks, clothing change, careful washing and decontamination of equipment, and avoidance of contamination through the ventilation system. See also below under "premises". More detailed information may be obtained from published guides.

In the United Kingdom pharmaceutical manufacturing is controlled by the licensing requirements of the Medicines Act 1968. The Department of Health and Social Security issues a "Guide to Good Pharmaceutical Manufacturing Practice", also known as the "Orange Guide". The following outline is consistent with the second edition (1977).

Personnel and training. Sufficient personnel with adequate qualifications and training are required for each process or manufacturing stage and their duties and responsibilities should be clearly defined. The production manager and the quality controller should be different persons who are jointly responsible for the quality of products, but act independently. Responsible deputies should be appointed for key personnel. Training of all personnel should include the basic principles of good pharmaceutical practice together with special training for specific tasks. In addition to initial training, revision and extension will be required at appropriate intervals.

Protective garments, including headgear, footwear, and gloves, should be worn in production areas, and high standards of hygiene should be observed. Especial care should be taken to prevent direct contact between the skin and raw materials, intermediate products, and finished medicines. Eating, drinking, and smoking should not be permitted in manufacturing and laboratory areas. The general standard of health of staff should be observed and persons with potentially infective conditions transferred to duties outside manufacturing or laboratory areas.

Documentation. Manufacture should be based on written instructions and records which should cover all procedures. Specifications for raw materials and packaging and a master formula document including methods of manufacture and packaging are needed for each product.

Detailed records should be kept of the manufacture and packing of each batch including all intermediate steps; all testing procedures including sampling of raw materials, intermediate and finished products, and packaging materials should follow written instructions. Analytical results should be fully recorded.

Premises. Premises should be built to reasonable standards so that contamination of the product by dust, flaking plaster, paint, etc. or by leakage of rainwater, is avoided, and that they are kept free from pests. Smooth impervious finishes are required, and suitable lighting and ventilation should be provided.

In premises where several products are manufactured buildings and ventilation systems should be arranged and plant installed so as to minimise the danger of cross-contamination from adjacent processes or through the ventilation system.

Apparatus. Suitable equipment should be installed to suit the processes being carried out. It should be cleaned and maintained as required so that it does not contaminate materials or products.

Procedure. Procedure should follow a master formula and method that have been devised after examination of the problems and of requirements such as batch reproducibility and stability.

Procedures should be kept under review and their

validity should be re-established after any changes that could affect the product, for example changes in supply of raw materials, major overhauls, changes of location, and modifications of equipment.

Raw materials. Raw materials should be allocated batch numbers and should not be used until authorised by the responsible quality controller after examination. They should be issued by a responsible person, and materials for a manufacturing procedure should be weighed or measured, filled into containers, and labelled in an area set aside for the purpose. Similar considerations apply to the storage and use of intermediate products.

Packaging and labelling. Precautions should be taken to avoid mistakes by using where possible roll-feed labels of a distinctive design for each product, and reconciling the number issued and used. Refinements intended to reduce error include on-line batch coding and the use of electronic code readers and label counters.

Storage and transport. The finished products should be stored under conditions that minimise deterioration, and should not be subjected to unacceptable extremes of temperature, light, moisture, or other adverse influences during transport.

Distribution records. The recipients of each batch should be recorded so that the material can be recalled if necessary.

Recall. A recall procedure should be prepared in case it should become necessary to recover stock of a product which has been found defective. The procedure should be capable of being put into operation immediately at any time and arrangements should provide for dealing with situations of varying urgency.

Small-scale Manufacture in Retail Pharmacy Business

Many of the problems above do not arise when small scale manufacture is performed as part of a retail pharmacy business, and in the United Kingdom a pharmacist does not require a licence under the Medicines Act for making his own medicines provided that they are sold or supplied from the pharmacy where they are made and provided that the products are not advertised. The Pharmaceutical Society of Great Britain has issued a short guide (*Pharm. J.*, ii/1971, 195) and the following is a revised version.

QUALITY CONTROL. A system of quality control is essential in the manufacture of medicinal products. The pharmacist himself will be responsible for this quality control and, although analytical testing is not a requirement for a product manufactured in a retail pharmacy business, the pharmacist should reasonably satisfy himself of the identity of the ingredients used and the quality of the final product. Where large quantities of medicines for sale in a pharmacy are prepared in a single batch consideration should be given to fuller analytical procedures to be carried out either on the premises or by a suitable laboratory.

SUITABILITY OF PREMISES. In many pharmacies the small-scale manufacture of products for sale in the pharmacy ("nostrums") will be carried out in the dispensary. (In the United Kingdom dispensaries will be the subject of regulations under Section 66 of the Medicines Act 1968.) In cases where small-scale manufacturing operations are carried out in a pharmacy in a place other than the dispensary the pharmacist must satisfy himself that the area is suitable for the operations involved. The pharmacist will have regard to the need to ensure that

(a) the area is free from offensive emissions, odours, and other possible sources of contamination, (b) the area is maintained in a clean and orderly condition and is adequately lit and ventilated, and (c) precautions are taken to protect against the entrance and harbouring of rodents, insects, birds, and other pests.

SUITABILITY OF EQUIPMENT. Equipment parts that come into contact with the materials being processed should not affect the ingredients or the product. The design of the apparatus should be such that it can be taken apart, if necessary, for cleaning. Where the same equipment is used to manufacture different formulations or to package different products it should be cleaned thoroughly when the processing of each batch is completed.

CONTROL OF RAW MATERIALS. In retail pharmacy business, raw materials used in manufacturing processes should be obtained under a warranty from the supplier. Pharmacists should reasonably satisfy themselves as to the identity of raw materials. All containers of raw materials received from manufacturers should carry an identifying batch reference mark. The pharmacist should confirm that such a mark is present or if it is not he should add his own batch mark. The date of receipt should also be marked on all containers of raw materials. Stocks of raw materials should be stored under appropriate conditions and batches used in order of purchase. The pharmacist must exercise his knowledge of the stability of materials and be prepared to destroy any that have been kept unused for unduly long periods.

MANUFACTURING OPERATIONS. The manufacturing process must be supervised by a pharmacist. Each batch of product should be manufactured in accordance with a working formula and method as described below under "records". Manufacturing operations should be conducted in a manner which avoids contamination of one product by another. Segregation should be practised to avoid mix-ups. Finally, the containers should be labelled appropriately.

STAFF. All staff employed on a process should wear clean protective garments appropriate to the process being carried out. A person known to be suffering from a disease in communicable form or to be the carrier of such disease or a person with open lesions on the exposed surface of the body must not be allowed to undertake manufacturing processes. Eating and smoking must not be allowed in the manufacturing area. Washing facilities must be provided and their use encouraged.

RECORDS. Adequate records should be kept to enable the raw materials used to be identified and to assist in the recall of the product if necessary. A written master formula, which lists the individual raw materials and quantities to be used for each batch size and a written manufacturing method should be kept for each product. A working formula should be made out and the process to be followed described for each batch of the product. This working document should be in accordance with the master formula and on it should be recorded at the time of manufacture: the supplier and identification mark of each raw material used; the quantities of each raw material used and any necessary checks made by the pharmacist; and the date of manufacture and batch identification mark of the product. Complete records of each batch manufactured should be retained in a suitable form for at least 2 years from the date of manufacture.

PACKAGING AND LABELLING. Containers should be those indicated in the entry for the type of product (mixture, liniment, lotion, etc.) and in agreement with the recommendations of the Council of the Pharmaceutical Society

(*Pharm. J.*, i/1972, 80). Any legal requirements such as the use of fluted bottles and child-resistant closures for certain types of product should be complied with. Containers should be labelled in accordance with legal requirements, such as, for the United Kingdom, the Medicines (Labelling) Regulations 1976 (S.I. 1726) and the Medicines (Labelling) Amendment Regulations 1977 (S.I. 996), and the label of the final packaged product should bear the batch identification mark. New labels must be printed when any change is made in the composition of a product. The filled containers of each batch should be labelled immediately after filling. Segregation should be practised to avoid mix-up.

STORAGE. Products should be correctly stored, particular attention being paid to the optimum temperature, protection from sunlight where the ingredients of a medicine are sensitive to light, and protection from atmospheric moisture if necessary.

Phenacetin

4'-Ethoxyacetanilide

NH·CO·CH₃

O·C₂H₅

$C_{10}H_{13}NO_2 = 179.2$

OTHER NAMES: Acetophenetidin; Aceto-*p*-phenetidide; Phenacetinum

A standard is given in the *European Pharmacopoeia Vol. I*

Description. Odourless, white, glistening, crystalline scales or fine, white, crystalline powder with a slightly bitter taste.

Solubility. Very slightly soluble in water; soluble, at 20°, in 20 parts of alcohol and in 20 parts of chloroform; very slightly soluble in glycerol.

Hygroscopicity. At relative humidities between about 15 and 90% the equilibrium moisture content at 25° is about 2%.

Identification. TESTS. 1. Mix about 100 mg with 1 ml of dilute hydrochloric acid, boil for 3 minutes, add 10 ml of water, cool, filter, and to the filtrate add a few drops of potassium dichromate solution; a violet colour is produced which changes rapidly to ruby-red.
2. Mix about 50 mg with 1 ml of dilute nitric acid and 1 ml of water, boil for 30 seconds, cool rapidly, and filter; a yellow crystalline precipitate is produced which, after washing with water and recrystallising from alcohol (95%), melts at about 102°.

MELTING-POINT. About 135°.

ULTRAVIOLET ABSORPTION. In alcohol (95%), maximum at 250 nm (E1%, 1cm = 877).

INFRA-RED ABSORPTION. Major peaks at 836, 1244, 1479, 1503, 1547, and 1657 cm⁻¹ (see Appendix 2a: Infra-red Spectra).

THIN-LAYER CHROMATOGRAPHY. See under Thin-layer Chromatography, System 3.

Determination in body fluids. GAS CHROMATOGRAPHY. In plasma: phenacetin and its metabolite paracetamol —W. A. Garland *et al.*, *J. pharm. Sci.*, 1977, **66**, 340.

HIGH PRESSURE LIQUID CHROMATOGRAPHY. In plasma or urine—G. G. Duggin, *J. Chromat.*, 1976, **121**, 156.

Metabolism. ABSORPTION. Readily absorbed after oral administration.

BLOOD CONCENTRATION. After an oral dose of 1.8 g, peak plasma concentrations of 1 to 25 μg/ml for phenacetin are attained within 2 hours and peak plasma concentrations of 5 to 18 μg/ml are attained for paracetamol, the major metabolite, within 3 to 4 hours; plasma concentrations appear to be lower in smokers than in non-smokers.

HALF-LIFE. Plasma half-life, 1 to 1.5 hours for phenacetin and 1.5 to 2 hours for the paracetamol derived from phenacetin.

DISTRIBUTION. Phenacetin diffuses throughout most body fluids; volume of distribution, 1 to 2 litres/kg; protein binding, about 30% bound to plasma proteins.

METABOLIC REACTIONS. Subject to extensive first pass metabolism; phenacetin is metabolised mainly in the liver to paracetamol and acetaldehyde by O-dealkylation; the paracetamol so formed is conjugated with sulphate or glucuronic acid (see under Paracetamol); other reactions are deacetylation to phenetidine (*p*-ethoxyaniline), N-, 2-, and α-hydroxylation forming mainly 2-hydroxyphenetidine and also 2-hydroxyphenacetin, sulphate conjugation of deacetylated metabolites, and glutathione conjugation to form S-(1-acetamido-4-hydroxyphenyl)-cysteine and its corresponding mercapturic acid. 2-Hydroxyphenetidine appears to be the nephrotoxic metabolite and is possibly involved in the formation of methaemoglobinaemia. As the dose is increased so the percentage of the dose which is deacetylated is increased producing proportionately more phenetidine and 2-hydroxyphenetidine; production of these metabolites is also increased by concomitant administration of aspirin, caffeine, and codeine. Phenacetin is not hepatotoxic despite being converted to paracetamol; this is because the enzyme systems which convert paracetamol to its toxic metabolite are also involved in the conversion of phenacetin to paracetamol and the two conversions therefore compete resulting in reduced paracetamol oxidation. Phenacetin metabolism is stimulated by cigarette smoking.

EXCRETION. 80 to 90% of a dose is excreted in the urine in 24 hours; 50 to 80% as the sulphate and glucuronic acid conjugates of paracetamol, 6 to 8% as 2-hydroxyphenetidine sulphate, about 2% as S-(1-acetamido-4-hydroxyphenyl)cysteine, about 0.3% as phenetidine and 2-hydroxyphenacetin, 0.2% as unchanged drug, and 2 to 3% as unconjugated paracetamol.

FURTHER INFORMATION. Comparison of metabolism of paracetamol and phenacetin—G. Margetts, *J. int. med. Res.*, 1976, **4**, *Suppl.* 4., 55; effect of smoking on metabolism—E. J. Pantuck *et al.*, *Clin. Pharmac. Ther.*, 1974, **15**, 9; effect of renal disease—L. F. Prescott, *Clin. Pharmac. Ther.*, 1969, **10**, 383; metabolism—N. T. Shahidi and A. Hemaidan, *J. Lab. clin. Med.*, 1969, **74**, 581 and R. L. Smith and J. A. Timbrell, *Biochem. J.*, 1972, **128**, 140P; pharmacokinetics—J. Raaflaub and U. C. Dubach, *Eur. J. clin. Pharmac.*, 1975, **8**, 261.

Actions and uses. Phenacetin is metabolised to paracetamol and has similar analgesic and antipyretic actions. It is used to relieve headache, toothache, and rheumatic and neuralgic pains, but is of little value for the relief of severe pain. The usual dose is 300 to 600 milligrams as a single dose. It is sometimes prescribed in admixture with caffeine, aspirin, or codeine, and such mixtures, in addition to causing the undesirable effects described below, may give rise to dependence. It has largely been replaced by safer analgesics.

Undesirable effects. Phenacetin alone or in conjunction with aspirin, when taken in large amounts over a prolonged period, may cause analgesic nephropathy. Prolonged use may also cause methaemoglobinaemia, sulphaemoglobinaemia, or haemolytic anaemia.

Precautions. The use of phenacetin for prolonged periods should be avoided.

Preparations

ASPIRIN, PHENACETIN, AND CODEINE TABLETS (*Syn.* Compound Codeine Tablets): for each tablet take:

Aspirin	250 mg
Phenacetin ..	250 mg
Codeine phosphate	8 mg

A standard for these tablets is given in the British Pharmacopoeia 1973
Containers and *Storage:* see the entry on Tablets for general information on containers and storage. Containers should be airtight and light resistant.
Dose: 1 or 2 tablets up to 4 times daily as necessary.
Advice for patients: the tablets should preferably be taken after meals. Use for prolonged periods should be avoided.

SOLUBLE ASPIRIN, PHENACETIN, AND CODEINE TABLETS (*Syn.* Soluble Compound Codeine Tablets): for each tablet take:

Aspirin, in fine powder	250 mg
Phenacetin	250 mg
Codeine phosphate	8 mg
Saccharin sodium	5 mg
Anhydrous citric acid	26 mg
Calcium carbonate	80 mg

A standard for these tablets is given in the British Pharmacopoeia 1973
Containers and *Storage:* see the entry on Tablets for general information on containers and storage. Containers should be airtight and light resistant.
Dose: 1 or 2 tablets up to 4 times daily as necessary.
Advice for patients: the tablets should be dissolved in water and taken preferably after meals. Use for prolonged periods should be avoided.

Phenazocine Hydrobromide

1,2,3,4,5,6 - Hexahydro - 8 - hydroxy - 6,11 - dimethyl - 3 - phenethyl-2,6-methano-3-benzazocinium bromide hemi-hydrate

$C_{22}H_{28}BrNO,\frac{1}{2}H_2O = 411.4$

OTHER NAME: *Narphen®*

A standard is given in the British Pharmacopoeia 1973

Description. An odourless white microcrystalline powder with a bitter taste.

Solubility. Soluble, at 20°, in 350 parts of water, in 45 parts of alcohol, and in 140 parts of chloroform; practically insoluble in ether.

Acidity. A 0.2% solution has a pH of 5 to 7.

Moisture content. 2 to 2.5%, determined by Fischer titration.

Stability. Phenazocine hydrobromide is stable in acid or neutral solution. Discoloration may occur in alkaline solutions in the presence of oxygen or of light.

Sterilisation. Solutions for injection are sterilised by heating in an autoclave or by filtration.

Storage. It should be protected from light.

Identification. TESTS. 1. Dissolve about 50 mg in 2 ml of *dilute sulphuric acid* and add 1 ml of a freshly prepared solution made by dissolving 700 mg of mercuric nitrate in 4 ml of water and adding 100 mg of sodium nitrite and filtering; no immediate red colour is produced. Heat for about 5 minutes; a yellow colour is produced.
2. Dissolve about 5 mg in 1 ml of water, add 1 drop of *dilute hydrochloric acid*, and a mixture of 1 ml of *potassium ferricyanide solution*, 1 drop of *ferric chloride test-solution*, and 4 ml of water; a green or bluish-green colour is produced within 15 minutes.

MELTING-POINT. About 164°.

ULTRAVIOLET ABSORPTION. In 0.01N hydrochloric acid, maximum at 278 nm (E1%, 1cm = 50); in 0.1N sodium hydroxide, maxima at 238 nm and 298 nm.

THIN-LAYER CHROMATOGRAPHY. See under Thin-layer Chromatography, System 7.

Actions and uses. Phenazocine is a synthetic analgesic which has many of the actions and uses described under Morphine Hydrochloride. Its analgesic action is greater than that of morphine, quicker in onset, and longer in duration. It is less likely to cause constipation than morphine and in equipotent analgesic doses causes less respiratory depression; tolerance develops more slowly and less completely.
Phenazocine, like morphine, is used for pre-operative medication, 1 to 2 milligrams of phenazocine hydrobromide being given by intramuscular injection 45 to 60 minutes before the operation.
For post-operative pain, 1 to 2 milligrams may be given by intramuscular injection.
The dose as a general analgesic is 1 to 3 milligrams by intramuscular injection; the total dose should not exceed 12 milligrams during 24 hours.
The usual dose by mouth is 5 milligrams.

Undesirable effects. Phenazocine, like morphine, is addictive, inducing euphoria and relieving the withdrawal syndrome in morphine addicts. Undesirable effects include nausea, vomiting, dizziness, and constriction of the pupils.

Contra-indications. Phenazocine is contra-indicated in coma, convulsive disorders, delirium tremens, hepatic insufficiency, myxoedema, and alcoholism.

Poisoning. Phenazocine is a potent respiratory depressant. This action may be antagonised by the intravenous injection of naloxone. The procedure described under Morphine Hydrochloride should be adopted.

Preparations

PHENAZOCINE INJECTION: a sterile solution of phenazocine hydrobromide, with 1.5% v/v of propylene glycol and suitable buffering agents, in water for injections. It is sterilised by heating in an autoclave or by filtration. The usual strength is 2 mg of phenazocine hydrobromide per ml.

A standard for this injection is given in the British Pharmacopoeia 1973
Containers and Labelling: see the entry on Injections for general information on containers and labelling.
Storage: it should be protected from light.

PHENAZOCINE TABLETS: available as tablets containing 5 mg of phenazocine hydrobromide.
A standard for these tablets is given in the British Pharmacopoeia 1973
Containers and Storage: see the entry on Tablets for general information on containers and storage. Containers should be airtight and light resistant.

Phenazone

2,3-Dimethyl-1-phenylpyrazol-5-one

$C_{11}H_{12}N_2O = 188.2$

OTHER NAMES: Antipyrine: Phenazonum
Auraltone® (with benzocaine); Sedonan® (with chlorbutol)

A standard is given in the European Pharmacopoeia Vol. III

Description. Odourless colourless crystals or white crystalline powder.

Solubility. Soluble, at 20°, in 1 part of water, of alcohol, and of chloroform, and in 50 parts of ether.

Acidity. A 5% solution has a pH of 5.8 to 7.

Moisture content. Not more than 1%, determined by drying at 60° in vacuo.

Dissociation constant. pK_a 1.5 (20°).

Incompatibility. It is incompatible with nitrites in acid solution and with tannic acid in aqueous solution. With sodium salicylate in the dry state it forms an oily liquid on exposure to air; it acts similarly with butylchloral hydrate and betanaphthol.

Identification. TESTS. 1. Dissolve about 100 mg in 10 ml of water containing 100 mg of sodium nitrite and add 1 ml of dilute sulphuric acid; a green colour is produced.
2. Dissolve about 2 mg in 2 ml of water and add 1 drop of ferric chloride test-solution; a deep red colour is produced. Add 0.5 ml of sulphuric acid; the colour changes to light yellow.

MELTING-POINT. About 111°.

ULTRAVIOLET ABSORPTION. In 0.1N hydrochloric acid, maximum at 231 nm (E1%, 1cm = 590); in 0.1N sodium hydroxide, maxima at 242 nm (E1%, 1cm = 485) and 256 nm (E1%, 1cm = 471); in alcohol (95%), maxima at 245 nm (E1%, 1cm = 495) and 272 nm (E1%, 1cm = 511).

INFRA-RED ABSORPTION. Major peaks at 770, 1324, 1484, 1577, 1591, and 1663 cm^{-1} (see Appendix 2a: Infra-red Spectra).

THIN-LAYER CHROMATOGRAPHY. See under Thin-layer Chromatography, System 3.

Determination in body fluids. GAS CHROMATOGRAPHY. In plasma—L. F. Prescott et al., J. Pharm. Pharmac., 1973, 25, 205.

Metabolism. ABSORPTION. Rapidly and completely absorbed after oral administration.

BLOOD CONCENTRATION. After an oral dose of 18 mg/kg, a plasma concentration of about 15 μg/ml is attained in 1 to 3 hours.

HALF-LIFE. The half-life is readily influenced by a number of factors; in normal subjects, the plasma half-life is about 11 to 15 hours but it is increased in subjects with renal function impairment or with hypothyroidism, and in subjects taking disulfiram, nortriptyline, allopurinol, or oral contraceptives; the half-life is decreased in subjects with hyperthyroidism, in subjects exposed to certain insecticides, and in subjects taking barbiturates or a combination of diphenhydramine and methaqualone; there appear to be variations due to age, the half-life being higher in older subjects, and according to sex, the half-life being higher in young males than in young females. The half-life of phenazone appears to reflect the rate of metabolism in the liver.

DISTRIBUTION. Evenly distributed throughout body water; volume of distribution, about 52 litres; secreted in saliva in concentrations similar to those in plasma; protein binding, bound to a small extent to plasma proteins.

METABOLIC REACTIONS. The rate of biotransformation is variable and appears to be genetically determined; metabolised by hydroxylation at the 4-position followed by glucuronic acid conjugation; demethylation also occurs; hydroxylation appears to be stimulated by phenobarbitone and other drugs including phenazone itself.

EXCRETION. 30 to 40% of a dose is excreted in the urine as the glucuronic acid conjugate, 5% is excreted unchanged, and about 6% is excreted as norphenazone.

FURTHER INFORMATION. Influences on half-life—J. Elfström et al., Eur. J. clin. Pharmac., 1976, 10, 63, R. J. Elin et al., Clin. Pharmac. Ther., 1975, 17, 447, K. O'Malley, Br. med. J., iii/1971, 607, M. M. Reidenberg and E. S. Vesell, Clin. Pharmac. Ther., 1975, 17, 650, C. J. van Boxtel et al., Eur. J. clin. Pharmac., 1976, 9, 327, and E. S. Vesell et al., Clin. Pharmac. Ther., 1975, 17, 48; metabolism in renal failure—M. Lichter et al., J. Pharmac. exp. Ther., 1973, 187, 612 and J. L. Maddocks et al., Br. J. clin. Pharmac., 1975, 2, 339; pharmacokinetics—P. B. Andreasen and E. S. Vesell, Clin. Pharmac. Ther., 1974, 16, 1059.

Actions and uses. Phenazone has analgesic and antipyretic properties and has been used for similar purposes to paracetamol. It is usually given as a single dose of 300 to 600 milligrams. Ear-drops containing approximately 5% of phenazone are used for the relief of painful ear conditions.
Phenazone is absorbed rapidly and completely; it is distributed throughout the body-water and is very slowly metabolised. It has therefore been used to estimate the body fluid volume. The half-life of phenazone may be used as a measure of liver function.

Undesirable effects. Nausea and rashes may occur.

Preparations

Preparations available include EAR-DROPS containing phenazone 5% with benzocaine 1% and ear-drops containing phenazone 5% with chlorbutol 1%.

Phenelzine Sulphate

Phenethylhydrazine hydrogen sulphate

$$C_6H_5\cdot[CH_2]_2\cdot NH\cdot NH_2, H_2SO_4$$

$C_8H_{14}N_2O_4S = 234.3$

OTHER NAME: *Nardil®*

A standard is given in the British Pharmacopoeia 1973

Description. A white powder or pearly platelets with a pungent odour.

Solubility. Soluble, at 20°, in 7 parts of water; very slightly soluble in alcohol; practically insoluble in ether and in chloroform.

Acidity. A 1% solution has a pH of 1.4 to 1.9.

Moisture content. Not more than 1%, determined by drying over phosphorus pentoxide *in vacuo*.

Storage. It should be stored in airtight containers, protected from light.

Identification. TEST. Dissolve about 100 mg in 5 ml of water, make alkaline with *sodium hydroxide solution*, and add 1 ml of *potassium cupri-tartrate solution*; a red precipitate is produced.

MELTING-POINT. About 166°.

ULTRAVIOLET ABSORPTION. In 0.1N sulphuric acid, weak maxima at 252 nm, 257 nm, and 263 nm, and an inflection at 247 nm.

Determination in body fluids. GAS CHROMATOGRAPHY. In urine—B. Caddy and A. H. Stead, *Analyst, Lond.*, 1977, **102**, 42.

Metabolism. ABSORPTION. Readily absorbed after oral administration.

DISTRIBUTION. Widely distributed throughout the body.

METABOLIC REACTIONS. Subject to polymorphic acetylation; in rats phenelzine is converted to phenylacetic acid and in addition to being an inhibitor of monoamine oxidase, it is also a substrate for that enzyme.

EXCRETION. About 1% of a dose is excreted unchanged in fast acetylators and about 2% is excreted unchanged in slow acetylators; phenylacetylglutamine has been identified as a urinary metabolite of phenelzine.

FURTHER INFORMATION. Acetylator phenotype and therapeutic effect—D. A. P. Evans *et al.*, *Clin. Pharmac. Ther.*, 1965, **6**, 430 and E. C. Johnstone *et al.*, *Br. J. clin. Pharmac.*, 1976, **3**, 355P; excretion in urine—B. Caddy *et al.*, *Br. J. clin. Pharmac.*, 1976, **3**, 633.

Actions and uses. Phenelzine is an antidepressant drug which inhibits monoamine oxidase and probably acts by influencing the metabolism of transmitter substances, such as noradrenaline and 5-hydroxytryptamine, in the brain.

Phenelzine appears to be of more value in the treatment of patients suffering from neurotic or reactive depressive illness than in the treatment of endogenous depression. After 3 or 4 days of treatment with phenelzine, patients have considerable relief of fatigue and tension, sleeping habits are improved and emotional control is regained. The usual dosage is the equivalent of 15 milligrams of the base by mouth 3 or 4 times a day, but for some patients only 15 milligrams a day may be required; 25 milligrams of phenelzine sulphate is approximately equivalent to 15 milligrams of phenelzine base. Such treatment is usually continued for one month; maintenance doses may be necessary for much longer periods. The drug should not be withdrawn abruptly because relapse may occur within a day or two.

Undesirable effects. The most frequently occurring undesirable effects are postural hypotension and attacks of giddiness, which usually disappear after suitable reduction in dosage. Dryness of the mouth, constipation, blurring of vision, rashes, headache, and liver damage may occur occasionally.

Precautions and drug interactions. As monoamine-oxidase inhibitors may potentiate the action of other drugs, caution should be exercised in giving phenelzine in conjunction with any other drug.

Amphetamine, atropine, carbamazepine, chloroquine, chlorpropamide, dexamphetamine, ephedrine, ethamivan, fenfluramine, guanethidine, insulin, mephentermine, methoxamine, methylamphetamine, morphine, orciprenaline, pethidine, phenmetrazine, phenylephrine, phenylpropanolamine, pseudoephedrine, tolbutamide, and tricyclic antidepressants such as amitriptyline, desipramine, imipramine, nortriptyline, protriptyline, and trimipramine should not be given at the same time as phenelzine.

There is a danger if reserpine is given to patients who are already undergoing treatment with a monoamine-oxidase inhibitor.

Certain foodstuffs contain pressor agents, such as tyramine, which may be formed by microbial decomposition from amino acids and may precipitate paroxysmal attacks in patients taking monoamine-oxidase inhibitors; the diet of such persons should therefore not include cheese, pickled herrings, broad bean pods, and certain protein extracts prepared from meat or yeast.

After the administration of phenelzine, an interval of about 2 weeks should be allowed to elapse before any of the drugs or foods listed above are given so as to ensure that the monoamine-oxidase inhibitor has been eliminated and that tissue levels of monoamine oxidase have returned to normal.

Preparation

PHENELZINE TABLETS: available as tablets containing phenelzine sulphate equivalent to 15 mg of phenelzine; they are sugar coated; the coat may be coloured.

A standard for these tablets is given in the British Pharmacopoeia 1973

Containers and *Storage:* see the entry on Tablets for general information on containers and storage. Containers should be airtight.

Labelling: the label on the container should state the amount of the medicament as the equivalent amount of phenelzine.

Advice for patients: treatment should not be discontinued without the advice of the prescriber. The tablets may affect mental concentration; persons affected should not drive or operate machinery.

Patients should be advised to avoid, during treatment and for 2 weeks thereafter, certain foodstuffs containing pressor agents such as cheese, pickled herrings, broad bean pods, and certain protein extracts prepared from meat or yeast, and medicines containing sympathomimetic drugs such as ephedrine, methoxamine, phenylephrine, phenylpropanolamine, and pseudoephedrine as found in cough and cold remedies, analgesics, and tonics. Warning cards containing this advice may be carried by the patient during treatment and shown when further medical or dental treatment is required or when other medicines are needed.

Phenethicillin Potassium

Potassium   (6*R*)-6-(2-phenoxypropionamido)penicillanate

$C_{17}H_{19}KN_2O_5S = 402.5$

OTHER NAME: *Broxil®*

A standard is given in the British Pharmacopoeia 1973

Description. A white fine crystalline powder with a slight sulphurous odour and a bitter taste.

Solubility. Soluble, at 20°, in 1.5 parts of water, in 85 parts of alcohol, and in 800 parts of dehydrated alcohol; very slightly soluble in chloroform; practically insoluble in ether.

Acidity or alkalinity. A 10% solution has a pH of 5.5 to 7.5.

Moisture content. Not more than 1.5%, determined by Fischer titration.

Specific rotation. +217° to +244°, determined on a 1% solution containing 0.2% of dipotassium hydrogen phosphate and 0.8% of potassium dihydrogen phosphate.

Dissociation constant. pK_a 2.7 (25°).

Stability. Solutions in water degrade slowly by hydrolysis, the pH of maximum stability being 6.5. Degradation is catalysed by monohydrogen phosphate ions but not by citrate or dihydrogen phosphate ions.

FURTHER INFORMATION. Stability in aqueous solution—M. S. Schwartz *et al.*, *J. pharm. Sci.*, 1962, **51**, 523.

Hygroscopicity. It absorbs insignificant amounts of moisture at 25° at relative humidities up to about 65%, but under damper conditions it absorbs significant amounts.

Storage. It should be stored in airtight containers.

Identification. TESTS. 1. Mix 2 mg with 2 mg of chromotropic acid sodium salt and 2 ml of sulphuric acid, and immerse in a suitable liquid at 150° for 4 minutes; the colour of the solution changes through yellow to yellowish-green to brownish-green and finally chars (distinction from certain other penicillins).

ULTRAVIOLET ABSORPTION. In 0.1N hydrochloric acid, maxima at 271 nm (E1%, 1cm = 44).

INFRA-RED ABSORPTION. Major peaks at 1237, 1328, 1493, 1513, 1610, and 1778 cm⁻¹ (see Appendix 2a: Infra-red Spectra).

Metabolism. ABSORPTION. Rapidly but variably absorbed after oral administration; phenethicillin is more resistant to acid hydrolysis and more completely absorbed than benzylpenicillin.

BLOOD CONCENTRATION. After oral doses of 125 mg and 250 mg respective peak serum concentrations of about 1 μg/ml and about 2.5 μg/ml are attained in 1 hour; peak serum concentrations are increased after concomitant treatment with chymotrypsin. After an intravenous dose of 500 mg, serum concentrations of about 9 μg/ml are obtained at 30 minutes falling to 2 μg/ml by 90 minutes.

HALF-LIFE. Serum half-life, 30 to 50 minutes.

DISTRIBUTION. Enters pleural, ascitic, pericardial, and synovial fluids and also the cerebrospinal fluid when the meninges are inflamed; phenethicillin crosses the placenta; *protein binding*, 70 to 85% bound to plasma proteins.

EXCRETION. About 60% of a dose is excreted in the urine in 24 hours, most of which is excreted in the first 6 hours; 30 to 35% is excreted in active form.

FURTHER INFORMATION. Absorption enhanced by chymotrypsin—S. Avakian and B. L. Kabacoff, *Clin. Pharmac. Ther.*, 1964, **5**, 716; blood concentrations—J. M. Bond *et al.*, *Br. med. J.*, ii/1963, 956; pharmacokinetics—C. M. Kunin, *Proc. Soc. exp. Biol. Med.*, 1961, **107**, 337.

Actions and uses. Phenethicillin has the actions and uses described under Phenoxymethylpenicillin. Although phenethicillin gives rise to higher blood levels than phenoxymethylpenicillin it is less potent as an antibiotic and the effect of the two substances is therefore similar.

The usual dose by mouth for an adult is the equivalent of 0.5 to 1.5 grams of phenethicillin daily in divided doses. Children under 1 year may be given the equivalent of 62.5 milligrams, 1 to 5 years 125 milligrams and 6 to 12 years 250 milligrams of phenethicillin; these doses should be repeated every 6 hours.

Precautions and contra-indications. As for Phenoxymethylpenicillin.

Preparations

PHENETHICILLIN CAPSULES: consisting of phenethicillin potassium, in powder, which may be mixed with a suitable inert diluent, enclosed in a hard capsule. The capsule shells may be coloured. Available as capsules containing phenethicillin potassium equivalent to 250 mg of phenethicillin.

A standard for these capsules is given in the British Pharmacopoeia 1973

Containers and *Storage:* see the entry on Capsules for general information on containers and storage.

Labelling: the label on the container should state the amount of the medicament as the equivalent amount of phenethicillin, the date after which the capsules are not intended to be used, and the conditions under which they should be stored.

Advice for patients: the capsules should be taken at regular intervals preferably half to 1 hour before meals. The prescribed course should be completed.

PHENETHICILLIN ELIXIR (*Syn.* Phenethicillin Syrup): a solution of phenethicillin potassium in a suitable coloured flavoured vehicle. It is prepared freshly by dissolving a powder consisting of the dry mixed ingredients in the specified volume of water for preparations. When a dose less than or not a multiple of 5 ml is prescribed, the elixir may be diluted, as described in the entry on Elixirs, with syrup. Available as a powder which, when reconstituted, provides an elixir containing phenethicillin potassium equivalent to 125 mg of phenethicillin in 5 ml.

A standard for this elixir is given in the British Pharmaceutical Codex 1973

Containers: see the entry on Elixirs for general information on containers.

Labelling: see the entry on Elixirs for general information on labelling. In addition, the label on the container of the dry powder should state the name as "Powder for Phenethicillin Elixir".

Storage: the elixir and the diluted elixir should be stored in a cool place and used within 1 week of preparation.

Advice for patients: see above under Phenethicillin Capsules.

PHENETHICILLIN TABLETS: available as tablets containing phenethicillin potassium equivalent to 250 mg of phenethicillin; peppermint oil may be added as a flavouring agent; they may be coloured.

A standard for these tablets is given in the British Pharmacopoeia 1973

Containers and *Storage:* see the entry on Tablets for general information on containers and storage. Containers should be airtight.

Labelling: the label on the container should state the amount of the medicament as the equivalent amount of phenethicillin, the date after which the tablets are not intended to be used, and the conditions under which they should be stored.

Advice for patients: see above under Phenethicillin Capsules.

Phenformin Hydrochloride

1-Phenethylbiguanide hydrochloride

$$\left[C_6H_5{\cdot}CH_2{\cdot}CH_2{\cdot}NH{\cdot}\overset{NH}{\overset{\|}{C}}{\cdot}NH{\cdot}\overset{NH}{\overset{\|}{C}}{\cdot}NH_2 \right] HCl$$

$C_{10}H_{16}ClN_5 = 241.7$

OTHER NAMES: *Dibotin®; Dipar®*

A standard is given in the British Pharmacopoeia 1973

Description. An odourless white crystalline powder with a bitter taste.

Solubility. Soluble, at 20°, in 8 parts of water and in 15 parts of alcohol; practically insoluble in ether and in chloroform.

Acidity. A 2.5% solution has a pH of 6 to 7.

Moisture content. Not more than 1%, determined by drying at 105°.

Identification. TESTS. 1. Dissolve about 25 mg in 5 ml of water, add 1.5 ml of *sodium hydroxide solution*, 1 ml of *1-naphthol solution*, and dropwise with shaking, 0.5 ml of *dilute sodium hypochlorite solution*; a red precipitate is produced which darkens on standing.

2. Mix equal volumes of a 10% solution of sodium nitroprusside, a 10% solution of potassium ferricyanide, and a 10% solution of sodium hydroxide and allow to stand for 20 minutes; dissolve about 10 mg of the sample in 10 ml of water and add 10 ml of the prepared solution; a wine-red colour is produced within 3 minutes.

MELTING-POINT. About 177°.

ULTRAVIOLET ABSORPTION. In water, maximum at 234 nm (E1%, 1cm = 600).

Determination in body fluids. ULTRAVIOLET SPECTRO-PHOTOMETRY. In whole blood or plasma—E. R. Garrett *et al., J. pharm. Sci.*, 1972, **61**, 1411. In urine—E. R. Garrett and J. Tsau, *J. pharm. Sci.*, 1972, **61**, 1404.

GAS CHROMATOGRAPHY. In plasma—S. B. Matin *et al., Analyt. Chem.*, 1975, **47**, 545. In serum or urine: phenformin and its metabolite 1-(4-hydroxyphenethyl)biguanide—M. Mottale and C. J. Stewart, *J. Chromat.*, 1975, **106**, 263.

Metabolism. ABSORPTION. Well absorbed after oral administration.

BLOOD CONCENTRATION. After an oral dose of 100 mg

as a sustained release preparation, peak plasma concentrations of about 150 ng/ml are attained in about 3 hours.

HALF-LIFE. Plasma half-life, about 5 hours for the α-phase, and 13 hours for the β-phase.

DISTRIBUTION. Accumulates in gastric juice and liver; secreted in saliva in concentrations paralleling those in plasma; *protein binding*, 12 to 20% bound to plasma proteins.

METABOLIC REACTIONS. Aromatic hydroxylation to form 1-(*p*-hydroxyphenethyl)biguanide.

EXCRETION. 30 to 50% of a dose is excreted unchanged in 36 hours.

FURTHER INFORMATION. Metabolism—P. J. Murphy and A. N. Wick, *J. pharm. Sci.*, 1968, **57**, 1125; pharmacokinetics—M. S. Alkalay *et al., J. clin. Pharmac.*, 1975, **15**, 446; plasma and urinary concentrations—S. B. Matin *et al., Analyt. Chem.*, 1975, **47**, 545; protein binding—E. R. Garrett *et al., J. pharm. Sci.*, 1972, **61**, 1411.

Actions and uses. Phenformin is an oral hypoglycaemic agent which, unlike the sulphonylureas, as described under Chlorpropamide, has an action that is independent of the pancreatic beta-cells. Although the precise mode of action of phenformin is not known, it is thought that its main activities are to control the glucose level of the blood by increasing its peripheral utilisation and to inhibit gluconeogenesis in the diabetic.

Unlike insulin, phenformin does not encourage lipogenesis. It reduces the blood-glucose level in diabetes and in cortisone-induced hyperglycaemia in pre-diabetes, but it has no effect on the blood-sugar level of normal persons except in the fasting state. It reduces the insulin requirements of young diabetics.

In a daily dosage of 50 to 100 milligrams, phenformin causes loss of weight in obese diabetics, whereas sulphonylureas usually give rise to a gain of weight.

Phenformin enhances fibrinolysis, particularly when it is given with oestrogens or anabolic steroids. It reduces the blood cholesterol in maturity-onset diabetes. In some diabetics it may cause ketosis.

Phenformin hydrochloride is absorbed after oral administration and its hypoglycaemic action lasts 6 to 8 hours; this period may be extended to 14 hours by the use of slow-release tablets or capsules. Because of its tendency to cause lactic acidosis phenformin is not used in patients who can be treated with sulphonylureas alone, but metformin, which has a lesser tendency to cause acidosis, is usually preferred when a biguanide hypoglycaemic agent is required.

As the mode of action of phenformin is different from that of the sulphonylureas, it is sometimes used in conjunction with one of them when neither drug is fully effective alone. Phenformin used by itself is not suitable for unstable or juvenile diabetics or for diabetic patients requiring large doses of insulin, but it is sometimes used in conjunction with insulin; it should never completely replace insulin in brittle cases.

Phenformin hydrochloride is given initially in doses of 25 milligrams in the morning or morning and evening and the dose increased by 25 milligrams at intervals of 2 or 3 days until the blood-glucose level is controlled. Doses of 100 milligrams per day should not normally be exceeded. A slow-release capsule of 50 milligrams may be given once or twice a day.

Undesirable effects. Phenformin may give rise to a metallic or bitter taste, anorexia, nausea, vomiting, and diarrhoea, particularly in patients on high dosage; these side-effects rarely necessitate withdrawal of the drug. Acute lactic acidosis is a rare but serious complication. Phenformin may reduce the patient's ability to compensate for acid loss, and may give rise to malabsorption of vitamin B_{12}.

Precautions and contra-indications. During stabilisation the urine should be tested frequently for glucose and ketones. Phenformin should not be used in severe renal disease, congestive heart failure, diabetic coma or the acute complications of diabetes, in pregnancy, before or after surgery, during acute infections, or in any condition likely to lead to hypertension.
Juvenile diabetics should never be treated with phenformin alone.
Hyperlactaemia may occur after ingestion of alcohol.

Poisoning. Hypoglycaemia should be treated by giving dextrose by mouth or, in serious cases, by the intravenous injection of a 20 to 50% solution of dextrose. Acidosis should be treated by the intravenous infusion of sodium bicarbonate solution.
When phenformin has been taken with a sulphonylurea the effects may be intensified, persist longer, and require treatment for a longer time.

Preparations

PHENFORMIN TABLETS: available as tablets containing 25 mg of phenformin hydrochloride.
A standard for these tablets is given in the British Pharmacopoeia 1973
Containers and *Storage:* see the entry on Tablets for general information on containers and storage. Containers should be airtight.
Advice for patients: the tablets should be taken at regular intervals preferably after meals. Treatment should not be discontinued without the advice of the prescriber. Alcohol should be avoided.

SLOW PHENFORMIN CAPSULES (*Syn.* Phenformin Slow Capsules): consisting of phenformin hydrochloride, in powder, which may be mixed with a suitable inert diluent in a slow-release formulation, enclosed in a hard capsule. The capsule shells may be coloured. Available as capsules containing 25 and 50 mg of phenformin hydrochloride.
Containers and *Storage:* see the entry on Capsules for general information on containers and storage.
Advice for patients: the capsules should be swallowed whole and the advice given under Phenformin Tablets should be followed.

OTHER PREPARATIONS available include TABLETS containing phenformin hydrochloride 50 mg in a slow-release formulation.

Phenindamine Tartrate

2,3,4,9 - Tetrahydro - 2 - methyl - 9 - phenyl - 1*H* - indeno-[2,1-*c*]pyridinium hydrogen tartrate

$C_{23}H_{25}NO_6 = 411.5$

OTHER NAME: *Thephorin*®

A standard is given in the British Pharmacopoeia 1973

Description. An almost odourless white voluminous powder with a bitter taste.

Solubility. Soluble, at 20°, in 70 parts of water and in 300 parts of alcohol; very slightly soluble in ether and in chloroform.

Acidity. A 1% solution has a pH of 3.4 to 3.9.

Moisture content. Not more than 1%, determined by drying at 105°.

Dissociation constant. pK_a 8.3 (25°).

Storage. It should be stored in airtight containers, protected from light.

Identification. TEST. Dissolve about 25 mg in 5 ml of sulphuric acid; an orange-brown colour is produced. Cautiously dilute by the addition of 20 ml of water; the colour is discharged.

MELTING-POINT. About 161°. It resolidifies at about 163° and remelts at about 168° with decomposition.

ULTRAVIOLET ABSORPTION. In water, maximum at 259 nm (E1%, 1cm = 220).

INFRA-RED ABSORPTION. Major peaks at 1302, 1340, 1365, 1381, 1411, and 1751 cm^{-1} (see Appendix 2a: Infra-red Spectra).

THIN-LAYER CHROMATOGRAPHY. See under Thin-layer Chromatography, System 4.

Actions and uses. Phenindamine has the actions and uses of the antihistamine drugs, as described under Promethazine Hydrochloride, but it has no marked anti-emetic effect. Unlike some other antihistamines, it does not usually produce drowsiness and may even be mildly stimulating. It has been used in the treatment of parkinsonism.
Phenindamine tartrate is given by mouth in a dosage of 25 to 50 milligrams once to 4 times a day. The dosage for a child 6 to 12 years is half the adult dose.

Undesirable effects. These occur frequently and may include dryness of the mouth, dizziness, and gastro-intestinal disturbances. Insomnia and convulsions may occur.

Poisoning. See under Promethazine Hydrochloride.

Preparation

PHENINDAMINE TABLETS: available as tablets containing 25 mg of phenindamine tartrate; they are sugar coated; the coat may be coloured.
A standard for these tablets is given in the British Pharmacopoeia 1973
Containers and *Storage:* see the entry on Tablets for general information on containers and storage. Containers should be airtight.
Advice for patients: the tablets should be taken before meals if the patient is inconvenienced by dryness of the mouth or after meals if there are gastro-intestinal disturbances. The tablets may affect mental concentration or occasionally cause drowsiness; persons affected should not drive or operate machinery. Alcohol should be avoided. To avoid insomnia doses should not be taken for several hours before bedtime.

Phenindione

2-Phenylindane-1,3-dione

$C_{15}H_{10}O_2 = 222.2$

OTHER NAMES: *Dindevan®*; Phenylindanedione

A standard is given in the British Pharmacopoeia 1973

Description. Almost odourless, tasteless, soft, white or creamy-white crystals.

Solubility. Very slightly soluble in water; soluble, at 20°, in 125 parts of alcohol, in 110 parts of ether, and in 6.5 parts of chloroform. Solutions are yellow to red in colour.

Moisture content. Not more than 1%, determined by drying at 105°.

Storage. It should be stored in airtight containers.

Identification. MELTING-POINT. About 149°.

ULTRAVIOLET ABSORPTION. In a solution prepared by dissolving the substance in alcohol (95%) with the aid of heat and diluting to volume with 0.1N sodium hydroxide, maxima at 278 nm (E1%, 1cm = 1375), and 330 nm (E1%, 1cm = 400).

Metabolism. ABSORPTION. Well absorbed after oral administration.

HALF-LIFE. Biological half-life, about 6 hours.

DISTRIBUTION. Secreted in milk and crosses the placenta.

Actions and uses. Phenindione is an anticoagulant which has actions and uses similar to those described under Warfarin Sodium. Warfarin is usually preferred to phenindione, as it is less liable to give rise to allergic and toxic effects. A therapeutic effect is obtained 24 to 36 hours after the initial oral dose has been given and ceases within 72 hours of the last dose.
Phenindione is given by mouth, usually in an initial dose of 200 to 300 milligrams; the daily maintenance dosage is 25 to 100 milligrams according to the prothrombin activity of the blood.

Undesirable effects. Rashes, pyrexia, and sore throat may occur. Kidney damage may occur in patients sensitive to phenindione; serious toxic effects are rare but may include liver damage, agranulocytosis, granulocytopenia, and eosinophilia. During treatment with phenindione the urine is sometimes coloured red but this is of no clinical significance.

Precautions and contra-indications; Drug interactions. As for Warfarin Sodium.

Preparation

PHENINDIONE TABLETS: available as tablets containing 10, 25, and 50 mg of phenindione; they may be coloured.
A standard for these tablets is given in the British Pharmacopoeia 1973
Containers and *Storage:* see the entry on Tablets for general information on containers and storage. Containers should be airtight.
Advice for patients: the tablets should be taken at regular intervals. Treatment should not be discontinued without the advice of the prescriber. Patients may carry an identification card giving details of their treatment and the name of the prescriber who should be contacted in the event of accident or illness. Patients should not take other medicines (including aspirin) without medical or pharmaceutical advice. Preparations containing liquid paraffin should also preferably be avoided. Phenindione may colour the urine red.

Phenobarbitone

5-Ethyl-5-phenylbarbituric acid

$C_{12}H_{12}N_2O_3 = 232.2$

OTHER NAMES: *Luminal®*; Phenobarb.; Phenobarbital; Phenobarbitalum
Belladenal® and *Fenobelladine®* (both with belladonna alkaloids); *Cantil with Phenobarbitone®* (with mepenzolate bromide); *Epanutin with Phenobarbitone®* (with phenytoin sodium); *Paminal®* (with hyoscine methobromide); *Peritrate with Phenobarbitone®* (with pentaerythritol tetranitrate); *Phenomet®* (with emetine hydrochloride); *Pro-Banthine with Phenobarbitone®* (with propantheline bromide); *Theogardenal®* and *Theominal®* (both with theobromine); *Veriloid VP®* (with *Veratrum viride* alkaloids)

A standard is given in the European Pharmacopoeia Vol. I

Description. An odourless, white, crystalline powder or colourless crystals, with a slightly bitter taste.

Solubility. Soluble, at 20°, in 1000 parts of water and in 10 parts of alcohol; soluble in ether, in chloroform, and in solutions of alkali hydroxides and carbonates.

Dissociation constant. pK_a 7.4 (25°).

Stability; Incompatibility. See under Barbiturates.

Identification. TESTS. It complies with general tests 1, 2, and 3 described under Barbiturates.

MELTING-POINT. About 176°.

ULTRAVIOLET ABSORPTION. See under Barbiturates.

INFRA-RED ABSORPTION. Major peaks at 1370, 1386, 1670, 1683, 1710, and 1770 cm^{-1} (see Appendix 2a: Infra-red Absorption).

THIN-LAYER CHROMATOGRAPHY. See under Thin-layer Chromatography, System 5.

Determination in body fluids. See under Barbiturates.

Metabolism (see also under Barbiturates). ABSORPTION. Readily absorbed after oral administration; food delays its absorption.

BLOOD CONCENTRATION. After an intramuscular dose of 10 mg/kg, plasma concentrations of 9, 12, and 13 μg/ml are attained in 30, 90, and 120 minutes respectively; during therapy with 90 to 300 mg/day, plasma concentrations of 7 to 17 μg/ml are attained; concentrations of greater than 20 μg/ml are necessary to eliminate or reduce seizures; peak concentrations appear to be reduced after the administration of pyridoxine.

HALF-LIFE. Serum half-life, up to about 75 hours in children and up to about 100 hours in adults; in the aged or in subjects with overdose the half-life may be increased, as in patients with cirrhosis of the liver in whom the half-life is increased to about 120 hours.

DISTRIBUTION. Crosses the placenta, is secreted in milk, and binds to red blood cells; cerebrospinal fluid concentrations reach about 50% of those in plasma; saliva concentrations parallel those in the plasma; *protein binding*, 20 to 40% bound to plasma proteins.

METABOLIC REACTIONS. *p*-Hydroxylation followed by sulphate conjugation; in dogs and horses, the glucuronide is formed in preference to the sulphate and in rats the 3,4-dihydroxyphenyl- and the 1-hydroxyethyl-metabolites have been isolated.

EXCRETION. About 70% of a dose of 1 to 3 mg/kg is excreted in the urine in 5 days; of the excreted material, one-third is unchanged drug and the remainder is 5-ethyl-5-(*p*-hydroxyphenyl)barbituric acid which is partly excreted as the sulphate ester. Urinary excretion of unchanged drug is increased when the urine is alkaline or when the urinary volume is increased. Small amounts of unchanged drug and metabolites are excreted in the bile. In patients with cirrhosis of the liver, urinary excretion of phenobarbitone is decreased to about 50% of the dose.

ENZYME INDUCTION. Most of the hepatic drug-metabolising enzymes are induced by phenobarbitone and thus the metabolism of a whole range of drugs is enhanced by phenobarbitone pretreatment; in animals, phenobarbitone enhances the metabolism of a number of drugs, including halothane, methoxyflurane, paracetamol, phenacetin, phenylbutazone, phenytoin, strychnine, and warfarin. Enzyme induction by phenobarbitone has been applied to the treatment of hyperbilirubinaemia in which phenobarbitone induces the activity of glucuronyl transferase which converts bilirubin to an excretable form by conjugation with glucuronic acid.

FURTHER INFORMATION. Brain and cerebrospinal fluid concentrations—F. Vajda *et al.*, *Clin. Pharmac. Ther.*, 1974, **15**, 597; effect of liver disease on metabolism—J. Alvin *et al.*, *J. Pharmac. exp. Ther.*, 1975, **192**, 224; effect of pyridoxine on blood concentrations—O. Hansson and M. Sillanpaa, *Lancet*, i/1976, 256; metabolism in children—L. K. Garrettson and P. G. Dayton, *Clin. Pharmac. Ther.*, 1970, **11**, 674; plasma and salivary concentrations—C. E. Cook *et al.*, *Clin. Pharmac. Ther.*, 1975, **18**, 742; urinary excretion—N. Kållberg *et al.*, *Eur. J. clin. Pharmac.*, 1975, **9**, 161.

Actions and uses. Phenobarbitone has the actions of long-acting barbiturates as described under Barbiturates. It has been used as a sedative in nervous and anxiety states, chorea, neurasthenia, climacteric disorders, dysmenorrhoea, and thyrotoxicosis, but has been largely replaced by other sedatives. It is also used in the treatment of migraine, and in epilepsy to diminish the frequency of attacks. The usual dose is 30 to 125 milligrams 3 times daily.

In anticonvulsant dosage, phenobarbitone does not act as a hypnotic, but should it become necessary, in order to control the fits, to increase the dosage to a level at which the patient would become drowsy, phenytoin or primidone may be used to supplement the action of the barbiturate instead of increasing the dosage.

Undesirable effects; Contra-indications; Dependence; Poisoning. See under Barbiturates.

Precautions. See under Barbiturates. Sudden withdrawal of phenobarbitone should be avoided as it may precipitate status epilepticus or confusional states. It should be used with caution in chronic airways obstruction.

Veterinary uses. Phenobarbitone has been used as a hypnotic and anticonvulsant in dogs and cats in doses of 6 to 12 milligrams per kilogram body-weight.

Preparations

PHENOBARBITONE ELIXIR:

Phenobarbitone	.. 3 g
Compound tartrazine solution	10 ml
Compound orange spirit	24 ml
Alcohol (90%)	400 ml
Glycerol	400 ml
Water, for preparations	to 1000 ml

Dissolve the phenobarbitone in the alcohol and add the glycerol, the compound orange spirit, the compound tartrazine solution, and sufficient of the water to produce the required volume. Add 25 g of sterilised purified talc, shake, allow to stand for a few hours, shaking occasionally, and filter.

When a dose less than or not a multiple of 5 ml is prescribed, the elixir may be diluted, as described in the entry on Elixirs, with syrup. The diluted elixir must be freshly prepared.

A standard for this elixir is given in the British Pharmaceutical Codex 1973

Containers: see the entry on Elixirs for general information on containers.

Storage: it should be protected from light.

Advice for patients: when used as an anticonvulsant agent, treatment should not be discontinued without the advice of the prescriber.

The elixir may cause drowsiness; persons affected should not drive or operate machinery. Alcohol should be avoided.

PHENOBARBITONE AND THEOBROMINE TABLETS: for each tablet take:

Phenobarbitone	30 mg
Theobromine	300 mg

Mix, and prepare by moist granulation and compression as described in the entry on Tablets.

A standard for these tablets is given in the British Pharmaceutical Codex 1973

Containers and *Storage:* see the entry on Tablets for general information on containers and storage. Containers should be airtight and light resistant.

Dose: 1 or 2 tablets.

Advice for patients: the tablets may cause drowsiness; persons affected should not drive or operate machinery. Alcohol should be avoided.

PHENOBARBITONE TABLETS (*Syn.* Phenobarbital Tablets): available as tablets containing 7.5, 10, 15, 30, 50, 60, 100, and 125 mg of phenobarbitone.

A standard for these tablets is given in the British Pharmacopoeia 1973

Containers and *Storage:* see the entry on Tablets for general information on containers and storage. Containers should be airtight.

Advice for patients: see above under Phenobarbitone Elixir.

OTHER PREPARATIONS available include CAPSULES containing phenobarbitone 60 mg in a slow-release formulation, capsules containing phenobarbitone 100 mg in a slow-release formulation, capsules containing phenobarbitone 50 mg with phenytoin sodium 100 mg; TABLETS containing phenobarbitone 15 mg with belladonna extract 15 mg, tablets containing phenobarbitone 50 mg with belladonna alkaloids 250 micrograms, tablets containing phenobarbitone 50 mg with belladonna alkaloids 250 micrograms in a slow-release formulation, tablets containing phenobarbitone 15 mg with emetine hydrochloride 100 micrograms, tablets containing phenobarbitone 30 mg with emetine hydrochloride 200 micrograms, tablets containing phenobarbitone 15 mg with mepenzolate bromide 25 mg, tablets containing phenobarbitone 15 mg with hyoscine methobromide 2.5 mg, tablets containing phenobarbitone 15 mg with pentaerythritol tetranitrate 10 mg, tablets containing phenobarbitone 15 mg with propantheline bromide 15 mg, and tablets containing phenobarbitone 15 mg with *Veratrum viride* alkaloids 2 mg.

Phenobarbitone Sodium

Sodium 5-ethyl-5-phenylbarbiturate

$C_{12}H_{11}N_2NaO_3 = 254.2$

OTHER NAMES: *Gardenal Sodium*®; Phenobarb. Sod.; Phenobarbital Sodium; Soluble Phenobarbitone *Garoin*® (with phenytoin sodium); *Parabal*® (as a complex with dihydroxyaluminium aminoacetate)

A standard is given in the British Pharmacopoeia 1973

Description. An odourless white hygroscopic powder with a bitter taste.

Solubility. Soluble, at 20°, in 3 parts of water and in 25 parts of alcohol; practically insoluble in ether and in chloroform.

Alkalinity. A 10% solution has a pH of not more than 11.

Moisture content. Not more than 7%, determined by drying at 130°.

Stability; Incompatibility. See under Barbiturates.

Sterilisation. Sterile solutions of phenobarbitone sodium were formerly prepared from the sterile powder immediately before use, by means of an aseptic technique, using water free from carbon dioxide. However, this procedure is now avoided by making use of the stabilising properties of propylene glycol to prepare a suitable solution which is sterilised by heating with a bactericide at 98° to 100° for 30 minutes. See also under Barbiturates.

Storage. It should be stored in airtight containers.

Identification. TESTS. Acidify an aqueous solution with *dilute hydrochloric acid* and extract with ether. The residue obtained after evaporation of the extract complies with general tests 1, 2, and 3 described under Barbiturates.

MELTING-POINT. The residue obtained in the test, above, after recrystallisation from alcohol (25%) melts at about 176°.

ULTRAVIOLET ABSORPTION. See under Barbiturates.

THIN-LAYER CHROMATOGRAPHY. See under Thin-layer Chromatography, System 5.

Determination in body fluids. See under Barbiturates.

Metabolism. See under Phenobarbitone and under Barbiturates.

Actions and uses. Phenobarbitone sodium has the actions and uses described under Phenobarbitone. 1.1 grams of phenobarbitone sodium is approximately equivalent to 1 gram of phenobarbitone. It may be given by mouth or by injection to produce a more rapid effect. The usual dose is 30 to 125 milligrams by mouth 3 times daily, or 50 to 200 milligrams, as a single dose, by intravenous, intramuscular, or subcutaneous injection. The usual dose by mouth for children is 3 to 5 milligrams per kilogram body-weight daily.

Undesirable effects; Contra-indications; Dependence; Poisoning. See under Barbiturates.

Precautions. As for Phenobarbitone.

Veterinary uses. Phenobarbitone sodium has been used as a hypnotic and anticonvulsant in dogs and cats in doses of 6 to 12 milligrams per kilogram body-weight.

Preparations

PHENOBARBITONE INJECTION: a sterile solution of phenobarbitone sodium, with not more than 0.02% of disodium edetate, in a mixture consisting of 90% v/v of propylene glycol and 10% v/v of water for injections. It is sterilised by heating with a bactericide. It contains 200 mg of phenobarbitone sodium per ml. For intravenous administration, 0.25 to 1 ml doses must be diluted to not less than 10 ml with water for injections immediately before use. Available in 1-ml ampoules.
A standard for this injection is given in the British Pharmacopoeia 1973
Containers and *Labelling:* see the entry on Injections for general information on containers and labelling.

PHENOBARBITONE SODIUM TABLETS (*Syn.* Soluble Phenobarbitone Tablets; Phenobarbital Sodium Tablets): the usual strengths are 30 and 60 mg of phenobarbitone sodium.
A standard for these tablets is given in the British Pharmacopoeia 1973
Containers and *Storage:* see the entry on Tablets for general information on containers and storage. Containers should be airtight.
Advice for patients: when used as an anticonvulsant agent, treatment should not be discontinued without the advice of the prescriber. The tablets may cause drowsiness; persons affected should not drive or operate machinery. Alcohol should be avoided.

OTHER PREPARATIONS available include TABLETS containing phenobarbitone sodium dihydroxyaluminium aminoacetate 250 mg (equivalent on a molecular basis to 10 mg of phenobarbitone sodium and stated to be therapeutically equivalent to 60 mg of phenobarbitone), and tablets containing phenobarbitone sodium 50 mg with phenytoin sodium 100 mg.

Phenol

Hydroxybenzene
$C_6H_5.OH = 94.11$

OTHER NAME: Carbolic Acid

A standard is given in the British Pharmacopoeia 1973

Description. Deliquescent, colourless or faintly pink, needle-shaped crystals or crystalline masses with a characteristic odour.

Solubility. Soluble, at 20°, in 12 parts of water; soluble in alcohol, in ether, in chloroform, in glycerol, in liquid paraffin, and in fixed and volatile oils; readily soluble in alkalis, forming solutions of alkali phenates.

At 20°, 100 parts of phenol is liquefied by the addition of 10 parts of water; this solution will dissolve about a further 30 parts of water, the solution remaining clear; on the further addition of water the liquid separates into two layers, one a solution of phenol in water and the other a solution of water in phenol, until about 1200 parts of water have been added, when a solution of phenol in water is formed.

Dissociation constant. pK_a 10 (25°).

Sterilisation. Oily solutions for injection are sterilised in hermetically sealed containers by dry heat.

Storage. It should be stored in airtight containers, protected from light, in a cool place.

Preparation and storage of solutions. See statement on aqueous solutions for antiseptics in the entry on Solutions.

Metabolism. ABSORPTION. Rapidly absorbed after oral administration and readily penetrates skin, mucous membranes, and other tissues.

METABOLIC REACTIONS. Hydroxylation and conjugation with glucuronic acid and sulphate.

EXCRETION. After an oral dose of 10 μg/kg, 90% is excreted in the urine in 24 hours mainly as sulphate (77%) with 16% as the glucuronide, and small amounts as conjugates of quinol and catechol metabolites.

FURTHER INFORMATION. Metabolism in animals—I. D. Capel, *Xenobiotica*, 1972, **2**, 25 and F. W. Oehme and L. E. Davis, *Toxic. appl. Pharmac.*, 1970, **17**, 283.

Actions and uses. Phenol is a bactericide which, in concentrated solution, is destructive to tissues. Its use as a germicide has largely declined in favour of more active and less toxic compounds, but it is effective against certain viruses.

When strong solutions of phenol are applied to the skin the area becomes white through precipitation of proteins, and a slough is formed. With continued application, phenol penetrates into the deeper tissues causing paralysis of sensory nerve endings and painless gangrene. If preparations containing phenol are applied to large wounds, phenol may be absorbed in amounts sufficient to produce toxic effects.

The antiseptic properties of phenol are greatly reduced, and the caustic action delayed, if it is dissolved in alcohol, glycerol, or fixed oils.

An aqueous solution containing 0.5% of phenol is used as a vehicle in some injections. A concentration of 1% of phenol in water will kill most vegetative bacteria within a few minutes.

Liquefied phenol has been used in dentistry as an analgesic for sensitive dentine and 5% solutions have been used to devitalise the pulp in deciduous teeth. Diluted solutions containing 0.2 to 0.5% of phenol, sometimes in the form of alkaline phenates, are used as astringent gargles and mouth-washes, but in these concentrations phenol can have little antibacterial action.

Phenol and glycerol injection is administered intrathecally for the relief of severe intractable pain and spasticity.

Phenol ear-drops are used in the treatment of otitis media and of boils in the ear.

Oily phenol injection is injected into the tissues around internal haemorrhoids as an analgesic thrombotic agent.

Phenol imparts to the urine a green tint, and this may happen even when phenol preparations are applied locally to the skin.

Aqueous solutions of phenol should be coloured with amaranth or other suitable red dye, unless otherwise ordered.

Poisoning. The stomach should be washed out with water and 500 millilitres of castor oil and 30 grams of sodium sulphate dissolved in 250 millilitres of water should be given by mouth. The usual supportive measures should be taken and special attention should be given to fluid and electrolyte balance.

Burns caused by phenol on the skin or mucous surfaces should be washed with large quantities of water and then swabbed with glycerol, alcohol, or oil to dissolve the phenol.

Preparations

ALKALINE PHENOL MOUTH-WASH:

Liquefied phenol	30 ml
Potassium hydroxide solution	30 ml
Amaranth solution	10 ml
Water for preparations	to 1000 ml

It should be diluted with 10 times its volume of warm water before use.

Containers and *Labelling:* see the entry on Mouth-washes for general information on containers and labelling.

Advice for patients: the diluted solution should be rinsed around the mouth 3 or 4 times daily as required. It should preferably not be swallowed. Prolonged use of the mouth-wash should be avoided.

LIQUEFIED PHENOL:

Phenol	800 g
Purified water, freshly boiled and cooled	to 1000 g

Melt the phenol by warming on a water-bath, add sufficient of the water to produce the required weight, and mix thoroughly.

When phenol is to be mixed with collodion, fixed oils or paraffins, melted phenol should be used and not liquefied phenol.

CAUTION. *Liquefied phenol is caustic.*

A standard for this solution is given in the British Pharmacopoeia 1973

Storage: it should be stored in airtight containers, protected from light. It may congeal or deposit crystals if stored at a temperature below 4°. If this occurs, it should be completely melted and mixed before use.

OILY PHENOL INJECTION (*Syn.* 5 per cent Phenol in Oil Injection):

Phenol	5 g
Almond oil	to 100 ml

Dissolve the phenol in the bulk of the almond oil, previously warmed, add sufficient of the oil to produce the required volume, filter, distribute into the final containers, seal the containers to give an airtight closure, and sterilise by dry heat.

Alternatively, sterilise sufficient of the almond oil by dry heat; by means of an aseptic technique, dissolve the phenol in the bulk of the warm sterile oil, add sufficient of the cold sterile oil to produce the required volume, distribute into the final sterile containers, and seal the containers. Available in 5-ml ampoules.

A standard for this injection is given in the British Pharmaceutical Codex 1973

Containers and *Labelling:* see the entry on Injections for general information on containers and labelling.

PHENOL AND GLYCEROL INJECTION (*Syn.* Phenol and Glycerin Injection):

Phenol	.. 5 g
Glycerol, previously dried at 120° for 1 hour	to 100 g

Dissolve the phenol in the glycerol, distribute the solution into dry ampoules, seal the ampoules, and sterilise by dry heat.

A standard for this injection is given in the British Pharmacopoeia 1973

Containers: see the entry on Injections for general information on containers.

Labelling: see the entry on Injections for general information on labelling. In addition, the label on the container should state the amount of the medicament as the percentage w/w of phenol.

Storage: it should be protected from light.

PHENOL EAR-DROPS:

Phenol glycerin	40 ml
Glycerol	to 100 ml

CAUTION. *Dilution with water renders this preparation caustic; it may be diluted with glycerol, if desired.*

A standard for these ear-drops is given in the British Pharmaceutical Codex 1973

Containers and *Labelling:* see the entry on Ear-drops for general information on containers and labelling.

Advice for patients: the preparation should be protected from water. The ear should be dried and the preparation applied undiluted.

PHENOL GARGLE (*Syn.* Carbolic Acid Gargle):

Phenol glycerin	50 ml
Amaranth solution	10 ml
Water for preparations	to 1000 ml

It should be diluted with an equal volume of warm water before use.

A standard for this gargle is given in the British Pharmaceutical Codex 1973

Containers and *Labelling:* see the entry on Gargles for general information on containers and labelling.

Advice for patients: the diluted solution should be used as described under Gargles. It should preferably not be swallowed. Prolonged use should be avoided.

PHENOL GLYCERIN:

Phenol	160 g
Glycerol	840 g

Dissolve the phenol in the glycerol, with the aid of gentle heat if necessary.

CAUTION. *Dilution with water renders this preparation caustic; it may be diluted with glycerol, if desired.*

A standard for this glycerin is given in the British Pharmaceutical Codex 1973

Storage: it should be stored in airtight containers.

POTASSIUM CHLORATE AND PHENOL GARGLE:

Potassium chlorate	30.00 g
Patent blue V (Colour Index No. 42051), food grade of commerce	0.01 g
Liquefied phenol	15.0 ml
Water for preparations	to 1000.0 ml

It should be diluted with 10 times its volume of warm water before use.

A standard for this gargle is given in the British Pharmaceutical Codex 1973

Containers and *Labelling:* see the entry on Gargles for general information on containers and labelling.

Storage: it should be protected from light.

Advice for patients: the diluted solution should be used as described under Gargles. It should preferably not be swallowed. Prolonged use should be avoided.

Phenolphthalein

3,3-Bis(4-hydroxyphenyl)phthalide

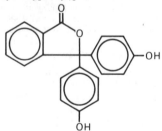

$C_{20}H_{14}O_4 = 318.3$

OTHER NAMES: *Kest®* (with magnesium sulphate); *Agarol®* and *Petrolagar Red Label®* (both with liquid paraffin)

A standard is given in the British Pharmacopoeia 1973

Description. An odourless, tasteless, white or yellowish-white, crystalline or amorphous powder.

Solubility. Very slightly soluble in water; soluble in alcohol and in ether; soluble in dilute solutions of alkali hydroxides forming a red solution.

Moisture content. Not more than 1%, determined by drying at 105°.

Dissociation constant. pK_a 9.7 (25°).

Hygroscopicity. It absorbs insignificant amounts of moisture at 25° at relative humidities up to about 90%.

Identification. MELTING-POINT. About 260°.

ULTRAVIOLET ABSORPTION. In methyl alcohol, maximum at 276 nm (E1%, 1cm = 145).

INFRA-RED ABSORPTION. Major peaks at 1178, 1220, 1240, 1265, 1278, and 1740 cm^{-1} (see Appendix 2a: Infra-red Spectra).

Actions and uses. Phenolphthalein is an irritant purgative which is usually taken at night to act in the morning. Some of it may be absorbed and excreted partly in the bile, so that purgative effects may continue for several days. It is excreted chiefly in the faeces, but some may be excreted by the kidneys, imparting a red colour to alkaline urine. Insignificant amounts are excreted in the milk. It is administered in tablets, either alone or with other purgatives, and in liquid paraffin mixture.

The usual dose of phenolphthalein for an adult is 50 to 300 milligrams, and the dose for children is one quarter to three quarters that for an adult.

Undesirable effects. Phenolphthalein may produce rashes and it has occasionally caused albuminuria and haemoglobinuria.

Preparations

LIQUID PARAFFIN AND PHENOLPHTHALEIN MIXTURE (*Syn.* Liquid Paraffin and Phenolphthalein Emulsion; Compound Liquid Paraffin Emulsion):

Phenolphthalein, microcrystalline	.. 3 g
Liquid paraffin mixture	to 1000 ml

Triturate the phenolphthalein with the liquid paraffin mixture.

It is essential to use phenolphthalein in which not more than an occasional particle has a diameter greater than

15 µm; larger particles tend to sediment in this mixture on storage and may prove difficult to redisperse uniformly by shaking the product. If a suitable microcrystalline grade is not obtainable, it may be prepared in small batches from ordinary grades by the following method: Dissolve the phenolphthalein, with the aid of gentle heat if necessary, in sufficient alcohol (95%) to give a 5% solution. Stir, by means of a high-speed stirrer, 25 times this volume of water in a suitable container, add slowly down the vortex the alcoholic phenolphthalein solution, and continue to stir for 5 minutes.

It is essential that an efficient stirrer is used in order to obtain particles of sufficiently small size.

Set the suspension aside for 1½ to 2 hours, collect the precipitated phenolphthalein on a suitable filter, such as a Whatman No. 42, and dry the phenolphthalein to constant weight at 80°. As phenolphthalein is slightly soluble in the diluted alcohol, a sufficient excess of phenolphthalein should be used and the quantity required for preparing the mixture should be weighed from the final dry powder.

A standard for this mixture is given in the British Pharmaceutical Codex 1973

Containers: see the entry on Mixtures for general information on containers. It should be supplied in wide-mouthed bottles.

Labelling: see the entry on Mixtures for general information on labelling. A direction to shake the bottle should be given on the label.

Dose: 5 to 20 millilitres.

Advice for patients: the mixture should not be taken within 30 minutes of mealtimes. It should not be used for longer than a few days without medical advice. The mixture may colour the urine red.

PHENOLPHTHALEIN TABLETS: the usual strength is 125 mg of phenolphthalein; they are made with chocolate basis.

A standard for these tablets is given in the British Pharmacopoeia 1973

Containers and *Storage:* see the entry on Tablets for general information on containers and storage. Containers should be airtight.

Advice for patients: the tablets should be chewed before being swallowed. They should not be used for longer than a few days without medical advice. They may colour the urine red.

OTHER PREPARATIONS available include a MIXTURE (emulsion) containing phenolphthalein 0.35% with liquid paraffin 7% and light liquid paraffin 18%, a mixture (emulsion) containing phenolphthalein 1.32% with liquid paraffin 31.9%; and TABLETS containing phenolphthalein 50 mg with magnesium sulphate 300 mg.

Phenolsulphonphthalein

4,4'-(3H-2,1-Benzoxathiol-3-ylidene)bisphenol 1,1-dioxide

$C_{19}H_{14}O_5S = 354.4$

OTHER NAME: Phenol Red

A standard is given in the British Pharmaceutical Codex 1973

Description. An odourless, bright to dark red, crystalline powder.

Solubility. Very slightly soluble in water; soluble, at 20°, in 350 parts of alcohol; soluble in solutions of alkali hydroxides and of alkali carbonates.

Sterilisation. Solutions for injection are sterilised by heating in an autoclave or by filtration.

Identification. TESTS. 1. Dissolve about 5 mg in 0.3 ml of 1N sodium hydroxide, add 2 ml of 0.1N bromine and 1 ml of *dilute hydrochloric acid*, shake well, allow to stand for 5 minutes, and make alkaline with 1N sodium hydroxide; an intense bluish-violet colour is produced. 2. When dissolved in solutions of alkali hydroxides or alkali carbonates, a violet-red to deep red colour is produced; the colour is changed to orange or yellow on the addition of a slight excess of acid and destroyed by warming with zinc powder.

Metabolism. ABSORPTION. Poorly absorbed after oral administration and absorption is further reduced when administered with viscous fluids; treatment with propantheline increases the extent of absorption from about 16% to about 25% of the dose.

DISTRIBUTION. *Protein binding*, bound to some extent to plasma proteins.

EXCRETION. Rapidly excreted, mainly in the urine, in normal subjects; small amounts are excreted in bile; probenecid decreases the rate of excretion of phenolsulphonphthalein; about 85% of a 6 mg dose administered intravenously is excreted in the urine in 6 hours with about 3% in bile in normal subjects; this is reduced in subjects with renal function impairment.

FURTHER INFORMATION. Effect of a viscous vehicle and an anticholinergic on bioavailability—J. J. Ashley and G. Levy, *J. pharm. Sci.*, 1973, **62**, 688.

Actions and uses. Phenolsulphonphthalein has been used as a test of renal function by estimating the rate of excretion in the urine after the intravenous injection of 6 milligrams, with 1.43 milligrams of sodium bicarbonate, in 1 millilitre of sodium chloride injection. With normal renal function, at least 50% is excreted in the urine in the first hour or 75% in the first and second hours. The concentration in the urine can be determined colorimetrically after making alkaline with sodium hydroxide solution.

Phenoxybenzamine Hydrochloride

N-Benzyl-N-(2-chloroethyl)-N-(1-methyl-2-phenoxyethyl)ammonium chloride

$C_{18}H_{23}Cl_2NO = 340.3$

OTHER NAME: *Dibenyline®*

A standard is given in the British Pharmacopoeia 1973

CAUTION. *Phenoxybenzamine hydrochloride in powder*

should not be allowed to come into contact with the eyes and skin as it may cause irritation.

Description. An odourless, tasteless, white crystalline powder.

Solubility. Very slightly soluble in water; soluble, at 20°, in 9 parts of alcohol and in 9 parts of chloroform; soluble in propylene glycol.

Stability of solutions. Neutral and alkaline solutions are unstable.

Identification. MELTING-POINT. About 138°.

INFRA-RED ABSORPTION. Major peaks at 698, 750, 1240, 1454, 1494, and 1598 cm^{-1} (see Appendix 2a: Infra-red Spectra).

Metabolism. ABSORPTION. Incompletely absorbed after oral administration.

DISTRIBUTION. Widely distributed throughout the body and may accumulate in body fat.

METABOLIC REACTIONS. *N*-Dealkylation, ether cleavage, and *p*-hydroxylation to produce, in rats, *N*-benzyl-*N*-(1-methyl-2-phenoxyethyl)amine(I), *N*-benzyl-*N*-(2-*p*-hydroxyphenoxy-1-methylethyl)amine(II), and 2-(benzylamino)propanol (III) and, in dogs, I, II, and *N*-(1-methyl-2-phenoxyethyl)amine(IV). In man, only II has so far been detected; I possesses weak α-adrenergic activity and IV possesses activity similar to but weaker than phenoxybenzamine.

EXCRETION. Excreted in the urine as unchanged drug and metabolites; about 80% of an intravenous dose is excreted in the urine in 24 hours.

FURTHER INFORMATION. Distribution—D. Masuoka *et al.*, *Acta pharmac. tox.*, 1967, **25**, 113; metabolism—D. R. Knapp *et al.*, *Drug Met. Disp.*, 1976, **4**, 164.

Actions and uses. Phenoxybenzamine has actions and uses similar to those described under Phentolamine Mesylate but its effect lasts longer than that of phentolamine, a substantial dose being capable of causing postural hypotension for up to 2 days.

Phenoxybenzamine is used to control hypertension caused by phaeochromocytomata and occasionally in the treatment of peripheral vascular disease. Its effect cannot be reversed by noradrenaline.

Phenoxybenzamine hydrochloride is given by mouth, usually commencing with 10 milligrams daily and increasing the dosage according to the response of the patient up to a total of 240 milligrams daily in divided doses. It may also be given by slow intravenous injection, well diluted with sodium chloride injection or dextrose injection (5%), in a daily dosage of 0.5 to 1 milligram per kilogram body-weight.

Preparations

PHENOXYBENZAMINE CAPSULES: consisting of phenoxybenzamine hydrochloride, in powder, which may be mixed with a suitable inert diluent, enclosed in a hard capsule. The capsule shells may be coloured. Available as capsules containing 10 mg of phenoxybenzamine hydrochloride.

A standard for these capsules is given in the British Pharmacopoeia 1973

Containers and *Storage:* see the entry on Capsules for general information on containers and storage.

Advice for patients: daily doses should preferably be taken at bedtime.

OTHER PREPARATIONS available include an INJECTION containing phenoxybenzamine hydrochloride 50 mg per ml in 2-ml ampoules.

Phenoxyethanol

2-Phenoxyethanol

$$C_6H_5 \cdot O \cdot CH_2 \cdot CH_2OH$$

$C_8H_{10}O_2 = 138.2$

OTHER NAMES: β-Phenoxyethyl Alcohol; *Phenoxetol*®

A standard is given in the British Pharmaceutical Codex 1973

Description. A colourless slightly viscous liquid with a faint pleasant odour.

Solubility. Soluble, at 20°, in 43 parts of water and in 50 parts of arachis and of olive oil; miscible with alcohol, with acetone, and with glycerol.

Weight per ml. At 20°, 1.105 to 1.110 g.

Preparation and storage of solutions. See statement on aqueous solutions of antiseptics in the entry on Solutions.

Identification. TEST. Mix 2 ml with a mixture of 4 g of potassium permanganate, 5.4 g of sodium carbonate, and 75 ml of water, shake until completely oxidised, filter, saturate the filtrate with sodium chloride, and acidify to litmus paper with hydrochloric acid; phenoxyacetic acid separates as soft crystals which, after recrystallising from water and drying, melt at about 99°.

Actions and uses. Phenoxyethanol has an antibacterial action against *Pseudomonas aeruginosa* and to a lesser extent against *Proteus vulgaris* and other Gram-negative organisms. Its action *in vitro* against *Ps. aeruginosa* is unaffected by the presence of 20% of serum.

Phenoxyethanol has been used, as a 2.2% solution or a 2% cream, in the local treatment of *Ps. aeruginosa* infections of superficial wounds, burns, and abscesses. The solution may be applied by irrigation or instillation, or as a wet dressing; it is best prepared by shaking the phenoxyethanol with hot water until dissolved, cooling, and adjusting to volume.

Phenoxyethanol has been used, in conjunction with penicillin, sulphonamides, acridine derivatives, or quaternary ammonium compounds, in the local treatment of mixed infections.

Phenoxymethylpenicillin

(6*R*)-6-(2-Phenoxyacetamido)penicillanic acid

$C_{16}H_{18}N_2O_5S = 350.4$

OTHER NAMES: Penicillin V; Phenoxymethylpenicillinum

A standard is given in the European Pharmacopoeia Vol. II

Description. A white finely crystalline powder.

Solubility. Very slightly soluble in water; soluble, at 20°, in 7 parts of alcohol; practically insoluble in fixed oils and in liquid paraffin.

Acidity. A 0.5% suspension has a pH of 2.4 to 4.

Specific rotation. +186° to +200°, determined on a 1% solution in n-butanol.

Dissociation constant. pK$_a$ 2.7 (25°).

Storage. It should be stored in airtight containers.

Identification. TEST. Mix 2 mg with 2 mg of chromotropic acid sodium salt and 2 ml of sulphuric acid, and immerse in a suitable liquid at 150° for 4 minutes; the solution remains colourless at first then changes through pink to purple and finally to dark blue (distinction from certain other penicillins).

INFRA-RED ABSORPTION. Major peaks at 1174, 1181, 1202, 1532, 1660, and 1754 cm^{-1} (see Appendix 2a: Infra-red Spectra).

Metabolism. ABSORPTION. Rapidly but incompletely absorbed after oral administration; calcium and potassium salts are better absorbed than the free acid; absorption appears to be reduced in subjects with coeliac disease; absorption appears to be more rapid in fasting than in non-fasting subjects.

BLOOD CONCENTRATION. After an oral dose of 125 mg, peak serum concentrations of 200 to 700 ng/ml are attained in 2 hours and after an oral dose of 500 mg, peak serum concentrations reach 2 to 5 μg/ml in 2 to 4 hours; following an intravenous dose of 500 mg, serum concentrations of about 8 μg/ml are obtained after about 30 minutes.

HALF-LIFE. Biological half-life, about 30 minutes.

DISTRIBUTION. Widely distributed throughout the body and enters pleural and ascitic fluids and also the cerebrospinal fluid when the meninges are inflamed; phenoxymethylpenicillin crosses the placenta and is secreted in the milk; *protein binding*, 50 to 80% bound to plasma proteins.

METABOLIC REACTIONS. Hydroxylation may occur.

EXCRETION. 20 to 35% of an oral dose is excreted in the urine in 24 hours and up to about 60% of a parenteral dose is similarly excreted; small amounts are excreted in bile; urinary excretion is blocked by probenecid.

FURTHER INFORMATION. Absorption and decomposition in body—K. Hellström *et al.*, *Clin. Pharmac. Ther.*, 1974, **16**, 826; bioavailability—T. Dimmling *et al.*, *Eur. J. clin. Pharmac.*, 1976, **10**, 55; pharmacokinetics—C. M. Kunin, *Proc. Soc. exp. Biol. Med.*, 1961, **107**, 337; salivary concentrations—C. F. Speirs *et al.*, *Br. J. Pharmac.*, 1971, **43**, 242.

Actions and uses. Phenoxymethylpenicillin is one of a group of penicillins that are stable in the acid of the stomach; therefore when they are given by mouth less is destroyed before absorption than with benzylpenicillin and the same blood level can be achieved with a small dose. In other respects these penicillins do not differ significantly in clinical effect from benzylpenicillin given orally; minor differences in protein binding, excretion rate, etc. are not of material importance in ordinary use. Being relatively insoluble, phenoxymethylpenicillin cannot be used parenterally and it should not be used topically.

Because absorption in patients who are acutely ill may be unreliable, phenoxymethylpenicillin should only be used in those who are taking food readily by mouth.

Phenoxymethylpenicillin is administered either as the free acid or as its calcium or potassium salt. It is best given half an hour before meals. Treatment started with an initial dose of benzylpenicillin by injection may be maintained with oral doses of 250 to 500 milligrams of phenoxymethylpenicillin every 4 to 6 hours for an adult. The usual dose for children up to 1 year is 62.5 milligrams; 1 to 5 years 125 milligrams, and 6 to 12 years 250 milligrams; these doses are repeated every 6 hours. Larger doses may cause diarrhoea.

Precautions and contra-indications. Phenoxymethylpenicillin should be used with caution in patients with an allergic diathesis. Its use should be avoided when there is a definite history of penicillin allergy as serious reactions have been reported.

Phenoxymethylpenicillin is secreted in the milk and should be used with caution in nursing mothers as it may provoke allergic reactions in the offspring.

Veterinary uses. Phenoxymethylpenicillin is used as an antibacterial, the usual dosage by mouth for all species being 5 to 10 milligrams per kilogram body-weight 3 times daily, but it should not be administered by mouth to adult ruminants.

Preparations

PHENOXYMETHYLPENICILLIN CAPSULES (*Syn.* Penicillin V Capsules): consisting of phenoxymethylpenicillin, of phenoxymethylpenicillin calcium, or of phenoxymethylpenicillin potassium, in powder, which may be mixed with a suitable inert diluent, enclosed in a hard capsule. The capsule shells may be coloured. Available as capsules containing 125 and 250 mg of phenoxymethylpenicillin or an equivalent quantity of the calcium or potassium salt.

A standard for these capsules is given in the British Pharmacopoeia 1973

Containers and *Storage:* see the entry on Capsules for general information on containers and storage.

Labelling: when the active ingredient is phenoxymethylpenicillin calcium or phenoxymethylpenicillin potassium, the label on the container should state the amount of the medicament as the equivalent amount of phenoxymethylpenicillin. In addition, the label on the container should state the date after which the capsules are not intended to be used, and the conditions under which they should be stored.

Advice for patients: the capsules should be taken at regular intervals, preferably half to 1 hour before meals. The prescribed course should be completed.

PHENOXYMETHYLPENICILLIN MIXTURE (*Syn.* Penicillin V Mixture): a suspension of phenoxymethylpenicillin, of phenoxymethylpenicillin calcium, or of phenoxymethylpenicillin potassium, in a suitable flavoured oily vehicle which may be coloured. When a dose less than or not a multiple of 5 ml is prescribed, the mixture may be diluted, as described in the entry on Mixtures, with fractionated coconut oil. The diluted mixture must be freshly prepared. Available as a mixture containing 125 mg of phenoxymethylpenicillin, or an equivalent amount of the calcium or potassium salt, in 5 ml.

A standard for this mixture is given in the British Pharmaceutical Codex 1973

Containers and *Labelling:* see the entry on Mixtures for general information on containers and labelling.

Storage: it should be stored in a cool place.

Advice for patients: see above under Phenoxymethylpenicillin Capsules.

PHENOXYMETHYLPENICILLIN TABLETS (*Syn.* Penicillin V Tablets): available as tablets containing 125, 250, and 300 mg of phenoxymethylpenicillin or an equivalent quantity of the calcium or potassium salt; they may be film coated.

A standard for these tablets is given in the British Pharmacopoeia 1973

Containers and *Storage:* see the entry on Tablets for general information on containers and storage. Containers should be airtight.

Labelling: when the active ingredient is phenoxymethylpenicillin calcium or phenoxymethylpenicillin potassium, the label on the container should state the amount of the medicament as the equivalent amount of phenoxymethylpenicillin. In addition, the label on the container should state the date after which the tablets are not intended to be used, and the conditions under which they should be stored.

Advice for patients: see above under Phenoxymethylpenicillin Capsules.

Phenoxymethylpenicillin Calcium

The dihydrate of the calcium salt of phenoxymethylpenicillin, or calcium (6*R*)-6-(2-phenoxyacetamido)penicillanate dihydrate.

$(C_{16}H_{17}N_2O_5S)_2Ca,2H_2O = 774.9$

OTHER NAMES: *Crystapen V®*; Penicillin V Calcium

A standard is given in the British Pharmacopoeia 1973

Description. A white finely crystalline powder which is odourless or has a slight characteristic odour and a slightly bitter taste.

Solubility. Slowly soluble, at 20°, in 120 parts of water; practically insoluble in fixed oils and in liquid paraffin.

Acidity or alkalinity. A 0.5% solution has a pH of 5 to 7.5.

Moisture content. Not more than 1.5%, determined by drying at 105°.

Storage. It should be stored in airtight containers.

Identification. TEST. It complies with the test given under Phenoxymethylpenicillin.

ULTRAVIOLET ABSORPTION. In water, weak maxima at 268 nm and 274 nm.

Metabolism. See under Phenoxymethylpenicillin.

Actions and uses. Phenoxymethylpenicillin calcium has the actions and uses described under Phenoxymethylpenicillin and is given in similar dosage. When given by mouth in equivalent doses it is absorbed more readily from the gastro-intestinal tract than the free acid and gives somewhat higher blood levels.

Precautions and contra-indications. As for Phenoxymethylpenicillin.

Veterinary uses. Phenoxymethylpenicillin calcium is used as an antibacterial, the usual dosage by mouth for all species being the equivalent of 5 to 10 milligrams of phenoxymethylpenicillin per kilogram body-weight 3 times daily, but it should not be administered by mouth to adult ruminants.

Preparations

PHENOXYMETHYLPENICILLIN CAPSULES; PHENOXYMETHYLPENICILLIN MIXTURE; PHENOXYMETHYLPENICILLIN TABLETS: see above under Phenoxymethylpenicillin.

Phenoxymethylpenicillin Potassium

The potassium salt of phenoxymethylpenicillin, or potassium (6*R*)-6-(2-phenoxyacetamido)penicillanate.

$C_{16}H_{17}KN_2O_5S = 388.5$

OTHER NAMES: *Apsin-VK®*; *Crystapen V®*; *CVK®*; *Distaquaine V-K®*; *Econocil-VK®*; *GPV®*; *Icipen®*; *Norcillin®*; Penicillin V Potassium; *Stabillin V-K®*; *Ticillin VK®*; *V-Cil-K®*

Tonsillin® (with benzalkonium chloride)

A standard is given in the British Pharmacopoeia 1973

Description. A white finely crystalline powder which is odourless or has a slight characteristic odour and a slightly bitter taste.

Solubility. Soluble, at 20°, in 1.5 parts of water; practically insoluble in ether, in fixed oils, and in liquid paraffin.

Acidity or alkalinity; Moisture content. As for Phenoxymethylpenicillin Calcium.

Storage. It should be stored in airtight containers.

Identification. TEST. It complies with the test described under Phenoxymethylpenicillin.

ULTRAVIOLET ABSORPTION. In water, weak maxima at 268 nm and 274 nm.

INFRA-RED ABSORPTION. Major peaks at 1215, 1245, 1333, 1500, 1609, and 1774 cm^{-1} (see Appendix 2a: Infra-red Spectra).

Metabolism. See under Phenoxymethylpenicillin.

Actions and uses. Phenoxymethylpenicillin potassium has the actions and uses described under Phenoxymethylpenicillin and is given in similar dosage. When given by mouth in equivalent doses it is absorbed more readily from the gastro-intestinal tract than the free acid and gives somewhat higher blood levels.

Precautions and contra-indications. As for Phenoxymethylpenicillin.

Veterinary uses. Phenoxymethylpenicillin potassium is used as an antibacterial, the usual dosage by mouth for all species being the equivalent of 5 to 10 milligrams of phenoxymethylpenicillin per kilogram body-weight 3 times daily, but it should not be administered by mouth to adult ruminants.

Preparations

PHENOXYMETHYLPENICILLIN CAPSULES: see above under Phenoxymethylpenicillin.

PHENOXYMETHYLPENICILLIN ELIXIR (*Syn.* Phenoxymethylpenicillin Solution; Phenoxymethylpenicillin Syrup; Penicillin V Elixir): a solution of phenoxymethylpenicillin potassium in a suitable coloured flavoured vehicle. It is prepared freshly by dissolving granules consisting of the dry mixed ingredients in the specified volume of water for preparations.

When a dose less than or not a multiple of 5 ml is prescribed, the elixir may be diluted, as described in the entry on Elixirs, with syrup.

Available as granules to prepare elixirs containing phenoxymethylpenicillin potassium equivalent to 62.5, 125, 150, and 250 mg of phenoxymethylpenicillin in 5 ml when reconstituted.

A standard for this elixir is given in the British Pharmaceutical Codex 1973

Containers: see the entry on Elixirs for general information on containers.

Labelling: see the entry on Elixirs for general information on labelling. In addition, the label on the container of the dry granules should state the name as "Granules for Phenoxymethylpenicillin Elixir".

Storage: the elixir and the diluted elixir should be stored in a cool place and used within 1 week of preparation.

Advice for patients: the elixir should be taken at regular intervals, preferably half to 1 hour before meals. The prescribed course should be completed.

PHENOXYMETHYLPENICILLIN MIXTURE; PHENOXYMETHYLPENICILLIN TABLETS: see above under Phenoxymethylpenicillin.

OTHER PREPARATIONS available include TABLETS containing phenoxymethylpenicillin potassium equivalent to 125 mg of phenoxymethylpenicillin with benzalkonium chloride 500 micrograms.

Phentolamine Mesylate

3 - [N - (2 - Imidazolin - 2 - ylmethyl) - p - toluidino]phenol methanesulphonate

$CH_3 \cdot SO_3H$

$C_{18}H_{23}N_3O_4S = 377.5$

OTHER NAMES: Phentolamine Methanesulphonate; *Rogitine®*

A standard is given in the British Pharmacopoeia 1973

Description. An odourless, slightly hygroscopic, white crystalline powder with a bitter taste.

Solubility. Soluble, at 20°, in 1 part of water, in 5 parts of alcohol, and in 700 parts of chloroform.

Incompatibility. It is incompatible with iron compounds.

Sterilisation. Solutions for injection are sterilised by filtration.

Storage. It should be stored in airtight containers, protected from light.

Identification. TESTS. 1. Dissolve about 500 mg in 5 ml of alcohol (95%) and 5 ml of 0.1N hydrochloric acid and add 2 ml of a 0.5% solution of ammonium vanadate; a light green precipitate is produced.
2. Dissolve about 100 mg in 40 ml of water, add 20 ml of a 20% solution of trichloroacetic acid, and allow to stand for 3 hours; a precipitate is produced which, after washing with water and drying at 105°, melts at about 138°.

MELTING-POINT. About 179°.

ULTRAVIOLET ABSORPTION. In water, maximum at 278 nm (E1%, 1cm = 247).

Metabolism. ABSORPTION. Rapidly absorbed after oral administration.

BLOOD CONCENTRATION. After oral administration, peak plasma concentrations are attained in 15 to 30 minutes and disappear as rapidly.

EXCRETION. About 10% of a dose is excreted in the urine in active form; in dogs, 50 to 65% is excreted in the urine in conjugated form following an oral dose and 30 to 50% is excreted in conjugated form following an intravenous dose.

Actions and uses. Phentolamine antagonises the vasoconstrictor effects of adrenaline and noradrenaline.
It has been used in the diagnosis of phaeochromocytomata, but the test is not considered satisfactory on account of the high incidence of false positives and it has been largely replaced by the direct estimation of circulating and excreted catecholamines. The diagnostic dose for an adult is 5 to 10 milligrams of phentolamine mesylate by intravenous injection; for a child it is 1 milligram. In patients with phaeochromocytomata, the blood pressure immediately falls, by at least 35/25 mm of mercury, into the normal range and remains depressed for several minutes. The maximum effect occurs within 2 minutes of the injection. The test may be vitiated by the simultaneous administration of other hypotensive agents.
Phentolamine has also been used, preoperatively and during operations for the removal of phaeochromocytomata, but phenoxybenzamine is usually preferred.

Undesirable effects. Moderate or light tachycardia may follow intramuscular injection, and intravenous injection may cause tachycardia with angina and, rarely, weakness, vertigo, and flushing.

Preparation

PHENTOLAMINE INJECTION: a sterile solution of phentolamine mesylate, with anhydrous dextrose and sodium metabisulphite, in water for injections. It is sterilised by filtration and distributed, by means of an aseptic technique, into sterile ampoules, the air in the ampoules being replaced with sterile nitrogen or other suitable gas, and the ampoules are sealed. Available in 1-ml ampoules containing 10 mg of phentolamine mesylate.
A standard for this injection is given in the British Pharmacopoeia 1973
Containers and *Labelling:* see the entry on Injections for general information on containers and labelling.
Storage: it should be protected from light.

Phenylbutazone

4-Butyl-1,2-diphenylpyrazolidine-3,5-dione

$C_{19}H_{20}N_2O_2 = 308.4$

OTHER NAMES: *Butacote®*; *Butazolidin®*; *Butazone®*; *Buvetzone®*; *Equi-Palazone®*; *Flexazone®*; *Oppazone®*; *Phenogel®*; Phenylbutazonum; *Prodynam®*; *Tetnor®*; *Zolaphen®*
Buta-Leucotrophin® (with cinchophen); *Delta-Butazolidin®* (with prednisone); *Parazolidin®* (with paracetamol)

A standard is given in the European Pharmacopoeia Vol. II

Description. An odourless white crystalline powder which is tasteless at first but has a bitter after-taste.

Solubility. Very slightly soluble in water; soluble, at 20°, in 28 parts of alcohol, in 15 parts of ether, and in 1.25 parts of chloroform; soluble in solutions of alkali hydroxides.

Dissociation constant. pK_a 4.4 (20°).

Stability of solutions. Aqueous solutions prepared by dissolving phenylbutazone in water with the addition of alkali hydroxide are slowly hydrolysed and oxidised by atmospheric oxygen.

Identification. TEST. Carry out the test described under Oxyphenbutazone; a red-brown precipitate is formed which dissolves in alcohol (95%) to give a red solution.

MELTING-POINT. About 105°.

ULTRAVIOLET ABSORPTION. In 0.01N sodium hydroxide, maximum at 264 nm (E1%, 1cm = 660).

INFRA-RED ABSORPTION. Major peaks at 697, 757, 1278, 1299, 1714, and 1755 cm^{-1} (see Appendix 2a: Infra-red Spectra).

THIN-LAYER CHROMATOGRAPHY. See under Thin-layer Chromatography, System 3.

Determination in body fluids. ULTRAVIOLET SPECTROPHOTOMETRY. In plasma—E. Jaehnchen and G. Levy, *Clin. Chem.*, 1972, **18**, 984.

GAS CHROMATOGRAPHY. In plasma or urine: phenylbutazone and oxyphenbutazone—R. B. Bruce *et al.*, *J. pharm. Sci.*, 1974, **63**, 446. In plasma: phenylbutazone and metabolites—Y. Tanimura *et al.*, *Chem. pharm. Bull.*, *Tokyo*, 1975, **23**, 651.

HIGH PRESSURE LIQUID CHROMATOGRAPHY. In plasma: phenylbutazone and oxyphenbutazone—N. J. Pound and R. W. Sears, *J. pharm. Sci.*, 1975, **64**, 284.

Metabolism. ABSORPTION. Readily though somewhat variably absorbed after oral administration; slowly absorbed after an intramuscular dose and well absorbed rectally; the rate of absorption of an oral dose appears to be decreased by the administration of tricyclic antidepressants.

BLOOD CONCENTRATION. During therapy with oral doses of 200 to 600 mg daily, peak plasma concentrations of 50 to 110 μg/ml are attained in 2 to 5 days; after a single oral dose of 200 mg, peak plasma concentrations of 20 to 40 μg/ml are attained in 2 to 6 hours; following an intramuscular dose, peak concentrations are attained in 6 to 10 hours.

HALF-LIFE. Plasma half-life, 1 to 7 days which is increased in subjects with renal failure, slightly increased in the aged, and decreased in subjects exposed to certain insecticides; in dogs, the half-life is dose-dependent.

DISTRIBUTION. Small amounts are secreted in the milk. *Protein binding*: extensively bound to plasma proteins; displaced from plasma proteins by indomethacin, sulphamethoxypyridazine, and tolbutamide; warfarin, chlorpropamide, and acetohexamide are displaced by phenylbutazone.

METABOLIC REACTIONS. The rate of metabolism appears to be genetically determined; the major reactions are aromatic hydroxylation to form oxyphenbutazone and (ω-1)-hydroxylation of the butyl side chain to form γ-hydroxyphenylbutazone; phenylbutazone and its metabolites do not appear to be conjugated.

EXCRETION. 10 to 20% of a dose is excreted as metabolites in the urine, mostly as the γ-hydroxymetabolite, with about 4% as oxyphenbutazone, and traces of unchanged drug.

FURTHER INFORMATION. Bioavailability studies—W. L. Chiou, *J. clin. Pharmac.*, 1972, **12**, 296, G. Lukas *et al.*, *J. clin. Pharmac.*, 1974, **14**, 397, G. R. Van Petten *et al.*, *J. clin. Pharmac.*, 1971, **11**, 177, and R. J. Withey *et al.*, *J. clin. Pharmac.*, 1971, **11**, 187; effect of dicophane on metabolism—A. Poland *et al.*, *Clin. Pharmac. Ther.*, 1970, **11**, 724; plasma half-life with impaired liver function—E. F. Hvidberg *et al.*, *Clin. Pharmac. Ther.*, 1974, **15**, 171; half-life variability— K. O'Malley *et al.*, *Br. med. J.*, iii/1971, 607; plasma concentrations of metabolites—K. K. Midha *et al.*, *J. pharm. Sci.*, 1974, **63**, 1234 and 1751; saturation of metabolism—I. J. McGilveray *et al.*, *Pharmacologist*, 1973, **15**, 213.

Actions and uses. Phenylbutazone is an anti-inflammatory agent that is similar in potency to aspirin. It exhibits uricosuric and sodium-retaining effects and it blocks iodine uptake by the thyroid and a variety of other intracellular enzymatic processes including mucopolysaccharide production. It is metabolised and excreted slowly and its therapeutic effect is therefore prolonged. It is used mainly to relieve symptoms of rheumatic disorders.

Phenylbutazone is given by mouth with meals in a dosage of 300 milligrams daily; larger doses should not be used except on the first day or two of treatment of acute conditions, when up to 600 milligrams may be given daily. The usual dose by mouth for children is 5 to 10 milligrams per kilogram body-weight daily.

Phenylbutazone may also be administered by rectum in suppositories in a dosage of 250 to 500 milligrams daily or by intramuscular injection in a dosage of 600 milligrams every 2 to 3 days.

Undesirable effects. Toxic effects occur frequently, even when the dosage does not exceed 400 milligrams daily, and may include oedema, rashes, gastric upset, and mucosal ulceration of the mouth, oesophagus, stomach, or duodenum, with haematemesis and melaena. Granulocytopenia is an indication to withdraw the drug as otherwise the condition may become irreversible.

Precautions and contra-indications. Blood dyscrasias due to phenylbutazone, though rare, are a significant cause of mortality. In patients who develop any intercurrent illness such as a serious infection, a blood count should be carried out and treatment with phenylbutazone discontinued immediately. Regular blood counts are however of no value in preventing serious incidents which occur particularly in the elderly.

Phenylbutazone should not be given to patients with cardiac failure, which may be aggravated by fluid retention; for the same reason it should be avoided in the elderly. Caution should be exercised when phenylbutazone is given to patients taking oral hypoglycaemic agents. The use of phenylbutazone with anticoagulants of the coumarin type should be avoided as it may displace them from protein binding sites with a consequent risk of haemorrhage.

It is contra-indicated in patients with renal or hepatic disease, peptic ulceration, blood dyscrasias, or sensitivity to pyrazoles.

Veterinary uses. Phenylbutazone is used as an analgesic and anti-inflammatory agent. The usual dose by mouth for horses is 4 to 8 milligrams per kilogram body-weight daily and for dogs 2 to 20 milligrams per kilogram body-weight daily.

Preparations

PHENYLBUTAZONE SUPPOSITORIES: prepared as described in the entry on Suppositories by incorporating phenylbutazone in a suitable basis. Available as suppositories containing 250 mg of phenylbutazone. *A standard for these suppositories is given in the British Pharmacopoeia 1973*
Containers and *Storage:* see the entry on Suppositories for general information on containers and storage.
Advice for patients: see the entry on Suppositories for general information on the use of suppositories.

PHENYLBUTAZONE TABLETS: available as tablets containing 100 and 200 mg and 2 g of phenylbutazone; they are film coated or sugar coated; they may be coloured; they need not be circular in shape.
A standard for these tablets is given in the British

Pharmacopoeia 1973 and in the British Pharmacopoeia (Veterinary)

Containers and *Storage:* see the entry on Tablets for general information on containers and storage. Containers should be airtight.

Advice for patients: the tablets should be taken after meals.

OTHER PREPARATIONS available include a veterinary POWDER in sachets containing phenylbutazone 1 g, a veterinary powder in sachets containing phenylbutazone 500 mg with cinchophen 1 g; TABLETS (enteric coated) containing phenylbutazone 100 and 200 mg, tablets containing phenylbutazone 50 mg with paracetamol 500 mg, and tablets containing phenylbutazone 50 mg with prednisone 1.25 mg.

Phenylephrine Hydrochloride

(R)-N-$(3,\beta$-Dihydroxyphenethyl)-N-methylammonium chloride

$C_9H_{14}ClNO_2 = 203.7$

OTHER NAMES: *Fenox®*; *Neophryn®*
Narex® (with chlorbutol); *Isopto Frin®* (with hypromellose); *Hayphryn®* (with thenyldiamine hydrochloride)

A standard is given in the British Pharmacopoeia 1973

Description. An odourless white crystalline powder with a bitter taste.

Solubility. Soluble, at 20°, in 2 parts of water, in 4 parts of alcohol, and in 2 parts of glycerol; practically insoluble in fixed oils.

Moisture content. Not more than 1%, determined by drying at 105°.

Specific rotation. −43° to −47°, determined on a 2% solution.

Dissociation constants. pK_a 8.9, 10.1 (20°).

Stability. In aqueous solution phenylephrine hydrochloride is gradually oxidised with the formation of coloured products; the rate of oxidation is greatest in alkaline solution. Depth of colour is not a reliable guide to the extent of oxidation. Discoloration is retarded by sodium metabisulphite and disodium edetate.

FURTHER INFORMATION. Stability in aqueous solutions —H. A. M. El-Shibini *et al.*, *Arzneimittel-Forsch.*, 1969, **19**, 676, 828, and 1613; R. T. Millard *et al.*, *J. Pharm. Pharmac.*, 1973, **25**, 24P; *Analytical Profiles of Drug Substances*, K. Florey (Ed.), Vol. 3, London, Academic Press, p. 483. Stability in intravenous infusions—C. R. Weber and V. Das Gupta, *J. Hosp. Pharm.*, 1970, **28**, 200.

Sterilisation. Solutions for injection are sterilised by filtration.

Storage. It should be stored in airtight containers, protected from light.

Identification. TESTS. 1. Dissolve about 10 mg in 1 ml of water and add 1 drop of *copper sulphate solution* and

1 ml of *sodium hydroxide solution*; a violet colour is produced. Add 1 ml of ether and shake; the ether layer remains colourless.

2. Dissolve about 300 mg in 3 ml of water, add 1 ml of *dilute ammonia solution* and induce crystallisation; a crystalline precipitate is produced which, after washing with ice-cold water and drying at 105° for 2 hours, melts at about 170°.

MELTING-POINT. About 142°.

ULTRAVIOLET ABSORPTION. In 1N sulphuric acid, maximum at 273 nm (E1%, 1cm = 96); in 0.1N sodium hydroxide, maxima at 238 nm (E1%, 1cm = 429) and 293 nm (E1%, 1cm = 147).

INFRA-RED ABSORPTION. Major peaks at 696, 784, 1273, 1305, 1462, and 1594 cm^{-1} (see Appendix 2a: Infra-red Spectra).

Determination in body fluids. GAS CHROMATOGRAPHY. In plasma—L. J. Dombrowski *et al.*, *J. pharm. Sci.*, 1973, **62**, 1761.

Metabolism. ABSORPTION. The hydrochloride is variably absorbed; corneal absorption is increased by raising the pH of the phenylephrine preparation with borate buffer.

EXCRETION. About 20 to 70% of an oral dose of the hydrochloride appears to be excreted in 24 hours.

FURTHER INFORMATION. Absorption from buffered eye-drops—E. S. N. Wang and E. R. Hammarlund, *J. pharm. Sci.*, 1970, **59**, 1559; sustained-release and plasma concentrations—R. L. Bogner and J. M. Walsh, *J. pharm. Sci.*, 1964, **53**, 617, and C. J. Cavallito *et al.*, *J. pharm. Sci.*, 1963, **52**, 259.

Actions and uses. Phenylephrine is a sympathomimetic drug which has actions similar to those described under Noradrenaline Acid Tartrate but it has weaker pressor activity and a longer duration of action than noradrenaline and lacks the cardiac and central adverse effects of adrenaline. After injection it produces peripheral vasoconstriction and increased arterial pressure; unlike adrenaline and ephedrine it also causes reflex bradycardia. The principal use of phenylephrine is in nasal congestion.

Phenylephrine is probably the safest vasoconstrictor to use with cyclopropane and other anaesthetics liable to cause cardiac irregularities. It is also a satisfactory vasoconstrictor for use with local anaesthetics. The initial dose is 5 milligrams of phenylephrine hydrochloride by subcutaneous or intramuscular injection, followed by supplementary doses of 1 to 10 milligrams if necessary. Alternatively, 5 to 20 milligrams may be given in 500 millilitres of sodium chloride injection or dextrose injection (5%) by slow intravenous infusion.

In treatment of peripheral vascular collapse, 500 micrograms may be given slowly by intravenous injection as a 0.02% solution, or 5 milligrams by intramuscular injection.

Solutions containing 0.25 to 0.5% of phenylephrine hydrochloride may be applied locally as vasoconstrictors in nasal congestion but excessive use may lead to a worsening of the condition.

For use in ophthalmology as a mydriatic and vasoconstrictor, solutions containing 5 to 10% are employed. If irritation occurs this can be prevented by the addition of a local anaesthetic.

Phenylephrine hydrochloride is occasionally used as an inhalation in bronchial asthma, in conjunction with a bronchodilator such as isoprenaline sulphate.

Undesirable effects. Parenteral administration produces a rise in blood pressure, with headache, palpitations, and vomiting. Extravasation of the injection may cause tissue necrosis.

The use of eye-drops containing a high concentration of phenylephrine may raise the blood pressure in babies.

Contra-indications. Parenteral administration of phenylephrine is contra-indicated in patients who are being treated with a monoamine-oxidase inhibitor such as isocarboxazid, nialamide, phenelzine, or tranylcypromine or within about 2 weeks of the discontinuation of such treatment. Phenylephrine should not be used parenterally in conjunction with tricyclic antidepressants such as amitriptyline, desipramine, imipramine, nortriptyline, protriptyline or trimipramine. The eye-drops should not be used in patients with glaucoma.

Preparations

PHENYLEPHRINE EYE-DROPS:

Phenylephrine hydrochloride	..	..	..	10.0 g
Sodium citrate	..	..	..	0.3 g
Sodium metabisulphite	..	..	..	0.5 g
Benzalkonium chloride solution		..	..	0.02 ml
Purified water	..	..	..	to 100.0 ml

Prepare by method B described in the entry on Eye-drops. *A standard for these eye-drops is given in the British Pharmaceutical Codex 1973*
Containers and *Labelling:* see the entry on Eye-drops for general information on containers and labelling.
Storage: it should be protected from light.

PHENYLEPHRINE INJECTION: a sterile solution of phenylephrine hydrochloride in water for injections. It is sterilised by filtration and distributed, by means of an aseptic technique, into sterile ampoules, the air in the ampoules is replaced by sterile nitrogen or other suitable gas, and the ampoules are sealed. For intravenous administration, an injection containing 10 mg of phenylephrine hydrochloride per ml should be diluted immediately before use.
A standard for this injection is given in the British Pharmacopoeia 1973
Containers and *Labelling:* see the entry on Injections for general information on containers and labelling.
Storage: it should be protected from light.

OTHER PREPARATIONS available include EYE-DROPS containing phenylephrine hydrochloride 0.12% with hypromellose 0.5%; NASAL DROPS containing phenylephrine hydrochloride 0.25%; a NASAL SPRAY containing phenylephrine hydrochloride 0.5%, a nasal spray containing phenylephrine hydrochloride 0.5% with chlorbutol 0.5%, and a nasal spray containing phenylephrine hydrochloride 0.5% with thenyldiamine hydrochloride 0.1%.

Phenylketonuria

Phenylketonuria is a genetically determined autosomal recessive disease in which there is a deficiency of the enzyme phenylalanine hydroxylase and a consequent inability to metabolise phenylalanine to tyrosine. Phenylalanine and its metabolites accumulate in the blood and lead to damage to the developing brain. Phenylketonuria may be detected by the presence of phenylpyruvic acid in the urine. It may be treated by a synthetic diet low in phenylalanine but complete in other nutrients. Phenylalanine should not be completely excluded from the diet as this may cause growth failure.

Phenylmercuric Acetate

A basic phenylmercuric acetate.
$C_8H_8HgO_2 = 336.7$

OTHER NAME: Phenylhydrargyri Acetas

A standard is given in the British Pharmaceutical Codex 1973

Description. An odourless white or creamy-white crystalline powder or small white prisms or leaflets.

Solubility. Soluble, at 20°, in 600 parts of water, in 24 parts of alcohol, and in 19 parts of acetone.

Storage. It should be protected from light.

Preparation and storage of solutions. See statement on aqueous solutions of antiseptics in the entry on Solutions.

Identification. TESTS. 1. To 5 ml of a saturated solution in water add 0.2 ml of *sodium sulphide solution*; a white precipitate is formed which turns black on boiling and allowing to stand.
2. To about 100 mg add 0.5 ml of nitric acid, warm gently until a dark brown colour is produced, and dilute with 10 ml of water; the odour of nitrobenzene is produced.
3. To about 100 mg add 0.5 ml of sulphuric acid and 1 ml of alcohol (95%) and warm; the odour of ethyl acetate is produced.

MELTING-POINT. About 151°.

Metabolism. DISTRIBUTION. In rats, subjected to enterohepatic circulation.

METABOLIC REACTIONS. In rats, cleavage to release benzene and inorganic mercury followed by oxidation to form phenol and quinol which are conjugated with glucuronic acid and sulphate.

EXCRETION. In rats, 2 to 5% of a dose is excreted unchanged in the urine, 34% as phenol conjugates, and about 2% as quinol conjugates; the major metabolite is the sulphate conjugate of phenol; inorganic mercury is excreted in the faeces; a certain amount of unchanged drug is excreted in the bile.

FURTHER INFORMATION. Metabolism in rats—J. W. Daniel *et al.*, *Biochem. J.*, 1972, **129**, 961.

Actions and uses. Phenylmercuric acetate has antibacterial, antifungal, and spermicidal properties similar to those described under Phenylmercuric Nitrate.

Phenylmercuric Nitrate

A basic phenylmercuric nitrate.
$C_{12}H_{11}Hg_2NO_4 = 634.4$

OTHER NAME: Phenylhydrargyri Nitras

A standard is given in the British Pharmacopoeia 1973

Description. Odourless white lustrous plates or crystalline powder, with a weakly metallic and astringent taste.

Solubility. Soluble, at 20°, in 1500 parts of water and in 1000 parts of alcohol; soluble in glycerol and in fixed oils; soluble in 160 parts of boiling water.

Moisture content. Not more than 1%, determined by drying over phosphorus pentoxide *in vacuo*.

Dissociation constant. pK_a 3.3 (20°).

Incompatibility. It is incompatible with chlorides, bromides, and iodides, with which it forms the less soluble halogen compounds.

Storage. It should be protected from light.

Preparation and storage of solutions. See statement on aqueous solutions of antiseptics in the entry on Solutions.

Identification. TESTS. 1. It complies with Test 1 described under Phenylmercuric Acetate.

2. Mix about 500 mg with 500 mg of zinc powder, 500 mg of reduced iron, and 5 ml of *sodium hydroxide solution*, and heat; ammonia is evolved.

MELTING-POINT. About 188°, with decomposition.

ULTRAVIOLET ABSORPTION. In water, weak maxima at 250 nm, 256 nm and 262 nm.

Actions and uses. Phenylmercuric nitrate has antibacterial and antifungal properties. It is used as a bactericide in a concentration of 0.001% in preparations for parenteral administration and in a concentration of 0.002% in some eye-drops, but its inclusion in eye-drops intended for use over long periods is not recommended. Phenylmercuric nitrate may be used in the process of sterilisation by heating with a bactericide, in which a solution or suspension of the medicament in a 0.002% solution of phenylmercuric nitrate in water for injections is heated in the final sealed containers at 98° to 100° for 30 minutes. It should not be used in solutions intended for intrathecal, intracisternal, or peridural injection, or in solutions intended for intravenous injection where the dose exceeds 15 millilitres.

Preparations of phenylmercuric nitrate have been used as chemical contraceptives. The spermicidal activity is much reduced in vaginal secretions of pH greater than 7.2.

Phenylpropanolamine Hydrochloride

1-Hydroxy-1-phenylprop-2-ylammonium chloride

$C_9H_{14}ClNO = 187.7$

OTHER NAMES: *Totolin®* (with guaiphenesin); *Triogesic®* (with paracetamol)

A standard is given in the British Pharmacopoeia 1973

Description. An odourless, white to creamy-white, crystalline powder with a bitter taste.

Solubility. Soluble, at 20°, in 2.5 parts of water and in 9 parts of alcohol; practically insoluble in ether and in chloroform.

Acidity. A 3% solution has a pH of 4.5 to 6.

Dissociation constant. pK_a 9.4 (20°).

Sterilisation. Solutions are sterilised by heating in an autoclave or by filtration.

Identification. TEST. Dissolve about 500 mg in 20 ml of water, add 10 ml of 1N sodium hydroxide, extract with three 25-ml portions of ether, wash each extract with the same 5 ml of water, dry the ether extracts over anhydrous sodium sulphate, filter, and evaporate to dryness; the residue, after drying at 80°, melts at about 102°.

MELTING-POINT. About 194°.

ULTRAVIOLET ABSORPTION. In 0.1N hydrochloric acid, weak maxima at 251 nm, 257 nm, and 262 nm.

INFRA-RED ABSORPTION. As phenylpropanolamine, major peaks at 703, 748, 1033, 1057, 1453, and 1492 cm^{-1} (see Appendix 2a: Infra-red Spectra).

Determination in body fluids. GAS CHROMATOGRAPHY. In plasma—L. Neelakantan and H. B. Kostenbauder, *J. pharm. Sci.*, 1976, **65**, 740.

Metabolism. BLOOD CONCENTRATION. After an oral dose of 50 mg, peak plasma concentrations of about 100 ng/ml are attained in 1 to 2 hours.

METABOLIC REACTIONS. In dogs, *p*-hydroxylation.

EXCRETION. About 90% of an oral dose is excreted in the urine.

FURTHER INFORMATION. L. Neelakantan and H. B. Kostenbauder, *J. pharm. Sci.*, 1976, **65**, 740.

Actions and uses. Phenylpropanolamine is a sympathomimetic amine with actions similar to those of ephedrine but it is somewhat more active as a vasoconstrictor and less active as a central stimulant and bronchodilator.

Phenylpropanolamine hydrochloride is given by mouth in doses of 25 to 50 milligrams for the symptomatic treatment of allergic conditions such as bronchial asthma or hay fever. It is applied as a 1 to 3% solution for the relief of nasal congestion.

Precautions and contra-indications. Phenylpropanolamine should be given with caution to hypertensive patients.

It should not be given to patients who are being treated with a monoamine-oxidase inhibitor, such as isocarboxazid, nialamide, phenelzine, or tranylcypromine, or within about 2 weeks of the discontinuation of such treatment.

Preparations

Preparations available include an ELIXIR containing phenylpropanolamine hydrochloride 3 mg with paracetamol 125 mg in 5 ml, diluent syrup or water for preparations, life of diluted elixir 14 days, an elixir containing phenylpropanolamine hydrochloride 7.5 mg with guaiphenesin 30 mg in 5 ml; and TABLETS containing phenylpropanolamine hydrochloride 12.5 mg with paracetamol 500 mg.

Phenytoin

5,5-Diphenylimidazolidine-2,4-dione

$C_{15}H_{12}N_2O_2 = 252.3$

OTHER NAMES: Diphenylhydantoin; *Epanutin®*

A standard is given in the British Pharmaceutical Codex 1973

Description. An odourless white crystalline powder.

Solubility. Very slightly soluble in water; soluble, at 20°, in 70 parts of alcohol, in 600 parts of ether, and in 500 parts of chloroform; soluble in solutions of alkali hydroxides.

Dissociation constant. pK_a 8.3.

Identification. TEST. Dissolve about 100 mg in a mixture of 0.5 ml of 1N sodium hydroxide and 2 ml of a 10% solution of pyridine, add a further 8 ml of the pyridine solution, shake, add 1 ml of *copper sulphate with pyridine solution*, and allow to stand for 10 minutes; a blue precipitate is produced.

MELTING-POINT. About 295°.

ULTRAVIOLET ABSORPTION. In methyl alcohol, maximum at 258 nm (E1%, 1cm = 29).

Determination in body fluids; Metabolism. See under Phenytoin Sodium.

Actions and uses. Phenytoin has the actions, uses, and undesirable effects described under Phenytoin Sodium; 0.9 gram of phenytoin is approximately equivalent to 1 gram of phenytoin sodium.

Precautions. As for Phenytoin Sodium.

Preparations

PHENYTOIN MIXTURE (*Syn.* Phenytoin Suspension): a suspension of phenytoin in a suitable coloured flavoured vehicle. When a dose less than or not a multiple of 5 ml is prescribed, the mixture may be diluted, as described in the entry on Mixtures, with syrup. The diluted mixture must be freshly prepared. Available as a mixture containing 30 mg of phenytoin in 5 ml.
A standard for this mixture is given in the British Pharmaceutical Codex 1973
Containers and *Labelling:* see the entry on Mixtures for general information on containers and labelling.
Advice for patients: the mixture should preferably be taken before meals; if there are gastro-intestinal disturbances the dose may be taken after meals. When initiating treatment there may be a time-lag of up to 2 weeks before a full therapeutic response is obtained. Treatment should not be discontinued without the advice of the prescriber.

OTHER PREPARATIONS available include TABLETS containing phenytoin 50 mg.

Phenytoin Sodium

The sodium derivative of 5,5-diphenylimidazolidine-2,4-dione

$C_{15}H_{11}N_2NaO_2 = 274.3$

OTHER NAMES: Diphenylhydantoin Sodium; *Epanutin®*; Phenytoinum Natricum; Soluble Phenytoin
Epanutin with Phenobarbitone®; *Garoin®* (with phenobarbitone sodium); *Mysoline with Phenytoin®* (with primidone)

A standard is given in the European Pharmacopoeia Vol. III Supplement

Description. An odourless, slightly hygroscopic, white, crystalline powder.

Solubility. Soluble in water and in alcohol; practically insoluble in ether and in chloroform.

Moisture content. Not more than 2.5%, determined by drying at 105°.

Stability. It absorbs carbon dioxide from the atmosphere with liberation of phenytoin.

Sterilisation. Solutions are sterilised by filtration.

Storage. It should be stored in airtight containers.

Identification. TESTS. 1. Dissolve about 100 mg in 10 ml of a 10% solution of pyridine, add 1 ml of *copper sulphate with pyridine solution* and allow to stand for 10 minutes; a blue precipitate is produced.
2. To a 5% solution add *dilute hydrochloric acid*; a white precipitate is produced which, after washing with water and drying at 105°, melts at about 295°.

Determination in body fluids. COLORIMETRY. In plasma, serum, or urine—W. A. Dill *et al.*, *J. Pharmac. exp. Ther.*, 1956, **118**, 270.

ULTRAVIOLET SPECTROPHOTOMETRY. In plasma, serum, or whole blood: includes a short review of methods with 25 references—J. E. Wallace and H. E. Hamilton, *J. pharm. Sci.*, 1974, **63**, 1795; A. J. Fellenberg *et al.*, *Clinica chim. Acta*, 1975, **59**, 155.

SPECTROFLUORIMETRY. In plasma—W. A. Dill *et al.*, *Clin. Chem.*, 1976, **22**, 908.

GAS CHROMATOGRAPHY. In serum—T. J. Giovanniello and J. Pecci, *Clinica chim. Acta*, 1976, **67**, 7. In plasma or urine—J. Gordos *et al.*, *J. Chromat.*, 1977, **143**(2), 171. In plasma: phenytoin and the major metabolite 5-(4-hydroxyphenyl)-5-phenylhydantoin—K. K. Midha *et al.*, *J. pharm. Sci.*, 1976, **65**, 1240. In plasma: comparison with a radioimmunoassay procedure—M. L'E. Orme *et al.*, *Clin. Chem.*, 1976, **22**, 246.

HIGH PRESSURE LIQUID CHROMATOGRAPHY. In plasma: phenytoin simultaneously with phenobarbitone—S. H. Atwell *et al.*, *J. pharm. Sci.*, 1975, **64**, 806. In urine: determination of the major metabolite 5-(4-hydroxyphenyl)-5-phenylhydantoin—J. Hermansson and K. Bo, *J. Chromat.*, 1977, **130**, 422.

Metabolism. ABSORPTION. Slowly but almost completely absorbed after oral administration; the rate of absorption is subject to individual variations and to bioavailability differences between formulations; intramuscular doses are more slowly absorbed than oral doses; large doses appear to be more slowly absorbed than small doses and this, in some cases, may result in therapeutic failure; the sodium salt is better absorbed than phenytoin itself.

BLOOD CONCENTRATION. Effective serum concentrations are in the range 10 to 20 μg/ml; at concentrations in the range 20 to 40 μg/ml, side-effects may occur and at concentrations above 40 μg/ml full toxic symptoms may appear; the serum or plasma concentration/time curve varies and after an oral dose more than one peak may be observed; during therapy with oral doses of 300 to 400 mg daily, steady-state serum concentrations of 10 to 20 μg/ml are attained after about 5 days; after an oral dose of 100 mg of the sodium salt, a peak plasma concentration of 1.5 to 3 μg/ml is attained in 3 to 6 hours which may be followed by a second peak after 10 to 12 hours; after an intramuscular dose of 500 mg of the sodium salt, a peak plasma concentration of about 4 μg/ml is attained at about 11 hours; following an intravenous dose of 250 mg of the sodium salt, a plasma concentration of about 5 μg/ml is obtained at 1 hour falling to about 2 μg/ml at 20 hours; administration of pyridoxine or folic acid appears to decrease plasma concentrations of phenytoin.

HALF-LIFE. Plasma half-life varies considerably and is in the approximate range of 7 to 40 hours; at doses above 100 mg, the half-life is dose dependent and is decreased by concomitant administration of disulfiram or carbamazepine.

DISTRIBUTION. Widely and rapidly distributed throughout the body; it is secreted in the milk, accumulates in red blood cells, and amounts secreted in saliva show a linear relationship to those in serum; cerebrospinal fluid concentrations may reach up to about 45% of those in serum; upon repeated intake phenytoin may accumulate; phenytoin is subject to enterohepatic circulation; volume of distribution, 0.4 to 1.8 litres/kg; *protein binding*, 70 to 90% bound to plasma proteins especially to albumin and thyroxine-binding globulins; protein binding varies according to plasma concentration of phenytoin and is decreased in hepatitis and in neonates; phenytoin binding is decreased by aspirin, salicylic acid, phenylbutazone, and sulphafurazole; the binding of warfarin and thyroxine is reduced by the presence of phenytoin; in renal function impairment, phenytoin binding varies according to the severity of the condition.

METABOLIC REACTIONS. Aromatic hydroxylation to form, in man, 5-(4-hydroxyphenyl)-5-phenylhydantoin (HPPH) and hydrolytic ring fission, in rats and dogs, to form diphenylhydantoic acid and α-aminodiphenylacetic acid; in dogs, *m*-hydroxylation occurs to a greater extent than *p*-hydroxylation; in rats a further hydroxylated metabolite has been identified, 5-(3,4-dihydroxy-1,5-cyclohexadien-1-yl)-5-phenylhydantoin (dihydrodiol), which is formed by oxidation of an aromatic double bond in one of the phenyl rings of phenytoin; the metabolite has also been identified in small amounts in the urine of man; hydroxylated metabolites are conjugated with glucuronic acid; the aromatic hydroxylation results in formation of optically active metabolites, and in man both the (+)- and (−)-forms of HPPH are produced with more of the (−)-metabolite than the (+)-metabolite appearing; in dogs, both the (+)- and (−)-forms of HPPH are produced but most of the *m*-hydroxylated metabolite is in the (+)-form; the metabolism of phenytoin is inhibited by chloramphenicol, disulfiram, dicoumarol, and isoniazid, whilst it is induced by phenobarbitone and phenytoin itself.

EXCRETION. Up to about 4% of a dose is excreted in the urine unchanged together with 50 to 90% as HPPH in free or conjugated form; the urinary excretion of HPPH is dependent on dose and as the dose is increased the percentage converted to HPPH is decreased; the excretion of unchanged drug is increased when the urine is alkaline; in rats and dogs, up to about 8% of a dose is excreted as diphenylhydantoic acid and up to about 30% is excreted as α-aminodiphenylacetic acid; small amounts are excreted as dihydrodiol in urine of both man and animals; up to about 15% of a dose may be excreted in the faeces.

FURTHER INFORMATION. Elimination in overdosed children—L. K. Garrettson and W. J. Jusko, *Clin. Pharmac. Ther.*, 1975, **17**, 481, and A. W. Pruitt *et al.*, *Clin. Pharmac. Ther.*, 1975, **18**, 112; influence of hepatitis on pharmacokinetics—T. F. Blaschke *et al.*, *Clin. Pharmac. Ther.*, 1975, **17**, 685; influence of disulfiram on pharmacokinetics—T. L. Svendsen *et al.*, *Eur. J. clin. Pharmac.*, 1976, **9**, 439; pharmacokinetics—J. D. Robinson *et al.*, *Br. J. clin. Pharmac.*, 1975, **2**, 345; plasma and salivary concentrations—C. E. Cook *et al.*, *Clin. Pharmac. Ther.*, 1975, **18**, 742; protein binding— G. D. Olsen *et al.*, *Clin. Pharmac. Ther.*, 1975, **17**, 677; reviews—*Antiepileptic Drugs*, D. M. Woodbury *et al.* (Eds), New York, Raven Press, 1972; stereoselectivity of hydroxylation—T. C. Butler *et al.*, *J. Pharmac. exp. Ther.*, 1976, **199**, 82; tissue binding to protein—M. A. Goldberg and T. Todoroff, *J. Pharmac. exp. Ther.*, 1976,

196, 579; transfer to intramuscular use—B. J. Wilder and R. E. Ramsey, *Clin. Pharmac. Ther.*, 1976, **19**, 360.

Bioavailability. Substituting the administration of one preparation of phenytoin by others in epileptic patients has resulted in the recurrence of seizures or in the development of toxic reactions. This loss in therapeutic control has been attributed to variations in formulation caused by differences in particle size, in solubility of the gelatin capsules used, and in the use of different excipients. Small particles are better absorbed than larger ones and when phenytoin is administered in a ground mixture with microcrystalline cellulose its absorption is further improved. When calcium sulphate is used as an excipient instead of lactose a reduction of about 70% in steady-state plasma concentration has been observed.

FURTHER INFORMATION. Bioavailability—S. Feldman *et al.*, *J. Am. pharm. Ass.*, 1975, **15**, 647; R. Gugler *et al.*, *Clin. Pharmac. Ther.*, 1976, **19**, 135; W. J. Jusko *et al.*, *J. Pharmacokinet. Biopharm.*, 1976, **4**, 327; B. E. Miles *et al.*, *Lancet*, i/1976, 255; P. Tammisto *et al.*, *Lancet*, i/1976, 254; K. Yamamoto *et al.*, *J. pharm. Sci.*, 1976, **65**, 1484.

Actions and uses. Phenytoin has an anticonvulsant action but relatively little hypnotic effect. It is used in the treatment of epilepsy and for this purpose has the advantage over phenobarbitone of being less likely to produce drowsiness and mental dullness. It is frequently effective in conjunction with phenobarbitone in patients in whom phenobarbitone alone causes too much depression. In changing from phenobarbitone or other sedatives to phenytoin, the transition should be made gradually with some overlapping of the use of the two drugs; too rapid withdrawal of phenobarbitone may lead to an increase in the frequency of seizures. Phenytoin is effective in controlling grand mal fits but is ineffective in petit mal.

The dosage for an adult is 50 to 100 milligrams of phenytoin sodium by mouth 3 times a day, increased if necessary to a maximum of 200 milligrams 3 times a day. A child over 6 years of age may be given 100 milligrams 3 or 4 times a day; younger children may be given 30 to 60 milligrams of phenytoin sodium 3 times a day.

Because phenytoin sodium is strongly alkaline, it may irritate the gastric mucosa; this may be avoided by giving the dose with a copious draught of water after meals, although it is more effective if given before meals.

Phenytoin sodium may be given by intramuscular or intravenous injection in doses up to 500 milligrams at a rate not exceeding 50 milligrams per minute. The corresponding dose for a child is up to 5 milligrams per kilogram body-weight.

Phenytoin is so poorly absorbed after intramuscular injection that loss of control may occur on changing from oral to intramuscular administration, and conversely toxic effects may be observed when changing from intramuscular to oral treatment. It is administered by slow intravenous infusion in the treatment of cardiac arrhythmias, the usual dose being 5 milligrams per kilogram body-weight.

Undesirable effects. Minor toxic effects such as dizziness, nausea, and rashes occur frequently, but may usually be overcome by reducing the dosage for a few days, after which they do not usually return on increasing the dosage to the original amount. Tenderness and hyperplasia of the gums may also occur.

Other toxic symptoms sometimes observed are fever, ataxia, diplopia, muscular tremors, hallucinations, and mental confusion. Leucopenia, exfoliative dermatitis, and purpura are more serious reactions which may be severe enough to necessitate the withdrawal of the drug. Nystagmus is a common sign of cerebellar disturbance due to phenytoin.

Phenytoin lowers the plasma folate concentration and may induce megaloblastic anaemia. Phenytoin may also reduce the serum calcium level and there is a possibility that osteomalacia may occur. Hirsutism may also occur.

Precautions. It should be used with caution in pregnancy and in nursing mothers, and its use in early pregnancy should be avoided unless the benefits outweigh the risks.

Drug interactions. The actions of phenytoin are enhanced by the simultaneous administration of isoniazid, sodium aminosalicylate, chloramphenicol, and disulfiram and decreased by reserpine, tricyclic antidepressants, phenobarbitone, and folic acid. The use of phenytoin in conjunction with digoxin should be avoided as it has been reported to cause brain damage.

Veterinary uses. Phenytoin sodium is used as an anticonvulsant, the usual dose by mouth for dogs being 10 to 20 milligrams per kilogram body-weight daily adjusted in accordance with the response.

Preparations

PHENYTOIN CAPSULES (*Syn.* Phenytoin Sodium Capsules; Soluble Phenytoin Capsules): consisting of phenytoin sodium, in powder, which may be mixed with a suitable inert diluent, enclosed in a hard capsule. Calcium sulphate should not be used as a diluent as it is known to impair the absorption of phenytoin sodium. Available as capsules containing 25, 50, and 100 mg of phenytoin sodium.
A standard for these capsules is given in the British Pharmacopoeia Addendum 1977 and in the British Pharmacopoeia (Veterinary)
Containers and *Storage:* see the entry on Capsules for general information on containers and storage.
Advice for patients: the capsules should be taken with a tumblerful of water, preferably before meals; if there are gastro-intestinal disturbances the dose may be taken after meals. When initiating treatment, there may be a time-lag of up to 2 weeks before a full therapeutic response is obtained. Treatment should not be discontinued without the advice of the prescriber.

PHENYTOIN INJECTION (*Syn.* Phenytoin Sodium Injection; Soluble Phenytoin Injection): a sterile solution of phenytoin sodium, with 40% v/v of propylene glycol and 10% v/v of alcohol, in water for injections. It is sterilised by filtration. Available in 5-ml ampoules containing 50 mg of phenytoin sodium per ml.
A standard for this injection is given in the British Pharmaceutical Codex Supplement 1976
Containers and *Labelling:* see the entry on Injections for general information on containers and labelling.
Storage: it should be stored at a temperature not exceeding 25°, protected from light. Solutions in which a haziness or precipitate develops should not be used.

PHENYTOIN TABLETS (*Syn.* Phenytoin Sodium Tablets; Soluble Phenytoin Tablets): available as tablets containing 30, 50, and 100 mg of phenytoin sodium; they are sugar coated.
A standard for these tablets is given in the British Pharmacopoeia 1973
Containers and *Storage:* see the entry on Tablets for general information on containers and storage. Containers should be airtight.

Advice for patients: see above under Phenytoin Capsules.

OTHER PREPARATIONS available include CAPSULES containing phenytoin sodium 100 mg with phenobarbitone 50 mg; TABLETS containing phenytoin sodium 100 mg with phenobarbitone sodium 50 mg, and tablets containing phenytoin sodium 100 mg with primidone 250 mg.

Pholcodine

O^8-(2-Morpholinoethyl)morphine monohydrate

$C_{23}H_{30}N_2O_4,H_2O = 416.5$

OTHER NAMES: Pholcodinum; *Sancos®* *Falcodyl®* and *Rubelix®* (both with ephedrine hydrochloride); *Pholcomed®* (with papaverine hydrochloride); *Pholtex®* (with phenyltoloxamine)

A standard is given in the European Pharmacopoeia Vol. III

Description. An odourless white crystalline powder with a very bitter taste.

Solubility. Soluble, at 20°, in 50 parts of water and in 3 parts of dehydrated alcohol; very slightly soluble in ether; soluble in chloroform, in acetone, and in dilute hydrochloric acid.

Moisture content. 3.9 to 4.5%, determined by drying at 105°.

Specific rotation. $-94°$ to $-98°$, determined on a 2% solution in alcohol (95%).

Dissociation constants. pK_a 8.0, 9.3 (37°).

Storage. It should be stored in airtight containers.

Identification. TEST. Dissolve about 50 mg in 1 ml of sulphuric acid and add 1 drop of *ammonium molybdate solution*; a pale blue colour is produced. Warm gently; the colour changes to deep blue. Add 1 drop of *dilute nitric acid*; the colour changes to brownish-red.

MELTING-POINT. About 99°, after sintering at about 95°.

ULTRAVIOLET ABSORPTION. In 0.1N hydrochloric acid, maximum at 283 nm (E1%, 1cm = 40).

THIN-LAYER CHROMATOGRAPHY. See under Thin-layer Chromatography, System 7.

Actions and uses. Pholcodine resembles codeine in suppressing cough and is used for the relief of unproductive cough. It has a less depressant effect on the respiratory centre than morphine and does not cause constipation.

The usual dose for an adult is up to 10 milligrams, and for a child up to 5 milligrams, as required to control the cough; these doses may be repeated up to 6 times a day.

Preparations

PHOLCODINE LINCTUS:

Strong pholcodine linctus	.. .. ..	500 ml
Syrup..		500 ml

When a dose less than or not a multiple of 5 ml is prescribed, the linctus may be diluted, as described in the entry on Linctuses, with syrup. It contains, in 5 ml, 5 mg of pholcodine.

A standard for this linctus is given in the British Pharmaceutical Codex 1973

Containers: see the entry on Linctuses for general information on containers.

Storage: it should be stored in a cool place.

Advice for patients: the linctus should be sipped and swallowed slowly. It should not be used for the suppression of productive cough. Treatment should not be continued for longer than a few days without medical advice.

STRONG PHOLCODINE LINCTUS:

Pholcodine .. .. 2 g
Citric acid monohydrate.. .. .. .. 20 g
Amaranth solution .. .. 2 ml
Compound tartrazine solution .. .. .. 20 ml
Chloroform spirit .. .. 150 ml
Syrup.. .. .. to 1000 ml

Dissolve the citric acid and the pholcodine each in a separate 75-ml portion of the chloroform spirit, mix the two solutions, add the amaranth solution, the compound tartrazine solution, and sufficient syrup to produce the required volume, and mix. When a dose less than or not a multiple of 5 ml is prescribed, the linctus may be diluted, as described in the entry on Linctuses, with syrup. It contains, in 5 ml, 10 mg of pholcodine.

A standard for this linctus is given in the British Pharmaceutical Codex 1973

Containers: see the entry on Linctuses for general information on containers.

Storage: it should be stored in a cool place.

Advice for patients: see above under Pholcodine Linctus.

OTHER PREPARATIONS available include a LINCTUS containing pholcodine 4 mg with ephedrine hydrochloride 4 mg in 5 ml; a linctus containing pholcodine 4 mg with ephedrine hydrochloride 6 mg in 5 ml, diluent syrup, life of diluted linctus 14 days; a linctus containing pholcodine 5 mg with papaverine hydrochloride 1.25 mg in 5 ml, diluent syrup, life of diluted linctus 14 days; a linctus containing pholcodine 19 mg with papaverine hydrochloride 5 mg in 5 ml, diluent syrup, life of diluted linctus 14 days; a linctus containing pholcodine 15 mg with phenyltoloxamine 10 mg (as ion-exchange resin complexes) in 5 ml, diluent syrup or tragacanth mucilage, life of diluted linctus 14 days; and PASTILLES containing pholcodine 4 mg with papaverine hydrochloride 1 mg.

Phosphoric Acid

Orthophosphoric acid
$H_3PO_4 = 98.0$

OTHER NAMES: Acidum Phosphoricum Concentratum; Concentrated Phosphoric Acid

A standard is given in the European Pharmacopoeia Vol. II

Phosphoric acid contains 85 to 90% w/w of H_3PO_4.

Description. A clear, colourless, corrosive, syrupy, odourless liquid. It may solidify at low temperatures forming colourless crystals which do not melt until the temperature reaches 28°.

Solubility. Miscible with water and with alcohol.

Weight per ml. At 20°, about 1.7 g.

Storage. It should be stored in glass containers.

Actions and uses. Dilute phosphoric acid is occasionally prescribed in mixtures containing vegetable bitters to stimulate appetite. Phosphoric acid is also used as an antoxidant synergist; it is usually effective in a concentration of 0.001 to 0.005%.

Photosensitivity

Photosensitivity is a condition in which there is abnormal reactivity of the skin to sunlight. Certain diseases such as porphyria or lupus erythematosus may be aggravated or precipitated by exposure to sunlight. Photosensitivity reactions may also be induced by drugs such as sulphonamides, sulphonylurea hypoglycaemics, tetracyclines (especially demeclocycline), chlorpromazine, and griseofulvin. Such patients may be affected by radiation of longer wavelengths than that responsible for sunburn.

Lesions vary from exaggeration of the normal reddening and tanning effects associated with strong sunlight to oedema, flaking, eczema, maculopapular eruptions, or urticaria. Discontinuation of the drug responsible is usually followed by resolution of the skin lesions. Screening agents may sometimes be required.

Phthalylsulphathiazole

4'-[N-(Thiazol-2-yl)sulphamoyl]phthalanilic acid

$C_{17}H_{13}N_3O_5S_2 = 403.4$

OTHER NAMES: Phthalylsulfathiazole; Thalazole®

A standard is given in the British Pharmacopoeia 1973

Description. Odourless, white or yellowish-white crystals or powder with a slightly bitter taste.

Solubility. Very slightly soluble in water and in chloroform; soluble, at 20°, in 600 parts of alcohol; soluble in aqueous solutions of alkali hydroxides and carbonates and in hydrochloric acid.

Moisture content. Not more than 2%, determined by drying at 105°.

Storage. It should be protected from light.

Identification. TESTS. 1. To about 2 g add 20 ml of sodium hydroxide solution, boil for 10 minutes, add 15 ml of hydrochloric acid, cool, and slowly add sodium bicarbonate solution until carbon dioxide ceases to be evolved and a white precipitate is produced; filter, recrystallise the precipitate from water and dry at 105°. The recrystallised material melts at about 200°, and complies with general test 1 described under Sulphonamides.

2. It complies with general test 2 described under Sulphonamides.

3. To about 100 mg add 50 mg of resorcinol and 1 ml of sulphuric acid, heat for 1 minute, cool, pour the solution into water and make alkaline with *sodium hydroxide solution*; a distinct green fluorescence is produced which disappears when the solution is acidified and reappears when the solution is again made alkaline.

MELTING-POINT. About 275°, with decomposition.

ULTRAVIOLET ABSORPTION. In 0.1N hydrochloric acid, maximum at 280 nm (E1%, 1cm = 380); in 0.1N sodium hydroxide, maximum at 263 nm (E1%, 1cm = 613); in alcohol (95%), maximum at 294 nm (E1%, 1cm = 686).

INFRA-RED ABSORPTION. Major peaks at 670, 1150, 1530, 1565, 1590, and 1722 cm^{-1} (see Appendix 2a: Infra-red Spectra).

THIN-LAYER CHROMATOGRAPHY. See under Thin-layer Chromatography, System 11.

Actions and uses. Phthalylsulphathiazole is a relatively insoluble compound which is only slowly broken down in the gastro-intestinal tract so that when it is given by mouth the bulk of the dose reaches the large intestine and is excreted in the faeces. A proportion of the dose is absorbed as sulphathiazole and in certain conditions, particularly where there is extensive ulceration of the intestinal mucosa, sufficient can be absorbed to cause systemic effects and renal tubular obstruction.

Phthalylsulphathiazole has the antibacterial actions of the sulphonamides, as described under Sulphadimidine, and is still sometimes used to treat bacterial dysentery and to reduce the bacterial flora of the large bowel before surgery.

It is given in a dosage of 5 to 10 grams daily in divided doses to adults. Children may be given 125 milligrams per kilogram body-weight daily divided into 4 to 6 doses.

Undesirable effects. Because of its effect on intestinal bacteria prolonged use may lead to overgrowth of *Candida* species.

Precautions. Vitamins of the B-group should be administered to replace those normally synthesised by sensitive gastro-intestinal organisms.

Veterinary uses. Phthalylsulphathiazole is an antibacterial used in the control of bowel infection. The usual dose for calves, pigs, lambs, dogs, and cats is 100 to 160 milligrams per kilogram body-weight daily for 3 or 4 days.

Preparation

PHTHALYLSULPHATHIAZOLE TABLETS: available as tablets containing 500 mg of phthalylsulphathiazole.
A standard for these tablets is given in the British Pharmacopoeia 1973
Containers and *Storage:* see the entry on Tablets for general information on containers and storage. Containers should be airtight and light resistant.
Advice for patients: the tablets should be taken at regular intervals. The prescribed course should be completed. The use of preparations containing liquid paraffin should be avoided.

Physostigmine

(3a*S*,8a*R*) - 1,2,3,3a,8,8a - Hexahydro - 1,3a,8 - trimethyl-pyrrolo[2,3-*b*]indol-5-yl methylcarbamate, an alkaloid obtained from the calabar bean, the seed of *Physostigma venenosum* Balfour (Fam. Leguminosae).

$C_{15}H_{21}N_3O_2 = 275.3$

OTHER NAME: Eserine

A standard is given in the British Pharmaceutical Codex 1973

Description. Odourless colourless crystals. It becomes pink on exposure to light and air.

Solubility. Soluble, at 20°, in 75 parts of water, in 10 parts of alcohol, in 30 parts of ether, and in 1 part of chloroform; soluble, on warming, in 100 parts of castor oil.

Specific rotation. −76° to −80°, determined on a 2% solution in chloroform.

Dissociation constants. pK$_a$ 1.8, 7.9 (25°).

Stability. See under Physostigmine Sulphate.

Sterilisation. Sterile oily solutions are prepared by an aseptic technique.

Storage. It should be stored in airtight containers, protected from light.

Identification. TESTS. It complies with the tests described under Physostigmine Salicylate.

MELTING-POINT. About 106°.

ULTRAVIOLET ABSORPTION. In 0.2N sulphuric acid, maxima at 246 nm (E1%, 1cm = 390) and 302 nm (E1%, 1cm = 96).

Metabolism. See under Physostigmine Salicylate.

Actions and uses. Physostigmine has the actions described under Physostigmine Salicylate. It has been used for the preparation of eye-drops containing up to 1% in sterile castor oil.

Physostigmine Salicylate

$C_{22}H_{27}N_3O_5 = 413.5$

OTHER NAMES: Eserine Salicylate; Eserinii Salicylas; Physostig. Sal.; Physostigminii Salicylas

A standard is given in the European Pharmacopoeia Vol. I

Description. Odourless colourless or faintly yellow crystals.

Solubility. Soluble, at 20°, in 90 parts of water and in 25 parts of alcohol.

Moisture content. Not more than 1%, determined by drying at 105°.

Specific rotation. −90° to −94°, determined on a 1% solution.

Stability. See under Physostigmine Sulphate.

Sterilisation. Solutions are sterilised by heating with a bactericide or by filtration. The pH of the solution should be kept below 4 and an antoxidant should be included.

Storage. It should be stored in airtight containers, protected from light. Solutions should be freshly prepared or, if kept, should be stored in hermetically sealed containers.

Identification. TESTS. 1. Mix about 5 mg with 0.3 ml of *dilute ammonia solution* and warm; a yellowish-red solution is produced. Evaporate the solution; a bluish residue remains which dissolves in alcohol (95%) producing a blue solution. Add acetic acid; the solution is blue by transmitted light and shows a red fluorescence which is intensified by dilution with water.
2. Dissolve about 50 mg in 5 ml of water and add 1N sodium hydroxide, dropwise; a white precipitate is produced which dissolves in excess of the reagent to give a red solution.

MELTING-POINT. About 185°.

Metabolism. ABSORPTION. Physostigmine and its salts are readily absorbed after oral administration or subcutaneous injection, or through mucous membranes, including the nasal mucosa after instillation of solutions in the eye.

METABOLIC REACTIONS. Rapidly hydrolysed by cholinesterases and most of a dose is so destroyed in about 2 hours.

EXCRETION. Very little of a dose appears to be excreted in the urine.

Actions and uses. Physostigmine inhibits cholinesterase activity and prevents the rapid destruction of acetylcholine, thereby enhancing its action. It increases salivary, gastric, and bronchial secretions and intestinal movements, slows the heart, and dilates peripheral blood vessels; these effects are antagonised by atropine. When applied to the eye, physostigmine constricts the pupil, reduces intra-ocular pressure if this is raised, and contracts the ciliary muscles.

Physostigmine salicylate is used chiefly as a miotic. The pupils begin to constrict within 20 minutes of its application and its effect lasts for about 12 hours. It is also used to counteract the dilatation of the pupil caused by homatropine or cocaine; in these circumstances it may, however, produce considerable irritation and pain due to spasm. It only partially reverses dilatation of the pupil by atropine. Physostigmine salicylate is also used to decrease intra-ocular pressure in glaucoma.

Undesirable effects. Physostigmine salicylate may give rise to nausea, vomiting, abdominal pain, and diarrhoea. It produces the nicotinic effects of acetylcholine; with large doses, muscular twitchings followed by muscular weakness and respiratory paralysis may occur.

Poisoning. The stomach should be washed out with water. Diazepam should be given, if necessary by intravenous injection, to control muscular twitching, and atropine may be given to relieve the muscarinic actions.

Physostigmine Sulphate

$C_{30}H_{44}N_6O_8S = 648.8$

OTHER NAMES: Eserine Sulphate; Physostig. Sulph.

A standard is given in the British Pharmacopoeia Supplement 1977

Description. An odourless, deliquescent, white, microcrystalline powder.

Solubility. Soluble, at 20°, in less than 1 part of water and of alcohol; very slightly soluble in ether.

Acidity. A 1% solution has a pH of 3 to 4.

Moisture content. Not more than 1%, determined by drying at 105°.

Specific rotation. −116° to −120°, determined on a 2% solution.

Stability. Physostigmine and its salts in the form of crystals or powder become pink on exposure to air and light; discoloration is most rapid for physostigmine sulphate which is deliquescent. In aqueous solutions of physostigmine salts physostigmine is hydrolysed to eseroline (a colourless phenolic compound) and methylcarbamic acid, which is rapidly decarboxylated to methylamine and carbon dioxide.

Eseroline is oxidised to the blood-red compound rubreserine and other coloured products such as eserine blue and eserine brown. The depth of colour is not a reliable guide to the extent of degradation by hydrolysis to products of negligible anticholinesterase activity. Hydrolysis is catalysed by hydrogen ions and by hydroxyl ions. At 25° solutions are most stable at pH 3.7; under these conditions the time for 10% of the physostigmine to be decomposed has been calculated to be 90 years. Solutions are much less stable if the pH is more than 5, and at pH 7.4 10% of the physostigmine is decomposed in about 2 weeks.

FURTHER INFORMATION. Stability in aqueous solution—I. Christenson, *Acta pharm. suec.*, 1969, **6**, 287; G. Fletcher and D. J. G. Davies, *J. Pharm. Pharmac.*, 1968, **20**, *Suppl.*, 108S; A. R. Rogers and G. Smith, *Pharm. J.*, ii/1973, 353. Anticholinesterase activity of physostigmine and its degradation products—B. A. Hemsworth and G. B. West, *J. pharm. Sci.*, 1970, **59**, 118.

Sterilisation. As for Physostigmine Salicylate.

Storage. It should be stored in airtight containers, protected from light.

Identification. TESTS. It complies with the tests described under Physostigmine Salicylate.

MELTING-POINT. About 146°.

Metabolism. See under Physostigmine Salicylate.

Actions and uses. Physostigmine sulphate has the actions, uses, and undesirable effects described under Physostigmine Salicylate. As the sulphate is more soluble than the salicylate and is compatible with a wider range of preservatives, it is now preferred for the preparation of eye-drops. Eye-drops containing up to 1% of physostigmine sulphate may be used in the treatment of glaucoma.

Poisoning. As for Physostigmine Salicylate.

Preparations

PHYSOSTIGMINE AND PILOCARPINE EYE-DROPS (*Syn.* Eserine and Pilocarpine Eye-drops): consisting of a sterile solution containing up to 0.5% of physostigmine sulphate and up to 4% of pilocarpine hydrochloride, with 0.2% of sodium metabisulphite and 0.02% of benzalkonium chloride solution, in purified water. It is prepared by method B or C described in the entry on Eye-drops. Strengths frequently prescribed are 0.25% of physostigmine sulphate with 2% of pilocarpine hydrochloride, and 0.5% of physostigmine sulphate with 4% of pilocarpine hydrochloride.

A standard for these eye-drops is given in the British Pharmaceutical Codex 1973

Containers: see the entry on Eye-drops for general information on containers. This solution is adversely affected by alkali.

Labelling: see the entry on Eye-drops for general information on labelling.

Storage: it should be protected from light.

Advice for patients: see the entry on Eye-drops for general information on the use of eye-drops. For the treatment of glaucoma when used in conjunction with neutral adrenaline eye-drops or similar preparations, physostigmine and pilocarpine eye-drops should be instilled first and neutral adrenaline eye-drops used 5 to 10 minutes later. Treatment should not be discontinued without the advice of the prescriber.

PHYSOSTIGMINE EYE-DROPS (*Syn.* Eserine Eye-drops; Physostigmine Sulphate Eye-drops): consisting of a sterile solution of physostigmine sulphate, with 0.2% of sodium metabisulphite and 0.02% of benzalkonium chloride solution, in purified water. It is prepared by method B or C described in the entry on Eye-drops. Available as eye-drops containing 0.25, 0.5, and 1% of physostigmine sulphate.

A standard for these eye-drops is given in the British Pharmacopoeia Addendum 1977 and in the British Pharmacopoeia (Veterinary)

Containers: see the entry on Eye-drops for general information on containers. This solution is adversely affected by alkali.

Labelling: see the entry on Eye-drops for general information on labelling.

Storage: it should be protected from light.

Advice for patients: see above under Physostigmine and Pilocarpine Eye-drops.

Phytomenadione

2-Methyl-3-phytyl-1,4-naphthoquinone

$C_{31}H_{46}O_2 = 450.7$

OTHER NAMES: *Aquamephyton®*; *Konakion®*; Phytonadione; Vitamin K_1

A standard is given in the British Pharmacopoeia 1973

Description. An almost odourless, clear, deep yellow oil.

Solubility. Practically insoluble in water; soluble, at 20°, in 70 parts of alcohol; soluble in ether, in chloroform, and in fixed oils.

Refractive index. 1.526 to 1.528.

Stability. It decomposes on exposure to sunlight.

Sterilisation. Dispersions for injection are sterilised by heating in an autoclave.

Storage. It should be stored in airtight containers, protected from light.

Identification. TEST. Mix 1 drop with 10 ml of methyl alcohol and 1 ml of a 20% solution of potassium hydroxide in methyl alcohol; a green colour is produced. Heat gently; the colour changes to purple and then to reddish-brown after standing.

ULTRAVIOLET ABSORPTION. In trimethylpentane, maxima at 243 nm (E1%, 1cm = 400), 249 nm (E1%, 1cm = 420), 261 nm (E1%, 1cm = 385), 270 nm (E1%, 1cm = 390), and 327 nm (E1%, 1cm = 70).

Metabolism. ABSORPTION. Readily absorbed after oral administration but requires the presence of bile salts; intramuscular doses are also well absorbed.

METABOLIC REACTIONS. Converted to a lactone which may be conjugated with glucuronic acid or possibly sulphate.

EXCRETION. Excreted as conjugates in urine, bile, and faeces.

Actions and uses. Phytomenadione is a naturally occurring vitamin K. The metabolic production by the liver of various coagulation factors (prothrombin and factors VII, IX, and X) is dependent upon vitamin K. In hypoprothrombinaemia the intravenous administration of phytomenadione causes a rise in the plasma-prothrombin level within 15 minutes and a reduction in the clotting-time. It acts more rapidly than the synthetic vitamin-K analogues and its effect is more prolonged.

Hypoprothrombinaemia may be caused by a variety of conditions including hepatocellular disease such as infectious hepatitis and advanced cirrhosis and intra-hepatic and extrahepatic biliary obstruction in which the absence of bile causes poor absorption of vitamin K. Dietary deficiency of vitamin K may also give rise to hypoprothrombinaemia but this is rare because the vitamin is synthesised by intestinal bacteria as well as being present in food, although some drugs such as neomycin may interfere with the bacterial synthesis. Hypoprothrombinaemia may also occur in newborn infants who have a deficiency of vitamin K for the first few days after birth as the vitamin is not synthesised in the sterile gut. Some drugs such as oral anticoagulants (but not heparin) interfere with the hepatic synthesis of prothrombin and other blood clotting factors.

Phytomenadione is used in the treatment of severe haemorrhage due to hypoprothrombinaemia caused by the above conditions, although it is not effective in hepatocellular disease.

It is given in doses of 5 to 20 milligrams by slow intravenous infusion; the dose may be repeated in a few hours. For less severe cases the same dose may be given intramuscularly or subcutaneously, or it may be given orally in initial doses of 5 to 10 milligrams, subsequently increased to 15 to 20 milligrams if necessary.

For the treatment of haemorrhagic disease of the newborn, 0.5 to 1 milligram is given intravenously or intramuscularly; for the prophylaxis of this condition the mother may be given 1 to 5 milligrams by injection 12 to 24 hours before expected delivery.

Undesirable effects. Excessive doses of phytomenadione may produce haemolytic anaemia, hyperbilirubinaemia, and kernicterus in the newborn, particularly in premature infants.

The administration of large doses of phytomenadione in an attempt to correct hypoprothrombinaemia associated with severe liver disease may further depress the prothrombin level.

The intravenous administration of phytomenadione injection may produce flushing, sweating, a sense of suffocation, and peripheral vascular failure. Intravenous injections should therefore be given very slowly.

Veterinary uses. Phytomenadione is used as an antidote to warfarin poisoning. The usual dose by mouth or by subcutaneous or intravenous injection for dogs and cats is 0.5 to 2 milligrams per kilogram body-weight daily.

Preparations

PHYTOMENADIONE INJECTION (*Syn.* Vitamin K₁ Injection): a sterile dispersion of phytomenadione, with suitable dispersing and stabilising agents, in water for injections. It is sterilised by heating in an autoclave. Available in 0.5-ml ampoules containing 1 mg of phytomenadione, and in 1-ml ampoules containing 10 mg of phytomenadione.

A standard for this injection is given in the British Pharmacopoeia 1973

Containers: see the entry on Injections for general information on containers.

Labelling: see the entry on Injections for general information on labelling. In addition, the label on the container should state that if separation has occurred or if oily droplets have appeared, the injection should not be used.

Storage: it deteriorates on exposure to light and should be stored in complete darkness. It should not be allowed to freeze. If separation has occurred or if oily droplets have appeared, the preparation is unsuitable for use.

PHYTOMENADIONE TABLETS (*Syn.* Vitamin K₁ Tablets): available as tablets containing 10 mg of phytomenadione; they are sugar coated.

A standard for these tablets is given in the British Pharmacopoeia 1973

Containers and *Storage:* see the entry on Tablets for general information on containers and storage. Containers should be airtight.

Advice for patients: the tablets should be chewed before being swallowed or allowed to dissolve slowly in the mouth.

Piles

see HAEMORRHOIDS

Pills

Pills are spherical or ovoid masses containing one or more medicaments. The active ingredients must be uniformly distributed throughout the mass, which should be of such a consistence that the pills retain their shape on keeping but are not so hard that they fail to disintegrate on ingestion. Very deliquescent substances should not be incorporated in pills.

Coatings may be applied to pills to mask the nauseous taste of medicaments and to improve their appearance and keeping properties. Pills may also be enteric coated. The materials and methods used for enteric coating must prevent disintegration of the pill in the stomach but ensure disintegration when the pill reaches the alkaline medium of the small intestine.

Standards are not imposed for total weight or diameter of pills, but the diameter should not normally be less than 3 millimetres for pills weighing up to 60 mg and not normally more than 8 millimetres for pills weighing about 300 mg.

Containers and storage. The directions given in the entry on Tablets should be followed.

Pilocarpine Hydrochloride

($\alpha S, \beta R$)-α-Ethyl-β-(1-methylimidazol-5-ylmethyl)-γ-butyrolactone hydrochloride

$C_{11}H_{17}ClN_2O_2 = 244.7$

OTHER NAMES: *Isopto Carpine*®; Pilocarp. Hydrochlor.; *Sno-Pilo*®

A standard is given in the British Pharmacopoeia Addendum 1977

Description. Odourless, hygroscopic, colourless crystals or white crystalline powder.

Solubility. Soluble, at 20°, in less than 1 part of water, in 3 parts of alcohol, and in 360 parts of chloroform; practically insoluble in ether.

Acidity. A 0.5% solution has a pH of 3.8 to 5.2.

Moisture content. Not more than 1%, determined by drying at 105°.

Specific rotation. +89° to +93°, determined on a 2% solution.

Stability. Solutions of pilocarpine salts degrade by hydrolysis to pilocarpic acid and by epimerisation to isopilocarpine; the degradation products possess little miotic activity. Degradation is catalysed by hydrogen ions and by hydroxyl ions. Solutions are most stable at pH 4 to 5.

FURTHER INFORMATION. Stability in aqueous solution— P.-H. Chung *et al.*, *J. pharm. Sci.*, 1970, **59**, 1300; I. S. Gibbs and M. M. Tuckerman, *J. pharm. Sci.*, 1974, **63**, 276; M. A. Nunes and E. Brochmann-Hanssen, *J. pharm. Sci.*, 1974, **63**, 716. Stability in frozen solution— S. S. Larsen, *Dansk Tidsskr. Farm.*, 1971, **45**, 317.

Incompatibility. It is incompatible with chlorhexidine acetate and phenylmercuric salts.

Sterilisation. Solutions are sterilised by heating in an autoclave or by filtration.

Storage. It should be stored in airtight containers, protected from light.

Identification. TEST. It complies with the test described under Pilocarpine Nitrate.

MELTING-POINT. About 202°.

Actions and uses. Pilocarpine hydrochloride has the actions and uses of pilocarpine, as described under Pilocarpine Nitrate. The hydrochloride is now preferred to the nitrate for the preparation of eye-drops because it is compatible with a more useful range of preservatives.

Poisoning. Gastric lavage should be employed and atropine given subcutaneously.

Preparations

PHYSOSTIGMINE AND PILOCARPINE EYE-DROPS: see under Physostigmine Sulphate.

PILOCARPINE EYE-DROPS (*Syn.* Pilocarpine Hydrochloride Eye-drops): consisting of a sterile solution of pilocarpine hydrochloride, with 0.02% of benzalkonium chloride solution, in purified water. It is prepared by method A, B, or C described in the entry on Eye-drops. Available as eye-drops containing 1, 2, 3, and 4% of pilocarpine hydrochloride.

A standard for these eye-drops is given in the British Pharmacopoeia Addendum 1977 and in the British Pharmacopoeia (Veterinary)

Containers: see the entry on Eye-drops for general

information on containers. This solution is adversely affected by alkali.

Labelling: see the entry on Eye-drops for general information on labelling.

Advice for patients: see the entry on Eye-drops for general information on the use of eye-drops. For the treatment of glaucoma, when used in conjunction with neutral adrenaline eye-drops or similar preparations, pilocarpine eye-drops should be instilled first and neutral adrenaline eye-drops used 5 to 10 minutes later. Treatment should not be discontinued without the advice of the prescriber.

VISCOUS PILOCARPINE EYE-DROPS: consisting of a sterile solution containing up to 4% of pilocarpine hydrochloride, with 4% of polyvinyl alcohol, 0.02% of benzalkonium chloride solution, 0.46% of sodium acetate, and 0.2% of acetic acid, in purified water. The acidity of the solution is adjusted to pH 5.2 by the addition of 0.1N hydrochloric acid or 0.1N sodium hydroxide solution as appropriate. It is prepared by method A, B, or C described in the entry on Eye-drops. Available as eye-drops containing 0.5, 1, 2, 3, and 4% of pilocarpine hydrochloride.

Containers: see the entry on Eye-drops for general information on containers. This solution is adversely affected by alkali.

Labelling: see the entry on Eye-drops for general information on labelling.

Advice for patients: see above under Pilocarpine Eye-drops.

OTHER PREPARATIONS available include EYE-DROPS containing pilocarpine hydrochloride 0.5, 1, 2, 3 and 4% with hypromellose 0.5%.

Pilocarpine Nitrate

($\alpha S,\beta R$)-α-Ethyl-β-(1-methylimidazol-5-ylmethyl)-γ-butyrolactone nitrate, the nitrate of an alkaloid obtained from the leaves of *Pilocarpus microphyllus* Stapf (jaborandi) and other species of *Pilocarpus* (Fam. Rutaceae).

$C_{11}H_{17}N_3O_5 = 271.3$

OTHER NAMES: Pilocarp. Nit.; Pilocarpinii Nitras

A standard is given in the European Pharmacopoeia Vol. I

Description. Odourless colourless crystals or white crystalline powder.

Solubility. Soluble, at 20°, in 8 parts of water and in 160 parts of alcohol; very slightly soluble in ether and in chloroform.

Dissociation constants. pK_a 1.6, 7.1 (15°).

Stability. See under Pilocarpine Hydrochloride.

Incompatibility. It is incompatible with chlorhexidine acetate and solutions containing more than 1% are incompatible with benzalkonium chloride.

Sterilisation. Solutions are sterilised by heating in an autoclave or by filtration.

Storage. It should be protected from light.

Identification. TEST. Dissolve about 10 mg in 5 ml of water, add 2 drops of *dilute sulphuric acid*, 1 ml of *hydrogen peroxide solution*, 1 ml of chloroform, and 1 drop of *potassium chromate solution*, shake well and allow to separate; the chloroform layer is coloured bluish-violet and the aqueous layer remains yellow.

MELTING-POINT. About 176°, with decomposition.

Actions and uses. Pilocarpine has the muscarinic actions of acetylcholine, as described under Physostigmine Salicylate. Like physostigmine, it has been used to constrict the pupil and decrease the intraocular pressure in glaucoma and detachment of the retina, but it is only about half as active; for this purpose, a 1% solution may be used.

Its action on the eye is less complete and of shorter duration than that of physostigmine and a slight increase of intra-ocular pressure may occur at first.

It has been used to counteract some of the common side-effects of ganglion-blocking agents, such as dryness of the mouth, constipation, and impaired vision. It has been used to antagonise the effects of atropine on the eye but is relatively ineffective for this purpose.

Poisoning. Gastric lavage should be employed and atropine given subcutaneously.

Preparations

Preparations available include EYE-DROPS containing pilocarpine 1, 2, 3, and 4% in single-dose packs.

Pindolol

1-(Indol-4-yloxy)-3-isopropylaminopropan-2-ol

$C_{14}H_{20}N_2O_2 = 248.3$

OTHER NAMES: Prindolol; *Visken®*
Viskaldix® (with clopamide)

Metabolism. ABSORPTION. Readily absorbed after oral administration.

BLOOD CONCENTRATION. After an oral dose of 10 mg, peak plasma concentrations of 20 to 100 ng/ml are attained in 1.5 to 2 hours; after an intravenous infusion of 5 mg administered over 3 hours, plasma concentrations of about 30 ng/ml are attained at cessation of infusion falling to about 2 ng/ml about 12 hours later.

HALF-LIFE. Plasma half-life 3 to 4 hours; the half-life appears to be unaffected by renal disease.

DISTRIBUTION. Volume of distribution, 100 to 270 litres; *protein binding*, about 57% bound to plasma proteins at a drug concentration of 60 ng/ml.

METABOLIC REACTIONS. Glucuronic acid and sulphate conjugation; the extent of metabolism may possibly be increased in subjects with renal function impairment.

EXCRETION. About 40% of a dose is excreted unchanged in the urine along with small amounts in the faeces.

FURTHER INFORMATION. Pharmacokinetics—R. Gugler *et al., Eur. J. clin. Pharmac.,* 1974, **7**, 17; pharmacokinetics and renal impairment—E. E. Ohnhaus, *Br. J. Pharmac.,* 1973, **47**, 620P, E. E. Ohnhaus, *et al., Eur. J. clin. Pharmac.,* 1974, **7**, 25, and S. Øie and G. Levy, *Eur. J. clin. Pharmac.,* 1975, **9**, 115; plasma concentrations—R. Gugler *et al., Clin. Pharmac. Ther.,* 1975, **17**, 127.

Actions and uses. Pindolol is a beta-adrenoceptor

blocking agent with the actions described under Propranolol Hydrochloride but it is used mainly in the treatment of hypertension. The usual initial dose for this purpose is 5 milligrams 3 times daily which may be increased at weekly intervals to a maximum of 15 milligrams 3 times daily; when given in conjunction with a diuretic smaller doses are used. A response is obtained within 1 to 2 weeks of treatment but a maximum response may take several weeks to develop.

Pindolol is also used to reduce the incidence of attacks in angina pectoris and has been used for the prophylaxis of migraine. The usual dose is 2.5 to 5 milligrams up to 3 times daily according to the response.

Undesirable effects; Contra-indications. As for Propranolol Hydrochloride.

Preparations

Preparations available include TABLETS containing 5 and 15 mg of pindolol, and tablets containing pindolol 10 mg with clopamide 5 mg.

Piperazine Adipate

$C_{10}H_{20}N_2O_4 = 232.3$

OTHER NAMES: *Coopane®*; Piperazini Adipas

A standard is given in the European Pharmacopoeia Vol. III Supplement

Description. An odourless white crystalline powder with a slightly acid taste.

Solubility. Soluble, at 20°, in 18 parts of water; practically insoluble in alcohol.

Acidity. A 5% solution has a pH of 5 to 6.

Identification. TESTS. 1. It complies with Test 1 described under Piperazine Hydrate.
2. To 10 ml of a 5% solution add 5 ml of hydrochloric acid, extract with three 10-ml portions of ether, reserve the aqueous layer, and evaporate the ether extracts to dryness; the residue, after washing with a little water and drying at 105°, melts at about 152°.
3. Warm the aqueous layer reserved in Test 1 to remove dissolved ether, add 500 mg of sodium nitrite, heat to boiling and cool in ice for 15 minutes, scratching the walls of the container with a glass rod; the crystals, after washing with 10 ml of ice-cold water and drying at 105°, melt at about 159°.

MELTING-POINT. About 250°, with decomposition.

Determination in body fluids; Metabolism. See under Piperazine Hydrate.

Actions and uses. Piperazine adipate has the actions, uses and undesirable effects described under Piperazine Hydrate; 120 milligrams of piperazine adipate is approximately equivalent to 100 milligrams of piperazine hydrate.

Veterinary uses. Piperazine adipate is used for the treatment of nematode infections. The usual dose for *Ascaris* infections in horses and cattle is 200 milligrams per kilogram body-weight and in pigs 300 milligrams per kilogram body-weight. The usual dose for *Toxocara* and *Uncinaria* infections in dogs and cats is 100 milligrams per kilogram body-weight. The usual dose for poultry is 250 milligrams per kilogram body-weight for *Ascaridia* and 500 milligrams per kilogram body-weight for *Capillaria* infections. Piperazine adipate is administered by mouth as a single dose.

Preparation

PIPERAZINE ADIPATE TABLETS: available as tablets for veterinary use containing 450 mg of piperazine adipate. *A standard for these tablets is given in the British Pharmacopoeia 1973*
Containers and *Storage:* see the entry on Tablets for general information on containers and storage. Containers should be airtight.

Piperazine Citrate

A hydrated piperazine citrate containing a variable amount of water of hydration, corresponding to 5 or 6 molecules of water.

$C_{22}H_{46}N_6O_{14} = 642.7$

OTHER NAMES: *Ascalix®*; *Citrazine®*; *Helmezine®* (available only in certain overseas countries); Piperazini Citras; *Verocid®*
Antepar® (with piperazine hydrate)

A standard is given in the European Pharmacopoeia Vol. III Supplement

Description. An odourless, fine, white, granular powder.

Solubility. Soluble, at 20°, in 1.5 parts of water; very slightly soluble in alcohol and in ether.

Acidity. A 5% solution has a pH of 5 to 6.

Moisture content. 10 to 14%, determined by Fischer titration.

Storage. It should be protected from light.

Identification. TESTS. 1. It complies with Test 1 described under Piperazine Hydrate.
2. It complies with Test 3 described under Piperazine Adipate using about 200 mg dissolved in 5 ml of *dilute hydrochloric acid* in place of the aqueous layer.

MELTING-POINT. About 190°, after drying at 105°.

Determination in body fluids; Metabolism. See under Piperazine Hydrate.

Actions and uses. Piperazine citrate has the actions, uses, and undesirable effects described under Piperazine Hydrate; 125 milligrams of piperazine citrate is approximately equivalent to 100 milligrams of piperazine hydrate.

Veterinary uses. As for Piperazine Adipate.

Preparations

PIPERAZINE CITRATE ELIXIR:

Piperazine citrate ..	..	..	..	..	187.5 g
Peppermint spirit ..	..	..	..	..	5.0 ml
Green S and Tartrazine Solution		..	..	15.0 ml
Glycerol	..	..	..	..	100.0 ml
Syrup..	..	..	..	..	500.0 ml
Water for preparations	..	..	..	to 1000.0 ml

Dissolve the piperazine citrate in part of the water and add the green S and tartrazine solution, the glycerol, the syrup, the peppermint spirit, and sufficient water to produce the required volume, and mix. When a dose less than or not a multiple of 5 ml is prescribed, the elixir may be diluted, as described in the entry on Elixirs, with syrup. The diluted elixir must be freshly prepared.
It contains, in 5 ml, the equivalent of about 750 mg of piperazine hydrate.
A standard for this elixir is given in the British Pharmaceutical Codex 1973

Containers: see the entry on Elixirs for general information on containers.

Storage: it should be stored in a cool place, protected from light.

Advice for patients: the prescribed course should be completed.

PIPERAZINE CITRATE TABLETS: available as tablets containing 500 mg of piperazine citrate.

A standard for these tablets is given in the British Pharmacopoeia (Veterinary)

Containers and *Storage:* see the entry on Tablets for general information on containers and storage. Containers should be airtight.

OTHER PREPARATIONS available include an ELIXIR containing piperazine citrate 550 mg in 4 ml (in certain overseas countries only); and an elixir containing piperazine citrate with piperazine hydrate together equivalent to 750 mg of piperazine hydrate in 5 ml, diluent syrup, life of diluted elixir 14 days.

Piperazine Hydrate

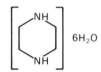

$C_4H_{10}N_2,6H_2O = 194.2$

OTHER NAMES: Piperazini Hydras
Antepar® (with piperazine citrate)

A standard is given in the European Pharmacopoeia Vol. III Supplement

Description. Colourless glassy deliquescent crystals with a faint characteristic odour.

Solubility. Soluble, at 20°, in 3 parts of water and in 1 part of alcohol; very slightly soluble in ether.

Dissociation constants. pK_a 5.6, 9.8 (25°).

Storage. It should be stored in airtight containers, protected from light.

Identification. TESTS. 1. Dissolve about 100 mg in 5 ml of water, add 500 mg of sodium bicarbonate, 0.5 ml of *potassium ferricyanide solution* and 0.1 ml of mercury, shake vigorously for 1 minute and allow to stand for 20 minutes; a reddish colour is slowly produced.
2. Dissolve about 200 mg in 3 ml of water, add 2 ml of *sodium hydroxide solution* and 0.5 ml of benzoyl chloride, shake vigorously for 15 minutes, cooling the tube in running water; a precipitate is produced which, after washing with *sodium carbonate solution*, recrystallising from alcohol (95%) and drying for 4 hours over phosphorus pentoxide *in vacuo*, melts at about 190°.

MELTING-POINT. About 43°.

Determination in body fluids. COLORIMETRY. In urine —S. Hanna and A. Tang, *J. pharm. Sci.*, 1973, **62**, 2024.

Metabolism. ABSORPTION. Piperazine and its salts are readily absorbed after oral administration.

EXCRETION. The adipate, citrate, and phosphate salts are all excreted in the urine at similar rates; wide variation in the rate of excretion occurs between individuals and 15 to 75% of a dose is excreted in the urine in 24 hours.

FURTHER INFORMATION. Urinary excretion—S. Hanna and A. Tang, *J. pharm. Sci.*, 1973, **62**, 2024 and E. W. Rogers, *Br. med. J.*, i/1958, 136.

Actions and uses. Piperazine is an anthelmintic which is effective against threadworms and roundworms. Roundworms are narcotised and unable to maintain their position in the gut of the host; they are expelled with the stools. Narcosis of roundworms takes at least five hours to develop; worms at all stages of maturity in the gut are affected, but larval forms in the tissues are not. The fact that piperazine does not stimulate the worms to muscular activity makes it the safest drug available for the treatment of heavy infections.

Little is known about the mode of action of piperazine on threadworms. It may act by blocking the action of acetylcholine. It has no significant action upon hookworms, whipworms, or tapeworms.

For the treatment of threadworm infections in an adult and in a child aged over 12 years, a daily dose equivalent to 2 grams of piperazine hydrate is given by mouth for one week. For a child aged from 7 to 12 years, the daily dose is 1.5 grams; for a child aged from 4 to 6 years, 1 gram; for a child aged from 2 to 3 years, 750 milligrams; and for a child aged from 9 to 24 months, 375 milligrams. The doses should preferably be divided and administered in 2 or 3 portions during the day. Re-infection should be prevented by treating any other infected members of the family and paying attention to personal hygiene.

For the treatment of roundworm infections, a single dose with the evening meal is usually sufficient to narcotise the worms, which are passed with the next stool. The dose for an adult is the equivalent of 4 grams of piperazine hydrate; for a child the doses are: up to 2 years 750 milligrams, 2 to 8 years 2.25 grams, 9 to 12 years 3 grams. If the patient has normal bowel movement, a purgative is not necessary; if the patient is constipated, a purgative should be given on the morning after the dose of the anthelmintic so that the worms are expelled before the effect of the drug wears off. In very sick children with heavy roundworm infections, piperazine should be given in divided doses as described for the treatment of threadworm infections. It is also necessary to correct fluid balance and electrolyte balance.

Piperazine is usually administered as the adipate, citrate, or phosphate; the equivalent of 100 milligrams of piperazine hydrate is contained in about 120 milligrams of adipate, 125 milligrams of citrate, and 104 milligrams of phosphate.

Undesirable effects. Piperazine salts rarely produce toxic effects unless prolonged treatment with large doses is given so that the drug accumulates in the tissues of the host; dizziness, paraesthesia, muscular incoordination, vomiting and blurred vision have been reported under these conditions. Toxic effects cease when treatment is discontinued. Convulsions have been reported in patients receiving piperazine in conjunction with phenothiazine.

Preparation

For an ELIXIR see above under Piperazine Citrate.

Piperazine Phosphate

$C_4H_{13}N_2O_4P,H_2O = 202.1$

OTHER NAMES: *Antepar®*; *Candizine®*; *Helmezine®* (available only in certain overseas countries)
Ancaris Thenium Compound® (with thenium closylate); *Pripsen®* (with sennosides A and B)

A standard is given in the British Pharmacopoeia 1973

Description. An odourless white crystalline powder with a slightly acid taste.

Solubility. Soluble, at 20°, in 60 parts of water; practically insoluble in alcohol.

Acidity. A 1% solution has a pH of 6 to 6.5.

Moisture content. 8 to 9.5%, determined by Fischer titration.

Identification. TESTS. 1. It complies with Test 1 described under Piperazine Hydrate.
2. It complies with Test 3 described under Piperazine Adipate using about 200 mg dissolved in 5 ml of *dilute hydrochloric acid* in place of the aqueous layer.

Determination in body fluids; Metabolism. See under Piperazine Hydrate.

Actions and uses. Piperazine phosphate has the actions, uses, and undesirable effects described under Piperazine Hydrate; 104 milligrams of piperazine phosphate is approximately equivalent to 100 milligrams of piperazine hydrate.

Veterinary uses. Piperazine phosphate is used for the treatment of nematode infections. The usual dose for *Ascaris* infections in horses and cattle is 185 milligrams per kilogram body-weight and in sheep and pigs 200 to 300 milligrams per kilogram body-weight. The usual dose for *Toxocara* and *Uncinaria* infections in dogs and cats is 80 to 125 milligrams per kilogram body-weight. The usual dose for poultry is 200 milligrams per kilogram body-weight for *Ascaridia* and 400 milligrams per kilogram body-weight for *Capillaria* infections. Piperazine phosphate is administered by mouth as a single dose.

Preparations

PIPERAZINE PHOSPHATE TABLETS: available as tablets containing 250 mg (for veterinary use), and in certain overseas countries 260 mg, of piperazine phosphate, and containing piperazine phosphate equivalent to 500 mg of piperazine hydrate; they may be coloured.
A standard for these tablets is given in the British Pharmacopoeia 1973
Containers and *Storage:* see the entry on tablets for general information on containers and storage. Containers should be airtight.
Advice for patients: the prescribed course should be completed.

OTHER PREPARATIONS available include POWDER containing piperazine phosphate 4 g with a standardised preparation of senna equivalent to 15.3 mg of sennoside B in each 10-g sachet.
Piperazine phosphate is an ingredient of compound thenium tablets.

Piperonyl Butoxide

5-[2-(2-Butoxyethoxy)ethoxymethyl]-6-propyl-1,3-benzodioxole

$C_{19}H_{30}O_5 = 338.4$

OTHER NAMES: *PB Dressing Cooper®* (with butyl aminobenzoate); *Dairy Flyspray Cooper®* and *Veterinary Insecticide Pybuthrin Cooper®* (both with pyrethrum)

A standard is given in the British Pharmacopoeia (Veterinary)

Description. A yellow or pale brown oily liquid with a faint and characteristic odour.

Solubility. Very slightly soluble in water; miscible with alcohol, with ether, with chloroform, with petroleum oils, and with liquefied aerosol propellants.

Weight per ml. At 20°, 1.050 to 1.065 g.

Refractive index. 1.497 to 1.512.

Identification. TESTS. 1. Dissolve about 100 μg in 0.1 ml of acetonitrile, add 10 mg of gallic acid, mix, add 3 ml of sulphuric acid to form a lower layer, allow to stand for 1 minute, and mix; a green colour is produced.
2. To 0.1 ml of a 0.05% solution in alcohol (95%) add 5 ml of a solution prepared by dissolving 25 mg of tannic acid in 20 ml of glacial acetic acid and adding 80 ml of phosphoric acid, shake vigorously for 1 minute and heat in a water-bath for 5 minutes; a blue colour is produced.

ULTRAVIOLET ABSORPTION. In dehydrated alcohol, maxima at 238 nm (E1%, 1cm = 150), and 290 nm (E1%, 1cm = 125).

Veterinary uses. Piperonyl butoxide is an acaricide which is also used for its synergistic effect with pyrethrins in insecticidal sprays. It acts by inhibiting the metabolism of pyrethins in the insect. The quantity used is between 1 and 10 times the amount of pyrethrins present.

Preparations

PIPERONYL BUTOXIDE APPLICATION:

Piperonyl butoxide	..	..	..	..	.. 5 g
Butyl aminobenzoate	..	..	..	..	.. 2 g
Dipropylene glycol, of commerce	..	..			93 g

Dissolve the piperonyl butoxide and the butyl aminobenzoate in the dipropylene glycol, and mix.
A standard for this application is given in the British Pharmacopoeia (Veterinary)
Containers and *Labelling:* see the entry on Applications for general information on containers and labelling.

OTHER PREPARATIONS available include a veterinary DUSTING-POWDER containing piperonyl butoxide 2.5% with pyrethrins 0.25%.
Piperonyl butoxide is an ingredient of compound pyrethrum spray.

Plague Vaccine

A suspension of suitable killed strains of *Pasteurella pestis*. It contains 0.5% of phenol, not more than 0.025% w/v of formaldehyde, and 3000 million bacteria (*P. pestis*) in 1 ml.

OTHER NAME: Plague/Vac

A standard is given in the British Pharmacopoeia 1973

Storage. It should be stored as described under Vaccines.

Actions and uses. Plague vaccine gives a useful degree of protection against attack. The vaccine is administered by subcutaneous or intramuscular injection of an initial dose of 0.5 millilitre followed by a second dose of 1 millilitre after an interval of 1 to 4 weeks. Persons exposed to infection should be given a reinforcing dose of 1 millilitre every year. The vaccine sometimes causes moderately severe local and general reactions which usually subside after 1 or 2 days.

Plasma, Dried Human

Prepared by drying a pool of the supernatant fluids which are separated, by centrifuging or by standing, from quantities of whole human blood.

OTHER NAME: Plasma Humanum Cryodesiccatum

A standard is given in the European Pharmacopoeia Vol. III

The supernatant fluid from each sample of whole human blood is siphoned through a closed system of sterile tubing by an aseptic technique and pooled with other supernatant fluids so that contributions from donors of A, O, and either B or AB groups are represented in approximately the ratio 9:9:2. In order to avoid untoward effects due to the products of bacterial growth, no individual contribution of plasma is used if there is any evidence of bacterial contamination and no pool is used unless it complies with the tests for sterility.

Not more than 10 separate donations of plasma should be pooled, unless an effective method of destroying the causative agent of serum hepatitis can be applied. The pool is dried either from the frozen state or by any other method which will avoid denaturing the proteins and will yield a product readily soluble in a quantity of water equal to the volume of the liquid from which the substance was prepared.

Description. A sterile pale to deep cream-coloured powder, which is completely soluble, at 15° to 20°, within 10 minutes, in a volume of water equal to the volume of water for injections stated on the label. Such a solution contains not less than 4.5% w/v of protein, and as shown by specific precipitation tests contains only human plasma proteins. Coagulation occurs when an aqueous solution of calcium chloride is added to the reconstituted plasma.

Storage. It should be stored in an atmosphere of nitrogen, in sterile containers sealed to exclude microorganisms and moisture, at a temperature below 25°, and protected from light.

It may be stored for several years in temperate and tropical climates if it is kept free from moisture. The only practical criterion of its fitness for use is complete solution within 10 minutes when reconstituted. If solution is incomplete or if a gel forms, the plasma should not be used, even though the expiry date has not been reached.

Actions and uses. Dried human plasma dissolved in a volume of water for injections, sodium chloride injection, or a solution containing 2.5% of anhydrous dextrose and 0.45% of sodium chloride, equivalent to the volume of the liquid plasma from which it was prepared, gives a reconstituted plasma which is mainly used for the restoration of plasma volume in patients suffering from burns, scalds, or crush injuries. It is also used in emergencies when whole human blood is not available, or while awaiting the results of compatibility tests.

Because of its keeping properties and ease of storage, dried human plasma is valuable as a transfusion medium in small hospitals without a blood bank and in isolated communities, but it should not be used in place of whole human blood merely for convenience.

The amount of plasma transfused and the rate at which it is given depend upon the patient's age and general condition, on the state of his circulatory system, and on the indication for its use.

Reconstituted dried human plasma should be used immediately after reconstitution and should be discarded if not used within 3 hours. The use of dried human plasma carries a risk of transmitting hepatitis, as explained in the entry on Blood Products.

Pneumonia

Pneumonia is inflammation of the lungs with the production of exudate which enters the alveoli causing consolidation. The lesions may be distributed in a lobar, segmental, or lobular manner and may be unilateral or bilateral. Most cases of pneumonia are due to infection with bacteria, some of which are capable of invading normal lung and some only able to invade the lung when the resistance to infection is lowered.

Common organisms which cause pneumonia include *Streptococcus pneumoniae* (the pneumococcus), *Staphylococcus pyogenes*, and *Klebsiella pneumoniae*. Pneumonia may also be caused by viruses, mycoplasma species, fungi, parasites, chemical or physical irritants, and allergic reactions in the lung.

Pneumonia is characterised by cough, pain, the production of sputum, dullness of the affected part of the chest to percussion, bronchial breathing, rapid shallow breathing, and diminished chest movements on the affected side. There is fever with rigors and other manifestations of toxaemia such as sleeplessness, headache, delirium, and weakness. Complications of pneumonia include pleural effusion, empyema, lung abscess, spontaneous pneumothorax, pericarditis, meningism, and meningitis.

Patients with pneumonia should be confined to bed and supportive treatment given. Chemotherapy is the most important part of treatment and brings about a rapid decline in temperature and resolution of the pneumonia. Before starting a course of a broad spectrum antibiotic, sputum samples should be taken to identify the organism responsible for the pneumonia and its sensitivity to antibiotics. When this has been determined, a more specific antibiotic may be substituted.

Podophyllum

The dried rhizome and roots of *Podophyllum peltatum* L. (Fam. Berberidaceae), a small herb with a long perennial rhizome, common in the eastern United States of America and eastern Canada.

OTHER NAMES: American Mandrake; Podoph.; Podophyllum Rhizome

A standard is given in the British Pharmaceutical Codex 1973

The rhizome is collected in the late summer, cut into pieces, and dried.

Constituents. Podophyllum contains the 3 closely related lignans, podophyllotoxin (up to about 1%) and α- and β-peltatins and their glycosides, all derivatives of naphthofuran which differ only in the number and position of the hydroxyl and methyl groups. It also contains another lignan (a deoxypodophyllin-1β-D-glucosopyranosyl ester), the flavonoids quercetin and astragalin (kaempferol 3-glucoside), starch, and resinous matter.

Podophyllotoxin is converted by alkalis into a salt of podophyllic acid, which readily loses water to form a crystalline lactone, picropodophyllin.

Podophyllum yields 2 to 8% or more of resin. The acid-insoluble ash is about 1 to 2.5% and the total ash about 4 to 7%. It yields to alcohol (90%) 11 to 16% of extractive. Up to 2% of foreign organic matter may be present.

Description. UNGROUND DRUG. *Macroscopical characters:* rhizome occurring in subcylindrical pieces about 50 to 100 mm or more long and about 5 mm thick; externally reddish-brown, smooth or slightly wrinkled longitudinally; at intervals of about 50 to 100 mm, rhizome enlarged for about 10 to 20 mm to a thickness of about 15 mm; upper surface of enlargement bearing a concave scar, left by the fall of the flowering stem, surrounded by several circular leaf scars; under surface of enlargement bearing up to 12 roots or root scars; roots, when present, cylindrical or flattened, about 1.5 mm thick, brown and brittle; fracture of rhizome short; smoothed, transversely cut surface white and starchy, unless rhizome has been dried at a temperature sufficient to gelatinise starch, when yellowish and horny; showing a thin cork and a circle of about 20 to 30 small oval vascular bundles situated about half-way between centre and circumference of rhizome.

It has a slight characteristic odour and a somewhat bitter and acrid taste.

Microscopical characters: the diagnostic characters are: rhizome: *epidermis* of longitudinally elongated tabular cells with dark *tannin* contents and brown suberised walls; *cork* in 1 to 3 layers, cells rectangular, about 2½ times as long as wide, those from enlarged regions more nearly isodiametric; *cortex* with outer collenchyma and wide zone of parenchyma; *pith* similar to cortical parenchyma, cells of both containing abundant *starch* granules, mostly compound with 2 to 4 to 15 components, some simple, 2 to 15 to 30 μm in diameter, and also cluster *crystals* of calcium oxalate often 60 to 100 μm in diameter, in idioblasts; vascular bundles with *vessels* with spirally thickened and pitted walls, pits elongated and bordered; bundles often accompanied by perimedullary *sclereids*, up to 630 μm long and with thick, pitted walls.

Root: *epidermis* slightly papillose and having somewhat thickened outer walls; *exodermis* with thin suberised walls; *cortical cells* parenchymatous, with pitted walls, containing *starch* granules and calcium oxalate *crystals* as in the rhizome; primary *xylem* strands 4 to 9; *pith* of thin-walled parenchyma and a central core of *sclereids*, each about 30 to 230 μm long with thick, pitted walls.

POWDERED DRUG. Powdered Podophyllum. A light brown powder possessing the diagnostic characters, odour, and taste of the unground drug.

Identification. TEST. Macerate 500 mg for 10 minutes with 10 ml of alcohol (95%), filter, and to the filtrate add 0.6 ml of *strong copper acetate solution*; a bright green colour, but no brown precipitate, is produced.

Uses. Podophyllum is used almost entirely for the preparation of podophyllum resin.

Podophyllum, Indian

The dried rhizome and roots of *Podophyllum emodi* Wall. ex Hook. f. et Thoms. (*P. hexandrum* Royle) (Fam. Berberidaceae), a plant growing in the temperate forests on the lower slopes of the Himalayas.

OTHER NAMES: Ind. Podoph.; Indian Podophyllum Rhizome; Podophyllum Emodi

A standard is given in the British Pharmaceutical Codex 1973

The roots form a large proportion of the drug and are mainly detached from the rhizome.

Constituents. Indian podophyllum contains the lignans, podophyllotoxin (1 to 4%) and its β-D-glucoside (0.5 to 1%), 4'-demethylpodophyllotoxin and its glucoside, and a deoxypodophyllin-1β-D-glucosopyranosyl ester, and the flavonoid astragalin (kaempferol 3-glucoside), but peltatins are absent.

Indian podophyllum yields 6 to 12% of resin, the composition of which is not identical with that from podophyllum. Up to 2% of foreign organic matter may be present.

Description. UNGROUND DRUG. *Macroscopical characters:* rhizome occurring in irregularly cylindrical or dorsiventrally flattened, contorted knotty pieces, yellowish-brown to earthy-brown; pieces about 20 to 40 mm long and 10 to 20 mm thick; upper surface with about 3 to 4 cup-shaped scars of aerial stems, under surface with numerous stout roots or circular root scars; fracture of rhizome short; smoothed, transversely cut surface pale brown and starchy, unless rhizome has been dried at a temperature sufficient to gelatinise starch, when horny; showing large central pith and a circle of about 20 radially elongated vascular bundles.

It has a slight characteristic odour and a somewhat bitter and acrid taste.

Microscopical characters: the diagnostic characters are: rhizome: *epidermis* absent; *cork* in up to 6 layers, cells polyhedral, not more than twice as long as wide; *cortex*, *medullary rays*, and *pith* parenchymatous, cells moderately thick-walled, with simple pits, and containing abundant *starch* granules, compound, usually 2 to 4 to 20 components, 2 to 7 to 34 μm in diameter, and cluster *crystals* of calcium oxalate, 20 to 30 to 60 μm in diameter; xylem *vessels* usually with elongated bordered pits; perimedullary groups of *sclereids*, up to 320 μm long with thick, pitted walls.

Root: *epidermis* slightly papillose and having very much thickened outer and anticlinal walls; *exodermis* suberised, with wavy walls; cortex very wide, parenchymatous, with *starch* granules but no calcium oxalate *crystals*; *xylem* in 4 to 9 primary strands; *pith* with large central core of *sclereids*, axially elongated or nearly isodiametric, walls very thick and pitted.

POWDERED DRUG. Powdered Indian Podophyllum. A light brown powder possessing the diagnostic microscopical characters, odour, and taste of the unground drug.

Identification. TEST. Macerate 500 mg for 10 minutes in 10 ml of alcohol (95%), filter, and to the filtrate add 0.6 ml of *strong copper acetate solution*; a brown precipitate, but no green colour, is formed.

Uses. Indian podophyllum is used almost entirely for the preparation of podophyllum resin.

Podophyllum Resin

The resin obtained from Indian podophyllum or more rarely from podophyllum.

OTHER NAMES: Podoph. Resin; Podophyllin *Posalfilin*® (with salicylic acid)

CAUTION. *Powdered podophyllum resin is strongly irritant and should be kept away from the eyes and tender parts of the skin.*

A standard is given in the British Pharmacopoeia 1973

It may be extracted by percolating with alcohol and

pouring the concentrated percolate into water acidified with hydrochloric acid. The precipitated resin is well washed and dried at a low temperature.

Constituents. Podophyllum resin contains podophyllotoxin, at least 40% in resin from Indian podophyllum and about 10% in resin from podophyllum, picropodophyllin and its glucoside, the flavonoids quercetin and astragalin (kaempferol 3-glucoside), and resinous substances.

Resin from Indian podophyllum contains in addition 4'-demethylpodophyllotoxin and its glucoside; that from podophyllum contains α- and β-peltatins.

Description. A light brown to greenish-yellow amorphous powder or brownish-grey masses with a characteristic odour and a bitter acrid taste.

Solubility. Very slightly soluble in cold water, but partly soluble in hot water, from which it is precipitated on cooling; soluble completely, or almost completely, in alcohol; partly soluble in ether, in chloroform, and in dilute ammonia solution.

Stability. It darkens on exposure to light or when heated above 25°.

Labelling. The label on the container states the botanical source.

Storage. It should be stored in airtight containers, protected from light.

Identification. TEST. The resin from podophyllum may be distinguished from that from Indian podophyllum by gently shaking 3 ml of a 13% w/v solution of the finely powdered resin in alcohol (60%) with 0.5 ml of 1N potassium hydroxide; the resin from podophyllum does not gelatinise, whereas that from Indian podophyllum forms a jelly on standing.

Actions and uses. Because of its cytotoxic action, podophyllum resin is used as a paint in the treatment of soft venereal and other warts.

Podophyllum resin has also been used as a purgative, in doses of 15 to 60 milligrams, but its use for this purpose constitutes an unnecessarily unpleasant treatment. It has been replaced by safer and more pleasant laxatives. It should not be given to children.

Undesirable effects. Powdered podophyllum resin is strongly irritant to the skin and mucous membranes.

Contra-indications. It should not be used in pregnancy.

Preparations

COMPOUND PODOPHYLLIN PAINT:

Podophyllum resin	150 g
Compound benzoin tincture	to 1000 ml

The compound benzoin tincture used in making this preparation may be prepared with industrial methylated spirit diluted so as to be of equivalent alcoholic strength, provided that the law and the statutory regulations governing the use of industrial methylated spirit are observed.

A standard for this paint is given in the British Pharmaceutical Codex 1973

Containers, Labelling, and *Storage:* see the entry on Paints for general information on containers, labelling, and storage.

Advice for patients: the paint should be applied carefully to the lesion, a dressing applied, and the paint washed off after 4 to 8 hours. Contact with normal skin should be avoided. It should not be applied to broken or inflamed skin or near to mucous membranes.

OTHER PREPARATIONS available include an OINTMENT containing podophyllum resin 20% with salicylic acid 25%.

Poisoning

Any substance which by its chemical action causes damage to structures, or disturbance of function when ingested, inhaled, or absorbed can act as a poison.

In the event of poisoning or suspected poisoning the patient should be advised to consult a medical practitioner as soon as possible. However, certain measures may be required immediately to limit the effects of the poison or to prevent serious illness or death. This includes the administration of specific antidotes which should always be readily available when dangerous poisons are being used.

It must be emphasised that early transfer to hospital is of the greatest importance in all cases of poisoning.

In the initial stages information about the poison and route of administration may not be available, and treatment should be supportive with particular attention being paid to respiratory failure and shock. When the nature and route of poisoning is known it may be possible with certain agents to take measures to prevent further absorption of the poison and to hasten its elimination from the body. In addition, for a few poisons a specific antidote is available. Information on the treatment of poisoning by specific drugs is given in the monographs on those drugs.

The agents most often used in self-poisoning are benzodiazepines, barbiturates, other hypnotics, aspirin, and antidepressants. It is becoming common for more than one drug to be taken, and often alcohol, which potentiates central nervous depression due to drugs, may have been ingested as well.

More information on diagnosis and treatment can be obtained from a Poisons Centre. The following are the telephone numbers of poisons information centres in the United Kingdom:

Belfast	0232-30503
Cardiff	0222-33101
Edinburgh	031-229-2477
Leeds	0532-32799
London	01-407-7600
Manchester	061-740-2254
Newcastle	0632-25131

Respiratory failure. This is often the greatest immediate emergency and it requires urgent treatment. Comatose patients should be laid on one side and the airway cleared. If breathing is too shallow for adequate gas exchange, immediate mouth-to-mouth respiration should be started and mechanically assisted ventilation substituted as soon as possible. The use of oxygen may be required, but it is important to realise that it is not a substitute for adequate ventilation. Its use is, of course, mandatory in poisoning with carbon monoxide or irritant gases. The use of respiratory stimulants was once widely advocated but their disadvantages are now felt to outweigh any possible benefits.

Shock. This by definition is a syndrome characterised by inadequate perfusion of the tissues. It is recognised clinically by poor skin circulation, tachycardia, low blood pressure, and inadequate urine output. The patient's legs should be raised and a blood volume expander such as whole human blood, plasma, or dextran injection infused intravenously until the circulation is restored. Progress is assessed by the condition of the skin circulation and by measurement of the pulse, central venous pressure, blood pressure, and urine output. Pressor drugs such as metaraminol tartrate can be used but great caution is necessary as, although they may raise the arterial blood pressure, they do not necessarily increase tissue flow, and indeed may cause renal vasoconstriction. Hypoxia is often associated with shock and should be treated with oxygen. If acidaemia persists after correction of shock and hypoxia, it may be controlled by infusion of sodium bicarbonate injection.

Prevention of further absorption of poison. The stomach is emptied to remove poison and also to protect unconscious patients against inhaling vomit. In a conscious child vomiting may be induced effectively by tickling the pharynx or by oral administration of ipecacuanha paediatric emetic draught, but if this is unsuccessful gastric lavage must be performed. This is particularly important where patients have swallowed salicylates as these drugs may remain unabsorbed for many hours. Certain berries may also remain in the stomach for many hours with resultant slow absorption of the toxins. With most other substances absorption is rapid and if lavage cannot be performed within 3 to 4 hours it is unlikely to be effective.

Great care must be taken when performing gastric lavage, and if the patient is not fully conscious a cuffed endotracheal tube must be inserted to protect the airway during washout. Tubes should not be passed in patients who have swallowed corrosives, owing to the danger of perforation. Petroleum products are best left in the stomach as attempts to remove them are likely to introduce some into the lungs where they cause more damage than if left in the gut.

Absorption may also be prevented by the administration orally of large doses of charcoal (up to 50 grams). This should not be given simultaneously with ipecacuanha paediatric emetic draught as it inactivates the latter.

Skin contamination is particularly dangerous with organophosphorus insecticides and certain other chemicals. Contaminated clothes should be removed and the skin washed with soap and water; in the case of phenol, 50% alcohol (and not water) should be used.

Transport to hospital. Early transport to hospital is advisable after immediate attention has been given to the airway, respiration, and shock. Gastric lavage should not be carried out until the patient reaches hospital. During transport supervision of respiration and the airway is essential. Information should be sent with the patient about the circumstances and what treatment may have been already given. If any vomit or urine sample is available this should be sent to aid identification of the poison.

Removal of poison from the blood stream. This can be attempted in two ways, either by diuresis when the substance is removed by the patient's own kidneys, or by dialysis. These techniques are not suitable for all poisons, in particular drugs which are rapidly metabolised or highly protein bound.

Forced diuresis. In patients with normal renal function intravenous infusion of fluids together with an osmotic diuretic (laevulose or mannitol) or frusemide may be used to create a copious diuresis. For maximum excretion of the poison the urinary pH should be adjusted to one at which the poison is highly ionised. The treatment must also be adjusted to the individual patient's response and the plasma electrolytes must be monitored. Careful watch must be kept for signs of heart failure and low urine output.

Forced diuresis is most useful as an alkaline diuresis for poisoning due to salicylates or phenobarbitone. For information on the use of forced diuresis for other drugs, see the specific monographs on the drugs concerned. If there is doubt about the effectiveness of forced diuresis for a particular poison, a poisons information centre should be consulted before the patient is exposed to an unnecessary risk.

Peritoneal dialysis and haemodialysis. These techniques may be useful for removing drugs which are normally excreted in the urine. Unlike forced diuresis they may be used when there is renal failure and/or fluid overload as it is possible to remove fluid from the body by using hyperosmotic dialysis solutions. Peritoneal dialysis is a simple technique which should prove practicable in most general hospitals whilst haemodialysis is restricted to specialised centres. Dialysis is thought to be useful in the treatment of poisoning with alcohols, amphetamines, phenobarbitone, borates, lithium salts, salicylates, and paraquat. Before dialysis is used for other poisons it is advisable to consult a poisons information centre.

Chelating and complexing agents. Many poisonous metallic ions may be rendered harmless and later removed from the body in the form of chelates and complexes. Antimony, arsenic, bismuth, gold, mercury, and thallium may be removed by dimercaprol, iron with desferrioxamine mesylate, and lead with sodium calciumedetate. Cyanide may be rendered harmless by cobalt edetate; alternatively the administration of sodium nitrite or amyl nitrite will induce the formation of methaemoglobin which removes cyanide from the circulation by the formation of cyanmethaemoglobin (see under Sodium Nitrite).

Specific antidotes. Overdosage with cholinesterase inhibitors such as organophosphorus compounds may be treated with atropine and pralidoxime, a specific reactivator of cholinesterase. Poisoning with opium alkaloids and with methadone or pethidine may be treated with opiate antagonists such as naloxone.

Poldine Methylsulphate

2-Benziloyloxymethyl-1,1-dimethylpyrrolidinium methylsulphate

$$\left[\begin{array}{c} CH_3 \quad CH_3 \\ N \\ CH_2 \cdot O \cdot CO \cdot C \cdot OH \end{array} \begin{array}{c} C_6H_5 \\ \\ C_6H_5 \end{array} \right] CH_3 \cdot SO_4^-$$

$C_{22}H_{29}NO_7S = 451.5$

OTHER NAME: *Nacton*®

A standard is given in the British Pharmacopoeia 1973

Description. An odourless white crystalline powder with a bitter taste.

Solubility. Soluble, at 20°, in 1 part of water and in 20 parts of alcohol; very slightly soluble in chloroform.

Acidity. A 1% solution has a pH of 5 to 7.

Stability. Aqueous solutions at a pH of less than 4.0

are stable for long periods when stored at a temperature not exceeding 30°. The rate of hydrolysis at the ester linkage increases with rise in pH and temperature and hydrolysis is rapid in solutions of pH greater than 7.0.

Identification. TEST. Dissolve about 2 mg in 10 ml of water, add 20 ml of *ammonium cobaltothiocyanate solution* and 5 ml of chloroform and shake well; a blue colour is produced in the chloroform layer.

MELTING-POINT. About 139°.

ULTRAVIOLET ABSORPTION. In water, weak maxima at 252 nm and 258 nm and inflections at 262 nm, 264 nm, and 268 nm.

INFRA-RED ABSORPTION. Major peaks at 701, 765, 1008, 1061, 1222, and 1751 cm^{-1} (see Appendix 2a: Infra-red Spectra).

Metabolism. ABSORPTION. Poorly absorbed after oral administration.

BLOOD CONCENTRATIONS. Plasma concentrations rapidly fall after intravenous administration to rats.

DISTRIBUTION. May be subject to enterohepatic cycling.

EXCRETION. Of an intraperitoneal dose given to rats, 70% is excreted in the faeces as unchanged drug and metabolites and about 11% is excreted in the urine; in rats, significant amounts are excreted in the bile.

FURTHER INFORMATION. Excretion—P. F. Langley *et al.*, *Biochem. Pharmac.*, 1966, **15**, 1821.

Actions and uses. Poldine is an anticholinergic drug with actions and uses similar to those described under Propantheline Bromide. Its effects are longer lasting than those of atropine.

A dosage of 2 to 6 milligrams every 6 hours may be required to reduce gastric secretion and spasm in ulcer patients; treatment should begin with the lower dose, which should be gradually increased until the symptoms are controlled.

Undesirable effects. Blurring of vision, constipation, hesitancy over micturition, and tachycardia may occur. If necessary the dose should be reduced progressively by 1 milligram until the undesirable effect is relieved.

Precautions and contra-indications. As for Atropine.

Preparation

POLDINE TABLETS: available as tablets containing 2 and 4 mg of poldine methylsulphate; they may be coloured.
A standard for these tablets is given in the British Pharmacopoeia 1973
Containers and *Storage:* see the entry on Tablets for general information on containers and storage. Containers should be airtight.
Advice for patients: the tablets should be taken between meals.

Poliomyelitis Vaccine (Inactivated)

An aqueous suspension of suitable strains of poliomyelitis virus, types 1, 2, and 3, grown in cultures of monkey kidney tissue and inactivated by a suitable method. When injected into animals, it stimulates the production of neutralising antibodies to poliomyelitis virus, types 1, 2, and 3, in the circulating blood.

OTHER NAMES: Poliomyelitis Vaccine (Killed); Pol/Vac (Inact); Vaccinum Poliomyelitidis Inactivatum

A standard is given in the European Pharmacopoeia Vol. II

Storage. It should be stored at 2° to 10°. Under these conditions it may be expected to retain its potency for 18 months.

Actions and uses. Poliomyelitis vaccine (inactivated) is used for active immunisation against poliomyelitis, although the live oral vaccine is often preferred.

The vaccine is administered by subcutaneous or intramuscular injection in 3 doses, each of 1 millilitre, with an interval of 6 to 8 weeks between the first and second doses and 4 to 6 months between the second and third. Reactions to the injection of the vaccine are negligible.

Poliomyelitis Vaccine (Oral)

An aqueous suspension of suitable live attenuated strains of poliomyelitis virus, types 1, 2, or 3, grown in suitable cell cultures; it may contain any one of the three virus types or combinations of them. It contains a stabilising agent.

OTHER NAMES: Poliomyelitis Vaccine (Live); Pol/Vac (Oral); Vaccinum Poliomyelitidis Perorale

A standard is given in the European Pharmacopoeia Vol. II

Storage. It should be stored at or below −20°. When thawed and kept at a temperature between 0° and 4° it should be used within 3 months. At higher temperatures it deteriorates rapidly and at ambient temperatures should be used within a few hours. When a stabiliser such as magnesium chloride or sucrose is present it may be stored for up to 6 months at 0° to 4° or 2 weeks at 25°.

Actions and uses. Poliomyelitis vaccine (oral) is used for active immunisation against poliomyelitis. It is given by mouth in the quantity indicated on the label as the dose either as 3 doses of a vaccine containing all 3 types (trivalent vaccine) at suitable intervals or as one dose of each of 3 monovalent vaccines containing virus types 1, 2, and 3 respectively at suitable intervals.

Suitable schedules for the immunisation of children and travellers are given under Vaccines.

Polyarteritis Nodosa

Polyarteritis nodosa is characterised by focal inflammatory lesions in small and medium-sized arteries. The lesion originates in the media as a cellular infiltration and fibrinoid necrosis, and spreads to the intima producing thrombosis and occlusion and to the adventitia where it results in bead-like nodes. It may appear as a fulminating disease, with prostration, fever, tachycardia, and wasting which is fatal in a few weeks, or the symptoms may remain localised. Most cases are fatal within a year. Polyarteritis nodosa is principally a vascular disease and its symptoms are due mainly to ischaemia or haemorrhage. It may give rise to symptoms in any system of the body. There are many related conditions, mainly localised to the lung and skin, which are benign.

Drugs such as penicillin and sulphonamides may sometimes precipitate polyarteritis nodosa. However, the aetiological factor is generally unknown and there is no specific treatment for the disease. Corticosteroids may be used to bring about a temporary improvement in the condition and control acute symptoms.

Polycythaemia

Polycythaemia is a condition in which there is a high red-cell count of the blood, accompanied by an increase in the haemoglobin and haematocrit values. Relative polycythaemia is seen in any condition which produces severe fluid loss and haemoconcentration, for example after severe burns. Polycythaemia may be secondary to any chronic disease which results in an increased erythropoiesis, for example chronic hypoxia due to lung disease or renal artery stenosis.

Polycythaemia vera is due to an abnormal proliferative activity of the bone marrow where all cellular components are increased (see under Myeloproliferative Diseases and Lymphoproliferative Diseases).

Substances used in the treatment of polycythaemia vera include busulphan, pyrimethamine, and sodium phosphate (^{32}P).

Polymenorrhagia

see under UTERINE BLEEDING, ABNORMAL

Polymenorrhoea

see under UTERINE BLEEDING, ABNORMAL

Polymyalgia

see GIANT-CELL ARTERITIS

Polymyositis

see under DERMATOMYOSITIS

Polymyxin B Sulphate

A mixture of the sulphates of certain antimicrobial polypeptides produced by the growth of certain strains of *Bacillus polymyxa* or obtained by any other means. It has a potency of not less than 6500 units per milligram calculated with reference to the dried substance.

OTHER NAMES: *Aerosporin*®; Polymyx. B Sulph.; Polymyxini B Sulphas

Polyfax® (with bacitracin zinc); *Otosporin*® (with hydrocortisone and neomycin sulphate); *Terramycin Ophthalmic Ointment with Polymyxin B Sulphate*®

A standard is given in the European Pharmacopoeia Vol. II

Description. An odourless, hygroscopic, white or creamy-white powder.

Solubility. Soluble in water; very slightly soluble in alcohol.

Acidity. A 2% solution has a pH of 5 to 7.

Moisture content. Not more than 6%, determined by drying over phosphorus pentoxide at 60° *in vacuo.*

Dissociation constant. pK_a 8.9.

Sterilisation. Solutions for injection are sterilised by filtration.

Storage. It should be stored in airtight containers, protected from light. If it is intended for parenteral administration the containers are sealed to exclude micro-organisms.

Labelling. If the material is intended for the preparation of injections the label states "Polymyxin B Sulphate for Injection". If the material is not intended for parenteral administration the label on the container states that the contents are not to be injected.

Identification. TEST. Dissolve about 2 mg in 5 ml of water, add 0.5 ml of a freshly prepared 0.1% solution of ninhydrin and 2 drops of pyridine, boil for 1 minute, and cool; a blue colour is produced.

Metabolism. ABSORPTION. Not absorbed after oral administration except in the newborn; it is also not absorbed by the skin or mucous membranes to any significant degree.

BLOOD CONCENTRATION. After an intramuscular dose of 2 to 4 mg daily, plasma concentrations of 1 to 8 μg/ml are attained; after single parenteral doses peak plasma concentrations are attained in 1 to 2 hours.

HALF-LIFE. Serum half-life, about 6 hours which may be increased to 2 to 3 days in subjects with renal function impairment.

DISTRIBUTION. After a parenteral dose, polymyxin B does not enter the cerebrospinal fluid, or the pleural or joint cavities; it does not cross the placenta and in subjects with renal function impairment will accumulate; similarly, accumulation occurs upon repeated dosage; *protein binding,* about 50% bound to plasma proteins.

METABOLIC REACTIONS. About 50% of its activity is lost in the presence of serum.

EXCRETION. After therapeutic parenteral doses, concentrations of 20 to 100 μg/ml are slowly attained in the urine; about 60% of a parenteral dose is ultimately excreted in the urine.

FURTHER INFORMATION. Dosage in renal failure—C. M. Kunin, *Ann. intern. Med.,* 1967, **67,** 151; review—A. Kucers and N. M. Bennett, Polymyxins, *The Use of Antibiotics,* 2nd Edn, London, Heinemann, 1975, p. 332; tissue binding and release in rabbits—W. A. Craig and C. M. Kunin, *J. Pharmac. exp. Ther.,* 1973, **184,** 757.

Actions and uses. Polymyxin B sulphate is active against nearly all Gram-negative bacteria with the exception of species of *Proteus* and *Neisseria*; Gram-positive bacteria and fungi are resistant. Its action is bactericidal. It is not absorbed from the gastro-intestinal tract.

Polymyxin B sulphate is administered by mouth or applied topically. For intestinal infections by sensitive bacteria it may be given in a dose of 1 000 000 units every 4 hours for adults or 40 000 units per kilogram body-weight for children. Very little is absorbed unless there is extensive ulceration.

Specific bacterial skin infections, especially of burns, may be treated topically with solutions containing 0.1 to 1.0%, applied as a wet dressing or a spray. Systemic toxicity may result from the treatment of large raw areas.

Polymyxin B sulphate is irritant to the tissues when administered systemically and colistin sulphomethate sodium which has a similar antibacterial spectrum is preferred. Polymyxin B sulphate may be given by intrathecal injection in a single dose of 10 000 to 50 000 units dissolved in 1 to 2 millilitres of sodium chloride injection for an adult or 5000 to 15 000 units in one millilitre for a child under 2 years, daily for a few days. Polymyxin B sulphate may be given by subconjunctival injection in doses of 10 000 to 250 000 units in 0.5 millilitre of lignocaine and adrenaline injection for the treatment of *Pseudomonas aeruginosa* infections of the eye.

Undesirable effects. Systemic toxicity may give rise to dizziness and paraesthesia, especially of the face. More serious but apparently reversible damage may occur to the renal tubules. These effects are only seen when polymyxin B sulphate is given by intramuscular or intravenous injection and not when given orally or intrathecally.

Drug interactions. When given parenterally polymyxin B sulphate potentiates the action of neuromuscular blocking agents, including other antibiotics with muscle relaxant effects such as kanamycin and streptomycin. It should not be given with cephaloridine, which increases its nephrotoxicity.

Preparations

HYDROCORTISONE, NEOMYCIN, AND POLYMYXIN EAR-DROPS: consisting of hydrocortisone, neomycin sulphate, and polymyxin B sulphate in an aqueous vehicle. It contains 10 mg of hydrocortisone, 3400 units of neomycin sulphate, and 10000 units of polymyxin B sulphate per ml.
Containers and *Labelling:* see the entry on Ear-drops for general information on containers and labelling.
Storage: it should be stored in a cool place, protected from light.
Advice for patients: the ear canal should be cleansed without the use of soap before the drops are instilled. The prescribed course should be completed.

POLYMYXIN AND BACITRACIN EYE OINTMENT: prepared by incorporating polymyxin B sulphate and bacitracin zinc in eye ointment basis, or any other suitable basis, by method B described in the entry on Eye Ointments. Available as an eye ointment containing 10000 units of polymyxin B sulphate and 500 units of bacitracin zinc per g.
Containers and *Labelling:* see the entry on Eye Ointments for general information on containers and labelling.
Storage: it should be stored in a cool place.
Advice for patients: see the entry on Eye Ointments for general information on the use of eye ointments. The prescribed course should be completed.

POLYMYXIN INJECTION (*Syn.* Polymyxin B Sulphate Injection): a sterile solution of polymyxin B sulphate in water for injections or in sodium chloride injection. It is prepared by dissolving the contents of a sealed container in water for injections or in sodium chloride injection shortly before use. Available as a powder in vials containing 500000 units of polymyxin B sulphate. *A standard for this injection is given in the British Pharmaceutical Codex 1973*
Containers and *Labelling:* see the entry on Injections for general information on containers and labelling.
Storage: the sealed container should be protected from light. The injection contains no bactericide and should be used as soon as possible after preparation, but solutions of polymyxin B sulphate may be expected to retain their potency for up to 24 hours after preparation provided they are stored at 2° to 10°.

OTHER PREPARATIONS available include an EYE OINTMENT containing polymyxin B sulphate 10000 units with oxytetracycline hydrochloride equivalent to 5 mg of anhydrous oxytetracycline per g; and an OINTMENT containing polymyxin B sulphate and bacitracin zinc in the same concentrations as in polymyxin and bacitracin eye ointment.

Polysorbate 20

A complex mixture of partial lauric esters of sorbitol and its mono- and di-anhydrides condensed with approximately 20 moles of ethylene oxide for each mole of sorbitol and its anhydrides.

OTHER NAMES: *Crillet 1®*; Polyoxyethylene (20) Sorbitan Monolaurate; Polysorbatum 20; *Tween 20®*

A standard is given in the European Pharmacopoeia Vol. III

Description. A clear, yellowish or brownish-yellow oily liquid with a characteristic odour and a bitter taste.

Solubility. Miscible with water, with alcohol, with ethyl acetate, and with methyl alcohol; soluble, at 20°, in 125 parts of cottonseed oil and in 200 parts of toluene; very slightly soluble in liquid paraffin.

Weight per ml. At 20°, about 1.10 g.

Acidity. A 5% solution has a pH of 5 to 7.

Moisture content. Not more than 3%, determined by Fischer titration.

Uses. Polysorbate 20 has the uses of the polysorbates, as described under Polysorbate 80. It is more hydrophilic than polysorbate 60 and polysorbate 80.
It is used alone or in conjunction with polysorbate 80 for the solubilisation of oils. It has also been used for the dispersion of coal tar in ointment bases.

Polysorbate 60

A complex mixture of partial stearic esters of sorbitol and its mono- and di-anhydrides condensed with approximately 20 moles of ethylene oxide for each mole of sorbitol and its anhydrides.

OTHER NAMES: *Crillet 3®*; Polyoxyethylene (20) Sorbitan Monostearate; Polysorbatum 60; *Tween 60®*

A standard is given in the European Pharmacopoeia Vol. III

Description. A yellowish-brown opaque semi-gel with a faintly sweet or oily odour and a slightly bitter taste. It becomes a clear oily liquid at temperatures above 24°.

Solubility. Soluble in water; miscible with acetone and with dioxan; soluble, at 20°, in 30 parts of cottonseed oil.

Weight per ml. At 20°, about 1.10 g.

Moisture content. Not more than 3%, determined by Fischer titration.

Uses. Polysorbate 60 has the uses of the polysorbates, as described under Polysorbate 80, from which it differs in solubility.

Polysorbate 80

A complex mixture of partial oleic esters of sorbitol and its mono- and di-anhydrides condensed with approximately 20 moles of ethylene oxide for each mole of sorbitol and its anhydrides.

OTHER NAMES: *Crillet 4®*; Polyoxyethylene (20) Sorbitan Mono-oleate; Polysorbatum 80; *Tween 80®*

A standard is given in the European Pharmacopoeia Vol. III

Description. A clear, yellowish or brownish-yellow oily

liquid with an odour characteristic of fatty acids and a slightly bitter taste.

Solubility. Miscible with water, with alcohol, with ethyl acetate, and with methyl alcohol; soluble, at 20°, in 125 parts of cottonseed oil; very slightly soluble in liquid paraffin.

Weight per ml. At 20°, about 1.08 g.

Acidity or alkalinity. A 5% solution has a pH of 6 to 8.

Moisture content. Not more than 3%, determined by Fischer titration.

Uses. Polysorbates are non-ionic surface-active agents. They are used in the preparation of emulsions, creams, ointments, and suppository bases.

When used alone, the polysorbates, being hydrophilic, yield oil-in-water emulsions, but emulsions and creams of varying character, including both oil-in-water and water-in-oil types, may be produced by incorporating varying proportions of sorbitan ether–esters. The emulsions are stable, being little affected by high concentrations of electrolytes or changes in pH.

Polysorbates are also used as solubilising agents for essential oils, oil-soluble vitamins, and phenobarbitone, and as wetting agents in suspensions for administration by mouth or injection.

Polythiazide

6-Chloro-3,4-dihydro-2-methyl-7-sulphamoyl-3-(2,2,2-trifluoroethylthiomethyl) - 2H - benzo - 1,2,4 - thiadiazine 1,1-dioxide

$C_{11}H_{13}ClF_3N_3O_4S_3 = 439.9$

OTHER NAME: *Nephril*®

A standard is given in the British Pharmacopoeia Addendum 1978

Description. A white crystalline powder with an alliaceous odour.

Solubility. Practically insoluble in water and in chloroform; soluble, at 20°, in 40 parts of alcohol.

Moisture content. Not more than 1%, determined by drying at 105°.

Identification. MELTING-POINT. About 209°.

ULTRAVIOLET ABSORPTION. In alcohol (95%), maxima at 270 nm (E1%, 1cm = 468) and 318 nm (E1%, 1cm = 63).

INFRA-RED ABSORPTION. Major peaks at 1071, 1120, 1162, 1326, 1345, and 1597 cm^{-1} (see Appendix 2a: Infra-red Spectra).

THIN-LAYER CHROMATOGRAPHY. See under Thin-layer Chromatography, System 6.

Metabolism. ABSORPTION. Well absorbed after oral administration.

METABOLIC REACTIONS. In dogs, hydrolytic ring fission to form 4-amino-6-chloro-3-N-methylsulphamoylbenzenesulphonamide and S-trifluoroethylthioglycollic acid.

EXCRETION. In dogs, about 80% is excreted in the urine

and 15 to 20% in the faeces in 5 days; in 24 hours about 30% is excreted as metabolites derived from hydrolysis.

FURTHER INFORMATION. Metabolism in the dog— R. Pinson et al., *J. mednl pharm. Chem.*, 1962, **5**, 491. Pharmacokinetic studies—D. C. Hobbs and T. M. Toomey, *Clin. Pharmac. Ther.*, 1978, **23**, 241.

Actions and uses. Polythiazide is a diuretic which has actions similar to those described under Chlorothiazide. For the treatment of oedema the usual dosage is 1 to 2 milligrams daily but up to 4 milligrams daily may be required in severe cases. For the treatment of mild or moderate hypertension the usual dose is 1 or 2 milligrams daily.

Undesirable effects; Precautions. As for Chlorothiazide.

Preparation

POLYTHIAZIDE TABLETS: available as tablets containing 1 mg of polythiazide.

A standard for these tablets is given in the British Pharmacopoeia Addendum 1978

Containers and *Storage:* see the entry on Tablets for general information on containers and storage. Containers should be airtight and light resistant.

Advice for patients: daily doses should preferably be taken in the morning. Treatment should not be discontinued without the advice of the prescriber.

Porphyria

The porphyrias are a group of disorders in which there are abnormalities of porphyrin metabolism, mainly due to inborn errors. The acute porphyrias (acute intermittent porphyria, variegate porphyria, and hereditary coproporphyria) may give rise to abdominal and limb pains, neuropsychiatric disturbances, and autonomic neuropathy; in the variegate and hereditary forms there may also be photosensitivity. Attacks may be spontaneous or follow the administration of porphyrinogenic drugs such as barbiturates, oestrogens, and progestogens; these drugs are usually microsomal enzyme inducers.

Symptoms of an acute attack are treated empirically using drugs known not to induce porphyria. Dihydrocodeine or pethidine may be given for the relief of pain and phenothiazine derivatives such as chlorpromazine and promazine may be used in psychiatric conditions. Hypertension and tachycardia may respond to propranolol, which is gradually withdrawn as recovery occurs. Severe constipation may be treated with neostigmine bromide. Carbohydrate loading by mouth or by intravenous infusion may be of value.

Cutaneous hepatic porphyria is often sporadic and is usually precipitated by chronic alcohol excess. This disease gives rise to cutaneous photosensitivity which responds to regular venesection. Erythropoietic protoporphyria, in which solar photosensitivity can be very severe, is treated with β-carotene which exerts a protective effect against skin damage.

Posology

Dosage schemes are given in the paragraphs on "Actions and uses" in the entries on medicinal substances. The doses are based on the opinions of medical and pharmaceutical experts and are intended for general guidance, but they should not be regarded as binding upon the

Table of Body-surface Area from Height and Weight (m²)

Weight (kg)

Height (m)	2.5	5	7.5	10	12.5	15	17.5	20	22.5	25	27.5	30	35	40	45	50	55	60	65	70	75	80	85	90	95	100	105	110	115	120
0.5	0.18	0.24																												
0.55	0.19	0.26	0.31																											
0.6	0.21	0.28	0.33	0.37																										
0.65	0.22	0.29	0.35	0.39																										
0.7	0.23	0.31	0.37	0.42	0.46																									
0.75		0.33	0.39	0.44	0.48	0.54																								
0.8			0.41	0.46	0.50	0.54																								
0.85				0.48	0.53	0.57																								
0.9				0.50	0.55	0.59	0.63	0.67																						
0.95				0.52	0.57	0.62	0.66	0.70																						
1.0				0.54	0.59	0.64	0.68	0.72	0.76																					
1.05				0.56	0.61	0.66	0.71	0.75	0.79	0.82	0.86																			
1.1					0.64	0.69	0.73	0.78	0.82	0.85	0.89	0.92																		
1.15						0.71	0.76	0.80	0.84	0.88	0.92	0.95	1.02																	
1.2						0.73	0.78	0.83	0.87	0.91	0.95	0.98	1.05																	
1.25							0.80	0.85	0.89	0.94	0.97	1.01	1.08	1.14																
1.3								0.88	0.92	0.96	1.00	1.04	1.11	1.17	1.24															
1.35								0.90	0.95	0.99	1.03	1.07	1.14	1.21	1.27	1.33														
1.4									0.97	1.02	1.06	1.10	1.17	1.24	1.30	1.36	1.42	1.47												
1.45									1.00	1.04	1.08	1.13	1.20	1.27	1.34	1.40	1.46	1.51	1.56											
1.5										1.07	1.11	1.15	1.23	1.30	1.37	1.43	1.49	1.55	1.60	1.65										
1.55											1.14	1.18	1.26	1.33	1.40	1.47	1.53	1.59	1.64	1.69	1.74									
1.6											1.16	1.21	1.29	1.37	1.44	1.50	1.56	1.62	1.68	1.73	1.78	1.83								
1.65												1.24	1.32	1.40	1.47	1.54	1.60	1.66	1.72	1.77	1.82	1.87								
1.7													1.35	1.43	1.50	1.57	1.63	1.70	1.75	1.81	1.86	1.92	1.96							
1.75														1.46	1.53	1.60	1.67	1.73	1.79	1.85	1.90	1.96	2.01	2.06	2.10					
1.8															1.56	1.64	1.70	1.77	1.83	1.89	1.94	2.00	2.05	2.10	2.15	2.20	2.24	2.28	2.33	
1.85																1.67	1.74	1.80	1.86	1.92	1.98	2.04	2.09	2.14	2.19	2.24	2.28	2.33	2.37	2.42
1.9																1.70	1.77	1.84	1.90	1.96	2.02	2.08	2.13	2.18	2.23	2.28	2.33	2.38	2.42	2.47
1.95																	1.80	1.87	1.94	2.00	2.06	2.12	2.17	2.22	2.28	2.33	2.38	2.43	2.47	2.51

prescriber. The statement "in accordance with the response of the patient" is made when the dose is too variable to be safely and usefully stated. When an unusually large dose appears to have been prescribed, it is the duty of the pharmacist to ensure that the prescriber's intention has been correctly interpreted.

Patients vary widely in their response to drugs. In most cases suggested dosage schemes are given but where the margin between therapeutic and toxic doses is narrow the actual dose must be calculated from body-weight or body-surface area. Because of the variable relationship between the size and weight of patients, it is sometimes more satisfactory to adjust dosage of medicines to body-surface rather than to weight. The average normal body-surface area for an adult man is 1.8 square metres. The table on p. 718 sets out the relationship between the height (in metres), weight (in kilograms), and body-surface area (in square metres). The values given are calculated from the formula of Dubois and Dubois,

body-surface (m²)
$$= \text{body-weight (kg)}^{0.425} \times \text{height (cm)}^{0.725} \times 0.007184$$

Paediatric Dosage

Where doses for children are given in the entries on medicinal substances they are usually divided into the following age groups: first 28 days (neonate), up to 1 year (infant), 1 to 5 years, and 6 to 12 years. Generally when a range of doses is stated for a given age range the lower dose applies at the lower age and the higher dose at the higher age limit, other doses being obtained by interpolation. Where no doses for children are specified they may be estimated by calculation.

Calculation of dosage. For many substances the dose for children can be calculated from the dose for an adult by taking into account age, body-weight, or body-surface.

Age. When basing dosage on age account should be taken of variations of development in children of a given age.

Body-weight. When using body-weight it should be noted that children vary in proportion of body fat which is relatively inactive in metabolism but may act as a reservoir for certain drugs.

Body-surface. Since body-surface area correlates fairly closely with metabolic active mass it should form the most accurate basis for assessment of dosage. The relationship between age, body-weight, body-surface, and dose is given in the table below (see also p. 718).

Age	Body-weight kg	Body-surface m²	Proportion of adult dose
2 weeks*	3.5	0.21	1/8
2 months*	4.5	0.28	1/6
4 months*	6.5	0.36	1/5
1 year	10	0.48	1/4
3 years	15	0.64	1/3
7 years	23	0.87	1/2
12 years	40	1.27	3/4
Adult	65	1.75	1

* The figures for infants relate to those born at full term and not prematurely. In the early post-natal period the doses may need to be halved or even further reduced according to the condition of the patient.

Factors requiring modification of dosage. Young children usually have a high proportion of water in the body (70 to 75% compared with 60% in adults). They also have a relatively greater body-surface than adults, and there are also differences in the distribution of drugs in the body. Doses may need modification when dehydration has occurred or in hepatic disease, hypothyroidism, renal impairment, or toxaemia.

Maturity of enzyme systems. Absorption may be influenced by the relative immaturity of the gastrointestinal tract, and this is particularly important because medicines for children are usually given by mouth. Metabolism and excretion of some drugs may differ from that in adults owing to immaturity of enzyme systems and differences in renal excretion and metabolic rate, especially in the newborn.

Physiological jaundice in the newborn is a sign that hepatic enzyme systems concerned with the conjugation of bilirubin and detoxication of various exogenous substances are impaired.

Problems associated with the use of medicines in infants. Impaired formation of the glucuronide of chloramphenicol is associated with the "grey syndrome" which may occur 3 to 4 days after initiation of treatment with chloramphenicol. Vitamin K, sulphonamides, and salicylates compete with unconjugated bilirubin for available binding sites on the serum albumin molecule and the increase in unbound bilirubin that results may cause kernicterus.

Young children are generally more tolerant of phenobarbitone than adults but may occasionally show behaviour disorders when phenobarbitone is administered to them. Children receiving steroid therapy may show an uncertain response owing to variable absorption of the corticosteroid and should be closely observed for infections which may produce severe reactions. Growing tissues may selectively incorporate certain drugs, and this is particularly marked in calcified tissue. Tetracyclines may be deposited in growing teeth (causing discoloration of enamel) and in growing bone.

Veterinary Dosage

Dosages quoted in the entries on substances used as veterinary medicines are primarily intended for guidance to the pharmacist and should not be regarded as binding upon the prescriber. They represent, unless otherwise stated, the usual quantity or range of quantities that is generally regarded as suitable. Unless another route is specified the doses are those for oral administration. The statement "in accordance with the response of the animal" is made when the dose is too variable to be safely and usefully stated. It should not be assumed that the statements indicate the greatest amounts that may be given; much depends on the species, breed, weight, and condition of the animal. When an unduly large amount appears to have been prescribed, it is the duty of the pharmacist to satisfy himself that the prescriber's intention has been correctly interpreted.

The quantities in the statements are usually given in terms of body-weight and apply to all species unless otherwise stated. The term "all species" is restricted to horses and cattle (500 kg), pigs (150 kg), sheep, goats, calves, foals (50 kg), dogs (10 kg), and cats (5 kg); the weights in the parentheses are the body-weights that have been used for calculating the stated doses. For heavier animals in each species doses may be proportionately more and sometimes a maximum dose is given.

For some substances the doses usually given over a stated period are specified, for example, "daily" (once in 24 hours), or "daily in divided doses" (at specified intervals more than once a day). In the absence of these or other indications of frequency, subdivision, or duration of action, the quantities are those generally suitable for administration on one occasion.

Postpartum Haemorrhage

Postpartum haemorrhage is significant blood loss (at least 500 ml) occurring after the birth of a baby. It may be haemorrhage from the placental site caused by an atonic uterus or retained products of conception, or it may be due to lacerations or hypofibrinogenaemia. It usually occurs soon after parturition and before complete delivery of the placenta but may occur as much as a month after delivery.

Postpartum haemorrhage may be prevented or controlled by the routine administration of oxytocin and ergometrine by injection at the time of placental separation to ensure uterine contraction. The placenta should be examined for completeness and any retained products of conception removed from the uterus.

If haemorrhage does occur the risk of serious blood loss may be reduced by bimanual uterine massage, injection of oxytocin, and repair of lacerations. Hypotension should be treated promptly to prevent pituitary necrosis.

Potassium Acetate

$CH_3.CO_2K = 98.14$

A standard is given in the British Pharmaceutical Codex 1973

Description. Odourless colourless crystals or a white crystalline powder.

Solubility. Soluble, at 20°, in less than 1 part of water and in 2 parts of alcohol.

Alkalinity. A 5% solution has a pH of 7.5 to 9.5.

Moisture content. Not more than 5%, determined by drying at 105°.

Storage. It should be stored in airtight containers.

Uses. Potassium acetate is a source of potassium ions and may be used to adjust the potassium content of solutions for haemodialysis.

Potassium Acid Tartrate

$C_4H_5KO_6 = 188.2$

OTHER NAMES: Pot. Acid Tart.; Potassium Hydrogen Tartrate; Purified Cream of Tartar

A standard is given in the British Pharmaceutical Codex 1973

Description. Odourless colourless crystals or white crystalline powder.

Solubility. Soluble, at 20°, in 190 parts of water; soluble in 16 parts of boiling water; practically insoluble in alcohol.

Hygroscopicity. It absorbs insignificant amounts of moisture at 25° at relative humidities up to about 90%.

Uses. Potassium acid tartrate has been used as a saline purgative. It is also a mild diuretic. The usual dose is 1 to 4 grams.

Potassium Bicarbonate

$KHCO_3 = 100.1$

OTHER NAMES: Pot. Bicarb.; Potassium Hydrogen Carbonate

A standard is given in the British Pharmaceutical Codex 1973

Description. Odourless, colourless monoclinic prisms or white granular powder.

Solubility. Soluble, at 20°, in 3 parts of water; very slightly soluble in alcohol.

Uses. Potassium bicarbonate is used in the preparation of effervescent tablets or mixtures for the prophylaxis or treatment of potassium deficiency.

Preparation

Potassium bicarbonate is an ingredient of effervescent potassium chloride tablets.

Potassium Bromide

$KBr = 119.0$

OTHER NAMES: Kalii Bromidum; Pot. Brom.

A standard is given in the European Pharmacopoeia Vol. I

Description. Odourless colourless crystals or white crystalline powder with a saline taste.

Solubility. Soluble, at 20°, in 1.6 parts of water and in 200 parts of alcohol; soluble in glycerol.

Moisture content. Not more than 1%, determined by drying at 130°.

Incompatibility. It is incompatible with oxidising agents and with salts of mercury and silver.

Actions and uses. Bromides are depressants of the central nervous system and are more effective as sedatives than as hypnotics. They may have to be administered for some days before the sedative effect is produced.

Mixtures containing bromides have been widely used as sedatives and anticonvulsants, but in view of their undesirable effects they have now been replaced by more effective substances such as chloral hydrate and benzodiazepines. The usual dose is 1 to 6 grams daily in divided doses.

Undesirable effects. During prolonged administration accumulation of bromide may occur, giving rise to symptoms of poisoning (bromism) which may consist of skin eruptions of various types, nausea and vomiting, mental dullness, lapses of memory, and even mental derangement. The symptoms usually subside when bromides are withheld and chlorides are administered.

Precautions. Special care should be taken in prescribing bromides for the aged or for patients suffering from impaired renal function or on a salt-restricted diet. Bromides should be avoided in nursing mothers as they may cause symptoms of bromism in the offspring.

Potassium Chlorate

$KClO_3 = 122.6$

A standard is given in the British Pharmaceutical Codex 1973

CAUTION. Potassium chlorate is liable to explode under

certain conditions and when mixing it with any dry substance friction and percussion should be avoided.

Description. Odourless colourless crystals or white powder.

Solubility. Soluble at 20°, in 14 parts of water and of glycerol; soluble in 2 parts of boiling water; very slightly soluble in alcohol.

Stability. Potassium chlorate is unstable and liable to explode when in contact with organic compounds or readily oxidisable substances such as charcoal, phosphorus, or sulphur, especially if heated or subjected to friction or percussion.

Storage and handling of tablets. Potassium chlorate tablets should not be allowed to come into contact with matches or surfaces containing phosphorus compounds and should be dispensed in bottles or boxes.

Actions and uses. Potassium chlorate is a sialogogue and mild astringent. It is used in the form of a gargle or in lozenges or tablets. The assumption that it has an antiseptic action is without rational basis.
The usual dose is 300 to 600 milligrams.

Undesirable effects. The internal administration of potassium chlorate may cause kidney damage or methaemoglobinaemia. In a susceptible person, it may produce acute haemolytic anaemia, giving rise to methaemoglobinuria.

Poisoning. The symptoms of acute poisoning by potassium chlorate are nausea, vomiting, abdominal pain, albuminuria, haematuria, and methaemoglobinaemia. Treatment consists in gastric lavage, maintenance of fluid output, and treatment of methaemoglobinaemia, for which methylene blue may not be suitable. Peritoneal dialysis or haemodialysis may be necessary to support renal function and may increase the rate of elimination of chlorate.

Preparation

POTASSIUM CHLORATE AND PHENOL GARGLE:

Potassium chlorate	30.00 g
Patent blue V (Colour Index No. 42051), food grade of commerce	0.01 g
Liquefied phenol	15.0 ml
Water for preparations	to 1000.0 ml

It should be diluted with 10 times its volume of warm water before use.
A standard for this gargle is given in the British Pharmaceutical Codex 1973
Containers and *Labelling:* see the entry on Gargles for general information on containers and labelling.
Storage: it should be protected from light.
Advice for patients: the diluted solution should be used as described under Gargles. It should preferably not be swallowed. Prolonged use should be avoided.

Potassium Chloride

KCl = 74.55

OTHER NAMES: Kalii Chloridum; *Kalium Durules®*; *Kay-Cee-L®*; *K-Contin®*; *Leo-K®*; *Ruthmol®*; *Selora®*; *Slow-K®*
Kloref® (with betaine hydrochloride and potassium bicarbonate); *Sando-K®* (with citric acid and potassium bicarbonate)

A standard is given in the European Pharmacopoeia Vol. I

Description. Odourless colourless crystals or white crystalline powder.

Solubility. Soluble, at 20°, in 3 parts of water; practically insoluble in dehydrated alcohol and in ether.

Moisture content. Not more than 1%, determined by drying at 130°.

Sterilisation. Solutions for injection are sterilised by heating in an autoclave or by filtration.

Actions and uses. Potassium ions play an important part in cellular metabolism. Their concentration is much higher in the cells than in the extracellular fluid, and there is an uptake of potassium during glycogen storage.
When administered by mouth, potassium salts are rapidly excreted in the urine and toxic concentrations are not usually achieved by this route even with large doses, but an excess of potassium ions, when injected intravenously, produces depression of the heart and may cause cardiac arrest. Electrocardiographic tracings show typical changes, but owing to the migration of potassium from the intracellular fluid to the serum during excretion, such changes are not always parallel with directly determined potassium concentrations.
Deficiency of potassium ions causes acute muscular weakness, paraesthesia, and cardiac arrhythmias. It is important to maintain the body-potassium in patients with diabetic acidosis, persistent diarrhoea and vomiting, following the abuse of purgatives, and during treatment with chlorothiazide and related diuretic substances.
When potassium supplements are given in conjunction with diuretic therapy, they should preferably be given on the day following that on which the diuretic is administered. The dose is determined by the physician in accordance with the needs of the patient.
Potassium chloride is used in doses of 2 to 10 grams orally daily for the treatment of cumulative digitalis poisoning.
In acute potassium deficiency, a solution of potassium chloride may be administered intravenously; administration should be slow in order to avoid toxic effects on the heart. The total amount of potassium chloride administered intravenously should not exceed 6 grams (80 millimoles) daily and the concentration of the solution should not exceed 3.2 grams (43 millimoles) per litre.
Compound sodium lactate injection is used in the treatment of acidosis.

Undesirable effects. Potassium salts by mouth are more irritant than the corresponding sodium salts; their low renal threshold for excretion promotes diuresis.
Tablets containing potassium salts may cause ulceration of the gastro-intestinal tract with bleeding and intestinal obstruction. Potassium chloride should therefore be given as a well-diluted solution or in the form of slow-release tablets.
Colonic irritation may occur during treatment with tablets containing potassium chloride together with a diuretic of the thiazide group.

Poisoning. Overdosage with potassium salts is usually due to inappropriate estimation of the dose, for example neglecting to allow for renal failure. The resulting hyperkalaemia should be treated with calcium gluconate injection (10%), 10 to 30 millilitres by slow intravenous injection, intravenous infusion of dextrose, and insulin injection subcutaneously. The cation-exchange resin, sodium polystyrene sulphonate, may be given by mouth in doses of 15 to 30 grams orally with water or sorbitol solution, or rectally in 2% methylcellulose mucilage. In severe cases of poisoning haemodialysis or peritoneal dialysis may be used.

Preparations

EFFERVESCENT POTASSIUM CHLORIDE TABLETS: containing potassium chloride and potassium bicarbonate, and either betaine hydrochloride or anhydrous citric acid, in an effervescent basis; they may contain suitable flavouring.

Formula A. Each tablet contains 600 mg of potassium chloride and 400 mg of potassium bicarbonate (providing 12 mmol of K^+ and 8 mmol of Cl^-), and 800 mg of citric acid.

Formula B. Each tablet contains potassium chloride 140 mg and potassium bicarbonate 455 mg (providing 6.7 mmol each of K^+ and Cl^-), and 740 mg of betaine hydrochloride.

The prescriber should state which formula should be supplied.

Containers and *Storage:* see the entry on Tablets for general information on containers and storage. Containers should be airtight.

Advice for patients: the tablets should be taken dissolved in water, preferably after meals.

POTASSIUM CHLORIDE AND DEXTROSE INJECTION: a sterile solution of potassium chloride and anhydrous dextrose or the equivalent amount of dextrose monohydrate for parenteral use, in water for injections. It is sterilised, immediately after preparation, by heating in an autoclave. The usual strength is 0.3% of potassium chloride (40 mmol each of K^+ and Cl^- per litre) and 5% of anhydrous dextrose.

A standard for this injection is given in the British Pharmacopoeia 1973

Containers: see the entry on Injections for general information on containers.

Labelling: see the entry on Injections for general information on labelling. In addition, the label on the container should state the amounts of the medicaments as the percentages w/v of potassium chloride and anhydrous dextrose.

When the injection is intended for intravenous infusion, the label should also state that rapid infusion may be harmful, the approximate concentrations, in millimoles per litre, of the potassium and the chloride ions, and the number of grams per litre of anhydrous dextrose.

Storage: it should be stored at a temperature not exceeding 25°.

POTASSIUM CHLORIDE AND SODIUM CHLORIDE INJECTION: a sterile solution of potassium chloride and sodium chloride in water for injections. It is sterilised by heating in an autoclave. The usual strength is 0.3% of potassium chloride and 0.9% of sodium chloride (40 mmol of K^+, 150 mmol of Na^+, and 190 mmol of Cl^- per litre).

A standard for this injection is given in the British Pharmacopoeia 1973

Containers: see the entry on Injections for general information on containers.

Labelling: see the entry on Injections for general information on labelling. In addition, the label on the container should state the amounts of the medicaments as the percentages w/v of potassium chloride and sodium chloride.

When the injection is intended for intravenous infusion, the label should also state that rapid infusion may be harmful, and the approximate concentrations, in millimoles per litre, of the potassium, sodium, and chloride ions.

POTASSIUM CHLORIDE, SODIUM CHLORIDE, AND DEXTROSE INJECTION: a sterile solution of potassium chloride, sodium chloride, and anhydrous dextrose or the equivalent amount of dextrose monohydrate for parenteral use, in water for injections. It is sterilised, immediately after preparation, by heating in an autoclave. It contains 0.18% of sodium chloride (30 mmol of Na^+ per litre) and 4% of anhydrous dextrose. The usual strengths of potassium chloride are those that provide between 10 and 40 mmol of K^+ per litre. The prescriber should state the strength of potassium chloride required in millimoles per litre.

A standard for this injection is given in the British Pharmacopoeia Addendum 1978

Containers: see the entry on Injections for general information on containers.

Labelling: see the entry on Injections for general information on labelling. In addition, the label on the container should state the amounts of the medicaments as the percentage w/v of potassium chloride, a sodium chloride content of 0.18% w/v, and an anhydrous dextrose content of 4% w/v, the concentration of potassium chloride in grams per litre and the approximate concentration of K^+ in millimoles per litre, a sodium chloride content of 1.8 g per litre equivalent to approximately 30 mmol of Na^+ per litre, the Cl^- content in millimoles per litre, and an anhydrous dextrose content of 40 g per litre.

The label should also state that rapid infusion may be harmful, and that solutions containing visible solid particles must not be used.

Storage: it should be stored at a temperature not exceeding 25°. On storage, separation of small solid particles from glass containers may occur. Solutions containing such particles must not be used.

POTASSIUM CHLORIDE TABLETS: available as tablets containing 500 mg.

A standard for these tablets is given in the British Pharmacopoeia 1973

Containers and *Storage:* see the entry on Tablets for general information on containers and storage. Containers should be airtight.

Labelling: the label on the container should state that the tablets should be dissolved in water before administration.

Advice for patients: the tablets should be taken dissolved in water preferably after meals.

SLOW POTASSIUM CHLORIDE TABLETS: they may be film coated or sugar coated and the coat may be coloured. They contain 600 mg of potassium chloride (providing 8 mmol of K^+) in a slow-release formulation.

Containers and *Storage:* see the entry on Tablets for general information on containers and storage. Containers should be airtight.

Advice for patients: the tablets should be swallowed whole with a tumblerful of water preferably after meals.

STRONG POTASSIUM CHLORIDE SOLUTION:

Potassium chloride	..	..	..	.. 15 g
Water for injections	..	..	..	.. to 100 ml

It is prepared as described in the entry on Solutions. It is distributed into ampoules and sterilised by heating in an autoclave. It contains, in 10 ml, approximately 20 mmol each of K^+ and Cl^-.

A standard for this solution is given in the British Pharmacopoeia 1973

Containers: see the entry on Injections for general information on containers. The solution should be supplied in ampoules which comply with the requirements of the European Pharmacopoeia for Glass Containers for Injectable Preparations.

Labelling: the label on the container should state the amount of the medicament as 20 mmol of K^+ and Cl^-

in 10 ml, and that it must be diluted before use with not less than 50 times its volume of sodium chloride injection or other suitable diluent.

OTHER PREPARATIONS available include an ELIXIR containing potassium chloride 75 mg (1 mmol of K$^+$) per ml; effervescent GRANULES containing potassium chloride 500 mg and potassium bicarbonate 1.35 g equivalent to 1.5 g of potassium chloride (20 mmol of K$^+$) with betaine hydrochloride 2.07 g per sachet; a POWDER containing potassium chloride 50%, with suitable flavouring agents, as a sodium-free "salt" substitute; a powder containing potassium chloride 92%, with suitable flavouring agents, as a sodium-free "salt" substitute; TABLETS containing potassium chloride 750 mg (10 mmol of K$^+$) in a slow-release formulation; and numerous diuretic preparations in which potassium chloride is an ingredient.

Potassium chloride is an ingredient of compound sodium chloride and dextrose powder, compound sodium lactate injection (see under Lactic Acid), haemodialysis solutions, and Ringer's solution for injection.

POTASSIUM CITRATE MIXTURE:

Potassium citrate	300 g
Citric acid monohydrate	50 g
Lemon spirit	5 ml
Quillaia tincture	10 ml
Syrup..	250 ml
Chloroform water, double-strength	300 ml
Water for preparations	to 1000 ml

It should be recently prepared. When a dose less than or not a multiple of 5 ml is prescribed, the mixture may be diluted, as described in the entry on Mixtures, with syrup.

A standard for this mixture is given in the British Pharmaceutical Codex 1973

Containers: see the entry on Mixtures for general information on containers.

Labelling: directions to shake the bottle and to dilute the dose well with water before administration should be given on the label.

Advice for patients: the mixture should be taken well diluted with water.

Potassium Citrate

$C_6H_5K_3O_7,H_2O = 324.4$

OTHER NAMES: Kalii Citras; Pot. Cit.

A standard is given in the European Pharmacopoeia Vol. III Supplement

Description. Odourless, slightly hygroscopic, white crystalline powder or granular crystals, with a fresh saline taste.

Solubility. Soluble, at 20°, in 1 part of water and in 2 parts of glycerol; very slightly soluble in alcohol.

Moisture content. 4 to 7%, determined by Fischer titration.

Storage. It should be stored in airtight containers.

Actions and uses. Potassium citrate has the actions of the alkali citrates and is used principally to make the urine alkaline, as described under Sodium Citrate. It is also a mild diuretic.

The usual dose for an adult is up to 10 grams daily in divided doses. Children under 1 year may be given 750 milligrams, 1 to 5 years 1.5 grams, and 6 to 12 years 3 grams; these doses may be given 3 times daily.

Preparations

POTASSIUM CITRATE AND HYOSCYAMUS MIXTURE:

Potassium citrate	300 g
Hyoscyamus tincture	200 ml
Citric acid monohydrate	50 g
Lemon spirit	5 ml
Quillaia tincture	10 ml
Syrup..	250 ml
Chloroform water, double-strength	200 ml
Water for preparations	to 1000 ml

It must be freshly prepared.

Containers: see the entry on Mixtures for general information on containers.

Labelling: directions to shake the bottle and to dilute the dose well with water before administration should be given on the label.

Dose: 10 millilitres, well diluted with water.

Potassium Gluconate

$$
\begin{array}{c}
\text{COO·K} \\
|\\
\text{HCOH} \\
|\\
\text{HOCH} \\
|\\
\text{HCOH} \\
|\\
\text{HCOH} \\
|\\
\text{CH}_2\text{OH}
\end{array}
$$

$C_6H_{11}KO_7 = 234.2$

OTHER NAME: *Katorin*®

A standard is given in the British Pharmaceutical Codex 1973

Description. An odourless white crystalline powder.

Solubility. Soluble, at 20°, in 3 parts of water; very slightly soluble in alcohol; practically insoluble in chloroform and in ether.

Moisture content. Not more than 2%, determined by drying at 105°.

Actions and uses. Potassium gluconate is almost tasteless and is therefore convenient for the oral administration of potassium supplements to patients undergoing diuretic therapy when there is danger of potassium depletion.

The usual dose is 5 to 10 grams (20 to 40 millimoles, or milliequivalents, of K$^+$).

Preparations

Preparations available include an ELIXIR containing potassium gluconate 3.3 g (14 mmol of K$^+$) in 10 ml.

Potassium Hydroxide

$KOH = 56.11$

OTHER NAME: Caustic Potash

A standard is given in the British Pharmacopoeia 1973

Potassium hydroxide is strongly alkaline and corrosive

and rapidly destroys organic tissues. It may be freed from carbonate by solution in alcohol, filtration, and evaporation.

Description. White sticks, pellets, or fused masses, which are dry, hard, and brittle, very deliquescent, and break with a crystalline fracture.

Solubility. Soluble, or almost completely soluble, in 1 part of water and in 3 parts of alcohol; very soluble in boiling dehydrated alcohol.

Hygroscopicity. When exposed to the air, it absorbs moisture and carbon dioxide.

Storage. It should be stored in airtight containers; if the containers are made of glass they should be closed by waxed corks or plastic-lined screw caps.

Actions and uses. Potassium hydroxide is a powerful caustic. A 2.5% solution in glycerol is used as a cuticle solvent.

Poisoning. Large draughts of water, or water containing vinegar, acetic acid, citric acid, or lemon juice should be given immediately, and followed by demulcent drinks and olive oil or arachis oil.
Burns due to potassium hydroxide should be flooded with water and then with dilute acetic acid.

Preparation

POTASSIUM HYDROXIDE SOLUTION (*Syn.* Potash Solution): an aqueous solution of potassium hydroxide. It contains 5% of total alkali, calculated as KOH.
A standard for this solution is given in the British Pharmacopoeia 1973
Storage: it should be stored in airtight containers of lead-free glass or of a suitable plastic.

Potassium Iodide

$KI = 166.0$

OTHER NAMES: Kalii Iodidum; Pot. Iod.
Chibret Iodo-chloride Collyrium® (with calcium chloride)

A standard is given in the European Pharmacopoeia Vol. I

Description. Odourless colourless crystals or white powder.

Solubility. Soluble, at 20°, in less than 1 part of water, in 23 parts of alcohol, and in 2 parts of glycerol.

Aqueous solutions. A marked fall in the temperature of the solution occurs when potassium iodide dissolves in water to form a strong solution; when sodium iodide dissolves a considerable rise in temperature occurs. Iodine readily dissolves in an aqueous solution of potassium iodide, forming a dark-brown solution containing potassium tri-iodide. Certain iodides, such as mercuric iodide, which are insoluble in water, also dissolve in an aqueous solution, double iodides being formed.

Alkalinity. Aqueous solutions may be slightly alkaline.

Moisture content. Not more than 1%, determined by drying at 105°.

Incompatibility. It is incompatible with salts of iron, bismuth, mercury, with potassium chlorate and other oxidising agents, and with strychnine hydrochloride, quinine sulphate, and other alkaloidal salts.

Storage. It should be stored in airtight containers, protected from light.

Actions and uses. Potassium iodide is rapidly absorbed

when given by mouth and is rapidly excreted, mainly by the kidneys but partly by the salivary, mucous, and other glands. Its secretion by the salivary glands is the cause of the persistent unpleasant taste.
It may be used for the prophylaxis and treatment of simple goitre, which is endemic in districts where the diet is deficient in iodides.
Potassium iodide is used in the pre-operative treatment of thyrotoxicosis in a dosage of 15 milligrams daily in divided doses. It is administered by mouth for 10 to 14 days prior to surgical operation on the thyroid in order to produce a firm texture suitable for operation. This treatment need not be given post-operatively and should not be continued for more than 3 weeks.
Potassium iodide has also been used as an expectorant. The usual dose for adults is 250 to 500 milligrams and for children 50 to 100 milligrams.
Potassium iodide is usually administered in mixtures or in solution, freely diluted, since concentrated solutions have an irritant action on the gastric mucosa.

Undesirable effects. Intolerance to iodides sometimes occurs, the symptoms being nasal catarrh, lachrymation, rashes of variable character, headache, and depression. Some patients showing idiosyncrasy to small doses appear to tolerate larger doses.

Precautions. Potassium iodide should not be administered during pregnancy and its use should be avoided in nursing mothers. It interferes with tests for thyroid function.

Veterinary uses. Potassium iodide is used in the treatment of actinobacillosis in cattle, the usual dose by mouth being up to 20 milligrams per kilogram body-weight twice daily. For the prevention and treatment of iodine deficiency it may be included in the diet at a dosage of 1 milligram per kilogram body-weight daily.

Preparations

Preparations available include EYE-DROPS containing potassium iodide 0.5% with calcium chloride 0.5%.
Potassium iodide is an ingredient of paediatric belladonna and ephedrine mixture.

Potassium Permanganate

$KMnO_4 = 158.0$

OTHER NAMES: Kalii Permanganas; Pot. Permang.

A standard is given in the European Pharmacopoeia Vol. II

Description. Dark purple or almost black crystals, often with a metallic lustre.

Solubility. Soluble, at 20°, in 16 parts of water.

Incompatibility. It is incompatible with iodides, reducing agents, and most organic matter.
An acidified solution in water is readily reduced by hydrogen peroxide, by easily oxidisable substances, and by organic matter.

Storage. It should be stored so as to avoid contact with organic substances.

Actions and uses. Potassium permanganate, because of its oxidising action, possesses disinfectant and deodorant properties. It is used as a 1 in 1000 solution in water as a cleansing application to ulcers or abscesses, 1 in 4000 as a gargle, mouth-wash, or vaginal irrigation, and 1 in 10000 to 1 in 5000 for application to weeping skin lesions and for urethral irrigation.
Potassium permanganate has been widely used as a

first-aid treatment in snake bite but it is of no value for this purpose although a solution will destroy any venom on the surface of the skin.

Solutions of potassium permanganate rapidly stain the skin brown; the stain can be removed by means of a dilute solution of oxalic or sulphurous acid.

Preparation

POTASSIUM PERMANGANATE SOLUTION:

Potassium permanganate .. .. 1 g
Water for preparations .. .. .. to 1000 ml

It must be freshly prepared. For application to weeping lesions or as a urethral irrigation it should be diluted with 7 times its volume of warm water before use. The diluted solution contains about 1 in 8000 of potassium permanganate.

Labelling: directions for diluting the solution should be given on the label.

Advice for patients: it should be diluted before use (see above). The solution stains the skin, hair, and fabric. The stain can be removed by washing with a dilute solution of oxalic acid or sulphurous acid.

Potassium Selenate

$K_2SeO_4 = 221.2$

OTHER NAME: *Dystosel*®

A standard is given in the British Pharmacopoeia (Veterinary)

Description. Odourless colourless crystals or white crystalline powder.

Solubility. Soluble, at 20°, in 1 part of water.

Veterinary uses. Potassium selenate is used in conjunction with alpha tocopheryl acetate in the prevention and treatment of vitamin-E deficiencies, particularly nutritional myopathies of young cattle and sheep. The usual dose by intramuscular injection for calves is 50 to 150 micrograms per kilogram body-weight and for lambs 10 to 30 micrograms per kilogram body-weight. These doses may be repeated if necessary after 2 to 4 weeks.

Preparations

Preparations available include a veterinary INJECTION containing potassium selenate equivalent to 1.5 mg of selenium with alpha tocopheryl acetate 68 units per ml in 50-ml vials.

Potassium Sorbate

Potassium 2,4-hexadienoate

$C_6H_7KO_2 = 150.2$

OTHER NAME: *Sorbistat-K*®

A standard is given in the British Pharmaceutical Codex 1973

Description. A white or creamy-white powder with a faint characteristic odour.

Solubility. Soluble, at 20°, in less than 1 part of water and in 70 parts of alcohol; very slightly soluble in acetone.

Moisture content. Not more than 1%, determined by Fischer titration.

Storage. It should be stored in airtight containers, protected from light, in a cool place.

Identification. ULTRAVIOLET ABSORPTION. In 0.01N hydrochloric acid, maximum at 264 nm (E1%, 1cm = 1780).

INFRA-RED ABSORPTION. Major peaks at 1005, 1386, 1397, 1550, 1602, and 1616 cm^{-1} (see Appendix 2a: Infra-red Spectra).

Uses. Potassium sorbate has the uses described under Sorbic Acid but it is more soluble in water.

Poultices

Poultices are thick pasty preparations, usually intended to be made extemporaneously for application to the skin with the object of reducing inflammation and allaying pain.

Povidone

Povidone is the pharmaceutical grade of polyvinylpyrrolidone, and consists of essentially linear polymers of 1-vinylpyrrolid-2-one. Variation in the degree of polymerisation results in the production of polymers with different chain lengths and consequently various molecular weights.

Polyvinylpyrrolidone is available commercially as a number of mixtures of polymers, each product having a particular mean molecular weight in the range 10000 to 700000.

$(C_6H_9NO)_n = 111.1 \times n$

OTHER NAMES: *Kollidon*®; *Plasdone*®; Polyvinylpyrrolidone; P.V.P.

A standard for non-injectable povidone is given in the British Pharmaceutical Codex 1973

Description. An odourless white or creamy-white powder.

Solubility. It is soluble in water, in a wide range of alcohols, aldehydes and ketones, amines, in ethylene glycol, and in certain chlorinated hydrocarbons, the solubility depending on the mean molecular weight; it is practically insoluble in most common hydrocarbons and ethers.

Viscosity of solutions. The viscosities of solutions increase with increasing molecular weight of the polymer, although the viscosities of aqueous solutions containing up to 10% of many grades do not differ significantly from water. The viscosity of solutions is not influenced by pH except in extreme cases; concentrated hydrochloric acid increases the viscosity but strong alkali will precipitate the polymer which redissolves on the addition of water. The viscosity of solutions decreases significantly with increase in temperature.

Povidone is often commercially designated with a "K number". This is a figure derived from the viscosity using the expression

$$\log Z = \frac{75k^2}{1+1.5k} + k$$

where Z = the relative viscosity defined as the flow time

in an Ostwald tube for a 1% solution divided by the flow time in the same tube for water. The K number = 1000*k*.

Moisture content. Not more than 5%, determined by Fischer titration.

Stability. Aqueous solutions of povidone are stable and can be stored for long periods in suitable containers. Such solutions should, however, be protected from moulds. The usual preservatives such as benzoic acid and hydroxybenzoate esters are suitable.

Hygroscopicity. Povidone is hygroscopic, significant amounts of moisture being absorbed even at low relative humidities; its equilibrium moisture content at 30, 50, and 70% relative humidity is 10, 20, and 40%, respectively.

Storage. It should be stored in airtight containers.

Identification. TESTS. 1. To 10 ml of a 2% solution add 20 ml of 1N hydrochloric acid and 5 ml of *potassium dichromate solution*; an orange-yellow precipitate is produced.
2. Add 5 ml of a 2% solution to 2 ml of *ammonium cobaltothiocyanate solution* which has been acidified with 5N hydrochloric acid; a pale blue precipitate is produced.
3. To 5 ml of a 0.5% solution add 4 drops of 0.1N iodine; a deep red colour is produced.

Metabolism. DISTRIBUTION. The higher molecular weight forms are stored in reticulo-endothelial tissues after injection.

METABOLIC REACTIONS. Does not appear to be metabolised after injection.

EXCRETION. The lower molecular weight forms are excreted in the urine and 60 to 70% of a dose is excreted in 1 to 3 days; small amounts are excreted in the faeces.

Uses. Povidone is used in concentrations up to 10% as a suspending and dispersing agent. It is also used in tablets as a binding, granulating, and film-coating agent, and for dispersing dyes in coloured tablets.
Povidone gives good adhesion for granulation and compression, but is readily soluble in water so that disintegration time is not increased. It can also be used in non-aqueous solutions as a granulating agent. The usual proportion of povidone required in granulation is 0.5 to 5%. The povidone in solution is added in small portions to the dry ingredients, mixing continuously, until the powder is uniformly coated. Alternatively, the povidone may be mixed in the dry state with the other ingredients and the mixture moistened with water or other solvent, or added to the moistened ingredients. 1 to 2% of povidone, dissolved in alcohol is used as an aid to the granulation of very light powders for the preparation of capsules.
Povidone is used for film coating tablets in conjunction with plasticisers such as macrogols, dimethyl, diethyl, and dibutyl phthalates, isopropyl myristate, polyvinyl alcohol, and glyceryl mono-oleate. A cross-linked insoluble polyvinylpyrrolidone is used as a tablet disintegrant.

Povidone-Iodine Solution

An aqueous solution of povidone-iodine, a complex produced by the interaction between iodine and polyvinylpyrrolidone. It contains 1% of available iodine, equivalent to about 10% of povidone-iodine.

OTHER NAMES: *Betadine*®; *Disadine*®; *Pevidine*®

A standard is given in the British Pharmacopoeia

Addendum 1977 and in the British Pharmacopoeia (Veterinary)

Description. A deep brown liquid with a characteristic odour.

Acidity. pH 3 to 5.5.

Storage. It should be stored in airtight containers, the materials of which are resistant to iodine.

Identification. TESTS. 1. Dilute 1 ml to 20 ml with water and to 1 ml of the dilution add a mixture of 1 ml of *starch mucilage* and 9 ml of water; a deep blue colour is produced.
2. Place 10 ml in a small flask and cover the mouth of the flask with filter paper moistened with starch mucilage; no blue colour develops on the paper within 1 minute.
3. Dilute 2 ml to 10 ml with water and add 0.1N sodium thiosulphate, dropwise, until the colour of the iodine is discharged. To 5 ml of this solution add 10 ml of 1N hydrochloric acid and 5 ml of *potassium dichromate solution*; a red precipitate is produced. To the remainder of the solution add 2 ml of *ammonium cobaltothiocyanate solution* which has been acidified with 5N hydrochloric acid; a blue precipitate is produced.

Uses. Povidone-iodine is an iodophore with a prolonged antibacterial and antifungal action due to the gradual release of iodine; it lacks the stinging and pronounced staining properties of iodine solutions.
A 10% solution is used for cleansing wounds and contaminated skin surfaces, and a 7.5% detergent solution is used in pre-operative scrubbing and disinfection of the surgeon's hands. Minor cuts or burns may be treated with an ointment containing 10% or a protective film formed from an aerosol spray containing 5%. A 1% solution is used as a mouth-wash and gargle for the treatment of infections of the mouth and throat.
Povidone-iodine is also used as pessaries containing 200 milligrams or a vaginal solution containing 10% for the treatment of vaginal candidiasis.

Precautions and contra-indications. It should not be used in patients who are hypersensitive to iodides. Application to large areas of broken skin should be avoided as excessive absorption of iodine may occur.

Preparations

Preparations available include an APPLICATION containing povidone-iodine 5% in an aerosol pack, an application containing povidone-iodine 4%, an application containing povidone-iodine 7.5%, an application containing povidone-iodine 4% with hydrous wool fat; a GARGLE and MOUTH-WASH containing povidone-iodine 1%; a GEL containing povidone-iodine 10%; an OINTMENT containing 10% of povidone-iodine; a PAINT containing povidone-iodine 10%; PESSARIES containing povidone-iodine 200 mg; a SOLUTION containing povidone-iodine equivalent to 0.75% of iodine, a solution containing povidone-iodine 10%; and a TINCTURE containing povidone-iodine equivalent to 1% of iodine.

Powders

OTHER NAME: Oral Powders

Powders are mixtures of powdered substances intended for administration by mouth. They are usually mixed with water before administration, but some oral powders for veterinary use are administered by mixing with animal rations. They consist of a powdered medicinal substance, or a mixture of powdered medicinal substances, sometimes with the addition of adjuvants such as diluents and dispersing agents.

Preparation of powders. Powders may be prepared by mixing the medicinal substance or substances, specified in the smallest quantity with gradually increasing quantities of the remaining material. After mixing, the product should be passed through a sieve of suitable mesh, usually No. 250, and triturated lightly, as partial separation of the ingredients may have occurred.

When the quantity of an ingredient is less than 60 milligrams or is such that it cannot be weighed conveniently on a dispensing balance, a suitable trituration is prepared by admixture with lactose or other suitable inert diluent, and a proportionately larger quantity of the triturate is weighed.

When a small quantity of a potent medicament is ordered by itself as a powder, it should be diluted by trituration with an amount of an inert diluent such as lactose so that the weight of the triturate to be taken as a dose is 120 milligrams: the triturate should then be supplied, suitably wrapped, as single doses. Powders are sometimes supplied in bulk with a direction to administer a given volume, such as a teaspoonful, as a dose. This method of presentation is unsuitable for powders containing potent ingredients as the dose varies according to the bulk density of the powder; in such cases doses should be individually weighed and wrapped as described above.

Effervescent powders dissolve with effervescence in water. They are intended to be dissolved in a tumblerful of water before administration.

Dispersible powders for veterinary use consist of the active ingredients, usually finely powdered, mixed with suitable non-toxic wetting, dispersing, or suspending agents. When stirred with water they mix readily, without persistent frothing, to form uniform suspensions which, if they separate on standing, do so only slowly, and are easily re-dispersed. They are used in preparing suspensions (drenches) for oral administration to animals.

Soluble powders for veterinary use are used to prepare medicated drinking water for administration to animals. This form of treatment is convenient for large flocks or herds.

Containers and storage. When dispensed for use in human medicine, powders should preferably be stored and supplied in white plain glass powder-jars with close-fitting lids. Deliquescent or volatile powders supplied as single doses should be doubly wrapped, the inner wrapper consisting of waxed or parchment paper; in exceptional cases, the wrapped powder should be enclosed in metal foil.

Individually wrapped powders should be enclosed in cartons or rigid slide boxes of paperboard or plastic material.

Powders, Particle Size and Classification of

The degree of comminution of a powder may be defined by means of a sieve number, indicating that the whole of the powder passes through the sieve described by that number. The numbers by which sieves are designated indicate the nominal aperture size, measured in millimetres for aperture sizes of 1 mm or greater and in micrometres (μm) for aperture sizes of less than 1 mm.

Such sieves comply with the requirements of British Standard 410: 1969.

Formerly, sieves were designated by the mesh count or mesh number which was the number of meshes per inch. The table below relates the sieve numbers now used to the mesh numbers formerly used. The relationship of the mesh number to the actual number of meshes per inch depends on the wire diameter and should be taken as an approximation.

Sieve number	Mesh number	Sieve number	Mesh number
mm		μm	
4.00	4	355	44
3.35	5	250	60
2.80	6	180	85
1.70	10	150	100
μm		125	120
710	22	106	150
500	30	75	200

Descriptive terms are used to indicate the degree of comminution of substances employed in the manufacture of pharmaceutical preparations, and these terms are defined as follows:

COARSE POWDER. A powder of which all the particles pass through a No. 1.70 sieve and not more than 40% pass through a No. 355 sieve.

MODERATELY COARSE POWDER. A powder of which all the particles pass through a No. 710 sieve and not more than 40% pass through a No. 250 sieve.

MODERATELY FINE POWDER. A powder of which all the particles pass through a No. 355 sieve and not more than 40% pass through a No. 180 sieve.

FINE POWDER. A powder of which all the particles pass through a No. 180 sieve.

VERY FINE POWDER. A powder of which all the particles pass through a No. 125 sieve.

ULTRA-FINE POWDER. A powder of which the maximum diameter of 90% of the particles is not greater than 5 μm and of which the diameter of none of the particles is greater than 50 μm.

Powders for Mixtures

Powders for mixtures are prepared by mixing together, by the general method described in the entry on Powders, the solid ingredients of mixtures in the proportions in which they occur in the preparations. Powders for mixtures may be in bulk, from which the appropriate quantity of powder is weighed in one operation, or in packs each containing sufficient powder for preparing a given volume of mixture.

There is a possibility of segregation of the constituents if powders for mixtures are stored for long periods or subjected to mechanical vibration. Care should therefore be taken to ensure homogeneity of powders for mixtures stored in bulk before weighing.

Labelling. The label on the container should state: (1) that the powder is for use in preparing a mixture; (2) the name of the mixture; and (3) the names and quantities of the remaining ingredients to be added to the powder in order to prepare the mixture.

Formulae for powders for mixtures are given under Kaolin, Magnesium Carbonate, and Magnesium Trisilicate.

Practolol

4'-(2-Hydroxy-3-isopropylaminopropoxy)acetanilide

$$NH \cdot CO \cdot CH_3$$

$$O \cdot CH_2 \cdot CH \cdot CH_2 \cdot NH \cdot CH(CH_3)_2$$
$$OH$$

$C_{14}H_{22}N_2O_3 = 266.3$

OTHER NAME: *Eraldin®*

A standard is given in the British Pharmacopoeia 1973

Description. An odourless fine white powder with a bitter taste.

Solubility. Soluble in 400 parts of water, in 40 parts of alcohol, and in 200 parts of chloroform.

Dissociation constant. pK_a 9.5 (20°).

Stability of solutions. Aqueous solutions are most stable at pH 6, and such solutions may be sterilised by heating in an autoclave and stored at room temperature, protected from light.

Hygroscopicity. It absorbs insignificant amounts of moisture at 25° at relative humidities up to about 80%.

Storage. It should be protected from light.

Identification. MELTING-POINT. About 142°.

ULTRAVIOLET ABSORPTION. In methyl alcohol, maximum at 248 nm (E1%, 1cm = 620).

INFRA-RED ABSORPTION. Major peaks at 820, 1241, 1296, 1508, 1527, and 1653 cm^{-1} (see Appendix 2a: Infra-red Spectra).

Determination in body fluids. SPECTROFLUORIMETRY. In blood or urine—G. Bodem and C. A. Chidsey, *Clin. Chem.*, 1972, **18**, 363.

GAS CHROMATOGRAPHY. In plasma or urine—J. P. Desager and C. Harvengt, *J. Pharm. Pharmac.*, 1975, **27**, 52.

Metabolism. ABSORPTION. Readily absorbed after oral administration.

BLOOD CONCENTRATION. Peak plasma concentrations are attained in 1 to 2 hours and after oral doses of 200, 400, and 800 mg reach 1 to 2 μg/ml, 1 to 3 μg/ml, and 4.5 to 6 μg/ml respectively; after an intravenous dose, concentrations at 1 to 2 hours are similar; after an intramuscular dose of 40 mg, a peak plasma concentration of about 0.8 μg/ml is attained in 1 hour; the peak concentration after oral administration to subjects with coeliac disease is delayed.

HALF-LIFE. Plasma half-life, 7 to 13 hours.

DISTRIBUTION. Rapidly distributed following intravenous administration; volume of distribution, about 1.7 litres/kg body-weight; *protein binding*, does not appear to be significantly bound to plasma proteins.

METABOLIC REACTIONS. Very little appears to be metabolised; in rats and dogs, about 9% is hydroxylated and about 4% is deacetylated.

EXCRETION. About 90% is excreted unchanged in urine in 24 hours; the urinary excretion of practolol is unaffected by changes in urinary pH.

FURTHER INFORMATION. Blood concentrations and effect on heart—S. G. Carruthers *et al.*, *Clin. Pharmac. Ther.*, 1974, **15**, 497, M. F. Cuthbert and R. F. Collins, *Br. J. clin. Pharmac.*, 1975, **2**, 49, and D. W. Schneck *et al.*, *Clin. Pharmac. Ther.*, 1972, **13**, 685; pharmacokinetics—G. Bodem and C. A. Chidsey, *Clin. Pharmac. Ther.*, 1973, **14**, 26; plasma concentrations in coeliac disease—R. L. Parsons and C. M. Kaye, *Br. J. clin. Pharmac.*, 1974, **1**, 348P.

Actions and uses. Practolol has actions similar to those described under Propranolol Hydrochloride but is more specific in inhibiting sympathetic stimulation of the heart and has less effect on respiratory function. It is therefore less likely to precipitate bronchospasm. Owing to the serious nature of its side effects practolol has been replaced by alternative beta-adrenergic blocking agents. It is not recommended for long-term therapy and is mainly used for emergency treatment of cardiac arrhythmias. The usual dose is 5 to 20 milligrams, according to the response of the patient, by slow intravenous injection.

Undesirable effects. These are described under Propranolol Hydrochloride. In addition rashes, diminished tear secretion, conjunctivitis, and sclerosing peritonitis may occur.

Preparation

PRACTOLOL INJECTION: a sterile solution of practolol, with citric acid, in water for injections. The acidity of the solution is adjusted to pH 6 by the addition of sodium hydroxide. It is sterilised by heating in an autoclave or by filtration. Available in 5-ml ampoules containing 2 mg of practolol per ml.

A standard for this injection is given in the British Pharmacopoeia 1973

Containers and *Labelling*: see the entry on Injections for general information on containers and labelling.

Pralidoxime Chloride

2-Hydroxyiminomethyl-1-methylpyridinium chloride

$$CH_3$$
$$N^+ \quad CH:N \cdot OH \quad Cl^-$$

$C_7H_9ClN_2O = 172.6$

Description. An odourless, white to pale yellow, crystalline powder.

Solubility. Soluble in 2 parts of water and in 100 parts of alcohol.

Acidity. A 1% solution has a pH of about 4.6.

Moisture content. Not more than 2%, determined by drying at 105°.

Identification. TESTS. 1. To 2 drops of a 20% solution add 1 ml of a 0.6% solution of ferric chloride; an amber-brown colour is produced.
2. To 0.5 ml of 2N sodium hydroxide add 1 ml of a 20% solution of the sample; a bright yellow colour is produced. The colour change is reversed by acidification with hydrochloric acid.

MELTING-POINT. About 220°, with decomposition.

ULTRAVIOLET ABSORPTION. In 0.1N hydrochloric acid, maxima at 242 nm and 292 nm; in 0.1N sodium hydroxide, maximum at 332 nm and an inflection at 280 nm.

Determination in body fluids. ULTRAVIOLET SPECTRO-PHOTOMETRY. In plasma or urine—J. R. May et al., J. pharm. Sci., 1965, **54**, 1508.

Actions and uses. Pralidoxime is a reactivator of cholinesterases which is used in conjunction with atropine in the treatment of poisoning by organophosphorus compounds with anticholinesterase activity. The effects of accumulated acetylcholine are reversed by the injection of atropine sulphate as described under Atropine, the administration of the atropine sulphate being repeated as necessary to maintain the reversal.

After initial atropinisation pralidoxime is given by intramuscular or slow intravenous injection or infusion of a solution of the mesylate in doses of 1 to 2 grams and the treatment repeated once or twice as necessary until the cholinesterases are fully reactivated and further treatment with atropine is not required. The usual dose of pralidoxime for children is 20 to 40 milligrams per kilogram body-weight.

Pralidoxime is effective in poisoning by many organophosphorus compounds but not against carbamate pesticides. It is ineffective when given 24 hours after exposure to an organophosphorus compound. Its effect should preferably be monitored by determinations of the blood cholinesterase concentration.

Undesirable effects. Pralidoxime may give rise to drowsiness, nausea, headache, dizziness, visual disturbances, tachycardia, hyperventilation, and muscular weakness. Large doses may cause transient neuromuscular blockade.

Supplies of pralidoxime chloride are available in the United Kingdom at certain hospitals; information on the availability of pralidoxime chloride and its suitability for the treatment of individual cases is available from the poisons information centres listed in the entry on Poisoning.

Prednisolone

11β,17α,21-Trihydroxypregna-1,4-diene-3,20-dione

$C_{21}H_{28}O_5 = 360.4$

OTHER NAMES: *Codelcortone®*; *Delta-Cortef®*; *Deltacortril Enteric®*; *Deltalone®*; *Delta Phoricol®*; *Deltastab®*; *Marsolone®*; *PreCortisyl®*; *Prednisolonum*; *Prednivet®* *Cordex-Forte®* (with aspirin); *Otopred®* (with chloramphenicol); *Dexolone®* (with dexamethasone acetate); *Opticortenol-S®* (with dexamethasone pivalate)

A standard is given in the European Pharmacopoeia Vol. II

Description. An odourless, hygroscopic, white, crystalline powder.

Solubility. Very slightly soluble in water; soluble, at 20°, in 27 parts of dehydrated alcohol; soluble in dioxan and in methyl alcohol.

Moisture content. Not more than 1%, determined by drying at 105°.

Specific rotation. +96° to +102°, determined on a 1% solution in dioxan.

Preparation of solid dosage forms. In order to achieve a satisfactory rate of dissolution, prednisolone in the form of an ultra-fine powder should be used.

Storage. It should be stored in airtight containers, protected from light.

Identification. TESTS. 1. It complies with Test 1 described under Betamethasone.
2. Dissolve about 200 μg in 1 ml of sulphuric acid; a wine-red colour is produced. Allow to stand for 1 minute and expose to ultraviolet radiation; the solution exhibits a deep yellow fluorescence.

MELTING-POINT. About 230°, with decomposition.

ULTRAVIOLET ABSORPTION. In alcohol (95%), maximum at 240 nm (E1%, 1cm = 415).

INFRA-RED ABSORPTION. Major peaks at 890, 1112, 1599, 1615, 1654, and 1708 cm^{-1} (see Appendix 2a: Infra-red Spectra).

THIN-LAYER CHROMATOGRAPHY. See under Thin-layer Chromatography, System 10.

Metabolism. ABSORPTION. Absorbed after oral administration.

HALF-LIFE. Biological half-life, about 3 hours.

DISTRIBUTION. *Protein binding*, about 50% bound to plasma proteins.

METABOLIC REACTIONS. Reduction to 20β-dihydroprednisolone, 20β-dihydroprednisone and hydrocortisone and conjugation occur to some extent.

EXCRETION. About 10 to 30% of a dose is excreted in the urine as unchanged prednisolone and the remainder as metabolites, 60 to 80% of which is conjugated; a dose is almost completely excreted in 3 days. Prednisolone is excreted in milk in insignificant amounts.

Actions and uses. Prednisolone has the actions and uses described under Cortisone Acetate but it is effective in about one-fifth to one-quarter of the dosage; in such dosage it has a weaker sodium-retaining effect than cortisone.

It is used especially for its anti-inflammatory action in the treatment of conditions where a cortisone-like action is required and, because of its weaker sodium-retaining action, it is usually to be preferred to cortisone in such conditions as rheumatoid arthritis, rheumatic fever, status asthmaticus, and ulcerative colitis. It is useful in the treatment of nephrotic oedema, as it produces diuresis. It is not used alone in the treatment of adrenal-deficiency states because of its weak salt-retaining effect.

Prednisolone is given by mouth, the dosage being adjusted to the needs of the patient and varying widely according to the disorder being treated.

In rheumatoid arthritis a single dose of 5 milligrams given by mouth at night will often ease night and early morning symptoms. For long-term suppressive treatment of rheumatoid arthritis the minimum dosage giving a satisfactory response should be used; not more than 7 milligrams daily should be given as otherwise the usual undesirable effects of long-term corticosteroid therapy will inevitably occur.

A somewhat higher regular maintenance dosage is usually necessary in the treatment of asthma, and prednisolone is also used in large daily doses such as 100 to 200 milligrams as an immunosuppressive agent for organ transplantation. In addition, single large doses such as 1 gram have been given intravenously in the form of soluble prednisolone compounds to prevent organ rejection after renal transplantation.

In conditions dangerous to life, such as pemphigus vulgaris, systemic lupus erythematosus, leukaemia, and acute haemolytic crises, high dosage, if necessary up to 100 milligrams daily, is permissible. In conditions such as status asthmaticus up to 60 milligrams daily may be given, although in severe crises intravenous administration of hydrocortisone or corticotrophin may be preferred.

Undesirable effects. These are the same as those described under Cortisone Acetate, the features of Cushing's syndrome becoming apparent on full dosage. Dyspepsia is common and peptic ulceration may occur.

Precautions and contra-indications. As for Cortisone Acetate.

Veterinary uses. Prednisolone is a glucocorticoid used to reduce inflammatory reactions especially dermatitis and tenosynovitis. The usual dose by mouth for all species is 250 to 500 micrograms per kilogram bodyweight 3 times a day. Prednisolone is also used in the treatment of bovine ketosis; the usual dose by intramuscular injection is 50 to 200 milligrams.

Preparations

PREDNISOLONE TABLETS: available as tablets containing 1 and 5 mg of prednisolone.
A standard for these tablets is given in the British Pharmacopoeia 1973
Containers and *Storage:* see the entry on Tablets for general information on containers and storage. Containers should be airtight and light resistant.
Advice for patients: in long-term use, treatment should not be discontinued without the advice of the prescriber. Patients may carry an identification card giving details of their treatment and the name of the prescriber, who should be contacted in the event of accident, feverish illness, diarrhoea, vomiting or alimentary disturbances. In short-term treatment, the prescribed course should be completed.

OTHER PREPARATIONS available include EAR-DROPS containing prednisolone 0.25% with chloramphenicol 1%; a veterinary INJECTION containing prednisolone 3 mg with dexamethasone acetate 1 mg per ml in 50-ml vials; a veterinary injection containing prednisolone 7.5 mg with dexamethasone pivalate 2.5 mg per ml in 20-ml vials; TABLETS (enteric coated) containing prednisolone 2.5 and 5 mg; and tablets containing prednisolone 1.5 mg with aspirin 300 mg.

Prednisolone Pivalate

$11\beta,17\alpha,21$-Trihydroxypregna-1,4-diene-3,20-dione 21-pivalate

$C_{26}H_{36}O_6 = 444.6$

OTHER NAMES: Prednisolone Trimethylacetate; *Ultracortenol*®; *Vecortenol*®

A standard is given in the British Pharmacopoeia 1973

Description. An odourless white crystalline powder.

Solubility. Very slightly soluble in water; soluble, at 20°, in 150 parts of alcohol and in 16 parts of chloroform.

Storage. It should be stored in airtight containers, protected from light.

Identification. TEST. It complies with Test 1 described under Betamethasone.

MELTING-POINT. About 229°.

INFRA-RED ABSORPTION. Major peaks at 1148, 1162, 1618, 1657, 1724, and 1740 cm^{-1} (see Appendix 2a: Infra-red Spectra).

THIN-LAYER CHROMATOGRAPHY. See under Thin-layer Chromatography, System 10.

Actions and uses. Prednisolone pivalate may be given as a microcrystalline suspension by intra-articular injection in rheumatoid and other forms of arthritis to reduce swelling and facilitate movement. For this purpose, 5 to 20 milligrams is given by intra-articular injection or by local infiltration.

Suspensions for injection are prepared by an aseptic technique.

Precautions and contra-indications. As for Cortisone Acetate.

Preparation

PREDNISOLONE PIVALATE INJECTION: a sterile suspension of prednisolone pivalate, in very fine particles, with suitable dispersing, stabilising, and buffering agents, in water for injections. It is prepared by means of an aseptic technique. Available in 1-ml ampoules containing 50 mg of prednisolone pivalate. Also available in 50-ml vials containing prednisolone pivalate 10 mg per ml.
A standard for this injection is given in the British Pharmacopoeia 1973
Containers: see the entry on Injections for general information on containers.
Labelling: see the entry on Injections for general information on labelling. In addition, the label on the container should state "For local injection only".
Storage: it should be stored at room temperature, protected from light.

Prednisolone Sodium Phosphate

Disodium 11β,17α,21-trihydroxypregna-1,4-diene-3,20-
dione 21-phosphate

$C_{21}H_{27}Na_2O_8P = 484.4$

OTHER NAMES: *Codelsol®*; *Prednesol®*; Prednisolone
Sod. Phos.; *Predsol®*
Predsol-N® (with neomycin sulphate)

A standard is given in the British Pharmacopoeia 1973

Description. An odourless hygroscopic white powder.

Solubility. Soluble, at 20°, in 3 parts of water and
in 1000 parts of alcohol; practically insoluble in
chloroform.

Alkalinity. A 0.5% solution has a pH of 7.5 to 9.

Moisture content. Not more than 8%, determined by
Fischer titration.

Specific rotation. +94° to +100°, determined on a 1%
solution.

Stability. Aqueous solutions having a pH of about 8.0
are stable if protected from light. Particular care must
be taken to prevent microbial contamination of the
solutions so as to avoid hydrolysis of the ester by
phosphatase which is a common product of microbial
metabolism.

Sterilisation. Solutions for injection are sterilised by
filtration.

Storage. It should be stored in airtight containers,
protected from light.

Identification. TEST. Dissolve about 2 mg in 2 ml of
sulphuric acid and allow to stand for 5 minutes; a wine-red
colour is produced (distinction from betamethasone
sodium phosphate).

ULTRAVIOLET ABSORPTION. In alcohol (95%), maximum
at 241 nm (E1%, 1cm = 282); in water, maximum at
247 nm (E1%, 1cm = 312).

INFRA-RED ABSORPTION. Major peaks at 990, 1059, 1114,
1600, 1614, and 1658 cm⁻¹ (see Appendix 2a: Infra-red
Spectra).

Actions and uses. Prednisolone sodium phosphate has
the actions, uses, and undesirable effects described
under Prednisolone. It is soluble in water and is used
in eye-drops and other preparations for topical therapy
in inflammatory or allergic conditions of the eye or skin.
It may be given by intravenous injection, in a dose
equivalent to 20 to 100 milligrams of prednisolone, when
a more rapid effect is required; 135 milligrams of prednisolone sodium phosphate is approximately equivalent
to 100 milligrams of prednisolone.
It is also given by intra-articular injection in rheumatoid
arthritis to relieve local pain and swelling in affected
joints.

Precautions and contra-indications. As for Cortisone
Acetate.

Preparations

PREDNISOLONE ENEMA (*Syn.* Prednisolone Sodium Phosphate Enema): an aqueous solution of prednisolone
sodium phosphate in a suitable buffered vehicle. It may
contain suitable stabilising agents and a preservative.
The solution is adjusted to pH 7 to 7.5. This preparation
is required to be retained in the colon and the vehicle
must be so formulated as to ensure that this requirement
is fulfilled. Available as an enema containing prednisolone sodium phosphate equivalent to 20 mg of prednisolone in 100 ml.
*A standard for this enema is given in the British
Pharmaceutical Codex 1973*
Containers: it should be supplied in a suitable disposable
plastic pack fitted with a rectal nozzle.
Storage: it should be stored at a temperature not
exceeding 25°, protected from light. Under these conditions, it may be expected to retain its potency for at
least 2 years.
Advice for patients: see the entry on Enemas for general
information on the use of enemas. It should preferably
be used at night.

PREDNISOLONE EYE-DROPS (*Syn.* Prednisolone Sodium
Phosphate Eye-drops): consisting of a sterile solution
containing prednisolone sodium phosphate, with a suitable preservative and stabilising agents, in purified
water.
A suitable solution may be prepared according to the
following formula:

Prednisolone sodium phosphate	0.518 g
Disodium edetate	0.01 g
Sodium acid phosphate	0.3 g
Sodium chloride	0.5 g
Benzalkonium chloride solution ..	0.02 ml
Sodium hydroxide..	a sufficient quantity
Purified water	to 100.0 ml

Dissolve the sodium acid phosphate, the prednisolone
sodium phosphate, the disodium edetate, and the sodium
chloride in 40 ml of the water and adjust to pH 8 by
adding, dropwise, a 4% solution of the sodium hydroxide
in the water. Add the benzalkonium chloride solution
mixed with 50 ml of the water, re-adjust, if necessary,
to pH 8 with a further addition of the sodium hydroxide
solution, add sufficient of the water to produce the
required volume, and mix. Transfer to the final containers, close the containers so as to exclude micro-
organisms, and sterilise by maintaining at 98° to 100° for
30 minutes.
This preparation is also used as ear-drops.
*A standard for these eye-drops is given in the British
Pharmaceutical Codex 1973*
Containers and *Labelling:* see the entry on Eye-drops
for general information on containers and labelling.
Storage: it should be protected from light.
Advice for patients: see the entry on Eye-drops for
general information on the use of eye-drops.

PREDNISOLONE SODIUM PHOSPHATE INJECTION: a sterile
solution of prednisolone sodium phosphate, with suitable
stabilising agents, in water for injections. It may contain
a suitable buffering agent. It is sterilised by filtration.
Available in 2-ml vials containing prednisolone sodium
phosphate equivalent to 16 mg of prednisolone per ml.
*A standard for this injection is given in the British
Pharmacopoeia 1973*

Containers: see the entry on Injections for general information on containers.

Labelling: see the entry on Injections for general information on labelling. In addition, the label on the container should state the amount of the medicament as the equivalent amount of prednisolone in a suitable dose-volume.

Storage: it should be stored in a cool place, protected from light.

OTHER PREPARATIONS available include EAR- and EYE-DROPS containing prednisolone sodium phosphate 0.5% with neomycin sulphate 0.5%; SUPPOSITORIES containing prednisolone sodium phosphate equivalent to 5 mg of prednisolone; and TABLETS containing prednisolone sodium phosphate equivalent to 5 mg of prednisolone.

Prednisone

17α,21-Dihydroxypregna-1,4-diene-3,11,20-trione

$C_{21}H_{26}O_5 = 358.4$

OTHER NAMES: *Decortisyl®*; *Deltacortone®*; *Marsone®*; Prednisonum
Delta-Butazolidin® (with phenylbutazone)

A standard is given in the European Pharmacopoeia Vol. II

Description. An odourless white crystalline powder.

Solubility. Very slightly soluble in water; soluble, at 20°, in 190 parts of alcohol, in 300 parts of dehydrated alcohol, and in 200 parts of chloroform.

Moisture content. Not more than 1%, determined by drying at 105°.

Specific rotation. +167° to +175°, determined on a 1% solution in dioxan.

Preparation of solid dosage forms. In order to achieve a satisfactory rate of dissolution, prednisone in the form of an ultra-fine powder should be used.

Storage. It should be protected from light.

Identification. TESTS. 1. It complies with Test 1 described under Betamethasone.

2. Dissolve about 200 μg in 1 ml of alcohol (95%), evaporate to dryness *in vacuo*, add 5 ml of 1N sodium hydroxide and heat at 70° for 30 minutes; not more than a slight yellow colour is produced (distinction from cortisone acetate).

3. Carry out Test 2 described under Prednisolone; a pale green fluorescence is produced.

MELTING-POINT. About 230°, with decomposition.

ULTRAVIOLET ABSORPTION. In alcohol (95%), maximum at 240 nm (E1%, 1cm = 415).

INFRA-RED ABSORPTION. Major peaks at 904, 1246, 1610, 1622, 1667, and 1709 cm⁻¹ (see Appendix 2a: Infra-red Spectra).

THIN-LAYER CHROMATOGRAPHY. See under Thin-layer Chromatography, System 10.

Determination in body fluids. HIGH PRESSURE LIQUID CHROMATOGRAPHY. In plasma—J. C. K. Loo and N. Jordan, *J. Chromat.*, 1977, **143**, 314.

Metabolism (see also under Prednisolone). ABSORPTION. Absorbed after oral administration.

HALF-LIFE. Biological half-life (for conversion to prednisolone), about 1 hour, which is increased in hepatic insufficiency.

Actions and uses. Prednisone is readily converted in the liver to prednisolone and there is no significant difference between the doses and effects of the two substances.

Undesirable effects. As for Prednisolone.

Precautions and contra-indications. As for Cortisone Acetate.

Preparations

PREDNISONE TABLETS: available as tablets containing 1 and 5 mg of prednisone.
A standard for these tablets is given in the British Pharmacopoeia 1973
Containers and *Storage:* see the entry on Tablets for general information on containers and storage. Containers should be airtight and light resistant.
Advice for patients: in long-term use, treatment should not be discontinued without the advice of the prescriber. Patients may carry an identification card giving details of their treatment and the name of the prescriber, who should be contacted in the event of accident, feverish illness, diarrhoea, vomiting, or alimentary disturbances. In short-term treatment, the prescribed course should be completed.

OTHER PREPARATIONS available include TABLETS containing prednisone 1.25 mg with phenylbutazone 50 mg.

Pre-eclampsia

see under TOXAEMIA OF PREGNANCY

Pregnancy

Pregnancy is the condition in which an embryo or foetus is developing in the body. Signs of pregnancy include cessation of menstruation, morning sickness, breast enlargement, and progressive enlargement of the abdomen.

For diseases associated with pregnancy see Choriocarcinoma, Postpartum Haemorrhage, and Toxaemia of Pregnancy. See also Abortion and Contraception.

The use of drugs in pregnancy. Many medicinal substances or their metabolites readily traverse the placenta and enter the foetal circulation. The foetus is especially sensitive to the actions of certain drugs and caution is therefore necessary when medicines are administered to pregnant patients, especially as the effect on the foetus has not been determined for many drugs. Particular caution should be exercised in the first three months.

Unless a patient's illness is likely to produce marked morbidity, the desirability of postponing treatment should be considered. While the paramount consideration must be the well-being of the patient, when treatment is to be given during pregnancy drugs known to be harmful to the foetus and any others that rational consideration indicates might be harmful should be avoided. There is a natural incidence of foetal abnormalities which may be increased by the action of teratogenic drugs (including rubella vaccine).

Experience with thalidomide showed that severe damage or death of the foetus occurred when it had been administered 1 to 14 days after conception and there was damage to the foetal nervous system at 13 to 25 days, the heart at 20 to 40 days, and limbs at 24 to 46 days. Drugs administered after the first trimester are unlikely to cause malformations but may affect the growth and function of tissues and organs.

Since most drugs, with exception of those of high molecular weight (above 1000) readily traverse the placenta, medicines given during the later stages of pregnancy may affect the foetus. In particular, substances that cause respiratory depression may reduce the chance of survival of the new-born, especially when birth is premature.

Drugs liable to give rise to congenital abnormalities

Anticonvulsants (cleft lip with or without cleft palate)
Androgens, progestogens, and oestrogens (masculinisation of the foetus and bone aging). Stilboestrol has been associated with vaginal carcinoma in adolescent girls whose mothers took the drug in pregnancy.
Corticosteroids (still birth, anencephaly or absence of brain, cleft palate, and low birth-weight)
Cytotoxic and immunosuppressant drugs (abortions and congenital malformations)
Rubella vaccine (congenital malformations)

Other drugs that should preferably be avoided during pregnancy

Analgesics and anaesthetics. Salicylates in high doses may give rise to neonatal haemorrhage. Phenacetin may cause methaemoglobinaemia. Certain local anaesthetics may cause methaemoglobinaemia and hypotension in the foetus. General anaesthetics may cause respiratory depression. The effects of narcotic analgesics are given under Tranquillisers (below).

Antibacterial agents. The following undesirable effects may occur. Aminoglycoside antibiotics such as gentamicin, kanamycin, neomycin, paromomycin, streptomycin, and vancomycin may give rise to foetal eighth cranial nerve damage and deafness. Chloramphenicol inhibits protein synthesis in dividing cells and when given in late pregnancy may give rise to a neonatal "grey syndrome" which may include hypothermia and circulatory failure. Isoniazid may cause encephalopathy. Nitrofurantoin may give rise to haemolytic reactions. Novobiocin and long-acting sulphonamides may cause severe neonatal jaundice. Tetracyclines may become incorporated in the skeleton with resultant discoloration and weakening of tooth enamel and retardation of bone growth.

Anticoagulants. Oral anticoagulant drugs carry a risk of haemorrhage at term. Their use should be discontinued at least a week before the expected date of birth. Heparin is a safer anticoagulant to use in late pregnancy.

Antihypertensives. Ganglion-blocking agents may give rise to neonatal hypotension and paralytic ileus. Reserpine may cause bradycardia, nasal congestion, and respiratory distress. Beta-adrenergic blocking agents such as propranolol may reduce cardiac output in the foetus. Diazoxide may cause alopecia.

Antimalarials. Chloroquine may cause foetal deafness. Retinal damage has been reported after long-term administration of chloroquine.

Antithyroid substances. These substances may give rise to foetal goitre or hypothyroidism. It is desirable to reduce the dosage progressively during pregnancy.

Diuretics. Thiazide and other diuretics may give rise to foetal jaundice and thrombocytopenia.

Oral antidiabetics. Oral antidiabetic agents may give rise to neonatal hypoglycaemia if given in sufficiently high dosage.

Tranquillisers. Phenothiazine derivatives such as chlorpromazine may cause retinal damage in the foetus when used in long-term treatment at high dosage. Lithium carbonate may give rise to foetal goitre. Sedatives depress neonatal activity and some, particularly barbiturates and morphine-like substances, depress respiration at birth. Diazepam in high dosage may cause lethargy and hypotonia in the offspring. Narcotic withdrawal symptoms may be fatal in babies born to drug addicts if not recognised.

Vitamins. High doses of vitamins administered in late pregnancy may result in the appearance of a withdrawal syndrome in the infant soon after birth. Thus maternal dosage with ascorbic acid gives rise to infantile scurvy and pyridoxine gives rise to convulsive seizures. Excessive dosage with vitamin D in pregnancy may cause mental retardation in the infant. Large doses of phytomenadione may cause severe jaundice.

Premixes

Premixes are medicinal substances or growth factors intimately mixed with a suitable diluent which is often a food or food product. They are formulated to mix readily with animal rations and are prepared as pellets, granules, or powder.

Premixes are intended to be mixed thoroughly, in appropriate proportions, with the basic feed and are used particularly in cases where continuous administration of medicinal substances or growth factors is necessary.

Preparations available as premixes fall into 6 groups: antibiotics, synthetic hormones, minerals, anti-infective agents, and water-soluble and oil-soluble vitamins.

Containers and storage. They should be stored in a cool dry place, protected from light. As premixes often have a food basis, precautions should be taken to prevent attack by insects or other animal pests and by moulds and bacteria.

Labelling. The label on the container should state (1) the names and proportions of the medicaments; (2) directions for the preparation of the medicated feed from the premix and the basic feed; (3) if applicable, the time which should elapse between the cessation of treatment with the diluted premix and slaughter of the animal for human consumption; and (4) any other special precautions associated with the use of the premix.

Preservatives

Preservatives are included in pharmaceutical preparations when it is necessary to combat the effects of contaminating micro-organisms which may be inherent in ingredients or introduced during production processes or during use by the patient. Preparations containing water are particularly susceptible to attack by microbial organisms and if growth is not checked adverse changes in the nature of the preparation may result.

Materials such as polysorbates and cetomacrogol used

in the formulation may themselves be contaminated as well as providing suitable substrates for the growth of micro-organisms.

Pharmaceutical preparations intended for parenteral and ophthalmic administration, for introduction into body cavities as irrigations, or for application to wounds must be specially prepared and sterilised. If presented in multi-dose containers an effective antimicrobial agent must be included in the formula.

Preservatives are also included in the formulation of other forms of medicines in which micro-organisms are capable of multiplying, in particular those intended for oral and topical administration and those which employ aqueous vehicles. The inclusion of a preservative in a formula is, however, no substitute for bacteriological cleanliness at the preparation stage during which every precaution should be taken to minimise contamination. The commonly occurring contaminants fall into two main categories: spoilage organisms and pathogenic organisms. A major source of spoilage contamination is water used in production processes. *Pseudomonas, Xanthomonas, Achromobacterium, Escherichia, Aerobacter,* and *Flavobacterium* spp. are generally known to proliferate in potable, distilled, and de-ionised waters. *Streptococcus, Bacillus, Staphylococcus* spp., yeasts and fungi, particularly *Aspergillus* spp. and *Penicillium* spp., frequently contaminate pharmaceuticals and may result in spoilage. Pathogenic and potentially harmful micro-organisms associated with pharmaceutical preparations include *Salmonella*, certain species of *Pseudomonas* (including *Ps. aeruginosa*), *Staphylococcus aureus*, and *Escherichia coli*.

An ideal preservative substance should possess effective antimicrobial activity against a broad spectrum of micro-organisms over a wide range of conditions of temperature and pH. It should be chemically stable in the systems in which it is used, readily soluble, free from toxicity and sensitising effects at the effective concentrations, and it should be compatible with the other components of the formulation. It should be free from objectionable odour, taste, or colour.

For emulsions, a low oil/water partition coefficient is required of the preservative. Many preservatives have partition coefficients which favour partition into the oily phase, for example chlorocresol, and in order to achieve antimicrobial efficacy in the aqueous phase they need to be present in considerably higher overall concentration in the product. Additional problems in the preservation of disperse systems may arise from adsorption of preservative from solution on to finely divided particles in suspension, thus depleting the aqueous phase of preservative.

Interaction between the preservative and other components of a formulation or between two incompatible preservatives may result in partial or complete inactivation of the preservative effect.

Similarly, interaction between the preservative and the container used for the preparation may markedly affect antimicrobial efficacy. Containers and closure materials such as plastics, some types of glass, and rubber may leach reactive substances into solutions stored in the container. In addition, sorption of materials may take place from the product into the walls of the container and into the closure. Interaction between preservatives in solution and chemicals in container material may take place with reduction in the antimicrobial efficacy of the preservative.

Preservative efficiency may be affected by micro-organisms inherently present in a preparation or by those introduced accidentally. Fungi and some species of *Pseudomonas* have the capacity to metabolise certain preservatives and where the preparation itself provides a good growth medium for the contaminating organism gross spoilage will occur and it may become actively infective. For example, it has been demonstrated that certain fungi and strains of *Pseudomonas* can actively metabolise *p*-hydroxybenzoate esters which were formerly used as preservatives for eye-drops.

All pharmaceutical preparations which require the inclusion of an antimicrobial agent should be subjected to suitable tests for preservative efficacy. There is no universally accepted standard method of testing. The normally accepted procedure is to challenge the particular preparation with standard inocula of organisms most likely to be encountered during production and use. The preparation, packed in its final container, is then stored under normal conditions and the microbial count is determined at intervals for an adequate period.

For injections, the British Pharmacopoeia 1973 requires the chosen bactericide to be capable of sterilising the injection within 3 hours of inoculation with 1×10^6 vegetative bacterial cells per ml.

The United States Pharmacopoeia XIX specifies inocula of both vegetative bacteria and fungal spores. The former must be reduced to a level of not more than 0.1% of their original value by the 14th day and the latter must not proliferate during the first 14 days; the concentration of each test micro-organism must remain at or below these levels during the remainder of the 28-day test period. For ophthalmic preparations, the preservative should be capable of sterilising an inoculum of 10^6 cells of *Pseudomonas aeruginosa*, preferably in 1 hour or less, whilst an emulsified preparation for dermatological use might be challenged with a mixed population of fungal spores, the preservative being required to reduce their number and prevent their germination.

No single preservative meets all the desirable criteria and selection becomes a matter of compromise. Efficient antimicrobial substances are likely to be highly active chemically and physiologically and so automatically provide constraints on their acceptability. Rarely, the medicament is itself sufficiently bactericidal and an additional preservative is unnecessary.

In some instances, combinations of preservatives or the inclusion of substances to enhance the antimicrobial activity of a particular preservative may have merit. For example the incorporation of phenethyl alcohol with either phenylmercuric nitrate or benzalkonium chloride reduces killing time and enables lower concentrations of bactericide to be used. Similarly phenethyl alcohol and disodium edetate under given conditions enhance the effects of chlorhexidine acetate and chlorocresol.

Preservatives commonly used in pharmaceutical products include alcohol, benzoic acid, benzyl alcohol, chlorbutol, chlorhexidine, chlorocresol, chloroform, glycerol, *p*-hydroxybenzoate esters, isopropyl alcohol, various mercurial compounds (including phenylmercuric nitrate, acetate, or borate, thiomersal, etc.), phenol, phenoxyethanol, quaternary ammonium compounds (such as cetrimide, benzalkonium chloride, and cetylpyridinium chloride), sorbic acid, sulphur dioxide, and sulphurous acid.

Further information on the use of preservatives is given in the entries on Eye-drops and Injections.

FURTHER INFORMATION. Contamination in pharmaceuticals: *Prevention of microbial contamination of medicinal products*, London, HM Stationery Office 1973, per *Pharm. J.,* i/1973, 271; *Microbial contamination of medicines administered to hospital patients*, Public Health Laboratory Service Working Party Report, HM

Stationery Office 1971, per *Pharm. J.*, ii/1971, 96; L. O. Kallings *et al.*, *Inquiry by the Royal Swedish Medical Board into Microbial Contamination*, Final Report, 1965; micro-organisms isolated from dregs of fluid medicaments—O. G. Clausen, *Pharm. Acta Helv.*, 1973, **48**, 622.
Review of available preservatives and their limitations: M. R. W. Brown and D. A. Norton, *J. Soc. cosmet. Chem.*, 1965, **16**, 369; J. H. S. Foster, *Mfg Chem.*, 1965, **36** (May), 45 and **36** (June), 43; R. M. E. Richards, *Australas. J. Pharm.*, 1967, **48**, 48 and 56.
Modification of preservative activity: phenethyl alcohol and organic mercurials—W. B. Hugo and J. H. S. Foster, *J. Pharm. Pharmac.*, 1963, **15**, 79; phenethyl alcohol with various bactericides—R. M. E. Richards and R. J. McBride, *J. Pharm. Pharmac.*, 1971, **23**, Suppl., 141S; chlorhexidine and chlorocresol with phenethyl alcohol and disodium edetate—R. M. E. Richards and R. J. McBride, *Pharm. J.*, i/1973, 118; polysorbate 80 and polymyxin B sulphate—R. M. E. Richards and M. R. W. Brown, *J. Pharm. Pharmac.*, 1964, **16**, 360; thiomersal and phenylmercuric nitrate with disodium edetate, thiosulphate, and metabisulphite—R. M. E. Richards and J. E. Reary, *J. Pharm. Pharmac.*, 1972, **24**, Suppl., 84P; polysorbate 80 and phenethyl alcohol with fentichlor—R. M. E. Richards and M. P. Hardie, *J. Pharm. Pharmac.*, 1972, **24**, Suppl., 90P; antimicrobial agents and preservatives in pharmaceutical and cosmetic products —*J. appl. Bact.*, 1978, **44**, Suppl.

Prilocaine Hydrochloride

2-Propylaminopropiono-*o*-toluidide hydrochloride

$C_{13}H_{21}ClN_2O = 256.8$

OTHER NAMES: *Citanest*®
Citanest with Octapressin® (with felypressin)

A standard is given in the British Pharmacopoeia 1973

Description. An odourless white crystalline powder with a bitter taste followed by numbness.

Solubility. Soluble, at 20°, in 5 parts of water and in 6 parts of alcohol; practically insoluble in ether.

Dissociation constant. pK_a 7.9 (25°).

Stability. Aqueous solutions are slowly hydrolysed to *o*-toluidine and 2-propylpropionic acid.

Incompatibility. It is precipitated from aqueous solutions under alkaline conditions when the concentration exceeds 5%.

Hygroscopicity. It absorbs insignificant amounts of moisture at relative humidities up to about 80%.

Sterilisation. Solutions for injection are sterilised by heating in an autoclave or by filtration.

Storage. It should be stored in airtight containers.

Identification. TEST. Dissolve about 250 mg in 10 ml of water and make alkaline with *dilute sodium hydroxide solution*; an oily liquid is produced. Dissolve the oil in 1 ml of alcohol (95%) and add 0.5 ml of a 10% solution of cobalt chloride and shake for 2 minutes; a bluish-green precipitate is produced.

MELTING-POINT. About 168°.

ULTRAVIOLET ABSORPTION. In 0.1N sulphuric acid, there is no significant absorption in the range 230 nm to 360 nm.

INFRA-RED ABSORPTION. Major peaks at 752, 763, 1299, 1471, 1538, and 1695 cm^{-1} (see Appendix 2b: Infra-red Spectra).

Metabolism. ABSORPTION. The absorption of prilocaine is delayed by adrenaline.

BLOOD CONCENTRATION. After the epidural administration of 10 to 30 ml of a 2% solution of prilocaine, maximum concentrations of 2 to 5 μg/ml are attained in the blood; after an intercostal injection of 40 ml of a 1% solution, maximum blood concentrations of 4 to 5 μg/ml are attained.

DISTRIBUTION. Prilocaine enters the cerebrospinal fluid.

METABOLIC REACTIONS. Hydrolysis and/or hydroxylation resulting in hydroxylated or deacetylated metabolites.

EXCRETION. About 35% of a dose is excreted in the urine as 4-hydroxy-2-methylaniline, 3% as 6-hydroxy-2-methylaniline, 1% as *o*-methylaniline, and less than 5% as unchanged drug.

Actions and uses. Prilocaine is a local anaesthetic with properties similar to those of lignocaine but it is less toxic and less liable to cause vasodilatation. It is used in dentistry and to produce infiltration and spinal anaesthesia. The total quantity of prilocaine hydrochloride should not exceed 400 milligrams unless adrenaline is present, when up to 600 milligrams may be given.
Injection solutions containing 0.5, 1.0, 1.5, and 4.0% of prilocaine hydrochloride, and 0.5% of prilocaine hydrochloride with adrenaline 1 in 250000, and 1.0% of prilocaine hydrochloride with adrenaline 1 in 200000 are available; solutions containing 3.0% of prilocaine hydrochloride with adrenaline 1 in 300000 or felypressin 0.03 unit per millilitre are available for dental purposes.

Undesirable effects. Like other local anaesthetics, prilocaine may stimulate the central nervous system.

Precautions and contra-indications. Overdosage may give rise to methaemoglobinaemia, and hence the use of prilocaine should be avoided in patients with anaemia. It should be used with caution in pregnancy as it may give rise to foetal methaemoglobinaemia.
Solutions containing adrenaline should not be used for inducing anaesthesia in digits because the profound ischaemia produced may lead to gangrene.

Preparations

Preparations available include an INJECTION containing prilocaine hydrochloride 5 mg per ml (0.5%) in 20- and 50-ml vials, an injection containing prilocaine hydrochloride 10 mg per ml (1%) in 20- and 50-ml vials, an injection containing prilocaine hydrochloride 40 mg per ml (4%) in 1.8- and 2.2-ml cartridges, an injection containing prilocaine hydrochloride 30 mg per ml (3%) with adrenaline 1 · in 300000 in 2-ml cartridges, an injection containing prilocaine hydrochloride 30 mg per ml with felypressin 0.03 unit per ml in 2-ml cartridges, an injection containing prilocaine hydrochloride 50 mg with dextrose 50 mg per ml in 2-ml ampoules; and a SOLUTION containing prilocaine hydrochloride 40 mg per ml (4%).

Primaquine Phosphate

8-(4-Amino-1-methylbutylamino)-6-methoxyquinoline di(dihydrogen phosphate)

$C_{15}H_{27}N_3O_9P_2 = 455.3$

A standard is given in the British Pharmacopoeia 1973

Description. An odourless orange-red crystalline powder with a bitter taste.

Solubility. Soluble, at 20°, in 16 parts of water; practically insoluble in alcohol, in ether, and in chloroform.

Acidity. A 1% solution has a pH of 2.5 to 3.5.

Stability. It is affected by light. Aqueous solutions are thermolabile; approximately half their activity is lost in 24 hours at 100°.

Hygroscopicity. It absorbs insignificant amounts of moisture at temperatures up to 37° at relative humidities up to about 80%.

Storage. It should be protected from light.

Identification. TESTS. 1. Dissolve about 10 mg in 5 ml of water and add 1 ml of a 5% solution of ammonium ceric sulphate in *dilute nitric acid*; a deep violet colour is produced immediately (distinction from chloroquine). 2. Dissolve about 100 μg in 1 ml of water and add 1 drop of *gold chloride solution*; a violet-blue colour is produced.

MELTING-POINT. About 200°.

ULTRAVIOLET ABSORPTION. In 0.01N hydrochloric acid, maxima at 265 nm (E1%, 1cm = 330) and 282 nm (E1%, 1cm = 327).

Metabolism. ABSORPTION. Readily absorbed after oral administration.

BLOOD CONCENTRATION. Peak plasma concentrations appear to be attained by about 6 hours.

METABOLIC REACTIONS. 6-*O*-Demethylation and oxidation at position 5 to form the 5,6-diol which is converted to an active quinone; *N*-dealkylation also occurs to form 8-amino-6-methoxyquinoline; the metabolism of primaquine is reduced by mepacrine.

EXCRETION. Little unchanged drug is excreted in the urine.

Actions and uses. Primaquine is an antimalarial drug which kills the exoerythrocytic stages of *Plasmodium vivax*, *P. ovale*, and *P. malariae* and the early pre-erythrocytic form of *P. falciparum*. It also kills gametocytes, or renders them incapable of development in the mosquito, but has little action on other erythrocytic stages and therefore should not be used alone in the treatment of a malarial attack. Primaquine is rapidly absorbed and metabolised.

Its chief use is for the radical cure of *P. vivax* infections in people returning from malarious areas. For this purpose, a short intensive course of treatment with a schizonticide such as chloroquine is given to kill any erythrocytic parasites, and this is followed by a course of fourteen daily doses of primaquine phosphate, each

equivalent to 15 milligrams of the base, by mouth, to kill the tissue forms; 15 mg of primaquine base is approximately equivalent to 26 mg of primaquine phosphate.

The corresponding dose for children under 1 year is the equivalent of 500 micrograms of primaquine base per kilogram body-weight daily, 1 to 5 years 4 to 6 milligrams daily, and 6 to 12 years 7 to 12 milligrams daily. For the prophylaxis of malaria these doses are doubled or quadrupled and given weekly.

Undesirable effects. The most common symptoms of overdosage are abdominal pain, methaemoglobinaemia, and, less frequently, haemolytic anaemia and methaemoglobinuria. Toxic effects occur most commonly in genetic groups with glucose-6-phosphate-dehydrogenase deficiency, a condition which is prevalent mostly among dark-skinned people.

Precautions. The blood of patients being treated with primaquine should be examined periodically for haemolysis and methaemoglobinaemia. Primaquine should be withdrawn if darkening of the urine occurs or if there is a sudden fall in the haemoglobin level.

Contra-indications. Primaquine is contra-indicated in acutely ill patients, those suffering from blood disorders, and those concurrently receiving potentially haemolytic drugs.

Poisoning. Methaemoglobinaemia may be treated by giving 200 milligrams of ascorbic acid 3 times daily after withdrawing primaquine.

Preparation

PRIMAQUINE TABLETS: available as tablets containing 13.2 mg of primaquine phosphate equivalent to 7.5 mg of primaquine; they are sugar coated; the coat may be coloured.

A standard for these tablets is given in the British Pharmacopoeia 1973

Containers and *Storage:* see the entry on Tablets for general information on containers and storage. Containers should be airtight.

Labelling: the label on the container should state the amount of the medicament as the equivalent amount of primaquine.

Advice for patients: the tablets should be taken at regular intervals, preferably after meals. For therapy, the prescribed course should be completed.

Primidone

5-Ethylperhydro-5-phenylpyrimidine-4,6-dione

$C_{12}H_{14}N_2O_2 = 218.3$

OTHER NAMES: *Mysoline®*
Mysoline with Phenytoin®

A standard is given in the British Pharmacopoeia 1973

Description. An odourless white crystalline powder with a slightly bitter taste.

Solubility. Very slightly soluble in water; soluble, at 20°, in 170 parts of alcohol; very slightly soluble in most organic solvents.

Identification. TESTS. 1. Dissolve about 100 mg in 5 ml of *chromotropic acid solution* and heat in a water-bath for 30 minutes; a pinkish-blue colour is produced.
2. It complies with general Test 1 described under Barbiturates.

MELTING-POINT. About 280°.

ULTRAVIOLET ABSORPTION. In alcohol (95%), weak maxima at 251 nm, 258 nm, and 264 nm.

Determination in body fluids. GAS CHROMATOGRAPHY. In serum: simultaneous determination of primidone with carbamazepine, phenobarbitone and phenytoin—C. V. Abraham and H. D. Joslin, *J. Chromat.*, 1976, **128**, 281. In plasma—R. N. Gupta *et al.*, *J. Chromat.*, 1977, **132**, 140. In serum: comparison of a gas chromatographic method with a radioimmunoassay method—L. Sun and E. R. Walwick, *Clin. Chem.*, 1976, **22**, 901.

Metabolism. ABSORPTION. Readily absorbed after oral administration.

BLOOD CONCENTRATION. After an oral dose of 500 mg, peak plasma concentrations of primidone are attained in about 3 hours; during therapy with daily doses of 0.25 to 1.25 g, mean serum concentrations of 3 to 15 μg/ml are attained.

HALF-LIFE. Plasma half-life for primidone, 3 to 25 hours, for phenobarbitone, 48 to 120 hours, and for phenylethylmalonamide, 24 to 48 hours.

DISTRIBUTION. Enters cerebrospinal fluid and is secreted in milk; active metabolites accumulate during chronic treatment; *protein binding*, not significantly bound to plasma proteins.

METABOLIC REACTIONS. Rapidly metabolised to phenobarbitone and to phenylethylmalonamide which are both active metabolites; aromatic hydroxylation to form *p*-hydroxyphenobarbitone also occurs followed by glucuronic acid conjugation; phenytoin stimulates the formation of phenobarbitone.

EXCRETION. In man 70% of a dose is excreted in the urine in 24 hours with 15% as phenobarbitone or its hydroxylated metabolite; in rabbits, 4% is excreted as phenobarbitone and *p*-hydroxyphenobarbitone, 48% is excreted as phenylethylmalonamide, and about 20% is excreted unchanged.

FURTHER INFORMATION. Metabolism: in rats—I. P. Baumel *et al.*, *J. Pharmac. exp. Ther.*, 1973, **186**, 305; to phenylethylmalonamide—I. P. Baumel *et al.*, *Archs Neurol.*, *Chicago*, 1972, **27**, 34; to phenobarbitone—J. Bogan and H. Smith, *J. Pharm. Pharmac.*, 1968, **20**, 64; urinary excretion in rabbits—J. M. Fujimoto *et al.*, *J. Pharmac. exp. Ther.*, 1968, **159**, 379; distribution in cerebrospinal fluid—J. W. Huisman, *Pharm. Weekbl. Ned.*, 1968, **103**, 573.

Actions and uses. Primidone is an effective anticonvulsant, particularly in grand mal and psychomotor attacks. It is used when adequate control is not obtainable with phenobarbitone and phenytoin. Any changeover of treatment should be gradual, both in introducing primidone and in withdrawing the previous treatment.
As primidone is partly metabolised to phenobarbitone in the liver the two substances should not be used in conjunction with each other because of the risk of excessive sedation.
The initial dosage for adults and children over 9 years is 500 milligrams by mouth daily in divided doses, increased by 250 milligrams at intervals of 3 days up to a total daily dosage of 1 to 2 grams; for children under 9 years these doses should be halved.

Undesirable effects. Toxic effects such as drowsiness, nausea, and rashes may occur, particularly during the first week of treatment, but are usually transient and the treatment may be continued, possibly with reduced dosage. Megaloblastic anaemia may occur.

Precautions. It should be used with caution in pregnancy and in nursing mothers. When it is used in early pregnancy there is an increased risk of congenital malformations in the foetus and the use of primidone should be avoided unless the benefit outweighs the risk.

Veterinary uses. Primidone is used in the treatment of epileptiform convulsions. The usual dose by mouth for dogs is 25 to 50 milligrams per kilogram body-weight daily in divided doses.

Preparations

PRIMIDONE MIXTURE (*Syn.* Primidone Suspension): a suspension of primidone in a suitable flavoured vehicle. When a dose less than or not a multiple of 5 ml is prescribed, the mixture may be diluted, as described in the entry on Mixtures, with syrup. The diluted mixture must be freshly prepared. If it is required to store a diluted mixture for more than 2 weeks, syrup should not be used as the diluent. A diluted mixture which is stable for 3 months may be prepared by using a diluent of the following composition:

Propyl hydroxybenzoate..	..	..	..	0.15 g
Methyl hydroxybenzoate	..	..	..	1.50 g
Sodium carboxymethylcellulose 50	..	..	10.00 g
Sucrose	..	..	..	..	200.00 g
Purified water, freshly boiled and cooled	..	..	..	to 1000.0 ml

Available as a mixture containing 250 mg of primidone in 5 ml.
A standard for this mixture is given in the British Pharmaceutical Codex 1973
Containers and *Labelling:* see the entry on Mixtures for general information on containers and labelling.
Advice for patients: when initiating treatment there may be a time-lag of up to 2 weeks before a full therapeutic response is obtained. The mixture may cause drowsiness and dizziness in the initial stages of treatment; persons affected should not drive or operate machinery. Alcohol should be avoided. Treatment should not be discontinued without the advice of the prescriber.

PRIMIDONE TABLETS: available as tablets containing 250 mg of primidone.
A standard for these tablets is given in the British Pharmacopoeia 1973
Containers and *Storage:* see the entry on Tablets for general information on containers and storage. Containers should be airtight.
Advice for patients: see above under Primidone Mixture.

OTHER PREPARATIONS available include TABLETS containing primidone 250 mg with phenytoin sodium 100 mg.

Probenecid

4-(Dipropylsulphamoyl)benzoic acid

$C_{13}H_{19}NO_4S = 285.4$

OTHER NAMES: *Benemid®*
Colbenemid® (with colchicine)

A standard is given in the British Pharmacopoeia 1973

Description. An odourless white crystalline powder with a slightly bitter taste becoming unpleasantly bitter.

Solubility. Practically insoluble in water; soluble in 25 parts of alcohol and in 12 parts of acetone; soluble in dilute solutions of alkali hydroxides and of sodium bicarbonate.

Identification. MELTING-POINT. About 199°.

ULTRAVIOLET ABSORPTION. In a mixture of 1 volume of 0.1N hydrochloric acid and 9 volumes of alcohol (95%), maxima at 225 nm and 248 nm (E1%, 1cm = 330).

INFRA-RED ABSORPTION. Major peaks at 1125, 1156, 1285, 1307, 1345, and 1683 cm^{-1} (see Appendix 2a: Infra-red Spectra).

Determination in body fluids. GAS CHROMATOGRAPHY. In urine: probenecid and its metabolites—W. D. Conway and S. Melethil, *J. Chromat.*, 1975, **115**, 222.

Metabolism. ABSORPTION. Rapidly and completely absorbed after oral administration; large doses are slowly absorbed.

BLOOD CONCENTRATION. After an oral dose of 2 g, peak plasma concentrations of about 80 μg/ml are attained in 1 to 5 hours; after an intramuscular dose of 2 g, plasma concentrations of 150 to 200 μg/ml are attained falling to 100 μg/ml after 7 hours; peak concentrations may take longer to appear in children.

HALF-LIFE. Plasma half-life, 4 to 17 hours.

DISTRIBUTION. Widely distributed throughout the body; *protein binding*, about 90% bound to plasma proteins.

METABOLIC REACTIONS. Side chain oxidation, glucuronic acid conjugation, and N-dealkylation; the major metabolite is the acyl glucuronide; low doses are more rapidly metabolised than high doses.

EXCRETION. About 75 to 90% of a dose is excreted in the urine; 3 to 35% is excreted unchanged, 5 to 42% is excreted as the acyl glucuronide, 15 to 25% is excreted as hydroxylated and carboxylic acid metabolites, and 4 to 8% is excreted as N-dealkylated metabolites; the excretion of unchanged probenecid is increased with increasing urinary pH values and urinary flow.

DRUG INTERACTIONS. Probenecid inhibits the tubular secretion of many drugs, for example, ampicillin, dopamine, indomethacin, and penicillin, and in animals appears to stimulate its own metabolism.

FURTHER INFORMATION. Metabolites—P. G. Dayton *et al.*, *Drug Met. Disp.*, 1973, **1**, 742 and Z. H. Israili *et al.*, *J. mednl Chem.*, 1972, **15**, 709; pharmacokinetics—P. G. Dayton *et al.*, *J. Pharmac. exp. Ther.*, 1963, **140**, 278; urinary excretion of probenecid and metabolites—

S. Melethil and W. D. Conway, *J. pharm. Sci.*, 1976, **65**, 861, J. M. Perel *et al.*, *Life Sci.*, 1970, **9**, 1337, and J. M. Perel *et al.*, *Eur. J. clin. Pharmac.*, 1971, **3**, 106.

Actions and uses. Probenecid is a uricosuric agent which is rapidly absorbed when given by mouth. In the treatment of gout it promotes excretion of urates by inhibiting tubular resorption, which results in a lowering of the elevated plasma-uric acid concentrations and a slow depletion of urate deposits (tophi) in the tissues.

Probenecid reduces tubular excretion of penicillins, thereby increasing the plasma concentrations up to tenfold. It is therefore used as an adjunct to therapy in conditions such as bacterial endocarditis, where very high concentrations of penicillins may be required. It may be used to reduce the rate of excretion of various penicillins, including ampicillin, benzylpenicillin, cloxacillin, methicillin, and phenoxymethylpenicillin, and it is also effective with cephalexin and cephalothin. The usual daily dose for this purpose is 2 grams of probenecid. Dosage is reduced in the elderly and in patients with renal impairment. Children over 2 years, weighing less than 50 kilograms may be given an initial daily dose of 25 milligrams per kilogram body-weight (or 700 milligrams per square metre body-surface), followed by 40 milligrams per kilogram body-weight daily (or 1.2 grams per square metre body-surface).

Probenecid has no analgesic action and is of no value in the treatment of acute gout although acute attacks usually diminish some weeks after beginning treatment with the drug.

Probenecid is used to reduce the frequency of acute attacks of gout and to prevent the formation of new tophi and reduce those already present. Acute attacks of gout may be precipitated in the first few weeks or months of treatment with probenecid, particularly with high dosage; it is therefore usual to start treatment with a dosage of 250 milligrams twice daily by mouth and to increase it gradually, usually to 1.5 to 2 grams daily. Colchicine, in a dosage of 500 micrograms once or twice daily, may be given concurrently with the aim of reducing the incidence of such attacks. The dosage should be uninterrupted, as any irregularity of dosage leads to reduced urate output and increased plasma-uric acid concentrations. The urine should be made alkaline in the initial stages of treatment and an adequate fluid intake ensured. Treatment must usually be continued for life. Aspirin, citrates, and salicylates should not be given with probenecid as they antagonise its uricosuric effect.

Undesirable effects. These are rare with a daily dosage of up to 1 gram, but with higher dosage, gastro-intestinal upsets, rashes, and, occasionally, drug fever and hypersensitivity reactions may occur.

Preparations

PROBENECID TABLETS: available as tablets containing 500 mg of probenecid.
A standard for these tablets is given in the British Pharmacopoeia 1973
Containers and *Storage:* see the entry on Tablets for general information on containers and storage. Containers should be airtight.
Advice for patients: the tablets should preferably be taken after meals. The prescribed course should be completed or, where applicable, treatment should not be discontinued without the advice of the prescriber. Adequate fluid intake should be maintained and preparations containing aspirin should be avoided.

OTHER PREPARATIONS available include TABLETS containing probenecid 500 mg with colchicine 500 micrograms.

Procainamide Hydrochloride

4-Amino-N-(2-diethylaminoethyl)benzamide hydrochloride

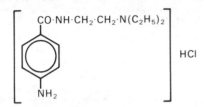

$C_{13}H_{22}ClN_3O = 271.8$

OTHER NAMES: *Procainamide Durules®; Pronestyl®*

A standard is given in the British Pharmacopoeia 1973

Description. An odourless, hygroscopic, white or yellowish-white, crystalline powder.

Solubility. Soluble, at 20°, in less than 1 part of water, in 2 parts of alcohol, and in 140 parts of chloroform; very slightly soluble in ether.

Acidity. A 10% solution has a pH of 5 to 6.5.

Moisture content. Not more than 1%, determined by drying at 105°.

Dissociation constant. pK_a 9.2 (20°).

Sterilisation. Solutions for injection are sterilised by heating in an autoclave or by filtration.

Storage. It should be stored in airtight containers.

Identification. MELTING-POINT. About 167°.

ULTRAVIOLET ABSORPTION. In 0.02N sodium hydroxide, maximum at 275 nm (E1%, 1cm = 600); in alcohol (95%), maximum at 286 nm (E1%, 1cm = 643).

INFRA-RED ABSORPTION. Major peaks at 1297, 1325, 1512, 1545, 1600, and 1639 cm^{-1} (see Appendix 2a: Infra-red Spectra).

THIN-LAYER CHROMATOGRAPHY. See under Thin-layer Chromatography, System 2.

Determination in body fluids. SPECTROFLUORIMETRY. In plasma: comparison with colorimetric and gas chromatographic methods—J. Sterling *et al.*, *J. pharm. Sci.*, 1974, **63**, 1744.

GAS CHROMATOGRAPHY. In plasma: procainamide and its metabolite N-acetylprocainamide—K. J. Simons and R. H. Levy, *J. pharm. Sci.*, 1975, **64**, 1967.

HIGH PRESSURE LIQUID CHROMATOGRAPHY. In plasma: procainamide and its metabolite N-acetylprocainamide—K. Carr *et al.*, *J. Chromat.*, 1976, **129**, 363.

Metabolism. ABSORPTION. Readily absorbed after oral administration.

BLOOD CONCENTRATION. During therapy with oral doses of 1 to 4 g of the hydrochloride daily, plasma concentrations of 2 to 10 µg/ml are attained; after intravenous doses of 0.5 to 1 g of the hydrochloride, concentrations of 5 to 20 µg/ml are reached within 30 minutes; after an intramuscular dose of 1 g, a plasma concentration of about 6 µg/ml is attained at 1 hour; therapeutic concentrations are in the range 4 to 8 µg/ml and toxic reactions may occur at concentrations over 15 µg/ml; after an oral dose of 6.5 mg/kg of procainamide, peak serum concentrations of the active N-acetylated metabolite reach about 1.8 µg/ml in rapid acetylators and about 0.4 µg/ml in slow acetylators.

HALF-LIFE. Plasma half-life, about 2.5 hours in rapid

acetylators and about 4.5 hours in slow acetylators; in subjects with heart disease or renal failure, the half-life may be increased.

DISTRIBUTION. Localised in the tissues especially in the kidneys, liver, lungs, spleen, and heart; volume of distribution, 1.7 to 2.3 litres/kg body-weight; *protein binding*, about 15% bound to plasma proteins.

METABOLIC REACTIONS. Polymorphic acetylation to form N-acetylprocainamide, which is an active metabolite, and hydrolysis to form p-aminobenzoic acid.

EXCRETION. About 70 to 90% of a dose is excreted in the urine in 72 hours, most of which is excreted in the first 8 hours; after an oral dose, 30 to 70% is excreted unchanged, 6 to 50% is excreted as N-acetylprocainamide, and 2 to 10% as 4-aminobenzoic acid; the urinary excretion of procainamide does not appear to be influenced by urinary pH or urinary flow.

FURTHER INFORMATION. Absorption from slow-release tablets—T. R. D. Shaw *et al.*, *Br. J. clin. Pharmac.*, 1975, **2**, 515; acetylator status—W. Campbell *et al.*, *Br. J. clin. Pharmac.*, 1976, **3**, 1023 and K. Frislid *et al.*, *Eur. J. clin. Pharmac.*, 1976, **9**, 433; metabolism—J. Dreyfuss *et al.*, *Clin. Pharmac. Ther.*, 1972, **13**, 366 and V. Giardina *et al.*, *Clin. Pharmac. Ther.*, 1976, **19**, 339; pharmacokinetics—C. Graffner *et al.*, *Clin. Pharmac. Ther.*, 1975, **17**, 414; polymorphic acetylation—M. M. Reidenberg *et al.*, *Clin. Pharmac. Ther.*, 1975, **17**, 722; renal elimination—R. L. Galeazzi *et al.*, *Clin. Pharmac. Ther.*, 1976, **19**, 55.
N-Acetylprocainamide: anti-arrhythmic potency—J. Elson *et al.*, *Clin. Pharmac. Ther.*, 1975, **17**, 134; in patients with renal failure—T. P. Gibson *et al.*, *Clin. Pharmac. Ther.*, 1976, **19**, 206; elimination after intravenous dose—C. Graffner, *J. Pharmacokinet. Biopharm.*, 1975, **3**, 69; pharmacokinetics—J. M. Strong *et al.*, *J. Pharmacokinet. Biopharm.*, 1975, **3**, 223.

Actions and uses. Procainamide has actions similar to those described under Procaine Hydrochloride, but its effects, particularly on the heart, are more sustained than those of procaine. Like quinidine, it diminishes the excitability, conductivity, and contractility of both atrium and ventricle, and increases the refractory period of the atrium.

Procainamide is used to reduce the risk of fibrillation during thoracic surgery and in the treatment of arrhythmias and extrasystoles, especially those provoked by anaesthetics. It is given by slow intravenous infusion (at a carefully controlled rate of 25 to 50 milligrams per minute) as a 2.5% solution of procainamide hydrochloride in doses of up to 1 gram. It may also be given by mouth; the dosage should rarely exceed 1 gram every 3 hours or 1 to 1.5 grams in a sustained release preparation 3 times daily.

Undesirable effects. Intravenous administration of procainamide may precipitate a grave fall in blood pressure. Large oral doses may cause such nausea that treatment has to be discontinued. A condition resembling lupus erythematosus may develop, especially when the procainamide is given orally over a long period.

Preparations

PROCAINAMIDE INJECTION: a sterile solution of procainamide hydrochloride, with 0.9% of benzyl alcohol and 0.1% of sodium metabisulphite, in water for injections. It is sterilised by heating in an autoclave or by filtration. Available in 10-ml vials containing 100 mg of procainamide hydrochloride per ml.

A standard for this injection is given in the British Pharmacopoeia 1973

Containers and *Labelling:* see the entry on Injections for general information on containers and labelling.

PROCAINAMIDE TABLETS: available as tablets containing 250 mg of procainamide.

A standard for these tablets is given in the British Pharmacopoeia 1973

Containers and *Storage:* see the entry on Tablets for general information on containers and storage. Containers should be airtight.

Advice for patients: the tablets should be taken at regular intervals. Treatment should not be discontinued without the advice of the prescriber.

SLOW PROCAINAMIDE TABLETS: available as tablets containing 500 mg of procainamide in a slow-release formulation.

Containers and *Storage:* see the entry on Tablets for general information on containers and storage. Containers should be airtight.

Advice for patients: the tablets should be swallowed whole and the advice given above under Procainamide Tablets followed.

Procaine Hydrochloride

2-Diethylaminoethyl 4-aminobenzoate hydrochloride

$C_{13}H_{21}ClN_2O_2 = 272.8$

OTHER NAMES: Procainii Chloridum
Willcain® (with adrenaline)

A standard is given in the European Pharmacopoeia Vol. I

Description. Odourless colourless crystals or white crystalline powder with a taste which is salty and bitter followed by a numbing sensation.

Solubility. Soluble, at 20°, in 1 part of water and in 25 parts of alcohol; very slightly soluble in chloroform; practically insoluble in ether.

Acidity. A 2% solution has a pH of 5 to 6.5.

Dissociation constant. pK_a 9.0 (25°).

Stability. In aqueous solution, procaine degrades by hydrolysis to 4-aminobenzoic acid and 2-aminoethanol. The 4-aminobenzoic acid is converted by decarboxylation to aniline which is then oxidised to various purple-coloured products. Hydrolysis of procaine is catalysed by hydrogen ions and by hydroxyl ions. At 25°, solutions are most stable at about pH 3.5.

FURTHER INFORMATION. T. Higuchi *et al.*, *J. Am. pharm. Ass., scient. Edn*, 1950, **39**, 405 and 411; H. W. Schmid, *Pharm. Acta Helv.*, 1961, **36**, 423; R. E. Thomas and M. Woodward, *Australas. J. Pharm.*, 1963, **44**, 590.

Sterilisation. Solutions for injection are sterilised by heating in an autoclave or by filtration.

Storage. It should be protected from light.

Identification. TESTS. 1. It complies with Test 2, described under Butyl Aminobenzoate (primary aromatic amines).

2. To a 10% solution add *sodium bicarbonate solution*; there is no change. Add *sodium hydroxide solution* or *sodium carbonate solution*; a colourless oily precipitate which becomes crystalline is produced which, after washing with water, drying at 100° and allowing to solidify, melts at about 60°.

MELTING-POINT. About 155°.

ULTRAVIOLET ABSORPTION. In alcohol (95%), maximum at 296 nm (E1%, 1cm = 773); in 0.1N sodium hydroxide, maximum at 267 nm (E1%, 1cm = 511).

INFRA-RED ABSORPTION. Major peaks at 772, 1116, 1174, 1272, 1607, and 1692 cm^{-1} (see Appendix 2a: Infra-red Spectra).

THIN-LAYER CHROMATOGRAPHY. See under Thin-layer Chromatography, System 2.

Metabolism. BLOOD CONCENTRATION. After an intravenous injection of 10 to 20 mg/kg, concentrations of 12 to 30 μg/ml are obtained in arterial blood within 5 minutes; concentrations of 7 to 17 μg/ml are obtained in the cerebrospinal fluid 5 minutes after the same dose.

HALF-LIFE. Serum half-life, less than 1 minute.

DISTRIBUTION. Procaine crosses the placenta together with its metabolite, 4-aminobenzoic acid.

METABOLIC REACTIONS. Hydrolysed by enzymes in the plasma and in various tissues to 4-aminobenzoic acid and diethylaminoethanol, both of which are further metabolised; procaine is rapidly and almost completely metabolised but in newborn infants, some uraemics, and patients with liver disease the rate of metabolism may be reduced.

EXCRETION. About 2% of a dose is excreted unchanged in the urine; 80 to 90% of the 4-aminobenzoic acid derived from procaine is excreted either unchanged or in conjugated form with 30% of the diethylaminoethanol.

Actions and uses. Procaine is a short-acting local anaesthetic. It is less toxic than cocaine, but because of its poor penetration of intact mucous membranes, it is useless for surface application. To prolong its effect, adrenaline, in a concentration of 1 in 400000 to 1 in 50000, is added to constrict the blood vessels at the site of injection.

Procaine and adrenaline injection is used for infiltration anaesthesia. Solutions containing adrenaline should not, however, be used for inducing anaesthesia in digits, because the profound ischaemia produced may lead to gangrene. Procaine and adrenaline injection should not be given by intravenous injection.

Procaine hydrochloride may be given intrathecally as a 2 to 10% aqueous solution or as a 5 to 10% solution in cerebrospinal fluid. A 5% aqueous solution is isotonic with blood serum; to increase its specific gravity for intrathecal injection, 5% of dextrose may be added. A 1% solution is used in caudal anaesthesia. For epidural anaesthesia the strength of the solution should not be more than 5%. In dental practice, procaine has been largely replaced by lignocaine for the production of local anaesthesia. It was formerly used as procaine and adrenaline injection; the effect of 1 to 2 millilitres appears in about 5 minutes and lasts for half to 2 hours.

Undesirable effects. Constant wetting of the skin with solutions of procaine hydrochloride may cause a dermatitis characterised by dryness and cracking of the skin.

Poisoning. Artificial respiration should be applied and diazepam administered intravenously to control the convulsions. The toxic action of procaine may be reduced by a preliminary dose of phenobarbitone or other barbiturate.

Preparations

PROCAINE AND ADRENALINE INJECTION (*Syn.* Strong Procaine and Adrenaline Injection):

Procaine hydrochloride	2.0 g
Adrenaline solution	2.0 ml
Chlorocresol	0.1 g
Sodium metabisulphite	0.1 g
Sodium chloride	0.5 g
Water for injections	to 100.0 ml

Dissolve the chlorocresol in about 90 ml of the water with the aid of gentle heat, cool, dissolve the procaine hydrochloride, the sodium metabisulphite, and the sodium chloride in the solution; add the adrenaline solution and sufficient of the water to produce the required volume. Distribute the solution into the final containers, seal the containers and sterilise by the process of heating with a bactericide. Alternatively, sterilise the solution by filtration; distribute, by means of an aseptic technique, into sterile final containers, and seal the containers.

A standard for this injection is given in the British Pharmacopoeia 1973

Containers: see the entry on Injections for general information on containers.

Labelling: see the entry on Injections for general information on labelling. In addition, the label on the container should state the amount of the medicament as "Procaine Hydrochloride 2%; Adrenaline, 1 in 50000".

Storage: it should be protected from light.

OTHER PREPARATIONS available include a veterinary INJECTION containing procaine hydrochloride 50 mg per ml (5%) with adrenaline 1 in 50000 in 50- and 250-ml bottles.

Procaine hydrochloride is an ingredient of lymecycline and procaine injection and tetracycline and procaine injection. It is also an ingredient of an injection and a veterinary injection containing oxytetracycline hydrochloride and a veterinary injection containing procaine penicillin.

Procaine Penicillin

The monohydrate of the procaine salt of benzylpenicillin.

$C_{29}H_{38}N_2O_6S,H_2O = 588.7$

OTHER NAMES: *Depocillin*®; *Duphapen*®; *Econopen*®; *Ethacilin*®; *Mylipen*®; *Penjectin*®; Procaine Benzylpenicillin; Procaine Penicillin G; *Willopen*® *Propen*® (with benethamine penicillin); *Depopen P*®, *Duphapen LA*®, *Duplocillin*®, *Ethacilin P–A*®, and *Lentrax*® (all with benzathine penicillin); *Bicillin*® (with benzylpenicillin); *Cepoxillin*® (with cephoxazole sodium); *Depomycin*®, *Duphapen-Strep*®, *Ilcocillin DryCow*®, *Milimycin*®, *Streptocillin*®, *Streptopen*®, and *Strypen*® (all with dihydrostreptomycin sulphate or streptomycin sulphate); *Mastikort 500/300*® (with neomycin sulphate); *Lenticillin*® (with procaine hydrochloride).

Triplopen® (with benethamine penicillin and benzylpenicillin); *Penidural-AP*® (with benzathine penicillin and benzylpenicillin)

A standard is given in the British Pharmacopoeia 1973

Description. A white crystalline powder.

Solubility. Soluble, at 20°, in 200 parts of water.

Acidity or alkalinity. A 30% suspension has a pH of 5 to 7.5.

Moisture content. Not more than 4.2%, determined by Fischer titration.

Storage. It should be stored in airtight containers at a temperature not exceeding 30°. If it is intended for parenteral administration, the containers should be sterile and sealed to exclude micro-organisms.

Labelling. If the material is not intended for parenteral administration, the label on the container states that the contents are not to be injected.

Identification. TESTS. 1. It complies with Test 1 described under Benzylpenicillin.
2. It complies with Test 2 described under Butyl Aminobenzoate (primary aromatic amines).

INFRA-RED ABSORPTION. Major peaks at 1124, 1176, 1266, 1613, 1695, and 1786 cm^{-1} (see Appendix 2b: Infra-red Spectra).

Metabolism. ABSORPTION. Slowly absorbed after intramuscular administration.

BLOOD CONCENTRATION. After an intramuscular dose of 300000 units of procaine penicillin, a peak serum concentration of benzylpenicillin of about 1.6 units/ml is attained in 1 to 3 hours falling to 0.4 unit/ml at 6 hours; serum concentrations are lower than those achieved after an equivalent dose of benzylpenicillin.

FURTHER INFORMATION. Absorption from intramuscular injection—F. H. Buckwalter and H. L. Dickison, *J. Am. pharm. Ass., scient. Edn*, 1958, **47**, 661; plasma concentrations of procaine after high doses—R. L. Green *et al.*, *New Engl. J. Med.*, 1974, **291**, 223.

Actions and uses. Procaine penicillin is a sparingly soluble salt of benzylpenicillin. It is administered intramuscularly to create a depot from which benzylpenicillin is slowly released into the blood stream. A dose of 300 to 900 milligrams may be expected to maintain an effective concentration in the blood for about 24 hours, so that injections need not be given more frequently than once a day; 300 milligrams of procaine penicillin is approximately equivalent to 200 milligrams of benzylpenicillin. Because of the relatively low blood-penicillin concentrations obtained it should be used only for the treatment of infections due to organisms that are highly sensitive to penicillin.

Procaine penicillin has the uses described under Benzylpenicillin; it is frequently mixed with benzylpenicillin, as in the fortified injection, the mixture being particularly useful at the beginning of the treatment.

Procaine penicillin is usually administered by intramuscular injection as an aqueous suspension.

Undesirable effects. Large doses given more frequently than once a day may give rise to undesirable effects due to the absorption of procaine and leave painful lumps at the injection site.

Precautions. The precautions against allergy described under Benzylpenicillin should be observed.

Veterinary uses. Procaine penicillin is a long-acting antibacterial agent. The usual daily dosage by intramuscular injection for horses, cattle, and pigs is 6 to 15 milligrams per kilogram body-weight, for foals, calves, piglets, and sheep 20 to 40 milligrams per kilogram body-weight, and for dogs and cats 30 to 200 milligrams per kilogram body-weight. Procaine penicillin is also used in cows by intramammary injection in a dose of 100 to 300 milligrams in each quarter, daily for 3 days.

Preparations

FORTIFIED PROCAINE PENICILLIN INJECTION: a sterile suspension of procaine penicillin, with suitable dispersing agents, in a solution of benzylpenicillin in water for injections. It may contain a suitable buffering agent. It is prepared by adding water for injections to the contents of a sealed container shortly before use. The medicaments in the sealed container are present in the ratio of 5 parts of procaine penicillin and 1 part of benzylpenicillin.

Available as a powder in vials containing 3 g (3 mega units) of procaine penicillin and 600 mg (1 mega unit) of benzylpenicillin.

A standard for this injection is given in the British Pharmacopoeia 1973

Containers: see the entry on Injections for general information on containers.

Labelling: see the entry on Injections for general information on labelling. In addition, the label on the container should state "For intramuscular injection only".

Storage: the sealed container should be stored at a temperature not exceeding 30°. The injection contains no bactericide and should be used as soon as possible after preparation but the injection may be expected to retain its potency for up to 7 days after preparation, or for up to 14 days if a buffering agent is present, provided it is stored at 2° to 10°.

PROCAINE PENICILLIN INJECTION (Syn. Procaine Benzyl-penicillin Injection): a sterile suspension of procaine penicillin, with suitable buffering and dispersing agents, in water for injections. Available in 10-, 30-, and 100-ml vials containing 300 mg (300000 units) of procaine penicillin per ml.

A standard for this injection is given in the British Pharmacopoeia 1973

Containers: see the entry on Injections for general information on containers.

Labelling: see the entry on Injections for general information on labelling. In addition, the label on the container should state "For intramuscular injection only".

Storage: it should be stored at a temperature not exceeding 20°, protected from light. Under these conditions it may be expected to retain its potency for 18 months.

OTHER PREPARATIONS: procaine penicillin is an ingredient of fortified benethamine penicillin injection and of fortified benzathine penicillin injection.

OTHER VETERINARY PREPARATIONS available include a sterile GEL containing procaine penicillin 10 mg (10000 units) with streptomycin sulphate, equivalent to 20 mg of streptomycin per ml, in 100-ml single-dose bottles; an INJECTION containing procaine penicillin 150 mg (150000 units) with benethamine penicillin 141.5 mg (150000 units) per ml in 30- and 100-ml vials, an injection containing procaine penicillin 150 mg (150000 units) with benzathine penicillin 113 mg (150000 units) per ml in 30-and 100-ml vials and in 50- and 100-ml bottles, an injection containing procaine penicillin 200 mg (200000 units) with neomycin sulphate equivalent to 100 mg of neomycin per ml in 100-ml vials, an injection containing procaine penicillin 300 mg (300000 units) with procaine hydrochloride 20 mg per ml in 30- and 90-ml vials; an INTRAMAMMARY INJECTION containing procaine penicillin 100 mg (100000 units) in each tube, an intramammary injection containing procaine penicillin 300 mg

(300000 units) in each tube in both normal and slow-release formulations, an intramammary injection containing procaine penicillin 250 mg (250000 units) with cephoxazole sodium equivalent to 250 mg of cephoxazole in each single-dose syringe, and an intramammary injection containing procaine penicillin 500 mg (500000 units) with neomycin sulphate equivalent to 300 mg of neomycin in each 4-g disposable syringe, and various injections and intramammary injections containing procaine penicillin with dihydrostreptomycin sulphate.

Procarbazine Hydrochloride

N-Isopropyl-α-(2-methylhydrazino)-p-toluamide hydrochloride

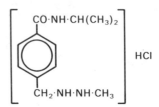

$C_{12}H_{20}ClN_3O = 257.8$

OTHER NAME: Natulan®

Description. A white to pale yellow crystalline powder with a slight odour.

Solubility. Soluble in water, in alcohol, in methyl alcohol, in ether, and in chloroform.

Identification. MELTING-POINT. About 223°, with decomposition.

ULTRAVIOLET ABSORPTION. Procarbazine in 0.1N sulphuric acid, maximum at 232 nm (E1%, 1cm = 497).

Metabolism. ABSORPTION. Readily and almost completely absorbed after oral administration.

BLOOD CONCENTRATION. Peak concentrations are attained in 30 to 60 minutes following an oral dose.

HALF-LIFE. Plasma half-life, 7 to 10 minutes.

DISTRIBUTION. Enters the cerebrospinal fluid rapidly; does not appear to show any special affinity to particular tissues.

METABOLIC REACTIONS. Rapidly metabolised by N-oxidation to N-isopropylterephthalamic acid and to hydrogen peroxide and hydroxyl radicals.

EXCRETION. Up to about 75% is excreted in the urine and 10% in the faeces; about 5% of a dose is excreted in the urine as unchanged drug; the remainder is excreted as metabolites.

FURTHER INFORMATION. Proceedings of Chemotherapy Conference on Procarbazine: Development and Applications, S. K. Cater (Ed.), Bethesda, Md., March 1975; B. Dewald et al., Biochem. Pharmac., 1968, 18, 2179; distribution and excretion—D. E. Schwartz et al., Arzneimittel-Forsch., 1967, 17, 1389.

Actions and uses. Procarbazine hydrochloride is a cytotoxic agent used in the treatment of Hodgkin's disease and other advanced reticuloses and solid tumours. It is often used alone or in conjunction with other cytotoxic drugs when the condition of the patient is no longer responsive to radiotherapy or to other antineoplastic agents.

The initial daily dose by mouth is usually the equivalent

of 50 milligrams of procarbazine increasing by 50 milligrams daily to a maximum daily dose of 250 to 300 milligrams which is continued until the greatest possible remission has been obtained. Treatment is then continued with a maintenance dose of 50 to 150 milligrams daily until a total of at least 6 grams has been administered. In children the initial dose is the equivalent of 50 milligrams of procarbazine daily increasing to 100 milligrams per square metre body-surface daily until a maximum response is obtained or leucopenia or thrombocytopenia arises.

Maintenance therapy may be resumed when the white-cell and platelet levels recover.

Undesirable effects. Anorexia, nausea, vomiting, and allergic skin reactions, may occur during the first few days of treatment. Stomatitis, diarrhoea, drowsiness, lethargy, depression, confusion, agitation, hallucinations, paraesthesias, peripheral neuropathy, leucopenia, and thrombocytopenia may also occur.

Precautions. Blood counts should be performed regularly.

Contra-indications. It is contra-indicated in severe leucopenia or thrombocytopenia and in patients with hepatic or renal damage.

Preparations

Preparations available include CAPSULES containing procarbazine hydrochloride equivalent to 50 mg of procarbazine.

Prochlorperazine Maleate

2-Chloro-10-[3-(4-methylpiperazin-1-yl)propyl]phenothiazine di(hydrogen maleate)

$C_{28}H_{32}ClN_3O_8S = 606.1$

OTHER NAMES: *Stemetil®*; *Vertigon®*

A standard is given in the British Pharmacopoeia 1973

Description. An almost odourless, white or pale yellow, crystalline powder with a slightly bitter taste.

Solubility. Very slightly soluble in water and in alcohol; practically insoluble in ether.

Moisture content. Not more than 1%, determined by drying at 105°.

Dissociation constant. pK_a 8.1 (24°).

Storage. It should be protected from light.

Identification. TESTS. 1. Dissolve about 5 mg in 2 ml of sulphuric acid and allow to stand for 5 minutes; a red colour develops.
2. Dissolve about 200 mg in a mixture of 3 ml of water and 2 ml of *sodium hydroxide solution*, and extract with three successive 3-ml portions of solvent ether; separate off the aqueous solution, add 2 ml of *bromine solution AsT*, warm in a water-bath for 10 minutes, boil, cool, add 2 drops of a solution of 10 mg of resorcinol in 3 ml of sulphuric acid and heat for 15 minutes in a water-bath; a bluish-black colour develops.

MELTING-POINT. About 200°.

ULTRAVIOLET ABSORPTION. In dehydrated alcohol containing 0.01% of *strong ammonia solution*, maxima at 258 nm (E1%, 1cm = 600) and 313 nm.

Determination in body fluids. ULTRAVIOLET SPECTROPHOTOMETRY. In blood, serum, or urine—J. E. Wallace and J. D. Biggs, *J. pharm. Sci.*, 1971, **60**, 1346.

Metabolism. METABOLIC REACTIONS. In rats, ring cleavage and *N*-dealkylation to form *N*-[3-(2-chloro-phenothiazin-10-yl)propyl]ethylenediamine.

EXCRETION. In rats, about 35% of a dose is excreted in the faeces in 24 hours; unchanged drug and metabolites are excreted in urine to some extent.

FURTHER INFORMATION. Tissue metabolites in rats and dogs—H. J. Gaertner *et al.*, *Drug Met. Disp.*, 1975, **3**, 437; tissue distribution and metabolism in rats—B. M. Philips and T. S. Miya, *J. pharm. Sci.*, 1964, **53**, 1098.

Actions and uses. Prochlorperazine has the actions and uses described under Chlorpromazine Hydrochloride but it is less sedating, more effective as an anti-emetic, and more liable to give rise to extrapyramidal side-effects. It is particularly effective for the prevention and relief of vomiting, for which it is given 3 times daily as a suppository or by mouth in a dose of 5 to 25 milligrams; it may be given by injection. It may also be effective in the treatment of Ménière's disease and other forms of vestibular disorder. In the treatment of psychiatric states it is given in a dosage of 15 to 100 milligrams daily in divided doses.

Undesirable effects. Prochlorperazine may give rise to parkinsonism, particularly in children, in whom severe dystonic reactions may occur. Drowsiness may occur in the early stages of treatment.

Preparations

PROCHLORPERAZINE SUPPOSITORIES: prepared as described in the entry on Suppositories by incorporating prochlorperazine in a suitable basis. Available as suppositories containing prochlorperazine equivalent to 5 and 25 mg of prochlorperazine maleate.
Containers and Storage: see the entry on Suppositories for general information on containers and storage. Containers should be light resistant.
Advice for patients: see the entry on Suppositories for general information on the use of suppositories. They may cause drowsiness; persons affected should not drive or operate machinery. Alcohol should be avoided.

PROCHLORPERAZINE TABLETS: available as tablets containing 5 and 25 mg of prochlorperazine maleate.
A standard for these tablets is given in the British Pharmacopoeia 1973
Containers and Storage: see the entry on Tablets for general information on containers and storage. Containers should be airtight and light resistant.
Advice for patients: the tablets may cause drowsiness; persons affected should not drive or operate machinery. Alcohol should be avoided.

OTHER PREPARATIONS available include CAPSULES containing prochlorperazine maleate equivalent to 10 and 15 mg of prochlorperazine in slow-release formulations.

Prochlorperazine Mesylate

2-Chloro-10-[3-(4-methylpiperazin-1-yl)propyl]phenothiazine dimethanesulphonate
$C_{22}H_{32}ClN_3O_6S_2 = 566.1$

OTHER NAMES: Prochlorperazine methanesulphonate; *Stemetil*®

A standard is given in the British Pharmacopoeia 1973

Description. An odourless white powder with a slightly bitter taste.

Solubility. Soluble, at 20°, in less than 0.5 part of water and in 40 parts of alcohol; very slightly soluble in chloroform; practically insoluble in ether.

Acidity. A 2% solution has a pH of 2 to 3.

Moisture content. Not more than 1%, determined by drying at 100° *in vacuo.*

Sterilisation. Solutions for injection are sterilised by heating in an autoclave in an atmosphere of nitrogen or other suitable gas.

Storage. It should be protected from light.

Identification. TESTS. 1. It complies with Test 1 described under Prochlorperazine Maleate.
2. Mix about 50 mg with 200 mg of powdered sodium hydroxide, heat to fusion and continue heating for a few seconds more; cool, add 0.5 ml of water and a slight excess of *dilute hydrochloric acid,* and warm; sulphur dioxide is evolved which turns starch-iodate paper blue.

MELTING-POINT. About 242°.

ULTRAVIOLET ABSORPTION. In dehydrated alcohol containing 0.01% of *strong ammonia solution,* maxima at 258 nm (E1%, 1cm = 628) and 313 nm.

INFRA-RED ABSORPTION. Major peaks at 758, 775, 1042, 1099, 1149, and 1220 cm^{-1} (see Appendix 2b: Infra-red Spectra).

Determination in body fluids; Metabolism. See under Prochlorperazine Maleate.

Actions and uses. Prochlorperazine mesylate has the actions, uses, and undesirable effects described under Prochlorperazine Maleate. It is administered by deep intramuscular injection in a dosage of 12.5 to 25 milligrams 2 or 3 times daily in the treatment of psychiatric disorders.
As an anti-emetic, 12.5 milligrams is given by intramuscular injection. For the treatment of acute alcoholism, it is given by intravenous injection in a dose of 100 milligrams.

Preparations

PROCHLORPERAZINE INJECTION: a sterile solution of prochlorperazine mesylate, with suitable buffering and stabilising agents, in water for injections free from dissolved air. It is distributed into the final containers, the air being replaced by nitrogen or other suitable gas, and the containers are sealed and sterilised by heating in an autoclave. Available in 1- and 2-ml ampoules containing 12.5 mg of prochlorperazine mesylate per ml. *A standard for this injection is given in the British Pharmacopoeia 1973*
Containers and *Labelling:* see the entry on Injections for general information on containers and labelling. *Storage:* it should be protected from light.

OTHER PREPARATIONS available include an ELIXIR containing prochlorperazine mesylate 5 mg in 5 ml, diluent syrup, life of diluted elixir 14 days.

Procyclidine Hydrochloride

1-(3-Cyclohexyl-3-hydroxy-3-phenylpropyl)pyrrolidinium chloride

$C_{19}H_{30}ClNO = 323.9$

OTHER NAME: *Kemadrin*®

A standard is given in the British Pharmacopoeia 1973

Description. A white crystalline powder with a faint odour and a bitter taste.

Solubility. Soluble, at 20°, in 40 parts of water and in 15 parts of alcohol; practically insoluble in ether and in acetone.

Acidity. A 1% solution has a pH of 4.5 to 6.5.

Sterilisation. Solutions are sterilised by heating in an autoclave or by filtration.

Identification. TEST. Dissolve about 250 mg in 10 ml of water, make alkaline by the addition of *dilute ammonia solution,* extract with three 10-ml portions of ether, dry the combined extracts over anhydrous sodium sulphate, filter, evaporate off the ether and scratch the residue to induce crystallisation; the residue melts at about 85°.

MELTING-POINT. About 226°.

ULTRAVIOLET ABSORPTION. In 0.1N hydrochloric acid or in alcohol (95%), weak maxima at about 254 nm, 258 nm, and 266 nm.

INFRA-RED ABSORPTION. Major peaks at 700, 746, 756, 1128, 1445, and 1467 cm^{-1} (see Appendix 2a: Infra-red Spectra).

THIN-LAYER CHROMATOGRAPHY. See under Thin-layer Chromatography, System 8.

Actions and uses. Procyclidine antagonises some of the actions of acetylcholine in a manner similar to that described under Atropine. It is used for the symptomatic treatment of parkinsonism. It decreases rigidity more than tremor and improves muscular co-ordination and mobility of the patient, but it has little effect on salivation.
The initial dosage by mouth is usually 2.5 milligrams of procyclidine hydrochloride 3 times a day and this is gradually increased by 2.5 milligrams a day until the optimum effect is obtained; 20 milligrams a day is often required and doses of up to 60 milligrams have occasionally been necessary. Post-encephalitic patients usually require larger doses than arteriosclerotic patients.
Procyclidine hydrochloride is usually administered by mouth but when necessary it may be given by intramuscular or intravenous injection in doses of 5 to 10 milligrams.
Solanaceous alkaloids and other drugs used for the relief of parkinsonism are sometimes given in conjunction with procyclidine.

Undesirable effects. Drowsiness, ataxia, giddiness, blurred vision, confusion, nausea, and vomiting may occur; they usually disappear when the dose is reduced.

Precautions and contra-indications. As for Atropine.

Preparations

PROCYCLIDINE INJECTION (*Syn.* Procyclidine Hydrochloride Injection): a sterile solution of procyclidine hydrochloride in water for injections. It is sterilised by heating in an autoclave or by filtration. Available in 2-ml ampoules containing 5 mg of procyclidine hydrochloride per ml.

A standard for this injection is given in the British Pharmaceutical Codex 1973

Containers and *Labelling:* see the entry on Injections for general information on containers and labelling.

Storage: it should be stored at a temperature not exceeding 25°. It should not be allowed to freeze.

PROCYCLIDINE TABLETS: available as tablets containing 5 mg of procyclidine hydrochloride.

A standard for these tablets is given in the British Pharmacopoeia 1973

Containers and *Storage:* see the entry on Tablets for general information on containers and storage. Containers should be airtight.

Advice for patients: the tablets should be taken after meals. Treatment should not be discontinued without the advice of the prescriber. The tablets may cause drowsiness; persons affected should not drive or operate machinery. Alcohol should be avoided.

Proflavine Hemisulphate

Acridine-3,6-diamine sulphate dihydrate

$C_{26}H_{24}N_6O_4S,2H_2O = 552.6$

OTHER NAMES: Neutral Proflavine Sulphate; Proflavine

A standard is given in the British Pharmaceutical Codex 1973

Description. An odourless hygroscopic orange to red crystalline powder.

Solubility. Soluble, at 20°, in 300 parts of water and in 35 parts of glycerol; soluble in 1 part of boiling water; very slightly soluble in alcohol; practically insoluble in ether and in chloroform.

Moisture content. 3 to 7%, determined by Fischer titration.

Storage. It should be stored in airtight containers, protected from light.

Preparation and storage of solutions. See statement on aqueous solutions of antiseptics, under Solutions.

Identification. TESTS. Dissolve about 100 mg in 30 ml of water and carry out the following tests.
1. Add 4 drops of the solution to a large volume of water; a greenish fluorescence is produced.
2. To 1 ml add 2 drops of sulphuric acid, an immediate precipitate of bright reddish-orange needles is produced.
3. To 2 ml add *sodium hydroxide solution*; a lemon-yellow precipitate is produced.
4. To 5 ml add 1 ml of 1N hydrochloric acid and 5 ml of a 10% solution of sodium nitrite and boil for 1 minute; a brown precipitate is produced. Filter the solution; the filtrate is yellow (distinction from certain other flavines).

Actions and uses. Proflavine and other acridine derivatives are slow-acting antiseptics which are effective against many Gram-positive and Gram-negative bacteria; they are used in the treatment of infected wounds. In the concentrations usually employed, they are not effective against *Proteus vulgaris*, *Pseudomonas aeruginosa*, and some strains of *Escherichia coli*. Their activity is not reduced by tissue fluids and serum, and, in concentrations of 0.01% or less, they do not interfere with the action of phagocytic cells.

For the dressing of wounds or burns, a 0.1% solution is used, but, if treatment is prolonged, weaker solutions or another antiseptic should be used, as the acridine derivatives tend to delay healing.

For the treatment of certain local infections of the external ear, mouth, throat, and skin, 0.1 to 1% w/v alcoholic or aqueous solutions are used.

Stains on the skin caused by acridine derivatives may be removed by washing with a dilute solution of sulphurous acid or of hydrochloric acid.

Preparation

PROFLAVINE CREAM (*Syn.* Flavine Cream; Proflavine Emulsion):

Proflavine hemisulphate	.. 1 g
Chlorocresol	.. 1 g
Yellow beeswax	25 g
Wool fat	50 g
Purified water, freshly boiled and cooled ..	250 g
Liquid paraffin	673 g

Dissolve the chlorocresol in 600 g of the liquid paraffin with the aid of gentle heat and add to the yellow beeswax and the wool fat previously melted together; cool, add, with continuous stirring, the proflavine hemisulphate dissolved in the water, followed by the remainder of the liquid paraffin, and stir gently until cold.

A standard for this cream is given in the British Pharmaceutical Codex 1973

Containers, Labelling, and *Storage:* see the entry on Creams for general information on containers, labelling, and storage.

Advice for patients: the cream stains the skin, hair, and fabric; the stain may be removed by washing with a dilute solution of sulphurous acid or of hydrochloric acid.

Progesterone

Pregn-4-ene-3,20-dione

$C_{21}H_{30}O_2 = 314.5$

OTHER NAMES: *Cyclogest*®; *Gestone*®; *Progestasert*®; Progesteronum

Gestin-E® (with alpha tocopherol); *Nymfalon*® (with chorionic gonadotrophin); *Implixa-BM*® (with oestradiol); *Paralut*® (with oestradiol benzoate).

A standard is given in the European Pharmacopoeia Vol. II

Description. Odourless colourless crystals or white or slightly yellowish-white crystalline powder.

Solubility. Practically insoluble in water; soluble, at 20°, in 8 parts of alcohol, in 16 parts of ether, in less than 1 part of chloroform, in 60 parts of arachis oil, in 60 parts of ethyl oleate, and in 100 parts of light petroleum.

Specific rotation. +186° to +194°, determined on a 1% solution in alcohol (95%).

Sterilisation. Oily solutions for injection are sterilised by dry heat.

Storage. It should be protected from light.

Identification. TEST. Mix about 20 mg with 75 mg of dinitrophenylhydrazine and 30 ml of alcohol (95%), heat under a reflux condenser for 15 minutes, add 1 ml of hydrochloric acid, heat under the reflux condenser for a further 15 minutes, and cool; a precipitate is produced which, after washing with 5-ml portions of alcohol (95%) followed by portions of a mixture of 1 volume of hydrochloric acid and 19 volumes of water until the washings are colourless, melts at about 270°.

MELTING-POINT. About 130°, or it may occur in a form which melts at about 121° due to polymorphism.

ULTRAVIOLET ABSORPTION. In dehydrated alcohol, maximum at 240 nm (E1%, 1cm = 540).

INFRA-RED ABSORPTION. Major peaks at 872, 1209, 1358, 1614, 1662, and 1700 cm^{-1} (see Appendix 2a: Infra-red Spectra).

THIN-LAYER CHROMATOGRAPHY. See under Thin-layer Chromatography, System 10.

Metabolism. ABSORPTION. Rapidly absorbed from all routes of administration; low doses are ineffective orally since progesterone is rapidly metabolised by the gastrointestinal mucosa and the liver.

BLOOD CONCENTRATION. Endogenous plasma concentrations in males and ovariectomised females, about 350 pg/ml; in normal females the endogenous plasma concentrations vary according to the stages of the menstrual cycle as follows: early follicular, about 800 pg/ml; mid-follicular, 350 to 500 pg/ml; late follicular, 1 to 2 ng/ml; early luteal, 1 to 2 ng/ml; mid-luteal, 8 to 20 ng/ml which then drops, at menstruation, to preovulatory concentrations; in pregnancy, concentrations gradually increase to about 120 to 200 ng/ml at 24 hours postpartum.

HALF-LIFE. After intravenous administration, 3 to 90 minutes.

DISTRIBUTION. Very little is bound to red blood cells; diffuses in small amounts into body fat from which it is slowly released; taken up by the uterus; secreted in the milk; subject to enterohepatic cycling; *protein binding*, extensively bound to plasma proteins and, in guinea pigs, bound to a specific globulin, "progesterone binding globulin".

METABOLIC REACTIONS. Rapidly metabolised by ring A reduction, hydroxylation at positions 6 and 16, reduction of the 20-keto group, and conjugation with glucuronic acid and sulphate; the hydroxylation reactions are stimulated by dicophane, chlordane, and phenobarbitone; differences in metabolism occur according to species and sex; metabolites include 5α- or 5β-pregnane-3α,20α-diols, pregnanolones and pregnanediones, along with 6α-hydroxy and 16α-hydroxy metabolites; intermediate metabolites in the formation of the ring A-reduced metabolites include 20α- and 20β-dihydroprogesterones, and 5α- and 5β-pregnenolones.

EXCRETION. About 50 to 60% of a dose is excreted in the urine as metabolites, about 10% is excreted in the faeces, and the fate of the remainder is unknown; 5 to 25% of the dose is excreted in the urine as pregnanediol, about 5% as pregnanolone, 2% as pregnanedione, 7% as 6α-hydroxy metabolites, 5% as 16α-hydroxy metabolites, and pregnanetriol; most of the metabolites are excreted as glucuronic acid conjugates with about 3% as sulphates; in pregnancy, small amounts of unchanged progesterone may be excreted in the urine.

FURTHER INFORMATION. Reviews—M. B. Aufrère and H. Benson, *J. pharm. Sci.*, 1976, **65**, 783 and K. Fotherby, *Vitamins and Hormones*, 1964, **22**, 153; F. A. Kincl, Chemistry and biochemistry of progesterone, *International Encyclopedia of Pharmacology and Therapeutics*, Sect. 48, M. Tausk (Ed.), Vol. 1, Oxford, Pergamon Press, 1971, p. 13.

Actions and uses. Progesterone, which is secreted by the corpus luteum, converts the proliferative endometrium to a secretory phase and, if pregnancy ensues, helps to maintain the decidua.

It is used in the treatment of functional uterine haemorrhage in a dosage of up to 10 milligrams daily in the second half of the menstrual cycle. Progesterone is administered by intramuscular injection and has been largely replaced by progestational compounds which are active when given by mouth and which have a less marked virilising action.

Progesterone has also been used in intra-uterine devices for the prevention of conception.

Precautions and contra-indications. It should not be used in pregnancy and should be used with caution in nursing mothers.

Veterinary uses. Progesterone is used to regulate the ovarian cycle. It is administered by subcutaneous or intramuscular injection of a solution in oil for the synchronisation of oestrus which occurs on withdrawal and also in the treatment of threatened abortion, the usual dose for all species being 200 to 500 micrograms per kilogram body-weight every 48 hours. It is also used in the treatment of habitual abortion in horses and cattle by implantation in a non-edible part of the body of 200 or 400 milligrams.

Preparations

PROGESTERONE IMPLANTS: available as implants containing 25, 50, and 100 mg of progesterone; they are sterile cylinders prepared by fusion or compression of progesterone without the addition of any other substance. They are distributed singly into sterile containers and the containers are then sealed to exclude microorganisms.

A standard for these implants is given in the British Pharmacopoeia (Veterinary)

Containers and *Labelling:* see the entry on Implants for general information on containers and labelling.

Storage: they should be protected from light.

PROGESTERONE INJECTION: a sterile solution of progesterone in ethyl oleate or other suitable ester, in a suitable fixed oil, or in any mixture of these. It may contain suitable alcohols. It is sterilised by dry heat.

Available in 1-ml ampoules and 10-ml vials containing 10 mg of progesterone per ml, in 1-ml ampoules and 10-and 50-ml vials containing 25 mg of progesterone per ml, and in 1- and 2-ml ampoules containing 50 mg of progesterone per ml.

A standard for this injection is given in the British Pharmacopoeia 1973

Containers: see the entry on Injections for general information on containers.

Labelling: see the entry on Injections for general information on labelling. In addition, the label on the package should state the composition of the solvent, and "For intramuscular injection only".

Storage: it should be protected from light. If solid matter separates on standing it should be redissolved by heating before use.

OTHER PREPARATIONS available include veterinary IMPLANTS containing progesterone 200 mg with oestradiol 20 mg; an INJECTION containing progesterone 12 mg with alpha tocopherol 100 mg per ml in 1-ml ampoules and 10-ml vials, a veterinary injection reconstituted from vials of powder containing progesterone 125 mg with chorionic gonadotrophin 3000 units, an injection containing progesterone 20 mg with oestradiol benzoate 2 mg per ml in 1-ml ampoules, an injection containing progesterone 50 mg with oestradiol benzoate 3 mg per ml in 1-ml ampoules; SUPPOSITORIES containing progesterone 200 and 400 mg; and an intra-uterine insert containing progesterone 38 mg in a slow-release formulation providing approximately 65 micrograms of progesterone per day.

Proguanil Hydrochloride

1-(4-Chlorophenyl)-5-isopropylbiguanide hydrochloride

$C_{11}H_{17}Cl_2N_5 = 290.2$

OTHER NAME: *Paludrine®*

A standard is given in the British Pharmacopoeia 1973

Description. An odourless white crystalline powder with a bitter taste.

Solubility. Soluble, at 20°, in 110 parts of water and in 40 parts of alcohol; very slightly soluble in ether and in chloroform.

Dissociation constants. pK_a 2.3, 10.4 (22.5°).

Hygroscopicity. It absorbs insignificant amounts of moisture at temperatures up to 37° at relative humidities up to about 80%.

Identification. TESTS. 1. It complies with Tests 1 and 2 described under Chlorproguanil Hydrochloride.
2. It complies with Test 1 described under Chlorhexidine Acetate.
3. To 15 ml of a saturated solution add 2 ml of *sodium hydroxide solution*, extract with 20 ml of ether, wash the ether extract with water and evaporate to dryness; the residue, after drying at 105°, melts at about 131°.

MELTING-POINT. About 245°.

Metabolism. ABSORPTION. Rapidly absorbed after oral administration.

BLOOD CONCENTRATION. Peak blood concentrations are achieved in about 5 hours.

DISTRIBUTION. Taken up by red blood cells; *protein binding*, about 75% bound to plasma proteins.

METABOLIC REACTIONS. Hydroxylation followed by cyclisation to cycloguanil which is an active metabolite.

EXCRETION. About 60% of a dose is excreted in the urine unchanged and about 30% is excreted as cycloguanil.

Actions and uses. Proguanil is used for the prevention and treatment of malaria. Its action is dependent upon the formation of an active metabolite, cycloguanil.

When used in the treatment of malaria caused by *Plasmodium falciparum*, proguanil kills parasites undergoing schizogony in the red blood cells and also the tissue forms. It thus acts as a causal prophylactic and effects a radical cure, so that attacks do not recur when treatment is stopped. In the treatment of malaria caused by *P. vivax*, proguanil kills the asexual parasites in the red blood cells, but will not always eradicate latent tissue infection, so that attacks may sometimes recur after treatment is stopped. Proguanil does not kill the gametocytes, but renders them noninfective for the mosquito while the drug is present in the blood.

Malaria parasites in the red blood cells are killed more rapidly by quinine, chloroquine, or mepacrine than by proguanil, which is therefore not the best drug to use for the treatment of acute malaria.

The prophylactic and suppressive dose for both vivax and falciparum malaria in non-immune subjects is 100 milligrams daily by mouth after food; twice this dose is necessary in highly endemic areas. The corresponding dose for children up to 1 year is 2.5 to 3 milligrams per kilogram body-weight, 1 to 5 years 25 to 50 milligrams daily, and 6 to 12 years 50 to 75 milligrams daily. Non-immune subjects should begin treatment a day before entry into a malarious region and continue until 1 month after leaving the area. Semi-immune individuals may be given 300 milligrams weekly or 200 milligrams twice weekly.

Acute attacks of vivax malaria are treated with an initial dose of 300 to 600 milligrams, followed by 300 milligrams daily for 5 to 10 days.

Strains of *Plasmodium* sometimes become resistant to proguanil; in such circumstances, chloroquine or mepacrine should be used for a time to prevent the transmission of resistant strains.

A dosage of 100 milligrams twice a week for 6 months following exposure to infection greatly reduces the chance of relapse in malaria caused by *P. vivax*.

Undesirable effects. These very rarely occur during the administration of therapeutic doses. Large doses may however cause vomiting, epigastric discomfort, renal irritation, and haematuria.

Preparation

PROGUANIL TABLETS: available as tablets containing 25 and 100 mg of proguanil hydrochloride.

A standard for these tablets is given in the British Pharmacopoeia 1973

Containers and *Storage:* see the entry on Tablets for general information on containers and storage. Containers should be airtight.

Advice for patients: the tablets should preferably be taken after meals. For prophylaxis, doses should be taken regularly during the period at risk and for 1 month thereafter. For therapy the prescribed course should be completed.

Promazine Hydrochloride

10-(3-Dimethylaminopropyl)phenothiazine hydrochloride

$$CH_2 \cdot CH_2 \cdot CH_2 \cdot N(CH_3)_2$$

HCl

$C_{17}H_{21}ClN_2S = 320.9$

OTHER NAMES: *Sparine®*
Tofranil with Promazine® (with imipramine hydrochloride)

A standard is given in the British Pharmacopoeia 1973

Description. An odourless, slightly hygroscopic, white crystalline powder.

Solubility. Soluble, at 20°, in 1 part of water and in 2 parts of alcohol and of chloroform.

Acidity. A 5% solution has a pH of 4.2 to 5.4.

Dissociation constant. pK_a 9.4 (25°).

Stability. It is affected by air and light and by traces of heavy metals. On decomposition, solutions may be coloured pink or red.

Sterilisation. Solutions for injection are sterilised by heating in an autoclave in an atmosphere of nitrogen or other suitable gas, or by filtration.

Storage. It should be stored in airtight containers, protected from light.

Identification. TESTS. 1. Dissolve about 5 mg in 2 ml of sulphuric acid and allow to stand for 5 minutes; an orange colour is produced.
2. Dissolve about 500 mg in 20 ml of water and add 0.5 ml of nitric acid; an orange precipitate is produced which rapidly turns brown. Add a further 2 ml of nitric acid; a yellow solution is produced.

MELTING-POINT. About 179°.

ULTRAVIOLET ABSORPTION. In 0.1N hydrochloric acid, maxima at 254 nm (E1%, 1cm = 1028) and 304 nm (E1%, 1cm = 137). In alcohol (95%), maxima at 254 nm (E1%, 1cm = 1050) and 305 nm (E1%, 1cm = 154).

INFRA-RED ABSORPTION. Major peaks at 751, 1234, 1250, 1287, 1339, and 1455 cm^{-1} (see Appendix 2a: Infra-red Spectra).

Metabolism. ABSORPTION. Well absorbed after oral administration but its absorption may be delayed by other compounds such as attapulgite, charcoal, or citrus pectin.

BLOOD CONCENTRATIONS. After an intravenous dose of 50 mg, plasma concentrations of about 0.5 μg/ml are obtained in 2 minutes falling to about 0.15 μg/ml by 5 minutes.

DISTRIBUTION. Enters the cerebrospinal fluid and crosses the placenta.

METABOLIC REACTIONS. Sulphoxide formation and demethylation; in dogs, the main metabolites are promazine sulphoxide, the monomethyl metabolite, and the monomethyl sulphoxide metabolite; glucuronic acid conjugation also appears to occur; promazine metabolism is reduced in pregnancy and in neonates and also by the administration of oral contraceptives, progesterone, and stilbamidine.

EXCRETION. In dogs and rats, about 50% of a dose is excreted in the urine in 24 hours with about 20 to 25% as unchanged drug; in 7 days about 75% is excreted in the urine and 25% is eliminated in the faeces.

FURTHER INFORMATION. Effects of adsorbents on absorption—D. L. Sorby, *J. pharm. Sci.*, 1965, **54**, 677, 1966, **55**, 504, and 1968, **57**, 1604; metabolism—A. H. Beckett *et al.*, *J. Pharm. Pharmac.*, 1964, **16**, 500, D. L. Shaw and J. A. Page, *Curr. ther. Res.*, 1960, **2**, 199, and S. S. Walkenstein and J. Seifter, *J. Pharmac. exp. Ther.*, 1959, **125**, 283; metabolism in neonates, and effects of oral contraceptives and pregnancy—J. S. Crawford and S. Rudofsky, *Br. J. Anaesth.*, 1966, **38**, 446.

Actions and uses. Promazine has actions, and undesirable effects similar to those described under Chlorpromazine Hydrochloride. It is little used as a tranquilliser but is of some value in elderly patients with minor psychiatric problems.

The usual dose is 50 to 800 milligrams by mouth or by intramuscular or intravenous injection daily in divided doses.

Poisoning. The procedure as described under Chlorpromazine Hydrochloride should be followed.

Preparations

PROMAZINE INJECTION: a sterile solution of promazine hydrochloride, with suitable buffering and stabilising agents, in water for injections free from dissolved air. It is distributed into the final containers, the air being replaced by nitrogen or other suitable gas, the containers are sealed and sterilised by heating in an autoclave. Alternatively, the solution is sterilised by filtration and distributed, by means of an aseptic technique, into sterile final containers, the air in the containers being replaced by sterile nitrogen or other suitable gas, and the containers are sealed.

Available in 1- and 2-ml ampoules containing 50 mg of promazine hydrochloride per ml.

A standard for this injection is given in the British Pharmacopoeia 1973

Containers and Labelling: see the entry on Injections for general information on containers and labelling.

Storage: it should be protected from light.

PROMAZINE TABLETS: available as tablets containing 25, 50 and 100 mg of promazine hydrochloride; they are sugar coated; the coat may be coloured.

A standard for these tablets is given in the British Pharmacopoeia 1973

Containers and Storage: see the entry on Tablets for general information on containers and storage. Containers should be airtight.

Advice for patients: the tablets may cause drowsiness; persons affected should not drive or operate machinery. Alcohol should be avoided.

OTHER PREPARATIONS available include CAPSULES containing promazine hydrochloride 50 mg with imipramine hydrochloride 25 mg.

Promethazine Hydrochloride

10-(2-Dimethylaminopropyl)phenothiazine hydrochloride

$C_{17}H_{21}ClN_2S = 320.9$

OTHER NAMES: *Phenergan®*; Promethazini Hydrochloridum
Sonergan® (with butobarbitone); *Pamergan®* (with pethidine hydrochloride)
A standard is given in the European Pharmacopoeia Vol. III

Description. An odourless, white or faintly yellowish, crystalline powder with a bitter taste.

Solubility. Soluble, at 20°, in less than 1 part of water, in 9 parts of alcohol, and in 2 parts of chloroform.

Acidity. A 10% solution has a pH of 3.5 to 5.

Dissociation constant. pK_a 9.1 (25°).

Stability. In aqueous solution promethazine hydrochloride is degraded by heat and light and degradation is more rapid in the presence of air or oxygen. Micelle formation, which occurs at concentrations above 0.5% of promethazine hydrochloride, decreases the degradation rate.
FURTHER INFORMATION. Stability in aqueous solution in the dark—B. J. Meakin *et al.*, *J. Pharm. Pharmac.*, 1978, **30**, 75.

Sterilisation. Solutions for injection are sterilised by heating in an autoclave in an atmosphere of nitrogen or other suitable gas.

Storage. It should be protected from light.

Identification. TESTS. 1. Dissolve about 5 mg in 2 ml of sulphuric acid and allow to stand for 5 minutes; a red colour is produced.
2. Dissolve about 20 mg in 5 ml of water and add 50 mg of lead dioxide; no red colour is produced but a blue colour slowly develops.
3. Dissolve about 50 mg in 5 ml of water and add 2 ml of nitric acid; a dark red colour develops which becomes yellowish.

MELTING-POINT. About 222°, with decomposition.

ULTRAVIOLET ABSORPTION. In 0.01N hydrochloric acid, maximum at 249 nm (E1%, 1cm = 915).

INFRA-RED ABSORPTION. Major peaks at 733, 758, 1129, 1229, 1336, and 1454 cm⁻¹ (see Appendix 2a: Infra-red Spectra).

THIN-LAYER CHROMATOGRAPHY. See under Thin-layer Chromatography, Systems 4 and 9.

Metabolism. BLOOD CONCENTRATION. After an intravenous dose, a peak plasma concentration may be attained in 1 to 2 hours.

HALF-LIFE. The plasma half-life after an intravenous dose is about 4 hours and the half-life determined from excretion data is about 8 hours; after an oral dose, the two corresponding half-lives are 7 and 10 hours respectively.

DISTRIBUTION. Volume of distribution about 170 litres; promethazine crosses the placenta; *protein binding*, about 90% bound to plasma proteins.

METABOLIC REACTIONS. Subject to extensive first pass metabolism; major reactions appear to be sulphoxidation and glucuronic acid conjugation; promethazine appears to induce pentobarbitone metabolism.

EXCRETION. About 2% of a dose is excreted in the urine unchanged; the major urinary metabolite is the sulphoxide.

FURTHER INFORMATION. Investigation of distribution, metabolism, and excretion in rats—W. Rusiecki and B. Wysocka-Paruszewska, *Dissnes pharm. Pharmac.*, 1969, **21**, 73; distribution and excretion in man—J. Quinn and R. Calvert, *J. Pharm. Pharmac.*, 1976, **28**, 59P.

Actions and uses. Promethazine is a powerful and long-acting antagonist of the H-1 receptor effects of histamine. The antihistamine drugs resemble each other in their effects of diminishing or abolishing most of the actions of histamine; they do not however antagonise its stimulant action on gastric secretion which is mediated by H-2 receptors. The action of histamine most readily affected is that on the involuntary muscle of the intestine, bladder, uterus and bronchioles; the vasodilator and vasoconstrictor actions of histamine are also antagonised. The dilatation and increased permeability of capillaries produced by histamine are prevented and the weals caused by intradermal injections of histamine are reduced by these drugs.
Anaphylactic reactions produced in animals and certain allergic reactions in man are modified by the antihistamine drugs, although larger doses are necessary for this purpose than are required to antagonise the effects of injected histamine. The histamine antagonists are not entirely specific, for when used in higher concentrations they may also antagonise the actions of acetylcholine and of adrenaline. Most of the histamine antagonists depress the central nervous system and cause drowsiness; they also produce local anaesthesia when applied locally or injected subcutaneously, but their administration by the latter route is not recommended, as irritation often results.
The antihistamine drugs are active when given by mouth. When assessing their activity, attention must be paid not only to the time taken for the drug to produce its maximum effect, but also to the duration of its action. The action of promethazine lasts for about 20 hours, and it may therefore be given less frequently than most other antihistamines. The daily dosage of promethazine hydrochloride required to maintain an effect against an intradermal injection of histamine in man is about one-fourteenth of that of mepyramine maleate.
The antihistamine drugs have been used in the treatment of allergic reactions of the skin and mucous membranes, such as acute urticaria, atopic dermatitis, allergic rhinitis, and hay fever. They are also used in treating allergic reactions caused by such drugs as the antibiotics and sulphonamides. Itching skin affections, such as atopic dermatitis, contact dermatitis, pruritus ani and vulvae, generalised pruritus, and insect bites, are often temporarily relieved either by giving antihistamines internally or by applying them externally in the form of an ointment or cream.
Topical application is not without risk, as skin sensitisation and dermatitis may result. Since the cause of the reaction is not removed, symptoms may reappear when the drug is stopped. In the treatment of chronic conditions, the general condition of the skin and mucous

membrane remains unaltered, although symptoms such as itching and sneezing may be relieved.

Certain types of bronchial asthma respond to treatment with the antihistamine drugs, but such treatment is unlikely to be effective during an acute attack unless supplemented by bronchodilators.

Some of the antihistamines have powerful anti-emetic properties and are used for the prevention and treatment of vomiting from various causes, including post-operative vomiting, irradiation sickness, drug-induced nausea, motion-sickness, vomiting of pregnancy, and Ménière's disease and other labyrinthine disturbances. Infection with the common cold is in no way influenced by these compounds.

Promethazine hydrochloride is administered by mouth, the usual daily dosage for an adult being 20 to 50 milligrams in single or divided doses. It may also be given by deep intramuscular injection in a dose not exceeding 50 milligrams.

The usual dose by mouth for motion sickness in children up to 1 year is 5 to 10 milligrams daily, 1 to 5 years 10 to 15 milligrams daily, and 6 to 12 years 15 to 25 milligrams daily. As a sedative, children up to 1 year may be given 2.5 to 5 milligrams and 1 to 5 years 5 to 10 milligrams; these doses may be given 3 times daily. The usual hypnotic dose for children up to 1 year is 5 to 10 milligrams and 1 to 5 years 15 to 20 milligrams.

Undesirable effects. Toxic effects commonly encountered with most of the antihistamine drugs are dryness of the mouth, throat, and nose, and abdominal pain with vomiting or diarrhoea.

Because the antihistamines may cause drowsiness and dizziness in some persons their use constitutes a danger to patients who drive vehicles or work with moving machinery. The danger is increased if alcohol is also taken.

Poisoning. Large doses of the antihistamines may cause convulsions and may precipitate fits in epileptics; if this stage is reached diazepam should be administered intravenously. Gastric lavage should be employed if the drug has recently been taken by mouth.

Veterinary uses. Promethazine hydrochloride is a tranquilliser and antihistamine which is used for the prevention and treatment of allergic conditions and of motion sickness in dogs; the effect of a single dose may persist for up to 24 hours. The usual dose by mouth for dogs is 2.5 to 10 milligrams per kilogram body-weight and for cats 10 to 40 milligrams per kilogram body-weight daily. The usual daily dose by intramuscular injection for horses and cattle is 0.5 to 1 milligram per kilogram body-weight, for sheep 2.5 to 10 milligrams per kilogram body-weight, for pigs 1 to 4 milligrams per kilogram body-weight, and for dogs 2.5 to 12.5 milligrams per kilogram body-weight.

Preparations

PROMETHAZINE ELIXIR: a solution of promethazine hydrochloride in a suitable coloured flavoured vehicle. When a dose less than or not a multiple of 5 ml is prescribed, the elixir may be diluted, as described in the entry on Elixirs, with syrup. The diluted elixir must be freshly prepared. Available as an elixir containing 5 mg of promethazine hydrochloride in 5 ml.

A standard for this elixir is given in the British Pharmaceutical Codex 1973

Containers and Labelling: see the entry on Elixirs for general information on containers and labelling.

Storage: it should be stored in a cool place protected from light.

Advice for patients: the elixir may cause drowsiness; persons affected should not drive or operate machinery. Alcohol should be avoided.

PROMETHAZINE HYDROCHLORIDE INJECTION: a sterile solution of promethazine hydrochloride, with suitable stabilising agents, in water for injections free from dissolved air. It is distributed into the final containers, the air being replaced by nitrogen or other suitable gas, and the containers are sealed and sterilised by heating in an autoclave. Available in 1- and 2-ml ampoules containing 25 mg of promethazine hydrochloride per ml, and in 10-ml ampoules containing 50 mg of promethazine hydrochloride per ml.

A standard for this injection is given in the British Pharmacopoeia 1973

Containers and Labelling: see the entry on Injections for general information on containers and labelling.

Storage: it should be protected from light.

PROMETHAZINE HYDROCHLORIDE TABLETS: available as tablets containing 10 and 25 mg of promethazine hydrochloride; they are sugar coated; the coat may be coloured.

A standard for these tablets is given in the British Pharmacopoeia 1973

Containers and Storage: see the entry on Tablets for general information on containers and storage. Containers should be airtight.

Advice for patients: see above under Promethazine Elixir.

OTHER PREPARATIONS available include an INJECTION containing promethazine hydrochloride 25 mg with pethidine hydrochloride 50 mg per ml in 2-ml ampoules; and TABLETS containing promethazine hydrochloride 15 mg with butobarbitone 75 mg.

Promethazine Theoclate

The 10-(2-dimethylaminopropyl)phenothiazine salt of 8-chlorotheophylline.

$C_{24}H_{27}ClN_6O_2S = 499.0$

OTHER NAME: *Avomine*®

A standard is given in the British Pharmacopoeia 1973

Description. An odourless white powder with a slightly bitter taste.

Solubility. Very slightly soluble in water; soluble, at 20°, in 70 parts of alcohol and in 2.5 parts of chloroform; practically insoluble in ether.

Storage. It should be stored in airtight containers, protected from light.

Identification. TESTS. 1. Dissolve about 5 mg in 2 ml of sulphuric acid and allow to stand for 5 minutes; a red colour is produced.

2. Mix about 400 mg with 10 ml of water, add 4 ml of dilute ammonia solution and extract with two 30-ml portions of ether, separate the aqueous layer, add to it 4 ml of hydrochloric acid, filter off the white precipitate, and wash it with water. The precipitate gives Test 2

described under Aminophylline, and, after fusion with anhydrous sodium carbonate and solution with *dilute nitric acid*, gives a white precipitate with *silver nitrate solution* which is soluble in *dilute ammonia solution*.

ULTRAVIOLET ABSORPTION. In dehydrated alcohol containing 0.01% of *strong ammonia solution*, maximum at 255 nm (E1%, 1cm = 786).

Metabolism. See under Promethazine Hydrochloride.

Actions and uses. Promethazine theoclate has the actions, uses, and undesirable effects of the antihistamine drugs, as described under Promethazine Hydrochloride; 1.5 grams of promethazine theoclate is approximately equivalent to 1 gram of promethazine hydrochloride. Promethazine theoclate is given by mouth for the prevention and relief of motion-sickness. The usual dose is 25 to 50 milligrams daily.

Poisoning. As for Promethazine Hydrochloride.

Preparation

PROMETHAZINE THEOCLATE TABLETS: available as tablets containing 25 mg of promethazine theoclate.
A standard for these tablets is given in the British Pharmacopoeia 1973
Containers and *Storage:* see the entry on Tablets for general information on containers and storage. Containers should be airtight and light resistant.
Advice for patients: the tablets may cause drowsiness; persons affected should not drive or operate machinery. Alcohol should be avoided.

Propanidid

Propyl 4-diethylcarbamoylmethoxy-3-methoxyphenyl-acetate

$$CH_2 \cdot CO \cdot O \cdot CH_2 \cdot CH_2 \cdot CH_3$$

$$O \cdot CH_3$$

$$O \cdot CH_2 \cdot CO \cdot N(C_2H_5)_2$$

$C_{18}H_{27}NO_5 = 337.4$

OTHER NAME: *Epontol®*

A standard is given in the British Pharmacopoeia 1973

Description. A pale, greenish-yellow, viscous, hygroscopic liquid with a slight odour.

Solubility. Very slightly soluble in water; miscible with alcohol, with ether, and with chloroform.

Identification. TEST. Mix 1 drop with a solution of 200 mg of hydroxylammonium chloride in 4 ml of 1N sodium hydroxide, boil for 30 seconds, cool, acidify with 5 ml of 1N sulphuric acid, and add 1 drop of a 1% solution of ferric chloride; an intense wine-red colour is produced.

ULTRAVIOLET ABSORPTION. In alcohol (95%), maximum at 280 nm (E1%, 1cm = 82).

Metabolism. BLOOD CONCENTRATION. After an intravenous dose of 7 mg/kg, serum concentrations of about 14 μg/ml are obtained at 1 minute falling to undetectable concentrations by 15 minutes.

DISTRIBUTION. Crosses the placenta; *protein binding,* bound to plasma proteins to some extent.

METABOLIC REACTIONS. Rapid hydrolysis by esterases in the plasma, hydrolysis of the amide moiety, and demethylation.

EXCRETION. Excreted in the urine as inactive metabolites.

FURTHER INFORMATION. Maternal plasma concentrations, umbilical vein concentrations, and plasma cholinesterase—J. S. Crawford, *Br. J. Anaesth.*, 1968, **40**, 713 and A. Doenicke *et al.*, *Br. J. Anaesth.*, 1968, **40**, 415.

Actions and uses. Propanidid is a short-acting anaesthetic for intravenous administration. It also has local anaesthetic activity. It is metabolised by esterases in the plasma and the liver.

The usual dose for the induction of anaesthesia is 100 to 750 milligrams by intravenous injection as a 5% solution and the resulting anaesthesia usually lasts for 3 to 6 minutes. Hyperventilation commonly occurs during induction and this may be followed by hypoventilation or apnoea. The action of suxamethonium may be enhanced and doses of the order of 8 to 10 milligrams per kilogram body-weight may depress the circulation. Propanidid has been used to produce ultra-light anaesthesia during conservative dental treatment but its use for this purpose has been questioned.

Undesirable effects. Flushing of the skin, urticaria, and hypotension may occur.

Preparations

Preparations available include an INJECTION containing propanidid 50 mg per ml in 10-ml ampoules.

Propantheline Bromide

NN-Di-isopropyl-*N*-methyl-*N*-2-(xanthen-9-ylcarbonyl-oxy)ethylammonium bromide

$$\left[\begin{array}{c} CH(CH_3)_2 \\ \overset{+}{|} \\ CO \cdot O \cdot CH_2 \cdot CH_2 \cdot N \cdot CH_3 \\ | \\ CH(CH_3)_2 \end{array} \right] Br^-$$

$C_{23}H_{30}BrNO_3 = 448.4$

OTHER NAMES: *Pro-Banthine®*
Pro-Banthine with Phenobarbitone®; *Pro-Banthine with Dartalan®* (with thiopropazate)

A standard is given in the British Pharmacopoeia 1973

Description. An odourless, slightly hygroscopic, white or yellowish-white powder with a very bitter taste.

Solubility. Soluble in water, in alcohol, and in chloroform; practically insoluble in ether.

Moisture content. Not more than 1.5%, determined by drying at 105°.

Storage. It should be stored in airtight containers.

Identification. TESTS. 1. Dissolve about 200 mg in 15 ml of water, add 2 ml of *sodium hydroxide solution*, boil for 2 minutes, cool slightly, add 5 ml of *dilute hydrochloric acid*, cool, and filter; a precipitate is produced which, after washing with water, recrystallising from alcohol (50%), and drying at 105° for 1 hour, melts at about 215°.

2. To about 10 mg of the crystals obtained in Test 1 add

5 ml of sulphuric acid; a bright yellow solution is produced which fluoresces strongly under ultraviolet radiation.

MELTING-POINT. About 159°.

ULTRAVIOLET ABSORPTION. In 0.1N hydrochloric acid, maxima at 244 nm (E1%, 1cm = 102) and 284 nm (E1%, 1cm = 61). In 0.1N sodium hydroxide, maxima at 252 nm (E1%, 1cm = 120) and 286 nm (E1%, 1cm = 60).

INFRA-RED ABSORPTION. Major peaks at 761, 1208, 1255, 1458, 1484, and 1733 cm^{-1} (see Appendix 2a: Infra-red Spectra).

THIN-LAYER CHROMATOGRAPHY. See under Thin-layer Chromatography, System 8.

Determination in body fluids. ULTRAVIOLET SPECTRO-PHOTOMETRY. In urine—M. Pfeffer et al., J. pharm. Sci., 1968, **57**, 1375.

GAS CHROMATOGRAPHY—MASS SPECTROMETRY. In urine—G. C. Ford et al., Biomed. Mass Spectrom., 1977, **4**, 94.

Metabolism. ABSORPTION. Propantheline undergoes decomposition in the intestine prior to the absorption of an oral dose; less than 50% of an oral dose is absorbed as intact drug.

DISTRIBUTION. Subject to enterohepatic circulation.

METABOLIC REACTIONS. Hydrolysed in the small intestine to xanthene carboxylic acid.

EXCRETION. After an oral dose, 50 to 65% of a dose is excreted in the urine in 24 hours; 1 to 10% is unchanged drug.

FURTHER INFORMATION. Absorption and metabolism— B. Beermann et al., Clin. Pharmac. Ther., 1972, **13**, 212; enterohepatic cycling—M. Pfeffer et al., J. pharm. Sci., 1968, **57**, 1375.

Actions and uses. Propantheline has the peripheral but not the central actions of atropine. It is administered, chiefly to reduce gastric secretion and intestinal mobility, in a dosage of 15 milligrams 3 times daily, with double the dose at bedtime. It has also been used to diminish biliary and ureteric spasm and to control excessive salivation, sweating, and nocturnal enuresis.

Undesirable effects. Hypotension, urinary retention, and constipation may occur. Propantheline has ganglion-blocking effects, but these are not important in therapeutic dosage. It is less liable than atropine to produce dryness of the mouth, tachycardia, and disturbances of vision.

Precautions and contra-indications. As for Atropine.

Preparations

PROPANTHELINE TABLETS: available as tablets containing 15 mg of propantheline bromide; they are sugar coated; the coat may be coloured.
A standard for these tablets is given in the British Pharmacopoeia 1973
Containers and Storage: see the entry on Tablets for general information on containers and storage. Containers should be airtight.
Advice for patients: the tablets should preferably be taken half an hour before meals. If there is dryness of the mouth the tablets may be taken after meals.

OTHER PREPARATIONS available include an INJECTION reconstituted from vials of powder containing propantheline bromide 30 mg; TABLETS containing propantheline bromide 15 mg with phenobarbitone 15 mg, and tablets containing propantheline bromide 15 mg with thiopropazate hydrochloride 3 mg.

Propellents

The three aerosol propellents dichlorodifluoromethane, dichlorotetrafluoroethane, and trichlorofluoromethane described below are those most commonly used in pharmaceutical aerosol formulations. As the names indicate, they are chlorofluorohydrocarbons (fluorinated hydrocarbons). They are non-inflammable when mixed with air at all concentrations, colourless, and virtually odourless, and have a low level of toxicity. It has been suggested that if the usage of these propellents were to be increased unduly it might result in depletion of the ozone layer of the stratosphere.

Dichlorodifluoromethane (PROPELLENT 12) is gaseous at room temperature and must be handled in a closed system under pressure or as a refrigerated liquid in an open system. Propellent 12 is the most volatile of the commonly used aerosol propellents and is used as the main source of pressure in pharmaceutical aerosol preparations. It is stable in the presence of water and has a vapour pressure of approximately 4.8 bars (70 p.s.i.g.) at room temperature. Normal pressure ranges are 1.4 to 3.5 bars (20 to 50 p.s.i.g.) for tinplate containers and up to 4.8 bars (70 p.s.i.g.) for aluminium containers and propellent 12 is therefore usually mixed with propellents 11 or 114 (or both) to give the required pressure in the formulation. The range of pressures which may be achieved with these mixtures is shown in TABLES 1 and 2, p. 753.
The presence of a miscible solvent such as alcohol in a propellent formulation will have the effect of reducing the overall pressure. In such cases propellent 12 may be used alone as the pressurising agent and the pressure of the mixture will have to be either obtained from standard tables or determined experimentally.
Apart from solvents, other factors such as emulsification of the propellent and partial solubility of the propellent in the formulation may affect the pressure and give the final formulation a different pressure from that of the propellents alone.
For further information on this propellent see the entry on Dichlorodifluoromethane.

Dichlorotetrafluoroethane (PROPELLENT 114) is gaseous at room temperature and must be handled either in a closed system under pressure or as a refrigerated liquid in an open system. Propellent 114 is stable in the presence of water and may be used in place of propellent 11 as a means of controlling the pressure in aqueous formulations.
For further information on this propellent see the entry on Dichlorotetrafluoroethane.

Trichlorofluoromethane (PROPELLENT 11) is the least volatile of the three propellents. It is liquid at room temperature and can be handled in open systems although care must be taken, by chilling or vapour retention, to prevent losses and exposure of personnel to the substance. Propellent 11 does not generate a significant pressure on its own and it is therefore used in combination with propellent 12 (or 12/114) in aerosol formulations. As it is liquid at room temperature and has good solvent properties, propellent 11 is very useful for preparing solutions or suspensions of active or other ingredients (concentrates) which are subsequently diluted with the pressurising propellent either in the aerosol can (pressure filling) or refrigerated prior to cold filling. Propellent 11 is unstable in the presence of water and must not be used in aqueous formulations. It is also unsuitable for formulations containing alcohol when used in aluminium containers. Propellent 114 is an alternative for controlling pressure.

For further information on this propellent see the entry on Trichlorofluoromethane.

Factors in the formulation of propellent mixtures. Properties of the propellent mixture other than those discussed above need to be taken into account when developing formulations. The propellent ratio will affect the type of spray which is produced by the aerosol. A formulation containing a large amount of propellent 12 will produce a rapidly evaporating "dry" spray whereas one containing a large proportion of propellent 11 will give a "wet" spray. Thus careful selection of propellent ratio will be important for all products where spray characteristics affect the efficacy and toxicity of the product. Space sprays (insecticides), surface sprays (antiseptics), and aerosol inhalations, for example, each require a different propellent mixture.

The density of the propellent blend is governed by the propellent ratio. Where possible it may be desirable to adjust the propellent ratio to give the optimum density for physical stability. For example, in suspension systems, the propellent ratio may be adjusted to allow the drug to sediment or float in the system. Suspension systems will generally need stabilising by suitable lipophilic surfactants, such as sorbitan esters, to avoid excessive claying or flocculation. Foam aerosols may be prepared by emulsifying a propellent of low volatility with an immiscible liquid phase by means of suitable excipients. If the propellent forms the disperse phase, stable viscous foams are produced. Foams which contain the propellent as the continuous phase break quickly to give wet, liquid preparations.

TABLE 1. Vapour Pressures of Mixtures of Propellents 12 and 11

	Parts by weight of propellent			
Propellent 12	100	75	50	25
Propellent 11	0	25	50	75
Vapour pressure of mixtures at 20°				
bar (10^5 pascal)	4.65	3.58	2.47	1:25
p.s.i.g.	67.6	52.0	35.9	18.1
Wt per ml at 20°				
g	1.329	1.373	1.415	1.454

TABLE 2. Vapour Pressures of Mixtures of Propellents 12 and 114

	Parts by weight of propellent			
Propellent 12	75	50	25	0
Propellent 114	25	50	75	100
Vapour pressure of mixtures at 20°				
bar (10^5 pascal)	3.88	3.00	1.99	0.82
p.s.i.g.	56.4	43.7	28.9	11.9
Wt per ml at 20°				
g	1.365	1.401	1.437	1.471

Propicillin Potassium

Potassium (6R)-6-(2-phenoxybutyramido)penicillanate

$C_{18}H_{21}KN_2O_5S = 416.5$

OTHER NAME: *Ultrapen®*

A standard is given in the British Pharmacopoeia 1973

Description. A white finely crystalline powder with a bitter taste.

Solubility. Soluble, at 20°, in 1.2 parts of water, in 25 parts of alcohol, and in 65 parts of dehydrated alcohol; very slightly soluble in ether and in chloroform.

Acidity. A 10% solution has a pH of 5 to 7.

Moisture content. Not more than 1%, determined by Fischer titration.

Specific rotation. +215° to +228°, determined on a 1% solution.

Dissociation constant. pK_a 2.7 (25°).

Stability. Aqueous solutions buffered with citrate show maximum stability at pH 6. Such solutions may be expected to lose not more than 10% of their potency when stored for 7 days at 25°.

Hygroscopicity. At relative humidities above about 50% it absorbs substantial amounts of moisture.

Storage. It should be stored in airtight containers at a temperature not exceeding 25°.

Identification. TEST. Mix 2 mg with 2 mg of chromotropic acid sodium salt and 2 ml of sulphuric acid, and immerse in a suitable liquid at 150° for 4 minutes; the colour of the solution changes through yellow to reddish-yellow and finally to yellowish-brown (distinction from certain other penicillins).

INFRA-RED ABSORPTION. Major peaks at 1220, 1316, 1493, 1613, 1667, and 1754 cm^{-1} (see Appendix 2b: Infra-red Spectra).

Metabolism. ABSORPTION. Propicillin is resistant to acid hydrolysis and is rapidly, though somewhat variably, absorbed after oral administration.

BLOOD CONCENTRATION. After oral doses of 125 to 250 mg, peak serum concentrations of 1 to 5 μg/ml are attained in about 1 hour; in the elderly, serum concentrations may be twice as high as those in younger subjects.

HALF-LIFE. Serum half-life, 0.5 to 1 hour.

DISTRIBUTION. Volume of distribution, about 29 litres; enters the cerebrospinal fluid when the meninges are inflamed; *protein binding*, about 90% bound to plasma proteins.

FURTHER INFORMATION. Plasma concentrations, protein binding, and urinary excretion—J. M. Bond et al., Br. med. J., ii/1963, 956.

Actions and uses. Propicillin has the actions and uses described under Phenoxymethylpenicillin.

Although propicillin potassium gives rise to higher blood levels than phenoxymethylpenicillin it is less potent as an antibiotic and the effect of the two substances is therefore similar. Although it is more resistant to staphylococcal penicillinase than phenoxymethylpenicillin, the difference is not sufficiently great to be of value in the treatment of penicillinase-producing staphylococcal infections.

It is given in a dosage of 0.5 to 1.5 grams of the equivalent of propicillin by mouth daily in divided doses. Children under 12 years may be given half the adult dose.

Precautions and contra-indications. As for Phenoxymethylpenicillin.

Preparation

PROPICILLIN TABLETS: available as tablets containing propicillin potassium equivalent to 250 mg of propicillin; peppermint oil may be added as a flavouring agent; they may be coloured.

A standard for these tablets is given in the British Pharmacopoeia 1973

Containers and *Storage:* see the entry on Tablets for general information on containers and storage. Containers should be airtight.

Labelling: the label on the container should state the amount of the medicament as the equivalent amount of propicillin, the date after which the tablets are not intended to be used, and the conditions under which they should be stored.

Advice for patients: the tablets should be taken at regular intervals preferably half to 1 hour before meals. The prescribed course should be completed.

Propranolol Hydrochloride

N-(2-Hydroxy-3-naphth-1-yloxypropyl)-N-isopropyl-ammonium chloride

$C_{16}H_{22}ClNO_2 = 295.8$

OTHER NAME: *Inderal®*

A standard is given in the British Pharmacopoeia 1973

Description. An odourless white powder with a bitter taste.

Solubility. Soluble, at 20°, in 20 parts of water and in 20 parts of alcohol; very slightly soluble in chloroform.

Acidity. A 1% solution has a pH of 5 to 6.

Dissociation constant. pK_a 9.5.

Stability. It is affected by light. In aqueous solutions, it decomposes with oxidation of the isopropylamine side-chain, accompanied by reduction in the pH and discoloration of the solution. Solutions are most stable at pH 3 and decompose rapidly when alkaline.

Hygroscopicity. It absorbs less than 1% of water at 25° at relative humidities up to 80%.

Sterilisation. Solutions for injection are sterilised by heating in an autoclave or by filtration.

Storage. It should be protected from light.

Identification. TEST. Dissolve about 200 mg in 6 ml of water, with the aid of heat if necessary, make alkaline with *sodium hydroxide solution*, extract with two 5-ml portions of ether, wash the combined extracts with water until free from alkali, dry over anhydrous sodium sulphate, and evaporate to dryness; the residue, after drying at 50° *in vacuo*, melts at about 94°.

MELTING-POINT. About 163°.

ULTRAVIOLET ABSORPTION. In methyl alcohol, maxima at 290 nm (E1%, 1cm = 210), 306 nm (E1%, 1cm = 125), and 319 nm (E1%, 1cm = 75).

Determination in body fluids. SPECTROFLUORIMETRY. In serum—P. K. Ambler *et al., Clinica chim. Acta,* 1974, **54**, 373. In plasma or urine—D. G. Shand *et al., Clin. Pharmac. Ther.,* 1970, **11**, 112.

GAS CHROMATOGRAPHY. In plasma: propranolol (also alprenolol and practolol) and metabolites—T. Walle, *J. pharm. Sci.,* 1974, **63**, 1885. In plasma—R. E. Kates and C. L. Jones, *J. pharm. Sci.,* 1977, **66**, 1490.

GAS CHROMATOGRAPHY—MASS SPECTROMETRY. In urine: simultaneous determination of (−)- and (+)-propranolol—H. Ehrsson, *J. Pharm. Pharmac.,* 1976, **28**, 662.

Metabolism. ABSORPTION. Almost completely absorbed after oral administration; buccal absorption of propranolol is pH-dependent.

BLOOD CONCENTRATION. After an oral dose of 80 mg, peak plasma concentrations of 30 to 200 ng/ml are attained in 1 to 2 hours in fasting subjects; after an intravenous dose of 300 μg/kg, plasma concentrations of greater than 100 ng/ml are attained; after oral doses of 120 and 320 mg daily, steady state plasma concentrations of 26 to 77 ng/ml are obtained. Plasma concentrations are increased in the elderly.

HALF-LIFE. Plasma half-life, 3 to 6 hours after oral administration and 2 to 4 hours after intravenous administration; in the elderly, the half-life is increased 2- to 3-fold. The half-life of the *l*-form of propranolol (3.2 hours) is longer than that of the *d*- and *dl*-forms (2.5 hours) as a consequence of decreased blood flow to the liver, caused by the *l*-form, which results in less drug being available for metabolism; the half-life of the major active metabolite, 4-hydroxypropranolol, after oral dosing, is less than that of the parent drug.

DISTRIBUTION. Extensively distributed throughout the body tissues and fluids; propranolol crosses the placenta, is taken up by the red cells, and is secreted in the milk, the amount secreted being dose dependent; volume of distribution, 150 litres; *protein binding*, 90 to 96% bound to plasma proteins.

METABOLIC REACTIONS. Extensively metabolised in the liver by ring hydroxylation, N-demethylation, oxidative deamination, and sulphate or glucuronic acid conjugation; the metabolites formed are determined by the route of administration; after oral administration propranolol undergoes extensive first pass metabolism and is hydroxylated to form the active metabolite, 4-hydroxypropranolol, as well as being metabolised by the other routes; after intravenous administration, no ring hydroxylation occurs; most of the metabolites are excreted as conjugates.

EXCRETION. Up to 90% of a dose is excreted in the urine and 1 to 4% is excreted in the faeces; of the material excreted in the urine, 20 to 40% is naphthoxylactic acid; other urinary metabolites include 4-hydroxypropranolol, N-desisopropylpropranolol, 1-α-naphthoxy-2,3-propyleneglycol and its ring hydroxylated form, α-naphthoxy-acetic acid, α-naphthol, and 1,4-dihydroxynaphthalene; urinary excretion of unchanged drug occurs to some extent and is influenced by urinary pH values, there being more excreted in acid urine.

DISEASE STATES. In coeliac disease and in liver disease, the placenta concentrations and half-lives of propranolol are increased and, in renal function impairment, the plasma half-life is decreased and the faecal excretion is increased.

FURTHER INFORMATION. Effect of age on plasma concentrations—C. M. Castleden et al., Br. J. clin. Pharmac., 1975, 2, 303; effect of route of administration on plasma concentration and effects—C. R. Cleaveland and D. G. Shand, Clin. Pharmac. Ther., 1972, 13, 181; pharmacokinetics in renal disease—D. T. Lowenthal et al., Clin. Pharmac. Ther., 1974, 16, 761, and F. D. Thompson et al., Br. med. J., ii/1972, 434; plasma concentrations and beta-blockade—D. G. McDevitt and D. G. Shand, Clin. Pharmac. Ther., 1975, 18, 708; urinary metabolites—T. Walle and T. E. Gaffney, J. Pharmac. exp. Ther., 1972, 182, 83.

Actions and uses. Propranolol has a specific blocking action on the adrenergic beta receptors and inhibits the sympathetic stimulation of the heart. It is used in the treatment of cardiac arrhythmias associated with heart disease, digitalis intoxication, or anaesthesia.

In urgent cases propranolol may be given intravenously in a dose of 1 milligram, dissolved in 1 millilitre of water, over a period of one minute, the injection being preceded, if the heart rate is already slow, by the intravenous administration of 1 to 2 milligrams of atropine; this dose may be repeated every 2 minutes until a response is observed or until 10 milligrams has been given to conscious patients or 5 milligrams to patients under anaesthesia.

In the treatment of arrhythmias, 10 to 40 milligrams may be given by mouth 3 or 4 times a day.

In patients with poor myocardial function it may be necessary to give digitalis at the same time. Propranolol may also be used in conjunction with digitalis in the treatment of auricular fibrillation.

Propranolol hydrochloride is used in the treatment of hyperthyroidism and somatic symptoms of anxiety, an initial dosage of 40 milligrams daily being gradually increased up to a maximum of 120 milligrams daily in divided doses.

The treatment of angina pectoris and arterial hypertension is started with a dosage of 80 milligrams by mouth daily in divided doses and increased at intervals of 3 days up to 160 milligrams daily, which may be further increased to 2 grams daily if necessary.

Propranolol hydrochloride is used in the treatment of cardiac arrhythmias and hyperthyroidism in children. The usual dosage is in the range 250 to 500 micrograms per kilogram body-weight 3 times a day by mouth ·or 25 to 50 micrograms per kilogram body-weight 3 or 4 times daily by slow intravenous injection.

Undesirable effects. Propranolol may precipitate cardiac failure in some patients and, if the failure persists after full digitalisation, propranolol must be withdrawn. It may also give rise to bronchospasm.

Nausea, vomiting, insomnia, lassitude, and mild diarrhoea may occur, but can usually be avoided by increasing the dose gradually during the first week of treatment.

Non-thrombocytopenic purpura, erythematous rash, and paraesthesiae of the hands may occur, but these reactions are rare. Propranolol may give rise to coldness of the extremities and sleep disturbances.

Contra-indications. It should not be given to patients with a history of bronchial asthma.

Preparations

PROPRANOLOL INJECTION: a sterile solution of propranolol hydrochloride, with citric acid, in water for injections. It is sterilised by heating in an autoclave or by filtration. Available in 1-ml ampoules containing 1 mg of propranolol hydrochloride.

A standard for this injection is given in the British Pharmacopoeia 1973

Containers and Labelling: see the entry on Injections for general information on containers and labelling.

PROPRANOLOL TABLETS: available as tablets containing 10, 40, 80, and 160 mg of propranolol hydrochloride; they may be coloured.

A standard for these tablets is given in the British Pharmacopoeia 1973

Containers and Storage: see the entry on Tablets for general information on containers and storage. Containers should be airtight.

Advice for patients: the tablets should preferably be taken before meals. Treatment should not be discontinued without the advice of the prescriber. The tablets may affect mental concentration; persons affected should not drive or operate machinery.

Propyl Gallate

Propyl 3,4,5-trihydroxybenzoate

$$CO·O·CH_2·CH_2·CH_3$$

HO — OH

OH

$C_{10}H_{12}O_5 = 212.2$

OTHER NAMES: Progallin P®; Tenox PG®
Tenox S-1® (with citric acid)

A standard is given in the British Pharmacopoeia 1973

Description. An odourless, white to creamy-white, crystalline powder with a slightly bitter taste.

Solubility. Soluble in 1000 parts of water, in 3 parts of alcohol, in 3 parts of ether, and in 2000 parts of arachis oil.

Moisture content. Not more than 1%, determined by drying at 105°.

Storage. It should be stored in airtight containers, protected from light, contact with metals being avoided.

Identification. TESTS. 1. Dissolve about 10 mg in 5 ml of hot water, cool, and add 5 ml of dilute ammonia solution; a red colour is produced which becomes brown on standing. Shake the solution; the red colour is restored.

2. Dissolve about 5 mg in 50 ml of water and add 1 drop of ferric chloride solution; a bluish-black colour is produced.

MELTING-POINT. About 148°.

ULTRAVIOLET ABSORPTION. In methyl alcohol, maximum at 275 nm (E1%, 1cm = 490).

Uses. Propyl gallate is used as an antioxidant for preserving oils and fats; it is also used to inhibit autoxidation of ether, paraldehyde, and similar substances which develop peroxides in the presence of oxygen.

Anhydrous oils and fats may contain up to 0.01% of propyl gallate and volatile oils up to 0.1%; propyl gallate is dissolved in fixed oils by warming the mixture to 70° to 80° and in solid fats by warming until the fat is just melted.

The formation of peroxides in ether is inhibited by 0.01% of propyl gallate and the oxidation of paraldehyde is retarded by 0.05%. The effectiveness of propyl gallate can be enhanced by the addition of an antoxidant synergist such as citric acid, phosphoric acid or lecithin. Other gallates (ethyl, octyl, and dodecyl) have similar uses. The choice of a particular gallate depends upon its solubility in the preparation.

Preparations

Preparations available include a SOLUTION containing propyl gallate 20% with citric acid 10% (in propylene glycol).

Propyl Hydroxybenzoate

Propyl 4-hydroxybenzoate

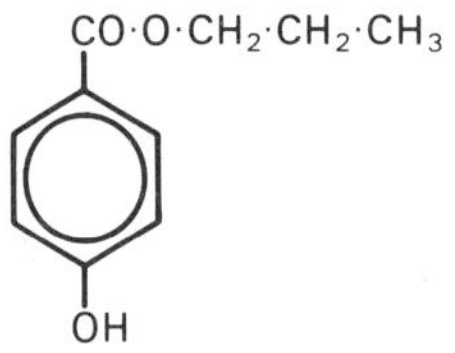

$$CO \cdot O \cdot CH_2 \cdot CH_2 \cdot CH_3$$

OH

$C_{10}H_{12}O_3 = 180.2$

OTHER NAMES: *Nipasol M®*; Propyl Parahydroxybenzoate; Propylis Parahydroxybenzoas; Propylparaben

A standard is given in the European Pharmacopoeia Vol. III

Description. An odourless, tasteless, white crystalline powder.

Solubility. Very slightly soluble in water; soluble, at 20°, in 3.5 parts of alcohol, in 3 parts of acetone, in 40 parts of fixed oils, and in 140 parts of glycerol; soluble in solutions of alkali hydroxides.

Dissociation constant. pK_a 8.4 (22°).

Identification. TEST. It complies with the test described under Methyl Hydroxybenzoate.

MELTING-POINT. About 96°.

ULTRAVIOLET ABSORPTION. In alcohol (95%), maximum at 258 nm.

INFRA-RED ABSORPTION. Major peaks at 1165, 1220, 1276, 1317, 1600, and 1665 cm⁻¹ (see Appendix 2a: Infra-red Spectra).

Uses. Propyl hydroxybenzoate is used as a preservative as described under Methyl Hydroxybenzoate. It is used in a concentration of 0.03% in conjunction with other hydroxybenzoates in aqueous preparations.

Propylene Glycol

Propane-1,2-diol

$$\begin{array}{c} OH \\ | \\ CH_3 \cdot CH \cdot CH_2OH \end{array}$$

$C_3H_8O_2 = 76.10$

OTHER NAME: Propyleneglycolum

A standard is given in the European Pharmacopoeia Vol. III

Description. An odourless, hygroscopic, clear, colourless, viscous liquid with a slightly sweet taste resembling that of glycerol.

Solubility. Miscible with water, with alcohol, with chloroform, and with acetone; soluble, at 20°, in 6 parts of ether; immiscible with light petroleum and with fixed oils.

Weight per ml. At 20°, 1.035 to 1.037 g.

Boiling-point. About 186°.

Refractive index. 1.431 to 1.433.

Sterilisation. It is sterilised by heating in sealed ampoules in an autoclave or by filtration.

Storage. It should be stored in airtight containers.

Uses. Propylene glycol is a useful solvent of low toxicity for some vitamins, barbiturates, and other substances which are insufficiently soluble in water or are unstable in aqueous solution.

It may be used, suitably diluted, in the preparation of injections and oral solutions and may be included in spray solutions to stabilise the droplet size. Examples of preparations in which propylene glycol is used are chloramphenicol ear-drops, digoxin injection, phenobarbitone injection, and benzoic acid solution.

Propylene glycol is also used as a solvent for topical corticosteroids in the formulation of ointments.

Veterinary uses. Propylene glycol is used in the treatment of bovine ketosis and pregnancy toxaemia of sheep. The usual dose by mouth for cattle is 200 to 300 millilitres and for sheep 60 to 100 millilitres; these doses are repeated daily for 3 or 4 days.

Propylhexedrine

2-Cyclohexyl-*N*,1-dimethylethylamine

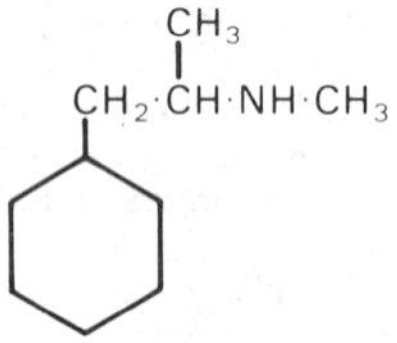

$$\begin{array}{c} CH_3 \\ | \\ CH_2 \cdot CH \cdot NH \cdot CH_3 \end{array}$$

$C_{10}H_{21}N = 155.3$

OTHER NAME: *Benzedrex®*

A standard is given in the British Pharmaceutical Codex 1973

Description. A clear colourless liquid with a characteristic amine-like odour.

Solubility. Miscible with alcohol, with ether, and with chloroform; soluble in dilute acids.

Weight per ml. At 20°, 0.853 to 0.861 g.

Dissociation constant. pK_a 10.7 (25°).

Storage. It should be stored in airtight containers.

Identification. TESTS. 1. Dissolve about 100 mg in a mixture of 3 ml of water and 0.2 ml of *dilute hydrochloric acid*. To 1 ml add 3 ml of *mercuric chloride test-solution*; a bulky white granular precipitate is produced (distinction from adrenaline, ephedrine, and phenylephrine).

2. To the remainder of the solution prepared in Test 1

add 20 ml of *trinitrophenol solution* and cool in ice; a precipitate is produced which, after washing with water, recrystallising from alcohol (20%), and drying for 2 hours at 80°, melts at about 107°.

BOILING-POINT. About 204°.

INFRA-RED ABSORPTION. Major peaks at 748, 1340, 1370, 1443, 1550, and 1663 cm^{-1} (see Appendix 2c: Infra-red Spectra).

Actions and uses. Propylhexedrine is a volatile sympathomimetic amine with a local vasoconstrictor action, but when inhaled it has little stimulating effect on the central nervous system.

It is used in inhalers, containing 250 milligrams, for the relief of congested nasal mucous membranes in hay fever, asthma, coryza, and vasomotor rhinitis and to relieve blockage of the eustachian tubes.

Propyliodone

Propyl 1,4-dihydro-3,5-di-iodo-4-oxopyrid-1-ylacetate

$$CH_2 \cdot CO \cdot O \cdot CH_2 \cdot CH_2 \cdot CH_3$$

$C_{10}H_{11}I_2NO_3 = 447.0$

OTHER NAME: *Dionosil®*

A standard is given in the British Pharmacopoeia 1973

Description. An odourless white crystalline powder.

Solubility. Very slightly soluble in water and in ether; soluble, at 20°, in 500 parts of alcohol and in 150 parts of chloroform.

Sterilisation. It is sterilised by dry heat.

Storage. It should be protected from light.

Identification. TESTS. 1. Heat with sulphuric acid; violet vapours are evolved.
2. Mix about 1 g with 10 ml of 1N sodium hydroxide, boil under a reflux condenser for 30 minutes, add 10 ml of water, and acidify to litmus paper with hydrochloric acid; a precipitate is produced which, after washing with water, melts at about 245°.

MELTING-POINT. About 188°.

ULTRAVIOLET ABSORPTION. In dehydrated alcohol, maxima at 239 nm (E1%, 1cm = 320) and 281 nm (E1%, 1cm = 260).

Metabolism. ABSORPTION. Upon instillation into the lungs, some of a dose may be swallowed and some expectorated; the remainder is hydrolysed in the lungs and absorbed.

METABOLIC REACTION. De-esterification to form di-iodopyridone-*N*-acetic acid.

EXCRETION. About 50% of a dose is excreted in the urine in 3 days as the de-esterified metabolite.

Actions and uses. Propyliodone is a contrast medium used in bronchography. It is a slightly soluble compound related to diodone and is rapidly eliminated from the lungs. It gives well-defined bronchograms, however, for at least 30 minutes.

It is used in either oily or aqueous suspension and is introduced either by a cannula through the cricothyroid membrane or by a catheter through the nose, the trachea and larynx having been previously anaesthetised by means of a local anaesthetic.

A dose of 300 milligrams for each year of age, up to a maximum of 9 grams for an adult, is usually adequate.

Undesirable effects. The toxicity of propyliodone is low, but it causes frequent coughing and for this reason adequate local anaesthesia of the trachea is essential.

Preparations

PROPYLIODONE INJECTION: a sterile suspension of propyliodone, with suitable dispersing and suspending agents, in water for injections. It may contain a suitable buffering agent and a bactericide. It is prepared by means of an aseptic technique. It contains 50% (500 mg per ml) of propyliodone. Available in 20-ml vials.

A standard for this injection is given in the British Pharmacopoeia 1973

Containers: see the entry on Injections for general information on containers.

Labelling: see the entry on Injections for general information on labelling. In addition, the label on the container should state the amount of the medicament as the percentage w/v of propyliodone.

Storage: it should be stored at 10° to 30°, protected from light.

PROPYLIODONE OILY INJECTION: a sterile suspension of propyliodone in arachis oil. It is prepared by means of an aseptic technique. It contains 60% (600 mg per ml) of propyliodone. Available in 20-ml vials.

A standard for this injection is given in the British Pharmacopoeia 1973

Containers: see the entry on Injections for general information on containers.

Labelling: see the entry on Injections for general information on labelling. In addition, the label on the container should state the amount of the medicament as the percentage w/v of propyliodone.

Storage: it should be stored at a temperature not exceeding 30°, protected from light.

Propylthiouracil

2-Mercapto-6-propylpyrimidin-4-ol

$$CH_3 \cdot CH_2 \cdot CH_2$$

$C_7H_{10}N_2OS = 170.2$

A standard is given in the British Pharmacopoeia 1973

Description. Odourless white or pale cream-coloured crystals or crystalline powder with a bitter taste.

Solubility. Very slightly soluble in water, in alcohol, in ether, and in chloroform; soluble in solutions of alkali hydroxides.

Dissociation constant. pK$_a$ 8.3 (20°).

Identification. TESTS. 1. To a boiling saturated solution add an equal volume of a freshly prepared solution containing 0.4% of sodium nitroprusside, 0.4% of hydroxylammonium chloride, and 0.8% of sodium carbonate; a greenish-blue colour is produced.

2. To about 25 mg add *bromine solution* dropwise until completely dissolved, cool, and add 10 ml of *barium hydroxide solution*; a white precipitate is produced.

MELTING-POINT. About 220°.

Determination in body fluids. COLORIMETRY. In serum —C. R. Ratliff *et al.*, *Clin. Chem.*, 1972, **18**, 1373.

Metabolism. ABSORPTION. About 50 to 90% of an oral dose is rapidly absorbed.

BLOOD CONCENTRATION. After an oral dose of 400 mg, a peak plasma concentration of 9 μg/ml is attained within 1 hour.

HALF-LIFE. After intravenous administration, the plasma concentration declines biphasically with a half-life of 6 minutes for the α-phase and 77 minutes for the β-phase.

DISTRIBUTION. The distribution of propylthiouracil fits a 2-compartment model and it is preferentially taken up by the thyroid with concentrations in the thyroid reaching 40 times that in the serum; volume of distribution, 22 litres.

EXCRETION. Very little unchanged drug is excreted in the urine; in rats, the major urinary metabolite appears to be a glucuronide.

FURTHER INFORMATION. Absorption, metabolism, and excretion in the rat—D. S. Sitar and D. P. Thornhill, *J. Pharmac. exp. Ther.*, 1972, **183**, 440; pharmacokinetics —W. D. Alexander *et al.*, *Br. med. J.*, ii/1969, 290 and J. Kampmann and L. Skovsted, *Acta pharmac. Tox.*, 1974, **35**, 361.

Actions and uses. Propylthiouracil is an antithyroid substance which has the actions, uses, and undesirable effects described under Carbimazole. For adults the controlling dosage is 200 to 600 milligrams daily; the maintenance dose is 50 to 200 milligrams daily. The dose for children is initially 150 to 300 milligrams per square metre body-surface daily in 3 divided doses, reducing according to the response.

Precautions. As for Carbimazole.

Preparation

PROPYLTHIOURACIL TABLETS: available as tablets containing 25 and 50 mg of propylthiouracil.
A standard for these tablets is given in the British Pharmacopoeia 1973
Containers and *Storage:* see the entry on Tablets for general information on containers and storage. Containers should be airtight.
Advice for patients: the tablets should be taken at regular intervals. Treatment should not be discontinued without the advice of the prescriber.

Prostaglandins

Prostaglandins occur in minute quantities throughout most mammalian tissues and have a wide spectrum of physiological and pharmacological effects. There are at least 14 naturally occurring prostaglandins and they are synthesised naturally via an unstable intermediate endoperoxide from unsaturated fatty acids found in cell membranes. Many physiological actions result from their ability to cause the contraction or relaxation of smooth muscle. The highest concentrations are found in organs of the female reproductive system and their secretions. Prostaglandins affect the male and female reproductive systems, the gastro-intestinal system, the cardiovascular system, the renal system, and the nervous system, and also affect many metabolic processes. Some prostaglandins of the E series are potent bronchodilators and most of those of the F series are potent bronchoconstrictors. Prostaglandin E_2 (dinoprostone; PGE_2) and prostaglandin $F_{2\alpha}$ (dinoprost; $PGF_{2\alpha}$) exert pharmacological actions on the reproductive system and are used in obstetrics for the induction of labour and therapeutic termination of pregnancy. They can stimulate the pregnant myometrium and are able, in appropriate dosage, to influence uterine activity at any stage of gestation. They are administered by the intravenous, intra-amniotic, extraamniotic, and oral routes. Other potential clinical uses of prostaglandins are as nasal decongestants, bronchial relaxants, and gastric antisecretory agents. They may also have useful antihypertensive and diuretic effects and are known to inhibit platelet aggregation and lipolysis. Prostaglandins may play a role in many types of inflammation and have been found in exudates from experimentally induced inflammation. Chronic inflammation in rheumatoid arthritis is characterised by a persistent mononuclear cell infiltrate in which macrophages producing substantial concentrations of prostaglandin activity occur.
Anaphylaxis is mediated by histamine SRS-A (slow reacting substance of anaphylaxis) and prostaglandins E_2 and $F_{2\alpha}$. SRS-A may release RCS (rabbit aorta contracting substance) and prostaglandins exert a negative feedback on further release of SRS-A. In therapeutic concentrations, analgesic drugs such as aspirin, indomethacin, fenoprofen, ibuprofen, mefenamic acid, and phenylbutazone inhibit the enzyme prostaglandin synthetase involved in the synthesis of prostaglandins from arachidonic acid and this potentiates SRS-A release. Aspirin, mefenamic acid, and indomethacin also antagonise the actions of RCS-releasing factor.

Protamine Sulphate Injection

A sterile solution in sodium chloride injection of protamine sulphate prepared from the sperm or mature testes of fish belonging to the family Clupeidae or Salmonidae.

A standard is given in the British Pharmacopoeia 1973

Description. A clear colourless solution.

Acidity. pH, 2.5 to 3.5.

Sterilisation. It is sterilised by filtration.

Storage. It should be stored at room temperature.

Actions and uses. Protamine sulphate is a specific antidote for heparin and is used to check haemorrhage caused by heparin overdosage. It is administered by slow intravenous injection, 5 millilitres of a 1% solution being injected over 10 minutes. If administered within 15 minutes of the injection of heparin, 1 milligram of protamine sulphate will neutralise the anticoagulant action of approximately 100 units of heparin; if a longer time has elapsed, less protamine sulphate is required especially as protamine sulphate itself has an anticoagulant action. Not more than 50 milligrams of protamine sulphate should be injected at any one time.

Undesirable effects. Intravenous injections of protamine sulphate, particularly if administered rapidly, may cause a sensation of warmth, flushing of the skin, hypotension, bradycardia, and dyspnoea.

Preparation

Available in 5-ml ampoules containing 10 mg of protamine sulphate per ml.

Prothionamide

2-Propylpyridine-4-carbothioamide

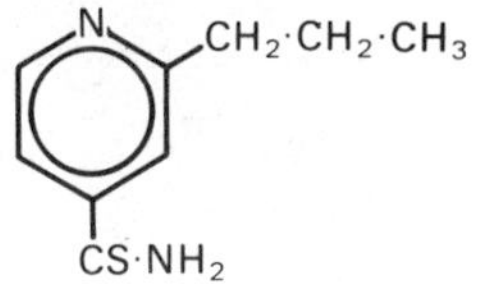

$C_9H_{12}N_2S = 180.3$

OTHER NAME: *Trevintix®*

A standard is given in the British Pharmaceutical Codex 1973

Description. Odourless yellow crystals or yellow crystalline powder.

Solubility. Practically insoluble in water; soluble, at 20°, in 30 parts of alcohol, in 300 parts of ether, in 200 parts of chloroform, and in 16 parts of methyl alcohol.

Moisture content. Not more than 1%, determined by drying at 105°.

Storage. It should be protected from light.

Identification. TESTS. 1. Heat about 100 mg with 5 ml of *sodium hydroxide solution*; vapours are evolved which turn red litmus paper blue.
2. Heat about 100 mg with 5 ml of 1N hydrochloric acid; vapours are evolved which blacken lead paper.
3. Dissolve about 10 mg in 5 ml of methyl alcohol and add 5 ml of 0.1N silver nitrate; a brownish-black precipitate is produced.

MELTING-POINT. About 141°.

ULTRAVIOLET ABSORPTION. In 0.1N sulphuric acid, maxima at 234 nm (E1%, 1cm = 414), 275 nm (E1%, 1cm = 331), and a shoulder at 315 nm (E1%, 1cm = 156).

INFRA-RED ABSORPTION. Major peaks at 826, 901, 1282, 1389, 1408, and 1587 cm^{-1} (see Appendix 2b: Infra-red Spectra).

Determination in body fluids. ULTRAVIOLET SPECTROPHOTOMETRY. In plasma—J. Pütter, *Arzneimittel-Forsch.*, 1972, **22**, 1027.

THIN-LAYER CHROMATOGRAPHY. In plasma or urine—M. Rossi and K. Ruebsamen, *J. Chromat.*, 1977, **132**, 562.

Metabolism. ABSORPTION. Well absorbed after oral administration.

BLOOD CONCENTRATION. After an oral dose of 500 mg, peak plasma concentrations of about 3 µg/ml for unchanged drug and 2.7 µg/ml for the sulphoxide metabolite are attained in 1 to 2 hours.

METABOLIC REACTIONS. Sulphoxidation.

EXCRETION. Excreted in the urine mainly as metabolites.

FURTHER INFORMATION. Plasma concentrations of prothionamide and its sulphoxide—J. Pütter, *Arzneimittel-Forsch.*, 1972, **22**, 1027.

Actions and uses. Prothionamide is a tuberculostatic agent with actions and uses similar to those of ethionamide but it causes a lower incidence of gastro-intestinal side-effects. Bacterial resistance develops simultaneously to both ethionamide and prothionamide and there is also some cross-resistance between them and thiacetazone.

The use of prothionamide is normally restricted to patients with infections that are resistant to other drugs.

It should always be given simultaneously with other tuberculostatic agents to delay the development of resistance.

The usual dose for an adult is 0.75 to 1 gram daily in single or divided doses. For children under 10 years of age the usual initial dose is 10 milligrams per kilogram body-weight daily, gradually increased, if tolerated, up to a maximum of 20 milligrams per kilogram body-weight daily.

Undesirable effects. These are as described under Ethionamide.

Precautions and contra-indications. Treatment should be discontinued if signs of liver damage occur. Prothionamide may cause damage to the foetus and should not be used in pregnancy unless no safer drug is available.

Preparation

PROTHIONAMIDE TABLETS: may be prepared by moist granulation and compression as described in the entry on Tablets. Available as tablets containing 125 mg of prothionamide; they may be coated with sugar or other suitable material.

A standard for these tablets is given in the British Pharmaceutical Codex 1973
Containers and Storage: see the entry on Tablets for general information on containers and storage. Containers should be airtight.
Advice for patients: the tablets should preferably be taken after meals and daily doses preferably at bedtime. Treatment should not be discontinued without the advice of the prescriber.

Protirelin

see under HYPOTHALAMIC RELEASING FACTORS

Protriptyline Hydrochloride

3-(5H-Dibenzo[a,d]cyclohepten-5-yl)propyl-N-methyl-ammonium chloride

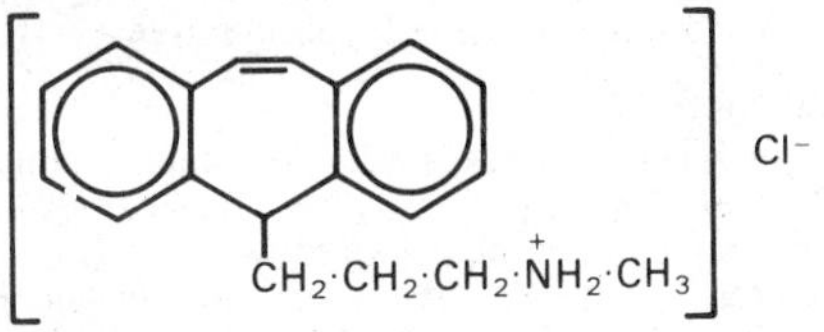

$C_{19}H_{22}ClN = 299.8$

OTHER NAME: *Concordin®*

A standard is given in the British Pharmacopoeia 1973

Description. An odourless white to yellowish-white powder with a bitter taste.

Solubility. Soluble, at 20°, in 2 parts of water, in 4.5 parts of alcohol, and in 3 parts of chloroform; practically insoluble in ether.

Acidity. A 1% solution has a pH of 5 to 6.5.

Identification. TEST. Dissolve about 50 mg in 3 ml of water and add 1 drop of a 2.5% solution of quinhydrone in methyl alcohol; a red colour gradually develops (distinction from amitriptyline).

MELTING-POINT. About 168°.

ULTRAVIOLET ABSORPTION. In a mixture containing 9

volumes of methyl alcohol and 1 volume of 1N hydrochloric acid, maximum at 292 nm (E1%, 1cm = 465).

INFRA-RED ABSORPTION. Major peaks at 750, 768, 792, 1434, 1464, and 1484 cm^{-1} (see Appendix 2a: Infra-red Spectra).

Metabolism. ABSORPTION. Well absorbed after oral administration.

BLOOD CONCENTRATION. During therapy with doses of 10 to 70 mg daily, plasma concentrations of 30 to 430 ng/ml are attained; after a single dose, peak concentrations are attained in 8 to 12 hours.

DISTRIBUTION. Taken up by many tissues; *protein binding*, about 92% bound to plasma proteins but the extent may be decreased by the presence of phenytoin.

METABOLIC REACTIONS. In dogs, *N*-demethylation; in rats, oxidation to form 10-hydroxy- and 10,11-dihydroxyprotriptyline and the 10,11-epoxide, with glucuronic acid conjugation of the hydroxy and dihydroxy metabolites.

EXCRETION. About 50% of a dose is excreted in the urine in 16 days with only small amounts being excreted unchanged; very little appears in the faeces.

FURTHER INFORMATION. 10,11-Epoxide excretion in rats– –V. Rovei *et al.*, *J. pharm. Sci.*, 1976, **65**, 810; metabolism and excretion—S. F. Sisenwine *et al.*, *J. Pharmac. exp. Ther.*, 1970, **175**, 51; plasma concentrations and excretion—K. D. Charalampous and P. C. Johnson, *J. clin. Pharmac.*, 1967, **7**, 93; steady-state concentrations in out-patients—J. T. Biggs *et al.*, *Am. J. Psychiat.*, 1975, **132**, 960.

Actions and uses. Protriptyline hydrochloride is a tricyclic antidepressant with actions and uses similar to those described under Amitriptyline Hydrochloride. It is, however, somewhat stimulant and may aggravate anxiety, tension, and insomnia. The usual dose is 15 to 60 milligrams daily in divided doses, reduced as depression becomes controlled. The last dose should be given no later than mid-afternoon.

Undesirable effects. As for Amitriptyline Hydrochloride but protriptyline has a stimulant effect and may give rise to insomnia.

Precautions and contra-indications; Drug interactions. As for Amitriptyline Hydrochloride.

Preparation

PROTRIPTYLINE TABLETS: available as tablets containing 5 and 10 mg of protriptyline hydrochloride; they are film coated; the coat may be coloured.
A standard for these tablets is given in the British Pharmacopoeia 1973
Containers and *Storage:* see the entry on Tablets for general information on containers and storage. Containers should be airtight.
Advice for patients: when initiating treatment there may be a time-lag of up to 1 week before a full therapeutic response is obtained. The tablets may affect mental concentration; persons affected should not drive or operate machinery. Alcohol should be avoided. To avoid insomnia doses should not be taken for several hours before bedtime. Direct exposure to sunlight should be avoided during treatment.

Proxymetacaine Hydrochloride

2-Diethylaminoethyl 3-amino-4-propoxybenzoate hydrochloride

$C_{16}H_{27}ClN_2O_3 = 330.9$

OTHER NAMES: *Ophthaine®*; Proparacaine Hydrochloride

A standard is given in the British Pharmaceutical Codex 1973

Description. An odourless white crystalline powder.

Solubility. Soluble, at 20°, in 30 parts of water and in 50 parts of alcohol.

Acidity. A 1% solution has a pH of 5.5 to 6.1.

Sterilisation. Solutions are sterilised by filtration in an atmosphere of nitrogen or other inert gas.

Storage. It should be stored in airtight containers.

Identification. TEST. Dissolve about 100 mg in 10 ml of water, heat to boiling, add, with stirring, 1 ml of a saturated solution of trinitrophenol in alcohol (20%), and allow to cool slowly; a precipitate is produced which, after washing with water and drying *in vacuo*, melts at about 119°.

MELTING-POINT. About 181°.

Actions and uses. Proxymetacaine is a local anaesthetic which is suitable for use in the eye. It has a potency somewhat greater than that of amethocaine.
The instillation of one drop of a 0.5% solution of proxymetacaine hydrochloride produces anaesthesia lasting about 15 minutes; deep anaesthesia, as required for cataract extraction, may be obtained by instilling one drop every 5 to 10 minutes until 5 to 7 drops have been administered.

Undesirable effects. Sensitivity reactions occur rarely.

Preparation

PROXYMETACAINE EYE-DROPS: consisting of a sterile solution containing 0.52% of proxymetacaine hydrochloride, with suitable preservatives, in purified water. It may contain glycerol. The air in the container should be replaced by nitrogen or other suitable gas.
A standard for these eye-drops is given in the British Pharmaceutical Codex 1973
Containers: see the entry on Eye-drops for general information on containers.
Labelling: see the entry on Eye-drops for general information on labelling. In addition, the label on the container should state the conditions under which it should be stored.
Storage: it should be protected from light. After the container has been opened for the first time, it should be stored at 2° to 10°. It should not be allowed to freeze. Solutions which have been discoloured should not be used.

Pruritus

Pruritus is a persistent itching which is not relieved by rubbing; it disturbs well-being by day and sleep by night. It may be due to atopy, or to persistent irritation of the skin in infections such as scabies, or hookworm. It may also be caused by obstructive jaundice or chronic renal failure.

Pruritus ani may be due to piles, anal fissures, threadworms, *Candida albicans*, or warts.

Pruritus vulvae may occur in glycosuria or as a result of *Candida albicans* infections which occur particularly in pregnancy or following the use of oral contraceptives or antibiotics. Pruritus may also occur without obvious cause.

Pruritus may be relieved by systemic use of antihistamines, including those with a marked sedative effect such as trimeprazine. Local applications containing phenol, crotamiton, or calamine may also be of value. General measures to reduce a tendency to itching include avoidance of extremes of temperature and rough clothing, reduction of exercise, and avoidance of alcohol.

Pruritus in the elderly may be related to dry skin and may be minimised by reducing the frequency of bathing, by bland applications, and by the use of emulsifying ointment in place of soap.

Pseudoephedrine Hydrochloride

$(+)$-$(\alpha S,\beta S)$-N-β-Hydroxy-α-methylphenethyl-N-methylammonium chloride, an alkaloid obtained from species of *Ephedra* (Fam. Ephedraceae).

$C_{10}H_{16}ClNO = 201.7$

OTHER NAMES: *d*-Isoephedrine Hydrochloride; *Sudafed®*
Actifed® (with triprolidine hydrochloride)

A standard is given in the British Pharmacopoeia 1973

Description. An almost odourless, white, crystalline powder with a bitter taste.

Solubility. Soluble, at 20°, in 1.6 parts of water, in 4 parts of alcohol, and in 60 parts of chloroform.

Acidity. A 5% solution has a pH of 5 to 6.

Specific rotation. +61° to +62.5°, determined on a 5% solution in a 2-dm tube.

Dissociation constant. pK_a 9.8.

Identification. TESTS. It complies with Tests 1 and 2 described under Ephedrine.

MELTING-POINT. About 184°.

ULTRAVIOLET ABSORPTION. See under Ephedrine.

INFRA-RED ABSORPTION. Major peaks at 704, 764, 1004, 1036, 1376, and 1456 cm^{-1} (see Appendix 2a: Infra-red Spectra).

Determination in body fluids. ULTRAVIOLET SPECTRO-

PHOTOMETRY. In plasma: phenylpropanolamine and ephedrine are stated to interfere—J. E. Wallace, *J. pharm. Sci.*, 1969, **58**, 1489.

GAS CHROMATOGRAPHY. In serum—L. M. Cummins and M. J. Fourier, *Analyt. Lett.*, 1969, **2**, 403.

Metabolism. ABSORPTION. Rapidly and completely absorbed after oral administration; aluminium hydroxide increases and kaolin decreases the rate of absorption.

BLOOD CONCENTRATION. After an oral dose of 180 mg, peak plasma concentrations of 500 to 900 ng/ml are attained in 1 to 3 hours; after an oral dose of 180 mg of a sustained release preparation, peak plasma concentrations of about 400 ng/ml are attained in 4 to 6 hours.

HALF-LIFE. Plasma half-life after an oral dose, 5 to 8 hours which may be increased in subjects with alkaline urine and decreased in subjects with acid urine.

DISTRIBUTION. Volume of distribution, 2 to 3 litres/kg body weight.

METABOLIC REACTIONS. *N*-Demethylation to a small extent.

EXCRETION. About 70% of a dose is excreted in the urine in 36 hours with less than 1% as norpseudoephedrine and the remainder as unchanged drug.

FURTHER INFORMATION. Cardiovascular effects and plasma concentrations—C. Bye *et al.*, *Eur. J. clin. Pharmac.*, 1975, **8**, 47; enhancement of absorption by aluminium hydroxide—R. L. Lucarotti *et al.*, *J. pharm. Sci.*, 1972, **61**, 903; influence of urinary pH on plasma half-life—R. G. Kuntzman *et al.*, *Clin. Pharmac. Ther.*, 1971, **12**, 62.

Actions and uses. Pseudoephedrine is a sympathomimetic amine with actions and undesirable effects resembling those of ephedrine. It is used as a bronchodilator and peripheral vasoconstrictor in preparations for the relief of nasal and bronchial congestion, particularly in bronchial asthma.

The usual dosage is 60 to 180 milligrams daily in divided doses. Children aged 2 to 5 years may be given 20 to 30 milligrams, and 6 to 12 years 30 to 45 milligrams, 2 or 3 times a day.

Precautions and contra-indications. Pseudoephedrine should be given with caution to hypertensive patients and those with prostatic enlargement. It should not be given to patients who are being treated with a monoamine-oxidase inhibitor, such as isocarboxazid, nialamide, phenelzine, or tranylcypromine, or within about 2 weeks of the discontinuation of such treatment.

Preparations

Preparations available include an ELIXIR containing pseudoephedrine hydrochloride 30 mg in 5 ml, diluent syrup, life of diluted elixir 14 days; an elixir containing pseudoephedrine hydrochloride 30 mg with triprolidine hydrochloride 1.25 mg in 5 ml, diluent syrup, life of diluted elixir 14 days; and TABLETS containing pseudoephedrine hydrochloride 60 mg, and tablets containing pseudoephedrine hydrochloride 60 mg with triprolidine hydrochloride 2.5 mg.

Psoriasis

Psoriasis is a chronic dermatosis of unknown cause characterised by sharply marginated reddened areas of skin with abnormal scaling. There is increased metabolic activity of the integument with excessive cellular proliferation which, when of sufficient magnitude, manifests itself as the characteristic lesion. The condition is genetically transmitted and appears on the scalp and in other areas which are exposed to trauma.

When psoriasis is mild, treatment may be unnecessary. In more troublesome cases treatment consists of the local application of preparations of salicylic acid, coal tar, dithranol, or other substances known to have a temporary beneficial effect. Corticosteroid creams or ointments are usually effective in the treatment of psoriasis but should be used with caution. Methotrexate has also been used in the treatment of severe forms of psoriasis. Attacks of psoriasis may be precipitated by emotional factors and by some drugs. Rest and the use of tranquillisers or hypnotics may be of prophylactic value. When psoriasis is accompanied by itching, this may be relieved by antihistamines.

Psychomotor Seizures

see under EPILEPSY

Psychoses

The psychoses are mental conditions characterised by disturbances in mental functions such as thinking or perception which cannot solely be explained as a response to experience and which are severe enough to distort the patients' appreciation of the real world and the relationship of events within it. They are often accompanied by delusions or hallucinations. The psychoses can be divided into the organic psychoses in which physical disease, either cerebral or general, underlies the mental state and the functional psychoses in which no such cause is apparent.

Organic Psychoses

Acute organic psychoses are characterised by clouding of consciousness and memory disturbance. They may be secondary to infectious toxaemias, endocrinological abnormalities, head injuries, etc. Treatment is aimed at the underlying condition. Chronic organic psychoses involve intellectual deterioration and memory loss and may be associated with brain tumours and other cerebral lesions, cerebrovascular disease, neurodegenerative disorders, or alcoholism.

Functional Psychoses

Manic-depressive psychosis is characterised by an excessive disturbance of mood. Apparent mental health lasting months or years is interspersed by periods of mania or profound depression. Mania is characterised by intense excitement and overactivity associated with a feeling of intense well-being and elevated mood. Depression is characterised by feelings of sadness accompanied by loss of interest in life (see the entry on Depression). Periods of mania may be treated with chlorpromazine or haloperidol and periods of depression may be treated with tricyclic antidepressants or monoamine-oxidase inhibitors. Alternatively, the excessive changes of mood may be lessened by long-term use of lithium carbonate.

Schizophrenia is a poorly defined collection of mental disorders in which characteristic disorders of thought, perception, emotion, and motor behaviour occur. In acute and severe cases these include thought disorder (inability to put thoughts together comprehensibly), a feeling of interference with thought processes, auditory hallucinations (voices), delusions of persecution, and blunting or inappropriateness of emotions. There may be derangement of personality and loss of contact with reality. Consciousness is unimpaired. In less severe, insidious, and chronic cases there may be fewer symptoms, hallucinations and delusions being most common. Both acute and chronic schizophrenia are treated with antipsychotic drugs such as butyrophenones, thioxanthenes, and phenothiazine derivatives. In some cases treatment may need to be long-term or life-long.

Psyllium

The dried ripe seed of *Plantago afra* L. (*P. psyllium*) or of *P. indica* L. (*P. arenaria* Waldst. et Kit.) (Fam. Plantaginaceae).

OTHER NAME: Flea seed

A standard is given in the British Pharmaceutical Codex 1973

The plants are annual herbs which are indigenous to the Mediterranean region (*P. afra*) and parts of Europe, Asia, and North Africa (*P. indica*).

Psyllium is produced mainly in southern France.

Constituents. Psyllium contains mucilage as its principal constituent, together with fixed oil and proteins. It yields about 2.5 to 4% of ash. Up to 3% of foreign organic matter may be present.

Description. UNGROUND DRUG. *Macroscopical characters:* **P. afra** seeds about 2 to 3 mm long and 0.8 to 1.2 mm wide, rounded-oblong in outline, dark reddish-brown, surface shining and glossy, very transparent and showing the embryo as a paler longitudinal area about one-third width of seed as seen through the outer layers; hilum pale coloured, in centre of concave surface, a slight transverse constriction across the centre of the convex surface; endosperm hard; embryo straight, almost as long as the seed, lying near the convex surface, and having two cotyledons and their contiguous flattened upper surfaces in the median plane; seeds becoming surrounded by a layer of colourless translucent mucilage when soaked in water.

P. indica seeds similar to those of *P. afra* but more elliptical in outline; blackish-brown in colour and not very transparent; surface rather dull; from 2 to 2.5 mm long and 1 to 1.5 mm wide at the centre; the furrow of the concave surface frequently extending to the extreme end of the seed.

The odour is not marked and the taste is mucilaginous.

Microscopical characters: the diagnostic characters are: *epidermis* with polyhedral cells, transparent and full of mucilage; *endosperm* composed of cells with thick, cellulose walls with numerous pits, cell contents granular; *embryo* of thin-walled polyhedral cells containing *fixed oil* and *aleurone grains.*

POWDERED DRUG. Powdered Psyllium. A light brown to brown powder possessing the diagnostic microscopical characters of the unground drug.

Adulterants and substitutes. The seeds of *P. lanceolata* L. are distinguished by their yellowish-brown colour, the dark furrow with a black central hilum, and the failure to produce any appreciable layer of mucilage when soaked in water; 100 seeds weigh about 0.16 g.

Actions and uses. Psyllium has the property of absorbing and retaining water and has therefore been used as a bulk-providing medium in the treatment of chronic constipation.

The usual adult dose is 5 to 15 grams; children may be given half the adult dose. It is taken with a draught of water.

Preparations of psyllium are also used to assist the production of a smooth solid faecal mass after colostomy.

Psyllium, on account of its content of mucilage, has been used as a demulcent.

Pulmonary Embolism and Infarction

Pulmonary embolism is the impaction in the pulmonary vascular bed of thrombus or other foreign matter which is brought to its site of lodgement by the blood stream. Its main complication is pulmonary infarction which is the necrosis of lung tissue resulting from interference with the blood supply. Most emboli arise from thrombosis in systemic veins (see venous thrombosis) but they may also be composed of air, fat, or malignant tissue.

The onset of pulmonary embolism is marked by sudden severe chest pain together with intense breathlessness. The heart rate is rapid and the cardiac output is reduced; signs of right heart failure may occur. There may also be restlessness, anxiety, or syncope. When pulmonary infarction also occurs it is characterised by haemoptysis, pleural effusion, and inflammation of the pleura with pain over the region involved.

When pulmonary embolism occurs without infarction, recovery is usually complete and occurs by organisation and recanalisation of the clot, whereas pulmonary infarction heals by fibrosis.

Pulmonary embolism may be associated with heart failure or it may be secondary to venous thrombosis occurring in other parts of the body, particularly in the legs, where it may be associated with postoperative immobility, pelvic disease, and operations. It is therefore important that these conditions should be treated so as to minimise the possibility of pulmonary embolism developing. Oestrogens administered to a patient may also predispose to development of pulmonary emboli.

Pulmonary embolism may be treated by surgical embolectomy or by intravenous administration of heparin, which prevents extension of the clot and limits the risk of further emboli being released from distant sources. Fibrinolytic agents such as streptokinase or urokinase may also be used. Heparin and fibrinolytic agents may be used in the acute phase, and followed by oral anticoagulants. Heparin administered subcutaneously has been used as a prophylactic against pulmonary embolism.

Pumilio Pine Oil

Obtained by distillation from the fresh leaves of *Pinus mugo* Turra var. *pumilio* (Haenke) Zenari (Fam. Pinaceae), a tree growing chiefly in the Austrian Alps, more especially in the Tyrol.

A standard is given in the British Pharmaceutical Codex 1973

Constituents. Pumilio pine oil consists largely of terpenes and sesquiterpenes, with up to 10% of bornyl acetate.

Description. A colourless or faintly yellow liquid with a pleasant and aromatic odour.

Solubility. Soluble, at 20°, in 10 parts of alcohol, with opalescence.

Weight per ml. At 20°, 0.858 to 0.870 g.

Refractive index. 1.470 to 1.480.

Optical rotation. −4° to −15°.

Adulterants and substitutes. Other commercially available oils are oil of Siberian fir from *Abies sibirica* Ledeb., which has a weight per ml at 20° of 0.900 to 0.920 g and contains 33 to 45% of esters, calculated as bornyl acetate, and oil of Scots pine, formerly from *P. sylvestris* L. but now distilled from the leaves and twigs of various conifers, which has a weight per ml at 20° of 0.860 to 0.870 g and contains 1.0 to 2.5% of esters, calculated as bornyl acetate.

Aromatic oil of pine, which is obtained as a by-product in the manufacture of steam-distilled wood turpentine in America, differs considerably in odour from the above oils, and consists largely of terpineol. It has a weight per ml at 20° of 0.927 to 0.942 g.

Storage. It should be stored in well-filled airtight containers, protected from light, in a cool place.

Actions and uses. Pumilio pine oil is pleasantly aromatic and is inhaled with steam, sometimes with the addition of menthol, eucalyptus oil, and compound benzoin tincture, to relieve cough and nasal congestion.

Preparations

It is an ingredient of compound thymol glycerin and zinc undecenoate dusting-powder.

Purgatives

see under CONSTIPATION

Purpura, Henoch-Schönlein

Henoch-Schönlein purpura (Allergic purpura; Anaphylactic purpura) is an acute or sometimes chronic vasculitis affecting primarily the skin, joints, or gastro-intestinal or renal systems. It is an allergic reaction which often follows an acute infection, especially of the upper respiratory tract by haemolytic streptococci, but it may also be due to food allergy or drug hypersensitivity. The vascular endothelium is damaged and becomes permeable to red cells resulting in a macular and papular rash with urticarial swellings. Symptoms include fever, malaise, joint pains due to effusion into joints, and bouts of abdominal pain with vomiting or bloody diarrhoea. Renal failure may sometimes occur.

No specific treatment is necessary for Henoch-Schönlein purpura as it resolves completely in 1 to 6 weeks, but any infections should be treated with appropriate antibacterial agents and patients who are severely ill may benefit from treatment with corticosteroids.

When Henoch-Schönlein purpura is due to food allergy or drug hypersensitivity, care should be taken not to repeat exposure to the allergen.

Pyelonephritis

see under URINARY TRACT INFECTIONS

Pyrazinamide

Pyrazine-2-carboxamide

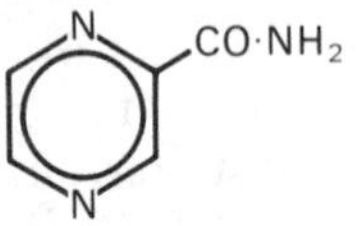

$C_5H_5N_3O = 123.1$

OTHER NAME: *Zinamide®*

A standard is given in the British Pharmacopoeia 1973

Description. An odourless, white, crystalline powder with a slightly bitter taste.

Solubility. Soluble, at 20°, in 60 parts of water and in 110 parts of alcohol; soluble in ether and in chloroform.

Storage. It should be stored in airtight containers.

Identification. MELTING-POINT. About 189°.

ULTRAVIOLET ABSORPTION. In water, maxima at 268 nm (E1%, 1cm = 655), and 310 nm (E1%, 1cm = 55).

INFRA-RED ABSORPTION. Major peaks at 1020, 1050, 1375, 1584, 1600, and 1685 cm^{-1} (see Appendix 2c: Infra-red Spectra).

Actions and uses. Pyrazinamide is a tuberculostatic drug with uses similar to those described under sodium aminosalicylate, but it is used only in infections that are resistant to other tuberculostatic drugs. Bacterial resistance to pyrazinamide may develop in 6 to 8 weeks and therefore it should always be used in conjunction with another drug to which the organism is sensitive.

The usual daily dosage for an adult is 20 to 35 milligrams per kilogram body-weight up to a maximum of 3 grams, given in 3 or 4 doses at equally spaced intervals. Children have been given 20 milligrams per kilogram body-weight (600 milligrams per square metre body-surface) daily divided into 3 or 4 doses, when there is no satisfactory alternative.

Undesirable effects. Signs of liver damage occur in a small proportion of patients taking 3 grams of pyrazinamide daily and jaundice occurs less frequently. Anorexia, malaise, nausea, vomiting, fever, arthralgia, difficulty in micturition, rashes, and photosensitivity may also occur.

Precautions and contra-indications. Pyrazinamide should not be given to patients with liver damage and tests for liver function should be made before commencing treatment and at frequent intervals during treatment. Care should be taken if the drug is given to patients with renal disease or a history of gout. If it is given to patients with diabetes mellitus it may cause difficulty in controlling the diabetes.

Preparation

PYRAZINAMIDE TABLETS: available as tablets containing 500 mg of pyrazinamide.
A standard for these tablets is given in the British Pharmacopoeia 1973
Containers and *Storage:* see the entry on Tablets for general information on containers and storage. Containers should be airtight.
Advice for patients: the tablets should be taken at regular intervals, preferably after meals. Treatment should not be discontinued without the advice of the prescriber.

Pyrethrum Flower

The dried flowerheads of *Chrysanthemum cinerariae-folium* Vis. (Fam. Compositae), a herbaceous perennial, indigenous to Yugoslavia, and cultivated chiefly in Kenya, Japan, Ecuador, and parts of east central Africa, Brazil, and the Indian subcontinent.

OTHER NAMES: Insect Flowers; Dalmatian Insect Flowers; Pyrethri Flos
Dairy Flyspray Cooper® and *Veterinary Insecticide (Pybuthrin) Cooper®* (both with piperonyl butoxide)

A standard is given in the British Pharmacopoeia (Veterinary)

Constituents. Pyrethrum flower owes its insecticidal properties to two groups of esters. One group consists of pyrethrin I and cinerin I, both of which have chrysanthemic acid (chrysanthemum monocarboxylic acid) as their acid component. The second group of esters consists of pyrethrin II and cinerin II, both of which have pyrethric acid (monomethyl ester of chrysanthemum dicarboxylic acid) as their acid component. The alcohol component of the pyrethrins is the keto-alcohol pyrethrolone, and that of the cinerins is the keto-alcohol cinerolone.

The pyrethrins and cinerins are soluble in alcohol, chloroform, and light mineral oils, are easily hydrolysed by weak alkalis, and are decomposed by heat and light. The combined content of the pyrethrins and cinerins varies from about 0.8 to 2% of which over 90% is contained in the cypselae, a little in the involucre and stem, and only traces in the corollas. The two groups of esters are generally present in approximately equal amounts, although flowers containing a larger proportion of either group occasionally occur. Chrysanthic acid, palmitic acid, linoleic acid, and a small amount of volatile oils are also present. Pyrethrum flower yields up to 1% of acid-insoluble ash.

Description. UNGROUND DRUG. *Macroscopical characters:* capitula occurring loose or compressed into masses, individual capitula being more or less flattened, about 6 to 12 mm in diameter, and commonly having a short piece of stalk attached; receptacle, usually about 5 to 10 mm in diameter, destitute of paleæ, almost flat, and surrounded by an involucre of 2 or 3 rows of brownish-yellow lanceolate bracts; ray florets number about 15 to 23, and disk florets about 200 to 300, ligulate corollas pale brownish and shrivelled, each being oblong in shape, about 16 mm long and showing 3 rounded apical teeth, the central one frequently being smaller in size than the lateral ones; about 17 veins in the middle region of the corolla; each disk floret has a yellow tubular corolla with 5 short lobes at the summit; each floret has an inferior 5-ribbed oblong cypsela, about 5 mm long, and surmounted by a membranous tubular calyx, about 1 mm in length; ovaries and lower part of the corollas covered with numerous scattered shining oil glands.
It has a faint characteristic odour and a slightly bitter taste.

Microscopical characters: the diagnostic characters are: loose, large-celled, lignified, moderately thick-walled, and pitted *parenchyma* of the receptacle; numerous spiny *pollen grains*, each with 3 pores and measuring about 34 to 40 μm in diameter; frequent ovoid-spherical glandular *trichomes*, each consisting of 3 to 4 tiers of 2 cells each; twisted T-shaped balance-hairs and lignified tissue from the involucral bracts; fragments of *ray florets*, showing cells of lower epidermis with wavy walls, and of upper epidermis with puckered papillæ;

fragments of the lobes of *disk florets*; portions of *stigmas* with papillose tips and, from the cypselæ, portions of brown *resin canals* and *sclerenchyma*, the cells of which contain diamond-shaped *crystals*, as also do the cells of the epidermis.

Adulterants and substitutes. The dried flowerheads of *C. roseum* Adam, from the Caucasus, and *C. marshallii* Aschers, from Iran, having red flowers, are occasionally met in commerce. They have more than 20, generally nearly 30, ray florets. The flowerheads of *C. leucanthemum* L. are sometimes substituted for pyrethrum flower; they are distinguished by the entire absence of calyx or pappus, by the 3 teeth terminating the strap of the somewhat lanceolate ligulate corolla, the central tooth being usually the largest, and by the presence of only 7 veins in the strap.

Storage. It should be stored in well-filled airtight containers, protected from light.

Actions and uses. Pyrethrum is an insecticide. Its action is due to the presence of its 4 constituents, pyrethrin I, pyrethrin II, cinerin I and cinerin II, all of which are rapidly toxic to flies when applied in a mineral-oil basis. Pyrethrum has no appreciable effect in insects as a stomach poison, but acts by contact, producing a characteristic effect on the nervous system, resulting in muscular excitation, convulsions, and paralysis.

On farms a spray containing 0.2% of pyrethrins in a kerosene basis is widely used for the control of flies on dairy cows and other livestock. It is usually sprayed about the sheds before milking and on each animal as it comes in at milking time.

Pyrethrum has a much quicker knock-down effect than dicophane or gamma benzene hexachloride, but it is less persistent and less stable. Its action can be enhanced by certain other substances such as piperonyl butoxide and bucarpolate (the piperonylic acid ester of the monobutyl ether of diethylene glycol). These synergists are frequently used in pyrethrum preparations, which may also include dicophane and gamma benzene hexachloride; such preparations combine a quick knock-down of the flies with a permanent effect. In the form of dusts, prepared by mixing pyrethrum extract with an inert powder such as talc, pyrethrum is widely used for the control of fleas on domestic animals and poultry.

Preparations

COMPOUND PYRETHRUM SPRAY:

Pyrethrum extract..	3.8 g
Piperonyl butoxide	7.6 g
Deodorised kerosene, of commerce	988.6 g

Mix and filter if necessary.
It contains about 0.09% w/w of pyrethrins and 0.76% w/w of piperonyl butoxide.
A standard for this spray is given in the British Pharmacopoeia (Veterinary)
Labelling: see the entry on Sprays for general information on labelling.

PYRETHRUM DUSTING-POWDER:

Pyrethrum extract..	16 g
Diatomite, in fine powder	300 g
Talc, in fine powder	684 g
Chloroform	a sufficient quantity

Dissolve the pyrethrum extract in the chloroform, and spray the solution on the diatomite and talc while mixing. Sift, and mix. It contains about 0.4% of pyrethrins.
A standard for this dusting-powder is given in the British Pharmacopoeia (Veterinary)

Labelling: see the entry on Dusting-powders for general information on labelling.

PYRETHRUM EXTRACT: prepared by exhausting pyrethrum flower, in coarse powder, by percolation with a hydrocarbon solvent. The solvent is removed from the percolate, which is concentrated at a low temperature. The content of pyrethrins in the extract is determined and, if necessary, the preparation is diluted with sufficient light liquid paraffin to produce an extract of the required strength. It may be decolorised. It contains about 25% w/w of pyrethrins of which not less than half is pyrethrin I.
A standard for this extract is given in the British Pharmacopoeia (Veterinary)
Description: a dark olive-green or brown viscous liquid, or, if decolorised, a pale orange liquid. It has a characteristic odour.
Weight per ml: At 20°, about 0.95 g.
Storage: it should be stored in well-filled airtight containers, protected from light. It should be thoroughly stirred before use.

OTHER PREPARATIONS available include a veterinary DUSTING-POWDER containing pyrethrins 0.25% with piperonyl butoxide 2.5%.

Pyridostigmine Bromide

3-Dimethylcarbamoyloxy-1-methylpyridinium bromide

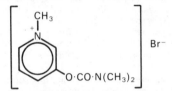

$C_9H_{13}BrN_2O_2 = 261.1$

OTHER NAMES: *Mestinon*®; Pyridostig. Brom.

A standard is given in the British Pharmacopoeia 1973

Description. A white deliquescent crystalline powder with an agreeable characteristic odour and a bitter taste.

Solubility. Soluble, at 20°, in less than 1 part of water and of alcohol and in 1 part of chloroform; very slightly soluble in ether and in light petroleum.

Moisture content. Not more than 2%, determined by drying at 105°.

Sterilisation. Solutions for injection are sterilised by heating in an autoclave or by filtration.

Storage. It should be stored in airtight containers, protected from light.

Identification. TEST. To about 100 mg add 0.6 ml of a 5% solution of sodium hydroxide; an orange colour is produced. Warm the solution; the colour becomes yellow and the vapour evolved turns moistened red litmus paper blue.

MELTING-POINT. About 154°.

ULTRAVIOLET ABSORPTION. In water, maximum at 269 nm (E1%, 1cm = 184).

INFRA-RED ABSORPTION. Major peaks at 680, 1010, 1163, 1259, 1515, and 1724 cm⁻¹ (see Appendix 2b: Infra-red Spectra).

Determination in body fluids. In plasma—K. Chan *et al.*, *J. Chromat.*, 1976, **120**, 349.

Metabolism. ABSORPTION. Poorly absorbed after oral administration.

BLOOD CONCENTRATION. In myasthenic subjects stabilised on intermittent oral doses of 60 mg, peak plasma concentrations of up to about 55 ng/ml are attained in 1 to 3 hours when determined by gas chromatographic techniques; after an oral dose of 120 mg, peak concentrations of up to 420 ng/ml have been determined by other less specific techniques.

HALF-LIFE. After oral administration, plasma half-life, about 4 hours and after intramuscular administration, about 1.5 hours.

DISTRIBUTION. In rats, crosses the placenta; pyridostigmine is secreted to some extent from the blood into the intestine.

METABOLIC REACTIONS. Hydrolysis to form 3-hydroxy-N-methylpyridinium; may be subject to first pass metabolism.

EXCRETION. About 2 to 16% of a dose is excreted in the urine unchanged and about 2.5% as 3-hydroxy-N-methylpyridinium; in rats given pyridostigmine by stomach tube, about 42% of a dose is excreted in the urine and about 38% is excreted in the faeces and intestinal contents.

FURTHER INFORMATION. Metabolism in man—S. M. Somani *et al.*, *Clin. Pharmac. Ther.*, 1972, **13**, 393; metabolism and excretion in rats—R. D. N. Birtley *et al.*, *Br. J. Pharmac.*, 1966, **26**, 393 and M. A. Husain *et al.*, *Br. J. Pharmac.*, 1968, **34**, 445; pharmacokinetics —H. E. Barber and G. R. Bourne, *Br. J. Pharmac.*, 1973, **48**, 329P; placental transfer in rats—J. B. Roberts *et al.*, *Br. J. Pharmac.*, 1970, **38**, 202; plasma concentrations in patients with myasthenia gravis—T. N. Calvey and K. Chan, *Clin. Pharmac. Ther.*, 1977, **21**, 187.

Actions and uses. Pyridostigmine has actions similar to those described under Neostigmine Methylsulphate but is only about one-fourth as active as neostigmine. Pyridostigmine is used in the treatment of myasthenia gravis; when given by mouth in doses of 60 to 240 milligrams of pyridostigmine bromide, it acts within 30 to 45 minutes and the effect lasts for 4 to 6 hours. It may also be given by subcutaneous or intramuscular injection in a dose of 1 to 5 milligrams.

Pyridostigmine does not always relieve the symptoms of myasthenia gravis as completely as neostigmine, but its prolonged effect often provides more sustained relief and it is therefore particularly suitable for treatment at night.

Undesirable effects. As for physostigmine salicylate. Pyridostigmine is less liable to cause nausea, vomiting, abdominal pain, and diarrhoea than neostigmine, but by increasing intestinal mobility it may cause disruption of intestinal suture lines.

Preparations

PYRIDOSTIGMINE INJECTION: a sterile solution of pyridostigmine bromide in water for injections. It is sterilised by heating in an autoclave or by filtration. Available in 1-ml ampoules containing 1 mg of pyridostigmine bromide.
A standard for this injection is given in the British Pharmacopoeia 1973
Containers and *Labelling:* see the entry on Injections for general information on containers and labelling.
Storage: it should be protected from light.

PYRIDOSTIGMINE TABLETS: available as tablets containing 60 mg of pyridostigmine bromide.

A standard for these tablets is given in the British Pharmacopoeia 1973
Containers and *Storage:* see the entry on Tablets for general information on containers and storage. Containers should be airtight and light resistant.

Pyridoxine Hydrochloride

4,5-Bis(hydroxymethyl)-3-hydroxy-2-methylpyridinium chloride

$C_8H_{12}ClNO_3 = 205.6$

OTHER NAMES: *Benadon®*; *Comploment®*; Vitamin B_6 *Ancoloxin®* (with meclozine hydrochloride)

A standard is given in the European Pharmacopoeia Vol. I

Description. An odourless white crystalline powder with a saline and bitter taste.

Solubility. Soluble, at 20°, in 5 parts of water and in 100 parts of alcohol; very slightly soluble in ether and in chloroform.

Acidity. A 5% solution has a pH of 2.3 to 3.5.

Dissociation constants. pK_a 5.0, 9.0 (25°).

Sterilisation. Solutions for injection are sterilised by heating in an autoclave or by filtration.

Storage. It should be protected from light.

Identification. TEST. To 2 drops of a 5% solution add 10 ml of a 5% solution of sodium acetate, 1 ml of water, and 1 ml of a 0.5% solution of dichloroquinonechloroimine in alcohol (95%), and shake; a blue colour is produced which rapidly fades and turns to brown. Repeat the test substituting 1 ml of a 3% solution of boric acid for the 1 ml of water; no blue colour is produced.

MELTING-POINT. About 205°, with decomposition.

ULTRAVIOLET ABSORPTION. In 0.1N hydrochloric acid, maximum at 290 nm (E1%, 1cm = 430); in 0.025M phosphate buffer solution pH 6.88, maxima at 254 nm (E1%, 1cm = 180), and 324 nm (E1%, 1cm = 350).

INFRA-RED ABSORPTION. Major peaks at 870, 1015, 1086, 1212, 1277, and 1540 cm⁻¹ (see Appendix 2c: Infra-red Spectra).

Metabolism. ABSORPTION. Readily absorbed after oral administration; absorption is decreased in gastrointestinal diseases and also in subjects taking isoniazid.

BLOOD CONCENTRATION. Endogenous blood concentrations are about 110 ng/ml.

METABOLIC REACTIONS. Converted to pyridoxal phosphate and to pyridoxic acid along with conjugation.

EXCRETION. Up to about 10% of a dose is excreted in the urine unchanged with 30 to 80% excreted as pyridoxic acid; in subjects with deficiency states the amount excreted may be reduced.

Actions and uses. Pyridoxine, pyridoxal, and pyridoxamine, which occur in foodstuffs, particularly in yeast, liver, cereals, and meat, are collectively known as vitamin B_6. In the body they are converted to pyridoxal phosphate, which is a coenzyme for a wide variety of metabolic transformations, including decarboxylation, transamination, racemization, and the metabolism of tryptophan, sulphur-containing amino acids, and hydroxyamino acids.

Pyridoxine plays a part in protein metabolism, the synthesis of fat from protein, haemopoiesis, and the nutrition of the skin. Convulsions and hypochromic anaemia have occurred in infants deficient in pyridoxine and in adults deprived of the vitamin. Lesions of the skin and mouth resembling those of ariboflavinosis and nicotinic acid deficiency have been observed in adults deprived of pyridoxine.

The daily requirement of pyridoxine in man is probably about 2 milligrams.

Pyridoxine has been used in the treatment of the nausea and vomiting of pregnancy and irradiation sickness, but the evidence of its value in these conditions is not impressive. The dosage of pyridoxine hydrochloride employed for this purpose has been purely empirical, quantities ranging from 20 to 100 milligrams daily having been given.

Pyridoxine, in doses of 50 milligrams daily, may be effective in relieving depression sometimes caused by oral contraceptives.

For convulsions in infants caused by pyridoxine deficiency, the dosage is 4 milligrams per kilogram body-weight daily for short periods. For the treatment of anaemia induced by pyridoxine deficiency in an adult, the dosage is 50 to 150 milligrams daily in divided doses.

Some types of megaloblastic anaemia, possibly due to pyridoxine deficiency, have responded to treatment with 100 to 200 milligrams of pyridoxine hydrochloride daily.

To prevent the possible occurrence of peripheral neuritis and anaemia in patients receiving isoniazid, pyridoxine is given in doses of 20 to 150 milligrams daily.

Drug interactions. Pyridoxine, even in small doses, blocks the action of levodopa.

Preparations

PYRIDOXINE TABLETS (*Syn.* Pyridoxine Hydrochloride Tablets; Vitamin B_6 Tablets): may be prepared by moist granulation and compression as described in the entry on Tablets. Available as tablets containing 10, 20, and 50 mg of pyridoxine hydrochloride.

A standard for these tablets is given in the British Pharmaceutical Codex 1973

Containers and *Storage*: see the entry on Tablets for general information on containers and storage. Containers should be airtight and light resistant.

OTHER PREPARATIONS available include TABLETS containing pyridoxine hydrochloride 100 mg in a slow-release formulation, and tablets containing pyridoxine hydrochloride 50 mg with meclozine hydrochloride 25 mg.

Pyridoxine hydrochloride is an ingredient of strong compound vitamin B tablets and of vitamins B and C injection (see under Riboflavine).

Pyrimethamine

5-(4-Chlorophenyl)-6-ethylpyrimidine-2,4-diamine

$C_{12}H_{13}ClN_4 = 248.7$

OTHER NAMES: *Daraprim*®
Supacox® (with amprolium hydrochloride, ethopabate, and sulphaquinoxaline); *Maloprim*® (with dapsone); *Fansidar*® (with sulphadoxine) (available only in certain overseas countries); *Whitsyn S*® (with sulphaquinoxaline)

A standard is given in the British Pharmacopoeia 1973

Description. An odourless, tasteless, white, crystalline powder.

Solubility. Practically insoluble in water; soluble, at 20°, in 200 parts of alcohol and in 125 parts of chloroform; soluble in warm, dilute, mineral acids.

Dissociation constant. pK_a 7.0 (20°).

Identification. TEST. Dissolve about 50 mg in 5 ml of *dilute sulphuric acid* and add 4 drops of *potassium mercuri-iodide solution*; a creamy-white precipitate is produced.

MELTING-POINT. About 240°.

ULTRAVIOLET ABSORPTION. In 0.005N hydrochloric acid, maximum at 272 nm (E1%, 1cm = 320); in alcohol (95%), maximum at 287 nm (E1%, 1cm = 365).

Determination in body fluids. THIN-LAYER CHROMATOGRAPHY. In plasma or urine—R. L. DeAngelis *et al.*, *J. Chromat.*, 1975, **106**, 41.

Metabolism. BLOOD CONCENTRATION. After an oral dose, a peak plasma concentration is attained in about 2 hours; during therapy with 50 mg daily, plasma concentrations of 0.3 to 0.6 μg/ml are attained.

HALF-LIFE. Plasma half-life, about 90 hours.

DISTRIBUTION. Secreted in milk.

EXCRETION. About 3% of a dose is excreted daily in the urine during the first week after administration.

FURTHER INFORMATION. Plasma concentrations and urinary excretion in falciparum malaria—M. H. Brooks *et al.*, *Clin. Pharmac. Ther.*, 1969, **10**, 85; persistent excretion—C. C. Smith and J. Ihrig, *Am. J. trop. Med.*, 1959, **8**, 60.

Actions and uses. Pyrimethamine is an antimalarial drug which has uses similar to those described under Proguanil Hydrochloride. It affects the nucleoprotein metabolism of the parasite by interference in the folic–folinic acid systems, and this action is exerted mainly at the time when the nucleus divides. It has little effect upon immature schizonts in the red corpuscles and is therefore slow to control a malarial attack; for this purpose it is better to use a rapidly acting drug such as chloroquine.

The chief value of pyrimethamine is as a suppressant. It usually kills the primary exoerythrocytic parasites of *Plasmodium vivax* and, if used regularly, will therefore prevent relapses of most strains of benign tertian malaria. Pyrimethamine also affects gametocytes, rendering them incapable of complete development in the mosquito.

Strains of *Plasmodium* occur which are resistant to pyrimethamine, and there is evidence that some strains of proguanil-resistant malaria in man are cross-resistant to pyrimethamine. This is a further reason for using a drug of a different type for the treatment of acute infections.

A dosage of 25 milligrams of pyrimethamine by mouth once weekly is usually adequate for the prophylaxis of all forms of malaria in an adult. For a child under 5 years a dosage of 6.25 milligrams, and for a child from 5 to 15 years 12.5 milligrams, is given once weekly. The drug is acceptable to children because it is tasteless.

Pyrimethamine is given together with chloroquine for the treatment of malarial fever during eradication campaigns; the chloroquine rapidly eliminates asexual parasites and the pyrimethamine helps to prevent transmission by the mosquito.

Sulphonamides and sulphones enhance the action of pyrimethamine, and combined courses of treatment may be used against chloroquine-resistant strains of malaria parasite.

In the treatment of toxoplasmosis 50 milligrams of pyrimethamine may be given daily together with 1 gram of sulphadiazine 6-hourly for 3 days followed by 25 milligrams of pyrimethamine daily in conjunction with 500 milligrams of sulphadiazine 8-hourly. This should be continued for 28 days provided the condition of the patient has improved within 2 weeks of initiating treatment.

The regimen for children in the treatment of toxoplasmosis is similar. Infants under 1 year may be given 100 milligrams per kilogram body-weight of sulphadiazine daily in divided doses together with 2 milligrams per kilogram body-weight of pyrimethamine daily for 3 days; the dose of pyrimethamine is then reduced to 1 milligram per kilogram body-weight daily for 28 days. In children over 1 year the dose of sulphadiazine may be based on the dosage scheme for sulphonamides described under Sulphadimidine. The usual dose of pyrimethamine is 25 milligrams daily for 3 days. Thereafter the dosage of sulphadiazine and pyrimethamine should be halved and treatment should be continued for a further 28 days.

Regular blood counts should be made throughout the treatment of toxoplasmosis. Calcium folinate may be given in a dosage of 1 milligram daily to infants and 5 to 15 milligrams to children and adults to reduce the toxicity of pyrimethamine.

Undesirable effects. No toxic effects have been observed during the administration of 25 milligrams of pyrimethamine once weekly. When 25 milligrams is given every day for long periods, depression of haemopoiesis is observed in some persons because of the antagonistic effect of the drug to folic acid. When treatment ceases, haemopoiesis is restored. Very large doses of pyrimethamine cause vomiting and convulsions.

Poisoning. The stomach should be washed out and an injection of calcium folinate given to counteract the effect of the drug upon the processes mediated by folic acid. Convulsions should be controlled by the injection of diazepam.

Veterinary uses. Pyrimethamine is administered to poultry in conjunction with other coccidiostats for the prophylaxis of coccidiosis. The usual concentration administered in the feed is 5 parts per million.

Preparations

AMPROLIUM, ETHOPABATE, SULPHAQUINOXALINE, AND PYRIMETHAMINE PREMIX: consisting of amprolium hydrochloride, ethopabate, sulphaquinoxaline, and pyrimethamine, mixed with a suitable diluent. It must be diluted before administration by mixing thoroughly with the feed.

Available as a premix containing 20% of amprolium hydrochloride, 1% of ethopabate, 12% of sulphaquinoxaline, and 1% of pyrimethamine.

A standard for this premix is given in the British Pharmacopoeia (Veterinary)

Containers and *Storage:* see the entry on Premixes for general information on containers and storage.

PYRIMETHAMINE TABLETS: available as tablets containing 25 mg of pyrimethamine.

A standard for these tablets is given in the British Pharmacopoeia 1973

Containers and *Storage:* see the entry on Tablets for general information on containers and storage. Containers should be airtight.

Advice for patients: for prophylaxis doses should be taken regularly during the period at risk, commencing one week before arrival in the risk area and for 4 weeks thereafter. For therapy the prescribed course should be completed.

OTHER PREPARATIONS available include an INJECTION (available only in certain overseas countries) containing pyrimethamine 10 mg with sulphadoxine 200 mg per ml in 2.5-ml ampoules; a veterinary SOLUTION containing pyrimethamine 9.1 mg with sulphaquinoxaline 30 mg per ml; TABLETS containing pyrimethamine 12.5 mg with dapsone 100 mg, and tablets (available only in certain overseas countries) containing pyrimethamine 25 mg with sulphadoxine 500 mg.

Pyrithidium Bromide

3-Amino-8-(2-amino-1,6-dimethyl-4-pyrimidinioamino)-6-(4-aminophenyl)-5-methylphenanthridinium dibromide

$C_{26}H_{27}Br_2N_7 = 597.4$

OTHER NAME: *Prothidium®*

A standard is given in the British Pharmacopoeia (Veterinary)

Description. An odourless, hygroscopic, brick-red to reddish-purple powder.

Solubility. Soluble, at 20°, in 40 parts of water and in 1900 parts of alcohol.

Acidity. A 2% suspension has a pH of 4 to 7.

Moisture content. Not more than 10%, determined by drying at 130°.

Identification. TESTS. 1. Dissolve about 50 mg in 20 ml of water, add 1 ml of hydrochloric acid, cool in ice, add 1 ml of *sodium nitrite solution*, and add to a cold solution of 100 mg of 2-naphthol in 20 ml of *dilute sodium hydroxide solution*; an intense dark blue colour or a purple precipitate is produced.
2. Mix about 100 mg with 5 mg of manganese dioxide and 1 ml of sulphuric acid and heat; bromine is evolved which gives a pink colour to a filter paper moistened with a 0.2% solution of fluorescein sodium in alcohol (95%).

ULTRAVIOLET ABSORPTION. In *dilute sulphuric acid*, maxima at 256 nm (E1%, 1cm = 425) and 313 nm (E1%, 1cm = 812).

Veterinary uses. Pyrithidium bromide is a trypanocide. A single dose of 2 milligrams per kilogram body-weight by subcutaneous or intramuscular injection is used to protect cattle for up to 6 months against *Trypanosoma congolense*, *T. vivax*, and mixed infections including *T. brucei*.

Preparation

PYRITHIDIUM SOLUTION-TABLETS FOR INJECTION: available as solution-tablets containing 500 mg of pyrithidium bromide.
A standard for these solution-tablets is given in the British Pharmacopoeia (Veterinary)
Labelling: the label on the container should state the amount of pyrithidium bromide in each solution-tablet, and that the solution for injection is prepared by dissolving the solution-tablet in boiling water and allowing to cool before administration.

Pyrophosphate Arthropathy

Pyrophosphate arthropathy (chondrocalcinosis) is a crystal deposition disease resembling gout in that acute attacks of synovitis occur as a result of deposition of crystals in the joint fluid. The crystals consist of calcium pyrophosphate dihydrate. It is the larger joints which are usually affected, particularly the knee. In addition to acute arthritis, pyrophosphate arthropathy may be associated with a chronic degenerative condition resembling osteoarthritis. It may be associated with hyperparathyroidism or haemochromatosis and may resolve when these conditions are treated.
Pyrophosphate arthropathy may be treated by aspiration of the joint and the injection of a suspension of a suitable corticosteroid into it. Anti-inflammatory agents such as aspirin, indomethacin, or phenylbutazone may also be of value.

Pyroxylin

Pyroxylin is a nitrated cellulose prepared by treating wood pulp or defatted cotton wool with a mixture of nitric and sulphuric acids under carefully controlled conditions. It is damped with not less than 25% w/w of isopropyl alcohol or industrial methylated spirit.

OTHER NAMES: Cellulose Nitrate; *Collodion 33042®*; *Necoloidine Solution 36059®*

A standard is given in the British Pharmacopoeia Addendum 1978

Pyroxylin is a mixture of nitrates of a polysaccharide of high molecular weight, $(C_6H_{10}O_5)_n$, consisting of at least 200 glycopyranose units. On this basis it has a composition corresponding to the introduction of 2 to 2½ nitrate groups per sugar unit.
The properties of nitrated cellulose, such as its solubility and the viscosity of its solutions, depend largely upon the number of nitrate groups introduced into the cellulose molecule, and this number depends upon the conditions of nitration, including the composition of the acid mixture and the temperature and length of time of nitration.
Nitrated celluloses which contain an average of more or less nitrate groups than pyroxylin are insoluble in a mixture of alcohol and ether; by this test gun-cotton, which contains an average of 3 nitrate groups per sugar unit, may be distinguished from pyroxylin.

Description. White cuboid granules or a white fibrous material which resembles·cotton wool but is harsher to the touch. It appears moist, smells strongly of the damping fluid, and is highly inflammable.

Solubility. Soluble, at 20°, in a mixture of 1 volume of alcohol (90%) and 3 volumes of ether, yielding an almost clear and colourless solution; soluble in acetone and in glacial acetic acid.

Storage. It should be kept in an airtight container, loosely packed, protected from light and stored in a cool place, remote from fire. The container should be suitably designed to disrupt should the internal pressure reach or exceed 200 lb per sq. in. The amount of damping fluid must not be allowed to fall below 25%; should this happen, the material should either be re-wetted or be used immediately for the preparation of collodion.

Uses. Pyroxylin is used in the preparation of collodions, which are convenient applications for the protection of small cuts and abrasions and for use as vehicles for drugs when prolonged local action is required.

Preparation

FLEXIBLE COLLODION:

Colophony	25 g
Castor oil	25 g
Collodion (see below)	to 1000 ml

Mix the ingredients and stir until the colophony has dissolved; allow any deposit to settle and decant the clear liquid. Collodion is prepared by adding 100 g of pyroxylin to 900 ml of a mixture of 3 volumes of solvent ether and 1 volume of alcohol (90%) and agitating continuously until dissolved. Sufficient of the mixed solvent is added to produce a solution having a kinematic viscosity of 405 to 700 centistokes. In making collodion the alcohol (90%) may be replaced by industrial methylated spirit diluted so as to be of equivalent alcoholic strength, provided that the law and the statutory regulations governing the use of industrial methylated spirit are observed.
When Collodion is prescribed or demanded, Flexible Collodion is supplied.
A standard for flexible collodion is given in the British Pharmacopoeia Addendum 1978
Storage: it should be stored in airtight containers in a cool place, remote from fire.
Advice for patients: the collodion should be painted onto the affected area and allowed to dry. Care should be. taken to keep well away from a naked flame while the collodion is being applied.

Flexible collodion is an ingredient of salicylic acid collodion.

Quassia

The dried stem-wood of *Picrasma excelsa* (Sw.) Planch. (Fam. Simarubaceae), a tree of moderate size indigenous to the West Indies and northern Venezuela but exported only from Jamaica.

OTHER NAME: Quassia Wood

A standard is given in the British Pharmaceutical Codex 1973

The trunks and larger branches are freed from the bark, cut into thin transverse slices or chips, and dried.

Constituents. Quassia contains about 0.2% of the bitter principles quassin (a lactone) and neoquassin (the hemiacetal of quassin) and a minute quantity of a yellow crystalline substance which exhibits a blue fluorescence in an acidified alcoholic solution. Quassia yields to water about 4 to 8% of extractive.

It yields up to 5% of ash and up to 2% of foreign organic matter may be present.

Description. UNGROUND DRUG. *Macroscopical characters:* transverse slices or chips; density about 0.54 to 0.56, pale yellow or sometimes bright yellow; diffuse porous, with false annual rings; tough, but easily split longitudinally; tangential surface ripple-marked.

It is odourless and has an intensely bitter taste.

Microscopical characters: the diagnostic characters are: *vessels* in groups of 2 to 11; walls with very numerous, minute bordered pits; vessel elements up to 200 μm wide and about 250 to 325 μm long, with transverse ends; *xylem fibres* about 750 to 900 μm long and 18 μm wide, with moderately thick walls having simple, oblique, slit-like pits; *xylem parenchyma* chiefly in interrupted tangential bands about 2 to 4 to occasionally 15 rows wide, some paratracheal parenchyma in 1 to several layers around parts of the vessels not adjacent to medullary rays; axial parenchyma in files about 4 cells long or up to 12 small cells each containing a prismatic *crystal* of calcium oxalate, 12 to 18 to 24 to 40 μm long; *medullary rays* storied, about 6 to 8 per mm of arc, mostly 2 to 4 cells wide, about 10 to 20% being uniseriate, some cells containing prisms of calcium oxalate and some cells of both parenchyma and rays containing small *starch* granules, about 4 to 12 μm in diameter, mostly simple and spherical or occasionally compound with 2 components.

POWDERED DRUG. Powdered Quassia. An odourless yellow to pale buff powder possessing the diagnostic microscopical characters and taste of the unground drug.

Adulterants and substitutes. Surinam quassia, from *Quassia amara* L. (Fam. Simarubaceae), is distinguished by the medullary rays which are mostly one cell wide, and by the absence of crystals of calcium oxalate; it contains quassin and neoquassin.

Exhausted quassia may be differentiated by the lower yield of aqueous extractive and by the less bitter taste. Quassia showing greyish patches is wood which has been attacked by fungus.

Actions and uses. Quassia is a bitter and, on account of its freedom from tannin, an infusion prepared from quassia, 1 to 100, may be given with salts of iron.

Preparations

Preparations available include a standardised SOLUTION containing quassin in industrial methylated spirit for use as a denaturant.

Quillaia

The dried inner part of the bark of *Quillaja saponaria* Molina, a tree indigenous to Chile and Peru, and cultivated in the Indian subcontinent, and of other species of *Quillaja* (Fam. Rosaceae).

OTHER NAMES: Panama Wood; Quillaia Bark; Quillaiae Cortex; Soap Bark

A standard is given in the British Pharmacopoeia 1973

Quillaia is exported only from Chile under the commercial designation of Valparaiso or San Antonio quillaia.

Constituents. Quillaia contains the colourless amorphous saponin glycosides, quillaic acid and quillaia-sapotoxin; they both impart to water the property of frothing, but the acrid taste and sternutatory effect are due to quillaiasapotoxin alone. Quillaia also contains sucrose and yields to alcohol (45 per cent) 28 to 40% of extractive.

It yields up to 1% of acid-insoluble ash and up to 2% of foreign organic matter may be present.

Description. UNGROUND DRUG. *Macroscopical characters:* pieces hard, tough, flat, up to about 1 m long, 100 to 200 mm broad and 3 to 6 to 10 mm thick; outer surface brownish-white bearing pale reddish-brown or blackish-brown streaks or patches of adherent outer bark; inner surface yellowish-white, smooth, and very hard; fracture splintery and laminated, the broken surface showing numerous large prisms of calcium oxalate as glistening points; smoothed, transversely cut surface appearing chequered, with delicate radial lines representing medullary rays and tangential lines formed by alternating tangential bands of phloem containing fibres.

It is sternutatory and has an acrid and astringent taste.

Microscopical characters: the diagnostic characters are: *outer bark*, when present, consisting of reddish-brown *cork cells* alternating with bands of brown parenchyma interspersed with numerous groups of *phloem fibres* and containing large prismatic *crystals* of calcium oxalate; *inner bark* composed of bands of tortuous *fibres* irregularly enlarged at intervals, about 500 to 1000 μm long and 20 to 50 μm wide, alternating with mixed *sieve tissue* and parenchyma; *medullary rays* mostly 3 to 4 but sometimes up to 6 cells wide with occasional subrectangular *sclereids* adjacent to the bundles of *phloem fibres*; *starch* grains 5 to 10 to 20 μm in diameter, and prismatic *crystals* of calcium oxalate, usually 50 to 170 μm long and up to 30 μm wide, present in the parenchymatous cells.

POWDERED DRUG. Powdered Quillaia. A pale buff powder with a pink tinge, possessing the diagnostic microscopical characters and taste of the unground drug; strongly sternutatory; forms a copious persistent froth when shaken with water.

Actions and uses. The saponins of quillaia in aqueous solution lower surface tension and the extract and tincture are used as emulsifying agents, especially for tar preparations and for volatile oils. Powdered quillaia has a powerful sternutatory action.

Preparations

QUILLAIA LIQUID EXTRACT:
Small-scale preparation

Quillaia, in moderately fine powder ..	..	1000 g
Alcohol (45%)		to 1000 ml

Exhaust the quillaia with the alcohol by percolation, reserving the first 850 ml of percolate; evaporate the subsequent percolate to the consistence of a soft extract, dissolve it in the reserved portion, and add sufficient of the alcohol to produce 1000 ml; allow to stand for not less than 24 hours, and filter.

Manufacture. Prepare the extract by the above method, appropriately scaled up, or by the alternative method described in the entry on Extracts.

A standard for this extract is given in the British Pharmaceutical Codex 1973

QUILLAIA TINCTURE:

Quillaia liquid extract	..	..	..	50 ml
Alcohol (45%)	..	..	..	to 1000 ml

Mix, allow to stand for not less than 12 hours, and filter.

A standard for this tincture is given in the British Pharmaceutical Codex 1973

Dose: 2.5 to 5 millilitres.

Quinalbarbitone Sodium

Sodium 5-allyl-5-(1-methylbutyl)barbiturate

$C_{12}H_{17}N_2NaO_3 = 260.3$

OTHER NAMES: Quinalbarb. Sod.; Secobarbital Sodium; Secobarbitalum Natricum; Secobarbitone Sodium; *Seconal Sodium®*
Tuinal® (with amylobarbitone sodium)

A standard is given in the European Pharmacopoeia Vol. II

Description. An odourless hygroscopic white powder with a bitter taste.

Solubility. Soluble, at 20°, in 3 parts of water and in 5 parts of alcohol; very slightly soluble in ether.

Alkalinity. A 10% solution has a pH of not more than 11.

Moisture content. Not more than 5%, determined by drying at 105°

Dissociation constant. pK_a 7.9 (25°).

Stability; Incompatibility. See under Barbiturates.

Storage. It should be stored in airtight containers.

Identification. TESTS. 1. Dissolve about 1 g in 100 ml of water, add 5 ml of *dilute acetic acid*, stir vigorously, add 200 ml of water, boil until the precipitate dissolves and no oily particles remain on the surface, allow to cool, induce crystallisation and allow to stand overnight; filter, wash the filter with water and dry the residue at 80°. The residue complies with general test 1 described under Barbiturates.

2. It complies with general test 3 described under Barbiturates.

3. An aqueous solution decolorises *potassium permanganate solution.*

MELTING-POINT. The residue obtained in Test 1 melts at about 96°.

ULTRAVIOLET ABSORPTION. (See also under Barbiturates.) In 0.1N sodium hydroxide, maxima at 219 nm (E1%, 1cm = 808) and 245 nm (E1%, 1cm = 273).

THIN-LAYER CHROMATOGRAPHY. See under Thin-layer Chromatography, System 5.

Determination in body fluids. See under Barbiturates.

Metabolism. (See also under Barbiturates.) ABSORPTION. About 90% of an oral dose is absorbed from the gastro-intestinal tract.

BLOOD CONCENTRATION. After an oral dose of about 3 mg/kg, a peak blood concentration of 2 μg/ml is obtained after 3 hours.

HALF-LIFE. Plasma half-life, about 30 hours.

DISTRIBUTION. *Protein binding,* about 70% bound to plasma proteins.

METABOLIC REACTIONS. Hydroxylation of both side chains at the C_5-position with further oxidation of the ω-position on the butyl side chain.

EXCRETION. Up to 10% of an oral dose is excreted unchanged in the urine; after a dose of 2 g, 50% is recovered in the urine as stereoisomers of 5-allyl-5-(3-hydroxy-1-methylbutyl)barbituric acid, and 5-(2,3-dihydroxypropyl)-5-(1-methylbutyl)barbituric acid; after a dose of 200 to 300 mg of the sodium salt, two diastereoisomeric forms of the following metabolites are excreted in the urine: 5-allyl-5-(3-hydroxy-1-methylbutyl)barbituric acid, 5-allyl-5-(1-methyl-3-oxobutyl)barbituric acid, 5-allyl-5-(3-carboxy-1-methylpropyl)barbituric acid, and 5 - (2,3 - dihydroxypropyl) - 5 - (1 - methylbutyl)barbituric acid.

FURTHER INFORMATION. Clearance from plasma—J. M. Clifford *et al., Clin. Pharmac. Ther.,* 1974, **16**, 376; metabolism—J. N. T. Gilbert *et al., J. Pharm. Pharmac.,* 1975, **27**, 343.

Actions and uses. Quinalbarbitone sodium is an intermediate-acting barbiturate, the actions and uses of which are described under Barbiturates. The usual hypnotic dose is 100 to 200 milligrams.

Undesirable effects; Precautions; Contra-indications; Dependence; Poisoning. See under Barbiturates.

Preparations

QUINALBARBITONE CAPSULES: consisting of quinalbarbitone sodium, in powder, which may be mixed with a suitable inert diluent, enclosed in a hard capsule. Available as capsules containing 50 and 100 mg of quinalbarbitone sodium.

A standard for these capsules is given in the British Pharmacopoeia 1973

Containers and *Storage:* see the entry on Capsules for general information on containers and storage.

Advice for patients: hypnotic doses should be taken half an hour before bedtime. The capsules may cause drowsiness on the following day; persons affected should not drive or operate machinery. Alcohol should be avoided.

QUINALBARBITONE TABLETS: the usual strengths are 50 and 100 mg of quinalbarbitone sodium; they are sugar coated.

A standard for these tablets is given in the British Pharmacopoeia 1973

Containers and *Storage:* see the entry on Tablets for general information on containers and storage. Containers should be airtight.

Advice for patients: see above under Quinalbarbitone Capsules.

OTHER PREPARATIONS available include CAPSULES containing quinalbarbitone sodium 50 mg with amylobarbitone sodium 50 mg, and capsules containing quinalbarbitone sodium 100 mg with amylobarbitone sodium 100 mg.

Quinidine Sulphate

The sulphate dihydrate of quinidine, (αS)-α-(6-methoxyquinolin-4-yl)-α-[(2R,4S,5R)-(5-vinylquinuclidin-2-yl)]-methanol, an alkaloid obtained from the bark of various species of *Cinchona*; the base is an optical isomer of quinine.

$C_{40}H_{50}N_4O_8S,2H_2O = 782.9$

OTHER NAMES: *Quinicardine*®
Kiditard® and *Kinidin*® (both are quinidine bisulphate); *Natisédine*® (quinidine phenylethylbarbiturate)

A standard is given in the British Pharmacopoeia 1973

Description. Odourless needle-like white crystals with a very bitter taste.

Solubility. Soluble, at 20°, in 80 parts of water and in 10 parts of alcohol.

Acidity. A 1% solution in water has a pH of 6 to 6.8.

Moisture content. 3 to 5%, determined by drying at 130°.

Specific rotation. About +278°, determined on a 3% solution in 0.1N hydrochloric acid.

Dissociation constants. pK_a 4.2, 8.8 (25°).

Stability. It darkens in colour on exposure to light. When heated, 1 molecule of water of crystallisation is lost at 100° and the second at 120°.

Sterilisation. Solutions for injection are sterilised by heating in an autoclave or by filtration.

Storage. It should be stored in airtight containers, protected from light.

Identification. TESTS. 1. To 5ml of a 0.1% solution add a few drops of *bromine solution* followed by 1 ml of *dilute ammonia solution*; an emerald-green colour is produced.
2. To a 0.5% solution add an equal volume of *dilute sulphuric acid*; a strong blue fluorescence is produced.
3. To 5 ml of a 1% solution add 1 ml of *silver nitrate solution* and stir with a glass rod; after a short interval a white precipitate, soluble in nitric acid, is produced (distinction from many other alkaloids).

ULTRAVIOLET ABSORPTION. Quinidine, in alcohol (95%), maxima at 236 nm (E1%, 1cm = 1110), 278 nm (E1%, 1cm = 132), and 332 nm (E1%, 1cm = 163).

Determination in body fluids. SPECTROFLUORIMETRY. In plasma—K. K. Midha *et al.*, *Can. J. pharm. Sci.*, 1977, **12**, 41.

GAS CHROMATOGRAPHY. In plasma—J. L. Valentine *et al.*, *J. pharm. Sci.*, 1976, **65**, 96.

THIN-LAYER CHROMATOGRAPHY. In plasma or serum—J. Christiansen, *J. Chromat.*, 1976, **123**, 57.

Actions and uses. Quinidine prolongs the refractory period of cardiac muscle and therefore reduces the rate at which successive contractions can take place.

Quinidine is used in the treatment of paroxysmal ventricular tachycardia, and of auricular fibrillation of recent origin in the absence of congestive heart failure; it is valuable in cases of thyrotoxicosis in which fibrillation persists after thyroidectomy.

A preliminary dose of 200 milligrams of quinidine sulphate is given by mouth in the morning and, if there are no signs of idiosyncrasy, 400 milligrams is given 4 hours later, followed by 600 milligrams after a further 4 hours. This treatment is continued as long as toxic symptoms do not occur, the maximum dosage being usually 3 grams a day. If there is no improvement after treatment for 10 days, the quinidine should be discontinued, as it is unlikely to be of any benefit. In successful cases, the change from auricular fibrillation to normal rhythm occurs suddenly and the dose should then be reduced gradually. It may be necessary to continue treatment with a dosage of 300 milligrams once or twice a day for a considerable time in order to maintain normal rhythm. For the prophylaxis of cardiac arrhythmias, 200 milligrams may be given 3 or 4 times a day.

Rarely, in an emergency, quinidine may be given by intravenous injection, but extreme care must be taken.

Undesirable effects. Occasionally, quinidine produces such effects as palpitation, headache, nausea, vomiting, dizziness, dimness of vision, scarlatiniform eruptions, and precordial pain.

Preparations

QUINIDINE SULPHATE TABLETS: they contain 200 mg of quinidine sulphate.

A standard for these tablets is given in the British Pharmacopoeia 1973

Containers and *Storage:* see the entry on Tablets for general information on containers and storage. Containers should be airtight and light resistant. The tablets should not be allowed to come into contact with metal.

Advice for patients: the tablets should be taken at regular intervals, preferably after meals. Treatment should not be discontinued without the advice of the prescriber.

SLOW QUINIDINE TABLETS: they contain 250 mg of quinidine bisulphate equivalent to 200 mg of quinidine sulphate in a slow-release formulation.

Containers and *Storage:* see the entry on Tablets for general information on containers and storage. Containers should be airtight and light resistant. The tablets should not be allowed to come into contact with metal.

Advice for patients: the tablets should be swallowed whole and taken at regular intervals, preferably after meals. Treatment should not be discontinued without the advice of the prescriber.

OTHER PREPARATIONS available include CAPSULES containing quinidine bisulphate 250 mg equivalent to 200 mg of quinidine sulphate in a slow-release formulation; and TABLETS containing quinidine phenylethylbarbiturate 100 mg.

Quinine Bisulphate

The hydrogen sulphate heptahydrate of quinine, (αR)-α-(6-methoxyquinolin-4-yl)-α-[(2S,4S,5R)-(5-vinyl-quinuclidin-2-yl)]methanol, an alkaloid obtained from the bark of various species of *Cinchona*.

$C_{20}H_{26}N_2O_6S,7H_2O = 548.6$

OTHER NAME: Quinine Acid Sulphate

A standard is given in the British Pharmacopoeia 1973

Description. Odourless colourless crystals or white crystalline powder with a very bitter taste. It is efflorescent in dry air.

Solubility. Soluble, at 20°, in 8 parts of water, giving a solution with a blue fluorescence, and in 50 parts of alcohol.

Acidity. A 1% solution has a pH of 2.8 to 3.4.

Moisture content. 19 to 24%, determined by drying at 60° *in vacuo*.

Specific rotation. About $-210°$, determined on a 3% solution in 0.1N hydrochloric acid.

Dissociation constants. pK_a 4.1, 8.5 (20°).

Hygroscopicity. It is efflorescent in dry air.

Storage. It should be stored in airtight containers, protected from light.

Identification. TESTS. It complies with Tests 1 and 2 described under Quinidine Sulphate.

ULTRAVIOLET ABSORPTION. See under Quinine Dihydrochloride.

Determination in body fluids; Metabolism. See under Quinine Dihydrochloride.

Actions and uses. Quinine bisulphate has the actions, uses, undesirable effects, precautions and contra-indications of quinine, as described under Quinine Dihydrochloride, and is used in the same dosage. It is used for the preparation of tablets.

Poisoning. As for Quinine Dihydrochloride.

Preparation

QUININE BISULPHATE TABLETS (*Syn.* Quinine Acid Sulphate Tablets): available as tablets containing 300 mg of quinine bisulphate; they are compression coated, film coated, or sugar coated. Sugar-coated tablets are supplied unless the contrary is indicated.

A standard for these tablets is given in the British Pharmacopoeia 1973

Containers and *Storage:* see the entry on Tablets for general information on containers and storage. Containers should be airtight and, for tablets which are not sugar coated, light resistant.

Advice for patients: the tablets should preferably be taken after meals. When used in the treatment of malaria, the tablets should be taken at regular intervals and the prescribed course completed. When used to treat night cramp, the dose should be taken at bedtime.

Quinine Dihydrochloride

The dihydrochloride of quinine.

$C_{20}H_{26}Cl_2N_2O_2 = 397.3$

OTHER NAME: Quinine Acid Hydrochloride

A standard is given in the British Pharmacopoeia 1973

Description. An odourless white powder with a very bitter taste.

Solubility. Soluble, at 20°, in less than 1 part of water, in 14 parts of alcohol, and in 7 parts of chloroform; practically insoluble in ether.

Acidity. A 3% solution has a pH of 2 to 3.

Moisture content. Not more than 3%, determined by drying at 105°.

Specific rotation. About $-225°$, determined on a 3% solution in 0.1N hydrochloric acid.

Sterilisation. Solutions for injection are sterilised by heating in an autoclave or by filtration.

Storage. It should be stored in airtight containers, protected from light.

Identification. TESTS. It complies with Tests 1 and 2 described under Quinidine Sulphate.

ULTRAVIOLET ABSORPTION. Quinine, in alcohol (95%), maxima at 236 nm (E1%, 1cm = 1110), 278 nm (E1%, 1cm = 133), and 332 nm (E1%, 1cm = 163).

Determination in body fluids. SPECTROFLUORIMETRY. In serum or urine—A. P. Hall *et al.*, *Clin. Pharmac. Ther.*, 1973, **14**, 580.

Metabolism. ABSORPTION. Readily absorbed after oral administration; magnesium and aluminium hydroxides decrease the amount absorbed after an oral dose by causing quinine to precipitate in the gastro-intestinal tract; rectally administered doses are poorly absorbed and intramuscular or subcutaneous doses of quinine salts are slowly absorbed.

BLOOD CONCENTRATIONS. Therapeutic plasma concentrations appear to be in the range 3 to 7 $\mu g/ml$; during therapy with oral doses of 500 to 650 mg daily, plasma concentrations of up to 12 $\mu g/ml$ may be attained; malarial infection inhibits hepatic metabolism and thus plasma concentrations resulting from a given dose will vary according to the severity of the infection.

HALF-LIFE. Plasma half-life, 6 to 9 hours which is increased to up to 15 hours in malarial infections and decreased to about 3 to 4 hours in patients being treated with antiepileptic drugs.

DISTRIBUTION. Crosses the placenta, is secreted in milk, saliva, and into the gastric juice, and is taken up by red blood cells and platelets; *protein binding*, highly bound to plasma proteins.

METABOLIC REACTIONS. Oxidation to form hydroxylated metabolites comprising mainly the 2-hydroxyquinoline and the 6-hydroxyquinoline derivatives.

EXCRETION. Following intravenous administration, and oral administration as tablets or as capsules, 18, 10 and 14% of these doses are excreted in the urine in 24 hours respectively; less than 5% of a dose appears to be excreted unchanged; during maintenance therapy, about 25% is excreted in the urine and less than 5% in the faeces in 24 hours; the urinary excretion of quinine is increased when the urine is acid; quinine is excreted to some extent in the bile.

FURTHER INFORMATION. Plasma concentrations and urinary excretion—M. H. Brooks *et al.*, *Clin. Pharmac. Ther.*, 1969, **10**, 85 and A. P. Hall *et al.*, *Clin. Pharmac. Ther.*, 1973, **14**, 580; quinine metabolism as an index of hepatic drug-metabolising capacity—C. Padgham and A. Richens, *Br. J. clin. Pharmac.*, 1974, **1**, 352P; metabolism impaired during malaria or fever—G. M. Trenholm *et al.*, *Clin. Pharmac. Ther.*, 1976, **19**, 459.

Actions and uses. Quinine suppresses the asexual cycle of development of malaria parasites in the erythrocytes. It has no action on the tissue forms of the malaria parasite and therefore will not prevent relapse of *Plasmodium vivax* infection; it also has no action on *P. falciparum* gametocytes and therefore does not prevent transmission of the infection by the mosquito.

Quinine is used in conjunction with primaquine in the radical cure of relapsing vivax malaria, and for the treatment of malaria due to strains of *P. falciparum* resistant to other antimalarial drugs.

Quinine dihydrochloride has been used to prevent and control overt attacks of malaria, but has now been largely superseded by less toxic and more effective antimalarial drugs. A dosage of 300 to 600 milligrams daily has been used as a suppressant. The equivalent dose for children up to one year is 7.5 to 15 milligrams per kilogram body-weight, 2 to 5 years 150 to 200 milligrams, and 6 to 12 years 300 to 450 milligrams.

For the treatment of an attack, 600 milligrams has been given by mouth 3 times a day for 4 days or until the symptoms are relieved; for this purpose, tablets containing the bisulphate are usually preferred. If vomiting prevents the retention of oral doses, a soluble salt of quinine may be given by intravenous injection or by slow intravenous infusion as described in the following paragraph. Intramuscular injections are slower in action than intravenous injections; they are painful and may cause tissue necrosis.

Quinine dihydrochloride is the salt usually employed for the preparation of injections. It is given by injection to patients with cerebral malaria, or when vomiting prevents the retention of the orally administered drug; 20 millilitres of a 3% solution may be given by slow intravenous injection or 200 millilitres of a 0.3% solution in warm sodium chloride injection may be given by slow intravenous infusion.

Quinine is no longer used for its antipyretic and analgesic properties.

A dose of 300 milligrams repeated if necessary has been used in the treatment of night cramps.

Undesirable effects. Therapeutic doses of quinine frequently produce mild toxic symptoms such as deafness, ringing in the ears, visual disturbances, and slight giddiness and tremors. Excessive doses may cause permanent deafness or blindness, and may also cause abortion in pregnant women.

The administration of quinine to a patient who has previously been suffering from a chronic and inadequately controlled malarial infection may precipitate an attack of blackwater fever.

Precautions. Particular care should be taken when administering quinine to patients with heart block or cardiac arrhythmias.

Contra-indications. Quinine is contra-indicated in patients sensitive to its action, in pregnancy near term unless absolutely necessary for the treatment of malaria, and in patients with optic neuritis.

Poisoning. Ingested quinine should be removed by gastric lavage or emesis followed by a saline cathartic. Fluids should be given by mouth or intravenously to promote renal excretion. Quinine is especially toxic to children.

Preparations

QUININE DIHYDROCHLORIDE INJECTION: a sterile solution of quinine dihydrochloride in water for injections. It is sterilised by heating in an autoclave or by filtration. It must be diluted before administration. A solution containing 300 mg of quinine dihydrochloride per ml should be diluted with at least 10 times its volume (and preferably more) of water for injections. Care must be taken to ensure slow intravenous injection.

A standard for this injection is given in the British Pharmacopoeia 1973

Containers: see the entry on Injections for general information on containers.

Labelling: see the entry on Injections for general information on labelling. In addition, the label on the container and the label on the package should state that the solution must be diluted before administration.

Storage: it should be protected from light.

QUININE DIHYDROCHLORIDE TABLETS (*Syn.* Quinine Acid Hydrochloride Tablets): may be prepared by moist granulation and compression as described in the entry on Tablets. Available as tablets containing 300 mg of quinine dihydrochloride; they may be sugar coated.

A standard for these tablets is given in the British Pharmaceutical Codex 1973

Containers and *Storage:* see the entry on Tablets for general information on containers and storage. Containers should be airtight and light resistant.

Advice for patients: the tablets should preferably be taken after meals. When used in the treatment of malaria the tablets should be taken at regular intervals and the prescribed course completed. When used to treat night cramp, the dose should be taken at bedtime.

Quinine Hydrochloride

The hydrochloride dihydrate of quinine.
$C_{20}H_{25}ClN_2O_2,2H_2O = 396.9$

OTHER NAME: Chininii Chloridum

A standard is given in the European Pharmacopoeia Vol. I

Description. Odourless, colourless, fine, silky, acicular crystals, often grouped in clusters, with a very bitter taste. On exposure to light it gradually becomes yellowish in colour. It is efflorescent in dry air.

Solubility. Soluble, at 20°, in 23 parts of water and in less than 1 part of alcohol; soluble in chloroform.

Moisture content. 6 to 10%, determined by drying at 105°.

Specific rotation. −240° to −258°, determined on a 2% solution in 0.1N hydrochloric acid.

Sterilisation. Solutions for injection are sterilised by heating in an autoclave or by filtration.

Storage. It should be stored in airtight containers, protected from light.

Identification. TESTS. It complies with Tests 1 and 2 described under Quinidine Sulphate.

ULTRAVIOLET ABSORPTION. See under Quinine Dihydrochloride.

Determination in body fluids; Metabolism. See under Quinine Dihydrochloride.

Actions and uses. Quinine hydrochloride has the

actions, uses, undesirable effects, precautions, and contra-indications of quinine, as described under Quinine Dihydrochloride and is used in the same dosage. It has been used in conjunction with urethane as a sclerosing agent in the treatment of varicose veins.

Poisoning. As for Quinine Dihydrochloride.

Preparations

Preparations available include TABLETS containing quinine hydrochloride 300 mg.

Quinine Sulphate

The sulphate dihydrate of quinine.
$C_{40}H_{50}N_4O_8S,2H_2O = 782.9$

A standard is given in the British Pharmacopoeia 1973

Description. Odourless, white, usually lustreless, acicular crystals with a very bitter taste.

Solubility. Soluble, at 20°, in 810 parts of water and in 95 parts of alcohol; very slightly soluble in ether and in chloroform; soluble in a mixture of 2 parts of chloroform and 1 part of dehydrated alcohol.

Acidity. A 1% suspension in water has a pH of 5.7 to 6.6.

Moisture content. 3 to 5%, determined by drying at 105°.

Specific rotation. About −240°, determined on a 3% solution in 0.1N hydrochloric acid.

Incompatibility. It is incompatible with alkalis and their carbonates, iodides, tannic acid, and mercuric chloride.

Storage. It should be stored in airtight containers, protected from light.

Identification. TESTS. 1. It complies with Test 1 described under Quinidine Sulphate.
2. To a few drops of a saturated solution add 1 drop of *dilute sulphuric acid*; a strong blue fluorescence is produced.

ULTRAVIOLET ABSORPTION. See under Quinine Dihydrochloride.

Determination in body fluids; Metabolism. See under Quinine Dihydrochloride.

Actions and uses. Quinine sulphate has the actions, uses, undesirable effects, precautions, and contra-indications of quinine, as described under Quinine Dihydrochloride, and is used in the same dosage. It may be given in tablets, but the bisulphate is usually preferred for this purpose. It is not sufficiently soluble for the preparation of injections and the dihydrochloride is more generally used.
The chief use of quinine sulphate is as a bitter.

Poisoning. As for Quinine Dihydrochloride.

Preparation

QUININE SULPHATE TABLETS: available as tablets containing 125, 200, and 300 mg of quinine sulphate; they are film coated or sugar coated. Sugar-coated tablets are supplied unless the contrary is indicated.
A standard for these tablets is given in the British Pharmacopoeia 1973
Containers and *Storage:* see the entry on Tablets for general information on containers and storage. Containers should be airtight and, for tablets which are not sugar coated, light resistant.
Advice for patients: the tablets should preferably be taken after meals. When used in the treatment of malaria the tablets should be taken at regular intervals and the prescribed course completed. When used to treat night cramp, the dose should be taken at bedtime.

Rabies

Rabies is an acute infectious disease of mammals characterised by central nervous system irritation which leads to paralysis and death. Man usually acquires the infection from the bite of a rabid dog, fox, or other animal.
The incubation period varies from 10 days to over a year, the length depending on the severity of the bite, its proximity to the head, and the quantity of virus injected. The virus travels along peripheral nerves and the spinal cord to the brain where it multiplies causing an encephalitis with multiple punctate haemorrhages. Some virus may pass along efferent nerves to salivary glands which then produce infective saliva.
Onset of the disease is marked by fever, heavy sweating, headache, malaise, and a sense of constriction in the throat. This is followed by restlessness, agitation, fear of water, paralysis, and convulsions which are invariably followed by death.
Because the incubation period of the disease is long, it is possible to vaccinate against rabies after exposure to an animal suspected of being rabid. For details of vaccination see Rabies Vaccine.

Rabies Antiserum

A preparation of rabies immunoglobulins or their derivatives, obtained by purification from native serum, which specifically neutralises rabies virus.

OTHER NAMES: Antirabies Serum; Immunoserum Antirabicum; Rab/Ser

A standard is given in the European Pharmacopoeia Vol. II

Actions and uses. Rabies antiserum is used for the prevention of rabies in patients who have received bites on areas of special danger, such as the head and the neck, from rabid animals or animals suspected of being rabid. It is given in conjunction with rabies vaccine.
The antiserum must be given as soon as possible after exposure, preferably within 24 hours. The dose is approximately 40 units per kilogram body-weight intramuscularly on the first day, followed by daily injections of rabies vaccine. Up to 5 millilitres of antiserum should, when feasible, be infiltrated around and under bites. The number of injections of vaccine will depend on the severity of the possible infection—see under Rabies Vaccine.
It is often useful to give the antiserum immediately and then start the vaccine treatment on the first sign of rabies in the biting animal. If signs suggestive of rabies are already present in the biting animal, then the antiserum must be given immediately, followed by the vaccine, which may be stopped on the fifth day after exposure if the animal is normal; the antiserum must not be given after the second day of vaccine treatment as it will interfere with the production of active immunity by the vaccine.
Two reinforcing doses of vaccine should be given on the tenth and twentieth days after completion of the primary course to overcome possible interference by passive antibody with active immune responses.

Serum reactions. See under Antisera.

Rabies Vaccine

Rabies Vaccine as described in the British Pharmacopoeia 1973 is a preparation of killed rabies fixed virus prepared in brain tissue. This vaccine and duck embryo vaccine, which has also been used, have been replaced by vaccine prepared in cell cultures. The vaccine available at present in the United Kingdom is prepared in human diploid cells, but vaccines prepared in other types of cell culture may also come into use.

Storage. The vaccine prepared in human diploid cells should be protected from light and stored at a temperature below 4°; it should not be allowed to freeze.

Actions and uses. Rabies vaccine is used for the immunisation of persons who because of their occupation or environment have special risk of infection with rabies. The quantity specified on the label as the dose is administered by subcutaneous injection. The primary course consists of 2 injections with an interval of 4 weeks. A further dose is given after 1 year after which doses may be given every 3 to 5 years. Rabies vaccination may also be used for post-exposure prophylaxis of rabies in patients who have been bitten by rabid animals or animals suspected of being rabid; in the latter case treatment is stopped if the animal is normal on the fifth day after exposure or attack or if acceptable laboratory findings are negative in the animal killed at the time of the attack. Infection cannot take place through unbroken skin, but it is possible through uninjured mucous membranes. Rabies antiserum may be administered before beginning treatment with the vaccine.

Before initiating antirabies treatment the following factors should be considered:

(1) Whether enzootic rabies exists in the country where the bite occurred or whether the biting animal has been recently imported from an enzootic area. Animals more likely to be infected than others are bats and carnivores (especially dogs, cats, skunks, foxes, coyotes, raccoons). Although rodents (squirrels, rats, and mice) are rarely infective, in enzootic areas any wild animal that bites or scratches, particularly those that escape, must be suspect.

(2) The circumstances of the biting incident. *Unprovoked* attacks mean that the animal is more likely to be rabid. Bites suffered while attempting to handle or feed apparently healthy animals may be regarded as *provoked*. The biting animal should be captured and confined under veterinary observation for signs of rabies for at least 10 days. Adult animals that have been adequately immunised with rabies vaccine are unlikely to develop rabies *or transmit virus.*

(3) The extent and location of bite wound. It is calculated that only 10 to 15% of human exposures to known rabid animals result in infection. Infection is more likely to occur after severe multiple or deep penetrating wounds or bites on the head, neck, or hands; it is less likely to occur after mild scratches, lacerations, or single bites on areas of the body other than the head, neck, or hands. Open wounds and abrasions suspected of being contaminated with saliva are also considered mild. Indirect contact or a lick on unabraded skin is not considered exposure.

Wounds should first be cleansed with a detergent to remove as much contamination as possible and treated with an antiseptic solution. Rabies antiserum may be administered by infiltration around the wounds. An injection of rabies vaccine may then be given subcutaneously and repeated on the 3rd, 7th, 14th, 30th and 90th days after exposure.

Patients who have been immunised against rabies prior to exposure require only 1 to 3 injections to boost the immune response.

Rabies Veterinary Vaccine, Inactivated

A fluid or freeze-dried preparation of a fixed strain of rabies virus, propagated in animal neural tissue or in cell culture and inactivated in such a manner that antigenic activity is retained.

A standard is given in the British Pharmacopoeia (Veterinary)

Storage. Fluid brain tissue vaccine should be protected from light and stored at 2° to 8° when it may be expected to retain its potency for 6 months. Phenolised suspensions should not be allowed to freeze. The dried vaccine should be stored at a temperature between −20° and −30°. It should be used immediately after reconstitution. Freeze-dried and fluid cell-culture vaccines should be protected from light and stored at 2° to 8° when they may be expected to retain their potency for 1 to 2 years, according to the manufacturer's indications. Dried vaccines should be used immediately after reconstitution.

Veterinary uses. It is administered by subcutaneous injection to horses, cattle, sheep, goats, dogs, and cats for prophylaxis of rabies. The use of rabies veterinary vaccine, inactivated, in the United Kingdom is restricted by the Agriculture Departments to quarantine kennels and for dogs and cats about to be exported.

Rabies Veterinary Vaccines, Living

Freeze-dried preparations of chick-embryo tissue or cell-culture liquid infected with a suitable attenuated strain of rabies virus.

A standard is given in the British Pharmacopoeia (Veterinary)

Storage. The dried vaccine should be protected from light, stored at 2° to 8° and used immediately after reconstitution.

Veterinary uses. It is administered by intramuscular injection for prophylaxis of rabies. Vaccine prepared from ERA or Vnukovo-32 strains of virus may be administered to all species except dogs less than 3 months old; vaccine prepared from the Flury HEP strain of virus may be administered to cattle, cats, and dogs of any age; vaccine prepared from the Flury LEP strain of virus may be administered only to dogs more than 3 months old; vaccine prepared from the Kelev strain of virus may be administered to cattle and to dogs less than 3 months old. The use of living rabies veterinary vaccines in the United Kingdom is restricted by the Agriculture Departments.

Radiation Sickness

see under NAUSEA AND VOMITING

Radiopharmaceuticals

Radiopharmaceuticals are medicinal products that are radioactive. They are used in numerous diagnostic procedures (organ uptake measurements, studies of the dynamics of physiological systems, and visualisation of organs or areas of the body) and as sources of radiation for therapeutic purposes. The number of diagnostic procedures has increased considerably in recent years, and the preparations used vary from simple solutions of inorganic salts to suspensions containing large organic molecules or complexes.

In general the radiopharmaceutical preparation, after assay of radioactivity and determination of the dose, is administered to the patient, usually by intravenous injection, less commonly by mouth, and occasionally by inhalation or some other route.

The chemical and physical properties of the radiopharmaceutical and the method of administration are chosen so that the labelled material either follows a particular anatomical or physiological pathway or is preferentially concentrated in an organ or other site of interest. Other substances may be administered in order to promote progress along the desired path or to inhibit movement of the radiopharmaceutical in some other pathway. For diagnostic purposes, measurements are made of the radiation emanating from the patient, or on plain or processed samples from the patient. The method and the frequency of measurement or sampling depend upon the type of investigation and the clinical information required.

Radiation Physics

Structure of the atom

Atoms consist of a central nucleus surrounded by a number of electrons which revolve in orbits. Most of the naturally occurring elements have a stable nucleus consisting of protons and neutrons in about equal numbers. The *proton* has a mass of 1 atomic unit and a positive charge equal to the charge on an electron. *Neutrons* also have a mass of 1 atomic unit but no charge. In a neutral atom the number of *electrons* is equal to the number of protons, which results in the overall charge of the atom being zero. The mass of the electron on the atomic mass scale is about 1/2000 part of that of either the proton or the neutron. Thus the major part of the mass of the atom lies in the nucleus.

The chemical identity of an atom is determined by the number of protons in the nucleus and this is called the *atomic number* (Z) of the atom. For the naturally occurring elements the atomic numbers range from 1 for hydrogen (one proton in the nucleus) to 92 for uranium (92 protons in the nucleus). The mass of an atom on the atomic mass scale is equal to the sum of the number of protons and the number of neutrons in the nucleus. This is called the *mass number* (A) of the atom (1 for hydrogen and 235 or 238 for uranium, depending on the neutron content).

In all elements it is possible to have several different numbers of neutrons in the nucleus, and in nature elements mostly occur as constant mixtures of various configurations. Thus although the atomic mass of any atom must be a whole number, the atomic mass (average) of an element need not be.

The different nuclear arrangements of any one element are known as *isotopes*.

If the nucleus of an atom has more or less neutrons than occur in any of its stable forms then that nucleus becomes unstable. Such an unstable nucleus is known as a *radioisotope* of that element and, since each atomic species is known as a *nuclide*, radioactive atomic species are also known as *radionuclides*. Any radioisotope tends to change into a more stable configuration by the process known as *radioactive decay*. In order to find a stable state the nucleus of the radioisotope must lose a charged particle, or capture an orbital electron and also lose its excess energy. The charged particles and energy emitted by a nucleus undergoing transformation is known as *nuclear radiation*. The resulting nucleus has a lower energy content than that of the parent radioactive nucleus; this energy appears as the energy of the emitted radiation.

All isotopic forms of an element (including the radioactive ones) are chemically indistinguishable, and as the nuclear radiation from each radioactive isotope has characteristic properties, radioisotopes have many varied applications as tracers in medicine and in other disciplines.

Radioactive decay

Radioisotopes decay in various ways, depending on their initial nuclear structure. Any given radioisotope disintegrates at a consistent rate, and the time taken for conversion of half of the number of atoms originally present is known as the *physical half-life* ($t_\frac{1}{2}$). Each radioisotope has a characteristic physical half-life and these range from fractions of a second to many years. Most radioisotopes used in medical diagnosis have half-lives in the range of minutes to months.

The proportion of atoms of any given radioisotope remaining unchanged after a period of time has elapsed is related exponentially to the time interval (*exponential decay*). Such a relationship is linear when log (activity) is plotted against time on graph paper and this forms the basis of a useful method for calculating activity at any time when the value is known at some other time.

Certain isotopes of high mass number decay by emission of *alpha particles*. These particles consist of two neutrons and two protons and hence have a mass of four atomic mass units and two units of positive charge. The alpha particle is identical with the nucleus of the helium atom.

Many radioisotopes decay by emission of *beta particles*; each carries a single unit of charge of either sign and has a mass equal to that of an electron. The negative beta particle (or *negatron*, denoted by the sign β^-) is identical with the electron; the positive beta particle is known as the *positron*, denoted by the sign β^+. With each beta particle emitted there is also a particle of zero charge called the *neutrino*. Because of its zero rest mass and lack of charge there is virtually no interaction between the neutrino and matter, and it is therefore of little material consequence. β^--decay normally occurs in atoms with an excess of neutrons and results in the conversion of a neutron into a proton. β^+-decay normally occurs when there is an excess of protons in the atom and a proton is effectively converted into a neutron. The two processes may, however, occur together in the same radioisotope.

Some radioisotopes having nuclei with an excess of protons decay by *electron capture* or *K-capture*. An electron from the innermost shell (the K-shell) is captured by the nucleus, thus converting a proton into a neutron. When the missing K-shell electron is subsequently replaced by a free electron the energy loss due to this action (the binding energy) results in the emission of the X-ray characteristic of the product atom.

Radioactive decay is frequently accompanied by the emission from the nucleus of electromagnetic radiation which carries away the excess energy that has not been removed by the particulate radiation; these emissions are known as *gamma rays*. A *metastable nucleus* (designated by "m") differs from its stable form only in having a slight excess of energy and decays by the emission of a gamma ray only, for example technetium-99m decays to technetium-99. This process of decay is called *isomeric transition*.

With many radioisotopes a proportion of the gamma rays emitted in the decay process interacts with an orbital electron (usually the K-shell electron). For any given radioisotope this fraction, called the *conversion ratio* is constant. A *conversion electron* is then emitted with the energy of the gamma ray less the binding energy of the electron. This process of electron emission is known as *internal conversion*. As in the case of electron capture the filling of the resulting vacant site in the K-shell results in the emission of the X-ray characteristic of the product nucleus. In some cases the energy may again be transferred to an electron which is emitted from the atom. This latter emission is known as an *auger electron*.

Nuclear Radiations

Alpha radiation consists of alpha particles, those emitted by a given isotope all having the same energy. Because of their relatively large charge and mass their passage through any absorbing material is accompanied by a great number of interactions in that material so that they rapidly lose their energy. Their range depends on the type of absorbing material and the energy of the particle, but it is always very short. The dense ionisation which they produce results in a high rate of tissue damage, and alpha-emitters are not used in radiopharmaceuticals.

Beta radiation consists of beta particles emitted as a result of radioactive decay. They have a continuous energy spectrum from zero up to a specific maximum energy for a given radioisotope. The balance of the energy for any beta particle which has less than its possible maximum is transferred to a neutrino. For general practical purposes the average energy of the β-particles of a given radioisotope can be taken approximately as one-third of the maximum energy.

Beta radiation is more penetrating than alpha radiation but its range of penetration is relatively short being of the order of millimetres in animal tissues, the absorption depending on the density and the atomic numbers of the atoms of the absorbing tissue. Since the range of beta particles is greater than that of alpha particles and their initial energy is less, the density of ionisation along the track is much lower.

As a beta particle is slowed down in an absorbing material some of its energy is converted into electromagnetic radiation which is known as *bremsstrahlung* or "braking radiation". This radiation has a continuous spectrum and the amount produced depends upon the magnitude of the atomic number of the absorbing material.

When a β^--particle is brought to rest it becomes a free electron and joins the population of free electrons in the same region. However, as a positron (β^+) comes to rest it unites with a free negative electron and both particles are destroyed with the production of two gamma-ray quanta of equal energy emitted in opposite directions. This process is called *annihilation* and the gamma rays are known as the *annihilation energy*. All positron emitters have annihilation energy photons (511 keV) in their emission.

Gamma radiation emitted as a result of radioactive decay consists of quanta of electromagnetic radiation (*photons*) whose energy is characteristic of their radioisotopic source. Photons are uncharged and are very penetrating.

In its passage through an absorbing material the intensity of the radiation falls exponentially with distance, and equal thicknesses of material reduce the intensity by equal fractions. A useful parameter that is used to measure absorption is the thickness of material required to reduce the intensity of the radiation to one half of its initial value. This is called the *half thickness* or *half value layer*, and the value depends on the density and atomic number of the material; the greater either of these, the smaller the half thickness.

In its passage through material gamma radiation undergoes absorption by the following three methods of interaction.

Compton scattering. The gamma ray is deflected and it loses some of its energy. The lost energy is imparted to an electron which is ejected from its parent atom.

Photoelectric absorption. All the energy of the gamma ray is imparted to a single electron which is again ejected from its parent atom. The frequency with which this process occurs depends upon the gamma-ray energy and the atomic number of the absorber.

Pair production. The gamma ray loses a fixed amount of energy to create an electron-positron pair and the excess energy is converted into the kinetic energy of these particles. These particles subsequently undergo the same fate as beta particles ejected from a radioactive nucleus. This process can only occur when the energy of the gamma ray exceeds a threshold value.

X-rays are physically identical with gamma rays, the only distinction being that gamma rays emanate from a nucleus which is undergoing a transformation whereas X-rays are produced either by causing a beam of electrons to strike a target or by the replacement of inner-shell electrons.

Methods of Detection of Radiation

All radiation detectors depend upon the interaction of radiation with matter. The radiation measurement is effectively a measure of this interaction or of secondary interactions. The most important interaction of radiation with matter is ionisation, that is the displacement of orbital electrons to form charged atoms or ions. This effect is used in two types of detector.

The *ionisation chamber* depends upon the ionisation by radiation of atoms of a gas between two electrodes. The ions are separated by an electric field so producing a very small electric current, typically of the order of 10^{-12} amperes. This current, called the *ionisation current*, is directly proportional to the intensity of the initial radiation and is independent of its type and its energy. The ionisation chamber is used for the measurement of gamma-emitting activity in a radioactive source and of radiation fields for protection purposes. In the first application the ionisation chamber is usually operated from electric mains and the sample to be measured is placed inside the chamber. In the second application the device may be portable and operated by batteries; it can be used to measure most types of radiation at the levels required for radiation protection.

The Geiger counter is similar to the ionisation chamber but the intensity of the electric field is increased so that the ions produced are accelerated and a cascade of secondary ionisation is produced. This results in a breakdown of the insulation of the gas and generates an electric pulse which can be detected. After each pulse the electric field is momentarily turned off to allow the ions to recombine and prepare the device for the next ionisation event. The period of time for which the field is turned off is called the *dead time* during which the device is refractory. Like the ionisation chamber, the Geiger counter measures the intensity of radiation but not its energy.

The Geiger counter may be used for the measurement of radioactivity or for the detection of radiation emanating from a patient, but generally it is used for the measurement of radiation for protection purposes, since it is more sensitive than the ionisation chamber.

The *scintillation counter* depends upon the emission of light by certain phosphors when exposed to radiation. Scintillations produced by interaction with radiation are detected and converted into electrical pulses by means of a photomultiplier tube; after suitable amplification the pulses are counted and their amplitude measured. The amplitude is proportional to the energy of the incident radiation, and so an energy spectrum may be obtained from a mixture of different incident radiations by means of a pulse-height analyser.

There are two main types of scintillation counter. In the first the phosphor, usually a thallium-activated sodium iodide crystal for gamma-ray detection, is attached to the photomultiplier, this complete unit being the scintillation detector. In the second form, which is used for measuring radioactive beta emitters, the radioactivity is mixed with a soluble type of phosphor and the solution then takes the place of the crystal. This technique is called *liquid scintillation counting* and it is one of the most sensitive methods of measuring beta radioactivity. The scintillation counter is the most widely used detector in clinical radioisotope work. It is available in many sizes (10 to 300 mm in diameter) and it is used for direct measurement on patients, for measurement of the radioactive content of samples, and for applications in radiation protection. It is the most sensitive of the radiation detectors.

Photographic film is affected by other radiation as well as light and gives a latent image that can be revealed by chemical development. It is used in diagnostic X-ray work and in radiation protection.

A small piece of wrapped film is enclosed in a plastic holder which has a number of radiation absorbers or filters. The device is worn or carried by a radiation worker and the exposure of the film gives a measure of the external radiation received by the worker. The filter system in the holder allows some assessment of the type of radiation which produced the exposure. This device is known as a *film badge*.

Radiation Protection

The object of radiation protection measures is to develop a healthy respect for radiation and radioactive procedures through knowledge and not fear of radiation and to reduce any risk due to its use to a minimum. A balance must be held between the benefits of using ionising radiation and the dangers involved, and it must be used in a controlled manner in order to minimise risks.

Hazards of radiation. Radiation has dangerous effects on biological systems. Locally induced ionisation in living cells promotes a number of irreversible changes. These changes may become manifest after a short period of time (hours or days) or they may take years to develop, or, as in the case of genetic changes, the effect will only be manifest in subsequent generations. It must be assumed that all effects of radiation on living systems are harmful and, in our present state of knowledge, it must be assumed that there is no threshold level for the onset of their effects.

In dealing with radioactive materials in pharmaceutical work, there are two types of hazard involved; those from the effects of external radiation on the body and those from contamination of the body with radioactive material.

To minimise hazards, a clean and safe working environment should be provided and checked by measurements of the degree of contamination and measurements of external radiation emitted from radioactive sources. To ensure that protection measures are adequate and to provide the means of assessing any necessary action in a radiation incident, assessments should be made of the radiation dose received by persons working with radiation or in an environment where radiation is being used and measurement should be made of their external and possibly internal contamination.

Radiation units and definitions

ACTIVITY. The activity of a radioactive material is the number of nuclear transformations or disintegrations that take place per unit of time. The traditional unit of activity is the *curie* (Ci), defined as 3.7×10^{10} disintegrations per second. The *becquerel* (Bq), 1 disintegration per second (equivalent to 2.7×10^{-11} Ci) has been assigned as the SI unit of activity. Because of the decay of radioactive material it is essential to state the time at which the activity is measured; the more rapid the decay the shorter the half-life and the more accurately the time should be specified.

ELECTRON VOLT (eV). Ionising radiation is a form of energy and the unit of measurement is the electron volt. The electron volt is the kinetic energy acquired by an electron when it is accelerated through a potential difference of 1 volt. It is a very small unit: $1 \text{ eV} = 1.60 \times 10^{-19}$ joule.

RAD (radiation absorbed dose). When ionising radiation passes through matter some of the energy of the radiation is absorbed. The rad is the traditional unit of absorbed dose, equivalent to 10^{-2} joules per kilogram. The *gray* (Gy), 1 joule per kilogram (equivalent to 100 rads) has been assigned as the SI unit of absorbed dose.

REM (rad-equivalent-man). When ionising radiation is absorbed in tissue the same absorbed dose may give rise to different biological effects depending on the type of radiation and the tissue. The unit of absorbed dose is modified to make allowance for the different effect by multiplying the dose in rads by a quality factor, that is, dose in rems equals dose in rads multiplied by the quality factor. For most radiations from radioisotopes the quality factor is equal to unity. The SI unit of dose is the joule per kilogram, equivalent to 100 rems.

Maximum permissible dose. Any exposure to radiation entails some risk but there are degrees of risk so low that the probability of radiation injury is very small. Such risks must be accepted if the benefits of using radiation are to be obtained. The limits judged to be acceptable are "maximum permissible doses" (MPD). The current Code of Practice (see below) specifies a level of MPD for whole body radiation for occupationally exposed workers of 5 rems per year.

There are restrictions on how this dose may be received and also a higher level of dose for individual organs or parts of the body. There are also permitted levels of ingested activity which are based on the MPD. The above level applies to occupationally exposed workers who are subject to special medical supervision and individual monitoring ("designated workers"); in the case of other workers the MPD is three-tenths of that for designated workers, and the limit for members of the public is one-tenth. These levels are the maximum permitted, but every effort should be made to keep exposure as far below these levels as possible.

Codes of practice. Detailed advice on radiation protection is contained in various codes of practice. The code currently used in hospitals in the United Kingdom is "Code of Practice for the Protection of Persons against Ionising Radiations arising from Medical and Dental Use", London, HM Stationery Office, 1972. These codes may in time be replaced or supplemented by guidelines or guidance notes.

The chapter on therapeutic and diagnostic uses of unsealed radiation sources gives guidance on various aspects of protection, and the Code also gives general advice on such matters as administrative arrangements and the duties of various protection officers. As is the case with most codes of practice on radiation usage the advice is based on recommendations of the International Commission on Radiological Protection (ICRP) and the International Atomic Energy Agency (IAEA).

Records are required to be kept of all unsealed sources received and issued, with signed receipts for the movement of sources, and of all radioactive waste materials disposed of, with dates and routes of disposal. There are further requirements for record keeping when radioactive material is administered to patients and also for radiation protection purposes. By careful cooperation the duplication of records can be avoided when there is close collaboration between a radiopharmacy and a department of nuclear medicine and when a system of recording has been designed to suit local conditions and to satisfy the recommendations of the Code of Practice. The above records are additional to those usually required in good pharmaceutical practice.

Waste disposal. In most countries the disposal of radioactive waste is subject to strict control and all users of radiopharmaceuticals must comply with the conditions that apply in their circumstances. The codes of practice give guidance on methods of waste disposal and restrictions to be observed. There are four main methods of disposal—by public sewerage system, by incineration, by normal solid waste collection, and by a national disposal system for toxic substances.

In any institution the permitted level of disposal by any of these routes is controlled by local conditions and agreed with a local inspectorate. The following general points apply particularly to hospitals.

The most favoured route of disposal is by the sewerage system, and the local inspectorate will usually agree to a high level of activity by this route because the radioactive waste rapidly becomes highly diluted. The disposal route to the main sewage outflow should however be as direct and short as possible. The only materials excluded from this route are radioactive solutions and solvents that are not miscible with water, for example fluid used for liquid scintillation counting. Small animal carcasses and even some solid waste may be disposed of if a suitable maceration system is installed. When a large incinerator system operating at a temperature of at least 600° is available, permission to use a moderate level of radioactive disposal by this means may be sought. Incineration is a useful method for the disposal of paper tissues, swabs, disposable apparatus, and certain carcasses. With suitable precautions it may also be used for the disposal of fluid used for liquid scintillation counting and vials; the main hazard from these items is the toxicity of the chemicals present and not the radioactivity.

If the normal solid waste collection system is to be used the active waste must be diluted with inactive waste below a specified level of activity, and there may be a limit to the quantity of radioactivity permitted in any item or container. If contaminated apparatus is to be disposed of it should be broken to prevent the possibility of salvage.

For the disposal of high activities of long-lived radioisotopic waste a national disposal system for toxic substances may have to be used. It is an expensive method and may require special licensing. It is not desirable to store radioactive waste except for short periods, and all contaminated materials should be disposed of as rapidly as possible.

Transport and storage of radioactive materials. In most countries there are detailed regulations governing the transport of radioactive materials and how they should be packaged in transit. Guidance must be obtained by consultation with the relevant authorities when radioactive material has to be transported between separate institutions.

For transport within an institution care must be taken to observe the following principles. The source must be sufficiently shielded to prevent the irradiation of the carrier or other persons. When unsealed sources are being transported the packaging and containers must be designed to minimise the risk of breakage and spillage of activity. Containers should be double walled and the outer container should be large enough to retain all the active contents in the event of an accident. Carrying apparatus should be clearly marked with radiation warning signs and all containers should be marked with their contents. Radioactive materials in transit must not be left unattended.

For the storage of unsealed sources all containers must be clearly marked with details of material and solvent, isotope, activity, date, and whether the contents are sterile. The storage place must be well shielded according to the type and activity of the isotope being stored. Access must be such that it helps to prevent the irradiation of workers removing individual items from the store. The contents of the store must be kept under constant review and expired materials must be removed and disposed of at the earliest opportunity. Consideration must be given to the storage of some materials at low temperature and when so required suitable refrigeration must be available. Access to the store by unauthorised persons must be prevented. The store should be locked or in a locked room. The fire prevention officer should be informed of the existence of the radioisotope store and given an estimate of its maximum contents.

Preparation and Dispensing of Radiopharmaceuticals

Laboratory facilities. These must be suitable for safe working with radioactive materials and also be adequately designed and equipped to carry out the appropriate pharmaceutical procedures, including where necessary the preparation of sterile materials.

For purposes of radiation protection all surfaces should be such that radioactive decontamination is easily undertaken, and all drainage should have a short route to the main sewer, with no open traps. Benches, where necessary, should be capable of carrying heavy lead shielding. Areas where radioisotopes are being handled should be marked and if more than one isotope is being used work areas should be separated. Unless a radiopharmacy has an exceptionally heavy work load (which may be the case if it serves several institutions), a laboratory equipped for the manipulation of such amounts of radioactivity as present a small degree of hazard may be satisfactory; such a laboratory is described in the U.K. Code of Practice for the Protection of Persons against Ionising Radiations arising from Medical and Dental Use under the classification grade C. For pharmaceutical purposes the facilities required depend to a large extent on the type of work undertaken. Where products are required to be sterile and can be sterilised before use (by autoclaving or membrane filtration) facilities should be to "clean area" standards as described in the U.K. Guide to Good Pharmaceutical Manufacturing Practice (1977). Where products are required to be sterile but cannot be sterilised before use they should be prepared under aseptic conditions in rooms designed for the purpose. Such a room should have an entry lobby with changing and washing facilities for staff; it should be designed to avoid microbial contamination and accumulation of dust and be easy to clean. Suitable ventilation should be provided.

Areas of extra containment will be required to reduce the danger of bacteriological contamination during manipulation. These areas may be provided by the use of balanced down-flow work stations (laminar flow cabinets) with the feature of venting to the outside atmosphere instead of to the room. In addition to protecting the product from microbial contamination, this type of cabinet also provides protection for the operator, since no radioactive material is allowed to escape from the cabinet into the room. Cabinets are best left in continuous operation but if they are switched off the working aperture should be closed; on restarting, time should be allowed for the air flow to discharge any loose particles from the inside of the cabinet before starting any manipulations. Since the interior of the cabinets is not inherently sterile it must be subjected to regular disinfection and cleaning.

Laboratory procedures. Staff working in a radiopharmaceutical laboratory should be adequately trained in radiological protection and in carrying out aseptic techniques. All procedures should be devised in consultation with a radiological protection adviser or other competent physicist and pharmacist, and a clinician with appropriate expertise should be involved when a new radiopharmaceutical is being prepared.

Legal requirements such as those of the U.K. Medicines Act 1968 and advisory statements such as Codes of Practice and advice of the Department of Health and Social Security Committee on Radiation from Radioactive Products should be implemented.

New procedures should include, where possible, dummy runs with non-radioactive materials in order to assess manipulations and probable hazards. Procedures adopted should allow containment of any spillage. This can be effected by working in trays lined with absorbent materials, but if these are used in a balanced down-flow cabinet care should be taken to ensure that the uniformity of the airflow is not destroyed. Spillage trays can usually be built into the cabinet. A well designed fume cupboard is a useful means of containment, but this does not always provide a pharmaceutically adequate environment.

Once procedures have been agreed a manual should be produced recording all working procedures from which practice should not deviate.

When they are working in the radiopharmaceutical laboratory, all staff should wear protective clothing including cap, overshoes, and gloves, and in an aseptic area they should change into sterile clothing. All clothing should be made of materials that do not shed fibres.

In all laboratory areas mouth pipetting, eating, drinking, smoking, and the application of cosmetics should be strictly forbidden. Routines for cleaning and maintenance of laboratories and equipment must be specified and made known to all the staff concerned.

In general, all procedures should be carried out as rapidly as possible to minimise exposure to radiation, since the radiation dose received by the operator is dependent on the time of exposure as well as the radioactivity present. Radiation dosage also decreases inversely with the square of the distance, and therefore radioactive materials should be kept at a distance from the operator and should not be handled directly, but rather with tongs or other remote handling devices. When drawing materials up in a syringe, distance can be provided by using a syringe larger than necessary (for example 10 ml rather than 5 ml). Specifically designed syringe shields may also be available, and should be used.

Local rules, which describe and explain radiation protection procedures as well as other safety procedures must be drawn up and read by all workers in the radiopharmacy. They must be fully reviewed and kept up to date in the light of new advice on problems arising as the nature of the work changes.

Many radiopharmaceutical preparations are administered by injection, and the same precautions to avoid microbial and other contamination are required as with other parenteral preparations.

Any operation likely to yield gas or vapour should be performed in a suitably vented fume or laminar flow cabinet which also prevents the escape of radioactive materials into the laboratory. Shielding should be designed in consultation with a radiation protection physicist, taking into account (i) the time that personnel are exposed to radiation, (ii) the working distance from the source of the radiations concerned (since intensity of radiation decreases as the square of the distance), and (iii) the nature of the absorbent material to be used. Gamma radiation is most effectively absorbed by materials of high atomic number, lead being the most useful for laboratory work. Materials of low atomic number are most suitable for beta radiation since they produce less bremsstrahlung radiation.

Data on shielding for beta radiation is given by L. Katz and A. S. Penfold (*Rev. Med. Phys.*, 1952, **24**, 28) and for gamma radiation in British Standard 4094 part 1 (1966).

Containers. Containers for radiopharmaceutical injections may be of the single-dose or multiple-dose type. If multiple-dose containers are used and the contents are not to be resterilised after each withdrawal, a suitable bactericide should be included. Many of the bactericides used in injections are broken down by radiation, sometimes with a deleterious effect on the preparation. The most commonly used bactericide is benzyl alcohol (0.9% v/v); phenol 0.5% and chlorocresol 0.1% may also be satisfactory. If no bactericide is incorporated in the formulation, withdrawal should be made under aseptic conditions and the container should be used only over a short period, such as 4 hours at laboratory temperature. Alternatively the container should be resterilised after each withdrawal.

Containers for radiopharmaceuticals should be labelled with the name of the preparation, the date, and the amount of activity in a specific volume at a stated time. Ideally, doses prepared for individual patients should be labelled to show the name of the patient.

Raw materials. For the preparation of radiopharmaceuticals raw materials are obtained from many sources and can be divided into two groups, those containing a radioisotope and those which are not radioactive. Non-radioactive materials should normally comply with recognised pharmaceutical standards. When material to pharmacopoeial or other recognised standards is not available other material may be used provided a careful check is made of the specification to ensure that it is of a suitable standard and that the material matches the specification. If doubt exists it may be necessary to perform toxicity tests on the material. Non-radioactive raw materials of a suitable quality can often be supplied by a hospital pharmacy.

Oral preparations. These preparations form a very small part of the work of most radiopharmaceutical laboratories. In their preparation normal pharmaceutical practice for the production of a preparation intended for oral administration should be followed.

Preparation of solutions and injections from generators. In most laboratories a radionuclide generator, prepared and supplied by a commercial manufacturer, is the main source of radionuclides. The most frequently used generator system is the ^{99}Mo/^{99m}Tc generator, but the ^{113}Sn/^{113m}In system is also used. The technetium-99m generator consists of a column of aluminium oxide on which is absorbed molybdate (^{99}Mo) ions, assembled under clean conditions, and sterilised by autoclaving. The daughter nuclide, technetium-99m, may be separated from the molybdenum-99 by eluting the column with sterile 0.9% sodium chloride solution. Generators are usually supplied as shielded, sterile columns together with sterile components to allow elution. These have to be used in accordance with the manufacturer's instructions to ensure a sterile eluate.

It is essential that the sterility of the generator system be maintained and therefore it should be housed under clean conditions in an area that is not used for other purposes. The environment provided by a laminar flow cabinet is ideal for housing generator systems, but if any extra shielding or equipment is introduced, the airflow pattern should be checked. Provided that the manufacturer's instructions for assembly have been followed, the storage conditions are good, and aseptic technique is used, the pertechnetate (^{99m}Tc) solution obtained on elution should be sterile. Similar principles apply to other generator systems.

Preparation of other radiopharmaceuticals for injection. These preparations include colloids and macroaggregates in suspension, labelled with a radioactive isotope. The preparations may be produced using commercial kits with tested ingredients which have been prepared in accordance with a manufacturing licence; in this case the manufacturer's directions should be followed. Preparations may also be made from other ingredients, in which case it is desirable to follow a method that has been adequately tested and evaluated, as for example, those that have been published in an authoritative periodical such as the *Journal of Nuclear Medicine* or the *British Journal of Radiology*. The required materials can often be provided in a suitable form by a hospital pharmacy sterile products department. Production should follow a written procedure and all stages should be checked by suitable quality control.

Quality Control of Radiopharmaceuticals

Quality control involves the monitoring of all aspects of the production of radiopharmaceuticals, including the quality of the raw materials used to make the preparation, the testing of the environment in which it is made, and the performance of the preparation itself. In some cases it is not possible to test the radiopharmaceutical fully before administration because of the short half-life of the radioisotope; reliance is placed on the procedure used and the in-process quality controls; these must, therefore, be carefully monitored by, among other things, retrospective tests on the preparations.

In addition to the usual test procedures (sterility, pyrogens, chemical purity, etc.) the following concepts are used in the examination of radiopharmaceuticals. *Radionuclidic purity* (or radioisotopic purity) is the proportion of the total activity that is present in the form of the specified radionuclide (or radioisotope). *Radiochemical purity* is the proportion of the specified radioisotope that is present in the stated chemical form. Since radionuclidic, radiochemical, and chemical purity may decrease with time it is essential to ensure that a dispensed radiopharmaceutical will be of satisfactory quality at the time it is intended to be used.

Analytical control involves the checking of raw material as previously mentioned and determination of the chemical and radiochemical purity of the radiopharmaceutical. Determination of chemical purity can be undertaken by routine chemical tests. Radiochemical purity of labelled products can usually be determined by a chromatographic method such as thin-layer chromatography or gel filtration. Radionuclidic purity of the isotope used should be checked by physical methods.

In-process control tests are carried out before the radiopharmaceutical is released for administration. In general, they consist of checking for the presence of any undesirable unbound radioactivity using a suitable chromatographic method. In the case of macroaggregated materials it includes checking the particle size of the preparation.

Generators. Routine testing of the sterility of generators should be undertaken as a check on the generator, its surroundings, and the technique of generator elution. This is best done by sending the final eluate of the generator for sterility testing. With generator systems there is the possibility of break-through of the parent nuclide. Where facilities are available therefore, the radionuclidic purity of the generator eluate should be checked by gamma-ray spectrometry or other physical measurements. This may have to be performed retrospectively.

Sterility and pyrogen tests. When working with radioisotopes having short half-lives, sterility testing cannot be undertaken before release of the product. Retrospective testing should be performed as it is the only method of assessing preparative procedures. It is not usually necessary to perform pyrogen tests frequently, but when new batches of materials or new procedures are being introduced, these tests must be included in the evaluation. The rabbit test may be supplemented by a rapid method for detecting the presence or absence of pyrogens using the limulus amoebocyte lysate test for endotoxin; this is of most benefit when intrathecal injections are being prepared since it can be completed before administration of the injection.

The *environment* of the radiopharmaceutical laboratory should be routinely tested for microbiological contamination. This can be done by exposing settle plates in the working areas and then incubating them appropriately. If there is evidence of undue contamination this should be investigated.

The performance of laminar flow cabinets should be monitored. Major testing should be undertaken by the manufacturers of the equipment, but the airflow pattern can be easily checked by using ventilation smoke tubes (and it is important to check airflow when large pieces of equipment are introduced into the cabinet) and the airspeed can be checked with an anemometer; unexpected changes in the reading on the anemometer indicate a fault in either the filter or the motors. Sterility of laminar flow cabinets should be checked using an air sampling method.

Clinical Uses of Radiopharmaceuticals

Radiopharmaceuticals are sometimes used therapeutically, as a source of appropriate radiation. Such uses are described under Gold (^{198}Au) Injection, Sodium Iodide (^{131}I) Solution, and Sodium Phosphate (^{32}P) Injection, and at the end of this chapter. The major use of radiopharmaceuticals is in diagnostic medicine, considered below.

Diagnosis with the Aid of Radiopharmaceuticals

General considerations make it necessary to avoid undue irradiation of patients and personnel. The choice of radiopharmaceutical in a particular case is therefore usually made by consultation between the clinician responsible for patient care during the tests and the responsible physicist and radiopharmacist. The preparation should be chosen to give a maximum of information for a minimum of body or organ exposure to radiation, having regard also to safety in other respects and performance as a diagnostic aid. Any published guidance on the amount of radioactivity to be used should be complied with and in the United Kingdom approval for the procedure must be sought from the Department of Health and Social Security Isotope Advisory Panel whether it is for routine, research, or an isolated case. Radioisotopes are used to make quantitative measurements of biochemical or physiological processes, or to determine the structure and distribution of normal processes and to detect any deviations from normal that may be indicative of disease. Assessments are made by serial measurement of radioactivity and its distribution with time in some part of the body, by measurements in samples such as blood, breath, or urine drawn from a body compartment, or by rendering visible the distribution of radioactivity within an organ or region of the body with the aid of a gamma scintillation camera or rectilinear scanner.

Labelled tracers and carrier-free materials. A material is stated to be *carrier-free* when the radioisotopic form is not accompanied by detectable amounts of the stable form of the element. Materials that are not carrier-free can only be used in diagnosis when the total amount of material used is insufficient to affect the biological system that is being investigated. *Tracers* are prepared by attaching a radioisotopic atom to a small proportion of the molecules of a compound; this is known as "*tagging*" or "*labelling*". Tracers may be used to study the metabolism of a pharmaceutical substance or other compound.

Compounds normally secreted by a certain route can be labelled and the secretion of the material and its passage can be followed. Changes in function, blockage to flow, or flow to abnormal anatomical or metabolic pathways can be detected. Some areas of the body maintain non-permeability to a tracer in the blood stream. If this barrier is destroyed by disease, the tracer can pass into areas that do not usually take it up (an important example is the impermeability of the blood-brain barrier).

Some abnormal tissue masses such as tumours or areas of sepsis may take up certain compounds markedly where no uptake is usually found. Some labelled compounds are used in procedures *in vitro* which involve only examination of a body fluid without administration of radioactivity to the patient; competitive protein-binding assays, including radioimmunoassays, measure minute amounts of substances often too small to be measured by chemical means. The labelled preparations are known as clinical reagents; they are not strictly radiopharmaceuticals since they are not administered to patients. So far these methods, which apply largely to endocrine function and metabolic processes, are adding diagnostic scope rather than replacing procedures *in vivo*. An exception is thyroid function measurement, where the use *in vivo* of iodine-131, which results in an undesirably high radiation dose to the thyroid gland, has been virtually eliminated.

Respiratory system. *Respiration* through the lungs may be studied with a radioactive gas such as xenon-133, and areas of abnormality shown on single breaths and by clearance of the inhaled gas. Reduced ventilation occurs in asthma, in heart disease, and in the presence of local lung lesions such as cysts. Inhalation of aerosols containing technetium-99m or indium-113m has been used to outline the bronchial trees and investigate ventilation of the lungs. Superior results have been reported in respiratory studies using the short-lived isotope krypton-81m produced in the cyclotron.

Arterial perfusion of the lungs may be studied by trapping radioactively labelled particles in the lung capillaries following injection into the blood stream. This technique reveals obstructions to the circulation from pulmonary emboli or early bronchial carcinoma when the chest X-rays are normal. Macroaggregated human serum albumin or microspheres of human serum albumin of average diameter 20 to 50 μm are used; extemporaneous labelling with technetium-99m is usually employed although a ready-prepared particulate injection labelled with iodine-131 [macrosalb (^{131}I) injection] has been used. The macroaggregated particles are broken down within a few hours of administration and although sensitisation to denatured human serum albumin is theoretically possible its actual occurrence has not been reported. The preparation should not be administered to patients with a right to left heart shunt since systemic emboli could occur. It should be avoided in severe pulmonary hypertension since the small amount of blockage of capillaries (normally up to 1%) might impose an undue strain on the heart.

Liver. Size and overall function may be studied by the intravenous injection of labelled colloidal particles 20 to 25 nm in diameter which become trapped in the Kupfer cells. Technetium-99m-labelled injections have now almost completely displaced other preparations such as gold-198 colloid. Space-occupying lesions such as secondary tumours, abscesses, or cysts may be detected if they are at least 1 cm in diameter. Reduction in liver function can be detected, for example in cirrhosis. In *obstructive jaundice* rose bengal sodium labelled with iodine-125 or iodine-131 may be used; it is normally excreted in the bile and its distribution can in some cases be used to distinguish intra- and extra-hepatic obstruction. This preparation permits liver function to be assessed more readily than with labelled colloid. Similar preparations labelled with technetium-99m may be used to investigate liver function and localise sites of biliary obstruction.

Pancreas. Since the pancreas takes up amino acids, selenomethionine (^{75}Se) may be used to study its activity. Selenomethionine is also taken up by the liver, and so a process of subtraction scanning is used in which a liver scan (obtained with a colloid labelled with a different nuclide, commonly technetium-99m) is compared with a selenomethionine scan. The method is not ideal and is liable to yield false positives.

In the diagnosis of *fat malabsorption* due to disease

states, triolein labelled with carbon-14 may be given by mouth when an unusually low amount of carbon-14 in the breath is indicative of fat malabsorption; confirmation of the diagnosis may be obtained by determining whether the abnormality is corrected by oral administration of pancreatic enzymes. In the examination of the *gut*, protein-losing gastroenteropathy may be detected by measurement of the abnormal increase in labelled plasma protein appearing in the gut after intravenous administration of chromic chloride (^{51}Cr) which links to the circulating caeruloplasmin when given by this route. The choice of a tracer that is not reabsorbed from the gut is necessary if the test is to be reliable, and stools have to be carefully collected and accurately assayed.

Urological system. Some structural information may be obtained by intravenous administration of chlormerodrin (^{197}Hg) injection or an appropriate technetium-99m labelled preparation which is retained specifically and then excreted by the kidney. In *renography*, if labelled material is administered by intravenous injection, its arrival in the kidney (related to adequacy of arterial inflow), passage through the kidney (related to the phases of excretion) and outflow from the kidney (related to the patency of outflow tracts) can all be measured. Time-related information, including glomerular filtration rate, can be much more useful than the purely visual display of kidney structure.

Residual urine volume remaining in the bladder after completion of micturition may be determined by following the excretion of a labelled substance such as sodium iodohippurate (^{125}I or ^{131}I) injection after intravenous administration. The *glomerular filtration rate* is useful in assessing overall renal function, and may be determined by measuring the rate of elimination of chromium (^{51}Cr) edetate from the circulation after intravenous injection, by using single or serial blood sampling, or even by external counting methods alone.

Thyroid. Functional studies of the gland may be carried out with the aid of radio-iodine, since the iodine is trapped in the gland for hormone synthesis. Iodine-132 is used when possible in preference to iodine-131, which gives a much greater radiation dose to the patient. Visualisation of the gland is best done with iodine-123 which gives excellent images with much less irradiation than with other radio-iodides. Technetium-99m (as pertechnetate) is also trapped in the thyroid but the fraction of the dose retained is much smaller and uptake in neighbouring tissues may sometimes obscure the image. However, since technetium-99m is more readily available than iodine-123 it is commonly used to visualise the gland.

Active *adrenal adenomas* have been visualised by their uptake of cholesterol which is a precursor for steroid synthesis and can be given labelled with radio-iodine. Preparations suitable for the visualisation of parathyroid, islet-cell, and other adenomata are not yet available.

Haematological processes have been widely investigated using tracer materials. *Red-cell survival*, which is reduced in haemolytic anaemias, is measured by labelling red cells with sodium chromate (^{51}Cr), injecting them intravenously and following their rate of disappearance from the circulation. *Iron absorption*, which may be altered in gut and other disorders, has been measured using tracer iron given with a meal. The kinetics of its metabolism may be assessed by correcting for the metabolism of absorbed tracer doses of iron-55 by an amount calculated from the disappearance of an intravenous tracer dose of iron-59 given simultaneously. The *circulating red-cell mass*, which is raised in polycythaemia, can be determined by injecting a quantity of the patient's own red cells that have been suitably labelled, and measuring the dilution after equilibration. Similarly, the circulating plasma volume and the total blood volume can be calculated from the dilution factor after labelled human serum albumin has been injected intravenously. *Splenic tissues* can be visualised by removing some red cells from the patient, damaging them chemically or by heating, and labelling with, for example, technetium-99m, and injecting them intravenously. These cells are rapidly trapped and destroyed in the spleen. Tracer colloid trapped by the reticuloendothelial system will also usually appear in the spleen as well as in the liver. The site and size of any splenic tissue can be determined whether it occupies the normal site or is in aberrant sites.

Vitamin-B$_{12}$ deficiency states can be assessed by comparing the absorption after oral administration of cyanocobalamin labelled with one tracer with that of cyanocobalamin labelled with a different tracer and bound before ingestion to the intrinsic factor that facilitates normal absorption. Both tracers are absorbed equally well in normal subjects. Free cyanocobalamin is absorbed poorly, but bound cyanocobalamin normally, in *pernicious anaemia*. Neither is absorbed normally in more generalised gut disorders.

Cardiovascular system. Some radiopharmaceuticals (for example preparations containing phosphate, as used for bone scanning) labelled with technetium-99m may be injected intravenously and used to detect areas of *cardiac infarction*. Cardiac muscle perfusion can be assessed by using tracers which are rapidly taken up and output of cardiac chambers may also be measured. Bolus injections of human serum albumin labelled with indium-113m or technetium-99m have been used successfully to outline larger arteries in sufficient detail to demonstrate blocked arteries (in the legs), cardiac shunts, arterio-venous malformation, and obstruction in the *cerebral circulation*. The large *placental blood pool* may be rendered visible after the intravenous injection of labelled human serum albumin or indium-113m chloride. The latter (as an acid solution from the indium-113m generator) binds irreversibly to transferrin in the blood stream. This forms the basis of a screening test to confirm or exclude the diagnosis of *placenta praevia* that may be used as an alternative to ultrasonic techniques.

Venous thrombosis can be detected after intravenous administration of iodine-125-labelled fibrinogen which is incorporated into forming clots, or technetium-99m-labelled urokinase which adheres to clots. Thrombosis can also be detected by isotope venography after injection of labelled preparations into the veins of the foot.

Brain. Scanning may be carried out using sodium pertechnetate (^{99m}Tc) or indium (^{113m}In) labelled chelate administered intravenously after the administration of potassium perchlorate (200 mg by mouth to adults) to prevent uptake in the choroid plexus.

The intact blood-brain barrier prevents the entry of the radioactive compounds into the brain tissue but they diffuse readily into lesions where localised breakdown of the barrier has occurred, thus rendering visible space-occupying intracranial lesions such as abscesses, most tumours, and vascular incidents.

Musculo-skeletal system. The whole skeleton can be visualised with a much smaller radiation dose than is used in radiological skeletal survey work. For this purpose labelled bone-seeking material is used. Technetium-99m is used as labelled complexes of phosphonate, polyphosphate, or pyrophosphate, while the short-lived fluorine-18, prepared carrier-free in the cyclotron, has been used as sodium fluoride solution. These preparations are administered by intravenous injection. Lesions such as those of *osteomyelitis*, and secondaries in bone and primary *bone tumours* can often be detected several months earlier than by X-rays. Active *joint disorders* can also be observed even when they are neither infected nor malignant. *Ischaemic areas* and areas of *Paget's disease* of bone can also be observed.

Preparations of bleomycin labelled with indium-111 or cobalt-57 have been used for the localisation of certain types of *tumour* but cannot be relied upon to detect all tumours present. Gallium-67 citrate has been used to detect *focal sepsis*, as may occur in pyrexia of unknown origin, and to detect tumours.

Current trends in the diagnostic use of radioisotopes include an increased usage of *short-lived radioisotopes* such as iodine-123 and other cyclotron-produced materials which extend the range of diagnostic capability. Equipment used for visualisation is being improved by the incorporation of computerised data-processing. New investigative imaging techniques using radioisotopes are being developed and dynamic functional studies and screening procedures are being developed to complement static visualisation techniques such as ultrasound and X-rays by computerised axial tomography.

Therapeutic Applications of Radioisotopes

Thyrotoxicosis in selected elderly patients may be treated with radio-iodine (^{131}I). Large doses of iodine-131 may be used to treat *thyroid cancers* that take up iodine. Phosphorus-32 has been used for the suppression of red-cell formation in the marrow of patients with *polycythaemia*. Colloidal gold (^{198}Au) and colloidal yttrium (^{90}Y) have been instilled into cavities such as those of the pleura and peritoneum when large volumes of fluid have collected because of widespread tumorous involvement of the membranes. Yttrium-90 has been injected into joint cavities in severe *rheumatoid arthritis* but its value has not been established. Other isotopes prepared in solid materials have been used for implantation into small organs such as the anterior pituitary, but such methods are being replaced by newer forms of external irradiation or other treatment. The therapeutic usage of radioisotopes is not large but the development of specific tumour-seeking radiopharmaceuticals could alter the situation.

Further Information

The Radiochemical Manual, 2nd Edn, Amersham, The Radiochemical Centre, 1966.

E. H. Belcher and H. Vetter, *Radioisotopes in Medical Diagnosis*, London, Butterworths, 1971.

D. E. Lovett, Radiopharmaceuticals, *Advances in Pharmaceutical Sciences*, H. S. Bean *et al.* (Eds), Vol. 4, London, Academic Press, 1974.

Codes of Practice

Code of Practice for the Carriage of Radioactive Materials by Road, Department of the Environment, HM Stationery Office, 1975.

Code of Practice for the Storage of Radioactive Material in Transit, Departments of the Environment and Employment, HM Stationery Office, 1972.

Code of Practice for the Protection of Persons against Ionising Radiations arising from Research and Teaching, HM Stationery Office, 1968.

Code of Practice for the Protection of Persons against Ionising Radiations arising from Medical and Dental Use, HM Stationery Office, 1972.

Rafoxanide

3'-Chloro-4'-(4-chlorophenoxy)-3,5-di-iodosalicylanilide

$C_{19}H_{11}Cl_2I_2NO_3 = 626.0$

OTHER NAMES: *Flukanide*®
Ranizole® (with thiabendazole)

A standard is given in the British Pharmacopoeia (Veterinary)

Description. A greyish-white to brown powder.

Solubility. Practically insoluble in water; soluble, at 20°, in 25 parts of acetone, in 40 parts of chloroform, in 200 parts of methyl alcohol, and in 35 parts of ethyl acetate.

Storage. It should be stored in airtight containers, protected from light.

Identification. TEST. Mix about 10 mg with 10 ml of alcohol (80%), add 2 drops of *ferric chloride test-solution*, and shake; a violet colour is produced.

MELTING-POINT. About 175°.

ULTRAVIOLET ABSORPTION. In 0.1N methanolic hydrochloric acid, maxima at 280 nm (E1%, 1cm = 243) and 335 nm (E1%, 1cm = 148).

INFRA-RED ABSORPTION. Major peaks at 1220, 1250, 1429, 1493, 1562, and 1587 cm^{-1} (see Appendix 2b: Infra-red Spectra).

Veterinary uses. Rafoxanide is used for the treatment of acute and chronic liver fluke infections in cattle and sheep. The usual dosage by mouth is 7.5 to 12 milligrams per kilogram body-weight as a single dose.

Preparations

RAFOXANIDE MIXTURE (*Syn.* Rafoxanide Suspension): an aqueous suspension of rafoxanide mixed with suitable suspending, dispersing, and preservative agents. Available as a mixture containing 2.27% of rafoxanide.

A standard for this mixture is given in the British Pharmacopoeia (Veterinary)

Containers and *Labelling:* see the entry on Mixtures for general information on containers and labelling.

THIABENDAZOLE AND RAFOXANIDE MIXTURE (*Syn.* Thiabendazole and Rafoxanide Suspension): an aqueous suspension of thiabendazole and rafoxanide mixed with suitable suspending and dispersing agents. Available as a mixture containing 13.3% of thiabendazole and 2.27% of rafoxanide.

A standard for this mixture is given in the British Pharmacopoeia (Veterinary)

Containers and *Labelling:* see the entry on Mixtures for general information on containers and labelling.

Raspberry Juice, Concentrated

Concentrated raspberry juice is prepared from the clarified juice of raspberries, *Rubus idaeus* L. (Fam. Rosaceae).

A standard is given in the British Pharmaceutical Codex 1973

Sufficient pectinase of commerce to destroy the pectin is stirred into pulped raspberries, the mixture allowed to stand for 12 hours, and the pulp pressed. The juice is clarified, sufficient sucrose added to adjust the weight per millilitre at 20° to 1.050 to 1.060 g, and the juice concentrated to one-sixth of its original volume. Sufficient sulphurous acid or sodium metabisulphite is added to preserve the product. The odour of the preservative may be apparent on first opening the container.

When 1 volume of concentrated raspberry juice is diluted with 5 volumes of water, a product equivalent to natural raspberry juice is obtained.

Storage. It should be stored in a cool place, protected from light.

Uses. Concentrated raspberry juice is used as a flavouring agent in elixirs and mixtures. It is an ingredient of paediatric paracetamol elixir and, in the form of raspberry syrup (see below), of paediatric kaolin mixture, paediatric succinylsulphathiazole mixture, and paediatric sulphadimidine mixture.

Preparation

RASPBERRY SYRUP (*Syn.* Syrupus Rubi Idaei): prepared by diluting 1 volume of concentrated raspberry juice with 11 volumes of syrup.

If it is prepared with precautions which will prevent fermentation and packed in such a manner as to preserve it in this condition, it need not be freshly prepared; once the container has been opened, however, it should be used within a few weeks.

If it is made without taking precautions to prevent fermentation, it must be freshly prepared.

A dye, or a mixture of dyes, may be added, provided that any dye used is of food grade of commerce and that its use for colouring food is permitted in the country concerned.

Raspberry syrup is intended only for flavouring pharmaceutical products. If it is used for other purposes it may not comply with the Preservatives in Food Regulations in respect of sulphur dioxide content.

A standard for this syrup is given in the British Pharmaceutical Codex 1973

Storage: it should be stored in a cool place, protected from light.

Rauwolfia Serpentina

The dried roots of *Rauwolfia serpentina* Benth. (Fam. Apocynaceae), an erect shrub growing in the Indian subcontinent, Burma, Thailand, and Java.

OTHER NAMES: *Hypercal®*; *Hypertane®*; *Hypertensan®*; *Raudixin®*; *Rauwiloid®*; Rauwolfia
Hypercal B® and *Hypertane Compound®* (both with amylobarbitone); *Rautrax Sine K®* (with hydroflumethiazide); *Pentoxylon®* (with pentaerythritol tetranitrate); *Rauwiloid + Veriloid®* (with alkaloids of *Veratrum viride*)

A standard is given in the British Pharmaceutical Codex 1973

Constituents. Rauwolfia serpentina contains numerous alkaloids, the most active as hypotensive agents being reserpine and its trimethoxycinnamate analogue, rescinnamine. Other indole alkaloids present include ajmaline (rauwolfine), ajmalinine, ajmalicine, isoajmaline (isorauwolfine), serpentine, rauwolfinine, and sarpagine. Up to 2% of foreign organic matter may be present.

Description. UNGROUND DRUG. *Macroscopical characters:* pieces about 80 to 150 mm long and 5 to 10 mm thick, some pieces as long as 400 mm and attaining a diameter of 20 mm; subcylindrical or slightly tapering, rather tortuous, rarely branched; rootlets usually absent; outer surface greyish to yellowish-brown, dull, with faint longitudinal ridges and a few small, circular root scars in a tetrastichous arrangement, somewhat scaly in the older pieces with small patches of exfoliating bark exposing the pale yellowish-white wood; fracture short; smoothed, transversely cut surface showing a large whitish, finely radiate, dense, and very finely porous xylem, occupying about three-quarters of the diameter, and a narrow yellowish-brown bark; starchy throughout. It is odourless and has a bitter taste.

Microscopical characters: the diagnostic characters are: *cork* stratified with about 2 to 7 alternating bands of smaller cells, in 3 to 7 rows, and larger cells in 1 to 3 rows; cells isodiametric in surface view, about 20 to 70 μm, the smaller, flattened cells about 5 to 20 μm and the larger cells about 40 to 75 μm in the radial direction; *phelloderm* of a few rows of parenchyma; *phloem* narrow, parenchymatous, with small scattered groups of sieve tissue; parenchyma filled with small *starch* granules, mostly rounded but a few muller-shaped or irregular, 5 to **8** to **12** to 20 occasionally 40 μm in diameter, some showing a hilum as a simple or radiate split; numerous cells of the phloem parenchyma starch-free but containing prismatic and conglomerate *crystals* of calcium oxalate; *xylem* with well-marked growth rings and a denser core about 0.5 mm wide and containing numerous small *vessels*, remaining secondary xylem very parenchymatous and with numerous *medullary rays*; parenchyma of xylem and medullary rays lignified, with numerous rounded simple pits and filled with small starch granules; *tracheids* and *vessels* in narrow interrupted radial rows, about 35 to 54 μm in diameter, with numerous bordered pits; *xylem fibres* few with small, slanting, slit-like pits; *latex cells* occasional, in medullary rays of phloem and in cortex of rhizome; *sclereids* and *phloem fibres* absent.

POWDERED DRUG. Powdered Rauwolfia Serpentina. An odourless brownish-grey powder possessing the diagnostic microscopical characters and taste of the unground drug.

Adulterants and substitutes. Roots from other species of *Rauwolfia* resemble those of *R. serpentina* in external characters; they are most readily distinguished by the microscopical characters of transverse sections. The root of *R. tetraphylla* L. has a uniform cork and abundant sclereids and fibres in the bark; its vessels are quite numerous, averaging about 75 μm in diameter; it contains reserpine, but no rescinnamine.

Actions and uses. Rauwolfia serpentina has the actions, uses, and undesirable effects described under reserpine. It is given by mouth as tablets of the powdered root in a dosage of 200 to 400 milligrams daily in divided doses for hypertension. Doses of 1 to 2 grams daily have been used in psychotic disturbances. Rauwolfia serpentina is also given as an extract containing the constituent alkaloids.

Preparations

Preparations available include TABLETS containing rauwolfia serpentina 50 mg, tablets containing rauwolfia serpentina total alkaloids 2 mg, tablets containing rauwolfia serpentina selected alkaloids 2 mg, tablets containing rauwolfia selected alkaloid hydrochlorides 2 mg, tablets containing rauwolfia serpentina 50 mg with hydroflumethiazide 50 mg, tablets containing rauwolfia serpentina total alkaloids 2 mg with amylobarbitone 15 mg, tablets containing rauwolfia serpentina selected alkaloids 2 mg with amylobarbitone 15 mg, tablets containing rauwolfia selected alkaloid hydrochlorides 1 mg with pentaerythritol tetranitrate 10 mg, and tablets containing rauwolfia selected alkaloid hydrochlorides 1 mg with veratrum viride alkaloids 3 mg.

Rauwolfia Vomitoria

The dried roots of *Rauwolfia vomitoria* Afz. (Fam. Apocynaceae), a bush or tree indigenous to tropical Africa from the Guinea coast to Mozambique.

OTHER NAME: African Rauwolfia

A standard is given in the British Pharmaceutical Codex 1973

Constituents. Rauwolfia vomitoria contains numerous alkaloids, the most active as hypotensive agents being the ester alkaloids reserpine (about 0.2%) and rescinnamine. Other alkaloids include reserpine N-oxide and seredine of the reserpine type, and ajmaline, alstonine, isoajmaline, isoreserpiline, raumitorine, rauvomitine, reserpiline, sarpagine, vomalidine, yohimbine, and α-yohimbine. Up to 2% of foreign organic matter may be present and it may yield up to 2% of acid-insoluble ash.

Description. UNGROUND DRUG. *Macroscopical characters:* roots occasionally branched, subcylindrical, very slightly tapering, up to about 300 mm long and 1.5 to 15 mm, rarely up to 90 mm, thick; outer surface greyish-brown, deeply longitudinally cracked or rubbed smooth, with a few oblique rootlet stumps; cork, if present, easily removed as flakes; fracture difficult, splintery in the wood, short in the bark; smoothed, transversely cut surface showing a narrow, pale brown bark, up to about 3 mm thick, and a buff or yellowish, finely radiate porous wood forming the majority of the drug.
It is odourless and has a bitter taste.

Microscopical characters: the diagnostic characters are: *cork* stratified with zones of flattened suberised cells, each 3 to 4 layers in radial width, alternating with zones of larger lignified cells, each from 1 to about 120 layers in radial width; cells isodiametric in surface view, about 10 to 55 μm, the flattened cells about 5 to 15 μm and the larger cells about 14 to 200 μm in the radial direction; *phelloderm* of about 5 to 16 layers of parenchyma and *sclereids* about 12 to 180 μm in width or length, singly or in small groups, occasionally containing prismatic *crystals* of calcium oxalate; *phloem* having scattered *secretion cells* with granular contents and isolated groups of *sclereids* forming in larger roots several discontinuous bands alternating with collapsed sieve tissue, *sieve elements* clearly defined in the inner region; phloem parenchyma with several cells containing prismatic or conglomerate *crystals* of calcium oxalate; *xylem* with numerous *vessels*, about 36 to 180 μm in diameter, solitary or paired, subcylindrical, walls with small bordered pits; vessel elements about 75 to 1200 μm long, lignified *tyloses* occasionally present in the older vessels; *fibres* numerous, about 200 to 1500 μm long and

up to 32 μm wide, with oblique, slit-like pits; *medullary rays* up to 3 cells wide, heterogeneous, with isolated groups of sclereids; *starch* granules in all parenchymatous tissues, rounded, 1 to 10 to 20 μm in diameter, with central hila or stellate clefts, also some 2- to 4-compound granules with muller-shaped components.

POWDERED DRUG. Powdered Rauwolfia Vomitoria. An odourless brownish-grey powder possessing the diagnostic microscopical characters and taste of the unground drug.

Adulterants and substitutes. The stems of *R. vomitoria* contain negligible quantities of reserpine and can be distinguished from the roots by the smoother cork, the presence of unlignified pericyclic fibres, a dense wood with marked growth rings and a central pith; xylem vessels, about 18 to 70 μm in diameter; latex canals occur in the pith and bark.
R. caffra Sond., which occurs in districts extending from the Cameroons to the Cape; the roots are similar, but the cork is unstratified and entirely lignified. Roots of other common African *Rauwolfia* species have smaller xylem vessels, their diameters not exceeding 125 μm.

Uses. Rauwolfia vomitoria is used almost entirely for the production of reserpine.

Raynaud's Disease

Raynaud's disease is a disease of small blood vessels in which vasospasm results in blanching, cyanosis, and numbing of the fingers and toes. It may be idiopathic or secondary to conditions such as occlusive artery disease or it may be caused by treatment with beta-adrenergic blocking agents. Attacks are precipitated by exposure to cold or by emotional upsets, and may last for minutes or hours. Ischaemia may lead to atrophy of the skin or small painful ulcers on the digital tips. Raynaud's disease is treated by protection from extremes of cold.
Smoking must be avoided as nicotine is a vasoconstrictor. The condition is widely treated with vasodilator drugs with varying success. Regional sympathectomy often alleviates the symptoms of Raynaud's disease, but sometimes only temporarily.

Renal Failure

Renal failure is the failure of the kidney to excrete metabolic waste products or to maintain plasma electrolytes at normal concentrations in the presence of normal dietary intake. It may be either acute or chronic. In either case it is characterised by the development of uraemia. Drugs which are excreted by the kidneys, for example many antibiotics, will remain in the body for longer than is normal and when used in renal failure their dosage will require adjustment as described below.

Uraemia is the clinical condition associated with advanced renal insufficiency and retention in the blood of nitrogenous waste products (azotaemia). At first there is lassitude, fatigue, and decreased neural acuity. Later there may be gastro-intestinal symptoms (anorexia, nausea, vomiting, and ulceration and bleeding from the gastro-intestinal tract), cardiovascular symptoms (hypertension, pericarditis and sodium and water retention leading to congestive heart failure), neuromuscular symptoms (muscular twitches, peripheral neuropathy, muscle cramp and convulsions), malnutrition leading to generalised wasting, yellow-brown discoloration of the skin, and pruritus.

Characteristic laboratory findings in uraemia include nitrogen retention, acidosis, and anaemia. Uraemia may be completely reversible when related to acute renal disease, or terminal as the end result of chronic renal disease. Peritoneal dialysis or haemodialysis will remove nitrogenous waste products from the circulation and delay the onset of uraemia.

Chronic renal failure or a chronic reduction in renal function is characterised by disturbance of the control of electrolyte balance and the progressive development of uraemia. At first, compensation for the loss of functioning nephrons may occur and the only sign of failure may be impaired powers of concentration and clearance, resulting in nocturia. Only when excretion fails to keep pace with production does the urea concentration rise.

Disturbance of electrolyte balance results in acidosis, with sodium and water depletion. Saline depletion leads to further impairment of glomerular filtration and blood urea rises more. The acidosis and hypovolaemia may be reduced by giving additional sodium bicarbonate.

In chronic renal failure there may be anaemia due to aplasia of bone marrow resulting from circulating toxic substances and impaired production of erythropoietin, defective coagulation, hypertension, hyperthyroidism, and gonadal depression.

Chronic renal failure may be caused by any disease which leads to widespread damage of renal tissue, for example renal tuberculosis, renal calculi, polycystic disease, progressive nephritis, diabetic renal disease, gout, renal lesions associated with collagen diseases (systemic lupus erythematosus, polyarteritis nodosa, etc.), obstruction in the urinary tract, or nephrotoxic substances such as phenacetin, methysergide, or heavy metals.

Chronic renal disease is treated by removal of the cause where possible and by treatment of metabolic disturbance. The diet should contain a minimum of protein and a maximum of carbohydrate to minimise urea production. There should be an adequate intake of salt and water, and hypertension should be treated. Care should be taken with the dosage of drugs used to treat urinary-tract infection since they may not be excreted normally; tetracyclines should be avoided since they increase protein catabolism. Where possible, long-term haemodialysis or renal transplantation are used to prevent the fatal outcome of chronic renal failure.

Acute renal failure or an acute severe reduction in renal function is characterised by an acutely rising blood urea, oliguria or anuria, and a failure to maintain electrolyte homeostasis. There may also be lumbar pain and tenderness, renal epithelial cells and casts in the urine sediment, or a moderate proteinurea. It is usually due to acute tubular necrosis such as may occur after crushing injuries, mismatched blood transfusions, major shock, burns, septicaemia, or poisoning by nephrotoxic substances.

Acute tubular necrosis is also liable to occur during or after major surgery unless blood pressure, blood volume, and fluid balance are maintained. Acute renal failure may also be due to urinary tract obstruction, acute glomerulonephritis, renal arterial embolism or renal artery or vein thrombosis. Acute renal failure due to hypovolaemia may resolve on restoration of fluid balance although if untreated may develop to acute tubular necrosis. Likewise, restoration of flow in the urinary tract or renal vessels may restore function. Acute glomerulonephritis and acute tubular necrosis are treated conservatively. Acute tubular necrosis is completely reversible but if it has extended to renal cortical necrosis it may be irreversible.

When acute tubular necrosis has occurred a diet containing no electrolyte or protein should be given, fluid intake should be restricted, and carbohydrate should be given to satisfy energy requirements.

Development of uraemia may be delayed by suppressing nitrogen catabolism with androgens such as norethandrolone or methandienone. Peritoneal dialysis may be required if uraemia occurs before kidney function returns. Glomerular filtration improves before tubular reabsorption and results in a diuretic phase during which it is important to prevent dehydration and sodium depletion. In some cases, especially where there is renal cortical necrosis, acute renal failure may progress to chronic renal failure.

Dosage for patients with impaired renal function. When drugs are administered to patients with impaired renal function the dosage may need to be modified to take into account the degree of renal impairment and the extent to which the drug and its active metabolities are excreted throughout the kidneys.

The glomerular filtration rate is a measure of renal impairment. It may be estimated by measuring the rate of elimination of creatinine from the plasma by the kidney (the creatinine clearance). The creatinine clearance is subject to wide biological variation but in normal adults is usually about 120 millilitres per minute, falling to 50 to 80 millilitres per minute in mild renal failure, 10 to 50 millilitres per minute in moderate renal failure, and less than 10 millilitres per minute in severe renal failure. If less than 25% of the drug is excreted through the kidney then, providing that its metabolites are non-toxic, there is little risk of accumulation in renal failure and dosage adjustment is not required. If 50% or more of the drug is excreted through the kidneys caution should be exercised during administration. Dosage should also be reduced if the drug itself is nephrotoxic, for example, for amphotericin. The initial dosage for patients with renal impairment is the same as that for normal patients and thereafter dosage is adjusted by increasing the intervals between doses or, if constant blood levels are necessary, by reducing the doses and maintaining the normal interval between them. Dosage of drugs in renal impairment may be calculated from the formula

$$D = \frac{D_n \times K}{K_n}$$

when D = dosage in renal impairment, D_n = dosage in normal patients, K = elimination rate constant in renal impairment, and K_n = elimination rate constant in normal patients.

The ratio of the elimination constants may be estimated by determinations of creatinine clearance values in the patient.

However, in renal impairment many factors may affect the rate of elimination and the dosage may be calculated more accurately from tables based on pharmacokinetic and clinical data for the actual drug. The following tables are based mainly on W. M. Bennett et al., Ann. intern. Med., 1977, **86**, 754.

TABLE 1 shows the increased dosage interval in hours for patients with various degrees of renal impairment. TABLE 2 shows the percentage of the normal dose to be administered at the normal intervals for such patients.

TABLE 1. Adjustment of Dosage Interval according to Degree of Renal Impairment

Drug	Normal to Mild	Moderate	Severe
	Dosage interval in renal impairment (Hours)		
Allopurinol	8	8 to 12	12 to 24
Amoxycillin	8	12	16[1]
Amphotericin B	24	24	36
Ampicillin	6	9	12 to 15[1]
Aspirin	4	4 to 6	Avoid
Azathioprine	24	24	24 to 36
Benzylpenicillin	8	8	8 to 12
Carbenicillin	4	6 to 12	12 to 16
Cephalexin	6	6	6 to 12
Cephalothin	6	6	8 to 12
Chlorothiazide	12	12	Avoid
Chlorpropamide	24 to 36	Avoid	Avoid
Chlorthalidone	24	24	48
Clofibrate	6 to 12	12 to 18	24 to 48
Colchicine	12	12	18
Co-trimoxazole	12	18	24
Cyclophosphamide	12	12	18 to 24
Diphenhydramine	6	6 to 9	9 to 12
Ethacrynic acid	6	6	Avoid
Ethambutol	24	24 to 36	48
Gentamicin	8 to 12	12 to 24	24 to 48
Guanethidine	24	24	24 to 36
Ibuprofen	6	8	12
Isoniazid	8	8	8 to 12
Kanamycin	8 to 24	24 to 72	72 to 96
Lincomycin	6	12	24
Lithium carbonate	8	Avoid	Avoid
Meprobamate	6	9 to 12	12 to 18
Methicillin	4	4	8 to 12
Methyldopa	6	9 to 18	12 to 24
Metronidazole	8	12	24
Minocycline	12	18 to 24	24 to 36
Neostigmine	6	6	12 to 18
Paracetamol	4 to 6	6	8[2]
Pentamidine	24	24 to 36	48
Phenformin	8	8	Avoid
Phenobarbitone	8	8	8 to 16
Phenylbutazone	8	8	Avoid
Primidone	8	8 to 12	12 to 24
Probenecid	12	Avoid	Avoid
Procainamide	3 to 4	6 to 12	8 to 24
Quinine	8	8 to 12	24
Spironolactone	6	6	Avoid
Streptomycin	12 to 24	24 to 72	72 to 96
Tetracycline	6 to 12	12 to 24	Avoid
Triamterene	12	12	Avoid
Trimethadione	8	8 to 12	12 to 14

1. Normal doses should be used in urinary tract infections.
2. Caution should be exercised because metabolites may accumulate.

TABLE 2. Adjustment of Dose at Constant Interval according to Degree of Renal Impairment

Drug	Dose interval Hours	Normal to Mild	Moderate	Severe
		Percentage of normal dose		
Cephaloridine	6	100 to 50	25	12.5
Cephradine	6	100	50	25
Digitoxin	24	100	100	50 to 75
Digoxin	24	100	25 to 75	10 to 25
Propranolol	6 to 8	100	100	50

TABLE 3. Drugs Requiring No Adjustment of Dosage

Amitriptyline	Dexamethasone	Methylprednisolone
Benzhexol	Dextropropoxyphene	Morphine
Bumetanide	Diazepam	Pentazocine
Chloramphenicol	Doxycycline	Pethidine
*Chlordiazepoxide	Erythromycin	Phenytoin
Chlorpheniramine	Frusemide	Prednisolone
Chlorpromazine	Haloperidol	Prednisone
Clindamycin	Hydrocortisone	Quinidine
Clonidine	Imipramine	Rifampicin
Cloxacillin	Indomethacin	Tolbutamide
Codeine	*Levodopa	Warfarin
Cortisone		

* Caution should be exercised because metabolites may accumulate.

Reserpine

Methyl 11,17α-dimethoxy-18β-(3,4,5-trimethoxybenzoyloxy)-3β,20α-yohimbane-16β-carboxylate *or* methyl O-(3,4,5-trimethoxybenzoyl)reserpate, an alkaloid obtained from the roots of species of *Rauwolfia* (Fam. Apocynaceae), mainly *R. serpentina* Benth. and *R. vomitoria* Afz., or prepared synthetically. The material obtained from natural sources may contain closely related alkaloids.

$C_{33}H_{40}N_2O_9 = 608.7$

OTHER NAMES: *Reserpine Dellipsoids D29®*; Reserpinum; *Serpasil®* *Abicol®* (with bendrofluazide); *Serpasil-Esidrex®* (with hydrochlorothiazide)

A standard is given in the European Pharmacopoeia Vol. III

Description. Odourless, almost tasteless, small, white to slightly yellow crystals or crystalline powder.

Solubility. Practically insoluble in water and in ether; very slightly soluble in alcohol and in methyl alcohol; soluble, at 20°, in 6 parts of chloroform and in 90 parts of acetone.

Specific rotation. −113° to −127°, determined on a 1% solution in chloroform.

Dissociation constant. pK_a 6.6 (25°).

Sterilisation. Solutions for injection are sterilised by filtration.

Storage. It should be stored in airtight containers, protected from light.

Identification. TESTS. 1. To about 1 mg add 2 drops of a 0.1% solution of sodium molybdate in sulphuric acid;

a yellow colour is produced which changes, within 2 minutes, to blue.

2. To about 1 mg add 4 drops of a freshly prepared 1% solution of vanillin in hydrochloric acid; a rose-pink colour is produced within 2 minutes.

3. Mix about 500 µg with 5 mg of dimethylaminobenzaldehyde and 4 drops of glacial acetic acid and 4 drops of sulphuric acid; a green colour is produced. Add 1 ml of glacial acetic acid; the colour changes to red.

MELTING-POINT. About 270°, with decomposition.

ULTRAVIOLET ABSORPTION. In alcohol (95%), maxima at 268 nm (E1%, 1cm = 275) and 291 nm (E1%, 1cm = 170).

Determination in body fluids. SPECTROFLUORIMETRY. In plasma or urine—T. T. Zsotér et al., Clin. Pharmac. Ther., 1973, **14**, 325.

Metabolism. ABSORPTION. Readily though somewhat erratically absorbed after oral administration; erratic absorption may be a consequence of drug precipitation; reserpine-povidone co-precipitates are rapidly and uniformly absorbed.

BLOOD CONCENTRATION. After an oral dose of 250 µg, peak plasma concentrations of 1.5 to 3 ng/ml are attained in 2 to 4 hours.

HALF-LIFE. Plasma half-life is extremely variable and may be up to 11 to 16 days.

DISTRIBUTION. Bound to red blood cells to some extent, secreted in milk, and crosses the placenta; protein binding, about 40% bound to plasma proteins.

METABOLIC REACTIONS. Rapidly and extensively metabolised by hydrolysis and O-demethylation; the major metabolites are tri-methoxybenzoic acid and methylreserpate with reserpic acid, syringomethyl reserpate, and syringic acid; metabolites may be conjugated with glucuronic acid or sulphate.

EXCRETION. About 60 to 75% of a dose is excreted in urine and faeces in 4 days; about 6% of a dose is excreted in the urine in 24 hours mainly as trimethoxybenzoic acid; unchanged reserpine is excreted in the faeces.

FURTHER INFORMATION. Absorption, excretion, and metabolism—A. R. Maass et al., Clin. Pharmac. Ther., 1969, **10**, 366; absorption of reserpine-povidone co-precipitates in rats—E. I. Stupak et al., J. Pharmacokinet. Biopharm., 1974, **2**, 511; excretion and metabolism in renal failure—T. T. Zsotér et al., Clin. Pharmac. Ther., 1973, **14**, 325.

Actions and uses. Reserpine has a central depressant action and produces sedation and a lowering of blood pressure accompanied by bradycardia. Its antihypertensive effect is due to the depletion of stores of catecholamines.

When given by mouth its effects are slow in onset, seldom appearing within 3 to 6 days of administration, and continue for some time after its withdrawal; it has a cumulative effect. Reserpine is of most value in younger patients with mild labile hypertension associated with tachycardia. In long-established hypertension it is best used in conjunction with more potent hypotensive drugs.

Patients vary in their response to reserpine and dosage must be adjusted to individual requirements. To control mild or moderate cases of hypertension, the dosage for an adult is in the range 100 to 500 micrograms, usually about 250 micrograms, daily by mouth. A thiazide diuretic may be given concurrently to potentiate the antihypertensive effect.

Reserpine is used in chronic psychoses. It has a tranquillising rather than hypnotic action with less somnolence than the barbiturates. Patients with chronic mental illness treated with reserpine often become relaxed, sociable, and cooperative.

In mild anxiety states, doses of 0.5 to 2 milligrams by mouth are usually adequate. In severe psychosis a daily dosage of 2 to 3 milligrams by mouth, in conjunction with 5 to 10 milligrams daily by intramuscular injection, may be given initially, the dosage being subsequently reduced according to the patient's response; the optimum dosage may vary widely between patients. Treatment may have to be continued over a long period and the drug should not be abruptly withdrawn.

Undesirable effects. Reserpine, even in the minimum therapeutic doses, may give rise to a number of toxic effects. Of these, the most common are nasal congestion, lethargy, drowsiness, peculiar dreams, vertigo, and gastro-intestinal upsets.

Dyspnoea and urticarial rash sometimes occur, and a few patients increase in weight.

Higher doses may cause flushing, injection of conjunctivae, insomnia, bradycardia, and occasionally parkinsonism and severe mental depression which may lead to suicide. Cases of oedema have also been reported.

Intramuscular or intravenous injection of reserpine may cause postural hypotension.

Toxic effects are usually transient and quickly disappear on reducing the dosage or discontinuing treatment.

Tolerance to reserpine does not develop and it does not appear to be habit-forming.

Precautions. Reserpine should be used with caution in depressive states. If it is used in conjunction with electroconvulsive therapy an interval of at least 7 days should be allowed to elapse between the last dose of reserpine and the commencement of the shock treatment.

Reserpine should also be given with caution to patients with cardiac arrhythmias, myocardial infarction or severe cardiac damage, bronchitis, asthma, or gastric ulcer. It may give rise to hypotension in patients undergoing anaesthesia.

Veterinary uses. Reserpine is used in turkeys as a tranquilliser to reduce stress during transportation. The usual dose is 100 parts per million in the feed.

Preparations

RESERPINE TABLETS: available as tablets containing 100 and 250 micrograms of reserpine; they may be coloured.

A standard for these tablets is given in the British Pharmacopoeia 1973

Containers and Storage: see the entry on Tablets for general information on containers and storage. Containers should be airtight and light resistant.

Advice for patients: daily doses should preferably be taken at bedtime. The tablets should be taken at regular intervals, preferably after meals. Treatment should not be discontinued without the advice of the prescriber. The tablets may cause drowsiness; persons affected should not drive or operate machinery. Alcohol should be avoided.

OTHER PREPARATIONS available include TABLETS containing reserpine 150 micrograms with bendrofluazide 2.5 mg, and tablets containing reserpine 150 micrograms with hydrochlorothiazide 10 mg.

Resistance to Antibiotics

Organisms that are normally sensitive to the action of an antibiotic may sometimes develop resistance to it. The organism may have developed the ability to destroy the antibiotic or to grow in its presence. Examples of the former type are penicillin-inactivating staphylococci, and chloramphenicol-acetylating staphylococci.

Mechanisms by which Resistance Develops

Selection. Resistant organisms may become apparent as a result of the destruction of sensitive strains by the antibiotic, allowing naturally resistant strains to colonise the patient. For example, penicillin therapy destroys much of the normal mouth flora and the mouth becomes colonised by penicillin-resistant organisms previously present in small numbers.

Mutation. A genetic mutation may occur during treatment and becomes apparent when the sensitive organisms are destroyed. Mutation occurs more readily with some antimicrobial agents than with others, and especially with streptomycin, rifampicin, and nalidixic acid.

Phage transduction. Certain organisms may acquire resistance as a result of the activity of phages (bacterial viruses) which incorporate a resistance present in one organism and when released carry the resistance over to an organism which was originally sensitive.

Transference. Resistance may be transferred from one bacterial genus to another as a result of an exchange of extra-chromosomal genetic particles (plasmids) during conjugation. This process occurs in many bacterial genera including most Gram-negative bacilli. It is most readily demonstrated among the Enterobacteriaceae. Resistance to a number of drugs including aminoglycosides, cephalosporins, chloramphenicol, fusidic acid, penicillins, and tetracyclines can be transmitted in this way. Resistance to several antibiotics may be transferred at one time. Resistance to other antibacterial agents such as sulphonamides and trimethoprim may also arise by transference.

Organisms carrying the plasmids or R-factor are very prevalent in the bowel of man and animals. Transference may occur in these sites, in burns, or in fluids being used for peritoneal dialysis.

Use in animals. The use of penicillin and tetracyclines in animal feeds increases the number of resistant organisms within the animal bowel and the existence of such organisms appears to increase the proportion of resistant organisms in man. The use of antibiotics in animal feeds was restricted in the United Kingdom following the adoption of recommendations of the report of the Swann Committee (Joint Committee on the use of Antibiotics in Animal Husbandry and Veterinary Medicine, Cmnd. 4190, H.M. Stationery Office, 1969).

Measures to Minimise the Spread of Resistance

The more frequently an antibiotic is used the greater the prevalence of bacteria resistant to that agent. For example, neomycin-resistant staphylococci appear when neomycin sprays or powders are widely used. The resistant organisms decrease in numbers when the use of the antibiotic is curtailed. When a resistance factor carrying resistance to several agents, for example ampicillin, carbenicillin, streptomycin, and tetracycline, is present in a hospital unit the resistant organisms may not disappear until the use of all these agents is stopped. Antibiotics should therefore not be used unless specifically indicated.

Since much antibiotic therapy is given in the absence of bacteriological studies in the individual patient, the current antibiotic sensitivity patterns of common organisms can provide a guide to the most suitable agent. Early treatment should be based on antibiotics that are most likely to succeed in a particular case, and should be modified as necessary when the results of sensitivity tests are available. This is particularly important in hospitals where the majority of resistant bacteria are found.

The pattern of resistance found among hospital organisms should influence the choice of antibacterials in general use. Periodic revision of prescribing policies is essential in limiting the spread of resistant organisms.

In long-term therapy, as in tuberculosis, two or more antibiotics or chemotherapeutic agents of different types should be given at the same time to delay the development of resistance.

Resorcinol

Benzene-1,3-diol

$C_6H_6O_2 = 110.1$

OTHER NAMES: Resorcin
Eskamel® (with sulphur)

A standard is given in the British Pharmacopoeia 1973

Description. Colourless acicular crystals or powder with a slight characteristic odour and a taste which is sweetish becoming bitter. When exposed to air and light it becomes pinkish in colour.

Solubility. Soluble, at 20°, in less than 1 part of water and in 1 part of alcohol; soluble in ether, in glycerol, and in fixed oils; very slightly soluble in chloroform and in carbon disulphide.

Dissociation constants. pK_a 9.5, 10.1 (20°).

Storage. It should be stored in airtight containers, protected from light.

Identification. TESTS. 1. Dissolve about 100 mg in 2 ml of *sodium hydroxide solution*, add 1 drop of chloroform, and heat; an intense crimson colour is produced. Add a slight excess of hydrochloric acid; the colour changes to pale yellow.
2. To 10 ml of a 1% solution add 2 drops of *ferric chloride test-solution*; a bluish-violet colour is produced. Add *dilute ammonia solution*; the colour changes to brownish-yellow (distinction from catechol and from quinol).

MELTING-POINT. About 110°. It sublimes on further heating.

Actions and uses. Resorcinol has antipruritic, exfoliative, and keratolytic properties. It is used as a lotion or ointment containing 2 to 5% for the treatment of acne and seborrhoea.

A 2.5% alcoholic solution has been used to remove dandruff, but may slightly discolour fair hair unless all traces of soap or alkali are removed before application.

Undesirable effects. Myxoedema has been reported as a result of prolonged application of resorcinol preparations to raw surfaces.

Precautions. Resorcinol should not be used over large

raw surfaces of skin, particularly in high concentrations.

Preparations

COMPOUND RESORCINOL OINTMENT:

Resorcinol	40 g
Cade oil	30 g
Zinc oxide, finely sifted	40 g
Bismuth subnitrate, finely sifted	80 g
Starch, finely sifted	100 g
Sodium metabisulphite	.. 2 g
Hard paraffin	20 g
Water for preparations	40 g
Wool fat	100 g
Yellow soft paraffin	548 g

Triturate the bismuth subnitrate, the zinc oxide, and the starch with a portion of the yellow soft paraffin until smooth and incorporate the wool fat and the melted hard paraffin; add the resorcinol and the sodium metabisulphite previously dissolved in the water, the cade oil, and the remainder of the soft paraffin, and mix.

A standard for this ointment is given in the British Pharmaceutical Codex 1973
Containers: see the entry on Ointments for general information on containers. Containers should prevent evaporation.
Advice for patients: the skin should be cleansed prior to application and the ointment should be applied sparingly to the affected area. Prolonged use should be avoided and its use should be discontinued if excessive drying or irritation of the skin occurs.
It should not be applied to broken or inflamed skin. It may discolour fair hair.

RESORCINOL AND SULPHUR PASTE:

Resorcinol, finely sifted	50 g
Precipitated sulphur	50 g
Zinc oxide, finely sifted	400 g
Emulsifying ointment	500 g

Triturate the zinc oxide, the resorcinol, and the precipitated sulphur with a portion of the emulsifying ointment until smooth and gradually incorporate the remainder of the emulsifying ointment.

A standard for this paste is given in the British Pharmaceutical Codex 1973
Containers and *Storage:* see the entry on Pastes for general information on containers and storage. It should be protected from light.
Advice for patients: see above under Compound Resorcinol Ointment, but it should be applied liberally to the affected area.

OTHER PREPARATIONS available include a CREAM containing resorcinol 2% with sulphur 8%.
Resorcinol is an ingredient of compound bismuth subgallate suppositories.

Reticulum Cell Sarcoma

see under LYMPHOPROLIFERATIVE DISEASES

Rheumatic Fever

Rheumatic fever is an acute or subacute inflammatory complication of group A streptococcal infections, characterised by arthritis, chorea, carditis, subcutaneous nodules, and erythema marginatum. It usually occurs 10 to 21 days after an upper respiratory tract infection and the first attack usually occurs before the age of 4 years. Only a minority of people with group A streptococcal infection develop rheumatic fever, but in those subjects it is liable to recur.

The arthritis of rheumatic fever is a febrile joint pain affecting most commonly the large joints and migrating from one joint to another (migratory polyarthritis). The joints are painful, tender, red, hot, and swollen. There may also be effusion into the joints.

The most dangerous site for the inflammatory reaction is in the cardiac valves where it causes rheumatic carditis. The mitral valve is the most commonly affected. Acute interstitial valvulitis occurs giving rise to oedema, thickening, fusion, retraction, and other destructive lesions of the valves. There may also be a pericardial rub, heart murmurs, cardiac enlargement, or congestive heart failure.

Sydenham's chorea often occurs late in the disease and may occur up to 6 months after the original streptococcal infection. It is insidious in onset and is characterised by irregular uncontrolled movements of the arm, leg, and other muscles. There may be only mild involuntary movements or violent continuous activity which may interfere with coordinated activity.

The treatment of the arthritis consists mainly of the relief of pain with salicylates. When carditis is present, treatment aims to suppress clinical inflammation whilst avoiding inflammatory rebound which often follows inflammation suppression. Inflammation may be controlled with salicylates but, when severe, corticosteroids may be necessary. There is no specific treatment for chorea, which recovers completely after 2 to 6 months. Bed rest to reduce external stimuli or tranquillisers of the phenothiazine group may be used for symptomatic treatment.

A course of treatment with benzylpenicillin may be useful in the acute disease to remove residual streptococci. After approximately two attacks of rheumatic fever, depending on the severity of the attacks, continuous anti-streptococcal prophylaxis with sulphonamides or penicillin should be maintained to prevent recurrent attacks. In patients with cardiac damage antibiotic prophylaxis may need to be continued up to the age of 18 years and may be required during dental extractions to prevent bacterial endocarditis.

Usually 2 grams of phenoxymethylpenicillin is given by mouth one hour before extraction or alternatively benzylpenicillin may be administered.

Rheumatoid Arthritis

Rheumatoid arthritis is a chronic inflammatory disease of the joints associated with changes in the connective tissues. The disease commonly commences in middle age and is more common in women than men. It is characterised by inflammation and deformation of the joints, the peripheral joints being mainly affected, and by swelling of the synovial membrane and periarticular tissues. Nodules surrounded by a loose capsule of fibrous tissue may occur in the subcutaneous tissues over pressure points and occasionally in the tendons. The erythrocyte sedimentation rate is raised, and a macroglobulin known as rheumatoid factor is often present.

In the earlier stages of the disease there is pain and stiffness of the joints, especially in the morning, and in later stages there may be structural changes leading to deformity and disability. The disease is chronic, with partial remissions and relapses.

Treatment includes rest and, if necessary, joints may be immobilised to reduce pain. Heat, cold, physiotherapy, hydrotherapy, electrotherapy, massage, and exercise may be of value. Pain and inflammation may be relieved by the use of aspirin or other analgesics and anti-inflammatory drugs. The systemic use of corticosteroids such as prednisolone is indicated in only a small minority of patients but hydrocortisone acetate and certain other corticosteroids may be given by intra-articular injection into affected joints.

Patients who do not respond to other treatment may be prescribed suitable courses of chloroquine, hydroxychloroquine, penicillamine, sodium aurothiomalate, or immunosuppressive drugs.

Rheumatoid Arthritis, Juvenile

Juvenile rheumatoid arthritis (Still's disease) is a chronic polyarthritis of childhood. Onset usually occurs at about 1 to 3 years or 10 to 15 years of age as a polyarthritis accompanied by systemic manifestations of malaise, irregular fever, and maculopapular rash. It may be accompanied by enlargement of lymph nodes and spleen and by iridocyclitis.

The pattern of joint involvement is similar to adult rheumatoid arthritis. Juvenile rheumatoid arthritis may remit in adolescence or it may progress to adult rheumatoid arthritis or ankylosing spondylitis. Flexion deformities of joints may be prevented by night-rest splinting and regular supervised exercise of all affected joints. Iritis may be treated by the application of eye-drops of atropine and corticosteroids. One of the analgesic, non-steroidal, anti-inflammatory agents and, occasionally, corticosteroids may also be required.

Rhinitis

see ALLERGIC RHINITIS AND HAY FEVER

Rhubarb

The rhizome of *Rheum palmatum* L. and possibly other species and hybrids of *Rheum* (Fam. Polygonaceae), excepting *R. rhaponticum* L., cultivated in China and Tibet, deprived of most of its bark, and dried.

OTHER NAMES: Rhei Rhizoma; Rheum

Peralvex® (with salicylic acid)

A standard is given in the British Pharmacopoeia 1973

Varieties. High-grade rhubarb, corresponding to that formerly known as Shensi rhubarb and now sometimes marketed as Chinghai rhubarb, has a bright yellow surface and shows distinct whitish reticulations which give rise to the characteristic "nutmeg" fracture, which exhibits a bright pink tint. Much of this material shows a single hole through which passed the cord by which the rhubarb was suspended during drying.

Another quality, similar to that formerly known as Canton rhubarb, may be poorly trimmed with greyish patches on the outer surface, is of a less agreeable odour and taste, and the whitish reticulations are much less distinct. The fracture of this rhubarb is more or less uniformly granular, shows no obvious marbling and can be of a paler pink colour than Chinghai. Inferior consignments will only contain a small proportion of rhubarb giving a pink fracture, the bulk of the pieces exhibiting a grey, mauve, or brown fracture. All Chinese rhubarb

is exported from Shanghai or Tientsin in wooden cases, lined with tin-plate, and containing 280 lb or 50 kg respectively, with the inferior grades sometimes packed in hessian bags. Such commercial designations as "East Indian", "Turkey", or "Muscovy" rhubarb are now rarely used; they referred to the route by which the drug once reached the European markets.

Constituents. Rhubarb contains a number of anthraquinone derivatives. Sennosides A, B, C, E, and F are present in Chinese rhubarb, sennoside A being present in a concentration of about 1.7%. Sennosides E and F are the oxalates of sennosides A and B respectively. Other anthraquinone derivatives are based on emodin, 6-methoxychrysophanol (physcione), chrysophanol, aloe-emodin (9,10-dihydro-1,8-dihydroxy-3-hydroxymethyl-9,10-dioxoanthracene), and rhein. These occur free and as the glycosides of their quinone, anthrone, or dianthrone forms.

Also present is an amorphous resin which on hydrolysis, yields rhein, chrysophanol, and other substances.

Rhubarb also contains cinnamic acid, gallic acid and tannins, rheinolic acid, volatile oil, starch and calcium oxalate.

Chinese Rhubarb yields to alcohol about 35 to 45% of extractive.

Up to 1% of acid-insoluble ash may be yielded and up to 1% of foreign organic matter may be present.

Description. UNGROUND DRUG. *Macroscopical characters:* pieces varying from subcylindrical and barrel-shaped to conical and plano-convex, or somewhat prismatic; often perforated with a hole; about 50 to 150 mm long and 30 to 100 mm wide; pieces usually covered with a bright brownish-yellow powder which on removal exposes the surface showing numerous longitudinal, dark reddish-brown lines or spots embedded in a whitish matrix; fracture granular and uneven; smoothed, transversely cut surface pinkish-brown or greyish; cambium line darker, near periphery (sometimes removed with external tissues on peeling); secondary phloem, when present, consisting of dark reddish-brown medullary rays containing colouring matter alternating with white lines of phloem parenchyma containing starch and calcium oxalate. Normal secondary xylem narrow, situated immediately to inner side of cambium, with an internal ring of more or less united star-like vascular strands consisting of dark red medullary rays radiating through central white phloem and peripheral xylem; these strands are known as star spots.

It has a characteristic, somewhat aromatic odour and a bitter slightly astringent taste.

Microscopical characters: the diagnostic characters are: *starch* granules, abundant in parenchyma, either simple or compound, with up to 5 components and showing a hilum usually in the form of a radiate split, individual granules about 4 to 18 μm, compound granules about 20 to 30 μm in diameter; large cluster *crystals* of calcium oxalate about 20 to 200 μm in diameter and frequently more than 100 μm; amorphous *yellow substance* insoluble in alcohol (90%) but soluble in water and in *chloral hydrate solution*, and becoming reddish-pink on treatment with *dilute ammonia solution* and deep red with solutions of caustic alkalis; *vessels* mostly with reticulately pitted walls giving no reaction for lignin; *cork* and *sclerenchyma* absent.

POWDERED DRUG: Powdered Rhubarb. An orange-yellow to yellowish-brown powder possessing the diagnostic microscopical characters, odour, and taste of the unground drug.

Adulterants and substitutes. Rhapontic rhubarb, the rhizome of *R. rhaponticum*, is imported from China and is known commercially as "Chinese rhapontica", although it may be offered by exporters as "Tai-Hwang" or "Tze-Hwang" rhubarb without indicating that it is of a rhapontic nature. The rhizome occurs as untrimmed pieces, sometimes split longitudinally, and has a distinctive, slightly sweet odour, which readily distinguishes it from the official drug.

Chinese rhapontica may be hollow in the centre and the radiate transverse section shows alternate paler and darker concentric circles and a diffuse ring of isolated star-spots.

It complies with the test for anthraquinone derivatives (see below) but may be distinguished by the following test. Macerate 500 mg of rhubarb in coarse powder or 500 mg of material peeled from the outside of the drug with 10 ml of alcohol (45%) for 15 to 20 minutes, shaking occasionally, and filter. Place 1 drop of the filtrate on a filter paper and examine under ultraviolet radiation, including radiation of wavelength 366 nm; it gives a distinct blue fluorescence which is intensified in colour by exposure to ammonia vapour (presence of rhapontic rhubarb).

Indian rhubarb, obtained from *R. emodi* Wall., occurs in cylindrical or irregular pieces, much shrunken, light in weight, and easily cut; sometimes with adherent bark, rather dark in colour, almost odourless, and taste bitter. It contains anthraquinone derivatives and yields about 25 to 30% of alcohol-soluble extractive.

Storage. It should be stored in airtight containers, protected from light.

Identification. TEST. Shake 100 mg, in powder or small pieces, with 10 ml of *ferric chloride solution* mixed with 5 ml of hydrochloric acid, and immerse in a water-bath for about 10 minutes; filter immediately, cool the filtrate, and extract with 10 ml of carbon tetrachloride; separate the carbon tetrachloride layer, wash with 5 ml of water, and shake with 5 ml of *dilute ammonia solution*; a rose-pink to cherry-red colour is produced in the ammoniacal layer (presence of anthraquinone derivatives).

Actions and uses. Rhubarb is a mild anthraquinone purgative which has actions and uses similar to those described under Senna Fruit. Its action differs from that of other anthraquinone-containing drugs in that the tannin present may exert an astringent action after purgation.

The usual adult dose is 0.2 to 1 gram; children may be given half the adult dose.

Preparations

AMMONIATED RHUBARB AND SODA MIXTURE (*Syn.* Mistura Rhei Ammoniata et Sodae; Rhubarb, Ammonia, and Soda Mixture):

Rhubarb, in powder	25 g
Sodium bicarbonate	80 g
Ammonium bicarbonate	20 g
Peppermint emulsion, concentrated	25 ml
Chloroform water, double-strength	500 ml
Water for preparations	to 1000 ml

It should be recently prepared.
A standard for this mixture is given in the British Pharmaceutical Codex 1973
Containers and *Labelling:* see the entry on Mixtures for general information on containers and labelling. A direction to shake the bottle should be given on the label.
Dose: 10 to 20 millilitres.

Advice for patients: the mixture should not be taken for longer than a few days without medical advice. It may colour the urine red.

COMPOUND RHUBARB POWDER (*Syn.* Gregory's Powder; Pulvis Rhei Compositus):

Rhubarb, in powder	250 g
Ginger, in powder	100 g
Heavy magnesium carbonate	325 g
Light magnesium carbonate	325 g

Mix, as described in the entry on Powders.
A standard for this powder is given in the British Pharmaceutical Codex 1973
Containers and *Storage:* see the entry on Powders for general information on containers and storage.
Dose: 0.5 to 5 grams.
Advice for patients: the powder should be taken mixed with a little water or other fluid. It should not be used for longer than a few days without medical advice. It may colour the urine red.

COMPOUND RHUBARB TINCTURE (*Syn.* Tinct. Rhei Co.):

Rhubarb, in moderately coarse powder	100.0 g
Coriander oil	0.03 ml
Cardamom oil	0.40 ml
Glycerol	100.00 ml
Alcohol (60%)	to 1000.00 ml

Prepare 850 ml of a tincture, using the rhubarb and a sufficient quantity of the alcohol, by the percolation process; add the coriander oil, the cardamom oil, the glycerol, and sufficient of the alcohol to produce 1000 ml. Mix. Filter, if necessary.
A standard for this tincture is given in the British Pharmacopoeia 1973
Dose: up to 15 ml daily, in divided doses.

OTHER PREPARATIONS available include a PAINT containing anthraquinone glycosides 5% with salicylic acid 1%.
Compound rhubarb tincture is an ingredient of compound figs syrup.

Riboflavine

3,10 - Dihydro - 7,8 - dimethyl - 10 - [(2S,3S,4R) - 2,3,4,5-tetrahydroxypentyl]benzopteridine-2,4-dione *or* 7,8-dimethyl-10-(D-ribit-1-yl)isoalloxazine

$C_{17}H_{20}N_4O_6 = 376.4$

OTHER NAMES: Lactoflavin; Riboflavinum; Vitamin B$_2$

A standard is given in the European Pharmacopoeia Vol. I

Description. A yellow to orange-yellow crystalline powder with a slight odour and a persistent bitter taste.

Solubility. Very slightly soluble in water and in alcohol; more soluble in saline solution and in a 10% solution of urea in water; practically insoluble in ether and in chloroform; soluble in dilute solutions of alkali hydroxides.

Acidity or alkalinity. A saturated solution has a pH of 5.5 to 7.2.

Moisture content. Not more than 1.5%, determined by drying at 105°.

Dissociation constants. pK_a 1.9, 10.2 (20°).

Stability. When dry it is not appreciably affected by diffused light, but in solution, especially in the presence of alkali, it deteriorates rapidly, the decomposition being accelerated by light.

FURTHER INFORMATION. Stability in aqueous solution —D. E. Guttman, *J. pharm. Sci.*, 1962, **51**, 1162; D. A. Wadke and D. E. Guttman, *J. pharm. Sci.*, 1964, **53**, 1073.

Sterilisation. Solutions for injection are sterilised by heating in an autoclave or by filtration.

Storage. It should be stored in airtight containers, protected from light.

Identification. TEST. Dissolve about 1 mg in 100 ml of water; the solution is a pale greenish-yellow colour by transmitted light, and by reflected light has an intense yellowish-green fluorescence which disappears on the addition of mineral acids or alkalis.

MELTING-POINT. About 280°.

ULTRAVIOLET ABSORPTION. In neutral, acid or alkaline solution, maxima at 266 nm, 375 nm, and 444 nm, but the absorbance varies with pH.

Determination in body fluids. ULTRAVIOLET SPECTRO-PHOTOMETRY. In urine—N. Wahba, *Analyst, Lond.*, 1969, **94**, 904.

THIN-LAYER CHROMATOGRAPHY. In urine—C. Haworth *et al.*, *Analyst, Lond.*, 1971, **96**, 432.

Metabolism. ABSORPTION. Readily absorbed after oral administration; absorption is influenced by gastric emptying rate and is slowed by anticholinergics although the total amount absorbed is increased; the presence of food and the concomitant administration of sodium alginate increases absorption; riboflavine appears to be absorbed by a specific absorption process in the proximal part of the small intestine and the absorption mechanism appears to have a limited capacity.

BLOOD CONCENTRATION. After an oral dose of 50 mg, a peak plasma concentration of up to 300 ng/ml is attained; endogenous plasma concentrations are less than 100 ng/ml.

DISTRIBUTION. Taken up by many tissues and by red blood cells and stored chiefly in the liver and kidneys; the distribution of riboflavine in the body is influenced by the presence of probenecid; riboflavine crosses the placenta, is secreted in milk and in the sweat; volume of distribution in anephric subjects, 30 to 50 litres; *protein binding*, about 60% bound to plasma proteins.

METABOLIC REACTIONS. In the body riboflavine is phosphorylated to form flavine mononucleotide (FMN) which is subsequently converted to flavine adenine dinucleotide (FAD); both flavines are important coenzymes in a wide variety of metabolic reactions especially in the oxidation of carbohydrates, amino-acids, aldehydes, and other compounds.

EXCRETION. After an intravenous dose, up to about 80 to 95% is excreted in the urine; after an oral dose, about 35% is excreted in the urine and this may be increased to about 50% in non-fasting subjects; the excretion of riboflavine is reduced by probenecid and increased if oral administration is preceded by a dose of bile salts.

FURTHER INFORMATION. Absorption, metabolism, and excretion of riboflavine phosphate (sodium salt)—W. J. Jusko and G. Levy, *J. pharm. Sci.*, 1967, **56**, 58; effect of age on absorption—W. J. Jusko et al., *J. pharm. Sci.*, 1970, **59**, 487; effect of anticholinergics on absorption— G. Levy et al., *J. pharm. Sci.*, 1972, **61**, 798; effect of probenecid—W. J. Jusko et al., *J. pharm. Sci.*, 1970, **59**, 566; absorption—B. Stripp, *Acta pharmac. tox.*, 1965, **22**, 353; pharmacokinetics—W. J. Jusko and G. Levy, *J. pharm. Sci.*, 1970, **59**, 765.

Actions and uses. Riboflavine, a member of the vitamin-B group, is a component of the coenzymes flavine mononucleotide and flavine adenine dinucleotide (see above under Metabolism), and has no known pharmacological actions.

The role of riboflavine in human nutrition is unknown, but it probably plays a part in the nutrition of mucous membranes and in protein metabolism. Riboflavine deficiency in man is characterised by a well-defined syndrome, the features of which are angular stomatitis, glossitis (magenta tongue), reddened, shiny, and denuded lips, seborrhoeic follicular keratosis of the nasolabial folds, nose, and forehead, and dermatitis of the ano-genital region. For normal health, an adult requires about 1.5 to 3 milligrams of riboflavine daily, children aged up to 1 year 500 micrograms, and other children and adolescents up to 2 milligrams. Requirements are increased in pregnancy and lactation.

There is little evidence that riboflavine is of therapeutic value except in the treatment of ariboflavinosis, for which a dosage of 2 to 10 milligrams daily is given according to the severity of the condition. Riboflavine is normally administered by mouth, but, if for any reason it cannot be absorbed or utilised by this route, it may be injected.

Veterinary uses. Riboflavine is used for the treatment of riboflavine deficiency in susceptible species. The usual dose is 100 to 200 micrograms per kilogram body-weight daily.

Preparations

Riboflavine is an alternative ingredient of vitamins B and C injection (see under Ascorbic Acid or Thiamine Hydrochloride), and an ingredient of compound vitamin B tablets, of strong compound vitamin B tablets (see under Thiamine Hydrochloride), and of vitamins capsules (see under Ascorbic Acid).

Riboflavine Phosphate (Sodium Salt)

Sodium 7,8-dimethyl-10-(D-ribit-1-yl)isoalloxazine 5'-phosphate dihydrate

$C_{17}H_{20}N_4NaO_9P,2H_2O = 514.4$

A standard is given in the British Pharmaceutical Codex 1973

Description. An odourless, hygroscopic, yellow to orange-yellow, crystalline powder.

Solubility. Soluble, at 20°, in 20 parts of water; very slightly soluble in alcohol; practically insoluble in ether and in chloroform.

Acidity. A 2% solution has a pH of 4 to 6.3.

Moisture content. 4 to 10%, determined by drying over phosphorus pentoxide at 100° *in vacuo.*

Specific rotation. +38° to +42°, determined on a 1.5% solution in 5N hydrochloric acid.

Dissociation constants. pK_a 2.5, 6.5, 10.3 (20°).

Stability; Sterilisation; Storage. See under Riboflavine.

Identification. TESTS. 1. To 1 ml of a 0.01% solution add 1 ml of 1N sodium hydroxide, expose the solution to ultraviolet radiation for 30 minutes, add sufficient acetic acid to make the solution acid to litmus paper, add 2 ml of chloroform and shake; the chloroform layer exhibits a yellow fluorescence.
2. Dissolve, with the aid of heat, about 100 mg in 1 ml of 5N hydrochloric acid, add 10 ml of alcohol (95%), cool in an ice-bath, induce crystallisation, and filter through a sintered-glass crucible (British Standard Grade No. 4); the residue, after washing with ether and drying, melts at about 200°.

ULTRAVIOLET ABSORPTION. In *solution of standard pH 7.0,* maxima at 266 nm (E1%, 1cm = 610), 372 nm, and 445 nm.

Actions and uses. Riboflavine phosphate (sodium salt) is a soluble compound of riboflavine which is used for the preparation of injections. It has the actions described under Riboflavine; 1.4 grams of riboflavine phosphate (sodium salt) is approximately equivalent to 1 gram of riboflavine.

Preparations

Riboflavine phosphate (sodium salt) is an alternative ingredient of vitamins B and C injection (see under Ascorbic Acid or Thiamine Hydrochloride).

Rickets

Rickets is a disease resulting from deficiency of vitamin D in infants and rarely from an inability of the renal tubules to absorb phosphate. The absorption of calcium and phosphate from the gut is decreased and there is a loss of calcium phosphate from the bones. There is broadening of the epiphysis of the long bones especially of the wrist and ankles, bending of the long bones, thinning of the skull and deformity of the thorax. Other features include decreased muscle tone, abdominal distension, and recurrent bronchitis. Treatment is described under Calciferol and Dihydrotachysterol; cod-liver oil, halibut-liver oil, concentrated vitamin D solution, and concentrated vitamins A and D solution are also used in the prevention and treatment of rickets.

Rifampicin

3-(4-Methylpiperazin-1-yliminomethyl)rifamycin SV

$C_{43}H_{58}N_4O_{12} = 823.0$

OTHER NAMES: *Rifadin®*; Rifampin; *Rimactane® Rifinah®* and *Rimactazid®* (both with isoniazid)

A standard is given in the British Pharmacopoeia Addendum 1978

Description. An odourless, brick-red to red-brown, crystalline powder.

Solubility. Very slightly soluble in water, in alcohol, in acetone, and in ether; soluble in chloroform and in methyl alcohol.

Acidity. A 1% suspension has a pH of 5 to 6.5.

Moisture content. Not more than 1%, determined by drying at 80°, *in vacuo.*

Storage. It should be stored in airtight containers in an atmosphere of nitrogen, in a cool place, protected from light.

Identification. TEST. Mix about 25 mg with 25 ml of water, shake for 5 minutes, filter, and to 5 ml of the filtrate add 1 ml of a 10% solution of ammonium persulphate in *solution of standard pH 7.4* and shake for a few minutes; the colour changes from orange-yellow to violet-red without the formation of a precipitate.

ULTRAVIOLET ABSORPTION. In *solution of standard pH*

7.4, broad, poorly defined maxima at 237 nm, 254 nm, 334 nm, and 475 nm.

Determination in body fluids. MICROBIOLOGICAL ASSAY. In saliva or serum—L. F. Devine *et al.*, *J. Am. med. Ass.*, 1970, **214**, 1055. REVIEW of methods for determining rifampicin in body fluids—G. Binda *et al.*, *Arzneimittel-Forsch.*, 1971, **21**, 1907.

Metabolism. ABSORPTION. Readily absorbed after oral administration; absorption may be reduced in non-fasting subjects and delayed by the presence of salicylates.

BLOOD CONCENTRATION. After oral doses of 150 to 600 mg, peak plasma concentrations of 2 to 9 μg/ml are attained in 2 to 4 hours; after a 900-mg dose, plasma concentrations of up to 27 μg/ml are attained in 2 to 4 hours; plasma concentrations are increased in subjects with renal or liver function impairment, in subjects given probenecid, and in fasting subjects; plasma concentrations also appear to be higher in female than in male subjects.

HALF-LIFE. Plasma half-life, 2 to 3 hours following doses up to 12 mg/kg; at doses above 16 mg/kg, the plasma half-life may be as long as 65 hours; during continuous therapy, the half-life may be reduced.

DISTRIBUTION. Widely distributed throughout the body and enters the cerebrospinal fluid when the meninges are inflamed; rifampicin is subject to enterohepatic circulation, is secreted in the milk, and crosses the placenta; it appears in inflammatory exudates and enters bone; *protein binding*, 75 to 88% bound to plasma proteins.

METABOLIC REACTIONS. Deacetylation to form the major metabolite, desacetylrifampicin, which has antibacterial properties; rifampicin induces the drug metabolising enzymes of the liver and may increase the metabolism of oral contraceptives, hydrocortisone, hexobarbitone, and tolbutamide as well as inducing its own metabolism.

EXCRETION. In 96 hours, up to about 45% of a dose may be excreted in the urine with the remainder eliminated in the faeces via excretion in the bile; 30 to 50% of the urinary excreted material is unchanged; the percentage of a dose excreted in the urine increases as the dose is increased.

FURTHER INFORMATION. Effect of probenecid on serum concentrations—R. J. Fallon *et al.*, *Lancet*, ii/1975, 792; effect of meals on absorption—D. I. Siegler *et al.*, *Lancet*, ii/1974, 197; induction of drug-metabolising enzymes—W. Zilly *et al.*, *Eur. J. clin. Pharmac.*, 1975, **9**, 219; pharmacokinetics, alone and with trimethoprim—J. M. T. Hamilton-Miller and W. Brumfitt, *J. antimicrob. Chemother.*, 1976, **2**, 181; pharmacokinetics—K. Winsel *et al.*, *Pharmazie*, 1976, **31**, 95; serum concentrations after oral administration—S. Virtanen and E. Tala, *Clin. Pharmac. Ther.*, 1974, **16**, 817.

Actions and uses. Rifampicin is an antibiotic which is effective against *Mycobacterium tuberculosis* and may be active when resistance to other drugs has developed. It is also active against a large number of Gram-positive and Gram-negative organisms including staphylococci and bacteroides and is occasionally used to treat infections with these organisms. It is excreted in the bile and has been used to treat biliary infections, but in general it is reserved for use in tuberculosis.

Rifampicin is bactericidal but should not be used alone in the treatment of tuberculosis because relatively rapid induction of bacterial resistance may occur. It is usually administered in conjunction with one or two other antitubercular drugs such as isoniazid, streptomycin, and ethambutol but not with aminosalicylic acid. It is

administered by mouth in a dose of 450 to 600 milligrams once daily (approximately 10 milligrams per kilogram body-weight, up to a maximum of 600 milligrams). Children may be given up to 20 milligrams per kilogram body-weight daily .

Undesirable effects. Gastro-intestinal disorders and rashes may occur and rarely acute renal failure, liver damage, thrombocytopenia, and purpura especially when a high dosage is being used.

Precautions. Rifampicin should be administered with caution in alcoholism, hepatic disease, and pregnancy.

Drug interactions. Rifampicin may reduce the activity of anticoagulants, corticosteroids, some oral hypoglycaemic drugs, anticonvulsants, and oral contraceptives.

Preparations

RIFAMPICIN CAPSULES: consisting of rifampicin, in powder, which may be mixed with a suitable inert diluent, enclosed in a hard capsule. The capsule shells may be coloured. Available as capsules containing 150 and 300 mg of rifampicin.

Containers and *Storage:* see the entry on Capsules for general information on containers and storage.

Advice for patients: the capsules should preferably be taken before breakfast or on an empty stomach. Treatment should not be discontinued without the advice of the prescriber. The urine, sweat, saliva, sputum, and tears may be coloured pink.

OTHER PREPARATIONS available include a MIXTURE containing rifampicin 100 mg in 5 ml; TABLETS containing rifampicin 150 mg with isoniazid 100 mg, and tablets containing rifampicin 300 mg with isoniazid 150 mg.

Rinderpest Vaccine, Living

A freeze-dried preparation of a live modified strain of rinderpest virus propagated in cell cultures or in goat, rabbit, or chick-embryo tissues.

A standard is given in the British Pharmacopoeia (Veterinary)

Storage. The dried vaccine should be protected from light and stored below $-20°$. If stored between $2°$ and $8°$ the dried vaccine cannot be expected to retain its potency for more than 6 months if prepared in cell culture, or for more than 3 months if prepared in tissues. The vaccine should be used immediately after reconstitution.

Veterinary uses. It is administered to cattle and buffaloes by subcutaneous injection for the prophylaxis of rinderpest.

Ringer's Solution for Injection

A sterile solution of 322 micrograms of calcium chloride (dihydrate), 300 micrograms of potassium chloride, and 8.6 mg of sodium chloride, per ml, in water for injections. Ringer-lactate solution for injection (Hartmann's solution for injection) is compound sodium lactate injection (see under Lactic Acid).

Ringer's solution for injection contains about 2.2 mmol of Ca^{2+}, 4 mmol of K^+, 147 mmol of Na^+, and 156 mmol of Cl^- per litre.

OTHER NAME: Compound Sodium Chloride Injection

Sterilisation. The solution is sterilised, immediately after preparation, by heating in an autoclave or by filtration.

Containers and Labelling. See the entry on Injections for general information on containers and labelling. The label on the container should state the content of calcium, potassium, sodium, and chloride in millimoles per litre.

Storage. The solution may, on storage, cause the separation of small solid glass particles from a glass container. A solution containing such particles must not be used.

Ringworm

see under TINEA INFECTIONS

Rosemary Oil

Obtained by distillation from the flowering tops or leafy twigs of *Rosmarinus officinalis* L. (Fam. Labiatae), an evergreen shrub indigenous to southern Europe, and growing abundantly on dry rocky hills in the Mediterranean regions.

OTHER NAME: Oleum Rosmarini

A standard is given in the British Pharmaceutical Codex 1973

Most rosemary oil is imported from Spain, the south of France, and other western Mediterranean countries, but that distilled in Great Britain is superior to the imported oil.

Constituents. Rosemary oil contains 2 to 5% of esters, notably bornyl acetate, and from 10 to 18% of free alcohols, including borneol and linalol. It also contains camphor, pinene, camphene, and cineole.

Description. A colourless or pale yellow liquid with the odour of rosemary.

Solubility. Soluble, at 20°, in 1 part of alcohol (90%).

Weight per ml. At 20°, 0.893 to 0.910 g.

Refractive index. 1.466 to 1.474.

Optical rotation. −5° to +10°.

Adulterants and substitutes. Camphor oil and eucalyptus have been used as adulterants, and the presence of either of these oils will raise the freezing-point of the complex of the oil with o-cresol above 39.8°.

Storage. It should be stored in well-filled airtight containers, protected from light, in a cool place.

Uses. Rosemary oil is used as a perfumery agent and is an ingredient of soap liniment.

Roundworm Infections

see ASCARIASIS

Rubella

Rubella (German measles) is a viral disease spread by droplet infection occurring mainly in older children, adolescents, and young adults during the spring and summer months. In children the disease is mild or occasionally symptomless. Pink discrete spots appear behind the ears and on the forehead spreading to the trunk and limbs, and there may be sore throat and swollen lymph nodes; in particular the occipital lymph nodes are enlarged and tender.

In adults onset may be rapid with fever and malaise; occasionally arthralgia and arthritis may be present. No specific treatment is required and the symptoms subside after 3 to 4 days. The incubation period is 14 to 21 days and the patients are infectious for 1 week before and 1 week after the appearance of the spots.

When the disease occurs in pregnant women during the first 3 to 4 months of pregnancy it increases the risk of congenital malformations of the foetus. It is therefore considered advisable to vaccinate girls (see immunisation schedules under Vaccines). Pregnant women who are in contact with cases of rubella should have blood taken for antibody tests, which will distinguish those already immune from those liable to contract the disease. Sequential studies are necessary in the latter group to determine if infection occurs. Reliance should not be placed upon human normal immunoglobulin for the prevention of abnormalities in the foetus of a non-immune woman exposed to the disease.

Rubella Vaccine (Live Attenuated)

An aqueous suspension of a suitable live attenuated strain of rubella virus grown in suitable cell cultures. It is prepared immediately before use by reconstituting the dried vaccine with a suitable sterile liquid; bactericides must not be added.

OTHER NAMES: Rubella Vaccine (Live); Rub/Vac (Live)

A standard is given in the British Pharmacopoeia 1973.

Storage. It should be stored at a temperature between 2° and 10°. Under these conditions it may be expected to retain its potency for 1 year.

The reconstituted vaccine should be used immediately after preparation.

Actions and uses. Rubella vaccine (live attenuated) is used for active immunisation against German measles. It is used to immunise girls aged 11 to 13 and also women of childbearing age who are not pregnant who have been shown by serological tests to be susceptible to rubella infections. It is administered by subcutaneous or intramuscular injection in a single dose of 0.5 millilitre. Susceptible subjects develop protective antibodies towards the end of the third week after vaccination.

Mild clinical effects lasting a day or two and consisting mainly of pyrexia, general irritability, and a transient rash develop in a minority of patients from 6 to 14 days after vaccination. Arthralgia occasionally occurs and is more likely to occur after rubella vaccination in adults than in children.

Suitable schedules for the immunisation of children are given under Vaccines.

Precautions and contra-indications. It is contraindicated in leukaemia, lymphoma, and other generalised malignant diseases, hypogammaglobulinaemia, acute febrile illness, and especially pregnancy.

It is important that any woman vaccinated is not pregnant and does not become pregnant for 8 weeks after vaccination.

Saccharin

1,2-Benzisothiazolin-3-one 1,1-dioxide

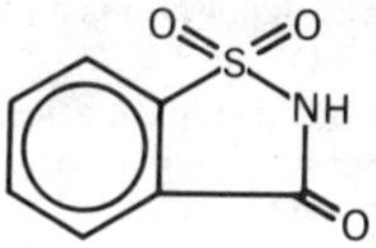

$C_7H_5NO_3S = 183.2$

A standard is given in the British Pharmacopoeia Addendum 1978

Description. White crystals or crystalline powder with an intensely sweet taste; odourless or with a faintly aromatic odour.

Solubility. Soluble, at 20°, in 290 parts of water, in 30 parts of alcohol, in 12 parts of acetone, and in 50 parts of glycerol; soluble in about 25 parts of boiling water; very slightly soluble in ether and in chloroform; soluble in dilute ammonia solution, in solutions of alkali hydroxides, and, with evolution of carbon dioxide, in solutions of alkali bicarbonates.

Moisture content. Not more than 1%, determined by drying at 105°.

Dissociation constant. pK_a 1.6 (25°).

Identification. TESTS. 1. Mix about 20 mg with 40 mg of resorcinol, add 10 drops of sulphuric acid, heat over a small flame until a dark green colour is produced, allow to cool, and add 10 ml of water and an excess of *sodium hydroxide solution*; a fluorescent green liquid is produced.
2. Dissolve about 100 mg in 5 ml of a 10% solution of sodium hydroxide, evaporate to dryness, fuse the residue over a small flame until ammonia is no longer evolved, allow to cool, dissolve in 20 ml of water, neutralise with *dilute hydrochloric acid*, filter, and to the filtrate add 1 drop of *ferric chloride test-solution*; a violet colour is produced.

MELTING-POINT. About 228°.

ULTRAVIOLET ABSORPTION. In 0.01N sodium hydroxide, maxima at 234 nm (E1%, 1cm = 351) and 268 nm (E1%, 1cm = 89), and an inflection at 284 nm.

Determination in body fluids. GAS CHROMATOGRAPHY. In plasma or urine—M. W. Couch *et al.*, *Biochem. Med.*, 1973, **8**, 362.

Metabolism. ABSORPTION. Rapidly absorbed after oral administration.

HALF-LIFE. Determined from urinary excretion data, about 10 hours.

DISTRIBUTION. Widely distributed throughout the body.

METABOLIC REACTIONS. Possible hydrolysis to form *o*-sulfamoylbenzoic acid which has been detected in the urine of monkeys but not in man.

EXCRETION. Up to about 95% of a dose is excreted in the urine in 72 hours; about 7% is excreted as a metabolite which may be *o*-sulfamoylbenzoic acid in conjugated form or may be unchanged drug which is bound to a normal urinary constituent.

FURTHER INFORMATION. Distribution and excretion in rats—H. B. Matthews *et al.*, *J. agric. Fd Chem.*, 1973, **21**, 916; metabolism and excretion—E. W. McChesney and L. Golberg, *Fd Cosmet. Toxicol.*, 1973, **11**, 403.

Actions and uses. Saccharin is a sweetening agent. It is usually accepted as being about 550 times sweeter than sugar.

Saccharin is used as a substitute for sugar, especially in diabetes mellitus and obesity, as it has no food value. It is excreted unchanged in the urine. It is preferably used as saccharin sodium, which is more soluble and comparatively free from the unpleasant after-taste of saccharin.

Saccharin Sodium

The dihydrate of the sodium derivative of saccharin.

$C_7H_4NNaO_3S,2H_2O = 241.2$

OTHER NAME: Soluble Saccharin

A standard is given in the British Pharmacopoeia Addendum 1978

Description. A white efflorescent crystalline powder, with an intensely sweet taste, even in dilute solution; odourless or with a faintly aromatic odour.

Solubility. Soluble, at 20°, in 1.5 parts of water and in 50 parts of alcohol.

Moisture content. 3 to 15%, determined by Fischer titration.

Sterilisation. Solutions for injection are sterilised by heating in an autoclave.

Storage. It should be stored in airtight containers.

Identification. TESTS. It complies with the Tests described under Saccharin.

INFRA-RED ABSORPTION. Major peaks at 678, 750, 1120, 1154, 1260, and 1646 cm^{-1} (see Appendix 2a: Infra-red Spectra).

Determination in body fluids; Metabolism. See under Saccharin.

Actions and uses. Saccharin sodium is used for the same purposes as saccharin. The addition of about 1% of a solution containing 10% of saccharin sodium is suitable for sweetening most liquid preparations.

Saccharin sodium has been used by intravenous injection to determine circulation time; a suitable dose is 2.5 grams in 5 millilitres of water for injections.

Salaam Attacks

see under EPILEPSY

Salbutamol

1-(4-Hydroxy-3-hydroxymethylphenyl)-2-(*tert*-butylamino)ethanol

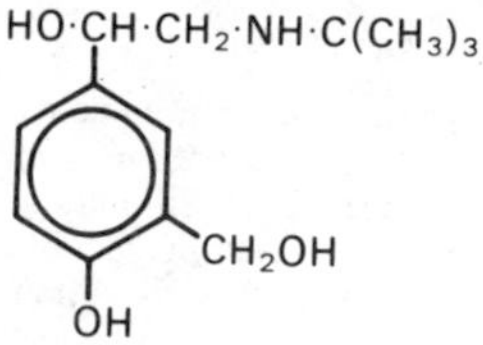

$C_{13}H_{21}NO_3 = 239.3$

OTHER NAME: *Ventolin*®

A standard is given in the British Pharmacopoeia 1973

Description. An odourless, almost tasteless, white, crystalline powder.

Solubility. Soluble, at 20°, in 70 parts of water and in 25 parts of alcohol; very slightly soluble in ether.

Storage. It should be protected from light.

Identification. TESTS. 1. Dissolve about 10 mg in 50 ml of a 2% solution of borax, add 1 ml of a 3% solution of 4-aminophenazone, 10 ml of a 2% solution of potassium ferricyanide, and 10 ml of chloroform, shake, and allow to separate; an orange-red colour develops in the chloroform layer.
2. To 2 ml of a 1% solution add 2 drops of *ferric chloride test-solution*; a reddish-orange colour is produced. Add *sodium bicarbonate solution*; the colour does not change.

MELTING-POINT. About 156°.

ULTRAVIOLET ABSORPTION. In 0.1N hydrochloric acid, maxima at 227 nm (E1%, 1cm = 323) and 278 nm (E1%, 1cm = 71). In 0.1N sodium hydroxide, maxima at 246 nm (E1%, 1cm = 469) and 297 nm (E1%, 1cm = 126).

INFRA-RED ABSORPTION. Major peaks at 1036, 1076, 1219, 1232, 1268, and 1337 cm^{-1} (see Appendix 2a: Infra-red Spectra).

Metabolism. ABSORPTION. Rapidly absorbed after oral administration and after inhalation; most of an inhaled dose is swallowed and more enters the lungs with positive intermittent breathing than by aerosol.

BLOOD CONCENTRATION. After an oral dose of 4 to 8 mg, peak plasma concentrations of about 23 ng/ml for unchanged drug and 50 to 100 ng/ml for unchanged drug plus metabolite are attained in 2.5 to 3 hours; after an inhaled dose of 80 μg, peak plasma concentrations of about 0.2 ng/ml for unchanged drug and about 1 ng/ml for drug plus metabolite are attained in about 3 hours; 2 hours after an intravenous dose of 200 μg, a plasma concentration of about 1 ng/ml is obtained for the unchanged drug and about 2 ng/ml for drug plus metabolite.

HALF-LIFE. Plasma half-life, 2 to 7 hours.

METABOLIC REACTIONS. Metabolised by first pass metabolism; the reactions and metabolites involved are not yet identified.

EXCRETION. About 75 to 95% of an oral dose is excreted in the urine and about 4% in the faeces in 3 days; after administration as an aerosol, up to 97% is excreted in the urine and up to about 11% in the faeces; after an intravenous dose about 80% is excreted in the urine and about 4% in the faeces; up to about 20% of an inhaled dose is lost in expired air and in the oral adapter; following oral administration or inhalation, 50 to 60% of the urinary excreted material is metabolised but after intravenous administration only about 27% is excreted in metabolised form.

FURTHER INFORMATION. Metabolism—M. E. Evans *et al.*, *Xenobiotica*, 1973, **3**, 113; metabolism and clinical pharmacology—S. R. Walker *et al.*, *Clin. Pharmac. Ther.*, 1972, **13**, 861.

Actions and uses. Salbutamol is a directly acting sympathomimetic amine with actions similar to those described under Isoprenaline Sulphate. Its main action, however, is on the adrenergic receptors in the bronchi and the respiratory tract rather than on the cardiac receptors. For this reason it induces bronchodilatation and inhibits bronchospasm in doses which do not produce marked cardiac acceleration. It is used in the treatment of asthma, chronic bronchitis, emphysema, and other bronchopulmonary disorders involving bronchospasm.
Salbutamol is administered as an aerosol inhalation in

doses of up to 200 micrograms 3 or 4 times daily. The usual dose for children is one inhalation of 100 micrograms 2 to 4 times daily.

Undesirable effects. Palpitations and tachycardia may occur in some patients.

Precautions and contra-indications. It is contra-indicated in patients with hypertension, myocardial insufficiency, and hyperthyroidism. The excessive use of sprays containing salbutamol should be avoided as it may lead to fatal results. Salbutamol should not be administered with non-selective beta-adrenoreceptor blocking drugs such as propranolol or oxprenolol.

Preparation

SALBUTAMOL AEROSOL INHALATION: a suspension of salbutamol, in powder of a suitable particle size, in a suitable mixture of aerosol propellents, which may contain a surface-active agent, stabilising agents, and other adjuvants. Available as an aerosol inhalation delivering 100 micrograms of salbutamol to the patient each time the valve is actuated.
A standard for this aerosol inhalation is given in the British Pharmaceutical Codex 1973
Containers, Labelling, and *Storage:* see the entry on Aerosol Inhalations for general information on containers, labelling, and storage.
Advice for patients: see the entry on Aerosol Inhalations for general information on the use of aerosol inhalations. The patient should be advised verbally to read the instructions enclosed with the product. If more than one inhalation is taken at a time at least 1 minute should elapse between the 2 inhalations and not less than 3 hours between any 2 doses. When used in conjunction with beclomethasone or another corticosteroid aerosol inhalation, salbutamol should be given first and the corticosteroid preparation used 5 minutes later. Excessive use of the preparation should be avoided.

Salbutamol Sulphate

1-(4-Hydroxy-3-hydroxymethylphenyl)-2-(*tert*-butyl-amino)ethanol hemisulphate
$C_{26}H_{44}N_2O_{10}S = 576.7$

OTHER NAME: *Ventolin®*

A standard is given in the British Pharmacopoeia 1973

Description. An odourless white powder with a slightly bitter taste.

Solubility. Soluble, at 20°, in 4 parts of water; soluble in alcohol, in ether, and in chloroform.

Storage. It should be protected from light.

Identification. TESTS. It complies with the Tests described under Salbutamol.

ULTRAVIOLET ABSORPTION. In 0.1N hydrochloric acid; maxima at 225nm (E1%, 1cm = 213) and 278 nm (E1%, 1cm = 60). In 0.1N sodium hydroxide, maxima at 245 nm (E1%, 1cm = 317) and 296 nm (E1%, 1cm = 111).

INFRA-RED ABSORPTION. Major peaks at 837, 976, 1027, 1076, 1111, and 1245 cm^{-1} (see Appendix 2a: Infra-red Spectra).

Metabolism. See under Salbutamol.

Actions and uses. Salbutamol sulphate has the actions described under Salbutamol. It is administered by mouth as tablets or as an elixir and is given in a dosage equivalent to 6 to 16 milligrams of salbutamol daily in divided doses. The usual dose for children by mouth is the equivalent of 300 micrograms of salbutamol per kilogram body-weight daily in divided doses. 1.2 milligrams of salbutamol sulphate is approximately equivalent to 1 milligram of salbutamol.

It may also be used as a respirator solution containing the equivalent of 0.5% salbutamol.

A solution for injection containing the equivalent of 50 or 500 micrograms or 1 milligram of salbutamol per millilitre is used in the treatment of severe bronchospasm or status asthmaticus. The usual dose by subcutaneous or intramuscular injection is the equivalent of 8 micrograms of salbutamol per kilogram body-weight every 4 hours, and by slow intravenous injection, 4 micrograms per kilogram body-weight, repeated as necessary.

A solution containing the equivalent of 10 micrograms of salbutamol per millilitre may be given by intravenous infusion in the treatment of status asthmaticus. The usual dose is 3 to 20 micrograms per minute. In addition, intravenous infusions of salbutamol sulphate are used in the management of uncomplicated premature labour of the third trimester. The initial dose is the equivalent of 10 micrograms of salbutamol per minute, increasing at 10-minute intervals until the strength, frequency, and duration of contraction are reduced. The infusion is maintained until contractions cease, then reduced at 6-hour intervals. Maintenance therapy may be continued thereafter with oral salbutamol as soon as is possible.

Undesirable effects. As for Salbutamol. In addition, oral administration may give rise to muscle tremors. The injection may give rise to nausea, vomiting, and headache.

Precautions and contra-indications. As for Salbutamol. In addition, parenteral salbutamol should not be administered during the first and second trimester òf pregnancy and should not be used in premature labour associated with toxaemia of pregnancy or antepartum haemorrhage.

Preparations

SALBUTAMOL TABLETS: available as tablets containing salbutamol sulphate equivalent to 2 and 4 mg of salbutamol; they may be coloured.
A standard for these tablets is given in the British Pharmacopoeia 1973
Containers and *Storage:* see the entry on Tablets for general information on containers and storage. Containers should be airtight.

OTHER PREPARATIONS available include CARTRIDGES (for use with an insufflation device) containing salbutamol sulphate equivalent to 200 and 400 micrograms of salbutamol; an ELIXIR containing salbutamol sulphate equivalent to 2 mg of salbutamol in 5 ml, diluent syrup, life of diluted elixir 14 days; an INJECTION containing salbutamol sulphate equivalent to 50 micrograms of salbutamol per ml in 5-ml ampoules, an injection containing salbutamol sulphate equivalent to 500 micrograms of salbutamol per ml in 1-ml ampoules, an injection (for intravenous infusion) containing salbutamol sulphate equivalent to 1 mg of salbutamol per ml in 5-ml ampoules; a SPRAY (for use diluted and undiluted with suitable nebulisers in respirator units) containing salbutamol sulphate equivalent to 5 mg of salbutamol per ml; and TABLETS containing salbutamol sulphate equivalent to 8 mg of salbutamol in a slow-release formulation.

Salicylic Acid

2-Hydroxybenzoic acid

$C_7H_6O_3 = 138.1$

OTHER NAME: Acidum Salicylicum

A standard is given in the European Pharmacopoeia Vol. III

Description. Almost odourless, colourless acicular crystals or white crystalline powder with a sweetish taste becoming acrid.

Solubility. Soluble, at 20°, in 550 parts of water and in 4 parts of alcohol; soluble in ether, in chloroform, and in solutions of ammonium acetate, sodium phosphate, potassium citrate, and sodium citrate.

Dissociation constants. pK_a 3.0, 13.4 (25°).

Incompatibility. It is incompatible with iron salts and with oxidising substances.

Identification. MELTING-POINT. About 160°.

ULTRAVIOLET ABSORPTION. In 0.1N sodium hydroxide, maximum at 298 nm (E1%, 1cm = 248). In alcohol (95%), maxima at 235 nm (E1%, 1cm = 450) and 303 nm (E1%, 1cm = 268).

INFRA-RED ABSORPTION. Major peaks at 756, 1209, 1240, 1292, 1441, and 1658 cm^{-1} (see Appendix 2a: Infra-red Spectra).

Actions and uses. Salicylic acid is a keratolytic substance with bacteriostatic and fungicidal properties.

It is used externally in dusting-powders, lotions, and ointments for the treatment of chronic ulcers, dandruff, and fungous infections of the skin. In the form of a paint in a collodion basis or as a plaster, it is employed to destroy warts or corns.

Preparations

AMMONIATED MERCURY, COAL TAR, AND SALICYLIC ACID OINTMENT (*Syn.* Unguentum Hydrargyri Ammoniati et Picis Carbonis cum Acido Salicylico):

Ammoniated mercury and coal tar ointment	980 g
Salicylic acid, in fine powder	20 g

Triturate the salicylic acid with a portion of the ammoniated mercury and coal tar ointment until smooth and gradually incorporate the remainder of the ointment.
A standard for this ointment is given in the British Pharmaceutical Codex 1973
Containers: See the entry on Ointments for general information on containers. Containers should prevent evaporation.
Advice for patients: the ointment should be applied sparingly to the affected area. It should not be applied to broken or inflamed skin; contact with the eyes should be avoided. Its use should be discontinued if excessive dryness or irritation occurs.

COAL TAR AND SALICYLIC ACID OINTMENT:

Prepared coal tar	20 g
Salicylic acid	20 g
Emulsifying wax	114 g
White soft paraffin	190 g
Coconut oil	540 g
Polysorbate 80	40 g
Liquid paraffin	76 g

Disperse the prepared coal tar in the polysorbate 80, incorporate the salicylic acid, and mix with the emulsifying wax, previously melted. Separately melt the white soft paraffin and the coconut oil, incorporate the liquid paraffin, warmed to the same temperature, and add, with stirring, to the other mixed ingredients. Mix thoroughly and stir until cold.

A standard for this ointment is given in the British Pharmaceutical Codex 1973

Containers: see the entry on Ointments for general information on containers.

Advice for patients: when used in scalp disorders a small amount of ointment should be rubbed gently into the roots of the hair. It should not be applied to broken or inflamed skin; contact with the eyes should be avoided. The ointment may stain skin, hair, and fabric. Its use should be discontinued if excessive dryness or irritation occurs.

SALICYLIC ACID AND MERCURIC CHLORIDE LOTION (*Syn.* Lotio Acidi Salicylici et Hydrargyri Perchloridi):

Salicylic acid	20 g
Mercuric chloride	1 g
Castor oil	10 ml
Acetone	125 ml
Alcohol (95%)	to 1000 ml

Dissolve the mercuric chloride and the salicylic acid in 500 ml of the alcohol, add the castor oil, the acetone, and sufficient of the alcohol to produce the required volume, and mix.

In making this preparation the alcohol (95%) may be replaced by industrial methylated spirit, provided that the law and the statutory regulations governing the use of industrial methylated spirit are observed.

A standard for this lotion is given in the British Pharmaceutical Codex 1973

Containers: see the entry on Lotions for general information on containers.

Labelling: see the entry on Lotions for general information on labelling. In addition, the label on the container should state "Caution. This preparation is inflammable. Do not use it or dry the hair near a fire or naked flame."

Storage: it should be stored in airtight containers, in a cool place.

Advice for patients: a small amount of the lotion should be rubbed gently into the roots of the hair and allowed to dry without the aid of heat. It should not be applied to broken or inflamed skin; contact with the eyes should be avoided. The lotion should be kept in the original container and contact with metals should be avoided.

SALICYLIC ACID AND SULPHUR CREAM (*Syn.* Salicylic Acid and Sulphur Application):

Salicylic acid, finely sifted	20 g
Precipitated sulphur, finely sifted	20 g
Aqueous cream	960 g

Triturate the salicylic acid and the sulphur with a portion of the aqueous cream until smooth and gradually add the remainder of the aqueous cream.

A standard for this cream is given in the British Pharmaceutical Codex 1973

Containers, Labelling, and *Storage:* see the entry on Creams for general information on containers, labelling, and storage.

Advice for patients: when used in scalp disorders a small amount of cream should be rubbed gently into the roots of the hair. When used in skin disorders, the cream should be applied sparingly to the affected area. It should not be applied to broken or inflamed skin; contact with the eyes should be avoided. Prolonged use should be avoided and treatment should be discontinued if excessive dryness or irritation occurs.

SALICYLIC ACID AND SULPHUR OINTMENT:

Salicylic acid, finely sifted	30 g
Precipitated sulphur, finely sifted	30 g
Oily cream	940 g

Triturate the salicylic acid and the precipitated sulphur with a portion of the oily cream until smooth and gradually incorporate the remainder of the oily cream.

A standard for this ointment is given in the British Pharmaceutical Codex 1973

Containers: see the entry on Ointments for general information on containers. Containers should prevent evaporation.

Advice for patients: the ointment should be applied sparingly to the affected area. It should not be applied to broken or inflamed skin; contact with the eyes should be avoided. Prolonged use should be avoided and treatment should be discontinued if excessive dryness or irritation occurs.

SALICYLIC ACID COLLODION:

Salicylic acid	120 g
Flexible collodion	to 1000 ml

A standard for this collodion is given in the British Pharmaceutical Codex 1973

Containers and *Storage:* it should be supplied in small coloured fluted glass bottles or jars with airtight closures and stored in a cool place.

Labelling: it should be labelled "For external use only".

Advice for patients: the collodion should be painted on to the wart or corn and allowed to dry. Contact with normal skin should be avoided. Care should be taken to keep well away from a naked flame while the collodion is being applied.

SALICYLIC ACID LOTION:

Salicylic acid	20 g
Castor oil	10 ml
Alcohol (95%)	to 1000 ml

Dissolve the salicylic acid in a portion of the alcohol, add the castor oil and sufficient of the alcohol to produce the required volume, and mix.

In making this preparation the alcohol (95%) may be replaced by industrial methylated spirit, provided that the law and the statutory regulations governing the use of industrial methylated spirit are observed.

A standard for this lotion is given in the British Pharmaceutical Codex 1973

Containers: see the entry on Lotions for general information on containers.

Labelling: see the entry on Lotions for general information on labelling. In addition, the label on the container should state "Caution. This preparation is inflammable. Do not use it or dry the hair near a fire or naked flame".

Advice for patients: a small amount of the lotion should be rubbed gently into the roots of the hair and allowed to dry without the aid of heat. It should not be applied to broken or inflamed skin; contact with the eyes should be avoided.

SALICYLIC ACID OINTMENT (*Syn.* Ung. Acid. Salicyl.):

Salicylic acid, finely sifted	..	..	20 g
Wool alcohols ointment ..	..	..	980 g

Melt the wool alcohols ointment, incorporate the salicylic acid, and stir until cold.

A standard for this ointment is given in the British Pharmacopoeia 1973

Containers: see the entry on Ointments for general information on containers.

Advice for patients: the ointment should be applied sparingly to the affected area. It should not be applied to broken or inflamed skin; contact with the eyes should be avoided. Prolonged use should be avoided and treatment should be discontinued if excessive dryness or irritation occurs.

ZINC AND SALICYLIC ACID PASTE (*Syn.* Lassar's paste):

Salicylic acid, finely sifted	..	..	20 g
Starch, finely sifted	..	..	240 g
Zinc oxide, finely sifted ..	..	..	240 g
White soft paraffin	..	..	500 g

Melt the white soft paraffin, incorporate the salicylic acid, the starch, and the zinc oxide, and stir until cold.

A standard for this paste is given in the British Pharmacopoeia 1973

Containers and *Storage:* see the entry on Pastes for general information on containers and storage.

Advice for patients: the paste should be applied liberally to the affected area. It should not be applied to broken or inflamed skin; contact with the eyes should be avoided. Prolonged use should be avoided and treatment should be discontinued if excessive dryness or irritation occurs.

OTHER PREPARATIONS: salicylic acid is an ingredient of compound benzoic acid ointment and of a number of other compound preparations.

Salmonella Infections

Typhoid Fever

Typhoid fever is an acute infectious disease due to *Salmonella typhi* and is characterised by high fever, abdominal pain and distension, constipation and later diarrhoea, splenomegaly, bradycardia, and the eruption of rose-coloured spots. Man is the only reservoir of infection and transmission occurs directly or indirectly by the faecal-oral route. The organisms pass through the mucous membrane of the gut and multiply in the mesenteric lymph nodes. Organisms are transported in the bloodstream to the liver, spleen, and other organs where they multiply further. Further bacteraemia distributes the organisms throughout the body and intestinal symptoms occur when the Peyer's patches of the small intestine are invaded. Hyperplasia and oedema of the Peyer's patches result in vascular obstruction, necrosis of the covering mucous membrane, and the formation of ulcers. Associated with ulceration is the risk of perforation of the bowel and of intestinal haemorrhage. The ulcers heal by scarring.

There is an incubation period of 10 to 14 days before the onset of symptoms which start gradually as a general malaise and lethargy and are followed by splenomegaly, rose-coloured spots, and fever. In the third week after onset of the disease either the symptoms begin to resolve or the patient is profoundly toxaemic with prostration, semiconsciousness, dehydration, and cyanosis. In the latter case recovery is unusual.

Typhoid fever is treated with a suitable antibacterial such as chloramphenicol, ampicillin, or co-trimoxazole. Corticosteroids may also be given to the severely-ill patient whose condition may improve greatly although theoretically there is an increased risk of gastro-intestinal perforation. Some patients have a relapse about 10 days after the cessation of specific treatment. A minority of patients develop a chronic carrier state with the intermittent excretion of *S. typhi* in the faeces or urine. The carrier state may not be susceptible to treatment with antibacterials (of which long-term high-dose ampicillin has been most effective). The residue of infection is usually in the gall bladder and cholecystectomy may be necessary.

Typhoid vaccine may be used to immunise travellers against typhoid infections.

Paratyphoid Fever

Paratyphoid fever is an acute infectious disease due to the Gram-negative bacillus *Salmonella paratyphi* A, B, or C. It has characteristics similar to those of typhoid fever but is usually milder and of shorter duration. It may be acute or insidious in onset and abdominal pain is more prominent than in typhoid fever. Severe headache may also occur. Without specific therapy the illness runs a 3- to 4-week course and although complications similar to those of typhoid fever may occur, they are uncommon. Treatment is the same as for typhoid fever.

Other Salmonella Infections

A large number of other species of *Salmonella* are pathogenic to man and cause an acute febrile gastro-intestinal illness accompanied by the passage of frequent stools. The whole gastro-intestinal tract is involved, the mucosa is hyperaemic, and Peyer's patches are prominent, although ulceration occurs only with severe infections. There is an incubation period of 12 to 24 hours followed by headache, malaise, nausea, vomiting, and diarrhoea. Abdominal pain occurs and may be severe; it is usually relieved by the passing of bowel motions. Dehydration is liable to occur and if severe may lead to a fall in urinary output, pre-renal uraemia, and ketosis, which leads to further nausea and vomiting.

The most important treatment in salmonella infections is adequate fluid and electrolyte replacement by mouth or, in severely dehydrated patients, by intravenous infusion. Antibiotics should be avoided as they do not shorten the illness and also hinder the elimination of organisms during convalescence, but in certain patients at risk of septicaemia, for example in neonates, elderly patients, and those with sickle-cell disease or immuno-deficiency states, antibiotics should be given. Treatment should be the same as that described under Typhoid Fever (above), using chloramphenicol or ampicillin; co-trimoxazole may also be used.

Sarcoma

see under NEOPLASTIC DISEASE

Sarcoma, Giant Follicular

see under LYMPHOPROLIFERATIVE DISEASE

Scabies

Scabies is an infection by the mite *Sarcoptes scabiei* which burrows through the skin and is spread by bodily contact. It causes an intense allergic itching beginning about one month after the initial infection.

Treatment consists of the application of an acaricidal preparation to the whole of the body surface. Preparations of benzyl benzoate, crotamiton, and gamma benzene hexachloride may be used. The application is usually repeated after 24 hours, and the residue is removed by washing on the following day. Contacts should be similarly treated. Secondary bacterial infections introduced by scratching in response to itching may require treatment with an antibiotic. The itch may persist for several weeks after treatment.

Schick Control

Schick test toxin that has been heated at 70° to 85° for not less than five minutes in order to destroy the specific toxin. Schick control is prepared from the same batch of Schick test toxin as that with which it is issued for use.

A standard is given in the European Pharmacopoeia Vol. III Supplement

Storage. As for Schick Test Toxin.

Actions and uses. Schick control is used in the Schick test to distinguish between the true Schick-positive reaction, due to the absence of diphtheria antitoxin in the blood, and a pseudo-reaction, due to susceptibility to non-specific substances.

Schick Test Toxin

A sterile filtrate from a culture in nutrient broth of *Corynebacterium diphtheriae* which, after being allowed to mature, is diluted so that the test dose is contained in 0.1 to 0.2 millilitre. To ensure stability the diluent is borate-boric acid buffer solution in saline isotonic with blood and containing a suitable bactericide.

OTHER NAME: Toxinum Diphthericum Diagnosticum

A standard is given in the European Pharmacopoeia Vol. III Supplement

Storage. Schick Test Toxin prepared with borate–boric acid buffer solution in saline and stored below 25° may be expected to retain its potency for 2 months; when stored at 2° to 8° it may be expected to retain its potency for 6 months when packed in containers of not more than 0.25 ml (individual dose) and for 2 years when packed into containers of not less than 1.5 ml.

Actions and uses. Schick test toxin is a reagent employed for the diagnosis of susceptibility to diphtheria. It is used in the Schick test, which consists in the intracutaneous injection of a specified amount of diphtheria toxin, known as the Schick dose; administration is followed by reactions which are readily recognised and can be used as a test for the presence or absence of a certain amount of diphtheria antitoxin.

The flexor surface of the forearms is a convenient site for the Schick test. The skin is first cleansed with alcohol, which is allowed to dry, or with soap and water, and 0.2 millilitre of Schick test toxin is then injected intracutaneously into the left arm, while 0.2 millilitre of Schick Control is injected intracutaneously into the right arm. The reactions to these injections may be read after an interval of 24 to 48 hours, although 5 to 7 days are necessary to detect late reactors and to reconsider earlier doubtful readings.

If it is possible to take a reading on only one occasion, this should be done not earlier than the fourth day and not later than the seventh. In most cases any pseudo-reaction will have subsided by this time.

The reactions which can be distinguished in the test are as follows:

A *positive* Schick reaction, indicating that the patient is susceptible to diphtheria, is shown by a red flush about 10 to 15 millimetres in diameter in the skin at the site of administration on the test arm, but no reaction on the control arm. The reaction fades slowly during the second week after injection, showing superficial desquamation and brown pigmentation.

A *negative* Schick reaction, indicating that the patient is immune to diphtheria, is one in which there is no redness on either arm.

A *negative-and-pseudo* Schick reaction, or "pseudo-reaction", indicating that the patient is immune to diphtheria, is shown by a flush which develops rapidly in 24 hours, equally or nearly equally, on each arm. It is less circumscribed than the positive reaction, fades more rapidly, and may leave some pigmentation but little or no desquamation. It is produced in some immune patients, particularly children over 10 years of age and adults, who are sensitive to constituents of the test material other than the specific toxin.

A *combined* or *positive-and-pseudo* Schick reaction, indicating that the patient is susceptible to diphtheria, is one in which a pseudo-reaction develops rapidly on both arms, but as this fades the positive reaction develops on the test arm. In this way, the test arm tends to acquire the characters of a true positive reaction, while the reaction on the control arm is fading.

All doubtful reactors should be regarded as positive, except well-marked pseudo-reactors, who are almost invariably immune. The latter are usually older children and adults who have been exposed to diphtheria infection; the exposures which have sensitised them have presumably led also to the development of specific antitoxin.

Infants born of immune mothers have an inherited immunity for the first few months of life; they do not respond very well to the vaccine on account of interference from the passive antitoxin.

Children between the ages of 6 months and 10 years who have not been given diphtheria toxoid are mostly Schick-positive and the Schick test is not considered essential for children up to 8 to 10 years old.

Above 10 years of age the state of immunity varies greatly and the test should always be performed.

Schistosomiasis

Schistosomiasis (Bilharziasis) is a chronic parasitic infection caused by trematodes of the genus *Schistosoma* which occur in certain tropical and subtropical regions. All types of infection give rise to a similar initial syndrome which is characterised by skin irritation as larvae pass through the skin, and a transient papular rash, followed by fever, cough, liver enlargement and tenderness, splenomegaly, and urticaria. Thereafter infection with *S. haematobium* is localised in the bladder and is characterised by frequency of micturition, dysuria, haematuria, ureteral obstruction, hydronephrosis, and calcification of the bladder; it may lead to squamous cell carcinoma of the bladder.

Infection with *S. mansoni* is localised in the inferior mesenteric vein and is sometimes asymptomatic but may result in the formation of granulomatous polyps of the large intestine accompanied by the appearance of blood in the faeces, iron-deficiency anaemia, and liver fibrosis with portal hypertension; it may also cause granulomatous lesions elsewhere in the body, for example in the spinal cord.

Infection with *S. japonicum* is localised in the superior and inferior mesenteric veins and results in chronic ill health with enlargement of the liver, fever, upper abdominal pain, cough, dyspnoea, urticaria, diarrhoea, and hepatic fibrosis. It may also cause cerebral granulomata resulting in encephalitis or epilepsy.

Infection is acquired by wading in or drinking fresh water containing larvae that have matured in snails that act as the intermediate host; the snails acquire their infection from the numerous eggs that are voided in the faeces and urine of infected human subjects.

Drug treatment may be used to kill the infecting schistosomes and thus eliminate eggs from the excreta. Control measures include treatment of infected persons, sanitation, provision of safe drinking water, prohibition of bathing in infected areas, and elimination of the host snails by means of molluscicides such as copper salts or sodium pentachlorophenate.

Drugs used in the treatment of schistosomiasis include antimony sodium tartrate and niridazole; lucanthone, sodium antimonylgluconate, and stibocaptate are also used.

Schizophrenia

see under PSYCHOSES

Sciatica

Sciatica is severe pain experienced along the course and distribution of the sciatic nerve, that is in the buttocks, back of thigh and calf, and outer side of the calf and foot. It is usually due to a prolapsed lower lumbar intervertebral disk causing irritation and compression of one or more nerve roots of the cauda equina. There is often a history of injury to the back from lifting weights or sudden movement. The pain usually begins in the small of the back (lumbago) and extends along the course of the sciatic nerve. The pain is severe and aggravated by stooping, coughing or turning in bed. After several weeks the pain usually subsides without operative removal of the protruding mass. Until then analgesics should be given. If pain does not subside or the patient's work is too heavy, the protruding mass should be removed surgically.

Sciatic pain may also be referred from other structures within the nerve distribution of the spinal segments from which the sciatic nerve arises, for example arthritis of the hip or sacroiliac joints. This pain is usually abolished by cure of the primary disease process.

Scleroderma

see SYSTEMIC SCLEROSIS

Scorpion Venom Antiserum

A preparation containing the specific globulins or their derivatives that neutralise the activity of the venom of one or more types of scorpion.

OTHER NAME: Antiscorpion Serum

A standard is given in the British Pharmacopoeia Addendum 1978

Storage. It should be protected from light and stored at 2° to 8°. It should not be allowed to freeze.

Actions and uses. Scorpions are widespread in tropical and subtropical areas and their venoms vary in potency and toxicity. *Buthus occitanus* occurs widely in North Africa, the Middle East, and some parts of Southern Europe, *B. maurus* occurs in the Sudan, *B. judaicus* in Syria, Turkey, and Iran, and *B. tamulus* in India; *Leiurus quinquestriatus* is common in Egypt, the Sudan, and the Middle East; *Androctonus australis* occurs in North West Africa and *A. crassicauda* in Turkey and Syria; various species of *Palamneus* are found in India. The venom of Central and South American scorpions is much more potent and toxic and is frequently lethal. The most important are *Tityus* and *Centruroides* species.

Some of the venoms of scorpions are antigenically similar and antisera produced against these may neutralise the venoms of several different species of scorpions.

The intensity of pain caused by a scorpion sting varies according to the site of sting, the species of scorpion, and the amount of venom injected. The pain may last for between 6 and 48 hours but is usually intense for the first 6 to 10 hours and rigors, sweating, and symptoms of shock are very common. The sting is not usually fatal in the African and Middle East areas but children and debilitated people may die; death frequently results from the sting of South and Central American scorpions.

An antiserum suitable for the species of scorpion prevalent in the area can prevent the symptoms and reduce the pain in a short time.

The quantity stated on the label as the dose is injected into or around the site of the sting or intramuscularly into a suitable proximal position.

Serum Reactions. See under Antisera.

Scurvy

Scurvy is due to a deficiency of ascorbic acid. It is characterised by a tendency to haemorrhage caused by an inability to form adequate amounts of intercellular material. In adults the onset is usually insidious and is marked by pallor and lassitude. The usual signs are subcutaneous ecchymoses, ulceration and haemorrhage of the gums, anaemia, debility, and failure of wounds to heal. In infants subperiosteal haemorrhage and pain and tenderness of the legs may occur.

Treatment is described under Ascorbic Acid.

Secbutobarbitone

5-*sec*-Butyl-5-ethylbarbituric acid

$C_{10}H_{16}N_2O_3 = 212.2$

OTHER NAME: Butabarbital

A standard is given in the British Pharmacopoeia 1973

Description. An odourless, fine, white, microcrystalline powder with a bitter taste.

Solubility. Soluble, at 20°, in 1400 parts of water, in 12 parts of alcohol, in 30 parts of chloroform, and in 30 parts of ether; soluble in aqueous solutions of alkali hydroxides and carbonates.

Dissociation constant. pK_a 8.0 (20°).

Stability; Incompatibility. See under Barbiturates.

Identification. TESTS. It complies with general tests 1 and 3 described under Barbiturates.

MELTING-POINT. About 166°.

ULTRAVIOLET ABSORPTION. See under Barbiturates.

INFRA-RED ABSORPTION. Major peaks at 1299, 1316, 1370, 1408, 1667, and 1754 cm^{-1} (see Appendix 2b: Infra-red Spectra).

Determination in body fluids. See under Barbiturates.

Metabolism. (See also under Barbiturates).

METABOLIC REACTIONS. Rapidly metabolised by ω- and $(\omega-1)$-oxidation of the methylpropyl side chain.

EXCRETION. About 40 to 60% of a dose is excreted in the urine, 5 to 9% as unchanged drug, 30% as 5-(2-carboxy-1-methylethyl)-5-ethylbarbituric acid, 3% as 2'-hydroxysecbutobarbitone, and 1% as 2'-oxosecbutobarbitone; larger amounts of unchanged drug may be excreted after excessive doses.

FURTHER INFORMATION. Metabolism—J. N. T. Gilbert et al., *J. Pharm. Pharmac.*, 1975, **27**, 923.

Actions and uses. Secbutobarbitone is an intermediate-acting barbiturate, the actions and uses of which are described under Barbiturates. The usual dose is 100 to 200 milligrams.

Undesirable effects; Precautions; Contra-indications; Dependence; Poisoning. See under Barbiturates.

Selenium Sulphide

$SeS_2 = 143.1$

OTHER NAMES: *Lenium*®; *Seleen*®; *Selsun*®

A standard is given in the British Pharmaceutical Codex 1973

Description. A bright orange to reddish-brown powder with a faint odour of hydrogen sulphide.

Solubility. Practically insoluble in water and in organic solvents.

Actions and uses. Selenium sulphide, although highly toxic if taken by mouth, is absorbed only in traces when applied to the skin, and is used as an application or cream, containing 2.5% in suspension, in the control of dandruff and seborrhoeic dermatitis of the scalp.

After the hair has been washed and rinsed, 5 to 10 millilitres of the application should be applied to the scalp together with a small volume of warm water to produce a lather. After rinsing, a second treatment should be made so that the time of exposure of the scalp to the action of the selenium sulphide is at least 5 minutes. The hair should then be thoroughly rinsed and all traces of the suspension removed from the hands and the finger nails. The application should be used twice a week, later once a week, and then less often as the condition is controlled.

Undesirable effects. Loss of hair has been reported from repeated use of selenium sulphide on the hair.

Precautions. Selenium sulphide should not be applied to inflamed or weeping areas because of the risk of cutaneous absorption. Care should be taken that it does not enter the conjunctival sac as it may cause keratitis and conjunctivitis.

Poisoning. Vomiting, anorexia, anaemia, and fatty degeneration of the liver may follow the ingestion of selenium sulphide.

The stomach should be emptied, a saline purgative such as sodium or magnesium sulphate should be given, and symptomatic treatment may be given as appropriate, but dimercaprol and disodium edetate should not be used.

Preparations

SELENIUM SULPHIDE SCALP APPLICATION (*Syn.* Selenium Sulphide Application): a suspension of selenium sulphide in a suitable liquid basis. Available as an application containing 2.5% of selenium sulphide and as an application for veterinary use containing 1% of selenium sulphide.

A standard for this application is given in the British Pharmaceutical Codex 1973

Containers: see the entry on Applications for general information on containers.

Labelling: the words "For external use only" and a direction to shake the bottle should be given on the label. In addition, the label on the container should state the directions for using the preparation, that the preparation should be kept away from the eyes, that the preparation should not be used within 2 days of the application of hair tints or permanent waving solutions, that the preparation should not be allowed to come into contact with metals, that all silver jewellery, hairpins, and other metal objects should be removed whilst using the preparation, and that the hands should be carefully washed after using the preparation.

Advice for patients: the hair should be washed with a bland soap (synthetic detergents should be avoided) and thoroughly rinsed prior to application. 5 to 10 millilitres of the preparation, with a little warm water should be rubbed into the hair and the roots of the hair; a lather is produced. The lather should be left on the hair for 2 to 3 minutes, rinsed, and the preparation applied for a second time. The hair should then be thoroughly rinsed or yellow or orange discoloration of fair hair may occur. The hands and fingernails should be carefully washed after using the preparation. See also under Labelling (above).

OTHER PREPARATIONS available include a CREAM containing selenium sulphide 2.5%.

L-Selenomethionine (^{75}Se) Injection

A sterile solution of L-selenomethionine (^{75}Se).

A standard is given in the British Pharmacopoeia 1973

CAUTION. *This material is radioactive and any regulations in force must be complied with*

Selenium-75 is a radioactive isotope of selenium which decays by electron capture with emission of γ-radiation mainly of energy 0.265 and 0.136 MeV. It has a half-life of 120 days. It may be prepared by neutron irradiation of natural selenium or selenium enriched in selenium-74. L-Selenomethionine (^{75}Se) may be prepared either by chemical synthesis or by the growth of certain micro-organisms in a medium containing selenite ion (^{75}Se).

Description. A clear colourless or faintly yellow liquid.

Acidity or alkalinity. pH 6 to 8.

Sterilisation. It is sterilised by heating in an autoclave.

Storage. It should be stored in an area assigned for the purpose. The storage conditions should be such that the maximum radiation-dose-rate to which persons may be exposed is reduced to an acceptable level. Glass containers may darken under the effects of radiation.

Labelling. The label of the container should state:
(1) the content of selenium-75 expressed in microcuries or millicuries at a given date,
(2) the volume of the injection,
(3) that the injection is radioactive, and
(4) either that the injection does not contain a bactericide or the name and proportion of any added bactericide.

Actions and uses. Selenomethionine (^{75}Se) is an amino acid in which a selenium-75 atom replaces a sulphur atom. Although it does not occur in nature it is metabolised similarly to methionine. The usual dose is 300 microcuries by intravenous injection. Its uptake and distribution in the body may be determined by scintiscanning or the use of the gamma-ray camera.
Scanning may be used in the detection of space-occupying lesions of the pancreas and in the investigation of pancreatitis. Since much larger amounts of selenomethionine are taken up by the liver and sometimes the spleen, special scanning techniques have been devised for examination of the pancreas. Special techniques are also available for the localisation of adenomata of the parathyroid.

Senega

The dried rootstock and root of *Polygala senega* L. or *P. senega* var. *latifolia* Torr. et Gray (Fam. Polygalaceae), a perennial herbaceous plant indigenous to southern Canada and the United States of America; it is also cultivated in Japan. Commercial supplies come mainly from Canada or Japan.

OTHER NAME: Senega Root

A standard is given in the British Pharmaceutical Codex 1973

Varieties. Canadian senega usually consists of a rootstock 10 to 40 mm wide, from which arises a tapering tap root, 3 to 6 mm in diameter, which frequently divides into two or more branches.
Japanese senega is obtained from young plants and is much smaller and more slender than the Canadian variety; it is paler in colour and the branched root bears numerous fine fibrous rootlets which form a tangled mass.

Constituents. Senega contains the saponin senegin which on hydrolysis with mineral acid yields 2 sapogenins, but on enzyme hydrolysis yields one sapogenin, praesenegin. The sugar components are less well known. It yields about 5% of ash, up to 3% of acid-insoluble ash, and up to 8% of sulphated ash; up to 2% of foreign organic matter and up to 2% of stems may be present.

Description. UNGROUND DRUG. *Macroscopical characters:* rootstock knotty, up to about 40 mm wide, bearing the remains of slender aerial stems and buds with purplish scale leaves, and a descending tap root, about 40 to 200 mm long and 2 to 6 mm wide just below the rootstock; tap root yellowish-brown, longitudinally or transversely wrinkled, usually tortuous with rather angular bends, on the concave side of which may occasionally be seen a distinct keel following a rapidly descending spiral; root bearing one or more spreading lateral roots and, in the Japanese variety, numerous fibrous rootlets about 0.5 to 2 mm thick and 40 to 100 mm long; fracture short and splintery in the wood, smooth in the bark; smoothed, transversely cut surface showing a thin layer of cork, a light brown bark, and a central whitish xylem traversed by almost imperceptible medullary rays; anomalous secondary thickening occurring, resulting in increased development of phloem in the keel region (where present) and in formation in the xylem of one or sometimes two wedge-shaped parenchymatous medullary rays with their apices adjacent to the primary xylem.
The drug imparts to water the property of frothing.
It has a characteristic odour, recalling that of wintergreen, and a taste which is sweetish at first becoming acrid.

Microscopical characters: the diagnostic characters are: root: *cork* of about 2 to 6 layers of yellowish-brown tabular cells; parenchyma containing droplets of *oil* but no *starch*; *xylem* consisting of numerous *tracheids* with pitted walls and fewer small *vessels*, with reticulately thickened or pitted walls, up to 65 μm in diameter and often with lateral perforations; primary xylem diarch; *fibres*, *sclereids*, and *crystals* absent.
Stem: *epidermis* of elongated subrectangular cells; *cortex* parenchymatous; *pericyclic fibres* unlignified, in a band; *phloem* of slender elements; *xylem* containing *tracheids* with pitted walls and *vessels* with pitted or reticulately or spirally thickened walls; *pith* parenchymatous.
Scale leaves: ovate, blunt, about 2 to 3 mm long, shortly ciliate with blunt unicellular *trichomes*, up to 115 μm long, often curved at the tip, walls striated, tip filled with a refractive deposit; *epidermal cells* with sinuous anticlinal walls; *stomata* anomocytic.

POWDERED DRUG. Powdered Senega. A grey powder possessing the diagnostic microscopical characters, odour, and taste of the unground drug. The powder is very irritating to the mucous membranes of the nose and throat.

Adulterants and substitutes. Indian or Pakistan senega consists of the roots of *Andrachne aspera* (L.) Spreng. (Fam. Euphorbiaceae), which are contorted, with 2 or 3 longitudinal ridges but no keel, a reddish-brown bark, and a normal whitish wood with up to 3 or 4 growth rings; fragments of the bark warmed with water acquire a reddish tint, whereas similar fragments of senega acquire a yellowish tint, similar delicate tints being imparted to the water; odourless.
Another Indian senega consists of the roots of *Glinus oppositifolius* (L.) A.DC. (Fam. Aizoaceae), the transversely cut surface of which shows a series of concentric rings of vascular tissue.

Actions and uses. The actions of senega are attributed to its saponin constituents, which, although not absorbed, are irritant to the gastric mucosa and give rise to a reflex secretion of mucus in the bronchioles.
Senega has been employed, usually with other expectorants, in the treatment of chronic bronchitis.

Senna Fruit

The dried fruits of *Cassia senna* L. (*C. acutifolia* Delile; *C. angustifolia* Vahl.) (Fam. Leguminosae), known in commerce as Alexandrian or Khartoum senna, which is indigenous to and cultivated in the Sudan, or Tinnevelly senna, which is cultivated largely in Southern India.

Small quantities of the fruits of both varieties are also exported from Eritrea.

OTHER NAMES: Alexandrian Senna Pods; *Bidrolar®*; Sennae Fructus; Sennae Fructus Acutifoliae; Sennae Fructus Angustifoliae; *Senokot®*; Tinnevelly Senna Pods; *X-Prep Liquid®*
Agiolax® (with ispaghula); *Pripsen®* (with piperazine phosphate)
A standard is given in the European Pharmacopoeia Vol. I

Varieties. Alexandrian senna pods are pale to greenish-brown, with a brown central zone where the positions of the seeds are indicated by slight swellings. The width of the pod varies from 20 to 25 mm. Tinnevelly senna pods are usually darker, slightly narrower (not more than 18 mm wide), and somewhat straighter than the Alexandrian, and the remains of the base of the style are usually more pronounced.
The testa of the seeds of Alexandrian senna is reticulately wrinkled and that of Tinnevelly seeds has transverse ridges.

Constituents. Senna fruit contains active constituents similar to those of the leaf. Commercial samples of Alexandrian pods contain about 2.5 to 4.5% of sennosides A and B [glucosides of stereoisomers of rhein dianthrone, 10,10'-bis(9,10-dihydro-1,8-dihydroxy-9-oxoanthracene-3-carboxylic acid)]; Tinnevelly pods contain about 1.2 to 2.5%.
Smaller quantities of the following anthraquinone glycosides are also present: sennosides C and D, based on the heterodianthrones of rhein and aloe-emodin [9,10-dihydro-10-(9,10-dihydro-1,8-dihydroxy-3-hydroxymethyl-9-oxoanthr-10-yl)-1,8-dihydroxy-9-oxoanthracene-3-carboxylic acid], rhein anthrone 8-glucoside, rhein 8-glucoside, rhein 8-diglucoside, aloe-emodin 8-glucoside, and aloe-emodin anthrone diglucoside.
Alexandrian senna pods yield to water about 35 to 40% of extractive, and Tinnevelly pods about 18 to 35%.
Up to 1% of foreign matter may be present and it may yield up to 6% of sulphated ash and up to 2% of acid-insoluble ash.

Description. UNGROUND DRUG. *Macroscopical characters:* fruit rounded-oblong to slightly reniform in shape, pale green to greenish-brown, texture parchment-like, laterally flattened, about 40 to 50 mm long and up to 25 mm wide; apex rounded, with a slightly projecting point formed by the base of the style; base cuspidate or shortly stalked; each pod containing about 6 to 7 flat obovate-cuneate hard seeds, about 5 to 6 mm long, having a wrinkled whitish-green surface and a short raised ridge on each side at the pointed end.
Average weight of a single senna pod is about 160 mg. It has a slight odour and taste.

Microscopical characters: the diagnostic characters are: pericarp: *epidermal cells* isodiametric, with thick outer walls; *stomata* occasional, paracytic or anomocytic; *trichomes* unicellular, warty; *endocarp* fibrous, *fibres* 5 to 7 μm wide and 0.5 to 1.4 mm long, in 2 to 4 layers crossing one another obliquely; walls thick, lignified; *mesocarp* parenchymatous, innermost layer, in contact with endocarp, with many cells containing a single prismatic *crystal* of calcium oxalate about 7 to 10 μm long; *vascular strands* of sutures each surrounded by a *crystal sheath* with prisms of calcium oxalate.
Seed coat: *epidermis* of small cells, *cuticle* thick, mucilaginous; *hypodermis* of palisade cellulosic *sclereids* followed to inner side by a layer of cells shaped like

inverted mushrooms, anticlinal walls of cells thickened, giving a horseshoe-shaped outline to intercellular spaces as seen in transverse section; these cells followed to inner side by parenchyma and then a similar layer of upright mushroom-shaped cells; *endosperm* composed of polyhedral cells with thick mucilaginous walls; *embryo* consisting of thin-walled tissue.

Adulterants and substitutes. Italian or dog senna pods, derived from *Cassia italica* (Mill.) Lam. ex F. W. Andr. (*Cassia obovata* Collad.), are about 35 to 55 mm long and 15 mm broad; they are reniform and strongly curved with rounded ends and contain about 8 to 10 seeds, the pericarp having a small crescent-shaped ridge over each seed.

Storage. Senna fruit should be protected from light.

Identification. TEST. It complies with the test given under Senna Leaf.

Actions and uses. Senna fruit is an anthraquinone purgative. The glycosides are absorbed from the intestinal tract and the active anthraquinones liberated in the course of their breakdown are excreted into the colon, which they then stimulate; the stomach and small intestine are not normally affected. As purgation occurs eight to ten hours after administration, senna preparations should preferably be given at bedtime.
The usual dose for an adult is 0.5 to 2 grams; children may be given half of the dose for an adult. Senna fruit was formerly administered in the form of an infusion, 4 to 12 pods being soaked in about 140 ml (5 fluid ounces) of warm water for about 12 hours. It has been largely replaced by standardised senna preparations.
Some of the anthraquinones are excreted by the kidneys, and the urine of patients taking senna preparations may acquire a marked yellow colour, which changes to red on the addition of an alkali. These compounds may also appear in other secretions, notably in the milk.

Preparations
SENNA LIQUID EXTRACT:
Small-scale preparation

Senna fruit, crushed	..	..	..	1000 g
Coriander oil	..	..	..	6 ml
Alcohol (90%)	..	..	..	250 ml
Chloroform water ..	..	..	a sufficient quantity
Purified water, freshly boiled and cooled	..	..	a sufficient quantity

Macerate the senna fruit in 5000 ml of the chloroform water for 8 hours, decant the clear liquid, and strain; repeat the process twice, using 2000 ml of the chloroform water for each maceration. Lightly press the marc, strain the expressed liquid, and mix it with the previously decanted liquids. Heat the liquid in a covered vessel for 3 minutes at 80°, allow to stand for 24 hours, and filter. Evaporate the filtrate to 750 ml under reduced pressure at a temperature not exceeding 60°, add the coriander oil dissolved in the alcohol and sufficient of the water to produce 1000 ml, allow to stand for not less than 24 hours, and filter.
Manufacture. Prepare the extract by the above method, appropriately scaled up.
A standard for this extract is given in the British Pharmaceutical Codex 1973
Dose: 0.5 to 2 millilitres.

SENNA TABLETS: available as tablets containing the powdered pericarp of senna fruit equivalent to 7.5 mg of total sennosides, calculated as sennoside B.

A standard for these tablets is given in the British Pharmacopoeia 1973

Containers and *Storage:* see the entry on Tablets for general information on containers and storage. Containers should be airtight.

Labelling: the label on the container should state the amount of the medicament in terms of total sennosides.

Advice for patients: the tablets should not be used for longer than a few days without medical advice. The urine may be coloured red.

OTHER PREPARATIONS available include an ELIXIR containing a biologically standardised extract of senna equivalent to 15 mg of sennosides A and B in 5 ml; an elixir containing a standardised preparation of senna equivalent to 7.5 mg of sennosides A and B, calculated as sennoside B, in 5 ml, diluent syrup, life of diluted elixir 14 days; an elixir containing a standardised extract of senna fruit equivalent to 142 mg of sennosides A and B, calculated as sennoside B, in 71 ml (single dose); GRANULES containing a standardised preparation of senna fruit equivalent to 5.5 mg of sennosides A and B, calculated as sennoside B, per g; granules containing senna fruit (Tinnevelly) 124 mg with ispaghula 542 mg per g; and a POWDER containing a standardised preparation of senna fruit equivalent to 15.3 mg of total sennosides, calculated as sennoside B, with piperazine phosphate 4 g in each 10-g sachet.

Senna liquid extract is an ingredient of compound figs syrup.

Senna Leaf

The dried leaflets of the paripinnate leaves of *Cassia senna* L. (*C. acutifolia* Delile; *C. angustifolia* Vahl.) (Fam. Leguminosae), known in commerce as Alexandrian or Khartoum senna, which is indigenous to and cultivated in the Sudan, or Tinnevelly senna, which is cultivated largely in Southern India. Small quantities of the leaflets of both varieties are also exported from Eritrea.

OTHER NAME: Sennae Folium

A standard is given in the European Pharmacopoeia Vol. I

Varieties. Alexandrian senna leaflets are pale greyish-green, ovate-lanceolate and usually slightly curved and twisted; they are brittle and often broken.

Tinnevelly senna leaflets are yellowish-green, lanceolate, flat and mostly unbroken. They are less pubescent than Alexandrian senna and are marked by occasional oblique and transverse lines produced by the hydraulic pressure used in packing the bales.

The vein islet number of Alexandrian senna is 25 to 30 and that of Tinnevelly senna is 20 to 23. The stomatal index of Alexandrian senna is 10 to 12.5 to 15 and that of Tinnevelly senna is 14 to 17.5 to 20.

Constituents. Senna leaf contains sennosides A and B [glucosides of stereoisomers of rhein dianthrone, 10,10'-bis(9,10 - dihydro - 1,8 - dihydroxy - 9 - oxoanthracene - 3-carboxylic acid)]; the aglycone of sennoside A is dextrorotatory, while that of sennoside B is the *meso*-form. Commercial samples of the leaf contain about 2 to 3% of the sennosides.

Smaller quantities of the following anthraquinone glycosides are also present: sennosides C and D, based on the heterodianthrones of rhein and aloe-emodin [9,10-dihydro - 10 - (9,10 - dihydro - 1,8 - dihydroxy - 3 - hydroxy-methyl - 9 - oxoanthr - 10 - yl) - 1,8-dihydroxy-9-oxoanthra-

cene-3-carboxylic acid], rhein anthrone 8-glucoside, rhein 8-glucoside, rhein 8-diglucoside, aloe-emodin 8-glucoside, and aloe-emodin anthrone diglucoside.

Senna leaf also contains rhein, aloe-emodin, kaempferol, and isorhamnetin in the free state and combined as glycosides. Myricyl alcohol, salicylic acid, phytosterolin, mucilage, resin, and calcium oxalate are also present.

Senna leaf yields to water about 30 to 40% of extractive. Up to 2% of stalks and 1% of foreign organic matter may be present, and up to 12% of sulphated ash and 2% of acid-insoluble ash may be yielded.

Description. UNGROUND DRUG. *Macroscopical characters:* leaflets lanceolate to ovate-lanceolate, about 20 to 50 mm long and 5 to 16 mm wide, pale greyish-green or yellowish-green, texture thin and brittle; asymmetrical and occasionally unequal at the base, covered with a very short fine pubescence, visible under a lens; margin entire and slightly revolute, apex acute and mucronate, petiole about 1 mm long, veins more distinct on under surface; rachis, when present, slender, about 70 to 100 mm long, with 4 to 6 pairs of leaflet scars and a longitudinal groove on the upper surface; young stem thicker and somewhat angled, bearing alternate leaf scars.

It has a slight characteristic odour and a taste which is at first mucilaginous then slightly bitter and unpleasant.

Microscopical characters: the diagnostic characters are: *epidermis* both surfaces with straight-walled polyhedral cells, many containing *mucilage* in the inner half, staining with *ruthenium red solution; stomata* paracytic, present on both surfaces; *trichomes* conical, unicellular, up to 250 μm long, frequently curved near the base, with thick warty walls; *mesophyll* isobilateral, with 1 layer of palisade cells below each epidermis, those beneath lower epidermis with wavy anticlinal walls; *veins* with upper and lower *bundle caps* composed of fibres, caps with outer sheath of parenchymatous cells, some of which contain a single prismatic *crystal* of calcium oxalate; cluster *crystals* of calcium oxalate present in some cells of the intercostal mesophyll.

POWDERED DRUG. Powdered Senna Leaf. A green to yellowish-green powder possessing the diagnostic microscopical characters, odour, and taste of the unground drug.

Adulterants and substitutes. Leaflets of *Cassia italica* (Mill.) Lam. ex F. W. Andr. (*Cassia obovata* Collad.), known as "dog senna", are distinguished by their obovate shape and, microscopically, by the papillose cells of the lower epidermis.

Leaflets of *C. montana* Hayne, which are darker in colour, have a rounded apex and a dark network of veins. Leaflets of *C. angustifolia*, growing wild in Arabia, known as Arabian or Mecca senna, are narrow, lanceolate, and usually discoloured.

Palthé senna, from *C. auriculata* L., consists of small oblong to obovate leaflets, which are coloured crimson by sulphuric acid (80% v/v).

Leaflets of *C. holosericea* Fresen. are small and hairy. Argel leaves, derived from *Solenostemma argel* Hayne (Fam. Apocynaceae), have been found admixed with Alexandrian senna, and occasionally the dehisced follicles and plumed seeds are also present; the texture of the leaves is thick and rigid; they are peculiarly curled, curved, or twisted; the surface is finely rugose and the veins are not evident; the leaf is equal at the base, the trichomes are three-celled, and the taste is distinctly bitter.

Storage. Senna leaf should be protected from light.

Identification. TEST. Heat about 25 mg, in fine powder with 50 ml of water and 2 ml of hydrochloric acid in a water-bath for 15 minutes; allow the mixture to cool, add 40 ml of ether, shake, allow to separate, and dry the ethereal layer with anhydrous sodium sulphate; evaporate 5 ml of the ethereal solution to dryness, allow the residue to cool, and add 5 ml of *dilute ammonia solution*; a yellow or, at most, orange colour is produced. Heat the solution on a water-bath for 2 minutes; a reddish-violet colour is produced.

Actions and uses. Senna leaf has the actions and uses described under Senna Fruit. The usual dose for an adult is 0.5 to 2 grams; children may be given half of the dose for an adult.

Serum, Dried Human

Prepared by drying a pool of the fluid which separates from human blood which has clotted in the absence of any anticoagulant.

A standard is given in the British Pharmacopoeia 1973

For the preparation of dried human serum, blood is collected by the method described under Whole Human Blood, except that the anticoagulant solution is omitted from the receiving vessel, from donors who fulfil the same requirements.

The blood is allowed to clot, and the serum is removed aseptically by siphoning through a closed system of sterile tubing. The serum is pooled with that from other samples of blood so that contributions from donors of A, O, and either B or AB groups are represented in approximately the ratio 9:9:2. In order to avoid untoward effects due to the products of bacterial growth, no individual contribution of serum is used if there is any evidence of bacterial contamination and no pool is used unless it complies with the tests for sterility.

Not more than 10 separate donations of serum are pooled. The pool is dried either from the frozen state or by any other method which will avoid denaturing the proteins and will yield a product readily soluble in a quantity of water equal to the volume of the liquid from which the substance was prepared.

Description. A sterile pale to deep cream-coloured powder or friable solid, which is completely soluble, at 15° to 20°, within 10 minutes, in a volume of water equal to the volume of water for injections stated on the label. Such a solution contains not less than 6.5% w/v of protein, and as shown by specific precipitation tests contains only human serum proteins. No coagulation occurs when an aqueous solution of calcium chloride is added to the reconstituted serum.

Storage. It should be stored, in an atmosphere of nitrogen, in sterile containers sealed to exclude micro-organisms and moisture, at a temperature below 25°, and protected from light.

It may be stored for several years in temperate and tropical climates if it is kept free from moisture. The only practical criterion of its fitness for use is complete solution within 10 minutes when reconstituted. If solution is incomplete or if a gel forms, the serum should not be used, even though the expiry date has not been reached.

Actions and uses. Dried human serum is used for the same purposes as those described under Dried Human Plasma and is reconstituted in a similar manner. Reconstituted serum should be used immediately after reconstitution and should be discarded if not used within 3 hours. The use of dried human serum carries a risk of transmitting hepatitis, as explained in the entry on Blood Products.

Sesame Oil

The fixed oil obtained by expression from the seeds of *Sesamum indicum* L. (Fam. Pedaliaceae), a plant grown in India, China, Japan, and most tropical countries; it may be refined.

OTHER NAMES: Gingelly Oil; Sesami Oleum; Teel Oil

A standard is given in the European Pharmacopoeia Vol. III Supplement

Constituents. Sesame oil consists of glycerides, the fatty acid constituents of which are chiefly oleic and linoleic acids, with small proportions of stearic, palmitic, and arachidic acids. It also contains about 1% of the lignan, sesamin, and a smaller amount of the closely related sesamolin.

Description. A pale yellow oil with a slight pleasant odour and a bland taste. It does not solidify when cooled to 0°.

Solubility. Very slightly soluble in alcohol; miscible with ether, with chloroform, and with light petroleum.

Weight per ml. At 20°, 0.916 to 0.919 g.

Refractive index. 1.472 to 1.476.

Sterilisation. It is sterilised by dry heat.

Storage. It should be stored in well-filled airtight containers, protected from light, in a cool place.

Identification. TEST. Shake 2 ml with 1 ml of a 1% solution of sucrose in hydrochloric acid; a pink or red colour is produced in the aqueous layer. A positive reaction to this test is still given after the oil has been heated to 250° but oils refined by certain commercial methods may give a reduced colour or no colour at all.

Uses. Sesame oil is used as a vehicle for oily injections. It has properties similar to those of olive oil and has been used instead of olive oil in the preparation of liniments, plasters, ointments, and soaps.

Shigella Infection

Bacillary dysentery (Shigellosis) is an acute infection of the bowel caused by Gram-negative organisms of the genus *Shigella*, and is characterised by the frequent passage of stools containing blood, pus, and mucus. It is transmitted by the faecal-oral route. It affects mainly the lower intestine, which is hyperaemic and oedematous and often has superficial mucosal ulcerations. After an incubation period of 1 to 4 days, onset is sudden, with fever, anorexia, diarrhoea, nausea or vomiting, abdominal pain, and tenesmus. The number of stools increases rapidly to 30 or 40 per day and the urgent desire to defaecate is practically continuous. The acute phase of the illness lasts for about a week and then gradually subsides, although some cases are fulminating and lead to death in a few hours.

Severe salt and water depletion occurs in shigellosis and there should be adequate fluid and electrolyte replacement by mouth where possible or, in the severely dehydrated patient, by intravenous infusion.

Antibacterial agents are not usually prescribed for the milder dysentery caused by *Shigella sonnei*, the form most usual in Britain, because they are liable to prolong the carrier state of the infection. Dysentery caused by *Shigella boydii, Shigella dysenteriae,* and *Shigella flexneri* is more severe and may be life threatening in debilitated persons. Treatment with antibacterials may then be required.

Antibacterial agents active against *Shigella* spp. include ampicillin, cephalosporins, chloramphenicol, colistin, gentamicin, kanamycin, streptomycin, sulphonamides, tetracyclines, and trimethoprim.

Shock

see under CIRCULATORY FAILURE

Silica in Dimethicone Suspension

A preparation containing 4.5 to 8% w/w of finely powdered silica in dimethicone 1000.

A standard is given in the British Pharmacopoeia (Veterinary)

Description. An almost odourless, tasteless, viscous, grey, translucent fluid.

Solubility. Immiscible with water; partly soluble in toluene, in xylene, in chlorinated hydrocarbons, and in solvent naphtha, leaving a residue of silica.

Veterinary uses. Silica in dimethicone suspension is administered by mouth or by injection into the cavity of the rumen in the form of an emulsion containing 1% for the treatment of frothy bloat in ruminants. The usual dose of silica in dimethicone suspension for cattle is 1 gram and for sheep and goats 250 milligrams.

Silver Nitrate

$AgNO_3 = 169.9$

OTHER NAME: Argenti Nitras

A standard is given in the European Pharmacopoeia Vol. I

Description. Odourless transparent colourless crystals or white crystalline powder.

Solubility. Soluble, at 20°, in less than 1 part of water and in 27 parts of alcohol; very slightly soluble in ether and in glycerol.

Acidity. A 4% solution has a pH of 5.4 to 6.4.

Incompatibility. It is incompatible with alkalis, halogen acids and their salts, phosphates, tannin, and astringent preparations.

Sterilisation. Solutions are sterilised by heating in an autoclave or by filtration.

Storage. It should be protected from light. Solutions should be freshly prepared and supplied in amber-coloured bottles.

Actions and uses. Silver nitrate is caustic, astringent, and bactericidal. It has been used as a caustic to destroy warts and other small skin growths.
Compresses soaked in a 0.5% solution of silver nitrate have been applied to severe burns to reduce infection. A 1% solution has been used locally in the eye for the prophylaxis of ophthalmia neonatorum.

Undesirable effects. Silver nitrate stains the skin black and prolonged use of solutions may cause permanent staining of the tissues.

Poisoning. A 1% solution of sodium chloride should be given and copious draughts of milk, demulcent drinks and, finally, a dose of castor oil. An analgesic such as morphine may be required for pain relief.

Preparations

SILVER NITRATE LOTION:

Silver nitrate   ..   ..   0.5 g
Purified water, freshly boiled and cooled   to 100.0 ml
It must be freshly prepared.
Containers: see the entry on Lotions for general information on containers.
Labelling: see the entry on Lotions for general information on labelling. In addition, a warning that the lotion will produce black stains on skin and fabric should be given on the label.
Storage: it should be protected from light.
Advice for patients: the lotion should be applied undiluted and discarded after use. It should not be used if a precipitate is present. The lotion will cause staining (see above under Labelling).

TOUGHENED SILVER NITRATE: prepared by fusing together 95 parts of silver nitrate and 5 parts of potassium nitrate and pouring the mixture into suitable moulds.
A standard for this preparation is given in the British Pharmacopoeia 1973
Storage: it should be protected from light.
Advice for patients: the tip of the preparation should be moistened by dipping in water and applied carefully to the lesion. Contact with normal skin should be avoided. It may produce black stains on skin and fabric.

Simmonds' Disease

see HYPOPITUITARISM

Sinusitis

Sinusitis, or inflammation of the nasal cavities, is characterised by head pains, especially of the face, and local tenderness. Symptomatic treatment, as described under Coryza, Acute, may be applied. If there is bacterial infection antibacterial agents may be used and surgical treatment may be necessary in prolonged or recurrent sinusitis.

Sleeping Sickness

see under TRYPANOSOMIASIS

Smallpox

Smallpox (Variola) is a communicable viral disease that was once endemic in some areas of Asia and Africa. It may affect people of all ages and is characterised by a severe illness and the formation of a pock-like rash. After an incubation period of 10 to 17 days there is sudden onset of severe constitutional illness with a rise in temperature, vomiting, and severe generalised aches and pains. After 2 to 3 days a rash develops starting first on the head, then the arms and trunk, and finally the legs and feet. The lesions appear mainly on skin which is normally exposed, and on bony prominences. The axilla is often free from lesions. The skin lesions are at first small pink macules but over the next 2 to 3 weeks they become hard and papular, then vesicular, then pustular and finally the pustules become hard dry crusts which may take several weeks to separate. All lesions tend to be at about the same stage of development at the same time.

When smallpox occurs in an individual who has previously been vaccinated, the illness is less severe, there are fewer eruptions, and these are smaller, shallower, and last for a shorter period of time. Protection against smallpox is conferred by vaccination, although this may wane after a period of time (see Smallpox Vaccine for details of vaccination). There is no specific treatment for smallpox, and treatment consists of relieving symptoms and preventing secondary bacterial infection of the vesicles. Methisazone may be used in the prophylaxis of smallpox in the contacts of people with known disease.

Since smallpox is no longer endemic routine vaccination is no longer recommended

Smallpox Vaccine

A preparation from the lesions produced on the skin of living animals, when it may be called "Vaccine Lymph"; alternatively, it may be prepared in chick chorio-allantoic membranes. It contains the living virus of vaccinia and produces the characteristic lesions of vaccinia virus when applied to a scarified area of the skin of man, calves, sheep, rabbits, or guinea-pigs.

OTHER NAMES: Liquid Smallpox Vaccine (Dermal); Vaccinum Variolae Fluidum Dermicum; Vaccinum Vacciniae; Var/Vac

A standard is given in the European Pharmacopoeia Vol. II

Storage. It should be protected from light and stored at a temperature above its freezing-point in accordance with instructions on the label. Under these conditions it may be expected to retain its potency for 12 months. When stored between 2° and 5°, it may be expected to retain its potency for 4 weeks.

Actions and uses. Smallpox vaccine is inoculated by multiple pressure or by a single linear scratch not more than 2 to 3 mm in length in a dosage of about 0.02 millilitre; it is not intended to be administered intradermally. The characteristic eruption of vaccinia is produced at the site of inoculation. As a result of this infection, immunity to smallpox develops. Generally all other preventive inoculations should be avoided within 3 weeks of primary vaccination. When a rapid programme of inoculations is necessary, vaccinations against yellow fever and smallpox may be done simultaneously at different sites. If this is not feasible an interval of at least 2 weeks should separate the respective vaccinations to minimise the likelihood of viral interference.

Routine vaccination against smallpox is no longer recommended but vaccination may be required for travellers to or from areas where smallpox cases have been reported. Successful vaccination confers immunity for at least 3 years.

Precautions and contra-indications. Important contra-indications to vaccination are the presence of eczema or a history of eczema, septic skin infections, leukaemia or other reticulo-endothelial malignancies, hypogammaglobulinaemia, and corticosteroid or other immunosuppressive treatment.

The danger of death following the vaccination of those suffering from allergic eczema is so great that such patients should not be vaccinated unless they are directly exposed to infection with smallpox. Equally at risk of potentially lethal eczema vaccinatum are eczematous persons who come into contact with recently vaccinated subjects.

If persons suffering from the conditions cited are vaccinated they should be given human antivaccinia immunoglobulin at the same time.

Additional contra-indications to vaccination include septic skin conditions and pregnancy. In the presence of suspected smallpox there are no absolute contra-indications to the immediate vaccination of close contacts.

Smallpox Vaccine, Dried

Dried smallpox vaccine is more stable than the liquid vaccine and is therefore particularly suitable when stocks need to be kept for long periods.

OTHER NAMES: Freeze-dried Smallpox Vaccine (Dermal); Vaccinum Variolae Cryodesiccatum Dermicum; Var/Vac

A standard is given in the European Pharmacopoeia Vol. II

Storage. It should be protected from light and stored continuously at a temperature below 5°. Under these conditions it may be expected to retain its potency for 3 years. The reconstituted vaccine may be kept for 7 days at a temperature between 2° and 10°.

Actions and uses. Dried smallpox vaccine has the actions and uses described under Smallpox Vaccine. The reconstituted vaccine is applied to the skin by scarification or by multiple pressure inoculation in a dose of 0.02 millilitre.

Snake Venom Antiserum

Native serum, or a preparation from native serum, containing the antitoxic globulins that have the power of neutralising the venom of one or more kinds of snake.

OTHER NAMES: Anti-Snakebite Serum; Antivenene; Antivenin; Antivenom; Antivenom Serum; Venom Antitoxin

A standard is given in the British Pharmaceutical Codex 1973

Storage. It should be stored as described under Antisera.

Actions and uses. The main toxic fractions of venom are neurotoxins, cytotoxins, including haemolysins, and coagulants. Neurotoxin predominates in the venom of elapine snakes (cobra, mamba, etc.) and cytotoxins and coagulants in viperine venoms (viper, adder, rattlesnake) but some viperine venoms, particularly those of certain rattlesnakes, are strongly neurotoxic.

No antiserum effective against all venoms is available because of the great immunological differences in the venoms of the snakes of different continents. The custom is for each country to prepare antisera able to neutralise the venoms of the indigenous snakes.

Specific monovalent antisera are prepared, but more commonly antivenin preparations are polyvalent, that is, they have a neutralising effect upon the venoms of more than one species. For example, in South Africa an antiserum is prepared primarily to neutralise the venoms of the Cape cobra, the ringhals, and the puff-adder and, in the Indian subcontinent, to neutralise those of the krait, cobra, Russell's viper, and the saw-scaled viper. The only poisonous snake found in Great Britain is the adder, or common viper, *Vipera berus.*

A bite by an elapine snake does not usually produce a severe local reaction, but death may ensue within a few minutes to several hours from the respiratory paralysis caused by the neurotoxin.

Viperine venom produces a severe local reaction, with pain, swelling, haemorrhage, and tissue damage, followed by generalised vascular injury, widespread internal haemorrhagic lesions, and blood loss, with resultant shock. Some viperine venoms, notably that of Russell's viper, contain powerful coagulants which may cause death by producing intravascular clotting.

Ideally, specific antiserum should be administered, but this requires that the reptile responsible for the bite is seen and identified accurately. If this is not possible it should always be assumed to be venomous and a large dose of polyvalent snake venom antiserum should be administered at the earliest possible moment, preferably intravenously; ideally, an intramuscular "trial dose" should be given half an hour before an intravenous injection, but in practice this is usually omitted owing to the urgency of the situation. In addition, as much antiserum as possible should be injected into and around the bitten area, the remaining antiserum being given subcutaneously or intramuscularly; the local injection of antiserum is particularly indicated in viperine bite. If improvement does not occur after an hour, a further dose should be given intravenously.

A scale of dosage cannot be laid down because the venoms of the snakes of different countries differ in toxicity and the antivenoms differ in potency; detailed instructions relating to dosage are issued with the antiserum.

It should be noted that the use of antisera entails the injection of large doses of globulins of animal origin, usually from horses, and that even when the globulins have been purified and pepsin-treated they will probably induce serum sickness. However, this is a transient disorder and preferable to the severe systemic disturbances, or death, caused by snake bite.

In Great Britain, the effect of an adder bite is not usually fatal in a healthy person. The use of snake venom antiserum is no longer recommended by the Department of Health and Social Security because the efficacy of the available antiserum against *Vipera berus* is unproved.

Serum Reactions. See under Antisera.

Soap, Soft

A soap made by the interaction of aqueous solutions of either potassium hydroxide or sodium hydroxide with a suitable vegetable oil or oils, or with fatty acids derived therefrom. The soap, if prepared from oil, contains the glycerol formed during saponification. It may be coloured with chlorophyll or not more than 0.015% of an innocuous green soap dye.

OTHER NAME: Sapo Mollis

A standard is given in the British Pharmacopoeia 1973

Description. A yellowish-white to green or brown unctuous substance.

Solubility. Soluble, at 20°, in 4 parts of water and in 1 part of alcohol; soluble in 1 part of boiling water. Some varieties of soft soap tend to separate as a gel from concentrated alcoholic solutions.

Uses. Soft soap is used to remove incrustations in chronic scaly skin diseases such as psoriasis and to cleanse the scalp before the application of antiseptic lotions. A solution in industrial methylated spirit, with the addition of solvent ether, is used to cleanse the skin. A solution of 1 part of soft soap in 20 parts of warm water is used as an enema.

Soft soap is liable to be heavily contaminated with micro-organisms.

Preparations

SOAP SPIRIT (*Syn.* Spiritus Saponatus):

Soft soap	..	..	..	..	..	650 g
Alcohol (90%)	..	..	..	..	to 1000 ml

Dissolve, and decant.

In making this preparation the alcohol (90%) may be replaced by industrial methylated spirit diluted so as to be of equivalent alcoholic strength, provided that the law and the statutory regulations governing the use of industrial methylated spirit are observed.

A standard for this spirit is given in the British Pharmaceutical Codex 1973

Advice for patients: when used in scalp disorders it is used instead of shampoo. Care should be taken to keep well away from a naked flame while the spirit is being applied.

OTHER PREPARATIONS: soft soap is an ingredient of turpentine liniment; soap liniment, which is made *in situ*, is described under Camphor.

Soda Lime

A mixture of sodium hydroxide, or sodium hydroxide and potassium hydroxide, with calcium hydroxide, prepared by fusion and subsequent granulation of the fused mass. It absorbs not less than 20% of its weight of carbon dioxide.

OTHER NAME: *Calona*®

A standard is given in the British Pharmacopoeia 1973

Description. Hard granules which may be white, or greyish-white, or coloured with an indicator to show their capacity for absorbing carbon dioxide; suitable indicators include phenolphthalein, potassium permanganate, and methyl violet.

Solubility. Partly soluble in water; almost completely soluble in dilute acetic acid.

Moisture content. 15 to 19%, determined by drying at 105°.

Storage. It should be stored in airtight containers.

Uses. Soda lime is used to absorb carbon dioxide in closed-circuit anaesthetic apparatus. Limits are specified for particle size to eliminate small granules, which cause excessive resistance to respiration, and large granules, which give inefficient absorption. The granules should be free from dust, which otherwise would be inhaled and cause irritation.

The containers for soda lime attached to the anaesthetic machines usually hold about 500 grams; if used continuously, this amount of soda lime will absorb carbon dioxide for 2 to 3 hours, in which time the granules will become coated with carbonate and further absorption prevented. After an interval of an hour, the soda lime will partially recover its absorptive capacity and may be used again. By using it intermittently in this way 500 grams of soda lime will provide efficient absorption for a total period of about 7 to 8 hours. The condition of the soda lime may be judged from the colour of the indicator which is usually incorporated.

Absorption of carbon dioxide by soda lime is accompanied by the evolution of heat, the temperature of the container usually reaching about 40°; if it becomes much hotter than this the soda lime should be discarded. It is preferable to change the soda lime container after each patient, as this allows the soda lime to cool and to recover. It is also advisable to moisten the soda lime with a few millilitres of water when filling the containers, as this increases the rate of absorption. Further moisture will be supplied by the water vapour exhaled by the patient.

Soda lime is similarly used to absorb carbon dioxide during determination of the basal metabolic rate.

Precautions. Soda lime must not be used with trichloroethylene, as this is decomposed by warm alkali into toxic products which give rise to lesions of the nervous system.

Sodium Acetate

$CH_3.CO_2Na,3H_2O = 136.1$

OTHER NAMES: Natrii Acetas; Sod. Acet.

A standard is given in the European Pharmacopoeia Vol. III Supplement

Description. Colourless crystals or a white crystalline powder which is efflorescent in warm air and has a cooling, saline, and slightly bitter taste; it may have a very faint odour of acetic acid.

Solubility. Soluble, at 20°, in less than 1 part of water and in 19 parts of alcohol.

Alkalinity. A 5% solution has a pH of 7.5 to 9.

Sterilisation. Solutions for injection are sterilised by heating in an autoclave or by filtration.

Uses. Sodium acetate is used as a source of sodium ions in preparing solutions for haemodialysis and intraperitoneal dialysis. It is preferred to sodium bicarbonate on account of its greater solubility.

Sodium Acid Citrate

$C_6H_6Na_2O_7,1\frac{1}{2}H_2O = 263.1$

OTHER NAMES: Disodium Hydrogen Citrate; Sod. Acid Cit.

A standard is given in the British Pharmacopoeia 1973

Description. An odourless white powder with a saline taste.

Solubility. Soluble, at 20°, in less than 2 parts of water; practically insoluble in alcohol.

Acidity. A 3% solution has a pH of 4.9 to 5.2.

Sterilisation. Solutions for injection are sterilised by heating in an autoclave or by filtration.

Actions and uses. Sodium acid citrate is an anticoagulant. It is used, generally in solution with dextrose, to prevent the clotting of blood intended for transfusion. For this purpose it is preferable to sodium citrate, as the dextrose-sodium acid citrate solution may be sterilised by heating in an autoclave with little danger of caramelisation. Sodium acid citrate solutions are less likely to damage the surface of glass containers with the production of glass spicules than sodium citrate solutions.

A suitable solution contains 1.7 to 2% of sodium acid citrate and 2.5% of dextrose in water for injections; 120 millilitres is sufficient to prevent the clotting of about 420 millilitres of blood. See also the entry on Anticoagulant and Preservative Solutions for Blood.

When very large blood transfusions are given, sufficient sodium acid citrate to affect the patient's coagulation mechanism may be inadvertently administered; in these circumstances heparinised blood should be used.

Sodium Acid Phosphate

$NaH_2PO_4,2H_2O = 156.0$

OTHER NAMES: *Fletchers' Disposable Phosphate Enema®*; *Practo-Clyss®*; Sod. Acid Phos.; Sodium Dihydrogen Phosphate
Beogex® (with sodium bicarbonate)

A standard is given in the British Pharmacopoeia 1973

Description. Odourless colourless crystals or white crystalline powder with an acid and saline taste.

Solubility. Soluble, at 20°, in 1 part of water; very slightly soluble in alcohol.

Stability. When heated, it loses its water of crystallisation at 100°, melts with decomposition at 205° forming sodium hydrogen pyrophosphate, $Na_2H_2P_2O_7$, and at 250° leaves a final residue of sodium metaphosphate, $NaPO_3$.

Actions and uses. Sodium acid phosphate is a saline purgative, the actions and uses of which are described under Magnesium Sulphate. It is also given to render the urine acid. It is administered by mouth in dilute aqueous solution in a dosage of 2 to 4 grams and as an enema.

Veterinary uses. Sodium acid phosphate is administered to render the urine acid. The usual dose by mouth for dogs and cats is 50 to 500 milligrams per kilogram body-weight daily.

Preparations

PHOSPHATES ENEMA (*Syn.* Sodium Phosphates Enema):
Formula A

Sodium acid phosphate	..	..	..	160 g
Sodium phosphate..	..	..	..	60 g
Purified water, freshly boiled and cooled	..	..	..	to 1000 ml

A suitable preservative may be added. Available in 120-ml units.

Formula B

Sodium acid phosphate	..	..	..	100 g
Sodium phosphate..	..	..	..	80 g
Purified water, freshly boiled and cooled	..	..	..	to 1000 ml

A suitable preservative may be added. Available in 128-ml units.

A standard for this enema is given in the British Pharmaceutical Codex 1973

Containers: both enemas should be supplied in a suitable disposable plastic pack fitted with a rectal nozzle.

Dose: Formula A—120 millilitres; *Formula B*—128 millilitres.

Advice for patients: see the entry on Enemas for general information on the use of enemas.

OTHER PREPARATIONS available include SUPPOSITORIES containing anhydrous sodium acid phosphate 700 mg with sodium bicarbonate 700 mg, and suppositories containing anhydrous sodium acid phosphate 1.32 g with sodium bicarbonate 1.08 g.

Sodium Alginate

Sodium alginate consists chiefly of the sodium salt of alginic acid.

OTHER NAMES: *Manugel®*; *Manutex®*
Alginate YZ® (with calcium alginate); *Ultrastat®* (with chlorhexidine hydrochloride); *Liquid Gaviscon®* (with sodium bicarbonate)

A standard is given in the British Pharmaceutical Codex 1973

Various grades of sodium alginate are available which yield aqueous solutions having viscosities covering the range of 20 to 400 centipoises in 1% solution at 20°.

Description. An odourless white or buff powder.

Solubility. Slowly soluble in water, forming a viscous solution; practically insoluble in alcohol, in ether, and in chloroform.

Moisture content. Not more than 22%, determined by drying at 105°.

Incompatibility. It is incompatible with acridine derivatives, crystal violet, calcium salts, phenylmercuric salts, alcohol in concentrations above 5%, and heavy metals.
Solutions are most stable between pH 4 and 10; alginic acid is precipitated below pH 3. Solutions should not be stored in metal containers.

Sterilisation. It is sterilised by heating in an autoclave. Solutions may be similarly sterilised, but some loss of viscosity occurs to an extent which varies according to the nature of the other substances present.

Labelling. The viscosity grade should be stated on the label.

Identification. TESTS. 1. It complies with Test 1 described under Alginic Acid.
2. To 5 ml of a 1% solution add 1 ml of *calcium chloride solution*; a voluminous gelatinous precipitate is produced.
3. To 10 ml of a 1% solution add 1 ml of *dilute sulphuric acid*; a heavy gelatinous precipitate is produced.

Uses. High and medium viscosity grades of sodium alginate are used for the preparation of gels, pastes, and creams and for thickening and stabilising emulsions. Medium viscosity sodium alginate is also used for its haemostatic properties as a surgical dressing. Low viscosity sodium alginate is used as a pharmaceutical adjuvant. A 1% solution has suspending properties similar to those of tragacanth mucilage and is a useful stabiliser of oil-in-water emulsions.
For the preparation of pastes and creams, 1 to 10% of sodium alginate is used according to the viscosity required; the addition of a trace of a soluble calcium salt increases the viscosity.
In preparing a solution, dispersion of the alginate may be aided by first mixing it with a suitable dispersing agent such as sugar, alcohol, glycerol, or propylene glycol. The solution should be prepared with a high-speed stirrer.

Preparations

Preparations available include an APPLICATION containing sodium alginate 7% with chlorhexidine hydrochloride 0.1%, in an aerosol pack; and a MIXTURE containing sodium alginate 500 mg with sodium bicarbonate 267 mg in 10 ml.

Sodium Aminosalicylate

Sodium 4-amino-2-hydroxybenzoate dihydrate

$C_7H_6NNaO_3,2H_2O = 211.1$

OTHER NAMES: Natrii Aminosalicylas; *Paramisan®*; Sod. Aminosal.; Sodium Para-aminosalicylate; Sodium PAS *Inapasade®* (with isoniazid)

A standard is given in the European Pharmacopoeia Vol. I

Description. Odourless white crystals or crystalline powder with a taste which is sweet, saline, and unpleasant.

Solubility. Soluble, at 20°, in 2 parts of water; soluble in alcohol; very slightly soluble in ether and in chloroform.

Acidity or alkalinity. A 2% solution has a pH of 6.5 to 8.5.

Moisture content. 16 to 17.5%, determined by drying at 105°.

Stability. Aqueous solutions are unstable and should be freshly prepared; oxidation and darkening in colour are retarded by adding 0.1% of sodium metabisulphite. Sodium aminosalicylate degrades by decarboxylation to 3-aminophenol which is then oxidised to various coloured products. Degradation is catalysed by hydroxide ions.

FURTHER INFORMATION. Stability in aqueous solution —K. H. Oberweger *et al.*, *Q. J. Pharm. Pharmac.*, 1948, **21**, 292; S. S. Kornblum and B. J. Sciarrone, *J. pharm. Sci.*, 1964, **53**, 935.

Storage. It should be stored in airtight containers, protected from light.

Actions and uses. Sodium aminosalicylate is used in the treatment of tuberculosis, but it has been largely replaced by more effective and better tolerated drugs. It is used in conjunction with other antituberculosis drugs, as the development of resistance by the infecting organisms is thereby delayed.
When taken by mouth it is rapidly absorbed, the maximum concentration in the blood being attained in about 1 hour, and is rapidly excreted, mainly by the kidneys. The greater proportion of a single dose is eliminated within 6 hours, and frequent doses are therefore necessary to maintain an adequate concentration in the blood. High concentrations are found in the lungs, liver, and kidneys; it also diffuses into the cerebrospinal fluid, pleural cavity, and aqueous humour.
The daily dosage of sodium aminosalicylate for an adult is usually 10 to 20 grams by mouth in divided doses; ideally, each dose is given at 4-hourly intervals, but for convenience it is usually given twice daily.
The usual dose for children is 200 to 300 milligrams per kilogram body-weight (8 grams per square metre body-surface) daily in divided doses.

Undesirable effects. Sodium aminosalicylate is liable to cause the usual undesirable effects of salicylates, such as drug fever, cutaneous eruptions, nausea, vomiting, diarrhoea, hypokalaemia with paralysis and cardiac arrhythmia, and jaundice; lymphadenopathy may sometimes occur.

Hypoprothrombinaemia may occur, but is of no clinical significance unless surgical procedures are to be undertaken.

Albuminuria, haematuria, and anuria have been reported.

Precautions. The urine of patients taking sodium aminosalicylate reduces Benedict's solution; this should be borne in mind when treating diabetic patients with the drug.

Patients hypersensitive to sodium aminosalicylate may also be hypersensitive to other compounds with a 4-aminophenyl group, including sulphonamides and certain hair dyes. Desensitisation may be attempted by reducing the dose of sodium aminosalicylate to that which avoids toxic symptoms and then increasing the dose each day within the limits of toleration until the desired daily quantity is again being given.

Preparations

SODIUM AMINOSALICYLATE AND ISONIAZID GRANULES: prepared by incorporating sodium aminosalicylate and isoniazid in a suitable basis and granulating the product. The granules may be coated and the coat may be coloured. Available as granules in sachets containing 50 mg of isoniazid with 2 g of sodium aminosalicylate, and 150 mg of isoniazid with 6 g of sodium aminosalicylate.
A standard for these granules is given in the British Pharmaceutical Codex 1973
Storage: they should be stored in airtight containers, in a cool place, protected from light.
Advice for patients: the granules should be placed on the tongue and swallowed with water, preferably after meals, or alternatively sprinkled on to cool food. Doses should be taken at regular intervals and treatment should not be discontinued without the advice of the prescriber.

SODIUM AMINOSALICYLATE AND ISONIAZID POWDER: consisting of sodium aminosalicylate and isoniazid mixed with a suitable coloured flavoured basis. The ingredients are usually in the proportion of 1 g of sodium aminosalicylate to each 25 mg of isoniazid.
Storage: it should be stored in airtight containers, in a cool place, protected from light.
Advice for patients: the powder should be taken dissolved in a little water or other fluid, preferably after meals. Doses should be taken at regular intervals and treatment should not be discontinued without the advice of the prescriber.

SODIUM AMINOSALICYLATE POWDER: consisting of sodium aminosalicylate. Available in 100-g containers.
Storage: it should be stored in airtight containers, in a cool place, protected from light.
Advice for patients: see above under Sodium Aminosalicylate and Isoniazid Powder.

Sodium Arsanilate

Sodium 4-aminophenylarsonate

$C_6H_7AsNNaO_3 = 239.0$

OTHER NAMES: Anhydrous Sodium Aminoarsonate; *Pro-Gen*®

A standard is given in the British Pharmacopoeia (Veterinary)

Description. An odourless hygroscopic white or creamy-white granular powder.

Solubility. Soluble, at 20°, in 3 parts of water and in 150 parts of alcohol; practically insoluble in chloroform and in ether.

Moisture content. Not more than 5%, determined by drying at 105°.

Identification. TESTS. It complies with Tests 1 and 2 described under Arsanilic Acid.

ULTRAVIOLET ABSORPTION. In water, maximum at 250 nm (E1%, 1cm = 656).

Veterinary uses. Sodium arsanilate is used for the prevention of enteric infections in pigs and poultry and for growth promotion. The usual dosage for pigs is 80 parts per million in the drinking water for 2 to 3 weeks and for poultry 160 parts per million in the drinking water for up to 7 days. For the treatment of scours, piglets up to 7 days may be given 8 milligrams, 8 to 14 days 16 milligrams and 15 to 21 days 24 milligrams. These doses may be given daily for 2 or 3 days.

Preparation

SODIUM ARSANILATE SOLUTION: an aqueous solution of sodium arsanilate. It contains a suitable thickening agent. It may contain a preservative and suitable colouring matter. Available in 150-ml bottles containing 8 mg of sodium arsanilate per ml.
A standard for this solution is given in the British Pharmacopoeia (Veterinary)
Labelling: the label on the container should state the amount of the medicament as the percentage w/v of sodium arsanilate, that animals should not be slaughtered for human consumption within 7 days after cessation of treatment, and that sodium arsanilate should not be given to pigs that are receiving any other arsenical compound.

Sodium Aurothiomalate

Sodium aurothiomalate consists chiefly of the disodium salt of aurothiomalic acid, $CO_2H.CH(S.Au).CH_2.$ CO_2H
$C_4H_3AuNa_2O_4S = 390.1$

OTHER NAMES: *Myocrisin*®; Sodium Aurothiosuccinate

A standard is given in the British Pharmacopoeia 1973

Description. A fine, pale yellow, hygroscopic powder with a faint odour.

Solubility. Soluble, at 20°, in less than 1 part of water; very slightly soluble in alcohol and in fixed oils.

Acidity. A 10% solution has a pH of 6 to 7.

Moisture content. Not more than 2%, determined by drying over phosphorus pentoxide *in vacuo.*

Sterilisation. Solutions for injection are sterilised by heating with a bactericide or by filtration.

Storage. It should be stored in airtight containers, protected from light.

Actions and uses. Compounds of gold, when given intramuscularly, are absorbed slowly and stored in the reticulo-endothelial cells. They are excreted slowly, mainly in the urine. No satisfactory explanation of their action has yet been found.

Sodium aurothiomalate is used in the treatment of rheumatoid arthritis. It is administered by deep intramuscular injection, usually as an aqueous solution, in an initial dose of 10 milligrams, followed at weekly intervals by 20, 30, 40, and 50 milligrams and continued with 50 milligrams weekly until a total of 1 gram has been given; thereafter 50 milligrams is given every other week. After prolonged remission the intervals between doses may be increased to 4 and then to 6 weeks.

An injection may cause transient exacerbation of rheumatoid symptoms necessitating a reduction in dosage. Significant improvement occurs in about 80% of patients after 6 to 12 weeks treatment, and such improvement may be maintained for several months without further treatment, but care should be taken to' minimise the possibility of relapses because a second course of treatment is unlikely to be effective.

Sodium aurothiomalate is also used in children in the treatment of juvenile rheumatoid arthritis, using a regimen similar to that described above and gradually increased to a maximum which is usually 10 milligrams for children under 25 kilograms body-weight, 20 milligrams from 25 to 50 kilograms body-weight, and 30 milligrams for children over 50 kilograms body-weight.

Undesirable effects. Toxic effects are relatively common, especially rashes. More serious reactions such as exfoliative dermatitis, toxic hepatitis, proteinuria, nephrotic syndrome, agranulocytosis, thrombocytopenia, and aplastic anaemia may occur.

Precautions. Patients should be examined regularly and full blood counts including platelets should be carried out at fortnightly intervals for 6 months and monthly thereafter. Urine should be examined for protein before each injection. The patient should be asked to report untoward symptoms such as fever, sore throat, skin reactions, pyrexia, or marked unexplained malaise, as they occur. If there is any sign of intolerance, treatment should be discontinued and dimercaprol or penicillamine may be administered.

Gold therapy should be discontinued during pregnancy and in nursing mothers.

Preparation

SODIUM AUROTHIOMALATE INJECTION: a sterile solution of sodium aurothiomalate in water for injections. It is sterilised by heating with a bactericide or by filtration. Available in 0.5-ml ampoules containing 1, 5, 10, 20, and 50 mg of sodium aurothiomalate (0.2%, 1%, 2%, 4%, and 10% respectively).

A standard for this injection is given in the British Pharmacopoeia 1973

Containers and *Labelling*: see the entry on Injections for general information on containers and labelling.

Storage: it should be protected from light.

Sodium Benzoate

$C_7H_5NaO_2 = 144.1$

OTHER NAME: Sod. Benz.

A standard is given in the British Pharmacopoeia 1973

Description. A white, amorphous, granular, flaky, or crystalline powder which is odourless or has a faint odour of benzoin and has an unpleasant, sweetish, and saline taste.

Solubility. Soluble, at 20°, in 2 parts of water and in 90 parts of alcohol.

Moisture content. Not more than 1.5%, determined by drying at 105°.

Incompatibility. It is incompatible with acids and with ferric salts.

Sterilisation. Solutions for injection are sterilised by heating in an autoclave or by filtration.

Actions and uses. Sodium benzoate, when given internally, is conjugated with glycine in the liver to form hippuric acid. This is the basis of a liver-function test. For the test, 6 grams dissolved in 200 millilitres of water is administered by mouth and the hippuric acid content of the urine is determined in specimens collected at suitable intervals. The test may also be carried out by the intravenous injection of 1.8 grams of sodium benzoate dissolved in 20 millilitres of water for injections. Sodium benzoate has also been used as a urinary antiseptic in a dosage of 0.3 to 2 grams given by mouth.

Preparations

Sodium benzoate is an ingredient of compound thymol glycerin, mouth-wash solution-tablets, and pastille basis (see the entry on Pastilles).

Sodium Bicarbonate

$NaHCO_3 = 84.01$

OTHER NAMES: Natrii Hydrogenocarbonas; Sod. Bicarb.; Sodium Hydrogen Carbonate
Beogex® (with sodium acid phosphate); *Liquid Gaviscon®* (with sodium alginate)

A standard is given in the European Pharmacopoeia Vol. I

Description. An odourless white crystalline powder.

Solubility. Soluble, at 20°, in 11 parts of water; practically insoluble in alcohol.

Stability. When heated it decomposes and, at 250° to 300°, is converted into anhydrous sodium carbonate. Solutions in water slowly decompose at ordinary temperatures with partial conversion into the normal carbonate; the decomposition is accelerated by agitation or warming.

Hygroscopicity. At relative humidities up to about 80%, the equilibrium moisture content at 25° is less than 1%, but at relative humidities above about 85%, it rapidly absorbs excessive amounts of moisture and this may be associated with decomposition by loss of carbon dioxide.

Sterilisation. Solutions are sterilised by heating in an autoclave or by filtration. When a solution is sterilised by heating in an autoclave, carbon dioxide is first passed through the solution in the final container, which is then hermetically sealed and not opened until at least 2 hours after the solution has cooled to room temperature.

Storage. Solutions, on storage, may cause separation of small solid glass particles from glass containers; solutions containing such particles must not be used.

Actions and uses. Sodium bicarbonate, and similar alkaline compounds, neutralise the acid secretion in the stomach. After absorption, the alkali carbonates increase the alkali reserve of the plasma and there is an increased excretion of urine, which is rendered less acid. Sodium bicarbonate is given by mouth in the treatment of hyperchlorhydria to relieve the pain and distension; it is given with bitters, such as gentian, 30 minutes before meals to neutralise excessive secretion in the stomach. It is also of value as an antacid in the treatment of dyspepsia and flatulence and of vomiting in children. The usual dose is 1 to 5 grams.

Solutions containing 1 to 4% of sodium bicarbonate are administered intravenously to correct sodium depletion; solutions containing up to 8.4% are used for the correction of metabolic acidosis caused by cardiac arrest. For its action in rendering mucus less viscid, sodium bicarbonate is added to spray solutions and washes for the throat and nose.

Sodium bicarbonate is an ingredient of compound sodium chloride mixture, which is taken as an expectorant. A weak solution (1 in 150) applied to the skin relieves itching, urticaria, and eczema.

Sodium bicarbonate eye lotion is used as a first-aid treatment for irrigating burns and injuries in the eye.

Veterinary uses. Sodium bicarbonate is an antacid. The usual dose for all species is 50 to 100 milligrams per kilogram body-weight.

Preparations

AMMONIATED RHUBARB AND SODA MIXTURE (*Syn.* Mistura Rhei Ammoniata et Sodae; Rhubarb, Ammonia, and Soda Mixture):

Rhubarb, in powder	..	..	..	25 g
Sodium bicarbonate	..	..	..	80 g
Ammonium bicarbonate ..	..	..	..	20 g
Peppermint emulsion, concentrated ..		..	25 ml
Chloroform water, double-strength	..	..	500 ml
Water for preparations	..	..	to 1000 ml

It should be recently prepared.

A standard for this mixture is given in the British Pharmaceutical Codex 1973

Containers and *Labelling:* see the entry on Mixtures for general information on containers and labelling. A direction to shake the bottle should be given on the label.

Dose: 10 to 20 millilitres.

Advice for patients: the mixture should not be taken for longer than a few days without medical advice. It may colour the urine red.

COMPOUND SODIUM BICARBONATE TABLETS (*Syn.* Soda Mint Tablets): for each tablet take:

Sodium bicarbonate	..	..	..	300 mg
Peppermint oil	..	..	..	.. 0.003 ml

A standard for these tablets is given in the British Pharmacopoeia 1973

Containers and *Storage:* see the entry on Tablets for general information on containers and storage. Containers should be airtight. The tablets should be stored in a cool place.

Advice for patients: the tablets should be allowed to dissolve slowly in the mouth. They should not be used for longer than a few days without medical advice.

SODIUM BICARBONATE EAR-DROPS:

Sodium bicarbonate	..	..	..	..	.. 5 g
Glycerol	..	..	..	..	.. 30 ml
Purified water, freshly boiled and cooled	..	..	..	..	.. to 100 ml

Dissolve the sodium bicarbonate in about 60 ml of the water, add the glycerol and sufficient of the water to produce the required volume, and mix.

The ear-drops should be recently prepared.

A standard for these ear-drops is given in the British Pharmaceutical Codex 1973

Containers and *Labelling:* see the entry on Ear-drops for general information on containers and labelling.

SODIUM BICARBONATE INJECTION: a sterile solution of sodium bicarbonate in water for injections. It may contain up to 0.01% of disodium edetate. It is sterilised by heating in an autoclave or by filtration. When it is sterilised by heating in an autoclave, it is placed in the final container and carbon dioxide is passed into the solution for 1 minute before sealing the container to form a gas-tight seal. The sealed container is not subsequently opened until at least 2 hours after the solution has cooled to room temperature. The usual strength is an injection containing 1.4% of sodium bicarbonate (167 mmol each of Na^+ and HCO_3^- per litre). Also available in 20- and 50-ml packs containing 5% of sodium bicarbonate.

A standard for this injection is given in the British Pharmacopoeia 1973

Containers: see the entry on Injections for general information on containers. Containers that have previously been subjected to heating in an autoclave should not be used.

Labelling: see the entry on Injections for general information on labelling. In addition, the label on the container should state the amount of the medicament as the percentage w/v of sodium bicarbonate.

When the injection is intended for intravenous infusion, the label on the container should also state the approximate concentrations, in mmol per litre, of Na^+ and HCO_3^-.

OTHER PREPARATIONS available include a MIXTURE containing sodium bicarbonate 267 mg with sodium alginate 500 mg in 10 ml; SUPPOSITORIES containing sodium bicarbonate 700 mg with anhydrous sodium acid phosphate 700 mg, and suppositories containing sodium bicarbonate 1.08 g with anhydrous sodium acid phosphate 1.32 g. Sodium bicarbonate is an ingredient of alkaline gentian mixture and of compound sodium chloride mixture.

Sodium Bromide

NaBr = 102.9

OTHER NAMES: Natrii Bromidum; Sod. Brom.

A standard is given in the European Pharmacopoeia Vol. III Supplement

Description. Odourless, small, colourless, transparent or opaque cubical crystals or, more generally, a white granular powder, with a saline and slightly bitter taste.

Solubility. Soluble, at 20°, in 1.5 parts of water and in 17 parts of alcohol.

Moisture content. Not more than 3%, determined by drying at 120°.

Incompatibility. It is incompatible with oxidising agents and with salts of mercury and silver.

Hygroscopicity. It absorbs moisture from the air but,

owing to the formation of $NaBr,2H_2O$, does not appear moist until over 20% of water has been absorbed.

Storage. It should be stored in airtight containers.

Actions and uses. Sodium bromide has the actions, uses, and undesirable effects described under Potassium Bromide. It is given in a dosage of 1 to 6 grams daily in divided doses.

Precautions. As for Potassium Bromide.

Sodium Butyl Hydroxybenzoate

Sodium butyl 4-hydroxybenzoate

$$CO \cdot O \cdot [CH_2]_3 \cdot CH_3$$

ONa

$C_{11}H_{13}NaO_3 = 216.2$

OTHER NAMES: *Nipabutyl Sodium®*; Sodium Butylparaben

A standard is given in the British Pharmacopoeia Addendum 1978

Description. An odourless hygroscopic white powder.

Solubility. Soluble, at 20°, in 1 part of water and in 10 parts of alcohol.

Alkalinity. A 0.1% solution has a pH of 9.5 to 10.5.

Moisture content. Not more than 5%, determined by Fischer titration.

Storage. It should be stored in airtight containers.

Identification. TESTS. 1. Dissolve about 500 mg in water, and acidify the solution with *dilute hydrochloric acid*; a white precipitate is produced which, after washing with water and drying, melts at about 69°.
2. The precipitate obtained in Test 1 complies with the test described under Methyl Hydroxybenzoate.

ULTRAVIOLET ABSORPTION. In alcohol (95%), maximum at 259 nm (E1%, 1cm = 750).

Uses. Sodium butyl hydroxybenzoate has preservative properties as described under Methyl Hydroxybenzoate and is used in place of butyl hydroxybenzoate when it is desirable to have a material which is more soluble in water.

Sodium Calciumedetate

The dihydrate of the calcium chelate of the disodium salt of ethylenediamine-*NNN'N'*-tetra-acetic acid.

$C_{10}H_{12}CaN_2Na_2O_8,2H_2O = 410.3$

OTHER NAMES: *Ledclair®*; *Sequestrene NA2Ca®*

A standard is given in the British Pharmacopoeia 1973

Description. A tasteless white or creamy-white powder with a slight odour.

Solubility. Soluble, at 20°, in 2 parts of water; very slightly soluble in alcohol; practically insoluble in ether and in chloroform.

Acidity or alkalinity. A 20% solution has a pH of 6.5 to 8.

Moisture content. 8 to 11%, determined by drying at 150°.

Dissociation constants. pK_a 2.0, 2.7, 6.2, 10.3 (20°).

Sterilisation. Solutions for injection are sterilised by heating in an autoclave or by filtration. Containers are made from lead-free glass.

Storage. It should be stored in airtight containers.

Actions and uses. The pharmacological action of sodium calciumedetate is due to its ability to exchange its calcium atom for lead ions in the blood, thereby forming a stable non-ionisable lead compound which is water-soluble and readily excreted unchanged by the kidneys. The exchange between the lead and calcium is preferential because other metals, such as iron, copper, and cobalt, are more strongly bound to tissue proteins. Sodium calciumedetate is therefore useful in the treatment of lead poisoning and lead encephalopathy.

Sodium calciumedetate is usually given by intravenous infusion as a 0.5 to 3% solution in sodium chloride injection or dextrose injection. The infusion fluid is usually administered over a period of 1 hour, to a maximum of 40 milligrams of the anhydrous salt per kilogram body-weight, twice daily for up to 5 days. The treatment may be repeated, if necessary, after an interval of 2 or 3 days.

Sodium calciumedetate given by mouth also produces a rapid excretion of lead in the urine, which continues for some days after the cessation of treatment; the usual dosage is the equivalent of 4 grams of the anhydrous salt daily in divided doses.

Undesirable effects. Although the toxicity of sodium calciumedetate is very low, there is evidence that the repeated administration of moderate doses may produce a toxic nephrosis which, however, clears up in a few days after the drug is withdrawn.

Veterinary uses. Sodium calciumedetate is used in the treatment of lead poisoning. The usual dose by intravenous injection for all species is the equivalent of 75 milligrams of anhydrous sodium calciumedetate per kilogram body-weight daily.

Preparations

SODIUM CALCIUMEDETATE INJECTION: a sterile solution of sodium calciumedetate in water for injections. It is sterilised by heating in an autoclave or by filtration. It contains sodium calciumedetate equivalent to 200 mg of anhydrous sodium calciumedetate per ml. Available in 5-ml ampoules.

A standard for this injection is given in the British Pharmacopoeia 1973
Containers: see the entry on Injections for general information on containers. Containers are made from lead-free glass.
Labelling: see the entry on Injections for general information on labelling. In addition, the label on the container should state the amount of the medicament

as the equivalent of anhydrous sodium calciumedetate in a suitable dose-volume. The label on the container or the label on the package should also state that the injection should be diluted with dextrose injection or with sodium chloride injection before administration.

SODIUM CALCIUMEDETATE TABLETS: they contain sodium calciumedetate equivalent to 500 mg of anhydrous sodium calciumedetate.
A standard for these tablets is given in the British Pharmacopoeia 1973
Containers and *Storage:* see the entry on Tablets for general information on containers and storage. Containers should be airtight.

Sodium Carbonate

$Na_2CO_3,10H_2O = 286.1$

OTHER NAMES: Natrii Carbonas Decahydricus; Sodium Carbonate Decahydrate

A standard is given in the European Pharmacopoeia Vol. II

Description. Odourless, colourless, transparent, efflorescent crystals or white crystalline powder, with an alkaline and salty taste.

Solubility. Soluble, at 20°, in 2 parts of water; practically insoluble in alcohol.

Storage. It should be stored in airtight containers.

Uses. Sodium carbonate is employed in the preparation of alkaline baths (250 g in 150 litres) and of surgical chlorinated soda solution (see below).

Preparation

SURGICAL CHLORINATED SODA SOLUTION (*Syn.* Dakin's Solution):

Boric acid	a sufficient quantity
Chlorinated lime	a sufficient quantity
Sodium carbonate..	a sufficient quantity
Purified water, freshly boiled and cooled	1000 ml

Determine the proportion of available chlorine in the chlorinated lime by the following method: triturate about 4 g, accurately weighed, with small portions of water, dilute the combined triturates to 1000 ml with water, shake well, and to 100 ml of the suspension add 3 g of potassium iodide in 100 ml of water and 5 ml of acetic acid, and titrate the liberated iodine with 0.1N sodium thiosulphate, each ml of which is equivalent to 0.003545 g of Cl. Prepare the solution by the following method, using the quantities of ingredient indicated in the table.

Available Chlorine in Chlorinated Lime	Chlorinated Lime	Sodium Carbonate	Boric Acid
%w/w	g	g	g
30	18.8	37.6	4.00
31	18.2	36.4	3.87
32	17.6	35.2	3.75
33	17.1	34.2	3.64
34	16.6	33.2	3.53
35	16.1	32.2	3.43
36	15.7	31.4	3.33
37	15.3	30.6	3.24
38	14.9	29.8	3.16
39	14.5	29.0	3.08
40	14.1	28.2	3.00

Dissolve the sodium carbonate in the water and add the solution, gradually and with constant trituration, to the chlorinated lime, previously powdered; shake occasionally during 20 minutes, allow to stand for a further 10 minutes, decant, and filter through a bleached filter; dissolve the boric acid in the filtrate.
It should be recently prepared.
A standard for this solution is given in the British Pharmaceutical Codex 1973
Storage: It should be stored in well-filled airtight bottles, in a cool place, protected from light.
Advice for patients: it has a bleaching action and will destroy most dyes.

Sodium Carboxymethylcellulose

The sodium salt of carboxymethylcellulose. It may be represented by the formula $[C_6H_{10-x}O_5(CH_2.CO_2Na)_x]_n$ where x represents the degree of substitution and n the number of anhydroglucose units in the molecule. The degree of polymerisation, n, affects the viscosity of the solution.

OTHER NAMES: *Cekol®*; *Cellulose Gum®*; *Cellosize CMC®*; *Courlose®*; *Edifas B®*; Sodium Cellulose Glycollate
Orabase® and *Orahesive®* (both with gelatin and pectin)

A standard is given in the British Pharmaceutical Codex 1973

Different grades of sodium carboxymethylcellulose are available which yield aqueous solutions having various viscosities covering the range 6 to 4000 centipoises (0.006 to 4 Pa.s) in 1% solution.

Description. An odourless, hygroscopic, white to cream-coloured powder.

Solubility. Soluble in water at all temperatures, giving a clear solution; practically insoluble in most organic solvents.

Moisture content. Not more than 10%, determined by drying at 105°.

Incompatibility. It is incompatible with strongly acid solutions and with soluble salts of iron and some other metals.

Hygroscopicity. It absorbs significant amounts of moisture at temperatures up to 37° at relative humidities of about 80%.

Sterilisation. Sodium carboxymethylcellulose can be sterilised in the dry state by maintaining at 160° for 1 hour, but this leads to a substantial decrease in viscosity and some deterioration in the properties of solutions prepared from the sterilised material.
Sterilisation of solutions by heating also causes some lowering of viscosity, but this is much less marked. When a solution is heated in an autoclave at 125° for 15 minutes and allowed to cool, the viscosity may be expected to decrease by about 25%; allowance should therefore be made for this when calculating the amount of sodium carboxymethylcellulose to be included in a preparation which is to be sterilised.

Identification. TESTS. Put about 2 g in a beaker, place a mechanical stirrer 25 mm above the surface, add 160 ml of water, stir for 30 minutes avoiding undue aeration of the solution, dilute to 200 ml with water and allow to stand for 16 hours. The solution complies with the following tests:
1. To 10 ml of the solution add *dilute hydrochloric acid*

to adjust to pH 0.5; a fine white precipitate is produced (distinction from methylcellulose).

2. Boil 10 ml of the solution for 5 minutes; no precipitate is produced (distinction from methylcellulose and ethylcellulose).

3. To 5 ml of the solution add 5 ml of hydrochloric acid, boil under a reflux condenser for 30 minutes, cool, neutralise to litmus paper with *sodium hydroxide solution*, and add 2 drops of this solution to 5 ml of hot *potassium cupri-tartrate solution*; a red precipitate is produced (presence of reducing sugar).

4. To 10 ml of the solution add 10 ml of a 1% solution of calcium chloride; no gelatinous precipitate is produced (distinction from sodium alginate).

5. The powder complies with Test 3 described under Methylcellulose (distinction from microcrystalline cellulose).

Uses. Sodium carboxymethylcellulose is used for suspending powders in aqueous preparations intended for external application or for oral or parenteral administration. It can also be used for stabilising emulsions and for dispersing the precipitate formed when resinous tinctures are added to water. For these purposes 0.25 to 1% of the medium-viscosity grades is usually adequate.

Higher concentrations, such as 4 or 6%, of the medium-viscosity grades produce gels which can be used as the basis for applications and pastes; glycerol is usually included in such preparations to prevent drying-out.

Aqueous preparations of sodium carboxymethylcellulose which are likely to be stored for long periods should contain a preservative. Medium- and high-viscosity grades of sodium carboxymethylcellulose, like those of methylcellulose, are used as bulk laxatives; for this purpose 4 to 10 grams is given daily in divided doses, each dose being taken with plenty of water.

Preparation

CARBOXYMETHYLCELLULOSE GELATIN PASTE: consisting of sodium carboxymethylcellulose, pectin, and gelatin in a suitable basis. Available as a paste containing 16.58% each of sodium carboxymethylcellulose, pectin, and gelatin, in a liquid paraffin-polyethylene basis.

Containers and *Storage*: see the entry on Pastes for general information on containers and storage. It may be packed in small collapsible tubes.

Advice for patients: it should be applied sparingly to the lesions after meals and at night.

Sodium Chloride

NaCl = 58.44

OTHER NAMES: Natrii Chloridum; *Slow Sodium*®; Sod. Chlor.; *Sterets Normasol*®
Dioralyte® (with dextrose, potassium chloride, and sodium bicarbonate)

A standard is given in the European Pharmacopoeia Vol. I

Description. Odourless, colourless, cubical crystals or white crystalline powder.

Solubility. Soluble, at 20°, in 3 parts of water, in 250 parts of alcohol, and in 10 parts of glycerol.

Moisture content. Not more than 1%, determined by drying at 130°.

Sterilisation. Solutions for injection are sterilised by heating in an autoclave or by filtration.

Storage. It should be stored in airtight containers. Solutions, on storage, may cause the separation of small solid glass particles from glass containers; solutions containing such particles must not be used.

Actions and uses. Sodium chloride is the most important salt for maintaining the osmotic tension of the blood and tissues; changes in osmotic tension influence the movement of fluids and diffusion of salts in the cellular tissues. Normal tissue fluid contains about 140 millimoles of sodium ions and about 100 millimoles of chloride ions per litre. About 5 to 12 grams of sodium chloride is taken daily in the food and a corresponding amount is excreted in the urine.

Excess of sodium chloride will act as a saline diuretic; when sodium chloride is absorbed from the intestine, or injected, the osmotic equilibrium of the blood is maintained by the excretion of the surplus salt and water by the kidneys. Sodium chloride in a dosage of 10 to 12 grams a day, by aiding excretion, is of value in the treatment of poisoning by bromides or iodides.

Solutions of sodium chloride, usually with the addition of dextrose, are given intravenously and sometimes by rectum to patients who are unable to take fluids by mouth. It may be necessary to give saline intravenously for 4 or 5 days until the patient can take fluids orally; if no fluid is taken by mouth, 3.5 litres is required daily in temperate climates and rather more in the tropics. This is best given as sodium chloride and dextrose injection. If the patient is not excreting chloride in his urine, his salt intake is insufficient. Sodium chloride injection has been used to combat dehydration, but it is found that the administration of large quantities may produce oedema, owing to accumulation of salt in the tissues.

Severe sweating, such as occurs when heavy work is done in a hot atmosphere, may cause a marked loss of sodium chloride, producing muscle cramps and involuntary tremors. This can be prevented or relieved by taking sufficient saline drink (a 0.5% salt solution is suitable) to compensate for the loss of sodium chloride in the sweat.

In Addison's disease the patient loses large quantities of sodium chloride in the urine owing to deficiency of adrenocortical hormones; such hormones, for example cortisone, may be given in replacement therapy. Additional salt is necessary to maintain the electrolyte balance. During replacement therapy with corticosteroids, care must be taken to ensure that abnormal retention of sodium chloride, with resultant oedema, does not occur.

Sodium chloride injection is often given parenterally for the treatment of shock and circulatory collapse, often in association with dextrose.

Sodium chloride injections may be given intraperitoneally to infants; for rectal administration half-strength saline is usually used, as it is more readily absorbed than normal saline.

The dietary intake of sodium chloride is restricted in cases of hypertension and oedema.

Preparations

COMPOUND SODIUM CHLORIDE AND DEXTROSE POWDER (*Syn.* Electrolyte Powder): for each powder take:

Sodium chloride, in powder	..	..	..	0.50 g
Dextrose (monohydrate), in powder	..	..	20.00 g
Potassium chloride, in powder	..	..	..	0.75 g
Sodium bicarbonate, in powder		..	..	0.75 g

Mix, as described in the entry on Powders, and dispense in airtight single-unit containers or wrap individually using an inner waxed paper or an outer covering of metal foil.

It contains in 1 litre, when reconstituted (see below), 35 mmol of Na^+, 20 mmol of K^+, 37 mmol of Cl^-, 18 mmol of HCO_3^-, and 200 mmol of dextrose. The total osmolarity is 310 mosmol per litre.

When Small Size Compound Sodium Chloride and Dextrose Powder is ordered, a powder of identical composition containing 8.8 g in each single-unit container is supplied; the powder is dissolved, as described under Uses, in sufficient water, recently boiled and cooled, to make 200 ml (7 fl. oz.) of solution.

Compound sodium chloride and dextrose powder, and small size compound sodium chloride and dextrose powder, may be flavoured.

A standard for this powder is given in the British Pharmaceutical Codex Supplement 1976

Labelling: directions for using the powder should be stated on the label or in a leaflet or card enclosed with the powders or single-dose units issued to the patient.

Uses: one powder or single-dose unit (22 g) is dissolved in sufficient water, recently boiled and cooled, to make 500 ml (17½ fl. oz.) of solution. Hygienic precautions should be taken throughout the preparation. Any portion of the solution remaining after 24 hours should be discarded.

The solution is administered by mouth as directed for rehydration and electrolyte replacement in the treatment of infantile diarrhoea. It is not intended for the preparation of injections.

COMPOUND SODIUM CHLORIDE MIXTURE:

Sodium chloride	20 g
Sodium bicarbonate	50 g
Chloroform water, double-strength	500 ml
Water for preparations	to 1000 ml

It should be recently prepared.

A standard for this mixture is given in the British Pharmaceutical Codex 1973

Containers and Labelling: see the entry on Mixtures for general information on containers and labelling.

Dose: 10 to 20 millilitres in a tumblerful of hot water, sipped slowly.

COMPOUND SODIUM CHLORIDE MOUTH-WASH:

Sodium chloride	15 g
Sodium bicarbonate	10 g
Peppermint emulsion, concentrated	25 ml
Chloroform water, double-strength	500 ml
Water for preparations	to 1000 ml

It should be diluted with an equal volume of warm water before use.

A standard for this mouth-wash is given in the British Pharmaceutical Codex 1973

Containers and Labelling: see the entry on Mouth-washes for general information on containers and labelling.

Advice for patients: the diluted solution should be rinsed around the mouth 3 or 4 times daily as required. It should preferably not be swallowed.

POTASSIUM CHLORIDE AND SODIUM CHLORIDE INJECTION: a sterile solution of potassium chloride and sodium chloride in water for injections. It is sterilised by heating in an autoclave or by filtration. The usual strength is 0.3% of potassium chloride and 0.9% of sodium chloride (40 mmol of K^+, 150 mmol of Na^+, and 190 mmol of Cl^- per litre).

A standard for this injection is given in the British Pharmacopoeia 1973

Containers: see the entry on Injections for general information on containers.

Labelling: see the entry on Injections for general information on labelling. In addition, the label on the container should state the amounts of the medicaments as the percentages w/v of potassium chloride and sodium chloride.

When the injection is intended for intravenous infusion, the label should also state that rapid infusion may be harmful, and the approximate concentrations, in millimoles per litre, of K^+, Na^+ and Cl^-.

POTASSIUM CHLORIDE, SODIUM CHLORIDE, AND DEXTROSE INJECTION: a sterile solution of potassium chloride, sodium chloride, and anhydrous dextrose or the equivalent amount of dextrose monohydrate for parenteral use, in water for injections. It is sterilised, immediately after preparation, by heating in an autoclave. It contains 0.18% of sodium chloride (30 mmol of Na^+ per litre) and 4% of anhydrous dextrose. The usual strengths of potassium chloride are those that provide between 10 and 40 mmol of K^+ per litre. The prescriber should state the strength of potassium chloride required in millimoles per litre.

A standard for this injection is given in the British Pharmacopoeia Addendum 1978

Containers: see the entry on Injections for general information on containers.

Labelling: see the entry on Injections for general information on labelling. In addition, the label on the container should state the amounts of the medicaments as the percentage w/v of potassium chloride, a sodium chloride content of 0.18% w/v, and an anhydrous dextrose content of 4% w/v, the concentration of potassium chloride in grams per litre and the approximate concentration of K^+ in millimoles per litre, a sodium chloride content of 1.8 g per litre equivalent to approximately 30 mmol of Na^+ per litre, the Cl^- content in millimoles per litre, and an anhydrous dextrose content of 40 g per litre.

The label should also state that rapid infusion may be harmful, and that solutions containing visible solid particles must not be used.

Storage: it should be stored at a temperature not exceeding 25°. On storage, separation of small solid glass particles from glass containers may occur. Solutions containing such particles must not be used.

SODIUM CHLORIDE AND DEXTROSE INJECTION: a sterile solution of sodium chloride, with anhydrous dextrose or the equivalent amount of dextrose monohydrate for parenteral use, in water for injections. It is sterilised, immediately after preparation, by heating in an autoclave. The usual strength is 0.18% of sodium chloride (30 mmol each of Na^+ and Cl^- per litre) with 4% of anhydrous dextrose.

A standard for this injection is given in the British Pharmacopoeia 1973

Containers: see the entry on Injections for general information on containers.

Labelling: see the entry on Injections for general information on labelling. In addition, the label on the container should state the amounts of the medicaments as the percentages w/v of sodium chloride and anhydrous dextrose. When the injection is intended for intravenous infusion, the label should also state the approximate concentrations, in millimoles per litre, of Na^+ and Cl^- ions and the number of grams per litre of anhydrous dextrose.

Storage: it should be stored at a temperature not exceeding 25°. On storage, the solution may cause separation of small solid glass particles from glass containers. Solutions containing such particles must not be used.

SODIUM CHLORIDE AND SODIUM CITRATE INJECTION: a sterile solution of sodium chloride and sodium citrate in water for injections. It is sterilised by heating in an autoclave or by filtration. It contains 5% (50 mg per ml) each of sodium chloride and sodium citrate.

A standard for this injection is given in the British Pharmacopoeia (Veterinary)

Containers and *Labelling:* see the entry on Injections for general information on containers and labelling.

Storage: the solution may, on storage, cause the separation of small solid glass particles from a glass container. A solution containing such particles must not be used.

SODIUM CHLORIDE EYE LOTION:

Sodium chloride	9 g
Purified water	to 1000 ml

Prepare as described in the entry on Eye Lotions. It should be used undiluted.

A standard for this eye lotion is given in the British Pharmaceutical Codex 1973

Containers and *Labelling:* see the entry on Eye Lotions for general information on containers and labelling.

Advice for patients: see the entry on Eye Lotions for general information on the use of eye lotions.

SODIUM CHLORIDE INJECTION: a sterile solution of sodium chloride in water for injections. It is sterilised by heating in an autoclave or by filtration. The usual strength is 0.9% of sodium chloride (150 mmol each of Na^+ and Cl^- per litre). When normal saline solution for injection is prescribed, sodium chloride injection of this strength is dispensed.

A standard for this injection is given in the British Pharmacopoeia 1973

Containers: see the entry on Injections for general information on containers.

Labelling: see the entry on Injections for general information on labelling. In addition, the label on the container should state the amount of the medicament as the percentage w/v of sodium chloride.

When the injection is intended for intravenous infusion, the label should also state the approximate concentrations, in millimoles per litre, of Na^+ and Cl^-.

Storage: the solution may, on storage, cause the separation of small solid glass particles from a glass container. A solution containing such particles must not be used.

SODIUM CHLORIDE SOLUTION (*Syn.* Normal Saline):

Sodium chloride	9 g
Purified water, freshly boiled and cooled	to 1000 ml

Dissolve, and filter.

CAUTION. *This solution should not be confused with normal sodium chloride solution which is used as a chemical reagent and contains 5.85% of sodium chloride.*

A standard for this solution is given in the British Pharmaceutical Codex 1973

Sterilisation: the solution may be sterilised by heating in an autoclave or by filtration.

Containers and *Labelling:* see the entry on Solutions for general information on containers and labelling.

SODIUM CHLORIDE TABLETS: available as tablets containing 300 mg of sodium chloride.

A standard for these tablets is given in the British Pharmacopoeia 1973

Containers and *Storage:* see the entry on Tablets for general information on containers and storage. Containers should be airtight.

Labelling: the label on the container should state that the tablets should be dissolved in water before administration.

Advice for patients: see above under Labelling.

OTHER PREPARATIONS available include EYE-DROPS containing sodium chloride 0.9% in 0.5-ml units; TABLETS containing sodium chloride 600 mg (providing approximately 10.3 mmol each of Na^+ and Cl^-) in a slow-release formulation, and tablets containing sodium chloride 450 mg with dextrose 200 mg.

Sodium chloride is an ingredient of many preparations, in particular haemodialysis solutions, intraperitoneal dialysis solution, and Ringer's solution for injection.

Sodium Chromate (^{51}Cr) Solution

A sterile solution of sodium chromate (^{51}Cr), made isotonic with blood by the addition of sodium chloride.

OTHER NAMES: Natrii Chromatis (^{51}Cr) Solutio Sterilisata; Sodium Chromate (^{51}Cr) Sterile Solution

A standard is given in the European Pharmacopoeia Vol. III

CAUTION. *This material is radioactive and any regulations in force must be complied with.*

Chromium-51 is a radioactive isotope of chromium which decays by electron capture with emission of γ-radiation of energy 0.320 MeV. It has a half-life of 27.7 days. It may be prepared by neutron irradiation of natural chromium enriched in chromium-50.

Description. A clear colourless or faintly yellow solution.

Acidity or alkalinity. pH 6 to 8.

Sterilisation. It is sterilised by heating in an autoclave.

Storage. It should be stored in an area assigned for the purpose. The storage conditions should be such that the maximum radiation-dose-rate to which persons may be exposed is reduced to an acceptable level. Glass containers may darken under the effects of radiation.

Labelling. The label on the container should state (1) the content of chromium-51 expressed in microcuries or millicuries at a given date and hour, (2) that the solution is radioactive, and (3) that it does not contain a bactericide.

The label on the package should state (1) the total volume in the container and (2) the content of total chromium.

Actions and uses. Sodium chromate (^{51}Cr) is used for labelling red blood cells. It crosses the red-cell membrane and becomes attached to the β-polypeptide chains of the haemoglobin molecules, from which it is only slowly eluted.

Doses of about 150 microcuries are used to determine the life span of red cells in the investigation of haemolytic anaemias. The γ-emission of sodium chromate (^{51}Cr) is of sufficiently high energy to permit the estimation of radioactivity at the body surface, thus enabling the sites of isotope accumulation due to red-cell destruction or pooling to be determined.

Sodium chromate (^{51}Cr) may also be used for labelling red blood cells in the investigation of haematological disorders and may be used for the detection of red-cell loss due to haemorrhage into the gastro-intestinal tract and for the determination of the circulating red-cell volume; doses of 50 microcuries may be used for these purposes.

Sodium Citrate

$C_6H_5Na_3O_7,2H_2O = 294.1$

OTHER NAMES: Natrii Citras; Sod. Cit.

A standard is given in the European Pharmacopoeia Vol. III

Description. Odourless, white, granular crystals or crystalline powder with a saline taste. In moist air it is slightly deliquescent and in warm dry air it is efflorescent.

Solubility. Soluble, at 20°, in less than 2 parts of water; practically insoluble in alcohol.

Moisture content. 11 to 13%, determined by Fischer titration.

Sterilisation. Solutions for injection are sterilised by heating in an autoclave or by filtration.

Storage. It should be stored in airtight containers. Solutions, on storage, may cause the separation of small solid glass particles from glass containers; solutions containing such particles must not be used.

Actions and uses. Sodium citrate is oxidised in the tissues and is partly excreted as carbon dioxide; it increases the alkali reserve and renders the urine less acid, having the ultimate effect of bicarbonates without their neutralising action upon gastric secretion. As the alkali citrates are absorbed more readily than the tartrates, their laxative action is less marked. Sodium citrate has been used to make the urine alkaline in the treatment of infections of the urinary tract and during treatment with some sulphonamides to prevent crystalluria. Up to 10 grams may be administered by mouth daily in divided doses. Children up to 1 year may be given 750 milligrams, 1 to 5 years 1.5 grams, and 6 to 12 years 3 grams; these doses may be given 3 times daily.

Sodium citrate was formerly added to milk in the feeding of infants and invalids to prevent the formation of large curds; for invalids, from 60 to 180 milligrams of sodium citrate has been added to each 40 millilitres of milk, and for infant feeding a solution containing 125 milligrams in 5 millilitres has been added to each feed.

Sodium citrate prevents the clotting of blood *in vitro*, a 2.5 to 3.8% solution being employed; a 3% solution is also used for washing out syringes and apparatus before collection of blood. Its use as an anticoagulant for whole human blood is described under Whole Human Blood but it has been largely replaced for this purpose by sodium acid citrate. See also the entry on Anticoagulant and Preservative Solutions for Blood.

Preparations

SODIUM CHLORIDE AND SODIUM CITRATE INJECTION: a sterile solution of sodium chloride and sodium citrate in water for injections. It is sterilised by heating in an autoclave or by filtration. It contains 5% (50 mg per ml) each of sodium chloride and sodium citrate.
A standard for this injection is given in the British Pharmacopoeia (Veterinary)

Containers and *Labelling:* see the entry on Injections for general information on containers and labelling.
Storage: the solution may, on storage, cause the separation of small solid glass particles from a glass container. A solution containing such particles must not be used.

SODIUM CITRATE MIXTURE:

Sodium citrate	300 g
Citric acid monohydrate	50 g
Lemon spirit	5 ml
Quillaia tincture	10 ml
Syrup..	250 ml
Chloroform water, double-strength	300 ml
Water for preparations	to 1000 ml

It should be recently prepared.
When a dose less than or not a multiple of 5 ml is prescribed, the mixture may be diluted, as described in the entry on Mixtures, with syrup.
A standard for this mixture is given in the British Pharmaceutical Codex 1973
Containers: see the entry on Mixtures for general information on containers.
Labelling: see the entry on Mixtures for general information on labelling. Directions to shake the bottle and to dilute the dose well with water before administration should be given on the label.
Advice for patients: the mixture should be taken well diluted with water.

SODIUM CITRATE TABLETS: available as tablets containing 125 mg of sodium citrate; they may contain up to 10% of starch as a disintegrating agent and up to 0.5% of magnesium stearate as a lubricant, but no other materials. They are intended for use in infant feeding.
A standard for these tablets is given in the British Pharmacopoeia 1973
Containers and *Storage:* see the entry on Tablets for general information on containers and storage. Containers should be airtight.
Labelling: the label on the container should state that the tablets should be dissolved in water before use.
Advice for patients: see above under Labelling. The resultant solution should be added to the feed.

STERILE SODIUM CITRATE SOLUTION FOR BLADDER IRRIGATION:

Sodium citrate	30 g
Dilute hydrochloric acid	2 ml
Purified water, freshly boiled and cooled	to 1000 ml

It is prepared as described in the entry on Solutions. Sterilise by heating in an autoclave or by filtration.
A standard for this solution is given in the British Pharmaceutical Codex 1973
Containers and *Labelling:* see the entry on Solutions for general information on containers and labelling.
Storage: it may, on storage, cause the separation of small solid glass particles from glass containers; solutions containing such particles must not be used.

Sodium Cromoglycate

Disodium 4,4'-dioxo-5,5'-(2-hydroxytrimethylenedioxy)di(chromene-2-carboxylate)

$C_{23}H_{14}Na_2O_{11} = 512.3$

OTHER NAMES: Cromolyn Sodium; Intal®; Lomusol®; Nalcrom®; Opticrom®; Rynacrom®
Intal Compound® (with isoprenaline sulphate)

A standard is given in the British Pharmacopoeia 1973

Description. An odourless, hygroscopic, white, crystalline powder which is tasteless at first, becoming slightly bitter.

Solubility. Soluble, at 20°, in 20 parts of water; practically insoluble in alcohol and in chloroform.

Moisture content. Not more than 10%, determined by drying at 100° *in vacuo*.

Dissociation constant. pK_a 2.5 (20°).

Storage. It should be stored in airtight containers.

Identification. TEST. To about 100 mg add 2 ml of water and 2 ml of *dilute sodium hydroxide solution* and boil for 1 minute; a yellow solution is produced. Add 0.5 ml of *diazoaminobenzenesulphonic acid*; a blood red colour is produced.

ULTRAVIOLET ABSORPTION. In *solution of standard pH 7.4*, maxima at 238 nm (E1%, 1cm = 600), and 326 nm (E1%, 1cm = 160).

INFRA-RED ABSORPTION. Major peaks at 1264, 1305, 1365, 1405, 1473, and 1635 cm^{-1} (see Appendix 2a: Infra-red Spectra).

Determination in body fluids. COLORIMETRY. In urine —S. H. Curry and G. G. Mills, *J. Pharm. Pharmac.*, 1973, **25**, 677.

Metabolism. ABSORPTION. Poorly absorbed after oral or subcutaneous administration; following inhalation, most of a dose is swallowed but that which enters the lungs is rapidly absorbed; the amount absorbed after inhalation appears to be affected by particle size and smaller particles are better absorbed than larger ones.

BLOOD CONCENTRATION. After inhalation, peak plasma concentrations are attained in about 15 minutes and reach about 10 ng/ml following a 20-mg dose and up to 300 ng/ml following a 60-mg dose.

HALF-LIFE. Plasma half-life, about 80 minutes.

METABOLIC REACTIONS. Sodium cromoglycate does not appear to be metabolised.

EXCRETION. After inhalation, up to about 3% of a dose is excreted unchanged in the urine in 24 hours and up to about 87% in the faeces in 3 days; after an oral dose, about 0.5% is excreted unchanged in the urine and after an intravenous dose, about 50% is excreted unchanged in the urine and about 50% is excreted unchanged in the faeces; sodium cromoglycate is excreted, to some extent, in the bile.

FURTHER INFORMATION. Effect of particle size on disposition after inhalation—S. H. Curry et al., *J. Pharm. Pharmac.*, 1974, **26**, *Suppl.*, 79P; plasma concentrations and excretion after inhalation—G. F. Moss et al., *Toxic.*

appl. Pharmac., 1971, **20**, 147 and S. R. Walker et al., *J. Pharm. Pharmac.*, 1972, **24**, 525; review of actions, uses, and pharmacokinetics—R. N. Brogden et al., *Drugs*, 1974, **7**, 164.

Actions and uses. Sodium cromoglycate is used in the prophylaxis of asthma. It appears to stabilise cells containing chemical mediators causing asthmatic attacks. It is ineffective when given by mouth for this purpose, and should be inhaled as a powder from a suitable inhaler. The usual dose is 20 milligrams every 3 to 12 hours for adults and children.
In addition to the cartridges (see below) it is available as a compound preparation containing isoprenaline to prevent bronchospasm due to inhalation of the powder; this preparation has the disadvantage that the bronchodilator effect of the isoprenaline frequently leads to incorrect use by the patient and prevents reliable assessment of the effect of the cromoglycate. Patients requiring an inhaled bronchodilator should use it 5 to 10 minutes before inhaling sodium cromoglycate to improve the penetration of the substance into the lungs. A nebuliser solution containing 1% of sodium cromoglycate is also available for use with a power-driven nebuliser.
Sodium cromoglycate is also used as a nasal insufflation for the prophylaxis of allergic rhinitis either as cartridges containing 10 milligrams of sodium cromoglycate powder for use with a suitable nebuliser or as a solution containing 2%. Adults and children may be given 10 milligrams of sodium cromoglycate powder or 2.6 milligrams as the solution into each nostril up to 6 times daily.
Sodium cromoglycate may be given orally in the treatment of ulcerative colitis. The usual adult dose is 200 milligrams 4 times daily. Children aged 2 to 14 years may be given 100 milligrams 4 times daily. For eye allergies eye-drops containing 2% of sodium cromoglycate are available.

Undesirable effects. Slight irritation of the throat and bronchi commonly occurs, especially during infective illnesses. Sudden withdrawal may precipitate asthma, particularly in cases where the use of sodium cromoglycate has permitted a reduction in corticosteroid dose.

Preparations

SODIUM CROMOGLYCATE CARTRIDGES: consisting of sodium cromoglycate, in powder of suitable particle size, mixed with an approximately equal quantity of lactose, enclosed in a hard capsule. The capsule shells may be coloured. They contain 20 mg of sodium cromoglycate. This preparation is entitled sodium cromoglycate inhalation in the British National Formulary 1976–78.
A standard for these cartridges is given in the British Pharmacopoeia 1973
Containers and *Storage:* see the entry on Capsules for general information on containers and storage. The cartridges should be stored at a temperature not exceeding 30°.
Labelling: the label on the container should state that each cartridge contains 20 mg of sodium cromoglycate, and that the cartridges are intended for use in an inhaler and are not to be swallowed.
Advice for patients: the cartridges should be used with a suitable inhaler and the contents inhaled through the mouth; they should not be swallowed. The patient should be advised to read the instructions on the leaflet enclosed with the product. When used in conjunction with salbutamol or other bronchodilator, the bronchodilator should be given first, and sodium cromoglycate car-

tridges used 5 minutes later. Treatment should not be discontinued without the advice of the prescriber.

SODIUM CROMOGLYCATE INSUFFLATION: consisting of sodium cromoglycate, in powder of suitable particle size, which may be mixed with a suitable inert diluent, enclosed in a hard capsule. The capsule shells may be coloured. Available as cartridges containing 10 mg of sodium cromoglycate.

Containers and *Storage:* see the entry on Capsules for general information on containers and storage. The cartridges should be stored at a temperature not exceeding 30°.

Labelling: the label on the container should state that each cartridge contains 10 mg of sodium cromoglycate, and that the cartridges are intended for use in an insufflator and are not to be swallowed.

Advice for patients: the cartridges should be used with a suitable insufflator and the contents insufflated into each nostril; they should not be swallowed. The patient should be advised to read the instructions on the leaflet enclosed with the product. Treatment should not be discontinued without the advice of the prescriber.

OTHER PREPARATIONS available include CAPSULES containing sodium cromoglycate 100 mg; CARTRIDGES (for use with a suitable inhaler) containing sodium cromoglycate 20 mg with isoprenaline sulphate 100 micrograms; EYE-DROPS containing sodium cromoglycate 2%; NASAL DROPS containing sodium cromoglycate 2%; a SPRAY (for use with a suitable power-driven nebuliser) containing sodium cromoglycate 10 mg per ml in 2-ml ampoules, and a spray containing sodium cromoglycate 2% (also supplied with a hand-pump to deliver approximately 2.6 mg of sodium cromoglycate per metered dose).

Sodium Diatrizoate

Sodium 3,5-diacetamido-2,4,6-tri-iodobenzoate

$C_{11}H_8I_3N_2NaO_4 = 635.9$

OTHER NAMES: *Hypaque 25/45®* *Gastrografin®*, *Hypaque 65/85®*, and *Urografin®* (all with meglumine diatrizoate)

A standard is given in the British Pharmacopoeia 1973

Description. An odourless white powder with a saline taste.

Solubility. Soluble, at 20°, in 2 parts of water; very slightly soluble in alcohol; practically insoluble in ether and in acetone.

Alkalinity. A 50% solution has a pH of 7 to 9.

Moisture content. 4.5 to 9% determined by Fischer titration.

Dissociation constant. pK_a 3.4 (20°).

Sterilisation. Solutions for injection are sterilised by heating in an autoclave or by filtration.

Storage. It should be protected from light.

Identification. TESTS. 1. Heat; violet vapours of iodine are evolved.

2. To about 20 mg add 5 ml of 1N sodium hydroxide, boil under a reflux condenser for 10 minutes, cool, add 5 ml of *dilute hydrochloric acid*, cool in ice for 5 minutes, add 4 ml of a 1% solution of sodium nitrite, cool in ice for 5 minutes, add 300 mg of sulphamic acid, swirl gently until effervescence ceases, and add 2 ml of a 0.4% solution of N-(1-naphthyl)ethylenediamine hydrochloride; an orange-red colour is produced.

3. Mix about 500 mg with 1 ml of sulphuric acid, heat on a water-bath until a pale violet solution is obtained, add 2 ml of alcohol (95%) and again heat; the odour of ethyl acetate is produced.

Actions and uses. Sodium diatrizoate is used as a contrast medium in diagnostic radiology for the examination of a wide range of systems of the body. For many purposes it has replaced diodone; in common with other tri-iodo-compounds it gives a higher degree of radio-opacity and is less toxic than diodone in similar concentration.

It is available in solutions containing 25 and 45%. Stronger solutions are available; these solutions consist of mixtures of the sodium and meglumine salts of diatrizoic acid and contain the equivalent of 65 and 85% of diatrizoates.

For intravenous pyelography, 20 millilitres of the 45% solution is usually sufficient, but if inadequate contrast is obtained larger volumes may be used. Usually, X-ray photographs can be obtained without preliminary preparation of the patient, but better results will be obtained if the patient avoids taking fluids for 12 hours prior to the examination and if a laxative is given on the night before to eliminate gas and faeces from the bowel. The total volume of medium should be injected in 1 to 3 minutes. Its excretion by the kidneys is almost immediately detectable by serial films. For retrograde pyelography the 25% solution is usually adequate.

For operative and post-operative cholangiography three successive injections of 4 millilitres of the 25% solution directly into the biliary system is usually sufficient for visualisation of the bile duct.

For translumbar aortography in adults where the injection is to be made immediately above the renal arteries, a single injection of between 20 and 30 millilitres of the 65% solution is used. The reason for this limitation of dosage is the nephrotoxic effect of larger doses. If, however, the injection is to be given some distance below the renal arteries, a quantity greater than 30 millilitres can be used with safety.

For angiocardiography, 1 millilitre of the 65 or 85% solution per kilogram body-weight is used. In calculating the volume, account must be taken of the dead space in the apparatus and pump which is used for the administration.

For peripheral arteriography and cerebral angiography a suitable concentration is 45%. In cerebral angiography an average of 8 millilitres should be used for each injection and a maximum of 80 millilitres should not be exceeded in any one complete investigation, because of the possibility of causing cerebral oedema. The injections are made into the common carotid artery or, for the study of the intracerebral structure, into the internal carotid artery.

Undesirable effects. The occasional undesirable reactions which may occur include nausea, vomiting, sensations of heat, weakness, headache, thirst, coughing, sneezing, itching, pallor, tachycardia, and hypotension. Urticarial rashes may occur and these can usually be relieved by the immediate intravenous injection of an antihistamine. In rare cases, profound shock leading to cardiac arrest may occur and supplies of adrenaline, oxygen, and a suitable corticosteroid for injection should be available.

Precautions. There is no wholly satisfactory test which will enable the radiologist to predict a severe reaction, but some workers make a preliminary sensitivity test by injecting intravenously 1 millilitre of medium and observing the patient for a period prior to the administration of the full injection.

Contra-indications. An idiosyncrasy to inorganic iodine does not necessarily contra-indicate the use of an organic compound of iodine. Sodium diatrizoate should not be used for pyelography in patients with multiple myeloma because renal failure may occur.

It should not be used for myelography or injected into the subarachnoid space.

It should not be used in patients with asthma or thyrotoxicosis and its use should be avoided during pregnancy.

Preparations

SODIUM DIATRIZOATE INJECTION: a sterile solution of sodium diatrizoate, with suitable buffering and stabilising agents, in water for injections. It is sterilised by heating in an autoclave or by filtration. Available in 20-ml ampoules and in 250-, 300-, and 350-ml infusion bottles containing 25% (250 mg per ml) of sodium diatrizoate, and in 20- and 30-ml ampoules containing 45% (450 mg per ml) of sodium diatrizoate.

A standard for this injection is given in the British Pharmacopoeia 1973

Containers: see the entry on Injections for general information on containers.

Labelling: see the entry on Injections for general information on labelling. In addition, the label on the container should state the amount of the medicament as the percentage w/v of sodium diatrizoate.

Storage: it should be protected from light.

OTHER PREPARATIONS available include an INJECTION containing sodium diatrizoate 3.9% with meglumine diatrizoate 26.1% (equivalent to 14.6% of iodine) in 10-ml ampoules and 250-ml bottles, an injection containing sodium diatrizoate 7.9% with meglumine diatrizoate 52.1% (equivalent to 29.2% of iodine) in 20-ml ampoules and 50-ml vials, an injection containing sodium diatrizoate 10% with meglumine diatrizoate 66% (equivalent to 37% of iodine) in 20-ml ampoules and 50-, 100-, and 200-ml vials, an injection containing sodium diatrizoate 25.23% with meglumine diatrizoate 50.46% (equivalent to 39% of iodine) in 20-ml ampoules, an injection containing sodium diatrizoate 28.33% with meglumine diatrizoate 56.67% (equivalent to 44% of iodine) in 20-ml ampoules, an injection containing sodium diatrizoate 40% with meglumine diatrizoate 18% (equivalent to 32.5% of iodine) in 20-ml ampoules and 50-ml vials; and a SOLUTION containing sodium diatrizoate 10% with meglumine diatrizoate 66%.

Sodium Fluoride

NaF = 41.99

OTHER NAMES: *En-De-Kay®*; *Fluor-a-day®*; *Hifluor®*; *Zymafluor®*

A standard is given in the British Pharmacopoeia 1973

Description. An odourless white powder.

Solubility. Soluble, at 20°, in 25 parts of water; practically insoluble in alcohol.

Storage. It should be stored in airtight containers.

Metabolism. ABSORPTION. Readily absorbed after oral administration but absorption may be reduced by the presence, in diet, of aluminium, calcium, or magnesium.

BLOOD CONCENTRATION. Normal fluoride plasma concentrations are in the range 140 to 190 ng/ml and may reach 260 ng/ml with larger intakes.

DISTRIBUTION. Rapidly and widely distributed in the body in both hard and soft tissues; about 96% of the fluoride in the body is located in hard tissues; soft tissues contain about 0.5 to 1.0 part per million of fluoride; fluoride is deposited in bones and teeth, crosses the placenta, is secreted in the milk, saliva, sweat, and tears, and is present in hair.

EXCRETION. About 10% of a dose is eliminated in the faeces and 60% is excreted in the urine; the remainder is retained in the body; in children up to 70% of a dose may be retained.

FURTHER INFORMATION. Review of the absorption, distribution, and excretion of fluoride—*Chronicle Wld Hlth Org.*, 1970, **24**, 271.

Actions and uses. Sodium fluoride is used for the prophylaxis of dental caries in communities where the intake of fluoride from drinking water and food is low. It may be added to water supplies to give a final concentration of 1 part of fluoride ion per million in temperate countries. This concentration is fairly critical as 1.5 parts of fluoride per million in drinking water may cause mottling of teeth.

A 2% solution of sodium fluoride in water may be applied to children's teeth, after preliminary cleansing, 3 times at intervals of 1 week at 3, 7, 10, and 13 years of age to correspond with tooth eruption. Alternatively, a paste containing 75% of sodium fluoride and 25% of glycerol is applied to the teeth, rubbed in for 1 minute, and removed by a mouth-wash.

The continued ingestion of excessive amounts of fluoride in food or drinking water during the period of tooth development leads to mottling of the tooth enamel.

Sodium fluoride is a constituent of some insecticides and rodenticides.

Undesirable effects. Sodium fluoride taken by mouth in quantities in excess of 250 milligrams causes nausea and vomiting, epigastric pain, and diarrhoea; large doses cause muscular weakness and clonic convulsions, followed by respiratory and cardiac failure, collapse, and death.

Poisoning. When sodium fluoride has been swallowed, the stomach should be washed out with a 1% solution of calcium chloride or with lime water. A saline purge speeds the elimination of the insoluble calcium fluoride formed.

If considerable absorption of fluoride has taken place, a 10% solution of calcium gluconate may be administered intravenously to control convulsions. Respiratory failure should be treated by oxygen and controlled respiration.

Preparations

Preparations available include a GEL containing sodium fluoride 1%; a MOUTH-WASH containing sodium fluoride 2%; a paediatric SOLUTION containing sodium fluoride 1.1 mg in each 10-drop dose; TABLETS containing sodium fluoride 550 micrograms equivalent to 250 micrograms of fluorine, and tablets containing sodium fluoride 2.2 mg equivalent to 1 mg of fluorine.

Sodium Fusidate

Sodium *ent*-16α-acetoxy-3β,11β-dihydroxy-4β,8β,14α-trimethyl-18-nor-5β,10α-cholesta-(17Z)-17(20),24-dien-21-oate, the sodium salt of fusidic acid, an antimicrobial substance produced by the growth of certain strains of *Fusidium coccineum* (K. Tubaki).

$C_{31}H_{47}NaO_6 = 538.7$

OTHER NAMES: *Fucidin*®
Fucidin H® (with hydrocortisone acetate)

A standard is given in the British Pharmacopoeia 1973

Description. An odourless, slightly hygroscopic, white, crystalline powder with a bitter taste.

Solubility. Soluble, at 20°, in 1 part of water and of alcohol, and in 350 parts of chloroform; very slightly soluble in ether and in acetone.

Alkalinity. A 1.25% solution has a pH of 7.5 to 9.

Moisture content. Not more than 1%, determined by Fischer titration.

Storage. It should be stored in airtight containers, protected from light.

Identification. INFRA-RED ABSORPTION. Major peaks at 1238, 1267, 1380, 1438, 1547 and 1706 cm^{-1} (see Appendix 2a: Infra-red Spectra).

Metabolism. ABSORPTION. Well absorbed after oral administration; topically administered doses penetrate the skin and the extent is increased when applied with dimethyl sulphoxide; cholestyramine reduces the absorption of sodium fusidate in rats and probably in man.

BLOOD CONCENTRATION. After an oral dose of 500 mg, a peak plasma concentration of about 30 μg/ml is attained in 2 to 4 hours; during therapy with oral doses of 1.5 g daily for 3 to 4 days, peak plasma concentrations of up to 200 μg/ml are attained.

HALF-LIFE. From urinary excretion data, 4 to 6 hours.

DISTRIBUTION. Widely distributed throughout the body but does not enter the cerebrospinal fluid; crosses the placenta and is secreted in the milk; *protein binding*, about 95% bound to plasma proteins.

EXCRETION. About 2% of a dose is excreted unchanged in the faeces; doses of sodium fusidate are excreted in the bile and, in small amounts, in the urine.

FURTHER INFORMATION. Concentrations in plasma and nasal secretions—J. E. Acornley *et al.*, *Br. J. Pharmac. Chemother.*, 1967, **31**, 210; concentrations in serum—W. Godtfredsen *et al.*, *Lancet*, i/1962, 928; concentrations in serum, aqueous humour, and vitreous body—J. Williamson *et al.*, *Br. J. Ophthal.*, 1970, **54**, 126; binding to albumins—F. Güttler *et al.*, *Br. J. Pharmac.*, 1971, **43**, 151; influence of cholestyramine on absorption in rats—W. H. Johns and T. R. Bates, *J. pharm. Sci.*, 1972, **61**, 735.

Actions and uses. Sodium fusidate is active against many Gram-positive bacteria and Gram-negative cocci. Nearly all strains of *Staphylococcus aureus* are inhibited by very low concentrations of sodium fusidate. The antibiotic is bacteriostatic, although in high concentrations it may be bactericidal. It is well distributed in all organs and tissue including bone, but excluding the cerebrospinal fluid.

Resistant strains of staphylococci may appear during treatment; this may be overcome by giving it with other antibiotics such as erythromycin or lincomycin.

Sodium fusidate is used mainly for the treatment of staphylococcal infections, particularly those due to penicillin-resistant strains. The dose of sodium fusidate is 1 to 2 grams daily in divided doses after meals; the total daily dose for children is 20 to 40 milligrams per kilogram body-weight. Twice these doses may be given in severe infections, which may also be treated with diethanolamine fusidate equivalent to 500 milligrams of fusidic acid given every 8 hours by intravenous infusion.

An ointment containing 2% of sodium fusidate is used for the treatment of skin infections.

Undesirable effects. Mild gastro-intestinal disturbances may occur, but these may be minimised if the dose is given with food. Rashes may also occur.

Preparations

FUSIDATE OINTMENT: a dispersion of sodium fusidate in a suitable basis. Available as an ointment containing 2% of sodium fusidate.
Containers: see the entry on Ointments for general information on containers.
Advice for patients: the ointment should be applied sparingly to the affected area. It should not be used near the eyes.

SODIUM FUSIDATE CAPSULES: consisting of sodium fusidate, in powder, which may be mixed with a suitable inert diluent, enclosed in a hard capsule. The capsule shells may be coloured. Available as capsules containing 250 mg of sodium fusidate.
A standard for these capsules is given in the British Pharmacopoeia 1973
Containers and *Storage:* see the entry on Capsules for general information on containers and storage.
Labelling: the label on the container should state the date after which the capsules are not intended to be used, and the conditions under which they should be stored.
Advice for patients: the capsules should be taken at regular intervals, preferably after meals. The prescribed course should be completed.

OTHER PREPARATIONS available include an OINTMENT containing sodium fusidate 2% with hydrocortisone acetate 1%; and TABLETS containing sodium fusidate 250 mg.

Sodium Hydroxide

NaOH = 40.00

OTHER NAMES: Caustic Soda; Sod. Hydrox.

A standard is given in the British Pharmacopoeia 1973

Description. White sticks, scales, pellets, or fused masses, which are dry, hard, and brittle, breaking with a crystalline fracture.

Solubility. Soluble, or almost completely soluble, at 20°, in 1 part of water; soluble in alcohol.
A solution free from carbonate may be prepared by dissolving sodium hydroxide in alcohol or in an equal weight of water, followed by filtration or decantation.

Hygroscopicity. When exposed to the air it rapidly absorbs moisture and liquefies, but subsequently becomes solid again, due to absorption of carbon dioxide and formation of sodium carbonate, and effloresces.

Storage. It should be stored in airtight containers; if the containers are made of glass they should be closed by waxed corks or plastic-lined screw caps.

Actions and uses. Sodium hydroxide is a powerful caustic. A 2.5% solution in glycerol is used as a cuticle solvent.

Sodium hydroxide is also used in a variety of pharmaceutical preparations, for example sodium hypochlorite solutions (see below).

Poisoning. Large draughts of water, or water containing vinegar, acetic acid, citric acid, or lemon juice should be given immediately, followed by demulcent drinks and olive oil or arachis oil.

Burns due to sodium hydroxide should be flooded with water and then with dilute acetic acid.

Sodium Hypochlorite Solutions

DILUTE SODIUM HYPOCHLORITE SOLUTION: a solution containing about 1% w/w of available chlorine.

It may be prepared by dilution of a strong sodium hypochlorite solution of known available chlorine content or by the electrolysis of a strong solution of sodium chloride.

It may contain stabilising agents and sodium chloride.

A standard for this solution is given in the British Pharmaceutical Codex 1973

Storage: it should be stored in well-filled airtight bottles, in a cool place, protected from light.

Uses: the uses of dilute sodium hypochlorite solution are described under Chlorinated Lime.

Advice for patients: for use as an antiseptic for wounds and as a cleansing agent. It has a bleaching action and will destroy most dyes.

STRONG SODIUM HYPOCHLORITE SOLUTION: prepared, in strengths of up to about 18% w/w of available chlorine, by absorption of chlorine in sodium hydroxide solution. It is often supplied as solutions of lower available-chlorine content. The solutions decrease in strength fairly rapidly and should be used as soon as possible. They may contain stabilising agents.

A number of preparations are available as solutions, or powder to prepare solutions, for example, *Chloros®, Deosan®, Diversol BX®, Hyposan®, Parozone®,* and *Voxsan®.*

A standard for this solution is given in the British Pharmaceutical Codex 1973

Containers and *Storage:* it should be stored in well-filled airtight bottles, closed with glass stoppers or suitable plastic caps, in a cool place away from acids, protected from light. It is particularly important that cool storage conditions are maintained, because containers may explode at higher temperatures.

It should not be stored for longer than a few months.

Labelling: the label on the container should state that the solution must be diluted before use, and the date after which the solution is not expected to comply with the relevant standard.

Advice for patients: for use only in diluted form as indicated above under Dilute Sodium Hypochlorite Solution.

Sodium Iodide

NaI = 149.9

OTHER NAMES: Natrii Iodidum; Sod. Iod.

A standard is given in the European Pharmacopoeia Vol. I

Description. Odourless colourless crystals or white crystalline powder with a saline and bitter taste.

Solubility. Soluble, at 20°, in less than 1 part of water, in 2 parts of alcohol, and in 1 part of glycerol.

AQUEOUS SOLUTIONS. A marked rise in the temperature of the solution occurs when sodium iodide dissolves in water to form a strong solution; when potassium iodide dissolves, a considerable fall in temperature occurs.

Moisture content. Not more than 5%, determined by drying at 105°.

Stability. Sodium iodide is deliquescent in moist air and decomposes, becoming yellow in colour owing to the liberation of iodine. It melts at dull red heat with some loss of iodine; at high temperatures it slowly volatilises.

A solution of sodium iodide in water gradually becomes coloured on exposure to light and air due to liberation of iodine.

Incompatibility. It is incompatible with salts of iron, bismuth, and mercury, with potassium chlorate and other oxidising agents, and with strychnine hydrochloride, quinine sulphate, and other alkaloidal salts.

Sterilisation. Solutions for injection are sterilised by heating in an autoclave or by filtration.

Storage. It should be stored in airtight containers, protected from light.

Actions and uses. Sodium iodide has actions, uses, and undesirable effects similar to those described under Potassium Iodide.

It is used for the prophylaxis of simple goitre, 0.01% of sodium iodide being added to table salt (iodised salt). Alternatively, for this purpose it may be given by mouth in a dosage of not more than 0.5 to 1 milligram daily, 5 to 10 milligrams once a week, or 200 milligrams daily for 10 days twice a year. It is also used, similarly to potassium iodide in the pre-operative treatment of patients with thyrotoxicosis for which purpose a dosage of 15 milligrams daily in divided doses may be given.

Sodium iodide has been used as an expectorant. The usual dose for an adult is 250 to 500 milligrams. Children may be given 50 to 100 milligrams.

Precautions. As for Potassium Iodide.

Veterinary uses. Sodium iodide is used in the treatment of actinobacillosis of cattle. The usual dose by intravenous injection is 50 to 100 milligrams per kilogram body-weight repeated weekly if necessary. It is contraindicated in late pregnancy.

Preparation

SODIUM IODIDE INJECTION: a sterile solution of sodium iodide, with up to 0.1% of sodium thiosulphate or other suitable reducing agent, in water for injections. It is sterilised by heating in an autoclave or by filtration. Available as an injection containing 80 mg of sodium iodide per ml.

A standard for this injection is given in the British Pharmacopoeia (Veterinary)

Containers and *Labelling:* see the entry on Injections for general information on containers and labelling.

Storage: it should not be allowed to come into contact with metals.

Sodium Iodide (^{125}I) Solution

Sodium Iodide (^{125}I) Solution is a solution suitable for oral administration containing sodium iodide (^{125}I); it also contains sodium thiosulphate or other suitable reducing agent.

OTHER NAME: Natrii Iodidi (^{125}I) Solutio

A standard is given in the European Pharmacopoeia Vol. III

CAUTION. *This material is radioactive and any regulations in force must be complied with.*

Iodine-125 is a radioactive isotope of iodine which decays by electron capture with emission of photons mainly of energy 0.028 MeV (X-radiation). It has a half-life of 60 days. It may be prepared by neutron irradiation of xenon-124.

Description. A clear colourless solution.

Alkalinity. pH 7 to 10.

Labelling. The label on the container should state:
(1) the content of iodine-125 expressed in microcuries or millicuries at a given date;
(2) that the solution is radioactive; and
(3) that the solution is not intended for parenteral administration.
The label on the package should state the total volume in the container.

Storage. It should be stored in an area assigned for the purpose. The storage conditions should be such that the maximum radiation-dose-rate to which persons may be exposed is reduced to an acceptable level.

Actions and uses. Sodium iodide (^{125}I) solution may be administered by mouth to study the uptake of iodine by the thyroid gland, but owing to the low energy of the radiation emitted by iodine-125 it is rarely used for this purpose.
Sodium iodide (^{125}I) solution, or a similar solution free from thiosulphate or other reducing agent, may be used for the radioactive labelling of albumin, fibrinogen, protein hormones, and other proteins which are to be administered to patients or used for assay procedures *in vitro.* Iodine-125 is preferred for this purpose to iodine-131 because of the reduced risk to workers carrying out diagnostic procedures and the reduced radiation dose to the patient. The dose of iodine-125 as sodium iodide solution or in the form of iodinated proteins is up to 100 microcuries.

Precautions and contra-indications. See under Sodium Iodide (^{131}I) Solution.

Sodium Iodide (^{131}I) Injection

A sterile solution containing sodium iodide (^{131}I); it also contains sodium thiosulphate and a suitable reducing agent.

A standard is given in the British Pharmacopoeia 1973

CAUTION. *This material is radioactive and any regulations in force must be complied with.*

Iodine-131 is a radioactive isotope of iodine which decays by emission of β^--radiation mainly having a maximum energy of 0.606 MeV with emission of γ-radiation mainly of energy 0.364 MeV. It has a half-life of 8.06 days. It may be prepared by neutron irradiation of tellurium-130.

Description. A clear colourless solution.

Alkalinity. pH 7 to 8.

Sterilisation. It is sterilised by heating in an autoclave.

Storage. It should be stored in an area assigned for the purpose. The storage conditions should be such that the maximum radiation-dose-rate to which persons may be exposed is reduced to an acceptable level. Glass containers may darken under the effects of radiation.

Labelling. The label on the container should state:
(1) the content of iodine-131 expressed in microcuries or millicuries at a given date and hour;
(2) that the injection is radioactive; and
(3) either that it does not contain a bactericide or the name and proportion of any added bactericide.
The label on the package should state the total volume in the container.

Actions and uses. Sodium Iodide (^{131}I) Injection has the actions and uses described under Sodium Iodide (^{131}I) Solution and is administered by intravenous injection in similar dosage.

Precautions and contra-indications. As for Sodium Iodide (^{131}I) Solution.

Sodium Iodide (^{131}I) Solution

Sodium Iodide (^{131}I) Solution is a solution suitable for oral administration containing sodium iodide (^{131}I); it also contains sodium thiosulphate or other suitable reducing agent.

OTHER NAMES: Natrii Iodidi (^{131}I) Solutio

A standard is given in the European Pharmacopoeia Vol. III

CAUTION. *This material is radioactive and any regulations in force must be complied with.*

Iodine-131 is a radioactive isotope of iodine which decays by emission of β^--radiation mainly having a maximum energy of 0.606 MeV with emission of γ-radiation mainly of energy 0.364 MeV. It has a half-life of 8.06 days. It may be prepared by neutron irradiation of tellurium-130.

Description. A clear colourless solution.

Alkalinity. pH 7 to 10.

Storage. It should be stored in an area assigned for the purpose. The storage conditions should be such that the maximum radiation-dose-rate to which persons may be exposed is reduced to an acceptable level. Glass containers may darken under the effects of radiation.

Labelling. The label on the container should state:
(1) the content of iodine-131 expressed in microcuries or millicuries at a given date and hour;
(2) that the solution is radioactive; and
(3) that the solution is not to be used for parenteral injection.
The label on the package should state the total volume in the container.

Actions and uses. Sodium Iodide (^{131}I) Solution is used for the oral administration of radioactive iodine-131. The volume containing the requisite dose is calculated from the content of radioactivity at a given time and date, as stated on the label, and from the rate of radioactive decay.
Doses of 2 to 10 microcuries, but occasionally up to 50 microcuries, are used to study the iodine uptake of the thyroid gland, the iodine-binding activity of the plasma, and the iodine-excretion rate in the diagnosis of hypo-

thyroidism or hyperthyroidism. Recent administration of any preparation containing iodine or thyroid hormone will, however, interfere with the iodine uptake of the gland. Doses of 100 to 200 microcuries are used to locate aberrant thyroid tissue, and to detect nodules in the thyroid gland which will take up iodine in greater or lesser amounts than the rest of the gland. Similar or smaller doses are sometimes used to determine the rate of iodine uptake of the thyroid in hyperthyroidism or of secondary deposits from a carcinoma of the thyroid, and to calculate the dose of Sodium Iodide (^{131}I) Solution required for the treatment of hyperthyroidism.

Doses of 1 to 15 millicuries, repeated if necessary, are given for the treatment of hyperthyroidism, but it is not normally regarded as the treatment of choice in patients less than 45 years old. This treatment carries a risk that permanent hypothyroidism may develop, perhaps months or even years after the treatment has ceased. Doses of 10 to 40 millicuries may be used in some patients with angina pectoris and heart failure to reduce the activity of the thyroid gland.

Doses of 60 to 150 millicuries are used for the treatment of carcinoma of the thyroid with secondary deposits, if these have been shown to take up significant amounts of iodine.

Precautions and contra-indications. The patient's urine must be monitored, because when doses greater than 1 millicurie are administered, significant amounts of iodine-131 may be excreted; it may be necessary to store the urine until its radioactivity is low enough for it to be disposed of in accordance with any regulations of the appropriate authorities.

The use of sodium iodide (^{131}I) solution is contra-indicated, even in diagnostic doses, during pregnancy and lactation. Foetal thyroid tissue takes up significant amounts of iodine-131 by the twelfth week of gestation and is highly susceptible to irradiation. Infants may receive dangerous amounts of radioactivity in the mother's milk. Children, too, are very sensitive to thyroid irradiation and should not be given radioactive iodine-131.

Sodium Iodohippurate (^{131}I) Injection

Sodium Iodohippurate (^{131}I) Injection is a sterile solution containing sodium o-iodohippurate (^{131}I).

OTHER NAME: Natrii Iodohippurati (^{131}I) Solutio Iniectabilis

A standard is given in the European Pharmacopoeia Vol. III Supplement

CAUTION. *This material is radioactive and any regulations in force must be complied with.*

Iodine-131 is a radioactive isotope of iodine which decays by emission of β^--radiation mainly having a maximum energy of 0.606 MeV with emission of γ-radiation mainly of energy 0.364 MeV. It has a half-life of 8.06 days. It may be prepared by neutron irradiation of tellurium-130.

Description. A clear colourless solution.

Acidity or Alkalinity. pH 6 to 8.5.

Stability. It decomposes with an accompanying decrease in radiochemical purity but should be issued in such a form that when stored as indicated below, the rate of decomposition, measured in terms of radiochemical purity, does not exceed 2% during a period of 10 days from the date stated on the label.

Sterilisation. It is sterilised by heating in an autoclave; benzyl alcohol 0.9% v/v is a suitable bactericide.

Storage. It should be stored in an area assigned for the purpose, protected from light, in a cool place. The storage conditions should be such that the maximum radiation-dose-rate to which persons may be exposed is reduced to an acceptable level. Glass containers may darken under the effects of radiation.

Labelling. The label on the container should state:
(1) the content of iodine-131 expressed in microcuries or millicuries at a given date and hour and;
(2) that the injection is radioactive.
The label on the package should state:
(1) the total volume of injection,
(2) the total content of sodium o-iodohippurate; and
(3) the name and proportion of any added bactericide.

Actions and uses. Sodium iodohippurate (^{131}I) is used in a test of renal function.

The material is selectively and rapidly excreted by the kidneys, and no tubular reabsorption takes place. In the standard technique for radioisotope renography its passage through the kidneys is detected by a pair of collimated scintillation counters, one located accurately over each kidney; sometimes a third similar counter is located over the bladder, so that the rise of radioactivity in the urine can be recorded graphically at the same time as records are made from each kidney, and in addition a fourth detector is sometimes placed over the head to enable a record of blood radioactivity to be made simultaneously. There are alternative techniques for obtaining the same information using a gamma-ray camera.

A suitable dose for this diagnostic procedure is about 20 microcuries administered intravenously in 1 to 2 millilitres of isotonic solution. The test is completed in 20 to 30 minutes.

Sodium iodohippurate is also used for the determination of effective renal plasma flow (ERPF) using about 20 microcuries administered intravenously.

Sodium Lauryl Sulphate

A mixture of the sodium salts of sulphated normal primary alcohols; these sulphated alcohols are sometimes incorrectly referred to as "sulphonated fatty alcohols". It consists chiefly of sodium lauryl sulphate, $C_{12}H_{25}O.SO_2.ONa$.

OTHER NAMES: *Cycloryl 580/585N/599®; Empicol LZ®; Maprofix Powder LK®; Sipon WD®*; Sod. Lauryl Sulph.; *Sulphonated Lorol Paste®*
Lanette Wax SXBP® (with cetostearyl alcohol)

A standard is given in the British Pharmacopoeia 1973

Description. White or pale yellow crystals or powder with a slight characteristic odour.

Solubility. Soluble in water, forming a turbid solution; partly soluble in alcohol.

Uses. Sodium lauryl sulphate is an anionic emulsifying agent. It is used in the preparation of emulsifying wax (see below) which is used as an emulsifying agent for producing oil-in-water creams. Such creams are stable over a wide pH range and suitable for the incorporation of anionic and non-ionic medicaments. For cationic medicaments, cetrimide emulsifying wax (see under Cetrimide) and cetomacrogol emulsifying wax (see under Cetomacrogol 1000) are more suitable emulsifying agents.

Sodium lauryl sulphate reduces surface tension and is used as a wetting agent and detergent. It is not affected by hard water on account of the solubility of the corresponding calcium and magnesium salts, and the addition of sodium lauryl sulphate to soap retards the formation of insoluble calcium soaps.

Aqueous solutions which are sufficiently concentrated to contain micelles will solubilise many water-insoluble materials.

Preparations

EMULSIFYING OINTMENT (*Syn. Ung. Emulsif.*):

Emulsifying wax	300 g
White soft paraffin	500 g
Liquid paraffin	200 g

Melt together and stir until cold.

Containers: see the entry on Ointments for general information on containers.

Emulsifying ointment is an ingredient of aqueous cream (see under Cetostearyl Alcohol).

EMULSIFYING WAX (*Syn.* Anionic Emulsifying Wax): containing cetostearyl alcohol and sodium lauryl sulphate or similar sodium salts of sulphated higher primary aliphatic alcohols. A satisfactory preparation may be prepared according to the following formula:

Sodium lauryl sulphate	10 g
Cetostearyl alcohol	90 g
Purified water	4 ml

Melt the cetostearyl alcohol and heat to about 95°, add the sodium lauryl sulphate, mix, and add the water; heat to 115° and maintain at this temperature, stirring vigorously, until frothing ceases and the product is translucent, and cool rapidly.

A standard for this emulsifying wax is given in the British Pharmacopoeia 1973

Sodium Metabisulphite

$Na_2S_2O_5 = 190.1$

OTHER NAME: Sodium Pyrosulphite

A standard is given in the British Pharmacopoeia 1973

Sodium metabisulphite usually contains small amounts of sodium sulphite and sodium sulphate.

Description. Colourless prismatic crystals or white or creamy-white crystalline powder with a sulphurous odour and an acid, saline taste.

Solubility. Soluble, at 20°, in 2 parts of water; less soluble in alcohol.

Stability. It is a powerful reducing agent, and on exposure to air and moisture it is slowly oxidised to sulphate, with disintegration of the crystals.

FURTHER INFORMATION. Stability of sulphurous acid salts—L. C. Schroeter, *J. pharm. Sci.*, 1963, **52**, 564, and 888.

Storage. It should be stored in airtight containers.

Uses. Sodium metabisulphite is an antioxidant and reducing agent and is widely employed in pharmaceutical preparations, especially in those containing substances which are readily oxidised to form coloured decomposition products. It is often used in a concentration of 0.1%, but concentrations of 0.01 to 1% have been employed.

In the formulation of a pharmaceutical preparation, the minimum concentration should be chosen which will give the desired antioxidant effect. A chelating agent such as sodium edetate is sometimes used in conjunction with sodium metabisulphite to remove heavy metallic ions which often catalyse oxidation reactions.

Sodium metabisulphite is usually employed as an antioxidant in acidic preparations; for alkaline preparations, sodium sulphite is usually preferred.

Sodium metabisulphite decomposes in air, especially on heating, and an appreciable amount may be lost during sterilisation before the substance has had time to exert its antioxidant effect; decomposition in solutions is accompanied by a fall in pH. Injections containing sodium metabisulphite should preferably be filled into containers in which the air has been replaced by an inert gas such as nitrogen.

Rubber caps used to close multidose containers should be pretreated with sodium metabisulphite solution if sodium metabisulphite is included in the contents of the containers.

Under certain conditions, sodium metabisulphite may react with adrenaline and other drugs which are derivatives of 2- or 4-hydroxybenzyl alcohol, and with some dyes and flavouring agents.

Sodium metabisulphite reacts with thiamine to form products with no vitamin activity.

Preparations containing sodium metabisulphite should be thoroughly tested to determine its effect on the active constituents and other ingredients.

Sodium metabisulphite is used as a preservative in acidic solutions and syrups, its antimicrobial action being due to the presence of sulphur dioxide liberated by the reaction between the metabisulphite and the acid.

FURTHER INFORMATION. A review of the uses of sulphurous acid salts as antioxidants—L. C. Schroeter, *J. pharm. Sci.*, 1961, **50**, 891. Properties, uses, toxicity, and limitations of sulphurous acid salts—L. C. Schroeter, *Sulfur Dioxide, Applications in Foods, Beverages, and Pharmaceuticals*, London, Pergamon Press, 1966. Review of uses and possible mutagenic effect—G. Smith and M. F. G. Stevens, *Pharm. J.* ii/1972, 570.

Sodium Methyl Hydroxybenzoate

Sodium methyl 4-hydroxybenzoate

$C_8H_7NaO_3 = 174.1$

OTHER NAMES: *Nipagin M Sodium*®; Sodium Methylparaben; Soluble Methyl Hydroxybenzoate

A standard is given in the British Pharmacopoeia 1973

Description. An almost odourless, hygroscopic, white, crystalline powder; it is tasteless but produces a slight burning sensation of the mouth and tongue, followed by local numbness.

Solubility. Soluble, at 20°, in 2 parts of water and in 50 parts of alcohol; practically insoluble in fixed oils.

Alkalinity. A 0.1% solution has a pH of 9.5 to 10.5.

Moisture content. Not more than 5%, determined by Fischer titration.

Storage. It should be stored in airtight containers.

Identification. TESTS. 1. Dissolve about 500 mg in 5 ml of water and acidify to litmus paper with hydrochloric acid; a precipitate is produced which, after washing with water and drying, melts at about 126°.
2. The precipitate produced in Test 1 complies with the Test described under Methyl Hydroxybenzoate.

Uses. Sodium methyl hydroxybenzoate is used in place of methyl hydroxybenzoate when it is desirable to have a material which is more soluble in water.

Sodium Nitrite

$NaNO_2 = 69.00$

A standard is given in the British Pharmaceutical Codex 1973

Description. Odourless, deliquescent, colourless or slightly yellow crystals or white or slightly yellow crystalline powder.

Solubility. Soluble, at 20°, in 1.5 parts of water and in 160 parts of alcohol.

Incompatibility. It is incompatible with oxidising agents, phenazone, and caffeine citrate.

Sterilisation. Solutions for injection are sterilised by heating in an autoclave or by filtration.

Storage. It should be stored in airtight containers.

Actions and uses. The actions and uses of sodium nitrite are similar to, but less marked than, those described under Glyceryl Trinitrate Solution. The onset of its effect is delayed for about 15 minutes and its actions last for about 1 hour. The usual dose is 30 to 120 milligrams by mouth.
Sodium nitrite occupies a special place in the treatment of cyanide poisoning; 10 millilitres of sodium nitrite injection is given intravenously during 3 minutes, followed after 5 minutes by 50 millilitres of sodium thiosulphate injection given intravenously during 10 minutes. The injections may be repeated in 2 hours if necessary. The sodium nitrite produces methaemoglobinaemia and the cyanide ions combine with the methaemoglobin to produce cyanmethaemoglobin, thus protecting essential enzymes from the cyanide ion. The cyanmethaemoglobin slowly dissociates, setting free cyanide, which is converted to thiocyanate by the sodium thiosulphate.
Sodium nitrite is added to aqueous antiseptic solutions to give a concentration of 1% in order to prevent rusting of surgical instruments.

Poisoning. The procedure as described under Glyceryl Trinitrate Solution should be adopted.
Methaemoglobinaemia severe enough to cause asphyxia may be reversed by the administration of methylene blue, 2 milligrams per kilogram body-weight, by mouth or by intravenous injection.

Preparation

SODIUM NITRITE INJECTION:

Sodium nitrite	..	..	..	..	.. 3 g
Water for injections	..	..	..	.. to 100 ml

Dissolve, and clarify by filtration. Sterilise by heating in an autoclave or by filtration.
A standard for this injection is given in the British Pharmaceutical Codex 1973
Containers: see the entry on Injections for general information on containers. The injection should be supplied in single-dose ampoules.
Labelling: see the entry on Injections for general information on labelling.

Sodium Nitroprusside

$Na_2[Fe(CN)_5NO],2H_2O = 298.0$

OTHER NAMES: *Acetest*®; *Nipride*®

A standard is given in the British Pharmacopoeia Addendum 1978

Description. Odourless reddish-brown crystals or powder.

Solubility. Soluble in water; very slightly soluble in alcohol and in chloroform.

Moisture content. 9 to 15%, determined by Fischer titration.

Stability. Solutions of sodium nitroprusside for injection should be prepared with dextrose injection (5%). No other diluent should be used when preparing solutions for intravenous infusion.

FURTHER INFORMATION. C. J. Vesey and G. A. Batistoni, *J. clin. Pharm.*, 1972, **2**, 105.

Storage. It should be stored in airtight containers, protected from light. When solutions are administered by intravenous infusion, the container should be wrapped in aluminium foil or other suitable material impervious to light.

Metabolism. ABSORPTION. After oral administration, sodium nitroprusside may be transformed, in the stomach or liver, to cyanide and thiocyanate which are absorbed.

BLOOD CONCENTRATION. After an intravenous infusion of 1.5 mg/kg administered over 2 hours, plasma-cyanide concentrations reach about 80 ng/ml (3 μmol per litre).

DISTRIBUTION. About 98% of the cyanide in the circulation, derived from sodium nitroprusside, is taken up by red blood cells.

METABOLIC REACTIONS. Converted to cyanide which is slowly detoxified, to form thiocyanate, by the action of tissue rhodanase.

EXCRETION. Slowly excreted as metabolites; some cyanide may be exhaled.

FURTHER INFORMATION. Relationship of dose and plasma thiocyanate and cyanide concentrations—C. J. Vesey *et al.*, *Br. med. J.*, iii/1975, 229 and C. J. Vesey *et al.*, *Br. J. Anaesth.*, 1976, **48**, 651.

Actions and uses. Sodium nitroprusside is a potent, rapid-acting hypotensive agent which produces vasodilatation and a fall in peripheral resistance by a direct action on the vessel wall. It is used mainly during hypertensive emergencies and for the production of controlled hypotension during anaesthesia.
Sodium nitroprusside is given by intravenous infusion and is fully effective within 1 to 2 minutes of administration. Blood pressure returns to pre-treatment levels within 10 minutes of the discontinuation of treatment.
Sodium nitroprusside is administered by intravenous infusion as a 0.005 or 0.01% solution in dextrose injection (5%). The rate of administration should be regulated with an infusion pump or similar device to allow precise measurement of the rate of flow; small changes in the rate of infusion produce large changes in blood pressure. As the response is variable, doses administered are titrated for each patient but the initial infusion rate for patients not receiving antihypertensive drugs is usually 0.5 to 1.5 micrograms per kilogram body-weight per minute (equivalent to 0.005 to 0.015 millilitre per kilogram body-weight per minute of the 0.01% solution). This dose is gradually adjusted, according to the re-

quirements of the patient, which are usually within the range 0.5 to 8 micrograms per kilogram body-weight per minute, but the rate of administration should not exceed 800 micrograms per minute.

For hypotensive anaesthesia up to 1.5 micrograms per kilogram body-weight per minute may be given.

If a response is not obtained in 10 minutes, administration of sodium nitroprusside should be discontinued. Oral antihypertensive agents should be substituted as soon as possible and treatment may be started whilst sodium nitroprusside is still being infused.

Undesirable effects. When used over short periods, undesirable effects are usually associated with too rapid a decrease in blood pressure and include drowsiness, palpitations, nausea, perspiration, behaviour disorders, and muscular twitches.

These effects may be controlled by stopping the infusion and restarting at a slower rate. With higher doses, accumulation of thiocyanate and cyanide, which are metabolic products of sodium nitroprusside, may occur and produce tachycardia, sweating, hyperventilation, cardiac arrhythmias, and metabolic acidosis. Sodium nitroprusside may also cause methaemoglobinaemia and cyanosis.

Precautions and contra-indications. Careful monitoring of blood pressure throughout the infusion is required. Sodium nitroprusside is metabolised to cyanide and thiocyanate and therefore monitoring of plasma levels for cyanide may be advisable. Plasma-cyanide concentrations should not be allowed to rise above 80 ng per ml (3 micromoles per litre).

In addition, the metabolites of sodium nitroprusside may interfere with iodine uptake and binding and vitamin-B_{12} metabolism. Sodium nitroprusside should therefore be avoided in patients with vitamin-B_{12} deficiency, Leber's optic atrophy, and liver damage.

Some workers have advocated the administration of high doses of hydroxocobalamin by injection, as an antidote to cyanide, before and during the administration of sodium nitroprusside, in such patients.

Caution should be exercised in patients with hypothyroidism and renal impairment. Patients receiving other antihypertensives and elderly patients may require lower doses of sodium nitroprusside. Compensatory hypertension such as arteriovenous shunt and coarctation of the aorta should not be treated with sodium nitroprusside.

Sodium nitroprusside solutions should be protected from light during administration and the solution discarded within 4 hours. Solutions which show more than a faint brown tint should not be used.

Poisoning. Cyanide intoxication may be treated with cobalt edetate intravenously; alternatively, sodium nitrite followed by sodium thiosulphate may be used. Hydroxocobalamin may also be of value.

Preparations

Preparations available include an INJECTION reconstituted from ampoules of powder containing sodium nitroprusside 50 mg supplied with 2-ml ampoules of dextrose injection 5%.

Sodium Perborate

$NaBO_2,H_2O_2,3H_2O = 153.9$

OTHER NAMES: *Bocasan®* (with sodium hydrogen tartrate)

A standard is given in the British Pharmaceutical Codex 1973

Description. Odourless, colourless, prismatic crystals or a white powder, stable in crystalline form.

Solubility. Soluble, at 20°, in 40 parts of water, with some decomposition.

Storage. It should be stored in airtight containers.

Actions and uses. Sodium perborate readily releases oxygen in contact with oxidisable matter and has been used in aqueous solution for purposes similar to those described under Hydrogen Peroxide Solution.

Mixed with 2 to 4 parts of calcium carbonate it has been employed also as a dentifrice, but frequent use may cause blistering and oedema.

Preparation

BUFFERED SODIUM PERBORATE MOUTH-WASH: consisting of a solution of sodium perborate, with sodium hydrogen tartrate, in water. It may contain suitable flavouring agents. It is prepared freshly by dissolving a powder consisting of the dry mixed ingredients in a suitable quantity of warm water. Available as a powder in sachets containing approximately 68% of sodium perborate monohydrate and approximately 29% of anhydrous sodium hydrogen tartrate with peppermint oil and menthol as flavouring agents.

Labelling: directions for preparing the mouth-wash should be given on the label.

Advice for patients: the contents of 1 sachet should be dissolved in half a tumblerful of warm water. The solution should be retained in the mouth for 2 to 3 minutes before spitting out. It should preferably not be swallowed.

Sodium Pertechnetate (^{99m}Tc) Injection

Sodium Pertechnetate (^{99m}Tc) Injection is a sterile solution containing technetium-99m in the form of pertechnetate ion and sufficient sodium chloride to make the solution isotonic with blood.

OTHER NAMES: Natrii Pertechnetatis (^{99m}Tc) Sine Fissione Formati Solutio Iniectabilis; Sodium Pertechnetate (^{99m}Tc) Injection (Non-fission)

A standard is given in the European Pharmacopoeia Vol. III

CAUTION. *This material is radioactive and any regulations in force must be complied with.*

Technetium-99m is a radioactive isotope of technetium which decays by isomeric transition with emission of γ-radiation of energy 0.140 MeV. It has a half-life of 6.0 hours. It may be prepared by elution of a column containing molybdenum-99 adsorbed on a suitable material such as alumina. Generators based on this principle are usually eluted once daily with sodium chloride injection, but may be eluted more frequently to give a lower concentration of technetium-99m in the eluate. Molybdenum-99 is prepared by neutron irradiation of natural molybdenum or molybdenum enriched in molybdenum-98.

Description. A clear colourless solution.

Acidity or alkalinity. pH 4 to 8.

Sterilisation. It is either prepared aseptically using a sterile generator or sterilised by heating in an autoclave or by filtration.

Storage. It should be stored in an area assigned for the purpose. The storage conditions should be such that the maximum radiation-dose-rate to which persons may be exposed is reduced to an acceptable level.

Labelling. The label on the container and the label on the package should state:
(1) the content of technetium-99m expressed in micro-curies or millicuries at a given date and hour;
(2) the volume;
(3) that the injection is radioactive; and
(4) the date and hour after which the injection is not intended to be used.

Actions and uses. Technetium-99m is the radionuclide that is most widely used for diagnostic procedures. Its monoenergetic 140 keV gamma rays, which are easily and efficiently collimated, and the absence of any beta radiation make it an almost ideal radiation source for external gamma scintigraphy with either rectilinear scanners or gamma-ray cameras.

Sodium pertechnetate, which is the form in which technetium-99m is obtained from a radionuclide generator, is selectively concentrated in various organs, including the brain, thyroid gland, and salivary glands, and in the choroid plexuses.

Sodium pertechnetate crosses the blood-brain barrier and is gradually taken up in many brain tumours. This property is utilised in the detection of both primary and secondary brain tumours. A short time after an injection, gamma scanning of the suspected area is begun. To avoid confusion, uptake in the choroid plexuses and glands is blocked by administering potassium perchlorate about an hour before the injection. The dosage required for brain scanning is usually of the order of 5 to 15 millicuries, for salivary gland scanning 2 millicuries and for thyroid scanning, 1 millicurie.

Other organs are visualised by technetium-99m scintigraphy with extemporaneously prepared injections in which sodium pertechnetate (^{99m}Tc) has been converted to a physical or chemical form which will localise in the organ concerned.

For external gamma scanning of the liver the ^{99m}Tc-radioactivity is required in the form of a colloid. A sulphur colloid or an antimony sulphide colloid is commonly used.

A suspension of particles having a diameter of 20 to 50 μm is used for lung scanning. It is usually prepared as a suspension of human albumin particles carrying ^{99m}Tc-activity.

An intravenous injection prepared by the addition of a chelating agent such as diethylenetriamine penta-acetic acid to sodium pertechnetate (^{99m}Tc) solution in the presence of a suitable buffer is used for scanning the kidneys and as an alternative to sodium pertechnetate injection for brain scanning.

For bone scanning, sodium pertechnetate (^{99m}Tc) solution is added to a preparation of a stannous salt and phosphonate, polyphosphate or pyrophosphate, which converts it to a form rapidly and selectively taken up by skeletal tissue after intravenous injection. Sodium pertechnetate (^{99m}Tc) has also been used to prepare labelled human albumin for blood pool studies, and particularly for placenta location.

Sodium Phosphate

$Na_2HPO_4,12H_2O = 358.1$

OTHER NAMES: Disodium Hydrogen Phosphate; *Fletcher's Disposable Phosphate Enema*®; Natrii Phos-

phas; *Phosphate-Sandoz Effervescent Tablets*®; *Practo-Clyss*®; Sod. Phos.

A standard is given in the European Pharmacopoeia Vol. II

Description. Odourless, colourless, transparent, strongly efflorescent crystals with a salty and slightly alkaline taste.

Solubility. Soluble, at 20°, in 5 parts of water; very slightly soluble in alcohol.

Moisture content. 57 to 61%, determined by drying at 130°.

Stability. When heated to 40° it fuses; at 100° it loses its water of crystallisation, and at dull-red heat it is converted into the pyrophosphate, $Na_4P_2O_7$.

Storage. It should be stored in airtight containers.

Actions and uses. Sodium phosphate is a saline purgative, the actions and uses of which are described under Magnesium Sulphate. After oral administration, a small proportion of the salt is absorbed and exerts a mild diuretic action. It is usually administered in solution. The usual adult daily dose is 2 to 16 grams.

Sodium phosphate, usually in conjunction with other phosphates to give solutions with an approximately neutral reaction, is administered in the treatment of calcium and phosphorus metabolic disorders.

Preparations

EFFERVESCENT PHOSPHATE TABLETS: available as tablets containing the equivalent of 500 mg of phosphorus, 481 mg of sodium (20.9 mmol of Na^+), and 123 mg of potassium (3.1 mmol of K^+).
Containers and *Storage:* see the entry on Tablets for general information on containers and storage. Containers should be airtight.
Advice for patients: the tablets should be dissolved in water before administration.

PHOSPHATES ENEMA: see under Sodium Acid Phosphate.

Sodium Phosphate (^{32}P) Injection

Sodium Phosphate (^{32}P) Injection is a sterile isotonic solution containing sodium phosphate (^{32}P) and added phosphate.

OTHER NAME: Natrii Phosphatis (^{32}P) Solutio Iniectabilis

A standard is given in the European Pharmacopoeia Vol. III

CAUTION. *This material is radioactive and any regulations in force must be complied with.*

Phosphorus-32 is a radioactive isotope of phosphorus which decays by emission of β^--radiation having a maximum energy of 1.709 MeV. It has a half-life of 14.3 days. It may be prepared by neutron irradiation of sulphur.

Description. A clear colourless solution.

Acidity or alkalinity. pH 6 to 8.

Sterilisation. It is sterilised by heating in an autoclave.

Storage. It should be stored in an area assigned for the purpose. The storage conditions should be such that the maximum radiation-dose-rate to which persons may be exposed is reduced to an acceptable level. Glass containers may darken under the effects of radiation.

Labelling. The label on the container should state:
(1) the content of phosphorus-32 expressed in micro-curies or millicuries at a given date and hour;

(2) that the injection is radioactive; and

(3) either that it does not contain a bactericide or the name and proportion of any added bactericide.

The label on the package should state:

(1) the total volume in the container; and

(2) the content of total phosphate.

Actions and uses. Sodium phosphate (^{32}P) injection is a solution suitable for the intravenous administration of radioactive phosphorus-32.

Phosphorus-32 has a half-life of just over 14 days, but because it is metabolised and excreted, its effective half-life in the human body is estimated to be only eight days. Phosphorus-32 is deposited in bone and nucleoprotein and rapidly dividing cells have a particular affinity for the element.

Sodium phosphate (^{32}P) injection is used for irradiating the body with β-rays. It is used as a palliative agent in the treatment of polycythaemia vera and its use may be preceded, if required, by phlebotomy. Initially, a single dose of 5 millicuries may be injected intravenously, followed, if necessary, by doses of not more than 3 or 4 millicuries at intervals of not less than two months. The full effect of treatment with radioactive phosphorus-32 may not be seen for three or four months but if the platelet count falls below 50000 per cubic millimetre, a remission, usually lasting for 4 months to 2 years, is likely to occur. Relapses may be treated with further courses of radioactive phosphorus-32 but an interval of at least 3 months should elapse between any two courses of the treatment.

In the treatment of chronic myeloid leukaemia, sodium phosphate (^{32}P) injection produces results resembling those obtained with X-ray treatment. An intravenous dose of 1 to 2 millicuries once a week may be required for 4 to 8 weeks to reduce the leucocyte count to about 10000 to 20000 per cubic millimetre. After a course of treatment, remissions last from 3 to 10 months in about half of the patients. Chronic lymphatic leukaemia does not respond so readily, and local irradiation of lymph nodes is sometimes more beneficial.

Radioactive phosphorus-32 has little effect during exacerbations in the course of chronic leukaemias and is of little value in the treatment of the acute leukaemias, Hodgkin's disease, and lymphosarcoma. In those reticuloses, however, in which the tumour is highly sensitive to irradiation, satisfactory results may be obtained by treatment with radioactive phosphorus-32.

Sodium phosphate (^{32}P) injection is of no value for the treatment of multiple myeloma or of most forms of carcinoma or sarcoma. Radioactive phosphorus-32 has also been used for the diagnosis and localisation of intraocular tumours and skin tumours.

Precautions and contra-indications. Significant amounts of radioactive phosphorus-32 are excreted in the urine and, after oral administration, in the faeces. The excreta must therefore always be monitored and, if necessary, stored until the radioactivity is low enough for it to be disposed of in accordance with any regulations of the appropriate authorities.

Because of its depressant effect on the red bone marrow, Sodium Phosphate (^{32}P) Injection, even in therapeutic doses, may produce aplastic anaemia, leucopenia, and thrombocytopenic purpura. Paradoxically, it has been reported that radioactive phosphorus-32, used for the treatment of polycythaemia vera, has induced leukaemia. Frequent examination of the blood during and after radioactive phosphorus-32 therapy is essential.

Symptoms of radiation sickness have followed its use. Special caution should be exercised when giving sodium phosphate (^{32}P) injection to leukaemic patients with an erythrocyte count of less than 2500000 per cubic millimetre. It is contra-indicated if the reticulocyte count, in the presence of significant anaemia, is less than 0.2% and also if the leucocyte count is less than 3000 per cubic millimetre or if the platelet count is less than 150000 per cubic millimetre.

Sodium Polymetaphosphate

A complex phosphate of sodium prepared by heating anhydrous sodium dihydrogen phosphate to a temperature above its melting-point, sufficient disodium hydrogen phosphate having been added to yield a product containing about 10% of tetrasodium pyrophosphate, $Na_4P_2O_7$, and cooling the melt rapidly. The presence of the pyrophosphate increases the pH of solutions to approximately 7. This substance has been called "sodium hexametaphosphate" but, in fact, it exists in much higher degrees of polymerisation.

OTHER NAME: *Calgon®*

A standard is given in the British Pharmaceutical Codex 1973

Description. Odourless, colourless, translucent, vitreous, deliquescent plates or powder.

Solubility. Slowly soluble in water; practically insoluble in alcohol.

Stability. Aqueous solutions of sodium polymetaphosphate slowly revert to orthophosphate; the rate of hydration is considerably increased by high temperatures and by the addition of sufficient acid or alkali.

Storage. It should be stored in airtight containers.

Uses. Sodium polymetaphosphate combines with calcium and magnesium ions to form complex soluble compounds and is therefore used, in a concentration of 1 in 600 to 1 in 300, to prevent the precipitation of calcium and magnesium compounds from water.

Sodium polymetaphosphate may also be used as a dusting-powder (5%) in hyperhidrosis and bromidrosis and as a prophylactic against mycotic infection of the toes.

Sodium Potassium Tartrate

$C_4H_4KNaO_6,4H_2O = 282.2$

OTHER NAMES: Rochelle Salt; Sod. Pot. Tart.

A standard is given in the British Pharmaceutical Codex 1973

Description. Odourless, colourless crystals or white crystalline powder.

Solubility. Soluble, at 20°, in 1.5 parts of water; very slightly soluble in alcohol.

Actions and uses. Sodium potassium tartrate is a saline purgative, the actions and uses of which are described under Magnesium Sulphate. It causes a watery evacuation of the bowel after 1 to 2 hours without producing irritation. The usual dose is 8 to 16 grams. Children may be given half of the adult dose.

The tartrates of the alkali metals are less readily absorbed than the citrates; their purgative action is therefore greater, while their diuretic action and effect in reducing the acidity of the urine are less pronounced.

Sodium Propionate

$C_3H_5NaO_2 = 96.06$

A standard is given in the British Pharmacopoeia Addendum 1977 and in the British Pharmacopoeia (Veterinary)

Description. Colourless, deliquescent crystals or white granular powder; odourless or with a slight characteristic odour.

Solubility. Soluble, at 20°, in 1 part of water and in 25 parts of alcohol.

Moisture content. Not more than 1%, determined by Fischer titration.

Storage. It should be stored in airtight containers.

Actions and uses. Sodium propionate is a fungicide which has been used in the treatment of superficial fungous infections, particularly dermatophytoses of the feet, groin, and mucous membranes. It is applied as a 10% ointment or dusting-powder, alone or in conjunction with other propionates, or with octoates or other fungicides. Solutions and jellies have also been used.

Veterinary uses. Sodium propionate is a glucogenic substance used in the treatment of bovine ketosis and pregnancy toxaemia in sheep. The usual dose by mouth for cattle and sheep is 500 milligrams per kilogram body-weight twice daily.

Sodium Propyl Hydroxybenzoate

Sodium propyl 4-hydroxybenzoate

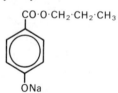

$C_{10}H_{11}NaO_3 = 202.2$

OTHER NAMES: *Nipasol M Sodium®*; Sodium Propylparaben; Soluble Propyl Hydroxybenzoate

A standard is given in the British Pharmacopoeia 1973

Description. An odourless, tasteless, hygroscopic, white crystalline powder.

Solubility. Soluble, at 20°, in 1 part of water, in 50 parts of alcohol, and in 2 parts of alcohol (50%); practically insoluble in fixed oils.

Alkalinity. A 0.1% solution has a pH of 9.5 to 10.5.

Moisture content. Not more than 5%, determined by Fischer titration.

Storage. It should be stored in airtight containers.

Identification. TESTS. 1. Dissolve about 500 mg in 5 ml of water and acidify to litmus paper with hydrochloric acid; a white precipitate is produced which, after washing with water and drying, melts at about 95°.
2. The precipitate produced in Test 1 complies with the Test described under Methyl Hydroxybenzoate.

Uses. Sodium propyl hydroxybenzoate is used in place of propyl hydroxybenzoate when it is desirable to have a material which is more soluble in water.

Sodium Salicylate

Sodium 2-hydroxybenzoate

COONa
OH

$C_7H_5NaO_3 = 160.1$

OTHER NAMES: *Entrosalyl (Standard)®*; Natrii Salicylas; Sod. Sal.

A standard is given in the European Pharmacopoeia Vol. III

Description. Almost odourless, colourless, small crystals or shiny flakes, or white crystalline powder, with a salty-sweet taste.

Solubility. Soluble, at 20°, in 1 part of water and in 11 parts of alcohol.

Incompatibility. It is incompatible with most acids and with solutions of some alkaloids. With alkali bicarbonates, a sodium salicylate solution gradually acquires a reddish-brown colour; if the prescriber will authorise the addition, sodium metabisulphite (0.1%) will retard this change. Sodium salicylate forms a deep purple solution with iron salts.

Actions and uses. Sodium salicylate has antipyretic and analgesic actions. When given by mouth, it is absorbed mainly through the intestine and is rapidly excreted; frequent doses are therefore required to maintain a satisfactory concentration in the blood. The usual dose is 0.6 to 2 grams.
Sodium salicylate is a gastric irritant and sodium bicarbonate is often given with it to reduce this effect; however, the bicarbonate also increases the rate of excretion and thus lowers the concentration of salicylate in the blood to less effective levels.
Sodium salicylate causes dilatation of the skin vessels and some perspiration and the increased loss of heat results in a fall in body temperature. The principal use of sodium salicylate is in the treatment of acute rheumatic fever; a dosage of 1.3 grams may be given by mouth every 2 hours, or 2 grams every 3 hours, until the temperature is reduced. For acute rheumatism, it is given in a daily dosage of 5 to 10 grams in divided doses.
Aspirin is preferable to sodium salicylate because it is a more effective analgesic.
The unpleasant taste of sodium salicylate may be disguised with orange peel infusion.

Undesirable effects. Some patients exhibit an idiosyncrasy to salicylates, as described under Aspirin. After large doses, most patients are liable to experience certain undesirable effects, which include headache, tinnitus, confusion, dimness of vision, excessive sweating, skin eruptions, and dyspnoea. Salicylates must be used with care in patients with acute renal disease. The prothrombin time may be prolonged after repeated large doses.

Poisoning. The procedure as described under Aspirin should be adopted.

Veterinary uses. Sodium salicylate is an analgesic and antipyretic. The usual dose by mouth for horses and cattle is 50 to 200 milligrams per kilogram body-weight and for pigs 10 to 20 milligrams per kilogram body-weight.

Preparations

SODIUM SALICYLATE MIXTURE:

Sodium salicylate	50 g
Sodium metabisulphite	1 g
Concentrated orange peel infusion	50 ml
Chloroform water, double-strength	500 ml
Water for preparations	to 1000 ml

It should be recently prepared.

A standard for this mixture is given in the British Pharmaceutical Codex 1973

Containers and *Labelling:* see the entry on Mixtures for general information on containers and labelling.

Advice for patients: the mixture should preferably be taken after meals.

STRONG SODIUM SALICYLATE MIXTURE:

Sodium salicylate	100 g
Sodium metabisulphite	1 g
Peppermint emulsion, concentrated	25 ml
Chloroform water, double-strength	500 ml
Water for preparations	to 1000 ml

It should be recently prepared.

A standard for this mixture is given in the British Pharmaceutical Codex 1973

Containers and *Labelling:* see the entry on Mixtures for general information on containers and labelling.

Advice for patients: the mixture should preferably be taken after meals.

OTHER PREPARATIONS available include TABLETS containing sodium salicylate 500 mg.

Sodium Stibogluconate

A pentavalent antimony compound of indefinite composition. It has been represented by the formula $C_6H_9Na_2O_9Sb$, but it usually contains less than 2 atoms of sodium for each atom of antimony.

OTHER NAME: *Pentostam®*

A standard is given in the British Pharmacopoeia 1973

Description. An odourless colourless powder consisting mainly of amorphous particles.

Solubility. Soluble in water; practically insoluble in alcohol and in ether.

Acidity. A 10% solution has a pH of 5 to 5.6.

Moisture content. 10 to 15%, determined by drying at 130° *in vacuo*.

Sterilisation. Solutions for injection are sterilised by heating in an autoclave or by filtration.

Storage. It should be stored in airtight containers.

Actions and uses. Sodium stibogluconate is used in the treatment of leishmaniasis. It is much less toxic than antimony sodium tartrate, and it forms a stable aqueous solution which is non-irritant. After parenteral administration a large proportion of the drug is excreted rapidly by the kidneys.

Sodium stibogluconate is administered by intramuscular or intravenous injection; a course of treatment usually consists of 6 to 10 daily injections, each of 6 millilitres of sodium stibogluconate injection. More than one course is usually necessary for the treatment of *Leishmania donovani* infections in East Africa, Ethiopia, and the Sudan. The interval between courses is 10 days.

For the treatment of oriental sore the injection may be infiltrated around the edges of the lesions, a total of not more than 2 millilitres being injected at one time, but intravenous or intramuscular injections combined with bland local dressings are generally more satisfactory.

Children tolerate larger doses of sodium stibogluconate than adults in proportion to body-weight. The dose for children by intravenous or intramuscular injection is 0.1 millilitre of stibogluconate injection per kilogram body-weight for 21 days.

Undesirable effects. Cardiac changes as described under Antimony Sodium Tartrate may rarely occur. Toxic effects, such as nausea, vomiting, or rigors, are rare.

Poisoning. As for Antimony Sodium Tartrate.

Preparation

SODIUM STIBOGLUCONATE INJECTION: a sterile solution of sodium stibogluconate in water for injections. It is sterilised by heating in an autoclave or by filtration. It contains the equivalent of 10% of total antimony (the equivalent of 600 mg of total antimony, or 2 g of sodium stibogluconate, in 6 ml). Available in 100-ml vials.

A standard for this injection is given in the British Pharmacopoeia 1973

Containers: see the entry on Injections for general information on containers.

Labelling: see the entry on Injections for general information on labelling. In addition, the label on the container should state the amount of the medicament as the equivalent amount of pentavalent antimony per ml.

Storage: it should be protected from light.

Sodium Sulphate

$Na_2SO_4,10H_2O = 322.2$

OTHER NAMES: Glauber's Salt; Natrii Sulfas Decahydricus; Sod. Sulph.; Sodium Sulphate Decahydrate

A standard is given in the European Pharmacopoeia Vol. I

Description. Odourless, colourless, transparent crystals or white crystalline powder with a saline, slightly bitter taste.

Solubility. Soluble, at 20°, in 2.5 parts of water, at 33°, in 0.3 part of water, and then decreasing with increase in temperature to 0.5 part at 100°; practically insoluble in alcohol. It readily forms a supersaturated solution when a saturated solution prepared at a temperature above 33° is cooled.

Moisture content. 52 to 57%, determined by heating for 1 hour at 30° followed by drying at 130°.

Stability. It rapidly effloresces in dry air and, when heated to a temperature of 33°, the crystals liquefy. The anhydrous salt fuses at red heat without decomposition.

Sterilisation. Solutions for injection are sterilised by heating in an autoclave or by filtration.

Storage. It should be stored in airtight containers.

Actions and uses. Sodium sulphate is a saline purgative, the actions and uses of which are described under Magnesium Sulphate. The usual dose for an adult is 5 to 15 grams; children may be given one to three quarters of the dose for an adult. A 12 to 25% solution is of value as a lymphagogue when applied to infected wounds.

Veterinary uses. Sodium sulphate is used as a laxative. The usual dose for horses, cattle, sheep, and pigs is 0.5 to 1 gram per kilogram body-weight.

Sodium Sulphate, Anhydrous

$Na_2SO_4 = 142.0$

OTHER NAMES: Anhyd. Sod. Sulph.; Dried Glauber's Salt; Dried Sodium Sulphate; Exsiccated Glauber's Salt; Exsiccated Sodium Sulphate; Natrii Sulfas Anhydricus

A standard is given in the European Pharmacopoeia Vol. I

Description. An odourless hygroscopic white powder.

Solubility. Soluble, at 20°, in 5 parts of water; practically insoluble in alcohol.

Moisture content. Not more than 5%, determined by drying at 130°.

Storage. It should be stored in airtight containers.

Actions and uses. Anhydrous sodium sulphate has the purgative actions of sodium sulphate. It is used for preparing effervescent granules and powders and in preparations for which the powdered crystals of sodium sulphate are not suitable. The usual dose is 1 to 8 grams.

Sodium Sulphite

$Na_2SO_3, 7H_2O = 252.1$

A standard is given in the British Pharmaceutical Codex 1973

Description. Odourless colourless monoclinic prisms.

Solubility. Soluble, at 20°, in 2 parts of water and in 28 parts of glycerol; practically insoluble in alcohol.

Stability. Sodium sulphite is efflorescent in air, becoming opaque and slowly oxidised to sulphate.
A solution in water is alkaline to litmus and is more rapidly oxidised than the solid salt. On boiling a saturated aqueous solution, the anhydrous salt separates out as a crystalline powder which redissolves on cooling.
On gently heating the salt, it softens but does not fuse; above 100° the crystals lose their water of crystallisation without melting or losing their shape; at a red heat the salt fuses, yielding an orange-red mixture of sodium sulphide and sodium sulphate.

Storage. It should be stored in airtight containers.

Uses. Sodium sulphite is used as an antoxidant and preservative in alkaline preparations, as described under Sodium Metabisulphite.

Sodium Thiosulphate

$Na_2S_2O_3, 5H_2O = 248.2$

OTHER NAMES: Natrii Thiosulfas; Sodium Hyposulphite

A standard is given in the European Pharmacopoeia Vol. III Supplement

Description. Odourless colourless monoclinic prisms. Efflorescent in warm dry air and slightly hygroscopic in moist air.

Solubility. Soluble, at 20°, in less than 1 part of water; practically insoluble in alcohol.

Stability. When rapidly heated it melts in its water of crystallisation at 50°; at 100° it loses all its water of crystallisation and at a red heat it is decomposed. It is slowly decomposed when boiled in aqueous solution.

Sterilisation. Solutions for injection are sterilised by heating in an autoclave in an atmosphere of nitrogen.

Storage. It should be stored in airtight containers.

Actions and uses. Sodium thiosulphate is used, in conjunction with sodium nitrite, in the treatment of cyanide poisoning; 10 millilitres of sodium nitrite injection is given intravenously during 3 minutes, followed after 5 minutes by 50 millilitres of sodium thiosulphate injection given intravenously during 10 minutes. The injections may be repeated in 2 hours if necessary.
The sodium nitrite produces methaemoglobinaemia and the cyanide ions combine with the methaemoglobin to produce cyanmethaemoglobin, thus protecting essential enzymes from the cyanide ions. The cyanmethaemoglobin dissociates, setting free cyanide, which is converted to thiocyanate by the sodium thiosulphate.
Sodium thiosulphate has also been used as a reducing agent in medicines, in concentrations of 0.01 to 1%.

Veterinary uses. Sodium thiosulphate is used in the treatment of cyanide poisoning. In horses and cattle 10 millilitres of a 20% solution of sodium nitrite is injected intravenously followed immediately without removing the needle by 40 to 50 millilitres of a 20% solution of sodium thiosulphate. In sheep 10 millilitres of a 10% solution of sodium nitrite and 20 millilitres of a 10% solution of sodium thiosulphate are used.

Preparation

SODIUM THIOSULPHATE INJECTION: a sterile solution of sodium thiosulphate in water for injections. The usual strength is 50% of sodium thiosulphate. A suitable preparation may be prepared according to the following formula:

Sodium thiosulphate	50 g
Water for injections	to 100 ml

Dissolve, and filter. Distribute the solution into single-dose containers, replace the air in the containers with nitrogen or other suitable gas, seal, and sterilise by heating in an autoclave.
A standard for this injection is given in the British Pharmaceutical Codex 1973 and in the British Pharmacopoeia (Veterinary)
Containers: see the entry on Injections for general information on containers. The injection should be supplied in single-dose containers.
Labelling: see the entry on Injections for general information on labelling.

Sodium Valproate

Sodium 2-propylpentanoate

$$CH_3 \cdot CH_2 \cdot CH_2 \cdot \underset{\underset{CH_2 \cdot CH_2 \cdot CH_3}{|}}{CH} \cdot COONa$$

$C_8H_{15}NaO_2 = 166.2$

OTHER NAMES: *Epilim®*; Valproate Sodium

Description. An odourless white crystalline powder with a saline taste.

Solubility. Soluble in water and in alcohol.

Determination in body fluids. GAS CHROMATOGRAPHY In plasma, saliva, or urine—C. J. Jensen and R. Gugler, *J. Chromat.*, 1977, **137**, 188.

Metabolism. ABSORPTION. Rapidly absorbed after oral administration; absorption is delayed in non-fasting subjects; the drug is converted to the free acid if taken on an empty stomach and may cause gastric irritation.

BLOOD CONCENTRATION. After an oral dose of 400 to 800 mg, peak plasma concentrations of 25 to 70 μg/ml are attained in 1 to 4 hours; during therapy with doses of 0.3 to 2.4 g daily, plasma concentrations range from 10 to 160 μg/ml; therapeutic plasma concentrations are in the range 50 to 100 μg/ml.

HALF-LIFE. Plasma half-life, 6 to 16 hours; the shorter half-lives may be obtained in epileptics undergoing therapy; in overdosage, the half-life may reach about 30 hours.

DISTRIBUTION. Volume of distribution, 0.15 to 0.4 litres/ kg; enters the cerebrospinal fluid in concentrations of about one-tenth of those in the plasma; secreted in milk and saliva but saliva concentrations do not correlate with plasma concentrations; in rodents, sodium valproate crosses the placenta and appears to be subject to enterohepatic circulation; *protein binding*, about 90% bound to plasma proteins.

METABOLIC REACTIONS. Rapidly metabolised in man probably by similar routes to those in rodents. Reactions include side-chain oxidation and glucuronic acid conjugation; the metabolism of sodium valproate is induced by phenytoin, primidone, phenobarbitone, and carbamazepine.

EXCRETION. In mice, about 70% of a dose is excreted in the urine in 24 hours; small amounts are excreted in the urine unchanged.

FURTHER INFORMATION. Review of pharmacokinetics, actions, and uses—R. M. Pinder *et al.*, *Drugs*, 1977, **13**, 81; pharmacokinetics in epileptic patients—F. Schobben *et al.*, *Eur. J. clin. Pharmac.*, 1975, **8**, 97.

Actions and uses. Sodium valproate has anticonvulsant actions and causes an increase in the concentration of gamma-aminobutyric acid in the brain. It may be used alone or in conjunction with other anticonvulsants in the treatment of petit mal and grand mal epilepsies and may have limited use in temporal lobe epilepsy.

Treatment is started with 200 milligrams 3 times daily, increasing after 3 days to 400 milligrams 3 times daily. If control is not obtained after 2 weeks, the dose may be increased further and another anticonvulsant given concomitantly; the dosage of both drugs is then adjusted to obtain optimum control. The initial dose for patients already receiving anticonvulsants is 200 milligrams 3 times daily increasing by 400 milligrams daily at 3-day intervals. Optimum control is usually obtained with doses of 0.8 to 1.4 grams of sodium valproate daily, but doses of 2.4 grams daily may be administered in very severe cases. The dose of other anticonvulsants may be reduced or gradually withdrawn depending on the patient's response.

If sedation is increased in patients receiving concomitant barbiturate treatment, the dose of barbiturate is gradually reduced as the dose of sodium valproate is increased.

The initial dosage given to children up to 3 years is 20 to 30 milligrams per kilogram body-weight daily and to children aged 4 to 15 years 400 to 600 milligrams daily.

Undesirable effects. Nausea, gastro-intestinal disturbances, and alopecia may occur.

Precautions. In women of child-bearing age and during pregnancy it should only be used for the treatment of epilepsy resistant to other treatment.

The testing of urine of diabetic patients may show a false positive as sodium valproate is partially excreted as ketone bodies by the kidneys.

Drug interactions. Sodium valproate may enhance the sedative actions of other anticonvulsants particularly the barbiturates and may also potentiate the actions of monoamine-oxidase inhibitors and other antidepressants.

Preparations

SODIUM VALPROATE TABLETS: available as tablets containing 200 and 500 mg of sodium valproate; they may be enteric coated and the coat may be coloured.

Containers and *Storage:* see the entry on Tablets for general information on containers and storage. Containers should be airtight.

Advice for patients: the tablets should preferably be taken after meals with non-aerated water. Enteric-coated tablets should be swallowed whole. When initiating treatment there may be a time-lag of up to 2 weeks before a full therapeutic effect is obtained. Treatment should not be discontinued without the advice of the prescriber.

OTHER PREPARATIONS available include an ELIXIR containing sodium valproate 200 mg in 5 ml, diluent syrup, life of diluted elixir 14 days. The syrup used as a diluent should not be preserved with metabisulphite.

Solubility

When a solid is placed in contact with a solvent, molecules or ions detach themselves from the surface of the solid and diffuse throughout the solvent. Some of the material returns to the surface of the solid and thus passes out of solution. The process continues until an equilibrium exists between the solid and the solvent. The resulting solution is a saturated solution, and the concentration of the solute is the solubility of the substance in the solvent at the temperature used.

Solubility statements in the Pharmaceutical Codex are intended only as information on approximate solubility. Where figures are stated they should not be regarded as precise because of the possibility of variations depending on the method and conditions of the determination. Where no temperature is given, statements of solubility apply at ordinary room temperature.

When the word "parts" is used in expressing the solubility of a substance, it means, unless otherwise stated, parts by weight (grams) of a solid in parts by volume (millilitres) of the solvent, or parts by volume (millilitres) of a liquid in parts by volume (millilitres) of the solvent, or parts by weight (grams) of a gas in parts by weight (grams) of the solvent.

In this edition of the Pharmaceutical Codex approximate figures are given for the solubility when a substance is soluble in less than 1000 parts of solvent. Some figures for much lower solubilities are given where these are known but, in general, when the solubility is less than 1 in 1000 parts, the expressions used are the same as those of the European Pharmacopoeia. Thus a solubility of about 1 in 1000 to 1 in 10000 is indicated by the expression "very slightly soluble", and solubilities lower than 1 in 10000 are indicated by the expression "practically insoluble".

Most of the substances have solubility statements for water, alcohol, ether, and chloroform. Other solvents are also included where they are considered to be useful for a particular substance. In these statements the word "water" refers to purified water, the word "ether" to solvent ether, and the word "alcohol", without qualification, to alcohol (95%).

Determination of Solubility

The simplest method of determining solubility for most compounds is to shake an excess of the substance with the solvent at the required temperature until equilibrium is reached. The concentration of the substance in the solution may then be determined by a suitable method, which may be a quantitative chemical or physical method, or may utilise a physical characteristic of the solution such as specific gravity or refractive index. In some cases it may be adequate to evaporate a measured volume of the solution and weigh the residue.

A variation of this method consists of preparing a number of mixtures containing varying quantities of the substance in a fixed volume of solvent and shaking them at the required temperature until equilibrium is reached. The solubility is then known to be in the range covered by two adjacent mixtures, in one of which the solid is completely dissolved and in the other of which a small amount of solid remains undissolved. This method is useful when there is not a suitable analytical method available or where the solvent is volatile.

The equilibrium state can be reached more quickly by heating an excess of solid with the solvent and then allowing the solution to cool to the required temperature. The cooling should take place in the presence of solid in order to avoid the formation of a supersaturated solution.

Solutions

Solutions are liquid preparations containing one or more soluble ingredients usually dissolved in water. They are intended for internal or external use or for instillation into body cavities. They are issued sterile or unsterilised, depending on the purpose for which they are intended.

Aqueous solutions of antiseptics are liable to become contaminated with resistant micro-organisms, and the following precautions should be taken.

Solutions should be prepared with freshly distilled or freshly boiled water and transferred to thoroughly cleansed containers (preferably sterile); closures of cork or containing cork liners must not be used; the contents should preferably not be used later than one week after the container has first been opened.

Solutions of antiseptics for application to broken skin or the eyes or for introduction into body cavities should be sterilised and supplied in a sterile condition (see below).

Sterile solutions. These include solutions for external application to wounds and abraded surfaces, anticoagulant solutions, bladder irrigations, intraperitoneal dialysis solutions, and concentrated solutions for the preparation of injections.

Preparation of sterile solutions. The apparatus used in the preparation of sterile solutions and the containers should be thoroughly cleansed before use. The medicament is dissolved in the solvent and the solution clarified by filtration, transferred to the final containers, which are then closed, and sterilised by heating in an autoclave or by heating with a bactericide. Alternatively, the solution is sterilised by filtration, and transferred by means of an aseptic technique to the final sterile containers, which are then closed to exclude micro-organisms.

Containers. Containers of sterile solutions should be readily distinguishable from containers used for intravenous fluids and should be closed so as to exclude micro-organisms. A readily breakable seal should cover the closure.

Labelling. The label on the sealed container of a sterile solution should state that the solution is sterile and that it is not to be used for injection.

Unsterilised solutions. These include solutions for internal administration, either alone or as ingredients of other preparations, solutions for external application to unabraded surfaces, and haemodialysis solutions. Precautions should be taken to minimise any microbial contamination during preparation.

Solution-tablets

Solution-tablets are compact products containing a medicament or a mixture of medicaments in compressed form and are intended, after being dissolved in water, to be used externally or on mucous surfaces. They are usually circular in shape with slightly convex surfaces, but solution-tablets containing poisons may be of a distinctive shape and coloured by the addition of a suitable dye.

Solution-tablets may be prepared by the methods described in the entry on Tablets, but any lubricant or diluent used should be readily soluble in water. Sodium chloride is normally used as a diluent, but solution-tablets containing this substance become less readily soluble on storage. Solution-tablets should be completely soluble in water.

Containers and storage. All solution-tablets should be stored and supplied in containers which provide adequate protection against crushing. In addition, solution-tablets which deteriorate if exposed to a moist atmosphere or to light should be stored and supplied in containers which are airtight or light resistant, or both. They should preferably be stored and supplied in amber glass bottles, jars, or vials, in amber or opaque plastic containers, or in cylindrical aluminium containers, suitably protected internally; lined screw-cap closures or plastic caps should be used.

Solution-tablets may also be packaged in strip foil, each tablet being separately sealed in a pocket of foil. This method gives good protection against ingress of moisture but effervescent solution-tablets so packed must have a very low initial moisture content.

Somatostatin

see under HYPOTHALAMIC RELEASING FACTORS

Sorbic Acid

Hexa-2,4-dienoic acid

$$CH_3 \cdot CH:CH \cdot CH:CH \cdot COOH$$

$C_6H_8O_2 = 112.1$

OTHER NAME: *Sorbistat®*

A standard is given in the British Pharmaceutical Codex 1973

Description. A white or creamy-white powder with a faint characteristic odour.

Solubility. Soluble, at 20°, in 700 parts of water, in 10 parts of alcohol, in 20 parts of ether, and in about 150 parts of fats and fatty oils.

Storage. It should be stored in airtight containers, in a cool place, protected from light.

Identification. TEST. To a saturated solution in water, add *bromine solution*, dropwise; the bromine solution is decolorised.

MELTING-POINT. About 135°.

ULTRAVIOLET ABSORPTION. In 0.1N hydrochloric acid, maximum at 264 nm (E1%, 1cm = 1880).

Uses. Sorbic acid has antifungal and antibacterial properties. In concentrations of 0.1 to 0.2% it is an effective preservative for acidic preparations; the optimum pH is 4.5. It is not effective above pH 6.5.
It is sometimes preferred to the hydroxybenzoate esters as a preservative in preparations containing non-ionic emulsifying agents but its use may give rise to skin irritation. Sorbic acid is irritant to the eyes.

Sorbitan Monolaurate

A mixture of the partial esters of sorbitol and its mono- and di-anhydrides with lauric acid.

OTHER NAMES: *Crill 1®*; *Span 20®*

A standard is given in the British Pharmaceutical Codex 1973

Description. An amber-coloured viscous liquid with a characteristic odour.

Solubility. Practically insoluble but dispersible in water; soluble at 20°, in 100 parts of cottonseed oil; very slightly soluble in ethyl acetate; miscible with alcohol.

Weight per ml. At 20°, about 1.00 g.

Uses. Sorbitan esters are non-ionic surface-active agents which are used in the preparation of emulsions, creams, and ointments. They are lipophilic in character and, when used alone, produce water-in-oil emulsions. They are also used in conjunction with suitable polysorbates, when, by appropriate choice of ester and concentration, the character of the emulsion can be varied and either water-in-oil or oil-in-water types may be obtained.
Sorbitan monolaurate is less lipophilic in character than the mono-oleate or the monostearate.

Sorbitan Mono-oleate

A mixture of the partial esters of sorbitol and its mono- and di-anhydrides with oleic acid.

OTHER NAMES: *Crill 4®*; *Span 80®*

A standard is given in the British Pharmaceutical Codex 1973

Description. An amber-coloured viscous liquid with an odour characteristic of fatty acids.

Solubility. Practically insoluble but dispersible in water; miscible with alcohol; practically insoluble in propylene glycol.

Weight per ml. At 20°, about 1.00 g.

Uses. Sorbitan mono-oleate has the uses of the sorbitan esters as described under Sorbitan Monolaurate. It is more lipophilic in character than the monolaurate, and is useful for the preparation of creams of the water-in-oil type; a small proportion of polysorbate 60 or polysorbate 80 may be added to reduce viscosity and to aid the formation of an emulsion, thus avoiding the necessity for passing the cream through a homogeniser or mill.

Up to 10% of sorbitan mono-oleate may be incorporated in paraffin-type bases to form anhydrous bases capable of absorbing large amounts of water.

Sorbitan Monostearate

A mixture of the partial esters of sorbitol and its mono- and di-anhydrides with stearic acid.

OTHER NAMES: *Crill 3®*; *Span 60®*

A standard is given in the British Pharmaceutical Codex 1973

Description. A pale yellow solid with a faint oily odour.

Solubility. Practically insoluble but dispersible in water; soluble, at 20°, in 120 parts of alcohol.

Setting-point. About 50°.

Uses. Sorbitan monostearate has the uses of the sorbitan esters, as described under Sorbitan Monolaurate. It has lipophilic properties similar to those of sorbitan mono-oleate.

Sorbitol

$$CH_2OH$$
$$H\!-\!C\!-\!OH$$
$$HO\!-\!C\!-\!H$$
$$H\!-\!C\!-\!OH$$
$$H\!-\!C\!-\!OH$$
$$CH_2OH$$

$C_6H_{14}O_6 = 182.2$

OTHER NAMES: *Howsorb®*; *Sorbex®*

A standard is given in the British Pharmacopoeia 1973

Description. An odourless, slightly hygroscopic, white, microcrystalline powder with a sweetish taste.

Solubility. Soluble, at 20°, in less than 1 part of water and in 25 parts of alcohol; practically insoluble in ether and in chloroform.

Moisture content. Not more than 1.5%, determined by Fischer titration.

Specific rotation. +13° to +16°, determined on a solution prepared by dissolving with 3 times its weight of borax in 1N sodium hydroxide.

Sterilisation. Solutions are sterilised by heating in an autoclave.

Storage. It should be stored in airtight containers.

Identification. TESTS. 1. Dissolve about 50 mg in 3 ml of water, add 3 ml of *catechol solution*, and pour the mixture into 6 ml of sulphuric acid; a pink colour is produced.
2. Heat about 1 g with a mixture of 1 ml of pyridine and 10 ml of acetic anhydride under a reflux condenser for 10 minutes, cool, add 25 ml of water, cool in ice, and filter; the residue, after recrystallisation from 10 ml of alcohol (95%), melts at about 100°.

MELTING-POINT. About 95°.

Metabolism. ABSORPTION. Almost completely absorbed after oral administration but at a slower rate than glucose.

BLOOD CONCENTRATION. After an oral dose of 35 g, blood concentrations of less than 30 μg/ml are obtained; after an oral dose of 50 g a concentration of about 90 μg/ml may be attained by 1 hour.

DISTRIBUTION. *Protein binding*, does not appear to be significantly bound to plasma proteins.

METABOLIC REACTIONS. Rapidly metabolised to fructose and glucose; at least 70% of an oral dose is metabolised to carbon dioxide.

EXCRETION. After an oral dose, less than 2% is excreted unchanged in the urine and 10% in the faeces; after rapid intravenous injection, about 30% of a dose is excreted in the urine whilst after a slow infusion about 6% is excreted; after application of an irrigation fluid containing sorbitol during transurethral resection of the prostate about 10% of the sorbitol is excreted in the urine in the 24 hours immediately following the operation.

FURTHER INFORMATION. Metabolism of ingested sorbitol—L. H. Adcock and C. H. Gray, *Biochem. J.*, 1957, **65**, 554; metabolism and excretion of intravenous sorbitol—P. A. Bye, *Br. J. Surg.*, 1969, **56**, 653; urinary excretion after use in transurethral irrigation—P. O. Madsen and K. G. Naber, *Investve Urol.*, 1974, **11**, 331; urinary excretion of hexitols in dogs—W. W. Smith *et al.*, *J. biol. Chem.*, 1940, **135**, 231.

Actions and uses. Sorbitol is administered by intravenous infusion in carbohydrate-deficiency states. It is usually given as 30% w/v solution at a rate not exceeding 2 millilitres per minute. According to the United Kingdom Labelling of Food Regulations 1970, 1 gram of sorbitol contributes 15.7 kilojoules (3.75 kilocalories), and a 30% solution therefore provides 4710 kilojoules (1125 kilocalories) per litre.

Sorbitol has also been used as an ingredient of some solutions for peritoneal dialysis.

Sorbitol may be used by diabetics in daily doses up to 30 grams as a substitute for sucrose. It is mildly laxative.

Sorbitol is stated to facilitate the absorption of paracetamol.

Some pharmaceutical uses of sorbitol are described below under Sorbitol Solution.

Preparations

SORBITOL INJECTION: a sterile solution of sorbitol in water for injections. It is sterilised by heating in an autoclave. The usual strength is 30% of sorbitol, providing 4710 kilojoules (1125 kilocalories) per litre.

A standard for this injection is given in the British Pharmacopoeia 1973

Containers: see the entry on Injections for general information on containers.

Labelling: see the entry on Injections for general information on labelling. In addition, the label on the container should state the amount of the medicament as the percentage w/v of sorbitol.

SORBITOL SOLUTION (*Syn.* Sorbitol Liquid): an aqueous solution containing 70% w/w of total solids consisting mainly of D-sorbitol $CH_2OH \cdot [CH \cdot OH]_4 \cdot CH_2OH$, which may be prepared by the catalytic hydrogenation of glucose.

Sorbitol solution is commonly available in two grades, a "crystallising" grade and a "non-crystallising" grade. The latter usually contains a small proportion of related products which help to retard crystallisation of the sorbitol under normal conditions of storage.

A standard for this solution is given in the British Pharmaceutical Codex 1973

Solubility: miscible with water.

Labelling: the label on the container should state whether the solution is the "crystallising" or "non-crystallising" grade.

Storage: it should be stored in airtight containers.

Uses: Sorbitol solution is used as a sweetening agent and vehicle in elixirs, linctuses, and mixtures; it has about half the sweetening power of syrup. When added to syrups containing sucrose it reduces their tendency to deposit crystals on storage; for this purpose, about 20 to 30% of sorbitol solution is usually sufficient.

Although the solubility of sorbitol is decreased in the presence of alcohol, sorbitol solution can usually be employed in elixirs and other preparations containing up to 40% v/v of alcohol.

It is used as a humectant in pharmaceutical and cosmetic creams and is an ingredient of some toothpastes. It is also employed as a plasticiser in the manufacture of gelatin capsules.

Spearmint Oil

Obtained by distillation from fresh flowering plants of *Mentha spicata* L. and *Mentha× cardiaca* (Gray) Bak. (Fam. Labiatae), grown in Europe and America, most of the oil of commerce being imported from north America.

OTHER NAMES: Oleum Menthae Crispae; Oleum Menthae Viridis

A standard is given in the British Pharmaceutical Codex 1973

Constituents. Spearmint oil contains 55 to 70% of (−)-carvone.

Description. A colourless, pale yellow, or greenish-yellow liquid when recently distilled, but becoming darker and viscous on keeping. The odour is that of spearmint.

Solubility. Soluble, at 20°, in 1 part of alcohol (80%). The solution may become opalescent on further dilution with alcohol (80%).

Weight per ml. At 20°, 0.917 to 0.934 g.

Refractive index. 1.484 to 1.491.

Optical rotation. −45° to −60°.

Storage. It should be stored in well-filled airtight containers, in a cool place, protected from light.

Actions and uses. The properties of spearmint oil resemble those of peppermint oil. It is used as a flavouring agent and carminative in doses of 0.05 to 0.2 millilitre.

Spectrophotometry

see under INFRA-RED and ULTRAVIOLET

Spirits

Spirits consist of medicinal substances or flavouring agents, usually of a volatile nature, dissolved in alcohol. Aromatic ammonia spirit is prepared by a process of distillation but most other spirits in current use (for example, lemon spirit) are prepared by simple solution in alcohol.

Spironolactone

7α - Acetylthio-3-oxo-17α-pregn-4-ene-21,17β-carbo-
lactone

$C_{24}H_{32}O_4S = 416.6$

OTHER NAMES: *Aldactone*®
Aldactide® (with hydroflumethiazide)

A standard is given in the British Pharmacopoeia 1973

Description. A buff-coloured powder which is odourless
or has a slight odour of thioacetic acid.

Solubility. Very slightly soluble in water; soluble, at 20°,
in 80 parts of alcohol, in 100 parts of ether, and in
3 parts of chloroform.

Specific rotation. −47.5° to −52.5°, determined on a
1% solution in dioxan.

Storage. It should be protected from light.

Identification. TEST. Mix about 10 mg with 2 ml of
sulphuric acid (50% v/v) and shake; an orange solution
with an intense yellowish-green fluorescence is produced. Heat the solution gently; the colour changes
to deep red and hydrogen sulphide is evolved. Pour
the solution into water; a greenish-yellow opalescent
solution is produced.

MELTING-POINT. About 205°.

ULTRAVIOLET ABSORPTION. In 0.1N hydrochloric acid,
maximum at 245nm (E1%, 1cm = 463); in 0.1N sodium
hydroxide, maxima at 249 nm (E1%, 1cm = 381), and
300 nm (E1%, 1cm = 162).

INFRA-RED ABSORPTION. Major peaks at 1115, 1127,
1170, 1185, 1676, and 1773 cm⁻¹ (see Appendix 2a:
Infra-red Spectra).

THIN-LAYER CHROMATOGRAPHY. See under Thin-layer
Chromatography, System 6.

Actions and uses. Spironolactone is a potassium-sparing
diuretic. It is a competitive inhibitor of the natural
corticosteroid hormone aldosterone, which promotes
retention of sodium and excretion of potassium by the
distal part of the distal tubules. It thus increases sodium
and reduces potassium excretion and so differs from
chlorothiazide and similar diuretics, which act on the
proximal part of the distal tubules and increase sodium
excretion but do not prevent excretion of potassium by
the distal tubules.

Provided that production of aldosterone is sufficiently
high, spironolactone is active when given by mouth to
patients on a low-salt diet. It is ineffective if aldosterone
output is low.

The use of spironolactone is justified in the treatment
of oedema when the condition is associated with excessive secretion of aldosterone. It is administered in
conjunction with chlorothiazide and similar diuretics to
reduce potassium loss while enhancing the excretion
of sodium. It is usually given by mouth in a dosage of
25 milligrams 4 times a day.

Undesirable effects. Spironolactone may give rise to
headache, gastro-intestinal disturbances, and, when
taken in large doses, drowsiness; skin rashes may
occasionally occur, but usually clear when the drug is
discontinued. Gynaecomastia may occur occasionally.

Precautions. Its use in nursing mothers should be
avoided as a metabolite (canrenone) is secreted in the
milk.

Preparations

SPIRONOLACTONE TABLETS: available as tablets containing 25 and 100 mg of spironolactone; peppermint oil is
added as a flavouring agent.
*A standard for these tablets is given in the British
Pharmacopoeia 1973*
Containers and *Storage:* see the entry on Tablets for
general information on containers and storage. Containers should be airtight and light resistant.
Advice for patients: daily doses should preferably be
taken in the morning and after meals. Treatment should
not be discontinued without the advice of the prescriber.
The tablets may cause drowsiness; persons affected
should not drive or operate machinery. Alcohol should
be avoided.

OTHER PREPARATIONS available include TABLETS containing spironolactone 25 mg with hydroflumethiazide
25 mg.

Spondylitis

see ANKYLOSING SPONDYLITIS

Sprays

Sprays are preparations of medicaments in aqueous,
alcoholic, or glycerol-containing media to be applied to
the nose or throat by means of an atomiser. The term
"Spray" is also applied to preparations such as compound pyrethrum spray which are intended to be used
as insecticidal sprays applied to walls and other
surfaces.
The choice of atomiser depends on the viscosity of the
liquid; the more viscous the liquid, the more powerful
the atomiser required.
Oily sprays have been used, but the oil retards the
ciliary action of nasal mucosa; drops of oil may enter
the trachea and cause lipoid pneumonia.

Containers. Sprays should be supplied in small,
coloured, fluted, glass bottles.

Labelling. The label on the container should state the
names and proportions of the medicaments, the directions for use, and any special precautions relevant to
the preparation.

Squill

The bulb of *Drimia maritima* (L.) Stearn [*Urginea
maritima* (L.) Baker] (Fam. Liliaceae). The plant is indigenous to the Mediterranean region.

OTHER NAME: Scilla

*A standard is given in the British Pharmaceutical
Codex 1973*

The bulbs are collected soon after the plant has flowered,
divested of their dry outer membranous coats, and
usually cut into transverse slices and dried. It is known
in commerce as white squill.

Constituents. Squill contains the glycosides scillarin A and scillarin B. The former is a pure crystalline glycoside, which gives on hydrolysis scillaridin A (bufa-3,5,20,22-tetraenolide) and a sugar, scillabiose (a glucosidorhamnoside). Scillarin B is a mixture of glycosides.

Squill also contains a small amount of glucoscillarin A, about 4 to 11% of mucilage, and a polyfructosan, sinistrin.

It yields to alcohol (60%) about 65 to 80% of extractive. It yields up to 1.5% of acid-insoluble ash.

Description. UNGROUND DRUG. *Macroscopical characters:* slices transverse, about 5 to 8 mm thick, occurring as straight or curved triangular pieces about 5 to 50 mm long and 3 to 8 mm wide at mid-point, tapering towards each end, yellowish-white, texture horny, somewhat translucent, breaking with an almost glassy fracture when quite dry, but readily absorbing moisture when exposed to the air and becoming tough and flexible; transversely cut surface showing a single row of prominent vascular bundles near the concave edge and numerous smaller bundles scattered throughout the mesophyll.

It is almost odourless and has a mucilaginous, acrid, and disagreeably bitter taste.

Microscopical characters: the diagnostic characters are: *epidermis,* cells polygonal and axially elongated, 1 to 2 times longer than wide, outer wall thick, stratified; *stomata* very rare, anomocytic, and nearly circular in outline, about 50 to 60 μm in diameter; *mesophyll* of colourless, thin-walled parenchyma containing very occasional *starch* granules, many cells containing bundles of acicular *crystals* of calcium oxalate embedded in *mucilage,* crystals up to about 1 mm long and about 1 to 15 μm wide; other cells containing *sinistrin; vascular bundles* collateral, scattered throughout the mesophyll; *xylem vessels* with spiral and annular wall thickening; *trichomes* absent.

POWDERED DRUG. Powdered Squill. A very hygroscopic white or yellowish-white powder possessing the diagnostic microscopical characters, odour, and taste of the unground drug.

Adulterants and substitutes. A red variety of *U. maritima* is used in French pharmacy in addition to the white variety; it has a more intensely bitter taste. This variety was formerly used for the manufacture of rat poison. It contains the toxic principle scilliroside, a glycoside similar to scillarin A.

Storage. It should be stored in a cool dry place. Powdered squill should be kept in a desiccated atmosphere.

Identification. TEST. The mucilage in the cells of the mesophyll stains red with *alkaline corallin solution* but gives no red colour with *ruthenium red solution* and no purple colour with *iodine water.*

Actions and uses. The glycosides of squill have an action upon the heart resembling that of digitalis, but are poorly absorbed from the gastro-intestinal tract and are less potent.

Squill irritates the gastric mucosa, and in large doses produces nausea and vomiting. In smaller doses (60 to 200 milligrams) it has a reflex expectorant action and its preparations are common constituents of cough mixtures.

Preparations

OPIATE SQUILL LINCTUS (*Syn.* Compound Squill Linctus; Gee's Linctus):

Squill oxymel	..	..	..	..	.. 300 ml
Camphorated opium tincture	..		..	..	300 ml
Tolu syrup ..	..	..	..	..	300 ml

Mix. Alternatively, disperse 900 mg of xanthan gum or 500 mg of powdered tragacanth in the camphorated opium tincture, add the squill oxymel and the tolu syrup, and mix. If xanthan gum is used, a high-speed stirrer is required in order to disperse the material.

When a dose less than or not a multiple of 5 ml is prescribed, the linctus may be diluted, as described in the entry on Linctuses, with syrup.

It contains, in 5 ml, about 800 micrograms of anhydrous morphine.

A standard for this linctus is given in the British Pharmaceutical Codex 1973

Containers: see the entry on Linctuses for general information on containers.

Dose: 5 millilitres.

Advice for patients: the linctus should be sipped and swallowed slowly. It should not be used for longer than a few days or given to children under 1 year without medical advice.

OPIATE SQUILL PASTILLES (*Syn.* Gee's Linctus Pastilles; Gee's Linctus): for each pastille take:

Squill liquid extract	..	..	..	.. 0.03 ml
Concentrated camphorated opium tincture ..	..	..	..	.. 0.075 ml
Cinnamic acid	..	..	..	.. 0.25 mg
Benzoic acid	..	..	..	.. 0.60 mg
Glacial acetic acid..	..	..	..	.. 0.02 ml
Purified honey	..	..	..	.. 0.20 ml

Each pastille contains the approximate equivalent of 2 ml of opiate squill linctus.

A standard for these pastilles is given in the British Pharmaceutical Codex 1973

Advice for patients: the pastilles should be allowed to dissolve slowly in the mouth. They should not be used for longer than a few days without medical advice.

PAEDIATRIC IPECACUANHA AND SQUILL LINCTUS:

Ipecacuanha tincture	..	..	..	20 ml
Squill tincture	..	..	..	30 ml
Compound orange spirit ..	..	..	..	1.5 ml
Blackcurrant syrup	..	..	..	500 ml
Syrup..	..	..	..	to 1000 ml

When a dose less than or not a multiple of 5 ml is prescribed, the linctus may be diluted, as described in the entry on Linctuses, with syrup.

A standard for this linctus is given in the British Pharmaceutical Codex 1973

Containers: see the entry on Linctuses for general information on containers.

Storage: it should be stored in a cool place.

Dose: CHILD: 5 millilitres.

Advice for patients: the linctus should be sipped and swallowed slowly. It should not be used for longer than a few days without medical advice.

PAEDIATRIC OPIATE SQUILL LINCTUS (*Syn.* Opiate Linctus for Infants):

Squill oxymel	60 ml
Camphorated opium tincture	60 ml
Tolu syrup	60 ml
Glycerol	200 ml
Syrup..	to 1000 ml

When a dose less than or not a multiple of 5 ml is prescribed, the linctus may be diluted, as described in the entry on Linctuses, with syrup.

It contains, in 5 ml, about 150 micrograms of anhydrous morphine.

A standard for this linctus is given in the British Pharmaceutical Codex 1973

Containers: see the entry on Linctuses for general information on containers.

Dose: CHILD: 5 to 10 millilitres.

Advice for patients: see above under Opiate Squill Linctus.

SQUILL LIQUID EXTRACT: *Small-scale preparation:*

Squill, or Indian squill, in coarse powder ..	1000 g
Alcohol (70%)	to 1000 ml

Exhaust the squill with the alcohol by percolation, reserving the first 850 ml of percolate; evaporate the subsequent percolate to the consistence of a soft extract, dissolve it in the reserved portion, add sufficient of the alcohol to produce 1000 ml, and filter.

Manufacture. Prepare the extract by the above method, appropriately scaled up, or by the alternative method described in the entry on Extracts.

A standard for this extract is given in the British Pharmaceutical Codex 1973

Dose: 0.06 to 0.2 millilitre.

SQUILL OXYMEL:

Squill, or Indian squill, bruised	50 g
Acetic acid	90 ml, or a sufficient quantity
Purified water, freshly boiled and cooled	250 ml
Purified honey	a sufficient quantity

Macerate the squill with the acetic acid and the water for 7 days, with occasional agitation, strain, and press out the liquid. Heat the mixed liquids to boiling, filter while hot, cool, and determine the concentration of acetic acid present in the solution. To the remainder of the solution add a sufficient quantity of the acetic acid to produce a solution containing approximately 8.5% w/v of acetic acid and mix. To every 3 volumes of this solution, add 7 volumes of the honey and mix thoroughly.

A standard for this oxymel is given in the British Pharmaceutical Codex 1973

Dose: 2.5 to 5 millilitres.

SQUILL SYRUP:

Squill vinegar	450 ml
Sucrose	800 g
Water for preparations	to 1000 ml

Dissolve the sucrose in the squill vinegar with the aid of gentle heat, strain, cool, add sufficient water to produce the required volume, and mix.

A standard for this syrup is given in the British Pharmaceutical Codex 1973

Dose: 2.5 to 5 millilitres.

SQUILL TINCTURE:

Squill, or Indian squill, bruised	100 g
Alcohol (60%)	1000 ml

Prepare by the maceration process.

A standard for this tincture is given in the British Pharmaceutical Codex 1973

Dose: 0.3 to 2 millilitres.

SQUILL VINEGAR (*Syn.* Acetum Scillae):

Squill, or Indian squill, bruised	100 g
Dilute acetic acid	1000 ml

Macerate the squill with the dilute acetic acid in a closed vessel for 7 days, shaking occasionally, strain, press the marc, and heat the combined liquids to boiling; allow to stand for not less than 7 days and filter.

A standard for this vinegar is given in the British Pharmaceutical Codex 1973

Dose: 0.6 to 2 millilitres.

Squill, Indian

The bulb of *Drimia indica* (Roxb.) J. P. Jessopp [*Urginea indica* (Roxb.) Kunth] (Fam. Liliaceae)

OTHER NAME: Urginea

A standard is given in the British Pharmaceutical Codex Supplement 1976

The plant is indigenous to India. The bulbs are collected soon after the plant has flowered, divested of their dry outer membranous coats, and usually cut into slices and dried.

Constituents. Indian squill contains cardioglycosides similar to those found in squill. It contains bufadienolides including scilliglaucosidin. It also contains about 35 to 40% of mucilage.

Indian squill yields to alcohol (60%) about 20 to 50% of extractive. It yields up to 6% of ash.

Description. UNGROUND DRUG. *Macroscopical characters:* curved or irregularly shaped strips, about 10 to 50 mm long, 3 to 10 mm wide, and 1 to 3 mm thick, frequently tapering towards the ends, occasionally grouped 3 or 4 together and attached to a portion of the axis; ridged in the direction of their length and varying in colour from pale yellowish-brown to buff; brittle when dry, but tough and flexible when damp. The pieces are darker in colour than squill.

It is odourless and has a bitter taste.

Microscopical characters: the diagnostic characters are: *epidermis,* cells tetrahedral to hexahedral, thin-walled, 3 to 5 times longer than wide, having a thick striated cuticle; *stomata* rare, circular in outline, 40 to 42 μm in diameter; *mesophyll* of thin-walled polyhedral cells containing *mucilage,* some cells containing bundles of acicular *crystals* of calcium oxalate 20 to 900 μm in length; *vascular bundles* collateral, scattered throughout the mesophyll; *xylem vessels* with spiral and annular wall thickening; *trichomes* and *starch* absent.

POWDERED DRUG. Powdered Indian Squill. A very hygroscopic buff-coloured powder possessing the diagnostic microscopical characters, odour, and taste of the unground drug.

Storage. It should be stored in a cool dry place. Powdered Indian squill should be kept in a desiccated atmosphere.

Identification. TEST. The mucilage contained in the cells of the mesophyll stains red with *alkaline corallin solution* and reddish-purple with *iodine water.*

Actions and uses. Indian squill has the actions and uses described under Squill.

Preparations

See above under Squill.

Stanolone

17β-Hydroxy-5α-androstan-3-one

$C_{19}H_{30}O_2 = 290.4$

OTHER NAMES: *Anabolex®*; Androstanolone

A standard is given in the British Pharmacopoeia Addendum 1975

Description. An odourless white powder.

Solubility. Very slightly soluble in water; soluble, at 20°, in 20 parts of alcohol and in 70 parts of ether.

Specific rotation. +25° to +31°, determined on a 5% solution in dioxan.

Storage. It should be protected from light.

Identification. MELTING-POINT. About 180°.

ULTRAVIOLET ABSORPTION. In alcohol (95%), maximum at 285 nm (E1%, 1cm = 0.66).

INFRA-RED ABSORPTION. Major peaks at 1027, 1046, 1064, 1277, 1444, and 1698 cm⁻¹ (see Appendix 2a: Infra-red Spectra).

THIN-LAYER CHROMATOGRAPHY. See under Thin-layer Chromatography, System 10.

Actions and uses. Stanolone is a steroid that has anabolic and, to a less extent, androgenic actions, and is used for purposes similar to those described for Methandienone. It is used to promote protein synthesis in debility states, post-operative recovery, convalescence, and osteoporosis.

The usual dosage for children up to 2 years is 12.5 milligrams daily for up to 15 days a month, and from 2 to 8 years 12.5 to 25 milligrams up to 15 days a month. Older children may be given 25 to 50 milligrams and adults 50 to 75 milligrams daily for not more than 21 days a month. The tablets should preferably be sucked or left to dissolve under the tongue.

Contra-indications. It should not be given to patients with prostatic carcinoma. It is contra-indicated in pregnancy owing to the possible virilising effects on a female foetus.

Preparation

STANOLONE TABLETS: available as tablets containing 25 mg of stanolone; they may contain peppermint oil.
A standard for these tablets is given in the British Pharmacopoeia Addendum 1975
Containers and *Storage:* see the entry on Tablets for general information on containers and storage. Containers should be airtight and light resistant.
Advice for patients: the tablets should preferably be allowed to dissolve slowly under the tongue. Alternatively, they may be crushed and taken in water or other fluid or mixed with food.

Starch

Polysaccharide granules obtained from the grains of maize, *Zea mays* L., of rice, *Oryza sativa* L., or of wheat, *Triticum aestivum* L. (*T. vulgare* Vill.) and other species of *Triticum* (Fam. Gramineae), or from the tubers of the potato, *Solanum tuberosum* L. (Fam. Solanaceae). Maize starch is also known as corn starch.

OTHER NAMES: Amylum; Amylum Maydis; Amylum Oryzae; Amylum Solani; Amylum Tritici; Maize Starch; Potato Starch; Rice Starch; Wheat Starch.

A standard is given in the European Pharmacopoeia Vol. I

Varieties. The diagnostic microscopical characters are:
Maize starch: polyhedral, subspherical or, occasionally, muller-shaped granules, about 5 to 10 to 20 to 30 μm in diameter; the hilum is represented by a central triangular or 2- to 5-rayed fissure, and striations are not visible; it shows a well-marked cross when viewed between crossed polars.
Rice starch: simple and compound granules; single granules are polyhedral and are usually 2 to 5 to 8 to 12 μm in diameter; the hilum is sometimes evident as a minute central point; spindle-shaped and lemon-shaped granules are absent (distinction from oat starch); the compound grains are ovate, usually about 12 to 30 μm long and 7 to 20 μm wide; they contain about 2 to 150 components.
Wheat starch: principally simple lenticular granules, which are circular, oval, or subreniform in outline; the hilum appears as a central point or, if the granule is on its edge, as a line; the granules are mostly simple, the smaller ones being usually 5 to 10 μm and the larger ones 20 to 25 or up to 50 μm in greatest width. A few compound granules of 2 to 4 components are present; there are always more than 400 granules per milligram having a maximum diameter exceeding 40 μm (distinction from barley starch). When viewed between crossed polars, a dull cross of the maltese shape is seen.
Potato starch (sometimes known as English arrowroot): ovoid, irregularly ovoid, or subspherical, and often somewhat flattened; the hilum is a point towards the narrower end of the granule, and has an eccentricity of ⅓ to ¼; the striations are well-marked and concentric; some rings appear darker than others. The granules are mostly simple, the subspherical ones measuring about 10 to 35 μm and the ovoid ones 30 to 100 μm. A few compound granules of 2 to 3 components are always present. The granules show a well-marked cross when viewed between crossed polars. Potato starch is easily distinguished from arrowroot and from other official starches by its rapid gelatinisation when mounted in a 0.9% w/v solution of potassium hydroxide in water.

Constituents. Starch contains amylose and amylopectin, both polysaccharides based on α-glucose; the proportions vary somewhat in different starches, but the ratio of amylose (β-amylose) to amylopectin (α-amylose) is usually about 1 to 4.
Amylose consists of linear chains of 250 to 300 1,4-linked α-glucose residues arranged in the form of a helix; amylopectin is also a polymer of α-glucose but the macromolecule is built up of branched chains of glucose units linked in both the 1,4 and 1,6 positions.
Amylopectin yields a gelatinous solution with water, whereas amylose yields a limpid solution which is coloured blue with iodine solution.
Starch yields up to 0.6% (maize starch, potato starch, and wheat starch), and up to 0.8% (rice starch) of sulphated ash; traces of cell debris may be present.

Description. An odourless fine white powder or irregular angular masses readily reducible to powder. The loss on drying at 100° to 105° is not more than 15% for maize, rice, and wheat starch, and not more than 20% for potato starch.

Solubility. Insoluble in cold water and in alcohol.

Adulterants and substitutes. Manihot (Manioc) starch, often known as cassava or tapioca starch, obtained from *Manihot esculenta* Crantz (Fam. Euphorbiaceae), occurs as a substitute and is described under Arrowroot. This cassava starch may be used as starch in tropical and subtropical parts of the world where official starches are not available.

Hygroscopicity. At relative humidities between about 25 and 55% the equilibrium moisture content of maize, rice, and wheat starches at 25° is between about 10 and 14% and that for potato starch between about 10 and 18%. At relative humidities above about 75%, all starches absorb substantial amounts of moisture.

Labelling. The label states the botanical source.

Storage. It should be stored in airtight containers, in a cool dry place.

Identification. TEST. When 1 g of starch is boiled with 50 ml of water and the mixture cooled, a mucilage is formed, which is coloured deep blue by *iodine solution*; the colour disappears on warming and reappears on cooling.

Actions and uses. Starch acts as an absorbent and is used as a dusting-powder for application to chafed or excoriated skin, either alone or mixed with zinc oxide or other similar substances.

Starch mucilage may be employed as an emollient for the skin and is the basis of some enemas; it may also be used as an antidote in the treatment of poisoning by iodine.

A poultice may be prepared by boiling 1 part of starch with 10 parts of water.

Starch is incorporated in some tablets as a disintegrating agent.

Preparations

ZINC, STARCH, AND TALC DUSTING-POWDER (*Syn.* Zinc Oxide and Starch Dusting-powder; Zinc Oxide, Starch, and Talc Dusting-powder):

Zinc oxide ..	..	..	..	..	..	250 g
Starch, in powder ..	..	..	..	..		250 g
Purified talc, sterilised	..	..	..	..		500 g

Prepare as described in the entry on Powders.

A standard for this dusting-powder is given in the British Pharmaceutical Codex 1973

Containers and *Labelling:* see the entry on Dusting-powders for general information on containers and labelling.

Advice for patients: the dusting-powder should be dusted lightly onto the affected area. It should not be applied to open wounds or to raw surfaces of a large area.

OTHER PREPARATIONS: starch is an ingredient of chlorphenesin dusting-powder, compound resorcinol ointment, compound zinc paste, talc dusting-powder, zinc and salicylic acid paste, and zinc undecenoate dusting-powder.

Status Epilepticus

see under EPILEPSY

Stearic Acid

A mixture of fatty acids, chiefly stearic and palmitic acids. It may contain a suitable antoxidant such as 0.005% of butylated hydroxytoluene.

OTHER NAMES: *Diadem®*; *Pristerene®*

A standard is given in the British Pharmaceutical Codex 1973

Stearic acid may be obtained by hydrolysis of various fats and subsequent removal of the liquid acids by cooling and filtration.

It may be powdered by sprinkling it with alcohol during trituration.

NOTE. Pure stearic acid, $C_{17}H_{35}.CO_2H = 284.5$, is obtained from an alcoholic solution of commercial stearic acid by fractional crystallisation, followed by conversion to magnesium stearate and subsequent acidification; it occurs in white shining flaky crystals or as a hard, somewhat glossy solid, melting at 69.3°.

Description. White greasy flaky crystals or hard masses showing signs of crystallisation. It is odourless or almost odourless.

Solubility. Insoluble in water; soluble at 20°, in 15 parts of alcohol; soluble in ether and in chloroform.

Labelling. The label on the container should state the name and proportion of any added antoxidant.

Uses. Stearic acid, partly neutralised with alkalis or triethanolamine, is used in the preparation of creams. In the form of a powder it has been used as a lubricant in making compressed tablets.

When partly neutralised, stearic acid forms a creamy basis with 5 to 15 times its weight of aqueous liquid and in this form it is sometimes used as the basis of vanishing creams; the proportion of alkali used largely determines the appearance and plasticity of the cream. After being neutralised and dissolved by heat in glycerol or alcohol, it will solidify when cold with at least 10 times its weight of liquid.

Sterculia

The gum obtained from *Sterculia urens* Roxb. and other species of *Sterculia* (Fam. Sterculiaceae). It is produced in India, Pakistan, and Africa.

OTHER NAMES: Indian Tragacanth; *Inolaxine®*; Karaya Gum; *Normacol Special®*; *Peridale®*; Sterculia Gum *Normacol Antispasmodic/Standard/X®* (with alverine citrate, frangula, or danthron respectively); *Normacol Diabetic®* is the sucrose-free form of *Normacol Standard®*

A standard is given in the British Pharmaceutical Codex 1973

Constituents. Sterculia yields on hydrolysis, among other products, galacturonic acid (about 43%), D-galactopyranose, L-rhamnopyranose, and acetic acid. Unlike tragacanth, sterculia does not contain methoxyl groups. When hydrolysed with phosphoric acid, the volatile acidity is about 14 to 16%, calculated as acetic acid. The drug contains no oxidase; it yields up to 7% of ash and up to 1% of acid-insoluble ash.

Description. UNGROUND DRUG. *Macroscopical characters:* irregular or vermiform pieces, about 5 to 20 mm thick; greyish or pinkish in colour; surface striated. It has the odour of acetic acid.

Microscopical characters: when powdered and mounted in alcohol, it appears as small, transparent, angular particles of various sizes and shapes; the particles lose their sharp edges when water is added and each gradually swells until a large, indefinite, almost structureless mass results; when mounted in *ruthenium red solution*, the particles are stained red; no starch granules visible when mounted in *iodine water*.

POWDERED DRUG. Powdered Sterculia. A white or buff-coloured powder possessing the diagnostic microscopical characters and odour of the unground drug.

Solubility. Partly soluble in water, in which it swells to a homogeneous, adhesive, gelatinous mass; insoluble in alcohol.

Storage. It should be stored in a cool dry place. Powdered sterculia should be stored in airtight containers.

Identification. TESTS. 1. Shake 1 g with 80 ml of water during 24 hours; a tacky and viscous granular mucilage is produced.
2. Boil 4 ml of the mucilage obtained in Test 1 with 0.5 ml of hydrochloric acid, add 1 ml of *sodium hydroxide solution*, filter, to the filtrate add 3 ml of *potassium cupri-tartrate solution* and heat; a red precipitate is formed.
3. Warm 500 mg with 2 ml of *sodium hydroxide solution*; a brown colour is produced.

Uses. Sterculia is used as a substitute for tragacanth in lozenges, pastes, and denture-fixative powders. It is also used as a bulk-forming laxative as it takes up water in the large intestine.
Sterculia gum is used as an adhesive for securing ileostomy and colostomy bags at stomata.

Preparations

Preparations available include veterinary CAPSULES containing sterculia 118 mg; GRANULES and veterinary granules containing sterculia 98%, granules containing sterculia 62% with alverine citrate 0.5%, granules containing sterculia 62% with frangula 8% (with and without sucrose); and a combination pack consisting of granules containing sterculia 62% with tablets containing danthron 200 mg.

Sterilisation

Sterilisation is the process of killing or removing microorganisms. It may be effected by killing the microorganisms by physical or chemical methods or by removing them by filtration.

Medicaments to be used for the preparation of sterile products should be stored in containers fitted with the type of stopper which prevents dust falling between the stopper and the neck and should be kept apart from materials used for normal manufacturing or dispensing purposes. The method of sterilisation chosen must not cause any important undesirable change in the materials (medicaments, vehicles, fabrics, apparatus, containers, wrappings) so that they remain suitable for their purpose. Failure to follow a recommended process meticulously involves the risk of producing either a non-sterile product or some deterioration of the material.

Observance of the principles of good manufacturing practice is an essential factor in the general organisation and control of the processes selected. It is desirable that all starting materials and apparatus used should be as free as possible from microbial contamination to minimise the risk that some organisms may survive or escape the process designed to kill or remove them.

Processes employing heat are the most reliable and are recommended whenever possible. Whichever method is chosen, the product should, if possible, be sterilised in its final container, thereby obviating the risk of contamination associated with the aseptic transference of a sterile material.

A product is accepted as sterile if, after it has been subjected to a properly applied sterilisation process, it complies with the test for sterility described in the European Pharmacopoeia or, in the case of surgical dressings, in the British Pharmaceutical Codex 1973.

The term "sterilised" is applied in the Codex to a product which has been subjected to a process of sterilisation and is sterile immediately on completion of the process; the term does not necessarily imply that the product is sterile subsequent to this.

In this chapter, methods of sterilisation and the techniques employed in aseptic processing are described first, followed by information on the application of these methods to the sterilisation of various types of material.

A. METHODS OF STERILISATION

Method 1. Dry Heat. The material is heated in a hot-air oven so that the whole of the load is kept at a specified minimum temperature for a stated time. In order to meet the required conditions, it is essential that the oven be provided with an efficient mechanical means for circulating the heated air; full details of the performance requirements of such ovens operating at temperatures between 140° and 180° are specified in British Standard 3421: 1961.

Various combinations of temperature and time are recommended depending on the material being sterilised; for example, the usual recommended minimum holding times and temperatures are: 150° for 1 hour for fixed oils, ethyl oleate, liquid paraffin, and glycerol; 160° for 1 hour or 180° for 11 minutes for glassware and other apparatus. The heating-up time of the material is not included in the periods stated.

Method 2. Heating in an Autoclave. The material is exposed to saturated steam at a selected temperature above 100° for an appropriate time in a suitable pressure apparatus (autoclave).

Full details of the construction and performance requirements of automatically controlled autoclaves suitable for sterilising different types of loads are given in British Standard 3970: 1966; similar considerations should be applied to non-automatic autoclaves. In order to meet any performance requirements, regular inspection and maintenance of an autoclave are essential.

The temperature–time combination used is selected having regard to the stability of the material being sterilised. Provided that the steam in the autoclave is saturated and free from air, the different temperatures may be attained by developing various specified pressures in the autoclave. It is preferable, however, to control the process by the temperature attained rather than by the pressure, as the presence of air in the autoclave results in a lower temperature than that expected under the correct conditions from the indicated pressure; in the case of porous materials, the air must be abstracted or displaced from the interstices in order to achieve sterilising conditions, as the presence of residual pockets of air within material may prevent contact between the steam and parts of the load.

Corresponding temperatures and steam pressures attained under the correct conditions, together with the recommended minimum holding times required to effect sterilisation, are given in TABLE A.

TABLE A

Temperature °C	Corresponding nominal pressure in excess of atmospheric		Recommended minimum holding time minutes
	bars	lbf/in²	
115° to 118°	0.70	10	30
121° to 124°	1.05	15	15
126° to 129°	1.40	20	10
134° to 138°	2.25	32	3

The period of heating must be sufficiently long to ensure that the whole of the material is maintained at the selected temperature for the appropriate recommended holding time. The time taken for the material to attain the sterilising temperature or to cool at the end of the holding time can vary considerably; it is dependent on a number of factors, including the size of the container and the thickness of its walls and the design, loading, and operation of the autoclave. It is necessary, therefore, that adequate tests be conducted to ensure that the procedure adopted is capable of sterilising the material and that the latter can withstand the treatment.

The process can be monitored by temperature-sensitive elements at different positions within the load.

Some indication that the heat treatment has been adequate can be gained by placing indicators at positions within the load where the required conditions are least likely to be attained. One such indicator is a Browne's tube which changes colour after the specified temperature has been maintained for a given time. Reliance should not be placed, however, on chemical indicators except when they suggest failure to attain sterilising conditions.

When it is inconvenient or impossible to use such means, the bactericidal efficiency of the process may be assessed by enclosing in different parts of the load small packets of material containing suitable heat-resistant spores, such as those of a suitable strain of *Bacillus stearothermophilus*; these are checked subsequently for the absence of viable test organisms.

Method 3. Heating with a Bactericide. This process is used for sterilising aqueous solutions and suspensions of medicaments that are unstable at the higher temperatures attained in the autoclaving process. It must not be used, however, if the preparation is to be administered parenterally by any route which contra-indicates the presence of a bactericide.

TABLE B

BACTERICIDES RECOMMENDED FOR METHOD 3

Name of bactericide	Concentration per cent w/v	Recommended by B.P. and Codex for parenteral use	by Codex for ophthalmic use
Benzalkonium chloride	0.01	No	Yes
Chlorhexidine acetate	0.01	No	Yes
Chlorocresol	0.2	Yes	No
Phenylmercuric acetate	0.002	Yes	Yes
Phenylmercuric nitrate	0.002	Yes	Yes
Thiomersal	0.01	No	Yes

In this process, one of the bactericides listed in TABLE B is included in the preparation to give the concentration recommended and the solution or suspension, in the final sealed container, is maintained at 98° to 100° for 30 minutes; this temperature can be conveniently attained by supporting the container in an atmosphere of steam produced above vigorously boiling water in a suitable container covered with a loose-fitting lid. The bactericide chosen must not interfere with the therapeutic efficacy of the medicament nor be the cause of any physical or chemical incompatibility in the preparation. For ophthalmic use, the choice is also governed by other considerations which are detailed in the entry on Eye-drops.

Method 4. Filtration. Liquids may be freed from vegetative organisms and spores by passage through a bacteria-proof filter.

This process has the advantage that the use of heat is avoided. It has the disadvantage, however, that there is always a risk that there may be an undetected fault in the apparatus or technique used, and because of this each batch of liquid sterilised by filtration must be tested for compliance with the test for sterility described in the European Pharmacopoeia.

The filters are made of cellulose derivatives or other suitable plastics, asbestos, porous ceramics, or sintered glass. Asbestos filters should not be used where alternatives are available. If asbestos filters are used, a filter made of another material which is able to trap asbestos fibres must be used downstream of the asbestos filter. The maximum pore size consistent with effective filtration varies with the material of which the filter is made and ranges from about 2 μm for ceramic filters to about 0.2 μm for plastic membrane filters. Methods of determining maximum pore diameter and uniformity of pore diameter are described in British Standard 1752: 1963. All filters must comply with the following test:

Assemble the filter into a filtering unit and sterilise the whole unit. Dilute an adequately large volume of a 24- to 48-hour culture of *Serratia marcescens* (*Chromobacterium prodigiosum*) in nutrient broth to 25 times its volume with nutrient broth and filter through the sterile apparatus, using a pressure of not less than 400 mm of mercury. By means of an aseptic technique, transfer 50 ml of the filtrate to a sterile container, close the container so as to exclude bacteria, and maintain at 25° for 5 days; no growth of *S. marcescens* or other micro-organism is visible in the sealed container.

Non-disposable filters should be tested periodically before use to ensure that their efficiency has not become impaired. An additional safeguard can be introduced by passing, after the filtration of a particular batch is finished, a test culture through the filter used and establishing that this filtrate is sterile.

Provided that a preparation is not to be administered parenterally by any route which contra-indicates the presence of a bactericide, a bactericide may be included in a concentration that prevents the growth of micro-organisms.

When required for use, the selected filter is attached to a filter flask, or other suitable receiver, having a bacteria-proof air-filter incorporated in the air exit. The receiver should preferably be fitted with a device to assist the aseptic transference (see Aseptic Technique, below) of the filtrate to the final sterile containers. All joints in the filtration system are made completely airtight and the assembled apparatus, suitably protected from re-contamination, is sterilised.

Filtration is best carried out with the aid of positive pressure, as this reduces the possibility of airborne contamination of the sterile filtered solution through leaks in the system; if the filtration is likely to take a long time and the preparation is susceptible to oxidation, nitrogen or other inert gas under pressure should be used rather than compressed air.

On completion of the filtration, the filtrate is transferred with aseptic precautions to the final sterile containers. Alternatively, the filtrate can be collected in the final sterile containers.

Small volumes of liquids, such as eye-drops, can be conveniently sterilised by this method by passage through a small filter disk which is either incorporated in a special filter-syringe or is enclosed in a suitable holder which can be attached to an ordinary hypodermic syringe.

Method 5. Exposure to Gaseous Ethylene Oxide.

Some materials which cannot be sterilised by dry heat or autoclaving may be sterilised by exposure to gaseous ethylene oxide. The method can be carried out at low temperatures and damages relatively few materials. It is, however, difficult to control, and the use of ethylene oxide should be considered only where the process is under the supervision of staff skilled in the method and having adequate facilities for bacteriological testing available.

Compared to other methods of sterilisation, the bactericidal efficiency of ethylene oxide is low and consequently particular attention should be paid to keeping microbial contamination of materials to be sterilised at a minimum.

Ethylene oxide forms explosive mixtures with air. This disadvantage can be overcome, either by using mixtures containing 10% of ethylene oxide in carbon dioxide or halogenated hydrocarbons, or by removing at least 95% of the air from the apparatus before admitting either ethylene oxide or a mixture of 90% ethylene oxide in carbon dioxide.

A suitable apparatus consists of a sterilising chamber capable of withstanding the necessary changes of pressure, fitted with an efficient vacuum pump and with a control system incorporating valves to regulate the introduction of the gas mixture and to maintain the desired gas pressure, a device to adjust the humidity within the chamber to the desired level, and, if required, a heating element with temperature controls.

The sterilising efficiency of the process depends upon (1) the partial pressure of ethylene oxide within the load, (2) the temperature of the load, (3) the state of hydration of the micro-organisms on the surfaces to be sterilised, and (4) the time of exposure to the gas.

All these factors must be closely controlled for successful sterilisation. The sensitivity of micro-organisms to ethylene oxide is dependent on their state of hydration. Organisms which have been dried are not only resistant to the process but are also slow to rehydrate. Because of this, it is not sufficient to rely solely on humidification of the atmosphere within the chamber during the sterilising cycle.

It has been found in practice that hydration and heating of the load can be more reliably achieved by conditioning it in a suitable atmosphere prior to commencing the sterilisation.

The bactericidal efficiency of the process is not assured simply by relying on physical monitoring of the above factors. Therefore, in addition, each sterilising cycle must be monitored by (1) the insertion of a minimum of 10 bacteriological test pieces into different parts of

the load most inaccessible to the ethylene oxide, and (2) sterility testing of random samples taken from the load.

Any failure in these tests indicates the need for reprocessing the load. The test pieces should consist of aluminium foil on which has been dried a suspension of at least 10^6 spores of *Bacillus subtilis* Camp Detrick strain NCTC 10073 (*B. subtilis* var. *niger*). Ethylene oxide is absorbed by some materials, and because of its toxic nature, great care must be taken to remove all traces of it after the sterilisation is finished; this can be achieved by drawing sterile air through the load.

Method 6. Exposure to Ionising Radiation.

Sterilisation may be effected by exposure to high-energy electrons from a particle accelerator or to gamma radiation from a source such as cobalt-60.

These types of radiation in a dosage of 2.5 megarads (25 kGy) have been shown to be satisfactory for sterilising certain surgical materials and equipment, provided that precautions have been taken to keep microbial contamination of the articles to a minimum. Other dosage levels may be employed provided that they have been authorised by the appropriate authority. Doses lower than 2.5 megarads may necessitate the use of additional controls to assess the adequacy of the procedure, including additional microbiological monitoring. This method can also be used for some materials which will not withstand the other sterilisation methods.

The method has the advantage over other "cold" methods of sterilisation in that bacteriological testing is not an essential part of the routine control procedure, as the process may be accurately monitored by physical and chemical methods. One method involves the measurement of induced colour change in irradiated plastics containing suitable dyes. *Perspex HX®* is suitable for this purpose. Sterilisation by exposure to ionising radiation also allows the use of a wider range of packaging materials than other methods.

B. ASEPTIC TECHNIQUE

Aseptic processing is a method of handling sterile materials by employing techniques which minimise the chances of microbial contamination. It is used in preparing products which, because of their instability, cannot be subjected to a final sterilisation process.

This technique is not easy to perform successfully and there is no certainty that the final product will, in fact, be sterile. Sterility in the final product can only be assumed if the material complies with the test for sterility described in the European Pharmacopoeia.

In the preparation of a sterile solution by this process, the medicament, preferably sterile, is dissolved or dispersed in the sterile vehicle and the product transferred to the final sterile containers, which are then sealed to exclude micro-organisms.

Aseptic techniques are especially important when carrying out the process of sterilisation by filtration (Method 4) and during the transference of sterile materials to the final sterile containers. In the particular case of the aseptic transference of liquids it is possible to assess whether or not asepsis is being achieved in the technique employed by transferring sterile bacteriological medium instead of the pharmaceutical liquid. The filled containers are closed and incubated at 32° for 7 days. Evidence of microbial growth in the incubated medium indicates that contamination has occurred during the transference. This type of process control should be used when setting up new aseptic liquid-filling processes and also as a periodic check that asepsis is being maintained. For success in aseptic processing, scrupulous care should be taken to reduce the risk of contamination of the materials being processed. If practicable, a room should be set aside for this work and a positive pressure maintained in it by introducing air which has been passed through a bacteria-proof filter. In addition, all manipulations should be carried out under a protective screen or in a current of sterile filtered air.

Likely sources of contamination include the hair, hands, clothing, and breath of the operator and the air impinging on exposed surfaces. The risk of contamination from these sources should be countered by accepted methods of cleansing and disinfection and by the use of protective clothing.

All working surfaces and the interior surfaces of screens should be disinfected; pressurised alcoholic sprays are convenient and effective for this purpose. If the screen is a sealed-cabinet type, gaseous ethylene oxide can be used; the air in the sealed cabinet is replaced by nitrogen or carbon dioxide and an effective concentration of ethylene oxide is introduced, allowed to remain for a specified period, and then removed by flushing the cabinet thoroughly with a sterile gas, initially either nitrogen or carbon dioxide and subsequently air. A minimum gaseous concentration of ethylene oxide of 10% v/v at normal pressure (equivalent to 200 mg per litre) maintained for at least 16 hours at 20° is recommended.

Sterile containers and equipment should be available in adequate quantity.

C. APPLICATION OF STERILISATION METHODS

Glass and Metal Apparatus

Apparatus should be freed from dirt and grease by washing with hot soapy water or other suitable detergent and thoroughly rinsed with purified water. New glass apparatus should be given a preliminary treatment with a mixture of sulphuric acid (46 parts by volume), sodium nitrate (6 parts), and water (46 parts). The apparatus is then wrapped in a suitable grade of paper or cloth and sterilised; it is not unwrapped until required for use.

Syringes are enclosed in glass or metal tubes.

Bottles or flasks should be closed with paper or metal foil caps or with some other suitable closure; if they are to be autoclaved, a small quantity of water should be placed in the vessels, or alternatively they should be closed with a steam-permeable closure.

Sterilisation is effected by autoclaving (Method 2), by heating at a temperature not lower than 160° for 1 hour or 180° for 11 minutes (Method 1), or by exposing to ionising radiation (Method 6).

Glass is likely to discolour and darken when sterilised by exposure to ionising radiation.

Rubber and Plastics

Natural rubber articles should be sterilised by autoclaving (Method 2); they must not be subjected to dry heat. If a long length of tubing is to be autoclaved, some water should be placed in it beforehand. Some synthetic rubbers, such as silicone rubber, have good heat resistance and may be sterilised by dry heat (Method 1) as well as by autoclaving (Method 2).

Rubber teats and closures should be made of high-quality materials which release negligible amounts of undesirable substances and absorb the minimum of materials from solutions in contact with them.

Before use, teats and closures should be washed with a suitable detergent, rinsed with purified water, and boiled in several changes of purified water. If they are to be used to close containers of a preparation which contains a bactericide, the teats or closures should first be placed in a closed container with a solution of the bactericide in purified water; the concentration of bactericide in the solution should be at least twice that used in the preparation and the volume of the solution sufficient to cover the articles and equivalent to not less than 2 millilitres for each gram of rubber. The closed container is then autoclaved at 115° to 116° for a time sufficient to ensure that the contents are maintained at this temperature for 30 minutes. The teats and closures are then stored in this autoclaved solution until required for use.

If the preparation with which the teats or closures are to be used also contains an antoxidant, the antoxidant is included, at double the concentration used in the preparation, in the bactericidal solution in which the teats and closures are heated and stored.

Rubber closures used for containers of oily injections should be made of oil-resistant material or should be prevented from coming into contact with the oil by the use of protective material.

Plastic containers and other items of medical and surgical equipment that are not thermostable may be sterilised by exposure to gaseous ethylene oxide (Method 5) or to ionising radiation (Method 6). With the latter method, degradation, discoloration, and darkening of some plastics may occur.

Pharmaceutical Containers

The methods of cleansing and sterilisation described for glass, rubber, and plastics are generally applicable to containers made of these materials, but the particular properties of each type of container should be established so that possible detrimental effects of sterilisation procedures can be minimised.

Glass containers for sterile products should not react with the medicament or affect its therapeutic properties, nor should they yield small solid particles. Soda-glass eye-drop bottles which have been specially treated to reduce the amount of alkali released when in contact with aqueous liquids should not be autoclaved more than once.

All containers should be capable of being sealed effectively to exclude micro-organisms. Tests for efficiency of closure of eye-drop bottles by rubber teats are described in British Standard 1679: Part 5: 1973.

SUBSTANCES AFFECTED BY ALKALI. The following are examples of substances that may, when in aqueous solution, be adversely affected by small amounts of alkali released by untreated soda-glass containers:

adrenaline acid tartrate	diphenhydramine
apomorphine	hydrochloride
hydrochloride	dipipanone hydrochloride
ascorbic acid	emetine hydrochloride
atropine sulphate	ergometrine maleate
calcium gluconate	ergotamine tartrate
carbachol	ethylmorphine
chlorhexidine acetate	hydrochloride
chlorhexidine gluconate	heparin
cocaine hydrochloride	histamine acid phosphate
corticotrophin	homatropine hydrobromide
cyanocobalamin	hydroxocobalamin
digoxin	hyoscine hydrobromide

isoniazid
lachesine chloride
levallorphan tartrate
levorphanol tartrate
mephenesin
methoxamine
 hydrochloride
morphine sulphate
nalorphine hydrobromide
neostigmine
 methylsulphate

noradrenaline acid
 tartrate
papaveretum
physostigmine sulphate
phytomenadione
pilocarpine hydrochloride
pyridostigmine bromide
pyridoxine hydrochloride
quinine dihydrochloride
strychnine hydrochloride
suxamethonium chloride
thiamine hydrochloride

Aqueous Solutions and Suspensions

Scrupulous attention should be paid to clean preparative methods and to the achievement of minimal contamination during preparation. The process of sterilisation by heating with a bactericide may fail if these precautions are not observed.

Solutions should be clarified by filtration before the preparation is filled into final containers, which are then sealed and sterilised by autoclaving (Method 2), by heating with a bactericide (Method 3), or by exposure to ionising radiation (Method 6).

The sterilisation method selected must take into account the stability of the preparation. The process of heating with a bactericide is used for aqueous preparations which are unstable at the higher temperatures attained in the process of heating in an autoclave, but it must not be used for the sterilisation of preparations to be administered by intrathecal, intracisternal, peridural, intraocular, or, if the volume of a single dose exceeds 15 millilitres and an individual entry describing a particular preparation does not indicate otherwise, intravenous injection. Vehicles for suspensions should be filtered before making the preparation.

Solutions may also be sterilised by filtration (Method 4) and then transferred aseptically to previously sterilised final containers which are then sealed to exclude micro-organisms.

Non-aqueous Liquids, Solutions, and Suspensions

Non-aqueous substances and preparations capable of withstanding fairly high temperatures may be sterilised in their final sealed containers, or in containers temporarily closed so as to exclude micro-organisms, by heating in a hot-air oven for a time sufficient to ensure that the whole of the contents is maintained at not less than 150° for 1 hour (Method 1).

This process is suitable for sterilising liquids, soft and hard paraffins, fixed oils, ethyl oleate, glycerol, waxes, and solutions or suspensions of stable substances in fixed oils or ethyl oleate. It must be emphasised, however, that when certain suspensions are sterilised in this way, the suspended substances may partly dissolve on heating and crystallise in large aggregates on cooling.

Sterile oily solutions or suspensions of substances which are incapable of withstanding the conditions of Method 1 are prepared aseptically, previously sterilised and cooled vehicle being used and the preparation being transferred aseptically to sterile final containers, which are then sealed to exclude micro-organisms.

Powders

Included among the procedures which may be satisfactory for the sterilisation of powdered substances are heating in a hot-air oven (Method 1), exposure to ethylene oxide (Method 5) or to ionising radiation (Method 6), and, if a suitable solvent is available, bacterial filtration (Method 4). The method selected must not cause decomposition or deterioration of the substance.

When dry heat is employed, the substance is spread in a thin layer in a suitable container, heated in a hot-air oven until the whole of the powder is at 150°, and then maintained at at least this temperature for 1 hour. Provided that it is not necessary to maintain asepsis, some substances may be heated to red heat in a muffle furnace.

If ionising radiation is used, the substance is exposed to gamma rays or accelerated electrons so that it is subjected to a dose of at least 2.5 megarads (25 kGy).

When filtration is used, the solution of the substance in a suitable inert solvent is filtered through a sterile bacteria-proof filter into previously sterilised containers and the solvent removed by an appropriate method to leave the residue in a suitable crystalline form or as a solid, which should, if necessary, be powdered. Aseptic precautions should be observed throughout.

Surgical Dressings

Surgical dressings are sterilised by autoclaving, dry heat, or exposure to ethylene oxide or ionising radiation, the choice depending on the nature of the dressing, with suitable modifications described below; any other method may be used provided that the finished sterilised dressing complies with the relevant standard. Sterilisation by any method may cause some deterioration in quality, and a dressing which complies with the appropriate standard before sterilisation may not do so afterwards; it may therefore be necessary to ensure that the sterile dressing is prepared from materials that are not too close to the minimum standard. Repeated sterilisation by autoclaving is likely to impair the absorbency of some materials, particularly cotton.

Packaging. Packaging suitable for sterile surgical dressings falls into two main categories depending upon the manner in which the dressing is intended to be used: (1) that suitable for dressings which are handled and applied with aseptic precautions, and (2) that suitable for dressings which, although not applied with aseptic precautions, are required to reach the user in a sterile condition.

The first category covers sterile dressings for use in operating theatres, hospital wards, clinics, etc., while the second category covers those intended, for example, for domestic use.

In both instances, the packaging must be adequate to maintain sterility of the dressing at least up to the time of opening the package. Dressings packed in such a manner may be labelled as "Sterile", and any dressing so labelled complies with the appropriate test for sterility.

The sterilisation process chosen governs both the choice of the wrapping material and the design of the pack. Double wrapping affords a distinct advantage over the use of a single wrapper for presenting a product in an aseptic manner, and when a surgical dressing or a composite pack (that is, a pack containing a variety of articles used in a single procedure) is to be used with aseptic precautions, double wrapping is essential. Both wrappers should be applied and the outer wrapper sealed before the package is sterilised. For such products, a packing carton or case is not a suitable outer wrapper. Packaging which maintains sterility of its contents during normal conditions may not do so if it becomes wet. It is important, therefore, that the outer wrapper chosen should, when wet, be as impervious as possible to the passage of micro-organisms in case the package is wetted inadvertently.

Methods. HEATING IN AN AUTOCLAVE (Method 2). Surgical dressings composed chiefly of cotton, rayon, or other cellulose material may be sterilised by the following method, which is designed to achieve efficient sterilisation and to deliver the sterilised dressings dry and ready for use.

A suitable apparatus consists of a sterilising chamber capable of withstanding the necessary changes in pressure and either insulated or surrounded by a steam jacket maintained at the sterilising temperature.

The chamber is provided with a suitable supply of steam under pressure which is dry but not superheated, a condensate discharge drain fitted with a near-to-steam trap, a thermometer to show the temperature in the coolest part of the chamber during the process, a pressure gauge, a pump capable of removing sufficient air from the load to ensure almost instantaneous penetration of the steam into the dressing, and a filter to allow sterile air to be admitted at the end of the process. A device is fitted which will detect the presence of sufficient residual air in the chamber to delay penetration of the steam and thereby interfere with the sterilising process. There must be no leaks in the valves or door seal of the chamber, and the chamber door must be adequately insulated. Full details of the construction and performance requirements of automatically controlled autoclaves suitable for sterilising porous loads are given in British Standard 3970: Part 1: 1966.

Steam is first admitted to the jacket, if one is provided. The dressings are placed in the sterilising chamber and so arranged by suitable packing that they can be permeated by steam. The chamber is closed, and air removed from the chamber by reducing the pressure. The removal of air during this part of the process may be assisted by the admission of steam, either as a series of pulses or a continuous flush.

Steam is then admitted until the chamber temperature reaches the chosen value, which is then maintained for the appropriate period, after which the steam is removed from the chamber and drying accomplished by reducing the pressure in the chamber.

Sterile air is then admitted through the filter, the chamber opened, and the dressings removed.

The whole process is usually automatically controlled. The sterilisation conditions used must be chosen with regard to the stability of the dressing. For materials which can withstand exposure to a temperature of 134° to 138° for 3 minutes, these conditions are usually chosen if suitable apparatus which can be carefully controlled is available. Most dressings are autoclaved at this temperature. However, dressings containing boric acid become tender at high temperatures, but they may be sterilised by using a temperature of 115° to 116° for 30 minutes; at this temperature the damage caused at higher temperatures is largely avoided.

Sterilisation can also be accomplished without the use of high vacuum by using steam to displace the air by the normal "downward displacement" method, but it requires extreme care and skill in packing the load and in carrying out the sterilisation process in order to effect the complete removal of air from all parts of the load and adequate penetration of the steam.

When surgical dressings are sterilised by heating in an autoclave the steam used should not contain more than 5% of entrained moisture.

DRY HEAT (Method 1). Dressings impregnated with soft paraffin may be sterilised by maintaining at a temperature not lower than 150° for 1 hour. It is essential that all parts of the dressing are maintained at this temperature.

EXPOSURE TO ETHYLENE OXIDE (Method 5). Wrappers enclosing the material must permit access of ethylene oxide, water vapour, and air, but prevent access of micro-organisms, and be able to withstand the changes of pressure in the chamber during sterilisation. After the sterilisation process, complete removal of ethylene oxide from the dressings by ventilation before final packing must be ensured, as prolonged contact with the skin, even in very low concentrations, may cause dermatitis or blistering.

EXPOSURE TO IONISING RADIATION (Method 6). This method is suitable for sterilising certain surgical dressings.

Some natural and synthetic fibres and plastics are likely to be degraded to a significant extent by repeated exposure to ionising radiation. With some materials, for example, cellulosic materials, major degradation occurs if they are autoclaved after they have been exposed to a sterilising dose of gamma radiation. There is also the possibility of toxicity developing in certain products if they are exposed to ethylene oxide after previous irradiation. Therefore no attempt should be made to resterilise a dressing which has been previously sterilised by exposure to ionising radiation.

Stilboestrol

(*E*)-α*β*-Diethylstilbene-4,4′-diol

$C_{18}H_{20}O_2 = 268.4$

OTHER NAMES: Diaethylstiboestrolum; Diethylstilbestrol; Diethylstilboestrol; *Pabestrol*® *Tampovagan Stilboestrol and Lactic Acid*®

A standard is given in the European Pharmacopoeia Vol. III

CAUTION. *Stilboestrol is a powerful oestrogen. Contact with the skin or inhalation of the dust should be avoided. Rubber gloves should be worn when handling the powder and, if the powder is dry, a face mask should also be worn.*

Description. An odourless white crystalline powder.

Solubility. Very slightly soluble in water; soluble, at 20°, in 5 parts of alcohol, in 3 parts of ether, and in 40 parts of arachis oil; soluble in solutions of alkali hydroxides.

Hygroscopicity. It absorbs insignificant amounts of moisture at 25° at relative humidities up to about 90%.

Sterilisation. Oily solutions for injection are sterilised by dry heat.

Storage. It should be protected from light.

Identification. TEST. Dissolve about 500 μg in 4 drops of glacial acetic acid, add 1 ml of phosphoric acid and heat on a water-bath for 3 minutes; a deep yellow colour is produced. Add 3 ml of glacial acetic acid; the colour almost disappears.

MELTING-POINT. About 172°.

ULTRAVIOLET ABSORPTION. In alcohol (95%), maximum at 241 nm (E1%, 1cm = 600).

INFRA-RED ABSORPTION. Major peaks at 833, 1176, 1205, 1250, 1428, and 1512 cm⁻¹ (see Appendix 2a: Infra-red Spectra).

THIN-LAYER CHROMATOGRAPHY. See under Thin-layer Chromatography, System 10.

Metabolism. ABSORPTION. Readily absorbed after oral administration.

DISTRIBUTION. In monkeys, volume of distribution at steady state, about 5 litres/kg; subject to enterohepatic circulation.

METABOLIC REACTIONS. In monkeys, rapidly metabolised in the liver and subject to first pass metabolism; mainly metabolised by glucuronic acid conjugation.

EXCRETION. After an intravenous dose to monkeys, 50 to 60% is excreted in the urine and 20 to 37% is excreted in the bile; in rats, most of a dose is excreted in the bile as the glucuronide whilst in the rabbit, about 70% of a dose is excreted as the glucuronide in the urine.

FURTHER INFORMATION. Absorption and enterohepatic circulation in young rats—L. J. Fischer et al., J. Pharmac. exp. Ther., 1973, **185**, 163; disposition in the rhesus monkey—E. J. Mroszczak and S. Riegelman, J. Pharmacokinet. Biopharm., 1975, **3**, 303.

Actions and uses. Stilboestrol has the actions, uses, and undesirable effects of the oestrogens, as described under Oestradiol Benzoate. Like the other synthetic oestrogens it is readily absorbed from the gastro-intestinal tract.

For the treatment of menopausal symptoms it is advisable to start with a low dosage, such as 100 micrograms by mouth 2 or 3 times a day, and subsequently to adjust the dosage to the minimum necessary to control the symptoms.

In the treatment of amenorrhoea due to ovarian insufficiency, 0.25 to 1 milligram is given daily during the proliferative phase of the menstrual cycle. Larger doses may be needed for such conditions as senile vaginitis and kraurosis vulvae.

For the suppression of lactation, 5 milligrams is given 2 or 3 times a day for 3 days and subsequently the dosage is gradually reduced.

For the palliative treatment of carcinoma of the prostate and mammary carcinoma, 10 to 20 milligrams or more is given daily.

Undesirable effects. As for Oestradiol Benzoate. In excessive dosage, stilboestrol may give rise to nausea and vomiting.

Stilboestrol may cause adenosis or virilisation of the foetus if given during pregnancy. Vaginal carcinomas may occur in the female offspring of mothers who received large doses of stilboestrol, usually to prevent miscarriage.

Veterinary uses. Stilboestrol is used as a growth promoter in cattle. It is administered by implantation in a non-edible part of the body in a dose of up to 50 milligrams.

Preparations

STILBOESTROL PESSARIES: for each pessary take:

Stilboestrol .. .. 0.5 mg
Propylene glycol .. .. 0.07 ml
Glycerol suppositories mass .. .. sufficient to fill
a 4-g mould

Prepare as described in the entry on Pessaries, dissolving the stilboestrol in the propylene glycol, with the aid of gentle heat, before incorporating in the melted glycerol suppositories mass.
A standard for these pessaries is given in the British Pharmaceutical Codex 1973
Containers and Storage: see the entry on Pessaries for general information on containers and storage.
Advice for patients: the pessaries should be inserted high into the vagina, preferably at night.

STILBOESTROL TABLETS (Syn. Diethylstilbestrol Tablets): available as tablets containing 100, 250, and 500 micrograms, and 1, 5, 25, and 100 mg of stilboestrol; they may be sugar coated and the coat may be coloured.
A standard for these tablets is given in the British Pharmacopoeia Addendum 1977
Containers and Storage: see the entry on Tablets for general information on containers and storage. Containers should be airtight and light resistant.
Advice for patients: the prescribed course should be completed or where applicable treatment should not be discontinued without the advice of the prescriber.

OTHER PREPARATIONS available include PESSARIES containing stilboestrol 500 micrograms with lactic acid 5%.

Stilboestrol Dipropionate

(E)-αβ-Diethylstilbene-4,4'-diyl dipropionate

$C_{24}H_{28}O_4 = 380.5$

OTHER NAME: Diethylstilboestrol Dipropionate

A standard is given in the British Pharmacopoeia (Veterinary)

Description. Odourless colourless crystals or white crystalline powder.

Solubility. Very slightly soluble in water; soluble in alcohol, in ether, and in fixed oils.

Sterilisation. Oily solutions are sterilised by dry heat.

Storage. It should be protected from light.

Identification. MELTING-POINT. About 105°.

ULTRAVIOLET ABSORPTION. In dehydrated alcohol, maximum at 238 nm (E1%, 1cm = 350).

Veterinary uses. Stilboestrol dipropionate is used in the treatment of infertility, uterine infections, and other gynaecological conditions. The usual dose in all species by intramuscular injection of an oily solution is 10 to 40 micrograms per kilogram body-weight. It is also administered to cattle by intra-uterine infusion as a single dose of 50 milligrams.

Preparation

STILBOESTROL DIPROPIONATE INJECTION: a sterile solution of stilboestrol dipropionate in ethyl oleate. It is sterilised by dry heat. Available in 10-, 25-, 30-, and 50-ml units containing 10 mg of stilboestrol dipropionate per ml.
A standard for this injection is given in the British Pharmacopoeia (Veterinary)
Containers and Labelling: see the entry on Injections for general information on containers and labelling.
Storage: it should be protected from light.

Still's Disease

see RHEUMATOID ARTHRITIS, JUVENILE

Stings

see INSECT BITES AND STINGS

Storax, Prepared

The purified balsam obtained from the trunk of *Liquidambar orientalis* Mill. (Fam. Hamamelidaceae), a tree indigenous to the south-west of Asiatic Turkey.

OTHER NAME: Styrax Praeparatus

A standard is given in the British Pharmaceutical Codex 1973

The secretion of the crude balsam, which is not a normal product of the tree, is induced by wounding the bark. The crude balsam forms an opaque greyish viscous liquid, which on standing separates into a supernatant aqueous liquid and a dark brown oleoresinous layer. It contains about 20 to 30% of water, together with fragments of bark and other extraneous material; from these it is purified by solution in alcohol, filtration, and evaporation.

Constituents. Prepared storax consists of a resin mixed with an oily liquid. The resin consists of compounds of unknown structure, including one or more resin alcohols which are partly free and partly esterified with cinnamic acid. The oily liquid contains styrene, vanillin, and free cinnamic acid, together with the ethyl, phenylpropyl, and cinnamyl esters of cinnamic acid.

Description. A brown viscous liquid which is transparent in thin layers. It has an agreeable and balsamic odour.

Solubility. Soluble in alcohol (90%), in carbon disulphide, in chloroform, and in glacial acetic acid; partly soluble in ether.

Adulterants and substitutes. American storax, or sweet gum, is a transparent viscous yellowish fluid obtained from *L. styraciflua* L. Partly exhausted storax is a balsam which has been partially deprived of its cinnamyl alcohol and cinnamic acid.

Factitious storax is also available.

Identification. TEST. Mix 1 g with 3 g of sand, add 5 ml of *potassium permanganate solution*, and warm gently; a distinct odour of benzaldehyde is produced.

Uses. Prepared storax is an ingredient of benzoin inhalation and of compound benzoin tincture.

Stramonium

The dried leaves or leaves and flowering tops of *Datura stramonium* L. (Fam. Solanaceae) and its varieties.

OTHER NAMES: Stramonii Folium; Stramonium Leaf; Thornapple Leaf

A standard is given in the European Pharmacopoeia Vol. I

The plants are annuals cultivated in the Balkans and the United States of America. The leaves and young shoots are collected while the plant is in flower, from about June to September.

Varieties. The leaves and stems of *D. stramonium* are green in colour and the corollas of the flowers are white when fresh and a pale buff colour when dry.

The stems and petioles and the main veins of the leaves of *D. stramonium* L. var. *tatula* (L.) Torr. vary in colour from a red tint to purple-black; the corollas are purplish blue when fresh and brown, sometimes with a purplish tint, when dry; the leaves are a somewhat darker green than those of *D. stramonium*.

D. stramonium L. var. *inermis* (Jacq.) Timm. and *D. stramonium* L. var. *godronii* Danert bear fruits devoid of spines.

Stramonium is sometimes imported in a broken (laminated) condition and is then frequently found to be adulterated.

Constituents. Stramonium contains 0.25 to 0.5% of alkaloids, which consist chiefly of (−)-hyoscyamine and (−)-hyoscine with a small amount of atropine [(±)-hyoscyamine]; about 30% of the alkaloids consist of (−)-hyoscine.

Up to 3% of stem with a diameter exceeding 5 mm may be present. It yields up to 20% of sulphated ash and up to 4% of acid-insoluble ash.

Description. UNGROUND DRUG. *Macroscopical characters:* leaves dark greyish-green and much shrivelled and twisted as a result of drying; when expanded, outline ovate or triangular-ovate, dentately lobed with an irregularly serrated margin, mostly 80 to 250 mm long and 70 to 150 mm broad; apex acuminate, base usually unequal; petiole often short and twisted; trichomes numerous on young leaves, older leaves almost glabrous; stems dichasially branched, slender with transverse and longitudinal wrinkles; flowers occurring solitarily at the forks, being about 75 mm long, erect and shortly pedicellate; corolla buff-coloured or brown, sometimes with a purplish tint, plicate and trumpet-shaped, but much twisted when dry; ovary superior, conical, spuriously tetralocular in the lower part, covered with short emergences, ovules numerous and campylotropous; immature fruit may be covered with numerous spinous emergences; seeds brown to black, flattened, subreniform, about 3 mm long, testa minutely pitted and vaguely reticulate, embryo curved in an oily endosperm.

It has a disagreeable and characteristic odour and a bitter and unpleasant taste.

Microscopical characters: the diagnostic characters are: leaf: *epidermis*, cells with a smooth *cuticle*, those of adaxial surface with straight or somewhat curved anticlinal walls and those of abaxial surface with sinuous anticlinal walls; *stomata* anisocytic, more numerous on abaxial epidermis; *trichomes* (a) *non-glandular*, straight or slightly curved, uniseriate, 3- to 5-celled, conical, with thin warty walls, the basal cell being largest and usually exceeding 50 μm in length and 35 μm in breadth, (b) *glandular*, usually curved and composed of short 1- or 2-celled stalk and 2- to 7-celled pyriform glandular head; *palisade cells* in 1 layer beneath the epidermis; *crystal layer* composed of cells most of which contain a single cluster crystal of calcium oxalate or occasional prisms or microsphenoidal crystals; *phloem* intraxylary in midrib.

Stem: *trichomes* as in leaf, but up to 800 μm long; *pericyclic fibres* occasional; *xylem fibres* and *vessels* numerous; *crystals* of calcium oxalate represented by cluster crystals in cells of *phloem* and pith and occasional microsphenoidal crystals.

Pollen grains: 60 to 80 μm in diameter, with 3 large pores and coarsely warty *extine*.

POWDERED DRUG. Powdered Stramonium. A greyish-green powder possessing the diagnostic microscopical characters, odour, and taste of the unground drug.

Adulterants and substitutes. Datura leaf, which contains about 0.5% of alkaloids, the majority being (−)-hyoscyamine, consists of the dried leaves and flowering tops of *D. innoxia* Miller and *D. metel* L., annual plants growing in the Indian subcontinent, although *D. innoxia* is indigenous to Mexico.

Datura leaves are about the same size as those of stramonium; those of *D. innoxia* are ovate to somewhat cordate; the margin entire, undulate or sometimes with 2 or 3 low teeth; both surfaces are densely pubescent; the trichomes are of 3 types, the most numerous being slender with a 2- to 4-celled uniseriate stalk and usually a unicellular glandular head, their length varying from 175 to 600 μm.

Leaves of *D. metel* are ovate to cordate and usually have 3 to 4 coarse teeth, but there are no small teeth in the sinuses; although glabrous to the unaided eye they have trichomes similar to those of stramonium, but the non-glandular trichomes are usually less than 35 μm in width at the base and the basal cell is rarely as long as 50 μm.

The leaves of *Xanthium strumarium* L. (Fam. Compositae), *Carthamus helenoides* Desf. (Fam. Compositae) and *Chenopodium hybridum* L. (Fam. Chenopodiaceae) have been recorded as adulterants.

Storage. It should be stored in a cool dry place, protected from light.

Actions and uses. The actions of stramonium are similar to those described under Belladonna Herb and Hyoscyamus. It has been used to control the salivation, muscular rigidity, and tremor of parkinsonism.

Stramonium is an ingredient of powders intended to be burnt and the fumes inhaled for the relief of asthma, but such a procedure often aggravates chronic bronchitis and is of little value in relieving asthma.

Precautions. The dose should not be increased too rapidly as this may lead to paralysis of accommodation.

Poisoning. As for Atropine.

Preparation

STRAMONIUM TINCTURE:

Stramonium, in moderately
coarse powder .. .. 100 g
Alcohol (45%) .. .. .. a sufficient quantity

Prepare about 900 ml of tincture by the percolation process and determine the proportion of alkaloids present in a portion of the percolate; if necessary, dilute the remainder of the percolate with sufficient of the alcohol to produce a tincture of the required strength. It contains, in 2 ml, 500 micrograms of the alkaloids of stramonium, calculated as hyoscyamine.

A standard for this tincture is given in the British Pharmacopoeia 1973

Dose: up to 6 ml daily, in divided doses.

Streptokinase

A protein obtained from culture filtrates of certain strains of haemolytic streptococcus group C, which has the property of activating human plasminogen to form plasmin. It is purified to contain not less than 600 units of streptokinase activity per microgram of bacterial protein nitrogen and then mixed with a suitable stabiliser and buffering agents. It is prepared by a process that yields a sterile product.

OTHER NAMES: *Kabikinase®*; *Streptase®* *Varidase®* (with streptodornase)

A standard is given in the British Pharmacopoeia Addendum 1975

Description. A white powder or friable solid.

Solubility. Soluble in water.

Acidity or alkalinity. A solution containing 5000 units per ml has a pH of 6.8 to 7.5.

Moisture content. Not more than 4%, determined by drying over phosphorus pentoxide *in vacuo*.

Storage. It should be stored in airtight containers, at a temperature of 2° to 8°, protected from light. Under these conditions it may be expected to retain its potency for 2 years.

Actions and uses. Streptokinase is an enzyme which converts plasminogen to plasmin, a fibrinolytic substance that causes dissolution of intravascular blood clots. It is used in the treatment of venous thrombosis, pulmonary embolism, occlusion of peripheral arteries, myocardial infarction, and clotting in haemodialysis shunts.

Streptokinase is administered by intravascular infusion of a solution in dextrose injection (5%) or sodium chloride injection. Most patients have a low titre of antibodies to streptokinase and respond to an initial dose of 250000 units administered over a period of half to one hour, followed by maintenance dosage at the rate of 100000 units per hour. Children and patients who have recently had a streptococcal infection or who have previously been treated with streptokinase may be subjected to a streptokinase resistance test and then given an initial dose, usually in the range 100000 to 600000 units, estimated to be sufficient to neutralise the circulating antibodies.

During maintenance therapy the thrombin clotting time should be kept within 2 to 4 times the normal value by adjustment of the dose if necessary.

When treatment with streptokinase is completed, anti-coagulant therapy with heparin and oral anticoagulants may be initiated to prevent the formation of further thrombi.

Solutions containing 5000 to 10000 units of streptokinase per millilitre with 1250 to 2500 units of streptodornase per millilitre are applied to suppurating surfaces to remove clotted blood and fibrinous matter.

Undesirable effects. Streptokinase may give rise to hyperpyrexia and anaphylactic reactions which may be treated with corticosteroids or an antihistamine. Haemorrhage may also occur, requiring treatment with aminocaproic acid.

Precautions. Streptokinase should not be given within 48 hours of surgery and should be used with caution in patients who have large raw areas as a result of surgery, in early pregnancy, and after parturition. It should also be used with caution in patients convalescing from streptococcal infections.

Contra-indications. Streptokinase is contra-indicated in haemorrhagic conditions, hypertension, streptococcal infections, and subacute bacterial endocarditis, and during menstruation. It should not be given to patients who have been treated with streptokinase within the preceding 3 months.

The unit is identical with the international unit of streptokinase activity (1964) and is contained in 2.090 μg of the standard preparation.

Preparations

STREPTOKINASE INJECTION: a sterile solution of streptokinase in water for injections. It is prepared by dissolving the contents of a sealed container in water for
injections immediately before use. Available as a powder
in vials containing 100 000, 250 000, 600 000, and 750 000
units of streptokinase.

*A standard for this injection is given in the British
Pharmacopoeia Addendum 1975*
Containers: see the entry on Injections for general
information on containers.
Labelling: see the entry on Injections for general information on labelling. In addition, the label on the sealed
container or the label on the package should state that
the preparation is antigenic.
Storage: the sealed container should be stored at a
temperature of 2° to 8°, protected from light. Under these
conditions it may be expected to retain its potency for
2 years. The injection decomposes on storage and should
be used immediately after preparation.

OTHER PREPARATIONS available include a SOLUTION
reconstituted from vials of powder containing streptokinase 100 000 units with streptodornase 25 000 units;
and TABLETS containing streptokinase 10 000 units with
streptodornase 2500 units.

Streptomycin Sulphate

The sulphate of *O*-2-deoxy-2-methylamino-α-L-gluco-
pyranosyl-(1→2)-*O*-5-deoxy-3-*C*-formyl-α-L-lyxo-
furanosyl-(1→4)-*N³N³*-diamidino-D-streptamine, an
antimicrobial base produced by certain strains of *Streptomyces griseus*.

$3H_2SO_4$

$C_{42}H_{84}N_{14}O_{36}S_3 = 1457.4$

OTHER NAMES: Streptomycini Sulfas; *Streptovex*®;
Stryzolin®
Crystamycin® (with benzylpenicillin); *Dimycin*® (with
dihydrostreptomycin sulphate); *Oroject NS*® (with neo-
mycin sulphate); *Streptopen*® (with procaine penicillin)
*A standard is given in the European Pharmacopoeia
Vol. II*

CAUTION. *Streptomycin may cause severe dermatitis in
sensitised persons, and pharmacists, nurses, and others
who handle the drug frequently should wear masks and
rubber gloves.*

Description. An almost odourless hygroscopic white
powder with a slightly bitter taste.

Solubility. Soluble in water; very slightly soluble in
alcohol, in ether, and in chloroform.

Acidity. A 25% solution has a pH of 4.5 to 7.

Moisture content. Not more than 7%, determined by
drying at 60° over phosphorus pentoxide *in vacuo.*

Stability. Aqueous solutions of streptomycin are stable
but some colour development can occur, which is
normally inhibited by the use of metal complexing agents
such as edetic acid and thiols.

Labelling. If the material is not intended for parenteral
administration, the label on the container states that the
contents are not to be injected.

Storage. It should be stored in airtight containers at
a temperature not exceeding 30°. If it is intended for
parenteral administration, the containers should be
sterile and sealed to exclude micro-organisms.

Identification. TESTS. 1. Mix a small quantity with 1N
sodium hydroxide, boil for a few minutes and add a slight
excess of hydrochloric acid and a few drops of *ferric
chloride solution*; an intense violet colour is produced.
2. Dissolve about 100 mg in 2 ml of water and add 1 ml
of *1-naphthol solution* and 2 ml of *dilute sodium hypochlorite solution*; a red colour is produced.

Determination in body fluids. COLORIMETRY. In serum
—E. Duda *et al., Biochem. Med.,* 1976, **15**, 330.

Metabolism. ABSORPTION. Poorly and irregularly absorbed after oral administration but rapidly absorbed after
intramuscular administration; subcutaneous doses are
initially more slowly absorbed than intramuscular doses
but after 2 hours follow a similar pattern.

BLOOD CONCENTRATION. After an intramuscular dose of
1 g, peak serum concentrations of 25 to 50 μg/ml are
attained in 0.5 to 2 hours, falling to 5 to 10 μg/ml at
12 hours; the minimum effective serum concentration
is about 7 μg/ml although, in severe infections or bacteraemia, concentrations of at least 14 μg/ml may be
necessary.

HALF-LIFE. Serum half-life, about 2.5 hours in young
adults; increased in the newborn and in adults over the
age of 40 years; in renal function impairment the half-life
may be increased to 2 to 5 days.

DISTRIBUTION. Widely distributed throughout the body
and enters pleural, peritoneal, and pericardial cavities,
bile, synovial fluid, milk, saliva, sweat, tears, and
aqueous and vitreous humours; it crosses the placenta,
does not enter red blood cells, and enters the cerebrospinal fluid when the meninges are inflamed; accumulates
in renal function impairment; *protein binding,* 25 to 30%
bound to plasma proteins.

EXCRETION. About 50 to 80% of a parenteral dose is
excreted in the urine unchanged in 24 hours; most of
an oral dose is eliminated in the faeces and about 1%
is excreted in the bile.

FURTHER INFORMATION. A. Kucers and N. M. Bennett, *The Use of Antibiotics*, 2nd Edn, London, Heinemann, 1975, p. 173.

Actions and uses. Streptomycin is an aminoglycoside antibiotic with a spectrum of antibacterial activity similar to that of gentamicin sulphate but it is more toxic and resistance develops more rapidly. Its clinical use depends on its bactericidal action against *Mycobacterium tuberculosis, Escherichia coli, Klebsiella pneumoniae, Brucella abortus*, and some species of *Proteus* and *Salmonella*.

It is used in the treatment of all forms of tuberculosis. Because relatively rapid induction of bacterial resistance may occur, streptomycin must always be used in conjunction with at least one other effective antituberculous drug.

The usual dose for an adult is 750 milligrams daily by intramuscular injection, but other dosage schemes such as 1 gram 2 or 3 times a week are also effective. Patients over 60 years should receive a reduced dosage, such as 500 milligrams daily, in divided doses, and the drug should preferably not be given to patients over 70 years. Dosage for small adults should be adjusted according to the body-weight of the patient. The dosage for children is 30 milligrams per kilogram body-weight daily, up to a maximum of 1 gram.

This treatment is suitable for the treatment of tuberculous meningitis provided that streptomycin is used in conjunction with drugs such as isoniazid which enter the cerebrospinal fluid; it is no longer considered to be generally essential to give streptomycin by intrathecal injection for this purpose. Streptomycin is sometimes given intrathecally in tuberculous meningitis to severely ill patients in single daily doses of 50 to 100 milligrams dissolved in 10 millilitres of sodium chloride injection or of the patient's own cerebrospinal fluid.

The corresponding dose for children is: for the newborn 5 milligrams; from 6 months to 1 year 10 milligrams; 2 to 3 years 15 milligrams; 4 to 9 years 15 to 30 milligrams; and 10 to 15 years 30 to 50 milligrams.

Streptomycin should not be given if there is meningeal irritation, as shown by an increase in polymorph cells in the cerebrospinal fluid.

It has been used for the treatment of non-tuberculous infections, particularly infections of the large bowel, cholecystitis, and peritonitis, but because of the rapid development of resistance and the prevalence of strains of bacteria that are already resistant it should only be used when the causative organisms are known to be sensitive to its action. It is given preferably with another antibiotic. In endocarditis caused by streptococci relatively resistant to penicillin the synergy frequently demonstrable between penicillin and streptomycin is clinically useful.

Undesirable effects. As for Gentamicin Sulphate, but the effects occur more frequently. Allergic reactions are relatively common, the usual symptoms being fever and rash occurring during the second week of treatment in patients who have not previously been treated with streptomycin or immediately after starting treatment in those patients who have previously been sensitised to the drug; desensitisation is possible but is rarely necessary because alternative drugs are available.

Damage to the auditory and vestibular divisions of the eighth cranial nerve occurs more readily than with gentamicin if the concentration of the drug in the tissues is allowed to rise slightly above the minimum that is necessary for effective therapy; vertigo, nausea, tinnitus, deafness, and nystagmus may arise suddenly and regress when the drug is withdrawn but permanent damage to hearing and balance may also develop insidiously during treatment or even some weeks afterwards. Damage to the renal tubules, bone marrow, and liver rarely occurs at the usual therapeutic levels.

Streptomycin may occasionally give rise to lupus erythematosus.

Precautions. As for Gentamicin Sulphate. The doses recommended for the treatment of tuberculosis are close to the toxic level and should be reduced if the blood-urea concentration is raised. As with other aminoglycosides monitoring of blood concentrations of the drug is advisable in the presence of renal impairment. In tuberculous patients over 60 years of age, the serum concentration of streptomycin 24 hours after injection should not exceed 1 microgram per millilitre.

Streptomycin impairs neuromuscular transmission and while this action is too weak to cause symptoms in normal subjects caution should be exercised in patients with myasthenia gravis.

Drug interactions. As for Gentamicin Sulphate. In addition, streptomycin may potentiate the neuromuscular blocking action of procainamide.

Veterinary uses. Streptomycin hydrochloride is an antibacterial agent. The usual dose by intramammary injection in cattle is the equivalent of 100 milligrams of streptomycin in each quarter. The usual dose by intramuscular or intravenous injection in horses, cattle, sheep, pigs, and dogs is the equivalent of 10 milligrams of streptomycin per kilogram body-weight.

Preparations

STREPTOMYCIN INJECTION: a sterile solution of streptomycin sulphate in water for injections. It is prepared by dissolving the contents of a sealed container in water for injections shortly before use. Available as a powder in vials containing streptomycin sulphate equivalent to 1 g of streptomycin.

Containers and *Labelling:* see the entry on Injections for general information on containers and labelling.

Storage: the sealed container should be stored at a temperature not exceeding 30°. The injection contains no bactericide and should be used as soon as possible after preparation but solutions of streptomycin sulphate may be expected to retain their potency for up to 1 month after preparation provided they are stored at a temperature not exceeding 4°, protected from light.

STREPTOMYCIN SULPHATE INJECTION: a sterile solution, with suitable stabilising agents, in water for injections. It may contain a suitable buffering agent. It is prepared by means of an aseptic technique. Available as an injection containing streptomycin sulphate equivalent to 50 mg of streptomycin per ml, and in 40- and 100-ml packs containing streptomycin sulphate equivalent to 250 mg of streptomycin per ml.

A standard for this injection is given in the British Pharmacopoeia 1973

Containers: see the entry on Injections for general information on containers.

Labelling: see the entry on Injections for general information on labelling. In addition, the label on the container should state the amount of the medicament as the equivalent amount of streptomycin in a suitable dose-volume.

Storage: it should be stored at a temperature not exceeding 20°, protected from light. Under these conditions it may be expected to retain its potency for 18 months.

OTHER PREPARATIONS available include a veterinary

sterile GEL containing streptomycin sulphate equivalent to 20 mg of streptomycin with procaine penicillin 10 mg (10000 units) per ml in 100-ml single-dose bottles; an INJECTION reconstituted from vials of powder containing streptomycin sulphate equivalent to 500 mg of streptomycin with benzylpenicillin sodium 300 mg (500000 units), a veterinary injection containing streptomycin sulphate equivalent to 500 mg of streptomycin with dihydrostreptomycin sulphate equivalent to 500 mg of dihydrostreptomycin in 3 ml in 30- and 100-ml vials; and a veterinary SOLUTION containing streptomycin sulphate equivalent to 1 g of streptomycin in 20 ml in 2-litre bottles, and a veterinary solution containing streptomycin sulphate 70 mg with neomycin sulphate 70 mg per ml.

Strongyloidiasis

Strongyloidiasis is a bowel infection caused by *Strongyloides stercoralis*, a worm which is about 2 mm long and has a life cycle similar to that of the hookworm (*Ancylostoma duodenale*). It lives in the small intestine where it produces non-infective rhabditiform larvae which pass out in the stools. These reproduce outside the body, or occasionally in the bowel, to produce infective filariform larvae. These re-enter man through either the skin of the feet or the mucosa or skin around the anus.

Infection with *Strongyloides stercoralis* may be symptomless or may result in pulmonary symptoms, intestinal malabsorption, abdominal pain, and diarrhoea. Larvae sometimes migrate throughout the body and may cause irritation; for example, larvae in the skin may give rise to intense pruritus and urticaria. If corticosteroid or immunosuppressive drugs are given for another illness, massive autoinfection occurs which may be fatal.

Strongyloidiasis may be treated with thiabendazole.

Strychnine Hydrochloride

The hydrochloride of an alkaloid obtained from the seeds of *Strychnos nux-vomica* L. and other species of *Strychnos* (Fam. Loganiaceae).

HCl, 2H₂O

$C_{21}H_{23}ClN_2O_2,2H_2O = 406.9$

OTHER NAME: Strych. Hydrochlor.

A standard is given in the British Pharmaceutical Codex 1973

Description. Colourless prismatic crystals or a white crystalline powder.

Solubility. Soluble, at 20°, in 40 parts of water and in 85 parts of alcohol; practically insoluble in ether.

Moisture content. 7 to 9%, determined by drying at 130°.

Dissociation constants. pK_a 2.3, 8.0 (25°).

Incompatibility. It is incompatible with alkali hydroxides and carbonates, aromatic ammonia spirit, bromides, and iodides.

Sterilisation. Solutions for injection are sterilised by heating in an autoclave or by filtration.

Identification. TESTS. 1. Dissolve about 100 μg in 4 drops of sulphuric acid and slowly move a small crystal of potassium dichromate through the solution; an intense violet colour is produced, which changes through red to yellow.

2. To about 500 μg add 4 drops of sulphuric acid, followed by 50 mg of ammonium vanadate, and stir; a deep violet colour is produced which changes to red. Add 1 ml of water; the colour changes to cherry-red.

ULTRAVIOLET ABSORPTION. In 0.1N sulphuric acid, maximum at 255 nm.

INFRA-RED ABSORPTION. Major peaks at 763, 1053, 1111, 1282, 1316, and 1667 cm⁻¹ (see Appendix 2b: Infra-red Spectra).

Determination in body fluids. ULTRAVIOLET SPECTROPHOTOMETRY. In blood and urine—J. Bogan *et al.*, *J. forens. Sci. Soc.*, 1966, **6**, 166.

Metabolism. ABSORPTION. Readily absorbed after oral or parenteral administration.

DISTRIBUTION. Rapidly enters the tissues and is taken up to some extent by red blood cells.

METABOLIC REACTIONS. Rapidly oxidised.

EXCRETION. About 20% of a dose is excreted unchanged in the urine.

Actions and uses. Strychnine stimulates all parts of the nervous system. It is rapidly absorbed from the gastrointestinal tract and is slowly excreted, so that its action may be cumulative. Its use as a therapeutic agent has now been largely abandoned.

Because of its bitter taste strychnine has been used as a stomachic and tonic, but there is no evidence to show that it is of special value for these purposes. It has also been used with cathartics, but its incorporation in purgative pills and tablets is without therapeutic justification and may cause fatal accidental poisoning, especially in young children.

Small doses of strychnine delay the onset of fatigue, but this delay is followed by a phase of depression of muscular activity. It has been used as an analeptic, but it stimulates the respiratory and cardiovascular centres only in convulsant doses.

Liquid medicines containing strychnine hydrochloride should be made slightly acid.

The usual dose by mouth is 2 to 8 milligrams.

Undesirable effects. Toxic doses of strychnine produce convulsions of all voluntary muscle. Since extensor muscles are generally the stronger, the body is arched backwards and assumes a position of generalised extension, the head is retracted, the feet are turned inwards, and the arms are extended. All forms of sensation are rendered more acute. Death results from spasm of the respiratory muscles.

Poisoning. The stomach should be emptied and washed out with water. An aqueous suspension of charcoal may be administered. An emetic should not be given owing to the danger of aspirating vomitus. Convulsions may be controlled by the intravenous injection of diazepam, 10 milligrams repeated every 30 minutes as required; alternatively a 5 or 10% solution of thiopentone sodium may be given by intravenous injection in conjunction with muscle relaxants such as tubocurarine chloride or gallamine triethiodide. The patient should be sheltered from external stimuli in a quiet darkened room. Artificial respiration or controlled respiration using oxygen is necessary if the respiratory muscles are fixed in spasm.

Styes

Styes are caused by staphylococcal infection of the follicle of an eyelash. There is a painful swelling of the eyelid which may discharge pus from the site of infection. Treatment consists of bathing the eyelid with warm water and the application of antibacterial eye ointments.

Succinylsulphathiazole

4'-(Thiazol-2-ylsulphamoyl)succinanilic acid mono-hydrate

$C_{13}H_{13}N_3O_5S_2, H_2O = 373.4$

OTHER NAMES: Succinylsulfathiazole; Succinylsulfa-thiazolum; *Sulfasuxidine®*
Cremosuxidine® and *Kaovax®* (both with kaolin)

A standard is given in the European Pharmacopoeia Vol. II

Description. Odourless, white or yellowish-white crystals or powder with a slightly bitter taste.

Solubility. Very slightly soluble in water and in acetone; soluble, at 20°, in 200 parts of alcohol; practically insoluble in ether and in chloroform; soluble in solutions of alkali hydroxides, and, with evolution of carbon dioxide, in solutions of alkali carbonates.

Moisture content. 4.0 to 5.5%, determined by drying at 105°.

Stability; Storage. See the entry on Sulphonamides.

Identification. TESTS. 1. To about 300 mg add 3 ml of *dilute sodium hydroxide solution* and 7 ml of water, heat on a water-bath for 1 hour, cool, and neutralise with *dilute hydrochloric acid*; a crystalline precipitate is produced which, after washing with water and drying at 105°, melts at about 200°, and complies with general test 1 described under Sulphonamides.
2. It complies with general test 2 described under Sulphonamides.
3. To about 500 mg add 10 ml of *dilute hydrochloric acid*, evaporate to dryness, add 5 ml of *dilute ammonia solution*, again evaporate to dryness, and maintain at 100° for 30 minutes, add 2.5 g of zinc powder, mix, transfer to a test-tube, place in the mouth of the tube a strip of filter paper freshly moistened with a 5% solution of dimethylaminobenzaldehyde in a mixture of 1 volume of hydrochloric acid and 20 volumes of alcohol (95%), and heat the tube gently over an open flame; the paper turns yellow.

MELTING-POINT. About 190°, with decomposition.

ULTRAVIOLET ABSORPTION. In 0.1N hydrochloric acid, maxima at 258 nm (E1%, 1cm = 547) and 280 nm (E1%,

1cm = 542); in 0.1N sodium hydroxide maximum at 258 nm (E1%, 1cm = 642); in alcohol (95%), maxima at 259 nm (E1%, 1cm = 568) and 288 nm (E1%, 1cm = 601).

THIN-LAYER CHROMATOGRAPHY. See under Thin-layer Chromatography, System 11.

Actions and uses. Succinylsulphathiazole has the actions and uses described under Phthalylsulphathiazole. The usual dose for adults is 10 to 20 grams daily in divided doses. For the treatment of bacillary dysentery, children aged 1 to 2 years may be given 1 gram of succinylsulphathiazole 4 times daily; 3 to 5 years, 2 grams 4 times daily; and over 5 years, 2 grams 6 times a day.

Undesirable effects. As for Phthalylsulphathiazole.

Preparations

PAEDIATRIC SUCCINYLSULPHATHIAZOLE MIXTURE:

Succinylsulphathiazole, in fine powder ..	100 g
Light kaolin or light kaolin (natural)	60 g
Compound tragacanth powder	10 g
Amaranth solution	10 ml
Benzoic acid solution	20 ml
Raspberry syrup '.	200 ml
Chloroform water, double-strength	500 ml
Water for preparations	to 1000 ml

Triturate the compound tragacanth powder, the succinyl-sulphathiazole, and the light kaolin with the raspberry syrup to form a smooth paste; add gradually, with constant stirring, the benzoic acid solution and the amaranth solution diluted with the double-strength chloroform water, and sufficient water to produce the required volume.
When prepared extemporaneously, it must be recently prepared, unless the kaolin has been sterilised.
Alternatively the compound tragacanth powder may be replaced by an equal quantity of sodium carboxymethyl-cellulose 50 and 20 grams of maize starch and the chloroform water, double-strength, by 50 ml of chloroform spirit. The mixture is prepared as follows: Stir a suspension of the starch in 125 ml of water into about 350 ml of boiling water. Maintain the temperature until the mixture becomes translucent, and cool rapidly. Triturate the sodium carboxymethylcellulose 50, the succinylsulphathiazole, and the light kaolin with the raspberry syrup to form a smooth paste; add gradually, with constant stirring, the starch mucilage, the benzoic acid solution, the amaranth solution, the chloroform spirit, and sufficient water to produce the required volume. It must be recently prepared.
A standard for this mixture is given in the British Pharmaceutical Codex 1973
Containers and *Labelling*: see the entry on Mixtures for general information on containers and labelling. A direction to shake the bottle should be given on the label.
Advice for patients: the mixture should be taken at regular intervals. The prescribed course should be completed. Adequate fluid intake should be maintained. The use of preparations containing liquid paraffin should be avoided.

SUCCINYLSULPHATHIAZOLE TABLETS: available as tablets containing 500 mg of succinylsulphathiazole.
A standard for these tablets is given in the British Pharmacopoeia 1973
Containers and *Storage*: see the entry on Tablets for general information on containers and storage. Containers should be airtight and light resistant.
Advice for patients: see above under Paediatric Succinylsulphathiazole Mixture.

OTHER PREPARATIONS available include a MIXTURE containing succinylsulphathiazole 500 mg with kaolin 500 mg in 5 ml, diluent syrup, life of diluted mixture 14 days; and a mixture containing succinylsulphathiazole 500 mg with kaolin 750 mg in 5 ml.

Sucrose

β-D-Fructofuranosyl-α-D-glucopyranoside, a sugar obtained from the juice of the sugar-cane, *Saccharum officinarum* L. (Fam. Gramineae), or of white-rooted varieties of the sugar-beet, *Beta vulgaris* (Fam. Chenopodiaceae).

$C_{12}H_{22}O_{11} = 342.3$

OTHER NAMES: Refined Sugar; Saccharum

A standard is given in the European Pharmacopoeia Vol. II

Description. Odourless, lustrous, dry, colourless crystals or white crystalline powder with a sweet taste.

Solubility. Soluble, at 20°, in less than 1 part of water and in 370 parts of alcohol.

Specific rotation. +66.2° to +66.8°, determined on a 20% solution.

Hygroscopicity. It absorbs insignificant amounts of moisture at 25° at relative humidities up to about 85%, but under damper conditions it absorbs substantial amounts.

Sterilisation. Solutions for injection are sterilised by heating in an autoclave or by filtration.

Identification. TEST. Dissolve about 25 mg in 5 ml of water and add 2 ml of *dilute sodium hydroxide solution* and 3 drops of *copper sulphate solution*; the solution is blue and clear. Boil; the solution remains clear. To the hot solution add 4 ml of *dilute hydrochloric acid* and 4 ml of *dilute sodium hydroxide solution*; an orange precipitate is produced immediately.

Actions and uses. Sucrose is used as a sweetening agent and as a demulcent. Solutions of sucrose in concentrations of less than 65% w/w ferment, but more concentrated solutions, such as syrups, have an osmotic pressure sufficiently great to inhibit the growth of most bacteria and fungi. The syrups may be used as flavouring agents.

Preparation

SYRUP:

Sucrose	667 g
Purified water	to 1000 g

Heat together until dissolved and add sufficient boiling purified water to produce 1000 g. A suitable preservative or mixture of preservatives may be added.
A standard for syrup is given in the British Pharmacopoeia 1973

Labelling: the label on the container should state the names and proportions of any added preservatives.
Storage: it should not be exposed to undue fluctuations in temperature.

Sulfa...

see under SULPHA...

Sulphacetamide Sodium

The monohydrate of the sodium derivative of N^1-acetylsulphanilamide.

$C_8H_9N_2NaO_3S,H_2O = 254.2$

OTHER NAMES: *Albucid®*; Soluble Sulphacetamide; Sulfacetamide Sodium; *Sulphacalyre®*; *Vasosulf®* *Cortucid®* (with hydrocortisone acetate); *Isopto Cetamide®* (with methylcellulose); *Sulfapred®* (with prednisolone sodium phosphate); *Ocusol®* (with zinc sulphate)

A standard is given in the British Pharmacopoeia 1973

Description. Odourless, white or yellowish-white crystals or microcrystalline powder, with a slightly bitter taste.

Solubility. Soluble, at 20°, in 1.5 parts of water; very slightly soluble in alcohol and in acetone.

Alkalinity. A 5% solution has a pH of 8 to 9.5.

Moisture content. 6 to 8%, determined by drying at 150°.

Dissociation constant. pK_a 5.4 (25°).

Stability; Sterilisation; Storage. See the entry on Sulphonamides.

Identification. TESTS. 1. Dissolve about 1 g in 10 ml of water, and add 2 ml of acetic acid; a white precipitate is produced which, after washing with water and drying at 105° for 4 hours, melts at about 183°, complies with general test 1 described under Sulphonamides, and when heated with a mixture of alcohol (95%) and sulphuric acid produces the odour of ethyl acetate.
2. It complies with general test 2 described under Sulphonamides.

ULTRAVIOLET ABSORPTION. In 0.1N hydrochloric acid, maximum at 271 nm (E1%, 1cm = 207); in 0.1N sodium hydroxide, maximum at 256 nm (E1%, 1cm = 626).

INFRA-RED ABSORPTION. Major peaks at 816, 1087, 1147, 1270, 1336, and 1550 cm^{-1} (see Appendix 2a: Infra-red Spectra).

THIN-LAYER CHROMATOGRAPHY. See under Thin-layer Chromatography, System 11.

Actions and uses. Sulphacetamide sodium has the actions of the sulphonamides, as described under Sulphadimidine. It is used chiefly for local application in infections and injuries of the conjunctiva.

In the treatment of acute conjunctivitis and in the prophylaxis of ocular infections after injuries or burns, a 10% solution is applied every 2 hours, or a 30% solution twice a day; alternatively, an ointment may be used.

Preparations

SULPHACETAMIDE EYE-DROPS: consisting of a sterile solution containing up to 30% of sulphacetamide sodium, with suitable preservatives and stabilising agents, in purified water. It is prepared by method A, B, or C described in the entry on Eye-drops.

A suitable solution may be prepared according to the following formula:

Sulphacetamide sodium ..	..	a sufficient quantity
Phenylmercuric acetate *or* nitrate	.. ..	0.002 g
Sodium metabisulphite ..	.. .. ..	0.100 g
Disodium edetate ..	.. ..	a sufficient quantity
Purified water	.. ..	to 100.0 ml

Disodium edetate 0.02% should be incorporated in solutions containing 10% of sulphacetamide sodium, and 0.05% of disodium edetate in solutions containing 30% of sulphacetamide sodium. The phenylmercuric acetate or nitrate may be replaced by 0.01% of thiomersal.

In making this preparation, precautions should be taken to minimise oxidation of the active ingredient. The purified water used should be freshly boiled and cooled, or alternatively, if the water is prepared by distillation, freshly distilled water may be used. The procedure adopted should be such that the amount of oxygen which dissolves in the solution during preparation is minimal. When the preparation is made by method A or C, a plain cap with an airtight seal should be used as the closure for the final container. A separate screw cap fitted with a teat and dropper, suitably wrapped and sterilised, should either be substituted for the plain cap by the pharmacist immediately before issue, care being taken to avoid contamination, or the wrapped sterile dropper assembly should be issued to the patient with instructions to exchange it for the plain cap on first using the eye-drops. When the preparation is made by method B, a sterile dropper assembly may be used as the closure for the final container, provided that the assembly prevents ingress of oxygen.

The precautions taken in preparing these eye-drops are necessary because, in addition to degradation by oxidation, some hydrolysis of the active ingredient to sulphanilamide occurs (see the entry on Sulphonamides).

When Weak Sulphacetamide Eye-drops are ordered or prescribed, a solution containing 10% of sulphacetamide sodium is supplied, and when Strong Sulphacetamide Eye-drops are ordered or prescribed, a solution containing 30% of sulphacetamide sodium is supplied.

Available as eye-drops containing 10, 15, 20, and 30% of sulphacetamide sodium.

A standard for these eye-drops is given in the British Pharmaceutical Codex 1973

Containers: see the entry on Eye-drops, as modified above, for general information on containers.

Labelling: see the entry on Eye-drops for general information on labelling. In addition, the label on the container should state that the eye-drops should be stored at room temperature and should not be allowed to freeze, and that the contents should be discarded 4 weeks after first opening the container.

Storage: it should be protected from light. Chemical stability of the drug in aqueous solution after opening

the container is limited and it deteriorates on storage. The eye-drops should therefore be used within 4 weeks of first opening the container.

It should be stored at room temperature. Storage at lower temperatures may result in formation of crystals. It should not be allowed to freeze.

Advice for patients: see the entry on Eye-drops for general information on the use of eye-drops. The prescribed course should be completed.

SULPHACETAMIDE EYE OINTMENT (*Syn.* Oculent. Sulphacetam.):

Sulphacetamide sodium, in No. 90 powder, sterile..	..	a sufficient quantity
Liquid paraffin ..	.. .. ..	10 g
Yellow soft paraffin ..	.. .. ..	90 g

Melt the yellow soft paraffin, add the liquid paraffin, filter the hot mixture through coarse filter paper placed in a heated funnel, and sterilise by dry heat at 150° for 1 hour; allow the basis to cool but maintain in a molten state. By means of an aseptic technique triturate the sulphacetamide sodium with a small portion of the melted basis until the mixture is smooth, gradually add the remainder of the melted basis and continue the trituration until the ointment is cold.

Available as an eye ointment containing 2.5 and 6% of sulphacetamide sodium.

A standard for this eye ointment is given in the British Pharmacopoeia 1973

Containers and *Labelling:* see the entry on Eye Ointments for general information on containers and labelling.

Advice for patients: see the entry on Eye Ointments for general information on the use of eye ointments. The prescribed course should be completed.

OTHER PREPARATIONS available include a CREAM (for use in the eye) containing sulphacetamide sodium 10% with hydrocortisone acetate 0.5%; EYE-DROPS containing sulphacetamide sodium 5% with zinc sulphate 0.1%, eye-drops containing sulphacetamide sodium 10% with prednisolone sodium phosphate 0.5%, and eye-drops containing sulphacetamide sodium 15% with methylcellulose 0.5%.

Sulphadiazine

N^1-(Pyrimidin-2-yl)sulphanilamide

$C_{10}H_{10}N_4O_2S = 250.3$

OTHER NAMES: *Debenal*®; Sulfadiazine
Coptin®, Co-trimazine, and *Tribrissen*® (all with trimethoprim)

A standard is given in the European Pharmacopoeia Vol. III

Description. Almost odourless, tasteless, white or yellowish-white or pinkish-white crystals or powder.

Solubility. Practically insoluble in water, in ether, and in chloroform; very slightly soluble in alcohol and in acetone; soluble in dilute mineral acids and in solutions of alkali hydroxides and carbonates.

Dissociation constant. pK$_a$ 6.5 (25°).

Stability; Sterilisation; Storage. See the entry on Sulphonamides.

Identification. TESTS. 1. It complies with the general tests described under Sulphonamides.
2. Gently heat about 1 g until a sublimate is formed; mix a small amount of the sublimate with 1 ml of a 5% solution of resorcinol in alcohol (95%) and add 1 ml of sulphuric acid; a deep red colour is produced. Carefully add 25 ml of ice-cold water followed by an excess of *dilute ammonia solution*; a blue or reddish-blue colour is produced.

MELTING-POINT. About 255°, with decomposition.

ULTRAVIOLET ABSORPTION. In 0.1N hydrochloric acid, maximum at 242 nm (E1%, 1cm = 597); in 0.1N sodium hydroxide, maxima at 240 nm (E1%, 1cm = 866) and 254 nm (E1%, 1cm = 876); in alcohol (95%), maximum at 274 nm (E1%, 1cm = 844).

INFRA-RED ABSORPTION. Major peaks at 683, 1159, 1328, 1444, 1494, and 1580 cm^{-1} (see Appendix 2a: Infra-red Spectra).

THIN-LAYER CHROMATOGRAPHY. See under Thin-layer Chromatography, System 11.

Metabolism (see also under Sulphonamides). ABSORPTION. Rapidly absorbed after oral administration.

BLOOD CONCENTRATION. After an oral dose of 1 g, peak blood concentrations of 20 to 40 μg/ml are attained within 3 to 4 hours; about 10 to 15% of the drug in the plasma is acetylated.

HALF-LIFE. Serum half-life, about 17 hours, which may be prolonged in renal function impairment.

DISTRIBUTION. The concentration of sulphadiazine in the cerebrospinal fluid may reach up to 80% of that in the blood; it is taken up by the red blood cells; accumulates in renal function impairment; *protein binding*, 20 to 60% bound to plasma proteins.

METABOLIC REACTIONS. Polymorphic acetylation and also glucuronic acid conjugation.

EXCRETION. About 80% of a dose is excreted in the urine in 2 to 3 days, about 45% being excreted in the first 24 hours; of the excreted material, about 45% is acetylated, about 50% is free drug, and about 4% is composed of glucuronic acid conjugates; urinary excretion is pH-dependent.

FURTHER INFORMATION. Excretion of metabolites in hepatitis and renal failure—S. T. Madsen, *Chemotherapia*, 1966, **11**, 1; kinetics of excretion in renal failure—E. E. Ohnhaus and P. Spring, *J. Pharmacokinet. Biopharm.*, 1975, **3**, 171; physical properties and protein binding—J. Rieder, *Arzneimittel-Forsch.*, 1963, **13**, 81, 89, and 95; plasma and urinary concentrations—J. Tuomisto and N.-E. Saris, *Annls Med. exp. Biol. Fenn.*, 1970, **48**, 38.

Bioavailability. Studies of the dissolution rates of proprietary formulations of sulphadiazine have shown that the time varies from 70 to 360 minutes for 50% of a tablet to dissolve. There was no correlation between dissolution rate and bioavailability but 2 of the proprietary brands showed decreased bioavailability. Microcrystalline powders appear to be better absorbed than ultrafine powders prepared by milling.

FURTHER INFORMATION. Bioavailability: influence of magnesium stearate—M. Ahmed and R. P. Enever, *J. Pharm. Pharmac.*, 1976, **28**, *Suppl.*, 5P; influence of particle size—per E. Nelson, *Clin. Pharmac. Ther.*, 1962, **3**, 673; studies with tablets—A. Maleque and K. Ahmad, *Bangladesh Pharm. J.*, 1974, **3** (4), 13 and G. R. Van Petten *et al.*, *J. clin. Pharmac.*, 1971, **11**, 27.

Actions and uses. Sulphadiazine has the actions of the sulphonamides as described under Sulphadimidine.
Sulphadiazine is effective in the treatment of infections due to haemolytic streptococci, pneumococci, meningococci, gonococci, *Escherichia coli*, and, to a lesser extent, staphylococci and the organisms of gas-gangrene. It is important to give sulphadiazine during the acute phase of the infection.
For systemic infections, sulphadiazine is usually given by mouth in an initial dose of 3 grams; the subsequent dosage should be 1 gram every 6 hours until the fever subsides or for a maximum of 7 days. This dosage is usually sufficient to produce a satisfactory blood level. For urinary tract infections, the initial dose is usually 2 grams; the subsequent dosage should be 0.5 to 1 gram every 6 to 8 hours. The dosage for children may be based on the scheme outlined under Sulphadimidine.
In severe meningitis, sulphadiazine is administered intravenously as sulphadiazine injection. It is necessary to maintain a blood concentration of 10 to 15 milligrams per 100 millilitres in this infection; for an adult a dosage of 1 to 1.5 grams every 4 hours is required. Sulphadiazine injection should therefore be given by intravenous infusion during the first 2 days of the infection, preferably diluted with sodium chloride injection or dextrose injection to give a concentration not exceeding 5% of sulphadiazine. It should never be given intrathecally. When it is given by intravenous injection, leakage into the subcutaneous tissues should be avoided, as the injection is strongly alkaline. Subsequently sulphadiazine should be given by mouth, the treatment being continued for 2 or 3 days after clinical recovery. Sulphonamide-resistant strains of meningococci are being increasingly recognised.
Sulphadiazine is used in conjunction with pyrimethamine in the treatment of toxoplasmosis, as described under Pyrimethamine.

Undesirable effects. The undesirable effects of the sulphonamides are described under Sulphadimidine. Sulphadiazine rarely causes toxic effects and is generally well tolerated, but anuria and haematuria must be guarded against and sufficient fluid should be given to maintain a large urinary output. The urine should be kept alkaline to prevent crystallisation of the acetyl derivative, which is less soluble than that of sulphadimidine.

Precautions; Contra-indications. As for Sulphadimidine.

Veterinary uses. Sulphadiazine is used in conjunction with trimethoprim as an antibacterial.

Preparations

SULPHADIAZINE AND TRIMETHOPRIM DISPERSIBLE POWDER: consisting of sulphadiazine and trimethoprim in the proportion of 5 parts to 1 part respectively mixed with suitable non-toxic wetting, dispersing, and suspending agents. Available as a dispersible powder containing 100 mg of sulphadiazine and 20 mg of trimethoprim per g.
A standard for this dispersible powder is given in the British Pharmacopoeia (Veterinary)
Labelling: the label on the container should state the amounts of the medicaments as the content of sulphadiazine and of trimethoprim, and the method of using the preparation.
Dose: HORSES, CATTLE, PIGS, and SHEEP: 25 mg of sulphadiazine and 5 mg of trimethoprim per kilogram body-weight daily, in divided doses.

SULPHADIAZINE AND TRIMETHOPRIM INJECTION: a sterile suspension of trimethoprim in a solution of the sodium derivative of sulphadiazine in water for injections free from dissolved air. It is prepared by the addition, by means of an aseptic technique, of sterile trimethoprim to a solution of sulphadiazine sodium previously sterilised by filtration. By means of an aseptic technique, the sterile preparation is distributed into sterile bottles, the air in the bottles being replaced by sterile nitrogen or other suitable gas, and the bottles are sealed.

Available in 50-ml vials containing 400 mg of sulphadiazine and 80 mg of trimethoprim per ml.

A standard for this injection is given in the British Pharmacopoeia (Veterinary)

Containers: see the entry on Injections for general information on containers.

Labelling: see the entry on Injections for general information on labelling. In addition, the label on the container should state the amounts of the medicaments as the amounts of sulphadiazine and trimethoprim in a suitable dose volume.

Storage: it should be protected from light.

Dose: FOR ALL SPECIES: by intramuscular injection, 12.5 mg of sulphadiazine and 2.5 mg of trimethoprim per kilogram body-weight daily, for up to 5 days.

SULPHADIAZINE AND TRIMETHOPRIM MIXTURE: an aqueous suspension of sulphadiazine and trimethoprim with suitable suspending and dispersing agents. It may contain suitable preservatives. Available as a mixture containing 50 mg of sulphadiazine and 10 mg of trimethoprim in 1.1 ml, and as a mixture containing 400 mg of sulphadiazine and 80 mg of trimethoprim per ml.

A standard for this mixture is given in the British Pharmacopoeia (Veterinary)

Containers and *Labelling:* see the entry on Mixtures for general information on containers and labelling.

Dose: PIGLETS: 25mg of sulphadiazine and 5 mg of trimethoprim per kilogram body-weight daily; POULTRY: 12.5 to 25 mg of sulphadiazine and 2.5 to 5 mg of trimethoprim per kilogram body-weight daily.

SULPHADIAZINE AND TRIMETHOPRIM TABLETS: available as tablets containing 100 mg of sulphadiazine and 20 mg of trimethoprim, tablets containing 400 mg of sulphadiazine and 80 mg of trimethoprim, and tablets containing 1 g of sulphadiazine and 200 mg of trimethoprim; they may be sugar coated; they may be coloured; the tablets need not be circular. Also available as tablets containing 410 mg of sulphadiazine and 90 mg of trimethoprim for use in human medicine.

A standard for these tablets is given in the British Pharmacopoeia (Veterinary)

Containers and *Storage:* see the entry on Tablets for general information on containers and storage. Containers should be airtight.

Labelling: the label on the container should state the amounts of the medicaments as the amounts of sulphadiazine and trimethoprim in each tablet.

Dose: FOR ALL SPECIES EXCEPT ADULT RUMINANTS: 25 mg of sulphadiazine and 5 mg of trimethoprim per kilogram body-weight daily in divided doses.

SULPHADIAZINE INJECTION: a sterile solution of the sodium derivative of sulphadiazine, with up to 0.1% of sodium thiosulphate, in water for injections free from dissolved air. It is distributed into ampoules, the air in the ampoules being replaced by nitrogen or other suitable gas, and the ampoules are sealed and sterilised by heating in an autoclave. Alternatively, the solution is sterilised by filtration, distributed, by means of an aseptic technique, into sterile ampoules, the air in the ampoules is replaced by sterile nitrogen or other suitable gas, and the ampoules are sealed.

Available in 4-ml ampoules containing sulphadiazine sodium equivalent to 250 mg of sulphadiazine per ml.

A standard for this injection is given in the British Pharmacopoeia 1973

Containers: see the entry on Injections for general information on containers.

Labelling: see the entry on Injections for general information on labelling. In addition, the label on the container should state the amount of the medicament as the equivalent amount of sulphadiazine in a suitable dose-volume.

Storage: it should be protected from light.

SULPHADIAZINE TABLETS: available as veterinary tablets containing 250 mg of sulphadiazine.

A standard for these tablets is given in the British Pharmacopoeia 1973

Containers and *Storage:* see the entry on Tablets for general information on containers and storage. Containers should be airtight and light resistant.

Advice for patients: the tablets should be taken at regular intervals. The prescribed course should be completed. Adequate fluid intake should be maintained. Direct exposure to sunlight should be avoided during treatment.

Sulphadimethoxine

N^1-(2,6-Dimethoxypyrimidin-4-yl)sulphanilamide

$C_{12}H_{14}N_4O_4S = 310.3$

OTHER NAMES: *Madribon®*; Sulfadimethoxine

A standard is given in the British Pharmacopoeia 1973

Description. An almost odourless, tasteless, white or creamy-white, crystalline powder.

Solubility. Very slightly soluble in water and in alcohol; soluble in dilute mineral acids and in solutions of alkali hydroxides and carbonates.

Dissociation constant. pK_a 5.9 (25°).

Stability; Storage. See the entry on Sulphonamides.

Identification. TESTS. It complies with the general tests described under Sulphonamides.

MELTING-POINT. About 201°.

ULTRAVIOLET ABSORPTION. In 0.1N hydrochloric acid, maximum at 278 nm (E1%, 1cm = 456); in 0.1N sodium hydroxide, maximum at 270 nm (E1%, 1cm = 851); in alcohol (95%), maximum at 274 nm (E1%, 1cm = 701).

INFRA-RED ABSORPTION. Major peaks at 1090, 1147, 1314, 1353, 1445, and 1590 cm^{-1} (see Appendix 2a: Infra-red Spectra).

THIN-LAYER CHROMATOGRAPHY. See under Thin-layer Chromatography, System 11.

Metabolism (see also under Sulphonamides). ABSORPTION. Readily absorbed after oral administration; absorption may be delayed but not reduced in non-fasting subjects.

BLOOD CONCENTRATION. After an oral dose of 2 g, peak plasma concentrations of up to 180 μg/ml for non-acetylated sulphonamide are attained within 4 to 6 hours; in the blood it is mostly in the unchanged form together with small amounts of acetyl and glucuronic acid conjugates.

HALF-LIFE. Serum half-life, 20 to 40 hours.

DISTRIBUTION. Cerebrospinal fluid levels reach about 50% of those in the blood; *protein binding*, about 90% bound to plasma albumin.

METABOLIC REACTIONS. Acetylation and N^1- and N^4-glucuronic acid conjugation.

EXCRETION. About 50% of a dose is excreted in the urine in 2 days and of the excreted material about 20% is acetylated, about 5% is the unchanged drug, and 60 to 80% is the N^1-glucuronide; small amounts of the N^4-glucuronide are also excreted and this may also be formed spontaneously in the urine; both sulphadimethoxine and an N^1-glucuronic acid conjugate are excreted in the bile in man.

FURTHER INFORMATION. Absorption, distribution, and excretion—T. Sakuma *et al.*, *Am. J. med. Sci.*, 1960, **142**, 92; effect of food on absorption—H. Macdonald *et al.*, *Chemotherapia*, 1967, **12**, 282; excretion of metabolites in hepatitis and renal failure—S. T. Madsen, *Chemotherapia*, 1966, **11**, 1; excretion of metabolites in dogs—A. Takaichi *et al.*, *Chem. pharm. Bull.*, Tokyo, 1971, **19**, 930; influence of protein binding on excretion—S. R. Walker, *J. Pharm. Pharmac.*, 1970, **22**, 574; species differences in metabolism—J. W. Bridges *et al.*, *Biochem. J.*, 1968, **109**, 851.

Actions and uses. Sulphadimethoxine is a long-acting compound which has the actions of the sulphonamides, as described under Sulphadimidine. When given by mouth it is rapidly absorbed and blood concentrations are maintained for at least 24 hours. It is highly protein bound, which influences the activity of the compound and affects its rate of excretion.

It is given in an initial dosage of 1 to 2 grams by mouth and subsequently in doses of 500 milligrams daily. The usual initial dose for children is 30 milligrams per kilogram body-weight followed by 15 milligrams per kilogram body-weight daily.

Undesirable effects. Headache and nausea may occur and, more rarely, blood dyscrasias and skin eruptions, the most serious of which is the Stevens-Johnson syndrome, a life-threatening variety of erythema multiforme.

Precautions. Treatment with sulphadimethoxine should be withdrawn if skin reactions occur and regular blood counts should be made during prolonged treatment. Patients with glucose-6-phosphate dehydrogenase deficiency should be observed for signs of haemolytic anaemia. Sulphadimethoxine is secreted in the milk in small amounts and should be used with caution in nursing mothers.

Contra-indications. As for Sulphadimidine.

Preparation

SULPHADIMETHOXINE TABLETS: available as tablets containing 500 mg of sulphadimethoxine.

A standard for these tablets is given in the British Pharmacopoeia 1973
Containers and Storage: see the entry on Tablets for general information on containers and storage. Containers should be airtight and light resistant.
Advice for patients: the tablets should be taken at regular intervals. The prescribed course should be completed. Adequate fluid intake should be maintained. Direct exposure to sunlight should be avoided during treatment.

Sulphadimidine

N^1-(4,6-Dimethylpyrimidin-2-yl)sulphanilamide

$C_{12}H_{14}N_4O_2S = 278.3$

OTHER NAMES: Sulfadimidine; Sulfadimidinum; Sulfamethazine; *Sulphamezathine®*; *Vesadin®*
Fortigro-S® (with carbadox); *Tylasul®* (with tylosin phosphate)

A standard is given in the European Pharmacopoeia Vol. I

Description. Odourless, white or creamy-white crystals or powder with a bitter taste.

Solubility. Very slightly soluble in water; soluble, at 20°, in 120 parts of alcohol; soluble in dilute mineral acids and in solutions of alkali hydroxides and carbonates.

Dissociation constant. pK_a 7.4 (25°).

Stability; Sterilisation; Storage. See the entry on Sulphonamides.

Identification. TESTS. 1. It complies with the general tests described under Sulphonamides.
2. Dissolve about 20 mg in a mixture of 10 ml of water and 2 ml of 0.1N sodium hydroxide and add 1 ml of *copper sulphate solution*; a pale green turbidity is produced which gradually changes to a brownish-grey suspension and finally settles as a reddish-brown precipitate.
3. Heat about 500 mg in a boiling-tube at 250°; the substance is decomposed into a brown residue and a white sublimate, with the evolution of fumes which turn moistened blue litmus paper red and lead acetate paper black. The sublimate melts at about 153°.

MELTING-POINT. About 198°.

ULTRAVIOLET ABSORPTION. In 0.1N hydrochloric acid, maxima at 244 nm (E1%, 1cm = 543), and 301 nm (E1%, 1cm = 248); in 0.1N sodium hydroxide, maximum at 258 nm (E1%, 1cm = 794); in alcohol (95%), maximum at 270 nm (E1%, 1cm = 791).

INFRA-RED ABSORPTION. Major peaks at 679, 863, 1147, 1303, 1595, and 1639 cm^{-1} (see Appendix 2a: Infra-red Spectra).

Metabolism (see also under Sulphonamides).

ABSORPTION. Rapidly absorbed after oral administration.

BLOOD CONCENTRATION. After an oral dose of 4 g, peak serum concentrations of about 110 μg/ml for non-acetylated sulphonamide are attained within 3 to 6 hours; large amounts of acetylated sulphadimidine are detectable in the blood.

HALF-LIFE. From urinary excretion data, 2 to 5 hours for rapid acetylators and 8 to 11 hours for slow acetylators.

DISTRIBUTION. Enters the cerebrospinal fluid to a lesser extent than sulphadiazine; accumulates in renal function impairment; *protein binding*, 60 to 80% bound to plasma proteins.

METABOLIC REACTIONS. Polymorphic acetylation.

EXCRETION. Slowly excreted in the urine and about 50% of a dose is excreted in 2 days; of the excreted material 40 to 70% is acetylated in slow acetylators and 80 to 95% is acetylated in rapid acetylators; urinary excretion of sulphadimidine appears to be pH-dependent.

FURTHER INFORMATION. Acetylator status: from sulphadimidine and isoniazid tests—G. A. Ellard and P. T. Gammon, *Br. J. clin. Pharmac.*, 1977, **4**, 5 and M. J. Mattila *et al.*, *Annls Med. exp. Biol. Fenn.*, 1969, **47**, 308; from sulphadimidine and procainamide tests—K. Frislid, *Eur. J. clin. Pharmac.*, 1976, **9**, 433; from sulphadimidine and sulphamethoxypyridazine tests—T. A. White and D. A. P. Evans, *Clin. Pharmac. Ther.*, 1968, **9**, 80; acetylator status and pharmacokinetics of sulphonamides—M. C. B. Van Oudtshoorn and F. J. Potgieter, *J. Pharm. Pharmac.*, 1972, **24**, 357; excretion in uraemic patients—W. R. Adam *et al.*, *Med. J. Aust.*, i/1973, 936, E. Fischer, *Lancet*, ii/1972, 210, and D. M. Williams *et al.*, *Lancet*, ii/1968, 1058.

Bioavailability. Differences in binding agents, compression, and formulation of sulphadimidine tablets results in variations in dissolution rate and also in absorption. Studies with tablets having dissolution rates of 1.5, 15 to 20, and 40 to 50 minutes showed distinct variations in bioavailability. Following the oral administration of 3 g of each formulation, the total urinary excretions, in 24 hours, are 89, 80, and 73% of the dose for the fast, intermediate, and slow dissolving tablets respectively. A similar variation is shown in the peak plasma concentrations.

Actions and uses. The actions of the sulphonamides, of which sulphadimidine may be taken as a typical example, are bacteriostatic rather than bactericidal and are considered to be due to the similarity of their chemical structure to that of *p*-aminobenzoic acid, a substance that is essential for the synthesis of folic acid by the bacterial cell which unlike mammalian cells is unable to absorb pre-formed folate. Sulphonamide competitively inhibits the responsible enzyme which then becomes incapable of its normal function.

Sulphonamides act on many species of bacteria, including streptococci and many Gram-negative rods such as *Escherichia coli* and *Proteus* spp. Resistance to sulphonamides has appeared rapidly in many strains and the main use of sulphonamides is now against organisms causing urinary tract infections.

The relative potencies of the sulphonamides used systemically appear to depend mainly on differences in solubility, absorption, and excretion rather than on any specificity. Infections due to the less susceptible organisms, such as pneumococci, respond best to those sulphonamides with which it is possible to maintain a high blood concentration.

When sulphonamides are used for the treatment of systemic infections, it is important to obtain rapidly an optimal concentration of the drug in the blood and to maintain this in order to prevent the development of resistant strains of the infecting organisms.

Sulphadimidine is rapidly absorbed from the gastrointestinal tract, so that with regular dosage by mouth the blood concentration can be readily maintained at 5 to 10 milligrams per 100 millilitres.

Sulphadimidine crosses the blood–brain barrier less easily than sulphadiazine; thus, while sulphadimidine is often the sulphonamide of choice in pneumococcal or streptococcal infections and in *Escherichia coli* infections of the urinary tract, sulphadiazine is usually preferred in meningeal infections.

Sulphonamides are concentrated in the urine. In the treatment of non-gonococcal genito-urinary infections, especially those due to *Esch. coli*, they are effective in relatively small doses.

For systemic infections, sulphadimidine should be given by mouth in an initial dose of up to 3 grams; the subsequent dosage should be 1 gram every 4 hours or 1.5 grams every 6 hours. For urinary tract infections, the initial dose is 2 grams; subsequent dosage should be up to 4 grams daily in divided doses.

Infants and children usually tolerate sulphonamides better than adults; for a child of average weight the recommended dosage is one-sixth the adult dose from 6 months to 1 year of age, one-third the adult dose from 1 to 5 years of age, one-half the adult dose from 6 to 12 years of age, and two-thirds the adult dose from 13 to 15 years of age.

Undesirable effects. A variety of toxic symptoms may follow the administration of sulphonamides. Nausea and vomiting are relatively common, but may be avoided by giving the drug in divided doses. Cyanosis, which may be due to methaemoglobinaemia, to sulphaemoglobinaemia, or to the action of an oxidation product, is occasionally seen; usually, however, it is not sufficiently severe to necessitate the suspension of treatment.

Skin rashes occur occasionally, and in such cases it is advisable to stop treatment and give abundant fluids; in general, patients undergoing sulphonamide therapy should avoid exposure to direct sunlight.

Sulphonamides applied to the skin are liable to give rise to sensitisation.

There is a danger of haematuria, due to the insolubility of the acetyl derivatives; it may occur whenever the fluid intake is restricted or the urine is acid. Granulocytopenia is rare, especially if the duration of a course of treatment does not exceed a week or 10 days and if an interval of several weeks is allowed between courses.

Sulphadimidine itself is well tolerated and serious toxic effects are infrequent. Nausea and vomiting seldom occur and the nausea is so slight as not to interfere with the continuation of treatment. Owing to the relatively high solubility of its acetyl derivative, even in acid urine, sulphadimidine is less likely to cause anuria and haematuria than sulphathiazole.

Precautions. During prolonged treatment regular examinations of the blood should be made. Patients with glucose-6-phosphate dehydrogenase deficiency should be observed for the symptoms of haemolytic anaemia. Sulphonamides are secreted in the milk in small amounts and should be used with caution in nursing mothers.

Contra-indications. Sulphonamides are contra-indicated in the presence of renal or hepatic disease and in hypersensitive patients.

Owing to the damger of kernicterus, sulphonamides are contra-indicated in premature and newborn babies and in pregnant women during the week before expected delivery.

Veterinary uses. Sulphadimidine is an antibacterial. The usual initial dose by mouth for all species is 200 milligrams per kilogram body-weight, and the maintenance dose is 100 milligrams per kilogram body-weight daily. It should not be administered by mouth to adult ruminants.

Preparations

PAEDIATRIC SULPHADIMIDINE MIXTURE:

Sulphadimidine, in fine powder	..	..		100 g
Compound tragacanth powder ..	..	..		40 g
Amaranth solution	..	..	..	10 ml
Benzoic acid solution	..	..	..	20 ml
Raspberry syrup ..	..	..	..	200 ml
Chloroform water, double-strength	..	..	500 ml
Water for preparations ..	..	..	to 1000 ml

Triturate the compound tragacanth powder and the sulphadimidine with the raspberry syrup to form a smooth paste; add gradually, with constant stirring, the benzoic acid solution and the amaranth solution diluted with the double-strength chloroform water, and sufficient water to produce the required volume. It must be recently prepared.

Alternatively, the compound tragacanth powder may be replaced by using 10 g of sodium carboxymethylcellulose 50 and 20 g of maize starch, and the double-strength chloroform water by 50 ml of chloroform spirit for each 1000 ml of mixture. The mixture is prepared as follows: Stir a suspension of the starch in 125 ml of water into about 350 ml of boiling water. Maintain the temperature until the mixture becomes translucent, and cool rapidly. Triturate the sodium carboxymethylcellulose 50 and the sulphadimidine with the raspberry syrup to form a smooth paste; add gradually, with constant stirring, the starch mucilage, the benzoic acid solution, the amaranth solution, the chloroform spirit, and sufficient water to produce the required volume.

It must be recently prepared.

When a dose less than or not a multiple of 5 ml is prescribed, the mixture may be diluted, as described in the entry on Mixtures, with chloroform water.

A standard for this mixture is given in the British Pharmaceutical Codex 1973

Containers and *Labelling:* see the entry on Mixtures for general information on containers and labelling. A direction to shake the bottle should be given on the label.

Advice for patients: the mixture should be taken at regular intervals. The prescribed course should be completed. Adequate fluid intake should be maintained. Direct exposure to sunlight should be avoided during treatment.

SULPHADIMIDINE TABLETS: available as tablets containing 500 mg of sulphadimidine, and as veterinary tablets containing 5 g of sulphadimidine.

A standard for these tablets is given in the British Pharmacopoeia 1973

Containers and *Storage:* see the entry on Tablets for general information on containers and storage. Containers should be airtight and light resistant.

Advice for patients: see above under Paediatric Sulphadimidine Mixture.

OTHER PREPARATIONS available include a PREMIX containing sulphadimidine 20 mg with tylosin phosphate equivalent to 20 mg of tylosin per g, and a premix containing sulphadimidine 100 mg with carbadox 50 mg per g.

Sulphadimidine Sodium

The sodium derivative of N^1-(4,6-dimethylpyrimidin-2-yl)sulphanilamide.

$C_{12}H_{13}N_4NaO_2S = 300.3$

OTHER NAMES: Sulfadimidine Sodium; *Sulphamezathine®; Vesadin®*

A standard is given in the British Pharmacopoeia 1973

Description. Odourless, hygroscopic, white or creamy-white crystals or powder with a bitter alkaline taste.

Solubility. Soluble, at 20°, in 2.5 parts of water and in 60 parts of alcohol.

Alkalinity. A 10% solution has a pH of 10 to 11.

Moisture content. Not more than 2%, determined by drying at 105°.

Stability; Sterilisation; Storage. See the entry on Sulphonamides.

Identification. TESTS. Acidify an aqueous solution with acetic acid; a white precipitate is produced which, after washing with water and drying at 105°, melts at about 198° and complies with the general tests described under Sulphonamides.

ULTRAVIOLET ABSORPTION. See under Sulphadimidine.

INFRA-RED ABSORPTION. An infra-red spectrum for Sulphadimidine is given in Appendix 2a (see under Sulphadimidine).

THIN-LAYER CHROMATOGRAPHY. See under Thin-layer Chromatography, System 11.

Metabolism. See under Sulphadimidine.

Actions and uses. Sulphadimidine sodium has the actions, uses, and undesirable effects described under Sulphadimidine, but it is administered by injection to patients in whom a satisfactory concentration of sulphadimidine cannot be obtained by oral administration.

The usual dose for an adult is 1 to 2 grams by intravenous or intramuscular injection. The dosage for children may be based on the scheme outlined under Sulphadimidine. It should not be given intrathecally.

Precautions; Contra-indications. As for Sulphadimidine.

Veterinary uses. Sulphadimidine Sodium is an antibacterial. The usual initial dose by intravenous injection for all species is 200 milligrams per kilogram body-weight, and the maintenance dose is 100 milligrams per kilogram body-weight daily. Similar doses may be given by intraperitoneal injection to cattle and sheep.

For the treatment of coccidiosis in poultry 2000 parts per million may be given in the drinking water for 5 days.

Preparation

SULPHADIMIDINE INJECTION: a sterile solution of sulphadimidine sodium prepared by the interaction of sulphadimidine and sodium hydroxide, with the equivalent of up to 0.1% of SO_2, in water for injections free from dissolved air. It is distributed into the final containers, the air in the containers being replaced by nitrogen or other suitable gas, and the containers are sealed and sterilised by heating in an autoclave. Alternatively, the solution is sterilised by filtration, distributed, by means of an aseptic technique, into sterile final containers, the air in the containers being replaced by sterile nitrogen or other suitable gas, and the containers are sealed.

Available in 3-ml ampoules, in 100- and 500-ml vials, and in 2-litre vials, containing 330 mg of sulphadimidine sodium per ml.

A standard for this injection is given in the British Pharmacopoeia 1973
Containers and Labelling: see the entry on Injections for general information on containers and labelling.
Storage: it should be protected from light.

Sulphadoxine

N^1-(5,6-Dimethoxypyrimidin-4-yl)sulphanilamide

$C_{12}H_{14}N_4O_4S = 310.3$

OTHER NAMES: Fanasil® (available only in certain overseas countries); Sulfadoxine
Borgal® and Trivetrin® (both with trimethoprim)

A standard is given in the British Pharmacopoeia Addendum 1977

Description. An odourless white or creamy-white crystalline powder.

Solubility. Very slightly soluble in water, in alcohol, and in methyl alcohol; practically insoluble in ether.

Sterilisation; Storage. See the entry on Sulphonamides.

Identification. TEST. It complies with general test 1 described under Sulphonamides.

MELTING-POINT. About 198°.

ULTRAVIOLET ABSORPTION. In 0.1N methanolic hydrochloric acid, maximum at 267 nm (E1%, 1cm = 550).

Metabolism (see also under Sulphonamides). ABSORPTION. Rapidly absorbed after oral or intramuscular administration.

BLOOD CONCENTRATION. After an oral dose of 1 g, plasma concentrations of about 110 μg/ml are found after one day, declining to about 40 μg/ml after 14 days.

HALF-LIFE. Serum half-life, about 180 hours, but may be up to 340 hours in newborn infants.

DISTRIBUTION. Enters the cerebrospinal, ascitic, and synovial fluids; crosses the placenta and is secreted in milk; protein binding, 78 to 97% bound to plasma proteins at concentrations of 20 to 250 μg/ml; in sheep, bound sulphadoxine is displaced by phenylbutazone.

METABOLIC REACTIONS. Acetylation and glucuronic acid or sulphate conjugation.

EXCRETION. About 30% of a dose is excreted in the urine in 4 to 7 days; of the urinary excreted material, about 30 to 60% is acetylated and 30 to 60% is non-acetylated of which up to 40% may be conjugated with glucuronic acid and up to 10% may be conjugated with sulphate.

FURTHER INFORMATION. Comparative studies in man and animals—E. Böhni et al., Chemotherapy, Basle, 1969, **14**, 195; blood concentrations, excretion, and response in falciparum malaria—M. H. Brooks et al., Clin. Pharmac. Ther., 1969, **10**, 85; influence of protein binding on excretion—S. R. Walker, J. Pharm. Pharmac., 1970, **22**, 574; displacement of protein-bound sulphadoxine by phenylbutazone—W. M. Wardell, Br. J. Pharmac., 1971, **43**, 325; metabolism and excretion—J. W. Bridges et al., Biochem. J., 1969, **111**, 167; metabolism and effects in infants—M. Vest, Schweiz. med. Wschr., 1966, **96**, 920.

Actions and uses. Sulphadoxine has the actions, uses, and undesirable effects of the long-acting sulphonamides, as described under Sulphadimethoxine. An initial dose of 2 grams followed by maintenance doses of 1 to 1.5 grams at intervals of one week is usually sufficient to maintain therapeutic blood concentrations. Children aged 2 to 5 years may be given one-quarter and children aged 5 to 8 one-half of the adult dosage.

Sulphadoxine is used for the treatment of meningococcal meningitis. For this purpose it is administered by deep intramuscular or slow intravenous injection of a solution of a soluble derivative in an initial dose of 2.5 grams followed if necessary by a second dose of 1.5 grams after an interval of 4 days; children may be given 60 milligrams per kilogram body-weight followed if necessary by 40 milligrams per kilogram body-weight after 4 days.

Sulphadoxine has been used in a single dose of 2 grams for the treatment of urinary-tract infections. In the long-term treatment of urinary-tract infections the usual dose is 2 grams weekly.

Sulphadoxine has also been given in conjunction with pyrimethamine in the treatment of malaria due to Plasmodium falciparum which is resistant to other therapy. A dose of 1 gram of sulphadoxine is followed by 500 milligrams on the following day and a single dose of 50 milligrams of pyrimethamine is also given.

Precautions. As for Sulphadimethoxine.

Contra-indications. As for Sulphadimidine.

Veterinary uses. Sulphadoxine is used in conjunction with trimethoprim as an antibacterial.

Preparations

SULPHADOXINE AND TRIMETHOPRIM INJECTION: a sterile solution of sulphadoxine and trimethoprim in the proportion of 5 parts to 1 part respectively in a suitable aqueous vehicle. The alkalinity of the solution is adjusted to approximately pH 10 by the addition of sodium hydroxide. It may contain 0.1% of lignocaine hydrochloride. It is distributed into the final containers, the air in the containers being replaced by nitrogen or other suitable gas, and the containers are sealed and sterilised by heating in an autoclave. Alternatively, the solution is sterilised by filtration, distributed, by means of an aseptic technique, into sterile final containers, the air in the containers being replaced by sterile nitrogen or other suitable gas, and the containers are sealed.

Available in 50-ml vials containing 62.5 mg of sulphadoxine, 12.5 mg of trimethoprim, and 1 mg of lignocaine hydrochloride per ml; and in 30- and 100-ml vials containing 200 mg of sulphadoxine and 40 mg of trimethoprim per ml.

A standard for this injection is given in the British Pharmacopoeia (Veterinary)
Containers: see the entry on Injections for general information on containers.
Labelling: see the entry on Injections for general information on labelling. In addition, the label on the container should state the amounts of the medicaments as the amounts of sulphadoxine and trimethoprim in a suitable dose-volume and, if present, the amount of lignocaine hydrochloride.

Storage: it should be stored at a temperature not exceeding 25°, protected from light.

Dose: ALL SPECIES: by intramuscular or intravenous injection, 12.5 mg of sulphadoxine and 2.5 mg of trimethoprim per kilogram body-weight.

SULPHADOXINE AND TRIMETHOPRIM TABLETS: available as tablets containing 250 mg of sulphadoxine and 50 mg of trimethoprim.

A standard for these tablets is given in the British Pharmacopoeia (Veterinary)

Containers and *Storage:* see the entry on Tablets for general information on containers and storage. Containers should be airtight and light resistant.

Labelling: the label on the container should state the amounts of the medicaments as the amounts of sulphadoxine and trimethoprim in each tablet.

Dose: FOALS, CALVES, PIGLETS, LAMBS, AND DOGS: 15 mg of sulphadoxine and 3 mg of trimethoprim per kilogram body-weight.

SULPHADOXINE TABLETS: available as tablets containing 500 mg of sulphadoxine (only in certain overseas countries).

Containers and *Storage:* see the entry on Tablets for general information on containers and storage. Containers should be airtight and light resistant.

Advice for patients: the tablets should be taken at regular intervals. Treatment should not be discontinued without the advice of the prescriber. Adequate fluid intake should be maintained. Direct exposure to sunlight should be avoided during treatment.

OTHER PREPARATIONS available include an INJECTION containing sulphadoxine 250 mg per ml in 10-ml ampoules.

Sulphafurazole

N^1-(3,4-Dimethylisoxazol-5-yl)sulphanilamide

$C_{11}H_{13}N_3O_3S = 267.3$

OTHER NAMES: *Gantrisin®*; Sulfafurazole; Sulfisoxazole

A standard is given in the British Pharmacopoeia 1973

Description. An odourless, white or yellowish-white, crystalline powder with a slight taste and a bitter after-taste.

Solubility. Very slightly soluble in water; soluble, at 20°, in 50 parts of alcohol, in 800 parts of ether, in 1000 parts of chloroform, and in 30 parts of a 5% solution of sodium bicarbonate.

Dissociation constant. pK_a 4.9 (25°).

Storage. See the entry on Sulphonamides.

Identification. TESTS. It complies with the general tests described under Sulphonamides.

MELTING-POINT. About 196°.

ULTRAVIOLET ABSORPTION. In 0.01N hydrochloric acid, maximum at 268 nm (E1%, 1cm = 480); in 0.1N sodium hydroxide, maximum at 254 nm (E1%, 1cm = 773); in alcohol (95%), maximum at 272 nm (E1%, 1cm = 713).

INFRA-RED ABSORPTION. Major peaks at 1092, 1166, 1349, 1436, 1598, and 1633 cm^{-1} (see Appendix 2a: Infra-red Spectra).

Metabolism (see also under Sulphonamides). ABSORPTION. Readily absorbed after oral administration; absorption is delayed by the presence of food.

BLOOD CONCENTRATION. After 2-g doses orally or intramuscularly, peak plasma concentrations of non-acetylated drugs of 120 to 180 μg/ml are attained within 1 to 4 hours; after an oral dose of 500 mg, a peak plasma concentration of about 40 μg/ml is attained in 2 to 3 hours.

HALF-LIFE. Serum half-life, about 6 hours, which is reduced to 4 hours when the urine is alkaline.

DISTRIBUTION. Distributed throughout the extracellular water; cerebrospinal fluid levels reach one third of those in the blood; *protein binding*, 85% bound to plasma proteins.

METABOLIC REACTIONS. Acetylation.

EXCRETION. Almost the entire dose is excreted in the urine in 2 days, 50 to 60% as non-acetylated sulphafurazole and about 30% as the acetylated metabolite; the urinary excretion is influenced by urinary pH and the drug is excreted more quickly when the urine is alkaline; probenecid appears to delay excretion.

FURTHER INFORMATION. Absorption and effect of food —H. Macdonald *et al., Chemotherapia*, 1967, **12**, 282; acetylation pattern in rapid and slow isoniazid acetylators—M. J. Mattila *et al., Annls Med. exp. Biol. Fenn.*, 1969, **47**, 308; effective plasma and urinary concentrations—J. Tuomisto and N.-E. Saris, *Annls Med. exp. Biol. Fenn.*, 1970, **48**, 38; saturable first-pass metabolism in rats—D. C. Bloedow and W. L. Hayton, *J. pharm. Sci.*, 1976, **65**, 334; pharmacokinetics—S. A. Kaplan *et al., J. pharm. Sci.*, 1972, **61**, 773 and E. Nelson and I. O'Reilly, *J. Pharmac. exp. Ther.*, 1960, **129**, 368; protein binding in tears—S. S. Chrai and J. R. Robinson, *J. pharm. Sci.*, 1976, **65**, 437; renal excretion—M. Cohen and R. Pocelinko, *J. Pharmac. exp. Ther.*, 1973, **185**, 703 and A. P. Goossens and M. C. B. van Oudtshoorn, *J. Pharm. Pharmac.*, 1970, **22**, 224.

Bioavailability. Two studies of bioequivalence of a number of different brands of sulphafurazole tablets showed all tablets to be bioequivalent.

FURTHER INFORMATION. Bioavailability of 11 products —G. W. A. Slywka *et al., J. pharm. Sci.*, 1976, **65**, 1494; bioavailability of 8 products—G. R. Van Petten *et al., J. clin. Pharmac.*, 1971, **11**, 35.

Actions and uses. Sulphafurazole has the actions and uses of the sulphonamides, as described under Sulphadimidine. In the treatment of systemic infections, an initial oral dose of 3 grams may be given followed by doses of up to 6 grams daily in divided doses.

Because of its relatively high solubility in urine (about 300 milligrams in 100 millilitres of urine at pH 6) it is especially useful in urinary tract infections and may be given as an initial oral dose of 2 grams followed by subsequent doses of up to 4 grams daily in divided doses. The dosage for children may be based on the scheme outlined under Sulphadimidine.

Undesirable effects. The undesirable effects of the sulphonamides are described under Sulphadimidine. Sulphafurazole is relatively free from toxic effects.

Precautions; Contra-indications. As for Sulphadimidine.

Preparation

SULPHAFURAZOLE TABLETS: available as tablets containing 500 mg of sulphafurazole.
A standard for these tablets is given in the British Pharmacopoeia 1973
Containers and *Storage:* see the entry on Tablets for general information on containers and storage. Containers should be airtight and light resistant.
Advice for patients: the tablets should be taken at regular intervals. The prescribed course should be completed. Adequate fluid intake should be maintained. Direct exposure to sunlight should be avoided during treatment.

Sulphaguanidine

2-(4-Aminobenzenesulphonyl)guanidine monohydrate

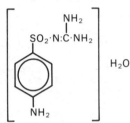

$C_7H_{10}N_4O_2S,H_2O = 232.3$

OTHER NAME: Sulfaguanidine

A standard is given in the British Pharmaceutical Codex 1973

Description. Odourless white crystals or powder, darkening slowly on exposure to light.

Solubility. Soluble, at 20°, in 1000 parts of water and in 250 parts of alcohol; soluble in 10 parts of boiling water; soluble in dilute mineral acids; very slightly soluble in acetone; practically insoluble in solutions of alkali hydroxides.

Moisture content. 6 to 8%, determined by drying at 105°.

Storage. See the entry on Sulphonamides.

Identification. TESTS. It complies with the general tests described under Sulphonamides.

MELTING-POINT. About 191°.

ULTRAVIOLET ABSORPTION. In alcohol (95%), maximum at 265 nm (E1%, 1cm = 899).

INFRA-RED ABSORPTION. Major peaks at 1084, 1130, 1236, 1500, 1529, and 1616 cm^{-1} (see Appendix 2a: Infra-red Spectra).

THIN-LAYER CHROMATOGRAPHY. See under Thin-layer Chromatography, System 11.

Metabolism (see also under Sulphonamides). ABSORPTION. Incompletely absorbed after oral administration; in rats, the absorption of sulphaguanidine is enhanced by bile salts.

BLOOD CONCENTRATION. After an oral dose of 7 g, peak blood concentrations of up to 40 µg/ml are attained within 2 to 4 hours; in the blood about 40% of the drug is acetylated.

DISTRIBUTION. *Protein binding,* about 8% bound to plasma proteins.

METABOLIC REACTIONS. Acetylation.

EXCRETION. Rapidly excreted in the urine; about 30% of the excreted material is the acetylated metabolite; large amounts are recovered in the faeces.

FURTHER INFORMATION. Effect of bile salts on absorption—K. Kakemi *et al., Chem. pharm. Bull., Tokyo,* 1970, **18**, 275 and 1034.

Actions and uses. Sulphaguanidine has the actions of the sulphonamides, as described under Sulphadimidine. It is not readily absorbed from the gastro-intestinal tract and is therefore used in the treatment of local intestinal infections, such as bacillary dysentery, although phthalylsulphathiazole and succinylsulphathiazole are now considered to be more effective, as the amounts of these drugs absorbed into the blood stream are much smaller.
In the treatment of dysentery doses of 3 grams are given 3 times a day for 3 days.
Sulphaguanidine may be of value in refractory cases of amoebic dysentery by controlling secondary bacterial infections, although some antibiotics are more effective in this respect.
In ulcerative colitis, sulphaguanidine may be absorbed into the blood stream in dangerous amounts; in this condition, therefore, the use of phthalylsulphathiazole is to be preferred.

Undesirable effects. As for Phthalylsulphathiazole. Toxic effects in conditions other than ulcerative colitis are slight, although rashes and haematuria have been reported.

Contra-indications. As for Sulphadimidine.

Preparation

SULPHAGUANIDINE TABLETS: may be prepared by moist granulation and compression as described in the entry on Tablets. Available as tablets containing 500 mg of sulphaguanidine.
A standard for these tablets is given in the British Pharmaceutical Codex 1973
Containers and *Storage:* see the entry on Tablets for general information on containers and storage. Containers should be airtight and light resistant.
Advice for patients: the tablets should be taken at regular intervals. The prescribed course should be completed. Preparations containing liquid paraffin should be avoided. Adequate fluid intake should be maintained. Direct exposure to sunlight should be avoided during treatment.

Sulphamerazine

N^1-(4-Methylpyrimidin-2-yl)sulphanilamide

$C_{11}H_{12}N_4O_2S = 264.3$

OTHER NAME: Sulfamerazine

A standard is given in the British Pharmacopoeia (Veterinary)

Description. An odourless, white or creamy-white, crystalline powder.

Solubility. Very slightly soluble in water and in chloroform; soluble, at 20°, in 550 parts of alcohol; soluble in dilute mineral acids and in aqueous solutions of alkali hydroxides and carbonates.

Dissociation constant. pK_a 7.1 (25°).

Storage. See the entry on Sulphonamides.

Identification. TEST. It complies with the general tests described under Sulphonamides.

MELTING-POINT. About 236°.

INFRA-RED ABSORPTION. Major peaks at 1149, 1316, 1389, 1493, 1562, and 1587 cm^{-1} (see Appendix 2b: Infra-red Spectra).

Determination in body fluids. HIGH PRESSURE LIQUID CHROMATOGRAPHY. In urine: sulphamerazine and its N^4-acetylated metabolite—J. P. Sharma *et al.*, *J. pharm. Sci.*, 1976, **65**, 1606.

Veterinary uses. Sulphamerazine is used as an antibacterial. The usual dose for dogs and cats is up to 100 milligrams per kilogram body-weight.

Sulphamethizole

N^1-(5-Methyl-1,3,4-thiadiazol-2-yl)sulphanilamide

$C_9H_{10}N_4O_2S_2 = 270.3$

OTHER NAMES: *Methisul®*; Sulfamethizole; *Urolucosil®*

A standard is given in the British Pharmacopoeia 1973

Description. Odourless colourless crystals or white or creamy-white powder with a slightly bitter taste.

Solubility. Very slightly soluble in water, in ether, and in chloroform; soluble, at 20°, in 25 parts of alcohol, and in 15 parts of acetone; soluble in 60 parts of boiling water, in solutions of alkali hydroxides, and in dilute mineral acids.

Dissociation constant. pK_a 5.3 (25°).

Storage. See the entry on Sulphonamides.

Identification. TESTS. It complies with the general tests described under Sulphonamides.

MELTING-POINT. About 209°.

ULTRAVIOLET ABSORPTION. In 0.1N hydrochloric acid, maximum at 268 nm (E1%, 1cm = 534); in 0.1N sodium hydroxide, maximum at 260 nm (E1%, 1cm = 696); in alcohol (95%), maximum at 284 nm (E1%, 1cm = 702).

INFRA-RED ABSORPTION. Major peaks at 699, 1084, 1134, 1152, 1549, and 1600 cm^{-1} (see Appendix 2a: Infra-red Spectra).

THIN-LAYER CHROMATOGRAPHY. See under Thin-layer Chromatography, System 11.

Metabolism (see also under Sulphonamides). ABSORPTION. Well absorbed after oral administration.

BLOOD CONCENTRATION. After an oral dose of 500 mg, peak concentrations in whole blood of about 20 μg/ml are attained for non-acetylated sulphonamide in about 2 hours.

HALF-LIFE. Serum half-life, about 2 hours.

DISTRIBUTION. Accumulates in renal function impairment; *protein binding*, about 90% bound to plasma proteins.

METABOLIC REACTIONS. Acetylation.

EXCRETION. In 5 hours 60% of a dose is excreted in the urine, 5 to 23% as the acetylated metabolite and in 15 hours excretion is complete; both unchanged drug and its acetylated metabolite are sufficiently soluble in urine to avoid crystalluria.

FURTHER INFORMATION. Blood concentrations—G. L. Mattok and I. J. McGilveray, *J. pharm. Sci.*, 1972, **61**, 746; metabolism and excretion—A. Takaichi *et al.*, *Chem. pharm. Bull.*, *Tokyo*, 1971, **19**, 937; pharmacokinetics in the elderly—E. J. Triggs *et al.*, *Eur. J. clin. Pharmac.*, 1975, **8**, 55; pharmacokinetics of renal excretion—R. Hori *et al.*, *J. pharm. Sci.*, 1976, **65**, 463.

Bioavailability. The bioavailabilities of tablet formulations from 3 manufacturers were not found to be significantly different.

FURTHER INFORMATION. Bioavailability—G. L. Mattok and I. J. McGilveray, *J. pharm. Sci.*, 1972, **61**, 746.

Actions and uses. Sulphamethizole has the actions, uses, undesirable effects, and contra-indications of the sulphonamides, as described under Sulphadimidine.
When given by mouth it is rapidly absorbed from the gastro-intestinal tract and rapidly excreted. It is used chiefly for the treatment of coliform infections of the urinary tract in a dosage of 100 to 200 milligrams by mouth 5 times a day for 5 to 7 days.
The usual dose for children is 50 to 100 milligrams 5 times daily.
The risk of crystalluria is low, and in temperate climates the fluid intake may be reduced to maintain the urinary concentration of the drug.

Precautions. As for Sulphadimidine.

Preparations

SULPHAMETHIZOLE TABLETS: available as tablets containing 100 mg of sulphamethizole.
A standard for these tablets is given in the British Pharmacopoeia 1973
Containers and Storage: see the entry on Tablets for general information on containers and storage. Containers should be airtight and light resistant.
Advice for patients: the tablets should be taken at regular intervals. The prescribed course should be completed. Direct exposure to sunlight should be avoided during treatment.

OTHER PREPARATIONS available include a MIXTURE containing sulphamethizole 100 mg in 5 ml, diluent syrup, life of diluted mixture 28 days.

Sulphamethoxazole

N^1-(5-Methylisoxazol-3-yl)sulphanilamide

$C_{10}H_{11}N_3O_3S = 253.3$

OTHER NAMES: *Gantanol®*; Sulfamethoxazole *Bactrim®*, Co-trimoxazole, and *Septrin®* (all with trimethoprim)

A standard is given in the British Pharmacopoeia 1973

Description. An odourless, white or yellowish-white, crystalline powder with a slight taste and a bitter after-taste.

Solubility. Very slightly soluble in water; soluble, at 20°, in 50 parts of alcohol and in 3 parts of acetone; soluble in solutions of alkali hydroxides.

Acidity. A 10% suspension has a pH of 4 to 6.

Dissociation constant. pK_a 5.6 (25°).

Storage. See the entry on Sulphonamides.

Identification. TESTS. 1. It complies with the general tests described under Sulphonamides.
2. Dissolve about 5 mg in 0.5 ml of 2N sodium hydroxide, add 5 ml of water and 100 mg of phenol, boil, cool, and add 1 ml of *dilute sodium hypochlorite solution*; a golden-yellow colour is produced immediately and persists.

MELTING-POINT. About 170°.

ULTRAVIOLET ABSORPTION. In 0.1N sodium hydroxide, maximum at 257 nm (E1%, 1cm = 684); in alcohol (95%), maximum at 270 nm (E1%, 1cm = 754).

INFRA-RED ABSORPTION. Major peaks at 685, 1145, 1160, 1368, 1599, and 1621 cm^{-1} (see Appendix 2a: Infra-red Spectra).

THIN-LAYER CHROMATOGRAPHY. See under Thin-layer Chromatography, System 11.

Metabolism (see also under Sulphonamides). ABSORPTION. Rapidly absorbed after oral administration.

BLOOD CONCENTRATION. After an oral dose of 800 mg, peak serum concentrations of 20 to 40 μg/ml for non-acetylated sulphonamide and about 80 μg/ml for total drug and metabolites appear after 2 to 4 hours and are maintained for a further 7 hours.

HALF-LIFE. Serum half-life, about 11 hours.

DISTRIBUTION. Widely distributed throughout the tissues; cerebrospinal fluid concentrations are lower than those in blood but are still therapeutically effective; crosses the placenta; secreted in milk and in saliva; *protein binding*, about 65% bound to plasma proteins.

METABOLIC REACTIONS. Acetylation; when sulphamethoxazole is administered in combination with trimethoprim its metabolism is unaffected.

EXCRETION. About 60% of a dose is excreted in the urine in 2 days and of the excreted material, about 50% is the N^4-acetylated metabolite and about 17% is the unchanged drug; the acetylated metabolite is relatively insoluble and crystalluria may occur; sulphamethoxazole is excreted in the bile and the biliary level may reach about 10% of that in the blood; the urinary excretion of sulphamethoxazole is increased when the urine is alkaline.

FURTHER INFORMATION. A. S. E. Fowle, Aspects of the pharmacokinetic behaviour of trimethoprim and sulphamethoxazole, *Trimethoprim/Sulphamethoxazole in Bacterial Infection; A Wellcome Foundation Symposium*, L. S. Bernstein and A. J. Salter (Eds), London, Churchill Livingstone, 1973, p. 63; dosage design—E. Kri ger-Thiemer and P. Bünger, *Chemotherapia, Basel*, 1965/66, **10**, 129; pharmacokinetics in children—M. I. Marks, *Can. med. Ass. J.*, 1975, **112**, 33S and C. M. Wilfert and L. T. Gutman, *Can. med. Ass. J.*, 1975, **112**, 73S; maternal and transplacental kinetics—D. W. J.

Reid *et al.*, *Can. med. Ass. J.*, 1975, **112**, 67S; effective plasma and urinary concentrations—J. Tuomisto and N.-E. Saris, *Annls Med. exp. Biol. Fenn.*, 1970, **48**, 38.

Bioavailability. Tablets, capsules, and suspensions containing sulphamethoxazole and trimethoprim in admixture exhibited similar bioavailability data with the exception that the suspension produced higher blood concentrations during the first 90 minutes.

FURTHER INFORMATION. Bioavailability—Y. Langlois *et al.*, *J. clin. Pharmac.*, 1972, **12**, 196.

Actions and uses. Sulphamethoxazole is an antibacterial agent with the actions of the sulphonamides as described under Sulphadimidine. Therapeutic blood concentrations are reached within 2 hours of administration of the drug and may be maintained by doses at intervals of 8 to 12 hours; peak concentrations are reached within 4 hours of administration.

Sulphamethoxazole has similar pharmacokinetic properties to trimethoprim and is used in conjunction with it under the name co-trimoxazole. Trimethoprim also acts on the folic acid pathway by inhibiting folic acid reductases and thus is able to act synergistically with sulphonamides to produce a bactericidal effect.

Co-trimoxazole is used in the treatment of many infections especially urinary-tract infections due to Gram-negative rods and respiratory infections due to pneumococci or *Haemophilus influenzae*. Species of *Klebsiella*, *Proteus*, *Salmonella* (including *S. typhi*), and *Shigella* are usually sensitive but *Pseudomonas* species and *Streptococcus faecalis* are less sensitive.

The usual initial oral dose of sulphamethoxazole is 2 grams, followed by 1 gram every 12 hours.

When given by mouth in conjunction with trimethoprim in the treatment of acute infections, the usual dosage is 800 milligrams of sulphamethoxazole with 160 milligrams of trimethoprim twice daily, which may be increased to thrice daily in severe infections. Lower doses such as 800 milligrams of sulphamethoxazole with 160 milligrams of trimethoprim daily in divided doses may be given in long-term treatment or in case of renal impairment. The dose for children is given under Paediatric Co-trimoxazole Mixture and Tablets, below.

For severe infections, sulphamethoxazole may be given in a dosage of 0.8 to 1.2 grams by intravenous infusion with 160 to 240 milligrams of trimethoprim in 250 to 500 millilitres of dextrose injection (5%) or sodium chloride injection over a period of 90 minutes every 12 hours. The usual dose for children up to 12 years is 30 milligrams per kilogram body-weight of sulphamethoxazole and 6 milligrams per kilogram body-weight of trimethoprim daily in divided doses. The infusion solution should be prepared immediately before use.

Undesirable effects. As for Sulphadimidine.

Precautions; Contra-indications. As for Sulphadimidine. When used in conjunction with trimethoprim for periods in excess of 1 month, the haemoglobin should be determined and a polymorph and platelet count performed monthly because of possible interference with folic acid metabolism. Sulphamethoxazole, when used in conjunction with trimethoprim, should be avoided during pregnancy. Infusions containing sulphamethoxazole and trimethoprim may give rise to pain and phlebitis.

Preparations

CO-TRIMOXAZOLE INJECTION: a sterile solution of the sodium derivative of sulphamethoxazole and trimethoprim in dextrose injection (5%) or sodium chloride injection. It is prepared immediately before use by diluting strong sterile co-trimoxazole solution (see below) with 25 to 35 times its volume of dextrose injection or sodium chloride injection.

Dose: for a solution containing 400 mg of sulphamethoxazole and 80 mg of trimethoprim in 5 ml, by intravenous infusion, 10 ml diluted before administration with 250 ml of diluent twice daily or 15 ml diluted before administration with 500 ml of diluent, twice daily.

CO-TRIMOXAZOLE MIXTURE (*Syn.* Trimethoprim and Sulphamethoxazole Mixture): a suspension of sulphamethoxazole and trimethoprim in a suitable flavoured vehicle. It contains 400 mg of sulphamethoxazole and 80 mg of trimethoprim in 5 ml.

When a dose less than or not a multiple of 5 ml is prescribed, the mixture may be diluted, as described in the entry on Mixtures, with syrup. The diluted mixture must be freshly prepared.

A standard for this mixture is given in the British Pharmaceutical Codex 1973

Containers and *Labelling:* see the entry on Mixtures for general information on containers and labelling.

Storage: it should be protected from light.

Dose: ADULT: 10 to 30 millilitres daily, divided into 2 or 3 doses.

Advice for patients: the mixture should be taken at regular intervals. The prescribed course should be completed. Adequate fluid intake should be maintained. Direct exposure to sunlight should be avoided during treatment.

CO-TRIMOXAZOLE TABLETS (*Syn.* Trimethoprim and Sulphamethoxazole Tablets): available as tablets containing 400 mg of sulphamethoxazole and 80 mg of trimethoprim, and as tablets containing 800 mg of sulphamethoxazole and 160 mg of trimethoprim; they may be film coated or sugar coated and the coat may be coloured; the tablets need not be circular in shape. Paediatric co-trimoxazole tablets are described below.

A standard for these tablets is given in the British Pharmacopoeia Addendum 1978

Containers and *Storage:* see the entry on Tablets for general information on containers and storage. Containers should be airtight.

Labelling: the label on the container should state the amounts of the medicaments as the amounts of sulphamethoxazole and trimethoprim in each tablet.

Dose: for tablets containing 400 mg of sulphamethoxazole and 80 mg of trimethoprim, 2 to 6 tablets daily.

Advice for patients: see above under Co-trimoxazole Mixture.

DISPERSIBLE CO-TRIMOXAZOLE TABLETS (*Syn.* Trimethoprim and Sulphamethoxazole Dispersible Tablets): available as tablets containing 400 mg of sulphamethoxazole and 80 mg of trimethoprim in a suitable basis; they may be coloured.

A standard for these tablets is given in the British Pharmacopoeia Addendum 1978

Containers and *Storage:* see the entry on Tablets for general information on containers and storage. Containers should be airtight.

Labelling: the label on the container should state the amounts of the medicaments as the amounts of sulphamethoxazole and trimethoprim in each tablet.

Dose: for tablets containing 400 mg of sulphamethoxazole and 80 mg of trimethoprim, 2 to 6 tablets daily in 2 or 3 divided doses.

Advice for patients: the tablets may be dispersed in water before administration or swallowed whole; advice as for Co-trimoxazole Mixture (above).

PAEDIATRIC CO-TRIMOXAZOLE MIXTURE (*Syn.* Paediatric Trimethoprim and Sulphamethoxazole Mixture): a suspension of sulphamethoxazole and trimethoprim in a suitable coloured flavoured vehicle. It contains 200 mg of sulphamethoxazole and 40 mg of trimethoprim in 5 ml.

When a dose less than or not a multiple of 5 ml is prescribed, the mixture may be diluted as described in the entry on Mixtures, with syrup. The diluted mixture must be freshly prepared.

A standard for this mixture is given in the British Pharmaceutical Codex 1973

Containers and *Labelling:* see the entry on Mixtures for general information on containers and labelling.

Storage: it should be protected from light.

Dose: CHILD: Twice daily: 6 weeks to 5 months, 2.5 millilitres; 6 months to 5 years, 5 millilitres; 6 to 12 years, 10 millilitres.

Advice for patients: see above under Co-trimoxazole Mixture.

PAEDIATRIC CO-TRIMOXAZOLE TABLETS (*Syn.* Paediatric Trimethoprim and Sulphamethoxazole Tablets): for each tablet take:

Sulphamethoxazole	..	..	..	..	100 mg
Trimethoprim	..	..	..	..	20 mg

Mix, and prepare by moist granulation and compression as described in the entry on Tablets; they may be film coated or sugar coated and the coat may be coloured; the tablets need not be circular in shape.

A standard for these tablets is given in the British Pharmacopoeia Addendum 1978

Containers and *Storage:* see the entry on Tablets for general information on containers and storage. Containers should be airtight.

Labelling: the label on the container should state the amounts of the medicaments as the amounts of sulphamethoxazole and trimethoprim in each tablet.

Dose: CHILD: Twice daily: 6 months to 5 years, 2 tablets; 6 to 12 years, 4 tablets.

Advice for patients: see above under Co-trimoxazole Mixture.

STRONG STERILE CO-TRIMOXAZOLE SOLUTION: a sterile solution of the sodium derivative of sulphamethoxazole, prepared by the interaction of sulphamethoxazole and sodium hydroxide, and trimethoprim, in the proportion of the equivalent of 5 parts of sulphamethoxazole to 1 part of trimethoprim, with 40% v/v of propylene glycol and suitable stabilisers, in water for injections. It is sterilised by heating in an autoclave.

Available in 5-ml ampoules containing the equivalent of 80 mg of sulphamethoxazole and 16 mg of trimethoprim per ml.

A standard for this solution is given in the British Pharmacopoeia Addendum 1978

Containers: see the entry on Injections for general information on containers.

Labelling: the label on the container should state "Strong Sterile Co-trimoxazole Solution", the amounts of the medicaments as the amounts of sulphamethoxazole and trimethoprim in a suitable volume, and that the solution must be diluted before use.

The label on the container or the label on the package should state "Strong Sterile Co-trimoxazole Solution for the preparation of Co-trimoxazole Injection", the amounts of the medicaments as the amounts of sulphamethoxazole and trimethoprim in a suitable volume, the name of any added preservative, that the solution must be protected from light, that the solution must be diluted with 25 to 35 times its volume of dextrose injection or sodium chloride injection, that the co-trimoxazole injection so prepared is administered by intravenous injection, and that the injection must be discarded if any visible particles appear.

Storage: it should be protected from light.

OTHER PREPARATIONS available include an INJECTION containing sulphamethoxazole 267 mg with trimethoprim 53 mg per ml in 3-ml ampoules; and TABLETS containing sulphamethoxazole 500 mg.

Sulphamethoxydiazine

N^1-(5-Methoxypyrimidin-2-yl)sulphanilamide

$C_{11}H_{12}N_4O_3S = 280.3$

OTHER NAMES: *Durenate*®; Sulfameter; Sulfamethoxydiazine

A standard is given in the British Pharmacopoeia 1973

Description. An odourless, white or yellowish-white, crystalline powder with a slightly bitter taste.

Solubility. Very slightly soluble in water, in alcohol, and in dilute hydrochloric acid; soluble in solutions of alkali hydroxides and carbonates.

Storage. See the entry on Sulphonamides.

Identification. TESTS. 1. It complies with the general tests described under Sulphonamides.
2. Mix about 10 mg with 2 ml of sulphuric acid and warm on a water-bath for 3 minutes; an intense violet fluorescence is produced.

MELTING-POINT. About 211°.

ULTRAVIOLET ABSORPTION. In 0.1N hydrochloric acid, maximum at 220 nm (E1%, 1cm = 591); in 0.1N sodium hydroxide, maximum at 245 nm (E1%, 1cm = 909); in alcohol (95%), maxima at 246 nm (E1%, 1cm = 893) and 262 nm (E1%, 1cm = 850).

INFRA-RED ABSORPTION. Major peaks at 1140, 1153, 1284, 1424, 1466, and 1597 cm^{-1} (see Appendix 2a: Infra-red Spectra).

THIN-LAYER CHROMATOGRAPHY. See under Thin-layer Chromatography, System 11.

Metabolism (see also under Sulphonamides). ABSORPTION. Well absorbed after oral administration.

BLOOD CONCENTRATION. After an oral dose of 0.5 to 1 g, peak blood concentrations of 30 to 90 µg/ml occur within 4 to 6 hours and fall to 10 to 20 µg/ml after 2 days.

HALF-LIFE. Serum half-life, 13 to 34 hours; from urinary excretion data, 29 to 58 hours.

DISTRIBUTION. *Protein binding,* about 80% bound to plasma proteins.

METABOLIC REACTIONS. Acetylation and glucuronic acid conjugation.

EXCRETION. About 70% of a dose is excreted in the urine

in 3 days, and of the excreted material, about 50% is unchanged drug, about 25% is acetylated, and about 20% is the glucuronic acid conjugate.

FURTHER INFORMATION. Acetylation pattern in rapid and slow isoniazid acetylators—M. J. Mattila *et al., Annls Med. exp. Biol. Fenn.*, 1969, **47**, 308; excretion of metabolites in hepatitis and renal failure—S. T. Madsen, *Chemotherapia,* 1966, **11**, 1.

Bioavailability. Differences in bioavailability observed for sulphamethoxydiazine tablets have been attributed to particle size, viscosity agents, and polymorphism. Two polymorphic forms have been studied, one of which is more soluble than the other, by administering them in solution. The more soluble form was more readily absorbed. In solution, the two forms interconvert but this interconversion may be eliminated by the addition of agents which increase viscosity. The presence of these agents tends to reduce absorption. Tablet formulations are absorbed more slowly than an oral suspension.

FURTHER INFORMATION. Bioavailability of 2 crystal forms—N. Khalafallah *et al., J. pharm. Sci.*, 1974, **63**, 861; gastro-intestinal absorption of 2 crystal forms— S. A. Khalil *et al., J. pharm. Sci.*, 1972, **61**, 1615.

Actions and uses. Sulphamethoxydiazine has the actions, uses, and undesirable effects of the long-acting sulphonamides, as described under Sulphadimethoxine. When given by mouth, it is rapidly absorbed from the gastro-intestinal tract and slowly excreted; the peak concentration in the blood is attained about 4 hours after administration and therapeutic blood concentrations may be maintained for up to 48 hours. An initial dose of 1 to 2 grams by mouth followed by 500 milligrams daily is usually sufficient to maintain a satisfactory blood concentration.

For severe infections, infants aged 3 months to 1 year may be given 40 milligrams per kilogram body-weight on the first day followed by 15 milligrams per kilogram body-weight daily. Children over 1 year may be given 30 milligrams per kilogram body-weight daily on the first day followed by 10 milligrams per kilogram body-weight daily.

Precautions. As for Sulphadimethoxine.

Contra-indications. As for Sulphadimidine.

Preparations

SULPHAMETHOXYDIAZINE TABLETS: available as tablets containing 500 mg of sulphamethoxydiazine.

A standard for these tablets is given in the British Pharmacopoeia 1973

Containers and *Storage:* see the entry on Tablets for general information on containers and storage. Containers should be airtight and light resistant.

Advice for patients: the tablets should be taken at regular intervals. The prescribed course should be completed. Adequate fluid intake should be maintained. Exposure to direct sunlight should be avoided during treatment.

OTHER PREPARATIONS available include a MIXTURE containing sulphamethoxydiazine 500 mg in 5 ml, diluent water for preparations, life of diluted mixture 14 days.

Sulphamethoxypyridazine

N^1-(6-Methoxypyridazin-3-yl)sulphanilamide

$C_{11}H_{12}N_4O_3S = 280.3$

OTHER NAMES: *Lederkyn®*; *Midicel®*; Sulfamethoxypyridazine

A standard is given in the British Pharmacopoeia 1973

Description. An odourless, white or yellowish-white, crystalline powder which is tasteless at first but has a bitter after-taste.

Solubility. Very slightly soluble in water and in alcohol; soluble, at 20°, in 25 parts of acetone; soluble in dilute mineral acids and in solutions of alkali hydroxides.

Dissociation constant. pK_a 7.2 (25°).

Storage. See the entry on Sulphonamides.

Identification. TESTS. It complies with the general tests described under Sulphonamides.

MELTING-POINT. About 181°.

ULTRAVIOLET ABSORPTION. In 0.1N sodium hydroxide, maximum at 250 nm (E1%, 1cm = 701); in alcohol (95%), maximum at 270 nm (E1%, 1cm = 739).

INFRA-RED ABSORPTION. Major peaks at 1130, 1159, 1324, 1470, 1480, and 1599 cm^{-1} (see Appendix 2a: Infra-red Spectra).

THIN-LAYER CHROMATOGRAPHY. See under Thin-layer Chromatography, System 11.

Metabolism (see also under Sulphonamides). ABSORPTION. Rapidly absorbed after oral administration; absorption is delayed by the presence of food.

BLOOD CONCENTRATION. After an oral dose of 4 g, peak blood concentrations of 110 to 180 μg/ml of total sulphonamide are attained within 5 hours; this level is maintained for approximately 3 hours and then slowly falls to about 30 μg/ml after 4 days; up to 15% of the drug in the blood may be in the acetylated form.

HALF-LIFE. Serum half-life, about 37 hours.

DISTRIBUTION. Small amounts of the drug may be taken up by the red blood cells; *protein binding*, about 85% bound to plasma proteins.

METABOLIC REACTIONS. Polymorphic acetylation and also glucuronic acid conjugation.

EXCRETION. About 45% of a dose is excreted in the urine in 2 days, about 65% as the N^4-acetylated conjugate, about 13% as glucuronide conjugates, and about 22% as unchanged drug; significant amounts are secreted in bile; urinary excretion appears to be pH-dependent.

FURTHER INFORMATION. Absorption and effect of food —H. Macdonald *et al.*, *Chemotherapia*, 1967, **12**, 282; acetylation—T. A. White and D. A. P. Evans, *Clin. Pharmac. Ther.*, 1968, **9**, 80; excretion of metabolites in hepatitis and renal failure—S. T. Madsen, *Chemotherapia*, 1966, **11**, 1.

Actions and uses. Sulphamethoxypyridazine has the actions, uses, and undesirable effects of the long-acting sulphonamides, as described under Sulphadimethoxine. As it is very soluble in neutral or acid urine, it is given by mouth in the treatment of urinary tract infections.

The usual initial dose for adults is 1 to 2 grams, with a subsequent dosage of 500 milligrams daily. Children may be given an initial dosage of 30 milligrams per kilogram body-weight followed by 15 milligrams per kilogram body-weight daily.

Precautions. As for Sulphadimethoxine.

Contra-indications. As for Sulphadimidine.

Veterinary uses. Sulphamethoxypyridazine is administered in the form of its sodium derivative, the usual dose for all species being 25 milligrams per kilogram body-weight daily by subcutaneous, intraperitoneal, or intravenous injection.

Preparations

SULPHAMETHOXYPYRIDAZINE INJECTION: a sterile solution of the sodium derivative of sulphamethoxypyridazine, prepared by the interaction of sulphamethoxypyridazine and sodium hydroxide, with up to 0.4% of sodium thiosulphate, in water for injections free from dissolved air. It is sterilised by filtration, distributed, by means of an aseptic technique, into sterile bottles, replacing the air in the bottles by sterile nitrogen or other suitable gas, and the bottles are sealed. Available in 100- and 250-ml bottles containing the equivalent of 250 mg of sulphamethoxypyridazine per ml.

A standard for this injection is given in the British Pharmacopoeia (Veterinary)

Containers: see the entry on Injections for general information on containers.

Labelling: see the entry on Injections for general information on labelling. In addition, the label on the container should state the amount of the medicament as the equivalent amount of sulphamethoxypyridazine in a suitable dose-volume.

Storage: it should be protected from light.

SULPHAMETHOXYPYRIDAZINE TABLETS: available as tablets containing 500 mg of sulphamethoxypyridazine; they may be coloured.

A standard for these tablets is given in the British Pharmacopoeia 1973

Containers and *Storage:* see the entry on Tablets for general information on containers and storage. Containers should be airtight and light resistant.

Advice for patients: the tablets should be taken at regular intervals. The prescribed course should be completed. Adequate fluid intake should be maintained. Exposure to direct sunlight should be avoided during treatment.

Sulphanilamide

4-Aminobenzenesulphonamide

$C_6H_8N_2O_2S = 172.2$

OTHER NAME: Sulfanilamide

A standard is given in the British Pharmacopoeia (Veterinary)

Description. An odourless white crystalline powder.

Solubility. Soluble, at 20°, in 170 parts of water; very slightly soluble in alcohol; practically insoluble in ether and in chloroform; soluble in solutions of alkali hydroxides.

Dissociation constant. pK_a 10.4 (20°).

Storage. See the entry on Sulphonamides.

Identification. TESTS. It complies with the general tests described under Sulphonamides.

MELTING-POINT. About 165°.

ULTRAVIOLET ABSORPTION. In 0.1N sodium hydroxide, maximum at 254 nm (E1%, 1cm = 1402); in alcohol (95%), maximum at 263 nm (E1%, 1cm = 1106).

INFRA-RED ABSORPTION. Major peaks at 1099, 1149, 1299, 1316, 1613, and 1639 cm^{-1} (see Appendix 2b: Infra-red Spectra).

THIN-LAYER CHROMATOGRAPHY. See under Thin-layer Chromatography, System 11.

Veterinary uses. Sulphanilamide is an antibacterial which may be administered by mouth to horses. The usual initial dose is 200 milligrams per kilogram body-weight followed by a maintenance dosage of 100 milligrams per kilogram body-weight twice daily. Foals, calves, and lambs may be given an initial dose of 150 milligrams per kilogram body-weight followed by 50 milligrams per kilogram body-weight 3 times daily. Treatment should not be continued for more than 7 days. Sulphanilamide powder is also applied topically as an antibacterial dressing for wounds.

Sulphapyrazole

N^1-(3-Methyl-1-phenylpyrazol-5-yl)sulphanilamide

$C_{16}H_{16}N_4O_2S = 328.4$

OTHER NAMES: Sulfapyrazole; Sulfazamet; *Vesulong*®

A standard is given in the British Pharmacopoeia (Veterinary)

Description. An odourless, white or creamy-white, crystalline powder.

Solubility. Practically insoluble in water; soluble in alcohol and in methyl alcohol; very slightly soluble in chloroform.

Storage. See the entry on Sulphonamides.

Identification. TEST. It complies with general test 1 described under Sulphonamides.

MELTING-POINT. About 185°.

Veterinary uses. Sulphapyrazole is a long-acting antibacterial. The usual dose by mouth or by intramuscular or slow intravenous injection of a solution of the sodium

salt for all species is 20 to 40 milligrams per kilogram body-weight daily.

It should not be administered by mouth to adult ruminants.

Preparations

Preparations available include a veterinary INJECTION containing sulphapyrazole 200 mg per ml in 500-ml vials; and veterinary TABLETS containing sulphapyrazole 500 mg.

Sulphapyridine

N^1-(Pyrid-2-yl)sulphanilamide

$C_{11}H_{11}N_3O_2S = 249.3$

OTHER NAMES: *M & B 693*®; Sulfapyridine

A standard is given in the British Pharmacopoeia 1973

Description. An odourless, white or yellowish-white, crystalline powder with a very slightly bitter taste.

Solubility. Very slightly soluble in water; soluble in 100 parts of boiling water; soluble, at 20°, in 400 parts of alcohol and in 65 parts of acetone; soluble in dilute mineral acids and in aqueous solutions of alkali hydroxides.

Dissociation constant. pK_a 8.4 (25°).

Storage. See the entry on Sulphonamides.

Identification. TESTS. It complies with the general tests described under Sulphonamides.

MELTING-POINT. About 192°.

ULTRAVIOLET ABSORPTION. In 0.1N hydrochloric acid, maxima at 240 nm (E1%, 1cm = 393), and 310 nm (E1%, 1cm = 380); in 0.1N sodium hydroxide, maximum at 246 nm (E1%, 1cm = 812); in alcohol (95%), maximum at 270 nm (E1%, 1cm = 857).

INFRA-RED ABSORPTION. Major peaks at 768, 949, 1078, 1127, 1264, and 1585 cm^{-1} (see Appendix 2a: Infra-red Spectra).

THIN-LAYER CHROMATOGRAPHY. See under Thin-layer Chromatography, System 11.

Metabolism (see also under Sulphonamides). ABSORPTION. Slowly and inconsistently absorbed after oral administration.

BLOOD CONCENTRATION. Peak serum concentrations of sulphapyridine are attained within 1 to 2 hours; in the blood 30 to 70% of the drug is acetylated; peak serum concentrations of total sulphapyridine metabolites of 50 to 60 μg/ml (expressed as sulphapyridine) are attained in 3 to 5 hours.

HALF-LIFE. Serum half-life for total sulphapyridine metabolites, about 8 hours.

DISTRIBUTION. The cerebrospinal fluid concentration is about 50% of that in the blood; *protein binding*, 10 to 45% bound to plasma proteins.

METABOLIC REACTIONS. Polymorphic N^4-acetylation;

hydroxylation, which may also be polymorphic, of the 5 position of the pyridine ring which is then conjugated with glucuronic acid.

EXCRETION. Urinary excretion is irregular with up to 80% of a dose being excreted in 3 to 4 days, mostly as the acetylated metabolite with small amounts of the glucuronide; small amounts of unchanged drug and the acetylated metabolite are excreted in the bile.

FURTHER INFORMATION. Acetylation and deacetylation —H. Schröder, *J. Pharm. Pharmac.*, 1971, **25**, 591; metabolism and excretion—H. Schröder and D. E. S. Campbell, *Clin. Pharmac. Ther.*, 1972, **13**, 539.

Actions and uses. Sulphapyridine has the actions of the sulphonamides as described under Sulphadimidine. It is now rarely used in medicine except in the treatment of patients with dermatitis herpetiformis which has not responded to dapsone.
It is given by mouth in a dosage of 3 to 4 grams daily until no further blisters develop and then in a dosage of 0.5 to 1 gram daily.

Undesirable effects. As for Sulphadimidine. Toxic symptoms are common and fever and rashes are more frequent than with the other sulphonamides. Agranulocytosis occasionally occurs. Sulphapyridine may cause deposition of crystals of an acetyl derivative in the urinary tract with consequent haematuria or anuria.
These risks are greater than with the other sulphonamides and may be reduced by maintaining a high fluid intake during treatment with the drug and by the administration of alkalis.

Precautions; Contra-indications. As for Sulphadimidine.

Preparations

SULPHAPYRIDINE TABLETS: available as tablets containing 500 mg of sulphapyridine.
A standard for these tablets is given in the British Pharmacopoeia 1973
Containers and *Storage:* see the entry on Tablets for general information on containers and storage. Containers should be airtight and light resistant.
Advice for patients: the tablets may be chewed or crushed and swallowed with water. Doses should be taken at regular intervals. The prescribed course should be completed. Adequate fluid intake should be maintained. Direct exposure to sunlight should be avoided during treatment.

OTHER PREPARATIONS available include veterinary TABLETS (oblong) containing sulphapyridine 5 g.

Sulphaquinoxaline

N^1-(Quinoxalin-2-yl)sulphanilamide

$C_{14}H_{12}N_4O_2S = 300.3$

OTHER NAMES: *Embazin®*; Sulfaquinoxaline
Saquadil® (with diaveridine); *Whitsyn S®* (with pyrimethamine); *Pancoxin®* (with amprolium hydrochloride and ethopabate); *Supacox®* (with amprolium hydrochloride, ethopabate, and pyrimethamine)

A standard is given in the British Pharmacopoeia (Veterinary)

Description. An odourless tasteless yellow powder.

Solubility. Practically insoluble in water, and in ether; very slightly soluble in alcohol; soluble in dilute mineral acids and in solutions of alkali hydroxides.

Moisture content. Not more than 1%, determined by drying at 105°.

Dissociation constant. pK_a 5.5 (20°).

Storage. See the entry on Sulphonamides.

Identification. TESTS. It complies with the general tests described under Sulphonamides.

MELTING-POINT. About 250°, with decomposition.

ULTRAVIOLET ABSORPTION. In 0.01N sodium hydroxide, maximum at 252 nm (E1%, 1cm = 1100).

Veterinary uses. Sulphaquinoxaline is used for the prevention and treatment of coccidiosis. The usual prophylactic dose for poultry is 125 parts per million in the feed for the first 8 weeks of life. The usual dose for the treatment of coccidiosis in poultry is 500 parts per million in the feed for 7 days.

Preparations

AMPROLIUM, ETHOPABATE, AND SULPHAQUINOXALINE PREMIX: consisting of amprolium hydrochloride, ethopabate, and sulphaquinoxaline, mixed with a suitable diluent. It must be diluted before administration by mixing thoroughly with the feed.
Available as a premix containing 20% of amprolium hydrochloride, 1% of ethopabate, and 12% of sulphaquinoxaline.
A standard for this premix is given in the British Pharmacopoeia (Veterinary)
Containers and *Storage:* see the entry on Premixes for general information on containers and storage.

AMPROLIUM, ETHOPABATE, SULPHAQUINOXALINE, AND PYRIMETHAMINE PREMIX: consisting of amprolium hydrochloride, ethopabate, sulphaquinoxaline, and pyrimethamine, mixed with a suitable diluent. It must be diluted before administration by mixing thoroughly with the feed.
Available as a premix containing 20% of amprolium hydrochloride, 1% of ethopabate, 12% of sulphaquinoxaline, and 1% of pyrimethamine.
A standard for this premix is given in the British Pharmacopoeia (Veterinary)
Containers and *Storage:* see the entry on Premixes for general information on containers and storage.

DIAVERIDINE AND SULPHAQUINOXALINE PREMIX: consisting of diaveridine and sulphaquinoxaline mixed with a suitable diluent. It must be diluted before administration by mixing thoroughly with the feed. Available as a premix containing 3.3% of diaveridine and 18.7% of sulphaquinoxaline.
A standard for this premix is given in the British Pharmacopoeia (Veterinary)
Containers and *Storage:* see the entry on Premixes for general information on containers and storage.

SULPHAQUINOXALINE SODIUM SOLUTION: an aqueous solution of the sodium derivative of sulphaquinoxaline, prepared by the interaction of sulphaquinoxaline and sodium hydroxide. Available as a solution containing the equivalent of 96 mg of sulphaquinoxaline per ml.

A standard for this solution is given in the British Pharmacopoeia (Veterinary)

Labelling: the label on the container should state the amount of the medicament as the equivalent amount of sulphaquinoxaline in a suitable dose-volume.

OTHER PREPARATIONS available include a PREMIX containing sulphaquinoxaline 22.5%; a SOLUTION containing sulphaquinoxaline 16 mg with diaveridine 14 mg per ml, and a solution containing sulphaquinoxaline 30 mg with pyrimethamine 9.1 mg per ml.

Sulphasalazine

4 - Hydroxy - 4' - (pyrid - 2 - ylsulphamoyl) azobenzene - 3 - carboxylic acid

$C_{18}H_{14}N_4O_5S = 398.4$

OTHER NAMES: *Salazopyrin®*; Salazosulfapyridine; Sulfasalazine

Description. An odourless yellow or brownish-yellow powder.

Solubility. Practically insoluble in water, in ether, and in chloroform; soluble in 2900 parts of alcohol; soluble in solutions of alkali hydroxides.

Storage. See the entry on Sulphonamides.

Identification. TESTS. 1. Mix about 20 mg with 5 ml of water and add *dilute sodium hydroxide solution*, dropwise with shaking, until the substance has dissolved; an intense orange-red to blood-red colour is produced.
2. To about 1 g add 3 ml of *stannous chloride solution*, allow to stand for 16 hours, add 15 ml of water, centrifuge, and reserve the supernatant liquid. Wash the residue with several portions of water and add 4 drops of *ferric chloride test-solution* to the washings; an intense violet colour is produced.
3. Pass a stream of hydrogen sulphide through the supernatant liquid reserved in Test 2 until precipitation is complete, filter, boil the filtrate to remove excess hydrogen sulphide, cool in ice, add 5 ml of *sodium nitrite solution*, again cool in ice, and add 5 ml of the cooled solution to 2 ml of *2-naphthol solution*; an intense red colour is produced.

MELTING-POINT. About 240°, with decomposition.

INFRA-RED ABSORPTION. Major peaks at 769, 1075, 1124, 1176, 1639, and 1667 cm^{-1} (see Appendix 2b: Infra-red Spectra).

Determination in body fluids. ULTRAVIOLET SPECTROPHOTOMETRY. In serum or urine—M. Sandberg and K.-A. Hansson, *Acta pharm. suec.*, 1973, **10**, 107.

SPECTROFLUORIMETRY. In serum or urine: determination

of free and acetylated 5-aminosalicylic acid—K.-A. Hansson, *Acta pharm. suec.*, 1973, **10**, 153.

Metabolism (see also under Sulphonamides). ABSORPTION. The unchanged drug is partially absorbed after oral administration and the remainder is metabolised by the gut flora to sulphapyridine and 5-aminosalicylic acid; sulphapyridine is well absorbed but 5-aminosalicylic acid is only absorbed to a small extent; sulphasalazine absorption is reduced by concomitant administration of ferrous sulphate.

BLOOD CONCENTRATION. After an oral dose of 4 g, sulphasalazine is detectable in the serum in 1.5 hours and peak concentrations of about 26 μg/ml are reached within 3 to 5 hours; after an oral dose of 4 g daily for 10 days, steady state serum concentrations of 5 to 45 μg/ml are attained for sulphasalazine, 40 to 90 μg/ml for sulphapyridine and its metabolites, and less than 2 μg/ml for 5-aminosalicylic acid and its metabolites.

HALF-LIFE. Serum half-life after a single oral dose, about 6 hours.

METABOLIC REACTIONS. The unabsorbed portion of the dose is metabolised by the gut flora, located in the colon, which cleave the azo linkage of the drug to form sulphapyridine and 5-aminosalicylic acid. Both of these metabolites, upon absorption, are further metabolised; sulphapyridine is either hydroxylated at the 5-position or acetylated; both of these reactions are polymorphic; the hydroxylated metabolites ultimately appear in the blood and urine as *O*-glucuronides; the 5-aminosalicylic acid moiety is further metabolised by acetylation. The absorbed sulphasalazine is not metabolised further in the body but may enter the enterohepatic circulation and be further metabolised by the gut flora; concomitant administration of antibiotics may decrease the population of gut flora and therefore alter the extent of sulphasalazine cleavage.

EXCRETION. Up to about 10% of a dose is excreted in the urine as unchanged drug; of the sulphapyridine formed, 60% is excreted in the urine as sulphapyridine and its metabolites and 25% in the faeces as sulphapyridine; of the 5-aminosalicylic acid formed, about 20% is excreted in the urine as 5-aminosalicylic acid and its metabolites and most of the remainder is eliminated in the faeces unchanged; no unchanged drug is eliminated in the faeces of normal subjects but in patients with ulcerative colitis, up to 7% of a dose may be eliminated unchanged by this route.

FURTHER INFORMATION. Clinical pharmacokinetics—K. M. Das and R. Dubin, *Clin. Pharmacokinet.*, 1976, **1**, 406; acetylation polymorphism in patients with ulcerative colitis and Crohn's disease—K. M. Das and M. A. Eastwood, *Clin. Pharmac. Ther.*, 1975, **18**, 514; metabolism in healthy subjects and patients with ulcerative colitis—H. Schröder *et al.*, *Clin. Pharmac. Ther.*, 1973, **14**, 802.

Actions and uses. Sulphasalazine is a sulphonamide derived from sulphapyridine and aminosalicylic acid. It is used in the treatment of ulcerative colitis and related conditions, either alone or in conjunction with corticosteroids or surgery.

The usual dosage in an acute attack or relapse is the maximum tolerated dose of 1 to 2 grams 4 to 6 times a day for 3 weeks, after which the dose should be progressively reduced as the condition improves, to a maintenance dosage of 500 milligrams 3 or 4 times daily. Children may be given 60 milligrams per kilogram body-weight daily in divided doses in an acute attack or relapse, reducing to a maintenance dose of 20 to 30 milligrams per kilogram body-weight daily in divided doses.

Sulphasalazine is administered by rectum in suppositories in the treatment of proctitis. The usual dosage is 1 gram night and morning for 2 to 3 weeks in an acute attack or relapse, dosage being gradually decreased as the condition improves. In proctocolitis sulphasalazine may be administered by mouth and in addition 0.5 to 1 gram may be given by rectum night and morning. Doses by rectum for children should be reduced in proportion to body-weight.

Undesirable effects. As for Sulphadimethoxine. In addition hypersensitivity reactions involving the lung may occur.

Precautions. As for Sulphadimethoxine. In addition sulphasalazine should not be used in patients sensitive to salicylates. Sulphasalazine may cause kernicterus in premature and newborn babies and in pregnant women during the week before term and should only be used when the benefit outweighs the risk.

Preparations

SULPHASALAZINE TABLETS: available as tablets containing 500 mg of sulphasalazine; they may be enteric coated. *Containers* and *Storage:* see the entry on Tablets for general information on containers and storage. Containers should be airtight and light resistant.
Advice for patients: the tablets should be taken at regular intervals preferably after meals; enteric-coated tablets should be swallowed whole. Treatment should not be discontinued without the advice of the prescriber. Adequate fluid intake should be maintained. The urine may be coloured orange-yellow.

OTHER PREPARATIONS available include SUPPOSITORIES containing sulphasalazine 500 mg.

Sulphathiazole

N^1-(Thiazol-2-yl)sulphanilamide

$C_9H_9N_3O_2S_2 = 255.3$

OTHER NAMES: Sulfathiazole; *Thiazamide®*
Amethozol® (with amethocaine); *Sulfex®* (with hydroxyamphetamine hydrobromide)

A standard is given in the British Pharmaceutical Codex 1973

Description. An odourless white crystalline powder.

Solubility. Very slightly soluble in water and in alcohol; soluble in dilute mineral acids and in solutions of alkali hydroxides and carbonates.

Dissociation constant. pK_a 7.1 (25°).

Sterilisation; Storage. See the entry on Sulphonamides.

Identification. TESTS. 1. It complies with the general tests described under Sulphonamides.
2. Heat about 50 mg in a dry tube; a brown to red colour

is produced; on further heating, the odours of ammonia, aniline, and hydrogen sulphide are produced.

MELTING-POINT. About 201°.

ULTRAVIOLET ABSORPTION. In 0.1N hydrochloric acid, maximum at 282 nm (E1%, 1cm = 563); in 0.1N sodium hydroxide, maximum at 259 nm (E1%, 1cm = 803); in alcohol (95%), maxima at 261 nm (E1%, 1cm = 687) and 290 nm (E1%, 1cm = 887).

THIN-LAYER CHROMATOGRAPHY. See under Thin-layer Chromatography, System 11.

Determination in body fluids. HIGH PRESSURE LIQUID CHROMATOGRAPHY. In urine: sulphathiazole and its N^4-acetylated metabolite—J. P. Sharma *et al.*, *J. pharm. Sci.*, 1976, **65**, 1606.

Actions and uses. Sulphathiazole has the actions and uses of the sulphonamides, as described under Sulphadimidine. It is the only sulphonamide which has any effect in staphylococcal infections; it is also effective in the treatment of infections due to β-haemolytic streptococci, pneumococci, and gonococci.

When given by mouth, sulphathiazole is rapidly absorbed, and the maximum concentration in the blood, 5 to 10 milligrams per 100 millilitres, is attained in about 4 to 6 hours. It does not readily cross the blood–brain barrier into the cerebrospinal fluid and is therefore unsuitable for the treatment of meningeal infections. It is more rapidly excreted than sulphadimidine or sulphadiazine, a single dose being almost completely excreted in 24 hours.

In the treatment of pneumococcal pneumonia and other respiratory-tract infections, as well as of localised staphylococcal infections such as otitis media and tonsillitis, it is usual to give an initial dose of 3 grams, followed by 1 gram every 4 hours until the temperature has remained normal for 3 days. The dosage for a child should be based on the scheme outlined under Sulphadimidine.

Undesirable effects. As for Sulphadimidine. Toxic symptoms are common; the most usual undesirable effect is drug fever, and rashes are more frequent than with the other sulphonamides. Agranulocytosis occasionally occurs.

Sulphathiazole is excreted partly as the insoluble crystalline acetyl derivative and this occasionally causes blocking of the renal tubules and anuria, while milder degrees of renal damage may be indicated by haematuria. These risks, which are greater with sulphathiazole than with other sulphonamides, may be reduced to a minimum by maintaining a high fluid intake during treatment with the drug and by the administration of alkalis.

Precautions. As for Sulphadimidine. In addition great care should be taken in its administration in hot climates. If haematuria develops administration of the drug must be discontinued.

Contra-indications. As for Sulphadimidine.

Preparations

SULPHATHIAZOLE TABLETS: may be prepared by moist granulation and compression as described in the entry on Tablets. Available as tablets containing 500 mg of sulphathiazole.
A standard for these tablets is given in the British Pharmaceutical Codex 1973
Containers and *Storage:* see the entry on Tablets for general information on containers and storage. Containers should be airtight and light resistant.
Advice for patients: the tablets should be taken at

regular intervals. The prescribed course should be completed. Adequate fluid intake should be maintained. Direct exposure to sunlight should be avoided during treatment.

OTHER PREPARATIONS available include a veterinary ear or eye OINTMENT containing sulphathiazole 10% with amethocaine 0.5%; and NASAL DROPS containing sulphathiazole 5% with hydroxyamphetamine hydrobromide 1%.

Sulphinpyrazone

1,2 - Diphenyl - 4 - (2 - phenylsulphinylethyl)pyrazolidine-3,5-dione

$C_{23}H_{20}N_2O_3S = 404.5$

OTHER NAMES: *Anturan*®; Sulfinpyrazone

A standard is given in the British Pharmacopoeia Addendum 1977

Description. An odourless white powder with a bitter taste.

Solubility. Practically insoluble in water and in light petroleum; soluble, at 20°, in 40 parts of alcohol, in 750 parts of ether, and in 2 parts of chloroform; soluble in aqueous solutions of alkali hydroxides.

Dissociation constant. pK_a 2.8 (22°).

Identification. TEST. Dissolve about 10 mg in 3 ml of acetone and add 1 drop of *ferric chloride solution* and 3 ml of water; a wine-red colour is produced.

MELTING-POINT. About 133°.

ULTRAVIOLET ABSORPTION. In 0.01N sodium hydroxide, maximum at 260 nm (E1%, 1cm = 550).

INFRA-RED ABSORPTION. Major peaks at 688, 742, 750, 1305, 1716, and 1750 cm^{-1} (see Appendix 2a: Infra-red Spectra).

Determination in body fluids. HIGH PRESSURE LIQUID CHROMATOGRAPHY. In serum—T. Inaba *et al.*, *J. Chromat.*, 1975, **104**, 165. In plasma or urine—J.-B. Lecaillon and C. Souppart, *J. Chromat.*, 1976, **121**, 227.

Metabolism. ABSORPTION. Readily absorbed after oral administration.

BLOOD CONCENTRATION. After an oral dose of 200 mg, peak plasma concentrations of 13 to 22 μg/ml are attained in 1 to 2 hours.

HALF-LIFE. Plasma half-life, about 3 hours.

DISTRIBUTION. *Protein binding*, appears to be about 98% bound to plasma proteins.

METABOLIC REACTIONS. *p*-Hydroxylation of one of the phenyl rings, hydroxylation at position 4, oxidation of the sulphinyl group, and glucuronic acid conjugation; the metabolites so formed include 1-*p*-hydroxyphenyl-2 - phenyl - 4 - (2 - phenylsulphinylethyl)pyrazolidine - 3,5-dione, 1,2-diphenyl-4-(2-phenylsulphonylethyl)pyrazolidine-3,5-dione, and 4-hydroxy-1,2-diphenyl-4-(2-phenyl-sulphinylethyl)pyrazolidine-3,5-dione.

EXCRETION. About 90% of a dose is excreted in the urine

in 4 days and up to about 10% in the faeces; 50 to 55% is excreted unchanged, 8 to 9% is excreted as the *p*-hydroxy metabolite, 2 to 3% is excreted as the sulphone, 0.5 to 1% is excreted as the 4-hydroxy metabolite and about 30% is excreted as the glucuronides of the unchanged drug and of the sulphone; the urinary excretion of sulphinpyrazone is decreased by the administration of probenecid.

FURTHER INFORMATION. Biotransformation and pharmacokinetics—W. Dieterle *et al.*, *Eur. J. clin. Pharmac.*, 1975, **9**, 135.

Actions and uses. Sulphinpyrazone is a uricosuric agent which is used in the treatment of gout to deplete the tissues of urates, to reduce the plasma-uric-acid concentration by increasing urinary urate excretion, and to diminish the incidence of acute attacks. Its effectiveness is reduced in the presence of citrates and salicylates.

Sulphinpyrazone is also used to reduce platelet adhesiveness in some vascular disorders.

Sulphinpyrazone may be given in conjunction with other uricosuric agents such as probenecid or with allopurinol when one drug alone has proved inadequate.

The usual dosage is 300 to 600 milligrams daily, given in divided doses every 6 to 12 hours, but at the beginning of treatment acute episodes may be precipitated and it is safer to begin with a reduced dosage of 100 to 200 milligrams daily.

Colchicine, in a dosage of 500 micrograms once or twice daily, may be given concurrently with the aim of reducing the incidence of such attacks. The urine should be made alkaline in the initial stages of treatment and an adequate fluid intake ensured.

Treatment must be continued for many months or years before the tophaceous deposits are very much reduced, and regular dosage is essential. In such prolonged treatment, the possibility that blood dyscrasias may occur should be borne in mind.

Precautions. It should not be used in patients who are sensitive to phenylbutazone or other pyrazoles. Salicylates should not be used concurrently.

Contra-indications. Sulphinpyrazone should not be used in the treatment of acute gout. It is contra-indicated in patients with impaired renal function, severe hepatic disease, and active peptic ulcer.

Preparation

SULPHINPYRAZONE TABLETS: available as tablets containing 100 mg of sulphinpyrazone; they are film coated; the coat may be coloured.

A standard for these tablets is given in the British Pharmacopoeia Addendum 1977

Containers and *Storage:* see the entry on Tablets for general information on containers and storage. Containers should be airtight.

Advice for patients: the tablets should preferably be taken after meals. The prescribed course should be completed or, where applicable, treatment should not be discontinued without the advice of the prescriber. Adequate fluid intake should be maintained and preparations containing aspirin should be avoided.

Sulphobromophthalein Sodium

Disodium 5,5′ - [4,5,6,7 - tetrabromo - 3 - oxo - 1(3H) - iso-benzofuranylidene]bis(2-hydroxybenzenesulphonate)

$C_{20}H_8Br_4Na_2O_{10}S_2 = 838.0$

OTHER NAMES: B.S.P.; S.B.P; Sulfobromophthalein Sodium

A standard is given in the British Pharmacopoeia 1973

Description. An odourless, hygroscopic, white, crystal-line powder with a bitter taste.

Solubility. Soluble, at 20°, in 12 parts of water; prac-tically insoluble in alcohol and in acetone.

Moisture content. Not more than 5%, determined by drying at 105°.

Sterilisation. Solutions for injection are sterilised by filtration.

Storage. It should be stored in airtight containers.

Metabolism. BLOOD CONCENTRATION. 10 minutes after an intravenous dose of 5 mg/kg, the amount of sulpho-bromophthalein in the plasma is about 1% of the dose in 100 ml of plasma, falling to about 0.1% in 100 ml by 40 to 60 minutes; in subjects with liver function impair-ment the plasma concentration remains above 0.1% in 100 ml even after 2 hours; the amount of drug remaining in the plasma after the 40- to 60-minute period is a reflection of liver function.

DISTRIBUTION. Distributed throughout the blood circu-lation; *protein binding*, appears to be extensively bound to plasma proteins.

METABOLIC REACTIONS. Metabolised in the liver, pos-sibly by conjugation via the glutathione pathway.

EXCRETION. Almost completely excreted in the bile in 30 to 60 minutes; in liver disease the rate of excretion will vary according to the severity of the condition.

FURTHER INFORMATION. Kinetic analysis of effect of carbon tetrachloride on sulphobromophthalein retention in rats—G. Giorgi and G. Segre, *J. Pharmacokinet. Biopharm.*, 1973, **1**, 217; species variation in metabolism, storage, and excretion—C. D. Klaassen and G. L. Plaa, *Am. J. Physiol.*, 1967, **213**, 1322; metabolism in rats and in man—J. I. Meltzer *et al.*, *Proc. Soc. exp. Biol. Med.*, 1959, **100**, 174; computer simulation of kinetics in rats—B. Montandon *et al.*, *J. Pharmacokinet. Biopharm.*, 1975, **3**, 277; elimination kinetics during continuous infusion—K. Winkler and C. Gram, *Acta med. scand.*, 1965, **178**, 439.

Actions and uses. Sulphobromophthalein sodium is used for testing the functional capacity of the liver, particularly of its reticuloendothelial cells. After intra-venous injection the dye combines with plasma proteins, but it is normally rapidly removed from the blood and excreted in the bile.

The test is usually performed in the morning after the patient has had a fat-free breakfast; no food must be given during the test. A dose of sulphobromophthalein sodium, usually 5 milligrams per kilogram body-weight, is given very slowly as a 5% solution by intravenous injection over a period of about 3 minutes. When fluid retention is present, the dose to be given should be calculated from the patient's ideal weight obtained from tables. Forty-five minutes after the injection, 10 milli-litres of blood is collected from another vein and allowed to clot, special care being taken to avoid haemolysis, and the amount of dye remaining in the serum is determined colorimetrically. In patients with normal liver function not more than 7% of the dye is present in the blood 45 minutes after the injection.

The test should not be performed on patients with a history of drug sensitivity, because of the risk of severe allergic reactions. The 5% solution may yield, on standing, a deposit which may not be readily observed. Immediately before use, therefore, the ampoules con-taining the solution must be immersed in boiling water for 20 minutes, well shaken, and cooled to body temperature.

Sulphonamides

The group of antimicrobial drugs known as "sulphon-amides" or "sulpha" drugs is restricted to N-substituted derivatives of the parent substance sulphanilamide (4-aminobenzenesulphonamide), in which one of the hy-drogen atoms on the sulphonamido group is variously substituted. The second hydrogen atom is sufficiently acidic to form stable salts.

Occasionally there may be an acyl substituent at the N^4 (anilino) function, but in the great majority of these drugs this function is unsubstituted.

The group of drugs known as "sulphonamides" does not subsume numerous other medicinal derivatives of benzenesulphonamide, which generally have different therapeutic actions.

Stability. Exposure to light and heat, especially in the presence of traces of heavy metals, causes sulphon-amides to darken in colour, the intensity of the change depending on the circumstances.

The presence of oxygen and moisture may accelerate the effects of heat and light and, in particular, aqueous solutions of the sodium derivatives, such as sulphacet-amide sodium, require stabilisation by the addition of a suitable antoxidant such as 0.1% of sodium metabi-sulphite. Additional precautions necessary are the use of deoxygenated water as solvent, and minimising ingress of oxygen and light during preparation of the solution. Ideally, the air in the container should be replaced by nitrogen or other suitable gas and this is normally done for solutions to be administered parenterally. For eye-drops, such as sulphacetamide eye-drops, the formula-tion is usually such that the small amount of oxygen in the air-space above the liquid is acceptable and replacing the air with nitrogen is not necessary.

The action of heavy metal ions is reduced by incorporating a suitable chelating agent, such as disodium edetate, in solutions of soluble sulphonamides in water. For a 10% solution of sulphacetamide sodium, for example, 0.02% of disodium edetate is used.

The presence of carbon dioxide may also affect solutions of sodium derivatives of sulphonamides. For example, when solutions of sulphadimidine sodium are exposed to air, carbon dioxide is absorbed and sulphadimidine is precipitated. In this particular case, aqueous solutions are most stable at pH 10 to pH 11 and a fall below pH 10 will also result in precipitation of sulphadimidine.

It is possible to sterilise some sulphonamides by dry heat with minimal degradation provided that all moisture is removed first (see below).

Hydrolysis of water-soluble sulphonamides may occur, especially when heated. For example, sulphacetamide sodium is hydrolysed in aqueous solution to sulphanilamide, a process accelerated by the presence of sodium metabisulphite. It is thus necessary to restrict the concentration of this antoxidant to limit the formation of sulphanilamide. Even so, some crystals of this substance may be deposited in solutions if stored at low temperatures. Hence, in formulations of sulphonamides in aqueous solution, a balance has to be struck to keep both oxidative and hydrolytic effects to a minimum.

Hygroscopicity. Sulphonamides other than the water-soluble derivatives are not hygroscopic. Sulphadimidine sodium absorbs significant amounts of moisture at 25° at a relative humidity of 78%.

Sterilisation. Some sulphonamides may be sterilised by dry heat when they are required in a sterile condition for local application.

The material is first reduced to a fine powder and dried at 100° and then sterilised by dry heat in the final sealed containers; the sterilised powders should not show more than a slight discoloration. This method may be used to sterilise sulphadiazine, sulphadimidine, sulphanilamide, and sulphathiazole.

Aqueous solutions of soluble sulphonamides are sterilised by heating in an autoclave, by heating with a bactericide, or by filtration. The appropriate precautions given above under Stability should be observed. When sterilisation is by filtration, and nitrogen or other suitable gas is used to replace the air in the final container, the gas should be sterile.

Storage. Sulphonamides should be protected from light and should preferably be stored in airtight containers.

Identification. GENERAL TESTS. 1. Dissolve about 100 mg in 2 ml of *dilute hydrochloric acid*, with the aid of heat if necessary, cool in ice, add 4 ml of a 1% solution of sodium nitrite, and pour the mixture into 2 ml of *2-naphthol solution* containing 1 g of sodium acetate; a bright orange-red precipitate is produced (presence of primary aromatic amine).

2. Dissolve about 50 mg in 5 ml of 0.1N sodium hydroxide and add 1 drop of a 1% solution of copper sulphate; a precipitate is produced the colour of which varies with the substance being tested, as shown in the table, below.

Colour	Substance
blue	sulphacetamide sulphaguanidine sulphanilamide
green	phthalylsulphathiazole sulphafurazole sulphamethizole sulphamethoxazole
green turning to brownish-green	sulphapyridine
green turning to dark brown	sulphamerazine
yellowish-green	sulphadimethoxine sulphaquinoxaline
greyish-green	succinylsulphathiazole
greenish-brown	sulphamethoxypyridazine
orange-brown	sulphasalazine
purple-brown	sulphamethoxydiazine sulphathiazole
brown turning to purple-brown	sulphadiazine

MELTING-POINT. The melting-points of a number of sulphonamides are given in the following table.

165° Sulphanilamide	198° Sulphadoxine
170° Sulphamethoxazole	201° Sulphathiazole
181° Sulphamethoxy- pyridazine	201° Sulphadimethoxine
	209° Sulphamethizole
183° Sulphacetamide	211° Sulphamethoxy- diazine
185° Sulphapyrazole	
*190° Succinylsulpha- thiazole	236° Sulphamerazine
	*240° Sulphasalazine
191° Sulphaguanidine	*250° Sulphaquinoxaline
192° Sulphapyridine	*255° Sulphadiazine
196° Sulphafurazole	*275° Phthalylsulpha- thiazole
198° Sulphadimidine	

* with decomposition

ULTRAVIOLET ABSORPTION; INFRA-RED ABSORPTION. Details for individual sulphonamides are given in the appropriate monographs.

THIN-LAYER CHROMATOGRAPHY. See under Thin-layer Chromatography, System 11.

Determination in body fluids. COLORIMETRY. In biological fluids and tissues—A. C. Bratton and E. K. Marshall, *J. biol. Chem.*, 1939, **128**, 537.

GAS CHROMATOGRAPHY. In blood, plasma, serum, or urine: sulphonamides and their N^4-acetyl metabolites —E. Roeder and W. Stuthe, *Z. analyt. Chem.*, 1974, **271**, 281.

Metabolism. The sulphonamides may be divided into 3 groups depending on the degree of absorption and rate of excretion, and these groups correspond with their pharmacological action.

Sulphonamides which are readily absorbed, distributed throughout the body, and slowly excreted are described as long- or intermediate-acting, for example, sulphamethoxydiazine, sulphadoxine, and sulphamethoxazole. The serum elimination half-lives of the drugs in this group vary from 10 to 12 hours for the intermediate-acting and from 17 to 200 hours for the long-acting sulphonamides.

Sulphonamides which are readily absorbed, and distributed throughout the body, but are rapidly excreted, are short-acting, for example sulphadimidine, sulphadiazine, and sulphafurazole. This group has serum half-lives in the range 4 to 7 hours.

Those sulphonamides which are poorly absorbed and are excreted almost entirely in the faeces are used only for the treatment of infections of the gastro-intestinal tract, for example phthalylsulphathiazole and succinylsulphathiazole.

The sulphonamides are usually given orally as the free

drug but occasionally they are given intravenously as the sodium salt or, as in the case of sulphacetamide sodium, applied locally.

ABSORPTION. Sulphonamides, with the exception of those which are insoluble, are readily absorbed from the small intestine and to some extent from the stomach following oral administration. The presence of food delays but does not reduce the amount of absorption.

DISTRIBUTION. The absorbed sulphonamides are well distributed throughout the body tissues and may be detected in saliva and sweat, and in cerebrospinal, ocular, peritoneal, pleural, synovial, and other fluids. All of the sulphonamides are bound to plasma protein to some extent. Both unchanged drugs and acetylated metabolites are bound and the binding affinity is often greater for the acetylated metabolites. Many drugs such as phenylbutazone, probenecid, sulphinpyrazone, indomethacin, and coumarin anticoagulants will displace the sulphonamides from the protein.

Absorbable sulphonamides readily cross the placental barrier and are also found in small amounts in the milk of lactating mothers.

METABOLIC REACTIONS. The absorbable sulphonamides are metabolised to inactive products by the following principal routes: oxidation of the heterocyclic substituent if present, or of the benzene ring; acetylation of the N^4- or N^1-amino groups; and conjugation with sulphuric acid or glucuronic acid at the N^1-, N^4-positions, or at the hydroxyl groups formed by oxidation of the ring structures. The extent of these reactions varies considerably between the sulphonamides and between individuals but the major reaction is N^4-acetylation. Rates of acetylation appear to be genetically determined since there are two distinguishable groups of individuals who acetylate sulphonamides either slowly or rapidly. The liver is the major site of metabolism but N^4-glucuronide formation may occur spontaneously in the urine.

The N^4-acyl sulphonamides which are not absorbed are hydrolysed to some extent by intestinal flora and the resultant free sulphonamide moieties are absorbed.

EXCRETION. The sulphonamides are excreted mainly in the urine but small amounts are also excreted in the bile. Renal excretion is dependent upon glomerular filtration and upon active transport in the proximal tubule.

Many sulphonamides and their acetylated metabolites are poorly soluble in water and precipitate out in the urine. The resulting crystalluria may cause renal damage. Most of the short-acting sulphonamides are excreted within 24 hours whilst the long acting drugs are excreted over periods of up to several weeks. Small amounts of unchanged sulphonamides are excreted with their acetylated metabolites in the bile. Some sulphonamides, excreted in slightly higher quantities in bile, are excreted as conjugates with glucuronic acid.

Sulphur, Precipitated

S = 32.06

OTHER NAMES: *Benoxyl with Sulphur*® and *Vanair*® (both with benzoyl peroxide); *Eskamel*® (with resorcinol)

A standard is given in the British Pharmacopoeia 1973

Description. *Macroscopical:* a soft, pale greyish-yellow or greenish-yellow, odourless powder, free from grittiness.

Microscopical: minute, colourless *spherules*, about 1.5 to 11 μm in diameter, a few occurring singly or in small groups of 2 to 20, but the majority in large irregular clumps of about 100 or more, each clump consisting of spherules of different sizes, the larger ones being less numerous; *crystalline particles* are absent.

When mounted in cresol and examined in polarised light on a dark field, precipitated sulphur assumes a brilliant golden tint with numerous bright green and red points.

Solubility. Practically insoluble in water and in alcohol; almost completely soluble in carbon disulphide, the solution depositing the insoluble variety of sulphur on exposure to light; soluble in hot aqueous solutions of alkali hydroxides with the formation of polysulphides and thiosulphates.

Melting-point. About 115°, forming a yellow mobile liquid which becomes dark and viscous on heating at about 160°.

Actions and uses. Precipitated sulphur is a mild antiseptic and parasiticide.

Preparations of sulphur are applied externally in the treatment of acne. It has also been used in a dose of 1 to 4 grams as a mild laxative.

Preparations

COMPOUND SULPHUR LOTION:

Precipitated sulphur	40 g
Quillaia tincture	5 ml
Glycerol	20 ml
Alcohol (95%)	60 ml
Calcium hydroxide solution	to 1000 ml

Disperse the precipitated sulphur in the alcohol and the glycerol previously mixed, add the quillaia tincture and sufficient of the calcium hydroxide solution to produce the required volume, and mix.

In making this preparation the alcohol (95%) may be replaced by industrial methylated spirit, provided that the law and the statutory regulations governing the use of industrial methylated spirit are observed.

Containers and *Labelling:* see the entry on Lotions for general information on containers and labelling.

Advice for patients: the skin should be cleansed prior to application and the lotion applied sparingly to the affected area. Prolonged use should be avoided and treatment should be discontinued if excessive dryness or irritation of the skin occurs.

RESORCINOL AND SULPHUR PASTE:

Resorcinol, finely sifted	50 g
Precipitated sulphur	50 g
Zinc oxide, finely sifted	400 g
Emulsifying ointment	500 g

Triturate the zinc oxide, the resorcinol, and the precipitated sulphur with a portion of the emulsifying ointment until smooth and gradually incorporate the remainder of the emulsifying ointment.

A standard for this paste is given in the British Pharmaceutical Codex 1973

Containers and *Storage:* see the entry on Pastes for general information on containers and storage. It should be protected from light.

Advice for patients: the skin should be cleansed prior to application and the paste applied to the affected area. Prolonged use should be avoided and treatment should be discontinued if excessive drying or irritation of the skin occurs. It should not be applied to broken or inflamed skin. It may discolour fair hair.

SALICYLIC ACID AND SULPHUR CREAM (*Syn.* Salicylic Acid and Sulphur Application):

Salicylic acid, finely sifted	..	..	..		20 g
Precipitated sulphur, finely sifted	..	..			20 g
Aqueous cream	..	..	..	..	960 g

Triturate the salicylic acid and the sulphur with a portion of the aqueous cream until smooth and gradually add the remainder of the aqueous cream.

A standard for this cream is given in the British Pharmaceutical Codex 1973

Containers, Labelling, and *Storage:* see the entry on Creams for general information on containers, labelling, and storage.

Advice for patients: when used in scalp disorders a small amount of cream should be rubbed gently into the roots of the hair. When used in skin disorders, the cream should be applied sparingly to the affected area. It should not be applied to broken or inflamed skin; contact with the eyes should be avoided. Prolonged use should be avoided and treatment should be discontinued if excessive dryness or irritation of the skin occurs.

SALICYLIC ACID AND SULPHUR OINTMENT:

Salicylic acid, finely sifted	..	..	..		30 g
Precipitated sulphur, finely sifted	..	..			30 g
Oily cream ..	..	..	..	..	940 g

Triturate the salicylic acid and the precipitated sulphur with a portion of the oily cream until smooth and gradually incorporate the remainder of the oily cream.

A standard for this ointment is given in the British Pharmaceutical Codex 1973

Containers: see the entry on Ointments for general information on containers. Containers should prevent evaporation.

Advice for patients: the ointment should be applied sparingly to the affected area. It should not be applied to broken or inflamed skin; contact with the eyes should be avoided. Prolonged use should be avoided and treatment should be discontinued if excessive dryness or irritation of the skin occurs.

SULPHUR OINTMENT (*Syn.* Ung. Sulphur.):

Precipitated sulphur, finely sifted	..	..	100 g
Simple ointment prepared with white			
soft paraffin	..	..	..	..	..	900 g

Triturate the precipitated sulphur with a portion of the simple ointment until smooth and gradually incorporate the remainder of the simple ointment.

A standard for this ointment is given in the British Pharmacopoeia 1973

Containers: see the entry on Ointments for general information on containers.

Advice for patients: see above under Compound Sulphur Lotion.

OTHER PREPARATIONS available include a CREAM containing sulphur 2% with benzoyl peroxide 5%, a cream containing sulphur 2.5% with benzoyl peroxide 10%, a cream containing sulphur 5% with benzoyl peroxide 10%, a cream containing sulphur 8% with resorcinol 2%; a LOTION containing sulphur 2% with benzoyl peroxide 5%, and a lotion containing sulphur 5% with benzoyl peroxide 2%.

Sulphur, Sublimed

S = 32.06

OTHER NAMES: Flowers of Sulphur
Dome-Acne® (with resorcinol monoacetate or salicylic acid)

A standard is given in the British Pharmaceutical Codex 1973

Description. *Macroscopical:* a fine, yellow, slightly gritty powder with a faint and not unpleasant odour.

Microscopical: yellowish *spherules,* about 5 to 40 μm in diameter, a very few isolated, but mostly in fairly large clumps of about 50 to 100 or more; occasional *semicrystalline lumps,* about 150 μm in diameter, occur and result from a somewhat higher temperature in the cooling chamber.

When mounted in cresol and examined in polarised light on a dark field, sublimed sulphur shines brightly with a dull golden-yellow colour.

Solubility. Practically insoluble in water and in alcohol; it is only partially soluble in carbon disulphide and is thereby distinguished from crushed lump sulphur which is completely soluble.

Melting-point. About 115°, forming a yellow mobile liquid which becomes dark and viscous on heating at about 160°.

Actions and uses. Sublimed sulphur has actions and uses similar to those described under Precipitated Sulphur. The usual dose is 1 to 4 grams.

Preparations

Preparations available include an APPLICATION containing sulphur 2% with salicylic acid 2%; a CREAM and a LOTION each containing sulphur 4% with resorcinol monoacetate 3%.

Sulphurated Potash

A mixture of potassium polysulphides and other potassium compounds, including sulphite and thiosulphate, prepared by fusing 2 parts of potassium carbonate with 1 part of sublimed sulphur.

OTHER NAMES: Liver of Sulphur; Potassa Sulphurata

A standard is given in the British Pharmaceutical Codex 1973

Description. Solid fragments, externally greenish-yellow, internally pale liver-brown rapidly changing to greenish-yellow on exposure to air; odour that of hydrogen sulphide.

Solubility. Almost completely soluble, at 20°, in 2 parts of water.

Stability. It readily absorbs moisture and carbon dioxide from the air and undergoes oxidation.

Incompatibility. It is incompatible with acids.

Storage. It should be stored in airtight containers.

Actions and uses. Sulphurated potash is used in the preparation of zinc sulphide lotion which has been used as a peeling agent in the treatment of acne.

Preparation

ZINC SULPHIDE LOTION (*Syn.* Sulphurated Potash and Zinc Lotion; Sulphurated Potash Lotion):

Zinc sulphate	..	..	..	..	50 g
Sulphurated potash		..	..	..	50 g
Concentrated camphor water	..	..	..	25 ml
Water for preparations	..	..	..	to 1000 ml

Dissolve the sulphurated potash and the zinc sulphate each in 450 ml of the water, add the solution of the sulphurated potash to the solution of the zinc sulphate, and stir; add sufficient water to produce almost the required volume, add gradually the concentrated camphor water, shaking thoroughly after each addition, and sufficient water to produce the required volume, and mix. It must be freshly prepared.

Containers and *Labelling:* see the entry on Lotions for general information on containers and labelling.

Advice for patients: the skin should be cleansed prior to application and the lotion applied sparingly to the affected area. Prolonged use should be avoided.

Sulphuric Acid

$H_2SO_4 = 98.07$

A standard is given in the British Pharmaceutical Codex 1973

Impure sulphuric acid of commerce, known as concentrated oil of vitriol, "C.O.V.", contains about 95 to 98% w/w of H_2SO_4; brown oil of vitriol, "B.O.V.", contains 75 to 85% w/w of H_2SO_4.

Nordhausen or fuming sulphuric acid, known commercially as "oleum", is prepared by the addition of sulphur trioxide to sulphuric acid and is available containing various proportions of SO_3.

Battery or accumulator acid is pure sulphuric acid diluted with distilled water to a specific gravity ranging from 1.20 to 1.26.

When diluting sulphuric acid, the acid should be added slowly, with constant stirring, to the water.

Description. A colourless corrosive liquid of oily consistency, evolving much heat when added to water.

Weight per ml. At 20°, about 1.84 g.

Storage. It should be stored in airtight containers.

Actions and uses. Sulphuric acid is a powerful corrosive which chars organic substances. In contact with the skin or mucous membrane it causes intense pain and rapid destruction of tissue.

Poisoning. A stomach tube or emetics should not be used. The acid must be neutralised as quickly as possible. Calcium hydroxide in water and magnesium hydroxide mixture are good antidotes; carbonates should be avoided if possible, as they lead to the liberation of carbon dioxide and the consequent risk of perforation. After neutralisation of the acid, demulcents such as milk, raw eggs, or a vegetable oil such as olive oil should be given and shock should be treated by warmth and intravenous infusions if required. Morphine should be given for the relief of pain.

Sulphuric acid burns should be treated by immediately flooding with water, followed by the application of sodium bicarbonate or chalk in powder, or by the application of sodium bicarbonate or saline packs.

Preparation

DILUTE SULPHURIC ACID: may be prepared by adding 104 g of sulphuric acid gradually, with constant stirring and cooling, to 896 g of purified water, freshly boiled and cooled.

A standard for dilute sulphuric acid is given in the British Pharmaceutical Codex 1973

Actions and uses: dilute sulphuric acid has actions similar to those of other dilute mineral acids. It has occasionally been used in mixtures containing vegetable bitters to stimulate the appetite but this use is difficult to justify. The usual dose is 0.3 to 5 millilitres, well diluted.

Poisoning: the procedure described under Sulphuric Acid should be adopted.

Sulthiame

4 - (Tetrahydro - 2*H* - 1,2 - thiazin - 2 - yl)benzenesulphonamide *SS*-dioxide

$C_{10}H_{14}N_2O_4S_2 = 290.4$

OTHER NAMES: *Ospolot*®; Sultiame

A standard is given in the British Pharmacopoeia 1973

Description. An odourless white crystalline powder with a slightly bitter taste.

Solubility. Very slightly soluble in water; soluble, at 20°, in 350 parts of alcohol, in 500 parts of ether, and in 700 parts of chloroform.

Identification. TEST. In a wide test-tube mix about 50 mg with 1 ml of *strong hydrogen peroxide solution* and 1 drop of *ferric chloride solution*, controlling the reaction by cooling with water if necessary; the colour changes from bright red to light yellow. Add 3 ml of water, 1 ml of *dilute hydrochloric acid* and 0.5 ml of *barium chloride solution*; a white precipitate is produced.

MELTING-POINT. About 186°.

ULTRAVIOLET ABSORPTION. In methyl alcohol, maximum at 246 nm (E1%, 1cm = 400).

INFRA-RED ABSORPTION. Major peaks at 889, 1138, 1158, 1172, 1293, and 1327 cm⁻¹ (see Appendix 2a: Infra-red Spectra).

Determination in body fluids. GAS CHROMATOGRAPHY. In plasma—L. P. Hackett and L. J. Dusci, *Clinica chim. Acta*, 1976, **66**, 443.

Metabolism. ABSORPTION. Readily though somewhat variably absorbed after oral administration.

BLOOD CONCENTRATION. During therapy with oral doses of 3 to 14 mg/kg daily, serum concentrations of 2 to 13 μg/ml are attained; after a single dose, peak serum concentrations are attained in 1 to 5 hours.

DISTRIBUTION. Sulthiame does not appear to accumulate upon repeated administration.

EXCRETION. About 17 to 70% is excreted in the urine as unchanged drug and active metabolites in 24 hours; 10 to 15% is eliminated in the faeces; during long-term therapy, 30% of a daily dose is excreted in the urine unchanged in 24 hours.

FURTHER INFORMATION. Metabolic studies—S. Diamond and L. Levy, *Curr. ther. Res.*, 1963, **5**, 325; blood and urinary concentrations—O. V. Olesen, *Acta pharmac. tox.*, 1968, **26**, 22 and K. J. Simons and R. H. Levy, *J. pharm. Sci.*, 1972, **61**, 1252; a possible interaction of sulthiame and phenytoin—P. N. Patsolos *et al.*, *Proc. analyt. Div. chem. Soc.*, 1975, **12**, 270.

Actions and uses. Sulthiame is an anticonvulsant of low toxicity which is more effective in controlling myoclonic seizures, focal epilepsy, and hyperkinetic behaviour than in influencing grand mal; it is not recommended for the treatment of petit mal. In changing from other anticonvulsants to sulthiame, the transition should be gradual. Sulthiame inhibits the metabolism of primidone and phenobarbitone and so enhances the anticonvulsant action when given in conjunction with these substances. The usual adult dose is 200 milligrams 3 times daily, but, when other therapy has already been instituted, 100 milligrams may be given twice daily as the initial dosage. For children the usual dosage is 10 to 15 milligrams per kilogram body-weight daily in divided doses, but one-third of this dosage should be given initially when other drugs are already being given.

Undesirable effects. The most usual undesirable effects are anorexia, ataxia, and paraesthesia which often disappear in a few days.

Poisoning. Symptoms of overdosage include vomiting, severe headache, vertigo, hyperventilation, and acidosis. Crystalluria may occur but can be prevented by correcting the acidosis and making the urine alkaline.

Preparations

SULTHIAME TABLETS: available as tablets containing 50 and 200 mg of sulthiame; they are film coated.
A standard for these tablets is given in the British Pharmacopoeia 1973
Containers and *Storage:* see the entry on Tablets for general information on containers and storage. Containers should be airtight.
Advice for patients: when initiating treatment there may be a time-lag of up to 2 weeks before a full therapeutic response is obtained. Treatment should not be discontinued without the advice of the prescriber. The tablets may cause drowsiness; persons affected should not drive or operate machinery. Alcohol should be avoided.

OTHER PREPARATIONS available include a MIXTURE containing sulthiame 50 mg in 5 ml, diluent tragacanth mucilage, life of diluted mixture 14 days (for storage of diluted mixtures for more than 14 days, the hydroxybenzoate-sodium carboxymethylcellulose 50 diluent described under Primidone for primidone mixture, or similar, is suitable).

Sunburn

Sunburn results from excessive exposure of the skin to strong sunlight and consists of a painful reddening followed by blistering. If large areas are burned there will be malaise, nausea, and vomiting as seen with other first-degree burns.

Prevention of Sunburn. Ultraviolet radiation of wavelength 290 to 320 nm is mainly responsible for the production of sunburn. In pale-skinned individuals reddening begins 2–8 hours after exposure. Tanning, which is stimulated by radiation of somewhat longer wavelengths, occurs after about 2 days and is accompanied by formation of melanin and thickening of the stratum corneum, thus providing temporary protection against radiation similar to that possessed by dark-skinned persons.
Sunburn may be prevented by avoiding exposure of the skin to the sun, or by increasing exposure to the sun gradually. Alternatively, sunscreens such as aminobenzoic acid lotion and similar preparations which absorb radiation at the harmful wavelengths may be used.

Treatment of Sunburn. Calamine lotion may be used to reduce irritation in mild cases and corticosteroid creams or crotamiton lotion for the more severely afflicted. Antihistamines may be used systemically but when applied topically they are liable to cause skin sensitisation. These treatments are not suitable for weeping and raw areas with severe blistering, for which antiseptic dressings are usually required. Titanium dioxide or zinc oxide paste are suitable for drying up small areas of exudation especially on the nose or lips or other small areas particularly vulnerable. In severe cases systemic corticosteroids may be required.

Suppositories

Suppositories are solid unit-dosage forms which are suitably shaped for rectal administration; they may either melt at body temperature or dissolve or disperse in the mucous secretions of the cavity.

Shapes and sizes. Suppositories are conical, cylindrical, or torpedo-shaped and are usually made in moulds which contain approximately 1 or 2 grams; if no size is stated 1-gram suppositories are supplied. For glycerol suppositories, a 4-gram mould is also used.
In veterinary medicine, suppositories are generally only administered to smaller animals; the usual weights are 1 or 2 grams, and the 1-gram size is supplied if no size is stated.

Absorption. Drugs are frequently administered in suppositories to exert local effects and occasionally to produce systemic action. One possible hazard of this form of medication is that proctitis, that is, inflammation of the rectum or anal area, may result from the irritant effect of some drugs.
Locally-acting drugs include astringents (bismuth subgallate and hamamelis), local anaesthetics (cinchocaine and benzocaine), evacuants (bisacodyl), and corticosteroids (hydrocortisone). Systemic action may also be achieved by administration of drugs in suppositories, for example ergot alkaloids, barbiturates, aminophylline, and chlorpromazine.
Suppositories may be convenient for pre-operative medication, for administration to children, and for drugs liable to cause nausea when administered orally.
Among factors which affect the rate of drug absorption from suppositories are the environmental conditions within the rectum, blood circulation, the pH of rectal fluids, and the physiological state of the rectal mucosa. Physico-chemical characteristics of the drug which influence absorption are the degree of dissociation, the lipid solubility, and the particle size; other important factors are the presence of surface-active agents and the drug concentration. Comparisons have been made between blood concentrations obtained *in vivo* by the administration of drugs by rectal, oral, and intravenous routes but results have been conflicting.

FURTHER INFORMATION. Effect of surface-active agents on drug release from suppository bases—N. A. Allawala and S. Riegelman, *J. Am. pharm. Ass., scient. Edn*, 1953, **42**, 267; M. Kata, *Pharmazie*, 1969, **24**, 395; J. M. Plaxco *et al.*, *J. pharm. Sci.*, 1967, **56**, 809; C. W. Whitworth and J. P. Larocca, *J. Am. pharm. Ass., scient. Edn*, 1959, **48**, 353; drug release from suppositories—J. Anschell and H. A. Lieberman, *Drug Cosmet. Ind.*, 1965, **97**, 341 and 507; Z. Hanko *et al.*, *Farmacia*, 1969, **17**, 705, per *Int. pharm. Abstr.*, 1970, **7**, 2939; R. Malati and T. V. Lehit, *J. Pharm. Pharmac.*, 1970, **22**, 427; N. Senior, *Pharm. J.*, i/1969, 703 and 732; W. H. Thomas and R. McCormack, *J. Pharm. Pharmac.*, 1971, **23**, 490; A. Wiess and B. Sciarrone, *J. pharm. Sci.*, 1969, **58**, 980; effect of pH on absorption—L. S. Schanker, *J. Pharmac. exp. Ther.*, 1959, **126**, 283; absorption *in vivo* of salicylates from theobroma oil and macrogol suppositories—U. Samelius and A. Astrom, *Acta pharmac. tox.*, 1958, **14**, 240; sulphasomidine absorption in rabbits and urinary excretion in human subjects—L. Pennati and K. Steiger-Trippi, *Pharm. Acta Helv.*, 1958,

33, 663; T. W. Schwartz and K. Bichsel, *Pharm. Acta Helv.*, 1963, **38**, 861; effect of sodium lauryl sulphate on absorption *in vivo* of aprobarbitone sodium—K. Ulrich and C. F. Wiese, *Arch. Pharm. Chemi*, 1967, **74**, 921; effect of four bases on absorption of salicylates—W. Lowental and J. F. Borzellaca, *J. pharm. Sci.*, 1965, **54**, 1790 and 1966, **55**, 151; absorption rates of soluble barbiturates from theobroma and macrogol bases—W. H. Hasler and G. J. Sperandio, *J. Am. pharm. Ass., pract. Edn*, 1953, **14**, 26; comparison of routes of administration of theophylline preparations—H. P. M. Kerkhoffs and T. Huizinga, *Pharm. Weekbl. Ned.*, 1967, **102**, 1183 and 1255.

Suppository bases. Ideally, the basis should melt or otherwise deform or dissolve to release its drug content at 37°; it should be non-irritating, non-toxic and non-sensitising; it should be compatible with a wide range of drugs and be readily moulded or formed into stable, rigid shapes which maintain uniform drug-release characteristics on storage.

Theobroma oil softens and melts between 30° and 35°. It is a mixture of solid and liquid triglycerides, chiefly 2-oleopalmitostearin and 2-oleodistearin.

Theobroma oil has the disadvantage that there is only a small amount of shrinkage on solidification which gives poor moulding properties. It exists in four polymorphic forms with different melting-points, and to minimise the formation of the unstable low melting-point forms, theobroma oil should only be heated for short periods and the temperature kept below 36°. When the melting-point of theobroma oil has been reduced by the addition of drugs such as volatile oils and chloral hydrate, it may be raised by the addition of 3 to 5% of beeswax.

Theobroma oil has a low absorptive capacity for water. Absorption can be improved by adding surface-active agents, such as cholesterol 2%, wool fat 5 to 10%, or polysorbates 5 to 10%. However, drug-basis interaction and changes in absorption characteristics may be induced at the same time.

Hard-fat alternatives to theobroma oil. Esterified, hydrogenated, or fractionated vegetable oils together with synthetic triglyceride mixtures have been produced commercially as alternatives to theobroma oil. Most of the synthetic bases have the advantage of freedom from polymorphism and the risk of rancidity; they usually require no mould lubricant and are available in various grades with different melting ranges and physico-chemical characteristics. They include *Extracoa®* and *Supercoa®* (grades of fractionated palm kernel oil) and various fatty bases marketed under the names Adeps Solidus, *Estarinum®*, *Massuppol®*, *Novata®*, *Suppocire®*, *Wecobee®*, and *Witepsol®*.

Glycerol suppository basis. The formula for this basis is given under Glycerol Suppositories in the entry on Glycerol. This water-soluble basis which contains glycerol 70% and gelatin 14% dissolves slowly in the mucous secretion. Factors which influence the dissolution rate of glycerol-gelatin basis in body fluid are the relative proportions of the basic constituents, the type of gelatin used, and its reaction with the active drug. Because glycerol is hygroscopic the basis requires protection from heat and moisture. The basis may also support microbial growth and the inclusion of preservatives may be necessary; methyl and propyl hydroxybenzoates have been recommended.

Gelatin is available in a number of grades and unless the correct type is used, there may be an incompatibility. There are two pharmaceutical grades which may be used to overcome this problem. Type A is prepared from an acid-treated precursor and is most effective at a pH of about 3.2. It is cationic and will be compatible with substances such as boric acid, lactic acid, and bismuth subnitrate. Type B is prepared from a limed precursor, its most effective pH is between 7 and 8, and it is anionic. It can therefore be used with ichthammol and zinc oxide.

Macrogols (polyethylene glycols). Water-soluble macrogols of various molecular weights have been blended to produce suppository bases which differ in their melting-point ranges, physical characteristics, and dissolution rates. Macrogols have the advantage of stability, inertness, high water capacity, and freedom from rancidity; they are useful as vehicles for drugs such as chloral hydrate and ichthammol which tend to lower the melting-points of other bases. Usually no mould lubricant is required but suppositories may be brittle unless the molten basis is poured into the mould at as low a temperature as possible. Brittleness can be reduced by the addition of surface-active agents or plasticisers such as castor oil or propylene glycol.

Macrogol bases are available which melt above body temperature; they offer less risk of leakage from body cavities and present fewer storage problems than lower melting-point bases. Because macrogol bases usually dissolve readily in the body fluids their drug release rates tend to differ from those obtained from fatty or glycerol bases. Substances which are incompatible with macrogols include tannic acid, benzocaine, clioquinol, quinine salts, silver salts, and sulphonamides.

Typical mixtures of macrogols are shown below. Dehydration of the rectal mucosa with consequent irritant effects can arise from the administration of macrogol bases formulated without water. Such irritant effects can be reduced by immersing the suppository in water before insertion or by the application of coatings of cetyl or stearyl alcohol, though these may retard dissolution.

Macrogol suppository bases. The following combinations of macrogols have appeared in the literature.*

1. Macrogol 1000 .. .. 96%
   Macrogol 4000 .. .. 4%

A low melting point basis which is useful if relatively rapid dissolution is desired. It may require refrigeration during the summer months.

2. Macrogol 1000 .. .. 75%
   Macrogol 4000 .. .. 25%

A more stable formulation than Basis 1; can be used if the suppository is to be subjected to extreme storage conditions.

3. Macrogol 1540 .. .. 70%
   Macrogol 6000 .. .. 30%

The melting-point of this basis is high enough to compensate for the lowering of melting-point by chloral hydrate, ichthammol, camphor, etc.

4. Macrogol 6000 .. .. 50%
   Macrogol 1540 .. .. 30%
   Macrogol 400 .. .. 20%

A good general purpose basis.

5. Macrogol 6000 .. .. 50%
   Macrogol 1540 .. .. 30%
   Water and medicament 20%

Contains water to facilitate the incorporation of medicaments soluble in water but not in macrogols.

* Bases 1 to 4—A. P. Collins *et al.*, *Am. prof. Pharm.*, 1957, **23**, 231. Bases 5 and 6—W. H. Hassler and G. J. Sperandio, *J. Am. pharm. Ass., pract. Edn*, 1953, **14**, 26.

6. Macrogol 6000 .. .. 47%
    Macrogol 4000 .. .. 33%
    Water and medicament 20%

Similar to Basis 5, but with a higher melting point.

Other bases. Hydrophilic or water-dispersible bases have been formulated which contain mainly non-ionic surface-active agents, either alone or mixed with vegetable oils or waxy solids.

Suppositories made by compression from effervescent bases which release carbon dioxide in the presence of moisture are used to induce peristalsis in the lower bowel.

FURTHER INFORMATION. Hydrophilic bases containing methylcellulose and sodium carboxymethylcellulose —W. D. Walkling, *Diss. Abstr.*, 1967, **27**, 4007B.

Coatings. Layered suppositories with an outer shell which melts at 37° to 38° and an inner core with a lower melting-point have been prepared as a means of controlling the rate of absorption and in order to separate incompatible drugs.

Coatings consisting of materials such as cetyl alcohol, macrogols, or polyvinyl alcohol and polysorbates have been applied by dipping to increase the disintegration time, to act as lubricants, and to prevent adhesion on storage.

FURTHER INFORMATION. Preparation of two-layer suppositories—N. Sharova *et al.*, *Farmatsiya (Moscow)*, 1969, **18**, 21, per *Chem. Abstr.*, 1969, **71**, 15991p.

Rectal (soft) gelatin capsules. This new unit-dosage form consists of the medicament and basis enclosed in a soft gelatin capsule shell of suitable size and shape. The contents should be solid at room temperature, as with conventional suppositories. Vegetable oils, solid fats, and their derivatives, together with surfactants such as glyceryl monostearate and polysorbates may be used in formulations. Rectal absorption studies demonstrate that efficient drug release and systemic absorption is achieved. Hydrophilic materials such as propylene glycol and macrogols of low molecular weight cannot be used as they may soften the capsule shell.

Rectal (soft) gelatin capsules are suitable for use in tropical climates, provided they are hermetically sealed. Special machinery is used for the production of these capsules.

Methods of preparation of suppositories

Although cold compression has been used on a small scale, the most common method of small- or large-scale preparation is by pouring the melted mass into suitable moulds. Traditionally, plated metal or stainless steel moulds have been used but these are being replaced, to some extent, by cheaper disposable moulds of plastic materials in which the suppositories are cast and remain enclosed until removal by the patient.

Moulds can be pre-formed from semi-rigid films of polyvinyl chloride or polyethylene or from aluminium; more rigid plastic moulds are also available. After sealing within such moulds, suppositories will withstand tropical conditions or high storage temperatures without distortion. When selecting packaging of this type, care must be taken to ensure that the plastic material is compatible with and impermeable to both the active constituents and other ingredients in the suppository. Metal foils may not be suitable for suppositories containing acidic substances.

Lubricants. The adhesion of theobroma oil to metal moulds can be minimised by the application of lubricants or release agents such as alcoholic solutions of soft soap and glycerin, silicones, and sodium lauryl sulphate in aqueous solution or in propylene glycol. The silicones can be applied, on the large scale, by a spraying technique. For macrogol-based suppositories a mineral oil may be used while for glycerol-gelatin bases vegetable oil or liquid paraffin is suitable.

Displacement value. Because the density of the medicament affects the amount of basis required for each suppository it is necessary to make an allowance for each medicament in terms of the particular basis; this allowance is termed the "displacement value".

Displacement values, that is the quantity of medicament which displaces one part of theobroma oil, are shown below. The same figure may be used for other fatty bases. For glycerol suppository basis, about 1.2 grams occupies the same volume as 1 gram of theobroma oil.

Medicament	Displacement Value
Aloin	1.3
Alum	1.8
Aminophylline	1.3
Aspirin	1.1
Barbitone	1.2
Barbitone sodium	1.2
Beeswax, white	1.0
Belladonna extract	1.3
Bismuth subgallate	2.7
Bismuth subnitrate	5.0
Camphor	2.0
Castor oil	1.0
Chloral hydrate	1.4
Cinchocaine	1.5
Cinchocaine hydrochloride	1.0
Cocaine hydrochloride	1.4
Codeine phosphate	1.1
Digitalis leaf	1.6
Dimenhydrinate	1.3
Diphenhydramine hydrochloride	1.3
Eucalyptus oil	1.0
Glycerol	1.6
Hamamelis dry extract	1.5
Hydrocortisone (or acetate)	1.5
Ichthammol	1.0
Menthol	0.7
Morphine hydrochloride	1.6
Morphine sulphate	1.6
Opium, powdered	1.5
Paraffin	1.0
Pentobarbitone sodium	1.2
Pethidine hydrochloride	1.6
Phenobarbitone sodium	1.2
Phenobarbitone	1.1
Podophyllum resin	1.3
Potassium iodide	4.5
Procaine hydrochloride	1.2
Quinalbarbitone sodium	1.2
Quinine hydrochloride	1.1
Resorcinol	1.5
Salicylic acid	1.3
Sulphathiazole	1.6
Sulphur	1.6
Tannic acid	1.3
Vegetable extracts	1.5
Zinc oxide	4.7
Zinc sulphate	2.4

A displacement value of 1.0 is generally adopted for liquids. Each mould should be calibrated with the particular basis before the displacement due to the medicament is calculated.

Moulding

Theobroma oil suppositories. The appropriate quantity of basis is melted over a water-bath by the application of as little heat as possible and the medicament is dissolved or incorporated. When almost at the solidification point, the uniform mass is poured into the lightly lubricated mould which is overfilled to allow for contraction on cooling. On solidification, the excess mass is trimmed off and after further cooling the suppositories are removed.

Synthetic bases and macrogol suppositories. A procedure similar to the above is adopted though it may not be necessary to include a lubricant.

Glycerol suppository basis. After incorporation or dissolution of the medicament the melted basis should be stirred as little as possible to avoid the formation of unsightly air bubbles. Ideally, the mould cavities are not overfilled since the cooled mass does not contract.

Incorporation of medicaments. Insoluble drugs are finely powdered and levigated with a little of the melted basis; immiscible liquids are treated similarly. The mixture is then added to the bulk of the melted basis. Soluble solids in powder, and miscible liquids are added directly to the basis. Special care is required in the case of suppositories containing chloral hydrate, in both theobroma oil and synthetic bases. When the liquid content is sufficiently high to reduce the rigidity of the suppository, an inert powder such as starch or magnesium oxide may be introduced. If the plasticity of the suppository mass is reduced due to the inclusion of a high concentration of powders it may be restored by the addition of a small amount of vegetable oil. The use of water for this purpose in fatty bases can lead to drug interaction or crystallisation, microbial spoilage, or rancidity of the basis.

FURTHER INFORMATION. Formulation of chloral hydrate suppositories—D. D. Breimer *et al., Pharm. Weekbl. Ned.,* 1973, **108**, 1101; H. L. M. Cox, *Pharm. Weekbl. Ned.,* 1971, **106**, 530; G. E. Schumacher, *Am. J. Hosp. Pharm.,* 1966, **23**, 110.

Testing. A close relationship has not yet been established between test methods for suppositories *in vitro* and *in vivo,* and pharmacopoeial tests are usually limited to appearance, disintegration, uniformity of weight, and drug content. Other tests which may be applied are the determination of softening and liquefaction temperatures, hardness, and friability.

FURTHER INFORMATION. Content uniformity of suppositories—I. Setnikar and F. Fountain, *J. pharm. Sci.,* 1970, **59**, 1319; weight uniformity specifications—I. Setnikar and V. Pietra, *J. pharm. Sci.,* 1969, **58**, 112; identification of analgesics, antipyretics and hypnotics in suppositories by thin-layer chromatography—F. Schmidt, *Pharm. Ztg, Berlin,* 1969, **114**, 1523.

Containers. Suppositories should be supplied in rigid, shallow boxes of paperboard, metal, or plastic materials. The boxes should be partitioned or lined with waxed paper. When intended for use in tropical or subtropical climates or when containing volatile ingredients, suppositories should be wrapped separately in waxed paper, in metal foil, or enclosed in a suitable form of strip packing. Glycerol suppositories and macrogol bases of low molecular weight are hygroscopic and should be suitably protected.

Storage. They should be stored in a refrigerator or in a cool place.

Labelling. When dispensed, suppositories should be labelled with directions to the patient with regard to unwrapping, the route of administration, and the need for low temperature storage.

Use of suppositories. Suppositories should be inserted as high as possible in the rectum. They may be retained in position by crossing the legs or lying on the side. If necessary they may be lubricated with a small quantity of olive oil before insertion.

Suramin

The symmetrical 3″-urea of the sodium salt of 8-(3-benzamido-4-methylbenzamido)naphthalene-1,3,5-trisulphonic acid.

$C_{51}H_{34}N_6Na_6O_{23}S_6 = 1429.2$

OTHER NAME: Suramin Sodium

A standard is given in the British Pharmaceutical Codex 1973

Description. An odourless hygroscopic white, pinkish-white or faintly cream-coloured powder.

Solubility. Soluble, at 20°, in less than 1 part of water; very slightly soluble in alcohol; practically insoluble in ether and in chloroform.

Moisture content. Not more than 10%, determined by Fischer titration.

Storage. It should be stored in airtight containers, in a cool place, protected from light.

Identification. TEST. Mix about 50 mg with a mixture of 1 ml of water and 1 ml of sulphuric acid, boil for 5 minutes, cool, add 20 ml of water and 20 mg of sodium nitrite, allow to stand for 1 minute, add 200 mg of urea, shake and allow to stand for 2 minutes, and then add 4 drops of this solution to a solution of 10 mg of N-(1-naphthyl)ethylenediamine hydrochloride and 500 mg of sodium acetate in 5 ml of acetic acid; a magenta colour is produced.

Metabolism. BLOOD CONCENTRATION. After intravenous administration, high concentrations are achieved in plasma which fall rapidly; low concentrations are maintained for 10 to 12 weeks.

DISTRIBUTION. Does not enter tissues readily but high concentrations are obtained in the kidneys; *protein binding,* highly bound to plasma proteins.

METABOLIC REACTIONS. Does not appear to be metabolised.

Actions and uses. Suramin is effective against the early stages of trypanosomiasis, particularly in patients infected with *Trypanosoma rhodesiense*. It does not cross the blood-brain barrier and is valueless in more advanced stages of trypanosomiasis in which the central nervous system is involved.

Suramin is also of value in the treatment of onchocerciasis.

Before starting a course of treatment, the patient's tolerance to suramin should be tested by a dose of 200 milligrams given intravenously. If no untoward reactions occur within 24 to 48 hours, a further dose of 1 gram is given and repeated weekly, usually until 5 grams has been given. A dosage of 2 grams weekly for 5 weeks has also been given. The urine should be tested before each dose is given and if protein is present the dosage should be reduced or administration delayed. The interval between doses may be shortened if no proteinuria develops.

Subcutaneous injection of suramin is painful and liable to produce necrosis.

Suramin is also used prophylactically against trypanosomiasis, a dose of 2 grams conferring protection for at least 3 months.

In onchocerciasis, suramin is effective against the adult parasites but it has little action on the microfilariae of *Onchocerca volvulus* except in high concentrations. It is usually given after a course of diethylcarbamazine.

The dose corresponding to an adult dose of 1 gram is, for children under 1 year, up to 25 milligrams per kilogram body-weight, 1 to 5 years 250 to 400 milligrams, and 6 to 12 years 450 to 700 milligrams.

Undesirable effects. Suramin may produce toxic effects, the chief of which is damage to the kidneys; the occurrence of proteinuria indicates the need for caution in further treatment. Other toxic reactions include vomiting, rashes, peripheral neuritis, amblyopia, shock, loss of consciousness, urticaria, paraesthesia, and photophobia.

Precautions. As with pentamidine, it is important to detect the more advanced infections and to treat them with a drug such as melarsoprol. Suramin should not be given to patients who have been shown to be intolerant to a test dose or those who have renal disease.

Preparation

SURAMIN INJECTION: a sterile solution of suramin in water for injections. It is prepared by dissolving the contents of a sealed container in water for injections immediately before use.

A standard for this injection is given in the British Pharmaceutical Codex 1973

Containers and *Labelling:* see the entry on Injections for general information on containers and labelling.

Storage: the sealed container should be stored in a cool place, protected from light. The injection decomposes on storage and should be used immediately after preparation.

Surgical Dressings

In this entry, surgical dressings are subdivided into six main categories according to their uses, and these categories are further subdivided into sections containing materials having a similar type of construction, as follows:

Absorbents
  Fabric Absorbents
  Fibrous Absorbents
  Fabric and Fibrous Combined Absorbents
  Medicated Absorbents

Wound Dressings
  Wound Dressing Pads
  Non-adherent Wound-contact Dressings
  Self-adhesive Dressing Pads
  Standard Dressings
  Other Wound Dressings

Bandages
  Retention Bandages
  Non-adhesive Support and Compression Bandages
  Adhesive Support and Compression Bandages
  Medicated Bandages

Surgical Adhesive Tapes
  Woven Tapes
  Non-woven Tapes
  Plastic Film Tapes
  Non-stitch Adhesive Sutures

Protectives

Plasters
  Unmedicated Plasters
  Medicated Plasters

To find information on articles suitable for a particular purpose, the appropriate category should be determined and a selection made from the items listed. To locate information when the name of the article or dressing is known, the main index should be used.

Sterilisation. Information on the sterilisation of surgical dressings is given in the entry on Sterilisation.

Packaging. All dressings should be packed in a well-closed package, which protects the contents from contamination with extraneous solids and does not allow the contents to be released unintentionally under normal conditions of handling, storage, and transport.

In addition, and in accordance with the requirements of the user, dressings may be packed in a sealed package. This is a well-closed package which is sealed in such a manner that the seal must be broken, and be seen to be broken, before the contents are used; the seal is not replaceable. If the product is labelled "sterile", the package must also exclude micro-organisms. Special considerations applicable to sterile surgical dressings are given in the entry on Sterilisation.

Waxed paper should not be used for any wrapping in contact with gauze products, lint products or cotton wool, as it reduces the absorbency of the material.

Labelling. The label on the outer wrapper of a package of a sterile surgical dressing should state: "Sterile. This package shall not be issued nor the contents used if the wrapper(s) or seal is broken".

In addition, if the inner wrapper encloses more than one dressing, the label on the outer wrapper should also state: "Unused contents should be discarded as non-sterile". If the product is dyed, the colour should be stated on the label.

Storage. Surgical dressings should be stored in a cool, dry, well-ventilated place.

The initial absorbency of surgical dressings is generally lost or much diminished after long storage or exposure to heat or damp. When stored under suitable conditions in temperate climates there is usually little loss of absorbency within 2 years of the date of manufacture, but occasionally the loss is more rapid.

Absorbents

Absorbents may be classified into three types: (i) fabric absorbents, such as gauze and lint; (ii) fibrous absorbents, such as cotton wool and cellulose wadding; and (iii) absorbents made of a combination of these materials.

Some absorbents may be medicated and many are available sterile.

Fabric Absorbents

GAUZE consists of either cotton cloth of plain weave (Absorbent Cotton Gauze; Absorbent Gauze; Gauze; Unmedicated Gauze; Tela Gossypii Absorbens) or a mixed cotton and viscose cloth of plain weave, containing up to 45% of viscose, in which the warp or the weft threads may be either 100% cotton or of blended composition; the weft threads may also be of 100% viscose. (Cotton and Viscose Gauze; Cotton and Rayon Gauze). Gauze is usually supplied in pieces, 900 mm wide, in various lengths and folded into convenient sizes. Standards for eight types of cotton gauze, differing in the number of threads per cm² (that number being the basis for the type number) and weight per unit area, are given in the European Pharmacopoeia, Volume II; the type designated "13 light" is the one generally used in the United Kingdom. The other seven European types are all less open and heavier than the British product.

A standard for Cotton and Viscose Gauze is given in the Supplement 1976 to the British Pharmaceutical Codex 1973.

Both Absorbent Cotton Gauze and Cotton and Viscose Gauze are available with a radio-opaque member incorporated in their construction to facilitate their detection if inadvertently left in the body during surgical procedures. The radio-opaque member may be a mono- or multi-filament; the image produced by a multifilament is less clear than that produced by a monofilament, but the better handling properties of a product containing a multifilament member may be preferred in certain procedures. A standard for X-ray-detectable Absorbent Gauze is given in the British Pharmaceutical Codex 1973. When Absorbent Cotton Gauze, Absorbent Gauze, Gauze or Unmedicated Gauze is prescribed or demanded, Cotton and Viscose Gauze may be supplied.

Gauze absorbs water and fluids readily, but its absorbency may be reduced considerably by medication, by prolonged storage, by exposure to elevated temperatures and by contact with waxed paper packaging. On sterilisation, it may shrink a little and discolour slightly.

Gauze is used in a number of simple and compound absorbent products. The simple absorbents fall into two broad categories: (i) those of the "swab" type, produced by folding and sometimes stitching, such as swabs, pads, strips, and pledgets, and (ii) those consisting of plain material, such as packs and ribbon. For information on compound absorbent products see under Fabric and Fibrous Combined Absorbents, below.

Gauze swabs consist of gauze folded into squares or rectangles in such a manner that the cut edges of the cloth are not exposed. They are available commercially in various sizes, ranging from 50 mm square to 200 mm square, and in various plies from 4 to 32; unusual sizes are produced extemporaneously to meet specific requirements. They are normally supplied in "tied 5's" to facilitate the checking of used swabs in operating theatres.

Gauze pads are swabs in the form of large squares or rectangles which have been stitched on the three open sides; a length of tape is stitched on to one corner in order to facilitate recovery of pads after use.

Gauze strips are rectangles of folded gauze stitched on the three open sides.

Pledgets are small squares of gauze, folded and stitched, or rolled, to form tight pads or balls.

Gauze packs consist of gauze, cut from large pieces and folded or rolled to give 8 plies, 2 to 3 m long and 100 to 200 mm wide. Absorbent ribbon gauze is described below.

All these products are available with a radio-opaque member incorporated in their construction.

Some of the products are available coloured with a suitable non-toxic blue or green dye in order to distinguish those used by anaesthetists from those used by surgeons.

Standards covering gauze swabs, pads, and strips are given in the British Pharmaceutical Codex 1973 under the titles Gauze Pad and X-ray-detectable Gauze Pad.

Uses. Gauze in its various forms is used pre-operatively, during operations, and post-operatively. In routine pre-operative preparation of a patient, the extent of which will depend upon the nature of the surgery, a defined area of the skin is swabbed with coloured antiseptic solution by means of a folded swab held in a swab holder; usually, two applications of distinctively coloured solution are made, the colour distinguishing the prepared area from the rest of the body. For this application, Absorbent Lint (see below), *Regal*® swabs (see under Fabric and Fibrous Combined Absorbents, below), and polyurethane sponge cubes are sometimes used instead.

If radio-opaque swabs are used, they are either removed from the operating theatre when preparation is complete, or hung on a swab rack and an entry made on the swab-count board to the effect that those swabs have been used at preparation.

Non-radio-opaque products are either used in a preparation area outside the operating theatre or kept on a separate preparation trolley which is removed from the theatre on completion of the preparation.

During surgery, gauze is used for several purposes. For absorbing blood and other body fluids, small swabs of low ply are used for superficial work and in the primary stages of surgery; larger unstitched swabs are used in cavities. Low-ply swabs are unsuitable for use in swab holders, as the metal jaws may protrude through the material and traumatise tissues. Generally, the higher-ply, and therefore bulkier, swabs are to be preferred because they are equally satisfactory whether they are hand held or grasped in holders. Gauze strips, 100 mm long and 25 mm wide, are frequently used in ear, nose, throat, and ophthalmic surgery.

To prevent damage to tissues and organs that may be obscuring or obstructing the operation site and to improve access to the area, gauze pads or packs are inserted into the cavity in a procedure known as "packing off". When a pack is used, sufficient is left outside the cavity to facilitate removal. The pads used are generally 12-ply and are 225 or 450 mm square; the attached tape is left outside the cavity and an artery forcep clipped to the free end.

If the packing off is carried out with dry dressings and there is a limited amount of body fluid present, the dressing may continue its primary function of absorption and cause excessive drying of the tissues and organs. If these are to be exposed for any length of time, the pads are immersed in warm sterile saline and squeezed out before insertion into the cavity; the damp dressings will now prevent undue drying out but will continue to absorb excess fluids. Damp pads may also be positioned between tissues and retractor blades to prevent pressure trauma.

Pads are also used to apply warmth to tissues and organs which become devitalised due to restriction of their blood supply. If there is any doubt regarding their viability, it is normal practice to apply pads which have been immersed in hot sterile saline solution and wrung out; the application of heat is also used to produce vasodilatation on a bleeding surface in order to identify the larger vessels that can be ligated. Heat is also applied in the same manner to the uterus after Caesarean section to assist contraction and retraction.

Small swabs and pledgets are applied directly to produce haemostatis and thus keep the operation site unobstructed by blood. The blood flow may be stopped either by direct application of pressure or, as in middle-ear surgery, the material is first saturated with adrenaline solution before positioning. Small swabs and pledgets are also frequently used to assist in dissection of tissues; they are wrapped round fingers or grasped in swab holders and used to cleave the muscle in the process of blunt dissection. For fine dissection, pledgets are held in artery forceps, care being taken to ensure that the ends of the forceps do not protrude beyond the material. For post-operative packing, packs or ribbon gauze are used to prevent the accumulation of haematomata, to keep "dead space" to a minimum and to allow cavity drainage. Ribbon gauze, 250 mm wide and with a radio-opaque multifilament member, is used together with a roll of radio-opaque gauze 150 mm wide; the end of the gauze is left outside the body and the gradual withdrawal of the pack allows the natural reduction of the cavity. To guard against the risk of adhesion and infection caused by "bacterial wicking", the gauze is sometimes impregnated with sterile liquid paraffin, proflavine emulsion or, rarely, eusol-liquid paraffin.

ABSORBENT RIBBON GAUZE (Unmedicated Ribbon Gauze) consists of cloth of plain weave, in which the warp threads are of cotton and the weft threads are of cotton or viscose, or of a combined cotton and viscose yarn. It is supplied in ribbons of various widths and lengths, with fast selvedges, and is available with and without a radio-opaque member. The cloth is less open in construction than Absorbent Gauze (13 Light), and the yarn is heavier than that in the corresponding type of European gauze; in other respects, its properties are similar to those described for Gauze (see above). Standards are given in the British Pharmaceutical Codex 1973 under the titles Absorbent Ribbon Gauze and X-ray-detectable Absorbent Ribbon Gauze.

Uses. Absorbent ribbon gauze, without a radio-opaque member, is used in one continuous length, usually 5 to 15 mm wide, to pack sinus, dental, and throat cavities; sufficient material must be left outside the cavity to facilitate its removal.

Material containing viscose swells as it absorbs fluids and this must be taken into account when packing in order to avoid the development of intracavity pressure and resulting pain to the patient.

Ribbon gauze, suitably medicated, may be used for pre-operative nasal packing. It is also used to pack infected open wounds to assist healing; for this purpose, it may be impregnated with euflavine, acriflavine, or eusol preparations. For other uses see under Gauze (above).

ABSORBENT LINT (Lint; Plain Lint; White Lint) consists of cloth of plain weave in which the warp threads are of cotton and the weft threads are of cotton or viscose, or of a combined cotton and viscose yarn; on one side of the cloth, a nap has been raised from the warp yarns. A standard is given in the British Pharmaceutical Codex 1973.

It absorbs water and fluids readily, but its absorbency may be reduced considerably by medication, by prolonged storage, by exposure to elevated temperatures, and by contact with waxed paper packaging.

Uses. Lint, in its unmedicated form, is used as an external absorbent and protective dressing, and is used widely in first-aid treatment in the home. Traditionally, it has been used as a wound dressing with the unlinted side in contact with the wound, the linted surface offering a large surface area for evaporation of water from wound exudate. However, the use of non-adherent materials is generally preferred.

ABSORBENT MUSLIN (Bleached Muslin) is a bleached cotton cloth of plain weave. A standard is given in the British Pharmaceutical Codex 1973.

Absorbent muslin is occasionally used in the treatment of extensive burns and as a wet dressing. It is a component of Eye Pad with Bandage (see under Wound Dressings: Standard Dressings).

OTHER FABRIC ABSORBENTS include the following proprietary products. *Sofnet®* swabs consist of a non-woven viscose fabric folded into pieces of various dimensions. They are occasionally used in error as a simple wound dressing. They have a lower total absorbent capacity than gauze but absorb more quickly because of the random orientation of their fibres. They can replace gauze swabs for general-purpose swabbing and cleansing procedures.

Sponcel® consists of cellulose sponge in the form of sheets and thin bands. It is used to absorb at small sites in surgery. The material is not radio-opaque and tends to lose particles; special precautions must therefore be taken when it is used in surgical procedures.

Neuropatties (*Cottonoid®*; *Macron®*; *Plintine®*; *Steripon®*) are small squares or strips of non-woven absorbent viscose material in various sizes with a thread stitched through the fabric and left long. They are used as "spot absorbents", particularly in neurosurgery. They are often moistened with sterile sodium chloride solution before application. The threads are left outside the surgical area to facilitate recovery.

Fibrous Absorbents

ABSORBENT COTTON WOOL (Absorbent Cotton; Lanugo Gossypii Absorbens) is prepared from cotton, which consists of the epidermal trichomes of *Gossypium herbaceum* L. and other cultivated species of *Gossypium* (Fam. Malvaceae). The seeds are removed mechanically and the trichomes freed from fatty matter by treatment with alkali, bleached, washed, and mechanically loosened and separated to form a fleecy mass of soft white filaments which consist almost entirely of cellulose. A standard is given in the European Pharmacopoeia, Vol. II.

Cotton wool absorbs water and fluids readily, but its absorbency may be reduced considerably by medication, by prolonged storage, by exposure to elevated temperatures, and by contact with waxed paper packaging. It may be attacked by moulds when stored under conditions which allow the moisture in the product to exceed about 9%.

Cotton wool is available in a number of different grades. The better grades are those which conform to the specification of the European Pharmacopoeia Vol. II. Lower quality materials, with a shorter staple length and more neps, are generally less resilient and contain more dust; these grades include those often described as "hospital quality" and "general purpose". Cotton wool is available in the form of rolled sheets or as balls, and the grade and form chosen will depend on the use to which it is to be put.

Cotton wool of European Pharmacopoeia quality should be used for procedures such as cleansing and swabbing wounds, pre-operative skin preparation, and the application of medicaments to the skin. It is sufficiently resilient to provide an effective pad for use over dressings to protect the wound and to absorb wound exudate. For insertion into orifices such as the ear and nose, for application to the eye and throat and for the preparation of swabs for taking specimens, it is advisable to use cotton wool with a longer average staple length than the minimum specified (10 mm). For these purposes and for cleansing, it is used in the form of balls.

Lower-grade materials should not be used in any situation where the loss of fibres may be detrimental to the patient, such as for cleansing wounds, or where the creation of dust may cause an environmental hazard, as in a ward for respiratory diseases; they may be used as general purpose absorbents, for swabbing, and for routine cleansing of incontinent patients.

ABSORBENT VISCOSE WADDING (Lanugo Cellulosi Absorbens) consists of bleached new fibres of regenerated cellulose or of delustred regenerated cellulose obtained by the viscose process and cut to a suitable staple length. A standard is given in the European Pharmacopoeia Vol. II.

Viscose wadding has a high rate of absorption, but unless mixed with cotton tends to be somewhat slippery in use and to collapse when wet with the resultant loss of previously retained fluid. It is therefore used for the same purposes as the lower-grade cotton wools, with the important advantage that it is generally free of dust and loose fibres. It is not suitable for use in situations where it is necessary for absorbent material to be retained in place for any length of time.

CELLULOSE WADDING is made entirely from high-grade bleached wood pulp, which consists of delignified disintegrated timber. It consists almost entirely of pure cellulose and is produced in a multiple laminate form. A standard is given in the British Pharmaceutical Codex 1973.

Cellulose wadding is used as an absorbent and protective pad. It can be used in large pieces to absorb large volumes of fluid in incontinence. It should not be used directly on wounds, but if required for that purpose, it should be enclosed in a non-adherent cover. Like viscose wadding it has a tendency to collapse when wet, with the resultant loss of previously retained fluid.

Fabric and Fibrous Compound Absorbents

GAUZE AND CELLULOSE WADDING TISSUE (Cellulose Tissue) consists of a thick layer of cellulose wadding enclosed in gauze in tubular form. A standard is given in the British Pharmaceutical Codex 1973.

It is used as an absorbent and protective pad. When used as a would dressing, a non-adherent layer must be placed between the pad and the wound. It has a high absorbency and, because of its thickness, it has the additional property of insulation, which raises the temperature at the skin surface and thus accelerates the rate of healing. There is a tendency for the cellulose wadding to collapse when very wet, and on a weeping surface it may become a semi-solid wet mass; gauze and cotton tissue is therefore preferred in cases where there is much exudate.

GAUZE AND COTTON TISSUE (Absorbent Gauze Tissue; Gauze Tissue; Gamgee Tissue) consists of a thick layer of absorbent cotton wool enclosed in gauze in tubular form. A standard is given in the British Pharmaceutical Codex 1973.

It has the same uses as gauze and cellulose wadding

tissue, but it has the advantage of having a higher absorbent capacity and is less likely to collapse when very wet. It is therefore preferred in place of gauze and cellulose wadding tissue for weeping surfaces, such as burns. It is also softer in use and thus conforms more readily to the wound surface. Like gauze and cellulose wadding tisue, it should not be used in direct contact with the wound surface, but should be placed on a non-adherent layer.

NON-WOVEN FILMATED SWABS (Regal® swabs) consist of a non-woven viscose fabric, folded into pieces of various dimensions and containing a fibrous insert which increases their total absorbent capacity. They can be used for general swabbing and cleansing, but should not be used as a wound dressing because of the possible shedding of loose fibres or adhesion to the wound.

Medicated Absorbents

EUFLAVINE LINT consists of absorbent lint impregnated with about 0.2% of euflavine. A standard is given in the British Pharmaceutical Codex 1973.

It is an antiseptic absorbent and protective dressing, used for the first-aid treatment of mild burns, and is a component of Medicated Lint Finger Dressing and of Medicated Lint Dressing (see under Wound Dressings: Standard Dressings). The absorbency of the lint is reduced by the impregnation with euflavine.

CAPSICUM COTTON WOOL (Capsicum Cotton) consists of absorbent cotton wool impregnated with capsicum oleoresin and methyl salicylate; it is dyed orange-brown. It contains about 0.05% of capsaicin and, when freshly prepared, about 1% of methyl salicylate. A standard is given in the British Pharmaceutical Codex 1973.

It is used as a counter-irritant on undamaged skin, and also in the treatment of certain rheumatic conditions. The counter-irritant effect may be increased by moistening the cotton wool slightly, thus allowing better penetration of the capsaicin into the skin. Care must be taken in handling the material to keep particles away from eyes and mucous membranes.

Wound Dressings

Wound dressings may be conveniently classified into four general types: (i) wound dressing pads; (ii) non-adherent wound-contact dressings; (iii) self-adhesive dressings pads; and (iv) the Standard Dressings. In addition to these four types, there are a number of other miscellaneous wound dressings.

Wound Dressing Pads

These dressings consist of sleeved and unsleeved absorbent pads; the sleeve may be a woven or non-woven fabric which may or may not have the property of non-adherence. The dressings can be applied to wound surfaces and retained in position with a surgical adhesive tape or with a stretch or non-stretch bandage.

Proprietary products of this type include Surgipad®, which is composed of a pad consisting of a mixture of cotton and viscose fibres enclosed in a sleeve of non-woven viscose gauze net, and A.D. Wool®, which is almost identical to Surgipad® but has a lower absorptive capacity. A.D. Cellulose® is another similar product, but it has bleached, layered, cellulose wadding within the sleeve. All of these products absorb fluids quickly, but they should not be used where there is the possibility of the wound drying out and causing adherence of the dressing to the wound surface and consequent trauma when the dressing is removed.

A further group of wound dressing pads include in their construction a non-adherent or partially non-adherent wound-facing layer. *Perfron®* consists of a sleeve of non-woven viscose gauze net, the surface of which has been coated in polypropylene, and which encloses an absorbent pad consisting of layers of cotton fibres interleaved with layers of semi-bleached permeable crepe cellulose tissue. It is highly absorbent with slow "strike through" and minimum adherence. It is therefore suitable for use where there is much exudation from the wound.

Melolin® is a non-sleeved, perforated-film absorbent dressing, and consists of an absorbent pad of mixed acrylic and cotton fibres, faced on one side by absorbent cotton gauze and on the other by a perforated polymeric film. It is positioned so that the polymeric film is in contact with the wound. It has low absorptive capacity, and is particularly useful as a dressing for a dry suture line, and also for treating small and difficult areas such as fingers, where the dressing is easily adjusted to fit the wound surface.

Non-adherent Wound-contact Dressings

In cases where the dressing pad does not have a non-adherent outer layer or where a large area is to be covered by an absorbent, such as gauze and cotton tissue, these non-adherent dressings are intended to be placed directly on the wound to prevent adhesion of the dressing pad which is used with them and the consequent damage to the wound which occurs when an adhering pad is removed. Proprietary preparations of this type include *Alutex®*, which is a viscose laminate cross-stitched with a perforated aluminium film which is placed in contact with the wound, *Micropad®*, which consists of a thin absorbent pad with a polymeric surface which is placed in contact with the wound, and *N-A®* wound dressing which consists of a warp-knitted viscose fabric. Tulle dressings, a number of which are medicated, are included in this group of non-adherent dressings. These medicated dressings must be carefully selected for good wound management.

PARAFFIN GAUZE DRESSING (*Jelonet®*; Paraffin Tulle Gras; *Paranet®*; *Paratulle®*; *Unitulle®*) consists of bleached leno cloth of cotton or viscose, or of combined cotton and viscose yarn, impregnated with yellow or white soft paraffin in such a way that the threads are coated but the spaces in between the threads are free. When the dressing is required for use in tropical or sub-tropical countries, the soft paraffin may be replaced by a mixture of hard and soft paraffins. A standard is given in the British Pharmaceutical Codex 1973.

Paraffin gauze dressing is available as a unit-packed sterile piece, 100 mm square, or in multiple packs containing 5 to 36 pieces; a sterile strip, 7 m × 100 mm, is also available. In the single-piece packs, the dressing is sandwiched between two packing leaves and this facilitates aseptic handling of the dressing. Preferably, the dressing should be taken from a freshly opened pack which contains only a sufficient number of pieces for use on a single occasion. If, however, any dressings in a multiple pack remain unused, they can be re-sterilised; if they are not re-sterilised, they should be discarded. A disadvantage of large multiple packs is that during storage there is a tendency for the soft paraffin to gravitate to the bottom of the pack, overloading the lower pieces and leaving the upper pieces deficient of soft paraffin. The soft paraffin prevents the dressing from adhering to the wound and is also semi-occlusive. The dressing is used primarily in the treatment of burns

and scalds, in which the protective function of the epidermis is lost and water vapour can escape. The dressing functions by reducing the transepidermal water loss whilst the water barrier layer, situated in the stratum corneum, is reforming.

The dressing can also be used as the wound-contact layer in lacerations, abrasions, bites, puncture wounds, and crash injuries, and also in ulcerative conditions, such as varicose, diabetic, or tropical ulcers, and bedsores, where, as a packing material, it is believed to promote granulation. Post-operatively, it is used as a vaginal or penile dressing, and for sinus packing.

Paraffin gauze dressing, heavily impregnated with soft paraffin, is used in the tailoring and transfer of skin grafts. The dressing is spread on the cutting board and the skin to be transplanted is laid on the dressing and cut to size. The cut skin and dressing are then transferred to the recipient area. In this case, the "tackiness" of the soft paraffin is used to facilitate the handling of grafts.

CHLORHEXIDINE GAUZE (TULLE) DRESSING (*Bactigras®*) is a leno cotton gauze impregnated with soft paraffin; it contains 0.5% of chlorhexidine acetate. It is available as a unit-packed sterile piece, 100 mm square. It is used in the same way as paraffin gauze dressing with the added advantage that the chlorhexidine inhibits the growth of many wound-infecting micro-organisms.

SODIUM FUSIDATE GAUZE (TULLE) DRESSING is a leno cotton gauze impregnated with a white soft paraffin and wool fat basis; it contains 2% of sodium fusidate. It is available as a unit-packed sterile piece, 100 mm square.

COD-LIVER OIL AND HONEY GAUZE (TULLE) DRESSING is a cotton gauze impregnated with a cod-liver oil and honey cream; it contains 1% of hexachlorophane. It is used in the treatment of bed sores and varicose ulcers.

FRAMYCETIN SULPHATE GAUZE (TULLE) DRESSING (*Soframycin Unitulle®*; *Sofra-tulle®*) is a lightweight leno gauze impregnated with soft paraffin; it contains 1% of framycetin sulphate. It is available as a unit-packed sterile piece, 100 mm square. This dressing is used in the same way as paraffin gauze dressing, with the added advantage that the presence of the non-systemic, broad-spectrum antibiotic helps to reduce wound infection. It is therefore used in the treatment of secondary infected skin conditions, eczema, dermatitis, and herpes, and on colostomies, ileostomies, and tracheostomies. In use the dressing is placed in contact with the wound and covered with an absorbent wound dressing retained in place by a bandage. The dressing must not be used on patients known to be allergic to aminoglycoside antibiotics.

SCARLET RED GAUZE DRESSING is a fine-mesh gauze impregnated with a blend of lanolin, olive oil, and soft paraffin; it contains 5% of scarlet red. It is used in certain skin infections.

Self-adhesive Dressing Pads

These are also known as *strip dressings*. They consist of an absorbent pad attached directly to the adhesive surface of a backing which extends beyond the edges of the pad; the pad and the adhesive margin are covered with a protective film. They are frequently supplied sterile and individually wrapped. These dressing pads have the advantage of partially sealing the wound from the atmosphere, thus reducing infection by producing a clean environment in the wound area. However, they have the disadvantage that the low absorptive capacity will not remove excess exudate from the wound and this could reduce the rate of healing. The adhesive backing must be capable of transmitting water vapour from the skin surface to which it is attached, otherwise the healthy skin area may be damaged. Large self-adhesive dressing pads are used post-operatively as clean suture-line dressings. Proprietary products of this type include *Airstrip®*, which consists of a *Melolin®* pad positioned on adhesive microporous plastic tape, *Dermicel®*, which consists of a pad of synthetic rubber foam faced with a layer of viscose non-woven gauze, coated with polyethylene along the fibre but rendered porous at the interstices of the fabric, the pad being attached to an acetate taffeta backing coated with an acrylic adhesive so that the polyethylene-coated gauze is the surface applied to the wound, and *Microdon®*, which consists of a pad of viscose fibre, enclosed in a non-woven viscose sleeve, attached to a transparent microporous tape.

PERFORATED PLASTIC WOUND DRESSING (Porous Plastic Dressing; *Steripad®*) consists of an absorbent pad fixed to a perforated plastic self-adhesive backing so as to leave a margin of adhesive surface surrounding the pad. The pad and adhesive margin are covered with a protector which is removed before application of the dressing. The pad is medicated with an antiseptic and dyed yellow if necessary with a non-toxic dye; the antiseptic and dye may be omitted if the dressing is supplied sterile. A standard is given in the British Pharmaceutical Codex 1973.

This dressing is used as a protective covering for wounds. It is permeable to air and water vapour, and is used in situations where permeability is required, or where impermeability is not a necessary factor for wound healing or for avoidance of contamination.

WATERPROOF PLASTIC WOUND DRESSING (Occlusive Plastic Dressing) is of the same construction as perforated plastic wound dressing, except that the backing is waterproof and not perforated. A standard is given in the British Pharmaceutical Codex 1973.

It is used as a protective covering for wounds when an occlusive dressing is required in order to ensure that the wound does not become contaminated with micro-organisms or dust particles. It also prevents micro-organisms in the wound from being transmitted beyond the wound dressing.

WATERPROOF MICROPOROUS PLASTIC WOUND DRESSING (Microporous Plastic Dressing; Semipermeable Plastic Dressing; *Airstrip®*) is constructed as for perforated plastic wound dressing, except that the backing is not perforated, but instead is semi-permeable and waterproof. A standard is given in the British Pharmaceutical Codex 1973.

It is used as a protective covering for wounds when a waterproof dressing is required, but it allows the passage of air and water vapour to and from the wound and skin surface, thus facilitating healing.

Standard Dressings

PLAIN LINT FINGER DRESSING (Standard Dressing No. 7) consists of a sterile unmedicated open-ended finger stall formed by a tube of lint, with raised surface on the outside, and attached obliquely to an open-wove bandage. A standard is given in the British Pharmaceutical Codex 1973.

The dressing is used as a wound dressing for fingers and toes. Care must be taken when removing the dressing, as the lint may adhere to the wound.

PLAIN LINT DRESSING (Standard Dressings Nos. 8 & 9) consists of an unmedicated pad of cotton wool faced with a rectangular piece of lint, with raised surface

inwards, and attached lengthwise to an open-wove bandage; the dressing is sterile.

The dressing is available in two sizes: in the medium size (No. 8), the pad is 75 mm by 100 mm, and in the large size (No. 9), 100 mm by 150 mm. A standard is given in the British Pharmaceutical Codex 1973.

The medium-size dressing is used as a wound dressing for hands and feet, and the large dressing for larger areas. Care must be taken when removing these dressings, as the lint may adhere to the wound.

MEDICATED LINT FINGER DRESSING (Standard Dressing No. 10) is a medicated version of Plain Lint Finger Dressing with euflavine lint or other medicated lint in place of plain lint. A standard is given in the British Pharmaceutical Codex 1973.

The dressing is used for the first aid treatment of mild burns of fingers and toes.

MEDICATED LINT DRESSING (Standard Dressings Nos. 11 & 12) are medicated versions of Plain Lint Dressing with euflavine lint or other medicated lint in place of plain lint. A standard is given in the British Pharmaceutical Codex 1973.

The dressings are used for the first aid treatment of mild burns of the hands, feet, and larger areas.

PLAIN WOUND DRESSING (Standard Dressings Nos. 13, 14, & 15) consists of an unmedicated pad, comprising a piece of cotton wool enclosed in gauze, attached to an open-wove bandage; the dressing is sterile.

The dressing is available in three sizes: in the small size (No. 13) the pad is 75 mm by 100 mm, in the medium size (No. 14), 100 mm by 150 mm, and in the large size (No. 15), 150 mm by 200 mm. A standard is given in the British Pharmaceutical Codex 1973.

The dressings are used as protective and absorbent dressings for wounds. On removing the dressing from its package, the rolled bandage can be retained in one hand, while the loose end of the bandage, which is wound round the pad, can be unwound with the other hand and pulled, resulting in the sterile pad face being presented for direct application to the wound with the minimum of handling. Care must be taken in removing these dressings, as the gauze may adhere to the wound.

FOMENTATION DRESSING (Standard Dressing No. 2) consists of a piece of polyethylene film, 150 mm square, and a sterilised inner package comprising a piece of lint, 300 mm square, cotton wool, and an open-wove bandage. A standard is given in the British Pharmaceutical Codex 1963.

The dressing can be used as a fomentation dressing with magnesium sulphate paste or kaolin poultice, or as a wet dressing formed by soaking the lint in any one of many preparations; the polyethylene film is placed over the dressing after application to prevent drying out.

ELASTIC ADHESIVE WOUND DRESSING (Standard Dressings Nos. 3, 4, & 5) consists of a fabric pad, comprising a piece of lint wrapped in muslin bandage, fixed to a rectangular piece of extension plaster so as to leave a margin of adhesive surface surrounding the pad. The elasticity of the plaster is unidirectional across the narrow width of the pad. The pad and adhesive margin are covered with a protector, which is removed before application. The pad is medicated with an antiseptic and dyed yellow, if necessary, with a non-toxic dye; the antiseptic and dye may be omitted if the dressing is supplied sterile.

The dressing is available in three sizes: in the small size (No. 3), the pad is 20 mm by 25 mm, in the medium size (No. 4), 10 mm by 50 mm (*Elastoplast®*) or 30 mm by

50 mm, and in the large size (No. 5), 35 mm by 60 mm. A standard is given in the British Pharmaceutical Codex 1963.

These dressings are used as a protective covering for small wounds. The former extra large size (No. 6) has been replaced by Self-adhesive Dressing Pads (see above).

EYE PAD WITH BANDAGE (Standard Dressing No. 16) consists of an oval pad of cotton wool 50 mm by 75 mm, faced on both sides with muslin and attached lengthwise to an open-wove bandage; the dressing is sterile. The pad must be fibre-fast, as the loss of fibre in the area of the eye can be dangerous. A standard is given in the British Pharmaceutical Codex 1973.

The dressing is used as a protective covering for the eye but not for the application of medicaments.

Other Wound Dressings

Opsite® DRESSING consists of an adhesive-coated polyurethane film, which is permeable to water vapour, supplied in "dressing size" pieces. It is applied directly to the wound without the use of an absorbent pad.

PLASTIC SPRAY DRESSINGS (*Nobecutane®*; *Octaflex®*) are aerosol preparations of acrylic polymers which can be sprayed directly on to a suture line to form a film which is permeable to water vapour. They are sometimes used for dry suture line dressings in combination with an acrylic adhesive tape. A solvent is supplied for removal of the acrylic skin.

DISPOSABLE POLYETHYLENE OCCLUSIVE DRESSINGS consist of polyethylene (150 gauge) in the form of arm and leg sleeves, foot bag, shorts, torso vest, and trousers. They are used as occlusive dressings in conjunction with medicated creams for the treatment of dermatological conditions.

STERILE DRESSING PACK (*Propax®*) contains 1 absorbent gauze tissue pad, consisting of cotton wool in an open-ended gauze sleeve, 4 absorbent gauze swabs, 4 large cotton wool balls, 1 absorbent paper towel consisting of cellulose wadding, and 1 water-repellent paper sheet which is used as the inner wrapper to enclose the other items; the pack is supplied sterile. The wrapper is folded in such a way that when it is opened it forms a sterile field for the enclosed dressings which can then be used without the inside of this field being touched by hand. The pack is used mainly for wound cleansing in community nursing, the precise method of using the components being generally detailed in a document on nursing procedure issued by each Area Health Authority. It should be noted that there is no dressing in the pack and in practice it is necessary to supply a supplementary pack which includes a low-exudate or high-exudate wound dressing.

MULTIPLE DRESSING PACKS are available which contain cotton wool, gauze, and open-wove bandages and are used mainly for cleansing purposes; they may be supplemented by a selected wound dressing.

Multiple Dressing Pack No. 1 contains 25 g of Absorbent Cotton Wool, 1 piece of Absorbent Cotton Gauze 900 mm × 1 m, and 3 Open-wove Bandages 50 mm × 5 m.

Multiple Dressing Pack No. 2 contains 100 g of Absorbent Cotton Wool, 3 pieces of Absorbent Cotton Gauze each 900 mm × 1 m, 2 Open-wove Bandages 50 mm × 5 m, and 1 Open-wove Bandage 75 mm × 5 m.

Bandages

Bandages may be classified into three types depending upon their function: (i) retention bandages; (ii) support and compression bandages, which may be non-adhesive or adhesive; and (iii) medicated bandages.

Retention Bandages

OPEN-WOVE BANDAGE (White Open-wove Bandage; Cambric Bandage) consists of cloth of plain weave, in which the warp threads are of cotton and the weft threads are of cotton or viscose, or of a combined cotton and viscose yarn. The cloth differs from European bandage cloths which have a construction and properties similar to those of gauze, in that it has a higher warp thread count and is made with heavier yarns. A standard is given in the British Pharmaceutical Codex 1973.

It is used mainly to protect absorbent dressings and to hold them in place. The heavy weft of the bandage gives a degree of support and also produces partial restriction of movement, which can assist in rapid healing of the wound. The bandage is available in a number of widths. A wide bandage is sometimes used as a support for slight sprains and strains; for this purpose, it is immersed in cold water before application to the injured joint. The cooling by evaporation helps to reduce the swelling, and the partial shrinkage of the bandage during drying increases the support provided. The mechanical strength of this bandage is sufficient for it also to be used to secure splints and to produce traction. The European absorbent bandages are not uncommonly used as direct wound dressings, but this usage is not appropriate with British bandages.

TRIANGULAR CALICO BANDAGE consists of a piece of unbleached calico in the form of a right-angled isosceles triangle. A standard is given in the British Pharmaceutical Codex 1973.

The bandage is used as a sling. If it is likely to come into contact with areas of broken skin, it should be sterilised before use. Disposable triangular bandages made of paper are also available

DOMETTE BANDAGE consists of union fabric of plain weave, in which the warp threads are of cotton or viscose, or of a combined cotton and viscose yarn, and the weft threads are of wool. A standard is given in the British Pharmaceutical Codex 1973.

It is used mainly for orthopaedic purposes, especially in cases where a high degree of warmth, protection, and support is required, those qualities being provided by the heavy wool weft.

COTTON CONFORMING BANDAGE (*Crinx®*; *Kling®*) consists of cotton cloth of plain weave, suitably treated in order to impart elasticity in both the weft and warp directions A standard is given in the British Pharmaceutical Codex 1973.

The fact that it has elasticity in both directions gives this bandage the ability to conform with the surface to which it is applied, and hence it is used to retain dressings in difficult positions such as on joints and other positions which would otherwise require the use of adhesive tape. An additional advantage over open-wove bandage (see above) is that a slight pressure is produced which maintains the dressing in close contact with the wound.

LIGHTWEIGHT CRÊPE BANDAGE (*Varicrepe®*; *Elvic®*; *Rayvic®*) consists of fabric of plain weave in which the warp threads are of cotton or of a combined cotton and viscose yarn and the weft threads are of cotton or viscose. Its stretch characteristics are comparable to other crêpe bandages. The bandage is generally used for holding dressings in place and for providing light support. Because of its stretch, it is easy to apply, even around awkward joints.

POLYAMIDE STRETCH BANDAGE (Nylon Stretch Bandage; *Nylex®*; *Slinky®*) consists of fabric of plain weave in which the warp threads are of crimped polyamide and the weft threads of viscose. The bandage is generally used for holding dressings in place and for light support. It possesses good stretch characteristics equal to those of a crêpe bandage but lasting considerably longer. It is thin and does not slip.

TUBULAR BANDAGE (*Tubegauz®*; *Tubinette®*; *Tubiton®*) consists of seamless tubular fabric woven from cotton, viscose, or combined cotton and viscous yarn. It is used for holding dressings in place and is available in a number of sizes appropriate for use on fingers, toes, limbs, head, and body. It is particularly useful for the small fingers and toes of children where the use of an ordinary strip bandage is impracticable. A special applicator is provided which facilitates positioning of the bandage.

TUBULAR ELASTIC NET BANDAGES (*Netelast®*; *Surgifix®*; *Setonet®*) are available in different sizes. Because of their tubular structure, they are equally suitable for retaining dressings on small limbs such as fingers and on the largest areas such as the trunk and abdomen. They have the advantage of applying continuous but elastic pressure to the entire surface of the dressing while producing a minimum occlusion of the undressed area.

TUBULAR STOCKINETTE BANDAGE (Elasticated Tubular Bandage; Elasticated Surgical Tubular Stockinette; *Tubigrip®*) consists of seamless tubular stockinette of close weave, knitted with a combined cotton and viscose yarn and in which is interspersed a rubber thread, which is covered with synthetic yarn in order to reduce adverse skin reaction. It is available in a number of sizes appropriate for use on hands, limbs, and body.

It may be used as a dressing cover and it also has the facility to exert and maintain an even pressure over the part enclosed without restricting movement, and hence provides support. It may be used in place of crêpe bandage (see under Non-adhesive Support and Compression Bandages, below), with the advantage that it can be applied by an untrained person or reapplied, without loss of performance, by the patient after bathing or sleeping.

SURGICAL STOCKINETTE (Cotton Surgical Tubular Stockinette) consists of seamless tubular stockinette, knitted with cotton yarn in plain weave or rib weave. It is available in a number of sizes. The bandage has low elasticity and is used to protect the skin prior to the application of plaster casts or adhesive bandages. It can also be used as a sleeve to protect bedding and clothing from ointments and creams.

Non-adhesive Support and Compression Bandages

The two-way-stretch bandages, described above, are used to retain a dressing in position. One-way-stretch bandages, which stretch along the bandage length, may also be used for the retention of dressings, but they have the additional function of giving support or applying pressure to the bandaged area. The choice of bandage will depend upon the purpose for which it is required. A light-weight bandage with low elasticity will give the minimum of support and compression; both support and compression increase with weight and elasticity, so that

a heavy-weight fabric with high elasticity will give maximum support to a limb and will act as a pressure bandage. The uses can be grouped in ascending order of support and compression requirements, and matched against existing one-way-stretch bandages. In practice, conditions may require the use of either greater support or greater compression, and this can be obtained by careful selection of the bandage and by modifying the tension under which the bandage is applied.

Use	*Suggested bandage*
Dressing retention with light support and pressure	Crêpe Bandage
Mild strains and sprains	Cotton Crêpe Bandage
Compression bandaging over paste dressings for varicose ulcers	Cotton Stretch Bandage
Dressing retention with pressure	Cotton and Rubber
Strains and sprains	Elastic Net Bandage
Medium support	Crêpe Bandage
Varicose conditions	
Pressure bandaging (with or without dressing)	
Firm support	Elastic Web Bandage
Support after removal of plaster	Cotton Elastic Bandage
Muscle trauma	
Joint effusions	

CRÊPE BANDAGE consists of characteristic fabric of plain weave, in which the warp threads are of cotton and of wool and the weft threads are of cotton. Its stretch characteristics are a function of its structure. A standard is given in the British Pharmaceutical Codex 1973

The bandage is used in the treatment of mild sprains and strains and in other conditions in which light support is required; it may be used for this purpose in conjunction with other surgical appliances. It is also used for correctional purposes and as a compression bandage, for instance over paste bandages in the treatment of varicose ulcers. Much of the elasticity of the bandage is lost during use, but it can be largely restored by washing the bandage in hot soapy water.

COTTON CRÊPE BANDAGE (*Elastocrepe®*) consists of characteristic fabric of plain weave, in which the warp threads are of cotton and the weft threads are of cotton or viscose, or of a combined cotton and viscose yarn. Like crêpe bandage its elasticity is produced by its structure. A standard is given in the British Pharmaceutical Codex 1973.

The bandage is used for the same purposes as crêpe bandage (see above) but it does not have the weight and the insulation property provided by the wool content of crêpe bandage.

COTTON STRETCH BANDAGE consists of characteristic fabric of plain weave, in which both the warp and the weft threads are of cotton. A standard is given in the British Pharmaceutical Codex 1973.

This is a lighter bandage than either crêpe bandage or cotton crêpe bandage (see above) but is used for the same purposes. It is also used in place of open-wove bandage for retaining dressings in position when the added functions of compression, support or immobilisation are required. In use, there is less likelihood of this bandage slipping than there is with open-wove bandage.

COTTON AND RUBBER ELASTIC NET BANDAGE (Cotton and Elastic Net Bandage; *Lastonet®*) consists of characteristic net fabric of lace construction, in which the warp threads are of a combined cotton and rubber yarn and the weft threads are of cotton. A standard is given in the British Pharmaceutical Codex 1973.

This bandage is used for the same purposes as crêpe bandage (see above), but it has a higher elasticity and therefore gives greater compression. The bandage retains its elasticity in use and can be left in position for a long period of time without reduction in performance.

COTTON AND RUBBER ELASTIC BANDAGE (Cotton Elastic Bandage; *Elastoweb®*) consists of characteristic fabric of plain weave, in which the warp threads are of cotton and combined cotton and rubber yarn, and the weft threads are of cotton. A standard is given in the British Pharmaceutical Codex 1973.

This is a heavy bandage and is used primarily to produce an even compression over a fairly large area; it may also be used to give support. It has the advantage over other stretch bandages that it will retain its compression and elastomeric properties over a long period of time and after a number of washings. It also has an advantage over elastic stocking in that the tension may be adjusted to suit the individual case. The degree of compression required will vary with the site and the nature of the wound, and care must be taken that the bandage is applied evenly in order to ensure that high-pressure areas do not develop with resulting local trauma. The bandage should be applied in such a way that the amount of overlap is approximately the same throughout the process. The bandage may have a stitched foot-loop at one end which assists in starting the bandaging process in the correct position at the base of the toes.

ELASTIC WEB BANDAGE is similar in construction to cotton and rubber elastic bandage (see above) but is of a heavier weight; running down the centre it has a coloured thread, which may be red or blue, and it may have a stitched foot-loop at one end. The red-line bandage is a heavier weight and has a higher elasticity than the blue-line bandage. It is used for the same purposes as cotton and rubber elastic bandage and is applied in the same way; the coloured thread acts as a margin to aid in achieving even overlap during bandaging.

COHESIVE BANDAGE and POLYURETHANE FOAM BANDAGE. The cohesive bandage *Coban®* has the advantage that it clings to itself and does not allow any slip to occur during use. Polyurethane foam bandage also has some cohesive properties and will also stretch in all directions so that it conforms more evenly than the traditional crêpe. It is soft in contact with the skin and non-occlusive.

Adhesive Support and Compression Bandages

There are two types of these bandages: (i) diachylon bandages, which are warmed before application, and (ii) self-adhesive bandages.

NOTE: All adhesive stretch bandages can cause damage to the skin on removal, and alternatives to direct contact with the skin have been suggested. The limb can be protected with a white open-wove bandage or tubular stockinette over which the adhesive bandage is then applied. Alternatively, the adhesive bandage can be reversed and applied with the adhesive layer away from the skin. Both of these methods result in a lowering of the performance of the bandage.

DIACHYLON ELASTIC ADHESIVE BANDAGE (Elastic Diachylon Bandage; (*Lestreflex®* Plain) consists of elastic cloth spread evenly with a diachylon mass, which is composed of lead soaps of the higher fatty acids to which suitable adhesives are added. The bandage is occlusive. A standard is given in the British Pharmaceutical Codex 1973.

The bandage is used to apply compression in the treatment of chronic leg ulcers in ambulant patients, and for the continuous pressure and support required for the treatment of varicose veins. The bandage is warmed before application in order to produce adhesion; it may be necessary to depilate the skin and ensure that it is dry to secure adequate adhesion. The application must be carried out with care and under experienced supervision in order to avoid pain and skin damage. The bandage can be unrolled without difficulty, thus making it easier than with the rubber-based adhesive bandages to apply with an evenly distributed pressure; it can also be removed more easily without pulling unduly the hair on the skin surface.

This bandage is useful in the treatment of patients who are sensitive to zinc oxide or to rubber adhesive bandages. However, if the bandage is intended to be used for an extended period of time, the sensitivity of the patient to diachylon mass should be determined by a patch test.

VENTILATED DIACHYLON ELASTIC ADHESIVE BANDAGE (Ventilated Elastic Diachylon Bandage; *Lestreflex®* Ventilated) consists of elastic cloth spread evenly with a diachylon mass so as to leave strips of unspread fabric along its length. A standard is given in the British Pharmaceutical Codex 1973.

The bandage is used for the same purposes and in the same way as diachylon elastic adhesive bandage. The unspread fabric allows ventilation.

ZINC OXIDE ELASTIC SELF-ADHESIVE BANDAGE (Elastic Adhesive Bandage; *Elastoplast®*; *Flexoplast®*; *Zopla-Band®*) consists of elastic cloth spread evenly with a self-adhesive plaster mass containing natural rubber, resins, and zinc oxide. A standard is given in the British Pharmaceutical Codex 1973.

This bandage is used for the same purposes as diachylon bandage (see above), but the lighter weight of the material facilitates its use in the treatment of conditions where support or compression is required, such as fractured ribs and clavicles, swollen or sprained joints, varicose veins, and leg ulcers. It is also used to secure dressings and appliances.

When the bandage is being unwound from the roll, it becomes stretched, because of self adhesion, and care must be taken to ensure that the bandage is not applied in the stretched state otherwise damage may occur to the skin during the elastic recovery of the bandage. This risk may be minimised by applying several strips of a narrow bandage rather than using one wide bandage; alternatively, a wide bandage may be torn or cut longitudinally. The narrow strips also mould better to the curve of the body than does a wide bandage.

When support strapping is required, the first bandage strips should be applied parallel to the muscle fascia, tendon, or ligament in order to give an anchorage; the direction in which subsequent strips are applied depends upon the lesion and the site. Removal of the bandage should be performed along its length and can be assisted by application of an organic solvent or light oil; it is preferable to push the skin away from the bandage rather than to pull the strip from the skin, as this results in less epithelial damage (see also NOTE under Adhesive Support and Compression Bandages, above). Patch sensitivity tests should be carried out if the bandage is to be used for an extended period of time.

HALF-SPREAD ZINC OXIDE ELASTIC SELF-ADHESIVE BANDAGE (Semi-spread Elastic Adhesive Bandage; Half-spread Elastic Adhesive Bandage; *Flexoplast®*) is elastic adhesive bandage with half the width of fabric unspread. A standard is given in the British Pharmaceutical Codex 1973. It is used in the same way as zinc oxide self-adhesive bandage.

VENTILATED ZINC OXIDE ELASTIC SELF-ADHESIVE BANDAGE (Ventilated Elastic Adhesive Bandage; *Flexplast®*) is elastic adhesive bandage in which the adhesive mass is spread evenly so as to leave strips of unspread fabric along its length.

A standard is given in the British Pharmaceutical Codex 1973.

It is used in the same way as zinc oxide self-adhesive bandage.

POROUS FLEXIBLE ADHESIVE BANDAGE (*Poroplast®*) consists of an elastic cloth spread evenly with a porous, pressure-sensitive, adhesive mass containing titanium dioxide; the mass does not contain either natural rubber or zinc oxide, and this reduces the likelihood of skin response in sensitive patients. It is used for the same purposes as zinc oxide self-adhesive bandage, but as it is lighter and its porosity is slightly greater, it can remain on the skin for a longer period of time.

EXTENSION PLASTER (Extension Strapping; Orthopaedic Strapping; *Elastoplast®*; *Zopla®*) consists of elastic cloth which stretches only across its width, spread evenly with a self-adhesive plaster mass containing zinc oxide. A standard is given in the British Pharmaceutical Codex 1973.

It is a medium-weight bandage and is used for the support of slight sprains which are not immobilised, of joints and limbs after the removal of plaster casts, and of fractured ribs. It is used most frequently for traction bandaging.

Medicated Bandages

These consist of a cotton bandage impregnated with a medicament formulated in a moist paste. They are used in the treatment of dermatological conditions and gravitational ulcers. They bring the medicated paste in direct contact with the affected area and may be left in position for periods of time up to several weeks. They are maintained in position by a support or compression bandage.

Prior to the application of paste bandages, the area around the ulcer should be carefully cleansed to remove pus and debris. It is recommended that the unstable skin surrounding the ulcer be protected by a barrier such as compound benzoin tincture.

The bandage is applied with the leg raised and the heel supported and positioned at an angle of 90° to the leg; this position is maintained during the entire bandaging procedure, which includes not only the application of the paste bandage but also the application of the pressure bandage. The paste bandage is applied starting from the toes, care being taken to prevent the formation of wrinkles in the bandage. For ease of application, the bandage may be cut into convenient length strips rather than applied in one continuous length. If necessary, the bandage may be applied in 6 or 8 layers over the ulcer to form an absorbent pressure pad, any folds in the bandage being positioned at the side of the leg and not over the crest of the tibia. With the foot in the position described, the support or compression bandage is now applied, commencing at the base of the toes. The next bandage turn should be as wide as possible and cover the foot and overlap the heel; a minimum number of turns around the foot is recommended to facilitate the replacement of a shoe. From this point, the bandage is now taken around the ankle and the leg, maintaining an even tension as for the first turn.

In pressure bandaging, the "figure 8" technique should not be used to secure the bandage around the ankle, as the downward pressure may cause damage to the skin over the anterior tibial tendon of the ankle. Once the bandaging has been completed, the bandage should be retained in position with a strip of self-adhesive plaster. The pressure, which should not be excessive, will vary with the state of the limb; an oedematous leg will need the maximum of tension, whilst a thin leg will require the minimum.

Pain will occur if the bandage is applied either too loosely or too tightly. If applied loosely, it allows the veins to distend and the swelling to return. It can also slide down the leg and produce excoriation of the skin in the ankle area. Too tight a bandage will cause persistent pain which will become worse when the patient retires to bed. This could result in damage to the underlying tissues if the excessive pressure is not relieved.

The bandage is normally changed after 3 to 7 days.

The change may be more frequent depending upon the amount of discharge, odour, or pain in the individual patients. As healing progresses, the time between redressing may become as long as a fortnight or a month.

HYDROCORTISONE AND SILICONE BANDAGE (*Cortacream®* Bandage) consists of a cotton bandage impregnated with a cream containing hydrocortisone acetate 1% and silicone fluid 10%, in an emulsified basis. It is suitable for the treatment of infantile eczema and certain irritating skin disorders.

ZINC PASTE BANDAGE consists of open-wove cotton cloth impregnated with a paste containing zinc oxide; the paste may be gelatinous (*Viscopaste®*; *Zincaband®*) or non-gelatinous (*Viscopaste BP7®*). A bandage with a gelatinous or Unna-type paste dries rapidly to form a thin shell. A standard is given in the British Pharmaceutical Codex 1973.

This bandage is used to support and prevent the swelling of fractured limbs after the removal of plaster casts and to support varicose veins. It is also used in the treatment of ulcers, varicose eczemas, phlebitis, and oedema of the legs.

ZINC PASTE AND COAL TAR BANDAGE (*Coltapaste®*; *Tarband®*) consists of open-wove cotton cloth impregnated with a paste containing zinc oxide and prepared coal tar. A standard is given in the British Pharmaceutical Codex 1973.

This bandage is used in the treatment of skin disorders arising as a complication of leg ulcers and of other skin affections, such as varicose eczema of the dry type, localised neurodermatitis and chronic simple prurigo of the limbs, verrucous lichen planus of the legs, and seborrhoeal infantile and chronic vesicular eczemas of palms and fingers.

ZINC PASTE AND ICHTHAMMOL BANDAGE (*Icthopaste®*; *Icthaband®*) consists of open-wove cotton cloth impregnated with a paste containing zinc oxide and ichthammol. A standard is given in the British Pharmaceutical Codex 1973.

This bandage is used in the treatment of varicose and gravitational ulcers. It can also be used as a bland dressing in the treatment of weeping eczemas, and as a protective barrier to fragile skin in compression bandaging.

ZINC PASTE, URETHANE, AND ICHTHAMMOL BANDAGE (*Uraband®*) consists of open-wove cotton cloth impregnated with a paste containing urethane and ichthammol.

It is used for the same purposes as zinc paste and ichthammol bandage, the addition of urethane being intended to encourage granulation of wounds.

ZINC PASTE, CALAMINE, AND CLIOQUINOL BANDAGE (Zinc Paste, Calamine, and Iodochlorhydroxyquinoline Bandage; *Quinaband®*) consists of open-wove cotton cloth impregnated with a paste containing zinc oxide, calamine, and clioquinol.

It is used for the same purposes as zinc paste bandage, with the advantage that it has an antibacterial agent for use on infected surfaces.

ZINC PASTE, URETHANE, AND CALAMINE BANDAGE (*Calaband®*) consists of open-wove cotton cloth impregnated with zinc oxide, urethane, and calamine. It is used for the same purposes as zinc paste, urethane, and ichthammol bandage, to which it is preferred in cases where there is a large fluid loss from the eczematous region.

Surgical Adhesive Tapes

Surgical adhesive tapes consist of a backing material which is coated, or partially impregnated, on one side with an adhesive mass. The backing material may be a woven textile, a non-woven textile, or a plastic film, and the adhesive mass may be based on rubber or on an acrylic copolymer. Different combinations of backing material and adhesive give products having different permeabilities; these include: (i) permeable tapes which are permeable to air, water, and bacteria; (ii) semipermeable tapes which are permeable to air and water vapour only; and (iii) occlusive tapes which are impermeable to air, water, water vapour, and bacteria.

Tape selection. The selection of a suitable adhesive tape requires consideration, not only of permeability and waterproofness, but also of the nature of the skin to which it is to be attached and the length of time it is intended to be left in position.

For an infant's skin and where the tape is only to be attached for a short period, the most suitable tape would be a microporous acrylic viscose tape which has good but not excessive adhesion, is hyporeactive, and has a comparatively short wear-time. In contrast, the exfoliating skin of a geriatric patient would require a tape with much higher adhesion.

For securing tubing during parenteral therapy, an acrylic non-woven tape with non-occlusive properties would be suitable; it would not interfere with the normal skin function and would leave little or no residue on the skin or equipment after its removal. When an adhesive tape is used to hold a dressing in position, repeated wound dressing can be a problem; epithelial damage may occur due to repeated removal of the tape, and therefore a tape should be chosen which is permeable, is hyporeactive, and has good adhesion and low extensibility. Alternatively, a "Montgomery strap" can be used. To prepare this, a piece of tape is folded back for a short distance with adhesive surfaces together, a small hole is cut in the folded portion, and the hole threaded with a cotton ribbon. Several of these adhesive strips are positioned on either side of a dressing with folded ends in juxtaposition and two opposing strips are brought together over the dressing and the cotton ribbons tied. The dressing can then be changed without removing the adhesive tapes from the skin surface.

In operating theatres, the use of adhesive tapes is usually restricted to the final dressing of the wound or to the retention of cannulae. If adhesive tapes are to be sterilised for this purpose they must not be left on the spool but should be cut into short pieces and attached to silicone release paper prior to processing. The orthopaedic use of adhesive tapes to reduce movement and to give support is limited to the heavier cloth tapes; alternatively, adhesive bandages (see under Adhesive Support and Compression Bandages) are used. Surgical adhesive tapes may be conveniently classified into three general types: (i) woven textile tapes; (ii) non-woven textile tapes; and (iii) plastic film tapes.

Woven Tapes

ZINC OXIDE SELF-ADHESIVE·TAPE (Zinc Oxide Self-adhesive Plaster; Adhesive Plaster; Zinc Oxide Plaster; *Band-Aid®*; *Elastoplast®*; *Paragon®*; *Thompson Tape®*; *Zopla®*) consists of a viscose or cotton cloth, or mixed cotton and viscose cloth, evenly spread with an adhesive mass which may include either a natural elastomer of para or pale crêpe rubber, or a synthetic elastomer of isobutylene alkyl-acrylate polymers, together with colophony resin or esterified resins, antoxidants, plasticisers, and other ingredients such as zinc oxide, starch, and talc. A standard for Zinc Oxide Self-adhesive Plaster is given in the British Pharmaceutical Codex 1973.

The adhesive mass is occlusive unless the tape has been mechanically pierced. The nature of the mass is liable to produce adverse skin reactions, and long-term use of the product should not be considered unless the patient has undergone a patch test to establish the absence of sensitivity.

Zinc oxide tape is used to secure dressings and to immobilise small areas. Because it has a woven textile base, and hence a certain amount of elasticity, the minimum of tension should be used when applying the tape. If the tape is put in position in a stretched state, then during elastic recovery a transverse tension will be produced on the skin surface, and this may, in some circumstances, produce an epithelial slip with blistering of the skin beneath the tape.

ACRYLIC ADHESIVE TAPE consists of a viscose taffeta cloth spread evenly with an adhesive mass which is an acrylic copolymer in which the balance between adhesion and cohesion is dependent upon the choice and control of the polymerisation conditions during manufacture. The polymer will permit the passage of air and water vapour, and the tape is therefore semipermeable under normal conditions of use. Proprietary preparations of this type include *Dermicel®*.

Acrylic tape is used to secure dressings and is particularly useful in cases where the patient is known to be sensitive to the adhesive mass of zinc oxide tape. The tape has a certain amount of elasticity and should be applied with the minimum of tension for the reasons described under Zinc Oxide Self-adhesive Tape, above. In general, acrylic tape leaves less residue on the skin surface and causes less damage on removal than zinc oxide tape.

Non-woven Tapes

These consist of a backing material of non-woven synthetic fibres, laid in a net or randomly and bonded in or on an evenly spread non-occlusive acrylic adhesive mass. They are permeable to air and water vapour, and this results in the maintenance of the normal environment at the skin surface beneath the tape. These tapes are comparatively simple to handle, are light in weight, and have good adhesion. Their tensile strength is not as high as that of the woven textile tapes, but the cohesive characteristics allow them to be removed from the skin without leaving debris on the surface. Proprietary preparations of this type include *Chirotape®*, *Hypal®*, and *Micropore®*. *Dermilite®* is a paper tape with similar characteristics.

Non-woven textile tapes are used for retaining dressings in position, and also as skin closures for small incisions.

Plastic Film Tapes

Plastic film tapes consist of either a perforated or a non-perforated plastic film which has been spread with either a copolymer adhesive or with a natural or synthetic rubber-based adhesive. The backing material may vary from polyethylene to a range of impermeable plastic films. The choice of film depends upon the porosity and degree of adhesion required by the user. They are used as the backing material in Self-adhesive Dressing Pads (see under Wound Dressings).

WATERPROOF PLASTIC SELF-ADHESIVE TAPE (Waterproof Plastic Self-adhesive Plaster; Plastic Adhesive Strapping; Waterproof Strapping; *Adaptopruf®*; *Aquatape®*; *Elastoplast®* waterproof plastic strapping; *Fast Aid®*; *Setonplast®* plastic adhesive strapping; *Sleek®* plastic adhesive strapping; *Zincoplast®* Waterproof) consists of an extensible water-impermeable plastic film spread evenly with a self-adhesive plaster mass. A standard for Waterproof Plastic Self-adhesive Plaster is given in the British Pharmaceutical Codex 1973.

It is used to secure dressings and appliances, and to cover a site of infection when total exclusion of water, water vapour, and air is required. This type of product has particular application in the food industry in order to cover wounds during the manipulation of foodstuffs, as the occlusive nature of the tape prevents transmission of organisms from infected wounds. It is also used as the backing material in Waterproof Plastic Wound Dressing (see under Wound Dressings).

WATERPROOF MICROPOROUS PLASTIC SELF-ADHESIVE TAPE (Waterproof Microporous Plastic Self-adhesive Plaster; Semipermeable Waterproof Plaster; Semipermeable Waterproof Tape; *Airstrip®*) consists of an extensible plastic film which is made impermeable to water but permeable to air and water vapour, spread with a self-adhesive mass. A standard for Waterproof Microporous Plastic Self-adhesive Plaster is given in the British Pharmaceutical Codex 1973.

It is used as the backing material in Waterproof Microporous Plastic Wound Dressing (see under Wound Dressings).

PERFORATED PLASTIC SELF-ADHESIVE TAPE (Perforated Plastic Self-adhesive Plaster; Porous Plastic Plaster; *Dermiclear®*; *Transpore®*) consists of an extensible perforated plastic film spread with a self-adhesive mass made permeable to air and water vapour. A standard for Perforated Plastic Self-adhesive Plaster is given in the British Pharmaceutical Codex 1973.

It is used to secure dressings and appliances, and to cover sites of infection when a completely permeable plaster which will not lose its adhesive properties when immersed in water is required. It is also used as the backing material in Perforated Plastic Wound Dressing (see under Wound Dressings).

POLYETHYLENE NON-POROUS SYNTHETIC ADHESIVE TAPE consists of an extensible, impermeable polyethylene film spread with a single-ingredient copolymer adhesive. The material is occlusive and is used to isolate the wound from the external environment, to secure dressings and appliances, and to cover sites of infection where total exclusion of water and water vapour is required.

Non-stitch Adhesive Sutures

STERILE SKIN CLOSURES are suitably shaped pieces of adhesive tape which are used to hold the two edges of a wound together after subcuticular stitching, thus allowing healing without the use of surface sutures. They may also be used to prevent spreading of the scar after removal of skin sutures. One type consists of a dumbbell-shaped piece of adhesive tape to which, at the narrowest part of the dumbbell is attached a small piece of lint or cotton gauze. A second type consists of a butterfly-shaped piece of adhesive tape which allows tension to be applied in such a way as to draw each edge of the wound together before being maintained in position by a secondary adhesive tab. Products include *Netaseal®* and *Dumb-bell®*.

ADHESIVE OPERATION SITE DRAPE consists of a large sheet of polyethylene coated with a layer of acrylic adhesive or a semipermeable adhesive-coated polyurethane film (*Opsite®*). It is placed over the previously cleansed and dried area of the skin prior to surgery. The surgical procedure continues without removing the drape, the edges of the wound being immediately protected by the adhering drape material. The same material is also available in smaller pieces as a direct wound dressing and as a means of closing a wound in place of sutures.

Protectives

ANTI-DECUBITUS PADS (Fleecy Pads) consist of high-pile polyester fibre pads with a plastic or fabric or plastic-coated fabric backing.

They are used in the prevention and treatment of decubitus ulcers (pressure sores) by placing them beneath those areas of the body which are subject to the highest pressure. The fibre mass allows the passage of urine, thus ensuring that the incontinent patient remains dry. Pads should be laundered frequently and, if necessary, sterilised. The formation of decubitus ulcers on heels and elbows can be prevented by using tubular bandages lined with fleecy pad.

ANIMAL WOOL FOR CHIROPODY (Animal Wool Long Strand; Lamb's Wool for Chiropody) is obtained from the sheep, *Ovis aries* L. (Fam. Bovidae); foreign substances and grease are removed by scouring, washing, and combing. It is very hygroscopic, absorbing up to 50% of moisture, and is usually supplied as a yellowish-white, continuous, slightly twisted, coherent sliver. A standard is given in the British Pharmaceutical Codex 1973.

Animal wool for chiropody is used for protective purposes, to assist in the retention of dressings on toes, and also as a substitute for felt or rubber padding when these are known to produce an adverse response in the patient.

FOAM-PADDED ELASTICATED SURGICAL TUBULAR STOCKINETTE (*Tubipad®*) consists of Tubular Stockinette Bandage (see under Bandages) lined with foam and is available in different limb and body sizes.

It is used to relieve pressure and eliminate friction on pressure-sensitive areas, or to hold a dressing in place over an existing pressure sore whilst reducing further damage. The porosity of the foam lining allows normal water loss from the skin surface.

OILED SILK consists of silk fabric which has been evenly

proofed with drying oils or synthetic resins so that the material is impervious to water. A standard is given in the British Pharmaceutical Codex 1973.

It is used as a protective layer to prevent wet dressings and fomentations from drying out and to protect adjacent clothing. An alternative material is oiled nylon.

ORTHOPAEDIC WADDING consists of a fibrous mass of cotton, or of cotton and viscose, which has been formed into a thin felt and made into rolls. It is used beneath either extension strapping or plaster of paris bandage to protect the skin surface from undue abrasion and, if required, to increase compression on a selected area. Proprietary products of this type include *Orthoban®*, *Sofban®*, and *Velban®*.

POLYURETHANE FOAM (SURGICAL) consists of polyurethane foam in various thicknesses with either a plain or an adhesive backing.

It is soft and resilient and is used for padding purposes and for lining plaster casts. It is especially useful for increasing the efficiency of pressure bandaging by placing it on top of a paste bandage and securing it with a diachylon bandage. The positioning will depend upon the condition being treated; it may be applied either directly above the ulcer or above the varicose vein causing the ulcer, and hence pressure can be increased on the area where it is required without increasing the overall pressure on the limb. *Polyfoam®* is a proprietary product of this type.

VACCINATION PADS consist of either square pads of lint enclosed in unmedicated gauze with elastic self-adhesive straps attached diagonally, or round pads made of a ring of adhesive felt backed by a disc of lint and covered with a plastic self-adhesive plaster. The first type is available in two sizes, one about 38 mm square for children, and the other about 50 mm square for adults; the second type is available in one size only. The pads are used mainly for protection and should be removed with care if adhesion occurs. The second (circular) type is of particular use in preventing adhesion of the lint to the vaccination surface. Proprietary products include *Helvia®* pads (square) and *Wades®* pads (circular).

Plasters

Unmedicated Plasters

PLASTER OF PARIS BANDAGE (*Gypsona®*) consists of cotton cloth impregnated with a mixture of dried calcium sulphate, consisting of both the amorphous and crystalline forms, and suitable adhesives so that the mixture is adherent to the fabric. The bandage is soaked in water before application.

The setting time of the bandage may be varied by the incorporation of various modifiers. A standard is given in the British Pharmaceutical Codex 1973.

Plaster of Paris bandage is used for the immobilisation of fractures, or of diseased bones and joints, for the correction and prevention of deformities, and for immobilisation in the treatment of burns and soft tissue injuries. Various application techniques are used, and the bandage should only be applied by experienced personnel. The bandage is used in the form of padded or unpadded casts, strengthening slabs, plaster beds, and removable splints.

Padding is used in all conditions where swelling is either present or is expected, and also where the bones in the limb are superficial or the limb itself is thin; bony prominences around joints may also need protection. For the purpose of padding, orthopaedic wadding (see under

Protectives) may be applied to the full length of the limb to be plastered, with minimal overlapping to prevent uneven layering.

Other padding materials used include tubular stockinette (see under Bandages), which can be folded back to protect the edge of the cast, and felt in rings or strips, which can be used to give special protection to bony prominences. Unpadded casts are applied either directly to the skin or on top of a fine stockinette lining; care must be taken that no plaster abrasions occur and that the blood circulation is not impaired.

Medicated Plasters

BELLADONNA SELF-ADHESIVE PLASTER (Belladonna Plaster) consists of a suitable cloth spread evenly with a self-adhesive plaster mass which contains an extract of *Atropa belladonna* herb or root and is covered with a removable protective film. A standard is given in the British Pharmaceutical Codex 1973.

The plaster is used as a counter-irritant in the treatment of rheumatism, lumbago, neuralgia, and similar conditions. It is applied, after removal of the protective film, to the pre-washed and dried skin, and is removed by soaking or immersion in warm water, followed by gentle stripping.

SALICYLIC ACID SELF-ADHESIVE PLASTER (Salicylic Acid Plaster) consists of a suitable cloth spread with a self-adhesive plaster mass which contains up to 40% of salicylic acid and is covered with a removable protective film. A standard is given in the British Pharmaceutical Codex 1973.

The plaster is used as a keratolytic agent in the removal of warts, corns, and verrucas. It is placed, after removal of the protective film, in direct contact with the area to be treated, care being taken to restrict the salicylic acid coating to the wart, corn, or verruca. It must not be used on hypersensitive skin areas. It is removed by gently soaking the material away from the skin surface.

Suxamethonium Bromide

2,2'-Succinyldioxybis(ethyltrimethylammonium) dibromide dihydrate

$[(CH_3)_3N\cdot[CH_2]_2\cdot O\cdot CO\cdot[CH_2]_2\cdot CO\cdot O\cdot[CH_2]_2\cdot N(CH_3)_3]^{2+}\ 2Br^-, 2H_2O$

$C_{14}H_{30}Br_2N_2O_4, 2H_2O = 486.2$

OTHER NAMES: *Brevidil M®*; Succinylcholine Bromide

A standard is given in the British Pharmacopoeia 1973

Description. An almost odourless, white or creamy-white powder with a slightly saline taste.

Solubility. Soluble, at 20°, in less than 1 part of water and in 5 parts of alcohol; practically insoluble in ether and in chloroform.

Acidity. A 1% solution has a pH of 4 to 5.

Moisture content. 6 to 8%, determined by drying at 105°.

Incompatibility. In solution, suxamethonium bromide is rapidly destroyed by alkalis and therefore should not be mixed with thiopentone sodium.

Storage. It should be protected from light.

Identification. TEST. Dissolve about 100 mg in 10 ml of water and add 10 ml of *dilute sulphuric acid* and 30 ml of *ammonium reineckate solution*; a pink precipitate is produced which, after standing for 30 minutes, washing with water, with alcohol (95%), and with ether, and drying at 80°, melts at about 180°.

MELTING-POINT. About 225°.

Metabolism. See under Suxamethonium Chloride.

Actions and uses. Suxamethonium bromide has the actions, uses, and undesirable effects described under Suxamethonium Chloride. The usual dose by intravenous injection for an adult is 0.5 to 1 milligram of the base per kilogram body-weight; 1.67 milligrams of suxamethonium bromide is approximately equivalent to 1 milligram of the cation.

Precautions; Poisoning. As for Suxamethonium Chloride.

Preparation

SUXAMETHONIUM BROMIDE INJECTION (*Syn.* Succinylcholine Bromide Injection): a sterile solution of suxamethonium bromide in water for injections. It is prepared by dissolving the contents of a sealed container in water for injections immediately before use. Available as a powder in ampoules containing 67 mg of suxamethonium bromide, equivalent to 40 mg of cation.
A standard for this injection is given in the British Pharmacopoeia 1973
Containers and *Labelling:* see the entry on Injections for general information on containers and labelling.
Storage: the sealed container should be protected from light. The injection decomposes on storage and should be used immediately after preparation.

Suxamethonium Chloride

2,2′-Succinyldioxybis(ethyltrimethylammonium)   dichloride dihydrate

$[(CH_3)_3N \cdot [CH_2]_2 \cdot O \cdot CO \cdot [CH_2]_2 \cdot CO \cdot O \cdot [CH_2]_2 \cdot N(CH_3)_3]^{2+}$ $2Cl^-$, $2H_2O$

$C_{14}H_{30}Cl_2N_2O_4, 2H_2O = 397.3$

OTHER NAMES: *Anectine*®; Succinylcholine Chloride; Suxamethonii Chloridum

A standard is given in the European Pharmacopoeia Vol. I

Description. An almost odourless, white, crystalline powder with a salty taste.

Solubility. Soluble, at 20°, in 1 part of water; soluble in alcohol; practically insoluble in ether.

Acidity. A 1% solution has a pH of 4 to 5.

Moisture content. 8 to 10%, determined by Fischer titration.

Incompatibility. In solution, suxamethonium chloride is rapidly destroyed by alkalis and therefore should not be mixed with thiopentone sodium.

Sterilisation. Solutions for injection are sterilised by heating with a bactericide or by filtration.

Storage. It should be protected from light.

Identification. TEST. It complies with the test described under Suxamethonium Bromide.

MELTING-POINT. About 160°.

Metabolism. ABSORPTION. Suxamethonium salts are slowly and incompletely absorbed after oral administration and are usually administered intravenously.

DISTRIBUTION. Crosses the placenta in small amounts.

METABOLIC REACTIONS. Hydrolysed in plasma and body tissues to form choline and succinylmonocholine; the latter is further hydrolysed to choline and succinic acid; succinylmonocholine   has   weak   muscle-relaxing properties.

EXCRETION. Less than 3% of a dose is excreted unchanged in the urine.

FURTHER INFORMATION. Plasma-cholinesterase activity and the action of suxamethonium in animals—F. Hobbiger and A. W. Peck, *Br. J. Pharmac.*, 1970, **40**, 775; hydrolysis of suxamethonium in blood—H. Holst-Larsen, *Br. J. Anaesth.*, 1976, **48**, 887.

Actions and uses. Suxamethonium chloride is a short-acting relaxant of voluntary muscle. It produces muscular paralysis by a depolarisation of the neuromuscular end-plate. This effect is increased rather than antagonised   by   the   anticholinesterase   drugs,   such   as neostigmine.

Suxamethonium chloride given intravenously in a dose of 30 to 60 milligrams to an adult will produce an immediate but short-lasting muscular relaxation with respiratory paralysis. The onset of relaxation is preceded by diffuse incoordinated muscular contractions which are painful; pain may also be experienced during recovery. The administration of suxamethonium chloride should therefore always be preceded by an intravenous anaesthetic such as thiopentone sodium.

The contractions occur in about 15 seconds after administration of the suxamethonium and last for about 20 seconds, their disappearance indicating the onset of paralysis. In the majority of patients, paralysis lasts for 2 to 6 minutes, after which time muscle power returns and becomes normal in a further 3 or 4 minutes.

Suxamethonium chloride is given intravenously, in single doses, for short operative manipulative procedures, such as endotracheal intubation, for the prevention of traumatic complications in electro-convulsion therapy, and in the symptomatic treatment of convulsions of tetanus. For long operations, repeated intravenous doses may be given; no cumulative effect or tachyphylaxis occurs. Alternatively, it may be given as a 1 in 1000 solution by continuous intravenous infusion, by which means the degree of relaxation can easily be controlled.

The dose of suxamethonium is often given in terms of the base; 1.37 milligrams of suxamethonium chloride is approximately equivalent to 1 milligram of the base.

Suxamethonium chloride may be used with any of the commonly employed anaesthetics.

Undesirable effects. Bradycardia and hypertension may occur, but these are of no significance except during electroconvulsive therapy or after severe burns when cardiac arrest has been attributed to them.

In normal persons, suxamethonium chloride is rapidly inactivated by cholinesterase enzymes, but occasionally paralysis may be prolonged and this is usually associated with low serum-cholinesterase activity which may occur in carcinoma of the bronchus, liver disease, malnutrition, and poisoning due to organophosphorus compounds, or as a result of genetic factors.

Pain in the muscles of the chest, shoulder, and neck sometimes follows the administration of suxamethonium chloride, particularly in patients who are ambulant shortly after its use.

Precautions. Respiratory paralysis will occur with adequate muscular relaxation and facilities for controlled respiration should be available when the drug is used.

In therapeutic doses, suxamethonium chloride does not cause liberation of histamine and it has no significant effect on the cardiovascular or any other system.

With high doses, especially when given by intravenous infusion, there may be a rise in blood pressure due to the stimulatory action of suxamethonium chloride on the sympathetic ganglia (nicotinic action); this may be counteracted by the administration of ganglion-blocking drugs, such as pentolinium tartrate.

Poisoning. Respiratory depression should be combated by controlled respiration, an insufflator or closed-circuit anaesthetic machine being used.

Preparation

SUXAMETHONIUM CHLORIDE INJECTION (*Syn.* Succinyl-choline Chloride Injection): a sterile solution of suxamethonium chloride in water for injections. It is sterilised by heating with a bactericide or by filtration. Available in 2-ml ampoules containing 50 mg of suxamethonium chloride per ml, equivalent to 36.5 mg of cation.

A standard for this injection is given in the British Pharmacopoeia 1973
Containers: see the entry on Injections for general information on containers.
Labelling: see the entry on Injections for general information on labelling. In addition, the label on the package should state the date of preparation.
Storage: it should be stored at as low a temperature as possible above its freezing-point and not exceeding 4°. Under these conditions it may be expected to retain its potency for 2 years.

Swine Erysipelas Antiserum

Serum of horses or other suitable animals immunised with antigens of *Erysipelothrix rhusiopathiae* or a preparation from the serum containing substances which specifically protect animals against *E. rhusiopathiae.*

OTHER NAME: Erysipelothrix Rhusiopathiae Antiserum

A standard is given in the British Pharmacopoeia (Veterinary)

Storage. It should be protected from light and stored at 2° to 8°. Liquid preparations should not be allowed to freeze.

Veterinary uses. It is used by subcutaneous injection in a dose of 0.2 millilitre per kilogram body-weight for protection of pigs against swine erysipelas, and by subcutaneous injection in a dose of 1 to 1.2 millilitres per kilogram body-weight for the treatment of infected pigs.

Swine Erysipelas Vaccine, Inactivated

A culture, in a suitable medium, of virulent immunogenic strains of *Erysipelothrix rhusiopathiae*, inactivated in such a manner that immunogenic activity is retained.

OTHER NAME: Erysipelothrix Rhusiopathiae Vaccine, Inactivated

A standard is given in the British Pharmacopoeia (Veterinary)

Storage. The vaccine should be protected from light and stored at 2° to 8°.

Veterinary uses. It is administered by intramuscular injection for prophylaxis of swine erysipelas in pigs and disease caused by *Erysipelothrix rhusiopathiae* in turkeys.

Swine Erysipelas Vaccine, Living

A culture, in a suitable medium, of a smooth strain or strains of *Erysipelothrix rhusiopathiae* that are not pathogenic to mice.

OTHER NAME: Erysipelothrix Rhusiopathiae Vaccine, Living

A standard is given in the British Pharmacopoeia (Veterinary)

Storage. The vaccine should be protected from light and stored at 2° to 8° when it may be expected to retain its potency for 4 weeks.

Veterinary uses. It is administered by intramuscular injection for prophylaxis of swine erysipelas in pigs and disease caused by *Erysipelothrix rhusiopathiae* in turkeys.

Sympathomimetics

A sympathomimetic agent is a substance that acts on the effector cells of the sympathetic nervous system and mimics the effect of sympathetic nerve stimulation.

Direct-acting sympathomimetic agents act directly on the adrenergic receptors. They may be selective in their action and can be used to stimulate specific tissues innervated by the sympathetic nervous system. For a more detailed account see Adrenergic Receptors.

Indirect-acting sympathomimetic agents act by releasing noradrenaline from storage sites in adrenergic nerve endings. Thus their effects on the sympathetic nervous system are more generalised.

Direct-acting sympathomimetics include adrenaline, isoprenaline, noradrenaline, orciprenaline, salbutamol, and terbutaline.

Indirect-acting sympathomimetics include amphetamine and dexamphetamine.

Sympathomimetics with a combination of direct and indirect action include ephedrine, mephentermine, metaraminol, methoxamine, phenylephrine, phenylpropanolamine, and pseudoephedrine.

Syphilis

Syphilis is a venereal disease due to infection with *Treponema pallidum*. It is usually passed on by sexual contact. If untreated, syphilis passes through three distinct stages. After an incubation period of 2 to 6 weeks primary syphilis characterised by the formation of a hard chancre (ulcer or nodule) occurs at the site of entry of the organism.

The usual site is the glans or prepuce of the male or the cervix or vaginal introitus of the female although sometimes it is in the anus or rectum. There is lymph-node enlargement and the chancre discharges serum which is highly infective.

After about 2 months the chancre heals, but there is then a general systemic illness—secondary syphilis. It is usually mild with a generalised rash, sore throat, headache, and generalised lymphadenitis. The rash is very variable but is often macular at first followed by a papular rash a few weeks later. Infective condylomata may occur later, especially in moist regions such as the perineum. After 1 to 2 months the rash usually disappears but may reappear at any time.

In the third stage painless destructive lesions can occur in any part of the body and symptoms may occur from

1 to 30 years after the initial infection. These lesions may occur in the aorta and large vessels, the meninges at the base of the brain, the skin, or elsewhere. Neurosyphilis usually occurs 1 to 10 years after primary infection and results in general paralysis and tabes dorsalis.

Diagnosis of syphilis depends on serological tests or in the primary stage identification of the organism in infected areas.

For the treatment of primary and early secondary syphilis benzylpenicillin is administered in the form of long-acting injections for up to 20 days; other antibiotics such as erythromycin and tetracycline are occasionally used in penicillin-hypersensitive patients. Tertiary syphilis is also treated with penicillins, but treatment may be needed for longer. Serological tests should be carried out at intervals to ensure that the disease has been eradicated.

Congenital syphilis sometimes occurs in infants born of infected mothers. Signs similar to those of adult syphilis are seen in the child in the first few years of life. It is treated by penicillins as for adult syphilis.

Syrups

Syrups are concentrated aqueous solutions of sucrose or other sugars to which medicaments or flavourings may be added. Glycerol, sorbitol, or other polyhydric alcohols are sometimes added in small amounts to medicated syrups to retard crystallisation of sucrose or to increase the solubility of other ingredients.

Medicated syrups provide a convenient form of stock solution of certain drugs for use in extemporaneous preparations.

Flavouring syrups are not usually medicated but contain various aromatic or pleasantly flavoured substances and are intended to be used as vehicles or flavours for extemporaneous preparations. They are of particular use in masking the disagreeable taste of bitter or saline drugs.

Dilute solutions of sucrose will support the growth of moulds, yeasts, and other micro-organisms. The apparatus used in the preparation of syrups should therefore be thoroughly cleansed before use. Water for preparations should be used and care should be taken to avoid contamination during preparation. Growth of micro-organisms is usually retarded when the concentration of sucrose is higher than 65% w/w, but at this strength crystallisation of the sucrose may occur.

Dilution of syrups. Unless otherwise indicated in the individual monograph, when a dose ordered or prescribed is less than or not a multiple of 5 millilitres, the syrup should be diluted appropriately with syrup, so that the dose to be measured by the patient is one 5-ml spoonful or multiple thereof.

Storage. Syrups should be recently prepared unless special precautions have been taken to prevent their contamination. Fruit syrups may be stored for longer periods if they have been heated to boiling point and filled into sterile bottles, which are then sealed to exclude micro-organisms.

Systemic Lupus Erythematosus

Systemic lupus erythematosus is a chronic disease in which many autoimmune phenomena develop. The most common autoimmune phenomenon is the formation of abnormal immunoglobulins which behave like antibodies to nucleoprotein. These are called antinuclear antibodies. There is also fibrinoid degeneration of collagen and intercellular connective tissues and vasculitis.

The disease occurs predominantly in young women and onset may be precipitated by exposure to sunlight, infection, or administration of drugs such as sulphonamides. Lesions may occur in any part of the body and may persist or recur for years.

Systemic lupus erythematosus may result in malaise, fever, arthralgia, progressive renal disease leading to renal failure, diffuse myocarditis leading to congestive heart failure, splenomegaly, lymph node enlargement, pneumonitis, thrombocytopenia, epilepsy, or psychoses. Symmetrical erythematous lesions occur on the skin, particularly of the face; when these occur in isolation, the disease is called discoid or cutaneous lupus erythematosus. The course of systemic lupus erythematosus is commonly chronic with relapses and remissions. The erythrocyte sedimentation rate is always raised.

Large doses of corticosteroids with or without immunosuppressive agents may be required to alleviate this condition and chloroquine may also be of value. Exacerbations of systemic lupus erythematosus may be reduced by the elimination of emotional stress, physical fatigue, and other predisposing factors such as exposure to sunlight; the use of drugs liable to precipitate an attack should be avoided. Non-steroidal anti-inflammatory drugs are used to control symptoms such as arthralgia.

Systemic Sclerosis

Systemic sclerosis (Scleroderma) is a disease in which deposition of collagen and obliterative lesions of small arteries result in a diffuse indurative change in the skin and subcutaneous tissues and sometimes in the viscera, especially the gastro-intestinal tract, lungs, kidneys, and heart. Raynaud's phenomenon may occur at first, to be later followed by the formation of hard waxy plaques in the skin which become firmly attached to underlying structures. The viscera may be affected by the sclerosing process at any stage of the disease. Visceral complications include dysphagia, intestinal malabsorption, and dyspnoea due to pulmonary fibrosis. Polyarthritis and heart failure may also occur.

There is no specific treatment for systemic sclerosis but penicillamine may be useful in the active phase of the disease. Non-steroidal anti-inflammatory drugs are used for pain relief but steroids should be avoided.

Tablets

Tablets are solid single-dose forms which comprise medicament(s), usually with excipients, compressed or moulded into circular shapes with flat or convex faces, or other suitable shapes. They are formulated to release the active ingredients in a way that will achieve the desired effect, and their quality is controlled by a number of standard tests which may include uniformity of weight and content, hardness, friability, disintegration, and dissolution.

Compressed Tablets

Compressed tablets are formed from a granulated preparation of the active ingredients by compaction using punches in suitable dies. The medicinal substances may be converted into dry free-flowing granules by one of the following processes.

Dry granulation processes are of value for medicaments

which are heat- or moisture-sensitive; two methods are used, direct compression and granulation by preliminary compression. A few medicaments (mainly inorganic salts) exhibit adequate flow, cohesive, and disintegrant properties and can be compressed directly into tablets, but in most instances, and especially when the dose of the medicament is small, diluents have to be added to produce a blend which is compressible and yet has disintegrant properties. A number of direct compression diluents have been developed; examples are lactose (spray dried and anhydrous grades), dicalcium phosphate dihydrate, microcrystalline cellulose, special grades of starch, and crystallisation products from sucrose-dextrin mixtures.

Granulation by preliminary compression is a more traditional process by which the medicament, blended with appropriate adjuvants in powder form, is precompressed in a heavy tablet machine or between rollers under controlled pressure. The "slugs" or cakes which form are broken into granules of appropriate size distribution by milling and screening. Granulation by preliminary compression is particularly suitable for preparing granules which are sensitive to moisture, and the process is frequently used in a controlled environmental area of low humidity.

Moist granulation. Cohesion of the powdered medicament and additives is achieved by the incorporation of an inert binder. The binder may be mixed, in the dry state, with the other components and takes effect only on the addition of a liquid; alternatively, the binder, dissolved or suspended in a suitable liquid, is dispersed throughout the powdered components. In either instance, the amount of liquid added and the efficiency of the mixing process should be such that the powder is moistened, not wetted, and is cohesive but does not adhere to the mesh when pressed through a sieve. By using as the moistening agent an anhydrous solvent, the moist granulation method may be used with materials that are sensitive to water.

Granules are formed by passing the mass through screens or sieves and drying at a temperature below 60°. The dried granules are again passed through a sieve and blended to an appropriate size range for tabletting; lubricants may also be incorporated at this stage.

Excipients should be inert and are either mixed with medicaments or added to granules; they include diluents, binders, aids to disintegration, glidants, and lubricants. Colours, flavours and sweetening agents are permitted for some preparations.

The most common of the *diluents* is lactose but sucrose, dextrose, starch, calcium phosphate, and sodium chloride are also widely used. Sucrose, dextrose, and starch serve additionally as *binders*; acacia, tragacanth, gelatin, cellulose derivatives, and alginates are also used as binders. They may be dissolved or dispersed in water, alcohol, or isopropyl alcohol.

Traditionally, starch and, more recently, modified starches, have been used as *disintegrating agents*; among other disintegrants are microcrystalline cellulose and alginates.

Glidants are substances added to enhance the flow properties of granules. The term *lubricant* is confined to materials such as stearic acid and stearates which are mixed with or sprayed on to granules to facilitate release of tablets from the punches and dies after compression.

Moulded tablets or tablet triturates are small disks which usually contain a potent medicament diluted with

lactose, sucrose, dextrose or mannitol, or a mixture of these diluents. The finely powdered components are moistened with alcohol (60%) or other suitable liquid, and tablets are formed by pressing the soft mass into a previously calibrated mould of metal, plastic, or rubber. After ejection from the mould, the tablets are dried at room temperature.

Effervescent tablets are compressed tablets which, on addition to water, release carbon dioxide formed by chemical reaction between citric or tartaric acid and carbonates or bicarbonates. They provide rapid disintegration and dissolution of the medicinal substances and, by adjustment of the acid content, palatability can be improved. Granulation is achieved either by the careful incorporation of controlled amounts of water followed by drying or by the use of a non-aqueous granulating liquid such as alcohol.

Chewable tablets should be rapidly disintegrated in the mouth by chewing; they can usually be taken without water. Mannitol is the diluent most frequently adopted for chewable tablets but sorbitol, lactose, dextrose, and glycine have also been used.

Buccal and sublingual tablets contain medicaments intended to be absorbed directly through the oral mucosa. They are held in the buccal pouch or beneath the tongue and are designed to dissolve slowly in most instances, to enable systemic absorption by this route to be completed.

Boluses are tablets weighing 5 g or more used in veterinary medicine.

Sustained-release tablets or slow tablets are usually formulated to provide an initial dose of the medicament and to release slowly further amounts to maintain a therapeutic response over a period of several hours. An advantage of sustained-release tablets is the reduction that can be achieved in the frequency of administration. On the other hand the substance may remain in the body for an unduly extended period when the preparation is withdrawn. Sustained-release tablets may be formulated to reduce the rate of release of medicinal substances such as potassium chloride which in high concentrations are irritant to the gastro-intestinal mucosa.

Many methods are used to achieve controlled release of medicinal substances; for example, the tablet may be prepared from coated granules, or the active substance in fine particles may be embedded in a hydrophobic matrix. Other techniques involve the use of inert porous carriers or the coating of inner cores of the medicinal substance with a resistant film; in other tablets a resistant core may be coated with an outer layer from which the initial dose of the medicinal substance is rapidly released. Ion-exchange resins are also used to form drug-resinates from which the drug is slowly displaced in the body by interaction with the ions in the gastro-intestinal fluids.

Layer tablets may be used to separate incompatible ingredients.

Coated Tablets

Coatings may be applied to tablets to protect the active ingredients from light and the atmosphere; coatings may also mask unpleasant tastes and odours or prevent contact with a substance of an irritant or potentially sensitising nature. The purpose of enteric coating is to control the location of drug release in the body whereas in sustained-release tablets the aim is to control the rate of release by suitable coatings on either the granules or the tablet cores.

The main coating processes are pan coating, compression coating, and air-suspension coating.

Pan coating is the traditional method in which tablet cores are rotated in a suitably-shaped bowl or cylinder of copper or stainless steel. Successive coats are formed in thin-layers by the application of a solution or suspension of the coating substance in a suitable liquid.

Compression coating is a high-speed technique by which the coating substance, in the form of dry granules, is compressed around the tablet core using punches and dies.

In the *air-suspension coating* method the tablet cores are fluidised and cycled by an upward current of air inside a cylindrical vessel and then sprayed with the coating substance dissolved or suspended in a volatile liquid.

Coating Composition

Sugar coating in a pan involves the addition of a series of coatings to the tablet cores. The application of a waterproofing coat of shellac, ethylcellulose, a silicone fluid, or other suitable sealant may be necessary to protect the core from the moisture in the subsequent coats; this is followed by subcoats and smoothing coats predominantly of sugar with starch or other suitable substances. The coating is applied by the addition of syrup, suitably coloured if required, and water is removed by forcing a current of hot air through the tablets. It is desirable that when tablets are coloured the process should be carefully controlled to ensure uniformity. Finally the coating is polished. Sugar coats may also be applied by compression coating.

Compression coating is a dry process which may be useful for moisture-sensitive substances, or to separate incompatible medicaments; it is also used for some types of sustained-release tablets. The materials used in granules for the coating can vary considerably but lactose and calcium phosphate are commonly used.

Film coatings can be applied rapidly by the air suspension technique or more slowly by either spraying or pouring in a coating pan. Vinyl polymers which include povidone and polyvinyl alcohol, cellulose derivatives including cellacephate, and natural gums and resins are used in film coats. Macrogols or phthalates are added as plasticisers and the vehicles are usually mixtures of non-aqueous volatile solvents.

Enteric coating is usually applied as a film by spraying in a pan or by the air-suspension technique; compression coating may be a suitable method for waxy or lipid materials. An enteric coat is required to resist the gastric fluid and to permit penetration of the intestinal fluid. Although various approaches have been followed to achieve the enteric effect the most common is to use pH-sensitive materials. Cellacephate, which is widely used, is soluble in fluids of pH 6 or above and is also digested by enzymes in the intestinal fluid. Anionic polymers of methacrylic acid have been introduced which, in thin films, swell and become permeable at pH values between 5.5 and 8; by using mixtures of these materials, control can be exercised over the conditions under which film disruption occurs.

Extemporaneous preparation of tablets. Compressed tablets are mainly manufactured on the large scale using multi-punch rotary tablet presses. Single-punch machines are used for small-scale production or when heavy compaction pressures are required.

Extemporaneous preparation of tablets to special formulations by compression or by moulding may occasionally be feasible where the necessary equipment is available, but it is often more practicable to dispense the substances in the form of hard capsules, provided that the prescriber agrees and there is little risk of alteration in the therapeutic efficacy of the medicine.

Identification. Pharmacists are sometimes shown tablets of unknown composition and asked to identify them. Unless imprinted codes or words are present on the tablets, positive identification is not usually possible without extensive work. Some information may be obtained from the appearance of the tablet and by comparison with samples of known identity. In the case of uncoated tablets the diameter may be measured and compared with tables of tablet diameters such as that given below. Occasionally simple chemical tests may give useful information, but care should be taken to avoid undue reliance on these procedures. Useful references include an illustrated guide to the identification of British proprietary tablets and capsules which is included in the *Chemist and Druggist Directory*, Benn Publications, London, published annually. Imprints that are used to mark tablets and capsules from British, European, and North American sources are indexed in W. A. L. Collier, *Imprex* (Index of Imprints used on Tablets and Capsules), 6th Edn, D. Ferrier Ltd, Edinburgh, 1976.

Administration of tablets. Tablets for oral administration are usually intended to be swallowed whole with a drink of water. For children or persons unable to swallow tablets whole, oral tablets may be crushed and moistened with water or a suitable liquid before administration, but this procedure cannot be adopted with enteric-coated or sustained-release tablets or those containing irritant substances. Some tablets are intended to be chewed rather than swallowed. Sublingual and buccal tablets are intended to be dissolved slowly under the tongue or between the cheek and gums. Soluble tablets and effervescent tablets are dissolved in water to make solutions for oral administration. Large tablets containing insoluble materials may be required to be mixed with water to form a suspension for administration.

Containers and storage. All tablets should be stored and supplied in containers which provide adequate protection against crushing. Airtight and light-resistant containers should be used when their need is indicated in individual entries. Tablets should be stored at room temperature unless otherwise stated in the entry describing a particular preparation, or on the label.

Suitable containers for dispensing tablets include tablet bottles, jars, or vials made from amber glass or amber or opaque plastic. Screw caps, if fitted, should be of metal or plastic with suitable liners; close-fitting plastic caps may also be used. Cylindrical aluminium containers are also suitable; they should be lined with paper or the internal surface should be coated with inert lacquer and fitted with either an aluminium screw cap or a close-fitting plastic cap. The appropriate British Standards are: for glass containers, BS 1679: Part 2, 1965; for plastic containers, BS 1679: Part 4, 1969; and for metal containers, BS 1679: Part 3, 1965. Tablets packaged in strip or blister packs should be dispensed in containers of the types described above, or in paperboard cartons or wallets which conform to BS 1679, Part 1, 1976.

Labelling. If the tablets are enteric-coated or a sustained-release formulation this should be stated. Special instructions to the patient with regard to the administration of the tablets should be given when required.

Tablet Diameters

In the following list, * indicates compression coated tablets. The names used correspond to the titles of tablets described in the relevent entries.

Tablet	Strength
Tablet diameter (mm) 5.0	
Acetomenaphthone	5 mg
Codeine Phosphate	15 mg
Colchicine	250 mcg
Dienoestrol	100 mcg
Ephedrine Hydrochloride	7.5 mg, 15 mg
Ergometrine	125 mcg
Ethinyloestradiol	10 mcg
Folic Acid	100 mcg
Glyceryl Trinitrate	300 mcg
Hyoscine	300 mcg, 400 mcg
Liothyronine	5 mcg
Morphine Sulphate	10 mg, 15 mg
Nicoumalone	1 mg
Papaveretum	10 mg
Phenobarbitone	15 mg
Phenobarbitone Sodium	15 mg
Proguanil	25 mg
Propylthiouracil	25 mg
Stilboestrol	100 mcg
Thiamine Hydrochloride	1 mg
Thyroid	30 mg
Tablet diameter (mm) 5.5	
Acetomenaphthone	10 mg
Amylobarbitone	15 mg, 30 mg, 50 mg
Atropine Sulphate	300 mcg
Belladonna and Phenobarbitone	—
Bendrofluazide	2.5 mg
Betamethasone Sodium Phosphate	250 mcg
Codeine Phosphate	30 mg
Colchicine	500 mcg
Dapsone	50 mg
Dienoestrol	300 mcg
Digitalis, Prepared	30 mg
Digitoxin	100 mcg
Digoxin	62.5 mcg, 125 mcg
Ephedrine Hydrochloride	30 mg
Ergometrine	250 mcg
Ethinyloestradiol	20 mcg
Folic Acid	5 mg
Glyceryl Trinitrate	500 mcg
Hydrocortisone [LOZENGES]	2.5 mg
Hyoscine	600 mcg
Ipecacuanha and Opium	60 mg
Isoniazid	25 mg
Liothyronine	20 mcg
Morphine Sulphate	30 mg
Nicotinic Acid	25 mg
Phenindione	10 mg
Phenobarbitone	30 mg
Phenobarbitone Sodium	30 mg
Prednisolone	1 mg
Prednisone	1 mg
Pyridoxine	10 mg
Reserpine	100 mcg
Riboflavine	1 mg
Sodium Citrate	60 mg
Stilboestrol	250 mcg
Thiamine Hydrochloride	3 mg
Thyroxine	50 mcg
Tablet diameter (mm) 6.0	
Dexamethasone (Veterinary)	250 mcg

Tablet	Strength
Diameter 6.0 mm (continued)	
Frusemide	20 mg
Medroxyprogesterone (Veterinary)	5 mg
Tablet diameter (mm) 6.5	
Acepromazine (Veterinary)	10 mg
Acetarsol	60 mg
Amylobarbitone	60 mg
Amylobarbitone Sodium	60 mg
Ascorbic Acid	5 mg
Atropine Sulphate	400 mcg
Bendrofluazide	5 mg
Betamethasone	250 mcg
Betamethasone Sodium Phosphate	500 mcg
Bethanidine	10 mg
Butobarbitone	60 mg
Chlorproguanil	20 mg
Dexamethasone	500 mcg, 750 mcg
Dextromoramide	5 mg
Dichlorphenamide	50 mg
Dienoestrol	1 mg
Digitoxin	200 mcg
Dimethisterone	5 mg
Ephedrine Hydrochloride	50 mg
Ergometrine	500 mcg
Ethisterone	5 mg
Ethyloestrenol (Veterinary)	500 mcg
Ferrous Succinate	100 mg
Fludrocortisone	100 mcg, 1 mg
Glyceryl Trinitrate	600 mcg
Hydroflumethiazide	25 mg
Methotrexate	2.5 mg
Methylprednisolone	4 mg
Methyltestosterone	5 mg
Methylthiouracil	50 mg
Morphine Sulphate	60 mg
Nicotinamide	50 mg
Nicotinic Acid	50 mg
Norethandrolone	10 mg
Pethidine	25 mg
Phenazocine	5 mg
Phenobarbitone	60 mg
Phenobarbitone Sodium	60 mg
Phenoxymethylpenicillin Potassium	62.5 mg
Phytomenadione	5 mg
Prednisolone	5 mg
Prednisone	5 mg
Prochlorperazine	5 mg
Propranolol	10 mg
Propylthiouracil	50 mg
Reserpine	250 mcg
Riboflavine	3 mg
Salbutamol	2 mg
Stilboestrol	500 mcg
Thiacetazone	25 mg
Thiamine Hydrochloride	5 mg
Thyroid	60 mg
Thyroxine	100 mcg
Tablet diameter (mm) 7.0	
Ascorbic Acid	25 mg
Atropine Sulphate	500 mcg, 600 mcg
Benztropine	2 mg
Betamethasone	500 mcg
Carbamazepine	100 mg
Carbimazole	5 mg
Chlorpheniramine	4 mg
Chlorpropamide	100 mg
Chlorthalidone	50 mg, 100 mg
Codeine Phosphate	60 mg

Diameter 7.0 mm (continued)

Tablet	Strength
Cyclopenthiazide	500 mcg
Dapsone	100 mg
Dienoestrol	5 mg
Digitalis, Prepared	60 mg
Digoxin	250 mcg
Dihydrocodeine	10 mg
Ephedrine Hydrochloride	60 mg
Ethacrynic Acid	50 mg
Ethinyloestradiol	50 mcg
Ferrous Fumarate	200 mg
Fluoxymesterone	5 mg
Guanethidine	10 mg
Haloperidol	1.5 mg
Hydrochlorothiazide	25 mg
Isoprenaline, Slow	30 mg
Lincomycin (Veterinary)	100 mg
Liothyronine	25 mcg
Meclozine	25 mg
Methandienone	5 mg
Methoserpidine	5 mg, 10 mg
Methyltestosterone	10 mg
Metoclopramide	10 mg
Nicoumalone	4 mg
Norethisterone	5 mg
Oxymetholone	50 mg
Oxyphencyclimine	5 mg
Pentobarbitone	100 mg
Phenindione	25 mg
Phenobarbitone	100 mg
Phenobarbitone Sodium	100 mg
Polythiazide	1 mg
Pyridoxine	20 mg
Reserpine	500 mcg
Sodium Citrate	125 mg
Stilboestrol	1 mg
Thiamine Hydrochloride	10 mg
Tolazoline	25 mg
Triprolidine	2.5 mg

Tablet diameter (mm) 7.5

Tablet	Strength
Co-trimoxazole:	
Trimethoprim }	20 mg
Sulphamethoxazole }	100 mg
Cyclizine	50 mg
Mercaptopurine	50 mg
Methadone	5 mg
Methylamphetamine	5 mg
Pyrimethamine	25 mg

Tablet diameter (mm) 8.0

Tablet	Strength
Acepromazine (Veterinary)	25 mg
Amylobarbitone	100 mg
Antazoline	100 mg
Ascorbic Acid	50 mg
Aspirin	150 mg
Aspirin Soluble, Paediatric	—
Atropine Sulphate	1 mg
Azathioprine	50 mg
Benzhexol	2 mg
Clonidine	100 mcg
Cortisone	5 mg
Co-trimoxazole:	
Trimethoprim }	20 mg
Sulphamethoxazole }	100 mg
*Cyclophosphamide	10 mg
Cyproheptadine	4 mg
Debrisoquine	10 mg, 20 mg
Dexamphetamine	5 mg
Diazepam	2 mg, 5 mg, 10 mg

Diameter 8.0 mm (continued)

Tablet	Strength
Dichloralphenazone	150 mg
Diethylcarbamazine	50 mg, 100 mg
Digitalis, Prepared	100 mg
Ethambutol	100 mg
Ethinyloestradiol	1 mg
Ethisterone	10 mg
Frusemide	40 mg
Griseofulvin	125 mg
Guanethidine	25 mg
Hydrochlorothiazide	50 mg
Hydroflumethiazide	50 mg
Isocarboxazid	10 mg
Isoniazid	50 mg
Isoprenaline	10 mg
Levorphanol	1.5 mg
Mepacrine	100 mg
Methoin	100 mg
Methyltestosterone	25 mg
Methylthiouracil	100 mg
Nicotinic Acid	100 mg
Nitrofurantoin	50 mg
Oxymetholone	5 mg
Pentaerythritol	10 mg, 30 mg
Pethidine	50 mg
Phenformin	25 mg
Phenindione	50 mg
Phenobarbitone	125 mg
Phenobarbitone Sodium	125 mg
Phenolphthalein	60 mg
Phenoxymethylpenicillin Potassium	125 mg
Poldine	2 mg
Proguanil	100 mg
Quinidine Sulphate	125 mg
Quinine Bisulphate	125 mg
Reserpine	1 mg
Sodium Citrate	200 mg
Stilboestrol	5 mg
Thiacetazone	50 mg
Thiamine Hydrochloride	25 mg
*Thiopropazate	5 mg
Thyroid	125 mg
Triamcinolone	1 mg, 2 mg
Vitamin B Compound	—
Warfarin	1 mg, 3 mg, 5 mg, 10 mg, 20 mg

Tablet diameter (mm) 8.5

Tablet	Strength
Aminophylline	100 mg
Amylobarbitone	200 mg
Benzylpenicillin	125 mg
Bethanidine	50 mg
*Busulphan	500 mg
Butobarbitone	100 mg
Cascara	—
*Chlorambucil	2 mg
Chlorcyclizine	50 mg
Chloroquine Sulphate	200 mg
Clefamide	250 mg
Cortisone	25 mg
Dihydrocodeine	30 mg
Dimenhydrinate	50 mg
Ferrous Sulphate	200 mg
Hydrocortisone	20 mg
*Melphalan	2 mg
Meprobamate	200 mg
Methallenoestril	3 mg
Orphenadrine Citrate, Slow	100 mg
Phenethicillin	125 mg

Diameter 8.5 mm (continued)

Tablet	Strength
Phenoxymethylpenicillin	62.5 mg
Phenoxymethylpenicillin Calcium	62.5 mg
Prochlorperazine	25 mg
Procyclidine	5 mg
Promethazine Theoclate	25 mg
Propicillin	125 mg
Propranolol	40 mg
Quinidine Sulphate	200 mg
Salbutamol	4 mg
Senna	7.5 mg
Sodium Bicarbonate, Compound	—
Sodium Chloride	300 mg
Spironolactone	25 mg
Stilboestrol	25 mg
*Thiopropazate	10 mg
Trifluomeprazine Maleate (Veterinary)	10 mg
*Trimipramine	10 mg

Tablet diameter (mm) 9.0

Tablet	Strength
Alprenolol	50 mg
Carbamazepine	200 mg
Ethyloestrenol	2 mg
Neostigmine	15 mg
Pyridoxine	50 mg
Stanolone	25 mg
Sulphamethizole	100 mg
Thiacetazone	75 mg
Thiamine Hydrochloride	50 mg

Tablet diameter (mm) 9.5

Tablet	Strength
Allopurinol	100 mg
Ammonium Chloride	300 mg
Amphetamine Sulphate	5 mg
Amylobarbitone Sodium	200 mg
Ascorbic Acid	100 mg
Azathioprine	100 mg
Benzhexol	5 mg
Carbenoxolone	50 mg
Chloroquine Phosphate	250 mg
Chlorpropamide	250 mg
Clomiphene	50 mg
Cyclobarbitone	200 mg
Cyloserine	250 mg
Dicyclomine	10 mg
Ethisterone	25 mg
Ipecacuanha and Opium	300 mg
Isoniazid	100 mg
Megestrol Acetate (Veterinary)	5 mg
Methyltestosterone	50 mg
Methylthiouracil	200 mg
Nialamide	25 mg
Nitrofurantoin	100 mg
Novobiocin (Sodium)	250 mg
Phenolphthalein	125 mg
Phenoxymethylpenicillin	125 mg
Phenoxymethylpenicillin Calcium	125 mg
Primidone	250 mg
Pyridostigmine	60 mg
Sodium Citrate	300 mg
Stilboestrol	100 mg
Thyroid	200 mg
Triamcinolone	4 mg
Yeast	300 mg

Tablet diameter (mm) 10.0

Tablet	Strength
Clonidine	300 mcg
Diethylcarbamazine (Veterinary)	200 mg
Glutethimide	250 mg

Diameter 10.0 mm (continued)

Tablet	Strength
*Melphalan	5 mg
Phenoxymethylpenicillin Potassium	250 mg
Sulphadoxine ⎫ (Veterinary)	250 mg
Trimethoprim ⎭	50 mg

Tablet diameter (mm) 10.5

Tablet	Strength
Acetarsol	250 mg
Aminophylline	200 mg
Amodiaquine	200 mg
Ampicillin	125 mg
Aspirin	300 mg
Aspirin, Compound	—
Aspirin and Caffeine	—
Barbitone Sodium	300 mg
Benzylpenicillin	250 mg
*Busulphan	2 mg
Calcium Lactate	300 mg
Calcium Sodium Lactate	300 mg
Carbromal	300 mg
*Chlorambucil	5 mg
Chlorotrianisene	24 mg
*Cyclophosphamide	50 mg
Di-iodohydroxyquinoline	300 mg
Iopanoic Acid	500 mg
Isoprenaline	20 mg
*Novobiocin (Sodium)	125 mg
Phenmetrazine	25 mg
Phenobarbitone and Theobromine	—
Phenoxymethylpenicillin	250 mg
Phenoxymethylpenicillin Calcium	250 mg
Phenoxymethylpenicillin Potassium	300 mg
Piperazine Adipate	300 mg
Piperazine Citrate (Veterinary)	250 mg
Piperazine Phosphate	260 mg
Potassium Chloride	500 mg
Procainamide	250 mg
Quinidine Sulphate	300 mg
Sodium Chloride	600 mg
Thiamine Hydrochloride	100 mg
*Trimipramine	25 mg

Tablet diameter (mm) 11.0

Tablet	Strength
Acetazolamide	250 mg
Aspirin	450 mg
Aspirin and Codeine	—
Barbitone Sodium	450 mg
Bunamidine (Veterinary)	100 mg
Calcium Sodium Lactate	450 mg
Chlorothiazide	500 mg
*Choline Theophyllinate	100 mg
Co-trimoxazole:	
Trimethoprim ⎫	80 mg
Sulphamethoxazole ⎭	400 mg
Disulfiram	200 mg
Dydrogesterone	10 mg
Ethionamide	250 mg
Lithium Carbonate	250 mg
Megestrol Acetate (Veterinary)	20 mg
Meprobamate	400 mg
Methyprylone	200 mg
Naproxen	250 mg
Neomycin	350000 units
Nialamide	100 mg
Orciprenaline	20 mg
Phenethicillin	250 mg
Proguanil	300 mg
Propicillin	*125 mg, 250 mg
Propranolol	80 mg
Sodium Calciumedetate	500 mg

Diameter 11.0 mm (continued)

Tablet	Strength
Sodium Valproate	200 mg
Thenium Closylate Compound (Veterinary)	—
Thymoxamine	40 mg
Thyroid	300 mg

Tablet diameter (mm) 11.5

Thiambutosine	500 mg

Tablet diameter (mm) 12.0

Benzylpenicillin	300 mg
Di-iodohydroxyquinoline	650 mg
Nitrazepam	5 mg, 10 mg
*Propicillin	250 mg

Tablet diameter (mm) 12.5

Ascorbic Acid	200 mg
Aspirin	500 mg, 600 mg
Aspirin, Phenacetin and Codeine	—
Aspirin and Codeine, Soluble	—
Benzocaine, Compound [LOZENGES]	—
Bunamidine (Veterinary)	200 mg
Calcium and Vitamin D	—
Calcium Lactate	600 mg
*Choline Theophyllinate	200 mg
Colistin	0.25, 1.5 mega-units
Co-trimoxazole:	
Trimethoprim ⎱	80 mg
Sulphamethoxazole ⎰	400 mg
Dichloralphenazone	650 mg
Dichlorophen	500 mg
Diloxanide Furoate	500 mg
Ethotoin	500 mg
Ipecacuanha and Opium	600 mg
Isoniazid	200 mg
Lithium Carbonate, Slow	400 mg
Magnesium Carbonate, Compound	—
Metronidazole	200 mg
Nalidixic Acid	500 mg
Niclosamide	500 mg
Paracetamol	500 mg
Phenolphthalein	250 mg
Phthalylsulphathiazole	500 mg
Piperazine Adipate (Veterinary)	450 mg
Piperazine Citrate (Veterinary)	500 mg
Probenecid	500 mg
*Prothionamide	125 mg
Pyrazinamide	500 mg
*Quinine Bisulphate	300 mg
Soluble Aspirin	—
Soluble Aspirin, Phenacetin and Codeine	—
Succinylsulphathiazole	500 mg
Sulphadiazine	500 mg
Sulphadiazine ⎱ (Veterinary)	400 mg
Trimethoprim ⎰	80 mg
Sulphadimethoxine	500 mg
Sulphadimidine	500 mg
Sulphafurazole	500 mg
Sulphaguanidine	500 mg
Sulphamethoxydiazine	500 mg
Sulphamethoxypyridazine	500 mg
Sulphapyridine	500 mg
Sulphathiazole	500 mg

Tablet diameter (mm) 13.0

Co-trimoxazole, Dispersible:	
Trimethoprim ⎱	80 mg
Sulphamethoxazole ⎰	400 mg

Diameter 13.0 mm (continued)

Tablet	Strength
Ethambutol	400 mg
Levodopa	500 mg
Sulphadoxine	500 mg
Tolbutamide	500 mg

Tablet diameter (mm) 13.5

Sulphasalazine	500 mg

Tablet diameter (mm) 14.0

Formaldehyde [LOZENGES]	—
Phenolphthalein	300 mg

Tablet diameter (mm) 16.0

Aluminium Hydroxide	—
Aluminium Phosphate	—
Amphotericin [LOZENGES]	10 mg
Benzalkonium [LOZENGES]	—
Bunamidine (Veterinary)	400 mg
Calcium Gluconate	—
Liquorice [LOZENGES]	—
Magnesium Trisilicate, Compound	—
Penicillin [LOZENGES]	1000 units

Tablet diameter (mm) 19.0

Bismuth, Compound [LOZENGES]	—
Calcium Gluconate, Effervescent	—
Thiabendazole	500 mg

Tablet diameter (mm) 22.0

Potassium Chloride, Effervescent, Formula A	

Tablet diameter (mm) 25.4

Phosphate, Effervescent	500 mg

Tachycardia

see under CARDIAC ARRHYTHMIAS

Taeniasis

see under TAPEWORMS

Talc, Purified

A purified native magnesium silicate corresponding approximately to the formula $Mg_6(Si_2O_5)_4(OH)_4$. It contains a small amount of aluminium silicate.

OTHER NAMES: Powdered Talc; Purified French Chalk; Talc; Talcum.

A standard is given in the European Pharmacopoeia Vol. III

Description. *Macroscopical characters:* An odourless, tasteless, light, homogeneous, almost white powder which is greasy to the touch.

Microscopical characters: irregular, sharply angled particles, either as small flakes or as pieces with jagged and laminated ends, up to 135 μm in length or width, the smaller ones about 3 to 5 μm. It does not stain with *safranine solution* or *alcoholic methylene blue solution*; mounted in cresol or chloral hydrate, it shines brightly on a dark field between crossed polars (distinction from magnesium trisilicate).

Moisture content. Not more than 1%, determined by drying at 180°.

Hygroscopicity. It absorbs insignificant amounts of moisture at 25° at relative humidities up to about 90%.

Sterilisation. It is sterilised by heating at a temperature not lower than 160° for sufficient time to ensure that the whole of the powder is maintained at this temperature for 1 hour or it may be sterilised by exposure to ethylene oxide under suitable conditions.

Actions and uses. Purified talc is used in massage and as a dusting-powder to allay irritation and prevent chafing; it is usually mixed with starch and zinc oxide. Purified talc used in dusting-powders should be sterilised. It is unsuitable for dusting surgical gloves, since it may cause foreign-body granulomata. Purified talc is also used to clarify liquids and as a lubricant in making tablets.

Preparations

TALC DUSTING-POWDER:

Purified talc, sterilised	900 g
Starch, in powder	100 g

Prepare as described in the entry on Powders.
A standard for this dusting-powder is given in the British Pharmaceutical Codex 1973
Containers and *Storage:* see the entry on Dusting-powders for general information on containers and storage.
Advice for patients: the dusting-powder should be dusted lightly onto the affected area. It should not be applied to open wounds or to raw surfaces of a large area.

ZINC, STARCH, AND TALC DUSTING-POWDER (*Syn.* Zinc Oxide and Starch Dusting-powder; Zinc Oxide, Starch, and Talc Dusting-powder):

Zinc oxide	250 g
Starch, in powder	250 g
Purified talc, sterilised	500 g

Prepare as described in the entry on Powders.
A standard for this dusting-powder is given in the British Pharmaceutical Codex 1973
Containers and *Storage:* see the entry on Dusting-powders for general information on containers and storage.
Advice for patients: see above under Talc Dusting-powder.

OTHER PREPARATIONS: purified talc is an ingredient of chlorphenesin dusting-powder.

Tannic Acid

Tannic acid may be obtained from oak galls by subjecting them to a process of fermentation and extracting with water-saturated ether.

OTHER NAME: Tannin

A standard is given in the British Pharmacopoeia 1973

Tannic acid is not a carboxylic acid; on hydrolysis with dilute sulphuric acid it yields gallic acid and glucose, and this decomposition indicates that its minimum complexity is represented by a pentadigalloylglucose, $C_{76}H_{52}O_{46}$, a formula which is in accordance with its slightly acid reaction and dextrorotation.

Many commercial samples of tannic acid contain gallic acid, the presence of which reduces the solubility and may be detected by the production of a pink colour on the addition of a 5% solution of potassium cyanide. These varieties of tannic acid are used in dyeing and in the manufacture of ink and are not suitable for medicinal use; they occur in coarse powder or lumps, darker in colour than the official substance.

Description. Yellowish-white or light-brown glistening scales, light masses, or impalpable powder with a characteristic odour.

Solubility. Soluble, at 20°, in less than 1 part of water and of alcohol; very slightly soluble in ether, in chloroform, and in light petroleum; soluble in acetone, slowly soluble in 1 part of glycerol.

Moisture content. Not more than 9%, determined by drying at 105°.

Stability. Aqueous solutions decompose on storage.

Incompatibility. It is incompatible with salts of iron, lead, antimony, and silver, and with alkaloids, albumen, and gelatin.

Identification. TESTS. 1. A precipitate is produced when a solution is added to either a solution of gelatin or a solution of albumen.
2. To a solution add *ferric chloride test-solution*; a bluish-black colour is produced. Add *dilute sulphuric acid*; the colour disappears and a yellowish-brown precipitate is produced.
3. A solution in water is dextrorotatory and acid to methyl red.

Actions and uses. Tannic acid precipitates proteins and forms insoluble complexes with many heavy metals, alkaloids, and glycosides.
Tannic acid has little action on intact skin, but on abraded surfaces it forms a hard coagulum and on this account has been employed in the treatment of burns; it is now seldom used for this purpose because the coagulum causes contractures and, moreover, sufficient tannic acid may be absorbed from large areas to cause damage to the liver.
The astringent action on the mucous membrane of the gastro-intestinal tract exerted by the combined tannic acids in catechu and in similar drugs has been used for the symptomatic management of diarrhoea. In lozenges, gargles, or sprays, tannic acid is used as an astringent for the mucous membrane of the mouth and throat.

Undesirable effects. Fatal hepatotoxic manifestations have followed the administration of barium sulphate enemas containing tannic acid, which has been added to improve the clarity of X-ray photographs.

Tapeworms

Tapeworms (Cestodes) are segmented helminths which occupy the gastro-intestinal tract in their adult form, and as larvae invade the tissues, most cestodes have a different host for their larval stage. Most human cestode infections are due to intestinal infection with the adult form of the worm, but some are due to infection with the larval form.
The commonest tapeworm which infects the human gastro-intestinal tract is the beef tapeworm (*Taenia saginata*). It is acquired by eating under-cooked beef containing the larval form which matures to the adult form in the human gastro-intestinal tract. The adult worm may measure up to 7 m in length. Other adult tapeworms infecting man include the pork tapeworm (*Taenia solium*), the fish tapeworm (*Diphyllobothrium latum*), and the dwarf tapeworm (*Hymenolepis nana*).
Symptoms of infection include abdominal discomfort, a large appetite, diarrhoea, and the passage of mature segments of the worm from the anus. Malabsorption and

vitamin B_{12} deficiency may also occur with less common species.

The larval forms of several tapeworms, for example *Echinococcus granulosus* and *Taenia solium* may invade the tissues of man, resulting in cysts containing the larvae anywhere in the body. There is no effective way of eliminating the larvae apart from surgery.

Drugs used in the treatment of adult cestode infections include dichlorophen, hexylresorcinol, male fern, mepacrine, and niclosamide.

Tar

The bituminous liquid obtained by the destructive distillation of the wood of the Scots pine, *Pinus sylvestris* L., and other trees of the family Pinaceae; it is known in commerce as Stockholm tar.

OTHER NAMES: Pix Liquida
Tardrox® (with halquinol)

A standard is given in the British Pharmacopoeia 1973

Constituents. Tar contains many substances, including hydrocarbons, which are chiefly terpenoid in character, and phenols, most of which are high-boiling dihydric phenols and their methyl ethers.

Description. A dark brown or almost black semi-liquid substance with a strong, characteristic, empyreumatic odour.

It is transparent in thin layers if free from water.

When stored for some time it separates into a layer which is granular in character due to minute crystallisation of catechol, resin acids, etc., and a surface layer of a syrupy consistence.

Solubility. Very slightly soluble in water; soluble, at 20°, in 10 parts of alcohol (90%); soluble in ether, in chloroform, and in fixed and volatile oils.

Identification. TESTS. 1. Mix 1 g with 20 ml of water, shake for 5 minutes, and separate the aqueous liquid, filtering with the aid of kieselguhr if necessary; to a portion of the aqueous liquid add 3 drops of a 0.1% solution of ferric chloride; a red colour is produced.

2. The aqueous liquid obtained in Test 1, is acid to *litmus solution* (distinction from coal tar).

Actions and uses. Tar has antipruritic properties, but its action is less marked than that of coal tar. It has been applied as an ointment in the treatment of chronic skin diseases, especially psoriasis and eczema.

Preparations

Preparations available include a CREAM containing tar 1% with halquinol 1.5%.

Tar, Coal

A product obtained by the destructive distillation of bituminous coal at about 1000°.

OTHER NAME: Pix Carbonis

A standard is given in the British Pharmaceutical Codex 1973

Constituents. The chief constituents are benzene, phenols, naphthalene, and pitch, together with small quantities of basic compounds such as pyridine and quinoline.

Description. A thick, nearly black, viscous liquid with a strong, penetrating, characteristic odour. On exposure to air, it gradually becomes more viscous.

Solubility. Very slightly soluble in water; partly soluble in alcohol, in ether, in chloroform, and in volatile oils.

Weight per ml. At 20°, about 1.15 g

Identification. TESTS. 1. A saturated solution in water is alkaline to *litmus solution* (distinction from tar obtained from wood or lignite, or by the destructive distillation of bituminous coal at temperatures below 600°).

2. Shake about 500 mg with 10 ml of light petroleum (boiling-range, 40° to 60°) and allow to stand; a greenish-blue colour is produced in the light petroleum layer.

Actions and uses. Coal tar has actions and uses similar to those described under Prepared Coal Tar. It is sometimes preferred to prepared coal tar but it is liable to be more irritating to the skin.

Undesirable effects. Coal tar may irritate the skin and produce acneform eruptions.

Preparations

COAL TAR PAINT (*Syn.* Pigmentum Picis Carbonis):

Coal tar		100 g
Acetone ⎱ of each equal		
Industrial methylated spirit ⎰ volumes		to 1000 ml

Dissolve.

This preparation was previously prepared with a vehicle consisting of equal volumes of acetone and benzene, nitration grade of commerce.

Containers, Labelling, and *Storage:* see the entry on Paints for general information on containers, labelling, and storage. In addition, the label on the container should state "This preparation is inflammable. Keep away from a naked flame".

Advice for patients: the undiluted solution should be applied to the lesions. Contact with normal skin should be avoided. It should not be applied to broken or inflamed skin, near the eyes or mucous membranes. The solution stains the skin, hair, and fabric. See also above under Labelling.

ZINC AND COAL TAR PASTE (*Syn.* Zinc Oxide and Coal Tar Paste; White's Tar Paste):

Zinc oxide, finely sifted		60 g
Coal tar		60 g
Emulsifying wax		50 g
Starch		380 g
Yellow soft paraffin		450 g

Melt the emulsifying wax at 70° and add the coal tar, followed by 225 g of the yellow soft paraffin; stir at 70° until completely melted and add the remainder of the yellow soft paraffin. When completely melted, cool to 30°, add the zinc oxide and the starch, with constant stirring, and mix until cold.

A standard for this paste is given in the British Pharmaceutical Codex 1973

Containers and *Storage:* see the entry on Pastes for general information on containers and storage.

Advice for patients: the paste should be applied liberally and carefully to the lesions with a suitable applicator. It should not be applied to broken or inflamed skin. It stains the skin, hair, and fabric.

Tar, Coal, Prepared

Prepared coal tar is a product obtained by heating commercial coal tar in a shallow vessel for 1 hour at 50° with frequent stirring.

OTHER NAME: Pix Carbonis Praeparata

A standard is given in the British Pharmacopoeia 1973

Constituents. The constituents are those of coal tar, with a smaller proportion of the more volatile constituents.

Description. A nearly black viscous liquid with a strongly empyreumatic odour; in very thin layers it is brown.

Solubility. Very slightly soluble in water; partly soluble in alcohol (90%) and in ether; soluble in chloroform.

Identification. TEST. Shake about 500 mg with 10 ml of light petroleum (boiling-range, 40° to 60°); a blue fluorescence is produced.

Actions and uses. Prepared coal tar has antipruritic properties. It is used in the form of ointments and lotions in the treatment of pruritus, psoriasis, eczema, and other skin affections.

Preparations

AMMONIATED MERCURY AND COAL TAR OINTMENT (*Syn.* Unguentum Hydrargyri Ammoniati et Picis Carbonis; Unguentum Picis Carbonis Compositum):

Ammoniated mercury, finely powdered	25 g
Strong coal tar solution	25 g
Yellow soft paraffin	950 g

Triturate the ammoniated mercury with a portion of the yellow soft paraffin until smooth, mix with the remainder of the yellow soft paraffin, and incorporate the strong coal tar solution.

A standard for this ointment is given in the British Pharmaceutical Codex 1973

Containers: see the entry on Ointments for general information on containers. Containers should prevent evaporation.

Advice for patients: the ointment should not be applied to broken or inflamed skin. It stains the skin, hair, and fabric.

AMMONIATED MERCURY, COAL TAR, AND SALICYLIC ACID OINTMENT (*Syn.* Unguentum Hydrargyri Ammoniati et Picis Carbonis cum Acido Salicylico):

Ammoniated mercury and coal tar ointment	980 g
Salicylic acid, in fine powder	20 g

Triturate the salicylic acid with a portion of the ammoniated mercury and coal tar ointment until smooth and gradually incorporate the remainder of the ointment.

A standard for this ointment is given in the British Pharmaceutical Codex 1973

Containers: see the entry on Ointments for general information on containers. Containers should prevent evaporation.

Advice for patients: the ointment should be applied sparingly to the affected area. It should not be applied to broken or inflamed skin; contact with the eyes should be avoided. The ointment stains the skin, hair, and fabric. Prolonged use should be avoided and its use should be discontinued if excessive dryness or irritation of the skin occurs.

CALAMINE AND COAL TAR OINTMENT (*Syn.* Compound Calamine Ointment; Unguentum Sedativum):

Calamine, finely sifted	125 g
Strong coal tar solution	25 g
Zinc oxide, finely sifted	125 g
Hydrous wool fat	250 g
White soft paraffin	475 g

Melt together the hydrous wool fat and the white soft paraffin, incorporate the calamine, the zinc oxide, and the strong coal tar solution, and stir until cold.

A standard for this ointment is given in the British Pharmaceutical Codex 1973

Containers: see the entry on Ointments for general information on containers. Containers should prevent evaporation.

Advice for patients: the ointment stains the skin, hair, and fabric. It should not be applied to broken or inflamed skin or near the eyes.

COAL TAR AND SALICYLIC ACID OINTMENT:

Prepared coal tar	20 g
Salicylic acid	20 g
Emulsifying wax	114 g
White soft paraffin	190 g
Coconut oil	540 g
Polysorbate 80	40 g
Liquid paraffin	76 g

Disperse the prepared coal tar in the polysorbate 80, incorporate the salicylic acid, and mix with the emulsifying wax, previously melted. Separately melt the white soft paraffin and the coconut oil, incorporate the liquid paraffin, warmed to the same temperature, and add, with stirring, to the other mixed ingredients. Mix thoroughly and stir until cold.

A standard for this ointment is given in the British Pharmaceutical Codex 1973

Containers: see the entry on Ointments for general information on containers.

Advice for patients: when used in scalp disorders a small amount of ointment should be rubbed gently into the roots of the hair. It should not be applied to broken or inflamed skin; contact with the eyes should be avoided. The ointment stains the skin, hair, and fabric. Prolonged use should be avoided and it should be discontinued if excessive dryness or irritation of the skin occurs.

COAL TAR AND ZINC OINTMENT:

Strong coal tar solution	100 g
Zinc oxide, finely sifted	300 g
Yellow soft paraffin	600 g

Mix the zinc oxide with the strong coal tar solution, triturate with a portion of the yellow soft paraffin until smooth, and gradually incorporate the remainder of the yellow soft paraffin.

A standard for this ointment is given in the British Pharmaceutical Codex 1973

Containers: see the entry on Ointments for general information on containers. Containers should prevent evaporation.

Advice for patients: the ointment should not be applied to broken or inflamed skin. It stains the skin, hair, and fabric.

COAL TAR PASTE (*Syn.* Pasta Picis Carbonis):

Strong coal tar solution	75 g
Compound zinc paste	925 g

Triturate the strong coal tar solution with a portion of the compound zinc paste until smooth and gradually incorporate the remainder of the paste.

A standard for this paste is given in the British Pharmaceutical Codex 1973

Containers and Storage: see the entry on Pastes for general information on containers and storage. Containers should prevent evaporation.

Advice for patients: the paste should be applied liberally and carefully to the lesions with a suitable applicator. It should not be applied to broken or inflamed skin. It stains the skin, hair, and fabric.

COAL TAR SOLUTION (*Syn.* Liq. Pic. Carb.):

Prepared coal tar	200 g
Quillaia, in moderately coarse powder ..	100 g
Alcohol (90%)	to 1000 ml

Macerate the prepared coal tar and the quillaia with 800 ml of the alcohol in a closed vessel for 7 days, shaking occasionally; filter, pass through the filter sufficient of the alcohol to produce the required volume, and mix.

In making this preparation, the alcohol (90%) may be replaced by industrial methylated spirit, diluted so as to be of equivalent alcoholic strength, provided that the law and the statutory regulations governing the use of industrial methylated spirit are observed.

A standard for this solution is given in the British Pharmacopoeia 1973

Advice for patients: the undiluted solution should be applied to the lesions. Contact with normal skin should be avoided. It should not be applied to broken or inflamed skin or near to the eyes or mucous membranes. The solution stains the skin, hair, and fabric.

STRONG COAL TAR SOLUTION (*Syn.* Liquor Picis Carbonis Fortis):

Prepared coal tar	400 g
Quillaia, in moderately coarse powder ..	100 g
Alcohol (95%)	to 1000 ml

Macerate the prepared coal tar and the quillaia with 800 ml of the alcohol in a closed vessel for 7 days, shaking occasionally; filter, pass through the filter sufficient of the alcohol to produce the required volume, and mix.

In making this preparation, the alcohol (95%) may be replaced by industrial methylated spirit, provided that the law and the statutory regulations governing the use of industrial methylated spirit are observed.

This preparation cannot be mixed with alcohol to prepare coal tar solution, as precipitation occurs on dilution.

A standard for this solution is given in the British Pharmaceutical Codex 1973

Advice for patients: see above under Coal Tar Solution.

OTHER PREPARATIONS: a number of preparations containing prepared coal tar or extracts and fractions derived therefrom are available.

Tartaric Acid

(2*R*,3*R*)-2,3-Dihydroxybutane-1,4-dioic acid

$$
\begin{array}{c}
COOH \\
| \\
H-C-OH \\
| \\
HO-C-H \\
| \\
COOH
\end{array}
$$

$C_4H_6O_6 = 150.1$

OTHER NAME: Acidum Tartaricum

A standard is given in the European Pharmacopoeia Vol. III

Description. Odourless colourless crystals or white powder with a strongly acidic taste.

Solubility. Soluble, at 20°, in less than 1 part of water and in 2.5 parts of alcohol; very slightly soluble in ether.

Dissociation constants. pK_a 3.0, 4.4 (25°).

Hygroscopicity. It absorbs insignificant amounts of

moisture at relative humidities up to about 65%, but at relative humidities above about 75%, it is deliquescent.

Storage. It should be stored in airtight containers.

Actions and uses. Tartaric acid is a purgative which has actions similar to those described under Sodium Potassium Tartrate. It is a constituent of effervescent powders and granules and of cooling drinks and should be taken well diluted with water.

Approximately neutral solutions are formed when 10 parts of tartaric acid are mixed in solution with 11 parts of ammonium bicarbonate, 6½ parts of magnesium carbonate, 13¼ parts of potassium bicarbonate, or 11¼ parts of sodium bicarbonate.

The usual dose for an adult is 0.3 to 2 grams. Children may be given one- to three-quarters of the dose for an adult.

Tartaric acid is also used in concentration of 0.05 to 0.5% to enhance the effects of antoxidants.

Preparations

Tartaric acid is an ingredient of effervescent calcium gluconate tablets and of aluminium acetate solution.

Tartrazine Solution, Compound

OTHER NAME: Liquor Flavus

A solution containing 0.75% of tartrazine, food grade of commerce, and 0.1% of sunset yellow FCF, food grade of commerce, with 20% of chloroform spirit and 25% of glycerol, in purified water.

Uses. Compound tartrazine solution is used in colouring medicines.

Sensitivity to tartrazine may occur and occasionally give rise to hypersensitivity reactions, especially in subjects who are sensitive to aspirin.

Preparations

Compound tartrazine solution is an ingredient of codeine linctus, diabetic codeine linctus, diamorphine linctus, ephedrine elixir, isoniazid elixir, methadone linctus, neomycin elixir, noscapine linctus, paediatric compound tolu linctus, phenobarbitone elixir, pholcodine linctus, and strong pholcodine linctus.

Tartrazine is an ingredient of strong cetrimide solution, and of green S and tartrazine solution.

Terbutaline Sulphate

N-*tert*-Butyl-*N*-[2-(3,5-dihydroxyphenyl)-2-hydroxy-ethyl]ammonium sulphate

$$
\left[HO\cdot CH\cdot CH_2\cdot \overset{+}{N}H_2\cdot C(CH_3)_3 \right]_2 SO_4^{2-}
$$

$C_{24}H_{40}N_2O_{10}S = 548.6$

OTHER NAMES: *Bricanyl*®; *Filair*®
Bricanyl Compound/Expectorant® (with guaiphenesin)

Description. An odourless, white to greyish-white, crystalline powder with a bitter taste.

Solubility. Soluble in 4 parts of water; very slightly

soluble in alcohol; practically insoluble in ether and in chloroform.

Dissociation constants. pK_a 8.7, 10.0, 11.0 (20°).

Melting-point. About 255°.

Metabolism. ABSORPTION. Partially absorbed after oral administration.

BLOOD CONCENTRATION. After an oral dose of 5 mg of the sulphate, peak serum concentrations of about 3 to 6 ng/ml are attained in 1 to 3 hours; after the administration of 220 μg of the sulphate from an aerosol, a peak plasma concentration of up to 4 ng/ml is attained in 1 to 4 hours.

HALF-LIFE. Serum half-life, 3 to 4 hours.

DISTRIBUTION. Small amounts are secreted in the milk.

METABOLIC REACTIONS. Subject to first pass metabolism mainly by sulphate conjugation; glucuronic acid conjugates are formed to some extent but the drug does not appear to be methylated.

EXCRETION. After an oral dose, up to about 50% is excreted in the urine, mostly as the sulphate, whilst after an intravenous or subcutaneous dose, up to about 90% may be excreted in the urine, mostly as unchanged drug; after administration by aerosol, about 3 to 35% is excreted in the urine, 2 to 37% in the faeces and up to about 30% of the dose appears to be retained in the aerosol mouthpiece.

FURTHER INFORMATION. Metabolism—D. S. Davies *et al.*, *Br. J. clin. Pharmac.*, 1974, **1**, 129 and H. T. Nilsson *et al.*, *Xenobiotica*, 1972, **2**, 363; metabolism and activity of terbutaline and its prodrug ibuterol—Y. Hörnblad *et al.*, *Eur. J. clin. Pharmac.*, 1976, **10**, 9; the fate of inhaled tritiated terbutaline—H. T. Nilsson *et al.*, *Eur. J. clin. Pharmac.*, 1976, **10**, 1.

Actions and uses. Terbutaline sulphate is a directly acting sympathomimetic amine with bronchodilator actions and uses similar to those of salbutamol. It is used in the treatment of asthma, chronic bronchitis, emphysema, and other bronchopulmonary disorders involving bronchospasm.

The dose by mouth for adults is 3 to 5 milligrams 3 times daily, for children aged up to 1 year, 0.75 to 1.5 milligrams 3 times daily, 1 to 5 years 1.5 to 3 milligrams 3 times daily, and 6 to 12 years 3 to 5 milligrams 3 times daily.

Adults may be given 250 micrograms 4 times daily by subcutaneous injection, increasing to 500 micrograms 4 times daily if necessary, and children aged 2 to 10 years may be given 10 micrograms per kilogram body-weight by subcutaneous injection, up to a maximum of 300 micrograms.

The dose for adults and children by inhalation is 200 to 500 micrograms as required, not more than 8 inhalations of 200 or 250 micrograms being administered in any period of 24 hours.

Undesirable effects. As for Salbutamol. In addition, oral administration may give rise to muscle tremors.

Precautions and contra-indications. As for Salbutamol.

Preparations

Preparations available include an AEROSOL INHALATION delivering terbutaline sulphate 200 micrograms per metered dose; an aerosol inhalation delivering terbutaline sulphate 250 micrograms per metered dose; an ELIXIR containing terbutaline sulphate 1.5 mg in 5 ml, diluent water for preparations, life of diluted elixir

14 days; an elixir containing terbutaline sulphate 1.5 mg with guaiphenesin 66.5 mg in 5 ml, diluent water for preparations, life of diluted elixir 14 days; an INJECTION containing terbutaline sulphate 500 micrograms per ml in 1-ml ampoules; a SPRAY (for use diluted with sodium chloride injection or water for injections with suitable nebulisers in respirator units) containing terbutaline sulphate 10 mg per ml; TABLETS containing terbutaline sulphate 5 mg; and tablets containing terbutaline sulphate 2.5 mg with guaiphenesin 100 mg.

Terpineol

A mixture of isomers in which $(\pm)$-α-terpineol largely predominates.

$C_{10}H_{18}O = 154.3$

A standard is given in the British Pharmaceutical Codex 1973

Description. A colourless, slightly viscous, optically inactive liquid, which may deposit crystals; it has a pleasant odour.

Solubility. Very slightly soluble in water; soluble, at 20°, in 2 parts of alcohol (70%); soluble in ether.

Weight per ml. At 20°, 0.931 to 0.935 g.

Refractive index. At 20°, 1.4825 to 1.4855.

Actions and uses. Terpineol has antibacterial properties and is a useful solvent. It prevents the crystallisation of chloroxylenol from chloroxylenol solution; solvents such as alcohol do not have this effect.

Testosterone

17β-Hydroxyandrost-4-en-3-one

$C_{19}H_{28}O_2 = 288.4$

OTHER NAME: *Testoral*®

A standard is given in the British Pharmacopoeia 1973

Description. An odourless white crystalline powder.

Solubility. Very slightly soluble in water; soluble, at 20°, in 5 parts of alcohol and in 150 parts of ethyl oleate.

Specific rotation. +106° to +112°, determined on a 1% solution in dehydrated alcohol.

Storage. It should be protected from light.

Identification. TEST. Mix about 100 mg in a stoppered tube with 3 ml of dehydrated pyridine and 0.6 ml of acetic anhydride, and heat on a water-bath for 3 hours; add water, dropwise, until crystals begin to form, slowly add a further 15 ml of water, allow to stand until precipitation is complete, collect the precipitate on a sintered glass crucible and wash with water until the washings are neutral to *methyl red solution*; the residue, after recrystallisation from alcohol (95%) with addition of a few drops of water if necessary to aid crystallisation, and drying at 105°, melts at about 140°.

MELTING-POINT. About 154°.

ULTRAVIOLET ABSORPTION. In alcohol (95%), maximum at 240 nm (E1%, 1cm = 560).

INFRA-RED ABSORPTION. Major peaks at 871, 1057, 1066, 1236, 1615, and 1660 cm⁻¹ (see Appendix 2a: Infra-red Spectra).

THIN-LAYER CHROMATOGRAPHY. See under Thin-layer Chromatography, System 10.

Metabolism. ABSORPTION. Readily absorbed after oral administration; it is absorbed through the skin and buccal mucosa; parenteral doses are readily absorbed but esters are more slowly absorbed.

BLOOD CONCENTRATION. Circulating plasma concentrations of testosterone in normal men and women are about 4 to 7 ng/ml and 0.3 to 0.8 ng/ml respectively; in prepubertal boys, plasma concentrations are less than 1 ng/ml; concentrations in men are subject to cyclical variations; in pregnant women, plasma concentrations are increased; in men, plasma concentrations of dihydrotestosterone, the active form of testosterone, are about 10% of those of testosterone itself.

HALF-LIFE. The plasma half-life has been variously reported as 10 to 20 minutes and 60 to 80 minutes.

DISTRIBUTION. Subject to enterohepatic circulation; *protein binding*, about 98% bound to plasma proteins, mainly to sex hormone binding globulin.

METABOLIC REACTIONS. Subject to first pass metabolism; rapidly metabolised by oxidation to androstenedione, which is reduced to epitestosterone, or by reduction at ring A to androstanediones followed by ketoreduction to androstanediols or androstanolones, and conjugation with glucuronic acid or sulphate; testosterone is also metabolised, mainly at target tissues, to dihydrotestosterone which is the active metabolite, and also directly to testosterone glucuronide or sulphate; hydroxylation at positions 6 and 19 may also occur.

EXCRETION. About 90% of a dose is excreted in the urine and 6% in the faeces; of the urinary excreted material, etiocholanolone and 3β-hydroxy-5α-androstan-17-one are the two major components, with small amounts of androsterone, 5α- and 5β-androstanediols, epitestosterone, and 6-hydroxy and 19-hydroxy metabolites; the majority of the urinary metabolites are excreted as conjugates.

FURTHER INFORMATION. A cycle of plasma testosterone in men—C. H. Doering *et al.*, *J. clin. Endocr. Metab.*, 1975, **40**, 492; K. Fotherby and F. James, Metabolism of synthetic steroids, *Advances in Steroid Biochemistry and Pharmacology*, M. H. Briggs and G. A. Christie (Eds), Vol. 3, London, Academic Press, 1972, p. 67; metabolism of testosterone in relation to thyroid states —L. Hellman and R. S. Rosenfeld, *J. clin. Endocr. Metab.*, 1974, **38**, 424; J. Jeffery and A. Klopper, Steroid metabolism in the foeto-placental unit, *Advances in Steroid Biochemistry and Pharmacology*, M. H. Briggs (Ed.), Vol. 2, London, Academic Press, 1970, p. 71; depression of plasma testosterone by acetylmethadol —J. H. Mendelson *et al.*, *Clin. Pharmac. Ther.*, 1976, **19**, 371; plasma concentrations of dihydrotestosterone in men—K. M. Pirke and P. Doerr, *Acta endocr. Copenh.*, 1975, **79**, 359; I. F. Sommerville and W. P. Collins, Indices of androgen production in women, *Advances in Steroid Biochemistry and Pharmacology*, M. H. Briggs (Ed.), Vol. 2, p. 267; *Testosterone*, Conference Proceedings 1967, J. Tamm (Ed.), Stuttgart, Georg Thieme Verlag, 1968.

Actions and uses. Testosterone is the androgenic hormone formed in the interstitial (Leydig) cells of the testes under the control of the anterior lobe of the pituitary gland. It controls the development and maintenance of the male sex organs and the male secondary sex characteristics. In small doses it increases the number of spermatozoa produced, but in large doses it inhibits the activity of the anterior lobe of the pituitary gland and suppresses the formation of spermatozoa. In under-developed or adolescent males, testosterone increases the size of the scrotum, phallus, seminal vesicles, and the prostate; libido and sexual activity may also be increased.

Testosterone is essential for the development of the secondary sex characteristics of the male—deep voice, facial and body hair, flat chest and pelvis, and aggressive drive. Testosterone also produces systemic effects such as increased nitrogen retention which leads to an increase in skeletal weight, water retention, increased vascularity of the skin, and increased growth of bone. Large and repeated doses given in early puberty may cause closure of the epiphyses and stop growth.

Testosterone inhibits the gonadotrophic activity of the anterior lobe of the pituitary gland, thereby suppressing ovarian activity and menstruation. Continued administration of large doses, in excess of about 300 milligrams monthly, to women produces symptoms of virilism, such as male-like hirsutism, deepening of the voice, atrophy of breast tissue and the uterine endometrium, and hypertrophy of the clitoris; libido is increased and lactation suppressed.

Testosterone and its derivatives are used in the male when the testes are absent or maldeveloped, when the sex organs are imperfectly developed as in eunuchoidism, and when the secondary sex characteristics are absent or their development is delayed. They are also used in the treatment of gynaecomastia. They are of no value in the treatment of sterility, unless this is due to sexual underdevelopment, or of undescended testicles, of impotence, or of prostatic hypertrophy.

Testosterone and its derivatives are used in the female in selected cases for the treatment of dysmenorrhoea, functional uterine bleeding (menorrhagia, metrorrhagia) and chronic mastitis, for relief of after-pains in labour, and for the palliative treatment of carcinoma of the breast in those patients beyond the scope of surgery or irradiation therapy.

Testosterone has been used for the suppression of post-partum breast engorgement. Small doses are used with oestrogens in the treatment of the climacteric.

Testosterone has been used in both the male and the female to increase weight in patients suffering from emaciation or wasting diseases, but less virilising anabolic agents such as norethandrolone are now preferred for this purpose.

To achieve a prolonged action, testosterone is implanted subcutaneously in a dose of 100 to 600 milligrams, for parenteral administration, testosterone propionate is generally used, and for oral use, methyltestosterone or fluoxymesterone.

Precautions. Patients under treatment with testosterone or its derivatives should be carefully watched for signs of oedema, and virilism.

The administration of testosterone and its derivatives should be avoided during pregnancy and in nursing mothers.

Veterinary uses. Testosterone is an androgen which may be used in male hypogonadism, including ageing, debility, decreased libido, and hormonal alopecia. In bitches it may be used for the suppression of pseudopregnancy and the treatment of oestrogen-dependent mammary tumours. In female calves and heifers it is given to promote growth.

Testosterone is administered by implantation. In animals that may be used for human consumption the implants should be inserted in non-edible parts of the body. The usual implantation dose for stallions, bulls, heifers, boars, and rams is 1 milligram per kilogram body-weight and for dogs and bitches 2.5 milligrams per kilogram body-weight.

Preparations

TESTOSTERONE IMPLANTS: consisting of sterile cylinders prepared by the fusion or heavy compression of testosterone without the addition of any other substance. They are distributed singly, by means of an aseptic technique, into sterile containers, and the containers are then sealed to exclude micro-organisms. Available as implants containing 25, 50, and 200 mg of testosterone. *A standard for these implants is given in the British Pharmacopoeia 1973*
Labelling: the label on the container should state the amount of the medicament as the nominal weight of testosterone.
Storage: they should be protected from light.

OTHER PREPARATIONS available include sublingual TABLETS containing testosterone 10 mg.

Testosterone Phenylpropionate

3-Oxoandrost-4-en-17β-yl 3-phenylpropionate

$C_{28}H_{36}O_3 = 420.6$

OTHER NAMES: *Androject®*
Durateston® (with testosterone decanoate, isohexanoate, and propionate); *Sustanon®* (with testosterone decanoate, isohexanoate, and propionate or with testosterone isohexanoate and propionate)

A standard is given in the British Pharmacopoeia 1973

Description. A white crystalline powder with a characteristic odour.

Solubility. Very slightly soluble in water; soluble, at 20°, in 40 parts of alcohol.

Specific rotation. +86° to +91°, determined on a 1% solution in dioxan.

Sterilisation. Oily solutions for injection are sterilised by dry heat.

Storage. It should be protected from light.

Identification. TEST. Dissolve about 25 mg in 1 ml of methyl alcohol, add 2 ml of *semicarbazide acetate solution,* heat under a reflux condenser for 30 minutes, and cool; a precipitate is produced which melts at about 218°.

MELTING-POINT. About 115°.

ULTRAVIOLET ABSORPTION. In alcohol (95%), maximum at 240 nm (E1%, 1cm = 395).

INFRA-RED ABSORPTION. Major peaks at 703, 1166, 1420, 1450, 1670, and 1734 cm⁻¹ (see Appendix 2a: Infra-red Spectra).

THIN-LAYER CHROMATOGRAPHY. See under Thin-layer Chromatography, System 10.

Metabolism. See under Testosterone.

Actions and uses. Testosterone phenylpropionate has the actions and uses described under Testosterone, but is more potent and has a longer duration of action. It is given by subcutaneous or intramuscular injection in a dosage of 10 to 50 milligrams every 4 to 14 days, according to the condition under treatment.

Precautions. As for Testosterone.

Veterinary uses. Testosterone phenylpropionate is an androgen which may be used in male hypogonadism, including ageing, debility, decreased libido, and hormonal alopecia. It may also be used in cases of feminisation in male animals and as an anti-oestrogen in female animals, for treatment of mammary tumours and pseudopregnancy, and for suppression of oestrus. It is administered as an oily injection and a single dose is effective for about 2 weeks. The usual dose by intramuscular injection for stallions, bulls, heifers, boars, and rams is 50 to 100 micrograms per kilogram body-weight and for dogs and bitches 500 micrograms per kilogram body-weight.

Preparations

TESTOSTERONE ESTERS INJECTION: a sterile solution of testosterone isohexanoate, testosterone phenylpropionate, and testosterone propionate, or these three esters together with testosterone decanoate, in a suitable oily vehicle. It is sterilised by dry heat.
Available in 1-ml ampoules containing testosterone isohexanoate 40 mg, testosterone phenylpropionate 40 mg, and testosterone propionate 20 mg, and in 1-ml ampoules containing testosterone isohexanoate 60 mg, testosterone decanoate 100 mg, testosterone phenylpropionate 60 mg, and testosterone propionate 30 mg.
Containers: see the entry on Injections for general information on containers.
Labelling: see the entry on Injections for general information on labelling. In addition, the label on the container should state "For intramuscular injection only".
Storage: it should be protected from light.

TESTOSTERONE PHENYLPROPIONATE INJECTION: a sterile solution of testosterone phenylpropionate in ethyl oleate or other suitable ester, in a suitable fixed oil, or in any mixture of these. It is sterilised by dry heat. Available in 10-ml vials containing 10 mg of testosterone phenylpropionate per ml.
A standard for this injection is given in the British Pharmacopoeia 1973
Containers: see the entry on Injections for general information on containers.
Labelling: see the entry on Injections for general information on labelling. In addition, the label on the container should state the composition of the solvent, and "For intramuscular injection only".
Storage: it should be protected from light.

OTHER PREPARATIONS available include a veterinary INJECTION containing testosterone decanoate 20 mg, with testosterone isohexanoate 12 mg, testosterone phenylpropionate 12 mg, and testosterone propionate 6 mg per ml in 10-ml vials.

Testosterone Propionate

3-Oxoandrost-4-en-17β-yl propionate

$C_{22}H_{32}O_3 = 344.5$

OTHER NAMES: Testosteroni Propionas; Virormone®
Durateston® and Sustanon® (both with other esters of
testosterone—see above under Testosterone Phenylpropionate)

A standard is given in the European Pharmacopoeia
Vol. II

Description. Odourless, colourless or at most slightly
yellowish-white crystals or white crystalline powder.

Solubility. Very slightly soluble in water; soluble, at 20°,
in 6 parts of alcohol, in 4 parts of acetone, in 35 parts
of arachis oil, and in 20 parts of ethyl oleate.

Specific rotation. +83° to +90°, determined on a 1%
solution in dioxan.

Sterilisation. Oily solutions for injection are sterilised
by dry heat.

Storage. It should be protected from light.

Identification. TESTS. 1. Dissolve about 1 mg in 1 ml of
sulphuric acid; the solution is colourless or yellowish.
Add 4 ml of water followed by 6 ml of sulphuric acid;
the solution becomes greenish-yellow with a green
fluorescence.
2. Mix about 150 mg with 6 ml of *alcoholic potassium
hydroxide solution*, boil for 30 minutes, dilute with water
and acidify with *dilute hydrochloric acid*; a precipitate
is produced which, after washing with water and drying
at 105°, melts at about 153°.

MELTING-POINT. About 120°.

ULTRAVIOLET ABSORPTION. In alcohol (95%), maximum
at 241 nm (E1%, 1cm = 485).

INFRA-RED ABSORPTION. Major peaks at 1231, 1243,
1271, 1613, 1669, and 1727 cm^{-1} (see Appendix 2a:
Infra-red Spectra).

THIN-LAYER CHROMATOGRAPHY. See under Thin-layer
Chromatography, System 10.

Metabolism. See under Testosterone.

Actions and uses. Testosterone propionate has actions
similar to those described under Testosterone. It is an
effective androgen for parenteral use, but is inactive
when given by mouth. It is given by intramuscular
injection in a dosage of 10 to 50 milligrams 2 or 3 times
a week for replacement therapy in the male; persistent
priapism is a sign of overdosage.
For the palliative treatment of carcinoma of the breast
beyond the aid of surgery, 100 to 300 milligrams a week
is given in divided doses. A dosage in excess of
300 milligrams monthly may produce virilism in the
female.

Precautions. As for Testosterone.

Veterinary uses. Testosterone propionate is used for
the same purposes as testosterone phenylpropionate and
is administered in similar dosage.

Preparations

TESTOSTERONE ESTERS INJECTION: see above under
Testosterone Phenylpropionate.

TESTOSTERONE PROPIONATE INJECTION: a sterile solution
of testosterone propionate in ethyl oleate or other
suitable ester, in a suitable fixed oil, or in any mixture
of these. It is sterilised by dry heat. Available in 1-ml
ampoules containing 5, 10, or 25 mg of testosterone
propionate, and in 1- and 2-ml ampoules containing
50 mg of testosterone propionate per ml.
A standard for this injection is given in the British
Pharmacopoeia 1973
Containers: see the entry on Injections for general
information on containers.
Labelling: see the entry on Injections for general
information on labelling. In addition, the label on the
container should state the composition of the solvent,
and "For intramuscular injection only".
Storage: it should be protected from light.

OTHER PREPARATIONS available include a veterinary
INJECTION containing the mixed testosterone esters (see
above under Testosterone Phenylpropionate).

Tetanus

Tetanus, or lock-jaw, is caused by *Clostridium tetani*,
an anaerobic spore-bearing organism present in soil and
animal faeces, which infects wounds and abscesses and
releases a potent neurotoxin.
The disease is characterised by initial restlessness,
muscle twitching, anxiety, and general malaise. Later,
stiffness of the neck and progressive muscle spasm
occur, followed by reflex convulsions initiated by minor
external stimuli. The reflex convulsions involve violent
contractions of all muscles, profuse sweating, and intense pain; the spasms end with a deep indrawing of
breath with the possibility of inhalation of oral and
pharyngeal secretion. If allowed to continue untreated,
the spasms lead to death due to exhaustion, cardiac
failure, or massive pulmonary collapse.
Neonatal tetanus occurs in some countries where neonatal hygiene is poor, especially where the umbilical
stump is contaminated with faeces or soil. This may be
prevented by adequate obstetric and neonatal hygiene.

Prophylaxis. Active immunisation as described under
Tetanus Vaccine may be carried out, or tetanus immunisation may be included in immunisation programmes
for children and travellers. Injured persons with wounds
at risk should receive adequate wound care, and suitable
antibiotics, such as benzylpenicillin or tetracyclines
should be given if it is thought that infection is present.
Primary immunisation should be given to non-immunised
patients who have wounds at risk from infection with
Clostridium tetani. Patients who have been actively
immunised and have wounds at risk should receive a
booster dose of tetanus toxoid.

Treatment. Circulating tetanus toxin is neutralised as
soon as possible with Human Tetanus Immunoglobulin.
Wounds infected with *Clostridium tetani* should be
opened to admit air and inhibit anaerobic growth; hyperbaric oxygen may be administered. The infection should
be treated by means of a suitable antibiotic such as
benzylpenicillin or tetracyclines. Muscle spasm and
convulsions may be controlled with antispasmodic
drugs, or if it is not possible to control convulsions in
this way curarisation may be used in conjunction with
intermittent positive pressure respiration.

Tetanus and Pertussis Vaccine

A mixture of tetanus formol toxoid and a suspension of killed *Bordetella pertussis*.

OTHER NAMES: Tetanus-Whooping-cough Prophylactic; TPer/Vac

A standard is given in the British Pharmacopoeia 1973

Storage. It should be stored as described under Vaccines.

Actions and uses. Tetanus and pertussis vaccine is used for active immunisation against tetanus and whooping-cough. Its use is limited to those cases where simultaneous immunisation with a diphtheria component is contra-indicated, as for instance when a child is known to be sensitive to diphtheria toxoid.

The vaccine is administered by intramuscular or deep subcutaneous injection as 3 doses each of 0.5 or 1 millilitre, as stated on the label as the dose, with an interval of 6 to 8 weeks between the first and second dose and 4 to 6 months between the second and third.

Tetanus Antitoxin

A preparation containing the specific antitoxic globulins or their derivatives that have the power of neutralising the toxin formed by *Clostridium tetani* and rendering it harmless to susceptible animals.

OTHER NAMES: Immunoserum Antitetanicum; Tet/Ser

A standard is given in the European Pharmacopoeia Vol. II

Storage. It should be stored as described under Antisera.

Actions and uses. Tetanus toxin has such an affinity for nerve cells that once it is present in the cells, antitoxin is unlikely to influence it. In the treatment of the acute disease antitoxin can be expected to neutralise only toxin which is still circulating.

For prophylactic use antitoxin may be injected into all non-immune or partially immunised persons as soon as possible after a wound. A suitable dose is 1500 units, or 3000 units in heavily infected wounds. It is doubtful if repeated doses are either useful or advisable; sensitivity to horse serum is rapidly induced and second or later doses of antitoxin may be so rapidly removed from the circulation as to render them useless.

In patients who have received horse serum of any kind on a previous occasion the first dose of antitoxin after wounding may similarly be rapidly eliminated and fail to give any protection. In such patients and in those who are hypersensitive to horse serum, bovine or ovine serum or human tetanus immunoglobulin may be safer.

When tetanus antitoxin in any form is given, the patient should also be given a dose of adsorbed tetanus vaccine and arrangements should be made to complete his active immunisation later.

If antitoxin is used in the treatment of tetanus, it should be given as early as possible. The maximum dose need not be more than 100000 units and repeated doses are unnecessary. Before surgical procedures involving old injured tissues, a similar dose may be given.

Precautions and contra-indications. Reactions to equine tetanus antitoxin are unfortunately common and often severe and opinion has turned against its routine use. Such reactions may be avoided by the use of human tetanus immunoglobulin.

Thorough wound toilet and the administration of peni-cillin for several days afterwards is now accepted as sound practice, though many would still give antitoxin in wounds thought to carry a high risk of tetanus. Whatever treatment is given, the opportunity should be taken to immunise the patient actively against tetanus with tetanus toxoid.

Serum reactions: See under Antisera.

Tetanus Antitoxin (Veterinary)

see CLOSTRIDIUM TETANI ANTITOXIN

Tetanus Toxoid (Veterinary)

see CLOSTRIDIUM TETANI VACCINE

Tetanus Vaccine

Prepared from tetanus toxin produced by the growth of *Clostridium tetani*. The toxin is converted to tetanus formol toxoid by treatment with formaldehyde solution.

OTHER NAMES: Tetanus Toxoid; Tet/Vac/FT

A standard is given in the British Pharmacopoeia 1973

Storage. It should be stored as described under Vaccines.

Actions and uses. Tetanus vaccine is used for active immunisation against tetanus. The vaccine is administered by intramuscular or deep subcutaneous injection in 3 doses each of 0.5 or 1 millilitre as stated on the label as the dose with an interval of 6 to 12 weeks between the first and second dose and 4 to 12 months between the second and third. This gives rise to the production of a considerable amount of tetanus antitoxin (immunoglobulin) in the blood. The antitoxin present in the blood after injection of the vaccine can usually be expected to persist for at least 5 years. A booster dose many years after the primary immunisation will stimulate the production of antibodies rapidly.

Immunisation of patients following injury must depend upon assessment of the risk associated with the type of wound involved. If the patient's immune status is known, it may already be adequate or require only the administration of a booster dose of vaccine. Non-immune subjects may require passive immunisation with human tetanus immunoglobulin, but the opportunity should also be taken to initiate the active immunisation of the subject.

When tetanus vaccine and human tetanus immunoglobulin are to be given at the same time, adsorbed tetanus vaccine should be used, the vaccine must not be injected into the same limb as the antitoxin, and the same syringe must not be used.

As a prophylactic for the routine immunisation of children, tetanus vaccine is often used in the form of the combined diphtheria, tetanus, and pertussis vaccine, with a booster dose of tetanus vaccine at school-leaving age; a suitable schedule is described under Vaccines.

Tetanus Vaccine, Adsorbed

Prepared from tetanus formol toxoid containing not less than 500 *flocculation equivalents* (500 Lf) per mg of protein nitrogen and a mineral carrier which may be aluminium hydroxide, aluminium phosphate, or calcium phosphate. It contains not more than 1.25 mg of Al or 1.3 mg of Ca in the recommended dose.

OTHER NAMES: Adsorbed Tetanus Toxoid; Tetanus Vaccine (Adsorbed); Tet/Vac/Ads; Vaccinum Tetanicum Adsorbatum

A standard is given in the European Pharmacopoeia Vol. III Supplement

Storage. It should be stored as described under Vaccines. Under these conditions it may be expected to retain its potency for 3 years.

Actions and uses. Adsorbed tetanus vaccine is used for the prophylaxis of tetanus as described under Tetanus Vaccine. The vaccine is administered by intramuscular or deep subcutaneous injection in 3 doses each of 0.5 or 1 millilitre as stated on the label as the dose with an interval of 6 to 12 weeks between the first and second dose and 4 to 12 months between the second and third.

Tetrachloroethylene

$CCl_2:CCl_2 = 165.8$

OTHER NAME: Perchloroethylene

A standard is given in the British Pharmacopoeia 1973

Tetrachloroethylene contains 0.01% w/w of thymol as a preservative.

Description. A colourless mobile liquid with a characteristic odour.

Solubility. Practically insoluble in water; soluble in alcohol; miscible with ether and with oils.

Weight per ml. At 20°, 1.620 to 1.626 g.

Boiling-point. About 120°.

Storage. It should be stored in airtight containers, protected from light.

Identification. TEST. To 5 ml in a stoppered cylinder add 5 ml of *bromine solution* and shake vigorously at intervals of 15 minutes during 1 hour; the colour of the bromine fades and a white turbidity is produced in the lower layer (distinction from chloroform and from carbon tetrachloride).

Metabolism. ABSORPTION. After oral administration, tetrachloroethylene does not appear to be absorbed to any significant extent; the drug is absorbed after inhalation.

Actions and uses. Tetrachloroethylene is given by mouth for the expulsion of hookworms; it is of little value against threadworms and is ineffective against liver flukes. The usual dose for an adult is 3 millilitres, and for a child 0.2 millilitre for each year of age up to 15 years.

The patient is usually given a saline purgative on an empty stomach, followed 2 hours later by the dose of tetrachloroethylene and then by a further dose of a saline purgative; purgation may however be omitted. If possible, the patient should be kept in bed during the treatment; food or alcohol should not be given. When large numbers of people are treated under field conditions, the dose of tetrachloroethylene is usually given at the same time as the saline purgative; if a second dose of tetrachloroethylene is necessary it should not be given until 10 days after the first dose. Tetrachloroethylene may be given without purgation and this is of advantage in anaemic patients, because the disturbance of the fluid balance brought about by saline purgatives is avoided; for such patients however, bephenium hydroxynaphthoate is to be preferred.

Undesirable effects. Toxic effects are rare; liver damage may occur occasionally, and a few patients may experience a transitory sensation of unsteadiness and vertigo after administration of the drug. Tetrachloroethylene may cause a burning sensation in the stomach, abdominal cramps, nausea, and vomiting.

Tetrachloroethylene is used as a solvent in industry. Prolonged inhalation of its vapour in concentrations of over 200 parts per million produces toxic effects on the central nervous system, kidneys and liver, initial symptoms including dizziness, excessive perspiration, nausea and vomiting, and stupor. Some deaths have occurred.

Precautions. Alcohol and fatty foods should not be taken just before or just after administration of tetrachloroethylene.

Dependence. Dependence of the barbiturate-alcohol type, as described under drug dependence, may occur in persons who habitually inhale small quantities of tetrachloroethylene vapour.

Poisoning. Industrial poisoning by tetrachloroethylene is treated by removal of the patient from the source of the vapour, by artificial respiration, and by the administration of oxygen.

Preparation

TETRACHLOROETHYLENE CAPSULES: consisting of tetrachloroethylene enclosed in a soft capsule. The usual strength is 1 ml of tetrachloroethylene.

A standard for these capsules is given in the British Pharmacopoeia 1973

Containers and Storage: see the entry on Capsules for general information on containers and storage. Containers should be light resistant. The capsules should be stored in a cool place.

Advice for patients: the dose should be taken on an empty stomach, preferably in the morning and the patient advised to rest in bed for about 4 hours after administration. Fatty foods and alcohol should be avoided for 24 hours before and after treatment.

Tetracosactrin Acetate

L-Seryl-L-tyrosyl-L-seryl-L-methionyl-L-glutamyl-L-histidyl-L-phenylalanyl-L-arginyl-L-tryptophylglycyl-L-lysyl-L-prolyl-L-valylglycyl-L-lysyl-L-lysyl-L-arginyl-L-arginyl-L-prolyl-L-valyl-L-lysyl-L-valyl-L-tyrosyl-L-proline hexa-acetate

OTHER NAMES: *Cortrosyn®*; Cosyntropin; *Synacthen®*; Tetracosactride

A standard is given in the British Pharmacopoeia 1973

Description. A white to yellow amorphous powder.

Solubility. Soluble in 70 parts of water.

Moisture content. 5 to 16%, determined by Fischer titration.

Specific rotation. −98° to −108°, determined on a 1% solution in water containing 1% v/v of glacial acetic acid.

Storage. It should be stored in airtight containers.

Metabolism. ABSORPTION. Appears to be well absorbed after intramuscular or subcutaneous injection or after nasal insufflation; oral doses appear to be inactivated.

Actions and uses. Tetracosactrin is a synthetic analogue of corticotrophin; it contains the first 24 of the 39 amino acids and has the complete therapeutic activity of the natural substance corticotrophin. It is used for the purposes described under Corticotrophin.

It may be administered by intravenous infusion of a solution in sodium chloride injection or dextrose injection (5%) over a period of 6 hours for therapeutic purposes. As a test for adrenocortical function tetracosactrin injection may be administered by intramuscular injection. The long-acting tetracosactrin zinc injection may be administered by intramuscular injection every 1 to 4 days. As a rough guide to dosage 1 milligram of tetracosactrin is equivalent to 100 to 150 units of corticotrophin zinc injection.

Undesirable effects. As for Corticotrophin. Occasionally, a local tissue reaction may occur following the use of the long-acting preparation.

Precautions and contra-indications. As for Corticotrophin.

Preparations

TETRACOSACTRIN INJECTION: a sterile aqueous solution of tetracosactrin acetate. Available in 1-ml ampoules containing tetracosactrin acetate equivalent to 250 micrograms of tetracosactrin.
Containers and *Labelling:* see the entry on Injections for general information on containers and labelling.
Storage: it should be protected from light.

TETRACOSACTRIN ZINC INJECTION: a sterile aqueous suspension of tetracosactrin acetate with zinc hydroxide and suitable stabilising agents. Available in 1-ml ampoules and 2-ml vials containing tetracosactrin acetate equivalent to 1 mg of tetracosactrin per ml.
A standard for this injection is given in the British Pharmacopoeia 1973
Containers: see the entry on Injections for general information on containers.
Labelling: see the entry on Injections for general information on labelling. In addition, the label on the container should state the amount of the medicament as the equivalent amount of tetracosactrin per ml, ''For subcutaneous or intramuscular injection only'', and that the container should be gently shaken before a dose is withdrawn.
Storage: it should be stored at a temperature between 2° and 15°. Under these conditions it may be expected to retain its potency for 3 years. It should not be allowed to freeze.

Tetracycline

A hydrated form of (4S,4aS,5aS,6S,12aR)-4-dimethyl-amino-1,4,4a,5,5a,6,11,12a-octahydro-3,6,10,12,12a-pentahydroxy-6-methyl-1,11-dioxonaphthacene-2-carboxamide.

$C_{22}H_{24}N_2O_8 = 444.4$

OTHER NAMES: *Achromycin®; Economycin®; Panmycin Aquadrops®; Steclin®; Tetrachel®; Tetracyn®; Tetrex®; Totomycin®*
Mysteclin® (with amphotericin or nystatin); *Albamycin-T Paediatric®* (with novobiocin calcium)

A standard is given in the British Pharmaceutical Codex 1973

Description. An odourless yellow crystalline powder.

Solubility. Very slightly soluble in water; soluble, at 20°, in 50 parts of alcohol; practically insoluble in ether and in chloroform; soluble in dilute acids and, with decomposition, in solutions of alkali hydroxides.

Acidity. A suspension prepared by shaking 100 mg with 10 ml of water has a pH of 3.5 to 6.

Moisture content. Not more than 13%, determined by drying at 105°.

Specific rotation. −260° to −280°, determined on a 1% solution in 0.1N hydrochloric acid.

Dissociation constants. pK_a 3.3 (acidic), 7.7 (acidic), 9.7 (basic) (25°).

Stability. See under Tetracycline Hydrochloride.

Storage. It should be stored in airtight containers, protected from light.

Labelling. The label on the container states that the contents are not to be injected.

Identification. TEST. To about 500 μg add 2 ml of sulphuric acid; an intense violet colour is produced. Add 1 drop of *ferric chloride solution*; the colour changes to brown or reddish-brown.

Metabolism. See under Tetracycline Hydrochloride.

Actions and uses. Tetracycline has the actions and uses described under Tetracycline Hydrochloride. It is used in the preparation of oral liquid preparations of the antibiotic; 1 gram of tetracycline (trihydrate) is approximately equivalent to 1 gram of tetracycline hydrochloride.
Salts of aluminium, calcium, iron, and magnesium, and antacids and milk, which may decrease the absorption of tetracyclines from the gut, should not be given with tetracycline.

Undesirable effects; Precautions and contra-indications; Drug interactions. As for Tetracycline Hydrochloride.

Preparations

TETRACYCLINE MIXTURE (*Syn.* Tetracycline Elixir; Tetracycline Syrup): a suspension of tetracycline in a suitable coloured flavoured vehicle.
When a dose less than or not a multiple of 5 ml is prescribed, the mixture may be diluted, as described in the entry on Mixtures, with syrup. The diluted mixture must be freshly prepared.
Available as a mixture containing tetracycline equivalent to 125 mg of tetracycline hydrochloride in 5 ml, and as a mixture for veterinary use containing tetracycline equivalent to 100 mg of tetracycline hydrochloride per ml.
A standard for this mixture is given in the British Pharmaceutical Codex 1973
Containers and *Labelling:* see the entry on Mixtures for general information on containers and labelling.
Storage: it should be stored in a cool place, protected from light.
Advice for patients: the mixture should be taken at regular intervals. Salts of aluminium, calcium, iron, and magnesium should not be taken within 1 hour of administration. This also applies to antacids and milk. The prescribed course should be completed.

TETRACYCLINE MOUTH-BATH: consisting of tetracycline mixture (see above) containing tetracycline equivalent to 125 mg of tetracycline hydrochloride in 5 ml.
Advice for patients: the dose should be retained in the mouth for 2 to 3 minutes then ejected.

OTHER PREPARATIONS available include CAPSULES containing tetracycline equivalent to 250 mg of tetracycline hydrochloride; granules to prepare a MIXTURE containing tetracycline 62.5 mg with novobiocin calcium equivalent to 62.5 mg of novobiocin in 5 ml when reconstituted, diluent water for preparations; and a mixture containing tetracycline equivalent to 125 mg of tetracycline hydrochloride with amphotericin 25 mg in 5 ml, diluent syrup, life of diluted mixture 2 months.

Tetracycline Hydrochloride

$(4S,4aS,5aS,6S,12aR)$-4-Dimethylamino-1,4,4a,5,5a,6,11,12a-octahydro-3,6,10,12,12a-pentahydroxy-6-methyl-1,11-dioxonaphthacene-2-carboxamide hydrochloride

$C_{22}H_{25}ClN_2O_8 = 480.9$

OTHER NAMES: *Achromycin®*; *Economycin®*; *Oppacyn®*; *Steclin®*; *Sustamycin®*; *Tetrachel®*; Tetracyclini Hydrochloridum; *Tetracyn®*; *Totomycin® Mysteclin®* (with amphotericin or nystatin); *Tetrabid®* (with fumaric acid); *Albamycin-T®* (with novobiocin sodium).

A standard is given in the European Pharmacopoeia Vol. II Supplement

Description. An odourless yellow crystalline powder with a bitter taste.

Solubility. Soluble, at 20°, in 10 parts of water, giving a clear solution which becomes turbid on standing, and in 100 parts of alcohol; very slightly soluble in ether, in chloroform, and in acetone; soluble in solutions of alkali hydroxides and carbonates.

Acidity. A 1% solution has a pH of 1.8 to 2.8.

Moisture content. Not more than 2%, determined over phosphorus pentoxide at 60° *in vacuo*.

Specific rotation. −239° to −258°, determined on a 1% solution in 0.01N hydrochloric acid.

Stability. In the form of powder or crystals, tetracycline and tetracycline hydrochloride darken in strong sunlight in a moist atmosphere. In aqueous solution, tetracycline and its hydrochloride degrade by epimerisation and other reactions to 4-epitetracycline, anhydrotetracycline, 4-epianhydrotetracycline, and other products. The major degradation product, 4-epitetracycline, has a very low antimicrobial activity; 4-epianhydrotetracycline is thought to be responsible for the renal dysfunction sometimes observed when degraded preparations of tetracycline are administered. Tetracycline is rapidly inactivated at a pH less than 2 and is slowly destroyed at pH 7 and above. The rate of degradation is increased in the presence of citric acid.

FURTHER INFORMATION. Epimerisation of tetracycline derivatives—D. A. Hussar *et al.*, *J. Pharm. Pharmac.*, 1968, **20**, 539; the kinetics of epimerisation—E. G. Remmers *et al.*, *J. pharm. Sci.*, 1963, **52**, 752; degradation products in fresh and aged tetracycline preparations—V. C. Walton *et al.*, *J. pharm. Sci.*, 1970, **59**, 1160; the kinetics of degradation at pH 1.5—P. H. Yuen and T. D. Sokoloski, *J. pharm. Sci.*, 1977, **66**, 1648.

Labelling. If the material is not intended for parenteral administration, the label on the container states that the contents are not to be injected.

Storage. It should be stored in airtight containers, protected from light.

Identification. TEST. To about 500 μg add 2 ml of sulphuric acid; a purplish-red colour is produced. Add 1 ml of water; the colour changes to deep yellow.

ULTRAVIOLET ABSORPTION. In 0.1N hydrochloric acid, maxima at 274 nm (E1%, 1cm = 387) and 360 nm (E1%, 1cm = 308); in 0.1N sodium hydroxide, maxima at 242 nm (E1%, 1cm=337) and 385 nm (E1%, 1cm=387).

INFRA-RED ABSORPTION. Major peaks at 1226, 1354, 1450, 1581, 1614, and 1664 cm^{-1} (see Appendix 2a: Infra-red Spectra).

Determination in body fluids. HIGH PRESSURE LIQUID CHROMATOGRAPHY. In urine—J. P. Sharma *et al.*, *J. pharm. Sci.*, 1977, **66**, 1319.

Metabolism. ABSORPTION. Incompletely and irregularly absorbed after oral administration; absorption is reduced by the presence of metal ions such as calcium, magnesium, aluminium, zinc, or iron, since these will form chelates or co-ordination compounds with tetracycline; milk and food also appear to reduce tetracycline absorption; the presence of phosphate may enhance tetracycline absorption; tetracycline is absorbed rectally. Therapeutic blood concentrations are achieved more readily by increasing the frequency of administration than by increasing the dose.

BLOOD CONCENTRATION. Therapeutic serum concentrations are in the range 2 to 5 μg/ml whilst toxic concentrations are approximately 12 μg/ml or over; during therapy with oral doses of 250 to 500 mg administered 4 times daily, serum concentrations of 1 to 4 μg/ml are maintained; after an intramuscular dose of 100 to 250 mg, peak serum concentrations of 2 to 4 μg/ml are attained in 1 to 2 hours; after an intravenous dose of 250 to 300 mg, serum concentrations of 5 to 30 μg/ml are obtained at 30 minutes.

HALF-LIFE. Serum half-life, about 9 hours.

DISTRIBUTION. Widely distributed throughout the body and readily enters most body fluids; appears to be subject to enterohepatic circulation; concentrations in cerebrospinal fluid are low and are much less than the corresponding concentrations in blood but are increased when the meninges are inflamed; tetracycline is secreted in milk and saliva and crosses the placenta; it is readily taken up by newly formed bones and teeth in which it forms a tetracycline-calcium orthophosphate complex; traces are detectable in the aqueous humour; it remains bound to malignant cells for a longer time than to non-malignant cells; *protein binding*, 20 to 70% bound to plasma proteins.

EXCRETION. Excreted in both urine and bile; after an oral dose, about 20% is excreted in the urine, mainly as unchanged drug; after intravenous doses, about 50% is excreted similarly; urinary excretion is increased when the urine is alkaline.

FURTHER INFORMATION. Absorption inhibited by zinc —K.-E. Anderson *et al.*, *Eur. J. clin. Pharmac.*, 1976, **10**, 59; the importance of 96-hour testing for inequivalence—C. M. Davis *et al.*, *Am. J. med. Sci.*, 1973, **265**, 69; plasma protein binding and lipophilic character— R. G. Green *et al.*, *J. Pharm. Pharmac.*, 1976, **28**, 514; pharmacokinetics of 4 tetracycline derivatives— R. Green *et al.*, *Eur. J. clin. Pharmac.*, 1976, **10**, 245; bioavailability of tetracycline products—M. C. Meyer *et al.*, *J. Pharmacokinet. Biopharm.*, 1974, **2**, 287 and T. Bergan *et al.*, *Acta pharmac. tox.*, 1973, **33**, 138.

Actions and uses. Tetracycline and its analogues are antibacterial agents which act by interfering with the synthesis of bacterial protein. Their action is bacterio-static. They are effective against a wide range of micro-organisms including Gram-positive and Gram-negative bacteria, rickettsiae, mycoplasmata, chlamydiae, and protozoa such as species of *Plasmodium*. Tubercle bacilli, fungi, and viruses are resistant. Resistance to tetracycline develops relatively slowly in susceptible organisms, but when it occurs there is often complete cross-resistance among all the members of the group.

The tetracyclines are widely used in general practice, mainly for the treatment of infections of the chest and soft tissues, and for superficial infections of acne vul-garis and acne rosacea. More specialised uses are con-cerned with the treatment of organisms other than common bacteria, for example brucellosis, psittacosis, lymphogranuloma venereum, Q fever, primary atypical pneumonia, typhus, and malaria.

All the tetracyclines are effective against the susceptible organisms indicated above, but tetracycline is the drug of choice in infections of the central nervous system and, like oxytetracycline, is preferred to chlortetracycline in the treatment of urinary-tract infections, especially when they are caused by *Klebsiella* species and *Escherichia coli*.

The usual dose of tetracycline hydrochloride by mouth for an adult is 250 to 500 milligrams every 6 hours, but up to 3 grams daily may be given in severe infections. In general, tetracyclines should not be given to children but when considered essential the usual dose by mouth is 2.5 to 7.5 milligrams per kilogram body-weight every 6 hours. Treatment should be continued for at least 48 hours after the patient's temperature has returned to normal and acute symptoms have subsided. In severe acute infections in adults, up to 1 gram may be given every 12 hours by slow intravenous infusion of a solution containing not more than 0.1%; the corre-sponding dose for children is 10 to 20 milligrams per kilogram body-weight daily in divided doses. Oral treat-ment should be substituted as soon as practicable because the injection may cause phlebitis.

Tetracyclines may be given by intramuscular injection, in a solution containing not more than 5%, in a dosage of 200 to 400 milligrams daily in divided doses for an adult and 5 milligrams per kilogram body-weight daily in divided doses for a child; as the injection is painful, procaine is usually included in the solution. Solutions for injection are prepared by an aseptic technique.

The tetracyclines are also applied topically in the treat-ment of some localised infections.

Undesirable effects. Treatment with tetracyclines may cause gastro-intestinal disturbances, with flatulence, nausea, vomiting, and diarrhoea.

Overgrowth of resistant organisms, such as *Candida* species and other fungi, may occur in the mouth and intestines, producing angular stomatitis, glossitis, and rectal and vaginal irritation; marked changes in the intestinal flora result from the destruction of susceptible organisms and facilitate the multiplication of resistant organisms, such as *Candida*, some strains of staphylo-cocci, and yeasts; the changed flora may also result in a deficiency of vitamins of the B group. The most serious toxic effect is the occurrence of staphylococcal entero-colitis, caused by organisms which have developed resistance; the onset of this condition is often sudden and it may end fatally. If this condition occurs, the tetracycline should be withdrawn and methicillin or cloxacillin given by injection in conjunction with ben-zylpenicillin, or vancomycin given by mouth, pending the results of sensitivity tests on the causative organism. Drug fever and allergic skin rashes occur on rare

occasions, but can usually be controlled by the adminis-tration of antihistamines. Tetracyclines (with the excep-tion of doxycycline) may cause a rise in blood urea and clinical deterioration in patients with renal impairment, and may cause liver damage especially during pregnancy; hepatotoxicity may occur on intravenous infusion. Benign intracranial hypertension may rarely occur but is reversed by discontinuing the administration of the tetracycline.

Precautions and contra-indications. Tetracyclines are contra-indicated in patients with renal impairment. Caution should be exercised when tetracyclines are administered in the presence of liver damage.

Tetracyclines readily cross the placental barrier and should not be given to pregnant women or to infants and children under 7 years, unless no other drug will control the infection, because they interfere with the growth and development of the teeth; the permanent front teeth may also be affected if tetracyclines are given to children up to 6 years and the permanent back teeth if tetracyclines are given to children up to 12 years. Tooth staining may occur. Tetracycline is secreted in the milk and should be used with caution in nursing mothers.

The antibiotics of the tetracycline group readily decom-pose on storage, especially in the presence of warmth and moisture, giving toxic decomposition products which cause nausea, glycosuria, proteinuria, and aminoaciduria.

Drug interactions. Iron salts reduce the absorption of tetracycline and alkalis lower the serum concentrations. Tetracycline potentiates the action of oral anticoagu-lants. Methoxyflurane administered to patients being treated with tetracycline may cause renal tubular necrosis.

Preparations

TETRACYCLINE AND PROCAINE INJECTION: a sterile solution of tetracycline hydrochloride and procaine hydrochloride, with suitable buffering and stabilising agents, in water for injections. It is prepared by dissolv-ing the contents of a sealed container in water for injections shortly before use. Available as a powder in vials containing 100 mg of tetracycline hydrochloride and 40 mg of procaine hydrochloride.

A standard for this injection is given in the British Pharmaceutical Codex 1973

Containers: see the entry on Injections for general information on containers.

Labelling: see the entry on Injections for general infor-mation on labelling. In addition, the label on the sealed container should state that the contents are to be used for intramuscular injection only.

Storage: the injection contains no bactericide and should be used as soon as possible after preparation but the injection may be expected to retain its potency for up to 24 hours after preparation, provided it is stored at 2° to 10°.

TETRACYCLINE CAPSULES: consisting of tetracycline hydrochloride, in powder, which may be mixed with a suitable inert diluent, enclosed in a hard capsule. The capsule shells may be coloured. Available as capsules containing 250 mg of tetracycline hydrochloride.

A standard for these capsules is given in the British Pharmacopoeia 1973

Containers and *Storage:* see the entry on Capsules for general information on containers and storage.

Labelling: the label on the container should state the date after which the capsules are not intended to be used, and the conditions under which they should be stored.

Advice for patients: the capsules should be taken at regular intervals and salts of aluminium, calcium, iron, and magnesium should not be taken within 1 hour of administration. The same applies to antacids and milk. The prescribed course should be completed.

TETRACYCLINE INJECTION: a sterile solution of tetracycline hydrochloride, with a suitable buffering agent, in water for injections. It is prepared by dissolving the contents of a sealed container, which includes the buffering agent, in water for injections, shortly before use. Available as a powder in vials containing 250 and 500 mg of tetracycline hydrochloride.

A standard for this injection is given in the British Pharmacopoeia 1973
Containers: see the entry on Injections for general information on containers.
Labelling: see the entry on Injections for general information on labelling. In addition, the label on the sealed container should state that the contents are to be used for intravenous injection only, in a well-diluted solution.
Storage: the sealed container should be protected from light. The injection contains no bactericide and should be used as soon as possible after preparation, but solutions of tetracycline hydrochloride may be expected to retain their potency for up to 72 hours after preparation, provided that they are stored at a temperature not exceeding 4°.

TETRACYCLINE TABLETS: available as tablets containing 250 mg of tetracycline hydrochloride; they are film coated or sugar coated; the coat may be coloured.
A standard for these tablets is given in the British Pharmacopoeia 1973
Containers and *Storage:* see the entry on Tablets for general information on containers and storage. Containers should be airtight.
Labelling: the label on the container should state the date after which the tablets are not intended to be used, and the conditions under which they should be stored.
Advice for patients: see above under Tetracycline Capsules.

OTHER PREPARATIONS available include CAPSULES containing tetracycline hydrochloride 250 mg in a slow-release formulation, capsules containing tetracycline hydrochloride equivalent to 125 mg of tetracycline with novobiocin sodium equivalent to 125 mg of novobiocin, capsules containing tetracycline hydrochloride 250 mg with fumaric acid 33 mg, capsules containing tetracycline hydrochloride 250 mg with nystatin 250 000 units; EYE-DROPS containing tetracycline hydrochloride 10 mg per ml (in an oily vehicle); an EYE OINTMENT containing tetracycline hydrochloride 10 mg per g; a MIXTURE containing tetracycline hydrochloride 125 mg in 5 ml, diluent syrup or water for preparations, life of diluted mixture 14 days; an OINTMENT containing tetracycline hydrochloride 30 mg per g; and TABLETS containing tetracycline hydrochloride 250 mg with nystatin 250 000 units.

Tetramisole Hydrochloride

(±)-2,3,5,6-Tetrahydro-6-phenylimidazo[2,1-*b*]thiazole hydrochloride

$C_{11}H_{13}ClN_2S = 240.8$

OTHER NAME: *Nilverm®* (this name is also applied to preparations of levamisole hydrochloride)

A standard is given in the British Pharmacopoeia (Veterinary)

Description. An odourless, white to pale cream-coloured, crystalline powder.

Solubility. Soluble, at 20°, in 5 parts of water and in 10 parts of methyl alcohol; very slightly soluble in ether and in acetone.

Dissociation constant. pK_a 7.8 (20°).

Identification. TEST. Dissolve about 50 mg in 20 ml of water and add 20 ml of *ammonium reineckate solution*; a pink precipitate is produced which, after washing with water and drying at 105°, melts at about 151°.

Veterinary uses. Tetramisole hydrochloride is used in the treatment of parasitic gastro-enteritis and parasitic bronchitis. The usual dose for cattle is 15 milligrams per kilogram body-weight up to a maximum of 4.5 grams, and for sheep, pigs, and goats 15 milligrams per kilogram body-weight, as a single dose.

Preparations

TETRAMISOLE MIXTURE (*Syn.* Tetramisole Solution): an aqueous solution of tetramisole hydrochloride, with suitable stabilising agents. It may contain suitable preservatives. Available as a mixture containing 3% of tetramisole hydrochloride.
A standard for this mixture is given in the British Pharmacopoeia (Veterinary)
Containers: see the entry on Mixtures for general information on containers.
Labelling: see the entry on Mixtures for general information on labelling. In addition, the label on the container should state that animals should not be slaughtered for human consumption within 7 days after cessation of treatment and that milk should not be drawn for human consumption within 24 hours after cessation of treatment.

OTHER PREPARATIONS available include GRANULES containing tetramisole hydrochloride 10%; a POWDER containing tetramisole hydrochloride 10%, and a powder containing tetramisole hydrochloride 17%.

Thenium Closylate

NN - Dimethyl - *N* - (2 - phenoxyethyl) - *N* - then - 2 - yl-ammonium 4-chlorobenzenesulphonate

$C_{21}H_{24}ClNO_4S_2 = 454.0$

OTHER NAMES: *Ancaris®* (with piperazine phosphate)

A standard is given in the British Pharmacopoeia (Veterinary)

Description. An odourless, white, crystalline powder with a slightly bitter taste.

Solubility. Soluble, at 20°, in 200 parts of water, in 25 parts of alcohol, and in 35 parts of chloroform; soluble in hot water, any excess forming an oily layer.

Moisture content. Not more than 1%, determined by drying at 60° *in vacuo*.

Identification. TESTS. 1. To about 200 mg add 2 ml of nitric acid, and shake; a greenish-black colour is produced which changes to deep red after allowing to stand for a few minutes.
2. Mix about 200 mg with *dilute sulphuric acid* and boil; a thiophene-like odour is produced.

MELTING-POINT. About 159°.

ULTRAVIOLET ABSORPTION. In 0.1N sulphuric acid, maxima at 223 nm (E1%, 1cm = 589), 268 nm (E1%, 1cm = 46), and 275 nm (E1%, 1cm = 36).

INFRA-RED ABSORPTION. Major peaks at 760, 1010, 1042, 1135, 1174, and 1210 cm^{-1} (see Appendix 2c: Infra-red Spectra).

Veterinary uses. Thenium closylate is used for the treatment of hookworm infections in dogs. Dogs over 4 kilograms body-weight may be given 2 doses each of the equivalent of 250 milligrams of thenium with an interval of 6 hours. Puppies may also be treated subject to careful control of the dose rate and diet.

Preparation

COMPOUND THENIUM TABLETS: available as tablets containing 216.25 mg of thenium closylate equivalent to 125 mg of thenium, and 260 mg of piperazine phosphate equivalent to 250 mg of piperazine hexahydrate.
A standard for these tablets is given in the British Pharmacopoeia (Veterinary)
Containers and *Storage:* see the entry on Tablets for general information on containers and storage. Containers should be airtight.
Labelling: the label on the container should state the amounts of the medicaments as the equivalent amounts of thenium and piperazine hexahydrate.

Theobroma Oil

The solid fat obtained from the crushed and roasted seeds of *Theobroma cacao* L. (Fam. Sterculiaceae), a tree cultivated in West Africa and other tropical areas; it is obtained as a by-product in the manufacture of cocoa.

OTHER NAMES: Cocoa Butter; Oleum Theobromatis

A standard is given in the British Pharmacopoeia 1973

Constituents. Theobroma oil consists chiefly of glycerides of stearic, palmitic, oleic, arachidic, and linoleic acids; 0.5 to 2% of theobromine is also present.

Description. A yellowish-white solid, becoming white on keeping. It has a faint agreeable odour resembling that of cocoa; it is sometimes deodorised. It is usually supplied in oblong cakes; it is brittle when cold and breaks with a smooth fracture which shows indications of crystalline structure; it becomes soft at 25°.

Solubility. Slightly soluble in alcohol; soluble in ether, in chloroform, in boiling dehydrated alcohol, and in light petroleum.

Melting-point. 31° to 34°.

Refractive index. At 40°, 1.456 to 1.458.

Adulterants and substitutes. Paraffin, stearin, tallow, Borneo tallow, and other fats have been reported as adulterants.

Uses. Theobroma oil is used for the preparation of suppositories, pessaries, and bougies. See also under Suppositories.

Theobromine

3,7-Dimethylxanthine, an alkaloid contained in the seeds of *Theobroma cacao* L. (Fam. Sterculiaceae).

$C_7H_8N_4O_2 = 180.2$

OTHER NAMES: Theobrominum
Theogardenal® and *Theominal®* (both with phenobarbitone); *Riddospas®* (with theophylline)

A standard is given in the European Pharmacopoeia Vol. II

Theobromine forms salts with alkali hydroxides and is not extracted from alkaline solution by shaking with immiscible solvents. It sublimes at about 290° without decomposition.

Description. An odourless white crystalline powder or rhombic needles with a bitter taste.

Solubility. Very slightly soluble in water, in alcohol, and in chloroform; practically insoluble in ether; soluble in solutions of alkali hydroxides and in dilute mineral acids.

Acidity. A solution prepared by boiling 1 g with 50 ml of water, cooling and filtering, has a pH of 5.5 to 7.

Dissociation constants. pK$_a$ < 1, 10.0 (25°).

Identification. TESTS. 1. It complies with Test 1 described under Aminophylline.
2. Dissolve, with the aid of gentle heat, about 20 mg in 2 ml of *dilute ammonia solution*, cool, and add 2 ml of *dilute silver nitrate solution*; the solution remains clear. Boil the solution gently for a few minutes; a white crystalline precipitate is produced.

ULTRAVIOLET ABSORPTION. In 0.1N hydrochloric acid, maximum at 274 nm (E1%, 1cm = 543); in alcohol (95%), maximum at 274 nm (E1%, 1cm = 524).

INFRA-RED ABSORPTION. Major peaks at 684, 1225, 1453, 1545, 1594, and 1680 cm^{-1} (see Appendix 2a: Infra-red Spectra).

THIN-LAYER CHROMATOGRAPHY. See under Thin-layer Chromatography, System 12.

Actions and uses. Theobromine has an action on the kidney similar to that described under Caffeine but has no stimulant effect upon the central nervous system. In the form of phenobarbitone and theobromine tablets, it has been employed to allay the nervous excitement and insomnia associated with hypertension, but this preparation has no advantage over other sedatives or phenobarbitone alone.
The usual dose of theobromine is 300 to 600 milligrams.

Undesirable effects. In large doses theobromine may cause nausea and loss of appetite.

Preparations

PHENOBARBITONE AND THEOBROMINE TABLETS: for each tablet take:

Phenobarbitone	..	..	..	..	30 mg
Theobromine	..	..	..	..	300 mg

Mix, and prepare by moist granulation and compression as described in the entry on Tablets.

A standard for these tablets is given in the British Pharmaceutical Codex 1973

Containers and *Storage:* see the entry on Tablets for general information on containers and storage. Containers should be airtight and light resistant.

Advice for patients: the tablets may cause drowsiness; persons affected should not drive or operate machinery. Alcohol should be avoided.

OTHER PREPARATIONS available include CAPSULES containing theobromine 150 mg with theophylline 150 mg; and SUPPOSITORIES containing theobromine 175 mg with theophylline 175 mg.

Theophylline

1,3-Dimethylxanthine, an alkaloid isomeric with theobromine.

$C_7H_8N_4O_2 = 180.2$

OTHER NAMES: Anhydrous Theophylline; *Nuelin®*; *Rona-Phyllin®*; *Rona-Slophyllin®*; *Theograd®*
Newmarket Cough Syrup® (with diphenhydramine hydrochloride); *Entair®* (with guaiphenesin); *Labophylline®* (with lysine); *Theo-Nar®* (with noscapine); *Riddospas®* (with theobromine)

A standard is given in the European Pharmacopoeia Vol. II

Theophylline is a weak base, forming salts with acids and soluble derivatives with alkali metals. It may be extracted from slightly acid solution by a mixture of isopropyl alcohol and chloroform.

Description. An odourless white crystalline powder with a bitter taste.

Solubility. Soluble, at 25°, in 120 parts of water and in 80 parts of alcohol; very slightly soluble in ether; soluble in solutions of alkali hydroxides.

Dissociation constants. $pK_a < 1$, 8.6 (25°).

Identification. TESTS. 1. It complies with Test 2 described under Aminophylline.
2. Dissolve about 10 mg in 10 ml of water, add 0.5 ml of a 5% solution of mercuric acetate, and allow to stand; a white crystalline precipitate is produced.
3. Dissolve about 200 mg in 5 ml of *potassium hydroxide solution* or *dilute ammonia solution*; a clear solution is produced (distinction from caffeine and theobromine).

MELTING-POINT. About 272°.

ULTRAVIOLET ABSORPTION. In 0.1N hydrochloric acid, maximum at 272 nm (E1%, 1cm = 530); in 0.01N sodium hydroxide, maximum at 277 nm (E1%, 1cm = 650).

INFRA-RED ABSORPTION. Major peaks at 744, 1189, 1445, 1565, 1665, and 1710 cm⁻¹ (see Appendix 2a: Infra-red Spectra).

THIN-LAYER CHROMATOGRAPHY. See under Thin-layer Chromatography, System 12.

Determination in body fluids. ULTRAVIOLET SPECTROPHOTOMETRY. In serum—J. Vasiliades and T. Turner, *Clinica chim. Acta*, 1976, **69**, 491.

GAS CHROMATOGRAPHY. In plasma—H. A. Schwertner *et al.*, *Analyt. Chem.*, 1976, **48**, 1875. In serum—J. D. Lowry *et al.*, *J. Chromat.*, 1977, **143**, 83.

HIGH PRESSURE LIQUID CHROMATOGRAPHY. In plasma—O. H. Weddle and W. D. Mason, *J. pharm. Sci.*, 1976, **65**, 865. In serum—M. J. Cooper *et al.*, *J. Chromat.*, 1977, **143**, 324.

THIN-LAYER CHROMATOGRAPHY. In plasma—B. Wesley-Hadzija and A. M. Mattocks, *J. Chromat.*, 1975, **115**, 501.

Metabolism. ABSORPTION. Erratically absorbed after oral administration or after administration as suppositories; theophylline salts are better absorbed than theophylline itself; rectal retention enemas are more consistently absorbed than suppositories; oral doses of theophylline may cause gastric irritation.

BLOOD CONCENTRATION. After an oral dose of 300 mg to adults, peak plasma concentrations of about 2 to 9 µg/ml are attained in 2 to 3 hours; higher peaks are attained after oral doses of theophylline with guaiphenesin, choline theophyllinate, or theophylline with monoethanolamine; after an oral dose of 312.5 mg of theophylline monoethanolamine to children aged 4 to 15 years, peak serum concentrations of 2 to 19 µg/ml are attained in 1 to 2 hours; after an intravenous dose of 3.2 mg/kg to children aged 1 to 4 years, plasma concentrations fall to about 5 µg/ml by 2 hours; therapeutic serum concentrations are in the range 5 to 9 µg/ml and toxic symptoms may begin to appear at concentrations of about 7 µg/ml but are well tolerated until concentrations reach about 20 µg/ml.

HALF-LIFE. Serum or plasma half-life, about 4.5 hours.

DISTRIBUTION. Rapidly and widely distributed throughout the tissues; volume of distribution, about 30 litres; saliva concentrations parallel those in the plasma; small amounts are excreted in the milk; *protein binding*, 20 to 60% bound to plasma proteins.

METABOLIC REACTIONS. Variably metabolised by N-demethylation and oxidation at position 8 to 1-methyluric acid, 1,3-dimethyluric acid, 3-methyluric acid, and uric acid.

EXCRETION. About 10% of an oral dose is excreted in the urine unchanged, with 35 to 50% as 1,3-dimethyluric acid, about 20% as 1-methyluric acid, and about 13% as 3-methyluric acid.

FURTHER INFORMATION. Effect of complexation with phenobarbitone on bioavailability—J. W. Bettis *et al.*, *Am. J. Hosp. Pharm.*, 1973, **30**, 240; effect of guaiphenesin and choline on blood concentrations—A. David and O. Morton, *Practitioner*, 1965, **194**, 511; serum concentrations and metabolism—J. W. Jenne *et al.*, *Clin. Pharmac. Ther.*, 1976, **19**, 375; disposition in children after intravenous injection—P. M. Loughnan *et al.*, *J. Pediat.*, 1976, **88**, 874; plasma and salivary concentrations—V. P. Shah and S. Riegelman, *J. pharm. Sci.*, 1974, **63**, 1283; influence of formulation on bioavailability—P. G. Welling *et al.*, *J. clin. Pharmac.*, 1976, **16**, 43; rectal administration and control of asthma—J. W. Yunginger *et al.*, *Ann. Allergy*, 1966, **24**, 469.

Actions and uses. Theophylline has actions resembling those of the other xanthine derivatives, caffeine and theobromine. Its diuretic action, although stronger than that of caffeine, is of short duration. It is a more powerful relaxant of involuntary muscle than theobromine or caffeine. It has only a slight stimulant action on the cerebrum. Because of its low solubility. theophylline itself is seldom used, its more soluble derivatives, such as aminophylline and choline theophyllinate, being preferred.

The usual dose of theophylline is 60 to 200 milligrams 3 or 4 times daily.

Undesirable effects. Theophylline may cause gastric irritation, nausea, and vomiting.

Preparations

AMINOPHYLLINE INJECTION (*Syn.* Theophylline and Ethylenediamine Injection): a sterile solution of aminophylline in water for injections free from carbon dioxide. It may be prepared by dissolving theophylline in a solution of ethylenediamine hydrate in water for injections free from carbon dioxide, 870 mg of theophylline being used for each g of aminophylline required. Ethylenediamine hydrate additional to that necessary for the formation of aminophylline may be added but the total amount of ethylenediamine, $C_2H_4(NH_2)_2$, should not exceed 251 mg for each g of anhydrous theophylline, $C_7H_8N_4O_2$, present.

It is sterilised by heating in an autoclave or by filtration. Exposure to carbon dioxide and contact with metals must be avoided throughout.

Available as a solution containing 25 mg of aminophylline per ml in 10-ml ampoules and as a solution containing 250 mg per ml in 2-ml ampoules.

A standard for this injection is given in the British Pharmacopoeia 1973

Containers and *Labelling:* see the entry on Injections for general information on containers and labelling; containers should be light resistant.

MERSALYL INJECTION (*Syn.* Mersalyl and Theophylline Injection):

Mersalyl acid	..	..	..	..	.. 9.56 g
Theophylline	..	..	..	..	.. 5 g
Sodium hydroxide..	..	..	..	.. 1 g

or a sufficient quantity

Water for injections .. .. to 100 ml

Suspend the mersalyl acid and the theophylline in about 80 ml of the water. Prepare an approximately 10% solution of the sodium hydroxide in water for injections and add to the suspension, stirring continuously, until solution is effected; adjust the alkalinity of the solution to pH 8 by the addition of a further quantity of the sodium hydroxide solution, add sufficient of the water to produce the required volume, mix, and clarify by filtration. Distribute the solution into ampoules, seal, and sterilise by heating with a bactericide, using phenylmercuric nitrate as the bactericide.

Alternatively, sterilise the solution by filtration; distribute, by means of an aseptic technique, into sterile ampoules, and seal.

The solution must not be allowed to come into contact with metal.

It contains 10% of $C_{13}H_{16}HgNNaO_6$. It contains, in 1 ml, 100 mg of mersalyl (the sodium salt of mersalyl acid) and 50 mg of theophylline.

A standard for this injection is given in the British Pharmacopoeia 1973

Containers: see the entry on Injections for general information on containers.

Labelling: see the entry on Injections for general information on labelling. In addition, the label on the container should state the amount of the medicament as 10% w/v of mersalyl.

Storage: it should be protected from light.

OTHER PREPARATIONS available include CAPSULES containing theophylline 60, 125, and 250 mg, in slow-release formulations; capsules containing theophylline 150 mg with guaiphenesin 90 mg; capsules containing theophylline 150 mg with theobromine 150 mg; an ELIXIR containing theophylline 80 mg in 15 ml, diluent syrup (up to a maximum of equal parts elixir and syrup), life of diluted elixir 14 days; a veterinary MIXTURE containing theophylline 3.5 mg with diphenhydramine hydrochloride 2.6 mg per ml; SUPPOSITORIES containing theophylline 175 mg with theobromine 175 mg; TABLETS containing theophylline 100, 125, and 200 mg; tablets containing theophylline 350 mg in a slow-release formulation; tablets containing theophylline 100 mg with lysine 74 mg; and tablets containing theophylline 200 mg with noscapine 30 mg in a slow-release formulation.

Theophylline Hydrate

1,3-Dimethylxanthine monohydrate

$C_7H_8N_4O_2,H_2O = 198.2$

OTHER NAME: Theophyllinum Monohydricum

A standard is given in the European Pharmacopoeia Vol. II

Description. An odourless, white, crystalline powder with a bitter taste.

Solubility. Soluble, at 25°, in 120 parts of water and in 80 parts of alcohol; very slightly soluble in ether; soluble in solutions of alkali hydroxides.

Moisture content. 8 to 9.5%, determined by drying at 105°.

Identification. TESTS. As for Theophylline.

MELTING-POINT. About 272°, after drying.

ULTRAVIOLET ABSORPTION. In 0.1N hydrochloric acid, maximum at 272 nm (E1%, 1cm = 523); in 0.1N sodium hydroxide, maximum at 277 nm (E1%, 1cm = 625).

INFRA-RED ABSORPTION; THIN-LAYER CHROMATOGRAPHY. As for Theophylline.

Determination in body fluids; Metabolism. As for Theophylline.

Actions and uses. Theophylline hydrate has the actions, uses, and undesirable effects described under Theophylline.

Thiabendazole

2-(Thiazol-4-yl)benzimidazole

$C_{10}H_7N_3S = 201.2$

OTHER NAMES: *Equizole®*; *Mintezol®*; Tiabendazole; *Thibenzole®*; *Thiprazole®*
Ranizole® (with rafoxanide)

A standard is given in the British Pharmacopoeia Addendum 1977 and the British Pharmacopoeia (Veterinary)

Description. An odourless white to cream-coloured powder.

Solubility. Practically insoluble in water; soluble, at 20°, in 150 parts of alcohol and in 300 parts of chloroform; very slightly soluble in ether; soluble in dilute mineral acids.

Identification. TEST. Dissolve about 5 mg in 5 ml of 0.1N hydrochloric acid, add 3 mg of *p*-phenylenediamine dihydrochloride, shake until dissolved, add 100 mg of zinc powder, mix, and allow to stand for 2 minutes; the odour of hydrogen sulphide is produced. Add 10 ml of *ferric ammonium sulphate solution*; a deep blue or blue-violet colour is produced.

MELTING-POINT. About 300°.

ULTRAVIOLET ABSORPTION. In 0.1N hydrochloric acid, maxima at 243 nm (E1%, 1cm = 587) and 302 nm (E1%, 1cm = 1225).

INFRA-RED ABSORPTION. Major peaks at 740, 902, 1306, 1358, 1404, and 1455 cm^{-1} (see Appendix 2c: Infra-red Spectra).

Determination in body fluids. SPECTROFLUORIMETRY. In plasma or urine: thiabendazole and metabolites— D. J. Tocco *et al.*, *J. Pharmac. exp. Ther.*, 1965, **149**, 263.

Metabolism. ABSORPTION. Readily absorbed after oral administration.

BLOOD CONCENTRATION. After an oral dose of 1 g, a peak plasma concentration of 2 to 6 μg/ml is attained in about 1 hour.

DISTRIBUTION. Small quantities are secreted in the milk of lactating animals.

METABOLIC REACTIONS. Hydroxylation at the 5-position followed by conjugation with glucuronic acid or sulphate.

EXCRETION. About 90% of a dose is excreted in the urine and 5% in the faeces in 48 hours; most of the urinary excreted material is conjugated 5-hydroxythiabendazole and less than 1% is unchanged drug or unconjugated 5-hydroxythiabendazole. A single dose is almost completely excreted in 5 days.

FURTHER INFORMATION. Absorption, metabolism, and excretion in man and laboratory animals—D. J. Tocco *et al.*, *Toxic. appl. Pharmac.*, 1966, **9**, 31.

Actions and uses. Thiabendazole is an anthelmintic which is administered orally and absorbed from the gastro-intestinal tract. Its principal use in human medicine is against *Strongyloides stercoralis* and *Trichuris trichiura*, and in creeping eruption (infection with larval forms of *Ancylostoma caninum* or *A. braziliense*). For infections with roundworm, threadworm, and hookworm in man other less toxic drugs are available, but it may be used for the treatment of multiple infections. It has been used against *Trichinella spiralis* but its action against the larval forms of this parasite in human tissue is uncertain. It is of value, however, in relieving the symptoms and reducing fever and eosinophilia during the invasive phase of the infection.

Thiabendazole is given in a dosage of 25 milligrams per kilogram body-weight twice daily for 2 or 3 days, or for mass therapy 50 milligrams per kilogram body-weight as a single dose for children and adults. A daily dosage of 3 grams should not be exceeded.

Undesirable effects. The incidence of undesirable effects is higher if a single dose rather than twice-daily dosage is given. Anorexia, nausea, vomiting, and epigastric discomfort may occur, and less commonly xanthopsia (yellow vision), pruritus, rashes, diarrhoea, headache, and drowsiness. Fever, chills, lymphadeno-

pathy, conjunctival infection, angioneurotic oedema, anaphylaxis, and erythema multiforme have been reported but may represent allergic response to dead parasites. A decrease in blood pressure and pulse rate may be noted. Crystalluria without haematuria has been reported but promptly disappears on discontinuing ingestion of the drug.

Some persons during treatment may excrete a metabolite that imparts to the urine an odour similar to that which may occur after ingestion of asparagus. The odour usually disappears not more than 24 hours after taking the last dose.

Precautions. Thiabendazole should be given with care to anaemic, dehydrated, and malnourished patients and to those with liver and kidney disorders. No teratogenic effect has been observed, but in the case of pregnant women, unless the symptoms produced by a helminthic infection are severe, it is in general best to postpone anthelmintic therapy until after parturition. It should preferably be avoided during breast feeding.

Veterinary uses. Thiabendazole is used for the treatment of gastrointestinal roundworm infections. The usual dose by mouth for horses is 45 milligrams per kilogram body-weight and for cattle 65 milligrams per kilogram body-weight as a single dose; these doses may be doubled in severe infections. The usual dose by mouth for sheep is 45 milligrams per kilogram body-weight for intestinal roundworms and 65 milligrams per kilogram body-weight for parasitic bronchitis; lambs may be given 90 milligrams per kilogram body-weight for nematodiriasis.

Preparations

THIABENDAZOLE AND RAFOXANIDE MIXTURE (*Syn.* Thiabendazole and Rafoxanide Suspension): an aqueous suspension of thiabendazole and rafoxanide mixed with suitable suspending and dispersing agents. Available as a mixture containing 13.3% of thiabendazole and 2.27% of rafoxanide.

A standard for this mixture is given in the British Pharmacopoeia (Veterinary)

Containers and *Labelling*: see the entry on Mixtures for general information on containers and labelling.

THIABENDAZOLE MIXTURE (*Syn.* Thiabendazole Drench; Thiabendazole Suspension): an aqueous suspension of thiabendazole mixed with suitable suspending and preservative agents. It may contain suitable colouring matter. Available as a mixture containing 13.3% of thiabendazole.

A standard for this mixture is given in the British Pharmacopoeia (Veterinary)

Containers: see the entry on Mixtures for general information on containers.

Labelling: see the entry on Mixtures for general information on labelling. In addition, the label on the container should state that the mixture should be administered undiluted. A direction to shake the bottle should be given on the label.

THIABENDAZOLE PELLETS: consisting of thiabendazole mixed with a suitable cereal diluent and made into pellets for administration by mouth. Available as pellets containing 4, 8.8, and 10.5% of thiabendazole.

A standard for these pellets is given in the British Pharmacopoeia (Veterinary)

Containers and *Storage:* they should be stored in airtight containers, in a cool place.

THIABENDAZOLE PREMIX: consisting of thiabendazole mixed with powdered soya bean meal or other suitable diluent. This preparation is not stable to hot pelleting processes. It must be diluted before administration by mixing thoroughly with the feed. Available as premixes containing 22.5 and 33.3% of thiabendazole.

A standard for this premix is given in the British Pharmacopoeia (Veterinary)
Containers and *Storage:* see the entry on Premixes for general information on containers and storage.

THIABENDAZOLE TABLETS: may be prepared by moist granulation and compression as described in the entry on Tablets. Available as tablets containing 500 mg of thiabendazole; they may contain suitable flavouring and sweetening agents; they may be coloured.

A standard for these tablets is given in the British Pharmacopoeia Addendum 1977
Containers and *Storage:* see the entry on Tablets for general information on containers and storage. Containers should be airtight.
Labelling: a direction to chew the tablets before they are swallowed should be given on the label.
Advice for patients: the tablets should be taken at regular intervals after meals. The prescribed course should be completed. The tablets may cause drowsiness; persons affected should not drive or operate machinery. Alcohol should be avoided. Adequate fluid intake should be maintained. Thiabendazole may impart an odour of asparagus to the urine. See also under Labelling above.

THIABENDAZOLE VETERINARY TABLETS: may be prepared by moist granulation and compression as described in the entry on Tablets. Available as tablets containing 500 mg and 2 g of thiabendazole; they need not be circular in shape.

A standard for these tablets is given in the British Pharmacopoeia (Veterinary)
Containers and *Storage:* see the entry on Tablets for general information on containers and storage. Containers should be airtight.

OTHER PREPARATIONS (all veterinary) available include a PASTE containing thiabendazole 44%, a paste containing thiabendazole 49.3%; PELLETS containing thiabendazole 4% with picadex 8%; a POWDER containing thiabendazole 33.3%, and a powder containing thiabendazole 58.4% with copper sulphate heptahydrate 1.96%.

Thiacetazone

4-Acetamidobenzaldehyde thiosemicarbazone

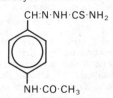

CH:N·NH·CS·NH$_2$

NH·CO·CH$_3$

$C_{10}H_{12}N_4OS = 236.3$

OTHER NAMES: Thioacetazone; *Thioparamizone®*

A standard is given in the British Pharmaceutical Codex 1973

Description. Odourless pale yellow crystals or crystalline powder.

Solubility. Very slightly soluble in water; soluble, at 20°, in 500 parts of alcohol and in 100 parts of propylene glycol.

Storage. It should be stored in airtight containers, protected from light.

Identification. TESTS. 1. Mix about 10 mg with 5 ml of 1N hydrochloric acid, boil for 3 minutes, cool, add sufficient water to produce 200 ml, mix 5 ml of this solution with 5 drops of *sodium nitrite solution* and add the mixture to 0.5 ml of *2-naphthol solution*; a red colour is produced.
2. Dissolve, with the aid of heat, about 10 mg in 1 ml of 6N sodium hydroxide, add 5 drops of *lead acetate solution*, and boil for 1 minute; a black precipitate is produced.

MELTING-POINT. About 227°, with decomposition.

ULTRAVIOLET ABSORPTION. In dehydrated alcohol, maximum at 328 nm (E1%, 1cm $=$ 1933).

INFRA-RED ABSORPTION. Major peaks at 1250, 1299, 1515, 1587, 1613, and 1667 cm^{-1} (see Appendix 2b: Infra-red Spectra).

Metabolism. BLOOD CONCENTRATION. After oral doses of 150 to 300 mg, peak serum concentrations of 1 to 9 μg/ml are attained in 4 to 5 hours; peak concentrations after larger doses are attained 1 to 2 hours later.

HALF-LIFE. Biological half-life, 8 to 12 hours.

DISTRIBUTION. Repeated doses may accumulate.

METABOLIC REACTIONS. Possible reactions include deacetylation to *p*-aminobenzoic acid thiosemicarbazone and also conversion to *p*-acetamidobenzoic acid.

EXCRETION. 20 to 40% of a dose is excreted in the urine in 24 to 48 hours.

FURTHER INFORMATION. Antitubercular activity and blood concentrations—G. A. Ellard *et al.*, *Tubercle*, 1974, **55**, 41; estimation in biological fluids by polarography—L. Molnár and H. Gergöová, *Arznei-mittel-Forsch.*, 1974, **24**, 1731; increased activity by administration at peak concentration—P. K. Sen *et al.*, *J. Indian med. Ass.*, 1973, **61**, 306; blood concentrations —P. K. Sen *et al.*, *Indian J. med. Res.*, 1974, **62**, 557; human pharmacology—G. Simmons *et al.*, *Am. Rev. Tuberc. Pulm. Dis.*, 1950, **62**, 128.

Actions and uses. Thiacetazone inhibits the growth of *Mycobacterium tuberculosis* and of *M. leprae* and is used in the treatment of tuberculosis and leprosy.
There are marked regional differences in the incidence of undesirable effects which seem to depend on the state of nutrition and presence of other endemic diseases in the populations concerned. In tolerant populations thiacetazone may be used in conjunction with streptomycin and isoniazid as a first choice in the treatment of susceptible infections. In most countries, however, its use is limited to the treatment of infections that are resistant to other drugs. Cross-resistance between thiacetazone and ethionamide or prothionamide may occur.
The usual adult dose in the treatment of tuberculosis is 150 milligrams, or 2 milligrams per kilogram body-weight, given daily in a single dose, but it is preferable to commence treatment with approximately one-tenth of the quantity and gradually increase the dose over a period of a week or 10 days to establish the maximum that the patient will tolerate.
Thiacetazone should always be given simultaneously with other drugs to delay the development of resistance. In the treatment of leprosy, the usual initial dose is 50 milligrams daily, gradually increasing over a period of 4 to 8 weeks to a total daily dose of 150 milligrams.

Undesirable effects. Allergic reactions commonly occur but are usually mild and subside rapidly when treatment is discontinued, but rashes and fever may be followed by the Stevens-Johnson syndrome, agranulocytosis, and similar serious or fatal responses if treatment is continued.

Dizziness, deafness, nausea, vomiting, and hepatitis may occur in patients being treated with thiacetazone in conjunction with other drugs. Displacement of streptomycin from protein binding sites or interference with renal excretion may be responsible for increased eighthnerve damage when thiacetazone is used in treatment schemes that include streptomycin.

Preparation

THIACETAZONE TABLETS: may be prepared by moist granulation and compression as described in the entry on Tablets. Available as tablets containing 75 mg of thiacetazone.

A standard for these tablets is given in the British Pharmaceutical Codex 1973

Containers and *Storage:* see the entry on Tablets for general information on containers and storage. Containers should be airtight and light resistant.

Advice for patients: the tablets should be taken at regular intervals. Treatment should not be discontinued without the advice of the prescriber.

Thiambutosine

1-(4-Butoxyphenyl)-3-(4-dimethylaminophenyl)thiourea

$C_{19}H_{25}N_3OS = 343.5$

OTHER NAME: *Ciba 1906®*

A standard is given in the British Pharmacopoeia 1973

Description. An odourless, white or creamy-white, crystalline powder with a bitter taste.

Solubility. Very slightly soluble in water; soluble, at 20°, in 300 parts of ether, and in 1.5 parts of chloroform; soluble in acetone.

Moisture content. Not more than 1%, determined by drying at 60° *in vacuo*.

Storage. It should be stored in airtight containers, protected from light.

Identification. TEST. Dissolve about 100 mg in 40 ml of methyl alcohol and add 40 ml of a saturated solution of picrolonic acid; a precipitate is produced which, after washing with water, methyl alcohol, and ether, melts at about 170°.

MELTING-POINT. About 125°.

ULTRAVIOLET ABSORPTION. In alcohol (95%), maximum at 270 nm (E1%, 1cm = 688).

Determination in body fluids. COLORIMETRY. In urine —G. A. Ellard and R. F. Naylor, *Lepr. Rev.*, 1961, **32**, 249.

Metabolism. ABSORPTION. Poorly absorbed after oral or intramuscular administration; intramuscular doses in arachis oil are better absorbed than aqueous doses.

HALF-LIFE. The half-life, determined from urinary excretion data, is 6 to 7 days for total *p*-dimethylaminodiphenylthioureas.

DISTRIBUTION. In dogs and rabbits, subject to enterohepatic circulation.

METABOLIC REACTIONS. In rabbits ω-oxidation of the butoxyl group to produce *p*-(3-carboxypropoxy)phenyl-*p'*-(dimethylamino)phenylthiourea followed by glucuronic acid conjugation; in man, the butoxyl group is rapidly metabolised to form *p*-dimethylaminodiphenylthioureas; desulphuration, demethylation, and the formation of a metabolite similar to that in the rabbit may also occur in man.

EXCRETION. Up to 75% of a dose is excreted in the urine and faeces with up to 40% appearing in the urine; biliary excretion occurs to a small extent.

FURTHER INFORMATION. Absorption, metabolism, and excretion: after injection—G. A. Ellard, *Lepr. Rev.*, 1966, **37**, 17; after oral administration—G. A. Ellard and R. F. Naylor, *Lepr. Rev.*, 1961, **32**, 249; metabolism in rabbits—R. L. Smith and R. T. Williams, *J. mednl pharm. Chem.*, 1961, **4**, 163.

Actions and uses. Thiambutosine, like dapsone, is given by mouth in the treatment of leprosy, but it causes less reaction than dapsone. It is particularly valuable in dimorphous cases with considerable tissue exacerbation and in tuberculoid cases.

It is used in a dosage of 500 milligrams daily, which is increased when necessary up to a maximum of 2 to 3 grams.

The initial daily dose for children under one year is 12.5 to 20 milligrams per kilogram body-weight, 1 to 5 years 125 to 200 milligrams, and 6 to 12 years 225 to 375 milligrams. Treatment may be continued for up to 2 years, after which time resistance may occur; thereafter dapsone can usually be given.

Thiambutosine has been used in conjunction with sulphones or with isoniazid, but it is more valuable when used alone in patients who react badly to dapsone. It has also proved useful in patients with severe neuritis who are sometimes intolerant of sulphones.

Undesirable effects. Antithyroid actions may occur with high dosage, but this is very rare. Occasional skin eruptions may occur, but usually it is not necessary to discontinue treatment.

Preparation

THIAMBUTOSINE TABLETS: available as tablets containing 500 mg of thiambutosine; they may be coloured.

A standard for these tablets is given in the British Pharmacopoeia 1973

Containers and *Storage:* see the entry on Tablets for general information on containers and storage. Containers should be airtight and light resistant.

Advice for patients: the tablets should be taken at regular intervals; treatment should not be discontinued without the advice of the prescriber.

Thiamine Hydrochloride

3-(4-Amino-2-methylpyrimidin-5-ylmethyl)-5-(2-hy-droxyethyl)-4-methylthiazolium chloride hydrochloride

$C_{12}H_{18}Cl_2N_4OS = 337.3$

OTHER NAMES: Aneurine Hydrochloride; *Benerva®*; Thiaminii Chloridum; Vitamin B_1
Parentrovite® (with other vitamins of the B group and vitamin C)

A standard is given in the European Pharmacopoeia Vol. I

Description. Colourless crystals or a white crystalline powder with a characteristic odour.

Solubility. Soluble, at 20°, in 1 part of water, in 100 parts of alcohol, and in 20 parts of glycerol; soluble in methyl alcohol; very slightly soluble in dehydrated alcohol, in ether, and in acetone.

Acidity. A 2.5% solution has a pH of 2.7 to 3.3.

Moisture content. Not more than 5%, determined by drying at 105°.

Dissociation constant. pK_a 4.8 (20°).

Stability. Solutions of pH 4 or less deteriorate only slowly, but neutral or alkaline solutions deteriorate rapidly, especially on exposure to air.

Sterilisation. Solutions for injection are sterilised by filtration.

Storage. It should be stored in airtight containers, protected from light, contact with metal being avoided.

Identification. TEST. Dissolve about 20 mg in 10 ml of water, add 1 ml of *dilute acetic acid* and 1.6 ml of 1N sodium hydroxide, heat on a water-bath for 30 minutes, cool, add 5 ml of *dilute sodium hydroxide solution*, 10 ml of *potassium ferricyanide solution* and 10 ml of n-butyl alcohol and shake vigorously for 2 minutes; the solvent layer exhibits an intense light blue fluorescence. Repeat the test using 0.9 ml of 1N sodium hydroxide and 200 mg of sodium sulphite instead of 1.6 ml of 1N sodium hydroxide; no fluorescence is produced.

MELTING-POINT. About 207°, with decomposition.

ULTRAVIOLET ABSORPTION. In alcohol (95%), maxima at 233 nm (E1%, 1cm = 380) and 267 nm (E1%, 1cm = 240).

INFRA-RED ABSORPTION. Major peaks at 1048, 1237, 1385, 1483, 1618, and 1660 cm^{-1} (see Appendix 2a: Infra-red Spectra).

Metabolism. ABSORPTION. Well absorbed after oral administration; absorption is retarded in non-fasting subjects.

BLOOD CONCENTRATIONS. Normal blood concentrations are about 10 to 15 ng/ml and concentrations of thiamine pyrophosphate in red blood cells are about 30 to 110 ng/ml.

DISTRIBUTION. Widely distributed throughout the body and secreted in milk.

METABOLIC REACTIONS. Converted to pyrimidine metabolites.

EXCRETION. Quantities in excess of the body's needs are excreted in the urine as unchanged drug and metabolites; excretion varies according to dietary thiamine content; normally 50 to 500 μg is excreted in the urine daily; excretion of less than 50 μg in 24 hours indicates a deficiency state; after an intramuscular dose of 350 μg per m^2 surface area, about 8% is excreted in 4 hours; after an intravenous dose of 1 mg, over 110 μg is excreted in 4 hours and after a similar dose administered orally, over 100 μg is excreted in 24 hours.

FURTHER INFORMATION. Absorption unaffected by a viscous vehicle—R. R. Hewitt and G. Levy, *J. pharm. Sci.*, 1971, **60**, 784.

Actions and uses. Thiamine, in the form of its pyrophosphate (co-carboxylase), is the prosthetic group for the enzymes involved in the decarboxylation of pyruvic and α-ketoglutaric acids. It therefore plays an important part in the intermediary metabolism of carbohydrate. In thiamine deficiency the oxidation of α-ketoacids is impaired and the blood pyruvate rises. Thiamine is devoid of pharmacological activity.

Thiamine is widely distributed in foods, the richest sources being whole grain, pulses, yeast, and pork. It is absorbed mainly from the small intestine, although there is some evidence that bacterial synthesis and absorption occur in the large intestine. Before utilisation, thiamine must be phosphorylated, a process which occurs in all nucleated cells, particularly in the liver, kidney, and white blood cells.

The optimum daily intake for an adult is 0.8 to 1.2 milligrams, for infants 400 micrograms, and for children and adolescents 0.5 to 1.4 milligrams. Requirements are directly related to the carbohydrate intake and metabolic rate and are increased in pregnancy, lactation, hyperthyroidism, pyrexia, exercise, and conditions causing increased metabolism or diuresis.

Thiamine has no therapeutic value apart from the treatment of thiamine deficiency. In beriberi there is a severe deficiency, not only of thiamine but of other factors of the vitamin-B group. Thiamine has been administered for the treatment of neuritis of varying etiology, but evidence of its value is lacking, unless the neuritis is due to thiamine deficiency.

There are a number of diseases in which thiamine deficiency may be caused by interference with its ingestion, absorption, and utilisation or by increasing its destruction or excretion. This is likely to occur, for example, in patients on restricted diets and in those suffering from gastro-intestinal diseases, some forms of mental disease, or alcoholism. Some cases of pregnancy neuritis may be due to thiamine deficiency. It is rational to supplement the diet in such cases not only with thiamine but also with other vitamins.

The prophylactic dose for adults and children is 2 to 5 milligrams daily and the therapeutic dose is 25 to 100 milligrams daily in divided doses. Thiamine is usually given by mouth; parenteral administration is usually unnecessary except for patients with impaired absorption or acute cardiac beriberi, when it may be given by subcutaneous or intramuscular injection.

Undesirable effects. Toxic effects have been produced by injections of 50 milligrams of thiamine hydrochloride. Large doses may also interfere with the metabolism of other vitamins of the vitamin-B group and may precipitate the symptoms of other deficiency states in poorly nourished patients. Except in the initial treatment of acute cardiac beriberi, there is no justification for the administration of single doses in excess of 10 milligrams.

Veterinary uses. Thiamine hydrochloride is used in the

treatment of bracken poisoning in horses, the usual dose by intramuscular or slow intravenous injection being 0.25 to 1.25 milligrams per kilogram body-weight repeated as required. Thiamine hydrochloride has also been used in the treatment of cerebrocortical necrosis in ruminants, the usual dose by intramuscular or slow intravenous injection being 5 to 10 milligrams per kilogram body-weight. A proportion of 1 to 3 parts per million may be added to the feed to prevent or treat thiamine deficiency in susceptible species.

Preparations

COMPOUND VITAMIN B TABLETS (*Syn.* Compound Aneurine Tablets; Compound Thiamine Tablets): for each tablet take:

Nicotinamide	15 mg
Riboflavine	1 mg
Thiamine hydrochloride	1 mg

Mix, and prepare by moist granulation and compression as described in the entry on Tablets.
A *standard for these tablets is given in the British Pharmaceutical Codex 1973*
Containers and *Storage:* see the entry on Tablets for general information on containers and storage. Containers should be airtight and light resistant and the tablets should not be in contact with metal.
Labelling: the label on the container should state the date after which the tablets are not intended to be used.
Dose: prophylactic, 1 or 2 tablets daily.

STRONG COMPOUND VITAMIN B TABLETS (*Syn.* Strong Compound Aneurine Tablets; Strong Compound Thiamine Tablets): for each tablet take:

Nicotinamide	20 mg
Pyridoxine hydrochloride	2 mg
Riboflavine	2 mg
Thiamine hydrochloride	5 mg

Mix, and prepare by moist granulation and compression as described in the entry on Tablets. The tablets may be coated with a chocolate-coloured coating of sugar or other suitable material.
A *standard for these tablets is given in the British Pharmaceutical Codex 1973*
Containers and *Storage:* see the entry on Tablets for general information on containers and storage. Containers should be airtight and light resistant and the tablets should not be in contact with metal.
Labelling: the label on the container should state the date after which the tablets are not intended to be used.
Dose: therapeutic, 1 or 2 tablets 3 times daily.

THIAMINE HYDROCHLORIDE INJECTION (*Syn.* Vitamin B_1 Injection): a sterile solution of thiamine hydrochloride in water for injections. It is sterilised by filtration. Available in 1-ml ampoules containing 25 and 100 mg of thiamine hydrochloride.
A *standard for this injection is given in the British Pharmacopoeia 1973*
Containers and *Labelling:* see the entry on Injections for general information on containers and labelling.
Storage: it should be protected from light.

THIAMINE HYDROCHLORIDE TABLETS (*Syn.* Vitamin B_1 Tablets): available as tablets containing 3, 10, 25, 50, 100, and 300 mg of thiamine hydrochloride.
A *standard for these tablets is given in the British Pharmacopoeia 1973*
Containers and *Storage:* see the entry on Tablets for general information on containers and storage. Containers should be airtight and light resistant and the tablets should not be in contact with metal.

VITAMINS B AND C INJECTION: a sterile solution of thiamine hydrochloride, pyridoxine hydrochloride, riboflavine or the equivalent amount of riboflavine phosphate (sodium salt), nicotinamide, and ascorbic acid (as the sodium salt), with anhydrous dextrose for the intravenous injection, or benzyl alcohol for the intramuscular injection, in water for injections. Stability during storage is achieved by dividing the ingredients between a pair of ampoules, one (number 1) containing the thiamine hydrochloride, the pyridoxine hydrochloride, the riboflavine and, in the intramuscular injections, the benzyl alcohol, and the other (number 2) containing the ascorbic acid, the nicotinamide, and, in the intravenous injection, the anhydrous dextrose. The air in the number 2 ampoule is replaced by nitrogen or other suitable gas.
The number 1 ampoules and the number 2 ampoules for intravenous injection are sterilised by heating in an autoclave. The number 2 ampoules for intramuscular injection are sterilised by heating with a bactericide; 0.2% chlorocresol is suitable. Alternatively, the solutions are sterilised by filtration.
The injection is prepared by mixing, immediately before use, the contents of a pair of ampoules.
When *Strong Vitamins B and C Injection for intravenous use* is ordered or prescribed, a pair of ampoules, one containing 250 mg of thiamine hydrochloride, 50 mg of pyridoxine hydrochloride, and 4 mg of riboflavine or the equivalent amount of riboflavine phosphate (sodium salt) in 5 ml, the other containing 500 mg of ascorbic acid (as the sodium salt), 160 mg of nicotinamide, and 1 g of anhydrous dextrose in 5 ml is supplied. The injection should not be added to intravenous infusion solutions but may be injected directly into the tubing of an intravenous giving set.
When *Strong Vitamins B and C Injection for intramuscular use* is ordered or prescribed, a pair of ampoules, one containing 250 mg of thiamine hydrochloride, 50 mg of pyridoxine hydrochloride, 4 mg of riboflavine or the equivalent amount of riboflavine phosphate (sodium salt), and 0.14 ml of benzyl alcohol in 5 ml, the other containing 500 mg of ascorbic acid (as the sodium salt) and 160 mg of nicotinamide in 2 ml, is supplied.
When *Weak Vitamins B and C Injection for intramuscular use* is ordered or prescribed, a pair of ampoules, one containing 100 mg of thiamine hydrochloride, 50 mg of pyridoxine hydrochloride, 4 mg of riboflavine or the equivalent amount of riboflavine phosphate (sodium salt), and 0.08 ml of benzyl alcohol in 2 ml, the other containing 500 mg of ascorbic acid (as the sodium salt) and 160 mg of nicotinamide in 2 ml is supplied.
A *standard for this injection is given in the British Pharmaceutical Codex 1973*
Containers: see the entry on Injections for general information on containers.
Labelling: see the entry on Injections for general information on labelling. In addition, the label on the container should state whether the injection is for intravenous or intramuscular use.
Storage: it should be stored in a cool place, protected from light.

OTHER PREPARATIONS: thiamine hydrochloride is an ingredient of vitamins capsules.

Thin-layer Chromatography

Thin-layer chromatography is a method of flat-bed chromatography which involves the passage of a solvent (mobile phase) across a uniform layer of a finely divided insoluble adsorbent (stationary phase). When different substances are applied to the adsorbent layer, they migrate across it at different rates with the passage of the solvent and are separated. As an analytical technique it was developed by Stahl in 1958, and it is now recognised as a rapid and extremely sensitive system for the identification of compounds and for the separation and detection of trace amounts of impurities.

Stationary phase. The most common adsorbents used are silica gel, kieselguhr, alumina, cellulose and cellulose derivatives, ion-exchange resins and polyamides. A thin layer of the appropriate adsorbent is supported on a rigid base of glass, plastics, or metal foil, and adherence to the base may be ensured by the inclusion of a binding agent such as calcium sulphate. As an aid to visualisation of the separated compounds, a fluorescence indicator may be mixed with the adsorbent.

The British and European Pharmacopoeias give directions for the spreading of plates extemporaneously, but pre-coated plates are commercially available and are generally to be preferred because they are usually more consistent with regard to physical properties and activity, provided that they have been stored correctly. The activity of a chromatoplate is influenced by the amount of moisture present, and the activity may be increased if necessary by heating the spread plate in an oven, usually at 110° for about 1 hour. During the heating process the plate should be placed in a vertical position. This heating and activation process is not applicable to partition (reverse phase) thin-layer chromatography.

Mobile phase. The choice of mobile phase, which may be a single solvent or a mixture of solvents, will depend on the polarity of the compounds to be separated and on the particular stationary phase which is being used. Information can often be obtained from the literature, but practical experience is of great benefit in the final choice.

Method. A development chamber or tank is prepared by placing sufficient of the mobile phase in it to produce a depth of 5 to 10 mm after which the chamber is sealed to establish vapour saturation (equilibration). In order to facilitate this process, the tank is usually lined with filter paper which dips into the mobile phase. Equilibration is usually established in one hour.

A volume of a solution, normally containing up to 10 μg of the substance under investigation in 1 to 20 μl of a suitable solvent, is applied to the stationary phase as a closely confined spot, preferably less than 5 mm in diameter and about 20 mm from the bottom edge of the chromatoplate. When several solutions of substances are applied to the same chromatoplate, the spots should be on a line, parallel to the bottom of the chromatoplate and usually at least 20 mm apart, although in some micro-methods this distance may be less. The solutions are applied with a micro-pipette (a melting-point capillary tube, drawn out at one end to a tip, is adequate for qualitative work), and are allowed to dry, either naturally or in a current of warm air from a blower. This latter method is necessary in order to maintain a minimal spot diameter if the larger volumes of solution are applied to the chromatoplate.

A line is scored across the chromatoplate, or a suitable mark is made, at an appropriate distance (usually 150 mm) from, and parallel to, the line of application, to indicate the extent to which the mobile phase should run. The chromatoplate is then placed vertically in the tank, ensuring that the line of application is above the solvent level. The tank is then sealed and allowed to stand, preferably in a constant temperature atmosphere, until

the solvent has travelled up the Plate to the predetermined level. The chromatoplate is then removed from the tank and the solvent allowed to evaporate, either in the air or under prescribed conditions of warming.

After drying, the separated components are visualised on the chromatoplate by the use of a suitable spray reagent. If the coating of the plate contains a fluorescence indicator, screened ultraviolet radiation (254 or 366 nm) may be used in addition to spraying for the detection of compounds; the former wavelength is used for compounds which quench the fluorescence of the indicator, and the latter wavelength for those compounds which fluoresce or can be induced to fluoresce. The use of fluorescence as a means of detection has the advantage that it is non-destructive.

The components of a mixture may not be completely separated by a single application of the above method and it may be advantageous, with some substances, to apply a "double-run" procedure. In this procedure the chromatoplate, after drying at the end of the first run, may be re-run either (a) in the same direction with the same mobile phase, or (b) at right-angles to the first run with the same or with a different mobile phase.

Evaluation. The movement of a compound across the chromatoplate can be expressed as an Rf (relative to front) value,

$$\text{where,} \quad \text{Rf} = \frac{\text{distance moved by compound}}{\text{distance moved by solvent front}}$$

This value is less than 1, and hence the value h.Rf ($= 100$ Rf) is often used in order to preclude the use of decimal fractions.

Rf values are affected by a number of factors (see below) and precisely controlled conditions are necessary in order to achieve reproducibility. For purposes of identification it is necessary to run a reference standard on the same chromatoplate as the sample. Preferably, the reference standard should be an authentic specimen of the compound. However, such specimens may not be readily available and the concept of relative Rf values may be used as an alternative.

When two compounds are run on the same chromatoplate, each will have its own Rf value, and if one of them (compound 1) is regarded as a standard or marker, the other (compound 2) can be assigned a relative Rf value (RRf),

$$\text{where,} \quad \text{RRf} = \frac{\text{Rf value of compound 2}}{\text{Rf value of compound 1}}$$

The relative Rf value is independent of the distance moved by the solvent front.

Suitable substances, as standards or markers, may be used in this way to determine RRf values for all the members of a chemically related group of compounds without reference to individual authentic specimens. Two or three markers suffice and these do not, necessarily, need to be related chemically to the compounds under investigation. A solution of mixed dyes can be used for this purpose.

Factors which Affect the Rf Value

The following are the most important factors which affect Rf values and which should be carefully controlled in order to achieve reproducibility.

STATIONARY PHASE. (1) The quality of the adsorbent, including batch variations and the presence or absence of impurities.

(2) The presence or absence of a binder, which may itself have adsorbent properties.

(3) The nature of the chromatoplate, including the evenness and thickness of the coating, and whether prepared extemporaneously or pre-coated.
(4) The degree of activation, which depends on pretreatment and storage.

MOBILE PHASE. (1) The composition and nature of the mobile phase, which is varied to achieve the correct polarity for the particular compound and chromatoplate.
(2) The degree of vapour saturation of the tank. Lack of equilibration usually results in the spots at the edge of the plate running faster than those in the middle of the plate, and also faster than those run in a saturated system.

TEMPERATURE. Precise control of temperature is not usually required because of the relatively short running times. However, large changes in temperature will significantly affect the running time. In general, the tank should be kept away from draughts and sources of heat, and out of direct sunlight.

TANK DIMENSIONS. The size of the tank is important, especially when mixed solvents are used as the mobile phase.

DEVELOPMENT DISTANCE. The normal practice is to allow the solvent front to move a distance of 150 mm. Variations in this distance will affect the distance moved by the compound.

WEIGHT LOADED ON TO THE CHROMATOPLATE. Loadings which are higher than normal give rise to lower Rf values and are usually accompanied by tailing of the spots.

Types of Thin-layer Chromatography

ADSORPTION THIN-LAYER CHROMATOGRAPHY. This is the most common physical process and depends on a surface activity phenomenon. As the mobile phase progresses up the stationary phase, both the solvent and the sample compete for the active adsorption sites on the surface. In the upper part of the plate there are fewer active sites due to adsorption of vapour and hence, for effective separation, overloading must be avoided.
The degree of adsorption is related to hydroxylation and hydrogen bonding effects, and varies according to the chemistry of samples and adsorbent. An example is the hydrogen bonding of silanol groups in silica gel with polar groups of adsorbed alkaloid molecules. Another important factor is acid-base interaction as, for instance, between silica gel and alkaloid molecules.

PARTITION OR REVERSE PHASE THIN-LAYER CHROMATOGRAPHY. This is an adaptation in which a liquid stationary phase (sometimes known as the impregnation liquid) is supported on the adsorbent layer. Buffer solutions are frequently employed and an immiscible solvent is used as the mobile phase. Partition chromatography using cellulose as the adsorbent is analagous to paper chromatography.

ION-EXCHANGE THIN-LAYER CHROMATOGRAPHY. This employs ion-exchangers such as DEAE-cellulose (diethylaminoethyl cellulose), ECTEOLA-cellulose (reaction product of epichlorhydrin, triethanolamine and alkali cellulose), and CM-cellulose (carboxymethylcellulose), or ion-exchange resins.

GEL THIN-LAYER CHROMATOGRAPHY. This uses a layer of *Sephadex*® (Pharmacia, Uppsala, Sweden), a cross-linked dextran which functions as a molecular sieve. The technique is useful for separating compounds of high molecular weight.

Thin-layer Chromatographic Systems

A number of thin-layer chromatographic systems suitable for use in the identification of specified drug substances are described below. The substances are divided into either chemical or pharmacological groups, and for each group appropriate systems are described. A general system (System 1), which can be used for all the substances, is also described. Rf values for System 1 are given alongside those for the specific systems for each group, for comparison purposes.
The Rf values which are quoted have been determined using the stated conditions; in all cases, commercial pre-coated plates were used. However, Rf values are subject to considerable variability and the values quoted are only intended as a guide to the approximate position on the chromatoplate at which a substance can be expected to appear, and as a means of choosing an appropriate system for the separation of the particular substances which are being examined.
For purposes of identification, a suitable reference substance should always be chromatographed on the same plate as the test substance (see under Evaluation, above).

NOTE. In the following tables the letter "s" after an Rf value indicates that streaking may occur.

System 1: General System

STATIONARY PHASE. Silica Gel 60F254, 0.25 mm.

MOBILE PHASE. Methyl alcohol, 100 volumes + *strong ammonia solution*, 1.5 volumes.

SAMPLE SOLUTION; VISUALISATION. For any particular group of substances, the sample solution and the visualisation reagents are the same as are stated for the alternative systems, following.

Rf VALUES. These are given in the tables of Rf values under the alternative systems, following.

System 2: Local Anaesthetics

System 2a: STATIONARY PHASE. Silica Gel 60F254, 0.25 mm, prepared with 0.1N sodium hydroxide.

MOBILE PHASE. Acetone.

SAMPLE SOLUTION. 0.1% in methyl alcohol; 1 and 10 μl applied to the chromatoplate.

VISUALISATION. (1) Examine under ultraviolet radiation, 254 nm. (2) Spray with *acidified iodoplatinate solution*.

System 2b: STATIONARY PHASE. Alumina (Type T) F254, 0.25 mm.

MOBILE PHASE. Chloroform.

SAMPLE SOLUTION; VISUALISATION. As for System 2a.

System 2c: STATIONARY PHASE. Alumina (Type E) F254, 0.25 mm.

MOBILE PHASE. Chloroform.

SAMPLE SOLUTION; VISUALISATION. As for System 2a.

Rf VALUES

| | *System Number* | | | |
	1	*2a*	*2b*	*2c*
Amethocaine Hydrochloride	0.62	0.18	0.24	0.34
Benzocaine	0.72	0.67	0.52	0.41
Cinchocaine Hydrochloride	0.68	0.32	0.14	0.60
Lignocaine Hydrochloride	0.74	0.62	0.51	0.60

	1	2a	2b	2c
Procainamide Hydrochloride	0.49	0.04	0.01	0.07
Procaine Hydrochloride	0.63	0.31	0.09	0.29

System 3: Analgesic and Anti-inflammatory Compounds

STATIONARY PHASE. Silica Gel 60F254, 0.25 mm.

MOBILE PHASES. *System 3a:* benzene, 120 volumes+ ether, 60 volumes+glacial acetic acid, 18 volumes+ methyl alcohol, 1 volume.

System 3b: butyl acetate, 6 volumes+chloroform, 4 volumes+formic acid, 2 volumes.

SAMPLE SOLUTION. 0.1% in alcohol (95%); 1 and 10 μl applied to the chromatoplate.

VISUALISATION. (1) Examine under ultraviolet radiation, 254 nm. (2) Spray with a 1% solution of potassium permanganate.

Rf VALUES

	System Number		
	1	3a	3b
Alclofenac	0.78	0.51	*
Aspirin	0.78	0.51	0.60
Baclofen	0.43 s	0.00	0.05
Benorylate	0.70	0.19	0.45
Fenoprofen Calcium	0.78	0.58	0.86
Flufenamic Acid	0.87	0.70	0.90
Ibuprofen	0.69 s	0.62	0.88
Indomethacin	0.75	0.51	0.78
Ketoprofen	0.74	0.52	0.77
Mefenamic Acid	0.86	0.73	0.92
Naproxen	0.85	0.53	0.81
Oxyphenbutazone	0.89	0.47	0.52
Paracetamol	0.72	0.13	0.34
Pentazocine Hydrochloride	0.63	0.01	0.16
Phenacetin	0.72	0.29	0.30
Phenazone	0.66	0.06	0.18
Phenylbutazone	0.77	0.70	0.91

* not detected

System 4: Antihistamines

STATIONARY PHASE. Silica Gel 60F254, 0.25 mm.

MOBILE PHASES. *System 4a:* benzene, 60 volumes+ dioxan, 35 volumes+*strong ammonia solution*, 5 volumes.

System 4b: glacial acetic acid, 30 volumes+alcohol (95%), 50 volumes+water, 20 volumes.

SAMPLE SOLUTION. 0.1% in alcohol (95%); it may be necessary to add water, dropwise, to aid solution; 1 and 10 μl applied to the chromatoplate.

VISUALISATION. (1) Examine under ultraviolet radiation, 254 nm. (2) Spray with *acidified iodoplatinate solution.*

Rf VALUES

	System Number		
	1	4a	4b
Antazoline Mesylate	0.31	0.30	0.72
Chlorpheniramine Maleate	0.45	0.50	0.35
Cyclizine Hydrochloride	0.70	0.69	0.72
Cyproheptadine Hydrochloride	0.66	0.69	0.72
Diphenhydramine Hydrochloride	0.60	0.70	0.69
Diphenylpyraline Hydrochloride	0.53	0.40	0.71
Mepyramine Maleate	0.62	0.48	0.35
Phenindamine Tartrate	0.72	0.54	0.72
Promethazine Hydrochloride	0.59	0.50	0.71
Trimeprazine Tartrate	0.65	0.68	0.70
Triprolidine Hydrochloride	0.53	0.39	0.54

System 5: Barbiturates

STATIONARY PHASE. Silica Gel 60F254, 0.25 mm.

MOBILE PHASES. *System 5a:* chloroform, 9 volumes+ acetone, 1 volume.

System 5b: isopropyl alcohol, 9 volumes+chloroform, 9 volumes+ammonia solution 25% w/w, 2 volumes.

SAMPLE SOLUTION. 0.1% in methyl alcohol; 1 and 10 μl applied to the chromatoplate.

VISUALISATION. (1) Examine under ultraviolet radiation, 254 nm. (2) Spray with *diphenylcarbazone solution,* followed by *mercury nitrate solution,* and then heat at 105° for 15 minutes.

Rf VALUES

	System Number		
	1	5a	5b
Amylobarbitone	0.82	0.28	0.60
Butobarbitone	0.85	0.24	0.57
Cyclobarbitone Calcium	0.85	0.22	0.50
Pentobarbitone Sodium	0.85	0.26	0.63
Phenobarbitone	0.82	0.18	0.32
Phenobarbitone Sodium	0.82	0.17	0.32
Quinalbarbitone	0.83	0.30	0.63

System 6: Diuretics

STATIONARY PHASE. Silica Gel 60F254, 0.25 mm.

MOBILE PHASES. *System 6a:* ethyl acetate, 4 volumes + benzene, 1 volume.

System 6b: ethyl acetate, 100 volumes+water, 1.5 volumes.

SAMPLE SOLUTION. 0.1% in methyl alcohol; 1 and 10 μl applied to the chromatoplate.

VISUALISATION. (1) Examine under ultraviolet radiation, 254 nm. (2) Spray with sulphuric acid (10% v/v), expose to nitrous fumes for 15 minutes, and then spray with an 0.5% solution of N-(1-naphthyl)ethylenediamine hydrochloride.

Rf VALUES

	System Number		
	1	6a	6b
Bendrofluazide	0.87	0.71	0.80
Chlorothiazide	0.88	0.06	0.29
Cyclopenthiazide	0.83	0.58	0.72
Ethacrynic Acid	0.86	0.00	0.02
Hydrochlorothiazide	0.78	0.18	0.47
Hydroflumethiazide	0.79	0.30	0.57

	1	6a	6b
Polythiazide	0.80	0.48	0.66
Spironolactone	0.78	0.48	0.60
Triamterene	0.45	0.00	0.02

System 7: Narcotic Analgesics and Related Substances

STATIONARY PHASE. Silica Gel 60F254, 0.25 mm.

MOBILE PHASES. *System 7a:* toluene, 50 volumes+ dioxan, 40 volumes+*strong ammonia solution*, 5 volumes+methyl alcohol, 5 volumes.

System 7b: alcohol (95%), 60 volumes+glacial acetic acid, 30 volumes+water, 10 volumes.

System 7c: toluene, 16 volumes+ethyl acetate, 4 volumes+diethylamine, 1 volume.

System 7d: methyl alcohol, 50 volumes+acetone, 50 volumes+*strong ammonia solution*, 1 volume.

SAMPLE SOLUTION. 0.1% in methyl alcohol; 1 and 10 µl applied to the chromatoplate.

VISUALISATION. (1) Examine under ultraviolet radiation, 254 nm. (2) Spray with *dilute potassium iodobismuthate solution*.

Rf VALUES

	System Number				
	1	7a	7b	7c	7d
Codeine Phosphate	0.35	0.28	0.24 s	0.14	0.30
Dextromethorphan Hydrobromide	0.29	0.52	0.43 s	0.39	0.20
Dextropropoxyphene Hydrochloride	0.72	0.72	0.67 s	0.60	0.68
Diamorphine Hydrochloride	0.47	0.40 s	0.28 s	0.32	0.40
Ethylmorphine Hydrochloride	0.37	0.28	0.27 s	0.15	0.30
Levallorphan Tartrate	0.68	0.60	0.75 s	0.31	0.65
Methadone Hydrochloride	0.58	0.70	0.62 s	0.61	0.48
Morphine Hydrochloride	0.52	0.10	0.30 s	0.02	0.30
Morphine Sulphate	0.38	0.10	0.29 s	0.02	0.30
Nalorphine Hydrobromide	0.68	0.15	0.55	0.02	0.71
Noscapine Hydrochloride	0.72	0.59	0.50	0.49	0.82
Papaverine Hydrochloride	0.72	0.50	0.40	0.32	0.79
Pethidine Hydrochloride	0.53	0.50	0.50	0.35	0.45
Phenazocine Hydrobromide	0.72	0.57	0.85	0.24	0.75
Pholcodine	0.32	0.15	0.05 s	0.07	0.25

System 8: Parasympatholytic Agents

STATIONARY PHASE. Silica Gel 60F254, 0.25 mm.

MOBILE PHASES. *System 8a:* chloroform, 5 volumes+ acetone, 4 volumes+diethylamine, 1 volume.

System 8b: n-butyl alcohol, 4 volumes+glacial acetic acid, 1 volume+water, 5 volumes.

SAMPLE SOLUTION. 0.1% in alcohol (95%); it may be necessary to add water, dropwise, to aid solution; 1 and 10 µl applied to the chromatoplate.

VISUALISATION. (1) Examine under ultraviolet radiation, 254 nm. (2) Spray with *acidified iodoplatinate solution*.

Rf VALUES

	System Number		
	1	8a	8b
Atropine Methonitrate	0.00	0.00	0.21
Atropine Sulphate	0.17	0.30	0.28
Benzhexol Hydrochloride	0.70	0.81	0.53
Benztropine Mesylate	0.12	0.48	0.42
Cyclopentolate Hydrochloride	0.67	0.72	0.33
Dicyclomine Hydrochloride	0.74	0.81	0.45
Homatropine Hydrobromide	0.18 s	0.33	0.25
Hyoscine Hydrobromide	0.62	0.50	0.25
Orphenadrine Citrate	0.58	0.65	0.38
Oxyphencyclimine Hydrochloride	0.02	0.19	0.32
Procyclidine Hydrochloride	0.51	0.72	0.43
Propantheline Bromide	0.01	0.01	0.26

System 9: Phenothiazines

System 9a: STATIONARY PHASE. Kieselguhr F254, 0.25 mm, impregnated with a mixture containing phenoxyethanol, 10 volumes+macrogol 400, 5 volumes+ acetone, 85 volumes.

MOBILE PHASE. Light petroleum (boiling-range 40° to 60°), 100 volumes+diethylamine, 2 volumes+phenoxyethanol, 8 volumes.

SAMPLE SOLUTION. 0.1% in chloroform; 1 and 10 µl applied to the chromatoplate.

VISUALISATION. (1) Spray with a 10% v/v solution of sulphuric acid in alcohol (95%). (2) Examine under ultraviolet radiation, 366 nm (see table of colours, below).

System 9b: STATIONARY PHASE. Kieselguhr F254, 0.25 mm, impregnated with a mixture containing phenoxyethanol, 2.5 volumes+formamide, 7.5 volumes+ acetone, 90 volumes.

MOBILE PHASE; SAMPLE SOLUTION; VISUALISATION. As for System 9a.

System 9c: STATIONARY PHASE. Silica Gel 60F254, 0.25 mm.

MOBILE PHASE. Benzene, 50 volumes+acetone, 10 volumes+*strong ammonia solution*, 5 volumes.

SAMPLE SOLUTION; VISUALISATION. As for System 9a.

Rf VALUES

	System Number		
	1	9a	9b	9c
Chlorpromazine Hydrochloride	0.52	0.72	1.00	0.74
Fluphenazine Hydrochloride	0.77	0.10	0.66 s	0.20
Perphenazine	0.71	0.03	0.38 s	0.14
Promethazine Hydrochloride	0.61	0.57	1.00	0.48
Thioridazine Hydrochloride	0.53	0.32	1.00	0.48
Trimeprazine Tartrate	0.62	0.82	1.00	0.58

TABLE 1. Rf Values for Steroids

	1	10a	10b	10c	10d	10e	10f	10g
				SystemNumber				
Alphadolone Acetate	0.89	0.99	0.80	0.89	0.45 s	0.05 s	0.59	0.22
Alphaxalone	0.86	0.99	0.90	0.90	0.72 s	0.05 s	0.60	0.22
Beclomethasone Dipropionate	0.90	0.99	0.89	0.90	0.42 s	0.01	0.75	0.38
Betamethasone	0.82	0.55	0.00	0.00	0.00	0.00	0.30	0.00
Betamethasone Sodium Phosphate	0.48	0.00	0.00	0.00	0.00	0.00	0.00	0.00
Betamethasone Valerate	0.90	0.98	0.20	0.15 s	0.02 s	0.00	0.58	0.27
Chlorotrianisene	0.90	0.98	0.98	0.98	0.92	0.99	0.88	0.77
Cortisone Acetate	0.78	0.96	0.55	0.00	0.00	0.00	0.72	0.28
Deoxycortone Acetate	0.75	1.0	0.98	0.98	0.95	0.45 s	0.86	0.52
Dexamethasone	0.71	0.60	0.00	0.00	0.00	0.00	0.32	0.08
Dienoestrol	0.75	0.85	0.34	0.30	0.05 s	0.00	0.72	0.25
Dimethisterone	0.76	0.99	0.91	0.91	0.95	0.55 s	0.80	0.42
Dydrogesterone	0.74	1.0	0.96	0.98	0.98	0.45 s	0.86	0.53
Ethinyloestradiol	0.73	0.87	0.40	0.31	0.40 s	0.07	0.72	0.30
Ethisterone	0.73	1.0	0.80	0.79	0.00	0.00	0.78	0.39
Ethyloestrenol	0.81	0.00	0.94	0.98	0.99	0.99	0.79	0.50
Ethynodiol Diacetate	0.80	0.98	0.95	0.98	0.99	0.99	0.83	0.61
Fludrocortisone Acetate	0.80	0.96	0.30	0.00	0.00	0.00	0.58	0.12
Fluocinolone Acetonide	0.78	0.92	0.10	0.22	0.01	0.00	0.42	0.08
Fluocortolone Hexanoate	0.81	0.99	0.88	0.90 s	0.00	0.00	0.79	0.39
Fluocortolone Pivalate	0.82	0.99	0.89	0.91	0.58	0.10	0.78	0.35
Fluoxymesterone	0.78	0.94	0.38	0.32	0.16 s	0.02	0.51	0.09
Hydrocortisone	0.76	0.57	0.08	0.25	0.00	0.00	0.27	0.02
Hydrocortisone Acetate	0.78	0.92	0.38	0.46	0.00	0.00	0.51	0.11
Hydrocortisone Hydrogen Succinate	0.79	0.05	0.00	0.00	0.00	0.00	0.08	0.00
Hydrocortisone Sodium Phosphate	0.35 s	0.00	0.00	0.00	0.00	0.00	0.00	0.00
Hydroxyprogesterone Hexanoate	0.80	1.0	0.99	0.99	0.90	0.31 s	0.81	0.55
Lynoestrenol	0.79	1.0	0.99	0.97	0.97	0.89	0.77	0.55
Medroxyprogesterone Acetate	0.78	1.0	0.98	0.98	0.85 s	0.35 s	0.80	0.50
Megestrol Acetate	0.77	1.0	0.98	0.98	0.85 s	0.46 s	0.80	0.50
Mestranol	0.82	0.98	0.90	0.90	0.90	0.72	0.86	0.52
Methallenoestril	0.84	0.90	0.70	0.68	0.54 s	0.11 s	0.79	0.18
Methandienone	0.80	0.98	0.87	0.81	0.61	0.20 s	0.65	0.10
Methylprednisolone	0.80	0.56	0.03	0.05 s	0.00	0.00	0.23	0.80
Methyltestosterone	0.81	1.0	0.91	0.90	0.71	0.25 s	0.70	0.16
Nandrolone Decanoate	0.85	1.0	0.97	0.99	0.95	0.69 s	0.88	0.49
Nandrolone Phenylpropionate	0.85	1.0	0.97	0.99	0.95	0.62 s	0.87	0.48
Norethandrolone	0.82	1.0	0.95	0.89	0.78	0.35 s	0.71	0.20
Norethisterone	0.82	1.0	0.87	0.78	0.63 s	0.20 s	0.71	0.22
Norethisterone Acetate	0.85	1.0	0.98	0.96	0.90	0.47 s	0.87	0.39
Norethynodrel	0.85	1.0	0.91	0.82	0.71	0.27 s	0.79	0.32
Oestradiol Benzoate	0.86	1.0	0.96	0.95	0.79	0.30 s	0.79	0.32
Oxymetholone	0.86	1.0	0.85	0.76	0.82	0.50 s	0.69	0.23
Prednisolone	0.81	0.56	0.02 s	0.03 s	0.00	0.00	0.20	0.00
Prednisolone Pivalate	0.87	0.98	0.44	0.56	0.00	0.00	0.69	0.04
Prednisolone Sodium Phosphate	0.46 s	0.00	0.00	0.00	0.00	0.00	0.00	0.00
Prednisone	0.81	0.74	0.10	0.25 s	0.00	0.00	0.41	0.00
Progesterone	0.75	0.95	0.99	0.98	0.95	0.82	0.81	0.20
Stanolone	0.76	0.98	0.90	0.91	0.72	0.60 s	0.78	0.11
Stilboestrol	0.77	0.79	0.18 s	0.38 s	0.03	0.00	0.65 s	0.10 s
Testosterone	0.74	0.98	0.90	0.86	0.63	0.24 s	0.60	0.07
Testosterone Phenylpropionate	0.78	0.99	0.99	0.97	0.98	0.91	0.86	0.28
Testosterone Propionate	0.83	0.99	0.99	0.99	0.98	0.92	0.78	0.12
Triamcinolone	0.70	0.18	0.00	0.00	0.00	0.00	0.09	0.00
Triamcinolone Acetonide	0.80	0.88	0.20	0.30 s	0.06	0.00	0.32	0.00

Colours for Phenothiazines

Substance	Colour after spraying	Fluorescence (366 nm) after spraying
Chlorpromazine Hydrochloride	purple	green-blue
Fluphenazine Hydrochloride	yellow-orange	—
Perphenazine	purple	green-blue
Promethazine Hydrochloride	purple	blue
Thioridazine Hydrochloride	blue	blue
Trimeprazine Tartrate	purple	blue

System 10: Steroids

Systems 10a and 10b: STATIONARY PHASE. Kieselguhr F254 impregnated with a mixture containing acetone, 9 volumes+formamide, 1 volume.

MOBILE PHASES. *System 10a:* chloroform.

System 10b: toluene, 3 volumes+chloroform, 1 volume.

SAMPLE SOLUTION. 0.1% in methyl alcohol; 1 and 10 μl applied to the chromatoplate.

VISUALISATION. (1) Examine under ultraviolet radiation, 254 nm. (2) Spray with a 10% solution of sulphuric acid in alcohol (95%) and heat the chromatoplate for 10 minutes at 105°. (3) Examine under ultraviolet radiation, 366 nm.

Systems 10c, 10d, and 10e: STATIONARY PHASE. Kieselguhr F254 impregnated with a mixture containing acetone, 9 volumes+propylene glycol, 1 volume.

MOBILE PHASES. *System 10c:* toluene.

System 10d: cyclohexane, 1 volume+toluene, 1 volume.

System 10e: cyclohexane, 1 volume+petroleum ether (boiling-range 40°/60°), 1 volume.

SAMPLE SOLUTION; VISUALISATION. As for Systems 10a and 10b.

Systems 10f and 10g: STATIONARY PHASE. Silica Gel 60F254.

MOBILE PHASES. *System 10f:* dichloromethane, 77 volumes+ether, 15 volumes+methyl alcohol, 8 volumes +water, 1.2 volumes.

System 10g: ethylene chloride, 95 volumes+methyl alcohol, 5 volumes+water, 0.2 volume.

SAMPLE SOLUTION; VISUALISATION. As for Systems 10a and 10b.

Rf VALUES. See p. 939.

System 11: Sulphonamides

STATIONARY PHASE. Silica Gel 60F254, 0.25 mm.

MOBILE PHASES. *System 11a:* chloroform, 4 volumes+methyl alcohol 1 volume.

System 11b: ethyl acetate, 9 volumes+methyl alcohol, 1 volume.

System 11c: acetone, 9 volumes+methyl alcohol, 1 volume.

SAMPLE SOLUTION. 1% in 0.1N sodium hydroxide; 1 and 10 μl applied to the chromatoplate.

VISUALISATION. (1) Examine under ultraviolet radiation, 254 nm. (2) Spray with a 1% solution of p-dimethyl-aminobenzaldehyde in a mixture of 90 volumes of alcohol (95%) and 10 volumes of hydrochloric acid. N-Substituted compounds may be detected by spraying with a 5% solution of copper sulphate.

Rf VALUES

	System Number			
	1	11a	11b	11c
Phthalylsulphathiazole	0.80	0.04	0.02	0.32
Succinylsulphathiazole	0.82	0.00	0.02	0.18 s
Sulphacetamide Sodium	0.81	0.10	0.44	0.62
Sulphadiazine	0.74	0.45	0.62 s	0.76
Sulphadimethoxine	0.80	0.63	0.77	0.82
Sulphadimidine	0.84	0.62	0.74	0.79
Sulphadimidine Sodium	0.84	0.62	0.74	0.79
Sulphaguanidine	0.73	0.28	0.33	0.78
Sulphamethizole	0.88	0.13	0.50	0.64 s
Sulphamethoxazole	0.89	0.42	0.79	0.82
Sulphamethoxydiazine	0.78	0.55	0.52	0.78
Sulphamethoxypyridazine	0.80	0.57	0.52	0.75
Sulphanilamide	0.70 s	0.45	0.57	0.77 s
Sulphapyridine	0.74	0.61	0.69	0.82
Sulphathiazole	0.80	0.42	0.58	0.80

System 12: Xanthines

STATIONARY PHASE. Silica Gel 60F254, 0.25 mm.

MOBILE PHASES. *System 12a:* chloroform, 9 volumes+alcohol (95%), 1 volume.

System 12b: chloroform, 8 volumes+carbon tetrachloride, 5 volumes+methyl alcohol, 1 volume.

SAMPLE SOLUTION. 0.1% in alcohol (95%), except for theobromine which is dissolved in *dilute sulphuric acid*; 1 and 10 μl applied to the chromatoplate.

VISUALISATION. (1) Examine under ultraviolet radiation, 254 nm. (2) Spray with a solution prepared by mixing 2 volumes of *iodine solution* with 1 volume of alcohol (95%) and 1 volume of a 25% w/w solution of hydrochloric acid.

Rf VALUES

	System Number		
	1	12a	12b
Aminophylline	0.78	0.36	0.25
Caffeine	0.60	0.49	0.38
Choline Theophyllinate	0.78	0.36	0.25
Theobromine	0.54	0.00	0.19
Theophylline	0.78	0.36	0.25

Thiomersal

The sodium salt of (2-carboxyphenylthio)ethylmercury.

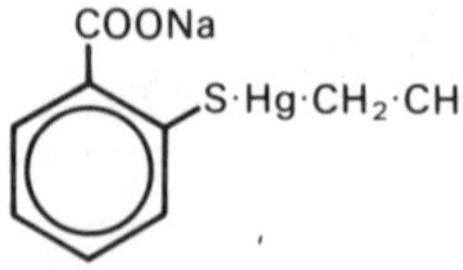

$C_9H_9HgNaO_2S = 404.8$

OTHER NAMES: *Merthiolate*®; Thimerosal; Thiomersalate

A standard is given in the British Pharmacopoeia 1973

Description. A light, cream-coloured, crystalline powder with a slight characteristic odour.

Solubility. Soluble, at 20°, in 1 part of water and in 8 parts of alcohol; very slightly soluble in ether.

Acidity or alkalinity. A 1% solution has a pH of 6 to 8.

Incompatibility. It is incompatible with acids, salts of heavy metals, and iodine, and it forms precipitates with many alkaloids.

The rate of oxidation of thiomersal in solution is greatly increased when traces of copper ions are present. In slightly acid solutions thiomersal is converted to *o*-(ethylmercurithio)benzoic acid which is soluble in about 3500 parts of water and so may be precipitated; solutions of the free acid undergo slow decomposition with the formation of insoluble products.

Sterilisation. Solutions are sterilised by heating in an autoclave or by filtration.

Storage. It should be protected from light.

Preparation and storage of solutions. See statement on aqueous solutions of antiseptics, in the entry on Solutions.

Identification. TESTS. 1. Dissolve about 100 mg in 10 ml of water and add 2 ml of *silver nitrate solution*; a white precipitate is produced.
2. Dissolve about 500 mg in 10 ml of water and add 2 ml of *dilute hydrochloric acid*; a white precipitate is produced which, after washing with water and drying over phosphorus pentoxide *in vacuo*, melts at about 110°.

Actions and uses. Thiomersal has an antibacterial action on some non-sporing organisms; it is also a fungicide. A 0.1% solution is used for the pre-operative sterilisation of the skin. A cream containing 0.1% is applied in mycotic infections of the skin.

Thiomersal is also used as a preservative in biological products, usually in a concentration of 0.01 to 0.02%. A concentration of 0.01% is also used as a preservative in certain eye-drops.

Preparations

Preparations available include a TINCTURE containing thiomersal 0.1%.

Thiopentone Sodium

A mixture of 6 parts of dried sodium carbonate and 100 parts of sodium 5-ethyl-5-(1-methylbutyl)-2-thiobarbiturate. The presence of sodium carbonate prevents the precipitation of free acid by atmospheric carbon dioxide.

$C_{11}H_{17}N_2NaO_2S = 264.3$

OTHER NAMES: *Intraval Sodium*®; *Pentothal*®; Soluble Thiopentone; Thiopent. Sod.; *Thiopentalum Natricum*

A standard is given in the European Pharmacopoeia Vol. II

Description. A hygroscopic yellowish-white powder with a characteristic alliaceous odour and a bitter taste.

Solubility. Soluble, at 20°, in 1.5 parts of water; partly soluble in alcohol; practically insoluble in ether.

Moisture content. Not more than 2.5%, determined by drying at 100° *in vacuo*.

Dissociation constant. pK_a 7.6 (20°).

Stability. Aqueous solutions decompose on keeping and solutions should not be used if they have become cloudy or a precipitate or crystals have formed. They may usually be stored for up to 24 hours without undue decomposition when the solvent is water and in the presence of sodium chloride but stability is reduced in the presence of dextrose and such a solution should be made immediately before use. See also under Barbiturates.

Incompatibility. See under Barbiturates.

Sterilisation. Sterile solutions of thiopentone sodium are prepared from sterile powder, by means of an aseptic technique. See also under Barbiturates.

Storage. It should be stored in airtight containers.

Identification. TESTS. 1. Dissolve about 250 mg in 5 ml of water, make acid with *dilute acetic acid*, filter, wash the filter with water, recrystallise the residue from water, and dry at 70°. The residue gives general test 1 described under Barbiturates.
2. Dissolve about 1 mg in 1 ml of 0.1N sodium hydroxide, add 1 mg of sodium nitroprusside, allow to stand for 15 minutes, and add 1 ml of *dilute hydrochloric acid*; a reddish-violet colour develops.

MELTING-POINT. The residue obtained in Test 1, above, melts at about 160°.

ULTRAVIOLET ABSORPTION. See under Barbiturates.

Determination in body fluids. See under Barbiturates.

Metabolism. (See also under Barbiturates). ABSORPTION. Thiopentone is administered by injection.

BLOOD CONCENTRATION. After an intravenous dose of 400 mg of thiopentone, plasma concentrations of about 25 μg/ml are attained within 5 minutes, falling to 5 μg/ml within 30 minutes.

HALF-LIFE. The plasma elimination half-life is 4 to 8 hours.

DISTRIBUTION. Brain concentrations of thiopentone reach about 10% of the dose within 1 minute and it is then rapidly distributed throughout the body, eventually accumulating in body fat; about 50% of a dose accumulates in this way after 30 to 90 minutes; the very short action of thiopentone is due to the brief α-phase half-life and the redistribution of the drug from the brain to other tissues. Thiopentone readily crosses the placental barrier; *protein binding*, about 70% bound to plasma albumin.

METABOLIC REACTIONS. ω-Hydroxylation, further oxidation, and some desulphuration; in animals, some ring fission.

EXCRETION. Only about 0.3% of a dose is excreted in the urine unchanged; after a dose of 2 to 4 g, 10 to 25% of the dose is excreted in the urine as 5-(3-carboxy-1-methylpropyl)-5-ethyl-2-thiobarbituric acid in 48 hours.

FURTHER INFORMATION. Effect of hepatic metabolism and injection site blood flow on uptake and distribution —L. J. Saidman and E. I. Eger, *Clin. Pharmac. Ther.*, 1973, **14**, 12.

Actions and uses. Thiopentone sodium is a very-short-acting thiobarbiturate, the actions and uses of which are described under Barbiturates. It is administered intravenously for the induction of general anaesthesia or for the production of complete anaesthesia of short duration. It is most useful for short operations, especially when inhalation anaesthetics are not available or are contra-indicated. In dental practice, it may be used for short easy extractions.

For inducing anaesthesia, 100 to 150 milligrams, as a 2.5 or, occasionally, 5% solution, is injected over 10 to 15 seconds; if relaxation has not occurred in about 30 seconds, a further 100 to 150 milligrams may be given. Injection should be given with the patient in the recumbent position and care should be taken to see that none of the solution is injected outside the vein, as it may cause tissue necrosis. For longer procedures, repeated or continuous administration may be used.

It may be administered by rectum as a basal anaesthetic in a dose of 40 milligrams per kilogram body-weight, with a maximum of 2 grams, dissolved in about 30 millilitres of purified water.

When used in pregnancy moderate doses of thiopentone sodium do not usually cause foetal depression.

Precautions and contra-indications. See under Barbiturates. Thiopentone should not be used in patients with impaired liver function or low blood pressure. The chief danger arising during anaesthesia with thiopentone is respiratory depression and means for treating respiratory failure should be at hand.

Veterinary uses. Thiopentone sodium is used as a general anaesthetic. The usual dose by intravenous injection for horses, cattle, sheep, and pigs is 10 to 15 milligrams per kilogram body-weight, for calves 15 to 20 milligrams per kilogram body-weight, and for dogs and cats 20 to 25 milligrams per kilogram body-weight.

Preparations

THIOPENTONE INJECTION: a sterile solution of thiopentone sodium in water for injections. It is prepared by dissolving the contents of a sealed container in water for injections shortly before use. Available as a powder in ampoules containing 0.5 and 1 g, and in bottles containing 2.5 and 5 g of thiopentone sodium.

A standard for this injection is given in the British Pharmacopoeia 1973
Containers and *Labelling:* see the entry on Injections for general information on containers and labelling.
Storage: the injection contains no bactericide and should be used as soon as possible after preparation but solutions of thiopentone sodium may be expected to retain their potency for up to 24 hours after preparation, provided they are stored at 2° to 10°.

Thioridazine Hydrochloride

10-[2-(1-Methylpiperid-2-yl)ethyl]-2-methylthiophenothiazine hydrochloride

$C_{21}H_{27}ClN_2S_2 = 407.0$

OTHER NAME: *Melleril*®

A standard is given in the British Pharmacopoeia 1973

Description. A white or cream-coloured crystalline powder with a slight odour and a very bitter taste.

Solubility. Soluble, at 20°, in 9 parts of water, in 10 parts of alcohol, and in 1.5 parts of chloroform; very slightly soluble in ether.

Acidity. A 10% solution has a pH of 3.5 to 4.5.

Dissociation constant. pK_a 9.5 (24°).

Storage. It should be stored in airtight containers, protected from light.

Identification. TESTS. 1. Dissolve about 5 mg in 2 ml of sulphuric acid and allow to stand for 5 minutes; a blue colour is produced.
2. Dissolve about 2 mg in 2 ml of water and add 2 ml of nitric acid; a blue colour and a transient white turbidity are produced.

MELTING-POINT. About 161°.

ULTRAVIOLET ABSORPTION. In 0.1N hydrochloric acid, maxima at 264 nm (E1%, 1cm = 822) and 313 nm (E1%, 1cm = 111); in alcohol (95%), maxima at 267 nm (E1%, 1cm = 925) and 313 nm (E1%, 1cm = 110).

INFRA-RED ABSORPTION. Major peaks at 754, 796, 1234, 1248, 1403, and 1455 cm^{-1} (see Appendix 2a: Infra-red Spectra).

THIN-LAYER CHROMATOGRAPHY. See under Thin-layer Chromatography, System 9.

Determination in body fluids. COLORIMETRY. In urine —H. K. Neve, *Acta pharmac. tox.*, 1961, **17**, 404.

ULTRAVIOLET SPECTROPHOTOMETRY. In urine—I. S. Forrest *et al.*, *Am. J. Psychiat.*, 1965, **121**, 1049.

GAS CHROMATOGRAPHY. In plasma: thioridazine and metabolites—E. C. Dinovo *et al.*, *J. pharm. Sci.*, 1976, **65**, 667; F. A. J. Vanderheeren *et al.*, *J. Chromat.*, 1976, **120**, 123.

Actions and uses. Thioridazine has a tranquillising action similar to that described under Chlorpromazine Hydrochloride but it has no therapeutically significant anti-emetic or hypothermic action and does not potentiate the action of anaesthetics.

Thioridazine is used mainly for the treatment of schizophrenia and for the control of mania and agitation. It may be used in the management of anxiety states and in children with behaviour problems. It is ineffective in severely depressed patients.

In severe mental illness the usual initial daily dosage for an adult is up to 600 milligrams of thioridazine hydrochloride by mouth; this is later reduced to a maintenance dosage of 100 to 200 milligrams daily. Dosage should not exceed 800 milligrams daily as otherwise pigmentary retinopathy may occur within 4 to 8 weeks of treatment. In treating children with behaviour problems, the basic dosage is 1 milligram per kilogram body-weight daily in divided doses.

Undesirable effects. The incidence of extrapyramidal side-effects is low. Amenorrhoea, galactorrhoea, hypotension, ventricular arrhythmias and, rarely, oedema, weight gain, blood dyscrasias, and photo-allergic and phototoxic reactions may occur.

Poisoning. As for Chlorpromazine Hydrochloride.

Preparation

THIORIDAZINE TABLETS: available as tablets containing 10, 25, 50, and 100 mg of thioridazine hydrochloride; they are sugar coated.

A standard for these tablets is given in the British Pharmacopoeia 1973

Containers and *Storage:* see the entry on Tablets for general information on containers and storage. Containers should be airtight.

Advice for patients: daily doses should preferably be taken at bedtime. The tablets may cause drowsiness; persons affected should not drive or operate machinery. Alcohol should be avoided.

Thiotepa

Phosphorothioic tri(ethyleneamide) *or* tri(aziridin-1-yl)phosphine sulphide

$C_6H_{12}N_3PS = 189.2$

A standard is given in the British Pharmacopoeia 1973

Description. Fine white crystalline flakes with a faint odour.

Solubility. Soluble, at 20°, in 8 parts of water, in 2 parts of alcohol, and in 2 parts of chloroform.

Moisture content. Not more than 2%, determined by Fischer titration.

Melting-point. About 54°.

Storage. It should be stored in airtight containers, at a temperature between 2° and 10°. At higher temperatures, it polymerises and becomes inactive.

Metabolism. ABSORPTION. Incompletely and variably absorbed after oral administration; intramuscular doses are also variably absorbed.

EXCRETION. Traces of unchanged drug along with tri-ethylenephosphoramide are excreted in the urine.

Actions and uses. Thiotepa, a cytotoxic alkylating agent with actions similar to those of mustine, is believed to act by releasing ethyleneimine radicals which have a marked cytotoxic effect on rapidly dividing cells by inhibiting nucleic acid synthesis. Like other drugs of this type, thiotepa prevents mitosis and damages the chromosomes.

Thiotepa is one of the less toxic alkylating agents and, although it produces destruction of tissues composed of rapidly dividing cells such as the bone marrow, the gastro-intestinal mucosa, and the gonads, cells with a low rate of mitosis are less affected. There is no selective uptake of thiotepa by any organ or tissue and it is rapidly broken down and excreted.

Thiotepa is used for the palliative treatment of widespread malignant disease, particularly carcinoma of the breast and ovary, chronic leukaemia, lymphosarcoma, reticulosarcoma, and Hodgkin's disease. It has also been used for the treatment of advanced malignant disease of the lung, gastro-intestinal tract, and genito-urinary and central nervous systems, although with less benefit. Remissions have been obtained in some cases of malignant melanoma.

Local instillation is sometimes employed to prevent the reaccumulation of fluid in patients with malignant pleural effusions and ascites. For the latter purpose thiotepa is preferred to mustine as it is not vesicant.

Thiotepa has been used in combination with the surgical ablation of malignant tumours to prevent the spread of tumour cells.

Thiotepa may be administered by intramuscular, intravenous, intra-arterial, intrapleural, or intraperitoneal injection, as well as by direct injection into the tumour mass. It can also be introduced directly into body cavities such as the bladder and pericardium. The dose must be adjusted according to the severity of the condition, the size and accessibility of the tumour, and the condition of the patient, and must be carefully controlled by repeated observations of the white-cell count.

As thiotepa can be given by a number of different routes according to the site, type, and grade of tumour, there is a wide range of dosage. For all routes of administration, except intravenous, the initial dose is 200 micrograms per kilogram body-weight daily, continued for 3 to 5 days. The maximum maintenance dose is 200 micrograms per kilogram body-weight every 1 to 3 weeks. It should be controlled by frequent white-cell counts; if the white-cell count is less than 3000 per cubic millimetre or the platelet count under 150000 per cubic millimetre, treatment should be stopped or the dose should be reduced. Half these doses should be employed if thiotepa is given intravenously.

As an adjunct to the surgery of malignant disease, 1 milligram per kilogram body-weight, divided into 3 equal doses, is given on the day of operation and on the first and second post-operative days. A dose of 10 to 60 milligrams may be injected into a tumour mass or, dissolved in 20 to 60 millilitres of fluid, it may be instilled into cavities at weekly intervals.

Undesirable effects. Vomiting, headache, and anorexia may occur. The main toxic effect is depression of the haemopoietic system, particularly of the white cells. Thrombocytopenia with haemorrhagic manifestations may occur.

These toxic effects are not related to the size of the dose and bone-marrow depression is unpredictably variable; for this reason alternative treatment may be preferred.

Precautions. Thiotepa should only be given to patients under close supervision. The blood of all patients receiving thiotepa should be examined weekly or more frequently if necessary.

Preparation

THIOTEPA INJECTION: a sterile solution of thiotepa, with sodium bicarbonate and sodium chloride, in water for injections. It is prepared by dissolving the contents of a sealed container, which includes the sodium bicarbonate and sodium chloride, in water for injections shortly before use. Available as a powder in vials containing 15 mg of thiotepa, 50 mg of sodium bicarbonate, and 80 mg of sodium chloride.

A standard for this injection is given in the British Pharmacopoeia 1973

Containers and *Labelling:* see the entry on Injections for general information on containers and labelling.

Storage: the sealed container should be stored at a temperature between 2° and 10°. The injection contains no bactericide and should be used as soon as possible after preparation, but solutions of thiotepa may be expected to retain their potency for up to 5 days after preparation provided they are stored at a temperature between 2° and 10°. If solid matter separates, the solution should not be used.

Threadworm Infection

see ENTEROBIASIS

Thrombin, Dried Human

A preparation of the enzyme which converts human fibrinogen into fibrin.

A standard is given in the British Pharmacopoeia 1973

Thrombin is obtained from liquid human plasma and may be prepared by precipitation with suitable salts and organic solvents under controlled conditions of pH, ionic strength, and temperature. The prothrombin of the human plasma is converted into thrombin in solution by the addition of a minimum amount of calcium ions and human thromboplastin. The solution is clarified by filtration and dried from the frozen state.

Description. A cream-coloured powder which is readily soluble in saline solution, forming a cloudy, pale yellow solution. It contains not less than 10 clotting doses per mg.

Storage. It should be stored, in an atmosphere of nitrogen, in sterile containers sealed to exclude micro-organisms and moisture, at a temperature below 25°, and protected from light.

Actions and uses. A solution of human thrombin in sodium chloride injection, prepared by means of an aseptic technique, is used in conjunction with human fibrinogen and human fibrin foam. When it is used with human fibrinogen, the strength of solution will depend upon the desired rapidity of clotting; when it is used with human fibrin foam, a solution containing 30 to 50 clotting doses per millilitre is employed. Solutions of human thrombin should never be injected.

The use of dried human thrombin carries the risk of transmitting hepatitis, as explained in the entry on Blood Products.

Thrombocythaemia, Primary

see under MYELOPROLIFERATIVE DISEASES

Thrombocytopenia

Thrombocytopenia is a deficiency of blood platelets which results in haemostatic failure and a prolonged bleeding time. It is characterised by bleeding into the skin with formation of petechiae and ecchymoses; bleeding from the nose, alimentary tract, kidneys, or uterus may also occur.

Thrombocytopenia due to a failure of production of platelets occurs in megaloblastic anaemia, aplastic anaemia, leukaemia, and neoplastic disease of the bone. Thrombocytopenia due to an excessive destruction of platelets may be idiopathic, when it is probably an auto-immune phenomenon, or it may occur after acute infections, as a result of hypersensitivity to drugs, in bone-marrow depression after treatment with immuno-suppressants such as azathioprine, or in certain conditions such as systemic lupus erythematosus.

Idiopathic (primary) thrombocytopenia may be treated with corticosteroids or by splenectomy. Treatment of secondary thrombocytopenia is aimed at the primary cause. In thrombocytopenia associated with surgery, platelets should be infused before and for two days after the operation. In drug hypersensitivity, rigid avoidance of all chemically related drugs is necessary.

Thrombophlebitis

see under VENOUS THROMBOSIS

Thrombosis, Coronary

see MYOCARDIAL INFARCTION

Thrombosis, Venous

see under VENOUS THROMBOSIS

Thrush

see CANDIDIASIS

Thymol

2-Isopropyl-5-methylphenol

$C_{10}H_{14}O = 150.2$

A standard is given in the British Pharmacopoeia 1973

Thymol may be prepared synthetically from piperitone, menthone, or *p*-cymene, or extracted from the volatile oils of *Thymus vulgaris* L., *Monarda punctata* L. (Fam. Labiatae), or *Trachyspermum ammi* (L.) Sprague (Fam. Umbelliferae). Thyme oil yields about 20 to 30% of thymol; the other two oils yield respectively about 60% and about 45 to 55%.

Description. Colourless crystals with a pungent, aromatic, thyme-like odour, and a pungent and aromatic taste.

Solubility. Soluble, at 20°, in 1000 parts of water and in less than 1 part of alcohol, of ether, and of chloroform.

Storage. It should be stored in airtight containers, protected from light.

Preparation and storage of solutions. See the statement on aqueous solutions of antiseptics in the entry on Solutions.

Identification. TESTS. 1. Mix 1 g with 5 ml of a 10% solution of sodium hydroxide and heat in a water-bath; a clear, colourless or pink solution is formed, which becomes darker on standing, and no oily drops separate. Add a few drops of chloroform and agitate the mixture; a violet colour is produced.

2. Dissolve a small amount in 1 ml of glacial acetic acid and add 3 drops of sulphuric acid and 1 drop of nitric acid; a green colour is produced.

3. It sinks in cold water but on heating to 45° it melts and rises to the surface.

Metabolism. BLOOD CONCENTRATION. After an oral dose of 1 g, a peak plasma concentration of about 600 ng/ml is attained in about 2.5 hours.

METABOLIC REACTIONS. Glucuronic acid conjugation.

EXCRETION. Excreted in the urine as unchanged drug and as the glucuronide conjugate.

FURTHER INFORMATION. Gas chromatographic determination—M. W. Noall *et al.*, *Analyt. Biochem.*, 1975, **69**, 10.

Actions and uses. Thymol is an ingredient of deodorant mouth-washes, toothpastes, and gargles. Compound thymol glycerin and similar preparations are used as deodorant mouth-washes and gargles, but are not effective as antiseptics.

Mixed with phenol and camphor, thymol is used in dentistry to prepare cavities and, mixed with zinc oxide, as a protective cap to the dentine prior to filling.

Thymol is added to trichloroethylene and tetrachloroethylene as an antoxidant in a concentration of 0.01%. Thymol is not suitable for use as a preservative because of its low solubility in water.

Preparations

COMPOUND THYMOL GLYCERIN:

Thymol	0.5 g
Glycerol	100 ml
Carmine	0.3 g
Menthol	0.3 g
Sodium metabisulphite	0.35 g
Sodium salicylate	5.2 g
Sodium benzoate	8.0 g
Sodium bicarbonate	10.0 g
Borax..	20.0 g
Methyl salicylate	0.3 ml
Pumilio pine oil	0.5 ml
Dilute ammonia solution..	0.75 ml
Cineole	1.3 ml
Alcohol (90%)	25 ml
Water for preparations	to 1000 ml

Dissolve the salts in 800 ml of the water and add the glycerol; dissolve the menthol, the thymol, the cineole, the methyl salicylate, and the pumilio pine oil in the alcohol, triturate with 25 g of sterilised purified talc or kaolin, add the mixture gradually to the solution of the salts, and filter. Dissolve the carmine by stirring it into the dilute ammonia solution, warm gently to dissipate most of the ammonia, mix the two solutions, add sufficient water to produce the required volume, and mix. In making this preparation the alcohol (90%) may be replaced by industrial methylated spirit diluted so as to be of equivalent alcoholic strength, provided that the law and the statutory regulations governing the use of industrial methylated spirit are observed.

A standard for this glycerin is given in the British Pharmaceutical Codex 1973

Containers and *Labelling:* see the entries on Gargles and Mouth-washes for general information on containers and labelling.

Storage: it should be protected from light.

Advice for patients: when used as a gargle or mouth-wash, it should be diluted with about 3 times its volume of warm water and the diluted solution should be used 3 or 4 times daily as required. It should preferably not be swallowed. Diluted solutions should be used immediately and any unused portion discarded. Prolonged use should be avoided.

MOUTH-WASH SOLUTION-TABLETS (*Syn.* Effervescing Mouth-wash Tablets; Solvellae pro Collutorio): for each solution-tablet take:

Menthol	0.81 mg
Thymol	0.81 mg
Sodium benzoate, in powder	32.4 mg
Tartaric acid, in powder..	259.2 mg
Sodium bicarbonate	324.0 mg
Saccharin	0.65 mg
Amaranth, food grade of commerce	2.62 mg
Eucalyptus oil	0.00296 ml
Lemon oil	0.00296 ml
Alcohol (95%)	a sufficient quantity
Water for preparations	a sufficient quantity

Dissolve the amaranth in a sufficient quantity of a mixture of equal parts of the alcohol and water. Prepare sodium bicarbonate granules by the moist granulation process described in the entry on Tablets, using a sufficient quantity of the amaranth solution as the liquid excipient. Mix the tartaric acid and the saccharin, and prepare granules by the moist granulation process, using the remainder of the amaranth solution as the liquid excipient. Dry the granules, and mix. Dissolve the menthol, the thymol, the eucalyptus oil, and the lemon oil in a sufficient quantity of the alcohol, mix with the dried granules, add the sodium benzoate, and compress.

A standard for these solution-tablets is given in the British Pharmaceutical Codex 1973

Containers and *Storage:* see the entry on Solution-tablets for general information on containers and storage.

Advice for patients: one solution-tablet should be dissolved in a tumblerful of warm water and the solution rinsed around the mouth 3 or 4 times daily as required. It should preferably not be swallowed. Prolonged use should be avoided.

Thymoxamine Hydrochloride

N-2-(4-Acetoxy-2-isopropyl-5-methylphenoxy)ethyl-NN-dimethylammonium chloride

$C_{16}H_{26}ClNO_3 = 315.8$

OTHER NAMES: Moxisylyte Hydrochloride; *Opilon*®

A standard is given in the British Pharmacopoeia Addendum 1975

Description. An odourless white crystalline powder.

Solubility. Soluble, at 20°, in 2.5 parts of water, in 11 parts of alcohol, and in 3 parts of chloroform; practically insoluble in ether and in light petroleum.

Acidity. A 5% solution in water has a pH of 4.5 to 5.5.

Storage. It should be protected from light.

Identification. TEST. Mix about 10 mg with 3 ml of *dilute hydrochloric acid*, boil for 15 minutes, cool, add dropwise sufficient *sodium hydroxide solution* to produce a turbidity, then slowly and with shaking add just sufficient *dilute hydrochloric acid* to redissolve the precipitate and then add 1 ml of *ferric chloride test-solution*; the colour changes to greenish-yellow and a yellow crystalline precipitate is produced.

MELTING-POINT. About 212°.

ULTRAVIOLET ABSORPTION. In 0.1N sulphuric acid, maximum at 275 nm (E1%, 1cm = 70) and an inflection at 280 nm.

INFRA-RED ABSORPTION. Major peaks at 1184, 1212, 1261, 1470, 1504, and 1761 cm^{-1} (see Appendix 2a: Infra-red Spectra).

Metabolism. ABSORPTION. Erratically absorbed after oral administration; buccal absorption of thymoxamine is pH-dependent and is increased at alkaline pH values.

BLOOD CONCENTRATION. After oral doses of 150 to 300 mg of the hydrochloride as capsules, plasma concentrations of up to 60 ng/ml are obtained in 30 to 90 minutes.

METABOLIC REACTIONS Deacetylation.

FURTHER INFORMATION. Influence of pH on absorption through the buccal mucosa—A. G. Arbab and P. Turner, *Br. J. Pharmac.*, 1971, **43**, 479P; blood concentrations by a spectrofluorimetric method—A. G. Arbab and P. Turner, *J. Pharm. Pharmac.*, 1971, **23**, 719; blood concentrations and improvement in specific airways conductance—J. P. Griffin *et al.*, *Lancet*, i/1972, 1288.

Actions and uses. Thymoxamine is an alpha-adrenergic blocking agent which acts by competing with noradrenaline at receptor sites. It causes dilatation of peripheral arterioles and improves the blood supply to the skin. It also has antihistaminic activity.

Thymoxamine is used with variable effectiveness in the treatment of peripheral ischaemia, chilblains, acrocyanosis, and erythrocyanosis; it is also used in the treatment of Raynaud's disease and of Ménière's disease due to vasospasm. It is used to prevent vasospasm during surgery.

Thymoxamine hydrochloride is administered by mouth in tablets, by intravenous or intra-arterial injection as a solution containing the equivalent of 5 or 15 milligrams of thymoxamine base per millilitre, or by intravenous infusion as a solution containing the equivalent of 30 milligrams of thymoxamine base in 500 millilitres of sodium chloride injection. 1.1 milligrams of thymoxamine hydrochloride is approximately equivalent to 1 milligram of thymoxamine base.

The usual dose by mouth is the equivalent of 40 milligrams of thymoxamine 4 times daily, increased, if necessary, to 80 milligrams 4 times daily. The usual dose by intramuscular injection or intravenous infusion is the equivalent of 100 micrograms of thymoxamine per kilogram body-weight daily, and by intra-arterial injection postoperatively into a distal artery, the equivalent of 5 milligrams.

Undesirable effects. Nausea, diarrhoea, headache, and flushing of the skin may occur. Sedation and nasal stuffiness may occur after intravenous administration.

Precautions. It should be given with caution to patients with coronary insufficiency or diabetes and to those being treated with tricyclic antidepressants.

Thymoxamine reduces arterial pressure in hypertensive patients and may potentiate the effects of antihypertensive drugs.

Poisoning. The effect of an excessive dosage of thymoxamine may be reversed by the administration of an intravenous infusion of noradrenaline.

Preparations

THYMOXAMINE TABLETS: available as tablets containing thymoxamine hydrochloride equivalent to 40 mg of thymoxamine; they may be coloured.
A standard for these tablets is given in the British Pharmacopoeia Addendum 1975
Containers and *Storage:* see the entry on Tablets for general information on containers and storage. Containers should be airtight and light resistant.

OTHER PREPARATIONS available include an INJECTION containing thymoxamine hydrochloride equivalent to 5 mg of thymoxamine per ml in 1-ml ampoules, and an injection containing thymoxamine hydrochloride equivalent to 15 mg of thymoxamine per ml in 2-ml ampoules.

Thyroid

The dried, powdered, defatted thyroid gland of the ox, sheep, or pig, diluted with lactose to the required strength. It contains 0.25% of iodine in thyroid combination.

OTHER NAMES: Dry Thyroid: *Thyroid Dellipsoids D 12*®; Thyroid Extract; Thyroid Gland; Thyroideum Siccum *Thyropit*® (with dry extract of pituitary anterior lobe)

A standard is given in the British Pharmacopoeia 1973

The organic iodine compounds present in thyroid occur in combination with protein as thyroglobulins, which are soluble in water. On drying the thyroid gland at a temperature of 40° or below, as much as 70% of the thyroglobulin remains unaltered and is therefore extractable by water.

If drying has been carried out at 100°, or by treatment with alcohol followed by drying at 60°, the thyroglobulins are almost completely denatured and made insoluble, and the product will not comply with the requirements of the British Pharmacopoeia.

Description. *Macroscopical characters:* a cream-coloured amorphous powder with a faint and meat-like odour and taste.

Microscopical characters: numerous highly refractive, smooth, vitreous, angular fragments of the colloid contents of the vesicles, having striated conchoidal surfaces and varying in size from about 10 by 15 μm to 95 by 140 μm; less conspicuous fragments of connective tissue, subcylindrical in shape, slightly undulate and having frayed fibrous ends; occasional irregularly ovoid particles composed of small vesicles adhering together and filled with their colloid contents; a few isolated epithelial cells, often with conspicuous nuclei and sparsely scattered fragments of striated muscle fibre. The colloid particles stain readily with *eosin solution* and with *iodine solution*.

Moisture content. Not more than 7.5%, determined by drying at 105°.

Storage. It should be stored in airtight containers, in a cool place.

Actions and uses. Thyroid has the actions, uses, and undesirable effects described under Thyroxine Sodium but thyroxine sodium is usually preferred since it has consistent hormonal properties.

The usual dose of thyroid is 30 to 250 milligrams daily; approximately 60 milligrams of thyroid is equivalent in therapeutic activity to 100 micrograms of thyroxine sodium.

Preparations

THYROID TABLETS: available as tablets containing 30, 60, and 125 mg of thyroid.

A standard for these tablets is given in the British Pharmacopoeia 1973

Containers and *Storage:* see the entry on Tablets for general information on containers and storage. Containers should be airtight. The tablets should be stored in a cool place.

Advice for patients: the tablets should be taken at regular intervals. Treatment should not be discontinued without the advice of the prescriber.

OTHER PREPARATIONS available include TABLETS containing thyroid 200 mg with pituitary (anterior lobe) dry extract 12 mg.

Thyrotoxicosis

see HYPERTHYROIDISM

Thyroxine Sodium

The sodium salt of 3-[4-(4-hydroxy-3,5-di-iodophenoxy)-3,5-di-iodophenyl]-L-alanine.

$C_{15}H_{10}I_4NNaO_4 = 798.9$

OTHER NAMES: *Eltroxin®*; Levothyroxine Sodium; L-Thyroxine Sodium; Thyroxinum Natricum

A standard is given in the European Pharmacopoeia Vol. III

Description. An odourless, almost white to pale brownish-yellow powder or a fine, slightly coloured, crystalline powder.

Solubility. Soluble, at 20°, in 600 parts of water and in 250 parts of alcohol; very slightly soluble in ether and in chloroform; soluble in solutions of alkali hydroxides.

Moisture content. 6 to 12%, determined by drying at 105°.

Specific rotation. +16° to +20°, determined on a 2% solution in a mixture of 1 volume of 1N hydrochloric acid and 4 volumes of alcohol (95%).

Storage. It should be stored in airtight containers, protected from light.

Identification. TEST. Dissolve about 5 mg in a mixture of 2 ml of alcohol (50%) and 1 drop of hydrochloric acid, add 1 drop of *sodium nitrite solution* and heat to boiling; a yellow colour is produced. Cool the solution and make alkaline by the addition of *dilute ammonia solution*; the colour changes to red.

ULTRAVIOLET ABSORPTION. In 0.1N sodium hydroxide, maximum at 325 nm (E1%, 1cm = 76).

Metabolism. ABSORPTION. Absorbed after oral administration.

BLOOD CONCENTRATION. Normal serum thyroxine concentrations are about 80 to 100 ng/ml.

HALF-LIFE. Serum half-life, 6 to 7 days, which may be increased in pregnancy or myxoedema and decreased in hyperthyroidism.

DISTRIBUTION. Rapidly taken up by the liver; crosses the placenta; insignificant amounts are secreted in the milk; subject to enterohepatic circulation; *protein binding*, almost completely bound to plasma proteins including a specific protein, thyroid binding globulin, which binds about 50 to 65% of the drug in blood.

METABOLIC REACTIONS. De-iodination to liothyronine, the principal active form of thyroxine, further de-iodination to metabolites such as thyroacetic acid (4-p-hydroxyphenoxyphenylacetic acid), and possibly cleavage of the ether linkage which, in rats, forms metabolites such as mono-iodotyrosine and di-iodotyrosine; conjugation with glucuronic acid and sulphate also occurs.

EXCRETION. About 30 to 55% of a dose is excreted in the urine and 20 to 40% in the faeces; of the urinary excreted material about 40% is thyroacetic acid and 20% is liothyronine.

FURTHER INFORMATION. Excretion of free and conjugated thyroxine—C. W. Burke *et al.*, *Lancet*, ii/1972, 1177 and C. S. Pittman *et al.*, *J. clin. Invest.*, 1972, **51**, 1759; effect of oestrogens on urinary excretion—V. Chan *et al.*, *Br. med. J.*, iv/1972, 619; effect of lithium on thyroid function—C. Child *et al.*, *Clin. Pharmac. Ther.*, 1976, **20**, 715; serum concentrations in patients given thyroxine —A. Kahn, *Can. med. Ass. J.*, 1973, **109**, 279.

Actions and uses. Thyroxine sodium produces an increase in oxygen consumption and an increase in general metabolism, with which are associated an increased excretion of nitrogen, calcium, and water in the urine and a decrease of body-weight.

Thyroxine sodium is indicated only in the treatment of thyroid-deficiency states; it should never be given to a patient with a normally functioning intact gland, as such administration diminishes the intrinsic secretion. A dosage of between 100 and 300 micrograms daily, varying according to the response of the patient, will restore most patients with myxoedema to normality and maintain them in a euthyroid state. Occasionally, higher doses may be necessary. After prolonged hypothyroidism, it is wise to restore a myxoedematous subject to normality only gradually, as some weeks are needed for mental and physical adaptation to the normal state.

Thyroxine sodium is used in the treatment of cretinism, the average dosage for a child of 6 months being 10 micrograms daily, increased to 100 to 200 micrograms daily at puberty. The only other indication for thyroid therapy, apart from primary and post-operative myxoedema, is hypothyroidism secondary to anterior pituitary destruction (Simmonds's disease). In these cases, however, thyroxine sodium is never administered alone, but only in conjunction with other hormones such as cortisone.

Obesity is not an indication for thyroxine administration,

unless accompanied by clear evidence of hypo-thyroidism.

Undesirable effects. Attempts to restore the patient to a normal state too rapidly may result in sweating, tachycardia, diarrhoea, restlessness, excitability, and cardiac arrhythmias, possibly with signs of cardiac strain or decompensation, particularly in the aged.

Even slight overdosage may induce angina pectoris in certain patients, with or without electrocardiographic abnormalities; pain in a limb and aggravation of symptoms due to pre-existing osteo-arthritis may also occur.

Veterinary uses. Thyroxine sodium is used for the treatment of thyroid hormone deficiency. The usual dose by mouth for cattle is 100 micrograms per kilogram body-weight daily and for dogs 5 micrograms per kilogram body-weight daily.

Preparation

THYROXINE TABLETS (*Syn.* L-Thyroxine Sodium Tablets): available as tablets containing 50 and 100 micrograms of thyroxine sodium.

A standard for these tablets is given in the British Pharmacopoeia 1973

Containers and *Storage:* see the entry on Tablets for general information on containers and storage. Containers should be airtight and light resistant.

Advice for patients: the tablets should be taken at regular intervals. Treatment should not be discontinued without the advice of the prescriber.

Tic Douloureux

see under NEURALGIA

Tinctures

Tinctures are alcoholic liquids usually containing, in comparatively low concentration, the active principles of crude drugs. They are generally prepared by maceration or percolation or obtained by dilution of the corresponding liquid or soft extract.

Maceration process. The solid ingredient(s) are placed in a closed vessel with the whole of the solvent and allowed to stand for 7 days with occasional stirring. The mixture is strained, the marc is pressed, and the combined liquids are clarified by filtration or by allowing them to stand and decanting.

Percolation process. The solid ingredient(s) are moistened evenly with a sufficient quantity of the solvent and allowed to stand for 4 hours in an airtight vessel. The damp mass is packed firmly in a suitable percolator, sufficient solvent is added to saturate the mass, and the top of the percolator is closed. When the liquid is about to drip, the lower outlet of the percolator is closed, sufficient additional solvent is added to give a shallow layer above the mass, and the mixture is allowed to macerate in the closed percolator for 24 hours. The percolation is then allowed to proceed slowly until the percolate measures about three-quarters of the required volume of the finished tincture. The marc is pressed, the expressed liquid mixed with the percolate, and sufficient solvent added to produce the required volume. The combined liquids are mixed and clarified by filtration or by allowing them to stand and decanting.

Tinea Infections

Tinea is infection of the skin and appendages caused by fungi of the genera *Epidermophyton, Microsporum*, and *Trichophyton.*

Athlete's foot (Tinea pedis) is characterised by maceration of the skin between the toes, often accompanied by inflammation, especially in hot weather. The feet may be cleansed by soaking in a mild antiseptic solution such as potassium permanganate (0.01%). If necessary, inflammation may be reduced by the application of a cream containing hydrocortisone together with a fungicide such as clioquinol. The usual treatment of this infection consists of local application of a fungicidal cream, lotion, or dusting-powder or compound benzoic acid ointment. The patient should take care not to expose other members of the household to the infection.

Ringworm of the scalp (Tinea capitis) manifests itself in children as round patches of partial baldness with surface scaling; the diseased stumps of hairs may fluoresce light green when viewed in filtered ultraviolet radiation. The condition is rare in adults; it occurs as scaling and baldness which progress slowly over the scalp. Systemic treatment with griseofulvin is effective.

Ringworm of the body (Tinea corporis) is characterised by clearly defined red annular lesions on the body. When the ringworm is due to infection from cattle it takes the form of less-well-defined reddish scaly plaques and is usually acutely inflamed. Treatment consists of griseofulvin by mouth. Pustules of cattle-type ringworm may be washed with a dilute antiseptic such as potassium permanganate (0.01%) and corticosteroid treatment may be required to reduce inflammation. Topical fungicidal preparations such as compound benzoic acid ointment may be applied locally.

Ringworm of the groin (Tinea cruris; Dhobie itch) is observed as a red scaly plaque and may be treated with griseofulvin by mouth. Topical fungicidal preparations may be applied locally but if compound benzoic acid ointment is used it is usually diluted to half the normal strength because of the sensitivity of the skin in the region of the groin.

Ringworm of the nails (Tinea unguium) is a condition in which the nails become thickened and discoloured and separate from the nail bed. The usual treatment is griseofulvin by mouth.

Titanium Dioxide

Titanium (IV) oxide
$TiO_2 = 79.90$

OTHER NAME: Titanium Oxide

A standard is given in the British Pharmacopoeia Addendum 1978

Titanium dioxide has a density of about 4.0; it forms titanates when fused with alkali hydroxides or carbonates.

Description. An odourless white amorphous powder.

Solubility. Practically insoluble in water, in hydrochloric acid, and in nitric acid; soluble in hydrofluoric acid and in hot sulphuric acid.

Actions and uses. Titanium dioxide has an action on the skin similar to that described under Zinc Oxide. It is used in the treatment of dermatoses with exudation and to relieve pruritus. It is an ingredient of face powders and other cosmetics and is used to prevent sunburn.

Titanium dioxide is also used to pigment and opacify hard gelatin capsules and also as a delustring agent for viscose and other man-made fibres.

Preparation

TITANIUM DIOXIDE PASTE:

Titanium dioxide	200 g
Chlorocresol	1 g
Red ferric oxide, of commerce	20 g
Light kaolin, or light kaolin (natural), sterilised	100 g
Zinc oxide, finely sifted	250 g
Glycerol	150 g
Water for preparations .. .. to	1000 g

Mix the ferric oxide, the light kaolin, the titanium dioxide, and the zinc oxide to form a homogeneous powder. Dissolve the chlorocresol in the glycerol, add the water, and gradually triturate the solution with the mixed powders to form a smooth paste.

A standard for this paste is given in the British Pharmaceutical Codex 1973

Containers and *Storage:* see the entry on Pastes for general information on containers and storage. It should not be allowed to come into contact with aluminium.

Tobramycin

6-*O*-(3-Amino-3-deoxy-α-D-glucopyranosyl)-2-deoxy-4-*O*-(2,6-diamino-2,3,6-trideoxy-α-D-*ribo*-hexapyranosyl)streptamine, an antibiotic substance produced by *Streptomyces tenebrarius*.

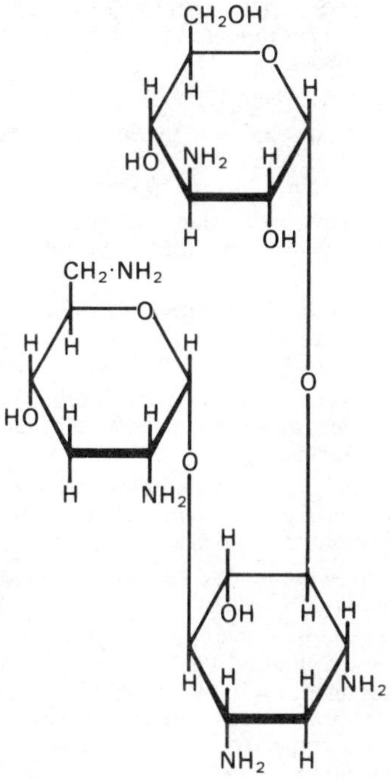

$C_{18}H_{37}N_5O_9 = 467.5$

OTHER NAME: *Nebcin*®

Description. A colourless hygroscopic crystalline powder.

Solubility. Soluble in water.

Storage. It should be stored in airtight containers.

Metabolism. ABSORPTION. Poorly absorbed after oral administration but readily absorbed after intramuscular injection.

BLOOD CONCENTRATION. After an intramuscular dose of 100 mg, peak plasma concentrations of 4 to 5 μg/ml are attained in 30 to 60 minutes; serum concentrations of 12 to 15 μg/ml may lead to toxic reactions.

HALF-LIFE. After an intramuscular dose, serum half-life, about 1.6 to 3 hours in normal subjects; in subjects with renal function impairment the half-life is greatly increased and may reach up to about 50 hours.

DISTRIBUTION. Volume of distribution, 17 to 25 litres; low concentrations are attained in the cerebrospinal fluid unless administered intrathecally or intraventricularly; crosses the placenta and is secreted in the saliva and, in small amounts, in the milk.

EXCRETION. About 60 to 90% of a dose is excreted in the urine unchanged in 72 hours.

FURTHER INFORMATION. Effect of renal impairment—L. D. Bechtol and H. R. Black, *Am. J. med. Sci.*, 1975, **269**, 317; new aminoglycosides compared—R. N. Brogden *et al.*, *Drugs*, 1976, **12**, 161; pharmacology and blood concentrations—B. R. Meyers and S. Z. Hirschman, *J. clin. Pharmac.*, 1972, **12**, 321; pharmacokinetics—C. Regamey *et al.*, *Clin. Pharmac. Ther.*, 1973, **14**, 396.

Actions and uses. Tobramycin is an aminoglycoside antibiotic and has a spectrum of antibacterial activity similar to that of gentamicin but it is more active against *Pseudomonas aeruginosa* and less active against *Staphylococcus epidermidis*. Some gentamicin-resistant strains of *Pseudomonas* may be sensitive to tobramycin. It may be administered as the sulphate by intramuscular injection or intravenous infusion in a concentration not exceeding the equivalent of 1 milligram of tobramycin per millilitre in dextrose injection (5%) or sodium chloride injection. It does not readily cross the blood-brain barrier and its use by the intrathecal or intra-cisternal route is not recommended except in life-threatening situations such as neonatal meningitis due to Gram-negative organisms.

It is excreted by glomerular filtration. In patients with normal kidney function the usual dose is the equivalent of 3 milligrams of tobramycin per kilogram body-weight daily increasing to 5 milligrams per kilogram body-weight daily in severe infections; it should be given in divided doses every 8 hours.

Undesirable effects; Precautions; Drug interactions. As for Gentamicin Sulphate.

Preparations

Preparations available include an INJECTION containing tobramycin sulphate equivalent to 10 mg of tobramycin per ml in 2-ml vials, and an injection containing tobramycin sulphate equivalent to 40 mg of tobramycin per ml in 1- and 2-ml vials.

Tocopheryl Acetate

see ALPHA TOCOPHERYL ACETATE

Tolazoline Hydrochloride

2-Benzyl-2-imidazoline hydrochloride

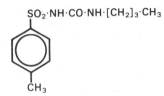

$C_{10}H_{13}ClN_2 = 196.7$

OTHER NAME: *Priscol®*

A standard is given in the British Pharmacopoeia 1973

Description. An odourless, white or creamy-white, crystalline powder.

Solubility. Soluble, at 20°, in less than 1 part of water, in 2 parts of alcohol, and in 2.5 parts of chloroform; practically insoluble in ether.

Acidity. A 1% solution has a pH of 5 to 7.

Dissociation constant. pK_a 10.6 (20°).

Sterilisation. Solutions for injection are sterilised by heating in an autoclave or by filtration.

Storage. It should be stored in airtight containers, protected from light.

Identification. TESTS. 1. Dissolve about 20 mg in 5 ml of water and add 2 ml of *ammonium reineckate solution*; a pink precipitate with a pearly lustre is produced.
2. Dissolve about 50 mg in 2 ml of water, add 10 ml of *trinitrophenol solution* and cool in ice; a precipitate is produced which, after washing with water, melts at about 147°.

MELTING-POINT. About 174°.

INFRA-RED ABSORPTION. Major peaks at 746, 1031, 1205, 1299, 1515, and 1613 cm⁻¹ (see Appendix 2b: Infra-red Spectra).

Actions and uses. Tolazoline causes marked dilatation of arterioles and capillaries, and increases the skin temperature to a greater extent and for a longer period than most other vasodilator drugs. It also stimulates gastric secretion.
Tolazoline antagonises those effects of noradrenaline and adrenaline that are attributed to alpha-receptor stimulation, but it has poor adrenergic-blocking activity and hence is of no value in the treatment of hypertension.
It is well absorbed after oral or parenteral administration and is rapidly excreted, mainly unchanged, in the urine. Tolazoline is used mainly for the treatment of peripheral vascular disorders due to arterial spasm or occlusion. In the treatment of Raynaud's disease, 25 to 50 milligrams of tolazoline hydrochloride may be given by mouth. It has been given by intramuscular or intravenous injection in doses of 10 to 20 milligrams and has also been applied topically in the treatment of local vascular disorders.

Undesirable effects. Tolazoline may produce nausea, vomiting, diarrhoea, and postural hypotension.

Contra-indications. It is contra-indicated in patients with coronary insufficiency or other severe heart disease and in cases of peptic ulceration.

Preparation

TOLAZOLINE TABLETS: available as tablets containing 25 mg of tolazoline hydrochloride.
A standard for these tablets is given in the British Pharmacopoeia 1973

Containers and *Storage:* see the entry on Tablets for general information on containers and storage. Containers should be airtight and light resistant.
Advice for patients: the tablets should preferably be taken after meals.

Tolbutamide

1-Butyl-3-tosylurea

$$SO_2 \cdot NH \cdot CO \cdot NH \cdot [CH_2]_3 \cdot CH_3$$

CH_3

$C_{12}H_{18}N_2O_3S = 270.3$

OTHER NAMES: *Rastinon®*; *Pramidex®*; Tolbutamidum

A standard is given in the European Pharmacopoeia Vol. II

Description. An almost odourless, white, crystalline powder.

Solubility. Practically insoluble in water; soluble, at 20°, in 10 parts of alcohol and in 3 parts of acetone; soluble in sodium hydroxide solution and in dilute mineral acids.

Dissociation constant. pK_a 5.3 (25°).

Identification. TESTS. 1. Mix 200 mg with 8 ml of sulphuric acid (50% w/w), boil for 30 minutes under a reflux condenser, cool, filter, and reserve the filtrate; the residue, after recrystallisation from hot water and drying at 105°, melts at about 136°.
2. Make the reserved filtrate in Test 1 alkaline with *sodium hydroxide solution* and heat; the odour of butylamine is produced.

MELTING-POINT. About 129°.

ULTRAVIOLET ABSORPTION. In alcohol (95%), maxima at 228 nm (E1%, 1cm = 500), 257 nm (E1%, 1cm = 22), 262 nm (E1%, 1cm = 26), and 274 nm (E1%, 1cm = 22).

INFRA-RED ABSORPTION. Major peaks at 813, 1087, 1149, 1316, 1538, and 1639 cm⁻¹ (see Appendix 2b: Infra-red Spectra).

Determination in body fluids. ULTRAVIOLET SPECTRO-PHOTOMETRY. In blood or urine—J. Shibasaki *et al.*, *Chem. pharm. Bull.*, Tokyo, 1973, **21**, 1747.

GAS CHROMATOGRAPHY. In plasma or urine; tolbutamide and metabolites—S. B. Matin and M. Rowland, *Analyt. Lett.*, 1973, **6**, 865.

HIGH PRESSURE LIQUID CHROMATOGRAPHY. In serum —D. J. Weber, *J. pharm. Sci.*, 1976, **65**, 1502; R. E. Hill and J. Crechiolo, *J. Chromat.*, 1978, **145**, 165.

Metabolism. ABSORPTION Readily absorbed after oral administration.

BLOOD CONCENTRATION. After an oral dose of 1 g, a peak serum concentration of 100 µg/ml is attained within 2 hours; after an intravenous dose of 1 g, plasma concentrations of 120, 90, and 70 µg/ml are obtained after 1, 4, and 7 hours respectively; effective concentrations are in the range 80 to 180 µg/ml.

HALF-LIFE. Variably reported to be 5 to 70 hours in plasma; the plasma half-life appears to be influenced by many factors and is decreased in subjects with hepatitis, asthma, and after prolonged tolbutamide therapy of diabetics; concomitant administration of other drugs such as sulphonamides, phenylbutazone, or dicoumarol also influences the half-life.

DISTRIBUTION. Volume of distribution, 10 to 20% of body-weight; saliva concentrations parallel those in the plasma; *protein binding*, about 90% bound to plasma proteins, which may be decreased in jaundice or after the administration of phenylbutazone or dicoumarol.

METABOLIC REACTIONS. Oxidation to form *p*-hydroxymethyl- and *p*-carboxy-metabolites; the rate of metabolism appears to be increased in alcoholic subjects.

EXCRETION. About 85% of an oral dose is excreted in urine as metabolites; two-thirds is excreted as the carboxy-metabolite and the remainder is excreted as the hydroxymethyl-metabolite.

FURTHER INFORMATION. Effect of oral and intravenous administration on plasma concentrations—P. B. Andreasen and E. S. Vesell, *Clin. Pharmac. Ther.*, 1974, **16**, 1059; inhibition of metabolism by sulphamethizole—B. Lumholtz *et al.*, *Clin. Pharmac. Ther.*, 1975, **17**, 731; comparison of salivary and plasma concentrations—S. B. Matin *et al.*, *Clin. Pharmac. Ther.*, 1974, **16**, 1052; effect of fasting on metabolism—M. Reidenberg and E. S. Vesell, *Clin. Pharmac. Ther.*, 1975, **17**, 650; serum concentrations—D. J. Weber, *J. pharm. Sci.*, 1976, **65**, 1502.

Actions and uses. Tolbutamide has the actions and uses described under Chlorpropamide. It is active when taken by mouth, but as it is excreted more rapidly than chlorpropamide it has a shorter duration of action. After a single dose, the blood-sugar level falls within 2 to 4 hours and the reduced level is maintained for 8 to 10 hours.

The usual initial daily dosage is 1.5 grams by mouth in divided doses. The dose and frequency of administration is subsequently adjusted to achieve a suitable balance adequate for controlling the blood-sugar level and preventing glycosuria; the maintenance dose is usually 0.5 to 1.5 grams daily in divided doses.

Tolbutamide, in the form of its sodium derivative, may also be given by intravenous injection in a dose of 1 gram for the diagnosis of insulinomas, but this is not without risk.

Undesirable effects. Rashes, gastro-intestinal disturbances, and intolerance to alcohol may occur and, rarely, blood dyscrasias and jaundice.

Precautions. Caution should be exercised in administering tolbutamide in conjunction with monoamine-oxidase inhibitors, oral anticoagulants, oxyphenbutazone, phenylbutazone, salicylates, and sulphonamides, which may enhance its activity. The activity of tolbutamide is also increased by hepatic or renal failure and by excessive alcohol intake.

Tolbutamide should preferably be avoided during pregnancy. It is secreted in the milk and may cause hypoglycaemia in breast fed infants.

Veterinary uses. Tolbutamide is used as an oral antidiabetic agent in dogs and cats, the usual dose being 10 to 30 milligrams per kilogram body-weight daily in divided doses.

Preparation

TOLBUTAMIDE TABLETS: available as tablets containing 500 mg of tolbutamide.

A standard for these tablets is given in the British Pharmacopoeia 1973

Containers and *Storage*: see the entry on Tablets for general information on containers and storage. Containers should be airtight.

Advice for patients: the tablets should preferably be taken after meals.

Treatment should not be discontinued without the advice of the prescriber. Intolerance to alcohol may occur.

Tolnaftate

O-Naphth-2-yl *N*-methyl-*m*-tolylthiocarbanilate

$C_{19}H_{17}NOS = 307.4$

OTHER NAMES: *Tinaderm*®
Tinaderm-M® (with nystatin)

A standard is given in the British Pharmacopoeia 1973

Description. An odourless white to creamy-white powder.

Solubility. Very slightly soluble in water and in alcohol; soluble, at 20°, in 55 parts of ether, in 3 parts of chloroform, and in 9 parts of acetone.

Identification. MELTING-POINT. About 110°.

ULTRAVIOLET ABSORPTION. In methyl alcohol, maximum at 257 nm (E1%, 1cm = 710).

INFRA-RED ABSORPTION. Major peaks at 752, 1163, 1176, 1205, 1370, and 1449 cm^{-1} (see Appendix 2b: Infra-red Spectra).

Actions and uses. Tolnaftate is an antifungal agent used for the topical treatment of ringworm and other skin infections due to *Epidermophyton floccosum*, *Microsporum audouinii*, *M. canis*, *Trichophyton mentagrophytes*, and *T. verrucosum*; infections due to *T. rubrum*, *T. tonsurans*, and *Malassezia furfur* may also respond. It is not active against species of *Candida* or bacteria.

Tolnaftate, like other topical agents, is not suitable for the treatment of tinea of the nails and scalp, but it may be used as an adjunct to systemic treatment with griseofulvin.

Since tolnaftate is not keratolytic, skin tolerance is very good but primary irritation and allergic sensitisation occasionally occur.

Tolnaftate is applied in the form of cream, dusting-powder, or solution containing 1%.

Preparations

TOLNAFTATE CREAM: a dispersion of tolnaftate in a suitable water-miscible basis. It contains 1% of tolnaftate.

Containers, Labelling, and *Storage:* see the entry on Creams for general information on containers, labelling, and storage.

Advice for patients: the cream should be rubbed lightly and sparingly onto the affected area. When used in conjunction with tolnaftate dusting-powder, the cream should be used first and the dusting-powder afterwards.

TOLNAFTATE DUSTING-POWDER: a dispersion of tolnaftate in a suitable dusting-powder basis. It contains 1% of tolnaftate.

Containers and *Labelling:* see the entry on Dusting-powders for general information on containers and labelling.

Advice for patients: the dusting-powder should be dusted lightly onto the affected area. See also under Tolnaftate Cream (above).

OTHER PREPARATIONS available include a CREAM containing tolnaftate 10 mg with nystatin 100000 units per g; and a SOLUTION containing tolnaftate 10 mg with butylated hydroxytoluene 1 mg per ml.

Tolu Balsam

A solid or semi-solid balsam obtained by incision from the trunk of *Myroxylon balsamum* (L.) Harms (Fam. Leguminosae), a tree indigenous to Columbia and adjoining regions in South America.

A standard is given in the British Pharmaceutical Codex 1973

Constituents. Tolu balsam contains 12 to 15% of free cinnamic acid, about 8% of free benzoic acid, a trace of vanillin, and about 7.5% of an oily liquid consisting of benzyl benzoate with a little benzyl cinnamate. The resin, of which the balsam contains about 80%, yields on saponification one or more resin alcohols, cinnamic acid, and a little benzoic acid.
Good fresh tolu balsam yields, when distilled with water, 1.5 to 3% of a very fragrant volatile oil.

Description. A soft, tenacious, brownish-yellow or brown, resinous solid when first imported, subsequently becoming harder and finally brittle; transparent in thin films; odour aromatic and vanilla-like; taste aromatic. When warmed and pressed between pieces of glass and examined with a lens, it exhibits crystals of cinnamic acid.

Solubility. Soluble in alcohol (90%), in ether, in chloroform, and in glacial acetic acid; partly soluble in carbon disulphide, the soluble portion consisting chiefly of cinnamic acid; very slightly soluble in light petroleum; partly soluble in solutions of caustic alkalis.

Adulterants and substitutes. Exhausted balsam may be detected by the deficiency of balsamic acids. Factitious tolu balsam made by adding synthetic balsamic acids to the exhausted balsam lacks the fragrance associated with the volatile oil.

Identification. TESTS. 1. Warm gently about 1 g, in powder, with 5 ml of *potassium permanganate solution*; the odour of benzaldehyde is produced.
2. To a solution in alcohol (90%) add *ferric chloride test-solution*; a green colour is produced.

Uses. Tolu balsam, in the form of tolu syrup, is frequently used to flavour cough mixtures.

Preparations

PAEDIATRIC COMPOUND TOLU LINCTUS:

Citric acid monohydrate .. .. 6 g
Benzaldehyde spirit .. .. 2 ml
Compound tartrazine solution .. .. .. 10 ml
Glycerol .. .. 200 ml
Invert syrup .. .. 200 ml
Tolu syrup .. .. to 1000 ml

When a dose less than or not a multiple of 5 ml is prescribed, the linctus may be diluted, as described in the entry on Linctuses, with syrup.
A standard for this linctus is given in the British Pharmaceutical Codex 1973
Containers: see the entry on Linctuses for general information on containers.

Storage: it should be stored in a cool place.
Dose: CHILD: 5 to 10 millilitres.
Advice for patients: the linctus should be sipped and swallowed slowly. It should not be used for longer than a few days or given to children under 1 year without medical advice.

TOLU SOLUTION:

Tolu balsam.. .. .. 50 g
Sucrose .. .. 500 g
Alcohol (90%) .. .. 300 ml
Water for preparations .. .. .. to 1000 ml

Dissolve the tolu balsam in 200 ml of the alcohol, add sterilised purified talc and 350 ml of the water heated to 70°, shake vigorously, and allow to stand for 24 hours. Filter, dissolve the sucrose in the filtrate with the aid of gentle heat, cool, add the remainder of the alcohol and sufficient water to produce the required volume, and mix.
A standard for this solution is given in the British Pharmaceutical Codex 1973

TOLU SYRUP:

Tolu solution .. .. 100 ml
Syrup.. .. .. to 1000 ml

Mix.
A standard for this syrup is given in the British Pharmaceutical Codex 1973

Tolu balsam is an ingredient of compound benzoin tincture; tolu syrup is an ingredient of methadone linctus, opiate squill linctus, paediatric belladonna and ipecacuanha mixture, paediatric ipecacuanha and ammonia mixture, and paediatric opiate squill linctus.

Tonsillitis

Tonsillitis is characterised by inflammation of the tonsils and pharynx, with tonsillar exudate and fever. The aetiological agent is often a virus but the commonest bacterial pathogen is the beta-haemolytic streptococcus. Symptomatic treatment is given and the infection is treated with a suitable antibacterial agent (a penicillin to which the infecting organism is sensitive).

Toxaemia of Pregnancy

The toxaemias of pregnancy (pre-eclampsia and eclampsia) are metabolic disturbances characterised by hypertension and proteinuria.
Pre-eclampsia occurs in late pregnancy and is characterised by hypertension and, in some cases, significant proteinuria. In severe cases oliguria, hypofibrinogenaemia, and cerebral or visual disturbances also occur. This condition may progress to eclampsia in which generalised convulsions are present.
Both pre-eclampsia and eclampsia carry a significant risk of death to both the mother and the foetus.
Pre-eclampsia may be controlled by salt restriction, rest, sedation, diuretics, and antihypertensives. Anticonvulsants may also be needed in eclampsia.
The toxaemias of pregnancy resolve spontaneously if pregnancy is terminated; induction of labour or caesarean section must therefore be considered if severe pre-eclampsia or eclampsia occur. Toxaemia does not necessarily recur in subsequent pregnancies unless there is underlying hypertensive disease.

Toxocara

Toxocara canis and *Toxocara catis* are animal round-worms similar to *Ascaris lumbricoides*. They may infect man and give rise to granulomatous inflammatory reactions. They are unable to develop to maturity in man but the larval lesions in the eye may result in blindness. Infections with these nematodes may be treated with diethylcarbamazine.

Tragacanth

The dried gummy exudation obtained by incision from *Astragalus gummifer* Labill. and some other species of *Astragalus* (Fam. Leguminosae), shrubs indigenous to Iran, Greece, Turkey, Iraq, and Syria; it is known in commerce as Persian tragacanth.

OTHER NAMES: Trag.; Tragacantha

A standard is given in the European Pharmacopoeia Vol. III

Some indication of the suspending properties of tragacanth may be obtained from the apparent viscosity of its mucilage; commercial samples vary considerably in this property.

Constituents. Tragacanth can be separated into 2 fractions, one termed tragacanthin, which is water soluble and the other termed bassorin which contains about 5% of methoxyl and which is insoluble but swells in water. Tragacanthin contains $(1 \rightarrow 4)$ linked α-D-galacturonic acid (43%) with C-3 side chains of D-xylose (40%), 2-O-α-L-fucopyranosyl-D-xylopyranose and 2-O-α-D-galactopyranosyl-D-xylopyranose. The galactoaraban portion of the gum contains highly branched $1 \rightarrow 6$, $1 \rightarrow 2$ linked D-galactose with side chains of L-arabinofuranose. The gum also contains 15% of moisture, and traces of starch and of altered cell-walls. It yields on hydrolysis, among other products, galacturonic acid, D-galactopyranose, L-arabinofuranose, and D-xylopyranose. Tragacanth has a volatile acidity of about 2 to 3%, calculated as acetic acid.

Up to 1% of foreign matter may be present and it may yield up to 4% of sulphated ash.

Description. UNGROUND DRUG. *Macroscopical characters:* thin, flattened, more or less curved, ribbon-like flakes, about 25 mm long and 12 mm broad; white or pale yellowish-white, horny, translucent, marked on flat sides with concentric ridges; fracture short.

It is odourless and almost tasteless.

Microscopical characters: the diagnostic characters are: when powdered and mounted in alcohol, it appears as small, transparent, angular particles of various sizes and shapes; the particles lose their sharp edges when water is added, each gradually swelling until large indefinite masses containing a few groups of small rounded starch granules result.

POWDERED DRUG. Powdered Tragacanth. A white powder possessing the diagnostic microscopical characters and taste of the unground drug; odourless.

Solubility. Partly soluble in water, in which it swells to a homogeneous, adhesive, gelatinous mass; practically insoluble in alcohol.

Adulterants and substitutes. "Vermicelli" tragacanth is composed of tears and vermiform pieces.

Smyrna tragacanth occurs in flakes, but is more opaque and less ribbon-like than the official drug; it contains appreciable quantities of starch.

Hog gum, or Caramania gum, occurs in yellowish or yellowish-brown, opaque tears or vermiform pieces; it is said to be obtained from a species of *Prunus* (Fam. Rosaceae).

Indian tragacanth (karaya gum) is described under Sterculia.

Ceratonia, or Carob gum, consisting of the endosperms of the seeds of *Ceratonia siliqua* L. (Fam. Leguminosae), occurs as translucent white oval concavo-convex disks containing about 58% of mannan and about 29% of galactan.

Storage. It should be stored in airtight containers. Powdered tragacanth should be similarly stored.

Identification. TESTS. 1. Warm with *sodium hydroxide solution*; a canary-yellow colour slowly develops.
2. Examine microscopically a small quantity mounted in *ruthenium red solution*; the particles do not acquire a pronounced pink colour (distinction from sterculia and agar).
3. To about 100 mg, in powder, add 1 ml of 0.02N iodine; the mixture acquires an olive-green colour (distinction from acacia and agar).

Uses. Tragacanth forms highly viscous solutions and gels even at relatively low concentrations; the viscosity of a 1% solution of a high grade sample may be over 3500 centipoises (3.5 pascal seconds). Gels are non-thixotropic and are stable at pH values as low as 2.5. In addition it is almost tasteless and non-toxic and, for these reasons, is widely used to modify the continuous phase of emulsions and suspensions for oral use in order to prevent creaming and settling respectively. Its colloidal nature also modifies the flocculation characteristics of such systems, increasing the sedimentation volume and assisting resuspension.

It is combined with acacia, sucrose, and starch to give an easily dispersible suspending agent suitable for extemporaneous use (compound tragacanth powder). Dispersion of tragacanth alone in water is facilitated by first wetting the gum with a little alcohol in which it is completely insoluble.

Tragacanth is also used in medicated and toilet creams and jellies containing glycerol. A thick mucilage is used as a drying application to the skin, for example as a basis for medicaments such as ichthammol, salicylic acid, resorcinol, and sulphur.

In dispensing lotions, creams, and jellies the tragacanth is first dispersed in a distributing agent, such as alcohol, essential oil, or glycerol, to prevent agglomeration on the addition of water. Tragacanth is used in the preparation of lozenges for its demulcent properties and as an excipient for pills and tablets. It is also used in obstetric creams and as the basis of lubricants for catheters and surgical instruments. The powder is used as an adhesive for dentures.

Like all natural gums, tragacanth is likely to be seriously contaminated with bacteria. Energetic methods to reduce contamination, such as irradiation and dry heat, may seriously impair the suspending properties of the gum. A suitable quality may, however, be achieved by gassing with ethylene oxide or slurrying with alcohol/water mixtures under appropriate conditions.

Preparation

COMPOUND TRAGACANTH POWDER (*Syn.* Pulv. Trag. Co.):

Tragacanth, finely powdered	..	..	..	150 g
Acacia, finely powdered ..	..	..	..	200 g
Starch, finely powdered ..	..	..	..	200 g
Sucrose, finely powdered	..	..	..	450 g

Mix.

Storage: it should be stored in airtight containers.

Tranexamic Acid

(Z)-4-Aminomethylcyclohexanecarboxylic acid

$C_8H_{15}NO_2 = 157.2$

OTHER NAMES: *Cyclokapron®*

Description. An odourless white crystalline powder.

Solubility. Soluble in 6 parts of water; very slightly soluble in alcohol; practically insoluble in ether and in chloroform.

Dissociation constants. pK_a 4.5, 10.5 (20°).

Actions and uses. Tranexamic acid has the actions and uses as described under Aminocaproic Acid but it has a more potent antifibrinolytic activity and a lower incidence of side-effects.

Tranexamic acid is used to prevent general fibrinolysis or local fibrinolysis in operations such as suprapubic prostatectomy.

It may be given by mouth or by slow intravenous injection or infusion. The usual dose by mouth or by injection is 15 milligrams per kilogram body-weight every 6 to 8 hours. The first doses may be given by intravenous infusion during an operation and in the immediate postoperative period, and treatment should be continued by mouth as soon as possible.

Tranexamic acid is also used to maintain postoperative haemostasis in constitutional bleeding disorders, as an adjunct to preoperative clotting factor therapy. For example, prior to dental extractions in haemophiliacs, the level of factor VIII in the patient is raised to 50% of normal by administration of human antihaemophilic fraction and tranexamic acid is administered by slow intravenous injection. The dosage is adjusted according to the requirements of the patient but is usually about 15 milligrams per kilogram body-weight. Dried human thrombin for topical use may be used to dry the socket and a tampon soaked in a sterile solution of tranexamic acid (100 milligrams per millilitre) may be inserted into the socket. Subsequently tranexamic acid is administered by mouth until healing is complete; the dosage is adjusted according to the needs of the patient but is usually about 30 milligrams per kilogram body-weight every 8 hours.

Sterile solutions of up to 100 milligrams per millilitre of tranexamic acid may be used topically, for example in bladder irrigation.

Undesirable effects. As for Aminocaproic Acid but less severe.

Contra-indications. As for Aminocaproic Acid.

Preparations

TRANEXAMIC ACID INJECTION: a sterile solution of tranexamic acid in water for injections. Available in 5-ml ampoules containing 100 mg of tranexamic acid per ml.
Containers and *Labelling:* see the entry on Injections for general information on containers and labelling.

TRANEXAMIC ACID TABLETS: available as tablets containing 500 mg of tranexamic acid.
Containers and *Storage:* see the entry on Tablets for general information on containers and storage. Containers should be airtight.
Advice for patients: the prescribed course should be completed.

Tranylcypromine Sulphate

(±)-*trans*-2-Phenylcyclopropylammonium sulphate

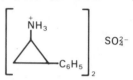

$C_{18}H_{24}N_2O_4S = 364.5$

OTHER NAMES: *Parnate®*
Parstelin® (with trifluoperazine hydrochloride)

A standard is given in the British Pharmacopoeia 1973

Description. A white crystalline powder which is odourless or has a faint odour of cinnamaldehyde and has an acid taste.

Solubility. Soluble, at 20°, in 20 parts of water; very slightly soluble in alcohol and in ether; practically insoluble in chloroform.

Dissociation constant. pK_a 8.2.

Identification. TEST. Suspend about 5 mg in 0.5 ml of alcohol (95%) and add 5 mg of ninhydrin; a purple colour is produced within 15 minutes.

ULTRAVIOLET ABSORPTION. In 0.2N sulphuric acid, maxima at 258 nm (E1%, 1cm = 14.4), 264 nm (E1%, 1cm = 16.2), and 271 nm (E1%, 1cm = 11.6).

INFRA-RED ABSORPTION. Major peaks at 694, 769, 962, 1020, 1111, and 1149 cm⁻¹ (see Appendix 2b: Infra-red Spectra).

Determination in body fluids. GAS CHROMATOGRAPHY. In serum or urine—R. C. Basalt *et al.*, *J. analyt. Toxic.*, 1977, **1**, 215.

Metabolism. METABOLIC REACTIONS. Glucuronic acid conjugation.

EXCRETION. After a 20-mg dose, 5 to 10% is excreted in the urine unchanged in 16 hours; in alkaline urine 1 to 2% is excreted unchanged in the urine in the same time period.

FURTHER INFORMATION. Influence of urinary pH on excretion—P. Turner *et al.*, *Nature*, 1976, **215**, 881.

Actions and uses. Tranylcypromine is a monoamine-oxidase inhibitor with actions and uses similar to those described under Phenelzine Sulphate. It is used in the treatment of depressive states, including endogenous, reactive, and psychoneurotic depression. It usually produces a response in susceptible patients within 3 days. The usual dosage is 20 milligrams daily in 2 doses by mouth, increased if necessary to 30 milligrams daily. For the intensive treatment of severe depression, a commencing dose of 40 milligrams daily may be given, increased at weekly intervals to a maximum of 60 milligrams daily; when a satisfactory response has been achieved, dosage may be reduced to a maintenance level of 20 milligrams daily. Unlike other monoamine-oxidase inhibitors, the effects of tranylcypromine persist for only 48 to 72 hours after the withdrawal of the drug.

Undesirable effects. The most frequently occurring reactions are insomnia, dizziness, muscular weakness, dryness of the mouth, and hypotension. In some patients, hypertension accompanied by severe headache may occur, requiring discontinuation of treatment with tranylcypromine and treatment with antihypertensive drugs such as phentolamine mesylate. Liver damage occurs less frequently than with phenelzine.

Precautions; Drug interactions. As for Phenelzine Sulphate.

Preparations

TRANYLCYPROMINE TABLETS: available as tablets containing tranylcypromine sulphate equivalent to 10 mg of tranylcypromine; they are sugar coated; the coat may be coloured.

A standard for these tablets is given in the British Pharmacopoeia 1973

Containers and *Storage:* see the entry on Tablets for general information on containers and storage. Containers should be airtight.

Labelling: the label on the container should state the amount of the medicament as the equivalent amount of tranylcypromine.

Advice for patients: daily doses should preferably be taken in the morning. Treatment should not be discontinued without the advice of the prescriber. The tablets may affect mental concentration; persons affected should not drive or operate machinery. To avoid insomnia, doses should not be taken for several hours before bedtime. Patients should be advised to avoid, during treatment and for 7 days thereafter, certain foodstuffs containing pressor agents such as cheese, pickled herrings, broad bean pods, and certain protein extracts prepared from meat or yeast. Medicines containing sympathomimetic substances such as ephedrine, methoxamine, phenylephrine, phenylpropanolamine, and pseudoephedrine, as found in cough and cold remedies, analgesics, and tonics, should also be avoided. Warning cards containing this advice may be carried by the patient during treatment and shown when further medical or dental treatment is required or when other medicines are needed.

OTHER PREPARATIONS available include TABLETS containing tranylcypromine sulphate equivalent to 10 mg of tranylcypromine with trifluoperazine hydrochloride equivalent to 1 mg of trifluoperazine.

Triamcinolone

9α-Fluoro-11β,16α,17α,21-tetrahydroxypregna-1,4-diene-3,20-dione

$C_{21}H_{27}FO_6 = 394.4$

OTHER NAMES: *Adcortyl®*; *Ledercort®*

A standard is given in the British Pharmaceutical Codex 1973

Description. An odourless white crystalline powder.

Solubility. Soluble, at 20°, in 500 parts of water and in 240 parts of alcohol; very slightly soluble in ether and in chloroform.

Moisture content. Not more than 2%, determined by drying at 60° *in vacuo*.

Specific rotation. +65° to +71°, determined on a 1% solution in dimethylformamide.

Identification. TESTS. 1. It complies with Test 2 described under Betamethasone.

2. Dissolve about 1 mg in 6 ml of alcohol (95%), add 5 ml of a 1% solution of di-t-butyl-*p*-cresol in alcohol (95%) and 5 ml of *dilute sodium hydroxide solution*, and heat on a water-bath under a reflux condenser for 20 minutes; a pinkish-lavender colour is produced.

MELTING-POINT. About 266°.

ULTRAVIOLET ABSORPTION. In alcohol (95%), maximum at 238 nm (E1%, 1cm = 380).

THIN-LAYER CHROMATOGRAPHY. See under Thin-layer Chromatography, System 10.

Metabolism. HALF-LIFE. Plasma half-life, in rats, 50 to 60 minutes and in dogs 100 to 150 minutes.

DISTRIBUTION. *Protein binding*, about 40% bound to plasma proteins.

METABOLIC REACTIONS. 6β-Hydroxylation.

EXCRETION. In dogs, 20% of an intravenous dose is excreted unchanged in the urine along with 25% as 6β-hydroxytriamcinolone and another 5% as an unidentified metabolite; excretion in man appears to be similar.

FURTHER INFORMATION. Metabolism in dogs—J. R. Florini *et al.*, *J. biol. Chem.*, 1961, **236**, 1038; plasma protein binding—J. R. Florini and D. A. Buyske, *J. biol. Chem.*, 1961, **236**, 247.

Actions and uses. Triamcinolone has the actions and uses described under Cortisone Acetate but has virtually no sodium-retaining effect. During the first days of administration it may even cause a loss of sodium from the body, and an initial mild diuretic action is sometimes observed. It is used, therefore, in all conditions for which cortisone is indicated, except in adrenocortical deficiency states, where some salt-retaining action is desirable.

It is given by mouth in a dosage slightly lower than that of prednisone or prednisolone, 4 milligrams of triamcinolone being approximately equivalent in glucocorticoid activity to 5 milligrams of prednisolone. The dosage is usually 4 to 48 milligrams daily in divided doses, but for extended use as an anti-inflammatory agent it should not exceed 6 milligrams daily.

Undesirable effects. These are as described under Cortisone Acetate but salt retention and oedema are unlikely to occur. The voracious appetite which occurs occasionally in patients during treatment with other cortisone analogues does not occur with triamcinolone. Dizziness, anorexia, somnolence, muscle weakness, and post-prandial flushing may occur.

Precautions and contra-indications. As for Cortisone Acetate.

Preparation

TRIAMCINOLONE TABLETS: may be prepared by moist granulation and compression as described in the entry on Tablets. Available as tablets containing 1, 2, and 4 mg of triamcinolone.

A standard for these tablets is given in the British Pharmaceutical Codex 1973

Containers and *Storage:* see the entry on Tablets for general information on containers and storage. Containers should be airtight.

Advice for patients: in long-term use, treatment should not be discontinued without the advice of the prescriber. Patients should carry an identification card giving details of their treatment and the name of the prescriber who should be contacted in the event of accident, feverish illness, diarrhoea, vomiting, or alimentary disturbances. In short-term treatment, the prescribed course should be completed.

Triamcinolone Acetonide

9α-Fluoro-11β,21-dihydroxy-16α,17α-isopropylidenedioxypregna-1,4-diene-3,20-dione

$C_{24}H_{31}FO_6 = 434.5$

OTHER NAMES: *Adcortyl®*; *Kenalog®*; *Ledercort®*; *Vetalog®*

Aureocort® (with chlortetracycline hydrochloride); *Remiderm®*, *Remotic®*, and *Vetalog Plus®* (all with halquinol); *Nystadermal®* (with nystatin); *Tricaderm®* (with salicylic acid)

A standard is given in the British Pharmacopoeia 1973

Description. An odourless white crystalline powder.

Solubility. Very slightly soluble in water; soluble, at 20°, in 150 parts of alcohol, in 40 parts of chloroform, and in 11 parts of acetone.

Moisture content. Not more than 1.5%, determined by drying at 60° *in vacuo.*

Storage. It should be protected from light.

Identification. TESTS. It complies with Tests 1 and 2 described under Betamethasone.

MELTING-POINT. About 277°.

ULTRAVIOLET ABSORPTION. In methyl alcohol, maximum at 238 nm (E1%, 1cm = 345).

INFRA-RED ABSORPTION. Major peaks at 902, 1060, 1082, 1609, 1618, and 1663 cm⁻¹ (see Appendix 2a: Infra-red Spectra).

THIN-LAYER CHROMATOGRAPHY. See under Thin-layer Chromatography, System 10.

Metabolism. ABSORPTION. Slowly though almost completely absorbed after intramuscular administration; absorbed to a small extent through the skin.

HALF-LIFE. Plasma half-life, 1 to 2 hours.

METABOLIC REACTIONS. Mainly 6β-hydroxylation; no significant hydrolytic cleavage of the acetonide occurs.

EXCRETION. Excreted in the urine mainly as the hydroxylated metabolites; excreted in the bile of dogs, monkeys, and rats.

FURTHER INFORMATION. Metabolism of triamcinolone acetonide 21-phosphate in animals—K. J. Kripalani *et al., J. pharm. Sci.,* 1975, **64**, 1351.

Actions and uses. Triamcinolone acetonide has the actions and uses of topically applied hydrocortisone but, being more potent, it is used in lower concentrations, usually 0.1%.

It is administered by intramuscular injection in doses of 40 to 100 milligrams, by intra-articular injection in doses of 2.5 to 15 milligrams, and by intradermal injection in doses of 2 to 3 milligrams in the treatment of inflammatory conditions.

Undesirable effects; Precautions and contra-indications. As for Cortisone Acetate.

Veterinary uses. Triamcinolone acetonide is a glucocorticoid used to reduce allergic and inflammatory reactions especially of the skin, muscle, and skeletal system. The usual dose as a sustained release preparation by subcutaneous or intramuscular injection is up to 40 micrograms per kilogram body-weight for horses and cattle and up to 200 micrograms per kilogram body-weight for dogs and cats. Triamcinolone acetonide is also administered by intra-articular injection, the dose depending on the animal and the response required, usually 5 to 20 milligrams for horses and 1 to 3 milligrams for dogs and cats.

Preparations

TRIAMCINOLONE CREAM (*Syn.* Triamcinolone Acetonide Cream): a dispersion of triamcinolone acetonide in a suitable water-miscible basis containing a mixture of methyl hydroxybenzoate and propyl hydroxybenzoate as the preservative system. It may also contain potassium sorbate.

When a strength less than that available from a manufacturer is prescribed, it may be diluted, taking hygienic precautions, with aqueous cream. The diluted cream must be freshly prepared.

Available as a cream containing 0.1% of triamcinolone acetonide.

A standard for this cream is given in the British Pharmaceutical Codex 1973

Containers, Labelling, and *Storage:* see the entry on Creams for general information on containers, labelling, and storage.

Advice for patients: the cream should be applied sparingly to the affected area.

TRIAMCINOLONE ACETONIDE INJECTION: a sterile suspension of triamcinolone acetonide, in very fine particles, with suitable dispersing agents, in water for injections, It is prepared by means of an aseptic technique. Available as an injection containing 2 mg of triamcinolone acetonide per ml, and in 5-ml vials containing 6 mg of triamcinolone acetonide per ml.

A standard for this injection is given in the British Pharmacopoeia (Veterinary)

Containers and *Labelling:* see the entry on Injections for general information on containers and labelling.

Storage: it should be stored at a temperature between 10° and 35°, protected from light.

TRIAMCINOLONE LOTION (*Syn.* Triamcinolone Acetonide Lotion): a dispersion of triamcinolone acetonide in a suitable lotion basis.

When a strength less than that available from a manufacturer is prescribed, it may be diluted, taking hygienic precautions, with a 3% solution of sodium carboxymethylcellulose (medium-viscosity grade) in water for preparations containing 0.2% of methyl hydroxybenzoate and 0.02% of propyl hydroxybenzoate. The diluted lotion must be freshly prepared.

Available as a lotion containing 0.1% of triamcinolone acetonide.

A standard for this lotion is given in the British Pharmaceutical Codex 1973
Containers and *Labelling:* see the entry on Lotions for general information on containers and labelling.
Advice for patients: the lotion should be applied sparingly to the affected area.

TRIAMCINOLONE OINTMENT: a dispersion of triamcinolone acetonide in a suitable anhydrous greasy basis.
When a strength less than that available from a manufacturer is prescribed, it may be diluted with a basis consisting of 1 part of wool fat and 9 parts of white soft paraffin.
Available as an ointment containing 0.1% of triamcinolone acetonide.
A standard for this ointment is given in the British Pharmaceutical Codex 1973
Containers and *Labelling:* see the entry on Ointments for general information on containers and labelling.
Advice for patients: the ointment should be applied sparingly to the affected area.

TRIAMCINOLONE DENTAL PASTE: a dispersion of triamcinolone acetonide in an adhesive gelatinous paste for application to oral surfaces.
Available as a dental paste containing 0.1% of triamcinolone acetonide.
A standard for this paste is given in the British Pharmaceutical Codex 1973
Containers and *Storage:* see the entry on Pastes for general information on containers and storage. It may be packed in small collapsible tubes.
Advice for patients: the paste should be applied without friction to the lesion after meals and at night and left to absorb moisture for 15 to 30 seconds. It may be applied on the tip of the finger or with the aid of an orange stick.

OTHER PREPARATIONS available include an APPLICATION containing triamcinolone acetonide 0.025% with chlortetracycline hydrochloride 1% in an aerosol pack, an application containing triamcinolone acetonide 4.95 mg with halquinol 31.2 mg in 75 g in an aerosol pack; a CREAM containing triamcinolone acetonide 0.025% with halquinol 0.75%, a cream containing triamcinolone acetonide 1 mg with chlortetracycline hydrochloride. 30 mg per g, a cream containing triamcinolone acetonide 1 mg with nystatin 100000 units per g; EAR-DROPS containing triamcinolone acetonide 0.025% with halquinol 0.75% in 0.3-ml single-dose units (capsules); an INJECTION containing triamcinolone acetonide 10 mg per ml in 5-ml vials, an injection containing triamcinolone acetonide 40 mg per ml in 1- and 2-ml disposable syringes; an OINTMENT containing triamcinolone acetonide 0.025% with halquinol 0.75%, an ointment containing triamcinolone acetonide 1 mg with chlortetracycline hydrochloride 30 mg per g, and an ointment containing triamcinolone acetonide 1 mg with nystatin 100000 units per g; a SOLUTION containing triamcinolone acetonide 0.2% with salicylic acid 2%; and a SPRAY containing triamcinolone acetonide 3.3 mg in 50 g.

OTHER VETERINARY PREPARATIONS available include an APPLICATION containing triamcinolone acetonide 1.65 mg with halquinol 10.4 mg in 25 g in an aerosol pack; and a CREAM containing triamcinolone acetonide 0.025% with halquinol 0.75%.

Triamterene

2,4,7-Triamino-6-phenylpteridine

$C_{12}H_{11}N_7 = 253.3$

OTHER NAMES: *Dytac*®
Dytide® (with benzthiazide); *Dyazide*® (with hydrochlorothiazide)

A standard is given in the British Pharmacopoeia 1973

Description. An odourless yellow crystalline powder which is tasteless at first becoming slightly bitter.

Solubility. Soluble, at 20°, in 1000 parts of water, in 3000 parts of alcohol, and in 4000 parts of chloroform; practically insoluble in ether.

Dissociation constant. pK_a 6.2.

Identification. TEST. Acidified solutions exhibit an intense bluish fluorescence.

ULTRAVIOLET ABSORPTION. In 0.1N hydrochloric acid, maxima at 228 nm (E1%, 1cm = 1618) and 360 nm (E1%, 1cm = 826); in 0.1N sodium hydroxide, maxima at 232 nm (E1%, 1cm = 1633), 270 nm (E1%, 1cm = 550), and 370 nm (E1%, 1cm = 741).

INFRA-RED ABSORPTION. Major peaks at 1355, 1424, 1536, 1574, 1584, and 1610 cm⁻¹ (see Appendix 2a: Infra-red Spectra).

THIN-LAYER CHROMATOGRAPHY. See under Thin-layer Chromatography, System 6.

Metabolism. ABSORPTION. Irregularly absorbed after oral administration; tablets appear to be better absorbed than capsules.

DISTRIBUTION. Widely distributed throughout the body; *protein binding*, about 65% bound to plasma proteins.

EXCRETION. About 10 to 90% of a dose is excreted in the urine in 24 hours.

FURTHER INFORMATION. Distribution and pharmacokinetics in rats—S. T. Kau and B. V. R. Sastry, *J. pharm. Sci.*, 1977, **66**, 53; diuretic effect and elimination—J. B. Lassen and O. E. Nielsen, *Acta pharmac. tox.*, 1963, **20**, 309; effectiveness of tablet and capsule formulations —P. J. Tannenbaum *et al.*, *Clin. Pharmac. Ther.*, 1968, **9**, 598.

Actions and uses. Triamterene is a potassium-sparing diuretic which exerts its effect directly on the distal part of the distal tubule. It increases sodium, chloride, and, to a lesser extent, bicarbonate excretion and thereby increases water diuresis. It is a weaker diuretic than the thiazides and it causes potassium retention rather than loss.
It is active when given by mouth, diuresis beginning after about 2 hours and reaching a peak level after about 4 to 8 hours; occasionally the maximum effect is not obtained until after 2 or 3 days' treatment.
Triamterene is used for the treatment of oedema, especially if due to corticosteroid treatment of secondary hyperaldosteronism. In conjunction with other diuretics it may be useful in patients who have become refractory to treatment. It does not activate latent diabetes mellitus and may be used in place of thiazide diuretics for diabetic patients.

Triamterene may be administered in doses of 100 milligrams, once or twice daily after meals. Maintenance doses may be administered on alternate days, with a thiazide diuretic on the days when triamterene is omitted, to prevent a rise in blood urea which may occur with prolonged daily dosage.

Undesirable effects. Triamterene may give rise to nausea, vomiting, mild diarrhoea, dryness of the mouth, headache, and muscle weakness; rashes may rarely occur.

Precautions. Triamterene may cause electrolyte imbalance and nitrogen retention. Periodic estimation of potassium and urea-nitrogen blood levels should be undertaken.

Preparations

TRIAMTERENE CAPSULES: consisting of triamterene, in powder, which may be mixed with a suitable inert diluent, enclosed in a hard capsule. The capsule shells may be coloured. Available as capsules containing 50 mg of triamterene.
A standard for these capsules is given in the British Pharmacopoeia 1973
Containers and Storage: see the entry on Capsules for general information on containers and storage.
Advice for patients: the capsules should preferably be taken after meals and daily doses preferably taken in the morning. Treatment should not be discontinued without the advice of the prescriber. A bluish colour may be imparted to the urine.

OTHER PREPARATIONS available include CAPSULES containing triamterene 50 mg with benzthiazide 25 mg; and TABLETS containing triamterene 50 mg with hydrochlorothiazide 25 mg.

Trichinosis

Trichinosis is an infection caused by *Trichinella spiralis*, a small roundworm 1 to 3 mm in length which inhabits the intestine. It produces larvae which invade the body and lodge in skeletal muscle. Infection is acquired by eating undercooked infected pork. The larvae from the pork mature and copulate in the jejunum. The mature adult produces larvae which burrow through the intestinal wall and are carried via the lymphatics and portal blood streams to skeletal muscle where they form cysts. Larvae which are carried elsewhere die and cause a foreign-body necrosis, with fever, malaise, periorbital oedema, severe headache, and photophobia. In addition they may cause signs and symptoms relating to the site at which the larvae have lodged, for example focal neurological signs.
If infection with *Trichinella spiralis* is suspected in the intestinal stage, piperazine may be used as treatment. In the later stages trichinosis may be treated with thiabendazole.

Trichloroacetic Acid

$CCl_3 . CO_2H = 163.4$

OTHER NAMES: Acidum Trichloraceticum; Trichloracetic Acid

A standard is given in the European Pharmacopoeia Vol. III

Description. Colourless very deliquescent crystals or crystalline masses with a slight characteristic pungent odour. It is very acid and corrosive.

Solubility. Soluble, at 20°, in about 0.1 part of water; soluble in alcohol and in ether.

Melting-point. About 56°.

Storage. It should be stored in airtight containers.

Actions and uses. Liquefied trichloroacetic acid, prepared by the addition of 10% by weight of water, is applied externally in the treatment of warts. A 10% aqueous solution has been used for application to corneal warts.

Trichloroethylene

$CHCl:CCl_2 = 131.4$

OTHER NAMES: Trichlorethylenum; *Trilene®*

A standard is given in the European Pharmacopoeia Vol. III

Trichloroethylene contains 0.01% w/w of thymol as a preservative; it may also contain not more than 0.001% w/w of a suitable blue colouring matter to distinguish it, when used for anaesthetic purposes, from chloroform, which it closely resembles in physical characteristics.

Description. A colourless or pale blue, transparent, mobile liquid with a characteristic odour resembling that of chloroform.

Solubility. Very slightly soluble in water; miscible with dehydrated alcohol, with ether, with chloroform, and with fixed and volatile oils.

Weight per ml. At 20°, 1.460 to 1.466 g.

Boiling-point. About 87°.

Stability. It is stable in the presence of moisture but undergoes decomposition on exposure to bright light in the presence of air.

Storage. It should be stored in airtight containers, in a cool place, protected from light.

Identification. TEST. It complies with the test described under Tetrachloroethylene (distinction from chloroform and from carbon tetrachloride).

Determination in body fluids. ULTRAVIOLET SPECTROPHOTOMETRY. In blood or urine—R. Bonnichsen and A. C. Maehly, *J. forens. Sci.*, 1966, **11**, 414.

INFRA-RED ABSORPTION. In blood—M. Feldstein, *J. forens. Sci.*, 1965, **10**, 207.

Metabolism. ABSORPTION. Well absorbed on inhalation.

BLOOD CONCENTRATION. During the administration of a 1% vapour, blood concentrations of 30 to 90 μg/ml are attained by 30 minutes.

DISTRIBUTION. Crosses the placenta.

METABOLIC REACTIONS. Metabolised to chloral hydrate, trichloroethanol, trichloroacetic acid, and to glucuronic acid conjugates; monochloroacetic acid is also a metabolite.

EXCRETION. Slowly excreted in the urine as metabolites; the major part of the dose is exhaled by the lungs.

FURTHER INFORMATION. Chloral hydrate as a transient metabolite of trichloroethylene—W. J. Cole *et al.*, *J. Pharm. Pharmac.*, 1975, **27**, 167; blood concentrations during major surgery—F. N. Prior, *Anaesthesia*, 1972, **27**, 379.

Actions and uses. Trichloroethylene is the least volatile of the liquid anaesthetics and is less potent than either chloroform or ether. It is non-irritant to mucous membranes and is non-inflammable when used with air or oxygen. It induces anaesthesia smoothly and rapidly.

Its main disadvantage is that it does not produce full muscular relaxation or deep anaesthesia and is therefore unsuitable for long operations and for those requiring complete relaxation. It may also increase the respiratory rate, inducing short jerky inspirations, and, like chloroform, may produce cardiac irregularities, such as auricular or ventricular extrasystoles.

Trichloroethylene is used by inhalation for analgesia in obstetrics, approximately 0.5% in air being recommended for this purpose; 1 millilitre is usually administered. It has been used by inhalation to alleviate the pain of trigeminal neuralgia.

Trichloroethylene has also been used to produce light anaesthesia, the vapour being mixed with air or nitrous oxide and oxygen. Owing to its low volatility it is difficult to administer on an open mask. For the induction of anaesthesia it may be given by means of suitable inhalers, some of which are for self-administration in obstetrics, by drawing air over the liquid in a bottle, or by means of a semi-closed apparatus.

In less pure form, trichloroethylene is used commercially in the dry-cleaning industry, for the degreasing of metals, and for oil and fat extraction. Improper working conditions may give rise to acute poisoning or narcosis which may be fatal, although temporary unconsciousness is a more common manifestation.

Precautions. Trichloroethylene must never be used in a closed-circuit apparatus, because the heat produced by the action of carbon dioxide and water vapour on the soda lime causes it to react with the soda lime to form dichloroacetylene, which may cause cranial palsies and may even be lethal. Adrenaline should never be administered at the same time as trichloroethylene owing to the danger of ventricular fibrillation.

Prolonged exposure to trichloroethylene vapour may cause cardiac irregularities and degenerative changes in the nervous system, particularly in the sensory fibres of the first and fifth cranial nerves. The maximum allowable concentration for an 8-hour daily exposure is 100 parts per million by volume.

Dependence. Dependence of the barbiturate–alcohol type, as described under Drug Dependence, may occur in persons who habitually inhale small quantities of trichloroethylene vapour.

Poisoning. Industrial poisoning by trichloroethylene is treated by removal of the patient from the source of the vapour, by artificial respiration, and by the administration of oxygen.

Trichlorofluoromethane

$CCl_3F = 137.4$

OTHER NAMES: *Arcton 11*®; Fluorotrichloromethane; *Isceon 11*®; Propellent 11; Refrigerant 11
Coolspray®, *Eleys Local Anaesthetic*®, *PR Spray*®, and *Skefron*® (all with dichlorodifluoromethane)

A standard is given in the British Pharmaceutical Codex 1973

Trichlorofluoromethane is liquid at ordinary temperatures, but because of its low boiling-point it is supplied as a liquefied gas under pressure in suitable metal containers.

Description. A clear, colourless, non-inflammable, volatile liquid with a faint, ethereal odour.

Solubility. In the liquid state: immiscible with water; miscible with dehydrated alcohol.

Weight per ml. At $-35°$, about 1.61 g; at 15°, about 1.50 g.

Boiling-point. About 23.7°.

Storage. It should be stored in suitable metal containers, in a cool place, away from any fire risk.

Metabolism. BLOOD CONCENTRATION. After administration by aerosol inhaler in metered doses of 25 mg, peak arterial concentrations of 0.5 to 4.5 and 0.2 to 2.0 $\mu g/ml$ are attained in 10 to 20 seconds after 2 and 1 metered doses respectively.

HALF-LIFE. In dogs, after an intravenous dose, the decline in blood concentration falls in a triphasic manner with half-lives of 3.2, 16, and 93 minutes for the individual phases.

DISTRIBUTION. In dogs, accumulates upon repeated doses; volume of distribution, approximately 6 times body-weight.

EXCRETION. Most of a dose is recovered in exhaled air within 1 hour.

FURTHER INFORMATION. Biotransformation and elimination in beagles—D. A. Blake and G. W. Mergner, *Toxic. appl. Pharmac.*, 1974, **30**, 396; blood concentrations in asthmatics from inhalation of aerosols—C. T. Dollery *et al.*, *Clin. Pharmac. Ther.*, 1974, **15**, 59 and J. W. Paterson *et al.*, *Lancet*, ii/1971, 565; pharmacokinetics in dogs—S. Niazi and W. L. Chiou, *J. pharm. Sci.*, 1975, **64**, 763.

Uses. Trichlorofluoromethane is used as a refrigerant and aerosol propellent, as described in the entry on Propellents.

Preparations

Preparations available include an APPLICATION containing trichlorofluoromethane with dichlorodifluoromethane in equal volumes, an application containing trichlorofluoromethane 77.5% with dichlorodifluoromethane 22.5%, and an application containing trichlorofluoromethane 85% with dichlorodifluoromethane 15% (all in aerosol packs).

Trichomoniasis

Trichomoniasis is an infection of the genital tract with the flagellate *Trichomonas vaginalis*. In males the infection is often symptomless, but may be characterised by a low-grade urethritis.

In females there may be thin, yellow, frothy discharge, inflammation of the vaginal wall, vulvitis, and painful micturition. The organism is recognised by microscopy of the discharge.

The infection may be treated orally with metronidazole or other 5-nitroimidazoles. The consort should be treated concurrently to prevent reinfection. If oral administration is contra-indicated pessaries containing acetarsol or mercurials may be used.

Trichuriasis

Trichuriasis is a large-bowel infection caused by the whipworm *Trichuris trichiura*, which is 30 to 50 mm long. Infection in man is acquired from polluted water or vegetables. The ova hatch in the small intestine and the worms fix themselves to the bowel wall by inserting their heads deep into the mucosa. They may cause vague abdominal pain and diarrhoea.

Another whipworm (common in the Philippines), *Capillaria philippinensis* which is a few mm long, causes severe malabsorption syndrome.

All whipworm infections may be treated with thiabendazole.

Triclofos Sodium

Sodium hydrogen 2,2,2-trichloroethyl phosphate

$$CCl_3 \cdot CH_2 \cdot O \cdot \overset{\displaystyle O}{\underset{\displaystyle OH}{\overset{\|}{\underset{|}{P}}} \cdot ONa}$$

$C_2H_3Cl_3NaO_4P = 251.4$

OTHER NAME: *Tricloryl®*

A standard is given in the British Pharmacopoeia 1973

Description. An odourless white hygroscopic powder with a saline taste.

Solubility. Soluble, at 20°, in 2 parts of water and in 250 parts of alcohol; very slightly soluble in ether.

Acidity. A 2% solution has a pH of 3 to 4.5.

Moisture content. Not more than 5%, determined by drying at 100° *in vacuo.*

Incompatibility. Aqueous solutions are incompatible with salts of heavy metals, calcium, magnesium, and alkaloids.

Storage. It should be stored in airtight containers.

Identification. TESTS. 1. Mix about 50 mg with 1 ml of sulphuric acid (50% v/v) and 1 ml of a 5% solution of potassium permanganate, heat in a water-bath for 5 minutes, add 7 ml of water and decolorise the solution with 1 ml of a 5% solution of oxalic acid; to 1 ml of the solution add 1 ml of pyridine and 1 ml of *sodium hydroxide solution* and heat in a water-bath for 1 minute with continuous stirring; a pink colour is produced in the pyridine layer.
2. Dissolve about 100 mg in 5 ml of water and add 2 ml of *silver nitrate solution*; a white precipitate, which is soluble in *dilute ammonia solution* and in *dilute nitric acid*, is produced.

INFRA-RED ABSORPTION. Major peaks at 709, 877, 926, 1099, 1124, and 1220 cm^{-1} (see Appendix 2b: Infra-red Spectra).

Metabolism. ABSORPTION. Rapidly hydrolysed in the stomach to trichloroethanol which is readily absorbed.

BLOOD CONCENTRATION. After an oral dose of 22 mg/kg, respective peak plasma concentrations of trichloroethanol and trichloroethanol glucuronide of about 8 and about 1 μg/ml are obtained; no unchanged triclofos is detectable in plasma.

HALF-LIFE. The plasma half-life for trichloroethanol is about 8 hours and for trichloroacetic acid, about 67 hours.

DISTRIBUTION. *Protein binding*, for trichloroethanol, about 35% and for trichloroacetic acid, about 95% bound to plasma proteins.

METABOLIC REACTIONS. Converted to trichloroethanol, which is conjugated with glucuronic acid, and also converted to trichloroacetic acid.

EXCRETION. About 12% of a dose is excreted as metabolites in the urine in 24 hours; possibly excreted as metabolites in bile.

FURTHER INFORMATION. Metabolism of chloral hydrate and triclofos—E. M. Sellers *et al., Clin. Pharmac. Ther.,* 1973, **14**, 147.

Actions and uses. Triclofos sodium has sedative and hypnotic actions similar to those of dichloralphenazone and other chloral compounds.

It is suitable for use as a sedative in domiciliary midwifery. The sedative dose is 500 milligrams once or twice daily and the hypnotic dose is 1 to 2 grams 30 minutes before bedtime. Doses should be taken with fluid since chloral is a gastric irritant.

The usual hypnotic dose for children up to 1 year is 100 to 250 milligrams, 1 to 5 years 250 to 500 milligrams, and 6 to 12 years 0.5 to 1 gram. For sedation children up to 1 year may be given doses of 100 milligrams, 1 to 5 years 250 milligrams, and 6 to 12 years 500 milligrams.

Undesirable effects. Flatulence, abdominal distension, nausea, headache, and rashes may rarely occur.

Dependence. It may give rise to dependence of the barbiturate–alcohol type, as described under Drug Dependence, and it may also enhance the effects of alcohol.

Drug interactions. It may increase the difficulty in controlling oral anticoagulant therapy by displacing the anticoagulants from binding sites.

Preparations

TRICLOFOS ELIXIR (*Syn.* Triclofos Syrup): a solution of triclofos sodium in a suitable coloured flavoured vehicle.

When a dose less than or not a multiple of 5 ml is prescribed, the elixir may be diluted, as described in the entry on Elixirs, with syrup. The diluted elixir must be freshly prepared.

Available as an elixir containing 500 mg of triclofos sodium in 5 ml.

A standard for this elixir is given in the British Pharmaceutical Codex 1973

Containers and *Labelling:* see the entry on Elixirs for general information on containers and labelling.

Storage: it should be stored in a cool place.

Advice for patients: hypnotic doses should be taken 30 minutes before bedtime. The elixir may cause drowsiness on the following day; persons affected should not drive or operate machinery. Alcohol should be avoided.

TRICLOFOS TABLETS: available as tablets containing 500 mg of triclofos sodium; they are film coated; the coat may be coloured.

A standard for these tablets is given in the British Pharmacopoeia 1973

Containers and *Storage:* see the entry on Tablets for general information on containers and storage. Containers should be airtight.

Advice for patients: the tablets should be swallowed whole with water. See also under Triclofos Elixir (above).

Triethanolamine

A variable mixture of bases consisting mainly of tri(2-hydroxyethyl)amine, $(CH_2OH \cdot CH_2)_3N$, together with di(2-hydroxyethyl)amine and smaller amounts of 2-hydroxyethylamine.

A standard is given in the British Pharmaceutical Codex 1973

Triethanolamine forms crystalline salts with mineral

acids, the hydrochloride and the hydriodide being sparingly soluble in alcohol. With the higher fatty or olefinic acids, it forms salts which are soluble in water and have the general characters of soaps.

Description. An odourless, clear, colourless or slightly yellow, hygroscopic liquid. It volatilises slowly at 100°.

Solubility. Miscible with water and with alcohol; very slightly soluble in ether.

Weight per ml. At 20°, 1.120 to 1.130 g.

Refractive index. At 20°, 1.482 to 1.485.

Dissociation constant. pK_a 7.8 (25°).

Storage. It should be stored in airtight containers.

Uses. Triethanolamine is chiefly used in combination with fatty acids such as stearic and oleic acids; equimolecular proportions of base and fatty acid form a soap which may be used as an emulsifying agent to produce fine-grained stable emulsions of the oil-in-water type with a pH of about 8. The emulsion is conveniently formed by adding, with constant stirring, a warm solution of the acid and other oil-soluble ingredients in the oil phase, to an aqueous solution of the triethanolamine and other water-soluble ingredients warmed to the same temperature; violent stirring should be avoided, as it may produce a persistent froth.

Although emulsions made with triethanolamine soaps are slightly more stable than those prepared with alkali soaps, they too break down in the presence of acids and high concentrations of ionisable salts.

For the emulsification of fixed oils, triethanolamine equal to 2 to 4% of the weight of oil, with 2 to 5 times as much fatty acid, is adequate; for liquid paraffin, the amount of triethanolamine should be increased to about 5% of the weight of liquid paraffin, with a proportionate increase in the weight of fatty acid.

Triethanolamine can also be used to neutralise carboxyvinyl polymers in the formation of aqueous gels containing glycerol or propylene glycol.

Preparations made with triethanolamine soaps are liable to darken on exposure to light.

Trifluomeprazine Maleate

10-(3-Dimethylamino-2-methylpropyl)-2-trifluoromethylphenothiazine hydrogen maleate

$C_{19}H_{21}F_3N_2S,C_4H_4O_4 = 482.5$

OTHER NAME: *Nortran*®

A standard is given in the British Pharmacopoeia (Veterinary)

Description. An odourless white crystalline powder.

Solubility. Very slightly soluble in water; soluble, at 20°, in 25 parts of alcohol and of chloroform; practically insoluble in ether.

Storage. It should be protected from light.

Identification. TESTS. 1. Dissolve about 20 mg in 2 ml of sulphuric acid; a pink to orange colour is produced. 2. Mix about 300 mg with 8 ml of water and 2 ml of *sodium hydroxide solution*, shake, add 10 ml of ether, shake, and allow to separate; to the aqueous layer add 2 ml of *bromine solution AsT*, warm in a water-bath for 10 minutes, boil, cool, and add 0.5 ml of the solution to a solution of 10 mg of resorcinol in 3 ml of sulphuric acid and heat in a water-bath for 15 minutes; a blue-black colour is produced.

MELTING-POINT. About 178°.

ULTRAVIOLET ABSORPTION. In 0.2N hydrochloric acid, maximum at 255 nm (E1%, 1cm = 600), and a less well-defined maximum at 305 nm.

Veterinary uses. Trifluomeprazine maleate is used as a tranquilliser and motion sickness remedy in dogs and cats. The usual dose is 0.5 to 2 milligrams per kilogram body-weight 2 to 4 times daily.

Preparation

TRIFLUOMEPRAZINE TABLETS: available as tablets containing trifluomeprazine maleate equivalent to 10 mg of trifluomeprazine.

A standard for these tablets is given in the British Pharmacopoeia (Veterinary)

Containers and *Storage:* see the entry on Tablets for general information on containers and storage. Containers should be airtight and light resistant.

Labelling: the label on the container should state the amount of the medicament as the equivalent of trifluomeprazine.

Trifluoperazine Hydrochloride

10-[3-(4-Methylpiperazin-1-yl)propyl]-2-trifluoromethylphenothiazine dihydrochloride

$C_{21}H_{26}Cl_2F_3N_3S = 480.4$

OTHER NAMES: *Stelazine*®
Amylozine® (with amylobarbitone); *Steladex*® (with dexamphetamine sulphate); *Stelabid*® (with isopropamide iodide); *Parstelin*® (with tranylcypromine sulphate)

A standard is given in the British Pharmacopoeia 1973

Description. An odourless, hygroscopic, white to pale yellow, crystalline powder with a bitter taste.

Solubility. Soluble, at 20°, in 2 parts of water; very slightly soluble in alcohol and in isopropyl alcohol; practically insoluble in ether.

Acidity. A 5% solution has a pH of 1.7 to 2.6.

Moisture content. Not more than 1%, determined by drying at 60° *in vacuo*.

Dissociation constant. pK_a 8.1 (24°).

Stability. In aqueous solution it is readily oxidised by atmospheric oxygen.

Sterilisation. Solutions for injection are sterilised by heating in an autoclave in an atmosphere of nitrogen or other suitable gas or by filtration.

Storage. It should be stored in airtight containers, protected from light.

Identification. TEST. Dissolve about 5 mg in 2 ml of sulphuric acid and allow to stand for 5 minutes; an orange colour is produced.

MELTING-POINT. About 240°.

ULTRAVIOLET ABSORPTION. In 0.1N hydrochloric acid, maxima at 257 nm (E1%, 1cm = 594) and 309 nm (E1%, 1cm = 77); in 0.1N sodium hydroxide, maximum at 258 nm (E1%, 1cm = 541).

INFRA-RED ABSORPTION. Major peaks at 1081, 1114, 1145, 1316, 1344, and 1426 cm⁻¹ (see Appendix 2a: Infra-red Spectra).

Determination in body fluids. SPECTROFLUORIMETRY. In urine: trifluoperazine and its sulphoxide—N. R. West *et al.*, *J. pharm. Sci.*, 1974, **63**, 417.

Metabolism. DISTRIBUTION. In rats, widely distributed with high concentrations appearing in the lungs, kidneys, and liver.

METABOLIC REACTIONS. In rats, ring cleavage, N-dealkylation, and sulphoxidation.

EXCRETION. In rats, about 10% of an intraperitoneal dose is excreted in the urine as the sulphoxide.

FURTHER INFORMATION. Tissue metabolites in rats—U. Breyer *et al.*, *J. pharm. Sci.*, 1974, **63**, 1842 and H. J. Gaertner *et al.*, *Drug Met. Disp.*, 1975, **3**, 437; nonpolar metabolites in rats—C. L. Huang and K. G. Bhansali, *J. pharm. Sci.*, 1968, **57**, 1511; tissue distribution in rats—J. E. Wallace and J. D. Biggs, *J. pharm. Sci.*, 1971, **60**, 1346.

Actions and uses. Trifluoperazine has the actions and uses described under Chlorpromazine Hydrochloride but it is effective in much smaller doses and may be effective in patients who do not respond to chlorpromazine. It acts rapidly in blocking conditioned responses and as an anti-emetic.

In psychotic patients, trifluoperazine may be stimulating rather than sedating, and the usual effective daily dosage by mouth is the equivalent of 15 to 30 milligrams of trifluoperazine, although higher dosage may be necessary. The equivalent of up to 5 milligrams daily may be given by intramuscular injection. In the treatment of psychoneurosis and nausea and vomiting, the equivalent of 2 to 4 milligrams daily is usually sufficient; 6 milligrams daily by mouth or 3 milligrams daily by intramuscular injection should not be exceeded.

Trifluoperazine is unlikely to produce hypotension or hypothermia or to enhance the actions of narcotics and analgesics and is not used for these purposes.

Undesirable effects. It may cause drowsiness, dizziness, and, occasionally, stimulation; it rarely gives rise to jaundice, blood dyscrasias, or galactorrhoea. High dosage may cause extrapyramidal symptoms, dystonias, and akathisia, particularly in children.

Poisoning. The procedure as described under Fluphenazine Hydrochloride should be followed. If necessary, hypotension may be treated by the intravenous infusion of noradrenaline.

Preparations

TRIFLUOPERAZINE TABLETS: available as tablets containing trifluoperazine hydrochloride equivalent to 1 and 5 mg of trifluoperazine; they are sugar coated; the coat may be coloured.

A standard for these tablets is given in the British Pharmacopoeia 1973

Containers and *Storage:* see the entry on Tablets for general information on containers and storage. Containers should be airtight.

Labelling: the label on the container should state the amount of the medicament as the equivalent amount of trifluoperazine.

Advice for patients: the tablets may cause drowsiness or occasionally affect mental concentration; persons affected should not drive or operate machinery. Alcohol should be avoided.

OTHER PREPARATIONS available include CAPSULES containing trifluoperazine hydrochloride equivalent to 2, 10, and 15 mg of trifluoperazine in slow-release formulations; capsules containing trifluoperazine hydrochloride equivalent to 2 mg of trifluoperazine with amylobarbitone 65 mg in a slow-release formulation; capsules containing trifluoperazine hydrochloride equivalent to 2 mg of trifluoperazine with dexamphetamine sulphate 10 mg in a slow-release formulation; an ELIXIR containing trifluoperazine hydrochloride equivalent to 1 mg of trifluoperazine in 5 ml, diluent syrup, life of diluted elixir 14 days; an elixir containing trifluoperazine hydrochloride equivalent to 1 mg of trifluoperazine with isopropamide iodide equivalent to 5 mg of isopropamide in 5 ml, diluent syrup, life of diluted elixir 14 days; an INJECTION containing trifluoperazine hydrochloride equivalent to 1 mg of trifluoperazine per ml in 1-, 2-, and 3-ml ampoules; a SOLUTION containing trifluoperazine hydrochloride equivalent to 10 mg of trifluoperazine per ml, diluents water for preparations and syrup, life of diluted solution 1 week and 3 months respectively (water containing a suitable preservative such as sodium benzoate 0.05% will permit storage of diluted solution for longer than 1 week); TABLETS containing trifluoperazine hydrochloride equivalent to 1 mg of trifluoperazine with isopropamide iodide equivalent to 5 mg of isopropamide; tablets containing trifluoperazine hydrochloride equivalent to 2 mg of trifluoperazine with isopropamide iodide equivalent to 7.5 mg of isopropamide; and tablets containing trifluoperazine hydrochloride equivalent to 1 mg of trifluoperazine with tranylcypromine sulphate equivalent to 10 mg of tranylcypromine.

Trimeprazine Tartrate

10 - (3 - Dimethylamino - 2 - methylpropyl) phenothiazine tartrate

$C_{40}H_{50}N_4O_6S_2 = 747.0$

OTHER NAMES: Alimemazine Tartrate; *Vallergan®*

A standard is given in the British Pharmacopoeia Addendum 1977

Description. An odourless, white or slightly cream-coloured powder; it darkens on exposure to light.

Solubility. Soluble, at 20°, in 4 parts of water, in 30 parts of alcohol, and in 4 parts of chloroform; very slightly soluble in ether.

Acidity. A 2% solution has a pH of 5 to 6.5.

Sterilisation. Solutions for injection are sterilised by heating in an autoclave in an atmosphere of nitrogen or other suitable gas.

Storage. It should be protected from light.

Identification. TESTS. 1. Dissolve about 5 mg in 2 ml of sulphuric acid and allow to stand for 5 minutes; a red colour is produced.
2. Dissolve about 500 mg in 10 ml of water and add 1 ml of nitric acid; a red colour is produced together with a white precipitate which rapidly redissolves. Warm the solution; the colour changes suddenly to dark green.
3. Dissolve about 500 mg in 5 ml of water, add 1.5 ml of *sodium hydroxide solution*, extract with two 10-ml portions of anaesthetic ether and to 2 ml of the aqueous layer add sufficient acetic acid to make it acid to litmus paper followed by 1 ml of *ammonium vanadate solution*; an orange-red colour is produced.

MELTING-POINT. About 161°.

ULTRAVIOLET ABSORPTION. In 0.1N hydrochloric acid, maxima at 252 nm (E1%, 1cm = 743) and 306 nm (E1%, 1cm = 104); in alcohol (95%), maxima at 256 nm (E1%, 1cm = 860) and 309 nm (E1%, 1cm = 128).

THIN-LAYER CHROMATOGRAPHY. See under Thin-layer Chromatography, Systems 4 and 9.

Metabolism. ABSORPTION. Readily absorbed after oral administration.

BLOOD CONCENTRATION. After oral doses of 5 and 15 mg, respective peak serum concentrations of about 0.1 and 0.4 μg/ml are attained in 3 to 6 hours for unchanged drug plus metabolites; after an oral dose of 15 mg as a sustained release preparation, peak serum concentrations of about 0.2 μg/ml are attained after about 6 hours for drug plus metabolites.

DISTRIBUTION. Widely distributed throughout the body. Small quantities are secreted in the milk.

EXCRETION. 70% of an oral dose is excreted in the urine in 48 hours.

FURTHER INFORMATION. Effect of sustained release on absorption and excretion—P. C. Johnson and Y. F. Masters, *J. Lab. clin. Med.*, 1962, **59**, 993.

Actions and uses. Trimeprazine has an antihistamine action resembling that of promethazine hydrochloride and an action on the central nervous system resembling that of chlorpromazine hydrochloride. Its most marked effect, however, is an antipruritic action.
For the relief of pruritus, trimeprazine tartrate is given by mouth, the usual daily dosage for an adult being 10 to 40 milligrams and for a child 7.5 to 25 milligrams, divided into 3 or 4 doses. It is also used for pre-operative medication of children, 2 to 5 milligrams per kilogram body-weight being given by mouth approximately one hour before operation. It may also be given for pre-operative medication by deep intramuscular injection in doses of 600 to 900 micrograms per kilogram body-weight about 1 to 2 hours before operation.

Undesirable effects. Trimeprazine frequently produces drowsiness; if this is pronounced, the dosage should be reduced or another antihistamine should be substituted. Other undesirable effects seen occasionally are dizziness, dryness of the mouth, allergic skin reactions and, rarely, agranulocytosis.

Poisoning. In acute poisoning the procedure as described under Chlorpromazine Hydrochloride should be adopted.

Veterinary uses. Trimeprazine tartrate is used as a tranquilliser and antihistamine in dogs and cats. The usual dose by mouth is 2 to 4 milligrams per kilogram body-weight as a tranquilliser or 1 milligram per kilogram body-weight as an antihistamine 3 or 4 times daily.

Preparations

PAEDIATRIC TRIMEPRAZINE ELIXIR (*Syn.* Trimeprazine Syrup): a solution of trimeprazine tartrate in a suitable coloured flavoured vehicle. It contains 7.5 mg of trimeprazine tartrate in 5 ml.
When a dose less than or not a multiple of 5 ml is prescribed, the elixir may be diluted, as described in the entry on Elixirs, with syrup. The diluted elixir must be freshly prepared.
A standard for this elixir is given in the British Pharmaceutical Codex 1973
Containers and *Labelling:* see the entry on Elixirs for general information on containers and labelling.
Storage: it should be protected from light.
Advice for patients: the elixir may cause drowsiness.

STRONG PAEDIATRIC TRIMEPRAZINE ELIXIR (*Syn.* Strong Trimeprazine Syrup): a solution of trimeprazine tartrate in a suitable coloured flavoured vehicle. It contains 30 mg of trimeprazine tartrate in 5 ml.
A standard for this elixir is given in the British Pharmaceutical Codex 1973
Containers and *Labelling:* see the entry on Elixirs for general information on containers and labelling.
Storage: it should be protected from light.
Advice for patients: the elixir may cause drowsiness.

TRIMEPRAZINE INJECTION: a sterile solution of trimeprazine tartrate, with suitable stabilising agents, in water for injections free from carbon dioxide. It is distributed into ampoules, the air in the ampoules being replaced by nitrogen or other suitable gas, and the ampoules are sealed and sterilised by heating in an autoclave. Available in 2-ml ampoules containing 25 mg of trimeprazine tartrate per ml.
A standard for this injection is given in the British Pharmaceutical Codex 1973
Containers and *Labelling:* see the entry on Injections for general information on containers and labelling.
Storage: it should be protected from light.

TRIMEPRAZINE TABLETS (*Syn.* Trimeprazine Tartrate Tablets): may be prepared by moist granulation and compression as described in the entry on Tablets. Available as tablets containing 10 mg of trimeprazine tartrate; they may be sugar coated and the coat may be coloured; a sealing coat of polyvinyl acetate may be applied before the sugar coat.
A standard for these tablets is given in the British Pharmacopoeia Addendum 1977
Containers and *Storage:* see the entry on Tablets for general information on containers and storage. Containers should be airtight.
Advice for patients: the tablets may cause drowsiness; persons affected should not drive or operate machinery. Alcohol should be avoided.

Trimethoprim

5-(3,4,5-Trimethoxybenzyl)pyrimidine-2,4-diamine

$C_{14}H_{18}N_4O_3 = 290.3$

OTHER NAMES: *Coptin®*, Co-trimazine, and *Tribrissen®* (all with sulphadiazine); *Borgal®* and *Trivetrin®* (both with sulphadoxine); *Bactrim®*; Co-trimoxazole, and *Septrin®* (all with sulphamethoxazole)

A standard is given in the British Pharmacopoeia 1973

Description. An odourless white powder with a very bitter taste.

Solubility. Very slightly soluble in water; soluble, at 20°, in 300 parts of alcohol, in 55 parts of chloroform, and in 80 parts of methyl alcohol; practically insoluble in ether.

Moisture content. Not more than 1%, determined by drying at 100° *in vacuo*.

Dissociation constant. pK_a 7.2.

Identification. MELTING-POINT. About 200°.

ULTRAVIOLET ABSORPTION. In 0.1N sodium hydroxide, maximum at 287 nm (E1%, 1cm = 245).

INFRA-RED ABSORPTION. Major peaks at 1126, 1421, 1458, 1470, 1596, and 1630 cm^{-1} (see Appendix 2c: Infra-red Spectra).

Determination in body fluids. SPECTROFLUORIMETRY. In blood or urine—S. A. Kaplan *et al.*, *J. pharm. Sci.*, 1970, 59, 358.

THIN-LAYER CHROMATOGRAPHY. In plasma or urine—C. W. Sigel and M. E. Grace, *J. Chromat.*, 1973, 80, 111.

POLAROGRAPHY. In blood or urine—M. A. Brooks *et al.*, *Analyt. Chem.*, 1973, 45, 263.

Metabolism. ABSORPTION. Readily absorbed after oral administration.

BLOOD CONCENTRATION. After an oral dose of 200 mg, peak plasma concentrations of about 2 µg/ml are attained in 3 to 4 hours; during therapy with 50-mg doses administered 4 times daily, steady-state plasma concentrations of about 2 µg/ml are attained after 2 to 3 days.

HALF-LIFE. Plasma half-life, 11 to 17 hours which is reduced in children to 2.5 to 5 hours.

DISTRIBUTION. Widely distributed throughout the body; secreted in body fluids, such as saliva and vaginal fluid and crosses the placenta; tissue concentrations are higher than those in plasma whilst cerebrospinal fluid concentrations are about 50% of those in plasma; *protein binding*, 30 to 70% bound to plasma proteins.

METABOLIC REACTIONS. Oxidation of the methylene group to a hydroxymethyl group, *N*-oxidation to form an oxide, *O*-demethylation, hydroxylation, and conjugation with glucuronic acid or sulphate.

EXCRETION. About 40 to 75% of a dose is excreted in the urine in 24 hours; of the urinary excreted material, 50 to 80% is excreted unchanged; urinary excretion of trimethoprim is pH-dependent and is increased in acid urine; some of a dose is excreted in the bile and a small amount in the milk.

FURTHER INFORMATION. Trimethoprim: antibacterial activity and potentiation of sulphonamides—S. R. M. Bushby and G. H. Hitchings, *Br. J. Pharmac. Chemother.*, 1968, 33, 72; metabolites in rat, dog, and man—D. E. Schwartz *et al.*, *Arzneimittel-Forsch.*, 1970, 20, 1867; trimethoprim 3-oxide as a urinary metabolite—C. W. Sigel and D. A. Brent, *J. pharm. Sci.*, 1973, 62, 694; pharmacokinetics—J. M. T. Hamilton-Miller and W. Brumfitt, *J. antimicrob. Chemother.*, 1976, 2, 181 and S. A. Kaplan *et al.*, *J. pharm. Sci.*, 1970, 59, 358; diffusion into vaginal fluid—T. A. Stamey and M. Condy, *J. infect. Dis.*, 1975, 131, 261. Co-trimoxazole: effects of urinary pH and renal impairment—W. A. Craig and C. M. Kunin, *Ann. intern. Med.*, 1973, 78, 491; bioavailability—Y. Langlois *et al.*, *J. clin. Pharmac.*, 1972, 12, 196; A. S. E. Fowle, Aspects of the pharmacokinetic behaviour of trimethoprim and sulphamethoxazole, *Trimethoprim/Sulphamethoxazole in Bacterial Infections*, L. S. Bernstein and A. J. Salter (Eds), London, Churchill Livingstone, 1973, p. 63; maternal and transplacental kinetics—D. W. J. Reid *et al.*, *Can. med. Ass. J.*, 1975, 112, 67S; pharmacokinetics in children—C. M. Wilfert and L. J. Gutman, *Can. med. Ass. J.*, 1975, 112, 73S.

Actions and uses. Trimethoprim is an antibacterial agent which is active against approximately the same range of organisms as the antibacterial sulphonamides. It inhibits bacterial dihydrofolate reductases which utilise as substrate the product of a reaction sensitive to the sulphonamides.

Trimethoprim is used mainly in admixture with sulphamethoxazole—see under Sulphamethoxazole.

It is also used in conjunction with a sulphonamide in the treatment of malaria due to susceptible strains of *Plasmodium falciparum* that are resistant to chloroquine. For this purpose doses of 0.5 to 1.5 grams of trimethoprim and 0.75 to 1.5 grams of sulfametopyrazine may be given over a period of 24 hours, or 10 milligrams of trimethoprim per kilogram and 20 milligrams of sulfametopyrazine per kilogram body-weight may be given as a single dose. When these doses are given, antiplasmodial blood concentrations of sulfametopyrazine may be expected to persist for 5 to 7 days.

Undesirable effects. Nausea may follow the administration of high doses of trimethoprim.

Precautions and contra-indications. Although the affinity of trimethoprim for mammalian dihydrofolate reductase is very low, repeated haematological determinations are required during prolonged therapy.

The use of trimethoprim in early pregnancy is not recommended. It should be used with caution in nursing mothers.

Veterinary uses. Trimethoprim is used in conjunction with sulphadiazine or sulphadoxine as an antibacterial.

Preparations

CO-TRIMOXAZOLE INJECTION: a sterile solution of the sodium derivative of sulphamethoxazole and trimethoprim in dextrose injection or sodium chloride injection. It is prepared immediately before use by diluting strong sterile co-trimoxazole solution (see below) with 25 to 35 times its volume of dextrose injection or sodium chloride injection.

Dose: for a solution containing 400 mg of sulphamethoxazole and 80 mg of trimethoprim in 5 ml, by intravenous infusion, 10 ml diluted before administration with 250 ml of diluent twice daily or 15 ml diluted before administration with 500 ml of diluent, twice daily.

CO-TRIMOXAZOLE MIXTURE (*Syn.* Trimethoprim and Sulphamethoxazole Mixture): a suspension of sulphamethoxazole and trimethoprim in a suitable flavoured vehicle. It contains 400 mg of sulphamethoxazole and 80 mg of trimethoprim in 5 ml. When a dose less than or not a multiple of 5 ml is prescribed, the mixture may be diluted, as described in the entry on Mixtures, with syrup. The diluted mixture must be freshly prepared.

A standard for this mixture is given in the British Pharmaceutical Codex 1973

Containers and *Labelling:* see the entry on Mixtures for general information on containers and labelling.

Storage: it should be protected from light.

Dose: ADULT: 10 to 30 millilitres daily, divided into 2 or 3 doses.

Advice for patients: the mixture should be taken at regular intervals. The prescribed course should be completed. Adequate fluid intake should be maintained. Direct exposure to sunlight should be avoided during treatment.

CO-TRIMOXAZOLE TABLETS (*Syn.* Trimethoprim and Sulphamethoxazole Tablets): available as tablets containing 400 mg of sulphamethoxazole and 80 mg of trimethoprim, and as tablets containing 800 mg of sulphamethoxazole and 160 mg of trimethoprim; they may be film coated or sugar coated and the coat may be coloured; the tablets need not be circular in shape.

Paediatric co-trimoxazole tablets are described below.

A standard for these tablets is given in the British Pharmacopoeia Addendum 1978

Containers and *Storage:* see the entry on Tablets for general information on containers and storage. Containers should be airtight.

Labelling: the label on the container should state the amounts of the medicaments as the amounts of sulphamethoxazole and trimethoprim in each tablet.

Dose: for tablets containing 400 mg of sulphamethoxazole and 80 mg of trimethoprim, 2 to 6 tablets daily.

Advice for patients: see above under Co-trimoxazole Mixture.

DISPERSIBLE CO-TRIMOXAZOLE TABLETS (*Syn.* Trimethoprim and Sulphamethoxazole Dispersible Tablets): available as tablets containing 400 mg of sulphamethoxazole and 80 mg of trimethoprim in a suitable basis; they may be coloured.

A standard for these tablets is given in the British Pharmacopoeia Addendum 1978

Containers and *Storage:* see the entry on Tablets for general information on containers and storage. Containers should be airtight.

Labelling: the label on the container should state the amounts of the medicaments as the amounts of sulphamethoxazole and trimethoprim in each tablet.

Dose: for tablets containing 400 mg of sulphamethoxazole and 80 mg of trimethoprim, 2 to 6 tablets daily.

Advice for patients: the tablets may be dispersed in water before administration or swallowed whole; advice as for Co-trimoxazole Mixture (above).

PAEDIATRIC CO-TRIMOXAZOLE MIXTURE (*Syn.* Paediatric Trimethoprim and Sulphamethoxazole Mixture): a suspension of sulphamethoxazole and trimethoprim in a suitable coloured flavoured vehicle. It contains 200 mg of sulphamethoxazole and 40 mg of trimethoprim in 5 ml.

When a dose less than or not a multiple of 5 ml is prescribed, the mixture may be diluted, as described in the entry on Mixtures, with syrup. The diluted mixture must be freshly prepared.

A standard for this mixture is given in the British Pharmaceutical Codex 1973

Containers and *Labelling:* see the entry on Mixtures for general information on containers and labelling.

Storage: it should be protected from light.

Dose: CHILD: Twice daily: 6 weeks to 5 months, 2.5 millilitres; 6 months to 5 years, 5 millilitres; 6 to 12 years, 10 millilitres.

Advice for patients: see above under Co-trimoxazole Mixture.

PAEDIATRIC CO-TRIMOXAZOLE TABLETS (*Syn.* Paediatric Trimethoprim and Sulphamethoxazole Tablets): for each tablet take:

Sulphamethoxazole	100 mg
Trimethoprim	20 mg

Mix, and prepare by moist granulation and compression as described in the entry on Tablets; they may be film coated or sugar coated and the coat may be coloured; the tablets need not be circular in shape.

A standard for these tablets is given in the British Pharmacopoeia Addendum 1978

Containers and *Storage:* see the entry on Tablets for general information on containers and storage. Containers should be airtight.

Labelling: the label on the container should state the amounts of the medicaments as the amounts of sulphamethoxazole and trimethoprim in each tablet.

Dose: CHILD: twice daily: 6 months to 5 years, 2 tablets; 6 to 12 years, 4 tablets.

Advice for patients: see above under Co-trimoxazole Mixture.

STRONG STERILE CO-TRIMOXAZOLE SOLUTION: a sterile solution of the sodium derivative of sulphamethoxazole, prepared by the interaction of sulphamethoxazole and sodium hydroxide, and trimethoprim, in the proportion of the equivalent of 5 parts of sulphamethoxazole to 1 part of trimethoprim, with 40% v/v of propylene glycol and suitable stabilisers, in water for injections. It is sterilised by heating in an autoclave.

Available in 5-ml ampoules containing the equivalent of 80 mg of sulphamethoxazole and 16 mg of trimethoprim per ml.

A standard for this solution is given in the British Pharmacopoeia Addendum 1978

Containers: see the entry on Injections for general information on containers.

Labelling: the label on the container should state "Strong Sterile Co-trimoxazole Solution", the amounts of the medicaments as the amounts of sulphamethoxazole and trimethoprim in a suitable volume, and that the solution must be diluted before use.

The label on the container or the label on the package should state "Strong Sterile Co-trimoxazole Solution for the preparation of Co-trimoxazole Injection", the amounts of the medicaments as the amounts of sulphamethoxazole and trimethoprim in a suitable volume, the name of any added preservative, that the solution must be protected from light, that the solution must be diluted with 25 to 35 times its volume of dextrose injection or sodium chloride injection, that the co-trimoxazole injection so prepared is administered by intravenous injection, and that the injection must be discarded if any visible particles appear.

Storage: it should be protected from light.

SULPHADIAZINE AND TRIMETHOPRIM DISPERSIBLE POWDER: consisting of sulphadiazine and trimethoprim in the proportion of 5 parts to 1 part respectively mixed with suitable non-toxic wetting, dispersing, and suspending agents. Available as a dispersible powder containing 100 mg of sulphadiazine and 20 mg of trimethoprim per g.

A standard for this dispersible powder is given in the British Pharmacopoeia (Veterinary)

Labelling: the label on the container should state the amounts of the medicaments as the content of sulphadiazine and of trimethoprim, and the method of using the preparation.

Dose: HORSES, CATTLE, PIGS, and SHEEP: 25 mg of sulphadiazine and 5 mg of trimethoprim per kilogram body-weight daily, in divided doses.

SULPHADIAZINE AND TRIMETHOPRIM INJECTION: a sterile suspension of trimethoprim in a solution of the sodium derivative of sulphadiazine in water for injections free from dissolved air. It is prepared by the addition, by means of an aseptic technique, of sterile trimethoprim to a solution of sulphadiazine sodium previously sterilised by filtration. By means of an aseptic technique, the sterile preparation is distributed into sterile bottles, the air in the bottles being replaced by sterile nitrogen or other suitable gas, and the bottles are sealed.

Available in 50-ml vials containing 400 mg of sulphadiazine and 80 mg of trimethoprim per ml.

A standard for this injection is given in the British Pharmacopoeia (Veterinary)

Containers: see the entry on Injections for general information on containers.

Labelling: see the entry on Injections for general information on labelling. In addition, the label on the container should state the amounts of the medicaments as the amounts of sulphadiazine and trimethoprim in a suitable dose volume.

Storage: it should be protected from light.

Dose: FOR ALL SPECIES: by intramuscular injection, 12.5 mg of sulphadiazine and 2.5 mg of trimethoprim per kilogram body-weight daily, for up to 5 days.

SULPHADIAZINE AND TRIMETHOPRIM MIXTURE: an aqueous suspension of sulphadiazine and trimethoprim with suspending and dispersing agents. It may contain suitable preservatives. Available as a mixture containing 50 mg of sulphadiazine and 10 mg of trimethoprim in 1.1 ml, and as a mixture containing 400 mg of sulphadiazine and 80 mg of trimethoprim per ml.

A standard for this mixture is given in the British Pharmacopoeia (Veterinary)

Containers and *Labelling:* see the entry on Mixtures for general information on containers and labelling.

Dose: PIGLETS: 25 mg of sulphadiazine and 5 mg of trimethoprim per kilogram body-weight daily; POULTRY: 12.5 to 25 mg of sulphadiazine and 2.5 to 5 mg of trimethoprim per kilogram body-weight daily.

SULPHADIAZINE AND TRIMETHOPRIM TABLETS: available as tablets containing 100 mg of sulphadiazine and 20 mg of trimethoprim, tablets containing 400 mg of sulphadiazine and 80 mg of trimethoprim, and tablets containing 1 g of sulphadiazine and 200 mg of trimethoprim; they may be sugar coated; they may be coloured; the tablets need not be circular. Also available as tablets containing 410 mg of sulphadiazine and 90 mg of trimethoprim for use in human medicine.

A standard for these tablets is given in the British Pharmacopoeia (Veterinary)

Containers and *Storage:* see the entry on Tablets for general information on containers and storage. Containers should be airtight.

Labelling: the label on the container should state the amounts of the medicaments as the amounts of sulphadiazine and trimethoprim in each tablet.

Dose: FOR ALL SPECIES EXCEPT ADULT RUMINANTS: 25 mg of sulphadiazine and 5 mg of trimethoprim per kilogram body-weight daily in divided doses.

SULPHADOXINE AND TRIMETHOPRIM INJECTION: a sterile solution of sulphadoxine and trimethoprim in the proportion of 5 parts to 1 part respectively in a suitable aqueous vehicle. The alkalinity of the solution is adjusted to approximately pH 10 by the addition of sodium hydroxide. It may contain 0.1% of lignocaine hydrochloride. It is distributed into the final containers, the air in the containers being replaced by nitrogen or other suitable gas, and the containers are sealed and sterilised by heating in an autoclave. Alternatively, the solution is sterilised by filtration, distributed, by means of an aseptic technique, into sterile final containers, the air in the containers being replaced by sterile nitrogen or other suitable gas, and the containers are sealed.

Available in 50-ml vials containing 62.5 mg of sulphadoxine, 12.5 mg of trimethoprim, and 1 mg of lignocaine hydrochloride per ml; and in 30- and 100-ml vials containing 200 mg of sulphadoxine and 40 mg of trimethoprim per ml.

A standard for this injection is given in the British Pharmacopoeia (Veterinary)

Containers: see the entry on Injections for general information on containers.

Labelling: see the entry on Injections for general information on labelling. In addition, the label on the container should state the amounts of the medicaments as the amounts of sulphadoxine and trimethoprim in a suitable dose volume and, if present, the amount of lignocaine hydrochloride.

Storage: it should be stored at a temperature not exceeding 25°, protected from light.

Dose: ALL SPECIES: by intramuscular or intravenous injection, 12.5 mg of sulphadoxine and 2.5 mg of trimethoprim per kilogram body-weight.

SULPHADOXINE AND TRIMETHOPRIM TABLETS: available as tablets containing 250 mg of sulphadoxine and 50 mg of trimethoprim.

A standard for these tablets is given in the British Pharmacopoeia (Veterinary)

Containers and *Storage:* see the entry on Tablets for general information on containers and storage. Containers should be airtight and light resistant.

Labelling: the label on the container should state the amounts of the medicaments as the amounts of sulphadoxine and trimethoprim in each tablet.

Dose: FOALS, CALVES, PIGLETS, LAMBS, and DOGS: 15 mg of sulphadoxine and 3 mg of trimethoprim per kilogram body-weight.

OTHER PREPARATIONS available include an INJECTION containing trimethoprim 53 mg with sulphamethoxazole 266 mg per ml in 3-ml ampoules.

Trimipramine Maleate

5 - (3 - Dimethylamino - 2 - methylpropyl) - 10,11 - dihydro-
5*H*-dibenz[*b,f*]azepine hydrogen maleate

$C_{24}H_{30}N_2O_4 = 410.5$

OTHER NAMES: *Surmontil®*; Trimipramini Maleas

*A standard is given in the European Pharmacopoeia
Vol. III*

Description. An odourless white crystalline powder with
a bitter taste followed by numbness.

Solubility. Soluble in water, in alcohol, and in chloroform; very slightly soluble in ether.

Storage. It should be protected from light.

Identification. TESTS. 1. Dissolve about 5 mg in 2 ml of
nitric acid; an intense blue colour is produced which
turns green on standing.
2. Triturate about 100 mg with 3 ml of water and 1 ml
of 10N sodium hydroxide, and extract with three 5-ml
portions of ether; to the aqueous solution add 2 ml of
bromine solution, heat in a water-bath for 10 minutes,
then boil, and cool; add 2 drops of this solution to a
solution of 10 mg of resorcinol in 3 ml of sulphuric acid,
heat on a water-bath for 2 minutes, and cool; a deep
blue colour is produced.

MELTING-POINT. About 142°.

ULTRAVIOLET ABSORPTION. In 0.1N hydrochloric acid,
maximum at 250 nm (E1%, 1cm = 215).

Determination in body fluids. GAS CHROMATOGRAPHY.
In serum—P. Hartvig *et al.*, *Analyt. Chem.*, 1976, **48**,
390.

Metabolism. ABSORPTION. Absorbed after oral
administration.

DISTRIBUTION. *Protein binding*, about 85% bound to
plasma proteins.

METABOLIC REACTIONS. Extensively metabolised.

EXCRETION. Slowly excreted in the urine.

Actions and uses. Trimipramine maleate is a tricyclic
antidepressant with actions and uses similar to those
described under Amitriptyline Hydrochloride, but its
sedative action is more pronounced. The usual dose is
the equivalent of 25 to 125 milligrams of trimipramine
daily in divided doses or as a single dose at bedtime.

Undesirable effects. As for Amitriptyline Hydrochloride. Changes in plasma transaminase may occur.

**Precautions and contra-indications; Drug inter-
actions.** As for Amitriptyline Hydrochloride.

Preparations

TRIMIPRAMINE TABLETS: available as tablets containing
trimipramine maleate equivalent to 10 and 25 mg of
trimipramine; they are compression coated.
*A standard for these tablets is given in the British
Pharmacopoeia 1973*

Containers and *Storage:* see the entry on Tablets for
general information on containers and storage. Containers should be airtight.
Advice for patients: daily doses should preferably be
taken at bedtime. When initiating treatment, there may
be a time-lag of up to 2 weeks before a full therapeutic
response is obtained. The tablets may cause drowsiness;
persons affected should not drive or operate machinery.
Alcohol should be avoided.

OTHER PREPARATIONS available include CAPSULES containing trimipramine maleate equivalent to 50 mg of
trimipramine.

Triprolidine Hydrochloride

(*E*)-2-[3-(Pyrrolidin-1-yl)-1-*p*-tolylprop-1-enyl]pyridine
hydrochloride monohydrate

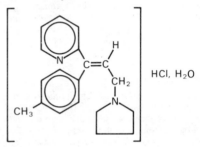

$C_{19}H_{23}ClN_2,H_2O = 332.9$

OTHER NAMES: *Actidil®*; *Pro-Actidil®*
Actifed® (with pseudoephedrine hydrochloride)

A standard is given in the British Pharmacopoeia 1973

Description. An odourless white crystalline powder with
a bitter taste.

Solubility. Soluble, at 20°, in 2 parts of water, in 1.5
parts of alcohol, and in less than 1 part of chloroform;
practically insoluble in ether.

Moisture content. 4.5 to 6%, determined by Fischer
titration.

Identification. TEST. Dissolve about 100 mg in 2 ml of
dilute hydrochloric acid and add 0.5 ml of *potassium
mercuri-iodide solution*; a pale yellow precipitate is
produced.

MELTING-POINT. About 119°.

ULTRAVIOLET ABSORPTION. In 0.1N hydrochloric acid,
maximum at 291 nm (E1%, 1cm = 294); in water, maxima
at 230 nm (E1%, 1cm = 495) and 276 nm (E1%,
1cm = 245).

INFRA-RED ABSORPTION. Major peaks at 772, 824, 1077,
1427, 1459, and 1580 cm⁻¹ (see Appendix 2a: Infra-red
Spectra).

THIN-LAYER CHROMATOGRAPHY. See under Thin-layer
Chromatography, System 4.

Actions and uses. Triprolidine hydrochloride has the
actions, uses, and undesirable effects of the antihistamine
drugs as described under Promethazine Hydrochloride.
It is effective when given by mouth and its action lasts
for about 12 hours. The usual dose for an adult is 5 to
15 milligrams daily in divided doses. Children under 1
year may be given 1 milligram 3 times daily, 1 to 6 years
2 milligrams 3 times daily and 7 to 12 years 3 milligrams
3 times daily.

Poisoning. As for Promethazine Hydrochloride.

Preparations

TRIPROLIDINE TABLETS: available as tablets containing 2.5 mg of triprolidine hydrochloride.

A standard for these tablets is given in the British Pharmacopoeia 1973

Containers and *Storage:* see the entry on Tablets for general information on containers and storage. Containers should be airtight.

Advice for patients: the tablets may cause drowsiness; persons affected should not drive or operate machinery. Alcohol should be avoided.

OTHER PREPARATIONS available include an ELIXIR containing triprolidine hydrochloride 2 mg in 5 ml, diluent syrup, life of diluted elixir 14 days; an elixir containing triprolidine hydrochloride 1.25 mg with pseudoephedrine hydrochloride 30 mg in 5 ml, diluent syrup, life of diluted elixir 14 days; TABLETS containing triprolidine hydrochloride 10 mg in a slow-release formulation; and tablets containing triprolidine hydrochloride 2.5 mg with pseudoephedrine hydrochloride 60 mg.

Tropical Sprue

Tropical sprue is a tropical disorder characterised by changes in the structure of the mucosa of the small intestine which result in malabsorption and the subsequent development of nutritional deficiencies. The onset of tropical sprue is characterised by diarrhoea, anorexia, and weight loss due to malabsorption. Later there may be megaloblastic anaemia and steatorrhoea.

Tropical sprue resembles coeliac disease, but does not respond to the withdrawal of gluten from the diet. The disorder usually responds to treatment with broad spectrum antibiotics and dietary measures. A high intake of protein, a normal fat intake, and supplementary folic acid are required.

Tropicamide

N-Ethyl-*N*-(pyrid-4-ylmethyl)tropamide

$$CH_2 \cdot N \cdot CO \cdot CH \cdot C_6H_5$$
with C_2H_5 and CH_2OH substituents

$C_{17}H_{20}N_2O_2 = 284.4$

OTHER NAME: *Mydriacyl®*

A standard is given in the British Pharmacopoeia 1973

Description. An odourless white crystalline powder.

Solubility. Soluble, at 20°, in 160 parts of water, in 3.5 parts of alcohol, and in 2 parts of chloroform.

Dissociation constant. pK_a 5.2.

Identification. TEST. Dissolve about 5 mg in 3 ml of a mixture of 9 ml of acetic anhydride, 1 ml of acetic acid and 100 mg of citric acid, and heat on a water-bath for 5 to 10 minutes; a reddish-yellow colour is produced.

MELTING-POINT. About 96°.

ULTRAVIOLET ABSORPTION. In 0.1N hydrochloric acid, maximum at 254 nm (E1%, 1cm = 180).

INFRA-RED ABSORPTION. Major peaks at 709, 761, 1266, 1419, 1601, and 1627 cm^{-1} (see Appendix 2a: Infra-red Spectra).

Actions and uses. Tropicamide has mydriatic and cycloplegic properties similar to those described under Atropine but it acts more quickly and its effect lasts for a shorter time.

The usual quantity required for refraction procedures is 2 drops of a 1% solution followed after 5 minutes by a further 2 drops; the duration of action may be extended by repeating the instillation of drops at intervals of 30 minutes.

For examination of the fundus 2 drops of a 0.5% solution may be used.

Precautions. As for Cyclopentolate Hydrochloride.

Preparation

TROPICAMIDE EYE-DROPS: consisting of a sterile solution of tropicamide, with 0.002% of phenylmercuric nitrate, in a suitable vehicle. Available as eye-drops containing 0.5 and 1% of tropicamide.

Containers and *Labelling:* see the entry on Eye-drops for general information on containers and labelling.

Advice for patients: see the entry on Eye-drops for general information on the use of eye-drops. Blurring of vision and sensitivity to light may occur for up to 8 hours after instillation of the drops.

Troxidone

3,5,5-Trimethyloxazolidine-2,4-dione

$C_6H_9NO_3 = 143.1$

OTHER NAMES: *Tridione®*; Trimethadione

A standard is given in the British Pharmacopoeia 1973

Description. Colourless granular crystals with a slightly camphoraceous odour.

Solubility. Soluble, at 20°, in 13 parts of water and in 2 parts of alcohol; soluble in ether and in chloroform.

Storage. It should be stored in airtight containers, in a cool place.

Identification. TESTS. 1. Dissolve about 100 mg in 5 ml of water and add 2 ml of *barium hydroxide solution*; a precipitate is immediately produced.

2. Mix about 500 mg with 4 ml of *sodium hydroxide solution*, heat on a water-bath for 30 minutes, evaporate to low bulk, cool in ice, and cautiously add hydrochloric acid until acid to litmus paper; to 10 drops of the solution add 2 drops of *ferric chloride test-solution*; a deep yellow colour is produced.

3. Extract the remainder of the solution obtained in Test 2 with three 10-ml portions of ether, evaporate the ether extracts, heat on a water-bath for 30 minutes and scratch the container to induce crystallisation; the residue, after recrystallisation from toluene, melts at about 80°.

MELTING-POINT. About 46°.

INFRA-RED ABSORPTION. Major peaks at 1100, 1296, 1395, 1445, 1732, and 1818 cm^{-1} (see Appendix 2a: Infra-red Spectra).

Metabolism. ABSORPTION. Readily absorbed after oral administration.

BLOOD CONCENTRATION. During prolonged therapy, plasma concentrations of 6 to 10 μg/ml are attained; after a single dose, peak concentrations are attained in 0.5 to 2 hours; control of seizures is attained with plasma concentrations of about 700 μg/ml for the active metabolite, dimethadione, which attains plasma concentrations about 20 times greater than those of troxidone following an oral dose of troxidone.

HALF-LIFE. Derived from urinary excretion data, 6 to 13 days for the active metabolite.

DISTRIBUTION. Widely and uniformly distributed throughout the body; volume of distribution, about 60% of body-weight; dimethadione accumulates upon repeated doses; protein binding, not significantly bound to plasma proteins.

METABOLIC REACTIONS. 3-Demethylation to form the active metabolite, dimethadione, which is not further metabolised.

EXCRETION. Slowly excreted in the urine mainly as dimethadione with about 2% appearing as unchanged drug in the first 8 hours; the urinary excretion of dimethadione is increased in alkaline urine.

FURTHER INFORMATION. Demethylation rate in dogs and mice—H.-H. Frey and R. Schulz, *Acta pharmac. tox.*, 1970, **28**, 477; O. Svensmark, Absorption, distribution, metabolism and excretion of antiepileptic drugs in man, *International Encyclopedia of Pharmacology and Therapeutics, Section 19, Vol. 1, Anticonvulsant Drugs*, J. Mercier (Ed.), Oxford, Pergamon, 1973; *Antiepileptic Drugs*, D. M. Woodbury *et al.* (Eds), New York, Raven Press, 1972.

Actions and uses. Troxidone prevents leptazol-induced convulsions in animals without causing general depression of the central nervous system, but does not control spontaneous convulsions in man.

Troxidone is used in the treatment of true petit mal epilepsy. The initial daily dosage for a child up to 2 years is 300 milligrams, from 2 to 6 years, 600 milligrams, and for an adult, 900 milligrams by mouth, in divided doses; if no toxic effects are observed, these doses may be increased, if necessary, at intervals of not less than a week up to a total daily dose of not more than twice these amounts.

The clinical improvement, usually observed within 1 to 4 weeks of beginning treatment, is accompanied by a marked reduction or disappearance of spike and wave formations in the electroencephalogram.

Undesirable effects. The most frequent undesirable effect is photophobia, which is usually experienced as a glare effect in brightly lit surroundings, and if this is severe and persistent the wearing of dark glasses may be necessary. Rashes, nausea, headache, fatigue, and muscular weakness occur occasionally.

Rarer but potentially fatal toxic effects are due to hypersensitivity reactions affecting the bone marrow, skin, kidney, and liver.

Precautions and contra-indications. Troxidone does not diminish the frequency or severity of convulsive seizures in patients with grand mal epilepsy and must not be used for the treatment of those patients, as it may precipitate status epilepticus. It does not relieve patients with psychomotor seizures, but in some of those patients it may augment the therapeutic action of phenytoin sodium.

It should only be used in pregnancy if the benefits outweigh the risks.

Preparations

PAEDIATRIC TROXIDONE TABLETS: may be prepared by moist granulation and compression as described in the entry on Tablets. Available as tablets containing 150 mg of troxidone; they may be cuboid in shape and contain suitable flavouring.

A standard for these tablets is given in the British Pharmaceutical Codex 1973

Containers and *Storage:* see the entry on Tablets for general information on containers and storage. Containers should be airtight and light resistant.

Labelling: a direction to crush or chew the tablets before they are swallowed should be given on the label.

Advice for patients: see above under Labelling. When initiating treatment there may be a time-lag of up to 4 weeks before a full therapeutic response is obtained. Treatment should not be discontinued without the advice of the prescriber. The tablets may cause drowsiness and sensitivity to light may occur in brightly lit surroundings; persons affected should wear dark glasses.

TROXIDONE CAPSULES: consisting of troxidone, in powder, which may be mixed with a suitable inert diluent, enclosed in a hard capsule. Available as capsules containing 300 mg of troxidone.

A standard for these capsules is given in the British Pharmacopoeia 1973

Containers and *Storage:* see the entry on Capsules for general information on containers and storage.

Advice for patients: when initiating treatment there may be a time-lag of up to 4 weeks before a full therapeutic response is obtained. Treatment should not be discontinued without the advice of the prescriber. The capsules may cause drowsiness; persons affected should not drive or operate machinery. Alcohol should be avoided. Sensitivity to light may occur in brightly lit surroundings, and the wearing of dark glasses may be necessary.

Trypanosomiasis

African trypanosomiasis (Sleeping sickness) is a chronic infection caused by flagellated protozoa of the genus *Trypanosoma* transmitted by various tsetse flies of the genus *Glossina*. In western areas of Africa infection is caused by *T. gambiense*. In eastern areas of Africa, the infection is more serious and is caused by *T. rhodesiense*.

In *T. gambiense* infection, a tender, small subcutaneous nodule appears at the site of the bite after 5 to 15 days. This primary chancre contains trypanosomes. After a few weeks there are bouts of irregular fever, sweating, fatigue, persistent headache and transitory swellings on the face. There is also enlargement of cervical lymph nodes and splenomegaly. This illness may subside but weeks or months later there is involvement of the central nervous system in the form of a chronic encephalopathy with personality change, headache, and general ill-health. The affected person loses interest and may be violent. Later this is followed by stupor and coma.

T. rhodesiense infection is similar, but the primary chancre is more evident and accompanied by a febrile illness which develops into an irregular fever with progressive weakness and anaemia with effusions into the serous cavities. This is followed by an acute or subacute encephalitis which may result in death within 6 to 9 months of the initial infection.

Suramin and pentamidine are effective against the try-panosome in the early stages before central nervous system involvement. For cerebral trypanosomiasis melarsoprol is required. Pentamidine is also used for prophylaxis.

American trypanosomiasis (Chagas' disease) is caused in Central and South America by infections with *T. cruzi*, a trypanosome similar to those involved in African trypanosomiasis. The insect vector is a blood-sucking reduviid bug. The acute infection may be symptomless or take the form of a general febrile illness, but long-term effects after 10 to 20 years may include chronic cardio-myopathy and megacolon.

No satisfactory treatment is available.

Tuberculin, Old

The heat-concentrated filtrate from a fluid medium on which the human or bovine strain of *Mycobacterium tuberculosis* has been grown. It contains 0.5% of phenol and not less than 100000 units in 1 ml.

OTHER NAME: Tuberculinum Crudum

A standard is given in the European Pharmacopoeia Vol. II

Storage. Old tuberculin should be protected from light and stored at 2° to 10°. Undiluted old tuberculin is stable for at least 8 years.

Diluted solutions of old tuberculin are much less stable, their stability depending upon their mode of preparation and the nature of the diluent. Diluted solutions should be kept in full containers and should be used as soon as possible after preparation. Once a container is opened any portion of the contents not used at once should be discarded.

Actions and uses. Old tuberculin is used as a diagnostic agent for tuberculosis.

A person showing a specific sensitivity to tuberculin is considered to have been infected with the tubercle bacillus, although the infection may be inactive. There is no significant difference between the active principle in preparations of the human type of *M. tuberculosis* and that in preparations of the bovine type.

Sensitivity tests to tuberculin can be performed in different ways, the intracutaneous test of Mantoux giving the most precise results. The diagnostic dose varies with the circumstances because of the great variation in sensitivity to tuberculin. In a full-scale test, the initial dose injected is 1 unit of either old tuberculin or tuberculin purified protein derivative in 0.1 millilitre. The test is read at 72 hours.

A positive reaction is characterised by an area of palpable infiltration of not less than 5 or 6 millimetres in diameter which may or may not be surrounded by erythema. Necrosis may occur in hypersensitive persons.

If the reaction is negative, the test is repeated with 10 units of tuberculin in 0.1 millilitre. If the second test is negative a final test may be made with 100 units in 0.1 millilitre before regarding the person as "Mantoux-negative". Frequently, where the sensitivity of the person is not expected to be unduly high, the initial test is with 5 or 10 units followed, if negative, by the test with 100 units. It is also common practice in epidemi-ological surveys to use a single test with 5 or 10 units.

A multiple-puncture (Heaf) method may be employed using a concentrated solution of tuberculin containing 100000 units in 1 millilitre. Results are obtained similar to those with a two-stage Mantoux test. The test is read at 3 to 7 days, preferably the latter.

In children aged less than 3 years, who have not been vaccinated with B.C.G. vaccine, a positive tuberculin reaction indicates an infection which should be sus-pected as active; between the ages of 3 and 5 years this inference is doubtful; in children over 5 years the possibility of active lesions must still be considered; in adolescence and adult life the diagnostic value of a positive reading is less than in childhood as the disease is less likely to be active.

A strong positive reaction in a person recently known to be negative signifies a recent tuberculous infection.

A negative reaction to 100 units in the Mantoux test, with some rare exceptions, excludes an active tubercu-lous infection. The test can be negative, however, when performed early in the infection before hypersensitivity to tuberculoprotein has developed, and also in certain very acute forms of the disease.

Temporary diminution of skin sensitivity to tuberculin may occur during an attack of measles or other viral infection, after ultraviolet light treatment, and during corticosteroid therapy.

CAUTION. As traces of tuberculin are apt to adhere to glassware, syringes used for tuberculin tests should not be used for other purposes.

Tuberculin Purified Protein Derivative

The active principle of old tuberculin prepared from the fluid medium on which the tubercle bacilli have been grown. The liquid contains 100000 units per ml and the freeze-dried powder contains 30000 units per mg. Not more than 0.5% of phenol is added. It is more constant in composition and potency than old tuberculin. The following dilutions are available: 1 in 100 (1000 units per ml; 100 units in 0.1 ml); 1 in 1000 (100 units per ml; 10 units in 0.1 ml); and 1 in 10000 (10 units per ml; 1 unit in 0.1 ml).

OTHER NAMES: Tuberculin P.P.D.; Tuberculini Deriva-tum Proteinosum Purificatum

A standard is given in the European Pharmacopoeia Vol. II

Storage. It should be protected from light and stored at 2° to 10°. Undiluted tuberculin purified protein deriv-ative in concentrated solution preserved with 0.5% of phenol is stable for 8 years and in the dried form the purified protein derivative will retain its potency indefinitely.

Diluted solutions are much less stable, their stability depending upon their mode of preparation and the nature of the diluent. Diluted solutions should be kept in full containers and should be used as soon as possible after preparation.

Once a container is opened any portion of the contents not used at once should be discarded.

Actions and uses. Tuberculin purified protein derivative has the actions and uses described under Old Tuberculin and is administered in similar dosage.

Veterinary uses. Tuberculin purified protein derivative is used for the diagnosis of tuberculosis in domesticated animals. In Great Britain the official test for the eradi-cation of bovine tuberculosis is the single-dose intra-dermal comparative test. Both mammalian and avian tuberculosis are injected separately in doses of 0.1 milli-litre into the neck. The reactions at each site are assessed by the increase in the thickness of the skin fold 72 hours after injection and by the character of the swelling.

CAUTION. As traces of tuberculin are apt to adhere to glassware, syringes used for tuberculin tests should not be used for other purposes.

Tuberculin purified protein derivative may produce toxic effects when inhaled, and care must be taken when handling the powder.

Tuberculosis

Tuberculosis is an acute or chronic communicable disease caused by *Mycobacterium tuberculosis*. It is characterised by inflammatory infiltrations, tubercle formation, caseation, fibrosis, and calcification. It usually affects the respiratory tract, but may involve any organ of the body. The human type of *Mycobacterium tuberculosis* is usually responsible for the disease but the bovine type is occasionally responsible, especially in countries where tuberculosis is still present in cattle. The tubercle bacillus usually enters the body by inhalation or ingestion and the most common site for tuberculosis in Britain is the lung.

The disease differs in its effects on patients meeting the disease for the first time and in those who already have some resistance due to a previous encounter with the organism. The former, or primary, tuberculosis occurs mainly in children and young adults and may spread via the bloodstream to produce tuberculosis at a distance from the initial lesion; the meninges, bones, and the genito-urinary tract may all be involved in this way.

Post-primary tuberculosis is usually a more circumscribed lesion which may extend by necrosis, ulceration, and cavitation to give extensive lesions. In the elderly and the debilitated the resistance to the tubercle bacilli may be lost and "miliary" spread via the bloodstream may occur as in primary tuberculosis.

B.C.G vaccination mimics the primary lesion of tuberculosis so that when a subject meets virulent tubercle bacilli the lesion, if any, is of post-primary type rather than the more dangerous primary type of tuberculosis. The development of resistance may be tested by a Heaf or Mantoux test which demonstrates hypersensitivity to protein of tubercle bacilli indicating previous exposure to the organism.

Progressive pulmonary tuberculosis is insidious in onset and is characterised by fatigue, weight loss, anorexia, fever, weakness, and malaise. There is also cough, production of sputum, haemoptysis, dyspnoea, and chest pain which is aggravated by respiratory effort.

When tuberculosis occurs in the gastro-intestinal tract it may cause ulceration, perforation, or obstruction. Tuberculosis in other organs leads to their destruction and symptoms associated with loss of their function. Healing of the tuberculous lesion may take place at any stage by resolution, fibrosis, and calcification. However, inactivated lesions may later extend due to re-infection or reactivation, especially after the administration of corticosteroids or immunosuppressives.

Treatment. Chemotherapy for about 1 year with two or three drugs is necessary to cure tuberculosis without the development of resistant strains of mycobacteria. Triple therapy should be used until the infection is controlled and the sensitivity of the mycobacteria to antibiotics has been determined. Treatment with two drugs to which the mycobacteria are sensitive is then continued for about 1 year. For over 20 years the standard initial

treatment of pulmonary tuberculosis has been triple therapy with streptomycin, aminosalicylic acid, and isoniazid followed by either aminosalicylic acid and isoniazid or streptomycin and isoniazid. Standard treatment may now begin with isoniazid, rifampicin, and usually ethambutol as the third drug, and continue with an appropriate pair of drugs when sensitivities are known. Other antitubercular drugs are less effective than the above five and should only be used to treat infection with mycobacteria that are resistant to the standard drugs.

In tuberculous meningitis triple therapy should always be used. When there is overwhelming or life-threatening tuberculous infection corticosteroids may be used to reduce inflammation. Prophylaxis is necessary when corticosteroids or immunosuppressive drugs are given to patients with evidence of old tuberculous lesions.

Drugs used in the treatment of tuberculosis include capreomycin sulphate, cycloserine, ethambutol, ethionamide, isoniazid, prothionamide, pyrazinamide, rifampicin, sodium aminosalicylate, streptomycin, thiacetazone, and viomycin.

Tubocurarine Chloride

The chloride of an alkaloid, (+)-tubocurarine, obtained from extracts of the stems of *Chondodendron tomentosum* Ruiz et Pav. (Fam. Menispermaceae) and possessing the specific biological activity of curare on neuromuscular transmission.

$C_{37}H_{42}Cl_2N_2O_6,5H_2O = 771.7$

OTHER NAMES: *Tubarine*®; Tubocurar. Chlor.; *d*-Tubocurarine Chloride; Tubocurarinii Chloridum

A standard is given in the European Pharmacopoeia Vol. I

Description. An odourless, white or slightly yellowish-white, crystalline powder.

Solubility. Soluble, at 20°, in 20 parts of water and in 30 parts of alcohol; soluble in solutions of alkali hydroxides; very slightly soluble in ether, in chloroform, and in acetone.

Acidity. A 1% solution has pH of 4 to 6.

Moisture content. 9 to 12%, determined by drying at 100° *in vacuo*.

Specific rotation. +210° to +218°, determined on a 1% solution.

Dissociation constants. pK$_a$ 8.0, 9.2 (22°).

Sterilisation. Solutions for injection are sterilised by heating in an autoclave in an atmosphere of nitrogen or other suitable gas.

Identification. TESTS. 1. Dissolve a few mg in 5 ml of water and add 1 ml of *potassium iodobismuthate solution*; an orange or orange-red precipitate is produced.
2. Dissolve about 10 mg in 1 ml of water and add a few drops of a 1.3% solution of ferric chloride; a green colour is produced. Warm the solution; the colour changes to brown.
3. Dissolve about 10 mg in 1 ml of water and add 1 ml of *mercury nitrate solution*; a cherry red colour is slowly produced.

MELTING-POINT. About 270°, with decomposition.

ULTRAVIOLET ABSORPTION. In water, maximum at 280 nm (E1%, 1cm = 118).

Metabolism. ABSORPTION. Slowly and incompletely absorbed after intramuscular injection; inactivated after oral administration.

BLOOD CONCENTRATION. After an intravenous dose of 300 μg/kg, serum concentrations of about 2 μg/ml are obtained at about 5 minutes falling to 25 to 83 ng/ml by 24 hours.

HALF-LIFE. Plasma half-life, about 13 minutes.

DISTRIBUTION. Widely distributed and concentrated at neuromuscular junctions; accumulates upon repeated dosage in renal function impairment; after therapeutic doses, does not cross the placenta but enters the cerebrospinal fluid in small amounts.

METABOLIC REACTIONS. Metabolism of tubocurarine occurs to a minor extent.

EXCRETION. About 30 to 70% of a dose is excreted unchanged in the urine in 3 to 6 hours.

FURTHER INFORMATION. Distribution and fate in dogs —E. N. Cohen *et al.*, *J. Pharmac. exp. Ther.*, 1965, **147**, 120; diffusion into cerebrospinal fluid—G. Devasankaraiah *et al.*, *Br. J. Pharmac.*, 1973, **47**, 787; effect of renal failure on duration of action—M. Gibaldi *et al.*, *Br. J. Anaesth.*, 1972, **44**, 163; serum concentrations by radioimmunoassay—P. E. Horowitz and S. Spector, *J. Pharmac. exp. Ther.*, 1973, **185**, 94.

Actions and uses. Tubocurarine produces relaxation of voluntary muscle by reducing its response to acetylcholine. When administered intravenously it produces first fatigue, then weakness, and, finally, paralysis of voluntary muscle, beginning in the eyes and spreading to the face, neck, limbs, abdomen, intercostal muscles, and diaphragm; recovery of muscle function occurs in the reverse order.
The effects of moderate doses are transient, owing to their rapid elimination and destruction. The peak effect is reached within 3 to 5 minutes of intravenous injection, and the effect begins to decline after about 20 minutes. When respiratory paralysis occurs, it will do so within 7 to 10 minutes of intravenous injection.
In the dosage used clinically, tubocurarine has no central stimulant, depressant, or analgesic action. Its action is antagonised by anticholinesterase drugs.
Tubocurarine chloride is used chiefly as an adjunct to anaesthesia to secure muscular relaxation in surgery. For this purpose, 10 to 20 milligrams of tubocurarine chloride is given by intravenous injection, followed, if necessary, as indicated by the degree of muscular relaxation, by further doses of 2 to 4 milligrams at intervals of about 30 minutes up to a total of 45 milligrams, provided that adequate methods for dealing with respiratory failure are

at hand. The usual dose for children is about 300 micrograms per kilogram body-weight.
It can be used with the usual anaesthetic agents, barbiturates, and intravenous analgesic drugs. In the presence of ether, however, the action of tubocurarine is enhanced; when ether is used as the anaesthetic, it is important, therefore, to reduce the dose of tubocurarine chloride to one-half to one-third of that used with other anaesthetics.
The additional doses of tubocurarine are sometimes given alternatively with small doses of a barbiturate during operation. Since precipitation may occur when a solution of tubocurarine chloride is mixed with certain barbiturates, admixture with these barbiturates must be avoided.
It is also used, usually by the intravenous route, to produce muscular relaxation before such procedures as bronchoscopy and laryngoscopy; 0.6 to 1.2 milligrams of atropine should be given to counteract the increased salivation caused by tubocurarine.
Tubocurarine has been used in certain neurological conditions for the symptomatic relief of hypertonia, tremor, and incoordination. It has also been used in tetanus and shock therapy to diminish the severity of the convulsions and to prevent fractures, and in the treatment of fractures and dislocations.

Undesirable effects. The chief dangers arising from the use of tubocurarine are respiratory failure and regurgitation of the stomach contents due to relaxation of the oesophageal muscle and sphincters.

Contra-indications. Tubocurarine is contra-indicated in patients with myasthenia gravis and in asthmatics, because it causes the release of histamine.

Poisoning. Neostigmine methylsulphate should be given intravenously in a dose of 5 milligrams after the intravenous injection of atropine sulphate 0.5 to 1 milligram; this dose of atropine may be repeated if necessary. Controlled respiration is essential until spontaneous breathing is resumed.

Preparation

TUBOCURARINE INJECTION:

Tubocurarine chloride	1 g
Water for injections, free from dissolved air	to 100 ml

Dissolve the tubocurarine chloride in the bulk of the water and clarify the solution by filtration. Add sufficient of the water to produce the required volume. Distribute the solution into ampoules, replace the air in the ampoules by nitrogen or other suitable gas, immediately seal the ampoules, and sterilise by heating in an autoclave.
It contains, in 1 ml, 10 mg of tubocurarine chloride.
Available in 1.5-ml ampoules.
A standard for this injection is given in the British Pharmacopoeia 1973
Containers and *Labelling*: see the entry on Injections for general information on containers and labelling.

Tumour

see under NEOPLASTIC DISEASE

Turner's Syndrome

A hereditary form of female hypogonadism (see under Hypogonadism).

Turpentine Oil

The oil obtained by distillation and rectification from turpentine, an oleoresin obtained from various species of *Pinus* (Fam. Pinaceae), notably *P. palustris* Mill. and *P. elliottii* Engelm. (*P. caribaea* Mor.) in North America and *P. pinaster* Ait. in southern Europe. The unrectified oil is the turpentine of commerce.

OTHER NAME: Oleum Terebinthinae

A standard is given in the British Pharmacopoeia 1973

French and Portuguese turpentine oils are always strongly laevorotatory, but American oils may be either laevo- or dextro-rotatory.

Constituents. Turpentine oil consists principally of pinenes, together with smaller amounts of other terpenes.

Description. It is a clear bright colourless liquid with a strong characteristic odour which becomes stronger and less pleasant on storage and exposure to air.

Solubility. Soluble, at 20°, in 7 parts of alcohol (90%) and in 3 parts of alcohol (95%); miscible with dehydrated alcohol, with ether, with chloroform, with carbon disulphide, and with glacial acetic acid.

Weight per ml. At 20°, 0.855 to 0.868 g.

Refractive index. 1.467 to 1.477.

Adulterants and substitutes. Petroleum, resin oil, and wood turpentine are common adulterants.
Petroleum may be detected by its effect in lowering the weight per ml, and also by the flash-point, which for pure turpentine oil is about 95°F.
White spirit, which is commonly used as a turpentine substitute, consists of petroleum fractions and has a flash-point of about 82°F.
Resin oil, a product of the destructive distillation of colophony, may be detected by the fatty stain which the adulterated oil leaves when evaporated from paper.
Wood turpentine, which is obtained by distilling the roots and stumps of various species of *Pinus*, has a higher weight per ml.
Sulphate turpentine, obtained during the manufacture of wood pulp by the sulphate process, resembles turpentine oil but contains sulphur compounds.

Stability. On prolonged exposure to the air, turpentine oil undergoes rapid change, especially in the presence of moisture; it becomes viscous and yellow and acquires an acid reaction, the weight per ml increases, the boiling-point rises, and the solubility in alcohol increases.

Storage. It should be stored in well-filled airtight containers, in a cool place, protected from light.

Actions and uses. Turpentine is applied externally in liniments as a counter-irritant and rubefacient.

Poisoning. Paediatric ipecacuanha emetic draught may be given and demulcent drinks may also be required, with magnesium sulphate to promote purgation and with morphine to relieve pain. It should be noted that emesis and gastric lavage are contra-indicated in poisoning with petroleum products commonly used as turpentine substitutes.

Veterinary uses. Turpentine oil is used in liniments as a counter-irritant and internally as a carminative and treatment for cattle bloat (ruminal tympany). The usual dose by mouth as a single dose for horses and cattle is 15 to 60 millilitres and for sheep 3 to 15 millilitres.

Preparations

TURPENTINE LINIMENT (*Syn.* Lin. Terebinth.):

Turpentine oil	650 ml
Camphor	50 g
Soft soap	75 g
Water for preparations	225 ml

Triturate the camphor with the soft soap until thoroughly mixed and gradually add the turpentine oil, triturating well after each addition. Transfer the mixture to a bottle with the aid of the water and shake thoroughly until a creamy emulsion is formed.
A standard for this liniment is given in the British Pharmacopoeia 1973
Containers and *Labelling:* see the entry on Liniments for general information on containers and labelling. A direction to shake the bottle should be given on the label.
Advice for patients: the liniment should be applied to the skin with considerable friction; it should not be applied to broken or inflamed skin or near the eyes or mucous membranes.

WHITE LINIMENT (*Syn.* Linimentum Album; White Embrocation):

Turpentine oil	250.0 ml
Ammonium chloride	12.5 g
Dilute ammonia solution..	45.0 ml
Oleic acid	85.0 ml
Water for preparations	625.0 ml

Mix the oleic acid with the turpentine oil, add the dilute ammonia solution mixed with an equal volume of the water, previously warmed, and shake. Dissolve the ammonium chloride in the remainder of the water, add to the emulsion, and mix.
A standard for this liniment is given in the British Pharmaceutical Codex 1973
Containers and *Labelling:* see the entry on Liniments for general information on containers and labelling. A direction to shake the bottle should be given on the label.
Advice for patients: see above under Turpentine Liniment.

Typhoid and Tetanus Vaccine

A mixture of a suspension of killed *Salmonella typhi* that are smooth and have the full complement of O, H, and Vi antigens and tetanus formol toxoid. It contains 1000 million or 2000 million typhoid bacilli (*S. typhi*) in 1 ml.

OTHER NAME: Typhoid/Tet/Vac

A standard is given in the British Pharmacopoeia 1973

Storage. It should be stored as described under Vaccines.

Actions and uses. Typhoid and tetanus vaccine may be used for primary immunisation.
The vaccine is used for reinforcing doses when it is advisable to boost the immunity against tetanus as well as typhoid. The vaccine is usually administered by subcutaneous injection in 2 doses of the volume stated on the label as the dose, separated by an interval of at least 4 to 6 weeks, the second dose being followed after an interval of preferably 4 to 6 months by a dose of tetanus vaccine or adsorbed tetanus vaccine. A single intramuscular dose of typhoid and tetanus vaccine is given as a reinforcing dose when required.

Typhoid Fever

see under SALMONELLA INFECTIONS

Typhoid Vaccine

A suspension of killed *Salmonella typhi* that are smooth and have the full complement of O, H, and Vi antigens. It contains not less than 500 million and not more than 1000 million typhoid bacilli (*S. typhi*) in 1 millilitre.

OTHER NAMES: Typhoid/Vac; Vaccinum Typhoidi

A standard is given in the European Pharmacopoeia Vol. II

Storage. It should be stored as described under Vaccines.

Actions and uses. Typhoid vaccine has been shown to be an effective prophylactic against typhoid fever, and as the value of paratyphoid vaccines has not been established, some practitioners prefer to prescribe simple typhoid vaccine and thus avoid injecting possible inert bacteria which may contribute to the reaction rate with typhoid-paratyphoid vaccines.

The vaccine is administered by subcutaneous injection in 2 doses of the volume stated on the label as the dose with an interval of 4 to 6 weeks between the doses. Immunity usually lasts for at least 2 years.

Suitable schedules for the immunisation of travellers are given under Vaccines. Local erythema, swelling, tenderness, pain, general malaise, nausea, and headache may sometimes occur after the subcutaneous injection of this vaccine.

Typhoid-paratyphoid Vaccines

Mixed suspensions of killed *Salmonella typhi*, *S. paratyphi* A, and *S. paratyphi* B. They may also contain Cholera Vaccine or Tetanus Vaccine as described below.

Typhoid-paratyphoid A and B Vaccine. OTHER NAMES: T.A.B. Vaccine; TAB/Vac

It contains 1000 million *S. typhi*, 500 or 750 million *S. paratyphi* A, and 500 or 750 million *S. paratyphi* B in 1 ml.

Intracutaneous Typhoid-paratyphoid A and B Vaccine. OTHER NAMES: Intracut. T.A.B. Vaccine; Intradermal Typhoid-paratyphoid A and B Vaccine; TAB/Vac (Intracutaneous)

It contains either 2500 million *S. typhi*, 1250 million *S. paratyphi* A, and 1250 million *S. paratyphi* B, or 2000 million *S. typhi*, 1500 million *S. paratyphi* A, and 1500 million *S. paratyphi* B in 1 ml (dose: 0.1 ml).

Typhoid-paratyphoid A and B and Cholera Vaccine. OTHER NAMES: T.A.B. and Cholera Vaccine; TABCho/Vac

It contains 1000 million *S. typhi*, 500 or 750 million *S. paratyphi* A, 500 or 750 million *S. paratyphi* B, and 8000 million cholera vibrios in 1 ml. The cholera component consists of equal parts of the two main serotypes, Inaba and Ogawa, of the classical biotype of *Vibrio cholerae*. This vaccine is suitable for use when an international certificate in respect of cholera vaccination is required.

Typhoid-paratyphoid A and B and Tetanus Vaccine. OTHER NAMES: T.A.B. and Tetanus Vaccine; TABT/Vac; Typhoid-paratyphoid A and B Vaccine-Tetanus Toxoid

It contains tetanus formol toxoid and 500 or 1000 million *S. typhi*, 250 or 500 million *S. paratyphi* A, and 250 or 500 million *S. paratyphi* B in 1 ml.

A standard is given in the British Pharmacopoeia 1973

The typhoid-paratyphoid components consist of vaccines prepared from strains of *S. typhi*, *S. paratyphi* A, and *S. paratyphi* B that are smooth and have the full complement of O and H antigens and, in the case of *S. typhi*, contain also the Vi antigen. Either a single strain or several strains of each species may be included.

Storage. They should be stored as described under Vaccines.

Actions and uses. Typhoid vaccine has been shown to be an effective prophylactic against typhoid fever. It is widely used in the form of Typhoid-paratyphoid A and B vaccine for the prevention of typhoid and paratyphoid fevers, although the value of the paratyphoid components has not been established.

Typhoid-paratyphoid A and B and cholera vaccine is used for primary immunisation against enteric fevers and cholera. Typhoid-paratyphoid A and B and tetanus vaccine is used for primary immunisation against enteric fevers and tetanus, for which 3 subcutaneous doses are required to immunise satisfactorily against tetanus, there being an interval of at least 4 to 6 weeks between the first and second doses and preferably 4 to 6 months between the second and third doses. These vaccines are seldom used for reinforcing doses as the intervals before a reinforcing dose is required for the various components do not correspond; it is preferable therefore to use the simple typhoid-paratyphoid, cholera, or tetanus vaccines separately for this purpose.

Typhoid-paratyphoid vaccines are usually administered by subcutaneous injection in 2 doses, using the volume stated on the label as the dose, preferably separated by an interval of 4 to 6 weeks; immunity usually lasts 2 to 3 years. When an epidemic or other major risk of infection arises it may be desirable to administer a reinforcing dose.

Suitable schedules for the immunisation of travellers are given under Vaccines.

Intracutaneous typhoid-paratyphoid vaccine is suitable for intracutaneous administration only. The dose is 0.1 millilitre and overdosage may give rise to an area of skin necrosis. The intracutaneous route is reliable only if the inoculation technique is satisfactory. Typhoid-paratyphoid vaccines prepared for subcutaneous injection are unsuitable for intracutaneous use.

Undesirable effects. Local erythema, swelling, tenderness, pain, general malaise, nausea, and headache may sometimes occur after subcutaneous or intramuscular injection of these vaccines.

Typhus Vaccine

A suspension of killed epidemic (Breinl strain) typhus rickettsiae which has been shown to protect susceptible animals against epidemic typhus.

OTHER NAME: Typhus/Vac

A standard is given in the British Pharmacopoeia 1973

Storage. It should be stored protected from light at 2° to 10°. It should not be allowed to freeze. Under these conditions it may be expected to retain its potency for one year.

Actions and uses. Typhus vaccine is of value in the prophylaxis of louse-borne typhus. The vaccine lessens the severity of the disease and the mortality rate, although it may not materially influence the attack rate. The primary course is 2 doses, each of 1 millilitre, for persons over the age of 9 years, given at intervals of 7 to 10 days. Children between the ages of 6 months and 4 years should have 0.2-millilitre doses and those between 4 and 9 years 0.5-millilitre doses.

Reinforcing doses of 1 millilitre should be given annually, except during an epidemic when they should be given every 3 months.

General reactions resulting from administration of the recommended doses are uncommon.

Ulcerative Colitis

Ulcerative colitis is a condition in which there are changes in the structure of the mucosa and submucosa of the wall of the colon, with widespread inflammation and superficial ulceration. It may vary in its form from mild diarrhoea to severe disease accompanied by toxaemia, dehydration, and malnutrition. The disease is usually characterised by attacks of diarrhoea with blood and mucus in the faeces; however when the disease is confined to the rectum there may be constipation. There is frequently tenesmus and pain before defaecation and there may be abdominal cramp caused by colonic spasm.

Symptomatic treatment may be required, parenterally if necessary, to correct deficiency of electrolytes, vitamins, minerals, and other nutrients. Blood transfusion is necessary for anaemic patients and antibacterial agents may be required for treatment of infections. Administration of corticosteroids by mouth or by rectum or injections of corticotrophin or tetracosactrin may be used to control the acute illness or exacerbation.

Prolonged administration of sulphasalazine by mouth or rectum is used to induce or maintain remissions and prevent exacerbation. Azathioprine has been used when other treatment has been unsuccessful.

Regular follow-up examinations should be made to detect the supervention of cancer of the colon. Surgery is required for cases not responsive to medical therapy.

Ultraviolet Spectrophotometry

Ultraviolet spectrophotometry is a technique for examining the absorption by chemical substances of radiation in the ultraviolet region. The usual wavelength range examined for analytical purposes is 230 nm to 360 nm. Absorption in the ultraviolet region is not usually specific for a particular substance. Absorption bands characteristic of certain absorbing structures ("chromophores") may be observed in the spectrum but it is not always possible to attribute the absorption bands to any particular absorbing species. Compounds of similar structure will have similar absorption characteristics and the absorption may be considerably affected by the polarity of the solvent or, in aqueous solution, by the pH. Thus the ultraviolet absorption characteristics cannot be used for the positive identification of a substance. However, consideration of the wavelengths of absorption maxima and of the corresponding specific extinction coefficients (see below) may give a useful indication of identity, especially when associated with other identification techniques. The absorption spectrum in the infrared region is more complex and gives more information about identity (see under Infra-red Spectrophotometry). The ultraviolet absorption of a substance is widely used in quantitative determinations. The amount of light absorbed is proportional to the concentration and to the thickness of the absorbing layer (Beer-Lambert Law), and the specific extinction coefficient (extinction of a 1-cm layer of a 1% solution) is expressed as

$$E(1\%, 1cm) = \frac{E}{cd}$$

where, E = the measured extinction, c = the concentration in %, and d = the thickness in centimetres of the absorbing layer.

The absorption is sometimes expressed as the molecular extinction coefficient

$$\epsilon = E(1\%, 1cm) \times \frac{\text{mol. wt}}{10}.$$

In these expressions, the symbol "E" may be replaced by the alternative symbol "A" (absorbance). The absorption of one component of a mixture can be measured provided that the other components do not absorb in the same region. Sometimes it may be possible to avoid interference by shifting the absorption of one component by a suitable adjustment of pH. The quantities of two components that absorb in the same region may be calculated from the absorption at two or more wavelengths within the absorbing region.

Ultraviolet spectrophotometers may be either manually operated single beam instruments or may be recording instruments having a double beam arrangement whereby a "blank" or reference solution may be scanned simultaneously with the sample. The double beam recording spectrophotometer is ideal for scanning the absorption spectrum, but various factors associated with automatic scanning such as the scan speed, the pen response, and the identification of wavelength on calibrated paper, will have an effect on the shape and intensity of the curve. It is therefore advisable to use a manually operated instrument for the measurement of extinction at a specific wavelength in quantitative measurements.

Ultraviolet data. Many of the entries on medicinal substances in this volume include data on ultraviolet absorption. Much of the information is based on laboratory determinations carried out especially for this publication, but some has been obtained from other published sources. Because of instrumental differences, and the possible effects of solvent and pH (noted above), E(1%, 1cm) values are subject to considerable variation, and the values quoted should not be taken as absolute. They are suitable as a guide in qualitative work but for quantitative work a reference specimen should be examined at the same time as the sample.

Undecenoic Acid

Undecenoic acid consists mainly of undec-10-enoic acid.

$$CH_2{:}CH{\cdot}[CH_2]_8{\cdot}COOH$$

$C_{11}H_{20}O_2 = 184.3$

OTHER NAMES: Acidum Undecylenicum; Undecylenic Acid

Mycota® (with dichlorophen or zinc undecenoate)

A standard is given in the European Pharmacopoeia Vol. III Supplement

Description. A colourless or pale yellow liquid or a white or very pale yellow crystalline mass with a characteristic odour.

Solubility. Practically insoluble in water; miscible with alcohol, with ether, with chloroform, and with fixed and volatile oils.

Refractive index. At 25°, 1.447 to 1.450.

Freezing-point. About 22°.

Storage. It should be stored in airtight containers, protected from light.

Actions and uses. Undecenoic acid is a fungicide used for the prophylaxis and treatment of superficial dermatophytoses of the head, ears, feet, axillae, and groin and of candidiasis and mycotic infections of the vulva and vagina.

For application to the skin, concentrations of 2 to 15% are used, sometimes in conjunction with zinc undecenoate, in ointments, emulsions, and dusting-powders.

For applications to mucous surfaces the concentration should not exceed 1% as stronger preparations may cause irritation.

Preparations

Preparations available include an APPLICATION containing undecenoic acid 2.5% with dichlorophen 0.25% in an aerosol pack; and a DUSTING-POWDER containing undecenoic acid 2% with zinc undecenoate 20%.

Undecenoic acid is an ingredient of zinc undecenoate dusting-powder and of zinc undecenoate ointment.

Undulant Fever

see BRUCELLOSIS

Units

see under WEIGHTS AND MEASURES

Uraemia

see under RENAL FAILURE

Urea

$$NH_2 \cdot CO \cdot NH_2$$

$CH_4N_2O = 60.06$

OTHER NAMES: *Aquadrate®*; *Calmurid®*; Carbamide; *Ureaphil®*; *Urevert®*
Alphaderm®, and *Calmurid HC®*, (both with hydrocortisone)

A standard is given in the British Pharmacopoeia 1973

Description. Odourless, colourless, transparent slightly hygroscopic, prismatic crystals with a cooling and saline taste.

Solubility. Soluble, at 20°, in 1 part of water and in 12 parts of alcohol; soluble in 1.5 parts of boiling alcohol; practically insoluble in ether and in chloroform.

Sterilisation. Solutions for injection are sterilised by filtration.

Storage. It should be stored in airtight containers.

Identification. TESTS. 1. Heat about 500 mg in a test-tube; it liquefies and ammonia is evolved. Continue heating until the liquid becomes turbid, cool, dissolve the liquid in a mixture of 10 ml of water and 0.5 ml of *sodium*

hydroxide solution, and add 1 drop of *copper sulphate solution*; a reddish-violet colour is produced.
2. Dissolve about 10 mg in 1 ml of water and add 1 ml of nitric acid; a white crystalline precipitate is produced.

MELTING-POINT. About 133°.

Metabolism. ABSORPTION. Absorbed after oral administration and also converted in the colon to ammonia, which is absorbed.

BLOOD CONCENTRATION. Normal concentrations in blood are about 300 μg/ml in adults and lower in infants; after an intravenous infusion of 0.24 to 1.5 g/kg as a solution containing 30% urea and 10% invert sugar, administered over a period of 10 minutes to several hours, plasma concentrations of 1 to 2 mg/ml are obtained at the end of infusion.

HALF-LIFE. Biological half-life, about 1 hour.

METABOLIC REACTIONS. Converted to ammonia in the colon.

EXCRETION. Normal urinary excretion is in the range 10 to 35 g in 24 hours; urea is not normally found in faeces.

FURTHER INFORMATION. O. Wrong, *Med. J. Aust.*, ii/1967, 281; P. R. Yarnell *et al.*, *Clin. Pharmac. Ther.*, 1972, **13**, 558.

Actions and uses. Urea exerts a diuretic action. When given by mouth, it is rapidly excreted and its excretion is accompanied by an increase in urinary output; the rate of excretion of 15 grams of urea administered in 100 millilitres of water is used as a test for renal function. The usual dose as a diuretic is 5 to 15 grams.

To produce decompression in concussion and cerebral injury, urea is administered by slow intravenous injection in a 30% solution in dextrose injection (5 or 10%). The dose is usually 40 to 90 grams of urea, but not exceeding 1.5 grams per kilogram body-weight, in 24 hours. The solution is irritant and care must be taken to avoid extravasation during injection.

A cream containing 10% of urea is used as a keratolytic in ichthyosis and other hyperkeratotic skin conditions.

Preparations

UREA CREAM: a dispersion of urea in a suitable basis. Available as a cream containing 10% of urea.
Containers, Labelling, and *Storage:* see the entry on Creams for general information on containers, labelling, and storage.
Advice for patients: the skin should be cleansed prior to application and the cream applied liberally to the affected area, left on the skin for 3 to 5 minutes, and then lightly rubbed in. Excess cream may be removed with a tissue.

UREA INJECTION: a sterile solution of urea in dextrose injection (5 or 10%). It is prepared by dissolving the contents of a sealed container, which also includes a small proportion of citric acid monohydrate, in the vehicle immediately before use. Available as a powder in units containing 40 to 90 g of urea.
A standard for this injection is given in the British Pharmacopoeia 1973
Containers and *Labelling:* see the entry on Injections for general information on containers and labelling.
Storage: the injection decomposes on storage and should be used immediately after preparation.

OTHER PREPARATIONS available include a CREAM containing urea 10% with hydrocortisone 1%; and a SOLUTION containing urea 20%.

Urethritis, Non-specific

Non-specific urethritis is an inflammation of the urethra which is transmitted by sexual intercourse but in which no infecting organism can be detected. It is attributed to strains of *Mycoplasma* or *Chlamydia*.

Non-specific urethritis is characterised by dysuria accompanied by a mucopurulent urethral discharge containing pus cells but no organisms. The incubation period is probably about 10 to 14 days and an attack may be precipitated by a large intake of alcohol. When severe, non-specific urethritis may be accompanied by abacterial or haemorrhagic cystitis. The infecting agents of non-specific urethritis may also cause abacterial cervicitis or proctitis.

It is treated by the avoidance of sexual intercourse and alcohol and the administration of tetracyclines.

Urinary-tract Infections

Urinary-tract infection may be present at any level of the urinary tract—urethra, bladder, ureters, pelvis, or the kidney itself—and symptoms are not a reliable guide to the localisation of infection. However, a rapid onset with pain in the loins, dysuria, fever, and leucocytosis indicates that the kidney is involved in the infection.

In general practice the usual infecting organism is *Escherichia coli* but infections acquired in hospital may be due to many other organisms.

Urinary-tract infection is very common in females. Symptoms, which are usually confined to the lower urinary tract, include frequent passing of urine, dysuria, and sometimes haematuria. Symptomless infection may also occur, especially during pregnancy.

Treatment of urinary-tract infection consists of bed rest and the use of antibacterial agents to which the infecting organisms are sensitive. If the urine is rendered alkaline, troublesome symptoms may subside before the infection is eliminated. Surgery may be required for obstructive lesions.

Urethritis is an inflammation of the urethra characterised by discharge of pus and dysuria. See the entries on Gonorrhoea and Urethritis, Non-specific.

Cystitis is an inflammation of the bladder which may be acute or chronic in nature. Symptoms include dysuria, frequency of passing urine, suprapubic pain, haematuria, fever, and general malaise. Acute attacks may occur in isolation with no indication of an underlying cause but more often they are the precursor of chronic infection. Infecting organisms and treatment are similar to those described under Pyelonephritis (below). Because many women with these symptoms do not have infected urine it is customary to culture the urine before using antibiotic therapy and in the interval symptomatic treatment may be all that is required. Antibiotics are sometimes given while awaiting results of urine culture.

Pyelonephritis. Acute pyelonephritis is an acute inflammation of the parenchyma and pelvis of the kidney, sometimes with pus formation, and one or both kidneys may be affected. It is due to an infection which may be associated with an obstruction of the urinary tract, the infection being due to *Escherichia coli*, or less commonly to species of *Streptococcus*, *Staphylococcus*, *Proteus*, *Klebsiella*, or *Pseudomonas*. Onset may be rapid, with pain in the loins, and sometimes dysuria, fever, and leucocytosis, or it may be insidious and characterised by lethargy and anorexia; symptomless pyelonephritis may also occur, especially during pregnancy.

Treatment consists of bed rest and the use of antibacterial agents to which the infecting organisms are sensitive. Surgery may be required for obstructive lesions. If the urine is rendered alkaline symptoms may subside before the infection is eliminated. Repeated attacks of acute pyelonephritis may lead to chronic pyelonephritis, a chronic inflammatory condition in which the kidneys are small and scarred. A similar condition may arise as a result of long-term administration of phenacetin.

Antibacterials used in the treatment of urinary tract infections include ampicillin, carbenicillin, cephalexin, co-trimoxazole, gentamicin, kanamycin, mandelic acid, nalidixic acid, nitrofurantoin, streptomycin, sulphonamides, and tetracyclines.

Urticaria

Urticaria is characterised by a transient redness and swelling of the skin which causes wheals in the dermis accompanied by an itching or stinging sensation. It is the result of localised oedema caused by an increase in permeability of the walls of blood vessels brought about by the release of histamine-like substances. Urticaria may be due to bites, stings, heat, friction, food or drug allergy, or intestinal parasites.

Where possible urticaria should be treated by removal of the underlying cause. Many cases respond to oral treatment with an antihistamine but refractory cases require investigation of the underlying allergic reactions and appropriate treatment. Cooling applications may also reduce irritation.

Uterine Bleeding, Abnormal

Bleeding from the female genital tract occurs normally in women of child-bearing age in a cyclical manner known as menstruation. All bleeding from the genital tract is abnormal in postmenopausal women. Abnormal uterine bleeding may be due to pathology in the uterus, ovary, pituitary, or hypothalamus or it may be attributable to psychological causes.

In *amenorrhoea* menstruation fails to commence at puberty (primary amenorrhoea) or is absent in a woman who has previously menstruated (secondary amenorrhoea).

In *polymenorrhoea* the blood loss at menstruation is normal, but it occurs at too frequent intervals.

In *menorrhagia* (*hypermenorrhoea*) the cycle of menstruation is of normal duration, but the amount of blood loss is excessive.

In *polymenorrhagia* the menstrual bleeding is excessive and the length of the cycle is reduced.

In *metrorrhagia* menstrual bleeding is irregular in amount, acyclic in nature, and often prolonged.

In *metropathia haemorrhagica* there is hyperplasia of the endometrium with irregular uterine haemorrhage.

Vaccines

Vaccines are preparations of antigenic materials that are administered with the object of inducing in the recipient a specific active immunity to infection or intoxication by the corresponding infecting agents. They may contain living or dead micro-organisms or bacterial toxins or toxoids or they may be purified products derived from bacteria. They may be simple vaccines prepared from one species only or mixed vaccines which are mixtures of two or more simple vaccines.

The methods of preparation are designed to ensure that the identity of the specific antigens is maintained and that no microbial contaminants are introduced. The final products are distributed under aseptic conditions into sterile containers which are then sealed to exclude extraneous micro-organisms. All forms, with the exception of certain living vaccines, comply with the test for sterility of the European Pharmacopoeia.

Bacterial vaccines may be prepared from one species only or may contain two or more different species or varieties. Each culture used for the preparation of bacterial vaccines is first carefully examined for its identity, antigenic properties, and purity. The culture is grown on a solid medium under appropriate conditions and is then washed off the medium with sodium chloride injection or other suitable solution; alternatively, it is grown in a fluid medium. The whole culture, or an extract or derivative of the culture, is used for preparing the vaccine.

In preparing sterile bacterial vaccines the bacteria are killed in such a manner that the antigenic potency of the product is not impaired. A suitable antibacterial substance, in a concentration sufficient to prevent the growth of micro-organisms, may be added to sterile bacterial vaccines and is invariably added to such vaccines when they are issued in multiple-dose containers.

Bacterial vaccines containing living bacteria are prepared from strains which are avirulent for man but which stimulate the production of antibodies active against pathogenic strains of the same species.

Bacterial vaccines are suspensions of varying opacity, usually white, in colourless or slightly coloured liquids. They may be standardised by determining the number of bacteria per ml, either by direct count in a counting chamber or by comparison of the opacity of the suspension with that of a preparation of standard opacity.

Bacterial toxoids are toxins or material derived therefrom, the specific toxicity of which has been reduced to a low level or completely removed by chemical or physical means without destroying the immunising potency.

Toxoids produced by the action of formaldehyde, the most commonly used detoxicating agent, are sometimes called *formol toxoids* or *anatoxins*.

Adsorbed toxoids may be prepared by adsorbing formol toxoids on a suspension of aluminium hydroxide, hydrated aluminium phosphate, or other suitable substance; the precipitate may be separated, washed, and suspended in a saline or other appropriate solution isotonic with blood.

Bacterial toxoids are clear colourless or yellow liquids, or suspensions of white or grey particles in colourless or yellow liquids. They comply with tests for minimum potency as immunising antigens.

Mixed vaccines are mixtures of two or more simple bacterial vaccines or bacterial toxoids. They are clear liquids or suspensions of varying opacity, usually white, in colourless or slightly coloured liquids.

Viral and rickettsial vaccines are prepared from infected tissue or blood obtained from artificially infected animals, from cultures in fertile eggs, or from cell or tissue cultures. The material may be inactivated by exposure to formaldehyde or by other suitable chemical or physical means. Living vaccines are usually prepared with attenuated antigenic strains of the specific organisms. A suitable antibacterial substance may be added to inactivated or living viral or rickettsial vaccines, provided that it has no action against the specific organisms.

Viral and rickettsial vaccines vary in appearance from clear colourless liquids to suspensions of varying opacity and colour.

Storage. Liquid bacterial vaccines, bacterial toxoids, and bacterial toxins should be protected from light and stored at 2° to 10° unless otherwise specified. They deteriorate at temperatures approaching 20°. Freeze-dried preparations should be stored below 20°. Unless otherwise specified, liquid vaccines should not be allowed to freeze.

Viral and rickettsial vaccines should be stored under the conditions described in the individual entries.

Age	Vaccine
During the first year of life, the first dose being given at an age of 3 months	diphtheria, tetanus, and pertussis
	poliomyelitis (oral)
NOTE. When oral poliomyelitis vaccine is given to infants, it should also be offered to unimmunised parents to protect them from the very small risk of contact vaccine-associated poliomyelitis.	Three doses, with an interval of 6 to 8 weeks between the first and second doses and 4 to 6 months between the second and third
During the second year of life	measles (live)
At entry to school or nursery school but allowing an interval of at least 3 years after completing the basic course	diphtheria and tetanus
	poliomyelitis (oral)
	or
	diphtheria, tetanus, and poliomyelitis
Eleven to thirteen years	bacillus Calmette-Guérin
NOTE. For tuberculin-negative children, normally at 13 years. B.C.G. vaccine should also be given at birth to children who come from environments where there is a high risk of contracting tuberculosis, and to tuberculin-negative contacts at any age. There should be an interval of at least 3 weeks between B.C.G. and rubella vaccination.	
Fifteen to nineteen years or on leaving school	{ poliomyelitis (oral or inactivated)
	{ tetanus
Girls eleven to thirteen years	rubella

NOTE. Where an age range is specific in the above table it includes the following birthday, that is, 11 to 13 years means from the eleventh to the fourteenth birthday.

Immunisation of Children

Protection against several infectious diseases in early life may be provided by active immunisation and the following scheme is based on recommendations of the United Kingdom Department of Health and Social Security (see TABLE opposite).

The *basic course* of immunisation against diphtheria, pertussis, tetanus, and poliomyelitis should begin at 3 months and be completed as soon as possible consistent with the likelihood of a good immunological response, that is, a second dose at 4½ to 5 months and a third dose at 8½ to 11 months of age.

If whooping-cough is prevalent, the intervals between the first and second and second and third doses may be reduced to 1 month; in addition, an immunising dose of diphtheria and tetanus vaccine, adsorbed should be given at age 12 to 18 months as otherwise the basic immunity to diphtheria and tetanus may be inadequate. *Reinforcement* of immunisation against diphtheria, tetanus, and poliomyelitis, should be given at school (or when appropriate nursery school) entry, and further reinforcement of immunisation against tetanus and poliomyelitis should be given at school-leaving age.

If the basic course has been interrupted it may be resumed without repetition of the earlier doses. If no immunisation has been given before entry to nursery or primary school, measles vaccine should be given followed by full courses of diphtheria and tetanus vaccine and poliomyelitis (oral) vaccine. Vaccines containing a pertussis component should not be given after the age of 3 years.

Routine vaccination against smallpox is not now recommended in the United Kingdom. Vaccination is still recommended for those at special risk, such as doctors, nurses, and other health service staff, and for travellers to areas of the world where smallpox is still occurring or where eradication programmes are in progress.

When anyone is vaccinated against smallpox, the possibility of accidental infection of eczematous members of the family must be borne in mind.

Routine vaccination against rubella is recommended for those women of childbearing age who are found to be seronegative. Women so vaccinated should be advised to avoid pregnancy for 8 weeks after vaccination because of possible harm to the foetus if pregnancy occurs within that period.

An interval of 3 weeks should normally be allowed to elapse between the administration of any two live vaccines.

Immunisation of Travellers

Two schedules are given as a guide to the inoculation of travellers. They may be amended according to the immunological history of the traveller and the time available before departure. When sufficient time is not available to follow the suggested procedures, the responses to some antigens may be suboptimal and there is a risk of undesirable reactions of various kinds.

For travellers who have to go abroad from time to time, the following schedule is recommended, provided that there is sufficient time before departure.

Week	Vaccine
1	yellow fever
4	smallpox (when required)
5	*read result of smallpox*
7	typhoid-paratyphoid A and B (1)
13	typhoid-paratyphoid A and B (2)

Travellers who have not received basic immunisation against poliomyelitis may be given three doses of poliomyelitis oral vaccine in weeks 10, 16, and 22. Immunisation against tetanus may be provided by using typhoid-paratyphoid A and B and tetanus vaccine in weeks 7 and 13 and tetanus vaccine in week 39.

When the schedule is completed, an occasional reinforcing dose may be all that is required before a subsequent journey. Reinforcing injections should be given as follows:

Vaccine	Frequency of reinforcing dose
yellow fever vaccine	every 10 years
typhoid-paratyphoid A and B vaccine	every year as long as the individual is at special risk; every 3 years in other circumstances
tetanus vaccine	every 5 years
smallpox vaccine (when required)	every 3 years

It should be noted that the International Certificate of Vaccination becomes valid, in respect of smallpox, 8 days after the date of a successful primary vaccination, or on the date of revaccination, and, in respect of yellow fever, 10 days after the first vaccination, or immediately on revaccination within 10 years. Only a limited number of countries now require a certificate of smallpox vaccination.

Vaccination against cholera is recommended for travellers to tropical and subtropical countries of Asia and Africa including the Mediterranean coast, and any other areas notified as infected. As the International Certificate of cholera vaccination is valid for a period of 6 months only, this vaccine has been omitted from the recommended schedule; the Certificate becomes valid 6 days after the first cholera vaccination and immediately on revaccination within 6 months. For the International Certificate cholera vaccine must contain the classical serotypes of Inaba and Ogawa and may also contain the El Tor biotypes; vaccine containing only El Tor biotypes is not recognised for this purpose. The International Certificate is no longer a requirement under international law but may be used as evidence of vaccination when required.

Alternative Schedule. For travellers who have little warning of their journey, the following alternative schedule may be adopted.

Day	Vaccine
1	cholera (1) and typhoid-paratyphoid A and B (1)
5	yellow fever and smallpox (at separate sites)
13	cholera (2)
	read result of smallpox
28	typhoid-paratyphoid A and B (2)

When smallpox vaccine and yellow fever vaccine must be given to the same person at short notice, the two vaccines may be given at the same time but at different sites; this is preferable to shortening the interval between the two vaccinations, a practice which might lead to interference between the two vaccines.

Travellers who have not received basic immunisation against poliomyelitis may receive poliomyelitis vaccine (oral) on days 1 and 28. Tetanus immunisation may be given by using typhoid-paratyphoid A and B and tetanus vaccine instead of the typhoid-paratyphoid vaccine. The third doses of poliomyelitis vaccine (oral) and tetanus vaccine will be required some months later to complete the primary courses of immunisation.

This alternative schedule is unsatisfactory from the immunological standpoint and longer intervals are desirable when the time is available.

Vancomycin Hydrochloride

The hydrochloride of an antibiotic produced by certain strains of *Streptomyces orientalis*.

OTHER NAME: *Vancocin*®

A standard is given in the British Pharmacopoeia 1973

Description. An odourless, light brown powder with a bitter taste.

Solubility. Soluble, at 20°, in 10 parts of water and in 700 parts of alcohol; very slightly soluble in ether and in chloroform.

Acidity. A 5% solution has a pH of 2.8 to 4.5.

Moisture content. Not more than 4.5%, determined by Fischer titration.

Storage. It should be stored in sterile containers, sealed to exclude micro-organisms.

Identification. TEST. Dissolve about 200 mg in 5 ml of water, add 1 ml of hydrochloric acid, heat in a water-bath for 10 minutes, dissolve the precipitate in the minimum of *sodium hydroxide solution*, add dropwise to the boiling solution 2.5 ml of *potassium cupri-tartrate solution* and filter; a red precipitate is obtained. Repeat the test omitting the sodium hydroxide solution; only a slight red precipitate is obtained.

ULTRAVIOLET ABSORPTION. In 0.1N sulphuric acid, maximum at 280 nm (E1%, 1cm = 34).

Metabolism. ABSORPTION. Not absorbed after oral administration and is administered intravenously.

BLOOD CONCENTRATION. After an intravenous dose of 500 mg, plasma concentrations of 5 to 10 μg/ml are obtained after 1 to 2 hours, falling to about 3 μg/ml by 6 hours.

HALF-LIFE. Plasma half-life, about 6 hours.

DISTRIBUTION. Widely distributed throughout the body and enters pleural, ascitic, pericardial, and synovial fluids and also, when the meninges are inflamed, the cerebrospinal fluid; accumulates in renal function impairment; may cross the placenta; *protein binding*, appears to be less than 10% bound to plasma proteins.

EXCRETION. Rapidly excreted, about 60% of a dose being excreted in the urine in 3 to 6 hours; nearly all the dose is eventually excreted in the urine with very little appearing in the faeces; small amounts may be secreted in the bile.

FURTHER INFORMATION. Dosage in renal failure—C. M. Kunin, *Ann. intern. Med.*, 1967, **67**, 151; renal excretion in renal disease—H. E. Nielsen *et al.*, *Acta med. scand.*, 1975, **197**, 261.

Actions and uses. Vancomycin is an antibiotic which is effective against Gram-positive cocci. It is given by intravenous injection, mainly in the treatment of systemic infections caused by staphylococci which are resistant to other antibiotics; it is also of value in the treatment of endocarditis and other infections caused by non-haemolytic streptococci resistant to penicillin.

The usual daily dosage for an adult is the equivalent of 2 grams of vancomycin given by slow intravenous infusion over a period of 24 hours, or 500 milligrams given by slow intravenous injection over a period of 20 to 30 minutes every 6 to 8 hours; the daily dosage for a child is 45 milligrams per kilogram body-weight.

When given by slow intravenous injection the dose of vancomycin hydrochloride is dissolved in 100 to 200 millilitres of sodium chloride injection or dextrose injection (5%); when given by intravenous infusion, the dose is dissolved in a larger volume. The solution is irritant and care should be taken to avoid extravasation during injection. To guard against accumulation, regular blood-level determinations should be made; a blood concentration of 10 to 20 micrograms per millilitre should be maintained.

Vancomycin hydrochloride is administered by mouth in the treatment of pseudomembranous colitis, the usual dosage being the equivalent of 500 milligrams of vancomycin every 6 hours.

Undesirable effects. Nausea, shivering, and rashes may occur. Impaired hearing is a more serious hazard, but is unlikely to occur unless treatment is prolonged or there is impairment of kidney function, when it is related to persistently high trough levels just before the next dose is due. Thrombophlebitis may occur at the site of injection and leakage from a vein may cause local necrosis. Vancomycin is nephrotoxic.

Precautions and contra-indications. The use of vancomycin should preferably be avoided in patients with renal disease but if its use is necessary, blood concentrations should be monitored.

Preparation

VANCOMYCIN INJECTION: a sterile solution of vancomycin hydrochloride in water for injections. It is prepared by dissolving the contents of a sealed container in water for injections immediately before use. Available as a powder in vials containing vancomycin hydrochloride equivalent to 500 mg (approximately 500 000 units) of vancomycin.

A standard for this injection is given in the British Pharmacopoeia 1973

Containers and *Labelling:* see the entry on Injections for general information on containers and labelling.

Storage: the injection decomposes on storage and should be used immediately after preparation.

Vanillin

4-Hydroxy-3-methoxybenzaldehyde

$C_8H_8O_3 = 152.1$

A standard is given in the British Pharmaceutical Codex 1973

Vanillin may be obtained from *Vanilla planifolia* Andrews or other species of *Vanilla* (Fam. Orchidaceae), or prepared synthetically.

Description. White or cream-coloured crystalline needles or powder with the characteristic odour of vanilla.

Solubility. Soluble, at 20°, in 100 parts of water and in 20 parts of glycerol; soluble in alcohol, in fixed and volatile oils, and in solutions of alkali hydroxides.

Storage. It should be stored in airtight containers, protected from light.

Identification. TESTS. 1. To 1 ml of a saturated solution add 1 ml of *lead acetate solution*; a white precipitate is produced which is soluble in hot water from which it separates in scales on cooling.
2. To 10 ml of a saturated solution add 4 drops of *ferric chloride test-solution*; a blue colour is produced. Heat at 80° for 3 minutes; the solution becomes brown. Cool; a white or almost white precipitate is produced.

MELTING-POINT. About 82°.

Metabolism. METABOLIC REACTIONS. In the rat, oxidation to vanillic acid, reduction to vanillyl alcohol, decarboxylation, demethylation, and glycine or glucuronic acid conjugation.

EXCRETION. In the rat, up to about 94% of a dose is excreted in the urine, mainly as vanillic acid and vanillyl alcohol with smaller amounts of vanilloylglycine, catechol, 4-methylguaiacol, 4-methylcatechol, guaiacol, protocatechuic acid, and about 7% as unchanged drug.

FURTHER INFORMATION. Metabolism of vanillin and isovanillin in rats—L. P. Strand and R. R. Scheline, *Xenobiotica*, 1975, 5, 49.

Uses. Vanillin is used as a flavouring agent and in perfumery.

Preparations

Vanillin is an ingredient of calcium gluconate tablets, liquid paraffin emulsion, and methylcellulose granules.

Varicella

see CHICKENPOX

Variola

see SMALLPOX

Vasopressin Injection

A sterile aqueous solution containing the pressor and antidiuretic principles, prepared by a process of fractionation, of the posterior lobe of mammalian pituitary bodies. It contains 20 units (pressor) per ml.

OTHER NAME: *Pitressin*®

A standard is given in the British Pharmacopoeia 1973

Description. A clear colourless liquid.

Acidity. pH 3 to 4.

Sterilisation. It is sterilised by filtration.

Storage. It should be stored at a temperature between 2° and 10°. Under these conditions it may be expected to retain its potency for 3 years from the date of manufacture. If stored at temperatures not exceeding 25°, it may be expected to retain its potency for 2 years from the date of manufacture.

Metabolism. BLOOD CONCENTRATION. Normal circulating concentrations of vasopressin are about 4 pg/ml which may be increased to 40 pg/ml during water deprivation; doses of 10 to 40 µg produce circulating concentrations 20 to 100 times greater than normal concentrations and are similar to those attained in severe shock.

DISTRIBUTION. Volume of distribution, 30 to 135 ml/kg body-weight.

METABOLIC REACTIONS. Deactivated by release of the C-terminal glycinamide moiety.

Actions and uses. Vasopressin injection has the pressor and antidiuretic actions of the posterior lobe of the pituitary gland but has practically no oxytocic activity. Vasopressin injection is used in the treatment of diabetes insipidus to control the polyuria. From 0.1 to 1 millilitre, equivalent to 2 to 20 units, is administered by subcutaneous or intramuscular injection. It must be given at least twice a day. It may also be given by intravenous injection but must be well diluted.

Vasopressin injection has been used to stimulate the muscle of the intestinal tract, but it has been superseded by cholinergic drugs because they are safer. It should not be used to raise the blood pressure.

Undesirable effects. The administration of vasopressin injection may be followed by marked pallor, nausea, eructation, cramp, and a desire to defaecate.

Contra-indications. It is contra-indicated in vascular disease, especially of the coronary arteries.

Venous Thrombosis

Venous thrombosis is the formation of a clot within a vein. It is characterised by oedema, pain, and congestion of superficial veins in the region of the thrombosis, together with fever and malaise. Thrombosis is usually due to stasis of blood associated with immobilisation such as occurs after abdominal surgery and chronic congestive heart failure. It may also be due to severe infection, neoplastic disease, or increased coagulability of the blood associated with the use of oral contraceptives containing oestrogens.

The veins of the leg are most commonly affected, and thrombosis in the inferior vena cava may lead to symptoms in both legs. Thrombosis in a vein results in inflammation (thrombophlebitis) and thrombosed veins may be palpated as tender hard cords. At first there is danger of movement of thrombus to the lung giving rise to pulmonary embolism, but soon after formation the clot becomes adherent to the walls of the vein and the risk of embolism is decreased. The organised thrombus may later be recanalised, restoring the blood flow through the vessel.

Venous thrombosis may be prevented by rhythmic calf compression during operation, elevation of the foot of the bed, and full length elastic stockings. Low-dose subcutaneous injections of heparin significantly reduce the risk of post-operative thrombosis and pulmonary embolism in certain operations. If venous thrombosis occurs, patients should rest in bed with the leg raised. The thrombus may be removed surgically to prevent pulmonary embolism. Treatment with anticoagulants should be started immediately to slow down propagation of the clot and reduce the risk of pulmonary embolism. Thrombosis may also occur in superficial veins where it may be felt as a linear cord. If it is inflamed the area round the thrombosis is painful, tender, erythematous, and warm.

Superficial venous thrombosis may sometimes recur in different areas in close succession (migratory thrombophlebitis) and this may indicate an underlying neoplasm. Superficial venous thrombosis is usually a self-limiting disease and responds promptly to analgesics, bed rest, and elevation of the affected limb. There is less risk of embolisation from superficial venous thrombosis than from deep vein thrombosis.

Verapamil Hydrochloride

5-[N-(3,4-Dimethoxyphenethyl)methylamino]-2-(3,4-dimethoxyphenyl)-2-isopropylvaleronitrile hydrochloride

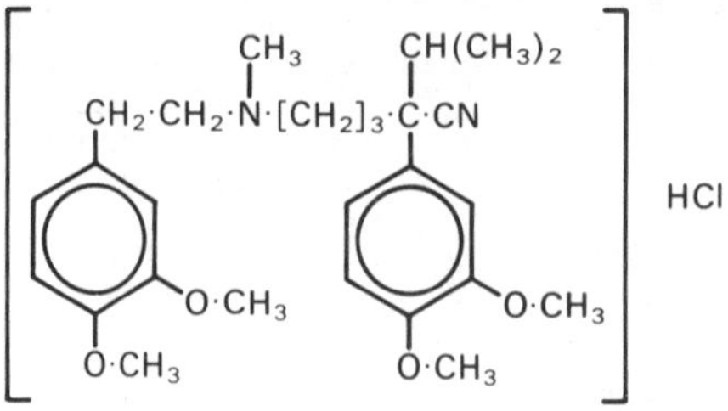

$C_{27}H_{39}ClN_2O_4 = 491.1$

OTHER NAME: *Cordilox®*

Description. A white odourless powder.

Solubility. Soluble in 20 parts of water, in 25 parts of alcohol, and in 1.5 parts of chloroform; practically insoluble in ether.

Acidity. A 5% solution has a pH of 4.5 to 6.5.

Identification. MELTING-POINT. About 146°.

ULTRAVIOLET ABSORPTION. In 0.1N hydrochloric acid, maxima at 228 nm (E1%, 1cm = 325), and 278 nm (E1%, 1cm = 114).

Determination in body fluids. SPECTROFLUORIMETRY. In plasma, serum, or urine—R. G. McAllister and S. M. Howell, *J. pharm. Sci.*, 1976, **65**, 431.

Metabolism. ABSORPTION. In dogs, readily absorbed after oral administration.

HALF-LIFE. In guinea-pigs, plasma half-life about 45 minutes.

DISTRIBUTION. Subject to enterohepatic circulation in dogs.

METABOLIC REACTIONS. In rats, O- and N-dealkylation; subject to first pass metabolism.

EXCRETION. Mainly in the faeces.

FURTHER INFORMATION. Tissue concentrations in guinea-pigs by fluorimetry—R. G. McAllister and S. M. Howell, *J. pharm. Sci.*, 1976, **65**, 431; review of uses—J. K. Vohra, *Drugs*, 1977, **13**, 219.

Actions and uses. Verapamil reduces the workload on the heart by reducing the oxygen requirements of the myocardium and by decreasing peripheral resistance. It may act by slowing calcium transport across myocardial membranes.

Verapamil is given by mouth to reduce and prevent the incidence of anginal attacks; verapamil may in addition be given intravenously in the treatment of cardiac arrhythmias. The usual initial adult dose of verapamil hydrochloride by mouth is 40 to 80 milligrams 3 or 4 times daily, which may be reduced to a maintenance dose of 40 milligrams 3 times daily.

In patients with angina pectoris who do not respond to oral verapamil and in patients with cardiac arrhythmias, 5 milligrams of verapamil hydrochloride may be administered by intravenous injection over 30 seconds, the patient's condition being monitored electrocardiographically. This dose may be given twice daily in angina. In cases of paroxysmal tachycardia, a further 5 milligrams of verapamil hydrochloride may be injected 5 to 10 minutes after the first dose if necessary. The corre-

sponding doses for children are: for the newborn 0.75 to 1 milligram; for children up to 5 years 2 to 3 milligrams, and 6 to 14 years 2.5 to 5 milligrams. Injection of verapamil should be discontinued as soon as the desired effect is observed.

Verapamil hydrochloride may also be administered by intravenous infusion, at a rate of 5 to 10 milligrams per hour; the usual daily dose is 25 to 100 milligrams.

Undesirable effects. Nausea and dizziness may occur after oral administration and flushing and dizziness after intravenous use. The injection may cause transient heart block, especially after rapid administration and, rarely, ventricular fibrillation may be precipitated. Allergic reactions occur frequently.

Precautions and contra-indications. Verapamil may precipitate cardiac failure and if this persists after full digitalisation, the verapamil should be withdrawn.

It should not be used in patients with recent myocardial infarction or complete heart block, and should be used with caution in hypotension, bradycardia, and conduction defects of the heart. It should not be given in conjunction with beta-adrenergic blocking agents.

Poisoning. The effects of verapamil may be reversed by the administration of adrenaline or orciprenaline by intravenous infusion or intracardiac injection or by the intravenous injection of 10 to 20 millilitres of calcium gluconate injection (10%). Symptomatic treatment and reversal of hypotension may also be required.

Drug interactions. It increases the effects of beta-adrenergic blocking agents, antifibrillants such as quinidine, and antihypertensives.

Preparations

Preparations available include an INJECTION containing verapamil hydrochloride 2.5 mg per ml in 2-ml ampoules; and TABLETS containing verapamil hydrochloride 40 and 80 mg.

Vinblastine Sulphate

The sulphate of an alkaloid occurring in *Catharanthus roseus* (L.) G. Don (*Vinca rosea* L.) (Fam. Apocynaceae).

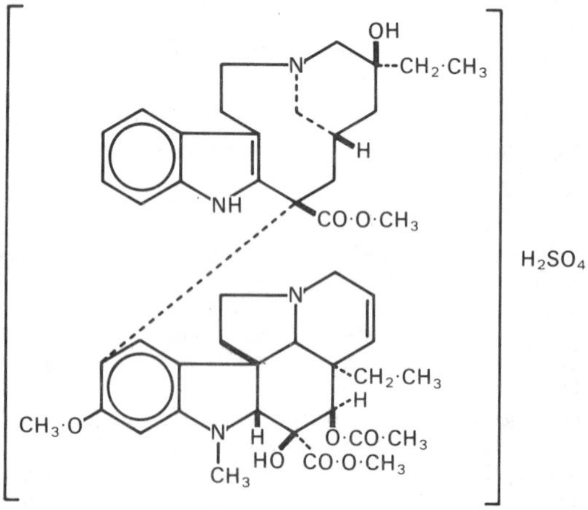

$C_{46}H_{60}N_4O_{13}S = 909.1$

OTHER NAME: *Velbe®*

A standard is given in the British Pharmacopoeia 1973

Description. An odourless, very hygroscopic, white to slightly yellow, amorphous or crystalline powder.

Solubility. Soluble, at 20°, in 10 parts of water, in 1200 parts of alcohol, and in 50 parts of chloroform; practically insoluble in ether.

Acidity. A 0.15% solution has a pH of 3.5 to 5.

Moisture content. Not more than 17%, determined by drying at 60° *in vacuo*.

Specific rotation. $-28°$ to $-35°$, determined on a 2% solution in methyl alcohol.

Dissociation constants. pK_a 5.4, 7.4.

Storage. It should be stored in airtight containers, at a temperature between 2° and 10°, protected from light.

Identification. TESTS. 1. To about 1 mg add 4 drops of a freshly prepared 1% solution of vanillin in hydrochloric acid and allow to stand for 1 minute; a pink colour is produced.
2. Mix about 500 μg with 5 mg of dimethylaminobenzaldehyde and 4 drops of glacial acetic acid, and add 4 drops of sulphuric acid; a reddish-brown colour is produced. Add 1 ml of glacial acetic acid; the colour changes to pink.

MELTING-POINT. About 284°, with decomposition.

ULTRAVIOLET ABSORPTION. In alcohol (95%), maxima at 246, 262, 287, and 296 nm.

Metabolism. BLOOD CONCENTRATION. After an intravenous dose of 15 mg, a plasma concentration of about 16 ng/ml is obtained at 24 hours; an additional dose of 15 mg at this time produces a plasma concentration of about 55 ng/ml 4 hours later.

HALF-LIFE. In whole blood, α-phase, about 4 minutes, and β-phase, about 190 minutes, for drug plus metabolites.

DISTRIBUTION. Rapidly distributed with high tissue binding; readily binds to platelets, red blood cells, and white blood cells; subject to enterohepatic circulation; volume of distribution, 86 to 111 litres; *protein binding*, binds in plasma to α- and β-globulins.

METABOLIC REACTIONS. In rats, deacetylation.

EXCRETION. In 72 hours, 25 to 40% of an intravenous dose is excreted in the faeces and 19 to 23% is excreted in the urine; most of the urinary excreted material is unchanged whilst that in the faeces is in the form of metabolites.

FURTHER INFORMATION. Pharmacokinetics of tritiated vinblastine—R. J. Owellen and C. A. Hartke, *Cancer Res.*, 1975, **35**, 975; radioimmunoassay—J. D. Teale *et al.*, *Br. J. clin. Pharmac.*, 1977, **4**, 169.

Actions and uses. Vinblastine sulphate is a cytotoxic drug that arrests cell growth at the metaphase. Its actions are more pronounced on the rapidly dividing cell than on the normal cell. In clinical dosage it depresses bone-marrow activity, affecting mainly the white cells, with relative sparing of the erythroid elements. The bone-marrow depression is reversible on stopping the drug.

Vinblastine sulphate suppresses the immune response and in high doses is neurotoxic. Like other cytotoxic drugs it is teratogenic.

Vinblastine sulphate is used mainly for the treatment of Hodgkin's disease and other lymphomas and choriocarcinoma. It is more likely to induce a remission in Hodgkin's disease than cyclophosphamide, although a combination of the two drugs with prednisolone is more effective than either drug alone. Some response has been reported in the treatment of inoperable solid tumours, such as those of the breast, female genital tract, lung, testis, and gastro-intestinal tract. The results are stated to be better if vinblastine sulphate is used in conjunction with other cytotoxic drugs, such as cyclophosphamide and chlorambucil.

Vinblastine sulphate is administered by the intravenous injection of a solution of 1 milligram per millilitre in water for injections or sodium chloride injection. It is given weekly, starting with a dose of 100 micrograms per kilogram body-weight, which is raised by weekly increments of 50 micrograms per kilogram body-weight. The dose should not be increased beyond that which reduces the white-cell count to 3000 per cubic millimetre. The maximum single dose in patients previously treated with cytotoxic agents or deep X-rays should not generally exceed 150 micrograms per kilogram body-weight; in previously untreated patients, higher doses may be tolerated. Higher doses are tolerated by children with leukaemia. The average weekly dose is 150 to 200 micrograms per kilogram body-weight.

Response to treatment may take 1 or 2 weeks, as in cases of Hodgkin's disease and choriocarcinoma, or may be delayed as long as 12 weeks in the case of solid tumours. Once a response has occurred a maintenance dose may be given indefinitely every 1 or 2 weeks. This is the maximum dose that the patient will tolerate without the production of serious leucopenia. White-cell counts should therefore be done before each injection and the dose of vinblastine sulphate adjusted so that the count does not fall below 4000 per cubic millimetre.

Vinblastine sulphate may also be administered in dextrose injection (5%) by intravenous infusion, by continuous intra-arterial infusion, and into body cavities. Withdrawal of the drug usually results in relapse within 3 weeks.

Undesirable effects. In general, these are dose-related. Effects on the haemopoietic system include neutropenia, and rarely thrombocytopenia, which may occur if vinblastine sulphate is given after courses of other cytotoxic drugs or after irradiation. Recovery occurs within 7 to 14 days of stopping the drug.

Other side-effects are epilation, nausea, vomiting, anorexia, diarrhoea, stomatitis, and urticaria.

The neurological manifestations, apart from bone-marrow depression, are the most serious side-effects. They include peripheral neuropathy, neuromyopathy, paraesthesia, loss of deep tendon reflexes, psychoses, and mental depression.

Dysfunction of the autonomic nervous system may also occur, with urinary retention, severe constipation leading to ileus, and parotid gland pain and tenderness.

Precautions. Vinblastine sulphate should be used with care in cachectic patients. Its use in pregnancy is not advised as it is teratogenic. Care should be used when it is injected intravenously as perivenous infiltration may cause cellulitis, phlebitis, and venous thrombosis.

Contra-indications. Vinblastine sulphate should not be given if the white-cell count is below 4000 per cubic millimetre, if bacterial infection is present, or if the bone marrow is infiltrated with neoplastic cells.

Preparation

VINBLASTINE INJECTION: a sterile solution of vinblastine sulphate in water for injections. It is prepared by dissolving the contents of a sealed container in water for injections shortly before use. Available as a powder in ampoules containing 10 mg of vinblastine sulphate.

A standard for this injection is given in the British Pharmacopoeia 1973

Containers and *Labelling:* see the entry on Injections for general information on containers and labelling.

Storage: the sealed container should be stored at a temperature between 2° and 10°, protected from light. The injection contains no bactericide and should be used as soon as possible after preparation, and in any case within 4 days. In the presence of a suitable bactericide such as phenol 0.5% it may be used for up to 1 month when stored at 2° to 10°.

Vincristine Sulphate

The sulphate of an alkaloid occurring in *Catharanthus roseus* (L.) G. Don (*Vinca rosea* L.) (Fam. Apocynaceae).

$C_{46}H_{58}N_4O_{14}S = 923.0$

OTHER NAME: *Oncovin®*

A standard is given in the British Pharmacopoeia 1973

Description. An odourless, very hygroscopic, white to slightly yellow, amorphous or slightly crystalline powder.

Solubility. Soluble, at 20°, in 2 parts of water, in 600 parts of alcohol, and in 30 parts of chloroform; practically insoluble in ether.

Acidity. A 0.1% solution has a pH of 3.5 to 4.5.

Moisture content. Not more than 12%, determined by drying at 40° *in vacuo*.

Dissociation constants. pK_a 5.0, 7.4.

Storage. It should be stored in airtight containers, at a temperature between 2° and 10°, protected from light.

Identification. TESTS. 1. To about 1 mg add 4 drops of a freshly prepared 1% solution of vanillin in hydrochloric acid and allow to stand for 1 minute; an orange colour is produced (distinction from vinblastine sulphate). 2. It complies with Test 2 described under Vinblastine Sulphate.

MELTING-POINT. About 277°.

ULTRAVIOLET ABSORPTION. In alcohol (95%), maxima at 255, 275, and 296 nm and an inflection at 290 nm.

Metabolism. BLOOD CONCENTRATION. After an intravenous dose of 2 mg, serum or plasma concentrations of about 100 to 400 ng/ml are obtained after 5 minutes, falling to less than 40 ng/ml by 10 minutes.

HALF-LIFE. Serum half-life, about 75 minutes.

FURTHER INFORMATION. Blood concentrations by bioassay with leucocytes—Y. Hirshaut *et al., Clin. Res.,* 1968, **16**, 360; radioimmunoassay—J. D. Teale *et al., Br. J. clin. Pharmac.,* 1977, **4**, 169.

Actions and uses. Vincristine sulphate is a cytotoxic drug which, like vinblastine sulphate, arrests mitosis in the metaphase. Although the depressant action of vincristine sulphate on the bone marrow is less than that of vinblastine sulphate, it has a more pronounced neurotoxic effect. In clinical dosage it may cause peripheral neuropathy, neuromuscular disturbances, and effects on the autonomic nervous system. It is administered intravenously. It is rapidly cleared from the blood and is excreted mainly through the bile.

Although the range of clinical activity resembles that of vinblastine sulphate, there are some differences. There is no cross-resistance between the two and vincristine sulphate is less effective in the treatment of Hodgkin's disease. It is more effective in the treatment of the acute leukaemias, particularly in children, but as it does not readily penetrate the blood–brain barrier, it should always be used with other oncolytic agents if the leukaemic process involves the central nervous system. Other conditions in which vincristine sulphate has produced remissions are lymphosarcoma, reticulum sarcoma, neuroblastoma, Wilms' tumour, and tumours of the brain, breast, and lung.

Vincristine sulphate is administered intravenously at weekly intervals, almost invariably in conjunction with other oncolytic drugs. For children with leukaemia the commencing weekly dose is 50 micrograms per kilogram body-weight with weekly increments of 25 micrograms per kilogram, until a maximum of 150 micrograms per kilogram is reached. After remission has occurred the dosage is reduced to a maintenance level of 50 to 75 micrograms per kilogram weekly. For adult leukaemia the weekly dose is from 25 to 75 micrograms per kilogram body-weight.

For other malignant conditions the dose is smaller, of the order of 25 micrograms per kilogram body-weight weekly until a remission occurs. The dose is then reduced to 5 to 10 micrograms per kilogram for as long as any anti-tumour effect can be observed.

Undesirable effects. These are dose-related and less likely to occur if the weekly dose is below 100 micrograms per kilogram body-weight.

The commonest adverse reactions are alopecia, neuromuscular and neurological disturbances, gastro-intestinal upsets, particularly abdominal colic, severe constipation, leucopenia, loss of weight, and dysuria. These effects may decrease or disappear on reducing the dose.

Precautions and contra-indications. Dosage is usually limited by neuromuscular rather than bone-marrow toxicity. Therefore regular examination of deep tendon reflexes should be carried out and the dose reduced if they are impaired. White-cell counts should also be made. Dosage should be reduced or temporarily omitted if infection is present.

Care should be taken to avoid extravasation during intravenous injection as this may cause phlebitis or cellulitis.

The concentration of the solution for injection should be from 10 to 100 micrograms per millilitre.

Preparation

VINCRISTINE INJECTION: a sterile solution of vincristine sulphate and lactose, in the proportion of 1 part and 10 parts respectively, in water for injections. It is prepared by dissolving the contents of a sealed container, which includes the lactose, in water for injections shortly before use. Available as a powder in ampoules containing 1 mg of vincristine sulphate and 10 mg of lactose, and in ampoules containing 5 mg of vincristine sulphate and 50 mg of lactose.

A standard for this injection is given in the British Pharmacopoeia 1973

Containers and *Labelling:* see the entry on Injections for general information on containers and labelling.

Storage: the sealed container should be stored at a temperature between 2° and 10°, protected from light. The injection contains no bactericide and should be used as soon as possible after preparation, and in any case within 24 hours. In the presence of a suitable bactericide such as benzyl alcohol 0.9% it may be used for up to 14 days when stored at 2° to 10°.

Vinyl Ether

Divinyl ether to which has been added about 4% v/v of dehydrated alcohol and not more than 0.01% w/v of phenyl-α-naphthylamine or other suitable stabiliser.

$$CH_2:CH \cdot O \cdot CH:CH_2$$

$C_4H_6O = 70.09$

A standard is given in the British Pharmacopoeia 1973

CAUTION. *Vinyl ether is inflammable and mixtures with oxygen or air at certain concentrations are explosive; it should not be used in the presence of a naked flame or of an electrical apparatus liable to produce a spark. Precautions should be taken against the production of static electrical discharge.*

On exposure to air and light, divinyl ether decomposes into formaldehyde and formic acid, ultimately polymerising to a jelly; decomposition is retarded by the presence of the stabiliser. The dehydrated alcohol is added to reduce the rate of evaporation of vinyl ether when used in anaesthesia and so reduce the possibility of ice formation on masks.

Description. A clear colourless liquid with a characteristic odour; it often has a slight purplish fluorescence which is due to the presence of the stabiliser.

Solubility. Soluble, at 20°, in 100 parts of water; miscible with alcohol, with ether, and with chloroform.

Weight per ml. At 20°, 0.770 to 0.778 g.

Boiling-point. About 29°.

Flash-point. Below −22 °F (closed-cup test).

Storage. It should be stored in airtight containers of not more than 200-ml capacity, in a cool place, protected from light. It should be used within 48 hours of first opening the container.

Identification. TESTS. 1. Mix 2 ml with 2 ml of *dilute sulphuric acid* and warm; the odour of acetaldehyde is produced.

2. Mix 2 ml with 2 ml of *bromine solution* and shake; the colour is immediately discharged.

Metabolism. Vinyl ether is rapidly absorbed. It is excreted in the urine in small amounts and through the lungs mainly as unchanged drug.

Actions and uses. Vinyl ether is a very volatile anaesthetic which has a potency about 4 times that of ether. It is more toxic and more rapid in action than ether and considerable care must therefore be exercised in its administration, as the stage of overdosage is very quickly reached. Recovery is very rapid. The degree of muscular relaxation induced by vinyl ether is more variable than that induced by ether and cannot be relied upon during surgical operations.

It is important to note that the eye signs which are usually depended upon in anaesthesia are entirely unreliable in the case of vinyl ether, and the extent of anaesthesia must be gauged by the rate, depth, and regularity of the respiration; overdosage is usually indicated by the development of cyanosis.

Other disadvantages of vinyl ether are the frequency with which excessive salivation occurs and the toxic effect on the liver.

Post-operative complications are rare, and nausea and vomiting relatively infrequent.

Vinyl ether is indicated for use in minor operative procedures of short duration. It has been used in dental surgery and in obstetrics. It is also useful as an induction anaesthetic and, in minimal doses, as an adjuvant to other anaesthetics; 1 part of vinyl ether with 3 parts of anaesthetic ether forms a mixture which gives a vapour of constant composition.

For short operations or as an induction anaesthetic, vinyl ether is commonly administered on an open mask or in an inhaler. For longer procedures the semi-closed or closed method is used, with admixture of nitrous oxide and oxygen.

Poisoning. In the event of poisoning resulting in collapse, the procedure described under Chloroform should be adopted.

Viomycin Sulphate

The sulphate of an antimicrobial substance produced by certain strains of *Streptomyces griseus* var. *purpureus*.

A standard is given in the British Pharmacopoeia 1973

Description. An odourless, somewhat hygroscopic, white powder with a slightly bitter taste.

Solubility. Soluble in water; very slightly soluble in alcohol and in ether.

Acidity. A solution containing 100 000 units per ml has a pH of 4.5 to 7.

Moisture content. Not more than 5%, determined by drying at 60° *in vacuo*.

Storage. It should be stored in airtight sterile containers, sealed to exclude micro-organisms, in a cool place.

Identification. TESTS. 1. Dissolve about 50 mg in 10 ml of water and to 5 ml of the solution add 1.5 ml of *sodium hydroxide solution*, 5 ml of a 0.1% solution of 1-naphthol in a 0.5% solution of sodium hydroxide, and 3 ml of *dilute sodium hypochlorite solution*; a red colour is produced.

2. To the remainder of the solution prepared in Test 1 add 1.5 ml of *sodium hydroxide solution* and, dropwise, a 0.5% solution of copper sulphate, stirring after each addition; a pale violet colour is produced.

ULTRAVIOLET ABSORPTION. In water, maximum at 268 nm.

Metabolism. ABSORPTION. Poorly absorbed after oral administration.

BLOOD CONCENTRATION. After an intramuscular dose peak concentrations are attained in 1 to 2 hours.

HALF-LIFE. 3 to 4 hours.

DISTRIBUTION. Does not appear to enter the cerebrospinal fluid.

EXCRETION. Excreted mainly in the urine.

Actions and uses. Viomycin is a polypeptide antibiotic which is active against *Mycobacterium tuberculosis*, including strains which are resistant to streptomycin. It is readily absorbed when given by intramuscular injection and is excreted mainly by the kidneys. Its action is bacteriostatic.

The main use of viomycin is in the treatment of all forms of tuberculosis when an antibiotic of the streptomycin group cannot be used because the organism is resistant or the patient hypersensitive. Like other antituberculous drugs, it has little effect when extensive caseation or fibrosis is present. As with streptomycin, treatment with viomycin should be combined with the administration of isoniazid or an aminosalicylate in order to minimise the emergence of resistant strains.

As viomycin penetrates the blood–brain barrier when the meninges are inflamed and is highly concentrated in the urine it is suitable for the treatment of meningitis and renal forms of tuberculosis. The usual adult dose is 1 mega unit (equivalent to 1 gram of viomycin) dissolved in not less than 2 millilitres of water for injections or sodium chloride injection 2 or 3 times a week in 2 equal doses, morning and evening. Treatment must be continued for 6 months or more. The usual dose for children is 30000 units (equivalent to 30 milligrams of viomycin) per kilogram body-weight 2 or 3 times a week.

Undesirable effects. Rashes, renal irritation, disturbances of electrolyte and fluid balances, abnormalities in the electrocardiogram, dizziness, and loss of hearing occur infrequently with normal dosage.

Precautions and contra-indications. Because of its potential toxicity, viomycin should not be used unless streptomycin is contra-indicated; it should not be used for patients with impaired kidney function.

If injections are given more frequently than recommended a check must be made on the electrolyte balance and kidney function.

Preparation

VIOMYCIN SULPHATE INJECTION: a sterile solution of viomycin sulphate in water for injections. It is prepared by dissolving the contents of a sealed container in water for injections shortly before use.

A standard for this injection is given in the British Pharmacopoeia 1973

Containers and *Labelling:* see the entry on Injections for general information on containers and labelling.

Storage: the injection contains no bactericide and should be used as soon as possible after preparation, but solutions of viomycin sulphate may be expected to retain their potency for up to 1 month after preparation, provided they are stored at a temperature between 2° and 10°.

Viprynium Embonate

6 - Dimethylamino - 2 - [2 - (2,5 - dimethyl - 1 - phenylpyrrol-3 - yl)vinyl] - 1 - methylquinolinium 4,4' - methylenebis(3-hydroxy-2-naphthoate)

$C_{75}H_{70}N_6O_6 = 1151.4$

OTHER NAMES: Pyrvinium Pamoate; *Vanquin®*; Viprynium Pamoate

A standard is given in the British Pharmacopoeia 1973

Description. An almost odourless, tasteless, bright orange-red to almost black, crystalline powder.

Solubility. Very slightly soluble in water, in alcohol, in ether, and in chloroform; soluble, at 20°, in 330 parts of methoxyethanol.

Moisture content. Not more than 6%, determined by drying at 130°.

Storage. It should be stored in airtight containers, protected from light.

Identification. TEST. Mix in a centrifuge tube about 50 mg of the sample, 1 ml of dimethylformamide, 5 ml of chloroform, and 5 ml of *sodium hydroxide solution*, stopper the tube, shake vigorously, and centrifuge until a clear aqueous phase is formed; the chloroform layer is deep red in colour and the yellowish aqueous layer exhibits a green fluorescence under ultraviolet radiation.

MELTING-POINT. About 206°, with decomposition.

ULTRAVIOLET ABSORPTION. In methoxyethanol, maxima at 358 nm (E1%, 1cm = 380) and 508 nm (E1%, 1cm = 750).

Actions and uses. Viprynium embonate is a dye which is used as an anthelmintic. It kills the worms by its action on their respiratory system. It is poorly absorbed.

It is administered by mouth as a single dose equivalent to 5 milligrams of the base per kilogram body-weight; 75 milligrams of viprynium embonate is approximately equivalent to 50 milligrams of viprynium base. It may be desirable to repeat the dose after 1 or 2 weeks. As the drug is virtually non-toxic it is desirable to treat all members of a family when one is infected as the worm eggs are readily transported from person to person.

Viprynium embonate stains the stools red and also stains any clothing with which it comes into contact. The tablets should be swallowed whole as otherwise the mouth is deeply stained.

Undesirable effects. Nausea and vomiting occasionally occur.

Preparations

VIPRYNIUM MIXTURE (*Syn.* Viprynium Suspension): a suspension of viprynium embonate in a suitable flavoured vehicle.

When a dose less than or not a multiple of 5 ml is prescribed, the mixture may be diluted, as described in the entry on Mixtures, with syrup. The diluted mixture must be freshly prepared.

Available as a mixture containing viprynium embonate equivalent to 50 mg of viprynium in 5 ml.

A standard for this mixture is given in the British Pharmaceutical Codex 1973

Containers and *Labelling:* see the entry on Mixtures for general information on containers and labelling.

Storage: it should be protected from light.

Advice for patients: viprynium colours the urine and stools and stains any fabric with which it comes into contact.

VIPRYNIUM TABLETS: available as tablets containing viprynium embonate equivalent to 50 mg of viprynium; they are film coated or sugar coated.

A standard for these tablets is given in the British Pharmacopoeia 1973

Containers and *Storage:* see the entry on Tablets for general information on containers and storage. Containers should be airtight.

Labelling: the label on the container should state the amount of the medicament as the equivalent of viprynium.

Advice for patients: the tablets should be swallowed whole. See also under Viprynium Mixture (above).

Viscose

Viscose is made from wood cellulose or cotton linters by solution in alkali and carbon disulphide, followed by reprecipitation of the cellulose in the form of a thread by forcing the solution of cellulose through fine holes in a metal plate into a coagulating fluid (viscose process).

OTHER NAMES: Rayon; Regenerated Cellulose

A standard is given in the British Pharmaceutical Codex 1973

Description. *Macroscopical characters:* white or slightly yellow, highly lustrous fibre, which burns without forming a bead or ash.

Microscopical characters: the fibres are solid and transparent with a diameter between about 10 and 20 μm and marked by longitudinal parallel lines distributed unequally over the width. Clearly visible in *chloral hydrate solution* and in *lactophenol*, almost invisible in cresol; transverse section rounded with an irregular crenate margin and invisible when viewed between crossed polars.

Solubility. Soluble in sulphuric acid (66% v/v); swollen by *ammoniacal copper oxide solution* and ultimately dissolved; insoluble in formic acid and in acetone; almost insoluble in *dilute sodium hydroxide solution.*

Moisture content. Not more than 13%, determined by drying at 105°.

Identification. TESTS. 1. Soak in *iodine water* for a few minutes, remove the excess of reagent by filter paper, and add 1 or 2 drops of sulphuric acid (66% v/v); the sample is stained blue.

2. Treat with *phloroglucinol solution,* followed by hydrochloric acid; no red colour is produced.

3. Treat with *iodinated zinc chloride solution;* a violet colour is produced.

Uses. Viscose is used for the preparation of viscose fabrics and absorbent viscose wadding.

Viscose, Delustred

Viscose which has been deprived of its sheen by dispersing finely divided titanium dioxide throughout the material during manufacture.

OTHER NAMES: Delustred Rayon; Delustred Regenerated Cellulose.

A standard is given in the British Pharmaceutical Codex 1973

Description. White matt fibre having the microscopical characters of viscose, with the addition of microscopic granular particles, of average diameter 0.25 to 1 μm, scattered throughout the material and appearing black by transmitted light.

Moisture content. Not more than 13%, determined by drying at 105°.

Identification. TESTS. 1. It complies with the tests described under Viscose.

2. Prepare a sulphated ash, dissolve it in 5 ml of sulphuric acid by warming gently, cool, pour the solution into 4 ml of water, filter, and add 4 drops of *hydrogen peroxide solution;* a yellow colour is produced (presence of titanium dioxide).

Uses. Delustred viscose is used for the preparation of viscose fabrics and absorbent viscose wadding.

Vitamin A Ester Concentrate

An ester or a mixture of esters of retinol, of natural or synthetic origin, or a solution of such ester or mixture of esters in arachis oil or other suitable vegetable oil; it may contain a suitable antoxidant or mixture of antoxidants.

A standard is given in the British Pharmacopoeia 1973

Description. A yellow oil or mixture of oil and crystalline material which when warmed yields a homogeneous yellow oil; it has a faint odour.

Solubility. Practically insoluble in water; soluble or partly soluble in alcohol; miscible with ether, with chloroform, and with light petroleum.

Storage. It should be stored in hermetically sealed containers in an atmosphere of nitrogen or other suitable gas, in a cool place, protected from light.

Metabolism. ABSORPTION. Readily absorbed after oral administration.

BLOOD CONCENTRATION. Serum-carotene concentrations are influenced by dietary intake but the normal range is approximately 0.5 to 2 μg/ml; vitamin A concentrations in normal subjects are approximately 0.2 to 0.5 μg/ml; after an oral dose of 13.8 mg of vitamin A acetate administered as a solution in oil or as microcapsules, respective peak plasma concentrations of 2.6 to 10.5 and 3.7 to 17 μg/ml are attained in 2 to 7 hours.

DISTRIBUTION. Stored in the liver, fat, and kidneys; crosses the placenta and is secreted in milk.

EXCRETION. Excreted in faeces and urine and about 15% of a dose is excreted in 24 hours.

FURTHER INFORMATION. Absorption in children with ascariasis—B. Sivakumar and V. Reddy, *J. trop. Med. Hyg.,* 1975, **78**, 114; bioavailability from oily solutions and microcapsules—P. Fascetti *et al., Boll. chim. farm.,* 1976, **115**, 108; plasma concentrations in the common dermatoses—P. D. Mier and J. J. M. A. Van Den Hurk, *Br. J. Derm.,* 1974, **91**, 155; depressed plasma concentrations of vitamin A and zinc in patients with alcoholic cirrhosis—J. C. Smith *et al., Lancet,* i/1975, 1251.

Actions and uses. Vitamin A ester concentrate has the actions, uses, and undesirable effects described under Concentrated Vitamin A Solution.

Vitamin A Solution, Concentrated

Concentrated vitamin A solution consists of a suitable fish-liver oil or blend of such oils, or a solution of a source of vitamin A in a vegetable oil such as arachis oil, prepared at a temperature not exceeding 60°. It contains approximately 50000 units of vitamin-A activity in 1 g (1.2 ml).

OTHER NAMES: *Ro-A-Vit*®
Rovigon® (with tocopheryl acetate)

A standard is given in the British Pharmaceutical Codex 1973

In preparing concentrated vitamin A solution, any suitable source of vitamin A may be used, such as fish-liver oil rich in the vitamin, a concentrate prepared therefrom, or synthetic vitamin A or its esters.

A concentrate may be prepared by molecular distillation from oils of suitable potency. It may also be prepared from fish-liver oils by saponifying with alcoholic potash, extracting the unsaponifiable matter with ether, evaporating off the ether, dissolving the residue in twice its weight of methyl alcohol, cooling to 0°, removing the cholesterol which crystallises out, and finally distilling off the methyl alcohol.

A concentrate so prepared from mammalian livers contains a very small amount of vitamin D, but may contain more vitamin A than a concentrate prepared in the same way from cod-liver oil. It is mixed with a suitable vegetable oil to give a solution of the required strength.

Description. A pale yellow or yellow oily liquid with a faint, but not rancid, odour.

Solubility. Very slightly soluble in alcohol; miscible with ether, with chloroform, and with light petroleum.

Storage. It should be stored in well-filled airtight containers, in a cool place, protected from light.

Actions and uses. Vitamin A maintains the development and normal function of epithelial tissue and plays an essential role in retinal function. The human requirements of Vitamin A cannot be accurately assessed, but are believed to be in the region of 5000 units daily, with an additional 1000 units during pregnancy and 3000 units during lactation. Children up to 1 year require 1500 units daily and other children and adolescents from 2000 to 5000 units. This vitamin is present in milk, butter, fish, vegetable oils, and most fats. Its precursor, carotene, is widely distributed in green vegetables, carrots, and tomatoes.

Deficiency of vitamin A leads to impaired dark-adaptation and atrophy of epithelial cells with differentiation into a stratified keratinising epithelium. In the eye, the conjunctiva is dry and wrinkled; there is also dryness of the cornea. This xerophthalmia may lead to secondary infection and panophthalmitis. Urinary calculi frequently accompany vitamin-A deficiency.

The earliest symptom indicating deficiency is night blindness, caused by failure of the retinal rods to resynthesise visual purple. Dryness and roughness of the skin may also occur. The epithelial changes may favour secondary infection, but the vitamin should not be called "anti-infective"; additional vitamin A given to persons who are not suffering from a deficiency of the vitamin does not increase their resistance to infection.

Deficient absorption of the precursors of vitamin A occurs in certain conditions, such as coeliac disease and sprue. Therapeutically, vitamin A may be administered in these conditions and when there is reason to suspect inadequate absorption of the fat-soluble vitamin due to defective absorption of fat.

Excessive use of liquid paraffin may inhibit absorption of appreciable amounts of vitamin A and its precursors from the small and large intestines.

A person suffering from vitamin A deficiency is prone to develop infections, particularly of the respiratory tract, and will benefit from the administration of vitamin A. But there is no evidence that vitamin A will influence the course of respiratory or other infections in a person receiving an adequate intake of vitamin A.

For the treatment of vitamin A deficiency, 25000 to 50000 units should be given daily until a clinical response is obtained.

For the treatment of xerophthalmia and keratomalacia associated with vitamin-A deficiency, the vitamin should be administered by intramuscular injection in daily doses of 50000 to 100000 units for 3 days, after which oral treatment suffices.

Undesirable effects. Signs of vitamin-A intoxication may occur if the intake is grossly excessive, e.g. 50000 units or more daily taken over long periods. The symptoms are a rough itching skin, dry coarse hair, tender firm deep swellings in the limbs, enlarged liver, a raised erythrocyte sedimentation rate, anaemia, and an increase in serum alkaline phosphatase.

Treatment consists in withdrawing the vitamin A, when most manifestations disappear within a week.

Preparations

VITAMINS A AND D CAPSULES: for each capsule take:

Vitamin D	.. 400 units
Vitamin-A activity	..4000 units

Mix the ingredients, with a suitable fixed vegetable oil if necessary, and enclose in a soft capsule. The capsule shells may be coloured.

A standard for these capsules is given in the British Pharmaceutical Codex 1973

Containers and *Storage:* see the entry on Capsules for general information on containers and storage. Containers should be light resistant.

Dose. 1 capsule daily.

Advice for patients: the capsules should not be taken for prolonged periods without medical advice.

VITAMINS CAPSULES: for each capsule take:

Vitamin D	.. 300 units
Vitamin-A activity	..2500 units
Riboflavine	.. 0.5 mg
Thiamine hydrochloride	.. 1.0 mg
Nicotinamide	.. 7.5 mg
Ascorbic acid	.. 15.0 mg

Mix the ingredients, with a suitable fixed vegetable oil if necessary, and enclose in a soft capsule. The capsule shells may be coloured.

A standard for these capsules is given in the British Pharmaceutical Codex 1973

Containers and *Storage:* see the entry on Capsules for general information on containers and storage. Containers should be light resistant.

Dose: prophylactic, 1 capsule daily; therapeutic, 2 capsules daily.

Advice for patients: the capsules should not be taken for prolonged periods without medical advice.

OTHER PREPARATIONS available include TABLETS containing vitamin A acetate equivalent to 50000 units of vitamin A, and tablets containing vitamin A 30000 units with tocopheryl acetate 70 mg.

Vitamin D Solution, Concentrated

Concentrated vitamin D solution consists of a suitable fish-liver oil or blend of such oils, or a solution of a source of vitamin D in a vegetable oil such as arachis oil, prepared at a temperature not exceeding 60°.

A standard is given in the British Pharmaceutical Codex 1973

Description. A pale yellow or yellow oily liquid with a faint, but not rancid, odour.

Solubility. Very slightly soluble in alcohol; miscible with ether, with chloroform, and with light petroleum.

Storage. It should be stored in well-filled airtight containers, in a cool place, protected from light.

Actions and uses. Concentrated vitamin D solution has the actions, uses, and undesirable effects described under Calciferol.

The usual prophylactic dose for an infant or adult is 0.04 millilitre, equivalent to approximately 400 units daily. The usual therapeutic dose for an infant or adult is 0.1 to 2 millilitres, equivalent to approximately 1000 to 20000 units daily.

In the treatment of hypoparathyroidism, a dosage of 5 to 20 millilitres, equivalent to approximately 50000 to 200000 units daily is given.

Precautions. As for Calciferol.

Preparations

VITAMINS A AND D CAPSULES; VITAMINS CAPSULES: See above under Concentrated Vitamin A Solution.

Vitamin Deficiencies

Vitamin deficiencies do not usually occur in persons living on a normal diet, but deficiency of the vitamin B group and of vitamin C and, less commonly, of other vitamins may occur in malnutrition, in alcoholics, in conditions of defective absorption such as coeliac disease and sprue, and in conditions with increased utilisation of vitamins, such as metabolic diseases, pregnancy, and lactation.

Vitamin A. Deficiency leads to impaired dark adaptation, xerophthalmia, and dryness and roughness of the skin. Treatment is described under Vitamin A Solution, Concentrated.

Sources of Vitamin A

Cod-liver Oil	Vitamins A and D Solution,
Halibut-liver Oil	Concentrated
Vitamin A Solution,	Vitamin A Ester
Concentrated	Concentrate

Vitamin B. Deficiency of vitamin B_1 gives rise to beri-beri. Treatment is described under Thiamine Hydrochloride. Deficiency of vitamin B_2 gives rise to ariboflavinosis, the distinctive features and treatment of which are described under Riboflavine. Deficiency of nicotinic acid gives rise to pellagra although deficiency of other B vitamins is also involved. Treatment is described under Nicotinic Acid.

Deficiency of vitamin B_6 gives rise to convulsions, anaemia, and skin conditions. The distinctive features and treatment of vitamin B_6 deficiency are described under Pyridoxine Hydrochloride.

Deficiency of vitamin B_{12} may give rise to pernicious anaemia or degenerative disease of the spinal cord and dementia. Treatment is described under Hydroxocobalamin.

Sources of Vitamins of the B group

Cyanocobalamin	Pyridoxine Hydrochloride
Hydroxocobalamin	Riboflavine
Malt Extract	Thiamine Hydrochloride
Nicotinamide	Yeast, Dried
Nicotinic Acid	

Vitamin C. Vitamin C affects the development of cartilage, bone, and teeth, the healing of wounds, and the absorption and utilisation of iron. Deficiency leads to scurvy of which a subclinical form is relatively common in elderly patients. Treatment is described under Ascorbic Acid.

Sources of Vitamin C

Ascorbic Acid	Black Currant

Vitamin D. Deficiency of vitamin D gives rise to rickets in the young and osteomalacia in adults. Treatment is described under Calciferol and Dihydrotachysterol.

Sources of Vitamin D

Calciferol	Vitamin D Solution,
Cod-liver Oil	Concentrated
Dihydrotachysterol	Vitamin A and D Solution,
Halibut-liver Oil	Concentrated

Vitamin K. Deficiency of vitamin K reduces the prothrombin level and the ability of the blood to clot. The treatment of haemorrhage due to low prothrombin level is described under Phytomenadione.

Sources of Vitamin K

Acetomenaphthone	Phytomenadione

Vitamins A and D Solution, Concentrated

Concentrated vitamins A and D solution consists of a suitable fish-liver oil or blend of such oils, or a solution of a source of vitamin A and a source of vitamin D in a vegetable oil such as arachis oil, prepared at a temperature not exceeding 60°.

OTHER NAMES: *Adexolin*® and *Esotone*® (both with ascorbic acid)

A standard is given in the British Pharmaceutical Codex 1973

Description. A pale yellow or yellow oily liquid with a faint, but not rancid, odour and a bland or slightly fishy taste.

Solubility. Very slightly soluble in alcohol; miscible with ether, with chloroform, and with light petroleum.

Storage. It should be stored in well-filled airtight containers, in a cool place, protected from light.

Actions and uses. Concentrated vitamins A and D solution is used as a dietary supplement to correct or prevent symptoms arising from a deficiency of these two vitamins. The usual daily dose is 0.06 to 0.6 millilitre of concentrated vitamins A and D solution, approximately equivalent to 2500 units to 25000 units of vitamin-A activity and 250 to 2500 units of antirachitic activity (vitamin D).

Undesirable effects. As for Calciferol and Concentrated Vitamin A Solution.

Preparations

CONCENTRATED VITAMINS SOLUTION: consisting of a solution containing 5250 units of vitamin-A activity,

1400 units of vitamin D, and 105 mg of ascorbic acid per ml.

Storage: it should be stored in airtight containers, in a cool place, protected from light.

Dose: CHILD: Up to 1 year, 5 drops daily; 1 to 5 years, 10 drops daily.

Advice for patients: the solution should not be taken for prolonged periods without medical advice.

VITAMINS A AND D CAPSULES: see above under Concentrated Vitamin A Solution.

OTHER PREPARATIONS available include CAPSULES containing vitamin-A activity 4000 units with calciferol 400 units; and TABLETS containing vitamin-A activity 4500 units, vitamin D 450 units, and ascorbic acid 30 mg.

Vitrellae

Vitrellae consist of thin-walled glass capsules containing a volatile medicament; they are protected by a wrapping of fabric or other suitable material. They are intended for use by crushing the glass and inhaling the vapour of a volatile medicament such as amyl nitrite.

The crushable glass should be completely enclosed in absorbent cotton wool, ensuring that no glass is exposed, a label placed on the cotton wool, and the whole fitted into a silk sleeve, the ends of which are tied with silk thread and trimmed. Alternatively, the glass capsule may be placed in a suitable tube, plugged at both ends, or enclosed completely in other suitable material which will not permit the escape of fragments of glass and will allow complete volatilisation of the medicament.

Vomiting

see NAUSEA AND VOMITING

Warfarin Sodium

The sodium derivative of 4-hydroxy-3-(3-oxo-1-phenyl-butyl)coumarin.

$C_{19}H_{15}NaO_4 = 330.3$

OTHER NAME: *Marevan*®

A standard is given in the British Pharmacopoeia 1973

Description. An odourless white crystalline powder with a slightly bitter taste.

Solubility. Soluble, at 20°, in less than 1 part of water and of alcohol; very slightly soluble in ether and in chloroform.

Alkalinity. A 1% solution has a pH of 7.2 to 8.3.

Moisture content. Not more than 2%, determined by Fischer titration.

Dissociation constant. pK_a 5.0 (20°).

Storage. It should be stored in airtight containers, protected from light.

Identification. TESTS. 1. Dissolve about 100 mg in 25 ml of water, add 2 drops of *dilute hydrochloric acid*,

and filter; a precipitate is produced which, after washing with water, melts at about 162°.

2. Dissolve about 1 g in 10 ml of water, add 5 ml of nitric acid, filter, and to the filtrate add 2 ml of 0.1N potassium dichromate and shake for 5 minutes; a light greenish-blue colour is produced.

ULTRAVIOLET ABSORPTION. In 0.1N sodium hydroxide, maximum at 308 nm (E1%, 1cm = 430).

INFRA-RED ABSORPTION. Major peaks at 763, 1031, 1538, 1613, 1667, and 1724 cm^{-1} (see Appendix 2b: Infra-red Spectra).

Determination in body fluids. SPECTROFLUORIMETRY. In plasma—D. S. Hewick and J. McEwen, *J. Pharm. Pharmac.*, 1973, **25**, 458.

GAS CHROMATOGRAPHY. In plasma—K. K. Midha *et al.*, *J. pharm. Sci.*, 1974, **63**, 1725; S. Hanna *et al.*, *J. pharm. Sci.*, 1978, **67**, 84.

HIGH PRESSURE LIQUID CHROMATOGRAPHY. In plasma —T. D. Bjornsson *et al.*, *J. pharm. Sci.*, 1977, **66**, 142; L. T. Wong *et al.*, *J. Chromat.*, 1977, **135**, 149.

Metabolism. ABSORPTION. Readily absorbed after oral administration; absorption is decreased by the presence of food.

BLOOD CONCENTRATION. After oral doses of 100 mg of each of the *R*- and *S*-enantiomers of warfarin, respective peak plasma concentrations of about 2.5 and 0.5 µg/ml are attained for the reduced metabolite (warfarin alcohol) in 24 to 48 hours whilst concentrations of the unchanged enantiomers of about 6 to 8 µg/ml are attained during the same period.

HALF-LIFE. Plasma half-life for the reduced metabolite of the *R*-enantiomer, 20 to 70 hours and of the *S*-enantiomer, 18 to 40 hours; the half-life is decreased in resistant subjects and in subjects with high alcohol intake.

DISTRIBUTION. Volume of distribution, 10 to 27% of body-weight; crosses the placenta and is secreted in milk; *protein binding*, about 97% bound to plasma proteins, the amount bound being decreased in the elderly; the bound drug is displaced by other drugs such as phenylbutazone, sulphaphenazole, and trichloroacetic acid.

METABOLIC REACTIONS. In rats and guinea-pigs, hydroxylation at positions 6, 7, 8 and at the *p*-position of the phenyl substituent, condensation to produce 3,4-dihydro - 2 - methyl - 4 - phenyl - 2*H*,5*H* - pyrano[3,2 - *c*][1]-benzopyran-5-one, and glucuronic acid conjugation; in man, the major metabolites are formed by reduction of the acetyl group to produce a 2-hydroxypropyl side chain; the hydroxyl group introduces an additional site for stereoisomerism; the *R*-form of warfarin is additionally metabolised in man to the 6-hydroxy metabolite whilst the *S*-form is metabolised to the 6- and 7-hydroxy metabolites; the metabolism of warfarin is stimulated by several other drugs such as barbiturates, phenazone, and dichloralphenazone.

EXCRETION. About 60 to 90% of an oral dose is excreted in the urine as metabolites.

FURTHER INFORMATION. Effect of food and drink on absorption—M. N. Musa and L. L. Lyman, *Curr. ther. Res.*, 1976, **20**, 630; prediction of absorption from dissolution rate—V. F. Smolen and R. Erb, *J. pharm. Sci.*, 1977, **66**, 297; bioavailability of commercial tablets —J. G. Wagner *et al.*, *J. pharm. Sci.*, 1971, **60**, 666; possible inhibition of metabolism by co-trimoxazole— J. M. Hansen *et al.*, *Br. med. J.*, ii/1975, 684 and C. Hassall *et al.*, *Br. med. J.*, ii/1975, 684; inhibition of metabolism by sulphamethizole—B. Lumholtz *et al.*, *Clin. Pharmac. Ther.*, 1975, **17**, 731; stimulation of metabolism by barbiturates—J. B. Whitfield *et al.*, *Br. med. J.*, i/1973, 316; pharmacokinetics of enantiomers —A. Breckenridge *et al.*, *Clin. Pharmac. Ther.*, 1974, **15**, 424, D. S. Hewick and J. McEwen, *J. Pharm. Pharmac.*, 1973, **25**, 458, and R. A. O'Reilly, *Clin. Pharmac. Ther.*, 1974, **16**, 348; plasma concentrations—T. D. Bjornsson *et al.*, *J. pharm. Sci.*, 1977, **66**, 142, D. G. Kaiser and R. S. Martin, *J. pharm. Sci.*, 1974, **63**, 1579; R. J. Lewis, *J. pharm. Sci.*, 1971, **60**, 1271, and J. G. Wagner, *J. pharm. Sci.*, 1971, **60**, 1272; protein binding—M. J. Hayes *et al.*, *Br. J. clin. Pharmac.*, 1975, **2**, 69; greater sensitivity to warfarin after acute myocardial infarction —A. M. M. Shepherd and I. H. Stevenson, *Br. J. clin. Pharmac.*, 1976, **3**, 347P.

Actions and uses. Warfarin sodium is a synthetic anticoagulant which prolongs the prothrombin time by inhibiting the formation of factor VII and of prothrombin. To obtain an immediate effect on blood coagulation, heparin must be given intravenously for the first 12 to 18 hours of warfarin therapy. During treatment the plasma-prothrombin activity should be determined frequently so that the daily dosage may be adjusted to the desired therapeutic level.

Warfarin sodium is used in those conditions in which it is desirable to lower the coagulability of the blood. It is used in the prophylaxis and treatment of thrombosis in veins or arteries of the extremities. It prevents further thrombosis where this has already occurred, thereby markedly reducing the risk of embolism. Because of the risk of haemorrhage, its use in the treatment of such conditions as cerebral thrombosis may be dangerous, but it is sometimes used in the treatment of post-operative venous thrombosis; therapy is continued until the patient is fully ambulant, which may be up to 3 months.

Warfarin sodium is given by mouth, the initial dose usually being 10 to 15 milligrams; in no circumstances should the initial dose exceed 50 milligrams. Subsequent doses of 3 to 10 milligrams should be given daily after the prothrombin time has begun to recede from its peak; the dosage must be adjusted in accordance with the prothrombin activity of the blood, which must be estimated periodically.

Early clinical signs of overdosage are mild bleeding from the gums or elsewhere and the presence of erythrocytes in the urinary deposit. Phytomenadione is the most effective antidote to overdosage; administration of water-soluble vitamin-K analogues and the transfusion of whole blood are less effective.

The usual dose of phytomenadione that is required is 2 to 10 milligrams by mouth. In severe hypoprothrombinaemia 10 to 20 milligrams of phytomenadione may be administered by slow intravenous injection in the form of phytomenadione injection, the dose depending on the degree of prothrombin time prolongation and the clinical urgency; overdosage may encourage thrombosis.

Sensitivity to warfarin sodium may develop during prolonged treatment and an alternative anticoagulant may have to be given.

In addition to its use in medicine, warfarin is also used as a rodenticide.

Undesirable effects. Rashes, pyrexia, diarrhoea, and sore throat may occur; liver damage may occur rarely.

Precautions and contra-indications. Warfarin sodium should be used with great caution in the presence of hepatic or severe renal disease and also in any condition where there is a risk of serious haemorrhage, such as a past history of peptic ulceration or uncontrolled hypertension. It should not be used within 3 days of parturition, or of surgical operation. Warfarin should be used with great caution in pregnancy, particularly in the first trimester. The risk of intra-uterine haemorrhage greatly increases in the late stages of pregnancy. If warfarin is given to nursing mothers the offspring should be carefully monitored as a prothrombin deficiency may result; if breast feeding is continued the offspring should be given vitamin K supplements.

Drug interactions. The effect of warfarin sodium may be modified by the concurrent administration of other drugs. Methandienone and other 17-alkylated steroids, clofibrate, phenylbutazone, and similar drugs may increase the anticoagulant effect by plasma protein displacement while barbiturates, dichloralphenazone, glutethimide, and meprobamate, by promoting metabolism of warfarin, may reduce its effect. Aspirin and other salicylates may increase the danger of haemorrhage during anticoagulant therapy. The absorption of warfarin sodium from the gastro-intestinal tract is reduced by preparations containing liquid paraffin and also by fat-rich meals.

Preparation

WARFARIN TABLETS: available as tablets containing 1, 3, 5, and 10 mg of warfarin sodium; they may be coloured.

A standard for these tablets is given in the British Pharmacopoeia 1973

Containers and *Storage:* see the entry on Tablets for general information on containers and storage. Containers should be airtight and light resistant.

Labelling: the label on the container should state the amount of the medicament as the equivalent amount of anhydrous, isopropyl alcohol-free warfarin sodium.

Advice for patients: the tablets should be taken at regular intervals. Treatment should not be discontinued without the advice of the prescriber. Patients may carry an identification card giving details of their treatment and the name of the prescriber who should be contacted in the event of accident or illness. Patients should not take other medicines, including aspirin, without medical or pharmaceutical advice. Preparations containing liquid paraffin should also preferably be avoided.

Warts

Warts are circumscribed, benign, virus-induced, epithelial growths of the skin and adjoining mucous membranes. They may be treated with caustic paints, collodions, or plasters containing salicylic acid or podophyllum resin. They may also be destroyed with carbon dioxide snow or liquid nitrogen or by electrodestruction. Many warts will, however, disappear in time without treatment.

Water

$H_2O = 18.02$

Three forms of water are used in pharmacy, namely water for preparations, purified water, and water for injections. Other forms such as sterilised water may be supplied for specific purposes. Potable water of satisfactory biological quality is available in many areas and may be used in preparations that are not intended to be sterile provided that the mineral impurities that it contains do not react with the medicaments or other ingredients; the use of this potable water is described under Water for preparations (below). Where potable water containing mineral substances is not acceptable purified water is used, but as it is usually contaminated with micro-organisms it is boiled or sterilised before use.

Distilled Water

Purified water (see below) is supplied when distilled water is ordered.

Purified Water (*Syn.* Aqua Purificata)

Water prepared from suitable potable water by distillation, by treatment with ion-exchange materials, or by any other suitable method.

A standard for purified water is given in the European Pharmacopoeia Vol. I

The ion-exchange materials used in the preparation of purified water are known as "de-ionising resins" and consist of hard organic polymer particles, each containing ionised functional groups of a single type distributed throughout the mass of the material. The potable water is passed through two columns containing a cation-exchange resin and an anion-exchange resin respectively, or through a single column containing a mixture of the two resins.

Resins which may be used include a strong cation exchanger containing sulphonic acid functional groups ($R.SO_3^-H^+$, where R stands for the resin structure) and a strong anion exchanger containing quaternary ammonium groups ($R.NZ_3^+OH^-$, where Z stands for an aliphatic group).

Micro-organisms may multiply in ion-exchange columns, but their growth can be minimised by using the column continuously and regenerating regularly after a thorough backwashing.

It is inadvisable to use the ion-exchange method for preparing purified water unless facilities are available for controlling the quality of the water.

Storage. It should be stored in airtight containers which do not alter the properties of the water.

Uses. Purified water is used as a solvent and vehicle. Aqueous preparations intended for parenteral injection should be prepared with water for injections.

Water for Injections (*Syn.* Aqua ad Iniectabilia; Aqua pro Injectionibus)

Sterilised distilled water free from pyrogens.

A standard for water for injections is given in the European Pharmacopoeia Supplement 1973
Water for injections may be prepared by distilling potable water from a neutral-glass or metal still fitted with an efficient device for preventing entrainment; the first portion of the distillate is rejected and the remainder is collected in suitable containers and immediately sterilised by heating in an autoclave or by filtration without the addition of a bactericide.

Water for injections free from carbon dioxide is prepared by boiling the distillate for ten minutes, cooling, and transferring to the final containers with as little exposure to air as possible and immediately sterilising by heating in an autoclave.

Uses. Water for injections is used in preparations intended for parenteral administration and in other sterile products. For these purposes it may be replaced by freshly distilled water, prepared by the process described under Water for Injections but omitting the sterilisation stage, provided that the final preparation is immediately sterilised.

When supplied in multidose containers, a suitable bactericide should be added, and the name and concentration of the bactericide given on the label. If it is to be used for the preparation of intrathecal injections or of intravenous injections with doses of more than 15 millilitres, a bactericide must not be added and the water should be distributed in single dose containers.

Water for Preparations

Potable or freshly boiled and cooled purified water.

Potable water is drawn freshly from a public supply ("mains" water) and must be suitable for drinking; water obtained from the supply via a local storage tank is unsuitable for this purpose. If such stored water is the only source of mains water, freshly boiled and cooled purified water should be used instead; this should also be used when the potable water in a district is unsuitable for a particular preparation.

Uses. Water for preparations is used in preparing medicines such as Mixtures that are not intended to be sterile but for which water of good bacteriological quality is required.

Waters, Aromatic

Aromatic waters are solutions, usually saturated, of volatile oils or other aromatic substances in water. Some of them have a mild therapeutic action, but they are mainly used for their flavouring properties in vehicles for the internal administration of medicaments. Hamamelis water is only used externally.

Preparation of aromatic waters. Aromatic waters are prepared by diluting the concentrated water with 39 times its volume of freshly boiled and cooled purified water. The aromatic waters thus prepared contain a small proportion, usually about 1.5% v/v, of alcohol (90%).

Weights and Measures

A. The International System of Units (SI)

The International System of Units has been generally accepted in the United Kingdom and certain other countries for use in medical sciences and pharmacy.
The base units of SI are:

metre (m) (length)
kilogram (kg) (mass)
second (s) (time)
ampere (A) (electric current)
kelvin (K) (thermodynamic temperature)
mole (mol) (amount of substance)
candela (cd) (luminous intensity)

The following units, derived from the base units, have special names.

hertz	$Hz = s^{-1}$	frequency
newton	$N = m\ kg\ s^{-2}$	force
pascal	$Pa = m^{-1}\ kg\ s^{-2}$	pressure
joule	$J = m^2\ kg\ s^{-2}$	energy
watt	$W = m^2\ kg\ s^{-3}$	power
coulomb	$C = s\ A$	electric charge
volt	$V = m^2\ kg\ s^{-3}\ A^{-1}$	electric potential difference
ohm	$\Omega = m^2\ kg\ s^{-3}\ A^{-2}$	electric resistance
siemens	$S = m^{-2}\ kg^{-1}\ s^3\ A^2$	electric conductance
farad	$F = m^{-2}\ kg^{-1}\ s^4\ A^2$	electric capacitance
becquerel	$Bq = s^{-1}$	activity of a radioactive source
gray	$Gy = J\ kg^{-1}$	absorbed dose of ionising radiation

Certain other units are not part of SI but will continue to be used in appropriate circumstances for the foreseeable future. They include:

minute	min ⎫	
hour	h	time
day	d ⎭	
litre	l	volume
degree Celsius	°C	temperature
electronvolt	eV	energy

The following units are in common use for various purposes and are expected to continue in use for a limited time. Some of them are used in the Codex and during the transitional period their SI equivalents are usually given.

ångström	Å	length
dyne	dyn	force
erg	erg	energy
stokes	St	kinematic viscosity
poise	P	dynamic viscosity
inch	in	length
pound (avoirdupois)	lb	mass
calorie	cal	energy
millimetre of mercury	mmHg	pressure
degree Fahrenheit	°F	temperature
curie	Ci	activity of a radioactive source
rad	rad	absorbed dose of ionising radiation
röntgen	R	exposure to ionising radiation

Decimal multiples and submultiples of units are denoted by the following prefixes. In practice, it is preferable to use only the thousandfold multiples, e.g. gram, milligram, microgram, nanogram.

Prefix	Symbol	Multiple or Submultiple
exa	E	10^{18} = 1 000 000 000 000 000 000
peta	P	10^{15} = 1 000 000 000 000 000
tera	T	10^{12} = 1 000 000 000 000
giga	G	10^{9} = 1 000 000 000
mega	M	10^{6} = 1 000 000
kilo	k	10^{3} = 1 000
hecta	h	10^{2} = 100
deca	da	10^{1} = 10
deci	d	10^{-1} = 0.1
centi	c	10^{-2} = 0.01
milli	m	10^{-3} = 0.001
micro	μ	10^{-6} = 0.000 001
nano	n	10^{-9} = 0.000 000 001
pico	p	10^{-12} = 0.000 000 000 001
femto	f	10^{-15} = 0.000 000 000 000 001
atto	a	10^{-18} = 0.000 000 000 000 000 001

Mass (Weights)

1 kilogram (kg) is the mass of the International Prototype Kilogram

1 gram (g)	= the 1000th part of 1 kilogram
1 milligram (mg)	= the 1000th part of 1 gram
1 microgram (μg)	= the 1000th part of 1 milligram
1 nanogram (ng)	= the 1000th part of 1 microgram

For the purpose of writing prescriptions the word "microgram" should be written in full; when an abbreviation is essential, the British Pharmacopoeia recommends that "mcg" should be used as the contrac-

tion. This divergence from the international practice is recommended to avoid the possibility of confusion between "μg" and "mg". Similar confusion may arise between the abbreviations "mg" and "ng".

Capacity (Volumes)

The litre (l) is now defined in the United Kingdom by the Units of Measurement Regulations 1976 (S.I. 1976: No. 1674) as 1 cubic decimetre, which represents a slight decrease from its former value of 1000.028 cubic centimetres. The litre is the accepted term for general use but should not be used for measurements of high precision.

1 litre (l)	= 1000 cm³
1 millilitre (ml)	= the 1000th part of 1 litre
1 microlitre (μl)	= the 1000th part of 1 millilitre

Length

1 metre (m) is the Metre as defined in the Weights and Measures (International Definitions) Order 1963

1 decimetre (dm)	= the 10th part of 1 metre
1 centimetre (cm)	= the 100th part of 1 metre
1 millimetre (mm)	= the 1000th part of 1 metre
1 micrometre (μm)	= the 1000th part of 1 millimetre
1 nanometre (nm)	= the 1000th part of 1 micrometre

Radioactivity

The curie (Ci) has been replaced as the unit of activity of radionuclides by the becquerel (Bq).

1 curie (Ci)	= 3.7×10^{10} disintegrations per second
	= 3.7×10^{10} becquerels
1 millicurie (mCi)	= 3.7×10^{7} becquerels
1 microcurie (μCi)	= 3.7×10^{4} becquerels

For further information on these units see under Radiopharmaceuticals.

B. Imperial System of Weights and Measures

The Imperial System is no longer used in medicine and pharmacy in the United Kingdom, but is still used for domestic and general trade purposes.

Mass (Weights)

1 pound (avoirdupois) (lb) is the Imperial Pound as defined in the UK Weights and Measures Act, 1963, Schedule 1

1 ounce (avoirdupois) (oz)	= the 16th part of 1 pound
	= 437.5 grains
1 grain (gr)	= the 7000th part of 1 pound

Capacity (Volumes)

1 gallon (gal) is now defined in the United Kingdom under the Units of Measurement Regulations 1976 (S.I. 1976: No. 1674) as 4.546 09 cubic decimetres.

1 pint (pt)	= the 8th part of 1 gallon
	= 20 fluid ounces
1 fluid ounce (fl oz)	= the 20th part of 1 pint
	= 8 fluid drachms
1 fluid drachm (fl dr)	= the 8th part of 1 fluid ounce
	= 60 minims
1 minim (min)	= the 60th part of 1 fluid drachm

RELATION OF CAPACITY TO WEIGHT

The following equivalents are stated to five significant figures:

1 minim	= the volume at 16.7° (62 °F) of 0.911 46 grain of water
1 fluid drachm	= the volume at 16.7° (62 °F) of 54.688 grains of water
1 fluid ounce	= the volume at 16.7° (62 °F) of 1 ounce (avoirdupois) or 437.5 grains of water
109.71 minims*	= the volume at 16.7° (62 °F) of 100 grains of water

* Usually taken as 110 minims

Length

1 yard (yd) is the Imperial Yard as defined in the Weights and Measures Act, 1963, Schedule 1
1 foot (ft) = the 3rd part of 1 yard
1 inch (in.) = the 12th part of 1 foot

C. SI Unit Equivalents of other Metric Units

Length

1 ångström (Å) = 10^{-10} metre = 10^{-1} nanometre (nm)
1 micron (μ) = 10^{-6} metre = 1 micrometre (μm)

Volume

1 millilitre (ml) = 1 cubic centimetre (cm³)
1 litre (l) = 1 cubic decimetre (dm³)

Energy

1 kilocalorie (kcal) = 4.1868×10^3 joules
1 erg (erg) = 10^{-7} joule
1 electronvolt (eV) = 1.6022×10^{-19} joule

Pressure

1 millimetre of mercury (mmHg) = 133.322 pascals
1 bar (bar) = 10^5 pascals

Viscosity, Dynamic

1 poise (P) = 10^{-1} pascal second (Pa s)
1 centipoise (cP) = 10^{-3} pascal second
  = 10^{-3} newton second per square metre (N s m^{-2})

Viscosity, kinematic

1 stokes (St) = 10^{-4} square metre per second (m² s^{-1})
1 centistokes (cSt) = 10^{-6} square metre per second

Temperature

1 degree Celsius (°C) = 1 kelvin (K)
1 degree Fahrenheit (°F) = $^5/_9$ kelvin

D. Imperial Equivalents of Metric and SI Units

Some figures have changed slightly as a result of the redefinition of the Imperial gallon in terms of the new litre (1 dm³).

Weights or Measures of Mass

1 picogram (pg) = 15.432×10^{-12} grain
1 nanogram (ng) = 15.432×10^{-9} grain
1 microgram (μg) = 15.432×10^{-6} grain
1 milligram (mg) = 0.015 432 grain
1 gram (g) = 15.432 grains
  = 0.032 15 ounce (apothecaries')
  = 0.035 27 ounce (avoirdupois)
1 kilogram (kg) = 2.204 6 pounds

Measures of Capacity

1 millilitre (ml) = 16.894 minims
1 litre (l) = 0.219 97 gallon
  = 1.759 75 pints
  = 35.195 1 fluid ounces

Measures of Length

1 ångström (Å) = 3.9370×10^{-9} inch
1 nanometre (nm) = 3.9370×10^{-8} inch
1 micrometre (μm) = 3.9370×10^{-5} inch
1 millimetre (mm) = 0.039 370 inch
1 centimetre (cm) = 0.393 70 inch
1 decimetre (dm) = 3.9370 inches
1 metre (m) = 39.370 inches
1 kilometre (km) = 0.621 37 mile

Pressure

1 bar (bar) = 14.50 pounds force per square inch (lbf/in²)

E. SI and Metric Equivalents of Imperial Weights and Measures

Weights or Measures of Mass

1 grain (gr) = 0.064 799 gram
1 ounce (avoirdupois) (437.5 gr) (oz) = 28.350 grams
1 ounce (apothecaries') (480 gr) = 31.104 grams
1 pound (lb) = 453.592 grams

Measures of Capacity

1 minim (min) = 0.059 194 millilitre
1 fluid drachm (fl dr) = 3.551 6 millilitres
1 fluid ounce (fl oz) = 28.413 millilitres
  = 0.028 413 litre
1 pint (pt) = 568.261 millilitres
  = 0.568 261 litre
1 gallon (gal) = 4.546 09 litres
1 gallon (US) = 3.785 41 litres
  = 0.832 674 gallon (UK)

Measures of Length

1 inch (in.) = 25.400×10^7 ångströms
  = 25.400×10^6 nanometres
  = 25.400×10^3 micrometres
  = 25.400 millimetres
1 foot (ft) = 304.80 millimetres
1 yard (yd) = 914.40 millimetres
1 mile = 1.609 3 kilometres

Pressure

1 pound force per square inch (lbf/in²) = 0.068 97 bar

Further Information. P. Anderton and P. H. Bigg, *Changing to the Metric System*, Ministry of Technology London, HM Stationery Office, 1965; The International System of Units (SI) 1970 (BS 3763: 1970); *The Use of SI Units*, British Standards Institution, PD 5686: 1972; D. A. Lowe, *A Guide to International Recommendations on Names and Symbols for Quantities and on Units of Measurement*, Geneva, World Health Organization, 1975; Report by the Symbols Committee of the Royal Society, *Quantities, Units, and Symbols*, 2nd Edn, London, The Royal Society, 1975; *SI, The International System of Units*, C. H. Page and P. Vigoureux (Eds), National Physical Laboratory, 3rd Edn, London, HM Stationery Office, 1977 (translation from French).

The use of SI units in medicine—D. N. Baron, *Br. med. J.*, iv/1974, 509.

The use of SI units in hospital laboratories—D. N. Baron *et al.*, *J. clin. Path.*, 1974, **27**, 590.

F. Atomic Weights of Elements

$^{12}C = 12$

Element	Atomic Number	Symbol	Atomic Weight
Aluminium	13	Al	26.98154
Antimony	51	Sb	121.75
Arsenic	33	As	74.9216
Barium	56	Ba	137.33
Bismuth	83	Bi	208.9804
Boron	5	B	10.81
Bromine	35	Br	79.904
Cadmium	48	Cd	112.41
Calcium	20	Ca	40.08
Carbon	6	C	12.011
Cerium	58	Ce	140.12
Chlorine	17	Cl	35.453
Chromium	24	Cr	51.996
Cobalt	27	Co	58.9332
Copper	29	Cu	63.546
Fluorine	9	F	18.998403
Gallium	31	Ga	69.72
Gold	79	Au	196.9665
Helium	2	He	4.00260
Hydrogen	1	H	1.0079
Indium	49	In	114.82
Iodine	53	I	126.9045
Iron	26	Fe	55.847
Krypton	36	Kr	83.80
Lanthanum	57	La	138.9055
Lead	82	Pb	207.2
Lithium	3	Li	6.941
Magnesium	12	Mg	24.305
Manganese	25	Mn	54.9380
Mercury	80	Hg	200.59
Molybdenum	42	Mo	95.94
Neon	10	Ne	20.179
Nickel	28	Ni	58.70
Nitrogen	7	N	14.0067
Osmium	76	Os	190.2
Oxygen	8	O	15.9994
Palladium	46	Pd	106.4
Phosphorus	15	P	30.97376
Platinum	78	Pt	195.09
Potassium	19	K	39.0983
Radium	88	Ra	226.0254
Rubidium	37	Rb	85.4678
Ruthenium	44	Ru	101.07
Selenium	34	Se	78.96
Silicon	14	Si	28.0855
Silver	47	Ag	107.868
Sodium	11	Na	22.98977
Strontium	38	Sr	87.62
Sulphur	16	S	32.06
Technetium	43	Tc	97
Thallium	81	Tl	204.37
Thorium	90	Th	232.0381
Tin	50	Sn	118.69
Titanium	22	Ti	47.90
Tungsten	74	W	183.85
Uranium	92	U	238.029
Vanadium	23	V	50.9414
Xenon	54	Xe	131.30
Yttrium	39	Y	88.9059
Zinc	30	Zn	65.38
Zirconium	40	Zr	91.22

Whipworm Infection

see TRICHURIASIS

Wild Cherry Bark

The dried bark of the wild or black cherry, *Prunus serotina* Ehrh. (Fam. Rosaceae), a tree widely distributed over North America.

OTHER NAMES: Prunus Serotina; Virginian Prune; Virginian Prune Bark

A standard is given in the British Pharmaceutical Codex 1973

The bark is collected in the states of Virginia, North Carolina, and Tennessee during the months of July to October, dried, and exported under the commercial designation of Thin Natural Wild Cherry Bark. The most esteemed bark is that collected in the autumn, preferably from young stems and branches.

Constituents. Wild cherry bark contains (+)-mandelonitrile glucoside (prunasin) and an enzyme system, which interact in the presence of water yielding benzaldehyde, hydrocyanic acid, and glucose. Benzoic, trimethylgallic, and *p*-coumaric acids and a small amount of volatile oil are present.

Other constituents are tannin, fatty acids, and resinous substances which yield β-methylaesculetin (scopoletin) on hydrolysis with acid. Good specimens of the drug yield 0.075 to 0.16% of hydrocyanic acid.

Wild cherry bark yields to alcohol (60%) 17 to 23% of extractive. The ash is about 3 to 4%, the acid-insoluble ash 0.2 to 0.6%, and the foreign organic matter 2%.

Description. UNGROUND DRUG. *Macroscopical characters:* irregular fragments or curved or channelled pieces up to 120 mm long and 50 mm wide and not more than 4 mm thick; young bark covered externally with a thin, smooth, reddish-brown to brownish-black papery cork sometimes exfoliated and revealing the smooth greenish-brown cortex, both cork and underlying cortex showing numerous, transversely elongated lenticels about 5 to 15 mm long; older bark darker and rougher; inner surface cinnamon-brown, showing fine wavy longitudinal striations anastomosing to form a fine reticulation with raised pale areas in the meshes, patches of narrowly lanceolate fissures, about 1.0 to 5.0 mm long, frequently present, reticulation less pronounced in young bark; fracture short, granular; smoothed, transversely cut surface with outer, thin, brown cork covering a narrow green cortex followed internally by a narrow line of pericyclic sclerenchyma and reddish-brown secondary phloem containing small groups of sclereids and traversed by numerous paler medullary rays.

It has a slight odour and when moistened develops a strong odour of benzaldehyde. The taste is astringent, aromatic, and bitter, resembling that of bitter almonds.

Microscopical characters: the diagnostic characters are: *phelloderm* and *cortex* parenchymatous, containing chlorophyll; *pericycle* consisting of an almost continuous zone of sclereids with very occasional *fibres*; sclereids, some branched, in numerous groups; *starch* granules about 5 to 9 μm in diameter, in cells of the *medullary rays; secondary phloem* and medullary rays with large, irregular fissures between them; *crystals* of calcium oxalate prismatic, 10 to 30 to 40 to 80μm long, and clusters, 10 to 18 to 30 μm wide, chiefly in cells of phloem bordering upon the fissures; typical *phloem fibres* absent.

POWDERED DRUG. Powdered Wild Cherry Bark. A light-brown powder possessing the diagnostic characters, odour, and taste of the unground drug.

Adulterants and substitutes. A form of the bark, known as "rossed" bark, sometimes occurs in commerce; this consists of bark from which the cortex, in addition to the cork, has been removed; its uniformly dark cinnamon-brown outer surface has a rough or rasped appearance and exhibits under a lens pale longitudinal strands of sclerenchymatous cells alternating with darker medullary rays.

Thick bark from the trunk and larger branches is characterised by numerous depressions on the outer surface and the absence of lenticels.

Barks from other species of *Prunus* are occasionally substituted for the official drug and may be recognised by the presence of fibres or by the taste, which is astringent and deficient in the flavour of bitter almond.

Storage. It should be stored in a cool dry place. Powdered wild cherry bark should be stored in airtight containers, in a cool place.

Identification. TEST. To 1 g, broken into small pieces or in powder, in a stoppered tube, add 1 ml of water, suspend a strip of filter-paper moistened with *trinitrophenol solution* above the liquid, stopper the tube, and allow to stand for 30 minutes; the paper becomes brick-red.

Actions and uses. In the form of the syrup, wild cherry bark has been used in the treatment of cough, but it has little therapeutic value. The chief use of wild cherry syrup is as a flavouring agent.

Preparation

WILD CHERRY SYRUP (*Syn.* Syrupus Pruni Serotinae; Virginian Prune Syrup):

Wild cherry bark, in moderately coarse powder	150 g
Sucrose	800 g
Glycerol	50 ml
Water for preparations	to 1000 ml

Percolate the wild cherry bark with water, collecting the percolate in a vessel containing the sucrose and the glycerol; continue the percolation until the total volume is 1000 ml, shake to dissolve the sucrose, without the aid of heat, and add sufficient water to produce the required volume.

A standard for this syrup is given in the British Pharmaceutical Codex 1973
Storage: it should be stored in a cool place
Dose: 2.5 to 10 millilitres.

Wilson's Disease

see under CIRRHOSIS OF THE LIVER

Wool Alcohols

Wool alcohols may be obtained by treating wool fat with alkali and separating the fraction containing cholesterol and other alcohols.

OTHER NAMES: *Argowax*®; *Hartolan*®; Wool Wax Alcohols

A standard is given in the British Pharmacopoeia 1973

Constituents. Wool alcohols is a crude mixture of steroid and triterpene alcohols, including 28 to 34% of cholesterol and 10 to 13% of isocholesterol.

Wool alcohols also contains 500 to 1000 parts per million of added antoxidant, either butylated hydroxyanisole or butylated hydroxytoluene.

Description. A somewhat brittle golden-brown solid with a smooth and shiny fracture and with a faint odour resembling that of wool fat.

Solubility. Practically insoluble in water; very slightly soluble in alcohol; completely soluble in 25 parts of boiling dehydrated alcohol; soluble in ether, in chloroform, and in light petroleum.

Melting-point. When warmed, it becomes plastic and melts at about 58°.

Storage. It should be stored in airtight containers, in a cool place protected from light.

Uses. Wool alcohols resembles wool fat in being a good emulsifying agent for water-in-oil emulsions. Emulsions made with it are usually preferred to those made with wool fat, since they do not darken on the surface or emit an objectionable odour in hot weather.

The proportion of water that can be incorporated in soft paraffin is increased threefold by the addition of 5% of wool alcohols. Such emulsions are not "cracked" by the addition of weak acids such as citric, lactic, or tartaric acid, and they may be improved and made more stable by the addition of cetostearyl alcohol.

Proportions of wool alcohols up to 2.5% may be added to oil-in-water emulsions in order to improve the texture, stability, and emollient properties.

Although wool alcohols may contain small amounts of phenolic antoxidants, higher concentrations of phenols may cause an incompatibility if included in emulsions containing wool alcohols.

Undesirable effects. Wool alcohols sometimes has a slightly irritant action and in rare instances may give rise to a bullous eruption. Occasional cases of skin sensitivity have occurred.

Preparations

OILY CREAM:

Wool alcohols ointment	500 g
Purified water	500 ml

Melt the wool alcohols ointment and add gradually, with constant stirring, the purified water previously boiled and cooled to 50°; mix vigorously until a smooth cream is obtained and stir until cold.

When oily cream is used in a white ointment, it should be prepared from wool alcohols ointment made with white soft paraffin; when used in a coloured ointment, it should be prepared from wool alcohols ointment made with yellow soft paraffin.

Containers and *Storage:* see the entry on Creams for general information on containers and storage. It should be stored in an airtight container made from non-absorbent material. If, on storage, some aqueous liquid separates, it is readily reincorporated by stirring.

WOOL ALCOHOLS OINTMENT (*Syn.* Ung. Alcoh. Lan.):

Wool alcohols	60 g
White soft paraffin or yellow soft paraffin	100 g
Hard paraffin	240 g
Liquid paraffin	600 g

Melt together and stir until cold.

In preparing wool alcohols ointment, the proportions of hard paraffin, soft paraffin, and liquid paraffin may be varied to produce wool alcohols ointment having suitable properties. When wool alcohols ointment is used in a white ointment, it should be prepared with white soft paraffin; and when used in a coloured ointment it should be prepared with yellow soft paraffin.

Containers: see the entry on Ointments for general information on containers.

Wool Fat

The purified anhydrous fat-like substance obtained from the wool of the sheep, *Ovis aries* L. (Fam. Bovidae).

OTHER NAMES: Adeps Lanae; Anhydrous Lanolin; *Corona®*; *White Swan®*; *Yeoman®*

A standard is given in the British Pharmacopoeia 1973

The natural grease is extracted from wool by scouring with dilute alkali with which it readily forms an emulsion; the emulsion is acidified and the wool fat separates as a distinct layer at the surface of the liquid. Purification may be effected by repeated treatment with water in a centrifuge.

Constituents. Wool fat consists mainly of fatty acid esters of cholesterol, lanosterol, and fatty alcohols, together with free alcohols, free fatty acids, and hydrocarbons.
Wool fat may also contain not more than 200 parts per million of added antioxidant, either butylated hydroxyanisole or butylated hydroxytoluene.

Description. A pale yellow tenacious unctuous substance with a slight characteristic odour.

Solubility. Practically insoluble in water; very slightly soluble in cold alcohol; soluble in 75 parts of boiling alcohol, depositing most of the wool fat as a flocculent precipitate on cooling; soluble in ether, in chloroform, in acetone, and in carbon disulphide.

Melting-point. About 39°.

Adulterants and substitutes. Paraffins and animal and vegetable fats and oils are possible adulterants.

Sterilisation. It is sterilised by dry heat.

Uses. Wool fat is used in the formulation of ointment bases. It can absorb about 30% of water and may be of value in stabilising water-in-oil emulsions. On storage, such emulsions are liable to darken on the surface. Occasional cases of skin sensitivity to wool fat have occurred.

Preparations

HYDROUS WOOL FAT (*Syn.* Adeps Lanae Hydrosus; Lanolin):

Wool fat	700 g
Purified water, freshly boiled and cooled	300 ml

Melt the wool fat and add the water gradually, with constant stirring.
A standard for hydrous wool fat is given in the British Pharmacopoeia 1973
Storage: it should be stored in airtight containers, in a cool place.

HYDROUS WOOL FAT OINTMENT (*Syn.* Unguentum Adipis Lanae Hydrosi):

Hydrous wool fat	500 g
Yellow soft paraffin	500 g

Melt together, and stir until cold.
Containers: see the entry on Ointments for general information on containers. Containers should prevent evaporation.

Wool fat is an ingredient of simple ointment (see under Paraffin, White Soft).

Xanthan Gum

A gum prepared by fermentation of dextrose solution with *Xanthomonas campestris* and subsequent purification. It consists of sodium, potassium, or calcium salts of a partially acetylated polysaccharide of high molecular weight containing D-glucose, D-mannose, and D-glucuronic acid units in the ratio 2.8:2:2; it also contains about 3% of pyruvate.

Description. A cream coloured powder.

Solubility. Soluble in hot or cold water.

Uses. Xanthan gum is used as a thickening and suspending agent but it is not generally suitable for use in the small-scale extemporaneous preparation of medicines. It is used as an alternative to tragacanth when it is desired to incorporate a suspending agent in the preparation of opiate squill linctus (see under Squill).
A 1% solution of xanthan gum has a viscosity of about 1000 centipoises (1 Pa s).

Xenon (^{133}Xe) Injection

Xenon (^{133}Xe) injection is a sterile solution of xenon-133 made isotonic with blood by the addition of sodium chloride.

A standard is given in the British Pharmacopoeia 1973

CAUTION. *This material is radioactive and any regulations in force must be complied with.*

Xenon-133 is a radioactive isotope of xenon which decays by emission of β^--radiation of maximum energy 0.346 MeV and γ-radiation mainly of energy 0.081 MeV. It has a half-life of 5.3 days. It may be prepared from the products of uranium fission.

Description. A clear colourless solution.

Acidity or alkalinity. pH 5.0 to 8.0.

Sterilisation. It is sterilised by heating in an autoclave.

Labelling. The label on the container should state (1) the content of xenon-133 expressed in microcuries or millicuries at a given date and hour, (2) the volume of the injection, (3) that the injection is radioactive, and (4) either that the injection does not contain a bactericide or the name and proportion of any added bactericide.

Containers. The injection should be supplied in a totally filled container, from which it can be extracted without the introduction of an air bubble, for example an injection cartridge; an air bubble if present should be less than 0.5% of the volume of the injection.

Storage. It should be stored in an area assigned for the purpose. The storage conditions should be such that the maximum radiation-dose-rate to which persons may be exposed is reduced to an acceptable level. Glass containers may darken under the effects of radiation.

Actions and uses. Xenon has a low solubility in blood plasma and when xenon (^{133}Xe) injection is administered intravenously its radioactivity is removed on first passing through the lungs. Xenon (^{133}Xe) injection is used for measurements of lung perfusion. The usual dose is 1 to 2 millicuries by intravenous injection. The radioactivity is examined by means of detectors placed over various regions of the lungs or by the use of the gamma-ray camera.
Xenon (^{133}Xe) injection is also administered intra-arterially or intravenously for cerebral and other regional blood flow studies and for circulation measurements. The usual dose is 300 microcuries. Blood flow in muscle and skin is determined after intramuscular or subcutaneous injection by recording the rate of disappearance of ^{133}Xe radioactivity from the relevant area.

Xylose

$C_5H_{10}O_5 = 150.1$

OTHER NAME: D-Xylose

A standard is given in the British Pharmacopoeia 1973

Description. Odourless colourless crystals or white crystalline powder with a slightly sweet taste.

Solubility. Soluble in less than 1 part of water; soluble in hot alcohol.

Specific rotation. $+18.5°$ to $+19.5°$, determined on a 10% solution containing 0.4% of *dilute ammonia solution.*

Metabolism. ABSORPTION. Incompletely absorbed after oral administration; there appears to be an inverse relationship between xylose absorption and serum immunoglobulin (IgG) concentrations; xylose absorption is reduced by administration of phenobarbitone and in cases of malabsorption.

BLOOD CONCENTRATION. Not normally present in blood; after an oral dose of 25 g, blood concentrations of over 250 $\mu g/ml$ are obtained in normal subjects.

HALF-LIFE. Biological half-life, about 1.5 hours.

METABOLIC REACTIONS. Metabolised to carbon dioxide and water.

EXCRETION. About 30% of an oral dose and 40 to 50% of an intravenous dose is excreted in the urine in 5 hours as unchanged drug.

FURTHER INFORMATION. Immunoglobulin concentrations and xylose absorption—G. C. Cook, *Br. med. J.,* iv/1974, 200; effect of gut motility on absorption—M. J. Kendall and L. Beeley, *Br. med. J.,* iii/1974, 471.

Actions and uses. Xylose is used orally in a dose of 25 grams to test the absorptive capacity of the intestinal mucosa. In normal subjects, at least 5 grams is excreted in the urine within 5 hours.

Yeast, Dried

Dried yeast consists of unicellular fungi belonging to the family Saccharomycetaceae, a sub-division of the Ascomycetales, which have been dried by a process which avoids decomposition of the vitamins present.

A standard is given in the British Pharmaceutical Codex 1973

The chief species of yeast used in the fermentation industries are *Saccharomyces cerevisiae* Meyen *emend.* Hansen, *S. carlsbergensis* Hansen, and *S. monacensis* Hansen, of which many different strains and races exist.

Constituents. Dried yeast contains vitamins of the B group, the amount in each gram being about 100 to 200 μg of thiamine hydrochloride, 300 to 600 μg of nicotinic acid, and 40 to 60 μg of riboflavine; it also contains pyridoxine, pantothenic acid, biotin, folic acid, vitamin B_{12}, *p*-aminobenzoic acid, and inositol, and is one of the richest known sources of the vitamin-B group. It contains about 46% of proteins, some of which

are combined with nucleic acid to form nucleins and nucleoproteins, and about 36% of carbohydrates.

A number of enzymes are present, including zymase, invertase, maltase, emulsin, and a proteolytic endotryptase.

Among other constituents are fat, choline, ergosterol, zymosterol, glycogen, various other carbohydrates, and glutathione.

It yields about 8.5% of ash.

Description. *Macroscopical characters:* a buff or brownish-buff, somewhat granular powder with a characteristic odour.

Microscopical characters: the diagnostic characters are: somewhat angular masses of loosely agglutinated, rounded or ovoid cells, or short-branched filaments composed of united cells; cells colourless, about 3 to 8 μm in diameter, containing a somewhat granular protoplasm with 1 or 2 vacuoles; cells occasionally containing 4 small spores formed under conditions of low nutrition, scanty moisture, and free aeration. Occasional starch grains may be present, derived from the filtration process.

Moisture content. Not more than 9%, determined by drying at 100°.

Storage. It should be stored in airtight containers.

Actions and uses. Dried yeast is a source of the vitamin-B group and has been used for the prevention and treatment of vitamin-B deficiency diseases. However it is doubtful whether sufficient of the vitamins present in yeast are absorbed from the human gut. As a dietary supplement, infants may be given 1 to 2.5 grams daily mixed with milk, children 4 to 6 grams daily, and adults 6 to 8 grams daily. In severe vitamin-B-deficiency diseases, such as beriberi, pellagra, or ariboflavinosis, doses of up to 30 grams daily may be given.

Undesirable effects. Large doses may cause diarrhoea.

Yellow Fever Vaccine

An aqueous suspension of chick-embryo tissue containing the attenuated yellow fever virus 17D strain which, although avirulent for man, is nevertheless highly immunogenic. The dry product is reconstituted immediately before use by dissolving the contents of a sealed container in saline or other appropriate solution so that the reconstituted vaccine is isotonic with blood.

OTHER NAME: Yel/Vac

A standard is given in the British Pharmacopoeia Addendum 1978

The potency of the vaccine is stated as the number of LD50 doses in 1 ml. The potency is determined in plaque-forming units and converted to mouse LD50 by an approved factor.

Storage. The dried vaccine should be protected from light and stored at approximately 0°. Under these conditions, it may be expected to retain its potency for one year; at lower temperatures it retains its potency for longer periods. At 20° it loses its potency within a few days.

The reconstituted vaccine should be used immediately after preparation.

Actions and uses. Yellow fever vaccine produces an active immunity which is usually established within 10 days of administration and persists for many years. Only one dose by subcutaneous injection is required for immunisation, but reinoculation every 10 years is desirable. One human dose is equivalent to not less than 1000 LD50 of vaccine.

Suitable schedules for the immunisation of travellers are given under Vaccines.

Undesirable effects and precautions. Reactions to the vaccine seldom occur. Allergic symptoms, which can usually be effectively controlled by the administration of adrenaline or an antihistamine, have been observed in persons sensitive to egg protein. Mild encephalitis occasionally occurs in infants under the age of 9 months and it is recommended that, when possible, vaccination against yellow fever should be postponed until an infant is at least 9 months old.

The precautions to be taken when vaccinating simultaneously against yellow fever and smallpox are described under Smallpox Vaccine.

Zinc Oxide

ZnO = 81.38

OTHER NAMES: *Pharmakon®*; Zinci Oxidum

A standard is given in the European Pharmacopoeia Vol. I

Zinc oxide forms cement-like products when mixed with a strong solution of zinc chloride or with phosphoric acid, owing to the formation of oxy-salts.

Commercial zinc oxide, manufactured for use as a pigment, is known as "zinc white".

Description. An odourless soft white or faintly yellowish-white powder.

Solubility. Practically insoluble in water; soluble in dilute mineral acids.

Hygroscopicity. When exposed to air it gradually absorbs moisture and carbon dioxide.

Sterilisation. It is sterilised by dry heat.

Actions and uses. Zinc oxide is applied externally, in dusting-powders, ointments, pastes, and lotions, as a mild astringent for the skin, as a soothing and protective application in eczema and as a protective for slight excoriations.

Preparations

COAL TAR AND ZINC OINTMENT:

Strong coal tar solution	100 g
Zinc oxide, finely sifted	300 g
Yellow soft paraffin	600 g

Mix the zinc oxide with the strong coal tar solution, triturate with a portion of the yellow soft paraffin until smooth, and gradually incorporate the remainder of the yellow soft paraffin.

A standard for this ointment is given in the British Pharmaceutical Codex 1973

Containers: see the entry on Ointments for general information on containers. Containers should prevent evaporation.

Advice for patients: the ointment should not be applied to broken or inflamed skin. It stains the skin, hair, and fabric.

COMPOUND ZINC PASTE (*Syn.* Zinc Paste):

Zinc oxide, finely sifted	250 g
Starch, finely sifted	250 g
White soft paraffin	500 g

Melt the white soft paraffin, incorporate the zinc oxide and the starch, and stir until cold.

A standard for this paste is given in the British Pharmacopoeia 1973

Containers and *Storage:* see the entry on Pastes for general information on containers and storage.

Advice for patients: the paste should be applied liberally to the affected area with a suitable applicator.

ZINC AND CASTOR OIL OINTMENT (*Syn.* Zinc and Castor Oil Cream; Zinc and Castor Oil):

Zinc oxide, finely sifted	75 g
Castor oil	500 g
Cetostearyl alcohol	20 g
White beeswax	100 g
Arachis oil	305 g

Triturate the zinc oxide with a portion of the castor oil until smooth and add the mixture to the remainder of the ingredients previously melted together; stir until the temperature is about 40°.

A standard for this ointment is given in the British Pharmacopoeia 1973

Containers: see the entry on Ointments for general information on containers.

ZINC AND COAL TAR PASTE (*Syn.* Zinc Oxide and Coal Tar Paste; White's Tar Paste):

Zinc oxide, finely sifted	60 g
Coal tar	60 g
Emulsifying wax	50 g
Starch	380 g
Yellow soft paraffin	450 g

Melt the emulsifying wax at 70° and add the coal tar, followed by 225 g of the yellow soft paraffin; stir at 70° until completely melted and add the remainder of the yellow soft paraffin. When completely melted, cool to 30°, add the zinc oxide and the starch, with constant stirring, and mix until cold.

A standard for this paste is given in the British Pharmaceutical Codex 1973

Containers and *Storage:* see the entry on Pastes for general information on containers and storage.

Advice for patients: the paste should be applied liberally and carefully to the lesions with a suitable applicator. It should not be applied to broken or inflamed skin. It stains the skin, hair, and fabric.

ZINC AND ICHTHAMMOL CREAM (*Syn.* Zinc Oxide and Ichthammol Cream):

Zinc cream	820 g
Ichthammol	50 g
Cetostearyl alcohol	30 g
Wool fat	100 g

Melt together the wool fat and the cetostearyl alcohol with the aid of gentle heat; triturate the warm mixture with the zinc cream until smooth and incorporate the ichthammol.

A standard for this cream is given in the British Pharmaceutical Codex 1973

Containers, Labelling, and *Storage:* see the entry on Creams for general information on containers, labelling, and storage.

Advice for patients: the cream should be rubbed lightly on the affected area. It should not be applied to broken skin.

ZINC AND SALICYLIC ACID PASTE (*Syn.* Lassar's Paste):

Salicylic acid, finely sifted	20 g
Starch, finely sifted	240 g
Zinc oxide, finely sifted	240 g
White soft paraffin	500 g

Melt the white soft paraffin, incorporate the salicylic acid, the starch, and the zinc oxide, and stir until cold.
A standard for this paste is given in the British Pharmacopoeia 1973
Containers and *Storage:* see the entry on Pastes for general information on containers and storage.
Advice for patients: the paste should be applied liberally and carefully to the lesions. It should not be applied to broken or inflamed skin; contact with the eyes should be avoided. Prolonged use should be avoided and its use should be discontinued if excessive dryness or irritation of the skin occurs.

ZINC CREAM:

Zinc oxide, finely sifted	320.0 g
Calcium hydroxide	0.45 g
Wool fat	80.0 g
Oleic acid	5.0 ml
Arachis oil	320.0 ml
Purified water, freshly boiled and cooled	to 1000.0 g

Mix the zinc oxide and the calcium hydroxide, triturate to a smooth paste with a mixture of the oleic acid and arachis oil, incorporate the wool fat, and gradually add, with continuous stirring, sufficient of the water to produce the required volume.
A standard for this cream is given in the British Pharmacopoeia 1973
Containers: see the entry on Creams for general information on containers.

ZINC OINTMENT (*Syn.* Ung. Zinc.):

Zinc oxide, finely sifted	150 g
Simple ointment	850 g

Triturate the zinc oxide with a portion of the simple ointment until smooth and gradually incorporate the remainder of the simple ointment.
A standard for this ointment is given in the British Pharmacopoeia 1973
Containers: see the entry on Ointments for general information on containers.

ZINC, STARCH, AND TALC DUSTING-POWDER (*Syn.* Zinc Oxide and Starch Dusting-powder; Zinc Oxide, Starch, and Talc Dusting-powder):

Zinc oxide	250 g
Starch, in powder	250 g
Purified talc, sterilised	500 g

Prepare as described in the entry on Powders.
A standard for this dusting-powder is given in the British Pharmaceutical Codex 1973
Containers and *Labelling:* see the entry on Dusting-powders for general information on containers and labelling.
Advice for patients: the dusting-powder should be dusted lightly onto the affected area. It should not be applied to open wounds or to raw surfaces of a large area.

OTHER PREPARATIONS
Zinc oxide is an ingredient of numerous other topical preparations.

Zinc Stearate

Zinc stearate consists chiefly of zinc stearate, $(C_{17}H_{35}.CO_2)_2Zn$, but contains a variable proportion of zinc palmitate, $(C_{15}H_{31}.CO_2)_2Zn$ and usually a small amount of zinc oleate, $(C_{17}H_{33}.CO_2)_2Zn$.

A standard is given in the British Pharmaceutical Codex 1973
Description. A light, white amorphous powder with a faint and characteristic odour.
Solubility. Practically insoluble in water, in alcohol, and in ether.
Actions and uses. Zinc stearate is used as a soothing and protective application in the treatment of skin inflammation. It is used either alone or combined with other powders or in the form of a cream.

Preparations
Zinc stearate is an ingredient of compound calamine application.

Zinc Sulphate

$ZnSO_4,7H_2O = 287.5$

OTHER NAMES: Zinci Sulfas; *Zincomed®*
Zincfrin® (with phenylephrine hydrochloride)

A standard is given in the European Pharmacopoeia Vol. I

Crude zinc sulphate is sometimes known as "white vitriol" or "white copperas".

Description. Odourless, efflorescent, colourless, transparent crystals or a white crystalline powder.
Solubility. Soluble, at 20°, in less than 1 part of water; practically insoluble in alcohol.
Acidity. A 5% solution has a pH of 4.4 to 5.6.
Incompatibility. It is incompatible with alkali carbonates and hydroxides and with astringent infusions and decoctions.
Sterilisation. Solutions are sterilised by heating in an autoclave or by filtration.
Storage. It should be stored in airtight containers.
Metabolism. ABSORPTION. Incompletely absorbed after oral administration and absorption is further reduced by the presence of phosphate, phytate, dairy products, or coffee in the diet, and also reduced in subjects with acrodermatitis enteropathica.

BLOOD CONCENTRATION. Normal plasma concentrations are in the range 0.7 to 1.5 $\mu g/ml$; following an oral dose of 50 mg to fasting subjects, peak plasma concentrations of about 2.5 $\mu g/ml$ are attained in 2 to 3 hours.

HALF-LIFE. Plasma half-life, about 3 hours; biological half-life for ^{65}Zn 250 to 500 days.

DISTRIBUTION. *Protein binding*, about 3% of ionic zinc in the blood is bound to low molecular weight serum proteins.

EXCRETION. After an intravenous dose, excreted mainly in the faeces.

FURTHER INFORMATION. Absorption and plasma concentrations—K.-E. Andersson *et al.*, *Eur. J. clin. Pharmac.*, 1976, **9**, 423; protein binding—T. J. Bradley and H. Sen, *J. Pharm. Pharmac.*, 1974, **26** *Suppl.*, 93P; retention of zinc-65 in patients with leg ulcers—T. Hawkins and J. Marks, *Lancet*, ii/1976, 319; absorption in acrodermatitis enteropathica—I. Lombeck *et al.*, *Lancet*, i/1975, 855; effect of foods on absorption—A. Pécoud *et al.*, *Clin. Pharmac. Ther.*, 1975, **17**, 469.

Actions and uses. Zinc sulphate is sometimes used to promote healing in granulating wounds in a dose of

220 milligrams 3 times a day. Higher doses of 0.6 to 2 grams, administered as a 1% solution were formerly used as an emetic.

Zinc sulphate is used externally in the form of astringent lotions for indolent ulcers and to assist granulation. Dilute aqueous solutions may be applied locally to relieve chronic inflammation of the cornea in conjunctivitis.

Poisoning. Alkali carbonate, milk, or white of egg should be administered liberally.

Preparations

COPPER AND ZINC SULPHATES LOTION (*Syn.* Copper and Zinc Lotion; Dalibour Water):

Copper sulphate	10 g
Zinc sulphate	15 g
Concentrated camphor water	25 ml
Water for preparations	to 1000 ml

Dissolve the copper sulphate and the zinc sulphate in 900 ml of the water, add the concentrated camphor water in small quantities, shaking vigorously after each addition, and add sufficient water to produce the required volume.

A standard for this lotion is given in the British Pharmaceutical Codex 1973

Containers and *Labelling:* see the entry on Lotions for general information on containers and labelling.

Advice for patients: the lotion may be applied on gauze as a wet dressing.

ZINC SULPHATE AND ADRENALINE EYE-DROPS:

Zinc sulphate	0.250 g
Adrenaline acid tartrate	0.090 g
Phenylmercuric acetate or nitrate	0.002 g
Sodium metabisulphite	0.050 g
Purified water	to 100.0 ml

Prepare by method A, B, or C described in the entry on Eye-drops.

It contains the equivalent of adrenaline, 1 in 2000.

A standard for these eye-drops is given in the British Pharmaceutical Codex 1973

Containers: see the entry on Eye-drops for general information on containers. This solution is adversely affected by alkali.

Labelling: see the entry on Eye-drops for general information on labelling.

Storage: it should be stored in a cool place, protected from light.

Advice for patients: see the entry on Eye-drops for general information on the use of eye-drops. With prolonged usage, staining of the sclera may occur. The eye-drops should not be used if the solution is discoloured.

ZINC SULPHATE EYE-DROPS: consisting of a sterile solution containing 0.25% of zinc sulphate, with 0.002% of phenylmercuric acetate or nitrate, in purified water. It is prepared by method A, B, or C described in the entry on Eye-drops.

A standard for these eye-drops is given in the British Pharmaceutical Codex 1973

Containers and *Labelling:* see the entry on Eye-drops for general information on containers and labelling.

Advice for patients: see the entry on Eye-drops for general information on the use of eye-drops.

ZINC SULPHATE LOTION (*Syn.* Lotio Rubra):

Zinc sulphate	10 g
Amaranth solution	10 ml
Water for preparations	to 1000 ml

A standard for this lotion is given in the British Pharmaceutical Codex 1973

Containers and *Labelling:* see the entry on Lotions for general information on containers and labelling.

ZINC SULPHATE MOUTH-WASH: consisting of zinc sulphate lotion (see above).

One part should be diluted with 4 parts of warm water before use.

Containers and *Labelling:* see the entry on Mouth-washes for general information on containers and labelling.

Advice for patients: the diluted solution should be rinsed around the mouth 3 or 4 times daily as required. It should preferably not be swallowed.

OTHER PREPARATIONS available include CAPSULES containing zinc sulphate 220 mg; and EYE-DROPS containing zinc sulphate 0.25% with phenylephrine hydrochloride 0.12%.

Zinc sulphate is an ingredient of zinc sulphide lotion.

Zinc Undecenoate

Zinc undec-10-enoate
$(C_{11}H_{19}O_2)_2Zn = 431.9$

OTHER NAMES: *Tineafax®*; Zinc Undecylenate; Zinci Undecylenas
Mycota® (with undecenoic acid)

A standard is given in the European Pharmacopoeia Vol. III Supplement

Description. A fine white powder.

Solubility. Practically insoluble in water and in alcohol.

Moisture content. Not more than 1.5%, determined by drying at 105°.

Melting-point. About 118°.

Actions and uses. Zinc undecenoate has a fungicidal action similar to that of undecenoic acid and is used for similar purposes. It is applied to the skin, usually in conjunction with undecenoic acid, in ointments and dusting-powders.

Preparations

ZINC UNDECENOATE DUSTING-POWDER:

Zinc undecenoate	100 g
Undecenoic acid	20 g
Pumilio pine oil	5 ml
Starch, in powder	500 g
Light kaolin, or light kaolin (natural), sterilised	to 1000 g

Triturate the pumilio pine oil and the undecenoic acid with most of the light kaolin, incorporate the starch, the zinc undecenoate, and the remainder of the light kaolin, sift, and mix.

A standard for this dusting-powder is given in the British Pharmaceutical Codex 1973

Containers and *Labelling:* see the entry on Dusting-powders for general information on containers and labelling.

Advice for patients: the dusting-powder should be dusted lightly onto the affected area after application of zinc undecenoate ointment. Treatment should be continued for 1 week after symptoms have disappeared.

ZINC UNDECENOATE OINTMENT (*Syn.* Ung. Zinc. Undecen.):

Zinc undecenoate, finely sifted	200 g
Undecenoic acid	50 g
Emulsifying ointment	750 g

Melt the emulsifying ointment, add the zinc undecenoate and the undecenoic acid, and stir until cold.

A standard for this ointment is given in the British Pharmacopoeia 1973

Containers: see the entry on Ointments for general information on containers.

Advice for patients: the ointment should be rubbed lightly onto the affected area. When used in conjunction with the dusting-powder, the ointment should be used first. Treatment should be continued for 1 week after symptoms have disappeared.

OTHER PREPARATIONS available include a DUSTING-POWDER containing zinc undecenoate 10%, and a dusting-powder containing zinc undecenoate 20% with undecenoic acid 2%.

Appendix 1

Reagent Solutions

Acetic Acid, Dilute: dilute glacial acetic acid with sufficient water to produce a solution containing 6% w/w of $C_2H_4O_2$.

Alum Solution: a 5% solution of alum.

Ammonia Solution, Dilute: dilute 375 ml of *strong ammonia solution* to 1000 ml with water. It contains approximately 10% w/w of NH_3.

Ammonia Solution, Strong: a solution containing 27 to 30% w/w of NH_3.

Ammonium Cobaltothiocyanate Solution: dissolve 37.5 g of cobalt nitrate and 150 g of ammonium thiocyanate in sufficient water to produce 1000 ml. It should be freshly prepared.

Ammonium Mercurithiocyanate Solution: dissolve 27 g of mercuric chloride and 30 g of ammonium thiocyanate in sufficient water to produce 1000 ml.

Ammonium Molybdate Solution: a 10% solution of ammonium molybdate.

Ammonium Reineckate Solution: a 1% solution of ammonium reineckate. It should be freshly prepared.

Ammonium Thiocyanate Solution: a 10% solution of ammonium thiocyanate.

Ammonium Vanadate Solution: dissolve, with the aid of heat, 5 g of ammonium vanadate in a mixture of 10 ml of *sodium hydroxide solution* and 90 ml of water, cool, and, if necessary, filter through glass wool.

Aniline Acetate Solution: a 25% solution of aniline in glacial acetic acid. It should be freshly prepared.

Antimony Trichloride Solution: to 100 ml of a 22% solution of antimony trichloride in alcohol-free chloroform add 2.5 ml of acetyl chloride, and allow to stand for half an hour.

Barium Chloride Solution: a 10% solution of barium chloride.

Barium Hydroxide Solution: a 3% solution of barium hydroxide.

Benzalkonium Chloride Solution: a solution containing 50% of a mixture of alkylbenzyldimethylammonium chlorides, calculated as $C_{22}H_{40}ClN$.

Borate Buffer Solution: dissolve 4 g of boric acid in a mixture of 27 ml of 1N sodium hydroxide and sufficient water to produce 100 ml.

Brine: a saturated solution of sodium chloride.

Bromine Solution: a saturated solution of bromine. It should be freshly prepared.

Bromine Solution AsT: a solution containing 30 g of bromine and 30 g of potassium bromide in sufficient water to produce 100 ml, and containing less than 1 part per million of arsenic.

Bromophenol Blue Solution: mix 100 mg of bromophenol blue with 3.0 ml of 0.05N sodium hydroxide and 5 ml of alcohol (90%), warm until dissolved and dilute to 250 ml with alcohol (20%).

Bromothymol Blue Solution: dissolve 100 mg of bromothymol blue in 3.2 ml of 0.05N sodium hydroxide and 5 ml of alcohol (90%), with the aid of heat, and dilute to 250 ml with alcohol (20%).

Calcium Chloride Solution: a 10% solution of calcium chloride.

Catechol Solution: a 10% solution of catechol. It should be freshly prepared.

Chloral Hydrate Solution: dissolve 50 g of chloral hydrate in 20 ml of water.

Chloramine Solution: a 2% solution of chloramine. It should be freshly prepared.

Chromic-sulphuric Acid Mixture: a saturated solution of chromium trioxide in sulphuric acid.

Chromotropic Acid Solution: dissolve 5 mg of chromotropic acid sodium salt in 10 ml of a mixture of 9 ml of sulphuric acid and 4 ml of water.

Cobalt Nitrate Solution: a 0.2% solution of cobalt nitrate in alcohol (95%).

Cobalt Thiocyanate Solution: dissolve 6.8 g of cobalt chloride and 4.3 g of ammonium thiocyanate in sufficient water to produce 100 ml.

Copper Acetate Solution, Strong: a 5% solution of copper acetate.

Copper Chloride Solution, Ammoniacal: dissolve 22.5 g of copper chloride in 200 ml of water and mix with 100 ml of *strong ammonia solution.*

Copper Oxide Solution, Ammoniacal: triturate 500 mg of copper carbonate with 10 ml of water and gradually add 10 ml of *strong ammonia solution.*

Copper Sulphate Solution: a 10% solution of copper sulphate.

Copper Sulphate with Pyridine Solution: dissolve 4 g of copper sulphate in 90 ml of water and add 30 ml of pyridine. It should be freshly prepared.

Corallin Solution, Alkaline: dissolve 5 g of corallin in 100 ml of alcohol (90%). Dissolve 25 g of sodium carbonate in 100 ml of water. When required, add 1 ml of the corallin solution to 20 ml of the sodium carbonate solution. The mixed solution must be freshly prepared.

Cupro-citric Solution: dissolve 25 g of copper sulphate,

50g of citric acid, and 144 g of anhydrous sodium carbonate in sufficient water to produce 1000 ml.

Cyanogen Bromide Solution: add, dropwise, a 10% solution of potassium cyanide to *bromine solution* until the colour disappears. It must be freshly prepared.

Diazoaminobenzenesulphonic Acid: dissolve, with the aid of heat, 200 mg of sulphanilic acid in 20 ml of 1N hydrochloric acid, cool to about 4°, add dropwise and with constant swirling 2.2 ml of a 4% solution of sodium nitrite, allow to stand in ice for 10 minutes, and add 1 ml of a 5% solution of sulphamic acid.

Dimethylaminobenzaldehyde Solution: dissolve 125 mg of dimethylaminobenzaldehyde in a cooled mixture of 65 ml of sulphuric acid and 35 ml of water, add 0.1 ml of *ferric chloride test-solution*, and allow to stand for 24 hours before use. It should be discarded when a yellow colour develops.

Dimethylaminobenzaldehyde Solution, Alcoholic: dissolve 1 g of dimethylaminobenzaldehyde in 30 ml of alcohol (95%) and add 180 ml of n-butyl alcohol and 30 ml of hydrochloric acid. It should be freshly prepared and must be discarded if a pink colour develops.

Dimethyl Yellow Solution: a 0.2% solution of dimethyl yellow in alcohol (90%).

Dinitrobenzoic Acid Solution: a 2% solution of dinitrobenzoic acid in alcohol (95%).

Dinitrophenylhydrazine Solution: dissolve 1.5 g of dinitrophenylhydrazine in 20 ml of sulphuric acid (50% v/v), dilute to 100 ml with water, and filter. It must be freshly prepared.

Diphenylcarbazone Solution: a 0.1% solution of diphenylcarbazone in alcohol (95%).

Eosin Solution: a 0.5% solution of eosin.

Ferric Ammonium Sulphate Solution: a 10% solution of ferric ammonium sulphate.

Ferric Chloride Solution: a solution containing 15% of $FeCl_3$.

Ferric Chloride Test-solution: a 5% solution of ferric chloride.

Ferrous Sulphate Solution: a 2% solution of ferrous sulphate in freshly boiled and cooled water. It should be freshly prepared.

Formaldehyde Solution: a solution containing 36% w/w of formaldehyde, CH_2O.

Glycerol, Dilute: a 33% solution of glycerol.

Glyoxal Solution: a 0.1% solution of glyoxal sodium bisulphite.

Gold Chloride Solution: a 2% solution of gold chloride.

Guaiacum Tincture: macerate 20 g of guaiacum resin with 100 g of alcohol (80%) for 10 days, with occasional shaking, and filter. It should be recently prepared.

Hydrochloric Acid, Dilute: a solution containing 10% w/w of HCl.

Hydrogen Peroxide Solution: a solution containing 6% w/v of H_2O_2 (" 20-volume ").

Hydrogen Peroxide Solution, Dilute: a solution containing 3% w/v of H_2O_2.

Hydrogen Peroxide Solution, Strong: a solution containing 30% w/w of H_2O_2 (" 100-volume ").

Iodine Solution: dissolve 2 g of iodine and 3 g of potassium iodide in sufficient water to produce 100 ml.

Iodine Water: mix 1 volume of 0.1N iodine with 4 volumes of water.

Iodoplatinate Solution, Acidified: dissolve 250 mg of platinic chloride and 5 g of potassium iodide in sufficient water to produce 100 ml, and add 2 ml of hydrochloric acid.

Lactophenol: dissolve 20 g of phenol in a mixture of 20 g of lactic acid, 40 g of glycerol, and 20 ml of water.

Lanthanum Nitrate Solution: a 5% solution of lanthanum nitrate.

Lead Acetate Solution: a 10% solution of lead acetate in carbon dioxide-free water.

Lithium and Sodium Molybdophosphotungstate Solution: dissolve 100 g of sodium tungstate and 25 g of sodium molybdate in 800 ml of water in a 1500-ml flask, add 50 ml of phosphoric acid and 100 ml of hydrochloric acid, and heat for 10 hours under a reflux condenser. Cool, add 150 g of lithium sulphate, 50 ml of water, and 0.2 to 0.3 ml of bromine, allow to stand for 2 hours, remove the excess bromine by boiling for 15 minutes without the condenser, cool, filter, and dilute to 1000 ml with water. It should be stored at a temperature not exceeding 4° and must not be used later than 4 months after preparation. It is golden yellow in colour and must not be used if any trace of green colour is present.

Litmus Solution: boil 25 g of litmus with 100 ml of alcohol (90%) under a reflux condenser for 1 hour, pour away the clear liquid, and repeat the operation twice using 75 ml. of alcohol (90%); digest the washed litmus with 250 ml of water and filter.

Magenta Solution, Decolorised: dissolve 1 g of basic magenta in 600 ml of water, cool in ice, add 20 g of sodium sulphite dissolved in 100 ml of water, cool in ice, add slowly with constant stirring, 10 ml of hydrochloric acid and dilute to 1000 ml. If the solution is turbid, it should be filtered, and if brown in colour it should be shaken with about 250 mg of decolorising charcoal and then filtered immediately. It may be necessary to add 2 or 3 ml of hydrochloric acid, followed by shaking, to remove any residual pink colour. After preparation it should be allowed to stand overnight before use; it should be protected from light.

Magnesium-ammonium Chloride Solution: dissolve 5 g of magnesium chloride and 10 g of ammonium chloride in sufficient water to produce 50 ml, make just alkaline with *strong ammonia solution*, allow to stand overnight, filter, just acidify the filtrate with *dilute hydrochloric acid*, add 0.5 ml of hydrochloric acid, and dilute to 100 ml with water.

Mercuric Chloride Test-solution: a 5% solution of mercuric chloride.

Mercury Nitrate Solution: Millon's Reagent: dissolve 3 ml of mercury in 27 ml of cold fuming nitric acid and dilute with an equal quantity of water. It must be recently prepared.

Methyl Orange Solution: a 0.04% solution of methyl orange in alcohol (20%).

Methyl Red Solution: dissolve 25 mg of methyl red in a mixture of 5 ml of alcohol (90%) and 0.95 ml of 0.05N sodium hydroxide, warming if necessary, and dilute to 250 ml with alcohol (50%).

Methylene Blue Solution: a 1% solution of methylene blue.

Methylene Blue Solution, Alcoholic: a 0.1% solution of methylene blue in alcohol (95%).

1-Naphthol Solution: dissolve 1 g of 1-naphthol in a solution of 6 g of sodium hydroxide and 16 g of anhydrous sodium carbonate in 100 ml of water. It must be freshly prepared.

2-Naphthol Solution: dissolve 5 g of freshly recrystallised 2-naphthol in 8 ml of *sodium hydroxide solution* and 20 ml of water and dilute to 100 ml with water. It must be freshly prepared.

Nitric Acid, Dilute: mix 106 ml of nitric acid with sufficient water to produce 1000 ml. It contains about 10% w/w of HNO_3.

Nitroaniline Solution, Diazotised: dissolve 400 mg of 4-nitroaniline in 60 ml of 1N hydrochloric acid, cool to 15°, and add a 10% solution of sodium nitrite in water until 1 drop of the mixture turns starch-iodide paper blue. It should be freshly prepared.

2-Nitrobenzaldehyde Solution: a 1% solution of 2-nitrobenzaldehyde in alcohol (50%).

Oxalic Acid and Sulphuric Acid Solution: a 5% solution of oxalic acid in a cooled mixture of equal volumes of sulphuric acid and water.

Phenol, Liquefied: a solution containing 80% w/w of phenol.

Phenolphthalein Solution: a 1% solution of phenolphthalein in alcohol (95%).

Phloroglucinol Solution: a 1% solution of phloroglucinol in alcohol (90%).

Phosphotungstic Acid Reagent: dissolve 25 g of sodium tungstate in 175 ml of water, add 18.75 ml of phosphoric acid, heat under a reflux condenser for 6 hours, and filter. It should be protected from light and stored at a temperature between 2° and 10°.

Phosphotungstic Acid Solution: dissolve 20 g of phosphotungstic acid and 5 g of sulphuric acid in sufficient water to produce 100 ml.

Potassium Chromate Solution: a 5% solution of potassium chromate.

Potassium Cupri-tartrate Solution: Fehling's Solution: *Solution No. 1:* dissolve 34.64 g of copper sulphate in 400 ml of water containing 0.50 ml of sulphuric acid and dilute to 500 ml with water.
Solution No. 2: dissolve 176 g of potassium sodium tartrate and 77 g of sodium hydroxide in sufficient water to produce 500 ml.
Mix equal volumes of the two solutions immediately before use.

Potassium Dichromate Solution: a 7% solution of potassium dichromate.

Potassium Ferricyanide Solution: wash about 1 g of potassium ferricyanide, in crystals, with water and dissolve the washed crystals in 100 ml of water. It should be freshly prepared.

Potassium Ferrocyanide Solution: a 5% solution of potassium ferrocyanide.

Potassium Hydroxide Solution: a 5% solution of potassium hydroxide.

Potassium Hydroxide Solution, Alcoholic: a 10% solution of potassium hydroxide in alcohol (95%). It should be recently prepared.

Potassium Hydroxide Solution in Aldehyde-free Alcohol: dissolve 40 g of potassium hydroxide in about 900 ml of aldehyde-free alcohol (95%) maintained at a temperature not exceeding 15°; when solution is complete, warm to 20° and dilute to 1000 ml with aldehyde-free alcohol (95%).

Potassium Iodide Solution: a 10% solution of potassium iodide.

Potassium Iodobismuthate Solution: dissolve 100 g of tartaric acid in 400 ml of water, add 8.5 g of bismuth oxide nitrate, shake for 1 hour, add 200 ml of a 40% solution of potassium iodide, shake well, allow to stand for 24 hours, and filter.

Potassium Iodobismuthate Solution, Dilute: dissolve 100 g of tartaric acid in 500 ml of water and add 50 ml of *potassium iodobismuthate solution.*

Potassium Mercuri-iodide Solution: Mayer's Reagent: add 1.36 g of mercuric chloride dissolved in 60 ml of water to a solution of 5 g of potassium iodide in 20 ml of water, mix, and dilute to 100 ml with water.

Potassium Mercuri-iodide Solution, Alkaline: Nessler's Reagent: dissolve 3.5 g of potassium iodide and 1.25 g of mercuric chloride in 80 ml of water, add a cold saturated solution of mercuric chloride, with constant stirring, until a slight red precipitate remains, dissolve 12 g of sodium hydroxide in the solution, add a little more of the saturated solution of mercuric chloride, dilute to 100 ml with water, allow to stand, and decant the clear liquid.

Potassium Permanganate and Phosphoric Acid Solution: dissolve 3 g of potassium permanganate in a mixture of 15 ml of phosphoric acid and 70 ml of water and dilute to 100 ml with water.

Potassium Permanganate Solution: a 1% solution of potassium permanganate.

Potassium Thiocyanate Solution: a 9.7% solution of potassium thiocyanate.

Resorcinol and Hydrochloric Acid Solution: a 1% solution of resorcinol in hydrochloric acid.

Ruthenium Red Solution: dissolve 8 mg of ruthenium red in 10 ml of *lead acetate solution.* It should be freshly prepared.

Safranine Solution: a saturated solution of safranine in alcohol (70%).

Semicarbazide Acetate Solution: triturate 2.5 g of semicarbazide hydrochloride with 3.3 g of sodium acetate, add 10 ml of methyl alcohol, mix, transfer to a flask with the aid of 20 ml of methyl alcohol, allow to stand at a temperature of about 4° for 30 minutes, filter, and dilute to 100 ml with methyl alcohol.

Silver Nitrate Solution: a 5% solution of silver nitrate. It should be freshly prepared.

Silver Nitrate Solution, Alcoholic: dissolve 4 g of silver nitrate in 10 ml of water and dilute to 100 ml with alcohol (95%).

Silver Nitrate Solution, Dilute: a 1.7% solution of silver nitrate. It should be freshly prepared.

Sodium Bicarbonate Solution: a 5% solution of sodium bicarbonate.

Sodium Carbonate Solution: a 10% solution of sodium carbonate.

Sodium Hydroxide Solution: a 20% solution of sodium hydroxide.

Sodium Hydroxide Solution, Dilute: a 5% solution of sodium hydroxide.

Sodium Hydroxide Solution, Strong: a 40% solution of sodium hydroxide.

Sodium Hypochlorite Solution: a solution containing 10 to 16% of available chlorine.

Sodium Hypochlorite Solution, Dilute: a solution containing 3.5% w/v of available chlorine.

Sodium Nitrite Solution: a 10% solution of sodium nitrite. It should be freshly prepared.

Sodium Nitroprusside Solution: a 1% solution of sodium nitroprusside. It should be recently prepared.

Sodium Sulphide Solution: a 10% solution of sodium sulphide.

Solution of Standard pH 2.0: mix 50 ml of 0.2M potassium chloride with 10.6 ml of 0.2N hydrochloric acid and dilute to 200 ml with freshly boiled and cooled water.

Solution of Standard pH 3.6: mix 50 ml of 0.2 M potassium hydrogen phthalate with 5.97 ml of 0.2 N hydrochloric acid and dilute to 200 ml with freshly boiled and cooled water.

Solution of Standard pH 4.0: mix 50 ml of 0.2M potassium hydrogen phthalate with 0.40 ml of 0.2N sodium hydroxide and dilute to 200 ml with freshly boiled and cooled water.

Solution of Standard pH 6.6: mix 50 ml of 0.2M potassium dihydrogen phosphate with 17.80 ml of 0.2N sodium hydroxide and dilute to 200 ml with freshly boiled and cooled water.

Solution of Standard pH 7.4: mix 50 ml of 0.2M potassium dihydrogen phosphate with 39.50 ml of 0.2N sodium hydroxide and dilute to 200 ml with freshly boiled and cooled water.

Solution of Standard pH 7.6: mix 50 ml of 0.2M potassium dihydrogen phosphate with 42.80 ml of 0.2N sodium hydroxide and dilute to 200 ml with freshly boiled and cooled water.

Solution of Standard pH 9.6: mix 50 ml of 0.2M boric acid-potassium chloride (containing 12.367 g of H_3BO_3 and 14.911 g of KCl per litre) with 36.85 ml of 0.2N sodium hydroxide and dilute to 200 ml with freshly boiled and cooled water.

Stannous Chloride Solution: dissolve 330 g of stannous chloride in 100 ml of hydrochloric acid and sufficient water to give a final volume of 1000 ml.

Starch Mucilage: triturate 0.5 g of starch with 5 ml of water, and add this, with constant stirring, to sufficient water to produce 100 ml; boil for a few minutes, cool, and filter. It should be recently prepared.

Sulphomolybdic Acid Solution: a 1% solution of ammonium molybdate in sulphuric acid.

Sulphomolybdic Reagent: a 0.5% solution of ammonium molybdate in sulphuric acid.

Sulphuric Acid, Dilute: mix carefully 104 g of sulphuric acid with 896 g of water and cool.

Tannic Acid Solution: a 10% solution of tannic acid.

Thymol Blue Solution: dissolve 100 mg of thymol blue in 4.3 ml of 0.05N sodium hydroxide and 5 ml of alcohol (90%), with the aid of heat, and dilute to 250 ml with alcohol (20%).

Titanous Chloride Solution: a 15% solution of titanous chloride, $TiCl_3$, in *dilute hydrochloric acid*. It must be protected from the atmosphere to avoid oxidation.

Trinitrophenol Solution: add 0.5 ml of *sodium hydroxide solution* to 100 ml of a saturated solution of trinitrophenol in water.

Xanthydrol Solution: dissolve 100 mg of xanthydrol in 80 ml of glacial acetic acid and mix with 20 ml of a 1% solution of hydrochloric acid in glacial acetic acid. It should be freshly prepared.

Zinc Chloride Solution, Iodinated: dissolve 20 g of zinc chloride and 6.5 g of potassium iodide in 10.5 ml of water, add 0.5 g of iodine, shake for 15 minutes, and filter, if necessary. It should be protected from light.

Appendix 2

Infra-red Spectra

This Appendix is divided into 3 sections in order to accommodate spectra determined on 3 different instruments. Spectra in Appendix 2a were determined on a Perkin Elmer 257 spectrophotometer, those in Appendix 2b on a Perkin Elmer 137, and those in Appendix 2c on a Unicam SP 200. Most of the spectra were determined in potassium bromide disks; a small number, all of them in Appendix 2b, were determined in a liquid paraffin mull and this is indicated on the appropriate spectra. Spectra in Appendixes 2a and 2c have a linear wavenumber scale and a logarithmic wavelength scale, whereas those in Appendix 2b have a logarithmic wavenumber scale and a linear wavelength scale.

Further information on infra-red data is given in the entry on Infra-red Spectrophotometry.

The spectra in Appendixes 2b and 2c have been provided by the Home Office Central Research Establishment, Aldermaston, and are Crown copyright.

Appendix 2a

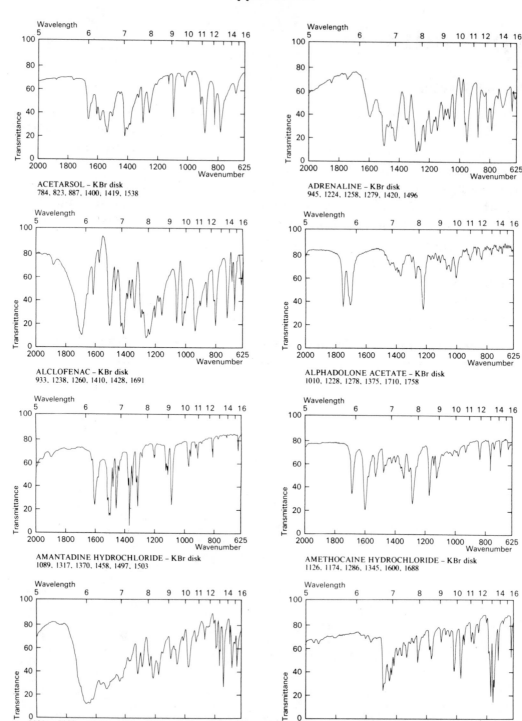

ACETARSOL – KBr disk
784, 823, 887, 1400, 1419, 1538

ADRENALINE – KBr disk
945, 1224, 1258, 1279, 1420, 1496

ALCLOFENAC – KBr disk
933, 1238, 1260, 1410, 1428, 1691

ALPHADOLONE ACETATE – KBr disk
1010, 1228, 1278, 1375, 1710, 1758

AMANTADINE HYDROCHLORIDE – KBr disk
1089, 1317, 1370, 1458, 1497, 1503

AMETHOCAINE HYDROCHLORIDE – KBr disk
1126, 1174, 1286, 1345, 1600, 1688

AMINOPHYLLINE – KBr disk
741, 1525, 1566, 1625, 1640, 1667

AMITRIPTYLINE HYDROCHLORIDE – KBr disk
746, 756, 770, 969, 1441, 1487

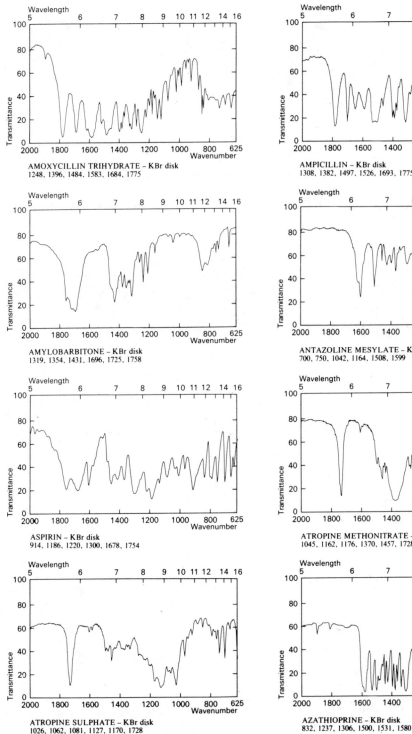

AMOXYCILLIN TRIHYDRATE – KBr disk
1248, 1396, 1484, 1583, 1684, 1775

AMPICILLIN – KBr disk
1308, 1382, 1497, 1526, 1693, 1775

AMYLOBARBITONE – KBr disk
1319, 1354, 1431, 1696, 1725, 1758

ANTAZOLINE MESYLATE – KBr disk
700, 750, 1042, 1164, 1508, 1599

ASPIRIN – KBr disk
914, 1186, 1220, 1300, 1678, 1754

ATROPINE METHONITRATE – KBr disk
1045, 1162, 1176, 1370, 1457, 1728

ATROPINE SULPHATE – KBr disk
1026, 1062, 1081, 1127, 1170, 1728

AZATHIOPRINE – KBr disk
832, 1237, 1306, 1500, 1531, 1580

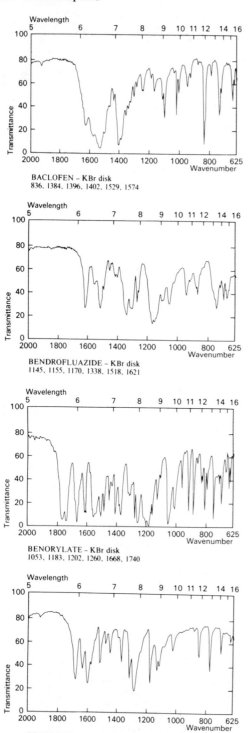

BACLOFEN – KBr disk
836, 1384, 1396, 1402, 1529, 1574

BENDROFLUAZIDE – KBr disk
1145, 1155, 1170, 1338, 1518, 1621

BENORYLATE – KBr disk
1053, 1183, 1202, 1260, 1668, 1740

BENZOCAINE – KBr disk
1128, 1175, 1282, 1314, 1599, 1681

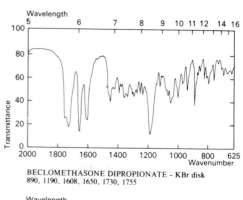

BECLOMETHASONE DIPROPIONATE – KBr disk
890, 1190, 1608, 1650, 1730, 1755

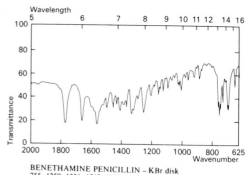

BENETHAMINE PENICILLIN – KBr disk
755, 1258, 1336, 1562, 1663, 1773

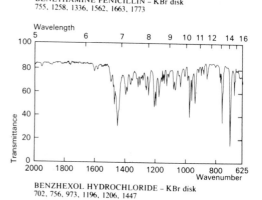

BENZHEXOL HYDROCHLORIDE – KBr disk
702, 756, 973, 1196, 1206, 1447

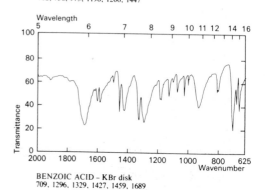

BENZOIC ACID – KBr disk
709, 1296, 1329, 1427, 1459, 1689

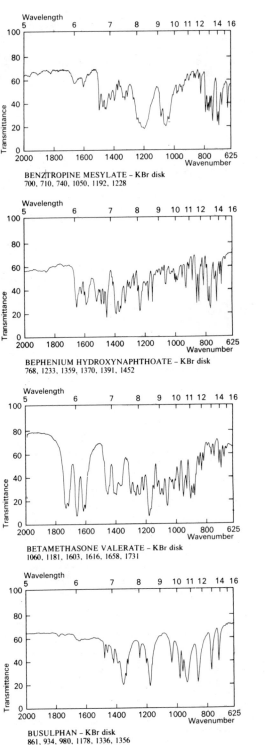

BENZTROPINE MESYLATE – KBr disk
700, 710, 740, 1050, 1192, 1228

BEPHENIUM HYDROXYNAPHTHOATE – KBr disk
768, 1233, 1359, 1370, 1391, 1452

BETAMETHASONE VALERATE – KBr disk
1060, 1181, 1603, 1616, 1658, 1731

BUSULPHAN – KBr disk
861, 934, 980, 1178, 1336, 1356

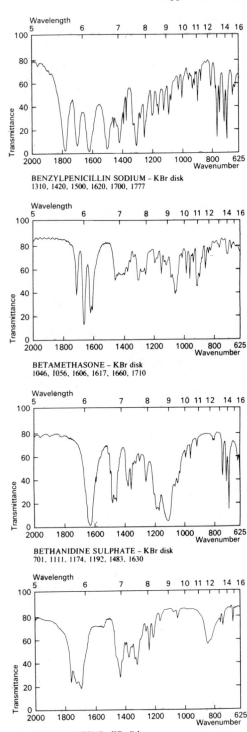

BENZYLPENICILLIN SODIUM – KBr disk
1310, 1420, 1500, 1620, 1700, 1777

BETAMETHASONE – KBr disk
1046, 1056, 1606, 1617, 1660, 1710

BETHANIDINE SULPHATE – KBr disk
701, 1111, 1174, 1192, 1483, 1630

BUTOBARBITONE – KBr disk
1323, 1337, 1435, 1696, 1727, 1760

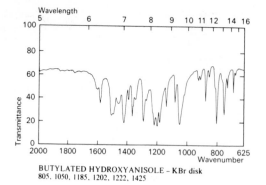

BUTYLATED HYDROXYANISOLE – KBr disk
805, 1050, 1185, 1202, 1222, 1425

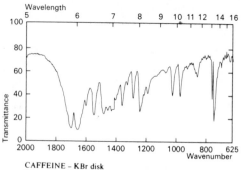

CAFFEINE – KBr disk
747, 1454, 1480, 1548, 1658, 1698

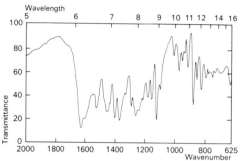

CARBIDOPA – KBr disk
1121, 1260, 1370, 1400, 1455, 1625

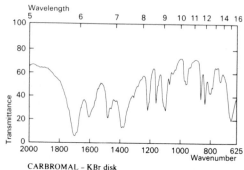

CARBROMAL – KBr disk
660, 1370, 1385, 1478, 1600, 1694

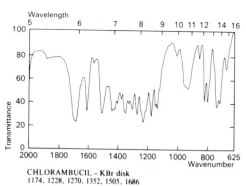

CHLORAMBUCIL – KBr disk
1174, 1228, 1270, 1352, 1505, 1686

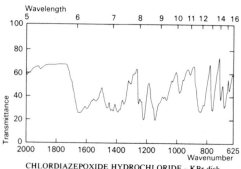

CHLORDIAZEPOXIDE HYDROCHLORIDE – KBr disk
845, 1146, 1222, 1394, 1425, 1650

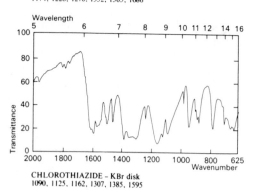

CHLOROTHIAZIDE – KBr disk
1090, 1125, 1162, 1307, 1385, 1595

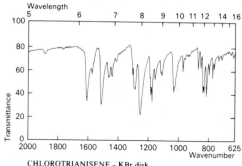

CHLOROTRIANISENE – KBr disk
813, 1174, 1184, 1250, 1510, 1606

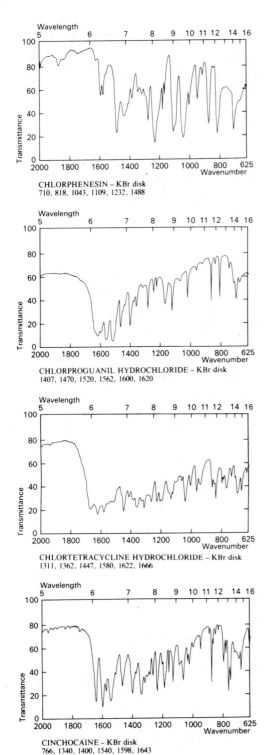

CHLORPHENESIN – KBr disk
710, 818, 1043, 1109, 1232, 1488

CHLORPROGUANIL HYDROCHLORIDE – KBr disk
1407, 1470, 1520, 1562, 1600, 1620

CHLORTETRACYCLINE HYDROCHLORIDE – KBr disk
1311, 1362, 1447, 1580, 1622, 1666

CINCHOCAINE – KBr disk
766, 1340, 1400, 1540, 1598, 1643

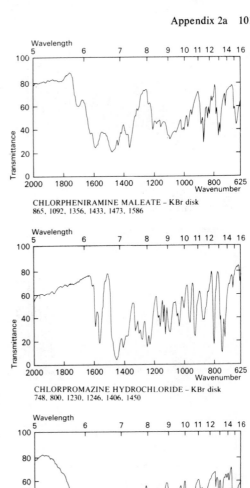

CHLORPHENIRAMINE MALEATE – KBr disk
865, 1092, 1356, 1433, 1473, 1586

CHLORPROMAZINE HYDROCHLORIDE – KBr disk
748, 800, 1230, 1246, 1406, 1450

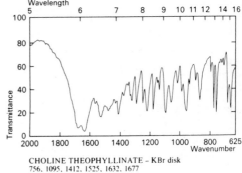

CHOLINE THEOPHYLLINATE – KBr disk
756, 1095, 1412, 1525, 1632, 1677

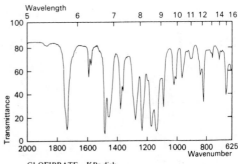

CLOFIBRATE – KBr disk
1140, 1175, 1238, 1282, 1486, 1735

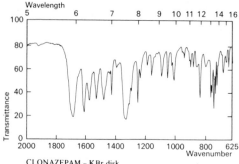

CLONAZEPAM – KBr disk
748, 1255, 1310, 1333, 1610, 1685

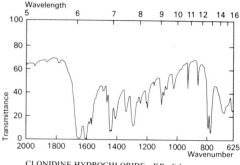

CLONIDINE HYDROCHLORIDE – KBr disk
775, 790, 1435, 1445, 1605, 1650

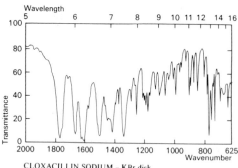

CLOXACILLIN SODIUM – KBr disk
1336, 1495, 1598, 1620, 1659, 1765

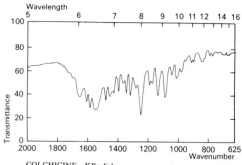

COLCHICINE – KBr disk
1090, 1250, 1485, 1550, 1578, 1610

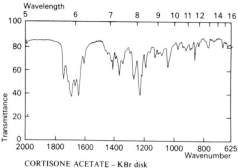

CORTISONE ACETATE – KBr disk
1235, 1279, 1650, 1675, 1700, 1753

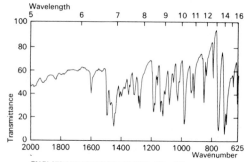

CYCLIZINE HYDROCHLORIDE – KBr disk
701, 716, 756, 984, 1449, 1496

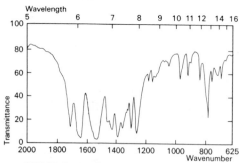

CYCLOBARBITONE CALCIUM – KBr disk
1260, 1357, 1389, 1429, 1537, 1645

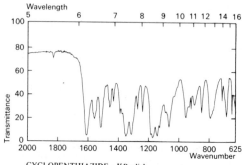

CYCLOPENTHIAZIDE – KBr disk
1138, 1168, 1181, 1309, 1345, 1605

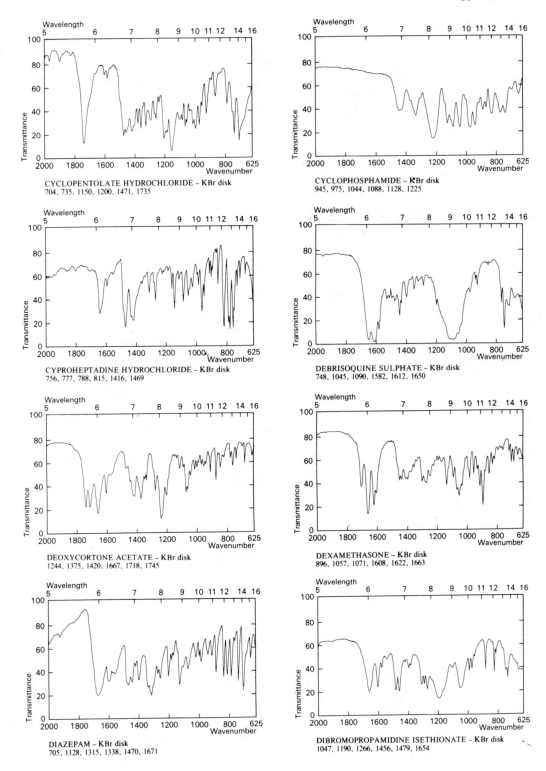

CYCLOPENTOLATE HYDROCHLORIDE – KBr disk
704, 735, 1150, 1200, 1471, 1735

CYCLOPHOSPHAMIDE – KBr disk
945, 975, 1044, 1088, 1128, 1225

CYPROHEPTADINE HYDROCHLORIDE – KBr disk
756, 777, 788, 815, 1416, 1469

DEBRISOQUINE SULPHATE – KBr disk
748, 1045, 1090, 1582, 1612, 1650

DEOXYCORTONE ACETATE – KBr disk
1244, 1375, 1420, 1667, 1718, 1745

DEXAMETHASONE – KBr disk
896, 1057, 1071, 1608, 1622, 1663

DIAZEPAM – KBr disk
705, 1128, 1315, 1338, 1470, 1671

DIBROMOPROPAMIDINE ISETHIONATE – KBr disk
1047, 1190, 1266, 1456, 1479, 1654

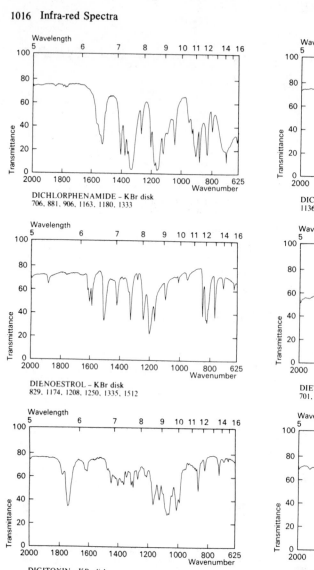

DICHLORPHENAMIDE – KBr disk
706, 881, 906, 1163, 1180, 1333

DICYCLOMINE HYDROCHLORIDE – KBr disk
1136, 1184, 1197, 1214, 1453, 1714

DIENOESTROL – KBr disk
829, 1174, 1208, 1250, 1335, 1512

DIETHYLPROPION HYDROCHLORIDE – KBr disk
701, 1230, 1287, 1383, 1443, 1682

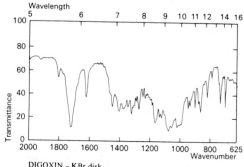

DIGITOXIN – KBr disk
990, 1010, 1058, 1072, 1125, 1740

DIGOXIN – KBr disk
1000, 1017, 1054, 1073, 1172, 1720

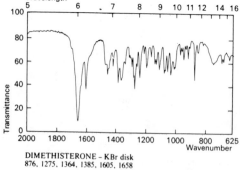

DIMETHISTERONE – KBr disk
876, 1275, 1364, 1385, 1605, 1658

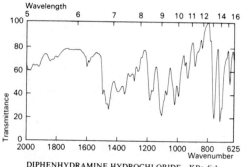

DIPHENHYDRAMINE HYDROCHLORIDE – KBr disk
713, 754, 1017, 1103, 1180, 1454

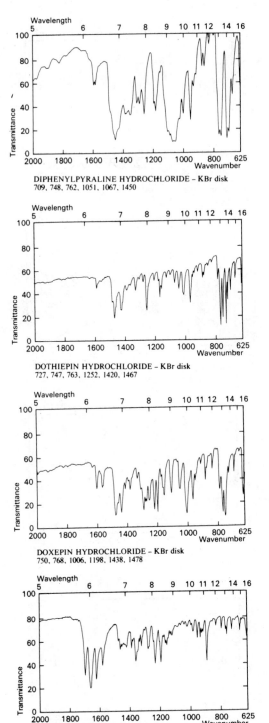

DIPHENYLPYRALINE HYDROCHLORIDE – KBr disk
709, 748, 762, 1051, 1067, 1450

DIPYRIDAMOLE – KBr disk
1010, 1214, 1354, 1436, 1464, 1526

DOTHIEPIN HYDROCHLORIDE – KBr disk
727, 747, 763, 1252, 1420, 1467

DOXAPRAM HYDROCHLORIDE – KBr disk
696, 710, 753, 1253, 1423, 1683

DOXEPIN HYDROCHLORIDE – KBr disk
750, 768, 1006, 1198, 1438, 1478

DOXYCYCLINE HYDROCHLORIDE – KBr disk
1220, 1244, 1462, 1580, 1613, 1660

DYDROGESTERONE – KBr disk
1197, 1232, 1581, 1622, 1660, 1697

EPHEDRINE HYDROCHLORIDE – KBr disk
699, 705, 754, 994, 1049, 1453

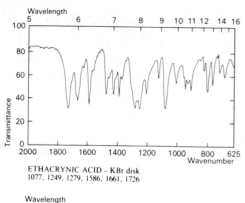

ETHACRYNIC ACID – KBr disk
1077, 1249, 1279, 1586, 1661, 1726

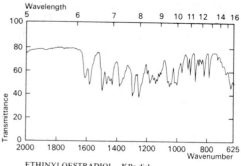

ETHINYLOESTRADIOL – KBr disk
645, 1055, 1259, 1301, 1388, 1501

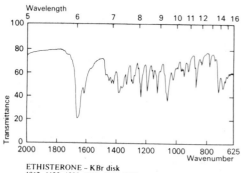

ETHISTERONE – KBr disk
1062, 1125, 1235, 1383, 1614, 1660

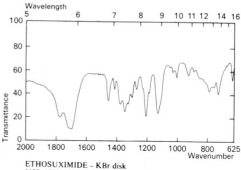

ETHOSUXIMIDE – KBr disk
1130, 1208, 1348, 1376, 1700, 1777

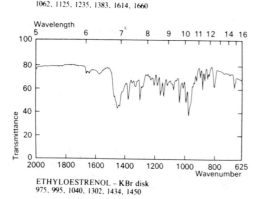

ETHYLOESTRENOL – KBr disk
975, 995, 1040, 1302, 1434, 1450

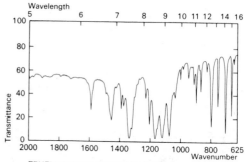

FENFLURAMINE HYDROCHLORIDE – KBr disk
748, 793, 1070, 1116, 1165, 1333

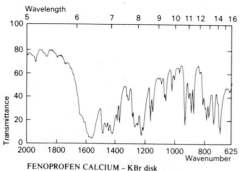
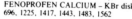

FENOPROFEN CALCIUM – KBr disk
696, 1225, 1417, 1443, 1483, 1562

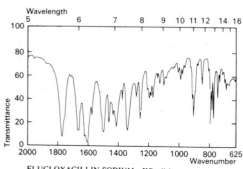

FLUCLOXACILLIN SODIUM – KBr disk
1337, 1495, 1603, 1622, 1660, 1767

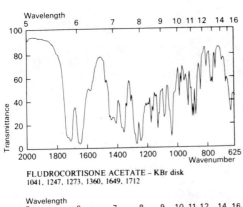

FLUDROCORTISONE ACETATE – KBr disk
1041, 1247, 1273, 1360, 1649, 1712

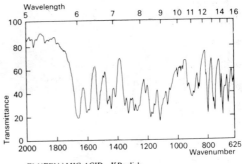

FLUFENAMIC ACID – KBr disk
698, 796, 1118, 1166, 1180, 1661

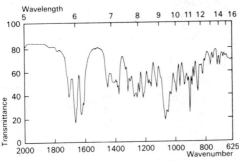

FLUOCINOLONE ACETONIDE – KBr disk
910, 1056, 1074, 1615, 1629, 1669

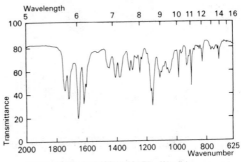

FLUOCORTOLONE HEXANOATE – KBr disk
1163, 1176, 1622, 1658, 1722, 1747

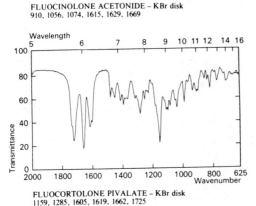

FLUOCORTOLONE PIVALATE – KBr disk
1159, 1285, 1605, 1619, 1662, 1725

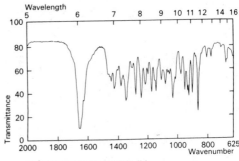

FLUOXYMESTERONE – KBr disk
867, 1036, 1247, 1350, 1627, 1654

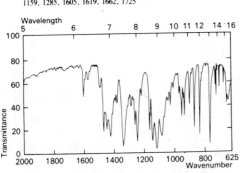

FLUPHENAZINE HYDROCHLORIDE – KBr disk
767, 1116, 1144, 1245, 1338, 1422

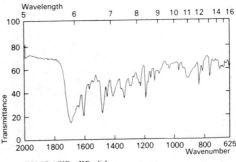

FOLIC ACID – KBr disk
1191, 1335, 1480, 1602, 1636, 1686

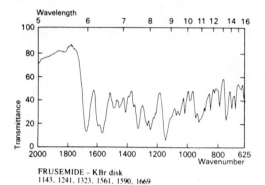

FRUSEMIDE – KBr disk
1143, 1241, 1323, 1561, 1590, 1669

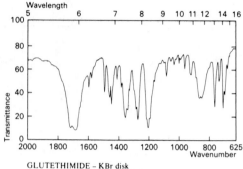

GLUTETHIMIDE – KBr disk
1200, 1270, 1336, 1352, 1680, 1713

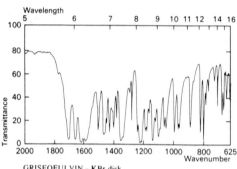

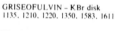

GRISEOFULVIN – KBr disk
1135, 1210, 1220, 1350, 1583, 1611

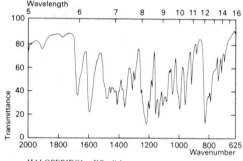

HALOPERIDOL – KBr disk
827, 998, 1137, 1158, 1218, 1598

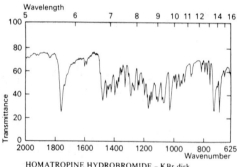

HOMATROPINE HYDROBROMIDE – KBr disk
697, 732, 1026, 1157, 1167, 1756

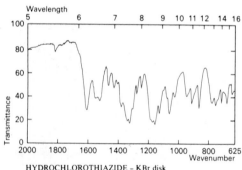

HYDROCHLOROTHIAZIDE – KBr disk
1062, 1128, 1157, 1172, 1324, 1340

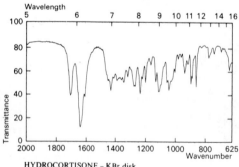

HYDROCORTISONE – KBr disk
1114, 1242, 1435, 1612, 1642, 1710

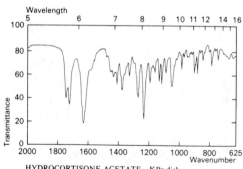

HYDROCORTISONE ACETATE – KBr disk
1233, 1272, 1377, 1629, 1723, 1745

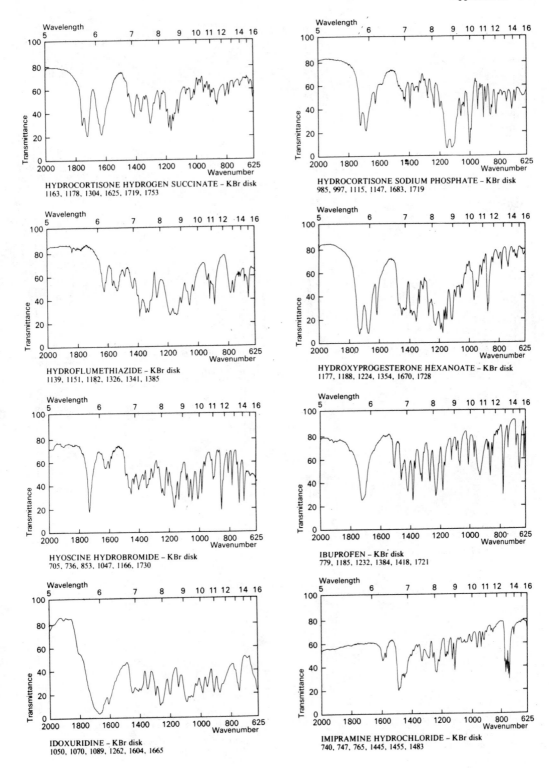

HYDROCORTISONE HYDROGEN SUCCINATE – KBr disk
1163, 1178, 1304, 1625, 1719, 1753

HYDROCORTISONE SODIUM PHOSPHATE – KBr disk
985, 997, 1115, 1147, 1683, 1719

HYDROFLUMETHIAZIDE – KBr disk
1139, 1151, 1182, 1326, 1341, 1385

HYDROXYPROGESTERONE HEXANOATE – KBr disk
1177, 1188, 1224, 1354, 1670, 1728

HYOSCINE HYDROBROMIDE – KBr disk
705, 736, 853, 1047, 1166, 1730

IBUPROFEN – KBr disk
779, 1185, 1232, 1384, 1418, 1721

IDOXURIDINE – KBr disk
1050, 1070, 1089, 1262, 1604, 1665

IMIPRAMINE HYDROCHLORIDE – KBr disk
740, 747, 765, 1445, 1455, 1483

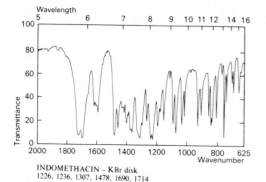

INDOMETHACIN – KBr disk
1226, 1236, 1307, 1478, 1690, 1714

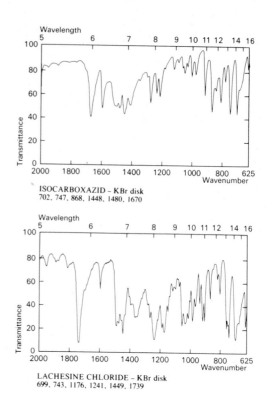

ISOCARBOXAZID – KBr disk
702, 747, 868, 1448, 1480, 1670

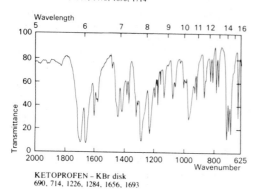

KETOPROFEN – KBr disk
690, 714, 1226, 1284, 1656, 1693

LACHESINE CHLORIDE – KBr disk
699, 743, 1176, 1241, 1449, 1739

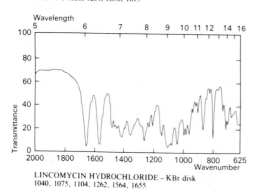

LINCOMYCIN HYDROCHLORIDE – KBr disk
1040, 1075, 1104, 1262, 1564, 1655

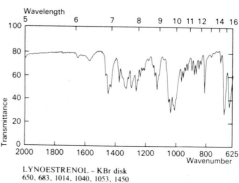

LYNOESTRENOL – KBr disk
650, 683, 1014, 1040, 1053, 1450

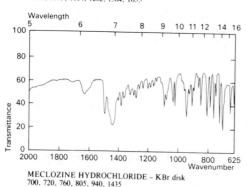

MECLOZINE HYDROCHLORIDE – KBr disk
700, 720, 760, 805, 940, 1435

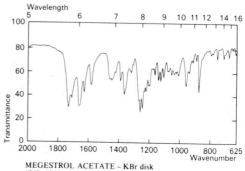

MEGESTROL ACETATE – KBr disk
1249, 1263, 1272, 1662, 1712, 1733

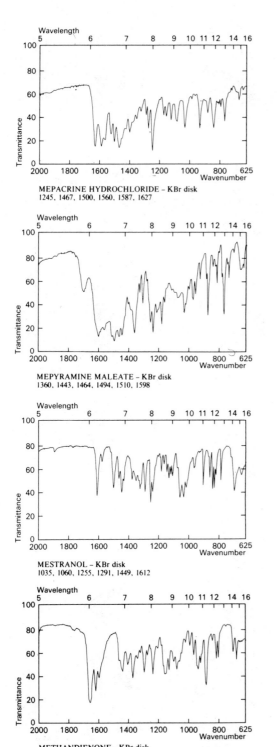

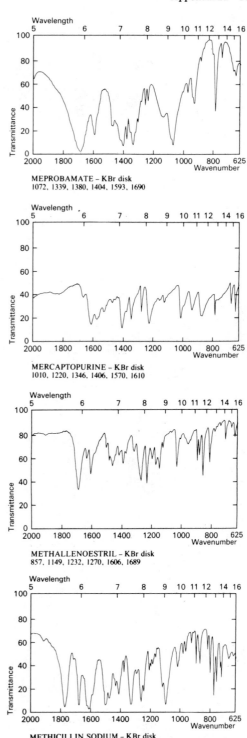

MEPACRINE HYDROCHLORIDE – KBr disk
1245, 1467, 1500, 1560, 1587, 1627

MEPROBAMATE – KBr disk
1072, 1339, 1380, 1404, 1593, 1690

MEPYRAMINE MALEATE – KBr disk
1360, 1443, 1464, 1494, 1510, 1598

MERCAPTOPURINE – KBr disk
1010, 1220, 1346, 1406, 1570, 1610

MESTRANOL – KBr disk
1035, 1060, 1255, 1291, 1449, 1612

METHALLENOESTRIL – KBr disk
857, 1149, 1232, 1270, 1606, 1689

METHANDIENONE – KBr disk
886, 1160, 1374, 1601, 1620, 1660

METHICILLIN SODIUM – KBr disk
1093, 1327, 1500, 1607, 1673, 1766

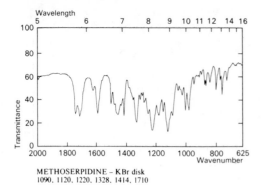

METHOSERPIDINE – KBr disk
1090, 1120, 1220, 1328, 1414, 1710

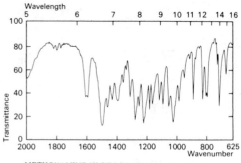

METHOXAMINE HYDROCHLORIDE – KBr disk
1022, 1179, 1219, 1276, 1461, 1496

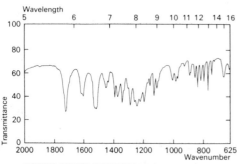

METHYLDOPATE HYDROCHLORIDE – KBr disk
1192, 1241, 1286, 1342, 1511, 1720

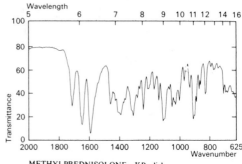

METHYLPREDNISOLONE – KBr disk
914, 1114, 1313, 1396, 1595, 1650

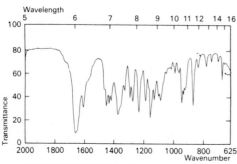

METHYLTESTOSTERONE – KBr disk
1160, 1239, 1377, 1454, 1612, 1664

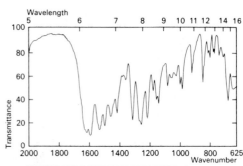

METOCLOPRAMIDE HYDROCHLORIDE – KBr disk
1254, 1311, 1496, 1530, 1590, 1614

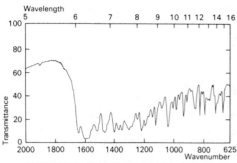

MINOCYCLINE HYDROCHLORIDE – KBr disk
1220, 1400, 1466, 1520, 1590, 1647

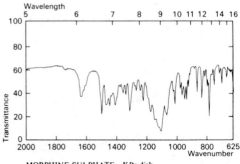

MORPHINE SULPHATE – KBr disk
786, 1070, 1108, 1175, 1313, 1500

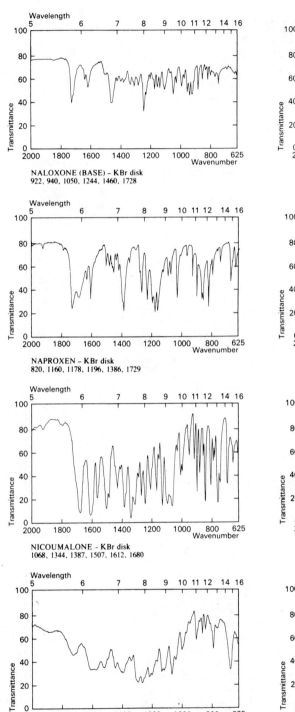

NALOXONE (BASE) – KBr disk
922, 940, 1050, 1244, 1460, 1728

NAPROXEN – KBr disk
820, 1160, 1178, 1196, 1386, 1729

NICOUMALONE – KBr disk
1068, 1344, 1387, 1507, 1612, 1680

NORADRENALINE ACID TARTRATE – KBr disk
1066, 1200, 1216, 1265, 1293, 1395

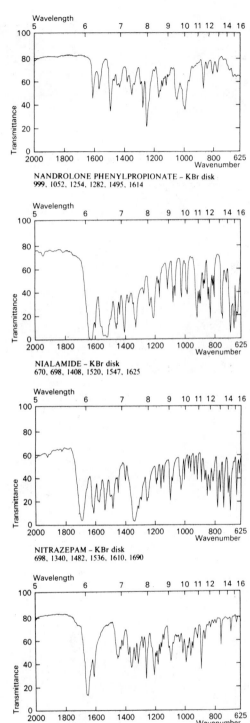

NANDROLONE PHENYLPROPIONATE – KBr disk
999, 1052, 1254, 1282, 1495, 1614

NIALAMIDE – KBr disk
670, 698, 1408, 1520, 1547, 1625

NITRAZEPAM – KBr disk
698, 1340, 1482, 1536, 1610, 1690

NORETHANDROLONE – KBr disk
894, 1210, 1263, 1583, 1612, 1650

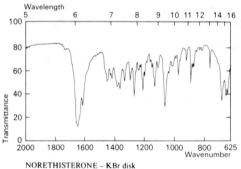

NORETHISTERONE – KBr disk
660, 689, 1068, 1272, 1617, 1649

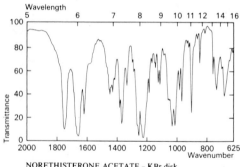

NORETHISTERONE ACETATE – KBr disk
1016, 1035, 1227, 1256, 1661, 1752

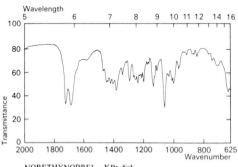

NORETHYNODREL – KBr disk
644, 1066, 1140, 1390, 1690, 1729

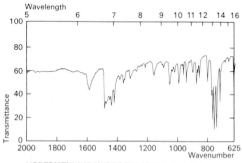

NORTRIPTYLINE HYDROCHLORIDE – KBr disk
742, 758, 769, 1442, 1476, 1488

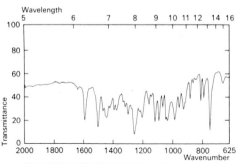

OXPRENOLOL HYDROCHLORIDE – KBr disk
750, 1037, 1092, 1120, 1258, 1500

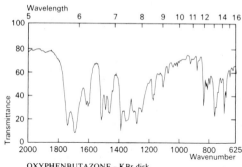

OXYPHENBUTAZONE – KBr disk
1277, 1350, 1383, 1513, 1685, 1736

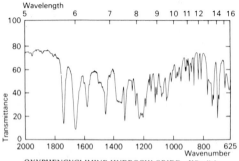

OXYPHENCYCLIMINE HYDROCHLORIDE – KBr disk
705, 1201, 1227, 1322, 1656, 1737

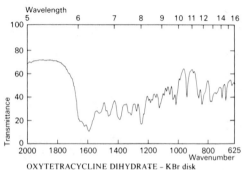

OXYTETRACYLINE DIHYDRATE – KBr disk
1243, 1312, 1386, 1462, 1590, 1622

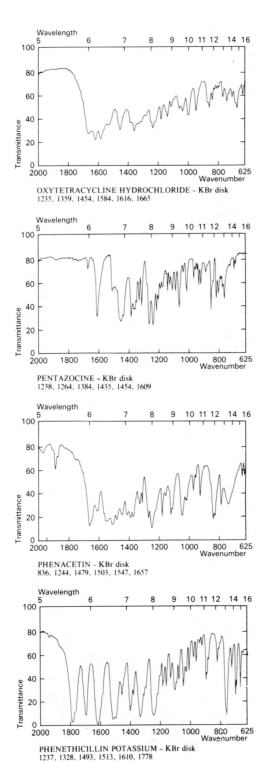
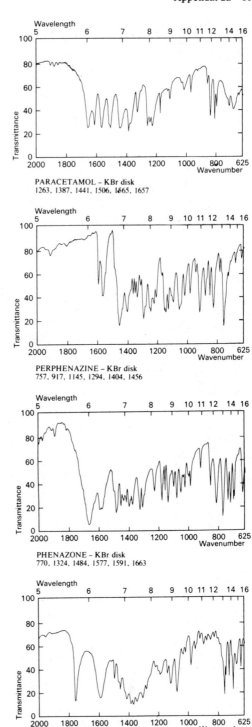

OXYTETRACYCLINE HYDROCHLORIDE – KBr disk
1235, 1359, 1454, 1584, 1616, 1665

PARACETAMOL – KBr disk
1263, 1387, 1441, 1506, 1565, 1657

PENTAZOCINE – KBr disk
1238, 1264, 1384, 1435, 1454, 1609

PERPHENAZINE – KBr disk
757, 917, 1145, 1294, 1404, 1456

PHENACETIN – KBr disk
836, 1244, 1479, 1503, 1547, 1657

PHENAZONE – KBr disk
770, 1324, 1484, 1577, 1591, 1663

PHENETHICILLIN POTASSIUM – KBr disk
1237, 1328, 1493, 1513, 1610, 1778

PHENINDAMINE TARTRATE – KBr disk
1302, 1340, 1365, 1381, 1411, 1751

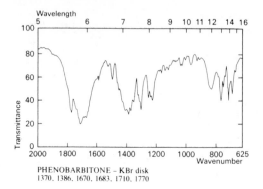

PHENOBARBITONE – KBr disk
1370, 1386, 1670, 1683, 1710, 1770

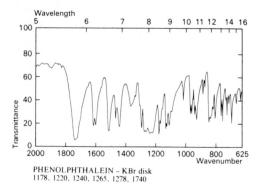

PHENOLPHTHALEIN – KBr disk
1178, 1220, 1240, 1265, 1278, 1740

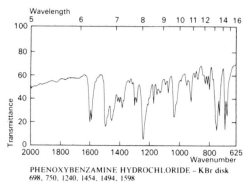

PHENOXYBENZAMINE HYDROCHLORIDE – KBr disk
698, 750, 1240, 1454, 1494, 1598

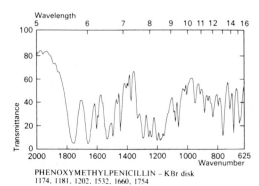

PHENOXYMETHYLPENICILLIN – KBr disk
1174, 1181, 1202, 1532, 1660, 1754

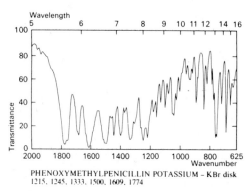

PHENOXYMETHYLPENICILLIN POTASSIUM – KBr disk
1215, 1245, 1333, 1500, 1609, 1774

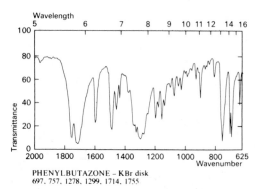

PHENYLBUTAZONE – KBr disk
697, 757, 1278, 1299, 1714, 1755

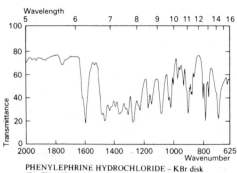
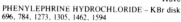

PHENYLEPHRINE HYDROCHLORIDE – KBr disk
696, 784, 1273, 1305, 1462, 1594

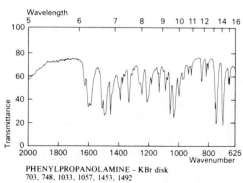

PHENYLPROPANOLAMINE – KBr disk
703, 748, 1033, 1057, 1453, 1492

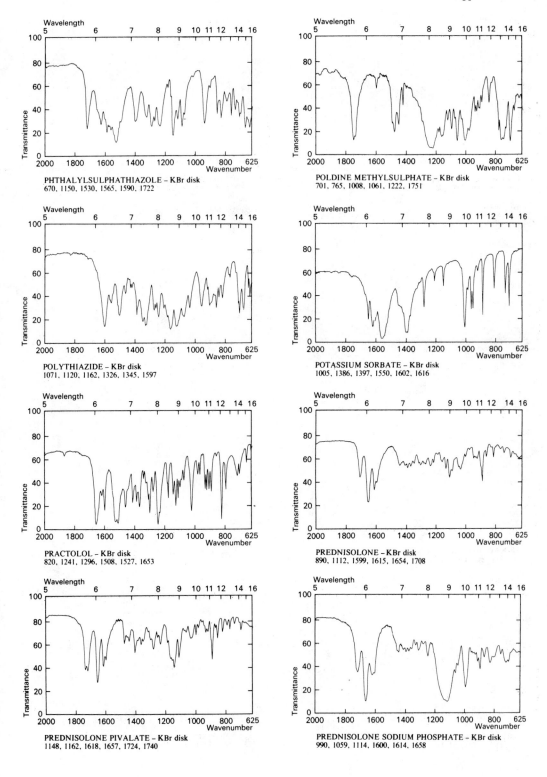

PHTHALYLSULPHATHIAZOLE – KBr disk
670, 1150, 1530, 1565, 1590, 1722

POLDINE METHYLSULPHATE – KBr disk
701, 765, 1008, 1061, 1222, 1751

POLYTHIAZIDE – KBr disk
1071, 1120, 1162, 1326, 1345, 1597

POTASSIUM SORBATE – KBr disk
1005, 1386, 1397, 1550, 1602, 1616

PRACTOLOL – KBr disk
820, 1241, 1296, 1508, 1527, 1653

PREDNISOLONE – KBr disk
890, 1112, 1599, 1615, 1654, 1708

PREDNISOLONE PIVALATE – KBr disk
1148, 1162, 1618, 1657, 1724, 1740

PREDNISOLONE SODIUM PHOSPHATE – KBr disk
990, 1059, 1114, 1600, 1614, 1658

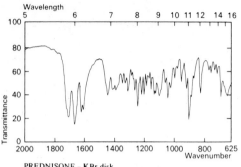

PREDNISONE – KBr disk
904, 1246, 1610, 1622, 1667, 1709

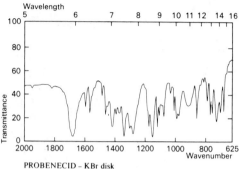

PROBENECID – KBr disk
1125, 1156, 1285, 1307, 1345, 1683

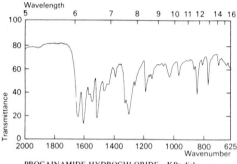

PROCAINAMIDE HYDROCHLORIDE – KBr disk
1297, 1325, 1512, 1545, 1600, 1639

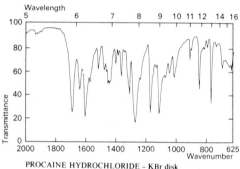

PROCAINE HYDROCHLORIDE – KBr disk
772, 1116, 1174, 1272, 1607, 1692

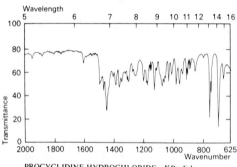

PROCYCLIDINE HYDROCHLORIDE – KBr disk
700, 746, 756, 1128, 1445, 1467

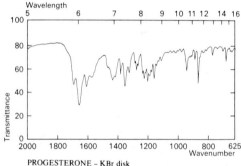

PROGESTERONE – KBr disk
872, 1209, 1358, 1614, 1662, 1700

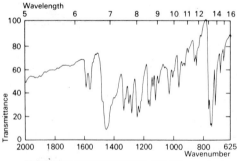

PROMAZINE HYDROCHLORIDE – KBr disk
751, 1234, 1250, 1287, 1339, 1455

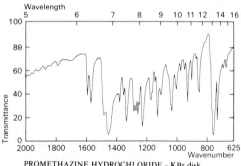

PROMETHAZINE HYDROCHLORIDE – KBr disk
733, 758, 1129, 1229, 1336, 1454

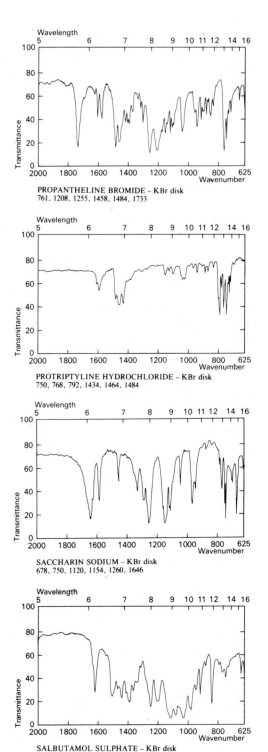

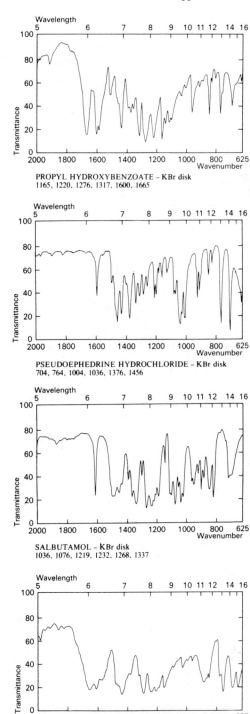

PROPANTHELINE BROMIDE – KBr disk
761, 1208, 1255, 1458, 1484, 1733

PROPYL HYDROXYBENZOATE – KBr disk
1165, 1220, 1276, 1317, 1600, 1665

PROTRIPTYLINE HYDROCHLORIDE – KBr disk
750, 768, 792, 1434, 1464, 1484

PSEUDOEPHEDRINE HYDROCHLORIDE – KBr disk
704, 764, 1004, 1036, 1376, 1456

SACCHARIN SODIUM – KBr disk
678, 750, 1120, 1154, 1260, 1646

SALBUTAMOL – KBr disk
1036, 1076, 1219, 1232, 1268, 1337

SALBUTAMOL SULPHATE – KBr disk
837, 976, 1027, 1076, 1111, 1245

SALICYLIC ACID – KBr disk
756, 1209, 1240, 1292, 1441, 1658

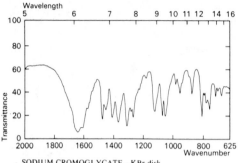

SODIUM CROMOGLYCATE – KBr disk
1264, 1305, 1365, 1405, 1473, 1635

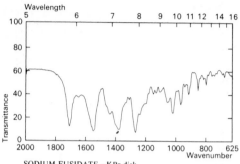

SODIUM FUSIDATE – KBr disk
1238, 1267, 1380, 1438, 1547, 1706

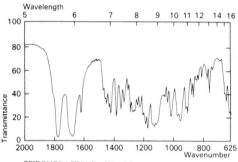

SPIRONOLACTONE – KBr disk
1115, 1127, 1170, 1185, 1676, 1773

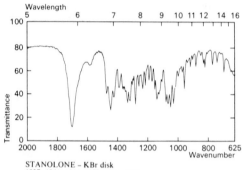

STANOLONE – KBr disk
1027, 1046, 1064, 1277, 1444, 1698

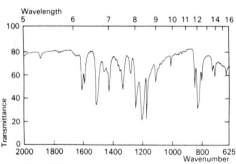

STILBOESTROL – KBr disk
833, 1176, 1205, 1250, 1428, 1512

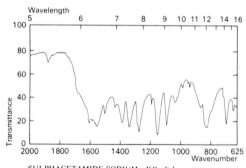

SULPHACETAMIDE SODIUM – KBr disk
816, 1087, 1147, 1270, 1336, 1550

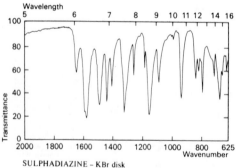

SULPHADIAZINE – KBr disk
683, 1159, 1328, 1444, 1494, 1580

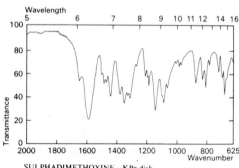

SULPHADIMETHOXINE – KBr disk
1090, 1147, 1314, 1353, 1445, 1590

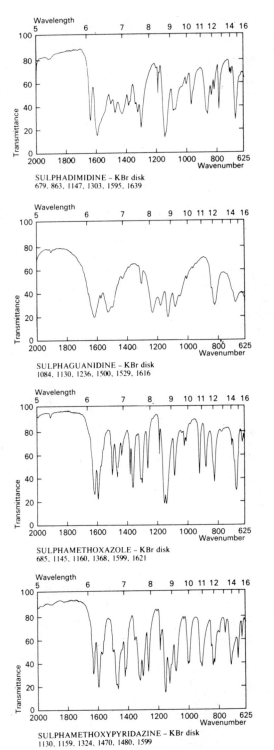

SULPHADIMIDINE – KBr disk
679, 863, 1147, 1303, 1595, 1639

SULPHAGUANIDINE – KBr disk
1084, 1130, 1236, 1500, 1529, 1616

SULPHAMETHOXAZOLE – KBr disk
685, 1145, 1160, 1368, 1599, 1621

SULPHAMETHOXYPYRIDAZINE – KBr disk
1130, 1159, 1324, 1470, 1480, 1599

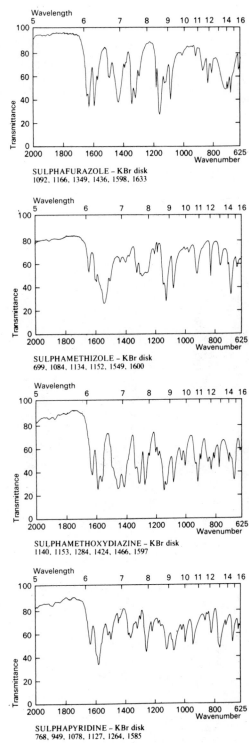

SULPHAFURAZOLE – KBr disk
1092, 1166, 1349, 1436, 1598, 1633

SULPHAMETHIZOLE – KBr disk
699, 1084, 1134, 1152, 1549, 1600

SULPHAMETHOXYDIAZINE – KBr disk
1140, 1153, 1284, 1424, 1466, 1597

SULPHAPYRIDINE – KBr disk
768, 949, 1078, 1127, 1264, 1585

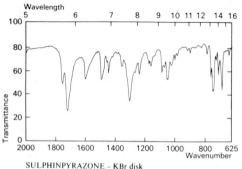

SULPHINPYRAZONE – KBr disk
688, 742, 750, 1305, 1716, 1750

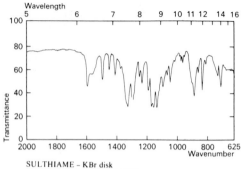

SULTHIAME – KBr disk
889, 1138, 1158, 1172, 1293, 1327

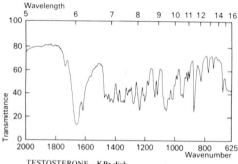

TESTOSTERONE – KBr disk
871, 1057, 1066, 1236, 1615, 1660

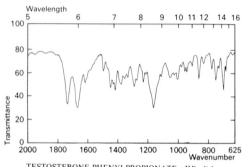

TESTOSTERONE PHENYLPROPIONATE – KBr disk
703, 1166, 1420, 1450, 1670, 1734

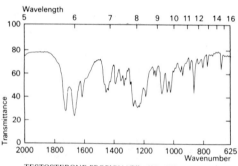

TESTOSTERONE PROPIONATE – KBr disk
1231, 1243, 1271, 1613, 1669, 1727

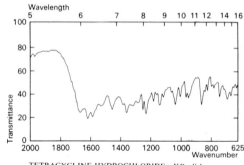

TETRACYCLINE HYDROCHLORIDE – KBr disk
1226, 1354, 1450, 1581, 1614, 1664

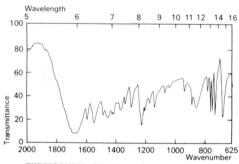

THEOBROMINE – KBr disk
684, 1225, 1453, 1545, 1594, 1680

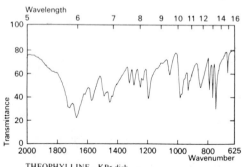

THEOPHYLLINE – KBr disk
744, 1189, 1445, 1565, 1665, 1710

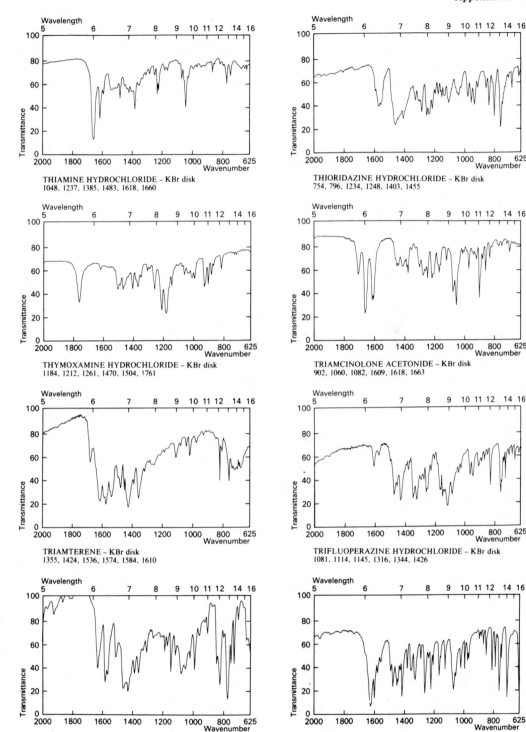

THIAMINE HYDROCHLORIDE – KBr disk
1048, 1237, 1385, 1483, 1618, 1660

THIORIDAZINE HYDROCHLORIDE – KBr disk
754, 796, 1234, 1248, 1403, 1455

THYMOXAMINE HYDROCHLORIDE – KBr disk
1184, 1212, 1261, 1470, 1504, 1761

TRIAMCINOLONE ACETONIDE – KBr disk
902, 1060, 1082, 1609, 1618, 1663

TRIAMTERENE – KBr disk
1355, 1424, 1536, 1574, 1584, 1610

TRIFLUOPERAZINE HYDROCHLORIDE – KBr disk
1081, 1114, 1145, 1316, 1344, 1426

TRIPROLIDINE HYDROCHLORIDE – KBr disk.
772, 824, 1077, 1427, 1459, 1580

TROPICAMIDE – KBr disk
709, 761, 1266, 1419, 1601, 1627

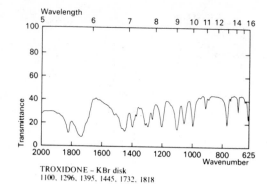

TROXIDONE – KBr disk
1100, 1296, 1395, 1445, 1732, 1818

Appendix 2b

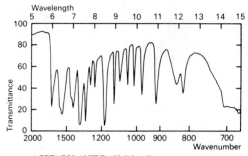

ACETAZOLAMIDE – Nujol mull
671, 704, 1176, 1316, 1538, 1667

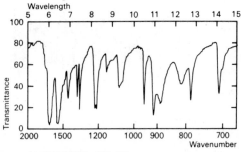

ALLOPURINOL – KBr disk
917, 1219, 1235, 1351, 1587, 1695

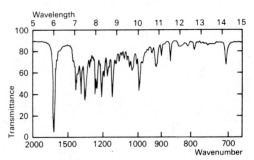

ALPHAXALONE – KBr disk
1149, 1219, 1266, 1351, 1389, 1695

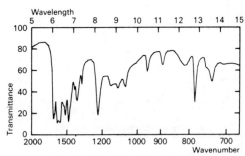

AMILORIDE HYDROCHLORIDE – KBr disk
1235, 1515, 1538, 1587, 1639, 1695

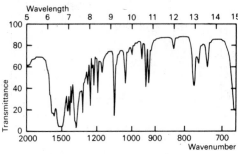

AMINOCAPROIC ACID – KBr disk
1099, 1316, 1370, 1449, 1538, 1613

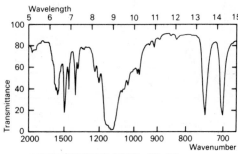

AMPHETAMINE SULPHATE – KBr disk
699, 741, 1111, 1389, 1493, 1562

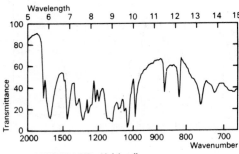

ASCORBIC ACID – Nujol mull
990, 1031, 1111, 1136, 1316, 1667

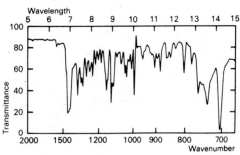

BIPERIDEN – Nujol mull
704, 735, 758, 1000, 1124, 1149

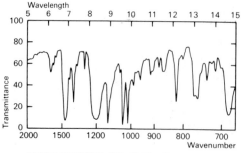

BRETYLIUM TOSYLATE – Nujol mull
680, 820, 1010, 1031, 1124, 1190

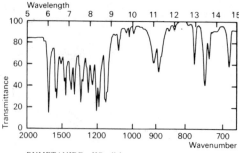

BUMETANIDE – KBr disk
1149, 1205, 1220, 1333, 1587, 1695

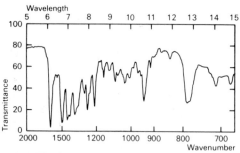

BUPIVACAINE HYDROCHLORIDE – KBr disk
1282, 1389, 1429, 1471, 1515, 1667

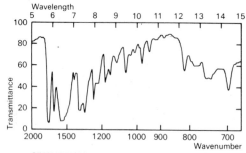

CEPHALEXIN – KBr disk
1266, 1351, 1389, 1587, 1695, 1754

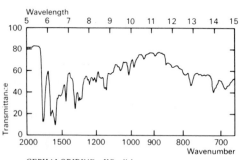

CEPHALORIDINE – KBr disk
1351, 1389, 1471, 1613, 1667, 1754

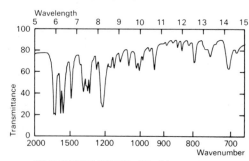

CEPHALOTHIN SODIUM – KBr disk
1235, 1333, 1515, 1613, 1639, 1695

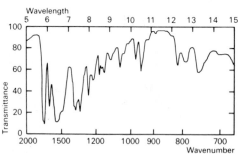

CEPHRADINE – KBr disk
1266, 1333, 1389, 1587, 1667, 1754

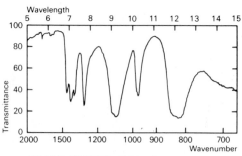

CHLORAL HYDRATE – Nujol mull
820, 971, 1087, 1299

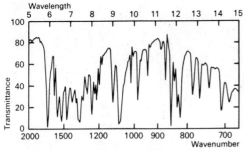

CHLORAMPHENICOL – Nujol mull
820, 847, 1075, 1515, 1562, 1695

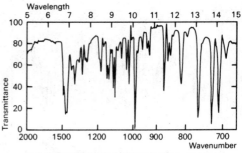

CHLORCYCLIZINE HYDROCHLORIDE – Nujol mull
704, 725, 758, 870, 990, 1087

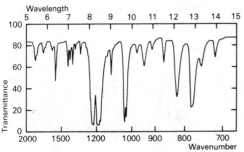

CHLORMETHIAZOLE EDISYLATE – KBr disk
781, 826, 1031, 1042, 1205, 1235

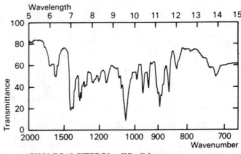

CHOLECALCIFEROL – KBr disk
893, 971, 1053, 1351, 1370, 1449

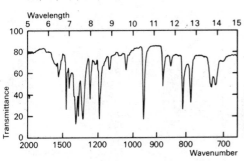

CLIOQUINOL – KBr disk
952, 1205, 1333, 1370, 1389, 1493

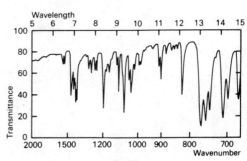

CLOTRIMAZOLE – KBr disk
709, 741, 752, 763, 1075, 1205

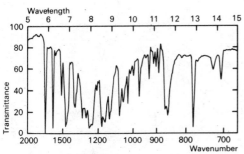

CYCLOMETHYCAINE SULPHATE – Nujol mull
775, 1176, 1235, 1250, 1613, 1724

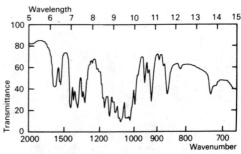

. CYTARABINE – KBr disk
. 1031, 1075, 1111, 1149, 1176, 1389

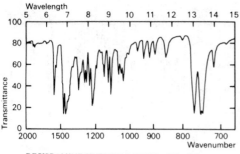

DESIPRAMINE HYDROCHLORIDE – KBr disk
741, 746, 763, 1235, 1449, 1471

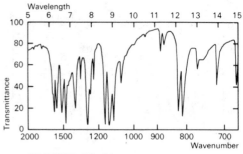

DIAZOXIDE – KBr disk
813, 1111, 1136, 1163, 1299, 1493

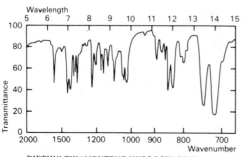

DIETHYLTHIAMBUTENE HYDROCHLORIDE – KBr disk
714, 741, 855, 1250, 1429, 1471

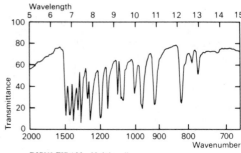

DISULFIRAM – Nujol mull
917, 962, 1149, 1190, 1266, 1515

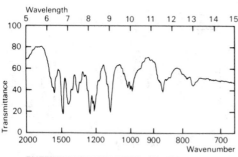

EMETINE HYDROCHLORIDE – KBr disk
1111, 1220, 1235, 1250, 1449, 1493

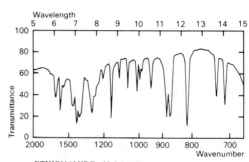

ETHIONAMIDE – Nujol mull
813, 870, 885, 1149, 1282, 1587

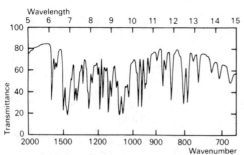

ETHYLMORPHINE HYDROCHLORIDE – Nujol mull
952, 1042, 1064, 1136, 1190, 1266

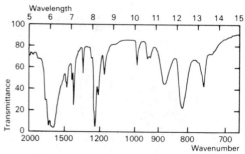

FLUOROURACIL – KBr disk
820, 1220, 1250, 1429, 1667, 1724

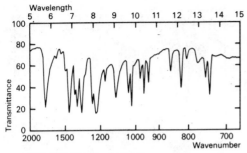

FURAZOLIDONE – Nujol mull
741, 1020, 1099, 1235, 1250, 1754

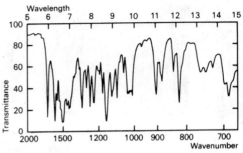

GLIBENCLAMIDE – KBr disk
1163, 1333, 1471, 1515, 1613, 1724

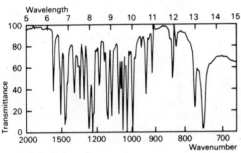

GUAIPHENESIN – Nujol mull
746, 1000, 1020, 1042, 1235, 1250

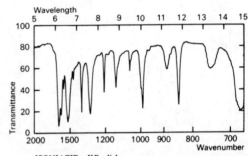

ISONIAZID – KBr disk
676, 1316, 1408, 1538, 1613, 1639

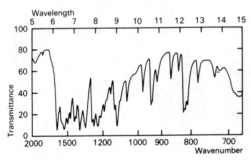

LEVODOPA – KBr disk
1124, 1250, 1351, 1389, 1562, 1639

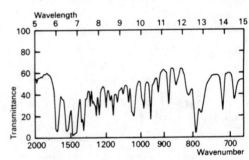

LIGNOCAINE HYDROCHLORIDE – Nujol mull
787, 952, 1031, 1149, 1538, 1639

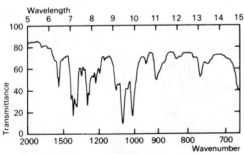

MANNOMUSTINE HYDROCHLORIDE – KBr disk
1010, 1064, 1299, 1389, 1429, 1449

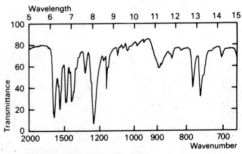

MEFENAMIC ACID – KBr disk
758, 1250, 1449, 1515, 1562, 1639

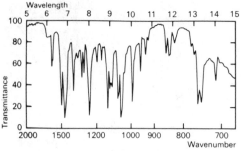

MEPHENESIN – Nujol mull
746, 758, 1053, 1124, 1250, 1515

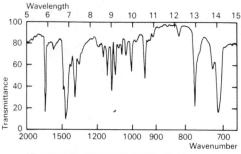

METHADONE HYDROCHLORIDE – Nujol mull
709, 769, 943, 1111, 1136, 1695

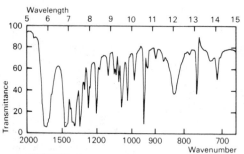

METHOHEXITONE – Nujol mull
943, 1042, 1205, 1250, 1316, 1695

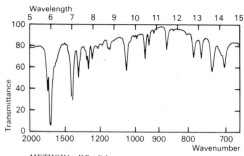

METHOIN – KBr disk
735, 1053, 1389, 1449, 1695, 1754

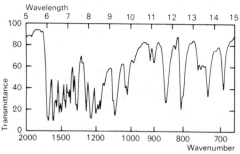

METHYL BENZOQUATE – KBr disk
1087, 1220, 1250, 1562, 1639, 1695

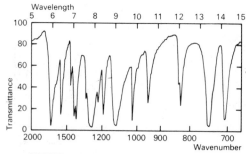

METHYL NICOTINATE – KBr disk
741, 1020, 1111, 1282, 1429, 1724

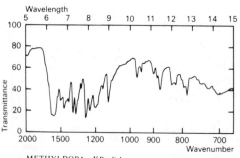

METHYLDOPA – KBr disk
1250, 1282, 1370, 1389, 1493, 1613

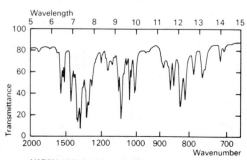

MICONAZOLE NITRATE – KBr disk
826, 1087, 1299, 1316, 1370, 1408

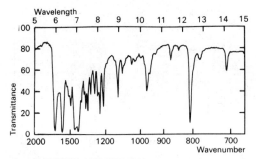

NALIDIXIC ACID – KBr disk
806, 1250, 1429, 1471, 1613, 1695

NICLOSAMIDE – KBr disk
1282, 1333, 1351, 1515, 1562, 1613

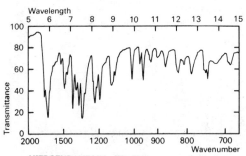

NITROFURANTOIN – KBr disk
1205, 1235, 1333, 1370, 1429, 1724

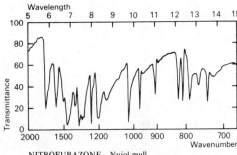

NITROFURAZONE – Nujol mull
971, 1020, 1205, 1250, 1587, 1724

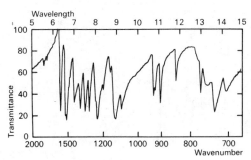

NITROXYNIL – KBr disk
730, 1124, 1250, 1316, 1333, 1538

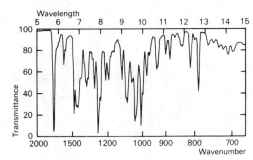

NOSCAPINE – Nujol mull
1010, 1042, 1087, 1282, 1493, 1754

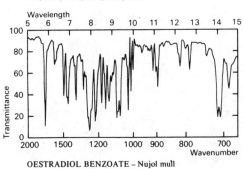

OESTRADIOL BENZOATE – Nujol mull
704, 709, 1075, 1220, 1250, 1724

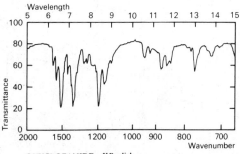

OXYCLOZANIDE – KBr disk
1163, 1205, 1408, 1471, 1538, 1587

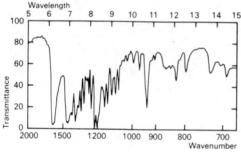

OXYMETHOLONE – Nujol mull
1149, 1190, 1220, 1235, 1316, 1613

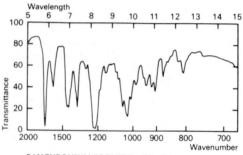

PANCURONIUM BROMIDE – KBr disk
1031, 1053, 1235, 1370, 1449, 1754

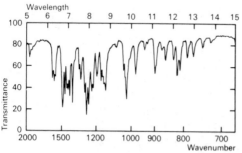

PAPAVERINE HYDROCHLORIDE – KBr disk
1020, 1266, 1282, 1408, 1429, 1515

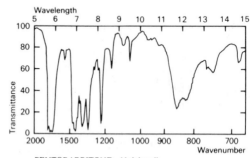

PENTOBARBITONE – Nujol mull
855, 1220, 1299, 1695, 1724, 1754

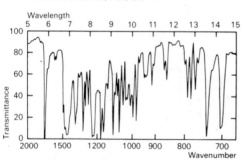

PETHIDINE HYDROCHLORIDE – Nujol mull
735, 1064, 1099, 1176, 1235, 1724

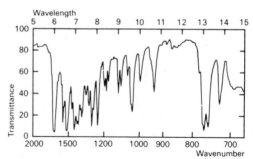

PRILOCAINE HYDROCHLORIDE – KBr disk
752, 763, 1299, 1471, 1538, 1695

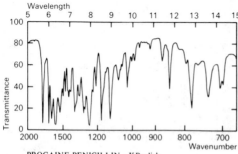

PROCAINE PENICILLIN – KBr disk
1124, 1176, 1266, 1613, 1695, 1786

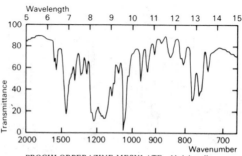

PROCHLORPERAZINE MESYLATE – Nujol mull
758, 775, 1042, 1099, 1149, 1220

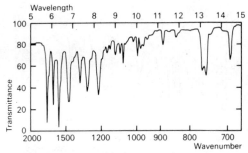

PROPICILLIN POTASSIUM – KBr disk
1220, 1316, 1493, 1613, 1667, 1754

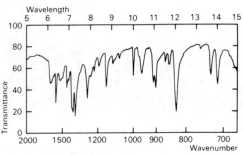

PROTHIONAMIDE – KBr disk
826, 901, 1282, 1389, 1408, 1587

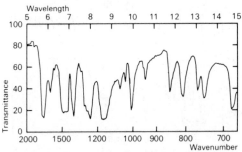

PYRIDOSTIGMINE BROMIDE – Nujol mull
680, 1010, 1163, 1250, 1515, 1724

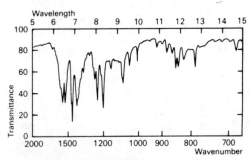

RAFOXANIDE – KBr disk
1220, 1250, 1429, 1493, 1562, 1587

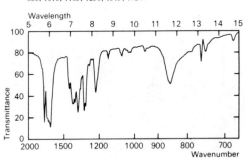

SECBUTOBARBITONE – KBr disk
1299, 1316, 1370, 1408, 1667, 1754

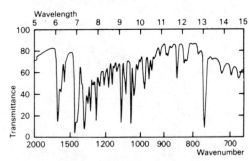

STRYCHNINE HYDROCHLORIDE – Nujol mull
763, 1053, 1111, 1282, 1316, 1667

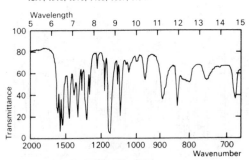

SULPHAMERAZINE – KBr disk
1149, 1316, 1389, 1493, 1562, 1587

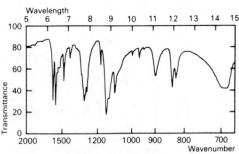

SULPHANILAMIDE – KBr disk
1099, 1149, 1299, 1316, 1613, 1639

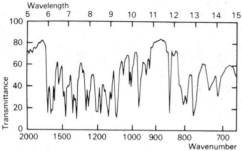

SULPHASALAZINE – Nujol mull
769, 1075, 1124, 1176, 1639, 1667

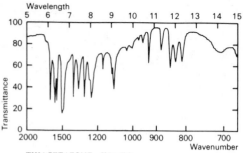

THIACETAZONE – KBr disk
1250, 1299, 1515, 1587, 1613, 1667

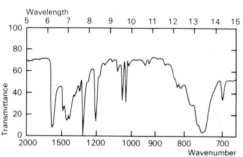

TOLAZOLINE HYDROCHLORIDE – Nujol mull
746, 1031, 1205, 1299, 1515, 1613

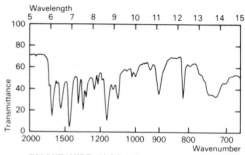

TOLBUTAMIDE – Nujol mull
813, 1087, 1149, 1316, 1538, 1639

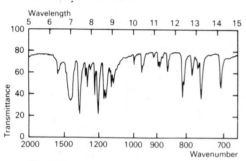

TOLNAFTATE – KBr disk
752, 1163, 1176, 1205, 1370, 1449

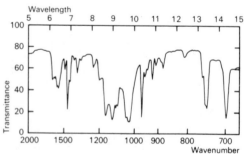

TRANYLCYPROMINE SULPHATE – Nujol mull
694, 769, 962, 1020, 1111, 1149

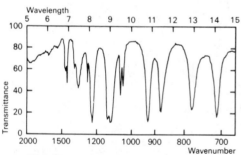

TRICLOFOS SODIUM – Nujol mull
709, 877, 926, 1099, 1124, 1220

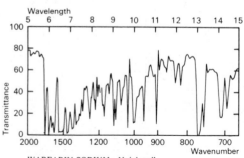

WARFARIN SODIUM – Nujol mull
763, 1031, 1538, 1613, 1667, 1724

Appendix 2c

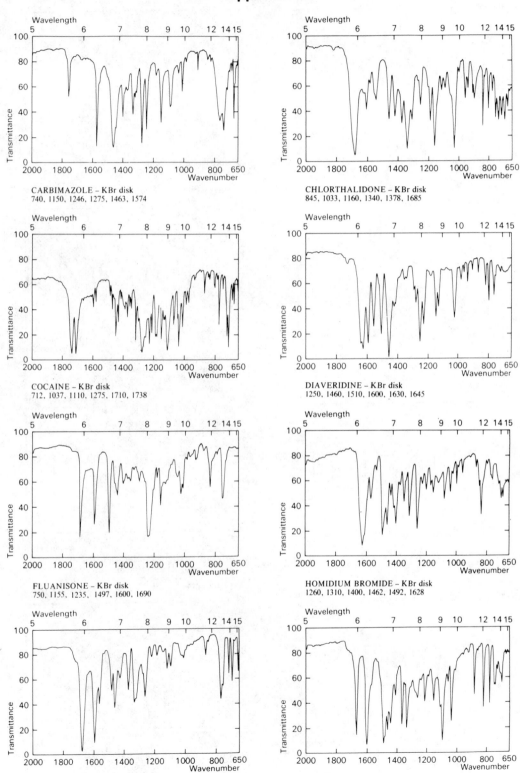

CARBIMAZOLE – KBr disk
740, 1150, 1246, 1275, 1463, 1574

CHLORTHALIDONE – KBr disk
845, 1033, 1160, 1340, 1378, 1685

COCAINE – KBr disk
712, 1037, 1110, 1275, 1710, 1738

DIAVERIDINE – KBr disk
1250, 1460, 1510, 1600, 1630, 1645

FLUANISONE – KBr disk
750, 1155, 1235, 1497, 1600, 1690

HOMIDIUM BROMIDE – KBr disk
1260, 1310, 1400, 1462, 1492, 1628

METHAQUALONE – KBr disk
770, 1335, 1465, 1565, 1600, 1680

METHISAZONE – KBr disk
1097, 1340, 1468, 1492, 1605, 1673

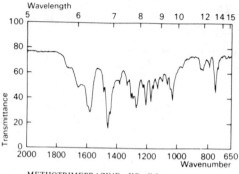

METHOTRIMEPRAZINE – KBr disk
1170, 1205, 1270, 1445, 1460, 1590

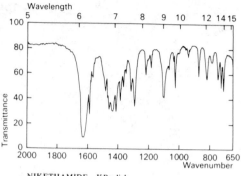

NIKETHAMIDE – KBr disk
1290, 1414, 1436, 1460, 1590, 1635

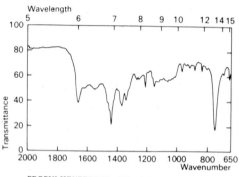

PROPYLHEXEDRINE – KBr windows
748, 1340, 1370, 1443, 1550, 1663

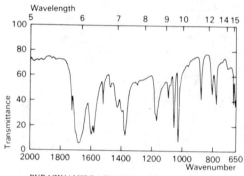

PYRAZINAMIDE – KBr disk
1020, 1050, 1375, 1584, 1600, 1685

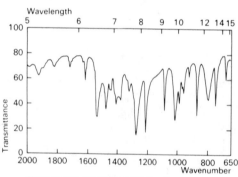

PYRIDOXINE HYDROCHLORIDE – KBr disk
870, 1015, 1086, 1212, 1277, 1540

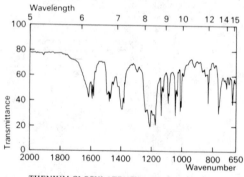

THENIUM CLOSYLATE – KBr disk
760, 1010, 1042, 1135, 1174, 1210

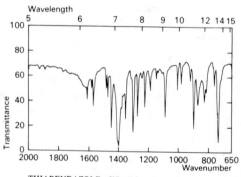

THIABENDAZOLE – KBr disk
740, 902, 1306, 1358, 1404, 1455

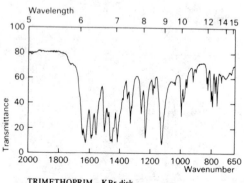

TRIMETHOPRIM – KBr disk
1126, 1421, 1458, 1470, 1596, 1630

Index

Entries are arranged alphabetically in word-by-word order; entries consisting of abbreviations represented by initial letters, e.g. ACTH, are treated as single words.
When an entry is followed by more than one page reference, the principal reference is printed in **bold** type.